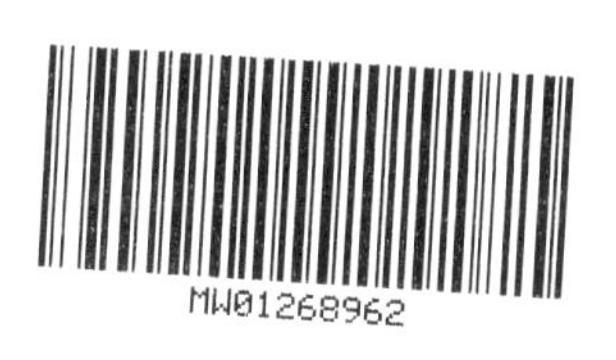
MW01268962

The ASCRS Textbook of Colon and Rectal Surgery

The ASCRS Textbook of Colon and Rectal Surgery

Second Edition

Editors

David E. Beck, MD, FACS, FASCRS
Patricia L. Roberts, MD, FACS, FASCRS
Theodore J. Saclarides, MD, FACS, FASCRS
Anthony J. Senagore, MD, FACS, FASCRS
Michael J. Stamos, MD, FACS, FASCRS
Steven D. Wexner, MD, FACS, FASCRS, FRCS, FRCS(Ed)

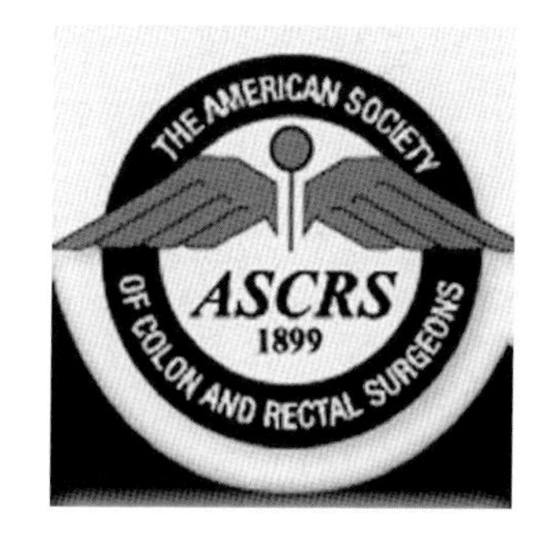

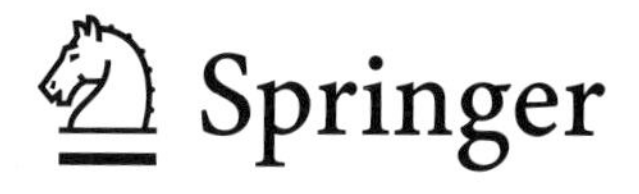

Editors
David E. Beck, MD, FACS, FASCRS
Department of Colon and Rectal Surgery
Louisiana State University Health Sciences Center
New Orleans, Louisiana, USA
dbeckmd@aol.com

Patricia L. Roberts, MD, FACS, FASCRS
Department of Colorectal Surgery
Lahey Clinic, Tufts University School of Medicine
Burlington, Massachusetts, USA
Patricia.l.roberts@lahey.org

Theodore J. Saclarides, MD, FACS, FASCRS
Section of Colon and Rectal Surgery,
Rush Medical Center,
Chicago, Illinois, USA
Theodore_Saclarides@rush.edu

Anthony J. Senagore, MD, FACS, FASCRS
Spectrum Health
Department of Surgery
Grand Rapids, Michigan, USA
asenagore@sbcglobal.net

Michael J. Stamos, MD, FACS, FASCRS
Department of Surgery
UCI Medical Center
Orange, California, USA
mstamos@uci.edu

Steven D. Wexner, MD, FACS, FASCRS, FRCS, FRCS(Ed)
Cleveland Clinic Florida
Department of Colorectal Surgery,
Weston, Florida, USA
wexners@ccf.org

ISBN 978-1-4419-1581-8 e-ISBN 978-1-4419-1584-9
DOI 10.1007/978-1-4419-1584-9
Springer New York Dordrecht Heidelberg London

Library of Congress Control Number: 2011926885

Printed on acid-free paper

Springer is part of Springer Science+Business Media (www.springer.com)

Foreword, 1st Edition

This text was developed under the aegis of the American Society of Colon and Rectal Surgeons (ASCRS). It represents an attempt to cover the field of colon and rectal surgery with input from expert surgeons who have, in one way or another, shown special interest or expertise in specific areas of the specialty.

The book will hopefully serve as a source of useful information and perhaps even guidance to surgeons whose practice is confined to the specialty of colon and rectal surgery, and also to general surgeons, surgery residents, and medical students with an interest in surgery.

The finished product represents significant efforts from authors who have taken time from their busy schedules to set into writing their often unique perspectives. I know for certain that no author of any chapter in this book has a light schedule, but that fact validates each author's selection for authorship.

Special acknowledgment is due the editors, Bruce Wolff, David Beck, John Pemberton, and Steven Wexner. This project simply would not have come together without their efforts on many levels.

Finally, Jim Fleshman must be singled out for special recognition. The idea of an ASCRS-sponsored text began with Jim – an idea that he advocated, developed, nurtured, and forced until it became realized in the substance you now hold.

Robert Fry, MD
Emilie and Roland deHellebranth
Professor of Surgery
Chief, Division of Colon and Rectal Surgery
The Hospital of the University of Pennsylvania

Foreword, 2nd Edition

The American Society of Colon and Rectal Surgeons (ASCRS) Textbook was originally conceived as a means of providing state of the art information to residents in training and fully trained surgeons seeking maintenance of certification and to support the mission of the ASCRS to continue to be the world's most established authority on colon and rectal disease. The second edition perpetuates these goals. This textbook has been significantly reorganized in response to the numerous important changes in our specialty. All chapters were rewritten and updated and new chapters have been added. While several authors from the first edition were retained, for the majority of chapters, new authors were selected. Most of these internationally acclaimed contributors are active members of the ASCRS who routinely contribute to our literature. These respected individuals have carefully crafted chapters which provide a comprehensive summary of the subject with an appropriate mixture of detailed personal experience and comprehensive literature review. This approach provides the reader with a very open-minded, evidence-based approach to all aspects of colorectal disease.

At the inception of the first edition, the editorial board was designed to be a rotating group of experts selected by the ASCRS Executive Council. As the two senior editors of this edition, it has been our distinct pleasure and honor to work with this edition's editorial board. They have sacrificed time and energy to achieve what we believe continues to be the standard in colon and rectal surgery. For the sake of ease of use and consistency, the Table of Contents correlates with the Core Curriculum established by the Association of Program Directors in Colon and Rectal Surgery and the key topics used by the American Board of Colon and Rectal Surgery. Furthermore, the Practice Parameters developed by the ASCRS Standards Committee have been incorporated into the text appendix. As occurred with the first edition, the proceeds from this textbook and any related publications will be utilized by the ASCRS Executive Council to sponsor the research and education efforts of the society.

The second edition continues to provide what the fellows and members of the ASCRS and trainees at all levels agree is the definitive source of knowledge in colon and rectal surgery. We are honored to have been a part of this ongoing monumental achievement and thank the leaders of the ASCRS for their continued support of the textbook. We thank our predecessors Bruce Wolf and Jim Fleshman, whose significant commitments as the co-senior editors of the first edition ensured the success of the textbook. We gratefully acknowledge our coeditors for their major contributions and rest comfortably as we leave the editorial board, knowing that future editions will continue to benefit from their dedication and expertise. We thank each chapter author and coauthor for their devotion to this task and to the mission of the ASCRS as without their individual and collective efforts the second edition would not be at such a tremendously high standard. We are grateful to the authors and coauthors of the first edition upon whose labors the foundation of this edition was easily laid. We also thank Sharon Beck for her support during this effort and our Developmental Editor Elektra McDermott for her extraordinary efforts which ensured the timely and professional completion of this second edition. Finally, we want to specially acknowledge the loss of our friend and colleague, W. Douglas Wong, past president of the ASCRS. During the production of this edition, Doug passed away after a courageous battle with a terrible disease. He made numerous major contributions to our specialty and to this textbook. Although Doug will be missed, his innovations and teachings will endure and continue to benefit surgeons and patients throughout the world.

David E. Beck, MD, FASCRS
Steven D. Wexner, MD, FASCRS
April 2011

Preface

Drs. David Beck and Steven Wexner (Senior Editors) as well as the other members of the editorial board, Drs. Patricia Roberts, Theodore Saclarides, Michael Stamos, and Anthony Senagore, are to be congratulated on their successful completion of the second edition of the American Society of Colon and Rectal Surgeons (ASCRS) Textbook. The table of contents has been changed to reflect recent changes in the Core Curriculum for training Residents in colon and rectal surgery and format changes have been made to improve the presentation of the material. At least one third of the material has been completely renewed to reflect advances in the science of our specialty.

The ASCRS Textbook has rapidly become a major resource for training, read by almost all trainees interested in our specialty. The purpose of the text was originally to provide a standardized reference for evidence-based recommendations, referenced to ASCRS practice parameter guidelines were available. The first edition has been downloaded onto the Web-based Colon and Rectal Education System as the reference for all the educational efforts of the ASCRS Continuing Medical Education Committee. Our society, as owners and editors of the ASCRS Textbook, can be proud to be one of the few national organizations with its own comprehensive textbook from which certification and recertification materials can be drawn. Using an entire society as the pool of authors, allows the ASCRS Textbook, as much as possible, to avoid personal bias in the materials presented.

The ASCRS Manual for Residents in training at all levels has also been released this past year. The current Editorial Board has condensed the material from each chapter of the first Edition of the ASCRS Textbook to provide students and residents rapid access to a succinct, distilled version of the ASCRS Textbook. The production of these two educational resources adds evidence that the ASCRS is "the" authority on colorectal disease and has within its membership individuals who can claim the status of "expert." Their contribution has made the ASCRS Textbook a success and should be considered a major selfless contribution to our society and specialty.

As time passes, our specialty and the body of knowledge surrounding it certainly change. The existence of this ASCRS Textbook and the mechanism which perpetuates it guarantees that we always have the most up-to-date information available to our members and trainees. The proceeds from the sale of the ASCRS Textbook also flow into the Education Foundation of the ASCRS to bring independence from outside sponsorship to our national meeting. The Executive Council of the ASCRS is fully supportive of this effort by the Editorial Board of the ASCRS Textbook and gratefully recognizes their contribution and that of the group of experts who provide new and updated chapters for each successive edition.

Please remember the sacrifice of time and effort that made this publication possible. Strive to add to the knowledge which one day changes our practice and our specialty. Use this ASCRS Textbook to show the world that the ASCRS is THE authority on colorectal disease as we improve patient care.

James W. Fleshman, MD
Senior Editor of the First Edition of the ASCRS Textbook of Colon and Rectal Surgery
Immediate Past President of the American Society of Colon and Rectal Surgeons
Professor of Surgery Washington University in St, Louis

Special Acknowledgement

Senior Editors from First Edition

Bruce G. Wolff
James W. Fleshman
David E. Beck
John H. Pemberton
Steven D. Wexner

Associate Editors from the First Edition

James M. Church
Julio Garcia-Aguilar
Patricia L. Roberts
Theodore J. Saclarides
Michael J. Stamos

Contents

Contributors

Nancy N. Baxter, MD, PhD
Associate Professor of Surgery, Department of Surgery, St. Michael's Hospital, University of Toronto, Toronto, ON, Canada

Jennifer S. Beatty, MD
Assistant Professor of Surgery, Division of Colon and Rectal Surgery, Creighton University School of Medicine, Omaha, NE, USA

Mitchell A. Bernstein, MD, FACS, FASCRS
Assistant Professor of Clinical Surgery; Senior Attending Department of Surgery, Program Director, Colon and Rectal Surgery Fellowship, Columbia University College of Physicians and Surgeons, New York, NY, USA; St. Luke's Roosevelt Hospital Center, New York NY, USA

Ronald Bleday, MD
Chair, Section of Colorectal Surgery, Department of Surgery, Brigham and Women's Hospital, Boston MA, USA

Jaime L. Bohl, MD
Staff Surgeon, Department of Colon and Rectal Surgery, Ochsner Clinic, New Orleans, LA, USA

Robin P. Boushey, BSc, MD, PhD, CIP, FRCSC
Assistant Professor of Surgery, Director, General Surgery Research, Site Lead, Colorectal Cancer Program Champlain LHIN, Investigator, Ottawa Regional Cancer Center, Affiliate Investigator, Ottawa Hospital Research Institute, Department of Surgery, The Ottawa Hospital – General Campus, Ottawa, ON, Canada

Nelya Brindzei, MD
Department of Surgery, Brigham and Women's Hospital, Boston, MA, USA

Peter A. Cataldo, MD
Professor of Surgery, Department of Surgery, Fletcher Allen Healthcare, Burlington, VT, USA

Christina Cellini, MD
Assistant Professor of Surgery, Division of Colorectal Surgery, University of Rochester, Strong Memorial Hospital, Rochester, NY, USA

Formosa Chen, MD
Department of Surgery, Ronald Regan UCLA Medical Center, Los Angeles, CA, USA

William T. Choctaw, MD, JD
Past Chief of Surgery, Department of Surgery, Citrus Valley Medical Center, Covina, CA, USA

James Church, MBChB, MMedSci, FRACS
Victor W. Fazio Chair in Colorectal Surgery, Department of Colorectal Surgery, Digestive Diseases Institute, Cleveland Clinic Foundation, Cleveland, OH, USA

Robert R. Cima, MD
Consultant, Associate Professor of Surgery, Mayo Clinic, Rochester, MN, USA

Conor P. Delaney, MD, MCh, PhD, FRCSI, FACS, FASCRS
Professor and Chief of Colorectal Surgery, Department of Surgery, University Hospital Case Medical Center, Cleveland, OH, USA

David W. Dietz, MD
Staff Surgeon, Department of Digestive Disease, Cleveland Clinic, Cleveland, OH, USA

Eric J. Dozois, MD
Associate Professor of Surgery, Department of Colon and Rectal Surgery, Mayo Clinic, Rochester, MN, USA

Nadav Dujovny, MD
Assistant Professor of Surgery, Ferguson Clinic, Spectrum Health Medical Group, Michigan State University, 4100 Lake Drive #205, Grand Rapids, MI 49546, USA

Kelli Bullard Dunn, MD
Associate Professor of Surgery, Roswell Park Cancer Institute and the University of Buffalo, State University of New York, Buffalo, NY, USA

Sharon L. Dykes, MD
Adjunct Instructor of Surgery, Division of Colorectal Surgery, University of Minnesota, Minneapolis, MN, USA

Jonathan E. Efron, MD
Associate Professor and Chair of the Ravitch Division, Department of Surgery, Johns Hopkins Hospital, Baltimore, MD, USA

David A. Etzioni, MD, MSHS
Associate Professor, Mayo Clinic College of Medicine, Senior Associate Consultant, Mayo Clinic Arizona, Department of Surgery, Phoenix, AZ, USA

John R. Fenyk Jr, MD
Professor of Medicine, Department of Dermatology, University of Minnesota Medical School, Minneapolis, MN, USA

Charles O. Finne III, MD
Adjunct Professor of Surgery, Division of Colon and Rectal Surgery, Department of Surgery, University of Minnesota Medical School, Minneapolis, MN, USA

Phillip Fleshner, MD, FACS, FASCRS
Director, Colorectal Surgery Residency; Clinical Professor of Surgery, Cedars-Sinai Medical Center, Los Angeles, CA, USA; UCLA School of Medicine, Los Angeles, CA, USA

Daniel M. Freeman, AB, JD
Academic Director, Public Law, Washington Semester Program,
American University, Washington, DC, USA

Susan L. Gearhart, MD
Assistant Professor of Colorectal Surgery, Department of Surgery,
Johns Hopkins Medical Institution, Baltimore, MD, USA

Lester Gottesman, MD, FACS, FASCRS
Associate Professor of Clinical Surgery, Columbia School of Physicians and Surgeons,
St. Luke's Roosevelt, Department of Colorectal Surgery, New York, NY, USA

Jose G. Guillem, MD, PhD
Attending Surgeon, Department of Colorectal Surgery,
Memorial Sloan-Kettering Cancer Center, New York, NY, USA

Brooke H. Gurland, MD
Staff Colon and Rectal Surgeon, Department of Colorectal Surgery,
Cleveland Clinic Foundation, Cleveland, OH, USA

Angelita Habr-Gama, MD, PhD, FACS (Hon), ASA (Hon), ESA (Hon)
Professor of Surgery; Director, University of São Paulo, Sao Paolo, Brazil;
Angelita & Joaquim Gama Institute, Sao Paolo, Brazil

Jason F Hall, MD
Assistant Professor of Surgery; Staff Surgeon, Department of Colon and Rectal Surgery,
Tufts University School of Medicine, Boston, MA, USA;
Lahey Clinic, Burlington, MA, USA

Maria Dolores Herreros Marcos, MD, PhD
Department of Colon and Rectal Surgery, Mayo Clinic, Rochester, MN, USA

Jon S. Hourigan, MD
Assistant Professor of Surgery, Section of Colorectal Surgery, Department of Surgery,
University of Kentucky, 800 Rose Street, C220 Lexington, KY 40536, USA

David B. Hoyt, MD, FACS
Executive Director, American College of Surgeons, Chicago, IL, USA

Tracy L. Hull, MD
Professor of Surgery, Department of Colon and Rectal Surgery,
Cleveland Clinic Foundation, Cleveland, OH, USA

Richard E. Karulf, MD
Clinical Professor, Division of Colon and Rectal Surgery, Department of Surgery,
University of Minnesota, Edina, MN, USA

José Marcio Neves Jorge, MD, PhD
Associate Professor, Department of Gastroenterology, Colorectal Division,
University of Sao Paolo, Sao Paolo, Brazil

Donald G. Kim, MD
Clinical Assistant Professor, Department of Surgery; Staff Colon and Rectal Surgeon,
Michigan State University College of Human Medicine, Lansing, MI, USA;
Ferguson Clinic, Grand Rapids, MI, USA

Clifford Y. Ko, MD, MS, MSHS, FACS, FASCRS
Professor of Surgery, Robert and Kelly Day Chair in Surgical Outcomes, Director, Center for Surgical Outcomes and Quality, Department of Surgery, Los Angeles, CA, USA

Ira J. Kodner, MD
Solon and Bettie Gershmen Professor of Colon and Rectal Surgery, Department of Surgery, Washington University School of Medicine, St. Louis, MO, USA

Walter A. Koltun, MD, FACS, FASCRS
Peter and Marshla Carlino Chair in Inflammatory Bowel Disease, Professor of Surgery, Chief, Division of Colon and Rectal Surgery, Department of Surgery, Penn State Milton S. Hershey Medical Center, Hershey, PA, USA

Hiroko Kunitake, MD
Department of Surgery, Massachusetts General Hospital, Boston, MA, USA

Elise Lawson, MD
Department of Surgery, Ronald Regan UCLA Medical Center, Los Angeles, CA, USA

Patrick Y. H. Lee, MD
Associate Clinical Professor; Consultant, Surgical Speciality/The Colon and Rectal Clinic, Oregon Health Sciences University, Portland, OR, USA

Michael E. Lekawa, MD, FACS
Professor and Chief, Division of Trauma and Critical Care, Director, Trauma Services, University of California, Irvine Medical Center, Orange, CA, USA

Marc A. Levitt, MD
Associate Professor, Colorectal Center for Children, Associate Professor, Division of Pediatric Surgery, Cincinanati Children's Hospital Medical Center, Cincinnati, OH, USA

Ann C. Lowry, MD
Adjunct Professor, Department of Surgery, Division of Colon and Rectal Surgery, University of Minnesota, St Paul, MN, USA

Martin Luchtefeld, MD
Chief of Colon and Rectal Surgery, Spectrum Health, Michigan Medical PC – Ferguson Clinic, Grand Rapids, MI, USA

Elisabeth C. McLemore, MD
Assistant Professor of Surgery, Colon & Rectal Surgery, Moores Cancer Center, University of California, San Diego, La Jolla, CA, USA

Robert D. Madoff, MD, FACS
Professor of Surgery, Department of Surgery, University of Minnesota, Minneapolis, MN, USA

Mari A. Madsen, MD
Clinical Chief, Division of Colon and Rectal Surgery, Cedars-Sinai Medical Center, West Hollywood, CA, USA

Floriano Marchetti, MD
Assistant Professor of Clinical Surgery, Program Director,
Colon and Rectal Surgery Residency Program, Department of Surgery,
University of Miami Miller School of Medicine, Miami, FL, USA

David A. Margolin, MD
Director, Colon and Rectal Surgery Research, Staff, Colon and Rectal Surgeon,
Department of Colon and Rectal Surgery, Ochsner Clinic Foundation,
New Orleans, LA, USA

Justin A. Maykel, MD
Assistant Professor of Surgery, Chief, Division of Colon and Rectal Surgery,
Department of Surgery, University of Massachusetts Medical Center, Worcester, MA, USA

Michael J. Meehan, BA, JD
Senior Director, Regional Hospitals Group, Cleveland Clinic Law Department,
Cleveland Clinic Foundation, Cleveland, OH, USA

Anders F. Mellgren, MD, PhD
Adjunct Professor of Surgery; Director, Department of Colon and Rectal Surgery,
University of Minnesota, Minneapolis, MN, USA;
Pelvic Floor Center, Minneapolis, MN, USA

Guillaum Meurette, MD
Chirurgie Digestive et Endocrine, Institut des Maladies de l'appareil Digestif,
Centre Hospitalo-Universitaire, Nantes, France

Steven Mills, MD, FASCRS
Assistant Clinical Professor of Surgery, Department of Surgery,
University of California, Irvine, Orange, CA, USA

Husein Moloo, MD, MSc, FRCSC
Assistant Professor of Surgery; Clinical Investigator,
Ottawa Hospital Research Institute, University of Ottawa, Ottawa, ON, Canada;
Department of Surgery, The Ottawa Hospital, Ottawa, ON, Canada

Harvey G. Moore, MD, FACS, FASCRS
Assistant Professor of Surgery, Department of Surgery,
New York University School of Medicine, New York, NY, USA

Zuri Murrell, MD, FACS
Attending Surgeon, Division of Colorectal Surgery, Cedars-Sinai Medical Center,
Los Angeles, CA, USA

Matthew Mutch, MD
Associate Professor of Surgery, Department of Surgery, Section of Colon and Rectal Surgery,
Barnes Jewish Hospital/Washington University School of Medicine, St. Louis, MO, USA

Harry T. Papaconstantinou, MD
Assistant Professor, Chief Section of Colon and Rectal Surgery,
Scott & White Memorial Hospital and Clinic, Temple, TX, USA;
Department of Surgery, Texas A & M University Health System, Temple, TX, USA

Alberto Peña, MD
Director, Colorectal Center for Children, Professor, Division of Pediatric Surgery
Cincinnati Children's Hospital Medical Center, Cincinnati, OH, USA

Janice F. Rafferty, MD
Professor of Surgery, Chief, Division of Colon and Rectal Surgery,
Department of Surgery, University of Cincinnati College of Medicine, Cincinnati, OH, USA

Nalini Raju, MD
General Surgery, Section of Colon and Rectal Surgery,
Stanford University School of Medical, Stanford, CA, USA

Jan Rakinic, MD
Associate Professor of Surgery, Chief, Section of Colorectal Surgery,
Department of Surgery, Southern Illinois University School of Medicine,
Springfield, IL, USA

Sonia Ramamoorthy, MD
Assistant Professor of Surgery, Colon and Rectal Surgery,
Rebecca and John Moores Cancer Center, La Jolla, CA, USA

Thomas E. Read, MD, FACS, FASCRS
Professor of Surgery; Staff Surgeon, Department of Colon and Rectal Surgery,
Program Director, Colon and Rectal Surgery Residency,
Tufts University School of Medicine, Boston, MA, USA;
Lahey Clinic Medical Center, Burlington, MA, USA

Craig A. Reickert, MD
Assistant Professor of Surgery, Wayne State University
School of Medicine, Detroit, MI, USA;
Department of Colon and Rectal Surgery, Henry Ford Hospital, Detroit, MI, USA

Dana R. Sands, MD, FACS, FASCRS
Director, Colorectal Physiology Center, Staff Surgeon, Department of Colorectal Surgery,
Cleveland Clinic Florida, Weston, FL, USA

Rocco Ricciardi, MD, MPH
Staff Surgeon, Assistant Professor of Surgery, Department of Colon and Rectal Surgery,
Lahey Clinic, Burlington, MA, USA

Lester Rosen, MD
Attending Surgeon, Department of Colon and Rectal Surgery,
Cleveland Clinic Florida, Weston, FL, USA

Joan Ryoo, MD
Department of General Internal Medicine/Health Services Research,
Ronald Regan UCLA Medical Center, Los Angeles, CA, USA

Bruce E. Sands, MD, MS
Associate Professor of Medicine; Acting Chief, Gastrointestinal Unit, Medical Co-director,
MGH Crohn's and Colitis Center, Harvard School of Medicine, Boston, MA, USA;
Massachusetts General Hospital, Boston, MA, USA

Laurence R. Sands, MD, MBA
Associate Professor of Clinical Surgery, Chief, Division of Colon and Rectal Surgery, Department of Surgery, University of Miami, Miller School of Medicine, Miami, FL, USA

David J. Schoetz Jr, MD
Chairman Emeritus, Department of Colon and Rectal Surgery; Professor of Surgery, Lahey Clinic, Burlington, MA, USA;
Tufts University School of Medicine, Boston, MA, USA

Mark Siegler, MD
Professor, Department of Medicine and Surgery, Lindy Bergman Distinguished Service Professor, Director, MacLean Center for Clinical Medical Ethics, Department of Medicine Ethics Center, University of Chicago, Chicago, IL, USA

Marc Singer, MD
Department of Surgery, Section of Colon and Rectal Surgery, NorthShore University Health System, Evanston, IL, USA

Michael J. Snyder, MD
Program Director, The University of Texas Health Sciences Center at Houston, Houston, TX, USA;
Department of Colon and Rectal Surgery, Methodist Hospital, Houston, TX, USA

Scott R. Steele, MD
Chief, Colon and Rectal Surgery
Department of Surgery, Madigan Army Medical Center, Tacoma, WA, USA

Sharon L. Stein, PhD
Department of General Surgery, University Hospital Case Medical Center, Cleveland, OH, USA

Scott A. Strong, MD
Department of Colon and Rectal Surgery, Cleveland Clinic Foundation, Cleveland, OH, USA

Ursula M. Szmulowicz, MD
Associate Staff, Department of Colorectal Surgery, Cleveland Clinic Foundation, Cleveland, OH, USA

J. Scott Thomas, MD
Assistant Professor, Department of Surgery, Section of Colon and Rectal Surgery, Scott & White Memorial Hospital and Clinic, Temple, TX, USA;
Texas A & M University Health System, Temple, TX, USA

Alan G. Thorson, MD
Clinical Associate Professor of Surgery; Program Director, Colon and Rectal Surgery, Creighton University School of Medicine, Omaha, NE, USA;
University of Nebraska College of Medicine, Omaha, NE, USA

Alan E. Timmcke, MD
Gastroenterologist, 1514 Jefferson Hwy, Jefferson, LA70121 USA

Melissa Times, MD
Assistant Professor of Surgery, Wayne State University
School of Medicine, Detroit, MI, USA;
Department of Colon and Rectal Surgery, Henry Ford Hospital, Detroit, MI, USA

Judith L. Trudel, MD, MSc, MHPE, FRCSC, FACS
Clinical Professor of Surgery, Department of Surgery, University of Minnesota,
St. Paul, MN, USA

Madhulika G. Varma, MD
Associate Professor, Chief, Section of Colorectal Surgery,
Department of Surgery, University of California, San Francisco, San Francisco, CA, USA

Carol-Ann Vasilevsky, MD, FRCSC, FACS
Assistant Professor of Surgery and Oncology, Division of Colorectal Surgery,
Jewish General Hospital, McGill University, Montreal, Quebec

Eric G. Weiss, MD
Vice Chairman, Colorectal Surgery, DIO/Chairman of Graduate Medical Education
and Program Director, Colorectal Surgery, Director of Surgical Endoscopy,
Cleveland Clinic Florida, Weston, FL, USA

Mark Lane Welton, MD, MHCM
Division of General Surgery, Section of Colon and Rectal Surgery, Stanford University
School of Medicine, Stanford, CA, USA

Charles B. Whitlow, MD
Staff Surgeon and Residency Program Director, Department of Colon and Rectal Surgery,
Ochsner Medical Center, New Orleans, LA, USA

Paul E. Wise, MD
Assistant Professor of Surgery, Director, Vanderbilt Hereditary Colorectal Cancer Registry,
Department of General Surgery, Vanderbilt University Medical Center, Nashville, TN, USA

W. Douglas Wong†, MD, FACS, FRSC(C)
Professor of Surgery; Chief, Colorectal Service,
Weill Medical College of Cornell University, New York, NY, USA;
Memorial Sloan-Kettering Cancer Center, New York, NY, USA

Tonia Young-Fadok, MD, MS, FACS, FASCRS
Professor of Surgery, Mayo Clinic College of Medicine, Chair,
Division of Colon and Rectal Surgery, Mayo Clinic Scottsdale, Phoenix, AZ, USA

1 Anatomy and Embryology

José Marcio Neves Jorge and Angelita Habr-Gama

Although much of our fundamental understanding of the anatomy of the colon, rectum, and anus comes from the efforts of researchers of the nineteenth and early twentieth centuries, comprehensive observations of this region had been made as early as 1543 by Andreas Vesalius through anatomic dissections.[1] However, anatomy of this region, especially that of the rectum and anal canal, is so intrinsically related to its physiology that much can be appreciated only in the living. Thus, it is a region in which the surgeon has an advantage over the anatomist through in vivo dissection, physiologic investigation, and endoscopic examination. However, anatomy of the pelvis is also challenging to the surgeon: the pelvis is a narrow space, packed with intestinal, urologic, gynecologic, vascular, and neural structures, all confined within a rigid and deep osseous–muscular cage. Therefore, detailed anatomy of this region is difficult to learn in the setting of an operating room and it demands not only observations in vivo, but historical reviews, anatomy laboratory studies, including dissections of humans and animals, with in-depth descriptions and drawings and sometimes associated with physiologic evaluation. Based on these studies, some controversial concepts of the anatomy, especially of the rectum and anal canal, have been actually changed.[2–8] In addition, virtual reality models have been designed to improve visualization of three-dimensional structures and more properly teach anatomy, pathology, and surgery of the anorectum and pelvic floor.[9]

Anatomy

Anus and Rectum

Anal Canal Structure, Anus, and Anal Verge

The anal canal is anatomically peculiar and has a complex physiology, which accounts for its crucial role in continence and, in addition, its susceptibility to a variety of diseases. The anus or anal orifice is an anteroposterior cutaneous slit that, along with the anal canal, remains virtually closed at rest, as a result of tonic circumferential contraction of the sphincters and the presence of anal cushions. The edge of the anal orifice, the anal verge or margin (anocutaneous line of Hilton), marks the lowermost edge of the anal canal and is sometimes the level of reference for measurements taken during sigmoidoscopy. Others favor the dentate line as a landmark because it is more precise. The difference between the anal verge and the dentate line is usually 1–2 cm. The epithelium distal to the anal verge acquires hair follicles, glands, including apocrine glands, and other features of normal skin, and is the source of perianal hidradenitis suppurativa, inflammation of the apocrine glands.

Anatomic Versus Surgical Anal Canal

Two definitions are found describing the anal canal (Figure 1-1). The "anatomic" or "embryologic" anal canal is only 2.0 cm long, extending from the anal verge to the dentate line, the level that corresponds to the proctodeal membrane. The "surgical" or "functional" anal canal is longer, extending for approximately 4.0 cm (in men) from the anal verge to the anorectal ring (levator ani). This "long anal canal" concept was first introduced by Milligan and Morgan[10] and has been considered, despite not being proximally marked by any apparent epithelial or developmental boundary, useful both as a physiologic and surgical parameter. The anorectal ring is at the level of the distal end of the ampullary part of the rectum and forms the anorectal angle, and the beginning of a region of higher intraluminal pressure. Therefore, this definition correlates with digital, manometric, and sonographic examinations.

Anatomic Relations of the Anal Canal

Posteriorly, the anal canal is related to the coccyx and anteriorly to the perineal body and the lowest part of the posterior vaginal wall in the female, and to the urethra in the male. The ischium and the ischiorectal fossa are situated on either side. The fossa ischiorectal contains fat and the inferior rectal

D.E. Beck et al. (eds.), *The ASCRS Textbook of Colon and Rectal Surgery: Second Edition*,
DOI 10.1007/978-1-4419-1584-9_1, © Springer Science+Business Media, LLC 2011

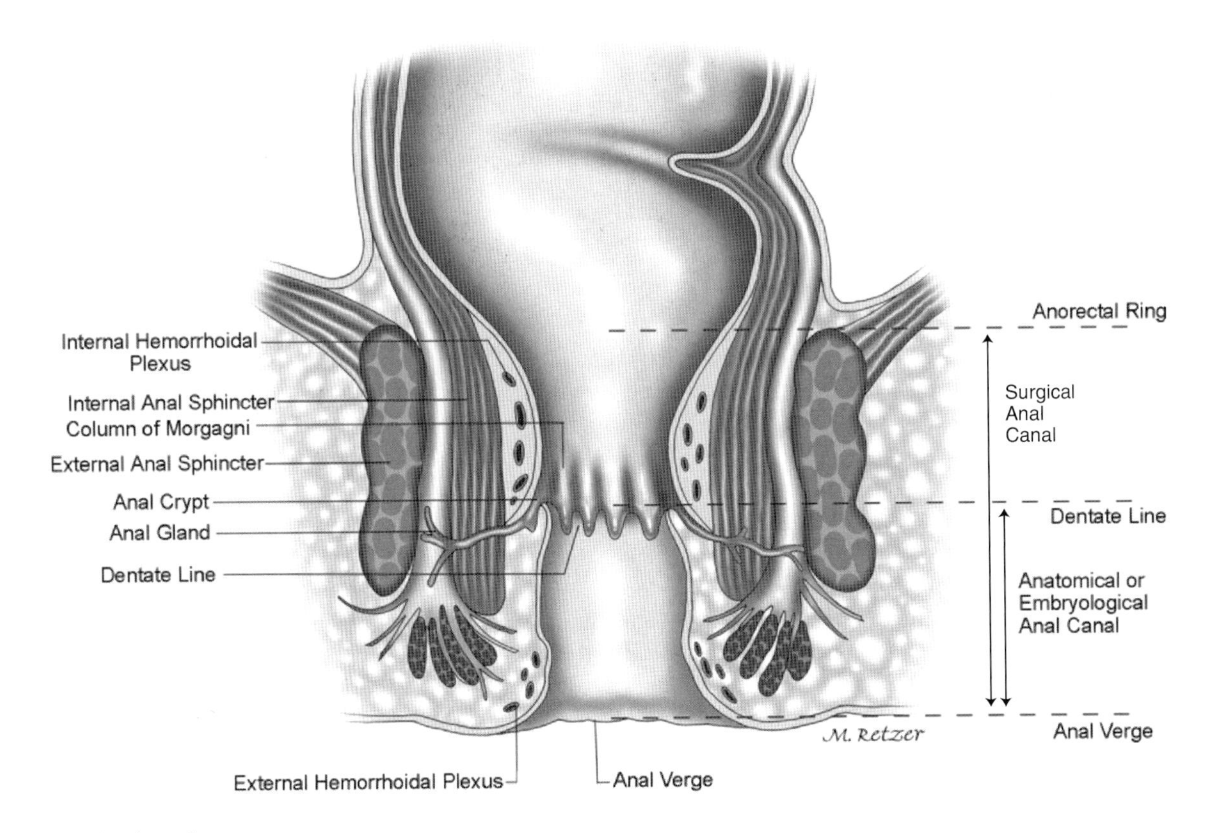

FIGURE 1-1. Anal canal.

vessels and nerves, which cross it to enter the wall of the anal canal.

Muscles of the Anal Canal

The muscular component of the mechanism of continence can be stratified into three functional groups: lateral compression from the pubococcygeus, circumferential closure from the internal and external anal sphincter, and angulation from the puborectalis (Figure 1-2). The internal and external anal sphincters, and the conjoined longitudinal are intrinsically related to the anal canal, and are addressed here.

Internal Anal Sphincter

The internal anal sphincter represents the distal 2.5- to 4.0-cm condensation of the circular muscle layer of the rectum. As a consequence of both intrinsic myogenic and extrinsic autonomic neurogenic properties, the internal anal sphincter is a smooth muscle in a state of continuous maximal contraction, and represents a natural barrier to the involuntary loss of stool and gas.

The lower rounded edge of the internal anal sphincter can be felt on physical examination, about 1.2 cm distal to the dentate line. The groove between the internal and external anal sphincter, the intersphincteric sulcus, can be visualized or easily palpated. Endosonographically, the internal anal sphincter is a 2- to 3-mm-thick circular band and shows a uniform hypoechogenicity.

External Anal Sphincter

The external anal sphincter is the elliptical cylinder of striated muscle that envelops the entire length of the inner tube of smooth muscle, but it ends slightly more distal than the internal anal sphincter. The external anal sphincter was initially described as encompassing three divisions: subcutaneous, superficial, and deep.[10] Goligher et al.[11] described the external anal sphincter as a simple, continuous sheet that forms, along with the puborectalis and levator ani, one funnel-shaped skeletal muscle. The deepest part of the external anal sphincter is intimately related to the puborectalis muscle, which can actually be considered a component of both the levator ani and the external anal sphincter muscle complexes. Others considered the external anal sphincter as being subdivided into two parts, deep (deep sphincter and puborectalis) and superficial (subcutaneous and superficial sphincter).[6,12,13] Shafik[14] proposed the three U-shaped loop system, but clinical experience has not supported this schema. The external anal sphincter is more likely to be one muscle unit, attached by the anococcygeal ligament posteriorly to the coccyx, and anteriorly to the perineal body, not divided into layers or laminae. Nevertheless, differences in

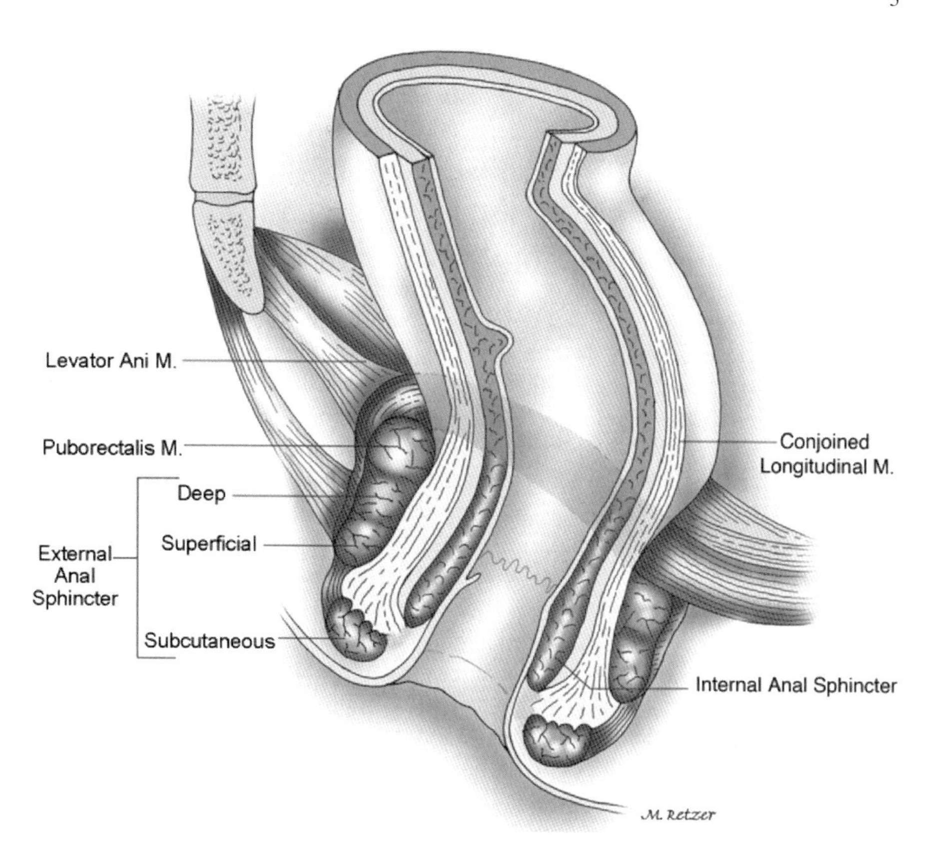

FIGURE 1-2. Muscles of the anal canal.

the arrangement of the external anal sphincter have been described between the genders.[15] In the male, the upper half of the external anal sphincter is enveloped anteriorly by the conjoined longitudinal muscle, whereas the lower half is crossed by it. In the female, the entire external anal sphincter is encapsulated by a mixture of fibers derived from both longitudinal and internal anal sphincter muscles.

Endosonographically, the puborectalis and the external anal sphincter, despite their mixed linear echogenicity, are both predominantly hyperechogenic, with a mean thickness of 6 mm (range, 5–8 mm). Distinction is made by position, shape, and topography. Recently, both anal endosonography and endocoil magnetic resonance imaging have been used to detail the anal sphincter complex in living, healthy subjects.[16–19] These tests provide a three-dimensional mapping of the anal sphincter; they help to study the differences in the arrangement of the external anal sphincter between the sexes and uncover sphincter disruption or defect during vaginal deliveries. In addition, there is some degree of "anatomical asymmetry" of the external anal sphincter, which accounts for both radial and longitudinal "functional asymmetry" observed during anal manometry.[20]

The automatic continence mechanism is formed by the resting tone, maintained by the internal anal sphincter, magnified by voluntary, reflex, and resting external anal sphincter contractile activities. In response to conditions of threatened incontinence, such as increased intraabdominal pressure and rectal distension, the external anal sphincter and puborectalis reflexively and voluntarily contract further to prevent fecal leakage. Because of muscular fatigue, maximal voluntary contraction of the external anal sphincter can be sustained for only 30–60 s. However, the external anal sphincter and the pelvic floor muscles, unlike other skeletal muscles, which are usually inactive at rest, maintain unconscious resting electrical tone through a reflex arc at the cauda equina level. Histologic studies have shown that the external anal sphincter, puborectalis, and levator ani muscles have a predominance of type I fibers, which are a peculiarity of skeletal muscles connecting tonic contractile activity.[21]

Conjoined Longitudinal Muscle

Whereas the inner circular layer of the rectum gives rise to the internal anal sphincter, the outer longitudinal layer, at the level of the anorectal ring, mixes with fibers of the levator ani muscle to form the conjoined longitudinal muscle. This muscle descends between the internal and external anal sphincter, and ultimately some of its fibers, referred to as the *corrugator cutis ani muscle*, traverse the lowermost part of the external anal sphincter to insert into the perianal skin. Some of these fibers may enter the fat of the ischiorectal fossa.[22] Other sources for the striated component of the conjoined longitudinal muscle include the puborectalis and deep external anal sphincter, the pubococcygeus and top loop of the external anal sphincter, and the lower fibers of the puborectalis.[7,23,24] In its descending course, the conjoined longitudinal muscle may give rise to medial extensions that cross the internal anal sphincter to contribute the smooth muscle of the submucosa (musculus canalis ani, sustentator tunicae mucosae, Treitz muscle, musculus submucosae ani).[25]

Possible functions of the conjoined longitudinal muscle include attaching the anorectum to the pelvis and acting as a skeleton that supports and binds the internal and external sphincter complex together.[22] Haas and Fox[26] consider that the meshwork formed by the conjoined longitudinal muscle may minimize functional deterioration of the sphincters after surgical division and act as a support to prevent hemorrhoidal and rectal prolapse. In addition, the conjoined longitudinal muscle and its extensions to the intersphincteric plane divide the adjacent tissues into subspaces and may actually have a role in the septation of thrombosed external hemorrhoids and containment of sepsis.[7] Finally, Shafik[23] ascribed to the conjoined longitudinal muscle the action of shortening and widening of the anal canal as well as eversion of the anal orifice, and proposed the controversial term evertor ani muscle. In addition to this primary function during defecation, a limited role in anal continence, specifically a potentialization effect in maintaining an anal seal, has also been proposed.[23]

Epithelium of the Anal Canal

The lining of the anal canal consists of an upper mucosal (endoderm) and a lower cutaneous (ectoderm) segment (Figure 1-1). The dentate (pectinate) line is the "sawtoothed" junction between these two distinct origins of venous and lymphatic drainage, nerve supply, and epithelial lining. Above this level, the intestine is innervated by the sympathetic and parasympathetic systems, with venous, arterial, and lymphatic drainage to and from the hypogastric vessels. Distal to the dentate line, the anal canal is innervated by the somatic nervous system, with blood supply and drainage from the inferior hemorrhoidal system. These differences are important when the classification and treatment of hemorrhoids are considered.

The pectinate or dentate line corresponds to a line of anal valves that represent remnants of the proctodeal membrane. Above each valve, there is a little pocket known as an anal sinus or crypt. These crypts are connected to a variable number of glands, in average 6 (range, 3–12).[27,28] The anal glands first described by Chiari in 1878[29] are more concentrated in the posterior quadrants. More than one gland may open into the same crypt, whereas half the crypts have no communication. The anal gland ducts, in an outward and downward route, enter the submucosa; two-thirds enter the internal anal sphincter, and half of them terminate in the intersphincteric plane.[28] Obstruction of these ducts, presumably by accumulation of foreign material in the crypts, may lead to perianal abscesses and fistulas.[30] Cephalad to the dentate line, 8–14 longitudinal folds, known as the rectal columns (columns of Morgagni), have their bases connected in pairs to each valve at the dentate line. At the lower end of the columns are the anal papillae. The mucosa in the area of the columns consists of several layers of cuboidal cells and has a deep purple color because of the underlying internal hemorrhoidal plexus. This 0.5- to 1.0-cm strip of mucosa above the dentate line is known as the anal transition or cloacogenic zone. Cephalad to this area, the epithelium changes to a single layer of columnar cells and macroscopically acquires the characteristic pink color of the rectal mucosa.

The cutaneous part of the anal canal consists of modified squamous epithelium that is thin, smooth, pale, stretched, and devoid of hair and glands. The terms pecten and pecten band have been used to define this segment.[31] However, as pointed out by Goligher, the round band of fibrous tissue called pecten band, which is divided in the case of anal fissure (pectenotomy), probably represents the spastic internal anal sphincter.[11,32]

Rectum

Both proximal and distal limits of the rectum are controversial: the rectosigmoid junction is considered to be at the level of the third sacral vertebra by anatomists but at the sacral promontory by surgeons, and likewise, the distal limit is regarded to be the muscular anorectal ring by surgeons and the dentate line by anatomists. The rectum measures 12–15 cm in length and has three lateral curves: the upper and lower are convex to the right and the middle is convex to the left. These curves correspond intraluminally to the folds or valves of Houston. The two left-sided folds are usually noted at 7–8 cm and at 12–13 cm, respectively, and the one on the right is generally at 9–11 cm. The middle valve (Kohlrausch's plica) is the most consistent in presence and location and corresponds to the level of the anterior peritoneal reflection. Although the rectal valves do not contain all muscle wall layers from a clinical point of view, they are a good location for performing a rectal biopsies because they are readily accessible with minimal risk of perforation.[13,33] The valves of Houston must be negotiated during proctosigmoidoscopy; they are absent after mobilization of the rectum, and this is attributed to the 5-cm length gained after complete surgical dissection. The rectal mucosa is smooth, pink, and transparent, which allows visualization of small and large submucosal vessels. This characteristic "vascular pattern" disappears in inflammatory conditions and in melanosis coli.

The rectum is characterized by its wide, easily distensible lumen, and the absence of taeniae, epiploic appendices, haustra, or a well-defined mesentery. The prefix "meso," in gross anatomy, refers to two layers of peritoneum that suspend an organ. Normally, the rectum is not suspended but entirely extraperitoneal on its posterior aspect, and closely applied to the sacral hollow. Consequently, the term "mesorectum" is anatomically inaccurate. An exception, however, is that a peritonealized mesorectum may be noted in patients with procidentia. But, the word "mesorectum" has gained widespread popularity among surgeons to address the perirectal areolar tissue, which is thicker posteriorly, containing terminal branches of the inferior mesenteric artery and enclosed by the fascia propria.[34,35] The "mesorectum" may be a metastatic site for a rectal cancer and is removed during surgery for rectal cancer without neurologic sequelae because no functionally significant nerves pass through it.

The upper third of the rectum is anteriorly and laterally invested by peritoneum; the middle third is covered by peritoneum on its anterior aspect only. Finally, the lower third of the rectum is entirely extraperitoneal because the anterior peritoneal reflection occurs at 9.0–7.0 cm from the anal verge in men and at 7.5–5.0 cm from the anal verge in women.

Anatomic Relations of the Rectum

The rectum occupies the sacral concavity and ends 2–3 cm anteroinferiorly from the tip of the coccyx. At this point, it angulates backward sharply to pass through the levators and becomes the anal canal. Anteriorly, in women, the rectum is closely related to the uterine cervix and posterior vaginal wall; in men, it lies behind the bladder, vas deferens, seminal vesicles, and prostate. Posterior to the rectum lie the median sacral vessels and the roots of the sacral nerve plexus.

Fascial Relationships of the Rectum

The parietal endopelvic fascia lines the walls and floor of the pelvis and continues on the internal organs as a visceral pelvic fascia (Figure 1-3A, B). Thus, the *fascia propria of the rectum* is an extension of the pelvic fascia, enclosing the rectum, fat, nerves, the blood, and lymphatic vessels. It is more evident in the posterior and lateral extraperitoneal aspects of the rectum.

The lateral ligaments or stalks of the rectum are distal condensations of the pelvic fascia that form a roughly triangular structure with a base on the lateral pelvic wall and an apex attached to the lateral aspect of the rectum.[32] Still a subject of misconception, the lateral stalks comprise essentially connective tissue and nerves, and the middle rectal artery does not traverse them. Branches, however, course through in approximately 25% of cases.[36] Consequently, division of the lateral stalks during rectal mobilization is associated with a 25% risk of bleeding. Although the lateral stalks do not contain important structures, the middle rectal artery and the pelvic plexus are both closely related, running, at different angles, underneath it.[37] One theoretical concern in ligation of the stalks is leaving behind lateral mesorectal tissue, which may limit adequate lateral or mesorectal margins during cancer surgery.[34,35,38]

The presacral fascia is a thickened part of the parietal endopelvic fascia that covers the concavity of the sacrum and coccyx, nerves, the middle sacral artery, and presacral veins. Operative dissection deep to the presacral fascia may cause troublesome bleeding from the underlying presacral veins. Presacral hemorrhage occurs as frequently as 4.6–7.0% of resections for rectal neoplasms, and despite its venous nature, can be life threatening.[39–41] This is a consequence of two factors: the difficulty in securing control because of retraction of the vascular stump into the sacral foramen and the high hydrostatic pressure of the presacral venous system. The presacral veins are avalvular and communicate via basivertebral veins with the internal vertebral venous system. The adventitia of the basivertebral veins adheres firmly to the sacral periosteum at the level of the ostia of the sacral foramina, mainly at the level of S3-4. With the patient in the lithotomy

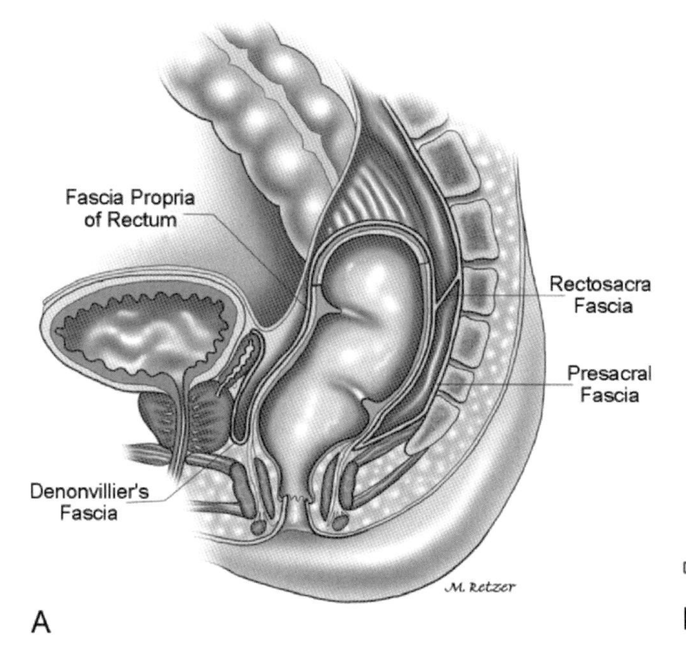

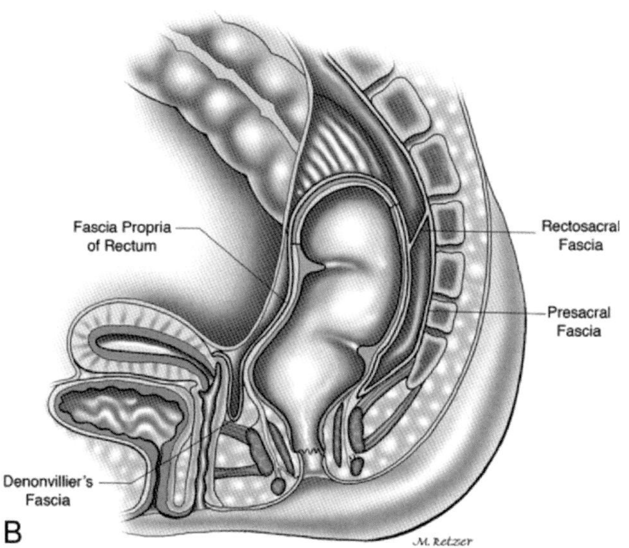

FIGURE 1-3. Fascial relationships of the rectum: **A** male, **B** female.

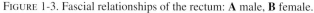

position, the presacral veins can attain hydrostatic pressures of 17–23 cm H_2O, two to three times the normal pressure of the inferior vena cava.[40]

The rectosacral fascia is an anteroinferiorly directed thick fascial reflection from the presacral fascia at the S-4 level to the fascia propria of the rectum just above the anorectal ring.[42] The rectosacral fascia, classically known as the fascia of Waldeyer, is an important landmark during posterior rectal dissection.[2,42]

The visceral pelvic fascia of Denonvilliers is a tough fascial investment that separates the extraperitoneal rectum anteriorly from the prostate and seminal vesicles or vagina.[43] Therefore, three structures lie between the anterior rectal wall and the seminal vesicles and prostate: anterior mesorectum, fascia propria of the rectum, and Denonvilliers' fascia. A consensus has generally been reached about the anatomy of the plane of posterior and lateral rectal dissection, but anteriorly, the matter is more controversial. The anterior plane of rectal dissection may not necessarily follow the same plane of posterior and lateral dissection, and the use of the terms close rectal, mesorectal, and extramesorectal have been recently suggested to describe the available anterior planes.[44] The close rectal or perimuscular plane lies inside the fascia propria of the rectum, and therefore it is more difficult and bloody than the mesorectal plane. The mesorectal plane represents the continuation of the same plane of posterior and lateral dissection of the rectum. This is a natural anatomic plane and consequently more appropriate for most rectal cancers. Finally, the extramesorectal plane involves resection of the Denonvilliers' fascia, with the exposure of prostate and seminal vesicles, and is associated with high risk of mixed parasympathetic and sympathetic injury because of damage of the periprostatic plexus.

Urogenital Considerations

Identification of the ureters is advisable to avoid injury to their abdominal or pelvic portions during colorectal operations. On both sides, the ureters rest on the psoas muscle in their inferomedial course; they are crossed obliquely by the spermatic vessels anteriorly and the genitofemoral nerve posteriorly. In its pelvic portion, the ureter crosses the pelvic brim in front of or a little lateral to the bifurcation of the common iliac artery, and descends abruptly between the peritoneum and the internal iliac artery. Before entering the bladder in the male, the vas deferens crosses lateromedially on its superior aspect. In the female, as the ureter traverses the posterior layer of the broad ligament and the parametrium close to the side of the neck of the uterus and upper part of the vagina, it is enveloped by the vesical and vaginal venous plexuses and is crossed above and lateromedially by the uterine artery.

Arterial Supply of the Rectum and Anal Canal

The superior hemorrhoidal artery is the continuation of the inferior mesenteric artery, once it crosses the left iliac vessels. The artery descends in the sigmoid mesocolon to the level of S-3 and then to the posterior aspect of the rectum. In 80% of cases, it bifurcates into right, usually wider, and left terminal branches; multiple branches are present in 17%.[45] These divisions, once within the submucosa of the rectum, run straight downward to supply the lower rectum and the anal canal. Approximately five branches reach the level of the rectal columns, and condense in capillary plexuses, mostly at the right posterior, right anterior, and left lateral positions, corresponding to the location of the major internal hemorrhoidal groups.

The superior and inferior hemorrhoidal arteries represent the major blood supply to the anorectum. In addition, it is also supplied by the internal iliac arteries.

The contribution of the middle hemorrhoidal artery varies with the size of the superior hemorrhoidal artery; this may explain its controversial anatomy. Some authors report the absence of the middle hemorrhoidal artery in 40–88%[46,47], whereas others identify it in 94–100% of specimens.[45] It originates more frequently from the anterior division of the internal iliac or the pudendal arteries, and reaches the rectum. The middle hemorrhoidal artery reaches the lower third of the rectum anterolaterally, close to the level of the pelvic floor and deep to the levator fascia. It therefore does not run in the lateral ligaments, which are inclined posterolaterally.[2] The middle hemorrhoidal artery is more prone to be injured during low anterior resection, when anterolateral dissection of the rectum is performed close to the pelvic floor and the prostate and seminal vesicles or upper part of the vagina are being separated.[37] The anorectum has a profuse intramural anastomotic network, which probably accounts for the fact that division of both superior and middle hemorrhoidal arteries does not result in necrosis of the rectum.

The paired inferior hemorrhoidal arteries are branches of the internal pudendal artery, which in turn is a branch of the internal iliac artery. The inferior hemorrhoidal artery arises within the pudendal canal and is throughout its course entirely extrapelvic. It traverses the obturator fascia, the ischiorectal fossa, and the external anal sphincter to reach the submucosa of the anal canal, ultimately ascending in this plane. Klosterhalfen et al.[4] performed postmortem angiographic, manual, and histologic evaluations and demonstrated that in 85% of cases the posterior commissure was less well perfused than were the other sections of the anal canal. In addition, the blood supply could be jeopardized by contusion of the vessels passing vertically through the muscle fibers of the internal anal sphincter with increased sphincter tone. The resulting decreased blood supply could lead to ischemia at the posterior commissure, in a pathogenetic model of primary anal fissure.

Venous Drainage and Lymphatic Drainage of the Rectum and Anal Canal

The anorectum also drains, via middle and inferior hemorrhoidal veins, to the internal iliac vein and then to the inferior vena cava. Although it is still a controversial subject, the presence of communications among these three venous systems may explain the lack of correlation between portal hypertension and hemorrhoids.[48] The paired inferior and middle hemorrhoidal veins and the single superior hemorrhoidal vein originate from three anorectal arteriovenous plexuses. The external hemorrhoidal plexus, situated subcutaneously around the anal canal below the dentate line, constitutes when dilated the external hemorrhoids. The internal hemorrhoidal plexus is situated submucosally, around the upper anal canal and above the dentate line. The internal hemorrhoids originate from this plexus. The perirectal or perimuscular rectal plexus drains to the middle and inferior hemorrhoidal veins.

Lymph from the upper two-thirds of the rectum drains exclusively upward to the inferior mesenteric nodes and then to the paraaortic nodes. Lymphatic drainage from the lower third of the rectum occurs not only cephalad, along the superior hemorrhoidal and inferior mesentery arteries, but also laterally, along the middle hemorrhoidal vessels to the internal iliac nodes. Studies using lymphoscintigraphy have failed to demonstrate communications between inferior mesenteric and internal iliac lymphatics.[49] In the anal canal, the dentate line is the landmark for two different systems of lymphatic drainage: above, to the inferior mesenteric and internal iliac nodes, and below, along the inferior rectal lymphatics to the superficial inguinal nodes, or less frequently along the inferior hemorrhoidal artery. In the female, drainage at 5 cm above the anal verge in the lymphatic may also spread to the posterior vaginal wall, uterus, cervix, broad ligament, fallopian tubes, ovaries, and cul-de-sac, and at 10 cm above the anal verge, spread seems to occur only to the broad ligament and cul-de-sac.[50]

Innervation of the Rectum and Anal Canal

Innervation of the Rectum

The sympathetic supply of the rectum and the left colon arises from L-1, L-2, and L-3 (Figure 1-4A, B). Preganglionic fibers, via lumbar sympathetic nerves, synapse in the preaortic plexus, and the postganglionic fibers follow the branches of the inferior mesenteric artery and superior rectal artery to the left colon and upper rectum. The lower rectum is innervated by the presacral nerves, which are formed by fusion of the aortic plexus and lumbar splanchnic nerves. Just below the sacral promontory, the presacral nerves form the hypogastric plexus (or superior hypogastric plexus). Two main hypogastric nerves, on either side of the rectum, carry sympathetic innervation from the hypogastric plexus to the pelvic plexus. The pelvic plexus lies on the lateral side of the pelvis at the level of the lower third of the rectum, adjacent to the lateral stalks.

The parasympathetic fibers to the rectum and anal canal emerge through the sacral foramen are called the nervi erigentes (S-2, S-3, and S-4). They pass laterally, forward, and upward to join the sympathetic hypogastric nerves at the pelvic plexus. From the pelvic plexus, combined postganglionic parasympathetic and sympathetic fibers are distributed to the left colon and upper rectum via the inferior mesenteric plexus, and directly to the lower rectum and upper anal canal. The periprostatic plexus, a subdivision of the pelvic plexus situated on Denonvilliers' fascia, supplies the prostate, seminal vesicles, corpora cavernosa, vas deferens, urethra, ejaculatory ducts, and bulbourethral glands. Sexual function is regulated by cerebrospinal, sympathetic, and parasympathetic components. Erection of the penis is mediated by both parasympathetic (arteriolar vasodilatation) and sympathetic inflow (inhibition of vasoconstriction).

All pelvic nerves lie in the plane between the peritoneum and the endopelvic fascia and are in danger of injury during rectal dissection. Permanent bladder paresis occurs in 7–59% of patients after abdominoperineal resection of the rectum[51]; the incidence of impotence is reported to range from 15 to 45%, and that of ejaculatory dysfunction from 32 to 42%.[52] The overall incidence of sexual dysfunction after proctectomy has been reported to reach 100% when wide dissection is performed for malignant disease[53–55]; however, this kind of procedure is unnecessary and these rates are much lower for benign conditions, such as inflammatory bowel disease (0–6%).[53,54,56,57] Dissections performed for benign conditions are undertaken closer to the bowel wall, thus reducing the possibility of nerve injury.[58]

Trauma to the autonomic nerves may occur at several points. During high ligation of the inferior mesenteric artery, close to the aorta, the sympathetic preaortic nerves may be injured. Division of both superior hypogastric plexus and hypogastric nerves may occur also during dissection at the level of the sacral promontory or in the presacral region. In such circumstances, sympathetic denervation with intact nervi erigentes results in retrograde ejaculation and bladder dysfunction. The nervi erigentes are located in the posterolateral aspect of the pelvis, and at the point of fusion with the sympathetic nerves are closely related to the middle hemorrhoidal artery. Injury to these nerves completely abolishes erectile function.[56] The pelvic plexus may be damaged either by excessive traction on the rectum, particularly laterally, or during division of the lateral stalks when this is performed close to the lateral pelvic wall. Finally, dissection near the seminal vesicles and prostate may damage the periprostatic plexus, leading to a mixed parasympathetic and sympathetic injury. This can result in erectile impotence as well as a flaccid, neurogenic bladder. Sexual complications after rectal surgery are readily evident in men but are probably underdiagnosed in women.[59]

Anal Canal

The internal anal sphincter is supplied by sympathetic (L-5) and parasympathetic nerves (S-2, S-3, and S-4) following the same route as the nerves to the rectum. The external anal sphincter is innervated on each side by the inferior rectal branch of the pudendal nerve (S-2 and S-3) and by the perineal branch of S-4. Despite the fact that the puborectalis

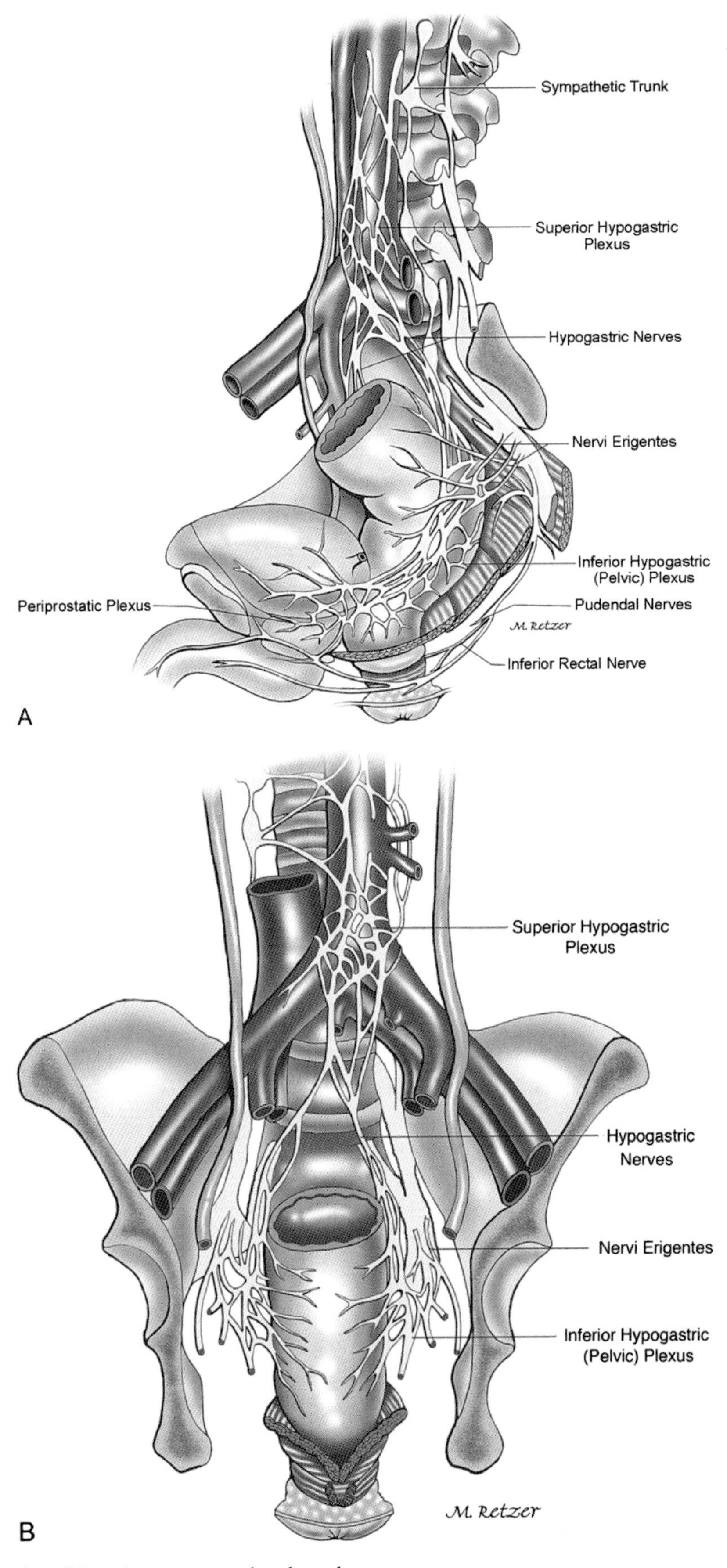

FIGURE 1-4. **A, B** Innervation of the colon, rectum, and anal canal.

and external anal sphincter have somewhat different innervations, these muscles seem to act as an indivisible unit.[14] After unilateral transection of a pudendal nerve, external anal sphincter function is still preserved because of the crossover of the fibers at the spinal cord level.

Anal sensation is carried in the inferior rectal branch of the pudendal nerve and is thought to have a role in maintenance of anal continence. The upper anal canal contains a rich profusion of both free and organized sensory nerve endings, especially in the vicinity of the anal valves.[60] Organized nerve endings include Meissner's corpuscles (touch), Krause's bulbs (cold), Golgi-Mazzoni bodies (pressure), and genital corpuscles (friction).

Anorectal Spaces

The potential spaces of clinical significance in close relation to the anal canal and rectum include: ischiorectal, perianal, intersphincteric, submucosal, superficial postanal, deep postanal, supralevator, and retrorectal spaces (Figure 1-5A, B).

The ischiorectal fossa is subdivided by a thin horizontal fascia into two spaces: the perianal and ischiorectal. The ischiorectal space comprises the upper two-thirds of the ischiorectal fossa. It is pyramid-shaped, situated on both sides between the anal canal and the lower part of the rectum medially, and the side wall of the pelvis laterally.[61] The apex is at the origin of the levator ani muscle from the obturator fascia; the base is the perianal space. Anteriorly, the fossa is bounded by the urogenital diaphragm and transversus perinei muscle. Posterior to the ischiorectal fossa is the sacrotuberous ligament and the inferior border of the gluteus maximus. On the superolateral wall, the pudendal nerve and the internal pudendal vessels run in the pudendal canal (Alcock's canal). The ischiorectal fossa contains fat and the inferior rectal vessels and nerves.

The perianal space surrounds the lower part of the anal canal and contains the external hemorrhoidal plexus, the subcutaneous part of the external anal sphincter, the lowest part of the internal anal sphincter, and fibers of the longitudinal muscle. This space is the typical site of anal hematomas, perianal abscesses, and anal fistula tracts. The perianal space is continuous with the subcutaneous fat of the buttocks laterally and extends into the intersphincteric space medially. The intersphincteric space is a potential space between the internal and external anal sphincters. It is important in the genesis of perianal abscess because most of the anal glands end in this space. The submucous space is situated between the internal anal sphincter and the mucocutaneous lining of the anal canal. This space contains the internal hemorrhoidal plexus and the muscularis submucosae ani. Above, it is continuous with the submucous layer of the rectum, and, inferiorly, it ends at the level of the dentate line.

The superficial postanal space is interposed between the anococcygeal ligament and the skin. The deep postanal space, also known as the retro-sphincteric space of Courtney, is situated between the anococcygeal ligament and the anococcygeal raphe. Both postanal spaces communicate posteriorly with the ischiorectal fossa and are the sites of horseshoe abscesses.

The supralevator spaces are situated between the peritoneum superiorly and the levator ani inferiorly. Medially, these bilateral spaces are limited by the rectum, and laterally by the obturator fascia. Supralevator abscesses may occur as a result of upward extension of a cryptoglandular infection or develop from a pelvic origin. The retrorectal space is located between the fascia propria of the rectum anteriorly and the presacral fascia posteriorly. Laterally are the lateral rectal ligaments and inferiorly the rectosacral ligament, and above the space is continuous with the retroperitoneum. The retrorectal space is a site for embryologic remnants and rare presacral tumors.

Pelvic floor Musculature

The muscles within the pelvis can be divided into three categories: (1) the anal sphincter complex; (2) pelvic floor muscles; and (3) muscles that line the sidewalls of the osseous pelvis.[61] Muscles in this last category form the external boundary of the pelvis and include the obturator internus and piriform. These muscles, compared with the other two groups, lack clinical relevance to anorectal diseases; however, they provide an open communication for pelvic infection to reach extrapelvic spaces. For example, infection from the deep postanal space, originated from posterior midline glands, can track along the obturator internus fascia and reach the ischiorectal fossa.

The anal sphincter and pelvic floor muscles, based on phylogenetic studies, derive from two embryonic cloaca groups, respectively, sphincteric and lateral compressor.[62] The sphincteric group is present in almost all animals. In mammals, this group is divided into ventral (urogenital) and dorsal (anal) components.[63] In primates, the latter components form the external anal sphincter. The lateral compressor or pelvicaudal group connects the rudimentary pelvis to the caudal end of the vertebral column. This group is more differentiated and subdivided into lateral and medial compartments only in reptiles and mammals. The homolog of the lateral compartment is the ischiococcygeus, and of the medial, pelvicaudal compartment, the pubococcygeus and ileococcygeus. In addition, most primates possess a variably sized group of muscle fibers close to the inner border of the medial pelvicaudal muscle, which attaches the rectum to the pubis. In humans, the fibers are more distinct and known as the puborectalis muscle.

Levator Ani

The levator ani muscle, or pelvic diaphragm, is the major component of the pelvic floor. It is a pair of broad, symmetric sheets composed of three striated muscles: ileococcygeus, pubococcygeus, and puborectalis (Figure 1-6A, B). A variable

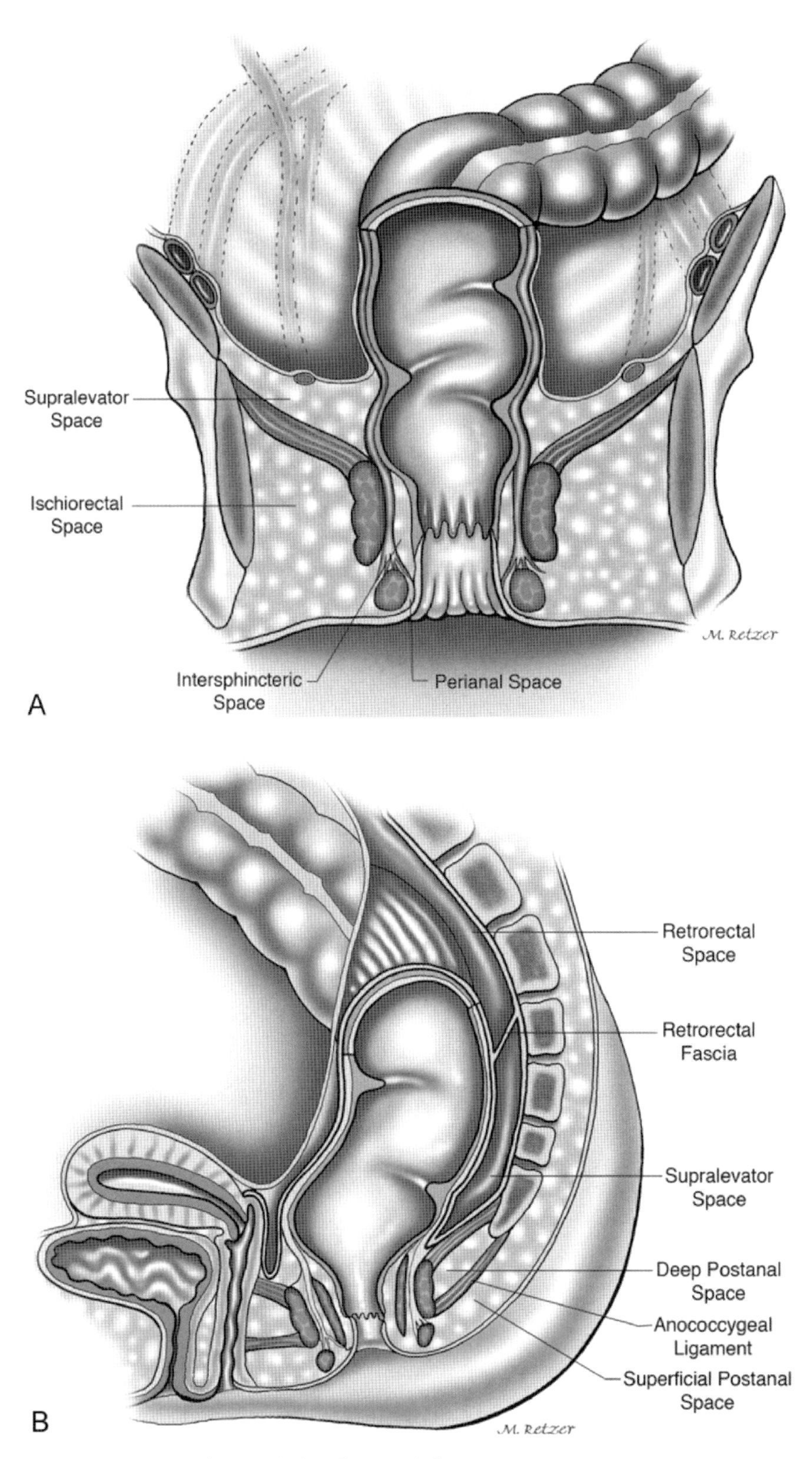

FIGURE 1-5. Paraanal and pararectal spaces. **A** Frontal view. **B** Lateral view.

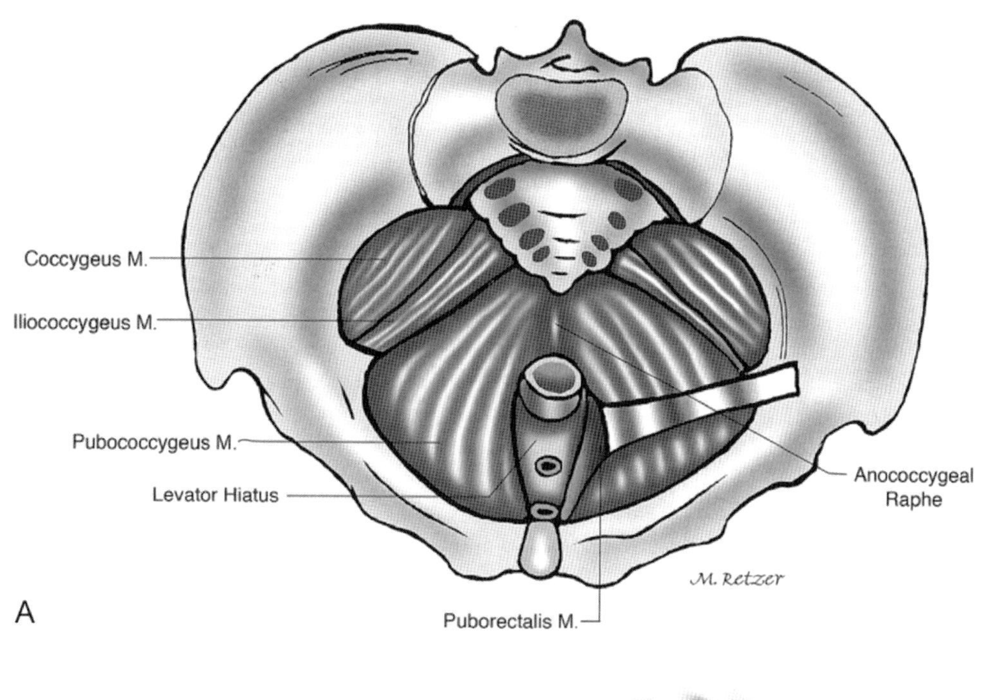

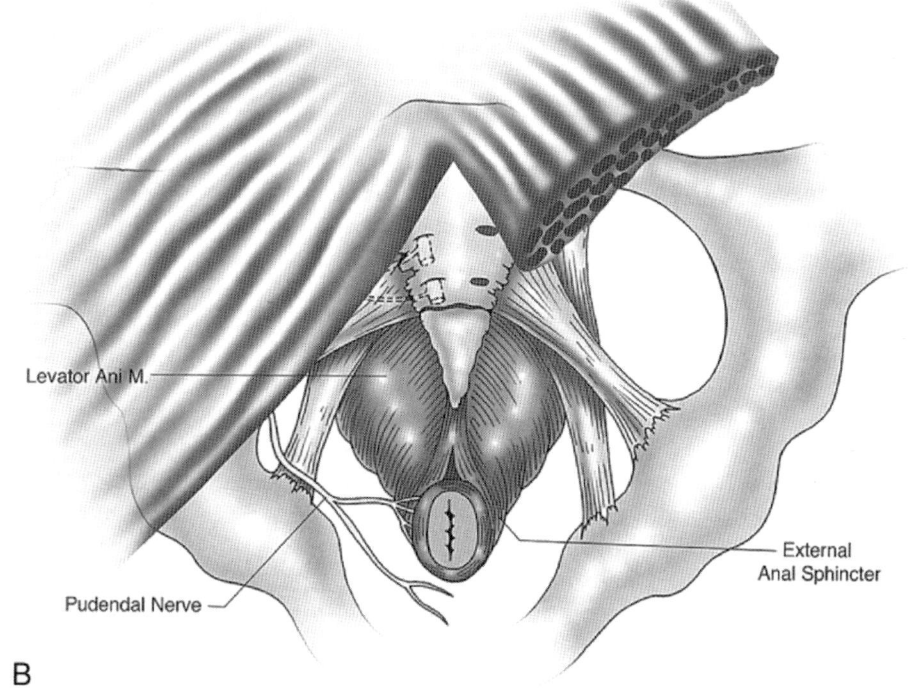

FIGURE 1-6. Levator ani muscle. **A** Superior. **B** Inferior surface.

fourth component, the ischiococcygeus or coccygeus, is rudimentary in humans and represented by only a few muscle fibers on the surface of the sacrospinous ligament. The levator ani is supplied by sacral roots on its pelvic surface (S-2, S-3, and S-4) and by the perineal branch of the pudendal nerve on its inferior surface. The puborectalis muscle receives additional innervation from the inferior rectal nerves.

The ileococcygeus muscles arise from the ischial spine and posterior part of the obturator fascia and course inferiorly and medially to insert into the lateral aspects of S-3 and S-4, the coccyx, and the anococcygeal raphe. The pubococcygeus arises from the posterior aspect of the pubis and the anterior part of the obturator fascia; it runs dorsally alongside the anorectal junction to decussate with fibers of the opposite side at the anococcygeal raphe and insert into the anterior surface of the fourth sacral and first coccygeal segments.

The pelvic floor is "incomplete" in the midline where the lower rectum, urethra, and either the dorsal vein of the penis in men, or the vagina in women, pass through it. This defect is called the levator hiatus and consists of an elliptic space situated between the two pubococcygeus muscles. The hiatal ligament, originating from the pelvic fascia, keeps the intrahiatal viscera together and prevents their constriction during contraction of the levator ani. A possible (but controversial) dilator function has been attributed to the anococcygeal raphe because of its crisscross arrangement.[14]

The puborectalis muscle is a strong, U-shaped loop of striated muscle that slings the anorectal junction to the posterior aspect of the pubis (Figure 1-7). The puborectalis is the most medial portion of the levator ani muscle. It is situated immediately cephalad to the deep component of the external sphincter. Because the junction between the two muscles is indistinct and they have similar innervation (pudendal nerve), the puborectalis has been regarded by some authors as a part of the external anal sphincter and not of the levator ani complex.[14,15] Anatomic and phylogenetic studies suggest that the puborectalis may be a part of the levator ani[63] or of the external anal sphincter.[24,62] Embryologically, the puborectalis has a common primordium with the ileococcygeus and pubococcygeus muscles, and it is never connected with the external anal sphincter during the different stages of development.[6] In addition, neurophysiologic studies have implied that the innervation of these muscles may not be the same because stimulation of the sacral nerves results in electromyographic activity in the ipsilateral puborectalis muscle but not in the external anal sphincter.[64] Currently, because of this controversy, the puborectalis has been considered to belong to both muscular groups, the external anal sphincter and the levator ani.[65]

The Anorectal Ring and the Anorectal Angle

Two anatomic structures of the junction of the rectum and anal canal are related to the puborectalis muscle: the anorectal ring and the anorectal angle. The anorectal ring, a term coined by Milligan and Morgan[10] is a strong muscular ring that represents the upper end of the sphincter, more precisely the puborectalis, and the upper border of the internal anal sphincter, around the anorectal junction. Despite its lack of embryologic significance, it is an easily recognized boundary of the anal canal appreciated on physical examination, and it is of clinical relevance because division of this structure during surgery for abscesses or fistula inevitably results in fecal incontinence.

The anorectal angle is thought to be the result of the anatomic configuration of the U-shaped sling of puborectalis muscle around the anorectal junction. Whereas the anal sphincters are responsible for the closure of the anal canal to retain gas and liquid stool, the puborectalis muscle and the anorectal angle are designed to maintain gross fecal continence. Different theories have been postulated to explain the importance of the puborectalis and the anorectal angle in the maintenance of fecal continence. Parks et al.[66] opined that increasing intraabdominal pressure forces the anterior rectal wall down into the upper anal canal, occluding it by

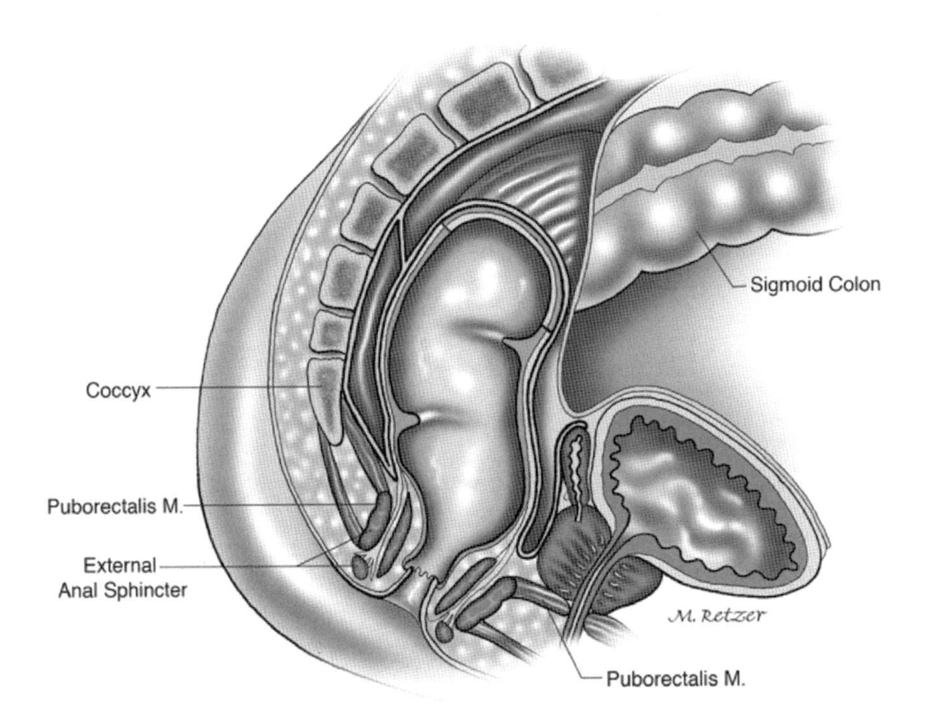

FIGURE 1-7. The anteriorly directed pull of the puborectalis contributes to the angulation between the rectum and anal canal, the anorectal angle.

a type of flap valve mechanism that creates an effective seal. Subsequently, it has been demonstrated that the flap mechanism does not occur. Instead, a continuous sphincteric occlusion-like activity that is attributed to the puborectalis is noted.[67,68]

Colon

General Considerations

The colon is a capacious tube that roughly surrounds the loops of small intestine as an arch. Named from the Greek *koluein* ("to retard"), the colon is variable in length, averaging approximately 150 cm, which corresponds to one-quarter the length of the small intestine. Its diameter can be substantially augmented by distension – it gradually decreases from 7.5 cm at the cecum to 2.5 cm at the sigmoid. In humans, the colon is described to be somewhere between the short, straight type with a rudimentary cecum, such as that of the carnivores, and a long sacculated colon with a capacious cecum, such as that of the herbivores.

Anatomic differences between the small and large intestines include position, caliber, degree of fixation, and, in the colon, the presence of three distinct characteristics: the taeniae coli, the haustra, and the appendices epiploicae. The three taeniae coli, anterior (taenia libera), posteromedial (taenia mesocolica), and posterolateral (taenia omentalis), represent bands of the outer longitudinal coat of muscle that traverse the colon from the base of the appendix to the rectosigmoid junction, where they merge. The muscular longitudinal layer is actually a complete coat around the colon, although it is considerably thicker at the taeniae.[69] The haustra or haustral sacculations are outpouchings of bowel wall between the taeniae; they are caused by the relative shortness of the taeniae, about one-sixth shorter than the length of the bowel wall.[13] The haustra are separated by the plicae semilunares or crescentic folds of the bowel wall, which give the colon its characteristic radiographic appearance when filled with air or barium. The appendices epiploicae are small appendages of fat that protrude from the serosal aspect of the colon.

Cecum

The cecum is the sacculated segment (Latin *caecus*, "blind") of the large bowel that projects downward as a 6- to 8-cm blind pouch below the entrance of the ileum. Usually situated in the right iliac fossa, the cecum is almost entirely or at least in its lower half, invested with peritoneum. However, its mobility is usually limited by a small mesocecum. The ileum terminates in the posteromedial aspect of the cecum; the angulation between these two structures is maintained by the superior and inferior ileocecal ligaments. These ligaments, along with the mesentery of the appendix, form three pericecal recesses or fossae: superior ileocecal, inferior ileocecal, and retrocecal. Viewed from the cecal lumen, the ileocecal junction is represented by a narrow, transversely situated, slit-like opening known as the ileocecal valve or the valve de Bauhin. At either end, the two prominent semilunar lips of the valve fuse and continue as a single frenulum of mucosa. A circular sphincter, the ileocecal sphincter, originates from a slight thickening of the muscular layer of the terminal ileum. A competent ileocecal valve is related to the critical closed-loop type of colonic obstruction. However, ileocecal competence is not always demonstrated on barium enema studies. Instead of preventing reflux of colonic contents into the ileum, the ileocecal valve regulates ileal emptying. The ileocecal sphincter seems to relax in response to the entrance of food into the stomach.[70] As in the gastroesophageal junction, extrasphincteric factors such as the ileocecal angulation apparently have a role in the prevention of reflux from the colon to the ileum.[71]

Appendix

The vermiform appendix is an elongated diverticulum that arises from the posteromedial aspect of the cecum about 3.0 cm below the ileocecal junction. Its length varies from 2 to 20 cm (mean, 8–10 cm), and it is approximately 5 mm in diameter. The appendix, because of its great mobility, may occupy a variety of positions, possibly at different times in the same individual. It has been estimated that in 85–95% of cases, the appendix lies posteromedial on the cecum toward the ileum, but other positions include retrocecal, pelvic, subcecal, preileal and retroileal.[72–74] The confluence of the three taeniae is a useful guide in locating the base of the appendix. The mesoappendix, a triangular fold attached to the posterior leaf of the mesentery of the terminal ileum, usually contains the appendicular vessels close to its free edge.

Ascending Colon

The ascending colon is approximately 15 cm long. It ascends, from the level of the ileocecal junction to the right colic or hepatic flexure, laterally to the psoas muscle and anteriorly to the iliacus, the quadratus lumborum, and the lower pole of the right kidney. The ascending colon is covered with peritoneum anteriorly and on both sides. In addition, fragile adhesions between the right abdominal wall and its anterior aspect, known as Jackson's membrane, may be present. Like the descending colon on its posterior surface, the ascending colon is devoid of peritoneum, which is instead replaced by an areolar tissue (fascia of Toldt) resulting from an embryologic process of fusion or coalescence of the mesentery to the posterior parietal peritoneum. In the lateral peritoneal reflection, this process is represented by the white line of Toldt, which is more evident at the descending-sigmoid junction. This line serves as a guide for the surgeon when the ascending, descending, or sigmoid colon is mobilized. At the visceral surface of the right lobe of the liver and lateral to the gallbladder, the ascending colon turns sharply medially and slightly caudad and ventrally to form the right colic (hepatic) flexure. This flexure is supported by the nephrocolic ligament and lies immediately ventral to the lower part of the right kidney and over the descending duodenum.

Transverse Colon

The transverse colon is approximately 45 cm long, the longest segment of the large bowel. It crosses the abdomen, with an inferior curve immediately caudad to the greater curvature of the stomach. The transverse colon is relatively fixed at each flexure, and, in between, it is suspended by a 10- to 15-cm-wide area which provides variable mobility; the nadir of the transverse colon may reach the hypogastrium. The transverse colon is completely invested with peritoneum, but the greater omentum is fused on its anterosuperior aspect. The left colic or splenic flexure is situated beneath the lower angle of the spleen and firmly attached to the diaphragm by the phrenocolic ligament, which also forms a shelf to support the spleen. Because of the risk of hemorrhage, mobilization of the splenic flexure should be approached with great care, preceded by dissection upward along the descending colon and medially to laterally along the transverse colon toward the splenic flexure. This flexure, when compared with the hepatic flexure, is more acute, higher, and more deeply situated.

Descending Colon

The descending colon courses downward from the splenic flexure to the brim of the true pelvis, a distance of approximately 25 cm.[32] Similarly to the ascending colon, the descending colon is covered by peritoneum only on its anterior and lateral aspects. Posteriorly, it rests directly against the left kidney and the quadratus lumborum and transversus abdominis muscles. However, the descending colon is narrower and more dorsally situated than the ascending colon.

Sigmoid Colon

The sigmoid colon is commonly a 35- to 40-cm-long, mobile, omega-shaped loop completely invested by peritoneum; however, it varies greatly in length and configuration. The mesosigmoid is attached to the pelvic walls in an inverted V shape, resting in a recess known as the intersigmoid fossa. The left ureter lies immediately underneath this fossa and is crossed on its anterior surface by the spermatic, left colic, and sigmoid vessels. Both the anatomy and function of the rectosigmoid junction have been matters of substantial controversy. As early as 1833, it was postulated that the sigmoid could have a role in continence as the fecal reservoir, based on the observation that the rectum is usually emptied and contracted.[74] Since then, a thickening of the circular muscular layer between the rectum and sigmoid has been described and diversely termed the sphincter ani tertius, rectosigmoid sphincter, and pylorus sigmoidorectalis, and it has probably been mistaken for one of the transverse folds of the rectum.[75–79] The rectosigmoid junction has been frequently regarded by surgeons as an indistinct zone, a region comprising the last 5–8 cm of sigmoid and the uppermost 5 cm of the rectum.[32,80] However, others have considered it a clearly defined segment because it is the narrowest portion of the large intestine; in fact, it is usually characterized endoscopically as a narrow and sharply angulated segment.[81] According to a study in human cadavers, the rectosigmoid junction, macroscopically identified as the point where the taenia libera and the taenia omentalis fuse to form a single anterior taenia and where both haustra and mesocolon terminate, is situated 6–7 cm below the sacral promontory.[5] With microdissection, this segment is characterized by conspicuous strands of longitudinal muscle fibers and the presence of curved interconnecting fibers between the longitudinal and circular muscle layers, resulting in a delicate syncytium of smooth muscle that allows synergistic interplay between the two layers. The rectosigmoid does not fit the anatomic definition of a sphincter as "a band of thickened circular muscle that closes the lumen by contraction and of a longitudinal muscle that dilates it"; however, this segment may be regarded as a functional sphincter because mechanisms of active dilation and passive "kinking" occlusion do exist.[81]

Blood Supply

The superior and inferior mesenteric arteries nourish the entire large intestine, and the limit between the two territories is the junction between the proximal two-thirds and the distal third of the transverse colon. This represents the embryologic division between the midgut and the hindgut. The superior mesenteric artery originates from the aorta behind the superior border of the pancreas at L-1 and supplies the cecum, appendix, ascending colon, and most of the transverse colon. After passing behind the neck of the pancreas and anteromedial to the uncinate process, the superior mesenteric artery crosses the third part of the duodenum and continues downward and to the right along the base of the mesentery. From its left side arises a series of 12–20 jejunal and ileal branches. From its right side arise the colic branches: middle, right, and ileocolic arteries. The ileocolic, the most constant of these vessels, bifurcates into a superior or ascending branch, which communicates with the descending branch of the right colic artery, and an inferior or descending branch, which gives off the anterior cecal, posterior cecal, and appendicular and ileal divisions.[82] The right colic artery may also arise from the ileocolic or middle colic arteries and is absent in 2–18% of specimens.[45,82,83] It supplies the ascending colon and hepatic flexure through its ascending and descending branches, both of them joining with neighboring vessels to contribute to the marginal artery. The middle colic artery is the highest of the three colic branches of the superior mesenteric artery, arising close to the inferior border of the pancreas. Its right branch supplies the right transverse colon and hepatic flexure, anastomosing with the ascending branch of the right colic artery. Its left branch supplies the distal half of the transverse colon. Anatomic variations of this artery include the absence in

4–20% of cases and the presence of an accessory middle colic artery in 10%; the middle colic artery can be the main supply to the splenic flexure in about 33% of cases.[82,84]

The inferior mesenteric artery originates from the left anterior surface of the aorta, 3–4 cm above its bifurcation at the level of L2-3, and runs downward and to the left to enter the pelvis. Within the abdomen, the inferior mesenteric artery branches into the left colic artery and two to six sigmoidal arteries. After crossing the left common iliac artery, it acquires the name superior hemorrhoidal artery (superior rectal artery). The left colic artery, the highest branch of the inferior mesenteric artery, bifurcates into an ascending branch, which runs upward to the splenic flexure to contribute to the arcade of Riolan, and a descending branch, which supplies most of the descending colon. The sigmoidal arteries form arcades within the sigmoid mesocolon, resembling the small-bowel vasculature, and anastomose with branches of the left colic artery proximally, and with the superior hemorrhoidal artery distally. The marginal artery terminates within the arcade of sigmoidal arteries. The superior hemorrhoidal artery is the continuation of the inferior mesenteric artery, once it crosses the left iliac vessels. The artery descends in the sigmoid mesocolon to the level of S-3 and then to the posterior aspect of the rectum. In 80% of cases, it bifurcates into right and left terminal branches; multiple branches are present in 17%.[45] These divisions, once within the submucosa of the rectum, run straight downward to supply the lower rectum and the anal canal.

The venous drainage of the large intestine basically follows its arterial supply. Blood from the right colon, via the superior mesenteric vein, and from left colon and rectum, via the inferior mesenteric vein, reaches the intrahepatic capillary bed through the portal vein.

Collateral Circulation

The anatomy of the mesenteric circulation is still a matter of controversy, and this may in part be related to the inherent confusion of the use of eponyms. The central anastomotic artery connecting all colonic mesenteric branches, first described by Haller[85] in 1786, later became known as the marginal artery of Drummond because this author was the first to demonstrate its surgical significance (1913).[86,87] Subsequently, discontinuity of the marginal artery has been shown at the lower ascending colon, and especially at the left colic flexure and the sigmoid colon. This potential hypovascularity is a source of concern during colonic resection. The splenic flexure comprises the watershed between midgut and hindgut supplies (Griffiths' critical point); this anastomosis is of variable magnitude, and it may be absent in about 50% of cases.[88] For this reason, ischemic colitis usually affects or is most severe near the splenic flexure.[89,90] Another potential area of discontinuity of the marginal artery is the Sudeck's critical point, situated between the lowest sigmoid and the superior hemorrhoidal arteries; however, surgical experience and radiological studies have both demonstrated adequate communications between these vessels.[91] There is also a collateral network involving middle hemorrhoidal, internal iliac, and external iliac arteries which could potentially prevent gangrene of the pelvis and even the lower extremities in case of occlusion of the distal aorta.[92,93]

The term arc of Riolan was vaguely defined as the communication between superior and inferior mesenteric arteries in the author's original work. Later, the eponym marginal artery of Drummond confused the subject.[94] In 1964, Moskowitz et al.[95] proposed another term, meandering mesenteric artery, and differentiated it from the marginal artery of Drummond. The meandering mesenteric artery is a thick and tortuous vessel that makes a crucial communication between the middle colic artery and the ascending branch of the left colic artery, especially in advanced atherosclerotic disease.[94] The presence of the meandering mesenteric artery indicates severe stenosis of either the superior mesenteric artery (retrograde flow) or inferior mesenteric artery (antegrade flow).

Lymphatic Drainage

The submucous and subserous layers of the colon and rectum have a rich network of lymphatic plexuses, which drain into an extramural system of lymph channels and follow their vascular supply.[50] Colorectal lymph nodes are classically divided into four groups: epiploic, paracolic, intermediate, and principal.[96] The epiploic group lies on the bowel wall under the peritoneum and in the appendices epiploicae; they are more numerous in the sigmoid and are known in the rectum as the nodules of Gerota. The lymphatic drainage from all parts of the colon follows its vascular supply. The paracolic nodes are situated along the marginal artery and on the arcades; they are considered to have the most numerous filters. The intermediate nodes are situated on the primary colic vessels, and the main or principal nodes on the superior and inferior mesenteric vessels. The lymph then drains to the cisterna chyli via the paraaortic chain of nodes. Colorectal carcinoma staging systems are based on the neoplastic involvement of these various lymph node groups.

Innervation

The sympathetic and parasympathetic components of the autonomic innervation of the large intestine closely follow the blood supply. The sympathetic supply of the right colon originates from the lower six thoracic segments. These thoracic splanchnic nerves reach the celiac, preaortic, and superior mesenteric ganglia, where they synapse. The postganglionic fibers then course along the superior mesenteric artery to the small bowel and right colon. The parasympathetic supply comes from the right (posterior) vagus nerve and celiac plexus. The fibers travel along the superior mesenteric artery, and finally synapse with cells in the autonomic plexuses within the bowel wall. The sympathetic supply of the left colon and rectum arises from L-1, L-2, and L-3.

Preganglionic fibers, via lumbar sympathetic nerves, synapse in the preaortic plexus, and the postganglionic fibers follow the branches of the inferior mesenteric artery and superior rectal artery to the left colon and upper rectum.

Embryology

Anus and Rectum

The distal colon, rectum, and the anal canal above the dentate line are all derived from the hindgut. Therefore, this segment is supplied by the hindgut (inferior mesenteric) artery, with corresponding venous and lymphatic drainage. Its parasympathetic outflow comes from S-2, S-3, and S-4 via splanchnic nerves.

The dentate line marks the fusion between endodermal and ectodermal tubes, where the terminal portion of the hindgut or cloaca fuses with the proctodeum, an ingrowth from the anal pit. The cloaca originates at the portion of the rectum below the pubococcygeal line, whereas the hindgut originates above it.

Before the fifth week of development, the intestinal and urogenital tracts terminate in conjunction with the cloaca. During the sixth to eighth weeks of fetal life, the urorectal septum or fold of Tourneux migrates caudally and divides the cloacal closing plate into an anterior urogenital plate and a posterior anal plate (Figure 1-8). Any slight posterior shift in the position of the septum during its descent reduces the size of the anal opening, giving rise to anorectal defects.

The cloacal part of the anal canal, which has both endodermal and ectodermal elements, forms the anal transitional zone after breakdown of the anal membrane.[73] During the tenth week, the anal tubercles, a pair of ectodermal swellings around the proctodeal pit, fuse dorsally to form a horseshoe-shaped structure and anteriorly to create the perineal body. The cloacal sphincter is separated by the perineal body into urogenital and anal portions (external anal sphincter). The internal anal sphincter is formed later (6th to 12th week) from enlarging fibers of the circular layer of the rectum.[6,97]

In the female, the fused Müllerian ducts that form the uterus and vagina move downward to reach the urogenital sinus about the sixteenth week. In the male, the site of the urogenital membrane is obliterated by fusion of the genital folds and the sinus becomes incorporated into the urethra. The sphincters apparently migrate during their development; the external sphincter grows cephalad and the internal sphincter moves caudally. Concomitantly, the longitudinal muscle descends into the intersphincteric plane.[6]

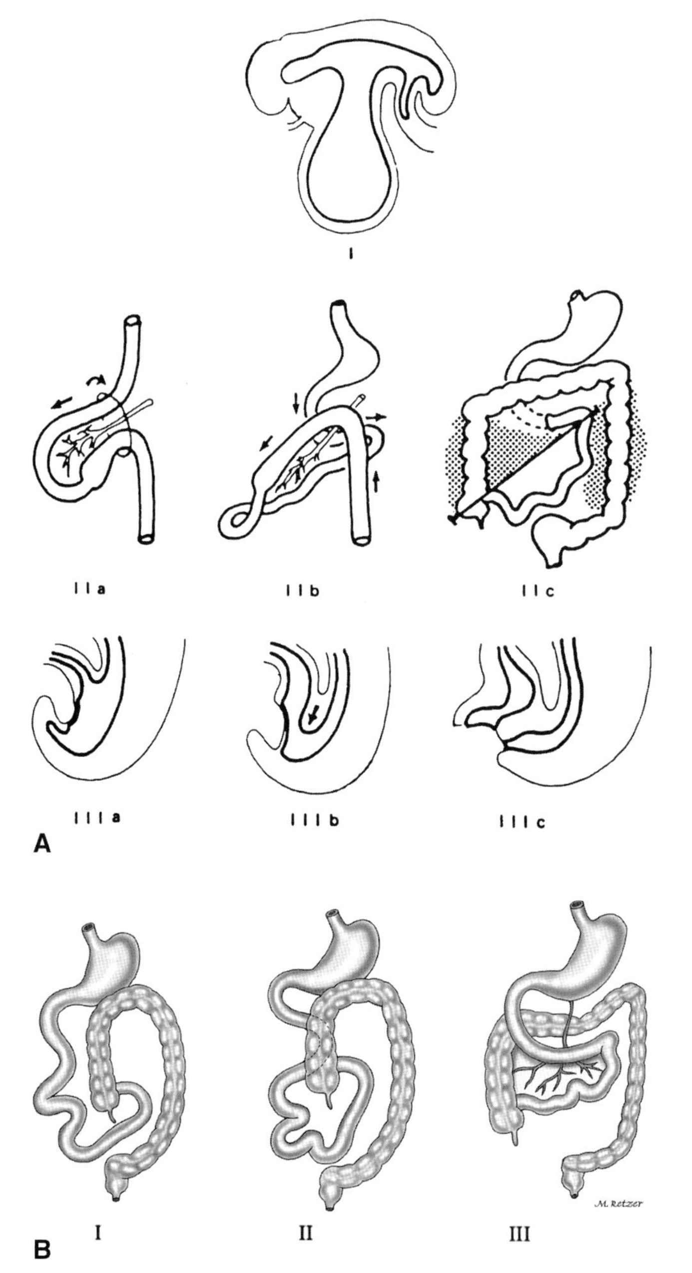

FIGURE 1-8. **A** Embryology of the large intestine. I. Sagittal section of early embryo with the primitive tube at the third week of development. II. Normal development of intestine. IIa: Midgut loop within the umbilical cord (physiologic herniation); IIb: midgut rotation and return to the abdomen; IIc: rotation complete with wide retroperitoneal fixation of small bowel mesentery as well as ascending and descending colon. III. Development of the anus and rectum. IIIa: The hindgut, tailgut, and the allantois form the cloaca; IIIb: at the sixth week, the urogenital septum grows to separate the hindgut posteriorally and the allantois anteriorally; IIIc: the rectum with the persistent anal membrane has been separated from the urogenital structures. **B** Malformations of the digestive systems. I, Nonrotation; II, incomplete rotation; III, reversed rotation.

Anorectal Malformations

The anorectal malformations can be traced to developmental arrest at various stages of normal maturation. The Duhamel's theory of "syndrome of caudal regression" is supported by the high incidence of spinal, sacral, and lower limb defects associated with these anomalies.[98] In fact, associated anomalies, most frequently skeleton and urinary defects, may occur in up to 70%.[99] Digestive tract, particularly

TABLE 1-1. Classification of anorectal malformations

A. Anal defects ("low" defects)
1. Anal stenosis
2. Membranous atresia (rare)
3. Anal agenesis
a. Without fistula
b. With fistula (ectopic anus)
B. Anorectal defects ("high" defects)
1. Anorectal agenesis
a. Without fistula
b. With fistula
2. Rectal atresia ("high" atresia)
C. Persistent cloaca
1. Rectal duplication
2. Developmental cysts

tracheoesophageal fistula or esophageal stenosis, cardiac, and abdominal wall defects may also occur in patients with anorectal anomalies. There is evidence for familial occurrence of anorectal defects; the estimated risk in a family of a second occurrence of some form of imperforate anus is up to 50 times the normal chance.[100]

The proposed classification systems for the congenital malformations of the anorectal region are usually either incomplete or complex. The most comprehensive system has been proposed by Gough[101] and Santulli[102] and takes into consideration whether the rectum terminates above (anorectal defects) or below (anal defects) the puborectalis sling (Table 1-1).

Anal Defects

Anal Stenosis

Some degree of stricture of the rectum is present in 25–39% of infants, and only about 25% of these shows some degree of disordered evacuation, but spontaneous dilation occurs between 3 and 6 months of age in the vast majority of patients.[103] Although stenosis has been attributed to excessive fusion of the anal tubercles, probably the cause is a posterior shift in the position of the urorectal septum during its descent at the sixth week of fetal life.[101]

Membranous Atresia

This defect, also known as "covered anus," is very rare. It is characterized by the presence of a thin membrane of skin between the blind end of the anal canal and the surface. Most cases occur in males and probably represent excessive posterior closure of the urogenital folds.[101]

Anal Agenesis

The rectum extends below the puborectalis and ends, either blindly, or more often, in an ectopic opening or fistula to the perineum anteriorly, to the vulva, or urethra. Regardless of the location of the ectopic orifice, the sphincter is present at the normal site.

Anorectal Defects

Anorectal Agenesis

Anorectal agenesis more often affects males and represents the most common type of "imperforate anus." The rectum ends well above the surface, the anus is represented by a dimple, and the anal sphincter is usually normal. This malformation is the result of excessive obliteration of the embryonic tailgut and the adjacent dorsal portion of the cloaca. The descending urorectal septum reaches the dorsal wall of the diminished cloaca, leaving a blindly ending colon above and an isolated rectal membrane below.

In most cases, there is a fistula or fibrous remnant connecting the rectal ending to the urethra or vagina. Fistulae represent areas in the septum where the lateral ridges have joined but failed to unite, although the more caudal union is complete. High fistulae, vaginal and urethral, with anorectal agenesis originate as early as the sixth or seventh week, whereas low fistulae (perineal) of anal ectopia originate in the eighth or ninth week of fetal life.

Rectal Atresia or "High Atresia"

Although considered clinically as an anorectal defect, embryologically this is the most caudal type of atresia of the large intestine. The rectum and anal canal are separated from each other by an atretic portion.

Persistent Cloaca

This is a rare condition that occurs only in female infants. It results from the total failure of the urorectal septum to descend, and therefore occurs at a very early stage of development (10-mm stage).

Colon and Small Bowel

The primitive gut tube develops from the endodermal roof of the yolk sac. At first, the primitive intestine is a straight tube suspended in a sagittal plane on a common mesentery. At the beginning of the third week of development, it can be divided into three regions: the foregut in the head fold, the hindgut with its ventral allantoic outgrowth in the smaller tail fold, and, between these two portions, the midgut, which at this stage opens ventrally into the yolk sac (Figure 1-8). The normal embryologic process of rotation of the intestinal tract includes three stages, as outlined below.

First Stage: Physiologic Herniation of the Primitive Digestive Tube

The first stage of rotation begins between the sixth and eighth weeks of intrauterine life, when the primitive intestinal tube elongates on its mesenteric around the superior mesenteric artery and bulges through the umbilical cord as a temporary physiologic herniation. This intraumbilical loop moves, at the eighth week of embryologic development, counterclockwise

90° from the sagittal to the horizontal plane. The anomalies of this stage are rare and include situs inversus, inverted duodenum, and extroversion of the cloaca.

Second Stage: Return of the Midgut to the Abdomen

The second stage of gut rotation occurs at the tenth week of intrauterine life. During this stage, the midgut loop returns to the peritoneal cavity from the umbilical herniation, and simultaneously rotates 180° counterclockwise around the pedicle formed by the mesenteric root. The prearterial segment of the midgut or duodenojejunal loop returns first to the abdomen, as the gut rotates counterclockwise. The duodenum comes to lie behind the superior mesenteric artery. The postarterial segment or cecocolic loop also reduces and comes to lie in front of the superior mesenteric artery. Anomalies of the second stage are relatively more common than the ones originated from the first stage and include nonrotation, malrotation, reversed rotation, internal hernia, and omphalocele.

Third Stage: Fixation of the Midgut

The third stage of gut rotation starts after return of the gut to the peritoneal cavity and ends at birth. The cecum, initially in the upper abdomen, descends, migrating to the right lower quadrant, as counterclockwise rotation continues to 270°. After completion of the sequential rotation of the gastrointestinal tract, in the latter weeks of the first trimester, the process of fixation initiates. Gradually, fusion of parts of the primitive mesentery occurs, with fixation of the duodenum, and the ascending and descending parts of the colon to the posterior abdominal wall in their final position. Anomalies of this stage are common and include mobile cecum, subhepatic or undescended cecum, hyperdescent of the cecum, and persistent colonic mesentery.

The midgut progresses below the major pancreatic papilla to form the small intestine, the ascending colon, and the proximal two-thirds of the transverse colon. This segment is supplied by the midgut (superior mesenteric) artery, with corresponding venous and lymphatic drainage.

The neuroenteric ganglion cells migrate from the neural crest to the upper end of the alimentary tract and then follow vagal fibers caudad. The sympathetic innervation of the midgut and likewise the hindgut originates from T-8 to L-2, via splanchnic nerves and the autonomic abdominopelvic plexuses. The parasympathetic outflow to the midgut is derived from the tenth cranial nerve (vagus) with preganglionic cell bodies in the brain stem.

The distal colon (distal third of the transverse colon), the rectum, and the anal canal above the dentate line are all derived from the hindgut. Therefore, this segment is supplied by the hindgut (inferior mesenteric) artery, with corresponding venous and lymphatic drainage. Its parasympathetic outflow comes from S-2, S-3, and S-4 via splanchnic nerves.

Abnormalities of Rotation

Nonrotation

In this condition, the midgut loop returns to the peritoneal cavity without the process of rotation, and, consequently, the entire small bowel locates on the right side of the abdomen, and the left colon is on the left side. This condition may be entirely asymptomatic and constitute a finding at laparotomies. However, it may complicate with volvulus affecting the entire small bowel. The twist of the entire midgut loop on its pedicle can occur, usually at the level of the duodenojejunal junction and the midtransverse colon because of the defective fixation of the mesenteric root.

Malrotation

In malrotation, the cecum fails to complete the 360° rotation around the superior mesenteric, and does not complete the migration process. As a result of this failure in the migration process, the malrotated cecum locates in the right upper quadrant and is fixed by lateral bands or adhesions. These bands can overlie the distal part of the duodenum and cause extrinsic compression.

Reversed Rotation

In this condition, the midgut rotates clockwise instead of counterclockwise; consequently, the transverse colon locates posteriorly and the duodenum anteriorly, in relation to the mesenteric artery.

Omphalocele

Omphalocele is the retention of the midgut in the umbilical sac as a result of failure of the gut to return to the peritoneal cavity.

Incomplete Attachment of Cecum and Mesentery

Under normal conditions, the cecum is almost entirely or at least in its lower half invested with peritoneum. However, its mobility is usually limited by a small mesocecum. In approximately 5% of individuals, the peritoneal covering is absent posteriorly; it then rests directly on the iliacus and psoas major muscles.[32] Alternatively, an abnormally mobile cecum-ascending colon, resulting from an anomaly of fixation, can be found in 10–22% of individuals.[104] In this case, a long mesentery is present, and the cecum may assume varied positions. This lack of fixation may predispose to the development of volvulus.

Internal Hernias Around the Ligament of Treitz

Both internal hernias and congenital obstructive bands or adhesions are causes of congenital bowel obstruction, and result from an anomaly during the process of fixation. This failure may occur when the fusion of mesothelial layers is incomplete or if it occurs between structures that are abnormally rotated. Retroperitoneal hernias can occur in any intraperitoneal fossae, particularly paraduodenal, paracecal, and intersigmoid. The most common internal hernias resulting from abnormal fixation of the colon are right and left paraduodenal hernias.[103]

Other Congenital Malformations of the Colon and Small Intestine

Proximal Colon Duplications

Duplication of the colon comprises three general groups of congenital abnormalities: mesenteric cysts, diverticula, and long colon duplication.[105]

Mesenteric cysts, similarly to the duplication cysts found at the retroperitoneum and the mediastinum, are lined by intestinal epithelium and a variable amount of smooth muscle. These cysts lie in the mesentery of the colon or behind the rectum, may be separable or inseparable from the bowel wall, and usually present, as the size increases, either as a palpable mass or intestinal obstruction. Diverticula are blind ending pouches of variable lengths and arise either from the mesenteric or the antimesenteric border of the bowel. They may have heterotopic gastric mucosa or pancreatic-type tissue. Long colon duplication or tubular duplication of the colon is the rarest form of duplication. Almost invariably, the two parts lie parallel, sharing a common wall throughout most of their length; frequently, it involves the entire colon and rectum. Often, there is an association of pelvic genitourinary anomalies.

Meckel's Diverticulum

Meckel's diverticulum is a remnant of the vitelline or omphalomesenteric duct, arising from the antimesenteric border of the terminal ileum, usually within 50 cm of the ileocecal valve.[73] Associated abnormalities include persistence of a fibrous band connecting the diverticulum to the umbilicus or a patent omphalomesenteric duct, the presence of ectopic mucosa or aberrant pancreatic tissue (in more than half of asymptomatic diverticula), and herniation of the diverticulum in an indirect inguinal hernia (Littré's hernia).

In most people, Meckel's diverticulum is asymptomatic, and according to autopsy series, it exists in 1–3% of the general population.[106] Surgical complications are more frequent in infants and children and include hemorrhage from ectopic gastric mucosa, intestinal obstruction resulting from associated congenital bands or ileocolic intussusception, diverticulitis, perforation, and umbilical discharge from a patent omphalomesenteric duct.

Atresia of the Colon

Colonic atresia is a rare cause of intestinal obstruction; it represents only 5% of all forms of gastrointestinal atresia. It is probably caused by a vascular accident occurring during intrauterine life.[104] Colonic atresia can be classified in three basic types: (1) incomplete occlusion of the lumen by a membranous diaphragm; (2) proximal end distal colonic segments that end blindly and are joined by a cord-like remnant of the bowel; and (3) complete separation of the proximal anal distal blind segments with the absence of a segment of megacolon.[107] Colonic atresia may be variable in length and can occur at any site in the colon, and its association with Hirschsprung's disease has been reported.[104]

Hirschsprung's Disease

Congenital megacolon is one of the most distressing of nonlethal anomalies, and was promptly attached to Hirschsprung's name after his description of autopsies of two infants who died from this condition in 1888.[108] However, it was recognized as early as 1825 in adults, and, in 1829, in infants.[109] This disease results from the absence of ganglion cells in the myenteric plexus of the colon caused by the interruption of migration of neuroenteric cells from the neural crest before they reach the rectum. The physiologic obstruction, more insidious than an anatomic atresia, results in proximal dilation and hypertrophy of the colon above. The extent of the aganglionosis is variable. The internal anal sphincter is involved in all cases, and the entire rectum in most cases. The disease is more common in males and its severity is related to the length of the aganglionic segment. Although most patients reach surgery before they are a year old, many are older, and a few reach adulthood. This topic is further discussed in Chap. 50.

References

1. Vesalii Bruxellensis Andreae, de Humani corporis fabrica. De Recti intestini musculis. 1st ed. 1543:228.
2. Church JM, Raudkivi PJ, Hill GL. The surgical anatomy of the rectum – a review with particular relevance to the hazards of rectal mobilisation. Int J Colorectal Dis. 1987;2:158–66.
3. Shafik A. A concept of the anatomy of the anal sphincter mechanism and the physiology of defecation. Dis Colon Rectum. 1987;30:970–82.
4. Klosterhalfen B, Vogel P, Rixen H, Mitterman C. Topography of the inferior rectal artery. A possible cause of chronic, primary anal fissure. Dis Colon Rectum. 1989;32:43–52.
5. Stoss F. Investigations of the muscular architecture of the rectosigmoid junction in humans. Dis Colon Rectum. 1990; 33:378–83.
6. Levi AC, Borghi F, Garavoglia M. Development of the anal canal muscles. Dis Colon Rectum. 1991;34:262–6.
7. Lunniss PJ, Phillips RKS. Anatomy and function of the anal longitudinal muscle. Br J Surg. 1992;79:882–4.
8. Tjandra JJ, Milsom JW, Stolfi VM, et al. Endoluminal ultrasound defines anatomy of the anal canal and pelvic floor. Dis Colon Rectum. 1992;35:465–70.
9. Dobson HD, Pearl RK, Orsay CP, et al. Virtual reality: new method of teaching anorectal and pelvic floor anatomy. Dis Colon Rectum. 2003;46:349–52.
10. Milligan ETC, Morgan CN. Surgical anatomy of the anal canal: with special reference to anorectal fistulae. Lancet. 1934;2:1150–6.

11. Goligher JC, Leacock AG, Brossy JJ. The surgical anatomy of the anal canal. Br J Surg. 1955;43:51–61.
12. Garavoglia M, Borghi F, Levi AC. Arrangement of the anal striated musculature. Dis Colon Rectum. 1993;36:10–5.
13. Nivatvongs S, Gordon PH. Surgical anatomy. In: Gordon PH, Nivatvongs S, editors. Principle and practice of surgery for the colon, rectum and anus. St. Louis, MO: Quality Medical Publishing; 1992. p. 3–37.
14. Shafik A. A new concept of the anatomy of the anal sphincter mechanism and the physiology of defecation. II. Anatomy of the levator ani muscle with special reference to puborectalis. Invest Urol. 1975;12:175–82.
15. Oh C, Kark AE. Anatomy of the external anal sphincter. Br J Surg. 1972;59:717–23.
16. Bollard RC, Gardiner A, Lindow S, Phillips K, Duthie GS. Normal female anal sphincter: difficulties in interpretation explained. Dis Colon Rectum. 2002;45:171–5.
17. Fritsch H, Brenner E, Lienemann A, Ludwikowski B. Anal sphincter complex: reinterpreted morphology and its clinical relevance. Dis Colon Rectum. 2002;45:188–94.
18. Morren GL, Beets-Tan RGH, van Engelshoven JMA. Anatomy of the anal canal and perianal structures as defined by phased-array magnetic resonance imaging. Br J Surg. 2001;88: 1506–12.
19. Williams AB, Bartram CI, Halligan S, Marshall MM, Nicholls RJ, Kmiot WA. Endosonographic anatomy of the normal anal compared with endocoil magnetic resonance imaging. Dis Colon Rectum. 2002;45:176–83.
20. Jorge JMN, Habr-Gama A. The value of sphincter asymmetry index in anal incontinence. Int J Colorectal Dis. 2000;15: 303–10.
21. Swash M. Histopathology of pelvic floor muscles in pelvic floor disorders. In: Henry MM, Swash M, editors. Coloproctology and the pelvic floor. London: Butterworth-Heinemann; 1992. p. 173–83.
22. Courtney H. Anatomy of the pelvic diaphragm and anorectal musculature as related to sphincter preservation in anorectal surgery. Am J Surg. 1950;79:155–73.
23. Shafik A. A new concept of the anatomy of the anal sphincter mechanism and the physiology of defecation. III. The longitudinal anal muscle: anatomy and role in sphincter mechanism. Invest Urol. 1976;13:271–7.
24. Lawson JON. Pelvic anatomy. II. Anal canal and associated sphincters. Ann R Coll Surg Engl. 1974;54:288–300.
25. Roux C. Contribution to the knowledge of the anal muscles in man. Arch Mikr Anat. 1881;19:721–3.
26. Haas PA, Fox TA. The importance of the perianal connective tissue in the surgical anatomy and function of the anus. Dis Colon Rectum. 1977;20:303–13.
27. Gordon PH. Anorectal anatomy and physiology. Gastroenterol Clin North Am. 2001;30:1–13.
28. Lilius HG. Investigation of human fetal anal ducts and intramuscular glands and a clinical study of 150 patients. Acta Chir Scand Suppl. 1968;383:1–88.
29. Chiari H. Über die Nalen Divertik Fel der Rectum-schleimhaut und Ihre Beziehung zu den anal fisteln. Wien Med Press. 1878;19:1482.
30. Parks AG. Pathogenesis and treatment of fistula-in-ano. BMJ. 1961;1:463–9.
31. Abel AL. The pecten band: pectenosis and pectenectomy. Lancet. 1932;1:714–8.
32. Goligher J. Surgery of the anus, rectum and colon. London: Bailliére Tindall; 1984. p. 1–47.
33. Abramson DJ. The valves of Houston in adults. Am J Surg. 1978;136:334–6.
34. Cawthorn SJ, Parums DV, Gibbs NM, et al. Extent of mesorectal spread and involvement of lateral resection margin as prognostic factors after surgery for rectal cancer. Lancet. 1990;335:1055–9.
35. Heald RJ, Husband EM, Ryall RD. The mesorectum in rectal cancer surgery – the clue to pelvic recurrence? Br J Surg. 1982;69:613–6.
36. Boxall TA, Smart PJG, Griffiths JD. The blood-supply of the distal segment of the rectum in anterior resection. Br J Surg. 1963;50:399–404.
37. Nano M, Dal Corso HM, Lanfranco G, Ferronato M, Hornung JP. Contribution to the surgical anatomy of the ligaments of the rectum. Dis Colon Rectum. 2000;43:1592–8.
38. Quirke P, Durdey P, Dixon MF, Williams NS. Local recurrence of rectal adenocarcinoma due to inadequate surgical resection. Histopathological study of lateral tumour spread and surgical excision. Lancet. 1986;1:996–8.
39. Jorge JMN, Habr-Gama A, Souza Jr AS, Kiss DR, Nahas P, Pinotti HW. Rectal surgery complicated by massive presacral hemorrhage. Arq Bras Circ Dig. 1990;5:92–5.
40. Wang Q, Shi W, Zhao Y, Zhou W, He Z. New concepts in severe presacral hemorrhage during proctectomy. Arch Surg. 1985;120:1013–20.
41. Zama N, Fazio VW, Jagelman DG, Lavery IC, Weakley FL, Church JM. Efficacy of pelvic packing in maintaining hemostasis after rectal excision for cancer. Dis Colon Rectum. 1988;31:923–8.
42. Crapp AR, Cuthbertson AM. William Waldeyer and the rectosacral fascia. Surg Gynecol Obstet. 1974;138:252–6.
43. Tobin CE, Benjamin JA. Anatomical and surgical restudy of Denonvilliers' fascia. Surg Gynecol Obstet. 1945;80:373–88.
44. Lindsey I, Guy RJ, Warren BF, Mortensen NJ. Anatomy of Denonvilliers' fascia and pelvic nerves, impotence, and implications for the colorectal surgeon. Br J Surg. 2000;87:1288–99.
45. Michels NA, Siddharth P, Kornblith PL, Park WW. The variant blood supply to the small and large intestines: its importance in regional resections. A new anatomic study based on four hundred dissections with a complete review of the literature. J Int Coll Surg. 1963;39:127–70.
46. Ayoub SF. Arterial supply of the human rectum. Acta Anat. 1978;100:317–27.
47. Didio LJA, Diaz-Franco C, Schemainda R, Bezerra AJC. Morphology of the middle rectal arteries: a study of 30 cadaveric dissections. Surg Radiol Anat. 1986;8:229–36.
48. Bernstein WC. What are hemorrhoids and what is their relationship to the portal venous system? Dis Colon Rectum. 1983;26:829–34.
49. Miscusi G, Masoni L, Dell'Anna A, Montori A. Normal lymphatic drainage of the rectum and the anal canal revealed by lymphoscintigraphy. Coloproctology. 1987;9:171–4.
50. Block IR, Enquist IF. Studies pertaining to local spread of carcinoma of the rectum in females. Surg Gynecol Obstet. 1961;112:41–6.
51. Gerstenberg TC, Nielsen ML, Clausen S, Blaabgerg J, Lindenberg J. Bladder function after abdominoperineal resection of the rectum for anorectal cancer. Am J Surg. 1980;91: 81–6.

52. Orkin BA. Rectal carcinoma: treatment. In: Beck DE, Wexner SD, editors. Fundamentals of anorectal surgery. New York: McGraw-Hill; 1992. p. 260–369.
53. Balslev I, Harling H. Sexual dysfunction following operation for carcinoma of the rectum. Dis Colon Rectum. 1983; 26:785.
54. Danzi M, Ferulano GP, Abate S, Califano G. Male sexual function after abdominoperineal resection for rectal cancer. Dis Colon Rectum. 1983;26:665–8.
55. Weinstein M, Roberts M. Sexual potency following surgery for rectal carcinoma. A follow-up of 44 patients. Ann Surg. 1977;185:295–300.
56. Bauer JJ, Gerlent IM, Salky B, Kreel I. Sexual dysfunction following proctectomy for benign disease of the colon and rectum. Ann Surg. 1983;197:363–7.
57. Walsh PC, Schlegel PN. Radical pelvic surgery with preservation of sexual function. Ann Surg. 1988;208:391–400.
58. Lee ECG, Dowling BL. Perimuscular excision of the rectum for Crohn's disease and ulcerative colitis. A conservative technique. Br J Surg. 1972;59:29–32.
59. Metcalf AM, Dozois RR, Kelly KA. Sexual function in women after proctocolectomy. Ann Surg. 1986;204:624–7.
60. Duthie HL, Gairns FW. Sensory nerve endings and sensation in the anal region in man. Br J Surg. 1960;47:585–95.
61. Kaiser AM, Ortega AE. Anorectal anatomy. Surg Clin North Am. 2002;82:1125–38.
62. Wendell-Smith CP. Studies on the morphology of the pelvic floor [Ph.D. thesis]. University of London; 1967.
63. Paramore RH. The Hunterian lectures on the evolution of the pelvic floor in non-mammalian vertebrates and pronograde mammals. Lancet. 1910;1(1393–1399):1459–67.
64. Percy JP, Swash M, Neill ME, Parks AG. Electrophysiological study of motor nerve supply of pelvic floor. Lancet. 1981;1:16–7.
65. Russell KP. Anatomy of the pelvic floor, rectum and anal canal. In: Smith LE, editor. Practical Guide to anorectal testing. New York: Igaku-Shoin; 1991. p. 744–7.
66. Parks AG, Porter NH, Hardcastle J. The syndrome of the descending perineum. Proc R Soc Med. 1966;59:477–82.
67. Bannister JJ, Gibbons C, Read NW. Preservation of faecal continence during rises in intra-abdominal pressure: is there a role for the flap valve? Gut. 1987;28:1242–5.
68. Bartolo DCC, Roe AM, Locke-Edmunds JC, Virjee J, Mortensen NJ. Flap-valve theory of anorectal continence. Br J Surg. 1986;73:1012–4.
69. Fraser ID, Condon RE, Schulte WJ, Decosse JJ, Cowles VE. Longitudinal muscle of muscularis externa in human and nonhuman primate colon. Arch Surg. 1981;116:61–3.
70. Guyton AC, editor. Textbook of medical physiology. Philadelphia: WB Saunders; 1986. p. 754–69.
71. Kumar D, Phillips SF. The contribution of external ligamentous attachments to function of the ileocecal junction. Dis Colon Rectum. 1987;30:410–6.
72. Wakeley CPG. The position of the vermiform appendix as ascertained by an analysis of 10, 000 cases. J Anat. 1983;67: 277–83.
73. Skandalakis JE, Gray SW, Ricketts R. The colon and rectum. In: Skandalakis JE, Gray SW, editors. Embryology for surgeons. The embryological basis for the treatment of congenital anomalies. Baltimore: Williams & Wilkins; 1994. p. 242–81.
74. O'Beirne J, editor. New views of the process of defecation and their application to the pathology and treatment of diseases of the stomach, bowels and other organs. Dublin: Hodges and Smith; 1833.
75. Hyrtl J. Handbuch der topographischen anatomie und ihrer praktisch medicinisch-chirurgischen anwendungen. II. Band, 4. Aufl. Wien: Braumüller; 1860.
76. Mayo WJ. A study of the rectosigmoid. Surg Gynecol Obstet. 1917;25:616–21.
77. Cantlie J. The sigmoid flexure in health and disease. J Trop Med Hyg. 1915;18:1–7.
78. Otis WJ. Some observations on the structure of the rectum. J Anat Physiol. 1898;32:59–63.
79. Balli R. The sphincters of the colon. Radiology. 1939; 33:372–6.
80. Ewing MR. The significance of the level of the peritoneal reflection in the surgery of rectal cancer. Br J Surg. 1952;39: 495–500.
81. Stelzner F. Die Verschlubsysteme am Magen-Darm-Kanal und ihre chirurgische Bedeutung. Acta Chir Austriaca. 1987;19:565–9.
82. Sonneland J, Anson BJ, Beaton LE. Surgical anatomy of the arterial supply to the colon from the superior mesenteric artery based upon a study of 600 specimens. Surg Gynecol Obstet. 1958;106:385–98.
83. Steward JA, Rankin FW. Blood supply of the large intestine. Its surgical considerations. Arch Surg. 1933;26:843–91.
84. Griffiths JD. Surgical anatomy of the blood supply of the distal colon. Ann R Coll Surg Engl. 1956;19:241–56.
85. Haller A. The large intestine. In: Cullen W, editor. First Lines of physiology. A reprint of the 1786 edition (Sources of Science 32). New York: Johnson; 1966. p. 139–40.
86. Drummond H. Some points relating to the surgical anatomy of the arterial supply of the large intestine. Proc R Soc Med Proctol. 1913;7:185–93.
87. Drummond H. The arterial supply of the rectum and pelvic colon. Br J Surg. 1914;1:677–85.
88. Meyers CB. Griffiths' point: critical anastomosis at the splenic flexure. Am J Roentgenol. 1976;126:77.
89. Landreneau RJ, Fry WJ. The right colon as a target organ of non-occlusive mesenteric ischemia. Arch Surg. 1990;125: 591–4.
90. Longo WE, Ballantyne GH, Gursberg RJ. Ischemic colitis: patterns and prognosis. Dis Colon Rectum. 1992;35:726–30.
91. Sudeck P. Über die Gefassversorgung des Mastdarmes in Hinsicht auf die Operative Gangran. Münch Med Wochenschr. 1907;54:1314.
92. Griffiths JD. Extramural and intramural blood supply of the colon. BMJ. 1961;1:322–6.
93. Lindstrom BL. The value of the collateral circulation from the inferior mesenteric artery in obliteration of the lower abdominal aorta. Acta Chir Scand. 1950;1:677–85.
94. Fisher DF, Fry WI. Collateral mesenteric circulation. Surg Gynecol Obstet. 1987;164:487–92.
95. Moskowitz M, Zimmerman H, Felson H. The meandering mesenteric artery of the colon. Am J Roentgenol. 1964;92: 1088–99.
96. Jameson JK, Dobson JF. The lymphatics of the colon. Proc R Soc Med. 1909;2:149–72.
97. Nobles VP. The development of the human anal canal. J Anat. 1984;138:575.
98. Duhamel B. From the mermaid to anal imperforation: the syndrome of caudal regression. Arch Dis Child. 1961;36:152–5.

99. Moore TC, Lawrence EA. Congenital malformations of rectum and anus. II. Associated anomalies encountered in a series of 120 cases. Surg Gynecol Obstet. 1952;95:281.
100. Anderson RC, Reed SC. The likelihood of congenital malformations. J Lancet. 1954;74:175–9.
101. Gough MH. Congenital abnormalities of the anus and rectum. Arch Dis Child. 1961;36:146–51.
102. Santulli TV, Schullinger JN, Amoury RA. Malformations of the anus and rectum. Surg Clin North Am. 1965;45:1253–71.
103. Brown SS, Schoen AH. Congenital anorectal stricture. J Pediatr. 1950;36:746–50.
104. Romolo JL. Congenital lesions: intussusception and volvulus. In: Zuidema GD, editor. Shackelford's surgery of the alimentary tract. Philadelphia: WB Saunders; 1991. p. 45–51.
105. McPherson AG, Trapnell JE, Airth GR. Duplication of the colon. Br J Surg. 1969;56:138.
106. Benson CD. Surgical implications of Meckel's diverticulum. In: Ravitch MM, Welch KJ, Benson CD, et al., editors. Pediatric surgery. 3rd ed. Chicago: Year Book; 1979. p. 955.
107. Louw JH. Investigations into the etiology and congenital atresia of the colon. Dis Colon Rectum. 1964;7:471.
108. Hirschsprung H. Fälle von angeborener Pylorusstenose beobachtet bei Säulingen. Jahrb Kinderh. 1888;27:61–9.
109. Finney JMT. Congenital idiopathic dilatation of the colon. Surg Gynecol Obstet. 1908:624–643.

2 Colonic Physiology

Ursula M. Szmulowicz and Tracy L. Hull

The human colon is a dynamic organ, involved in a vast array of functions, including the absorption of water and electrolytes, the salvage of unabsorbed nutrients, and the transport of luminal contents as feces. While not an organ essential for life, the colon still plays a major role in maintaining the overall health of the human body. Understanding these physiologic principles is integral to the successful treatment – both medical and surgical – of colonic disease.

Embryology

The embryology of the colon informs its anatomy. In the third and fourth weeks of gestation, the primitive intestine arises from the cephalocaudal and lateral folding of the dorsal surface of the endoderm-lined yolk sac, forming a straight tube situated posteriorly in the embryo.[1–3] Although the mucosa originates from the endoderm of the yolk sac, the muscular wall, connective tissue, and serosa have a mesodermal etiology.[4] By the fourth week of gestation, the gut tube develops into three distinct regions: the foregut, midgut, and hindgut.[4] The midgut begins immediately distal to the confluence of the common bile duct and the duodenum, extending to include the proximal two-thirds of the transverse colon. At the midgut, the primitive intestine maintains its connection to the yolk sac via the vitelline duct; failure of the vitelline duct to obliterate ultimately results in a Meckel's diverticulum or a vitelline cyst or fistula.[2,5] The hindgut reaches from the distal third of the transverse colon to the anal canal proximal to the dentate line. The midgut receives its vascular supply from the superior mesenteric artery and the hindgut from the inferior mesenteric artery.[6]

The colon gains its ultimate position by means of a series of rotations of the embryonic gut. During the fifth week of gestation, the midgut, particularly the future ileum, rapidly enlarges beyond the capacity of the abdominal cavity, culminating in its physiologic herniation through the umbilicus in the sixth week.[1] While exteriorized, this hairpin-shaped primary intestinal loop rotates 90° counterclockwise around an axis comprised of the superior mesenteric artery, as viewed from the front. Although the cranial limb of the herniated primary intestinal loop – the future small intestine – continues to elongate and organize into loops, the caudal limb – the proximal colon – remains mainly unaltered, its only adjustment involving the development of a cecal bud, a bulge from its antimesenteric border.[3] In the tenth week of gestation, the herniated intestine commences its return to the abdominal cavity, in the process completing an additional 180° counterclockwise rotation to finalize the disposition of the embryonic proximal jejunum on the left and the primitive colon on the right.[2] The cecum – the last component to reenter the abdomen – initially is located in the right upper quadrant but then migrates inferiorly to the right iliac fossa as the dorsal mesentery suspending the ascending colon shortens and then recedes.[4] As the cecal bud descends, the appendix appears as a narrow diverticulum.[2–7] The loss of the dorsal mesentery of the ascending and descending colon produces their retroperitoneal fixation, absent in the cecum, transverse colon, and sigmoid colon.[2]

Innervation

Colonic innervation emanates from two sources: the extrinsic and the intrinsic nerves. Extrinsic innervation involves the sympathetic and parasympathetic nerves of the autonomic nervous system, which are responsible for colonic motility and sensation. Intrinsic innervation arises from the poorly understood enteric nervous system.

The parasympathetic nerves primarily exert an excitatory affect upon colonic motility. The main parasympathetic neurotransmitters include acetylcholine and tachykinins such as substance P. The parasympathetic supply to the proximal colon originates from the posterior division of the vagus nerve – the tenth cranial nerve.[8,9] These parasympathetic fibers reach the colon by following the branches of the superior mesenteric artery: the ileocolic and middle colic arteries. The distal colon, however, receives its parasympathetic

D.E. Beck et al. (eds.), *The ASCRS Textbook of Colon and Rectal Surgery: Second Edition*,
DOI 10.1007/978-1-4419-1584-9_2, © Springer Science+Business Media, LLC 2011

input from the second to fourth sacral nerves, with the third sacral nerve the most dominant.[8,9] These pelvic splanchnic nerves – the nervi erigentes – emerge from the lateral horns of S2–4.[8,9] After exiting the spinal column, the preganglionic parasympathetic fibers travel superiorly and laterally, deep to the peritoneum, to join the inferior hypogastric plexus, located on the anterolateral pelvic wall, adjacent to the lateral ligaments at the level of the lower third of the rectum.[10] From the inferior hypogastric plexus, these parasympathetic fibers are distributed to the pelvic organs and to the distal colon as far proximal as the splenic flexure.[11] The preganglionic parasympathetic fibers ultimately synapse in the bowel wall at the ganglia within the myenteric plexus of Auerbach and Meissner's plexus.[12]

Unlike the parasympathetic nerves, the sympathetic system effects a tonic inhibition of the nonsphincteric colonic muscle and, thus, of colonic peristalsis.[11] Additionally, sympathetic fibers prevent epithelial secretion and reduce splanchnic blood flow.[9] However, the sympathetic supply is excitatory to sphincter muscles, particularly to the ileocecal junction and the internal anal sphincter.[9,11,13] The primary sympathetic neurotransmitter is norepinephrine.[8,11] The inhibition of colonic tone, although not fully understood, is believed to be mediated via α_2 adrenergic receptors.[14] In one study in humans, the α_2 agonist clonidine was determined to decrease fasting colonic tone, while the α_2 antagonist yohimbine increased it.[15] Stimulation of the α_2 adrenoreceptor also blocked the release of acetylcholine from the hyperpolarized parasympathetic neurons in the myenteric and pelvic plexi, thus arresting parasympathetic function.[11,15] In contrast, the in vivo administration of the α_1 agonist phenylephrine and the β_2 agonist ritodrine at the highest acceptable dosages had no impact upon colonic tone.[15] Yet, in an in vitro study, agonists of the β_1, β_2, and β_3 colonic adrenoceptors relaxed the human taenia coli; the circular muscular tone maximally diminished after treatment with the β_1 agonist.[16]

The preganglionic sympathetic effector cells are derived from the intermediolateral cell column (lateral horns) of the thoracic (T1–12) and, in particular, the lumbar spine (L1–2 or 3–4). The sympathetic nerve fibers leave the spinal column via the ventral spinal nerve roots (rami). These myelinated preganglionic fibers then exit from the ventral spinal nerve root as a white ramus communicans ("communicating branches") to merge with the paired sympathetic trunks (paravertebral ganglia), found along the entire length of the vertebral column. Once it has joined a sympathetic trunk, the preganglionic sympathetic nerve fiber either immediately synapses at that ganglion or it ascends or descends along the trunk before synapsing at another vertebral level, from the first cervical vertebra to the first coccygeal vertebra, along the sympathetic trunk.[17] A single preganglionic fiber synapses with 30 or more postganglionic fibers.[8] After synapsing, the unmyelinated postganglionic fibers depart the sympathetic trunk as a gray ramus communicans, reuniting with the ventral spinal ramus, after which it is distributed to the sweat glands and arrector pili muscles of the body wall and to the smooth muscle of the blood vessels throughout the body.[18] Yet, most preganglionic fibers – those innervating the abdominopelvic viscera – pass through the sympathetic trunk without synapsing, instead proceeding to the interconnected collateral (preaortic or prevertebral) ganglia that lie anterior to the aorta at its junction with its main vascular branches as part of a specific splanchnic ("visceral") nerve: the greater (T5–T9 or 10), lesser (T10–T11), least (T12), or lumbar (L1–2) splanchnic nerves.[12,17,19] While the midgut receives its sympathetic input from the lesser splanchnic nerve, the hindgut is supplied by the lumbar splanchnic nerve.[18] Once these preganglionic fibers synapse at a collateral ganglion, the postganglionic fibers follow the vasculature to the intestine, concluding in the enteric ganglia.[20] Some of the postganglionic fibers terminate instead on intestinal epithelial cells, whereby intestinal secretion is inhibited.[20] The midgut derivatives are primarily innervated by postganglionic fibers from the superior mesenteric ganglion and the hindgut structures, from the inferior mesenteric ganglion, although commingling between the ganglia is common.[8]

The intrinsic innervation of the colon – the enteric nervous system – is uniquely able to mediate reflex behavior independent of input from the brain or spinal cord.[21] This intrinsic network regulates the majority of colonic motility.[9] However, the activity of the enteric nervous system is impacted by the extrinsic nerves: the sympathetic, parasympathetic, and visceral afferent nerves.[8,11] This "little brain" employs the same modulators and neuro transmitters present in the central nervous system, including the excitatory acetylcholine, substance P, and neurokinin A and the inhibitory nitric oxide, adenosine triphosphate (ATP), vasoactive intestinal polypeptide (VIP), and pituitary adenyl cyclase-activating peptide.[9,13,21,22] The enteric nervous system acts through many different types of neurons, with their cell bodies amassed within neuronal plexi positioned either between the circular and longitudinal muscles (the myenteric plexus of Auerbach) or in the submucosal layer.[9] The submucosal plexi are comprised of Meissner's plexus, situated adjacent to the mucosa, and Schabadasch's plexus, which lies near the circular muscle.[9] Notably, the number of neurons in the enteric nervous system greatly exceeds that of the entire autonomic nervous system.[9] The myenteric plexus directs smooth muscle function while the submucosal plexus modulates mucosal ion transport and absorptive functions.[11] Moreover, the enteric network influences blood flow to the colon.[20] Control of colonic motor function via the enteric nervous system remains poorly understood at this time. However, a reflex arc is initiated by a mechanical (e.g., stretch), chemical, or other noxious stimulus, which activates an enteric primary afferent neuron; the impulse is carried to an enteric motor neuron – the effector cell – via an enteric interneuron, producing an excitatory or inhibitory effect.[9,20]

Colonic Function

Salvage, Metabolism, and Storage

Although digestion and absorption primarily take place in the stomach and small intestine, the colon still plays a major role in these operations. The colon processes various complex carbohydrates and, to a lesser extent, proteins that prove resistant to digestion and absorption in the more proximal intestine.[23,24] Unlike the small intestine, the colon salvages nutrients from these products via fermentation. Fermentation occurs by means of the saccarolytic and proteolytic members of the over 400 species of bacteria, the majority of which are obligate anaerobes, present within the colon.[25] Approximately 10% of ingested carbohydrates enter the cecum as undigested material.[11] Among the diverse end products of the bacterial fermentation of complex carbohydrates – mainly the soluble plant residues (fiber) – are the short-chain fatty acids, represented principally by butyrate (15%), propionate (25%), and acetate (60%).[26] Ingestion of a diet higher in complex carbohydrates, beans, resistant starches, and soluble fiber leads to a greater output of short-chain fatty acids than that of insoluble fibers. The composition of the bacterial microenvironment also influences the amount of synthesized short-chain fatty acids.[11,27] The nondigestible carbohydrate inulin – an extract of chicory – has been studied as a prebiotic, a food that selectively alters the admixture of the colonic bacterial flora; although its addition to the diet increased the proportion of beneficial bifidobacteria in the feces in various studies, its impact – whether healthful or harmful – upon other bacterial species could not be well gauged.[28] Bacterial fermentation of the complex carbohydrates primarily transpires in the ascending and proximal transverse colon. In contrast, the undigested dietary proteins that reach the colon, as well as proteins from mucous and sloughed epithelial cells, are fermented in the distal colon, primarily because the carbohydrates – the preferred nutrient of most bacteria – were previously exhausted in the proximal colon; the concentration of the short-chain fatty acids produced in the distal colon is 30% less than in the proximal colon.[27,29,30] However, a diet that includes prebiotics such as inulin results in a greater degree of saccarolytic fermentation in the distal colon due to the greater availability of these slowly fermentable, highly polymerized carbohydrates.[27] The fermented proteins are converted into short-chain fatty acids, branched chain fatty acids, and amines. In addition, the bacterial fermentation of undigested proteins generates ammonia, phenols, indoles, and sulfurs; these possibly toxic substances are considered potential etiologic agents for such diseases as colon cancer and ulcerative colitis.[27] Some of these proteolytic metabolites become a nitrogen source for bacterial growth.[29,31] The residual products of the bacterial fermentation of complex carbohydrates and proteins are absorbed or, like carbon dioxide, hydrogen, and methane, passed with the feces.[28] The dietary fats that reach the colon likely are not recovered in the colon but are expelled with the stool.[25]

The short-chain fatty acids occupy an integral position in colonic health. More than 95% of the short-chain fatty acids are created in and are immediately appropriated by the colon, with very little excreted in the feces.[25,27,32] An average of 400 mmol/day, with a range of 150–600 mmol/day, of short-chain fatty acids are produced in the colon.[33,34] This reclamation of undigested matter in the colon as short-chain fatty acids provides 5–15% of the total caloric needs of an individual.[27] These weak acids – the preeminent colonic anions – mainly remain dissociated in the colonic lumen until absorbed either in exchange for bicarbonate via a SCFA/HCO_3^- transport channel; by an active transport mechanism such as the sodium-coupled monocarboxylate transporter (SMCT1) or the monocarboxylate transporter isoform 1 (MCT1); or by diffusion in their lipid soluble form.[27] The sodium-coupled monocarboxylate transporter facilitates the conservation of sodium, chloride, and water in the colon.[27] Furthermore, the short-chain fatty acids are incorporated as the basic elements for mucin synthesis, lipogenesis, gluconeogenesis, and protein production. In particular, propionate combines with other three-carbon compounds in the liver to participate in gluconeogenesis. Acetate is used by the liver as a component to fashion longer-chain fatty acids and by the muscle as sustenance.[23,24]

Although the least abundant of the short-chain fatty acids, butyrate has the greatest import in colonic homeostasis. This short-chain fatty acid acts as the primary energy source for the colonocyte, supplying 70–90% of its energy requirements; these epithelial cells receive their nourishment solely from luminal substrates, not from the bloodstream.[20,23,24] Of the short-chain fatty acids, butyrate best promotes the absorption of water, sodium, and chloride from the colon, acting as an antidiarrheal agent.[27] This short-chain fatty acid also advances colonic cell proliferation and differentiation, repair, and immune function.[11,27,35] Butyrate has been shown to influence colon carcinogenesis: studies have revealed that fewer butyrate transporters were present in human colonic adenocarcinomas, resulting in a decrease in the utilization of the trophic butyrate in the malignant cells.[27] Moreover, in vitro studies of cancer cell lines identified apoptosis, nonproliferation, and differentiation after the administration of butyrate.[27] One method by which butyrate modulates gene expression and, thus, cancer growth likely arises from its ability to suppress histone deacetylase, thus encouraging the union of various transcription factors with nuclear DNA; to modify intracellular kinase signaling; and to inhibit nuclear factor-κB.[27]

In the colon, many metabolic processes are influenced by functional food components. These foods – the pre- and probiotics – alter the colonic microenvironment, adding to the impact of environmental factors and genetics.[33] As previously discussed, prebiotics – primarily nondigestable oligosaccharides (NDOs) – are slowly fermentable foods that selectively propagate microbial proliferation and/or activity.[36] These products are completely metabolized in the colon into short-chain fatty acids, energy, and lactic acid, leaving no nondigestable oligosaccharides in the stool.[33] In contrast, probiotics represent active bacterial cultures that benefit the host by replenishing the colonic microenvironment.[37] Synbiotics combine the action of pre- and probiotics.[33] Investigations of these functional foods have focused on the lactobacilli and bifidobacteria, the growth of which transforms the colonic milieu, augmenting the immune function of the gut-associated lymphoid tissue (GALT).[31,33] The effect of these supplements is thought to be attributable to an increased production of butyrate, changes in mucin production, or interference in the binding of pathogenic bacteria to the colonic mucosa.[27,38] Prebiotics are particularly associated with an elevation of the concentration of short-chain fatty acids.[33] To combat the rising incidence of antibiotic-resistant bacteria in hospitals, the World Health Organization has recommended the use of microbial interference therapies – nonpathogenic bacteria that eradicate pathogens – such as probiotics.[34] Currently, probiotics are prescribed in cases of disturbed microbial balance, such as antibiotic-associated diarrhea. In the future, pre- and probiotics may become important supplements regularly administered to patients to promote health and to prevent illness. These functional foods further present the possibility of reducing the potential of carcinogens to form cancers.[31,38]

While the colon is one organ, it demonstrates regional differences. As noted, the proximal and distal colon have different embryological origins, derived from the mid- and hindgut, respectively. In appearance, the proximal colon is more saccular and the distal colon, more tubular.[39] The short-chain fatty acids are principally synthesized in the more acidic environment of the proximal colon. The proximal colon serves as a reservoir, in contrast to the distal colon, which mainly performs as a conduit.[40] Yet, this truism is disputed by studies in which radiopaque markers were determined to have the same dwell time of approximately 11 h in the proximal, distal, and middle colonic segments, suggesting that the proximal colon does not preferentially operate as a receptacle for stool.[9] Also, the character of the luminal contents impacts transit times. Large volumes of liquid quickly pass through the ascending colon but remain within the transverse colon for as long as 20–40 h; in contrast, a solid meal is retained by the cecum and ascending colon for longer periods than a liquid diet.[9,41,42] The salvage of water and electrolytes is primarily accorded to the proximal colon, although the distal colon and rectum contribute to this task, albeit to a lesser extent.[43,44] In the event that a large amount of chyme is delivered to the colon, the distal colon and rectum may assist in the absorption of enough fluid to produce a solid stool.[41] The regional heterogeneity of the colon exhibits adaptability. After a right hemicolectomy, the transverse colon adjusts to become a neo-proximal colon; 6 months after the surgery, the progress of an ingested isotope from the small intestine through the shortened colon returns to the preoperative baseline.[45] The assumption of this role may ensue due to the greater concentrations of short-chain fatty acids to which the transverse colon is exposed following a right hemicolectomy, producing such changes as an increase in water and sodium retention.[30]

Transport of Water and Electrolytes

Among its roles in preserving intestinal homeostasis, the colon is also integral to water and electrolyte transport. The colon maintains an appropriate hydration and electrolyte balance by means of the absorption and secretion of intestinal water and electrolytes. The mucosal surface area available for these processes amounts to approximately 2,000 cm^2.[30] While the surface epithelial cells in the colon are primarily responsible for absorption, the crypt cells are involved in fluid secretion; however, crypt cells have been found to some degree to contribute to absorption.[11,30,46] After the liquid effluent from the small intestine has traversed the colon, fluid and electrolyte absorption and secretion as well as bacterial activity produce about 200 g of solid feces per day.[20]

The colon is extremely efficient at conserving intestinal water.[13] Water is passively absorbed along an osmotic gradient, enabled by a luminal sodium concentration lower than that of the epithelial cells; as such, the salvage of intestinal water relies upon sodium conservation.[11,30] Normally, the colon is presented with 1.5–2 L of water daily, as compared to the 9–10 L that pass through the small intestine; of this amount, 1.5–2 L are ingested, with the remainder originating from salivary, biliary, pancreatic, and intestinal secretions.[24,30] Approximately 90% of this water is reclaimed by the colon, leaving 100–150 mL in the feces.[20] The absorption of water primarily follows a paracellular pathway, although a transcellular route involves various protein channels: aquaporins 3, 4, 5, 8, and 9.[20] The ascending colon demonstrates the greatest absorptive capability, as the chyme resides within this segment the longest, thus maximizing its contact with the mucosa. As a consequence, diarrhea more consistently ensues after a right, as opposed to a left, hemicolectomy. Fluid retention is promoted by the antidiuretic hormone.[43] When challenged, the proximal colon, with the additional contribution of the sigmoid colon and rectosigmoid, is able to save a further 5–6 L of intestinal water daily.[47–49] Yet this facility is contingent upon the composition, rate of flow (less than 1–2 mL/min), and amount of the effluent. In the case that the absorptive capacity of the colon is exceeded, diarrhea results. Fluid secretion in the colon only transpires in the presence of diverse secretagogues, such as laxatives, bacterial endotoxins, hormones (e.g., VIP), and endogenous substances (e.g., bile acids).[43]

The colon is essential to the recovery of sodium. Under normal conditions, the colon principally absorbs sodium and chloride but secretes bicarbonate and potassium. The liquid chyme delivered to the colon contains 130–140 mmol/L of sodium whereas the concentration in stool is 40 mmol/L;

approximately 95% of the sodium transported into the colon is conserved.[29,43] If required, the colon is able to increase its salvage of sodium to 800 mmol/L/day.[43] The normal colon can prevent hyponatremia even despite a diet containing as little as 1 mEq of sodium daily; in contrast, the absence of a colon encourages dehydration and hyponatremia.[43] The transport mechanisms for sodium absorption, located on the luminal surface of the epithelial cells, vary throughout the colon: a Na^+/H^+ exchange channel in the proximal colon and an electrogenic sodium-specific channel (ENaC) in the distal colon and rectum.[20] The Na^+/H^+ exchange channels (NHE 2 and 3) are coupled to the Cl^--HCO_3^- exchange channels.[20] The activity of the electrogenic sodium-specific channel in the distal colon and rectum is requisite for the desiccation of stool.[20] These two types of transport channel allow for the passive diffusion of sodium into the colonic epithelial cells along an electrochemical gradient, consisting of a low intracellular sodium concentration (<15 mM) and a negative intracellular electrical potential difference as compared to the lumen.[30] This favorable electrochemical gradient is created by the active extrusion of sodium via the Na^+/K^+ ATPase pump on the basolateral membrane of the epithelial cell: three sodium ions are expelled in exchange for two potassium ions.[20,30] Aldosterone, a mineralocorticoid secreted by the adrenal gland in response to sodium depletion and dehydration, enhances fluid and sodium absorption in the colon.[46,50] The absorption of sodium is further promoted by somatostatin, α_2-adrenergic agents (e.g., clonidine), and the short-chain fatty acids.[11,24]

Like sodium, chloride is recovered from the colonic lumen. In the proximal colon, chloride is traded for bicarbonate via the Cl^--HCO_3^- exchange channel found on the luminal surface of the epithelial cells; the activity of this channel is linked to the Na^+/H^+ exchange protein.[20,29] However, chloride also is absorbed through a Cl^--HCO_3^- exchange channel that is not associated with sodium.[20] Chloride absorption is supported by an acidic luminal milieu; consequentially, the concomitant secretion of bicarbonate neutralizes organic acids within the colonic lumen.[24,43] The transport mechanism for bicarbonate secretion is poorly understood. Yet, bicarbonate, responsible for the alkalinity of the feces, is the primary electrolyte wasted in diarrhea.[20]

Potassium transport is primarily a passive process, following the movement of sodium across cell membranes. However, active potassium secretion occurs in the proximal colon and active absorption in the distal colon.[11,20] The H^+/K^+ ATPase actively conveys potassium into the epithelial cells of the distal colon and rectum.[20] A potassium channel is believed to facilitate active secretion in the proximal colon.[20] Potassium secretion, combined with potassium derived from bacteria and colonic mucous, may explain the relatively high concentration of this electrolyte – 50–90 mmol/L – in stool.[51,52]

The colon contributes to the metabolism of urea. Approximately 0.4–1 g of urea enters the colon in the small bowel effluent daily.[43] The urea is converted by the colonic microorganisms into ammonia, which is then passively absorbed by the surface epithelial cells.[29,43] Ammonia is also derived from dietary nitrogen, the sloughed mucosal lining, and bacterial waste. Only 1–3 mmol of ammonia is excreted with the feces. The majority of the ammonia that reaches the colon is returned via the enterohepatic circulation to the liver, where it is refashioned into urea.[30]

Colonic Motility

Methodology to Measure Colonic Transit

Although altered motility is thought to play a major role in various gastrointestinal disorders, surprisingly little is known about the subject. This lack of understanding arises in part from the inaccessibility of the colon, particularly the proximal colon, for direct study. Bowel questionnaires have been used to gain insight into colonic motility; however, interestingly, stool frequency – or the recollection of the patient of their stool frequency – and colorectal transit time, which represents 75% of total intestinal transit time, are poorly related.[41,53,54] Early evaluations using barium were also unable to achieve a precise measurement of colonic motility.[55] The initial techniques to determine colonic motility began with the calculation of colonic transit time.

Radiopaque Markers

One of the first methods to gauge colonic transit time involves radiopaque markers. This study, proposed by Hinton and colleagues in 1969 to assess severe constipation, follows the passage of the markers over sequential abdominal radiographs.[11,56] Total and regional colonic transit times are reflected by the number and the location of the markers.[11] For men, the average total colonic transit is 30.7 h (SD 3.0) and for women, 38.3 h (SD 2.9).[55] Currently, the commercially available Sitzmarks™ (Konsyl Pharmaceuticals, Easton, MD) are composed of a gelatin capsule containing 24 radioopaque PVC O-rings. Various protocols for the examination exist, all of which require the cessation of all laxatives 48 h prior to swallowing the markers. In one approach that focuses on total colonic transit, 5 days after taking the capsule, an abdominal radiograph is obtained. A normal study demonstrates evacuation of 80% of the markers. The retention of more than 20% of the markers suggests slow transit constipation. Some physicians give a single capsule on Sunday evening and obtain abdominal X-rays on days 1, 3, and 5. The film on the first day provides evidence that gastric and small motility are grossly normal if all the markers are in the colon.

In order to localize the markers to specific segments of the colon – right, left, and pelvis – another technique requires that the patient consume one capsule, after which abdominal radiographs are performed every other day until all 24 markers have been expelled. As an alternative, patients ingest single capsules on three successive days, with only one abdominal radiograph done on day 4 of the study so as to minimize radiation exposure.[57] The number of markers present equals the colonic transit time in hours. To better determine the distribution of the markers, some centers use capsules holding markers of different shape on each of the 3 days. An accumulation of the markers in the rectosigmoid indicates a dyssynergic defecation pattern.[58] The reliability of the technique is affected by patient compliance as well as by differences in the interpretation of the results.[59]

Scintigraphy

Some centers favor the more expensive colonic scintigraphy over the radiopaque marker method to measure colonic transit. As with the marker study, the protocols are not standardized among institutions. Although patients refrain from taking laxatives or opiates 24 h before the test, a normal diet is maintained throughout the study. The isotope is positioned in the cecum by the ingestion of a delayed release capsule or by orocecal intubation.[11] The delayed release capsule, coated with the pH-sensitive polymer methacrylate, is comprised of activated charcoal or polystyrene pellets labeled with either ^{111}In or ^{99m}Tc. The coating dissolves at the pH of 7.2–7.4 found in the distal ileum, after which the radioactive material is delivered into the colon.[40,60] Images are taken with a gamma camera at specified intervals, usually at 4, 24, and 48 h after consumption of the isotope, although this can be performed as frequently as twice daily.[11,61] Segmental transit is usually determined for the ascending, transverse, descending, and rectosigmoid regions of the colon. The proportion of the counts is calculated in each section and then multiplied by a weighing factor: 0 for the cecum, 1 for the ascending colon, 2 for the transverse colon, 3 for the descending colon, 4 for the rectosigmoid colon, and 5 for stool.[60] The results are expressed as the geometric center of the isotope mass at any given time point, with a low count indicating that the isotope is close to the cecum and a higher count that it has progressed more distally.[11,61] For clinical use, the total percentage of retained isotope as compared to normal data appears to be the most convenient reporting system. Scintigraphy correlates well with the radiopaque technique in assessing colonic transit, with a similar sensitivity in diagnosing patients with slow transit constipation.[60] The total exposure to radiation is also equivalent.[11] Due to its greater costs, in most cases scintigraphy serves as a research instrument.

Wireless Motility Capsule

The wireless motility capsule has been proposed as an alternative method to determine colonic transit time. This technique, already proven for the study of gastroparesis, uses a capsule containing miniature pressure, temperature, and pH measurement devices. The capsule is ingested, after which continuous recordings are obtained in an ambulatory setting, with the data captured over 5 days via a wireless instrument.[59] In one trial, the results from the capsule approach correlated well with those acquired from the radiopaque markers, with a similar sensitivity and specificity in detecting abnormal transit in those patients with constipation.[59] The capsule is able to gauge phasic colonic contractions but not colonic motor patterns.[62] This costly procedure is not widely employed but is attractive in that radiation exposure is avoided and patient compliance is facilitated.[59]

Techniques to Record Colonic Motility

Colonic motility remains a constantly evolving field of study. The techniques by which colonic motility are gauged rely upon the monitoring of electrical activity or of intraluminal pressure, using surface electrodes or a manometry or barostat apparatus, respectively.[11] This indirect assessment of colonic motility has been hindered by the instruments available for its measurement, the colonic anatomy, and the need for prolonged readings. Recordings are usually obtained over 6 h in the laboratory and over 24 h in an ambulatory setting due to the long colonic transit time, especially as compared to the small intestine.[62] Also, the methods suffer from an absence of standardization. Although evaluations of colonic motility had initially focused upon the easily accessed distal colon, subsequent trials have indicated that this segment is not representative of the proximal colon. Yet, placement of the intraluminal devices is difficult, requiring either oral or nasal intubation or colonoscopy; furthermore, application of the surface electrodes demands surgery. Additionally, the necessity to purge the colon of stool may impact the results, producing an increase in the number of high amplitude propagated contractions, although these findings are conflicting.[63,64] Determinations of colonic pressure are further influenced by artifact from extrinsic forces such as cough, straining, and sneezing.[62] Thus, most of these approaches rest in the researchers' domain and have not been assimilated into the standard clinical armamentarium. However, significant progress is being gained with these tools to understand the physiology and pathophysiology of colonic motility.

Manometry

Colonic manometry has been the more frequently employed method to measure phasic (brief) colonic contractions. However, few centers utilize this technique in regular practice. In this procedure, a flexible catheter – either a solid-state or a water-perfused catheter system – is inserted into the colon. It is argued that the water-perfused system increases the amount of fluid in the colon, thus altering the results. However, the solid-state catheters are fragile, expensive, and sensitive to corrosive damage from colonic irritants.[65] However, this nonperfused system is more convenient and portable, allowing for long-term and ambulatory recordings.[66] The validity of the readings depends upon the proper placement of the catheter. As noted, the introduction of the catheter occurs via an oral or nasal route, confirmed with fluoroscopy, or by colonoscopy. With endoscopy, the catheter is either carried along with the colonoscope in a piggyback fashion, grasped by biopsy forceps, or is threaded over a guidewire, deposited via the colonoscope, under fluoroscopic guidance. The tip of the catheter is stationed as far proximal as the transverse colon; with direct colonoscopic deployment, the proximal transverse colon is reached in all subjects, with the probe remaining in position in greater than 80% of cases.[65,67–69] To adhere to more physiologic conditions, unprepared colons are currently advocated, despite the impediment presented by the retained stool to the retrograde placement of the catheters; in some cases, enemas are instead used. Also, to prevent data artifact, minimal air is insufflated via the colonoscope and as much aspirated as possible during its withdrawal. The patients are often asked to maintain a diary to mark events such as bowel movements, flatus, and meals. Manometry is well able to detect the changes in intraluminal pressure after eating or the administration of a colonic stimulant (e.g., bisacodyl). However, these variations in pressure do not consistently correspond to contractions: in a study of colonic motility, the simultaneous use of manometry and colonoscopy indicated that a majority of pressure fluctuations perceived by the catheter reflected colonic relaxation, not contraction.[70] Furthermore, manometry does not reliably identify all contractions, some of which are not associated with an appreciable pressure deflection.[9,70] An investigation comparing the barostat with manometry suggested that the measurements obtained from manometry are also affected by the luminal diameter in which the tip of the device lies.[70] However, unlike the barostat, manometry recognizes patterns of motor activity due to the multiple recording sites along the catheter.[62]

Barometry

The colonic barostat device addresses the inability of manometry to record colonic tone, i.e., sustained contractions. As with manometry, it is utilized clinically in few centers. The instrument includes a compressible polyethylene balloon, placed within the colonic lumen, that is attached via tubing to a barostat – a cylinder containing a piston.[11] The balloon is maintained at a low constant pressure such that it is continuously in close contact with the colon wall in a single location.[71] Contraction of the colon constricts the balloon, reducing its volume by forcing air into the barostat; in contrast, colonic relaxation produces an increase in the volume of the balloon so as to sustain a constant pressure.[11] Changes in the volume of the balloon reflect colonic tone, although phasic contractions are also assessed.[72,73] However, patterns of colonic activity cannot be distinguished as measurements are obtained in only one site.[62] Unlike the manometry technique, the barostat system is capable of detecting contractions that do not produce a significant pressure change, even in colonic segments wider than 5.6 cm.[11]

Electrodes

Electrodes have also been applied for the study of colonic motility. These devices record the myoelectrical signals from the colon that result in muscular activity.[74,75] The electrodes are placed on the serosal surface via surgery or on the mucosa by colonoscopy. The technique is seldom used due to ethical concerns.

Peristalsis

Peristalsis represents the alternating waves of contraction and relaxation of the circular muscles of the colon wall. Fecal material is propelled antegrade through the colon by the contraction of the circular muscle proximal but the relaxation of the muscle distal to it, i.e., descending inhibition.[11] During peristaltic activity, the saccular haustra – the product of circular muscle contraction – recede and then reform, first proximal to and subsequently at the level of the transferred material, again giving rise to colonic segmentation.[9,41,76] The contribution of the longitudinal smooth muscle to colonic activity is unknown.[9] The average rate of antegrade colonic transit is approximately 1 cm/h.[9] The peristaltic reflex is thought to be initiated by luminal distention and, possibly, by chemical stimuli, which stimulate the enteric sensory neurons; ultimately, the enteric motor neurons – the effector cells – are activated via the intermediary of the enteric interneurons.[11] The interneurons may also directly detect changes in smooth muscle length.[77] The primary neurotransmitters involved in the peristaltic reflex include the excitatory acetylcholine and the inhibitory nitric oxide and adenosine triphosphate (ATP).[11] Although the enteric nervous network primarily controls peristalsis, the extrinsic nervous system modifies the reflex, with the sympathetic nerves suppressing and the parasympathetic nerves promoting motility, especially during defecation. Interestingly, the parasympathetic nerves also assist in the synchronization of descending inhibition. The antegrade movement of the fecal bolus is further dependent upon the radius of the colonic segment, the consistency of the feces, and the pressure differential between segments.

Colonic motility adheres to several patterns. Generally, contractions vary between tonic and phasic. The poorly understood tonic contractions are sustained events of slow onset, not necessarily inciting an elevation of the intraluminal pressure.[76] Bassotti et al. further classify the briefer phasic contractile episodes as high and low amplitude propagated contractions and as segmental contractions.[71,78]

High amplitude propagated contractions – also known as migrating long spike bursts, large bowel peristalsis, and giant migrating contractions – function to transport large volumes of feces over long distances.[71,78,79] These contractions are believed to be the manometric equivalent of mass movement – first identified on radiographic studies of the colon – whereby colonic contents are projected distally in seconds.[40,67,80,81] The high amplitude propagated contractions transpire between 2 and 24 times a day, with an average of approximately five to six times a day.[62,71] These contractions, with an amplitude of 100–200 mmHg (average of 100 mmHg), persist for 20–30 s.[62,71] The contraction usually begins in the proximal colon and is transmitted distally for 15 cm or longer, with the velocity gradually increasing to as fast as 1 cm/s as the impulse moves caudad.[11] A contraction that starts in the proximal colon is conveyed farther than that commencing in the distal colon: 50 cm from the cecum and 20 cm from the sigmoid colon.[9] More than 95% of these contractions proceed antegrade; however, only one-third of these contractions result in the transit of fecal material.[11,71,78] Moreover, not all instances of defecation, particularly those involving liquid stool, are incited by a high amplitude propagated contraction.[78] High amplitude propagated contractions are considered the probable origin of the pressure spikes that occur upon morning waking (35%) and after meals (50%).[71] The urge to defecate is likely attributable to these contractions.[71] Borborigmy is thought also to arise from high amplitude propagated contractions.[78] The impetus for these contractions is incompletely comprehended. These contractions are elicited by cholinergic medications (e.g., neostigmine), eating, colonic distention, short-chain fatty acids, and laxatives (e.g., bisacodyl).[11] However, only in 50% of cases does colonic distention produce propagating activity.[78] In patients with constipation, high amplitude propagated contractions are decreased in number, amplitude, extent, and speed.

The low amplitude propagated contractions are still less understood. These contractions (5–40 mmHg) – also referred to as long spike bursts – last for 3 s.[71] As with the high amplitude propagated contractions, these contractions are strongly related to meals and the sleep-wake cycle. There may be an association with the passage of flatus and, in particular, liquid stool.[82,83] Similar to the high amplitude propagated contractions, these contractions are likely provoked by colonic distention.[71] The mechanisms by which these two propagated contractions are regulated remain unclear. However, propulsive activity depends upon a functional enteric nervous system.[71]

Segmental contractions, presenting singly or in rhythmic or arrhythmic bursts, account for the majority of colonic activity, particularly at rest.[78] These contractions appear with an amplitude of 5–50 mmHg.[71] Found primarily in the ascending and transverse colon, this activity produces localized contractions of the circular and longitudinal muscles, in effect segregating the haustrae.[71] These segmental contractions, the correlate of myoelectical short spike bursts, result in the slow, sequential antegrade or retrograde movement of colonic contents among the haustra, allowing for mixing of the material.[13] Additionally, contact with the mucosal surface is maximized, which permits the absorption of intestinal water and electrolytes.[71] Only 6% of segmental contractions are rhythmic, with a frequency of 2–8 cycles per minute; however, in the rectosigmoid region, a slower interval of 3 cycles per minute is preeminent, possibly giving rise to a physiologic sphincter to aid in continence.[9,78,83]

Unlike other mammals, humans possess a colon in which cyclic motility is absent.[78] The human rectum, however, does display such cyclic activity, the rectal motor complex. The rectal motor complex is comprised of phasic contractions with amplitude of more than 5 mmHg. These phasic contractions appear at a cycle of 2–3 per minute, with each persisting for approximately 3 min. Yet, the interlude between these contractions ranges from 10 to 260 min. This phasic activity in the rectum and, potentially, the rectosigmoid may contribute to fecal continence, as it is correlated with an elevated anal canal pressure; this role is further suggested by the greater prominence of this activity at night.

Cellular Basis of Motility

Colonic motor activity is driven and coordinated by the interstitial cells of Cajal, the intestinal pacemaker cells.[84] In the absence of these cells, the intestinal smooth muscle is inactive.[85] The interstitial cells of Cajal arise from smooth muscle precursor cells; that is, the cells are of mesenchymal, not neuronal, origin.[86] These cells are classified by their location as ICC_{MY} – in the myenteric plexus, between the muscular layers; ICC_{SM} – in the submucosal surface of the circular muscle; and ICC_{IM} – within the circular and longitudinal muscles.[87] The interstitial cells of Cajal are linked to the individual smooth muscle cells via intracellular gap junctions; the similarly coupled smooth muscle cells function as a single unit, a syncytium.[9] The gap junctions allow for the passage of current – predominantly slow waves – from the interstitial cells of Cajal to the smooth muscle syncytium, leading to its depolarization.[86] The interstitial cells of Cajal are believed to be mechanosensitive, able to transduce stretch stimulus from the distended colonic lumen into electrical activity.[88] The ICC_{SM} – the primary pacemaker cells – continuously generate high amplitude slow waves, at a frequency of 2–4 per minute, within the circular muscle layer.[9] Unlike the other types of interstitial cells of Cajal, the ICC_{SM} are present only within the colon, solely in its proximal portion.[86] A slow wave of sufficient charge produces a smooth muscle action potential, allowing for an influx of calcium into the smooth muscle cells via the L-type calcium channels and, thus, a brief contraction.[76] The amplitude of the slow waves is greatest at the submucosal surface of the circular muscle, diminishing while traveling through the muscular wall.[89] Slow waves migrate antegrade and retrograde along short segments of the colon, rapidly in the circumferential and slowly in the longitudinal axis; as waves of different inception meet, their propagation ceases, giving rise to nonpropulsive mixing activity.[9,85] A second pacemaker site may involve the ICC_{MY}. In addition to the slow waves, the ICC_{MY} may initiate low amplitude myenteric potential oscillations (MPOs) at a frequency of 12–20 per minute, which are conveyed to the circular and longitudinal smooth muscle.[9] The MPOs possibly are the source of propagating contractions.[9] Moreover, the ICC_{MY} synchronize the activity of the circular and longitudinal layers of the smooth muscle.[86] As opposed to the ICC_{SM}, the ICC_{MY} are widespread throughout the colon.[86] The etiology of the intrinsic electrical activity of the ICC_{MY} and ICC_{SM} is uncertain but may involve calcium regulated nonselective cation channels or large-conductance chloride channels; the oscillations from the interstitial cells of Cajal remain even the absence of extrinsic neural input.[9] The ICC_{IM} are thought to mediate such extrinsic input – from the enteric and autonomic neural networks – upon smooth muscle function; the release of acetylcholine and nitric oxide from excitatory and inhibitory neurons, respectively, results in alterations in the activity of the ICC_{IM}.[9,88] Furthermore, the ICC_{IM} appear to augment the slow waves and MPOs from the ICC_{SM} and ICC_{MY}, respectively, as they are transmitted along the smooth muscle syncytium.[9] Much still remains to be elucidated about the cellular basis of colonic motility.

Characteristics of Colonic Motility in Health

Manometry studies have demonstrated a noncyclical pattern of colonic activity.[11] The variations in colonic activity are mirrored by changes in colonic tone.[83] The human colon follows a circadian rhythm in which sleep is associated with its relaxation and, thus, with a marked diminution of its pressure activity.[65,90] However, as previously noted, the rectum and rectosigmoid display continued phasic activity during the night. Immediately after morning waking, a two- to three-fold increase in colonic pressure activity – likely due to high amplitude propagated contractions – occurs, inciting an urge to defecate in some cases. A similar rise in colonic activity transpires during brief night-time arousals or during REM sleep.[71] The mechanism by which the colon rapidly responds to these alterations in wakefulness is unknown. During the day, the transverse and descending colon reveal more pressure activity than the rectosigmoid colon. Moreover, less activity is seen in the transverse and descending colon of women, as compared to men.[65]

Oral intake also impacts colonic activity. Within 1–3 min of the initial bites of a meal, long before the food reaches the colon, segmental contractions begin in the proximal and distal colon, persisting for 2–3 h.[65,91] This colonic motor response to eating, or gastrocolic reflex, also features a concomitant increase in the colonic smooth muscle tone, especially in the proximal colon, often affiliated with high amplitude propagated contractions.[39,41,71] The colon exhibits regional differences in its response to a meal: the proximal colon evinces a swifter but briefer duration of contractile activity than the distal colon.[71] Although infrequently identified during scintigraphic studies, retrograde propulsion most commonly appears after meals as well as during morning waking.[65] Colonic motility is instigated by a higher calorie meal (more than 500 kcal), fat, and, to a lesser degree, carbohydrates; in contrast, proteins inhibit motor function.[71] The colonic response to eating includes two phases: an initial stimulation of the gastro-duodenal wall mechano- and chemoreceptors and a subsequent activation of receptors in the colonic wall.[71] The means by which the gastrocolic reflex arises is unclear but may involve cholecystokinin, gastrin, serotoninergic input, or cholinergic stimuli. However, cholecystokinin antagonists do not block the reflex; also, infusions of high dose cholecystokinin have no effect upon colonic activity although pancreatic exocrine secretion and gallbladder contraction are maximally stimulated.[92] Interestingly, the colonic motor response to eating persists following a gastrectomy or spinal injury; yet, the colon must be in continuity for the reflex to take place.[71]

Stress, both physical and emotional, also influences colonic function. One study found that psychological stress induced a significant increase in propagating contractions, both in their frequency and amplitude, throughout the colon, even in the absence of an appreciable autonomic response.[93] Despite the withdrawal of the stressor, the augmented motor activity endured.[93] In contrast, physical stress, consisting of exposures to extremes of temperature, precipitated a significant elevation in the frequency and amplitude of simultaneous contractions, which ceased immediately after the activity stopped.[93] In some trials, low and high amplitude propagated contractions are stimulated by acute physical exercise.[71,94]

Defecation

The process of defecation involves the entire colon, not solely the anus and rectum. As already described, the majority of colonic activity – the segmental contractions – serve to retain fecal material so as to promote the salvage of intestinal water and electrolytes. However, periodically, colonic activity shifts in order to foster the expulsion of stool. Approximately 1 h prior to the act of defecation, an involuntary preexpulsive phase is initiated, in which the frequency and amplitude of antegrade nonpropagating and, particularly, propagating contractions steadily increase throughout the whole colon.[95] The early component of the preexpulsive phase – the first 15–60 min – is characterized by propagating contractions that initially arise from the proximal colon but subsequently from the distal colon; this initial sequence is thought to transport stool into the distal colon, thus stimulating distal colonic afferent nerves, which in turn provoke further propagating sequences.[9,95] During the late phase, consisting of the last 15 min, the point of origin of these contractions reverses from the distal to the proximal colon.[9,95] Scintigraphic studies reveal that, in one bowel movement, 20% of the ascending colon can be emptied; other evaluations indicate that nearly the entire colon may be evacuated of stool in a single defecatory action.[9,96] A number of investigations identified antegrade high amplitude propagated contractions in close temporal relation to defecation; yet, not all of these contractions necessarily precede or end in defecation.[78,97,98] However, at least one high amplitude propagated contraction of very high amplitude usually coincides with the urge to defecate.[95] While the early activity is unnoticed, the late phase is often associated with the urge to defecate that occurs prior to the voluntary act of fecal evacuation.[95]

Colonic Sensation

Colonic sensation has proved a complicated, poorly understood topic. The normal physiologic processes of the healthy colon are largely unnoticed, with only fullness and an urge to defecate consciously perceptible.[11] The colon itself contains no specialized sensory end organs.[41] However, naked nerve endings lie within the serosa, muscularis propria, and mucosa of the colon while Pacinian corpuscles are found in the mesentery.[9] Afferent nerve fibers reach the central nervous system via parasympathetic pathways and spinal afferent nerves, both of which display mechano- and chemosensitivity.[99] The parasympathetic fibers convey sensory information from the proximal colon via the vagus nerve to cell bodies in the nodose and jugular ganglia and, from the distal colon, by the pelvic splanchnic nerves.[13,41,99] The precise role of the parasympathetic afferent fibers remains unknown but likely involves unconscious reflex sensation, not painful stimuli.[9] Sensory input from the colon is chiefly detected by spinal afferent neurons, primarily by those with their cell bodies within the lumbar dorsal root ganglia.[8,9,99] These lumbar spinal afferent nerves travel with the sympathetic fibers within the lumbar splanchnic nerves from the colon by way of the inferior mesenteric ganglia.[9] The lumbar spinal afferent fibers conclude in sensory endings throughout the entire large intestine, whereby pain, colorectal distention, mesenteric traction, and noxious mucosal stimuli are discerned.[9] In contrast, the sacral spinal afferents, with their cell bodies in the sacral dorsal root ganglia of S2–4, are thought to be concerned with a sensation of rectal fullness and an urge to defecate.[9] These sacral spinal afferent fibers are borne along with the parasympathetic pelvic splanchnic nerves.[8]

Visceral pain sensation is carried by rapidly conducting Aδ fibers or by unmyelinated C fibers.[11] The Aδ fibers are associated with the more localized "discriminative" pain, which persists for as long as the stimulus, and the C fibers in the diffuse "affective-motivational" pain, which continues beyond the duration of the catalyst.[11] Sensory information is transported to the brain along the spinothalamic and spinoreticular tracts as well as by the dorsal column of the spinal cord.[11] The spinothalamic tracts specifically transmit sensation from the Aδ and C fibers to the somatosensory cortex via the lateral thalamic nuclei or to the frontal, parietal, and limbic regions by means of the medial thalamic nuclei, respectively.[11]

The modulation of visceral sensation occurs through several methods. Enteroenteric reflexes mediated by the spinal cord produce variations in the smooth muscle tone, leading to changes in the activation of the nerve endings in the intestine or mesentery.[100] The perception of visceral pain is influenced by descending noradrenergic and serotonergic pathways that emanate from the reticular formation, hypothalamus, and frontal cortex. These fibers project to the dorsal horn of the spinal cord, where they modify noxious input from the visceral afferent nerves.[13] This mechanism likely explains the experience of wounded soldiers who feel no pain in the midst of battle.[101] The intersection of visceral spinal afferent nerves with somatic afferent nerves in the dorsal horn of the spinal cord produces the phenomenon of referred pain, in which visceral sensation is consciously recognized as somatic pain, located in a dermatome of the same embryologic origin as the visceral structure: T8–T12 for the midgut and T12–L2 for the hindgut.[8,13,101] In addition, visceral afferent nerves from the colon relay information via collaterals to the reticular formation and thalamus, which induce alterations in affect, appetite, pulse, and blood pressure through autonomic, hypothalamic, and limbic system connections.[13,102]

Disturbances in Colonic Physiology

Physiology of Constipation

Constipation is a common complaint, with a prevalence of 2–28% among Western populations.[103] This disorder refers to infrequent bowel movements (fewer than three per week); hard or lumpy stools; incomplete evacuation; a sensation of anorectal obstruction; the need for manual maneuvers to facilitate defecation; and/or excessive straining.[104] Individuals with constipation are an incredibly heterogeneous group. Distinct subtypes of constipation exist, each requiring different treatment modalities; however, even within these subtypes, there may be wide variability in the clinical presentation and pathophysiologic etiology. The causes for constipation range from dietary, pharmacologic, structural, to systemic.

Many people become constipated due to dietary and lifestyle neglect. In the USA, fiber intake is overall low. Two primary roles of the colon, solidifying liquid chyme into stool and defecation, are dependent upon adequate dietary fiber: dietary fiber "normalizes" large bowel function.[105,106] In particular, the bulkier stool produced by fiber supplementation stimulates propulsive activity, thus decreasing colonic transit time.[103] The recommendation for adequate fiber intake ranges from 20 to 35 g/day for adults.[107] For an individual on a 1,500–2,000 kcal/day diet, in order to include 15 g of fiber, 11 servings of refined grains and 5 servings of fruits and vegetables must be consumed.[105] Fiber is classified as either soluble or insoluble, acting by differing mechanisms to increase stool weight. Soluble fibers such as oat bran provide rapidly fermentable material to the proximal colon, which allows for sustained bacterial growth.[108] The consequent higher bacterial content of the stool results in the greater fecal mass.[108] In an average bowel movement, 50% of the stool weight consists of bacteria.[103] Also, soluble fibers cause a rise in the excretion of lipid and fat, further boosting stool weight.[108] In contrast, poorly fermentable insoluble fibers such as wheat bran, cellulose, and lignin augment stool weight by providing more undigested plant material for evacuation.[108] One gram of wheat bran generates 2.7 g of stool.[103] Wheat bran also promotes fat excretion, but not to the extent of oat bran.[108] The outcomes of fiber supplementation as a treatment for constipation have yielded conflicting data.

Constipation may be seen more commonly in sedentary individuals. The Nurses Health Study suggested that those women who engaged in daily strenuous activity were 44% less likely to experience constipation than those who exercised less than once a week.[109] During exercise, phasic and propagating motor activity is diminished in the colon, with the effect more pronounced with more vigorous effort; however, after the physical exertion is completed, an increase in the frequency and amplitude of the propagating pressure waves is demonstrated, possibly due to the restoration of parasympathetic input.[68] This postexercise pattern may precipitate the propulsion of feces.[68] During or after exercise, individuals often report an urge to defecate or defecation itself.[109] In fact, abdominal cramps and diarrhea are frequently related by runners.[110,111] However, in a small study of the impact of regular exercise – 1 h a day, 5 days a week – upon chronic idiopathic constipation, there was no symptomatic improvement in the eight subjects after 4 weeks of increased activity.[112] Moreover, a small study examining colonic transit in otherwise sedentary men after mild exercise, consisting of 1 h of walking on a treadmill for 3 days/week, showed no significant difference in the passage of radiopaque markers as compared to baseline.[113]

Idiopathic slow transit constipation involves ineffectual colonic propulsion, resulting in a measurable delay in the movement of fecal material through the colon. The severity of the presentation is variable, with the most intractable cases referred to as colonic inertia. These patients with slow transit constipation, usually women, have fewer than one bowel movement per week, often in association with abdominal pain, a lack of an urge to defecate, malaise, fatigue, or bloating.[103] Little benefit is gained from dietary fiber supplementation, which, conversely, may cause worsened constipation, or from laxatives.[103] The symptoms often arise during puberty and steadily deteriorate over time.[103] Retarded colonic transit in these individuals is either pan-colonic or segmental.[60] Slow transit constipation is consistently affiliated with a blunted colonic motor response to eating (i.e., gastrocolic reflex), including both propulsive and segmental contractions.[60,64,83] In contrast, in patients with colonic inertia, there is *no* colonic response to a meal.[103] A significant decrease in the frequency as well as the amplitude of high amplitude propagated contractions is demonstrated in slow transit constipation, leading to reduced colonic propulsive activity.[41,64,71,114,115] Furthermore, the preexpulsive phase of the defecatory process is depressed.[103] Conflicting results have been obtained from investigations into excessive, disorganized rectosigmoid phasic activity – a "brake" to antegrade propulsion – as a factor in slow transit constipation.[60,64] Histological evaluations reveal a marked decrease in the population of myenteric plexus neurons; however, of the neurons present in the myenteric plexus, those that produce the potent inhibitory neurotransmitter nitric oxide are vastly predominant, especially as compared to controls.[116] Slow transit constipation also features a significant reduction in the interstitial cells of Cajal either throughout the colon or solely in the sigmoid colon.[84,117,118] Moreover, the morphology of the existing cells is seen to be strikingly abnormal, demonstrating few dendrites and an irregular surface.[103] Colonic transit studies of slow transit constipation reveal retention of more than 20% of the radiopaque markers 5 days after their ingestion.[103]

Obstructed Defecation

Obstructed defecation usually results from abnormalities in pelvic as opposed to colonic function. Typically, this disorder is associated with failure of the puborectalis muscle to relax during defecation, producing a functional – not a physical – obstruction.[11] Anatomic abnormalities also causing obstructed defecation include rectocele, enterocele, excessive perineal descent, and rectal intussusception. These patients report inordinate straining, incomplete evacuation, painful defecation, infrequent bowel movements, and digital anal disimpaction.[103] Among the diagnostic tests for obstructed defecation are anorectal manometry or electromyelography, balloon expulsion, barium defecography, and dynamic MRI. A defecogram may identify retention of 50–100% of the instilled barium in the rectum of patients with obstructive defecation.[58] Colonic transit studies in these patients demonstrate collection of six or more radiopaque markers in the distal colon, indicating partial evacuation of the rectum.[58,119] Two-thirds of patients with obstructive defecation may display a concurrent pattern of slow transit constipation.[58]

Obstructed defecation rarely arises from a colonic source – a sigmoidocele. In this variant, a redundant sigmoid colon descends into the rectovaginal pouch (of Douglas) during defecation, impinging upon the rectum during attempted evacuation.[120] In one study of 463 patients with constipation, fecal incontinence, or chronic idiopathic rectal pain, a sigmoidocele was diagnosed on defecography in 5.2%.[120] Defecography is the primary method of diagnosis of a sigmoidocele. The severity of a sigmoidocele is determined by the extent of its decline into the pelvis, as compared to the pubococcygeal and ischiococcygeal lines.[120]

While third degree sigmoidoceles likely benefit from a sigmoid colectomy, the significance and optimal management of first and second degree sigmoidoceles are not fully understood.[120] The clinician should also be cognizant of concomitant pelvic floor disorders in these patients.

Irritable Bowel Syndrome

Irritable bowel syndrome (IBS) is a functional disorder with multiple manifestations: constipation-predominant (IBS-C), diarrhea-predominant (IBS-D), and mixed (IBS-A). Irritable bowel syndrome is characterized by altered bowel habits and chronic, recurring abdominal pain directly related to defecation, in the absence of an anatomic abnormality.[54] Extracolonic complaints include lower back pain, lethargy, nausea, urinary symptoms, dyspareunia, and dysmenorrhea.[121] The etiology of irritable bowel syndrome is unclear but is believed to involve visceral hypersensitivity to intraluminal stimuli.[54] Aberrant motility, inflammation, anomalies in extrinsic autonomic innervation, abnormal brain–gut interaction, and the role of psychosocial factors have also been extensively investigated. Hormonal factors may be involved, as symptoms are often increased perimenstrually; however, the complaints persist even in the absence of menses.[122] The treatment of IBS is based on the nature and severity of symptoms. Education, reassurance, and the elimination of foods that incite the typical complaints are the initial interventions. In some patients, fiber supplementation exacerbates the IBS.[121] For those who do not respond to conservative measures, medication is considered. However, the pharmacologic therapy of IBS-A has not been well studied.

In approximately one-third of patients with irritable bowel syndrome, constipation is the main feature (IBS-C). Women are primarily affected by IBS-C. The majority of these patients demonstrate normal colonic transit and motility patterns, although there is a possible overlap with slow transit constipation.[123] Tegaserod, an agonist of the 5-HT$_4$ receptor that is involved in the metabolism of serotonin, showed promise as a treatment of IBS-C but was withdrawn by the Food and Drug Administration in 2007 due to a high incidence of myocardial infarction, stroke, and unstable angina.[124,125] In some studies, probiotics such as *Lactobacillus* and *Bifidobacterium* produce variable degrees of alleviation of IBS symptoms such as pain.[126] Lubiprostone (Amitiza®, Sucampo Pharmaceuticals, Inc., Bethesda, MD), a prostaglandin E1 analog, activates type 2 chloride channels on the apical membrane of colonic epithelial cells.[127,128] This medication promotes intestinal fluid secretion and, indirectly, colonic motility in patients with IBS-C.[128] Studies of lubiprostone revealed significant improvement in stool frequency and consistency, abdominal discomfort and pain, straining, and bloating.[128] Cholecystokinin, found in elevated levels in the plasma and sigmoid colon of IBS-C patients, has been implicated in the pathogenesis of IBS: infusion of cholecystokinin induces typical symptoms of irritable bowel syndrome.[129,130] However, in a randomized trial, the CCK-1 receptor antagonist dexloxiglumide led to no amelioration in IBS symptomology; moreover, overall colonic transit was unchanged, although emptying of the ascending colon was delayed.[130] However, a pilot study of a similar CCK-1 receptor antagonist, loxiglumide, yielded some improvement in IBS symptoms.[131] A randomized trial of neurotrophin-3, a protein growth factor integral to the development of the enteric nervous system, in constipated patients revealed more frequent spontaneous bowel movements, a more rapid colonic transit time, and a reduction in associated symptoms.[132] Approximately one-third of subjects experienced transient injection site reactions after subcutaneous administration.[132]

Diarrhea-predominant irritable bowel syndrome is encountered in approximately one-third of patients with IBS. The majority of men with irritable bowel syndrome experience the diarrhea-predominant type. This subtype is often affiliated with urgency and fecal incontinence.[121] IBS-D may follow an episode of acute gastroenteritis, pelvic surgery, or emotional stress.[11] Some patients with IBS-D display accelerated proximal colonic transit, with an increased frequency of high and low amplitude propagated contractions.[11,78] Additionally, the colonic motor response to eating is enhanced in a proportion of these patients, resulting in an intense urge to defecate and abdominal pain immediately after meals.[11] Rectal hypersensitivity is also a feature in some of these patients.[11] Antispasmodics such as hyoscine are prescribed for those with abdominal pain and bloating, especially after meals. Low-dose tricyclic antidepressants (e.g., amitriptyline) are added when the pain is more constant and even disabling; these medications function not as mood stabilizers but instead act directly on the gut and central pain processing.[121,124,133] Loperamide is an antidiarrheal agent safe for long-term use.[121] Diarrhea is effectively addressed by selective serotonin 5-HT$_3$ antagonists such as Alosetron. This drug was initially FDA approved in March 2000, only to be retracted due to reports of ischemic colitis, severe constipation, and even death.[134] In June 2002, it was adopted solely for women with chronic, severe IBS-D.[135] However, the medication may only be supplied by physicians participating in the Prometheus Prescribing Program, after the patient signs a patient–physician agreement.[135] Further investigation into these novel pharmaceuticals for IBS is required.

Ogilvie's Syndrome

Ogilvie's syndrome, initially described in 1948, is also known as acute colonic pseudo-obstruction. This disorder is characterized by an imbalance of autonomic innervation to the colon: the inhibitory sympathetic input exceeds that of the excitatory parasympathetic nerves.[136] A massively dilated colon – particularly the proximal colon – results from the consequent suppression of peristaltic activity.[136] The specific source for the initial motor disturbance that allows for this scenario is unknown.[136] One hypothesis ascribes this functional obstruction to impairment of the pelvic (parasympathetic) splanchnic nerves supplying the distal colon, giving rise to an atonic segment, lacking peristaltic function.[136] Acute colonic pseudo-obstruction has been reported concurrent with infectious or inflammatory (e.g., acute pancreatitis), cardiovascular (e.g., myocardial infarction), metabolic (e.g., hypokalemia), postoperative (e.g., spinal or pelvic surgery), posttraumatic, neurologic (e.g., Alzheimer's disease), respiratory (e.g., pneumonia), and neoplastic causes (e.g., metastatic disease); drugs (e.g., antidepressants); and old age.[136] As indicated by the law of LaPlace (wall stress = [(transmural pressure) × (radius)]/ wall thickness), the cecum is at greatest risk of perforation in light of its thin wall and large diameter.[137] Despite symptoms and signs consistent with a large bowel obstruction, no mechanical blockade is present. The management of Ogilvie's syndrome begins with eliminating the presence of a physical obstruction with a water-soluble contrast enema. In the majority of cases, colonic dilatation responds to conservative therapy, including nasogastric decompression, correction of fluid and electrolyte abnormalities, cessation of antimotility medications such as opiates, and remedy of the underlying illness.[138] In the absence of peritoneal signs or a cecal diameter greater than 12 cm on radiographic studies, conservative measures may be continued for 48–72 h. This approach is associated with a 14% mortality rate.[136] The colon may also be mechanically decompressed via colonoscopy, although, in one study, this difficult procedure in an unprepared colon was affiliated with a 1.7% morbidity and a 3.4% mortality rate; yet, colonoscopic decompression was successful in 79.3% of cases, albeit with a recurrence in 20% of patients.[139] Pharmacologic treatment has become the mainstay of management for acute colonic pseudo-obstruction if conservative measures fail. Neostigmine (2–2.5 mg IV over 1–60 min), an acetylcholinesterase inhibitor, provides a surfeit of acetylcholine to the enteric neurons and the neuromuscular junctions, thus inducing propagating contractions, specifically high amplitude propagating contractions, and the prompt evacuation of stool and flatus.[62,138,140] In a double-blind randomized trial, the initial clinical response to neostigmine was 91%, as compared to 0% among those receiving a placebo; colonic distention recurred in two patients (18%) given neostigmine, ultimately requiring a subtotal colectomy in one patient.[138] Administration of neostigmine may produce bradycardia, abdominal pain, vomiting, and excessive salivation.[138] Alternative, less-studied pharmacologic treatments are comprised of 5-HT_4 receptor agonists (e.g., cisapride), motilin receptor agonists (e.g., erythromycin), muscarinic receptor agonists (e.g., bethanechol), neurotrophins (e.g., NT-3), nitric oxide synthase inhibitors (e.g., nitro-L-arginine methyl ester), and somatostatin analogs (e.g., octreotide).[136] Surgical treatment – a cecostomy tube or a subtotal colectomy – is a final option if less invasive techniques are unsuccessful. Even in a nonemergent setting, surgery has a 30% mortality rate.[136] However, failure to decompress the colon may yield cecal ischemia and/or perforation in 14–40% of cases; the mortality of these patients increases to 40–50%.[136]

Implications of Colonic Physiology for the Surgeon

Why is an understanding of colonic physiology important for the surgeon? Knowledge of the embryologic development of the colon is essential when considering nerve preservation, vascular supply, and resection margins during colectomies. The poorly understood topic of colonic motility impacts surgeons, particularly in the phenomenon of postoperative ileus. In a murine model of postoperative ileus, a reduction in the number of interstitial cells of Cajal was evident on both sides of the colonic anastomosis within hours of the surgery; as a consequence, fewer slow waves were identified in that particular segment, possibly giving rise to postoperative ileus.[88] Various disorders of colonic motility may stem from abnormalities of the interstitial cells of Cajal. These cells are significantly depleted in the colons of patients with diverticulosis and with slow transit constipation.[141] As basic science research advances, the surgeon ultimately will be called upon to evaluate and apply novel pharmaceuticals to reduce the impact of postoperative ileus as well as to treat other disorders of colonic motility. Surgeons also will invariably be consulted to assess the suitability of surgical management for abnormalities of colonic motility such as colonic inertia and intractable constipation.

The resection of a portion or the entirety of the colon can have profound functional ramifications for the patient. Prior to a colectomy, the surgeon optimally should discuss these possible outcomes with the patient. Postoperatively, the physiologic consequences of a colectomy must be managed. For instance, a patient with a new ileostomy requires counseling regarding adequate fluid and salt intake to compensate for the loss of the colon. Furthermore, defecatory dysfunction – frequent bowel movements, urgency, or soiling – may occur after a low anterior resection. Subsequent to the procedure, injury of the parasympathetic pelvic splanchnic nerves due to dissection around the inferior mesenteric artery may produce a denervated colonic segment with an increased colonic transit time and a greater proportion of nonpropagating contractions.[142] The neorectum demonstrates a decline in compliance postoperatively, although the maximum tolerated volume returns to normal 6 months later.[143] Yet, the volume needed to elicit the recto-anal inhibitory reflex is persistently reduced even 1 year after surgery.[143]

Conclusion

The colon has proven an enigmatic organ. Its major roles – the salvage of intestinal water and electrolytes, the storage of fecal material, and the production of short-chain fatty acids – seem unambiguous. However, the mechanisms underlying its physiologic and pathophysiologic processes remain difficult to define. Although not essential for life, its normal function is integral to our well-being.

References

1. Larsen WJ. Development of the gastrointestinal tract. human embryology. New York: Churchill Livingstone; 1993. p. 205–34.
2. Sadler T. Langman's medical embryology. 10th ed. Philadelphia: Lippicott Williams & Wilkins; 2006.
3. Moore KL, Persaud TVN. The developing human: clinically oriented embryology. 7th ed. Philadelphia: Saunders; 2003.
4. Pokorny WJ, Rothenberg SS, Brandt ML. Growth and development. In: O'Leary JP, Capote LR, editors. The physiologic basis of surgery. 2nd ed. Philadelphia: Lippincott Williams & Wilkins; 1996. p. 61–6.
5. Wexner SD, Jorge JMN. Anatomy and embryology of the anus, rectum, and colon. In: Corman ML, editor. Colon and rectal surgery. 5th ed. Philadelphia: Lippincott Williams & Wilkins; 2005. p. 1–29.
6. Langmen J. Digestive system. In: Langmen J, editor. Medical embryology. 4th ed. Baltimore: Lippincott Williams & Wilkins; 1982. p. 212–33.
7. Cobb RA, Williamson RCN. Embryology and developmental abnormalities of the large intestine. In: Phillips SF, Pemberton JH, Shorter RG, editors. The large intestine: physiology, pathophysiology, and disease. New York: Raven Press; 1991. p. 3–12.
8. Moore KL, Dalley AF, Agur AMR. Clinically oriented anatomy. 6th ed. Philadelphia: Wolters Kluwer; 2010.
9. Cook IJ, Brookes SJ. Colonic motor and sensory function and dysfunction. In: Sleisenger & Fordtran's gastrointestinal and liver disease: pathophysiology, disease, management. 8th ed. Philadelphia: Saunders Elsevier; 2006.
10. Church JM, Raudkivi PJ, Hill GL. The surgical anatomy of the rectum – a review with particular relevance to the hazards of rectal mobilisation. Int J Colorectal Dis. 1987;2:158–66.
11. Bharucha AE, Camilleri M. Physiology of the colon and its measurement. In: Peters JH, Pemberton JH, Yeo CJ, Dempsey DT, Klein AS, editors. Shackelford's surgery of the alimentary tract. Philadelphia: Saunders; 2007.
12. Woodburne RT. The abdomen. In: Woodburne RT, editor. Essentials of human anatomy. 6th ed. New York: Oxford University Press; 1978. p. 363–464.
13. Camilleri M, Ford MJ. Review article: colonic sensorimotor physiology in health, and its alteration in constipation and diarrhoeal disorders. Aliment Pharmacol Ther. 1998;12:287–302.
14. Gillis RA, Dias Souza J, Hicks KA, et al. Inhibitory control of proximal colonic motility by the sympathetic nervous system. Am J Physiol. 1987;253:G531–9.
15. Bharucha AE, Camilleri M, Zinsmeister AR, Hanson RB. Adrenergic modulation of human colonic motor and sensory function. Am J Physiol. 1997;273:G997–1006.
16. Manara L, Croci T, Aureggi G, et al. Functional assessment of B adrenoceptor subtypes in human colonic circular and longitudinal (taenia coli) smooth muscle. Gut. 2000;47:337–42.
17. Anderson JE. Grant's atlas of anatomy. 7th ed. Baltimore: Lippincott Williams & Wilkins; 1978.
18. Hollinshead W, Rosse C. Textbook of anatomy. 4th ed. Philadelphia: Harper & Row; 1985.
19. Nivatvongs S, Gordon PH. Surgical anatomy. In: Gordon PH, Nivatvongs S, editors. Principles and practice of surgery for the colon, rectum, and anus. St. Louis: Quality Medical Publishing; 1992. p. 3–37.
20. Harrell LE, Chang EB. Intestinal water and electrolyte transport. In: Sleisenger & Fordtran's gastrointestinal and liver disease: pathophysiology, disease, management. 8th ed. Philadelphia: Saunders Elsevier; 2006.
21. Tack J, Vanden Berghe P. Neuropeptides and colonic motility: it's all in the little brain. Gastroenterology. 2000;119:257–60.
22. Mitolo-Chieppa D, Mansi G, Rinaldi R, et al. Cholinergic stimulation and nonadrenergic, noncholinergic relaxation of human colonic circular muscle in idiopathic chronic constipation. Dig Dis Sci. 1998;43:2719–26.
23. Rombeau JL. Rethinking the human colon: a dynamic metabolic organ. Contemp Surg. 2003;59:450–2.
24. Christl SU, Scheppach W. Metabolic consequences of total colectomy. Scand J Gastroenterol. 1997;32 Suppl 222:20–4.
25. Nordgaard I. Colon as a digestive organ: the importance of colonic support for energy absorption as small bowel failure proceeds. Dan Med Bull. 1998;45:135–56.
26. Tazoe H, Otomo Y, Kaji I, Tanaka R, Karaki S-I, Kuwahara A. Roles of short-chain fatty acids receptors, GPR41 and GPR43 on colonic functions. J Physiol Pharmacol. 2008;59 Suppl 2:251–62.
27. Hamer HM, Jonkers D, Venema K, Vanhoutvin S, Troost FJ, Brummer RJ. Review article: the role of butyrate on colonic function. Aliment Pharmacol Ther. 2008;27:104–19.
28. Flint HJ, Duncan SH, Scott KP, Louis P. Interactions and competition within the microbial community of the human colon: links between diet and health. Environ Microbiol. 2007;9:1101–11.
29. Schouten WR, Gordon PH. Physiology. In: Gordon PH, Nivatvongs S, editors. Principles and practice of surgery for the colon, rectum, and anus. St. Louis: Quality Medical Publishing; 1992. p. 39–79.
30. Sandle GI. Salt and water absorption in the human colon: a modern appraisal. Gut. 1998;43:294–9.
31. Priebe MG, Vonk RJ, Sun X, He T, Harmsen HJM, Welling GW. The physiology of colonic metabolism. Possibilities for interventions with pre- and probiotics. Eur J Nutr. 2002;41(Suppl):1101–8.
32. Topping DL. Short-chain fatty acids and human colonic function: roles of resistant starch and nonstarch polysaccharides. Physiol Rev. 2001;81:1031–64.
33. Hoyles L, Vulevic J. Diet, immunity and functional foods. In: Huffnagle GB, Noverr MC, editors. GI microbiota and regulation of the immune system. Austin: Landes Bioscience and Springer; 2008. p. 79–92.
34. Bengmark S. Colonic food: pre- and probiotics. Am J Gastroenterol. 2000;95(Suppl):S5–7.
35. Mortensen PB, Clausen MR. Short-chain fatty acids in the human colon: relation to gastrointestinal health and disease. Scand J Gastroenterol. 1996;216(Suppl):132–48.

36. Gibson GR, Roberfroid MB. Dietary modulation of the human colonic microbiota: introducing the concept of prebiotics. J Nutr. 1995;125:1401–12.
37. Fuller R. Probiotics in man and animals. J Appl Bacteriol. 1989;66:365–78.
38. Bengmark S. Pre-, pro- and synbiotics. Curr Opin Clin Nutr Metab Care. 2001;4:571–9.
39. Jouet P, Coffin B, Lemann M, et al. Tonic and phasic motor activity in the proximal and distal colon of healthy humans. Am J Physiol. 1998;274:G459–64.
40. Proano M, Camilleri M, Phillips SF, Brown ML, Thomforde GM. Transit of solids through the human colon: regional quantification in the unprepared bowel. Am J Physiol. 1990; 258:G856–62.
41. O'Brien MD, Phillips SF. Colonic motility in health and disease. Gastroenterol Clin North Am. 1996;25:147–62.
42. Kamath PS, Phillips SF, O'Connor MK, Brown ML, Zinsmeister AR. Colonic capacitance and transit in man: modulation by luminal contents and drugs. Gut. 1990;31:443–9.
43. Phillips SF. Functions of the large bowel: an overview. Scand J Gastroenterol. 1984;93(Suppl):1–12.
44. Devroede GJ, Phillips SF, Code CF, Lund JF. Regional differences in rates of insorption of sodium and water from the human large intestine. Can J Physiol Pharmacol. 1971; 49:1023–9.
45. Fich A, Steadman CJ, Phillips SF, et al. Ileocolic transit does not change after right hemicolectomy. Gastroenterology. 1992;103:794–9.
46. Cooke HJ. Regulation of colonic transport by the autonomic nervous system. In: Phillips SF, Pemberton JH, Shorter RG, editors. The large intestine: physiology, pathophysiology, and disease. New York: Raven Press; 1991. p. 169–79.
47. Hammer J, Phillips SF. Fluid loading of the human colon: effects of segmental transit and stool composition. Gastroenterology. 1993;7:543–51.
48. Phillips SF, Giller J. The contribution of the colon to electrolyte and water conservation in man. J Lab Clin Med. 1973;81:733–46.
49. Debongnie JC, Phillips SF. Capacity of the human colon to absorb fluid. Gastroenterology. 1978;74:698–703.
50. Binder HJ, Sandle GI, Rajendran VM. Colonic fluid and electrolyte transport in health and disease. In: Phillips SF, Pemberton JH, Shorter RG, editors. The large intestine: physiology, pathophysiology, and disease. New York: Raven Press; 1991. p. 141–68.
51. Giller J, Phillips SF. Electrolyte absorption and secretion in the human colon. Am J Dig Dis. 1972;17:1003–11.
52. Binder HJ, Sandle GI. Electrolyte absorption and secretion in mammalian colon. In: Johnson LR, editor. Physiology of the gastrointestinal tract. 2nd ed. New York: Raven Press; 1987. p. 1398–418.
53. Devroede G. Dietary fiber, bowel habits, and colonic function. Am J Clin Nutr. 1978;10 Suppl 31:157–60.
54. Keller J, Layer P. Intestinal and anorectal motility and functional disorders. Best Pract Res Clin Gastroenterol. 2009;23:407–23.
55. Keighley MRB, Williams NS. Anatomy and physiology investigations. In: Keighley MRB, Williams NS, editors. Surgery of the anus, rectum, and colon. 2nd ed. London: WB Saunders; 1999. p. 1–48.
56. Hinton JM, Lennard-Jones JE, Young AC. A new method for studying gut transit times using radiopaque markers. Gut. 1969;10:842–7.
57. Metcalf AM, Phillips SF, Zinsmeister AR, MacCarty RL, Beart RW, Wolff BG. Simplified assessment of segmental colonic transit. Gastroenterology. 1987;92:40–7.
58. Rao SSC. Constipation: evaluation and treatment of colonic and anorectal motility disorders. Gastroenterol Clin North Am. 2007;36:687–711.
59. Rao SSO, Kuo B, McCallum RW, et al. Investigation of colonic and whole-gut transit with wireless motility capsule and radiopaque markers in constipation. Clin Gastroenterol Hepatol. 2009;7:537–44.
60. Bharucha AE. Constipation. Best Pract Res Clin Gastroenterol. 2007;21:709–31.
61. Scott SM, Knowles CH, Newell M, Garvie N, Williams NS, Lunniss PJ. Scintigraphic assessment of colonic transit in women with slow-transit constipation arising de novo following pelvic surgery or childbirth. Br J Surg. 2001;88:405–11.
62. Camilleri M, Bharucha AE, Di Lorenzo C, et al. American Neurogastroenterology and Motility Society consensus statement on intraluminal measurement of gastrointestinal and colonic motility in clinical practice. Neurogastroenterol Motil. 2008;20:1269–82.
63. Lemann M, Flourie B, Picon L, et al. Motor activity recorded in the unprepared colon of healthy humans. Gut. 1995;37:649–53.
64. Rao SSC, Sadeghi P, Beaty J, Kavlock R. Ambulatory 24-hour colonic manometry in slow-transit constipation. Am J Gastroenterol. 2004;99:2405–16.
65. Rao SSC, Sadeghi P, Beaty J, Kavlock R, Ackerson K. Ambulatory 24-h colonic manometry in healthy humans. Am J Physiol Gastrointest Liver Physiol. 2001;280:G629–39.
66. Bassotti G, Chistolini F, Sietchiping-Nzepa F, Morelli A. Intestinal manometry: value and limitations. Diabetes Nutr Metab. 2004;17:33–7.
67. Bassotti G, Gaburri M. Manometric investigation of high-amplitude propagating contractive activity of human colon. Am J Physiol Gastrointest Liver Physiol. 1988;255:G660–4.
68. Rao SSC, Beaty J, Chamberlain M, Lambert P, Gisolfi C. Effects of acute graded exercise on human colonic motility. Am J Physiol Gastrointest Liver Physiol. 1999;276:G1221–6.
69. Narducci F, Bassotti G, Gaburri M, Morelli A. Twenty-four hour manometric recordings of colonic motor activity in healthy man. Gut. 1987;28:17–25.
70. Sasaki Y, Hada R, Nakajima H, et al. Difficulty in estimating localized bowel contraction by colonic manometry: A simultaneous recording of intraluminal pressure and luminal calibre. Neurogastroenterol Motil. 1996;8:247–53.
71. Bassotti G, Iantorno G, Fiorella S, Bustos-Fernandez L, Bilder C. Colonic motility in man: features in normal subjects and in patients with chronic idiopathic constipation. Am J Gastroenterol. 1999;94:1760–70.
72. Steadman CJ, Phillips SF, Camilleri M, et al. Variation of muscle tone in the human colon. Gastroenterology. 1991;101:373–81.
73. Steadman CJ, Phillips SF, Camilleri M, et al. Control of muscle tone in the human colon. Gut. 1992;33:541–6.
74. Sarna SK, Otterson MF. Myoelectric and contractile activities. In: Schuster MM, editor. Atlas of gastrointestinal motility in health and disease. Baltimore: Lippincott Williams & Wilkins; 1993. p. 3–42.

75. Dapoigny M, Trolese J-F, Bommelaer G, et al. Myoelectric spiking activity of right colon, left colon, and rectosigmoid of healthy humans. Dig Dis Sci. 1988;33:1007–12.
76. Brading AF, Ramalingam T. Mechanisms controlling normal defecation and the potential effects of spinal cord injury. Prog Brain Res. 2006;152:345–58.
77. Smith TK, Spencer NJ, Hennig GW, Dickson EJ. Recent advances in enteric neurobiology: mechanosensitive interneurons. Neurogastroenterol Motil. 2007;19:869–78.
78. Bassotti G, Germani U, Morelli A. Human colonic motility: physiological aspects. Int J Colorectal Dis. 1995;10:173–80.
79. Garcia D, Hita G, Mompean B, et al. Colonic motility: electric and manometric description of mass movement. Dis Colon Rectum. 1991;34:577–84.
80. Crowell MD, Bassotti G, Cheskin LJ, Schuster MM, Whitehead WE. Method for prolonged ambulatory monitoring of high-amplitude propagated contractions from colon. Am J Physiol. 1991;261:G263–8.
81. Bassotti G, Betti C, Fusaro C, Morelli A. Colonic high-amplitude propagated contractions (mass movements): repeated 24-h studies in healthy volunteers. J Gastrointest Motil. 1992;4:187–91.
82. Bassotti G, Clementi M, Antonelli E, Peli MA, Tonini M. Low-amplitude propagated contractile waves: a relevant propulsive mechanism of human colon. Dig Liver Dis. 2001;33:36–40.
83. Bassotti G, de Roberto G, Castellani D, Sediari L, Morelli A. Normal aspects of colorectal motility and abnormalities in slow transit constipation. World J Gastroenterol. 2005;11:2691–6.
84. Lyford GL, He CL, Soffer E, et al. Pan-colonic decrease in interstitial cells of Cajal in patients with slow transit constipation. Gut. 2002;51:496–501.
85. Sanders KM, Stevens R, Burke EP, Ward SM. Slow waves actively propagate at submucosal surface of circular layer in canine colon. Am J Physiol. 1990;259:G258–63.
86. Camborova P, Hubka P, Sulkova I, Hulin I. The pacemaker activity of interstitial cells of Cajal and gastric electrical activity. Physiol Res. 2003;52:275–84.
87. Takaki M. Gut pacemaker cells: the Interstitial Cells of Cajal (ICC). J Smooth Muscle Res. 2003;39:137–61.
88. Sanders K. Interstitial cells of Cajal at the clinical and scientific interface. J Physiol. 2006;576(3):683–7.
89. Rae MG, Fleming N, McGregor DB, et al. Control of motility patterns in the human colonic circular muscle layer by pacemaker activity. J Physiol. 1998;510:309–20.
90. Roarty TP, Suratt PM, Hellmann P, McCallum RW. Colonic motor activity in women during sleep. Sleep. 1998;21:285–8.
91. Duthie H-L. Colonic response to eating. Gastroenterology. 1978;75:527–9.
92. Niederau C, Faber S, Karaus M. Cholecystokinin's role in regulation of colonic motility in health and in irritable bowel syndrome. Gastroenterology. 1992;102:1889–98.
93. Rao SSC, Hatfield RA, Suls JM, Chamberlain MJ. Psychological and physical stress induce differential effects on human colonic motility. Am J Gastroenterol. 1998;93:985–90.
94. Cheskin LJ, Crowell MD, Kamal D, et al. The effects of acute exercise on colonic motility. J Gastrointest Motil. 1992;4:173–7.
95. Bampton PA, Kinning PG, Kennedy ML, Lubowski DZ, deCarle D, Cook IJ. Spatial and temporal organization of pressure patterns throughout the unprepared colon during spontaneous defecation. Am J Gastroenterol. 2000;95:1027–35.
96. Lubowski DZ, Meagher AP, Smart RC, Butler SP. Scintigraphic assessment of colonic function during defecation. Int J Colorectal Dis. 1995;10:91–3.
97. Hardcastle JD, Mann CV. Study of large bowel peristalsis. Gut. 1968;9:512–20.
98. Hardcastle JD, Mann CV. Physical factors in the stimulation of colonic peristalsis. Gut. 1970;11:41–6.
99. Blackshaw LA, Brookes SJH, Grundy D, Schemann M. Sensory transmission in the gastrointestinal tract. Neurogastroenterol Motil. 2007;19(Suppl):1–19.
100. Parkman HP, Ma RC, Stapelfeldt WH, Szurszewski JH. Direct and indirect mechanosensory pathways from the colon to the inferior mesenteric ganglion. Am J Physiol. 1993;265: G499–505.
101. Ganong WF. Cutaneous, deep, and visceral sensation. In: Ganong WF, editor. Review of medical physiology. 10th ed. Los Altos: Lange Medical Publishers; 1981. p. 97–106.
102. Ganong WF. The reticular activating system, sleep, and the electrical activity of the brain. In: Ganong WF, editor. Review of medical physiology. Los Altos: Lange Medical Publishers; 1981. p. 144–53.
103. Patel SM, Lembo AJ. Constipation. In: Feldman M, Freidman LS, Brandt LJ, editors. Sleisenger & Fordtran's gastrointestinal and liver disease: pathophysiology/diagnosis/management. 6th ed. Philadelphia: Saunders Elsevier; 2006.
104. McCullum IJD, Ong S, Mercer-Jones M. Chronic constipation in adults. BMJ. 2009;338:763–6.
105. Haack VS, Chesters JG, Vollendorf NW, Story JA, Marlett JA. Increasing amounts of dietary fiber provided by food normalizes physiologic response of the large bowel without altering calcium balance or fecal steroid excretion. Am J Clin Nutr. 1998;1998:615–22.
106. Harvey RF, Pamare EW, Heaton KW. Effects of increased dietary fibre on intestinal transit time. Lancet. 1973;1: 1278–80.
107. Pilch SM. Physiological effects and health consequences of dietary fiber. Bethesda: Life Sciences Research Office, Federation of American Societies for Experimental Biology; 1987.
108. Chen HL, Haack VS, Janecky CW, Vollendorf NW, Marlett JA. Mechanisms by which wheat bran and oat bran increase stool weight in humans. Am J Clin Nutr. 1998;68:711–9.
109. Dukas L, Willett WC, Giovannucci EL. Association between physical activity, fiber intake, and other lifestyle variables and constipation in a study of women. Am J Gastroenterol. 2003;98:1790–6.
110. Moses FM. Effect of moderate exercise on the gastrointestinal tract. Sports Med. 1990;9:159–72.
111. Riddoch C, Trinick T. Prevalence of running-induced gastrointestinal (GI) disturbances in marathon runner. Br J Sports Med. 1998;22:71–4.
112. Meshkinpour H, Selod S, Movahedi H, et al. Effects of regular exercise in management of chronic idiopathic constipation. Dig Dis Sci. 1998;43:2379–83.
113. Robertson G, Meshkinpour H, Vandenberg K, James N, Cohen A, Wilson A. Effects of exercise on total and segmental colon transit. J Clin Gastroenterol. 1993;16:300–3.
114. Krevsky B, Maurer AH, Fisher RS. Patterns of colonic transit in chronic idiopathic constipation. Am J Gastroenterol. 1989;84:127–32.

115. Hutchinson R, Notghi A, Harding LK, et al. Scintigraphic measurement of ileocecal transit in irritable bowel syndrome and chronic idiopathic constipation. Gut. 1995;36:585–9.
116. Cortesini C, Cianchi F, Infantino A, Lisa M. Nitric oxide synthase and VIP distribution in enteric nervous system in idiopathic chronic constipation. Dig Dis Sci. 1995;40:2450–5.
117. Wedel T, Spiegler J, Soellner S, et al. Enteric nerves and interstitial cells of Cajal are altered in patients with slow-transit constipation and megacolon. Gastroenterology. 2002;2002:1459–67.
118. Yu CS, Kim HC, Hong HK, et al. Evaluation of myenteric ganglion cells and interstitial cells of Cajal in patients with chronic idiopathic constipation. Int J Colorectal Dis. 2002;17:253–8.
119. Kuijpers HJ, Bleijenberg G, deMorree H. The spastic pelvic floor syndrome. Large bowel outlet obstructions caused by pelvic floor dysfunction: a radiological study. Int J Colorectal Dis. 1986;1:44–8.
120. Jorge JMN, Yung-Kang Y, Wexner SD. Incidence and clinical significance of sigmoidoceles as determined by a new classification system. Dis Colon Rectum. 1994;37:1112–7.
121. Shekhar C, Whorwell PJ. Tailor treatment to the patient in irritable bowel syndrome. Practitioner. 2008;252:23–9.
122. Agrawal A, Whorwell PJ. Review article: abdominal bloating and distention in functional gastrointestinal disorders – epidemiology and exploration of possible mechanisms. Aliment Pharmacol Ther. 2007;27:200–10.
123. Pemberton JH, Rath DM, Ilstrup DM. Evaluation and surgical treatment of severe chronic constipation. Ann Surg. 1991;214:403–11.
124. Drossman DA, Camilleri M, Mayer EA, Whitehead WE. AGA technical review on irritable bowel syndrome. Gastroenterology. 2002;123:2108–31.
125. Zelnorm (tegaserod maleate) Information. US Food and Drug Administration; 2009.
126. Eddins C, Gray M. Do probiotic or synbiotic preparations alleviate symptoms associated with constipation or irritable bowel syndrome? J Wound Ostomy Continence Nurs. 2007;34:615–24.
127. Lacy BE, Chey WD. Lubiprostone: chronic constipation and irritable bowel syndrome with constipation. Expert Opin Pharmacother. 2009;10:143–52.
128. Crowell MD. IBS: Lubiprostone: trials and tribulations. Nat Rev Gastroenterol Hepatol. 2009;6:259–60.
129. Zhang H, Yan Y, Shi R, Lin Z, Wang M, Lin L. Correlation of gut hormones with irritable bowel syndrome. Digestion. 2008;78:72–6.
130. Cremonini F, Camilleri M, McKinzie S, et al. Effect of CCK-1 antagonist, dexloxiglumide, in female patients with irritable bowel syndrome: a pharmacodynamic and pharmacogenomic study. Am J Gastroenterol. 2005;100:652–63.
131. Cann PA, Rovati LC, Smart HL, Spiller RC, Whorwell PJ. Loxiglumide, a CCK-A antagonist, in irritable bowel syndrome. A pilot multicenter clinical study. Ann NY Acad Sci. 1994;713:449–50.
132. Parkman HP, Rao SS, Reynolds JC, et al. Neurotrophin-3 improves functional constipation. Am J Gastroenterol. 2003;98:1338–47.
133. Jackson JL, O'Malley PG, Tomkins G, Balden E, Santoro J, Kroenke K. Treatment of functional gastrointestinal disorders with antidepressant medications: a meta-analysis. Am J Med. 2000;108:65–72.
134. Lotronex (alosetron hydrochloride) Tablets. 2008. http://www.accessdata.fda.gov/drugsatfda_docs/label/2008/021107s013lbl.pdf. Accessed 31 Oct 2009.
135. Medication Guide. http://www.fda.gov/downloads/Drugs/DrugSafety/ucm088624.pdf. Accessed 31 Oct 2009.
136. De Giorgio R, Barbara G, Stanghellini V, et al. Review article: the pharmacological treatment of acute colonic pseudo-obstruction. Aliment Pharmacol Ther. 2001;15:1717–27.
137. Murphy RA. Muscle. In: Berne RM, Levy MN, editors. Physiology. 3rd ed. St. Louis: Mosby Year Book; 1993. p. 281–324.
138. Ponec RJ, Saunders MD, Kimmey MB. Neostigmine for the treatment of acute colonic pseudo-obstruction. N Engl J Med. 1999;341:137–41.
139. Wegener M, Borsch G. Acute colonic pseudo-obstruction (Ogilvie's syndrome): Presentation of 14 of our own cases and analysis of 1027 cases reported in the literature. Surg Endosc. 1987;1:179–84.
140. Trevisani GT, Hyman NH, Church JM. Neostigmine: safe and effective treatment for acute colonic pseudo-obstruction. Dis Colon Rectum. 2000;43:599–603.
141. Bassotti G, Battaglia E, Bellone G, et al. Interstitial cells of Cajal, enteric nerves, and glial cells in colonic diverticular disease. J Clin Pathol. 2005;58:973–7.
142. Koda K, Saito N, Seike K, et al. Denervation of the neorectum as a potential cause of defecatory disorder following low anterior resection for rectal cancer. Dis Colon Rectum. 2005;48:210–7.
143. Williamson ME, Lewis WG, Finan PJ, et al. Recovery of physiologic and clinical function after low anterior resection of the rectum for carcinoma: Myth or reality? Dis Colon Rectum. 1995;1995:411–8.

3 Anorectal Physiology

Richard E. Karulf

Normal bowel continence and evacuation are complex processes that involve the coordinated interaction between multiple different neuronal pathways and the pelvic and perineal musculature.[1] The importance of the anatomic relationships of the pelvic floor in maintaining normal continence has been suggested since the 1950s.[2] However, the complex series of neural and behavioral-mediated interactions, combined with a lack of an ideal study to take all elements into account, makes complete understanding of anorectal anatomy and physiology's role in preserving continence difficult.[3] Complicating this are multiple other factors that play a role in normal regulation such as systemic disease, sphincter integrity, bowel motility, stool consistency, evacuation efficiency, pelvic floor stability, cognitive and emotional affects.[4]

The anus and rectum have been observed, dissected, measured, and recorded in every imaginable condition to try to explain their unique ability to voluntarily withhold and evacuate both solid stool and flatus. Conventional anorectal physiology testing using techniques such as manometry, endoanal ultrasound, electrophysiologic studies, and defecography help to elucidate anorectal structures and function. However, diagnostic dilemmas occur when patients report normal function with grossly abnormal test results or abnormal function with a normal test profile. Physicians with an in-depth knowledge of normal and abnormal anorectal physiology can apply results in a meaningful way to diagnose and direct therapy while searching for other, currently unmeasured, factors. This chapter reviews the current knowledge regarding muscular, neurologic, and mechanical factors.

Muscles of the Pelvic Floor and Sphincter Complex

Control of stool can be thought of as a pressure vector diagram, with continence represented as a balance of propulsive and resistive forces. Contraction of the muscles of the pelvic floor and sphincter complex provides resistance and tone is noted during periods of rest or deep sleep. Voluntary contraction of the puborectalis and external sphincter increase resistance and defers defecation. The anal sphincter is not a paired muscle structure, like the biceps and triceps in the arm; there is no extensor ani muscle. Evacuation occurs when propulsive forces (increased intra-abdominal pressure and peristalsis of the colon and rectum) overcome the resistance of the pelvic floor and sphincter muscles. Simple skeletal or smooth muscles alone cannot perform these functions.

The pelvic floor consists of a striated muscular sheet through which viscera pass. This striated muscle, the paired levator ani muscles, is actually subdivided into four muscles defined by the area of attachment on the pubic bone. The attachments span from the pubic bone, along the arcus tendineus (a condensation of the obturator fascia), to the ischial spine. The components of the levator ani are therefore named the pubococcygeus, ileococcygeus, and ischiococcygeus. The pubococcygeus is further subdivided to include the puborectalis. Between the urogenital viscera and the anal canal lies the perineal body. The perineal body consists of the superficial and deep transverse perinei muscles and the ventral extension of the external sphincter muscle to a tendinous intersection with the bulbocavernosus muscle.[5]

The fourth sacral nerve innervates the levator ani muscles. Controversy continues regarding the innervation and origin of the puborectalis muscle. Cadaver studies differ from in vivo stimulation studies as to whether the puborectalis muscle receives innervation only from the sacral nerve or also from the pudendal nerve. Comparative anatomy and histological studies of fiber typing also support the inclusion of the puborectalis muscle with the sphincter complex and not as a pelvic floor muscle. In addition, electromyography (EMG) studies of the external anal sphincter (EAS) and puborectalis muscle indicate that the muscles function together with cough and strain.[6]

The rectal smooth muscle consists of an outer muscularis mucosa, inner circular muscle, and the outer longitudinal layer. The inner circular muscle forms the valves of Houston proximally and distally extends down into the anal

D.E. Beck et al. (eds.), *The ASCRS Textbook of Colon and Rectal Surgery: Second Edition*,
DOI 10.1007/978-1-4419-1584-9_3, © Springer Science+Business Media, LLC 2011

canal becoming the internal anal sphincter (IAS). This is not a simple extension of muscle as there are histologic differences between the upper circular muscle and the IAS. For instance, the IAS is thicker than the circular muscle due to an increased number of smaller muscle cells. The outer longitudinal layer surrounds the sigmoid colon coalescing proximally into thicker bands called taenia coli. This same layer continues down to the anorectal junction where it forms the conjoined longitudinal muscle along with fibers from the pubococcygeus muscle. Distally, this muscle lies in the intersphincteric plane and fibers may fan out and cross both the internal and EAS muscles. In an ultrasound view of the anal canal, the longitudinal muscle is seen as a narrow hyperechoic line in the intersphincteric space.

The puborectalis muscle, EAS, and IAS muscles are easily viewed with endoanal ultrasound. In the hands of an experienced ultrasonographer, the technique is highly sensitive and specific in identifying internal and external sphincter defects.

External Anal Sphincter

Anatomical and sonographic studies indicate that the EAS begins development, along with the puborectalis muscle, at 9–10 weeks gestation. At 28–30 weeks it is mature and the anal sphincter then consists of three components, the striated puborectalis muscle, the smooth IAS muscle, and the smooth and striated EAS muscle.[7] Further differentiation of the EAS into two or three components is highly debated. In 1715, Cowper described it as a single muscle. Later, Milligan and Morgan promoted the naming of the components as subcutaneous, superficial, and deep. Recently, Dalley makes a convincing point that the three components can only be seen in the exceptionally dissected specimen and, in most cases, the muscle is one continuous mass and should be considered as such.[8]

The EAS is innervated bilaterally by the pudendal nerve arising from S2 to S4. Motorneurons arise in the dorsomedial and ventromedial divisions of Onuf's nucleus in the ventral horn of the spinal cord. Cross-over of the pudendal innervation was first suggested in studies by Swash and Henry on rhesus monkeys.[9] Hamdy and associates evaluated corticoanal stimulation of humans and found variable cross-over which was symmetric in some and either right- or left-sided dominant in others.[10] This has been offered as one possible explanation for the inconsistent relationship between unilateral pudendal neuropathy and fecal incontinence.

The EAS maintains tonic activity at rest due to monosynaptic spinal reflex. The tone can be abolished with spinal anesthesia and in conditions such as tabes dorsalis, where large-diameter afferent sensory fibers are destroyed, and over distension of the rectum, due to the inflation response. Maximum tone, due to phasic activity in the EAS, can be maintained for only about 1 min, before fatigue is encountered. Of interest, the only other striated muscles that maintain continuous low-level resting activity are the abductor of the larynx, the cricopharyngeus and the external urinary sphincter.[11]

Internal Anal Sphincter

The IAS is an involuntary, smooth muscle. It is the major source of anal resting pressure and is relatively hypoganglionic.[12] There are nerve fibers expected in an autonomic muscle – cholinergic, adrenergic, and nonadrenergic noncholinergic fibers. It receives sympathetic innervation via the hypogastric and pelvic plexus. Parasympathetic innervation is from S1, S2, and S3 via the pelvic plexus. There is considerable evidence that the sympathetic innervation is excitatory but conflicting information regarding the parasympathetic effect.[12] The IAS contributes 55% to the anal resting pressure. The myogenic activity that contributes 10 and 45% is due to the sympathetic innervation. The remainder of the resting tone is from the hemorrhoidal plexus (15%) and the EAS (30%).[13] Spinal anesthesia decreases rectal tone by 50% and the decreased resting tone seen in diabetic patients may be due to an autonomic neuropathy.[14]

The IAS has slow waves occurring 6–20 times each minute increasing in frequency toward the distal anal canal. Ultraslow waves occur less than two times a minute and are not present in all individuals occurring in approximately 5–10% of normal individuals. Ultraslow waves are associated with higher resting pressures, hemorrhoids, and anal fissures.[12] The occurrence of anal slow-wave activity with rectal pressure waves exceeding anal resting pressure suggests a role for anal slow waves in preserving continence.[15] Ultrasound examination of the anal canal shows the hypoechoic IAS ending approximately 10 mm proximal to the most distal portion of the hyperechoic EAS.

Sensory Factors

Many authors describe the important relationship between anorectal sensation and fecal continence. Conventional concepts of the sensory innervation of the rectum have been challenged by data from continent patients following sphincter saving surgery and ileal pouch-anal anastomosis (IPAA).

Anal canal sensation to touch, pinprick, heat, and cold are present from the anal verge to 2.5–15 mm above the anal valves. This sensitive area is thought to help discriminate between flatus and stool but local anesthesia does not obliterate that ability. The rectum is only sensitive to distention. Rectal sensation may be due to receptors in the rectal wall but also in the pelvic fascia or surrounding muscle. The sensory pathway for rectal distention is the parasympathetic system via the pelvic plexus to S2, S3, and S4. Below 15-cm rectal distention is perceived as flatus, but above 15-cm air distention causes a sensation of abdominal discomfort.

Anal canal sensation is via the inferior rectal branch of the pudendal nerve that arises from S2, S3, and S4. This is the first branch of the pudendal nerve and along with the second branch, the perineal nerve, arises from the pudendal nerve in the pudendal canal (Alcock's canal). The remainder of the pudendal nerve continues as the dorsal nerve of the penis or clitoris.[16]

Many articles report daytime continence following low rectal resections with coloanal or IPAA. The reports of nighttime soiling following these procedures suggest that the ability to interpret sensory input from the neo-rectum requires conscious thought and not simple reflex contraction and relaxation. It is not clear if the decreased continence rate at night is solely due to impaired sensation (and subsequent defective discrimination of solid stool and gas) or if other factors limit fine control.

Reflexes

There are a great number of reflexes that end with the name "... anal reflex." The reason for this is, in part, that the EAS is readily accessible and represents a convenient end point for recording during electrophysiological study. Consequently, there are a number of ways that one can assess the integrity of neurological connection through or around the spinal cord.[11]

Cutaneous-Anal Reflex

The cutaneous-anal reflex was first described by Rossolimo in 1891, as a brief contraction of the anal sphincter in response to pricking or scratching the perianal skin.[17] This is a spinal reflex that requires intact S4 sensory and motor nerve roots. Both afferent and efferent pathways travel within the pudendal nerve.[17] If a cauda equina lesion is present, this reflex will usually be absent. Henry et al. recorded the latency of the anal reflex in 22 incontinent patients as compared to 33 control subjects. The mean latency was 13.0 ms vs. 8.3 ms, respectively. The mean latency was within normal range in only three (14%) of the incontinent patients.[18] However, Bartolo et al. have suggested that latency measurement of the cutaneous-anal reflex may be an inadequate means of demonstrating nerve damage in patients with fecal incontinence.[19] From a practical standpoint, this is a sacral reflex that can be interrogated during physical examination by simply scratching of the perianal skin with visualization of contraction of the subcutaneous anal sphincter. The response to perianal scratch fatigues rapidly so it is important to test this as the first part of the sphincter examination.

Cough Reflex

Chan et al., using intercostal, rectus abdominis, and EAS electrodes, studied the latencies in response to voluntary cough and sniff stimulation. When compared to latencies from transcranial magnetic stimulation it appeared that the EAS response was consistent with a polysynaptic reflex pathway.[20] Visible contraction of the subcutaneous EAS as a consequence to cough and sniff stimulation is a simple nonintrusive validation of the pathways involved in the anal reflex. This response can also be displayed during anal sphincter manometry. Amarenco et al. demonstrated that the greater the intensity of the cough, the greater was the electromyographic response within the anal sphincter.[21] The reflex is preserved in paraplegic patients with lesions above the lumbar spine, but it is lost if the trauma involves the lumbar spine or with cauda equine lesions. The mechanism of the cough-anal reflex contributes to the maintenance of urinary and fecal continence during sudden increases in intra-abdominal pressure as might also be seen with laughing, shouting, or heavy lifting.

Bulbocavernosus Reflex

The bulbocavernosus reflex was first described by Bors and Blinn in 1959.[22] The bulbocavernosus reflex is the sensation of pelvic floor contraction elicited by squeezing the glans penis or clitoris.[23] The EAS is used as the end point, because it is easily accessed either for visual assessment or by concentric needle EMG recording. The BCR latency will be prolonged by various disorders affecting the S2–S4 segments of the spinal cord.

Rectal Anal Inhibitory Reflex

The rectoanal inhibitory reflex (RAIR) represents the relaxation of the IAS in response to distension of the rectum. This was first described by Gowers in 1877 and documented by Denny-Brown in 1935.[24,25] It is felt that this permits fecal material or flatus to come into contact with specialized sensory receptors in the upper anal canal.[26] This sampling process, the sampling reflex, creates an awareness of the presence of stool and a sense of the nature of the material present. It is felt that this process of IAS relaxation with content sampling is instrumental in the discrimination of gas from stool and the ability to pass them independently.[26] The degree to which IAS relaxation occurs appears to be related to the volume of rectal distension more so in incontinent patients than in constipated or healthy control patients.[27] Lower thresholds for the RAIR have been found to be associated with favorable response to biofeedback therapy in patients with fecal incontinence for formed stool.[28] The amplitude of sphincter inhibition is roughly proportional to the volume extent of rectal distension.

The RAIR is primarily dependent upon intrinsic nerve innervation in that it is preserved even after the rectum has been isolated from extrinsic influences, following transaction of hypogastric nerves and the presence of spinal cord lesions. The inhibition response is in part controlled by nonadrenergic, noncholinergic (NANC) mediators.[29] The reflex matures quite early in that it is generally present at birth and has been detected in 81% of premature infants older than 26 weeks postmenstrual age.[30] The reflex is destroyed in Hirschsprung's disease when myenteric ganglia are absent. In addition, the reflex is lost after circumferential myotomy and after generous lateral internal sphincterotomy.[31] Saigusa et al. found that at an average of 23 months following closure of ileostomy after IPAA, only 53% of patients maintained a positive RAIR as compared to 96% preoperatively. The incidence of nocturnal soiling was significantly greater, 72% in those who did not have preserved, or recovered RAIR as compared to those 40% who had postoperative preserved RAIR.[32]

The RAIR appears to be nearly abolished in the early postoperative period following LAR resection for cancer. In a study involving 46 patients, O'Riordain found that the RAIR that had been present in 93% of patients preoperatively was only present in 18% of patients 10 days following low anterior resection. However, at 6–12 months the RAIR was intact in 21% of patients and this increased to 85% after 2 years.[33] Similarly, van Duijvendijk et al., in a study of 11 patients, found the RAIR present in only 36% of patients after undergoing total mesorectal excision for carcinoma at 4 months postoperation. However, 81% of patients had a detectable RAIR at 12 months postsurgery.[26]

Loss of the RAIR is often a consequence of restorative proctocolectomy. Saigusa et al. found that the RAIR was present in only 53% of double-stapled IPAA patients at a mean of 23 months after closure of the ileostomy. Preservation of the RAIR correlated with less nocturnal soiling.[32]

The RAIR in children can be elicited even when general anesthetic agents or neuromuscular blockers are used. Glycopyrrolate, an anticholinergic appears to inhibit RAIR.[34,35]

Disturbances in the RAIR appear to be involved in the incontinence that is associated with systemic sclerosis. Heyt et al. found that 25 of 35 (71.4%) patients with systemic sclerosis demonstrated an impaired or absent RAIR compared with none of 45 controls. Impaired RAIR was closely correlated with fecal incontinence in that 11 of 13 (84%) of incontinent systemic sclerosis patients exhibited an impaired RAIR.[36]

Rectal Anal Excitatory Reflex

The rectal anal excitatory reflex (RAER) or inflation reflex is the contraction of the EAS in response to rectal distension. Rectal distension sensation is most likely transmitted along the S2, S3, and S4 parasympathetic fibers through the pelvic splanchnic nerves.[37] However, on the motor side, a pudendal nerve block abolishes the excitatory reflex suggesting that pudendal neuropathy may interfere with the RAIR. Common methodologies for assessing the integrity of the pudendal nerve involve both single fiber density (SFD) of the EAS and pudendal nerve terminal motor latency (PNTML). However, derangement of the distal RAER was shown by Sangwan et al. to compare favorably with these more traditional and discomforting methodologies as an indicator of neuropathic injury to the EAS. It would appear that patients that have both an abnormal PNTML and an abnormal distal RAER do not require further study with SFD.[38]

Mechanical Factors of Continence and Defecation

Anorectal Angle and Flap-Valve

As a part of the pelvic floor musculature, the puborectalis arises from the pubic bone and passes horizontally and posteriorly around the rectum as the most medial portion of the levator ani muscle. This forms a U-shaped sling around the rectum near its anatomic junction with the anus, pulling the rectum anteriorly, and giving rise to the so-called anorectal angle. There are differences of opinion as to whether the puborectalis and anorectal angle are truly important in maintaining continence. Unlike the fine control of the external and internal sphincter muscles, the puborectalis sling is felt to be more involved with gross fecal continence.[39] Parks postulated a mechanism by which this takes place.[40] As intra-abdominal pressure is increased – such as with sneezing, coughing, or straining – the force is transmitted across the anterior wall of the rectum at the anorectal angle. The underlying mucosa is opposed against the upper anal canal, creating a flap-valve mechanism that prevents stool from passing to the lower anal canal and preserving continence. Yet other authors have disputed this flap-valve mechanism and downplayed the role and reliability of measuring the anorectal angle. Bannister et al., in a study of 29 patients including 14 patients with incontinence, found no evidence of a flap-valve in the normal subjects by using manometric measurements during rising intra-abdominal pressures.[1] However, in the incontinent patients, the manometric pressures were consistent with a flap-valve. Yet subjects still had leakage of stool, questioning the contribution to overall continence. Bartolo and colleagues also used manometric and EMG measurements in 13 subjects both at rest and during Valsalva, demonstrating a similar rise in rectal and sphincter pressures and puborectalis EMG recordings.[19] Yet, with concomitant barium studies the anterior rectal wall separated from the mucosa, allowing contrast to fill the rectum. The authors proposed that the puborectalis functions more like a sphincter rather than contributing to the flap-valve mechanism.

Furthermore, quantifying the anorectal angle and relating that to patient symptoms has resulted in mixed views. One study noted significant interobserver variation in anorectal angle measurements between three interpreters but good intraobserver consistency, suggesting that variation in anorectal angle measurements may be due to subjective interpretation of the rectal axis along the curved rectal wall. In another study assessing the reproducibility of anorectal angle measurement in 43 defecating proctograms, the authors found significant intra- and interobserver variations, and concluded that the anorectal angle is an inaccurate measurement.[41] Jorge and associates measured the anorectal angle during rest, squeeze, and push in 104 consecutive patients and also found highly significant differences in each measurement category.[42]

Reservoir

As an additional part of the continence mechanism, the rectum must be able to function as a temporary storage site for liquid and solid stool. With passage of the fecal stream into the rectum, the pliable rectal walls are able to distend and delay the defecation sequence until an appropriate time. This process relies both on rectal innervation to sense and tolerate the rising volume of stool (capacity), as well as maintain a relatively low and constant pressure with increases in volume (compliance). Extremes of either of these components can lead to fecal incontinence through decreased accommodation or overflow states. Although decreased compliance has been demonstrated more often in patients with fecal incontinence, it has also been shown to occur as a normal consequence of aging.[43] In addition, Bharucha and associates in a study of 52 women with fecal incontinence demonstrated that the rectal capacity was reduced in 25% of women, and these lower volume and pressure thresholds were significantly associated with rectal hypersensitivity and urge fecal incontinence.[44] Furthermore, following low anterior resection for cancer, those patients with resultant lower rectal compliance and lower rectal volume tolerability (capacity) have been associated with higher rates of fecal incontinence.[45]

Normal Defecation

The awareness of the need to defecate occurs in the superior frontal gyrus and anterior cingulate gyrus. The process begins with movement of gas, liquid, or solid contents into the rectum. Distention of the rectum leads to stimulation of pressure receptors located on the puborectalis muscle and in the pelvic floor muscles, which in turn stimulate the RAIR. The IAS relaxes allowing sampling of contents. If defecation is to be deferred, voluntary contraction of the EAS and levator ani muscles occurs, and the rectum accommodates with relaxation after an initial increase in pressure. When the anal canal is deemed to have solid contents and a decision to defecate is made, the glottis closes, pelvic floor muscles contract, and diaphragm and abdominal wall muscles contract, all increasing abdominal pressure. The puborectalis muscle relaxes, resulting in straightening of the anorectal angle, and the pelvic floor descends slightly. The EAS relaxes and anal canal contents are evacuated. Upon normal complete evacuation, the pelvic floor rises and sphincters contract once more in a "closing reflex."

Pathologic Conditions

Incontinence

Incontinence is the inability to defer the passage of gas, liquid, or solid stool until a desired time. Numerous alterations in anorectal physiology can lead to incontinence and many patients have more than one deficit. Structural defects in the internal or EAS muscles occur due to obstetric injury, trauma, or anorectal surgery. The keyhole deformity is a groove in the anal canal allowing the seepage of stool or mucus. Originally described as a complication after the posterior midline fissurectomy or fistulotomy, it can also occur with lateral IAS defects. Intact sphincter muscles with impaired neurologic function, due to pudendal nerve damage or systemic disorders, such as diabetes, can also result in incontinence, especially if the impaired sphincter is further stressed by diarrhea or irritable bowel syndrome.

Abnormal rectal sensation can lead to incontinence in two ways. Conditions such as proctitis due to inflammation or radiation can result in hyperacute sensation. The rectum fails to accommodate and the reservoir function is impaired leading to urgency and frequent stools. Fragmentation of stools is commonly described by patients after low anterior resection, particularly if the pelvis has been radiated as in the case of adjuvant therapy for the treatment of rectal cancer. In the case of blunted sensation, due to a large rectocele, megarectum, or neurogenic disorders, the rectum becomes over distended and overflow incontinence occurs.

The majority of patients with rectal prolapse are incontinent. Chronic stretching of the anal sphincters from full thickness prolapse leads to a patulous anus through which gas and liquid stool easily leak. A reflex relaxation of the IAS may also occur as the rectal wall descends toward the anal canal. Patients with mucosal prolapse may have seepage of mucus or small amounts of liquid stool. Correction of the prolapse can resolve the incontinence if the anal sphincter tone sufficiently returns. Age and duration of prolapse can affect this.

Obstructed Defecation

Suspected Enterocele or Rectocele (Obstructed Defecation)

Patients with symptoms of enterocele or rectocele describe prolonged straining at defecation, with a sensation of partial or complete blockage (frequently a "closed trap door" preventing passage of stool). Defecography can demonstrate the presence of a rectocele or enterocele, suggest the presence of a peritoneocele, and clarify contributing disorders such as a nonrelaxing pelvic floor, rectal intussusception or prolapse, and potentially uterovaginal prolapse.

Rectocele

A rectocele is defined as greater than 2 cm of rectal wall outpouching or bowing while straining, and can precede or accompany rectal intussusception. The rectocele can prevent passage of stool both by obstructing the anal orifice and by acting as a diverticulum to sequester stool. Patients with rectoceles commonly complain of the need for frequent sequential episodes of defecation, and even for manual compression or splinting of the anterior perineum or posterior vagina in order to completely evacuate. Additionally, patients may experience incontinence with relaxation, leading to reduction of the rectocele and return of the sequestered stool to the lower rectum.

Van Dam and associates investigated the utility of defecography in predicting the outcome of rectocele repair.[46] Rectocele size, barium trapping, intussusception, evacuation, and perineal descent were measured during defecography exams of 74 consecutive patients with symptomatic rectoceles. The patients then underwent a transanal/transvaginal repair, followed by 6-month postoperative defecography and reassessment of the five most common presenting symptoms (excessive straining, incomplete evacuation, manual assistance required, sense of fullness, bowel movement less than three times per week). No postoperative defecograms demonstrated a persistent or recurrent rectocele; however, one-third of patients had a poor result based on persistent symptoms. There was no association between defecography measurements and outcome of the repair. Still, the authors concluded that defecography serves three major purposes in the evaluation of a rectocele: preoperative evidence of its presence and size, documentation of additional pelvic floor abnormalities, and an objective assessment of postoperative changes.

An abnormal increase in perineal descent (typically greater than 2 cm) has been described among both incontinent patients and continent patients who strain during defecation.[32,33] These conflicting data underscore the poorly understood relationship between neuropathic pelvic floor damage and symptomatology. Bartolo and associates evaluated patients with perineal descent using manometric, radiographic, and neurophysiologic studies.[47] When comparing 32 patients with incontinence and increased perineal descent with 21 patients with obstructed defecation and increased perineal descent, the authors found no significant difference in the extent of perineal descent or neuropathic damage to the EAS. Patients who were incontinent had lower manometric pressures (both resting and squeeze pressures) while those with obstructed defecation had normal manometric pressures. In a separate study, these authors also found that incontinent patients with increased perineal descent had severe denervation of both the puborectalis and the EAS compared to continent patients with increased perineal descent, who had partial denervation of the EAS only.[47] Miller and colleagues evaluated sensation in two similar patient groups.[48] Patients who were frankly incontinent actually had less perineal descent than continent patients with descent but had severely impaired anal sensation.

Berkelmans and others tried to determine if women with increased perineal descent and straining at stool were at risk for future development of incontinence.[49] The authors identified 46 women with perineal descent who strained during defecation but were continent. Twenty-four of the 46 were followed after 5 years and 13 of these (54%) had developed fecal incontinence, compared with 3 of 20 (15%) control patients. During their initial evaluation, the patients who previously strained and later developed incontinence had significantly greater perineal descent at rest and less elevation of the pelvic floor during maximal sphincter contraction than the women who strained but did not develop incontinence.

Thus, perineal descent may be a predictor of incontinence among patients with denervation of both the EAS and the puborectalis, and in patients with impaired anal sensation. Among patients with constipation, perineal descent and straining at stool may predict future fecal incontinence.

Dyskinetic Puborectalis

Dyskinetic puborectalis, paradoxical puborectalis, nonrelaxing puborectalis, and anismus are terms that describe the absence of normal relaxation of pelvic floor muscles during defecation, resulting in rectal outlet obstruction.[50] Once diagnosed, dyskinetic puborectalis is usually treated with biofeedback and bowel management. Patients who fail conservative treatment have been offered botulism toxin injections into the puborectalis muscle with limited success.[51]

Continence

The interplay of all the aforementioned anatomy and physiology ensures continence. It does not follow that a deficit in any one area ensures incontinence. Continence achieved in the ileoanal pouch patient is proof that the rectum is not essential. An intact and functional puborectalis muscle can provide continence in the pediatric imperforate anus patient, but incontinence can ensue during adulthood. Even profound deficits do not necessarily lead to incontinence if stool consistency is solid, while minor deficits can easily lead to incontinence to gas. To determine and treat abnormal fecal incontinence requires a systematic approach focusing on identifying the specific deficits present, applying appropriate testing to elucidate anal physiology and anatomy, and then directing therapy accordingly.

Summary

The unique physiology of the anus and rectum and the ability to master the complex task of fecal continence has many interesting facets. Understanding the anatomy, innervation, and reflexes of the pelvic floor and anal sphincters is the key to assessing disorders of continence. Further work in this area remains promising.

Acknowledgments. This chapter was written by Susan M. Parker and John M. Coller in the first edition of this textbook.

References

1. Bannister JJ, Gibbons C, Read NW. Preservation of faecal continence during rises in intra-abdominal pressure: is there a role for the flap-valve? Gut. 1987;28:1242–4.
2. Berglas B, Rubin IC. Study of the supportive structures of the uterus by levator myography. Surg Gynecol Obstet. 1953;97:677–92.
3. Cherry DA, Rothenberger DA. Pelvic floor physiology. Surg Clin North Am. 1988;68(6):1217–30.
4. Mavrantonis C, Wexner SD. A clinical approach to fecal incontinence. J Clin Gastroenterol. 1998;27(2):108–21.
5. Woodburne RT. Essentials of human anatomy. New York: Oxford University Press; 1994.
6. Henry MM, Swash M, editors. Coloproctology and the pelvic floor. Oxford: Butterworth-Heinemann Ltd; 1992. p. 3–249.
7. Bourdelat D, Muller F, Droulle P, Barbet JP. Anatomical and sonographical studies of the development of fecal continence and sphincter development in human fetuses. Eur J Pediatr Surg. 2001;11:124–30.
8. Dalley AF. The riddle of the sphincters. The morphysiology of the anorectal mechanism reviewed. Am Surg. 1987;53:298–306.
9. Wunderlich M, Swash M. The overlapping innervation of the two sides of the external anal sphincter by the pudendal nerves. J Neurol Sci. 1983;59:97–109.
10. Hamdy S, Enck P, Aziz Q, Uengoergil S, Hobson A, Thompson DG. Laterality effects of human pudendal nerve stimulation on corticoanal pathways: evidence for functional asymmetry. Gut. 1999;45(1):58–63.
11. Uher E, Swash M. Sacral reflexes: physiology and clinical application. Dis Colon Rectum. 1998;41:1165–77.
12. Penninckx F, Lestar B, Kerremans R. The internal anal sphincter: mechanisms of control and its roles in maintaining anal continence. Clin Gastroenterol. 1992;6:193–213.
13. Lestar B, Penninckx F, Kerremans R. The composition of anal basal pressure: an in vivo and in vitro study in man. Int J Colorectal Dis. 1989;4:118–22.
14. Sangwan Y, Solla J. Internal anal sphincter: advances and insights. Dis Colon Rectum. 1998;41:1297–311.
15. Sorensen SM et al. Scand J Gastroenterol. 1989;24:115–20.
16. Jorge JMN, Wexner S. Anatomy and physiology of the rectum and anus. Eur J Surg. 1997;163:723–31.
17. Rossolimo G. Der Analreflex, seine physiologie und pathologie. Neurologisches Centralblatt 1891;4:257–9.
18. Henry MM, Parks AG, Swash M. The anal reflex in idiopathic faecal incontinence: an electrophysiological study. Br J Surg. 1980;67:781–3.
19. Bartolo DC, Jarratt JA, Read NW. The cutaneo-anal reflex: a useful index of neuropathy? Br J Surg. 1983;70(11):660–3.
20. Chan CL, Ponsford S, Swash M. The anal reflex elicited by cough and sniff: validation of a neglected clinical sign. J Neurol Neurosurg Psychiatry. 2004;75(10):1449–51.
21. Amarenco G, Ismael SS, Lagauche D, Raibaut P, Rene-Corail P, Wolff N, et al. Cough anal reflex: strict relationship between intravesical pressure and pelvic floor muscle electromyographic activity during cough. Urodynamic and electrophysiological study. J Urol. 2005;173(1):149–52.
22. Bors E, Blinn K. Bulbocavernousus reflex. J Urol. 1959;82:128–30.
23. Podnar S. Electrodiagnosis of the anorectum: a review of techniques and clinical applications. Tech Coloproctol. 2003;7:71–6.
24. Gowers WR. The automatic action of the sphincter ani. Proc R Soc Lond B Biol Sci. 1877;26:77–84.
25. Denny-Brown D, Robertson EG. An investigation of the nervous control of defecation. Brain. 1935;58:256–310.
26. van Duijvendijk P, Slors F, Taat CW, Heisterkamp SH, Obertop H, Boeckxstaens GEE. A prospective evaluation of anorectal function after total mesorectal excision in patients with a rectal carcinoma. Surgery. 2003;133:56–65.
27. Duthie HL, Bennett RC. The relation of sensation in the anal canal to the functional anal sphincter: a possible factor in anal continence. Gut. 1963;4:179–82.
28. Chiarioni G, Bassotti G, Stanganini S, Vantini I, Whitehead WE. Sensory retraining is key to biofeedback therapy for formed stool fecal incontinence. Am J Gastroenterol. 2002;97(1):109–17.
29. Tomita R, Tanjoh K, Fujisaki S, Fukuzawa M. The role of nitric oxide (NO) in the human internal anal sphincter. J Gastroenterol. 2001;36(6):386391.
30. de Lorijn F, Omari TI, Kok JH, Taminiau AJM, Benninga MA. Maturation of the rectoanal inhibitory reflex in very premature infants. J Pediatr. 2003;143:630–3.
31. Lubowski DZ, Nichols RJ, Swash M, Jordan MY. Neural control of internal anal sphincter function. Br J Surg. 1987;74:668–70.
32. Saigusa N, Belin BM, Choi HJ, Gervaz P, Efron JE, Weiss EG, et al. Recovery of the rectoanal inhibitory reflex after restorative proctocolectomy: does it correlate with nocturnal continence? Dis Colon Rectum. 2003;46(2):168–72.
33. O'Riordain MG, Molloy RG, Gillen P, Horgan A, Kiran WO. Rectoanal inhibitory reflex following low stapled anterior resection of the rectum. Dis Colon Rectum. 1992;35(9):874–8.
34. Kaur G, Gardiner A, Duthie GS. Rectoanal reflex parameters in incontinence and constipation. Dis Colon Rectum. 2002;45(7):928–33.
35. Pfefferkorn MD, Croffie JM, Corkiins MR, Gupta SK, Fitzgerald JF. Impact of sedation and anesthesia on the rectoanal inhibitory reflex in children. J Pediatr Gastroenterol Nutr. 2004;38(3):324–7.
36. Heyt GJ, Oh MK, Alemzadeh N, Rivera S, Jimenez SA, Rattan S, et al. Impaired rectoanal inhibitory response in scleroderma (systemic sclerosis): an association with fecal incontinence. Dig Dis Sci. 2004;49(6):1040–5.
37. Rao SSC. Pathophysiology of adult fecal incontinence. Gastroenterology. 2004;126:S14–22.
38. Sangwan YP, Coller JA, Barrett RC, Murray JJ, Roberts PL, Schoetz Jr DJ. Prospective comparative study of abnormal distal rectoanal excitatory reflex, pudendal nerve terminal motor latency, and single fiber density as markers of pudendal neuropathy. Dis Colon Rectum. 1996;39:794–8.
39. Beck DE, Wexner SD. Fundamentals of anorectal surgery. 2nd ed. Philadelphia, PA: W.B. Saunders; 1998. p. 19–20.
40. Parks AG. Anorectal incontinence. Proc R Soc Med. 1975;68:681–90.
41. Jorgenson J, Stein P, King DW, Lubowski DZ. The anorectal angle is not a reliable parameter on defaecating proctography. Aust N Z J Surg. 1993;63(2):105–8.
42. Jorge JM, Wexner SD, Marchetti F, Rosato GO, Sullivan ML, Jagelman DG. How reliable are currently available methods of measuring the anorectal angle? Dis Colon Rectum. 1992;35(4):332–8.

43. Broen PM, Penninckx FM. Relation between anal electrosensitivity and rectal filling sensation and the influence of age. Dis Colon Rectum. 2005;48(1):127–33.
44. Bharucha AE, Fletcher JG, Harper CM, Hough D, Daube JR, Stevens C, et al. Relationship between symptoms and disordered continence mechanisms in women with idiopathic fecal incontinence. Gut. 2005;54(4):546–55.
45. Rasmussen O. Anorectal function. Dis Colon Rectum. 1994;37(4):386–403.
46. van Dam JH, Ginai AZ, Gosselink MJ, et al. Role of defecography in predicting clinical outcome of rectocele repair. Dis Colon Rectum. 1997;40(2):201–7.
47. Bartolo DC, Roe AM, Locke-Edmunds JC, Virjee J, Mortensen NJ. Flap-valve theory of anorectal continence. Br J Surg. 1986;73(12):1012–4.
48. Miller R, Bartolo DC, Cervero F, Mortensen NJ. Differences in anal sensation in continent and incontinent patients with perineal descent. Int J Colorectal Dis. 1989;4(1):45–9.
49. Berkelmans I, Heresbach D, Leroi AM, et al. Perineal descent at defecography in women with straining at stool: a lack of specificity or predictive value for future anal incontinence? Eur J Gastroenterol Hepatol. 1995;7(1):75–9.
50. Lowry AC, Simmang CL, Boulos P, et al. Consensus statement of definitions for anorectal physiology and rectal cancer: report of the Tripartite consensus conference on definitions for anorectal physiology and rectal cancer, Washington, D.C., May 1, 1999. Dis Colon Rectum. 2001;44(7):915–9.
51. Ron Y, Avni Y, Lukovetski A, et al. Botulinum toxin type-A in therapy of patients with anismus. Dis Colon Rectum. 2001;44(12):1821–6.

4 Physiologic Testing

Anders F. Mellgren

Functional anorectal symptoms are common and affect all ages of the population.[1] Normal anorectal physiologic function is complex and relies on a multiplicity of factors, including a intact anatomy and an intact link between somatic and visceral function of the anus rectum and colon. Consequently, a comprehensive evaluation of anorectal function demands a combination of several tests that complement each other. There is no single test that can comprehensively assess the function of the pelvic floor. In the clinical setting, physiologic testing should always be a complement to a proper patient history, physical examination, and frequently other tests including endoscopy and other imaging studies. The history may be complemented by use of questionnaires and quality of life instruments. The clinical utility of some physiologic testing is limited because of a lack of reference data from healthy individuals and lack of standardization.[2,3]

Several of the existing physiologic tests are proven to improve diagnostic yield and to directly influence clinical management.[4] This chapter describes the physiologic tests that are clinically available to assess functional disorders of the pelvic floor and colon (Table 4-1).

Anorectal Manometry

Indications

Anorectal manometry measures the pressures in the anal canal and the distal rectum. This test serves as one of the most accepted and widely used investigations to measure the function of the internal anal sphincter (IAS) and the external anal sphincter (EAS). Evaluation of sphincter function in patients with fecal incontinence is the primary indication for manometry. Other indications for anorectal manometry include screening for functional outlet obstruction (nonrelaxing pelvic floor), Hirschsprung's disease (absence of rectoanal inhibitory reflex (RAIR)), and damage to sacral reflex arc (absence of cough reflex). Manometry is also used for performing and predicting responses to biofeedback training and to objectively quantify pressure before and after surgical intervention.

Equipment and Testing

There are four essential components in anorectal manometry equipment: (1) a probe for measuring intraluminal pressure; (2) a pressure recording device (amplifier/recorder, pneumohydraulic pump, and pressure transducers); (3) a balloon for inflation inside the rectum; and (4) a monitor/printer/storage system.

The probes can be of different types, including solid state, water perfused, air charged, or microballoon.[5] The diameter of the probe should not exceed 5–6 mm and the probe usually includes sensors radially distributed to measure several pressures at each level. Calibration of the probe and the recorder is critical for accurately measuring and obtaining reproducible results. Bowel enema before the test is optional, but if formed stool is found at digital examination an enema is advisable to avoid interference with the testing. Any manipulation of the rectum, such as digital rectal examination or administration of enema prior to a test should be followed by a minimum of 5 min of rest to allow sphincter activity to return to baseline.[6]

The two most commonly used and clinically available tests for measuring anal canal pressures are the stationary pull-through and the dynamic pull-through technique. The stationary pull-through technique is today the recommended method of choice since the dynamic pull-through technique creates a reflex sphincter contraction due to the stimulation generated by the probe resulting in higher anal pressures. The stationary pull-through measures the resting pressure and the squeeze increase at 6, 5, 4, 3, 2, and 1 cm from the anal verge by extracting the probe in increments of 1 cm from the rectum to the anal verge. Allowing a waiting period between each measurement minimizes artifacts.

Anal Resting Tone

The anal resting reflects the tonic activity of the IAS (55%), the EAS (30%), and the anal cushions (15%).[7] The IAS has

D.E. Beck et al. (eds.), *The ASCRS Textbook of Colon and Rectal Surgery: Second Edition*,
DOI 10.1007/978-1-4419-1584-9_4, © Springer Science+Business Media, LLC 2011

TABLE 4-1. Anorectal and colonic physiologic tests

Type of test	Measured modality	Primary indication
Test of function		
Anorectal manometry	Function of anal sphincter Rectoanal reflexes Anorectal sensation Rectal compliance Rectal motor function and coordination (balloon expulsion test, defecatory maneuver)	Fecal incontinence, nonrelaxation of the pelvic floor, Hirschsprung's disease
Vector volume manometry	Pressure profile and function of the anal sphincter	Fecal incontinence, sphincter injury
Saline infusion test	Rectal continence	Incontinence
Perineometry	Position of the pelvic floor	Pelvic floor laxity
Pudendal nerve terminal motor latency (PNTML)	Pudendal nerve terminal motor latency	Pudendal nerve injury or neuropathy
Electromyography (EMG)	Muscle activation. Motor unit potentials and fiber density (needle EMG)	Sphincter injury, biofeedback, imperforate anus
Test of structure		
Endoanal ultrasound	Two-dimensional or three-dimensional assessment of the internal and external anal sphincter, pelvic floor, and rectum	Fecal incontinence, fistula, tumors
Endoanal magnetic resonance imaging (MRI)	Assessment of the internal and external anal sphincter, pelvic floor, and rectum	Fecal incontinence, fistula, tumors
Test of function and structure		
Dynamic defecography	Rectal evacuation and dynamic assessment of the rectum and vagina	Fecal outlet obstruction, pelvic prolapse
Dynamic MRI	Rectal evacuation and dynamic assessment of the pelvis	Fecal outlet obstruction, pelvic prolapse
Marker study	Global transit time	Constipation
Radionuclide gamma scintigraphy	Global segmental colon transit	Constipation
SmartPill®	Stomach emptying, small bowel transit, colonic transit	Constipation, functional disorders of the stomach and small bowel

an oscillating tonic activity with both slow waves of low amplitude[8,9] and ultraslow waves of high amplitude.[10]

The anal resting tone is usually measured at 6, 5, 4, 3, 2, and 1 cm from the anal verge with the stationary pull-through technique. The maximum resting pressure (MRP) is usually defined as the highest recorded resting pressure.[11] There is some radial asymmetry in pressures in the different parts of the anal canal[12] and therefore the pressures in the four quadrants is usually averaged to account for this asymmetry.[13] The pressure profiles in the anal canal vary also according to gender, age, and measuring technique (Figure 4-1). The length of the functional anal canal or high pressure zone is defined as the length of the anal canal with resting pressures exceeding 30% of the rectal pressure.[11]

Patients with fecal incontinence tend to have lower anal resting tone than do continent patients or normal controls.[14–16] The clinical value of measuring basal anal canal pressures alone is limited, since patients with low pressures may have normal continence and patients with incontinence may have normal pressures. There is also a lack of defined values of what is the normal range for the anal resting tone.

Squeeze Pressure

Squeeze increase of the anal canal pressure is generated by contraction of the EAS and can be calculated as the increase in pressure from the anal canal resting tone during maximal anal squeeze (Figure 4-2).[3,5]

The squeeze increase is usually measured at 6, 5, 4, 3, 2, and 1 cm from the anal verge with the stationary pull-through technique. The squeeze increase is obtained by asking the patient to maximally squeeze the sphincter at each level and hold this squeeze for 3 s. Instructing the patient to avoid contraction of accessory muscles, particularly the gluteal muscles, or to avoid increasing the intra-abdominal pressure reduces the risk of measuring false high squeeze increase. The maximum voluntary squeeze pressure (MSP) is usually defined as the highest pressure recorded above the baseline (zero) at any level of the anal canal during maximum squeeze effort.[11] An alternative measurement is the highest pressure recorded above the resting pressure during maximum squeeze effort. The latter pressure is thus the increment of pressure above the resting tone.

Decreased squeeze pressures are frequently correlated to injuries in the EAS, neurologic damage, or just poor patient compliance/voluntary control. If the latter problem is suspected, the results of decreased squeeze pressure should be interpreted in context with the EAS response to coughing (see the section "Cough Reflex").

The susceptibility for fatigue of the EAS can be estimated by measuring the patient's ability to sustain the squeeze effort over time. The squeeze duration is often reduced in patients

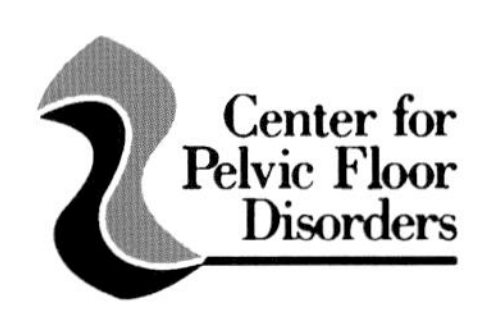

Anorectal Manometry Report:

Patient Name:
Patient ID#:
Referring Physician:
Physician:
Date of Test:

Radial Pressure Analysis

Resting Level

Resting Average (mmHg)

	Post	Right	Anter.	Left	Min	Max	Median	HPZ	Mean	M Z
6.0 cm	4	4	3	7	3	7	4		5	
5.0 cm	15	3	3	12	3	15	8		8	
4.0 cm	20	4	10	20	4	20	15		14	
3.0 cm	55	23	14	44	14	55	34		34	
2.0 cm	45	45	20	48	20	48	45	X	40	
1.0 cm	51	84	78	71	51	84	75	X	71	55.5

Squeeze Increase

Squeeze Increase (mmHg)

	Post	Right	Anter.	Left	Min	Max	Median	HPZ	Mean	M Z
6.0 cm	13	4	4	13	4	13	8		8	
5.0 cm	49	10	17	44	10	49	30		30	
4.0 cm	40	22	20	42	20	42	31		31	
3.0 cm	62	24	17	21	17	62	23		31	
2.0 cm	55	48	39	51	39	55	50	X	48	
1.0 cm	79	88	86	76	76	88	82	X	82	65

Sensation/RAIR

Sensation	Measured Values	Normal Values
First Sensation	50 ml	40-80 ml
Max Tolerable Volume	150 ml	120-180 ml

RAIR	Measured Values	Normal Values
RAIR present	50ml	
RAIR not present	ml	

FIGURE 4-1. Anorectal manometry report. Resting pressures and squeeze increases at different levels are found in the columns "Mean."

with incontinence.[17] The squeeze durability can be measured as a fatigue index (the coefficient of maximum squeeze pressure and the gradient of decay).[18]

Rectoanal Inhibitory Reflex

Rectal distension or attempted defecation results in a treatment inhibition of the tonic activity of the IAS and the consequent relaxation of this muscle. The RAIR is mediated via the myenteric plexus and it is modulated by the spinal cord.[19,20] This reflex facilitates rectal emptying and it is also believed to serve as a discriminatory function of the rectum, as it can facilitate discrimination of gas from fecal substance and allow rectal contents to be "sampled" by the sensory area of the anal canal. Concomitant with the relaxation of the IAS, there is sometimes a reflex EAS contraction during rectal distension that is automatic and not reflex mediated. By asking the patient to relax, this contraction sometimes can be limited.[21]

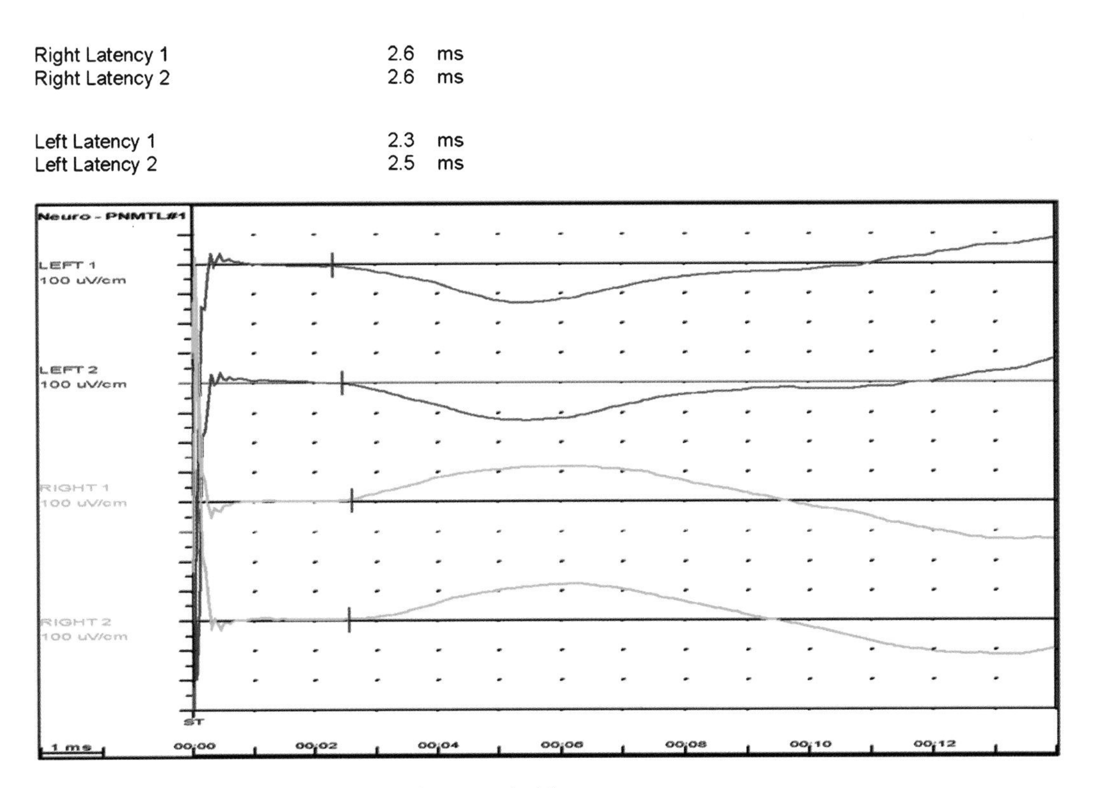

FIGURE 4-2. Pudendal nerve motor latency measure twice on each side.

The RAIR can be tested by inflation of a balloon in the whole distal rectum simultaneously measuring the pressure in the anal canal. The anal canal probe is usually positioned at the level of the highest recorded anal resting pressure, as this positioning facilitates the recording of a normal RAIR.

Presence of an intact RAIR is dependent on an intact myenteric plexus and is usually impaired in patients with Hirschsprung's disease.[22] An absence of RAIR may indicate a diagnosis of Hirschsprung's disease[23] and should be followed by a full-thickness rectal biopsy to confirm an agangliotic segment diagnostic of Hirschsprung's disease. Hirschsprung's disease is usually diagnosed in early childhood and therefore rarely newly discovered in adults. The prevalence and the clinical relevance of ultra short Hirschsprung's disease in adults is controversial.[24]

Cough Reflex

A normal response following a rapid increase in intra-abdominal pressure is a contraction of the EAS. This reflex, the cough reflex, maintains continence in case of a rapid increase in intra-abdominal pressure. The cough reflex can be assessed with a probe supplied with an intrarectal balloon (estimating the intra-abdominal pressure) and sensors located in the anal canal. If the increment of the anal canal pressure is higher than the rectal pressure, the reflex is considered to be normal. A sphincter defect or innervations injury may result in a weaker anal pressure increase and an abnormal cough reflex. Even though the clinical use of this test is limited, it can serve as an instrument to measure compliance in patients with attenuated voluntary squeeze pressures without evidence of spinal damage.[25]

Rectal Sensation and Compliance

Rectal sensation (and rectal compliance) can be measured by intermittent balloon distension in the distal rectum while simultaneously monitoring the patient's response. The first sensation, the first urge, and the maximal tolerable volume are usually recorded. Rectal compliance can also be assessed by measuring the pressure and volume relationship when a balloon is inflated in the rectum. This method is associated with a significant intersubjective variation, but some studies have demonstrated a good reproducibility of the recorded sensory thresholds.[26,27] Some data supports that the sensory perception of the rectal distension is directly related to the rectal wall tension. Reduced sensory threshold levels of the rectum (rectal hypersensitivity) in patients with fecal incontinence could indicate a presence of urge fecal incontinence and increased frequency of defecation,[28,29] whereas incontinent patients with increased sensory threshold levels (rectal hyposensitivity) may suffer from passive (overflow) incontinence.[30]

Vector Volume Manometry

Using a stationary pull-through technique and an eight-channel manometric catheter with radially oriented side holes, a three-dimensional picture of the pressure profile in the anal canal can be obtained. Pressure asymmetry corresponding to any sphincter defects can possibly be located by this method. The clinical utility of vector volume manometry today has largely been replaced by endoanal ultrasound.

Other Tests of Anorectal Function

Balloon Expulsion Test

Rectal expulsion ability can be evaluated by inflation of a water-filled rectal nonlatex balloon. The main purpose of this test is to identify patients with obstructed defecation [3]. Normal subjects can usually expel a balloon containing 50–150 mL, but patients suffering from constipation with megarectum are frequently unable to expel the balloon even though the intrarectal pressures are within the normal range.[31] A variation of the technique uses a detachable water or air-filled balloon that is inserted into the rectum. The patient is then allowed to sit on a commode in a private bathroom to pass it.[32] This method may be more physiological then trying to pass a balloon attached to a catheter in the lateral position.

There are several factors that may lead to over diagnosis of functional outlet obstruction, including the inability of the balloon to accurately mimic patient's stool, technical challenges to standardize the test, and embarrassment experienced by the patients in the test setting.[33,34] The volume of the balloon may also influence the ability to expel the balloon.[35] The utility of the balloon expulsion test alone is limited, but in addition to other physiologic tests it may assist in the evaluation of patients with a nonrelaxing pelvic floor.[36]

Saline Continence Test

The saline continence test evaluates the ability of the sphincters to remain continent at continuous infusion of saline into the rectum. The time and volume at first leak and total leaked volume are assessed. Approximately 1.5 L can be infused in normal subjects without any significant leakage.[37,38] Patients with fecal incontinence due to weak sphincter function or reduced rectal compliance usually starts leaking after infusion of 250–600 mL saline.[39] This test is used sparingly and may be useful for objectively evaluating patients with fecal incontinence or for assessing improvement to surgical or medical treatment.[37]

Perineometry

There is a relation between increased perineal descent (pelvic floor laxity) and fecal incontinence. The pelvic floor should descend <1.5 cm during normal defecation. The perineometer measures the level of the perineum with respect to the ischial tuberosities and is used to estimate the perineal descent.[40] This test has limited clinical utility because of poor reproducibility and comparatively more accurate radiologic methods for evaluating the movement of the pelvic floor are available.[41]

Neurophysiologic Tests

Pudendal Nerve Terminal Motor Latency

The pudendal nerve innervates the EAS, urethral sphincter, perineal musculature, mucosa of the anal canal, and the perineal skin. The nerve carries both afferent and efferent information originating from the nerve roots S2, S3, and S4 and travels along the lateral pelvic floor and exits the pelvis at the ischial spine into the pudendal canal (Alcock's canal).

Pudendal nerve terminal motor latency (PNTML) is measured with a disposable finger-mounted electrode (St Mark's electrode) with a distal stimulating electrode at the fingertip and a recording electrode located at the finger base. By placing the finger tip as close as possible to the pudendal nerve at the ischial spine, the nerve conduction velocity (latency) from the ischial spine to the EAS (at the finger base) can be measured. PNTML provides an estimation of the fastest conducting fibers in the pudendal nerve with a risk of showing a normal PNTML in a damaged nerve as long as some of the fast conducting fibers remain intact.[42]

The use of this test is controversial because of suboptimal test sensitivity and specificity.[43] However, knowledge of any existing neuropathy or injury of the pudendal nerve may be of importance before sphincter surgery or biofeedback. PNTML is therefore used as a complementary tool in the physiologic evaluation of anorectal function.[44] The American Gastroenterological Association does not recommend PNTML for evaluation of patients with fecal incontinence[2] on the basis of its unknown test reproducibility,[45] age-dependent results independent of continence status,[46] operator dependency[47] and high rate of false-negative result. However, the test is widely performed and relied upon by surgeons who operate on patients with fecal incontinence, constipation, and rectal prolapse.

Electromyography

Anal electromyography (EMG) can be used to sample the activity of striated pelvic floor muscles.[2,48,49] In the clinical setting, EMG is primarily used to identify EAS activity and whether appropriate sphincter relaxation and contraction exists. This information can be obtained using surface electrodes and can identify patients with nonrelaxing pelvic floor (Figures 4-3 and 4-4) and it is also used in biofeedback therapy. Needle EMG can also provide information about possible nerve injury (denervation–reinnervation potentials) and locate muscle in the EAS. The latter indication has today largely been replaced by endoanal ultrasound.

Surface electrodes (anal plug and skin electrodes) are associated with less patient discomfort and a lower risk of infection.[50,51] Surface electrodes are frequently used to measure

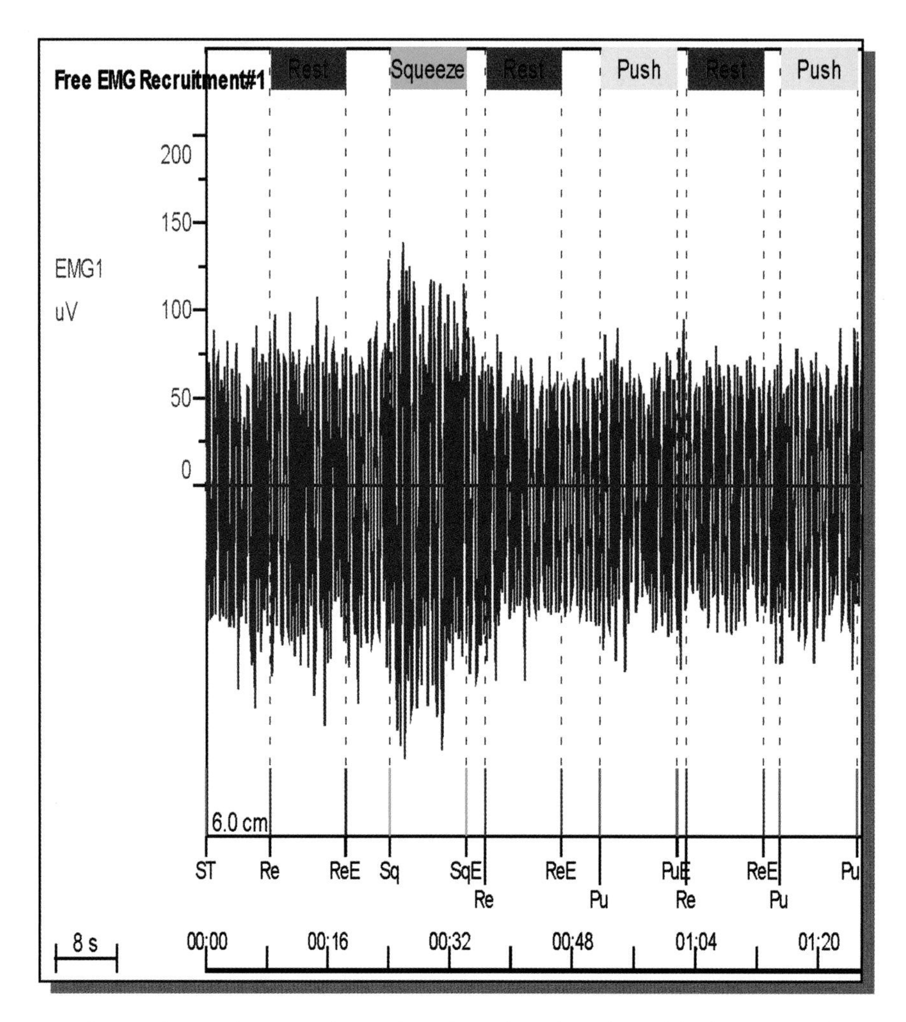

FIGURE 4-3. Electromyography recruitment demonstrating equivocal reaction, since the activity is unchanged at "push."

EAS activity to determine appropriate sphincter relaxation and contraction (Figure 4-5). Anal plug electrodes are frequently used in biofeedback training. Using this technique, patients suffering from fecal incontinence or nonrelaxing sphincter are be able to obtain a visual or audible signal as a response to sphincter contraction.

Needle electrodes can be either single-fiber electrodes or concentric needle electrodes. Single-fiber needle electrodes record a single motor unit at a time. Increased fiber density (motor unit grouping) can be detected as evidence of nerve denervation with reinnervation.[49,52] Single-fiber EMG results have shown a high degree of repeatability among independent investigators.[53] Concentric needle EMG, which measures approximately 30 motor units at a time, is useful for detecting polyphasic or prolonged duration of the motor unit potentials as evidence for reinnervation in the EAS.[49] In patients with fecal incontinence, high fiber density and longer motor unit potentials are more commonly detected in EMG than in controls,[42,54–56] but the extent of denervation measured by EMG in the EAS does not appear to influence the severity of incontinence.[57]

The clinical utility of EMG has diminished since mapping of the EAS has been replaced in many centers by endoanal ultrasound,[58] EAS is less painful and provides the examiner with a two- or three-dimensional picture of the anal canal and the anal sphincters.[59] According to the American Gastroenterological Association, EMG still has a role in confirming imperforate anus before surgical placement of the bowel if endoanal ultrasound is not possible or not available and in biofeedback therapy.[2] Many colorectal surgeons find that anal ultrasound compliments rather than replaces EMG. The former test offers gross anatomic information while the latter evaluation reveals more about function rather than structure.

Anatomic Assessment

Endoanal Ultrasound

Endoanal ultrasound is described in more detail in Chap. 7. Endoanal ultrasound is one of the most reliable tests in identifying anatomic defects (Figure 4-6) in the anal sphincters with a high sensitivity and specificity when conducted by experienced

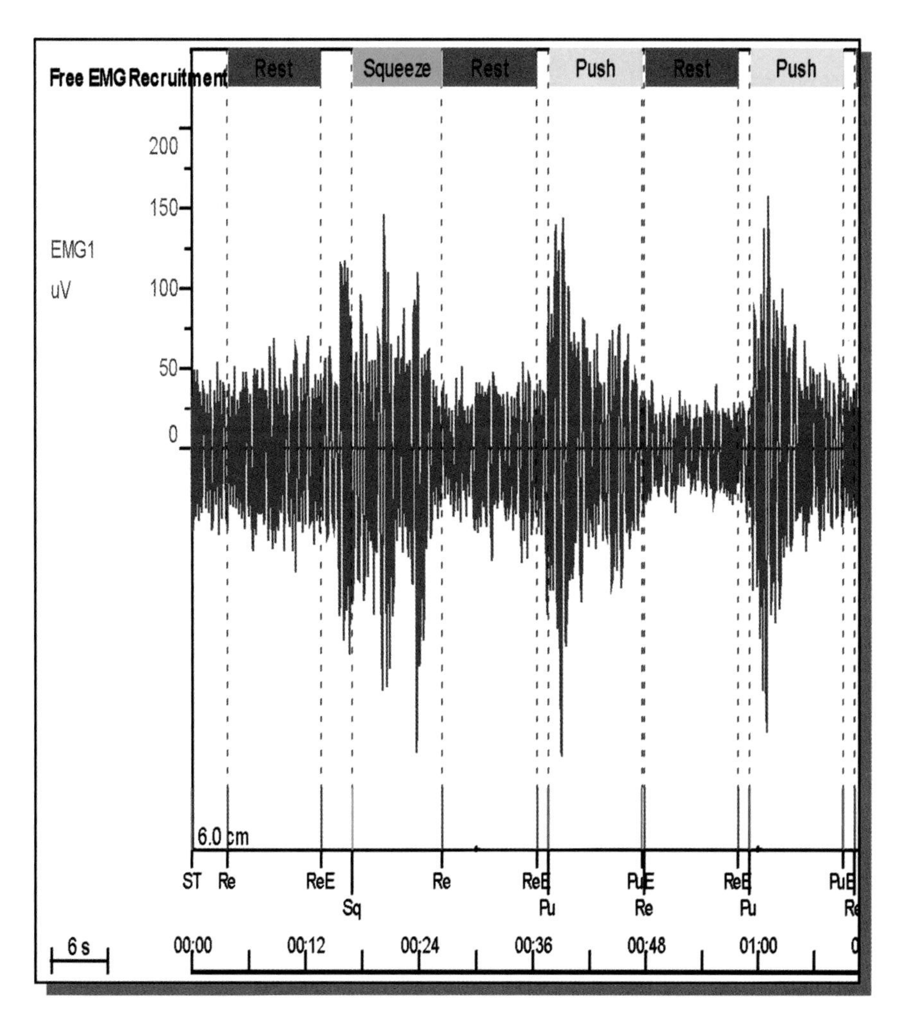

FIGURE 4-4. Electromyography recruitment demonstrates paradoxic reaction, since the activity is increased at "push."

investigators.[58–62] Usually, a 7- or 10-MHz frequency endoanal probe is used for imaging of the sphincters. The latter provides a higher resolution and hence a superior picture quality. The transducer provides a 360° view of the anal canal.

The main indication for endoanal ultrasound is to diagnose defects in the IAS and/or EAS.[62–64] A high correlation between histologic and intraoperative findings has been suggested.[58,65,66] The investigation and the interpretation of the procedure is operator dependent, especially considering evaluation of the EAS.[67] By using three-dimensional endoanal ultrasound, visualization of the EAS anatomy is facilitated and the diagnostic accuracy of detecting EAS abnormalities might improve[68] and anal EMG right at some point in the future be rendered superior.

Endoanal ultrasound can be used as a tool in selecting patients for surgical repair and for assessing the postoperative results.[69–71] Recently, ultrasound has been introduced to document other injuries in the pelvic floor and pelvic prolapse.

Magnetic Resonance Imaging

During the past two decades magnetic resonance imaging (MRI) has become increasingly used to image the anal canal and the pelvic floor muscles. Images can be generated either with use of an endoanal coil or use of an external phased array coil. These two techniques are comparable in diagnosing anal sphincter defects and EAS atrophy,[72] although MRI using an endoanal coil usually are restricted to specialized centers and might be associated with some discomfort when the coil is introduced.

There is no consensus regarding the use of MRI vs. endoanal ultrasound. Some authors recommend the use of endoanal ultrasound as the primary tool in the identification of sphincter injuries and to reserve MRI to be used as a complimentary technique to exclude patients with EAS atrophy in patients considered for surgical anal sphincter repair.[73]

Tests of Function and Structure

The dynamic nature of some of the anorectal disorders, such as rectal intussusception and rectal prolapse, requires a combination of dynamic and structural imaging modalities. Fluoroscopic defecography and MR defecography are methods that can be used to assess the dynamics of the pelvic floor function.

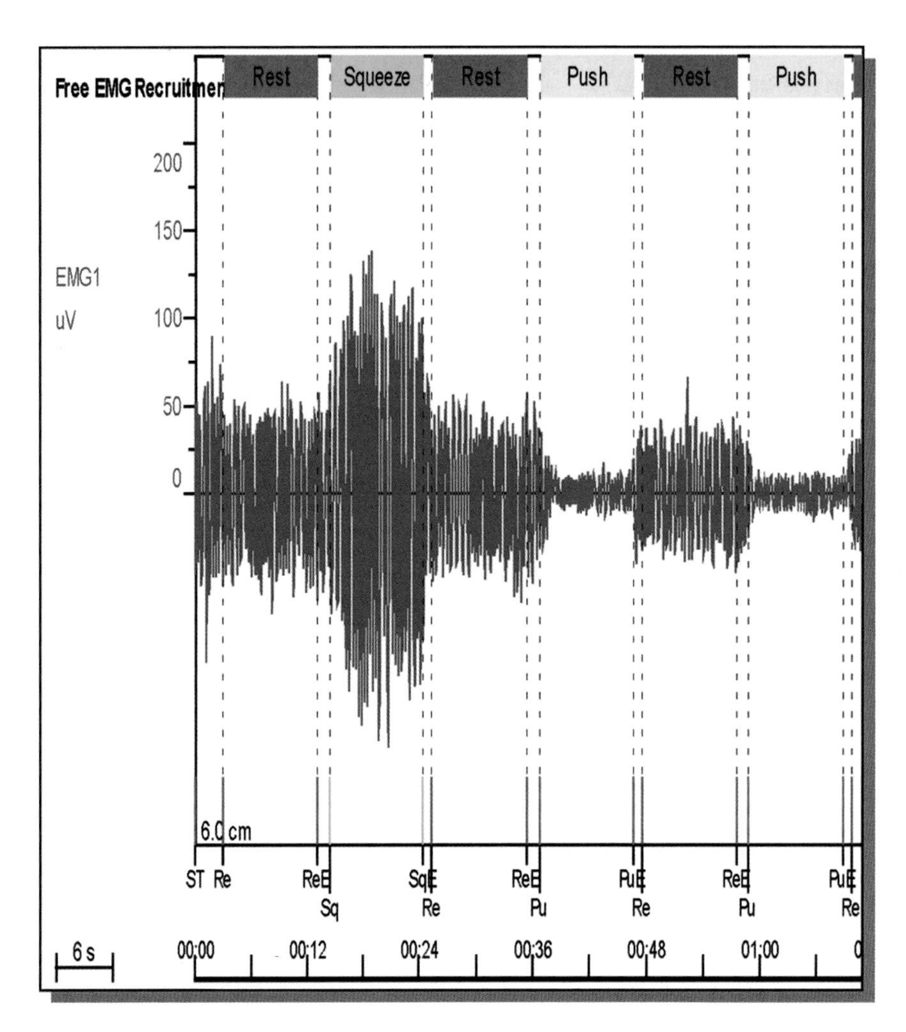

FIGURE 4-5. Electromyography recruitment demonstrates normal reaction, since the activity is increased at "squeeze" and decreased at "push."

Dynamic Fluoroscopic Defecography

Fluoroscopic defecography is a dynamic radiologic test providing morphologic information about the anal canal, rectum, vagina, and the pelvic floor during the defecation maneuver.[74–76] Defecography involves filling of the rectum and if possible also the vagina with contrast. Some centers advocate use of contrast in the small bowel, the bladder, and even the peritoneal cavity.[77,78] The primary indication for defecography is evaluation of patients with outlet obstruction and prolapse. The technique can visualize the defecation process, identify signs of nonrelaxation, and visualize various anatomic abnormalities.

It should be remembered that patients may feel embarrassed by the nature of the test. This reluctance may result in a false-positive test result of pelvic floor relaxation and a false-negative assessment of anatomic abnormalities because of insufficient rectal emptying.[32,79] Another limitation of defecography is an interobserver variation in interpreting results.[80,81] There is also high incidence of "abnormal findings" in both patients with symptoms[82] and in subjects without symptoms.[83]

Anorectal Angle and Rectal Emptying

The anorectal angle is the angle between the anal canal and rectum.[11] The action of the puborectalis muscle during straining decreases this angle from 75–90° in resting to 90–110°, and the angle increases to 110–180° at evacuation. The anorectal angle is believed to play a role in maintaining continence. The quantification of the anorectal angle in defecography has somewhat limited clinical value due to a high observer variation.[81,84]

The ability to relax the puborectalis muscle, and increase the anorectal angle, is pivotal for the evacuation process. A persistent contraction of the puborectalis muscle during the evacuation process is consistent with nonrelaxing pelvic floor, which is also named anismus or paradoxic contraction of the pelvic floor.[85]

Rectal emptying should be rapid (<30 s) and complete (<10% residual contrast). In patients with evacuation difficulties, emptying is frequently achieved in small portions. Perineal descent during emptying is measured relative to a line drawn in between the tip of the coccyx and the pubis bone (the pubococcygeal line). During squeezing the pelvic floor will rise and during straining and evacuation it will descend.

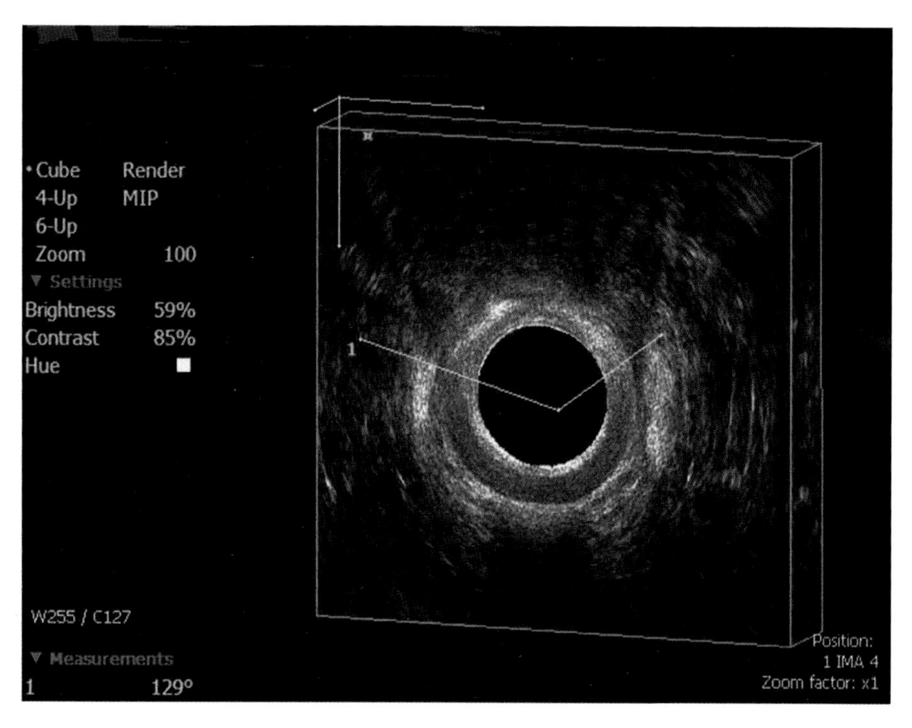

FIGURE 4-6. Sphincter defect in the anterior aspect.

Rectal Intussusception and Rectal Prolapse

Rectal intussusception is a circumferential infolding of the entire thickness of the rectal wall not extending beyond the anal verge, while a rectal prolapse is a protrusion of the entire thickness of the rectal wall extending through and beyond the anal verge.[86]

Rectal intussusception is difficult to diagnose at clinical examination. Defecography can sometimes help in the differentiation between a small rectal prolapse from large hemorrhoids, which sometimes can be difficult. A more important indication for defecography in patients with rectal prolapse at clinical examination is the ability to identify patients with concomitant enterocele or vaginal prolapse that may need surgical attention at the same time as the prolapse repair.

Rectocele

Rectocele is a herniation of the anterior rectal wall into the vagina. The bulge in the anterior part of the distal rectum should be ≥3 cm. Rectoceles are common in both patients and asymptomatic subjects. Barium trapping in the rectocele or facilitation of emptying by digital support of the posterior vagina wall is used by some surgeons to define surgical candidates for rectocele repair.

Peritoneocele, Enterocele, and Sigmoidocele

A peritoneocele is a peritoneal herniation extending the pouch of Douglas below the upper third of the vaginal length and at the same time increasing the distance between the rectum and vagina.[77,87] An enterocele is formed when small bowel descends into the peritoneocele and a sigmoidocele is formed when the sigmoid colon descends into the peritoneocele.[88]

Dynamic MR Defecography

The development of dynamic MR defecography has flourished after the development of fast MRI sequences enabling dynamic evaluation of the pelvic floor. A comprehensive evaluation of the anatomy and function can be obtained by repeating scans during rest, squeezing, straining, and evacuation. The best results are obtained when contrast (usually sonographic gel) is used and emptied. Several of the above-mentioned "abnormalities" are seen only if emptying is obtained.[89]

Dynamic MR defecography can be performed with open- or closed-configuration units. The open-configuration MRI unit, where the patient is sitting during the investigation, is superior to the closed-configuration unit. This equipment is, however, expensive and not readily available in most institutions. The image quality is usually also inferior in open-configuration units, when compared with closed-configuration units. However, closed unit MRI has the disadvantage of only permitting patients to be investigated in a supine position. The influence of having the patient emptying the rectum in the supine position is debated. Some studies report that this has limited influence on the results obtained, with the exception of identifying rectal intussusceptions.[90,91] Dynamic MRI defecography is a nonionizing investigation and provides the investigator with a dynamic picture of the complete pelvic floor and pelvic organs. This can be useful in preoperative planning since concomitant findings are common in patients with pelvic floor disorders. In one study, it was noted that dynamic MRI defecography changed the type of surgical therapy in 67% of evaluated patients with fecal incontinence.[92] Dynamic MRI defecography might be a more accurate tool to diagnose rectal intussusception than conventional defecography[93,94] and to differentiate mucosal prolapse from full-thickness intussusceptions.[95]

Gastrointestinal Transit Studies

Most of the previously mentioned tests are focused on evaluating the function and/or the anatomy of the rectum, the pelvic floor, and the surrounding organs. Transit studies provide an objective evaluation of the gastrointestinal motility, which is of paramount importance for stool consistency and in facilitating defecation through the "recto-colic reflex."[96] Marker studies and scintigraphy techniques provide estimation of transit times. Recently, a new technique with a wireless capsule (SmartPill®) has been introduced as an instrument for investigating gastrointestinal transit time.

Colonic Markers Study

The most commonly used method for diagnosing patients with slow transit constipation is based on (usually 24 markers) radio-opaque markers. This is a simple technique that requires the patient to ingest a capsule containing radio-opaque markers. Five days after the ingestion of the capsule, a plain supine radiograph is obtained to determine the position and the number of remaining markers.[97] The test is considered to be normal if five or fewer markers (≤20%) still are present in the colon. If more than five markers are present in the colon, the transit time is considered to be prolonged. If the markers are predominantly present in the distal colon, this may suggest a pelvic floor problem resulting in obstructed defecation. If the markers are more diffusely distributed in the colon, this finding may be a sign of gastrointestinal dysmotility or colon inertia.

Alternatives to the above-mentioned technique are used by some centers. Some use an image obtained on the seventh day and others ask the patient to ingest markers over a number of days.[98] An additional variation has the patient ingest markers on Sunday evening and obtain an abdominal X-ray on Monday morning, Wednesday, and Friday. The initial film serves as a gross screening test of gastric and small bowel motility. Patients with normal upper gastrointestinal motility will have all markers in the colon on this first film.

Small bowel transit can be evaluated with oral lactulose ingestion followed by measurement of breath hydrogen excretion. Basically the lactulose ferments in the cecum to release hydrogen allowing inexpensive, safe, rapid and reproducible measurement of orocecal transit time.[99]

Radionuclide Gamma Scintigraphy of the Colon

Radionuclide gamma scintigraphy of the colon is a more complex and expensive evaluation of the colonic transit time compared to colonic marker study and the technique is only available at specialized centers with access to nuclear imaging equipment. By ingestion of a radiolabeled isotope, the colon can be visualized with a gamma camera and frequent scans can be obtained. Scintigraphy provides a quantitative segmental picture of the colon and can potentially provide information about the variability of the motility in different colon segments.[100]

SmartPill®

SmartPill® is a wireless monitoring system built inside a pill that measures temperature, intraluminal pressure, and pH and is recorded by a portable receiver. The capsule is ingested by the patient and a drop in pH and a change in motility delineates the transition from the distal ileum into the cecum. From these data, whole gut transit and colonic transit can be separated and calculated. SmartPill has been compared with colonic scintigraphy and seems to be a promising tool to diagnose and evaluate patients suffering from slow transit constipation,[101,102] but more studies are needed to prove its clinical applicability and utility.

Acknowledgments. This chapter was written by Lee E. Smith and Garnet J. Blatchford in the first edition of this textbook.

References

1. Whitehead W, Wald A, Diamant N, Enck P, Pemberton J, Rao S. Functional disorders of the anus and rectum. Gut. 1999;45 Suppl 2:II55–9.
2. Diamant N, Kamm M, Wald A, Whitehead W. AGA technical review on anorectal testing techniques. Gastroenterology. 1999;116:735–60.
3. Rao S, Hatfield R, Soffer E, Rao S, Beaty J, Conklin J. Manometric tests of anorectal function in healthy adults. Am J Gastroenterol. 1999;94:773–83.
4. Scott S, Gladman M. Manometric, sensorimotor, and neurophysiologic evaluation of anorectal function. Gastroenterol Clin North Am. 2008;37:511–38. vii.
5. Rao S, Azpiroz F, Diamant N, Enck P, Tougas G, Wald A. Minimum standards of anorectal manometry. Neurogastroenterol Motil. 2002;14:553–9.
6. Corrazziari E. Anorectal manometry: a round table discussion. Gastroenterol Int. 1989;2:115–7.
7. Lestar B, Penninckx F, Kerremans R. The composition of anal basal pressure. An in vivo and in vitro study in man. Int J Colorectal Dis. 1989;4:118–22.
8. Sun W, Rao S. Manometric assessment of anorectal function. Gastroenterol Clin North Am. 2001;30:15–32.
9. Rasmussen O. Anorectal function. Dis Colon Rectum. 1994;37:386–403.
10. Read N, Sun W. Anorectal manometry. In: Henry M, Swash M, editors. Coloproctology and the pelvic floor. Oxford: Butterworth-Heinemann Ltd; 1992. p. 119–45.
11. Lowry A, Simmang C, Boulos P, Farmer K, Finan P, Hyman N, et al. Consensus statement of definitions for anorectal

physiology and rectal cancer: report of the tripartite consensus conference on definitions for anorectal physiology and rectal cancer, Washington, D.C., May 1, 1999. Dis Colon Rectum. 2001;44:915–9.
12. Taylor B, Beart RJ, Phillips S. Longitudinal and radial variations of pressure in the human anal sphincter. Gastroenterology. 1984;86:693–7.
13. Bharucha A. Fecal incontinence. Gastroenterology. 2003; 124:1672–85.
14. McHugh S, Diamant N. Anal canal pressure profile: a reappraisal as determined by rapid pullthrough technique. Gut. 1987;28:1234–41.
15. Read N, Harford W, Schmulen A, Read M, Santa Ana C, Fordtran J. A clinical study of patients with fecal incontinence and diarrhea. Gastroenterology. 1979;76:747–56.
16. Hiltunen K. Anal manometric findings in patients with anal incontinence. Dis Colon Rectum. 1985;28:925–8.
17. Telford K, Ali A, Lymer K, Hosker G, Kiff E, Hill J. Fatigability of the external anal sphincter in anal incontinence. Dis Colon Rectum. 2004;47:746–52. discussion 52.
18. Marcello P, Barrett R, Coller J, Schoetz DJ, Roberts P, Murray J, et al. Fatigue rate index as a new measurement of external sphincter function. Dis Colon Rectum. 1998;41:336–43.
19. Meunier P, Mollard P. Control of the internal anal sphincter (manometric study with human subjects). Pflugers Arch. 1977;370:233–9.
20. Gowers W. The automatic action of the sphincter ani. Proc R Soc Lond. 1878;26:77–84.
21. Whitehead W, Orr W, Engel B, Schuster M. External anal sphincter response to rectal distention: learned response or reflex. Psychophysiology. 1982;19:57–62.
22. Aaronson I, Nixon H. A clinical evaluation of anorectal pressure studies in the diagnosis of Hirschsprung's disease. Gut. 1972;13:138–46.
23. Meunier P, Marechal J, Mollard P. Accuracy of the manometric diagnosis of Hirschsprung's disease. J Pediatr Surg. 1978;13:411–5.
24. Wu J, Schoetz DJ, Coller J, Veidenheimer M. Treatment of Hirschsprung's disease in the adult. Report of five cases. Dis Colon Rectum. 1995;38:655–9.
25. Azpiroz F, Enck P, Whitehead W. Anorectal functional testing: review of collective experience. Am J Gastroenterol. 2002;97:232–40.
26. Sun W, Read N, Prior A, Daly J, Cheah S, Grundy D. Sensory and motor responses to rectal distention vary according to rate and pattern of balloon inflation. Gastroenterology. 1990;99:1008–15.
27. Varma J, Smith A. Reproducibility of the proctometrogram. Gut. 1986;27:288–92.
28. Sun W, Read N, Miner P. Relation between rectal sensation and anal function in normal subjects and patients with faecal incontinence. Gut. 1990;31:1056–61.
29. Chan C, Scott S, Williams N, Lunniss P. Rectal hypersensitivity worsens stool frequency, urgency, and lifestyle in patients with urge fecal incontinence. Dis Colon Rectum. 2005;48:134–40.
30. Gladman M, Scott S, Chan C, Williams N, Lunniss P. Rectal hyposensitivity: prevalence and clinical impact in patients with intractable constipation and fecal incontinence. Dis Colon Rectum. 2003;46:238–46.
31. Read N, Timms J, Barfield L, Donnelly T, Bannister J. Impairment of defecation in young women with severe constipation. Gastroenterology. 1986;90:53–60.
32. Beck DE. A simplified balloon expulsion test. Dis Colon Rectum. 1992;35:597–8.
33. Voderholzer W, Neuhaus D, Klauser A, Tzavella K, Müller-Lissner S, Schindlbeck N. Paradoxical sphincter contraction is rarely indicative of anismus. Gut. 1997;41:258–62.
34. Duthie G, Bartolo D. Anismus: the cause of constipation? Results of investigation and treatment. World J Surg. 1992;16:831–5.
35. López A, Holmström B, Nilsson B, Dolk A, Johansson C, Schultz I, et al. Paradoxical sphincter reaction is influenced by rectal filling volume. Dis Colon Rectum. 1998;41:1017–22.
36. Pezim M, Pemberton J, Levin K, Litchy W, Phillips S. Parameters of anorectal and colonic motility in health and in severe constipation. Dis Colon Rectum. 1993;36:484–91.
37. Rao S. Diagnosis and management of fecal incontinence. American College of Gastroenterology Practice Parameters Committee. Am J Gastroenterol. 2004;99:1585–604.
38. Haynes W, Read N. Ano-rectal activity in man during rectal infusion of saline: a dynamic assessment of the anal continence mechanism. J Physiol. 1982;330:45–56.
39. Read N, Haynes W, Bartolo D, Hall J, Read M, Donnelly T, et al. Use of anorectal manometry during rectal infusion of saline to investigate sphincter function in incontinent patients. Gastroenterology. 1983;85:105–13.
40. Henry M, Parks A, Swash M. The pelvic floor musculature in the descending perineum syndrome. Br J Surg. 1982;69:470–2.
41. Oettle G, Roe A, Bartolo D, Mortensen N. What is the best way of measuring perineal descent? A comparison of radiographic and clinical methods. Br J Surg. 1985;72:999–1001.
42. Cheong D, Vaccaro C, Salanga V, Wexner S, Phillips R, Hanson M, et al. Electrodiagnostic evaluation of fecal incontinence. Muscle Nerve. 1995;18:612–9.
43. Hill J, Hosker G, Kiff E. Pudendal nerve terminal motor latency measurements: what they do and do not tell us. Br J Surg. 2002;89:1268–9.
44. Wexner S, Marchetti F, Salanga V, Corredor C, Jagelman D. Neurophysiologic assessment of the anal sphincters. Dis Colon Rectum. 1991;34:606–12.
45. Bharucha A. Outcome measures for fecal incontinence: anorectal structure and function. Gastroenterology. 2004;126:S90–8.
46. Rasmussen O, Christiansen J, Tetzschner T, Sørensen M. Pudendal nerve function in idiopathic fecal incontinence. Dis Colon Rectum. 2000;43:633–6. discussion 6–7.
47. Madoff R, Parker S, Varma M, Lowry A. Faecal incontinence in adults. Lancet. 2004;364:621–32.
48. Scott M, Lunniss P. Investigations of anorectal function. London: Springer London; 2007.
49. Swash M. Electromyography in pelvic floor disorders. 2nd ed. Oxford: Butterworth-Heinemann Ltd; 1992.
50. Sørensen M, Tetzschner T, Rasmussen O, Christiansen J. Relation between electromyography and anal manometry of the external anal sphincter. Gut. 1991;32:1031–4.
51. Pinho M, Hosie K, Bielecki K, Keighley M. Assessment of noninvasive intra-anal electromyography to evaluate sphincter function. Dis Colon Rectum. 1991;34:69–71.
52. Neill M, Swash M. Increased motor unit fibre density in the external anal sphincter muscle in ano-rectal incontinence:

a single fibre EMG study. J Neurol Neurosurg Psychiatry. 1980;43:343–7.

53. Rogers J, Laurberg S, Misiewicz J, Henry M, Swash M. Anorectal physiology validated: a repeatability study of the motor and sensory tests of anorectal function. Br J Surg. 1989;76:607–9.
54. Bartolo D, Jarratt J, Read M, Donnelly T, Read N. The role of partial denervation of the puborectalis in idiopathic faecal incontinence. Br J Surg. 1983;70:664–7.
55. Rogers J, Levy D, Henry M, Misiewicz J. Pelvic floor neuropathy: a comparative study of diabetes mellitus and idiopathic faecal incontinence. Gut. 1988;29:756–61.
56. Womack N, Morrison J, Williams N. The role of pelvic floor denervation in the aetiology of idiopathic faecal incontinence. Br J Surg. 1986;73:404–7.
57. Infantino A, Melega E, Negrin P, Masin A, Carnio S, Lise M. Striated anal sphincter electromyography in idiopathic fecal incontinence. Dis Colon Rectum. 1995;38:27–31.
58. Burnett S, Speakman C, Kamm M, Bartram C. Confirmation of endosonographic detection of external anal sphincter defects by simultaneous electromyographic mapping. Br J Surg. 1991;78:448–50.
59. Sultan A, Kamm M, Talbot I, Nicholls R, Bartram C. Anal endosonography for identifying external sphincter defects confirmed histologically. Br J Surg. 1994;81:463–5.
60. Law P, Kamm M, Bartram C. A comparison between electromyography and anal endosonography in mapping external anal sphincter defects. Dis Colon Rectum. 1990;33:370–3.
61. Felt-Bersma R, van Baren R, Koorevaar M, Strijers R, Cuesta M. Unsuspected sphincter defects shown by anal endosonography after anorectal surgery. A prospective study. Dis Colon Rectum. 1995;38:249–53.
62. Felt-Bersma R, Cuesta M, Koorevaar M, Strijers R, Meuwissen S, Dercksen E, et al. Anal endosonography: relationship with anal manometry and neurophysiologic tests. Dis Colon Rectum. 1992;35:944–9.
63. Tjandra J, Milsom J, Schroeder T, Fazio V. Endoluminal ultrasound is preferable to electromyography in mapping anal sphincteric defects. Dis Colon Rectum. 1993;36:689–92.
64. Enck P, von Giesen H, Schäfer A, Heyer T, Gantke B, Flesch S, et al. Comparison of anal sonography with conventional needle electromyography in the evaluation of anal sphincter defects. Am J Gastroenterol. 1996;91:2539–43.
65. Deen K, Kumar D, Williams J, Olliff J, Keighley M. Anal sphincter defects. Correlation between endoanal ultrasound and surgery. Ann Surg. 1993;218:201–5.
66. Sentovich S, Wong W, Blatchford G. Accuracy and reliability of transanal ultrasound for anterior anal sphincter injury. Dis Colon Rectum. 1998;41:1000–4.
67. Emblem R, Dhaenens G, Stien R, Mørkrid L, Aasen A, Bergan A. The importance of anal endosonography in the evaluation of idiopathic fecal incontinence. Dis Colon Rectum. 1994;37:42–8.
68. Cazemier M, Terra M, Stoker J, de Lange de Klerk E, Boeckxstaens G, Mulder C, et al. Atrophy and defects detection of the external anal sphincter: comparison between three-dimensional anal endosonography and endoanal magnetic resonance imaging. Dis Colon Rectum. 2006;49:20–7.
69. Engel A, Kamm M, Sultan A, Bartram C, Nicholls R. Anterior anal sphincter repair in patients with obstetric trauma. Br J Surg. 1994;81:1231–4.
70. Sultan A, Kamm M, Hudson C, Bartram C. Third degree obstetric anal sphincter tears: risk factors and outcome of primary repair. BMJ. 1994;308:887–91.
71. Dobben A, Terra M, Deutekom M, Slors J, Janssen L, Bossuyt P, et al. The role of endoluminal imaging in clinical outcome of overlapping anterior anal sphincter repair in patients with fecal incontinence. AJR Am J Roentgenol. 2007;189:W70–7.
72. Terra M, Beets-Tan R, van der Hulst V, Dijkgraaf M, Bossuyt P, Dobben A, et al. Anal sphincter defects in patients with fecal incontinence: endoanal versus external phased-array MR imaging. Radiology. 2005;236:886–95.
73. Terra M, Beets-Tan R, van der Hulst V, Deutekom M, Dijkgraaf M, Bossuyt P, et al. MRI in evaluating atrophy of the external anal sphincter in patients with fecal incontinence. AJR Am J Roentgenol. 2006;187:991–9.
74. Ekberg O, Nylander G, Fork F. Defecography. Radiology. 1985;155:45–8.
75. Mahieu P, Pringot J, Bodart P. Defecography: I. Description of a new procedure and results in normal patients. Gastrointest Radiol. 1984;9:247–51.
76. Mahieu P, Pringot J, Bodart P. Defecography: II. Contribution to the diagnosis of defecation disorders. Gastrointest Radiol. 1984;9:253–61.
77. Bremmer S, Mellgren A, Holmström B, Udén R. Peritoneocele and enterocele. Formation and transformation during rectal evacuation as studied by means of defaeco-peritoneography. Acta Radiol. 1998;39:167–75.
78. Bremmer S, Mellgren A, Holmström B, López A, Udén R. Peritoneocele: visualization with defecography and peritoneography performed simultaneously. Radiology. 1997;202:373–7.
79. Schouten W, Briel J, Auwerda J, van Dam J, Gosselink M, Ginai A, et al. Anismus: fact or fiction? Dis Colon Rectum. 1997;40:1033–41.
80. Müller-Lissner S, Bartolo D, Christiansen J, Ekberg O, Goei R, Höpfner W, et al. Interobserver agreement in defecography – an international study. Z Gastroenterol. 1998;36:273–9.
81. Ferrante S, Perry R, Schreiman J, Cheng S, Frick M. The reproducibility of measuring the anorectal angle in defecography. Dis Colon Rectum. 1991;34:51–5.
82. Mellgren A, Bremmer S, Johansson C, Dolk A, Udén R, Ahlbäck S, et al. Defecography. Results of investigations in 2,816 patients. Dis Colon Rectum. 1994;37:1133–41.
83. Shorvon P, McHugh S, Diamant N, Somers S, Stevenson G. Defecography in normal volunteers: results and implications. Gut. 1989;30:1737–49.
84. Penninckx F, Debruyne C, Lestar B, Kerremans R. Observer variation in the radiological measurement of the anorectal angle. Int J Colorectal Dis. 1990;5:94–7.
85. Halligan S, Bartram C, Park H, Kamm M. Proctographic features of anismus. Radiology. 1995;197:679–82.
86. Bremmer S, Udén R, Mellgren A. Defaeco-peritoneography in the diagnosis of rectal intussusception and rectal prolapse. Acta Radiol. 1997;38:578–83.
87. Bremmer S. Peritoneocele. A radiological study with defaeco-peritoneography. Acta Radiol Suppl. 1998;413:1–33.
88. Jorge JM, Yang YK, Wexner SD. Incidence and clinical significance of sigmoidoceles as determined by a new classification system. Dis Colon Rectum. 1994;37(11):1112–7.

89. Vanbeckevoort D, Van Hoe L, Oyen R, Ponette E, De Ridder D, Deprest J. Pelvic floor descent in females: comparative study of colpocystodefecography and dynamic fast MR imaging. J Magn Reson Imaging. 1999;9:373–7.
90. Bharucha A. Update of tests of colon and rectal structure and function. J Clin Gastroenterol. 2006;40:96–103.
91. Fielding J, Griffiths D, Versi E, Mulkern R, Lee M, Jolesz F. MR imaging of pelvic floor continence mechanisms in the supine and sitting positions. AJR Am J Roentgenol. 1998;171:1607–10.
92. Hetzer F, Andreisek G, Tsagari C, Sahrbacher U, Weishaupt D. MR defecography in patients with fecal incontinence: imaging findings and their effect on surgical management. Radiology. 2006;240:449–57.
93. Lamb G, de Jode M, Gould S, Spouse E, Birnie K, Darzi A, et al. Upright dynamic MR defaecating proctography in an open configuration MR system. Br J Radiol. 2000;73:152–5.
94. Roos J, Weishaupt D, Wildermuth S, Willmann J, Marincek B, Hilfiker P. Experience of 4 years with open MR defecography: pictorial review of anorectal anatomy and disease. Radiographics. 2002;22:817–32.
95. Bharucha A, Fletcher J, Seide B, Riederer S, Zinsmeister A. Phenotypic variation in functional disorders of defecation. Gastroenterology. 2005;128:1199–210.
96. Shafik A. Recto-colic reflex: role in the defecation mechanism. Int Surg. 1996;81:292–4.
97. Martelli H, Devroede G, Arhan P, Duguay C, Dornic C, Faverdin C. Some parameters of large bowel motility in normal man. Gastroenterology. 1978;75:612–8.
98. Metcalf A, Phillips S, Zinsmeister A, MacCarty R, Beart R, Wolff B. Simplified assessment of segmental colonic transit. Gastroenterology. 1987;92:40–7.
99. Jorge JM, Wexner SD, Ehrenpreis ED. The lactulose hydrogen breath test as a measure of orocaecal transit time. Eur J Surg. 1994;160(8):409–16.
100. Lundin E, Karlbom U, Westlin J, Kairemo K, Jung B, Husin S, et al. Scintigraphic assessment of slow transit constipation with special reference to right- or left-sided colonic delay. Colorectal Dis. 2004;6:499–505.
101. Maqbool S, Parkman H, Friedenberg F. Wireless capsule motility: comparison of the SmartPill GI monitoring system with scintigraphy for measuring whole gut transit. Dig Dis Sci. 2009;54:2167–74.
102. Rao SS, Kuo B, McCallum RW, Chey WD, Dibaise JK, Hasler WL, et al. Investigation of colonic and whole gut transit with wireless motility capsule and radioopaque markers in constipation. Clin Gastroenterol Hepatol. 2009;7:537–44.

5 Endoscopy

Charles B. Whitlow

The large intestine from cecum to anus can be effectively and accurately examined as part of a complete physical examination. An ultimate diagnosis of large bowel diseases can only be made by direct observation of the abnormalities and, if indicated, a biopsy. Different equipment is designed and used for different purposes.

Anoscopy

Anoscopy is the examination of the anal canal. The lower part of the rectal mucosa, upper anal mucosa, anoderm, dentate line, internal and external hemorrhoids can be seen through this examination.

There are basically two types of anoscopes: Beveled type such as the Buie or Hirschman scope (Figure 5-1) and the lighted Welch-Allyn scope (Figure 5-2) that uses the same light source as the rigid proctosigmoidoscope. Another type is the side-opening Vernon-David scope with Hirschman handle (Figure 5-3). The Hinkel-James anoscope (Figure 5-4) is much longer than the Vernon-David scope and is suitable for patients with deep buttock cheeks.

Indication

Any anal and perianal diseases or conditions require a full examination of the anal canal. These include anal fissures, anal fistulas, anal Crohn's disease, anal tumors, hemorrhoids, anal condyloma, bright red rectal bleeding and pruritus ani. Anoscopy is frequently used in conjunction with colonoscopy, flexible sigmoidoscopy, and rigid proctosigmoidoscopy as part of the examination.

Contraindications

Patients who have severe anal pain such as an acute anal fissure or a perianal or intersphincteric abscess may not tolerate the examination. In general, if a patient can tolerate a digital examination, anoscopy can usually be done. A 2% lidocaine jelly should be used in patients with anal pain. Anal stricture or severe anal stenosis is another contraindication.

Preparation

No preparation is required.

Positioning

A prone jackknife position gives the best exposure. An alternative is the left-lateral recumbent (Simms) position.

Technique

The Vernon-David, which is a side-opening endoscope, gives the best examination. Inspection of the anal area should always precede any other examination and, for this, good lighting is essential. The cheeks of the buttock are gently spread to gain exposure. Skin tags, excoriation and change in color or thickness of the anal verge and perianal skin can be detected quickly. A scar, patulous, or irregularly shaped anus may give clues to the cause of anal incontinence. Particularly in multiparous women, the anal verge may be pushed down too far during straining – a feature of the perineal descent syndrome. When the anal verge is scratched or pricked with a needle, the external sphincter visibly contracts because of the anal reflex. It is useful for testing the sensibility of the anal canal, which may be absent in areas of previous scar or defect, or in patients with an underlying neuropathy.

The next step is to do a digital examination. The index finger should be well lubricated with a lubricant jelly, and the finger pressed on the anal aperture to "warn" the patient. Then the finger should be gradually inserted and swept all around the anal canal to detect any mass or induration. In men, the prostate should be felt. In women, the posterior vaginal wall should be pushed anteriorly to detect any evidence of a rectocele. Anal tone, whether tight or loose, can be easily estimated. A stricture or narrowing from scarring or a defect in the internal or external sphincters from a

D.E. Beck et al. (eds.), *The ASCRS Textbook of Colon and Rectal Surgery: Second Edition*,
DOI 10.1007/978-1-4419-1584-9_5, © Springer Science+Business Media, LLC 2011

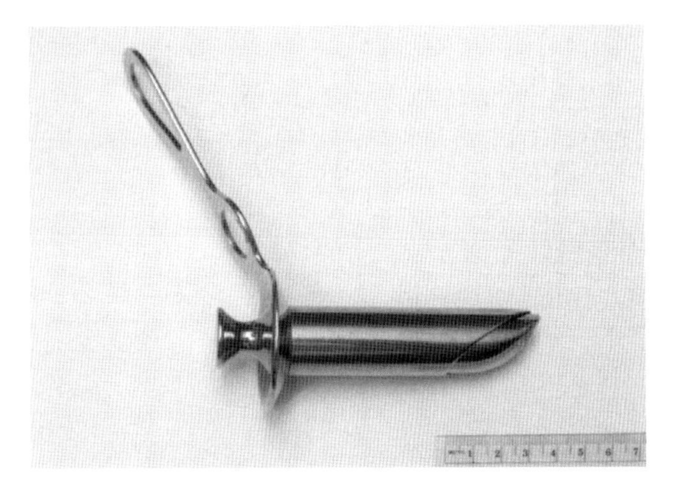

FIGURE 5-1. Buie anoscope.

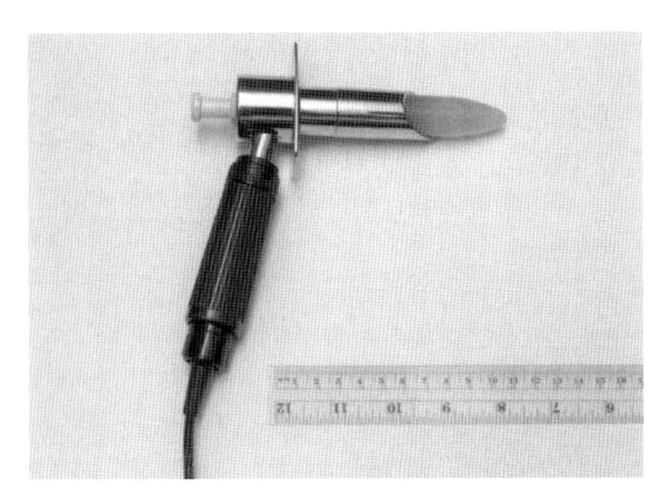

FIGURE 5-2. Lighted Welch-Allyn anoscope.

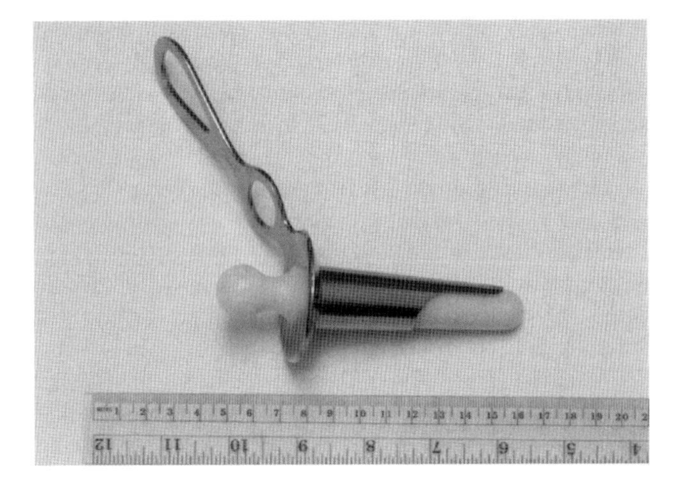

FIGURE 5-3. Vernon-David with Hirschman handle anoscope.

previous operation can be felt. A fibrous cord or induration in the anal area and the anal canal may indicate a fistulous tract. The external sphincter, puborectalis, and levator ani muscles can also be appreciated by digital examination.

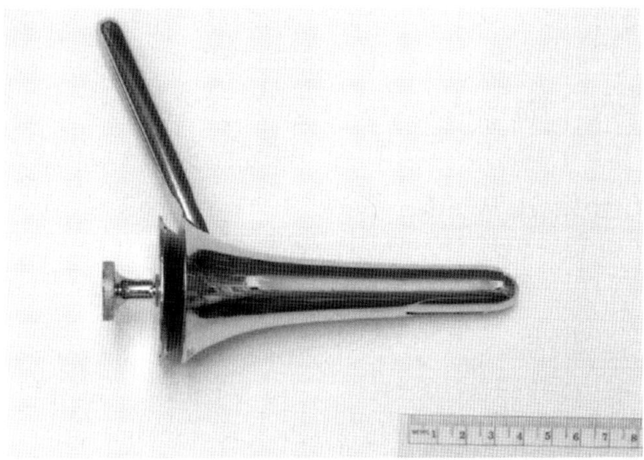

FIGURE 5-4. Hinkel-James anoscope.

When the puborectalis is pulled in the posterior quadrant, the anus will gape but will close immediately when the traction is released. Persistence of the gaping indicates an abnormal reflex pathway in the thoracolumbar region frequently seen in paraplegic patients. The finger should press gently on these muscles for signs of tenderness. When the person with good anal function is asked to contract the muscles, the examiner not only feels the squeeze of the muscle on the examining finger but also feels the finger pulled forward by the puborectalis muscle.

Insertion of the anoscope should always be done with the obturator in place. The obturator is removed during examination and reinserted to rotate the instrument to another area. In patients with redundant mucosa, reinsertion of the obturator may cause discomfort if the mucosa gets trapped between the obturator and the anoscope. However, if the beveled type of endoscope is used, the endoscope can be rotated without having to reinsert the obturator. If an inverted (jackknife) position is used, the examination table need not be tipped down more than 10–15°. If a left-lateral position is used, an assistant needs to pull up the right cheek of the buttock for exposure. During examination, the patient is asked to strain with the anoscope sliding out to detect any prolapse of the rectal mucosa and the anal cushion. Excoriation, metaplastic changes, and friable mucosa indicate a prolapsed hemorrhoid.

Biopsies may be taken via the anoscope. Care should be taken to have adequate lighting and suction as needed. Local anesthesia is necessary for biopsies of lesions in the anal canal, including the sensate area extending 1–2 cm proximal to the dentate line.

Complications

Anal tear, especially at the posterior midline, can occur in patients with anal stenosis. Additionally, friable hemorrhoids may bleed from contact with the anoscope.

Rigid Proctosigmoidoscopy

Three sizes of rigid proctosigmoidoscope are available (Figure 5-5). A 19 mm×25 cm scope is the standard size for a general examination and for polypectomy or electrocoagulation. A 15 mm×25 cm endoscope is an ideal size for general examination. It is much better tolerated by the patient, causing less spasm of the rectum and thus, minimal air insufflation, yet enables as adequate an examination as the standard-size endoscope. An 11 mm×25 cm endoscope should be available for examining the patient who has anal or rectal stricture, such as Crohn's disease. Some physicians and surgeons prefer a disposable standard-size rigid proctosigmoidoscope for routine examination.

Indications

Rigid proctosigmoidoscopy has largely been replaced by flexible sigmoidoscopy. However, rigid proctosigmoidoscopy is still useful in examination of the anorectum. One of its advantages is that any blood clots or stool can easily be washed out. In fact, in a patient who has massive gastrointestinal bleeding, a rigid proctosigmoidoscopy is the first line of examination to rule out the source of bleeding in the anorectum.

A rigid proctosigmoidoscopy is used when an abnormality of the anal canal and rectum is suspected such as nonspecific proctitis, radiation proctitis, anorectal ulcer, anorectal neoplasm, infectious proctitis, and anorectal Crohn's disease. Rigid proctosigmoidoscopy is also useful to identify the precise site and size of rectal neoplasm.

Contraindications

Patients with severe anal pain from an acute fissure, thrombosed external hemorrhoids, and perianal abscess may not allow an examination. The examination should be postponed to some other date. Anal stricture that will not allow the passage of the smallest size rigid proctosigmoidoscope is a contraindication to its use.

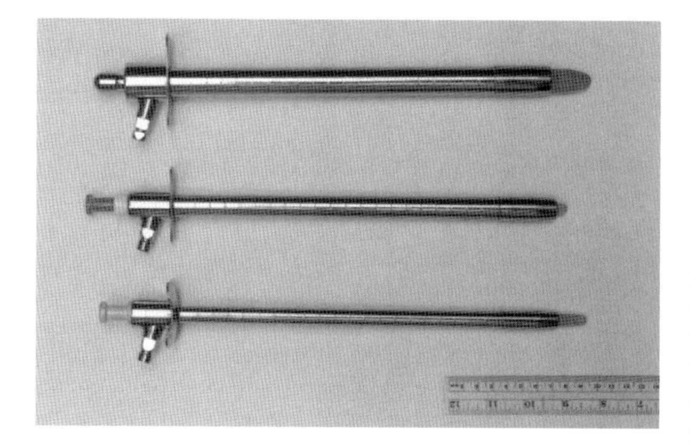

FIGURE 5-5. Rigid proctosigmoidoscope. *Top* 19 mm×25 cm, *middle* 15 mm×25 cm, *bottom* 11 mm×25 cm.

Patients with acute abdomen of any cause or a rectal or sigmoid anastomosis less than 2 weeks postoperatively should have a rigid proctosigmoidoscopy with caution.

Preparation

Two phosphate enemas should be given within 2 h of the examination. This is not necessary in a patient who has diarrhea or active bleeding. Sedation is unnecessary.

Positioning

A prone jackknife is the position of choice. However, the left-lateral position also gives an adequate examination and should be used in conditions such as pregnancy, severe hypertension, retinal detachment, or postoperative eye surgery and some apprehensive patients.

Technique

Although a standard proctosigmoidoscope is 25 cm in length, the average distance that the scope can be passed is 20 cm. In men, the scope can be passed to 21–25 cm half of the time, and in women, it can be passed that distance one-third of the time.[1] Rigid proctosigmoidoscopy is suitable only to examine the rectum and, in some patients, the distal sigmoid colon. The pain experienced from proctosigmoidoscopy is from stretching the mesentery of the rectosigmoid colon when the scope is pushed against the rectal wall, and from the air insufflation. When properly performed, rigid proctosigmoidoscopy should produce no pain or only mild discomfort. Most patients are fearful of the examination because of past bad experience with the procedure or from what they have heard. A few words of reassurance will be helpful.

With the obturator in place and held steady with the right thumb, the well-lubricated rigid proctosigmoidoscope is gently inserted into the anal canal, aiming toward the umbilicus for a distance of about 4–5 cm. Then the endoscope is angled toward the sacrum and advanced another 4–5 cm into the rectum. The obturator is removed and the bowel lumen is negotiated under direct vision. Air insufflation is limited to the amount necessary to open the lumen. When an angle is encountered, the endoscope is withdrawn 3–4 cm and then readvanced. This may be repeated several times to straighten the angulation. If further advancement is unsuccessful, the procedure is terminated at this point. Careful examination is done as the instrument is withdrawn. It is usually necessary to insufflate a small amount of air for good visualization of the lumen. The instrument should be rotated on withdrawal to ensure examination of the entire circumference. The mucosal folds in the rectum (valves of Houston) can be flattened with the tip of the endoscope to see the area immediately proximal to them. The length of insertion should be measured from the anal verge without stretching the bowel wall. The appearance of the mucosa and depth of insertion should be accurately described. If a lesion is seen, the size, appearance, location and level are recorded. If a biopsy is performed, the location, level, number of biopsies and whether electrocoagulation is necessary should be noted. During the entire procedure, suction and water irrigation should be available. A rigid cautery snare (Frankfelt snare) and cautery tip attachments are useful for excision or ablation of rectal neoplasms.

Complications

If not careful, the tip of the endoscope can tear the mucosa; a small or moderate amount of bleeding may occur. Abdominal pain and distention can occur from excessive air insufflation.

Perforation from diagnostic rigid proctosigmoidoscopy is extremely rare. Gilbertsen[2] reported an incidence of five perforations in 103,000 examinations. Nelson et al.[3] reported two perforations in over 16,000 examinations.

Flexible Sigmoidoscopy

The present day flexible sigmoidoscope is no longer fiberoptic but contains a videochip at the tip of the endoscope. This videochip transmits the image through the processing unit to the monitor. The flexible videosigmoidoscope is 60 cm in functional length (Figure 5-6). The entire sigmoid colon can be reached by the flexible sigmoidoscope in 45–85% of cases and in some cases the splenic flexure can also be visualized.[4,5] The discrepancies in success depend on patient selection and the experience of the endoscopist. For selective screening examination, flexible sigmoidoscopy has a three to six times greater yield than does rigid proctosigmoidoscopy in detecting colonic and rectal abnormalities, especially neoplasms.[6,7] Because of this higher yield and better exposure, many physicians have discarded rigid proctosigmoidoscopy.

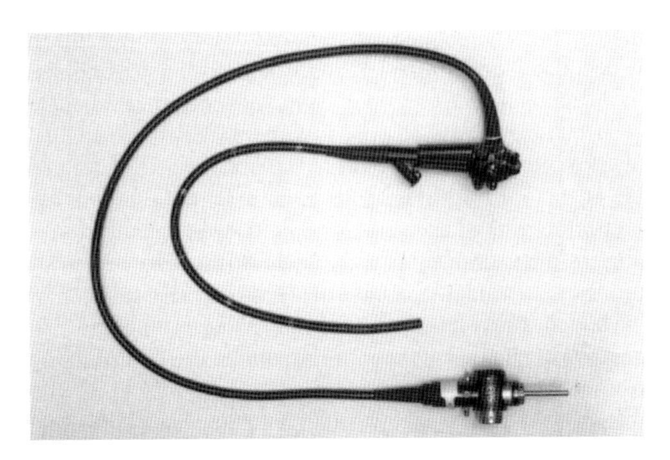

FIGURE 5-6. Flexible video sigmoidoscope.

Indications

The role of flexible sigmoidoscopy is difficult to define, because it can examine only the sigmoid colon and rectum in most cases. However, it is more convenient to use, and in many cases the entire colon need not be examined.

In acute diarrhea, flexible sigmoidoscopy can be used to rule out Clostridium difficile colitis, acute bacterial colitis, amebic colitis, and ischemic colitis particularly after aortic aneurysm repair. Flexible sigmoidoscopy is also an excellent tool to examine bright red rectal bleeding to detect its cause such as nonspecific proctitis, radiation proctitis, anorectal Crohn's disease, rectal ulcer, and also anorectal neoplasm. Additional common indications for flexible sigmoidoscopy include postoperative evaluation to look for anastomotic strictures and to detect local recurrence of neoplasms treated by transanal excision or radical excision. Flexible sigmoidoscopy is also used for colorectal cancer screening in conjunction with tests for fecal occult blood and to complement a barium enema examination. In this situation, CO_2 may be used for air insufflation if a barium enema is to follow.

Contraindications

Patient with severe anal pain from anal diseases may not tolerate the insertion of the scope. This also applies to anorectal stricture and colorectal anastomosis less than 2 weeks postoperatively. Other contraindications include acute sigmoid diverticulitis, toxic colitis, and patients with an acute abdomen.

Preparation

Bowel preparation with two fleet enemas given within 2 h of examination is adequate. The patient may eat normally. Patients with diarrhea do not require the enemas.

Positioning

Left-lateral recumbent or prone jackknife position.

Technique

Sedation is unnecessary. The anal canal is lubricated by digital examination. A well-lubricated flexible sigmoidoscope is then inserted. Advancement of the endoscope is performed under direct vision. Pushing the endoscope through a bend in the bowel is a poor technique. Instead, the endoscope should be withdrawn to straighten the bowel. The key to success is short withdrawal and advancement of the endoscope or a to-and-fro movement ("dithering"), together with rotating (torquing) the instrument clockwise and/or counter clockwise as needed. Use of air insufflation should be kept to a minimum. The procedure should be completed within 5–10 min. If a lesion is detected and proved by biopsy to be a neoplasm, a complete colonic investigation is indicated, ideally by total colonoscopy at some other date. A polyp up to 8 mm in size can be sampled and frequently completely excised with cold biopsy forceps. Alternatively, cautery forceps (hot biopsy) and fulguration can be used. To prevent possible explosion, due to hydrogen or methane gas in the lumen, air should be exchanged in the colon and rectum with repeated insufflation and suction. For larger polyps and in those cases when a full colonoscopy is planned, delay in treatment until time of colonoscopy with full bowel preparation is preferable.

Complications

Excessive air insufflation can cause acute abdominal distention and abdominal pain. This is best corrected by reinsertion of the endoscope and aspiration of air. Too rough and improper technique can cause perforation and other injuries, such as mucosal laceration with associated bleeding.

The most common site of perforation in flexible sigmoidoscopy is in the distal sigmoid colon where it is angulated from the relatively fixed rectum at promontory of the sacrum. Complications from flexible sigmoidoscopy are uncommon but can be serious. They can be immediately apparent or delayed. Gatto et al.[8] reported a large population-based cohort that consisted of a random sample of 5% of Medicare beneficiaries living in the region of the USA covered by the surveillance, epidemiology, and end results program registries between 1991 and 1998. There were 35,298 flexible sigmoidoscopies performed. The perforation rate within 7 days of the procedure was 0.9/1,000. Anderson et al.[9] evaluated the 10-year experience between 1987 and 1996 at Mayo Clinic, Scottsdale, Arizona. There were 49,501 flexible sigmoidoscopies performed. Two perforations occurred – one was in the cecum, most likely from excessive air. The other was in the sigmoid colon but was not detected until 17 days later as a pelvic abscess. Both required operation. There was no mortality. Levin et al.[10] analyzed 107,704 individuals who underwent 109,534 flexible sigmoidoscopic screenings as part of Colorectal Cancer Prevention Program from 1994 to 1996 at North California Kaiser Permanente Medical Care Program. There were two perforations, two episodes of diverticulitis requiring operation, two cases of bleeding requiring blood transfusion and one episode of unexplained colitis. In this study in multivariate models, complications were significantly more common in men than in women (odds ratio, 3.34; confidence interval 95%).

Ileoscopy

Examination of the small intestine via an ileostomy can be performed using a rigid proctosigmoidoscope or a flexible scope.

Indications

Indications for endoscoping the terminal ileum are few. Most of the time it is to rule out recurrent Crohn's disease or to find an abnormality in patients with high ileostomy output.

Contraindications

Stricture of the stoma.

Preparation

Bowel preparation is not required, but it is helpful if the patient has been on a clear liquid diet for 1 day. Sedation is not required.

Positioning

Supine.

Technique

The examination starts with a digital examination to gently dilate the stoma which is frequently slightly stenotic. The well-lubricated rigid scope is introduced directly into the ileostomy. The terminal ileum is quite active with frequent spasm. It requires more air insufflation than scoping the rectum. The distance traversed by the endoscope is usually limited to 12–15 cm. In patients with a large para-ileostomy hernia, the endoscope may usually not be passed beyond 10 cm.

Flexible ileoscopy is much easier to perform. The angulation of the small bowel can be straightened by push, pull, and rotation of the scope. A moderate amount of air insufflation is usually required.

Complications

The small bowel has thin walls and requires gentle maneuvering of the endoscope. Perforation can easily occur. If an angle cannot be straightened the procedure should be terminated.

Pouchoscopy

Kock Pouch or Continent Ileostomy

Indications

Although the ileoanal pouch has completely replaced the Kock pouch, there are still many patients with a Kock pouch. One of the most common problems that require endoscopy is the extrusion of the valve causing difficulty or impossibility of intubation to evacuate the stool. The examination is performed to help decompress the obstructed pouch and to place a draining tube. Other indications include Crohn's disease and complication of the pouch with fistulas and high output of the pouch.

Both rigid and flexible endoscopes can be used. Church et al.[11] advised using a pediatric flexible endoscope.

Contraindications

Stricture of the stoma. Unless the procedure is performed under a general anesthetic.

Preparation

Bowel preparation is unnecessary and sedation is not usually required. If possible, the pouch should be emptied or irrigated immediately prior to the examination. It is preferable if the patient has been on a clear liquid diet for 1 day prior to the procedure.

Positioning

Supine.

Technique

The endoscope can usually be passed easily into the pouch with inspection of the stoma being performed on insertion or withdrawal. The pouch can be lavaged as necessary.

A general inspection of the pouch is performed noting the mucosal appearance, the pouch size, distensibility and the status of suture lines. If possible, the afferent loop of ileum should be intubated, especially in patients presenting with pouch inflammation. The endoscope must be retroflexed within the pouch to check valve length and symmetry. A careful search for foreign material should be made, particularly around the base of the valve. If mesh was used to reinforce the nipple valve, a fistula may form at this area. In patients with slippage or extrusion of the valve, passing the endoscope will be difficult.

For an obstructed pouch from a slipped valve, Church et al.[11] used a flexible endoscope as an obturator to insert the rigid proctosigmoidoscope. The rigid endoscope is placed over the flexible endoscope, which is itself inserted into the pouch. Then the rigid endoscope is advanced over the flexible endoscope into the pouch. Now the flexible endoscope can be withdrawn and a drainage catheter inserted to temporarily relieve the obstruction. Another option is to pass a guide wire or forceps through the biopsy channel of the flexible endoscope that has been inserted through the valve into the pouch. The wire or forceps (with the handle removed) is then left in the pouch and the scope is withdrawn, a drainage catheter can then be passed into the pouch over the wire or forceps, and surgical repair of the nipple valve is almost always required.

Complications

Perforation can occur, particularly when there is an obstruction of the pouch.

Ileoanal Pouch

Examination of the ileoanal pouch is best performed using a flexible sigmoidoscope although a rigid proctoscope can also be used. Unless there is an anastomotic anal stricture, the examination is usually easy. The endoscope can be used to examine the entire pouch and usually the terminal ileum proximal to the pouch.

Indications

Examination of the pouch is indicated for patients with bleeding from the pouch, diarrhea, recent onset of fecal incontinence, obstructive symptoms, pouchitis, for surveillance follow-up examination to exclude neoplastic changes and to rule out Crohn's disease.

Contraindications

Severe anal or anastomotic stricture, unless the procedure is performed under general anesthetic.

Preparation

The patient is prepared by taking clear liquids for 1 day or administered a small enema before the examination. Sedation is not required.

Positioning

Left-lateral recumbent or prone jackknife position.

Technique

The examination starts with a digital examination to evaluate the anal canal and the anal anastomosis. If there is a stricture, it should first be dilated with a finger or with Hegar dilators.

The well-lubricated flexible sigmoidoscope or a colonoscope is introduced into the anal canal. The endoscope is advanced into the pouch. The terminal ileum proximal to the pouch can usually be intubated. The examiner should evaluate the mucosa of the pouch and anal canal for any edema of the mucosa, granularity, mucosal bleeding, contact bleeding, erosion, fibrin exudate, pattern of mucosal ulceration, plaque and mass. Abnormal mucosa should be biopsied. Only cold biopsy should be performed.

Complications

Tear of the anal canal can occur if there is stricture of the anus or anastomosis. Traumatic injury from the scope may cause moderate bleeding which usually stops spontaneously. A perforation can occur from the instrumentation or a biopsy.

Colonoscopy

With the many methods available for evaluation and often therapy of colorectal disorders, colonoscopy has emerged as the gold standard for diagnosis. It is also, in some areas, an increasingly frequent option for therapy, be it definitive or palliative.

Indications

Indications for diagnostic colonoscopy include: the evaluation of virtually all symptoms associated with potential benign or malignant, acute or chronic diseases of the colorectum; for resolution of abnormalities seen on other imaging modalities; for investigating otherwise unexplained symptoms such as anemia; the evaluation of chronic and acute bleeding per annum; for screening and surveillance of patients at high risk for colon adenomas or carcinoma; localization of nonpalpable lesions at open or laparoscopic operation. It is also increasingly possible to combine diagnostic colonoscopy and other imaging techniques such as ultrasound.

Contraindications

Contraindications to diagnostic colonoscopy may be classified as *absolute* or *relative*. Although colonoscopy is appropriately considered a minimally invasive procedure there are risks involved which may be avoided or, at least minimized, by careful patient selection and certainly these risks should be discussed prior to the performance of the procedure.

Absolute contraindications are as follows: suspected bowel perforation, established peritonitis, or fulminant colitis.

Relative contraindications include suspected ischemia and acute colitis, in either of which instance an experienced examiner may safely perform a limited examination. Patients with a recent anastomosis may be examined with caution. Active bleeding, once a relative contraindication to colonoscopy, is being used more and more in this setting. This is described in both the prepped and unprepped colon with low complication rates.[12] The author performs colonoscopy in acute lower gastrointestinal bleeding in patients who have evidence of ongoing bleeding and either a (1) negative nuclear medicine tagged red blood cell scan or (2) positive tagged red blood cell scans followed by negative mesenteric angiography.

Preparation

Preparation for colonoscopy, of necessity, should include preparation of the endoscopist, preparation of the patient in general and of the colon specifically. Several organizations have prepared and published guidelines for credentialing the individual who is permitted to perform colonoscopy in an institutional setting[13] and, in some institutions, Credentials Committees have been established which grant privileges. Although there is some controversy involving required numbers of experiences in training, all recommendations include the following elements: background knowledge of anatomy, physiology and pathology of the colon; familiarity with instruments and accessories used in endoscopy; some formal training; and quality assurance practices. The concept of proctoring has also been addressed by some.[14] Equipment for resuscitation should be available and individuals qualified to perform cardiopulmonary resuscitation should be present in the area where colonoscopy is performed. The necessity for qualified assistance during the performance of the procedure and for monitoring the patient's condition cannot be overstated.

Obtaining informed consent is an opportunity for discussing with the patient elements of the past and present medical history, especially medications and operative procedures, which may expose psychological concerns or the need to modify preparation or change medication, timing, and dosage. It is necessary to point out the potential hazards of colonoscopy, noting aspects of the process that might cause discomfort but it is also important to give reassurance that while the risk of complication is low the examiner is prepared for prompt management. The question of the need for antibiotic prophylaxis stems from concern that although diagnostic colonoscopy is a low-risk procedure for bacteremia, infection of damaged cardiac valves or implanted prosthesis is a risk. The American Heart Association (AHA) and the American Society for Gastrointestinal Endoscopy (ASGE) have issued guidelines stating that antibiotic prophylaxis is not required for gastrointestinal endoscopy solely for prevention of infectious endocarditis.[15,16] A separate scientific statement from the AHA does not recommend routine antibiotic prophylaxis in patients who have nonvalvular cardiovascular devices (including vascular grafts) and are undergoing gastrointestinal procedures.[17]

Preparation

Thorough mechanical preparation of the colon is absolutely essential for efficient, safe, and complete endoscopic examination. In addition, should perforation occur, the empty colon certainly poses less risk of significant peritoneal contamination. There are various forms of mechanical preparation possible, but the most thorough and safest current regimen involves the use of polyethylene glycol electrolyte lavage solutions. Other forms of preparation that are sometimes employed involve ingestion of a saline cathartic (usually sodium phosphate or magnesium citrate) as well as enemas. Sodium phosphate bowel preparations have been associated with acute phosphate nephropathy, which has lead to the discontinuation of most over the counter sodium phosphate preparations. A consensus statement from the ASGE, the American Society of Colon and Rectal Surgeons (ASCRS) and the Society of American Gastrointestinal and Endoscopic Surgeons (SAGES) from 2006 includes sodium phosphate bowel preparation in its "regimens of colon cleansing before colonoscopy." Contraindications include pediatric or elderly patients, patients with bowel obstruction, renal insufficiency or failure, congestive heart failure, or liver failure.[18] An addendum to this statement was published shortly after its release, which adds the "Food and Drug Administration (FDA) warning about oral sodium phosphate." This statement includes additional risk factors for acute phosphate nephropathy including "medications that affect renal perfusion or function…"[19]

Monitoring

Although the use of pulse oximetry, heart rate, and intermittent monitoring of blood pressure, as well as electrocardiography (if clinically indicated), have now become standard procedures, it is important for the assistant as well as the endoscopist to be aware of any changes in the patient's level of awareness, respirations, and abdominal distention.

Bleeding Prophylaxis

Although bleeding is rarely associated with diagnostic colonoscopy there are concerns about bleeding at or after colonoscopy, if biopsy or polypectomy are contemplated. This has led to modification of anticoagulation regimens and cessation of drugs which might alter platelet function. Recommendations for periprocedural management of anticoagulants must take into consideration the magnitude of risk of a thromboembolic event and its attendant morbidity/mortality vs. the risk of bleeding from the procedure and the morbidity/mortality from those events. Two resources have thorough discussions of these issues and recommendations for management.[20,21] A summarization of these recommendations are that patients who are on chronic warfarin, who are at high risk for a thromboembolic event, and who are undergoing a high risk procedure (e.g., colonoscopy with polypectomy), should be managed with discontinuation of warfarin, "bridging" anticoagulation with heparin (intravenous unfractionated heparin or subcutaneous low-molecular weight heparin), and postprocedural resumption of their oral anticoagulation. Recommendations from the American College of Chest Physicians for antiplatelet therapy (including clopidogrel) and are updated regularly and practitioners performing colonoscopy should familiarize themselves with these guidelines.[21]

Technique

For successful passage of the colonoscope to the most proximal desired anatomic region (cecum or anastomosis) it is imperative that a few principles be understood.[22] The examiner must appreciate that the colon is of variable length, that respiratory and peristaltic activity is in progress during the examination, and that some areas of the colon are more fixed (by normal anatomy, previous inflammation, or postoperative change). It is dangerous to proceed with introduction of the endoscope without knowing at all times the location of the lumen.

Before starting the examination the equipment should be checked to verify that it is in good working order that irrigation, suction, and air insufflation channels are open, and that the directional controls are in the unlocked position. With the patient in the left-lateral recumbent position, the examination is initiated by thoroughly inspecting the perianal area for fissures, fistulae, hemorrhoids, condylomata and rarer conditions such as melanoma, Bowen's disease, extramammary Paget's disease, squamous and anal gland carcinomas. Next, the lubricated gloved right index finger is inserted into the anus and a rectal exanimation carefully performed, paying special attention to the surface of the prostate gland in the middle aged and older male patient. With the right index finger still in the rectum, the endoscopist then holds the tip of the instrument in the left hand, places it at right angles to the right index finger and by effacing the sphincter with gentle pressure of the right index finger, the instrument tip can be gently inserted as the right index finger is withdrawn. The examiner then grasps the head of the instrument in the palm of the left hand, leaving the thumb and index finger free to manipulate the knobs for tip deflection with the former and the air and water insufflation as well as suction buttons with the other. The right hand is placed on the instrument shaft. With the instrument in the rectal ampulla it is usually necessary to insufflate the lumen with a small amount of air in order to visualize the direction of the lumen.

The main objective on insertion of the instrument is to reach the most proximal point desired in as expeditiously a fashion as possible, leaving detailed inspection until the process of withdrawal of the endoscope. However, detection of an abnormality on insertion may require a change in strategy. For example, it may be important to detect, localize, sometimes biopsy, or even remove a small lesion for fear of not being able to find it easily on withdrawal. In some circumstances at least localization and biopsy should be performed, even on insertion.

One of the earliest challenges to insertion is advancing the instrument into the descending colon. The unprepared examiner, looking at the stylized cartoons of many an endoscopy record form and even many anatomical and surgical textbooks may not recognize how long the sigmoid colon can be and how easy it may be to insert a considerable length of the instrument into it. Because the sigmoid is commonly not fixed, it accepts the instrument so readily that when the acute angle at the junction of the sigmoid and (fixed) descending colon is reached the inexperienced examiner may think that he has achieved insertion to the splenic flexure. Attempts at further insertion may be hindered then by the loop created in the sigmoid colon. Most of the time this frustrating situation may be entirely avoided by attempting to keep the sigmoid collapsed and shortened as early as possible. Some have found that a clockwise turn with the right hand on the shaft of the instrument and with jiggling of the shaft, as well as back and forth motion, will often allow the bowel to fall over the instrument, so to speak, allowing insertion with a less than one-to-one motion. It is this pleating or "accordioning" of the bowel over the instrument with alternating release that allows for efficient advancement and more than one-to-one motion. As a matter of fact, the recognition of this intermittent intussusception and reduction as part of the normal advancement of the instrument makes it understandable that, in estimating the extent of intubation or the location of a lesion, the least accurate determination is measuring on the shaft of the instrument.

Having entered the descending colon with the sigmoid shortened and "straight," it is usually quite easy to advance to and around the splenic flexure. Difficulty in intubation beyond the splenic flexure is more common when the patient has undergone previous operation within this area with adhesions in the left upper quadrant which may produce fixation. Alternatively, a high, acutely angulated flexure can cause difficulty. If the endoscopist recognizes the distal transverse colon by endoscopic anatomy or transmitted aortic pulsation, it is to be recalled that, like the sigmoid, the transverse colon is on a long mesentery and is rarely fixed. The hepatic flexure can be more easily reached by keeping the transverse colon as collapsed as possible.

The hepatic is often a more complicated flexure than is the splenic and one may wander a while before entering the distal ascending colon. However, once the latter has been entered and there has been no prior right abdominal operation (for example, cholecystectomy or appendectomy) the cecum is often rapidly reached by application of suction to collapse the bowel over the instrument. A change in position from lateral to supine may also be helpful. It is important to be fully cognizant of the vagaries of endoscopic anatomy in order to confirm cecal intubation – by visualization of the appendiceal orifice and the ileocecal valve. Looking for transillumination from the instrument tip through the abdominal wall in the right lower quadrant is, unfortunately, a trap for the unsophisticated endoscopist who uses it to verify cecal entry. It merely points out that the instrument tip is in the right lower quadrant but the endoscopic tip may be in any mobile part of the colon, for example, the transverse colon or even the sigmoid. In fact, the student of anatomy recognizes that the cecum is not always in the right lower quadrant. There are aids to overcoming obstacles to cecal intubation. One is changing the patient's position from left-lateral to supine if this was not done earlier. This maneuver can also be helpful when progress is impeded at the rectosigmoid junction or the flexures. A second common technique is attempting to keep the sigmoid in a straight position so that on further insertion the tip may progress proximally. Abdominal pressure by an assistant is often used in an attempt to keep the sigmoid from reforming a loop since once it has already been straightened. One should not expect or direct the assistant to reduce the loop by compression because this could theoretically lead to injury of the bowel wall. Rather, the sigmoid has to be straightened and then pressure may be used to keep the loop from being reformed. If one reviews a series of barium enema films or has acquaintance with the position of the omega loop of the sigmoid at abdominal operation it helps to understand these maneuvers. For those who have the capability of fluoroscopy in their endoscopy units, much can be learned and much assistance provided in this maneuver, especially in the individual's early endoscopic experience. For one, it is humbling to recognize how inaccurate one can be of the extent of insertion or the shape of the bowel with the endoscope inserted. There are two recent developments in endoscopic and related instrumentation which may facilitate overcoming the difficult sigmoid loop, still the most challenging aspect of diagnostic colonoscopy. One is the development in the design of some colonoscopes for the endoscopist to vary the stiffness of the endoscope to allow a previously shortened and straightened segment of bowel from reforming a loop. The assumption is that the endoscopist knows with certainty that the loop has been adequately reduced and that it is safe to insert a now more rigid instrument. Those who have expertise with fluoroscopy know that this can be a fallible assumption. Another development is an extracorporeal magnetic device that can track the course and shape of the endoscope during insertion.[23] If proven accurate this device could potentially obviate fluoroscopy for localization, reduction of difficult loops, and even allow for safer stiffening of the endoscope utilizing either a variable stiffness endoscope or the external splinting device introduced by Shinya in the early days of colonoscopy. Certainly, the external splinting device should never be used without the benefit of fluoroscopic assistance, because with an angulated segment of bowel, it is possible to damage the bowel wall if the mucosa is caught in the space between the edge of the splinting device and the shaft of the instrument. When using the external splinting device the fluoroscope is used to first verify that the tip of the instrument is just beyond the splenic flexure and acutely angled (Figure 5-7). The deflection knobs are then placed in the locked position and, as the instrument is withdrawn and the sigmoid loop straightened under fluoroscopic control, the external splint is advanced over the endoscope up to but not beyond the proximal descending colon.[22] One does not wish to advance it to the splenic flexure where the lienocolic ligament may be vulnerable to avulsion. An assistant has to keep

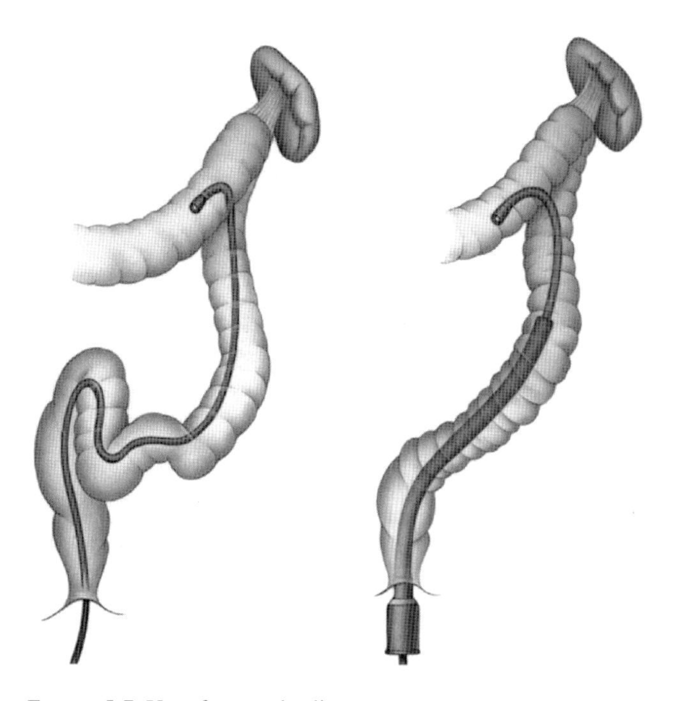

FIGURE 5-7. Use of external splint.

the splinting device fixed at the anus so that the examiner does not insert it further than desired during the remainder of the examination.

External manipulation may also be helpful in two other circumstances. Sometimes the transverse colon, having a long mesentery, may form a loop extending well into the pelvis. Reduction of this loop by withdrawing the instrument and utilizing suction will usually achieve rapid progress into the ascending colon. But one can sometimes keep the loop from reforming by having an assistant apply pressure from the right abdomen directed to the left upper quadrant (because the transverse colon mesentery is longer on the right and the loop is therefore more prominent in the right portion of the abdomen or pelvis). If the cecum is not fixed (as from prior operation, for example, appendectomy or pelvic surgery), it may be possible with gentle pressure or the abdominal wall to collapse it onto the tip of the instrument, remembering, however, that the cecum is not always in the right lower quadrant. Sometimes placing the patient in the prone position allows easier intubation of the cecum

On withdrawal of the instrument one has to be sure that the entire mucosa is visualized. The author has found it helpful to place the patient supine for withdrawal. This aids in localization as fluid will collect in the most dependent portions of the colon – cecum, hepatic and splenic flexure, and rectum. Additionally, fluid and solid matter will move with gravity, thereby exposing portions of the colonic wall that were obscured in the left-lateral position. As one withdraws the instrument and the bowel recedes inspection is accomplished, but it requires close attention since one can easily withdraw too rapidly as a previously accordioned segment escapes without the examiner's control. It may be necessary to go back over an area not adequately visualized initially. In this connection, adequate preparation is even more important at this time than on insertion. If liquid material is present but too thick to be aspirated by suction through the instrument channel one may purposefully change the patient's position to allow the fluid to shift to another area. Withdrawal through the sigmoid colon perforce requires more time and attention because there are more folds and recesses. While the experienced examiner can usually withdraw very slowly through the anal canal and thus visualize its entire circumference this is sometimes better if complemented by retroflexing the tip of the instrument in the anal ampulla to visualize the region of the dentate line (if the rectal ampulla is readily distensible). As the endoscope is withdrawn through each segment of the colon, it is useful to decompress each examined segment with suction so that at the conclusion of the examination the abdomen is minimally distended.

Normal Endoscopic Anatomy

Some segments of the colon are more readily recognized than others and one has to be careful not to be overconfident unless a classic appearance is present. On insertion it is important to first recognize the three rectal valves of Houston since the relationship of a lesion to them will have great relevance if surgical intervention is to be contemplated. Diverticula may be seen throughout the intraperitoneal colon but rarely below the peritoneal reflection. The descending colon, being fixed along the white line of Toldt will often present a long straight "tunnel view." Occasionally the splenic flexure is specifically recognized if there is an external bulging bluish mass indenting the colon, descending with respiration. More common in the sigmoid colon, diverticula may be seen throughout the length of the large intestine. Their orifices may be so wide that they may be mistaken for the bowel lumen. It is therefore safer to back away somewhat and have a longer view to be sure of the location of the lumen. In any one field of view, the diverticulum will of course be at right angles to the lumen (Figure 5-8). The transverse colon, on insertion, being suspended by the three taenia coli presents the appearance of an equilateral triangle (the so-called cathedral ceiling appearance). Quite commonly, the distal transverse colon can be identified in relation to the proximal since the point of maximal impulse of the aorta is transmitted through the diaphragm which overlies the distal transverse colon. Especially, in thin patients, the liver casts a broad flat bluish green cast outside the colon but since this may be seen for a variable distance from distal transverse colon to mid ascending colon, it is not particularly helpful with localization of a lesion. At the hepatic flexure the colon often assumes a spiral configuration which can cause the tenia to so approximate each other as to make the novice assume the cecum has been reached (what has been called "the fool's cecum" or "the faux cecum").

The interhaustral folds in the ascending colon are low in profile compared with those in the left colon. The ileocecal valve is most commonly recognized as an eccentric bulge with a sometimes visible umbilication. Because there is more adipose tissue in it the appearance is often a yellowish color compared with the pink of the rest of the colon. The ileocecal valve is rarely seen head on but it is, of course, more easily recognizable when it is. It is important to intubate proximal to the valve since the true caput of the colon may be at a variable distance from the ileocecal valve. As the three tenia merge at the caput(often appearing like the branches of a tree or a crow's foot), the appendiceal orifice is commonly recognized, even in the patient who has undergone previous appendectomy. Whenever possible, the ileocecal valve should be intubated and the granular appearance of the small bowel noted. Routine practice of this improves the endoscopists proficiency for cases when intubation of the small bowel is likely to be of most value, for example, in acute lower gastrointestinal bleeding and inflammatory bowel disease.

Abnormal Findings

Exophytic lesions are the easiest to visualize and recognize at colonoscopy, the most common being adenocarcinoma.

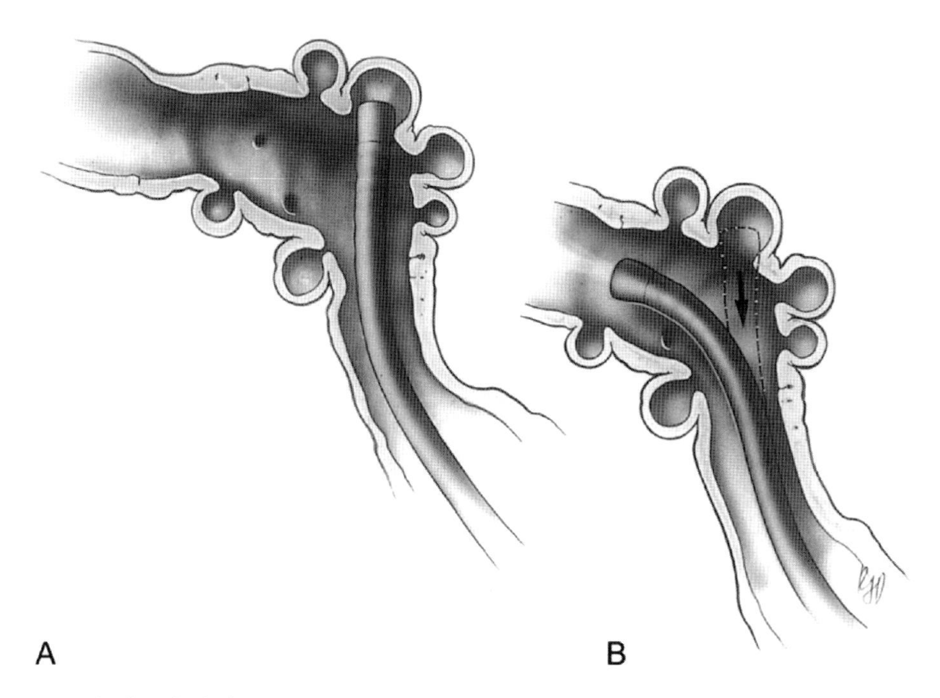

FIGURE 5-8. Finding lumen in diverticulosis.

All polypoid lesions of the colon may be visualized at colonoscopy and virtually all have distinguishing characteristics. Many are submucosal (lymphoid hyperplasia, stromal tumors, lipomas, carcinoids, endometriomas, hemangiomas, neurofibromas, or lymphoma). A few are metastatic from other organs (for example, prostate, pancreas, or kidney). The diagnosis of most of these lesions can be made by endoscopic visualization or sampling. Some, being of no clinical consequence, require only recognition (lymphoid, hyperplasia, and lipoma). Chromoendoscopy and narrow band imaging are techniques which may improve polyp detection rate and differentiation of polyp type. As of this writing, neither technique has demonstrated widespread benefit.[24–26] Additionally, a retroscope that fits through the working channel of the colonoscope has also been described, but its usefulness has yet to be proven.

In addition to lesions which protrude, there are numerous inflammatory or degenerative conditions which have a recognizable endoscopic appearance and many can be safely sampled if necessary. These include the various colitides (bacterial, viral, ulcerative, granulomatous), ischemia, radiation proctopathy (formerly called "proctitis") and melanosis coli. Melanosis coli, when marked, may help in visualization of adenomatous tissue since the pigment is not deposited in only normal mucosa. Areas of angiodysplasia (vascular ectasias, arteriovenous malformations) can be recognized on diagnostic colonoscopy but must be distinguished from bruises created from instrumentation or even preparation. The endoscopist has to recognize colonic anatomy disturbed by previous operation and therefore has to be familiar with the variety of intestinal anastomoses performed.

Areas of stenosis and stricture may be encountered secondary to benign conditions (previous resection and anastomosis, diverticulitis, colitis, radiation injury) or malignancy. Other rare findings to be recognized include colitis cystica profunda, pneumatosis, and Behçet's syndrome. The manner in which the nature of a lesion is established at diagnostic colonoscopy will vary. A tiny sessile lesion (for example, a diminutive polyp) may be removed in its entirety with the biopsy forceps for pathologic examination. A pedunculated lesion suspected of being a benign adenoma may be removed at the time of diagnostic examination by snare polypectomy. Larger sessile lesions may be elevated with submucosal injection with saline and then excised with a snare completely or piecemeal. Fulguration with monopolar cautery or argon plasma coagulator may be used to ablate tissue. A sessile lesion suspected of being a carcinoma may be biopsied at one or more sites or even partially removed with a snare and cautery to obtain a satisfactory specimen. A stricture may be sampled for possible malignant cells by advancing a cytology brush into the stricture ahead of the colonoscope (Figure 5-9). Malignant cells may thus be harvested even though the stricture cannot be traversed with the endoscope. A lesion which appears vascular and friable may be simply photographed. A submucosal lesion may be exposed by disrupting the overlying mucosa with sequential bites from a biopsy forceps. Lesions which are not located near a definitive landmark (cecum, ileocecal valve, rectum) and are likely to require colonic resection, should be marked with a submucosal (India ink) tattoo placed in all four quadrants of the colonic lume approximately 5 cm distal to the lesion.

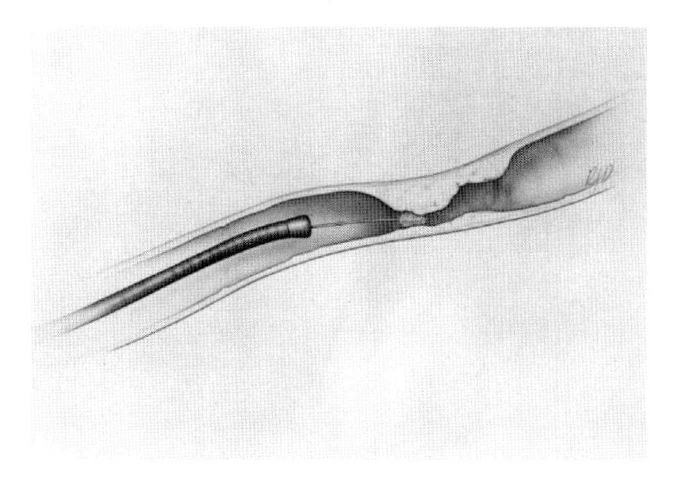

FIGURE 5-9. Cytology through stricture.

Complications

While colonoscopy is an overall safe procedure, it is invasive and adverse events do occur. The most common serious complication of diagnostic colonoscopy is perforation but the reported incidence of 0.03–0.7% and a mortality rate of 7–26% for patients who sustain a perforation.[27–30] Other reported complications include abdominal distension, dehydration, respiratory depression, vasovagal reaction, thrombo phlebitis, incarcerated hernia, splenic capsular tear and subcutaneous and/mediastinal emphysema and equipment failure.

In diagnostic colonoscopy, perforation may be instrumental (instrument, overtube, or accessory device), traction on a fixed segment of colon or over insufflation of a segment, especially a closed loop as may occur in patients with multiple strictures (inflammatory bowel disease) or as a consequence of prior radiation therapy and with hernia incarceration. Impaction of the instrument in a diverticulum with overdistention of the latter has also been a cause of perforation. As one studies the types of complications reported, it becomes clear that adequate training and experience should decrease these adverse events to a minimum. Because of perforation related to the use of coagulation ("hot") biopsy forceps and the low risk of bleeding from multiple forceps biopsies, there has been a falling off of usage of this instrument despite the advantages of obtaining a good specimen and simultaneously achieving hemostasis. Perforation during diagnostic colonoscopy tends to be detected earlier when it is from instrumental causes, whereas perforation from therapeutic procedures is frequently related to thermal injury and is often delayed. Indeed the management of perforation following colonoscopy is still controversial.[31,32] While there is universal agreement that perforation with generalized peritonitis suggests continuing contamination of the peritoneal cavity and therefore demands operation to halt the process, some feel that if the onset of symptoms is delayed and signs localized with a patient who is not septic (even with the demonstration of pneumoperitoneum) that nonoperative management may be undertaken. An uncommon presentation of a contained perforation may be the presence of retroperitoneal or mediastinal air and even subcutaneous emphysema which usually resolves without treatment.

Avoidance of perforation during diagnostic colonoscopy, related as it is to training, skill and experience may be best achieved by avoidance of dehydration and over sedation, discontinuation of the procedure if the preparation is poor, avoiding forceful instrument insertion, recognition of vulnerable bowel (inflammation, ischemia, narrowing, fixation); careful identification and avoidance of diverticular ostia, avoidance of bowing of the instrument, awareness of fixation from pelvic adhesions or tumor extending through and beyond the colon wall, insuring that abdominal and inguinal hernias remain reduced, avoiding over insufflation, and looping in the splenic flexure region. There should be constant identification of the location of the lumen with avoidance of "slide by" (sidewise passage of the instrument without direct visualization of the lumen). Colonoscopy during acute bleeding is technically more difficult and should not be attempted if one has not had adequate experience with routine diagnostic colonoscopy.

If perforation occurs, early diagnosis will ensure more efficient management. Undue and sustained pain (especially shoulder discomfort), absence of liver dullness on percussion, demonstration of pneumoperitoneum on upright chest film and subcutaneous emphysema, are all help in making the diagnosis. Signs and symptoms will in general be related to factors such as adequacy of bowel preparation, size of injury, and underlining pathologic state of the colon. For example, the ischemic colon or one involved with active colitis will be more vulnerable to instrumental injury. Surgical intervention is favored by most surgeons for early recognized perforation at diagnostic colonoscopy. There are, however, some patients with either a delayed perforation or one that has remained localized without symptoms or signs of diffuse peritonitis. Nonoperative management but continuing observation of this subset of patients may be entirely satisfactory. With early surgical intervention of a mechanical perforation, if technically feasible, primary closure with or without protective proximal stoma is the most desirable and usually is feasible. However, the surgeon must use good judgment in assessment of such factors as adequacy of tissue perfusion, degree of spillage, and colon tissue free of inflammation.

Acknowledgments. This chapter was written by Santhat Nivatvongs and Kenneth E. Forde in the first edition of this textbook.

References

1. Nivatvongs S, Fryd DS. How far does the proctosigmoidoscope reach? A prospective study of 1000 patients. N Engl J Med. 1980;303:380–2.
2. Gilbertsen VA. Proctosigmoidoscopy and polypectomy in reducing the incidence of rectal cancer. Cancer. 1974;34(Suppl):936–9.

3. Nelson RL, Abcarian H, Prasad ML. Iatrogenic perforation of the colon and rectum. Dis Colon Rectum. 1982;25:305–8.
4. Lehman GA, Buchner DM, Lappas JC. Anatomic extent of fiberoptic sigmoidoscopy. Gastroenterology. 1983;84:803–8.
5. Ott DJ, Wu WC, Gelfand DW. Extent of colonic visualization with fiberoptic sigmoidoscope. J Clin Gastroenterol. 1982;4:337–41.
6. Marks G, Boggs HW, Castro AF, Gathright JR, Ray JE, Salvati E. Sigmoidoscopic examinations with rigid and flexible fiberoptic sigmoidoscopes in the surgeon's office. A comparative prospective study of effectiveness in 1012 cases. Dis Colon Rectum. 1979;22:162–8.
7. Winnan G, Berci G, Parrish J, Talbot TM, Overholt BF, McCallum RW. Superiority of the flexible to the rigid sigmoidoscope in routine proctosigmoidoscopy. N Engl J Med. 1980;302:1011–2.
8. Gatto NM, Frucht H, Sundararajan V, Jacobson JS, Grann VR, Neugut AI. Risk of perforation after colonoscopy and sigmoidoscopy: a population-based study. J Natl Cancer Inst. 2003;95:230–6.
9. Anderson ML, Pasha TM, Leighton JA. Endoscopic perforation of the colon: lessons from a 10-year study. Am J Gastroenterol. 2000;95:3418–22.
10. Levin TR, Conell C, Shapiro JA, Chazan SG, Nadel MR, Selby JV. Complications of screening flexible sigmoidoscopy. Gastroenterology. 2002;123:1786–92.
11. Church JM, Fazio VW, Lavery IC. The role of fiberoptic endoscopy in the management of the continent ileostomy. Gastrointest Endosc. 1987;33:203–9.
12. Green BT, Rockey DC. Lower gastrointestinal bleeding – management. Gastroenterol Clin North Am. 2005;34:665–78.
13. Society of American Gastrointestinal Endoscopic Surgery (SAGES). Granting of privileges for gastrointestinal endoscopy by surgeons. Los Angeles, CA: SAGES; 1992.
14. Society of American Gastrointestinal Endoscopic Surgeons (SAGES). Framework for postresidency surgical education and training: a SAGES guideline. Surg Endosc. 1994;8:1137–42.
15. Wilson W, Taubert KA, Gewitz M, et al. Prevention of infective endocarditis. Guidelines from the American Heart Association. Circulation. 2007;116:1736–54.
16. American Society of Gastrointestinal Endoscopy Standards of Practice Committee. Antibiotic prophylaxis for GI endoscopy. Gastrointest Endosc. 2008;67:791–8.
17. Baddour LM, Bettmann MA, Bolger AF. Nonvalvular cardiovascular device-related infections. Circulation. 2003;108:2015–31.
18. Wexner SD, Beck DE, Baron TH. A consensus document on bowel preparation before colonoscopy: prepared by a task force from the American Society of Colon and Rectal Surgeons (ASCRS), The American Society for Gastrointestinal Endoscopy (ASGE), and The Society of American Gastrointestinal and Endoscopic Surgeons (SAGES). Dis Colon Rectum. 2006;49:792–809.
19. Wexner SD, Beck DE, Baron TH. *Addendum to* A consensus document on bowel preparation before colonoscopy: prepared by a task force from the American Society of Colon and Rectal Surgeons (ASCRS), The American Society for Gastrointestinal Endoscopy (ASGE), and The Society of American Gastrointestinal and Endoscopic Surgeons (SAGES). Surg Endosc. 2006;20:1161.
20. American Society of Gastrointestinal Endoscopy Standards of Practice Committee. Guideline on the management of anticoagulation and antiplatelet therapy for endoscopic procedures. Gastrointest Endosc. 2002;55:775–9.
21. Douketis JD, Berger PB, Dunn AS, et al. The perioperative management of antithrombotic therapy. American College of Chest Physicians evidence-based clinical practice guidelines (8th edition). Chest. 2008;133(Suppl):299s–339.
22. Forde KA. Technique of diagnostic colonoscopy. In: Greene FI, Ponsky JL, editors. Endoscopic surgery. Philadelphia, PA: Saunders; 1994. p. 219–34.
23. Shah SG, Pearson HJ, Moss S, et al. Magnetic endoscopic imaging: a new technique for localizing colonic lesions. Endoscopy. 2002;34:900–4.
24. Davila RE. Chromoendoscopy. Gastrointest Endosc Clin N Am. 2009;19:193–208.
25. Adler A, Aschenbeck J, Yenerim T, et al. Narrow-band versus white-light high definition television endoscopic imaging for screening colonoscopy: a prospective randomized trial. Gastroenterology. 2009;136:410–6.
26. Waye JD, Heigh RI, Fleisher DE, et al. A prospective efficacy evaluation of the third eye retroscope auxiliary endoscopy system. Gastrointest Endosc. 2008;67:Ab 101–2.
27. Ackroyd FW. Complications of flexible endoscopy. In: Greene FL, Ponsky JL, editors. Endoscopic surgery. Philadelphia, PA: Saunders; 1994. p. 440–1.
28. Korman LY, Overholt BF, Box T, et al. Perforation during colonoscopy in endoscopic ambulatory surgical centers. Gastrointest Endosc. 2003;58:554–7.
29. Wexner SD, Forde KA, Sellers G, et al. How well can surgeons perform colonoscopy? Surg Endosc. 1998;12:1410–4.
30. Lohsiriwat V, Sujarittanakarn S, Akaraviputh T, et al. What are the risk factors of colonoscopic perforation? BMC Gastroenterol. 2009;9:71.
31. Damore LJ, Rantis PC, Vernava AM, et al. Colonoscopic perforations. Dis Colon Rectum. 1996;39:1308–14.
32. Avgerinos DV, Llaguna OH, Lo AY, Leitman M. Evolving management of colonoscopic perforations. J Gastrointest Surg. 2008;12:1783–9.

6
Radiology

Jaime L. Bohl and Alan E. Timmcke

The aim of this chapter is to discuss the radiology studies that are diagnostic and therapeutic adjuncts to the Colon and Rectal surgeon's daily clinical practice. It is imperative that the Colon and Rectal surgeon use radiological studies as a way to narrow a differential diagnosis or treat a specific disease process. To achieve this goal, the surgeon must choose an appropriate radiological study based on the known strengths and limitations of each modality, the anticipated findings and the intended therapeutic outcomes.

Plain Films

The picture provided by plain films is the result of differential absorption of X-rays by various components of the abdominal wall, bony skeleton, and the intra-abdominal contents. In particular, it is the interface between organs with varying degrees of radiolucent fat and radio-opaque gas which overlay one another and produce diagnostic boundaries on the abdominal plain film. These interfaces delineate the liver edge, renal shadow, and psoas shadow and allow differentiation of the stomach, small bowel, and colon.[1]

In order to extract the maximal amount of information from an abdominal plain film, the position of the patient, the number of views needed and the known sensitivity of this modality for various diagnoses should be considered. An abdominal plain film is referred to as a KUB (kidneys, ureter, and bladder). An acute abdominal series is comprised of an upright chest, supine abdomen, and upright, decubitus or cross table lateral of the abdomen. The series of radiographs with the patient in various positions is meant to maximize the diagnostic yield of plain films. However, Mirvus et al. found that the upright abdominal view added little additional information and that the supine abdominal view in combination with the erect chest film identified 98% of imaging abnormalities.[2] Whether two or three abdominal films are obtained is of secondary importance. The most important goal is to image the entire abdominal cavity and ensure that the diagnostic question is addressed.

The American College of Radiology suggests the use of abdominal plain films for certain symptoms or diseases which may be encountered by the Colon and Rectal surgeon (Table 6-1). It is important to remember that plain films are not a screening tool and when used as such may contribute to increased radiation exposure for little diagnostic yield. If the clinical scenario suggests a diagnoses which is better imaged with a different radiologic modality, the alternate imaging study should be used as the initial or only examination for that patient.[3] As such, plain abdominal films are useful to the colon and rectal surgeon to identify foreign bodies, check the position of drains and catheters, evaluate changes or abnormalities in intestinal gas distribution and occasionally identify skeletal or mucosal changes associated with inflammatory bowel disease.

The most amount of information can be extracted from the abdominal plain film with a systematic diagnostic approach.[4] The first step is to identify abnormalities in the bony skeleton and abnormal intra-abdominal calcifications. This step rarely identifies a primary problem for the Colon and Rectal surgery patient but can diagnose secondary complications of a primary disease process. For example, plain films may provide information regarding the extraintestinal manifestations of IBD including sacroileitis, ankylosing spondylitis, and osteopenia secondary to chronic steroid use.[5] The second step to plain film examination is the identification of catheter, drain and foreign body location, and position. While the confirmation of appropriate intravascular catheter or intra-abdominal drain placement is self-evident, the evaluation of a rectal foreign body is not. Retained anal foreign bodies may migrate proximal to the anal sphincter as far up as the descending or sigmoid colon.[6] If there is proximal migration, the object may change axial position, induce bowel wall edema and become entrapped by the curvature of the rectum and sacrum. Plain abdominal films not only document the proximal extent of the object but can determine the number, size, and shape of the foreign body (Figure 6-1A and B). These evaluations assist the clinician in determining a plan for successful removal.

D.E. Beck et al. (eds.), *The ASCRS Textbook of Colon and Rectal Surgery: Second Edition*,
DOI 10.1007/978-1-4419-1584-9_6,

TABLE 6-1. Indications for abdominal radiography

Abdominal, flank, or pelvic pain
Vomiting
Abdominal distention, bloating, or increased girth
Evaluation for and follow-up of bowel obstruction or nonobstructive ileus
Constipation
Diarrhea
Palpable abdominal mass or organomegaly
Follow-up of the postoperative patient
Blunt or penetrating abdominal trauma
Search for foreign bodies
Assessment of the GI tract for residual contrast which can interfere with another imaging study
Evaluation of medical device position
Evaluation of pneumoperitoneum
Follow-up of contrast examinations of the gastrointestinal or urinary tracts

Additional steps for reading abdominal plain films depend on the determination of abdominal gas locations and patterns.[4] Gas collections may be extraperitoneal or intraperitoneal. Extraperitoneal collections in the soft tissue of the abdominal wall may reflect a necrotizing infection or recent intervention such as surgical incision. Intraperitoneal air may be located outside the intestinal lumen (free air), within the wall of the bowel or within the confines of the bowel wall. Appropriate localization of abdominal gas collections along with clinical correlation assists the clinician in distinguishing a benign condition from a surgical emergency.

Pneumoperitoneum or air outside the confines of the bowel wall is diagnostic of a perforated viscus and can be diagnosed with high sensitivity using an upright chest film.[7] However, if the patient has peritonitis or is extremely ill and cannot sit upright, a left lateral decubitus film can be obtained. The left lateral decubitus film in the expiratory phase or the upright chest in the midinspiratory phase have a high sensitivity and can be diagnostic of as little as 1 cm^3 of free intraperitoneal air.[8] The left lateral decubitus film is preferred to the right, because it allows air movement between the liver and right hemidiaphragm where it is easily imaged and not confused with the gastric bubble. It is important to maintain the left lateral decubitus position for at least 5–10 min prior to imaging in order to allow migration of air.[9]

Diagnostic signs of free intraperitoneal air have been widely recognized and described. Two signs that are most commonly present are right upper quadrant gas and Rigler's sign (Figure 6-2A and B).[10] A right upper quadrant gas sign is a triangular or linear gas collection which has an oblique (superomedial to inferolateral) orientation between the liver and right hemidiaphragm. Rigler's sign, outlining of both the mucosal and serosal sides of the bowel wall with associated bowel wall thickening (1–8 mm) is also indicative of free intraperitoneal air. Other less commonly seen diagnostic signs include the falciform ligament sign (a thin linear soft tissue density in the right upper quadrant caused by free intraperitoneal air lining both sides of the falciform ligament), the football sign (visualization of gas anterior to

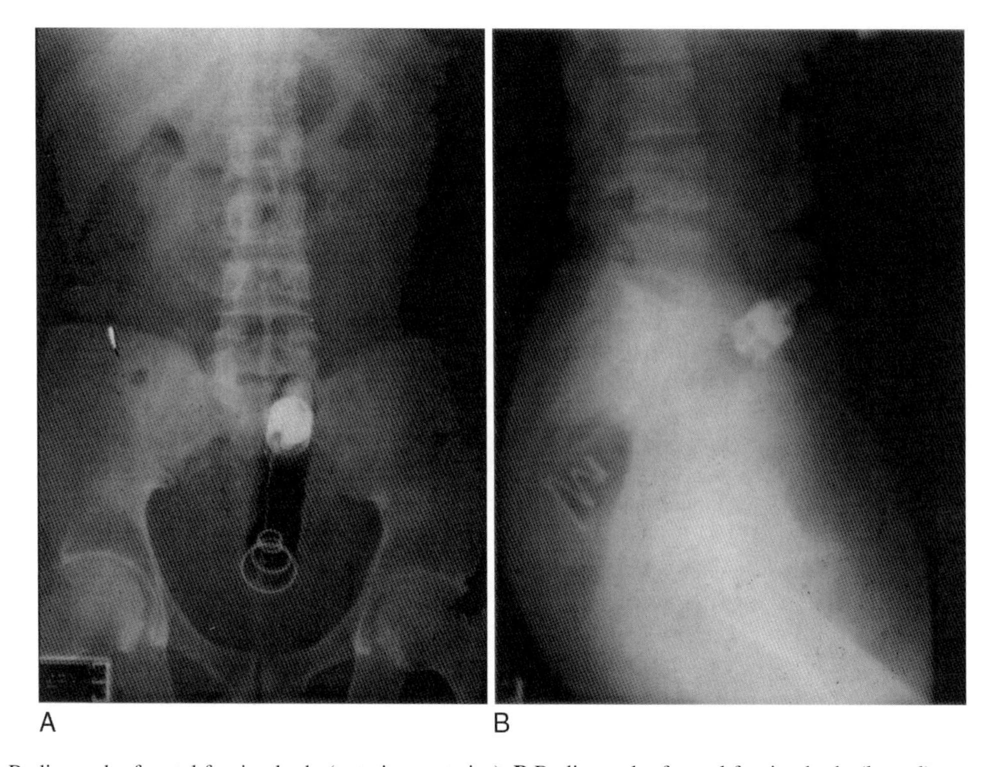

FIGURE 6-1. **A** Radiograph of rectal foreign body (anterior posterior). **B** Radiograph of rectal foreign body (lateral).

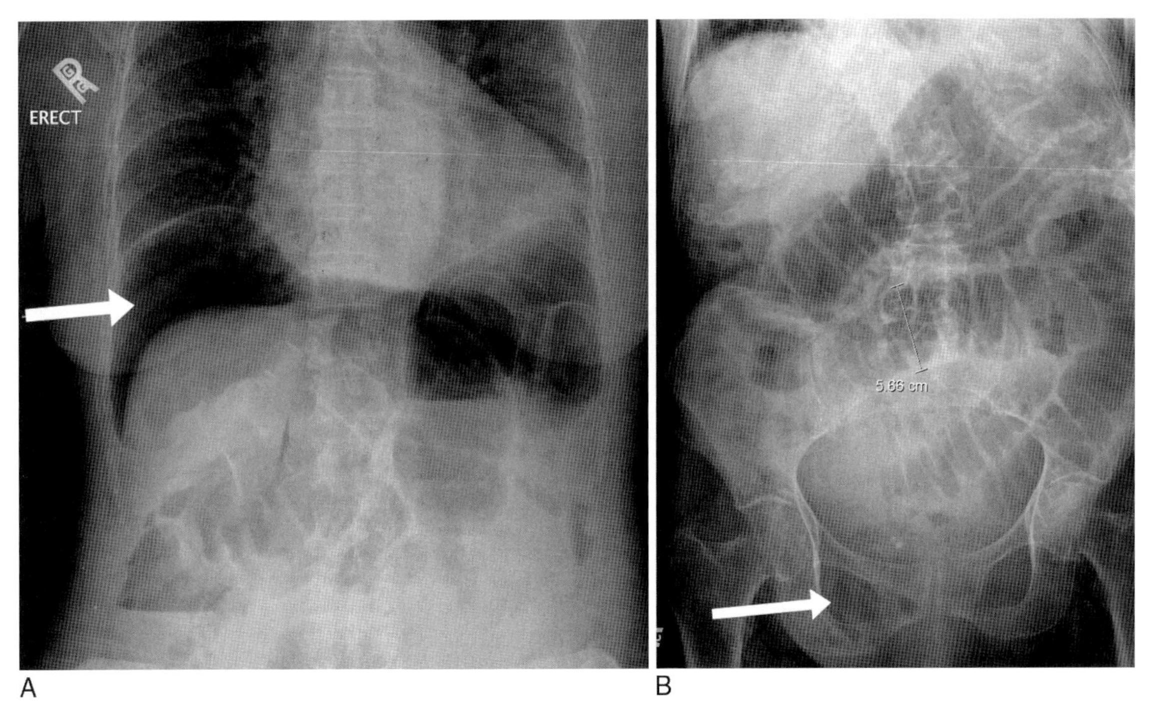

FIGURE 6-2. **A** Upright radiograph of the abdomen demonstrates a collection of air within the peritoneal space between the liver and the diaphragm. **B** Plain radiograph demonstrates the "Rigler" sign or "double lumen" sign (gas on both sides of the bowel wall).

loops of bowel within the central abdomen), and the inverted V sign (visualization of the medial umbilical folds in the pelvis). A diagnosis of free intraperitoneal air must always be correlated with the clinical condition of the patient. For instance, free intraperitoneal air can be a normal finding after surgery.[11] Free air is typically reabsorbed over several days following surgery but reabsorption may be delayed in the recumbent or thin patient. Increasing amounts of air imaged over time or in association with increasing abdominal pain may be indicative of an anastomotic leak or intestinal perforation. In addition, various conditions may be mistaken for free air. Chilaiditi syndrome is the interposition of the colon between the liver and diaphragm and can mimic the finding of pneumoperitoneum on plain abdominal films.[9]

Extralumenal air may also be located within a loculated abscess cavity, within solid organs that do not typically contain air, in the venous system or within the bowel wall. Portal venous air is peripherally located air which may have entered the portal venous system as a result of bowel ischemia and necrosis or a gas-producing bacteria. In contrast, pneumobilia or air within the biliary tract is centrally located and can result from a cholecystoduodenal fistula or from an endoscopic sphincterotomy. Finally, linear air within the bowel wall (pneumatosis intestinalis) may result from bowel ischemia and necrosis while cystic air collections within the bowel wall signify a benign condition called pneumatosis cystoides.[11]

Determination of intralumenal bowel gas patterns can help differentiate a small from large bowel obstruction or a bowel obstruction from a paralytic ileus. Bowel dilation is identified by the 3, 6, 9 rule. The small bowel is dilated when the diameter is 3 cm, the colon when it reaches 6 cm and the cecum when it dilates to 9 cm.[12] The small bowel can be differentiated from the colon by valvulae conniventes which cross the entire bowel loop and are more narrowly spaced compared to the haustra of the colon which are thicker, further apart, and only extend halfway across the colon diameter. In addition, dilated small bowel loops may form a stepladder appearance when dilated from obstruction (Figure 6-3). The valvulae conniventes may trap air between them as the obstructed small bowel fills with fluid giving a string of beads appearance. This finding is sensitive for a high-grade small bowel obstruction (SBO).[4] However, other signs of obstruction can be misleading. Air-fluid levels may be indicative of a SBO, gastroenteritis, or paralytic ileus. Ileus may be differentiated from obstruction by air found throughout the small bowel and colon (Figure 6-4). In contrast, a completely obstructed bowel may be void of air distal to the obstruction. In a partial or early bowel obstruction, distal air evacuation may not be present and the distinction between ileus and obstruction is impossible.[13]

Large bowel obstructions clinically appear like a distal SBO. On plain abdominal films the colon alone may be dilated if the ileocecal valve is competent (Figure 6-5). This causes the cecum to dilate. Acute cecal dilation beyond 12 cm places the patient at risk of perforation. In the setting of an incompetent ileocecal valve, air refluxes proximally into the small bowel which can make it difficult to distinguish between a paralytic ileus or distal bowel obstruction

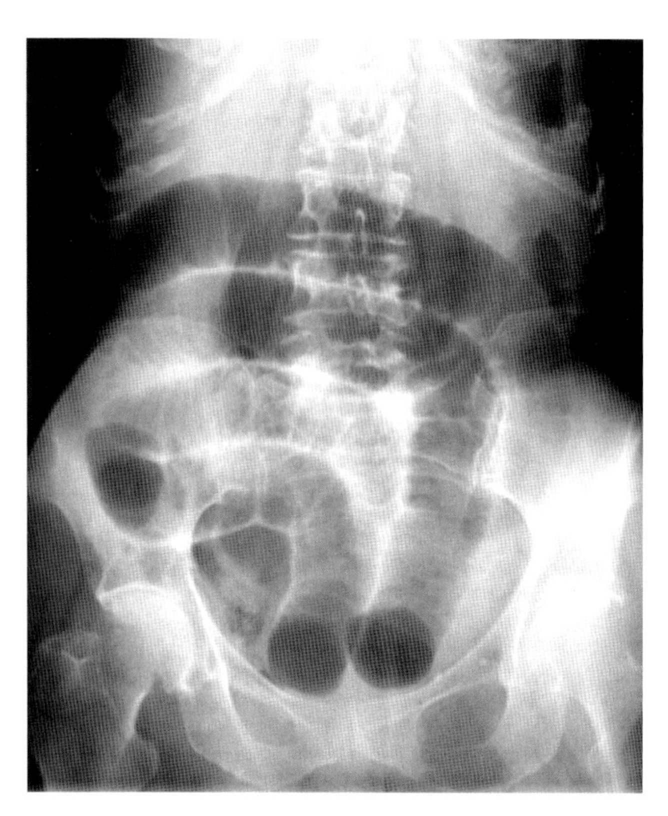

FIGURE 6-3. Plain film of small bowel obstruction with dilated small bowel loops, forming a stepladder.

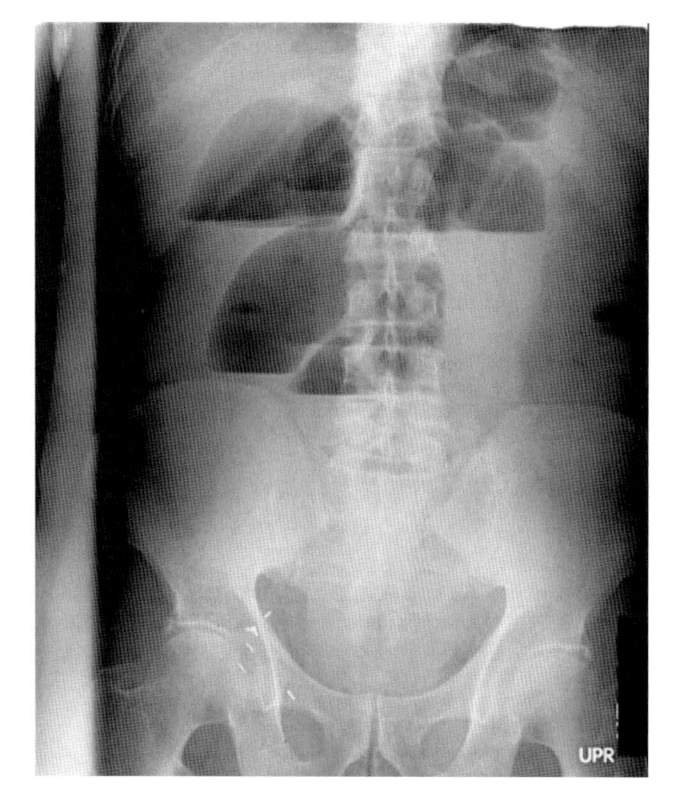

FIGURE 6-4. Small bowel obstruction air-fluid levels.

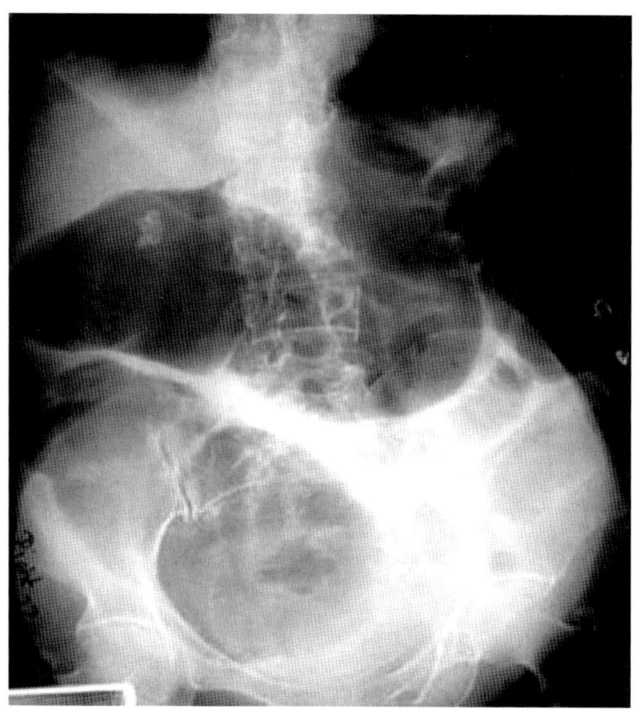

FIGURE 6-5. Large bowel obstruction secondary to sigmoid cancer. Competent ICV.

(Figure 6-6).[4] Volvulus in the cecum or sigmoid gives rise to a closed loop obstruction within the colon and can result in characteristic findings on abdominal plain films. The classic finding of a sigmoid volvulus is a U-shaped loop of colon projected toward the right upper quadrant in the shape of a "bent inner tube." In the middle of the sigmoid loop the medial walls of the obstructed sigmoid colon point into the pelvis (Figure 6-7). These findings are also associated with a dilated colon and small bowel proximal to the sigmoid. Cecal volvulus is characterized by a dilated cecum in the left upper quadrant with a "coffee bean" or "kidney" shape because of the medially placed ileocecal valve (Figure 6-8).[14,15]

Finally, the abdominal radiograph can reveal changes in mucosal contour and thickness. Normal bowel wall thickness is less than 2 mm. However, various forms of colitis may give rise to bowel wall thickening and mucosal irregularity. Thumbprinting is a radiographic sign that signifies bowel wall and mucosal edema, and in the setting of colon dilation may signify the presence of toxic megacolon with risk of impending perforation. Chronic mucosal inflammation may lead to haustral blunting and a tubular burned out colon from longstanding colitis (Figure 6-9).[4,5]

Abdominal plain films can yield a large amount of information if used in the appropriate clinical setting. In addition, they are inexpensive and can be performed at the patient's bedside. However, abdominal plain films are insensitive and other imaging modalities may be needed for definitive diagnosis.

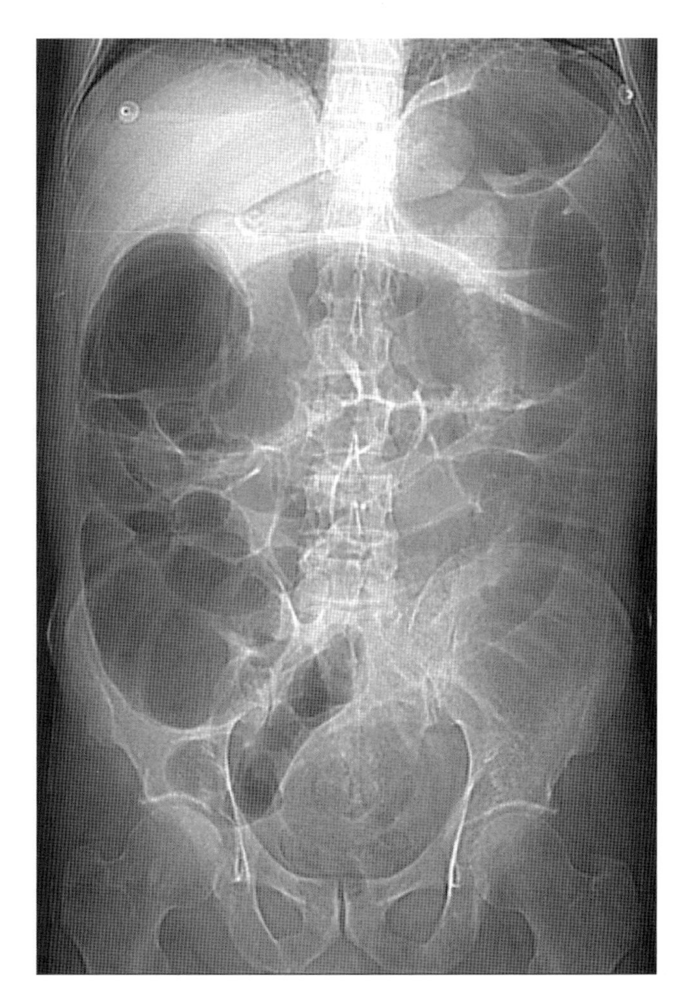

FIGURE 6-6. Large bowel obstruction secondary to sigmoid cancer. Incompetent ICV.

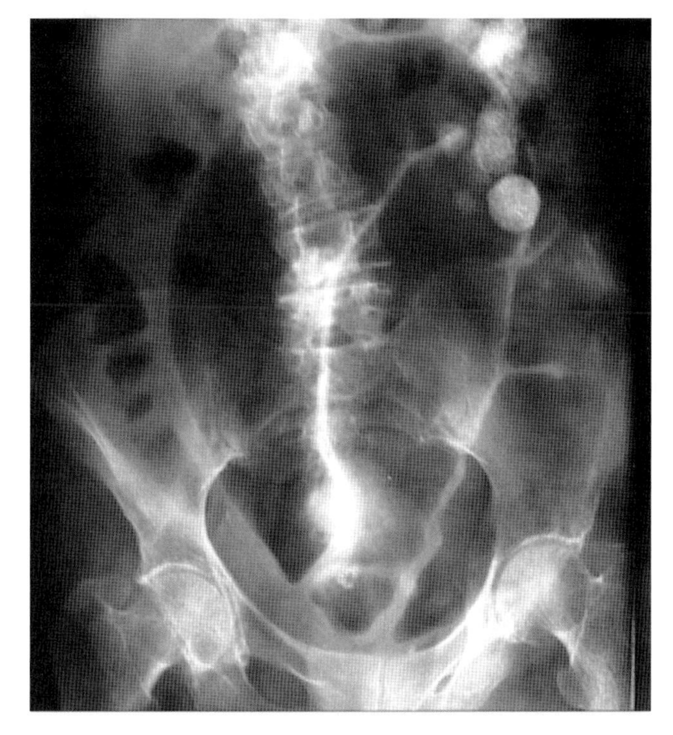

FIGURE 6-7. Plain film of sigmoid volvulus.

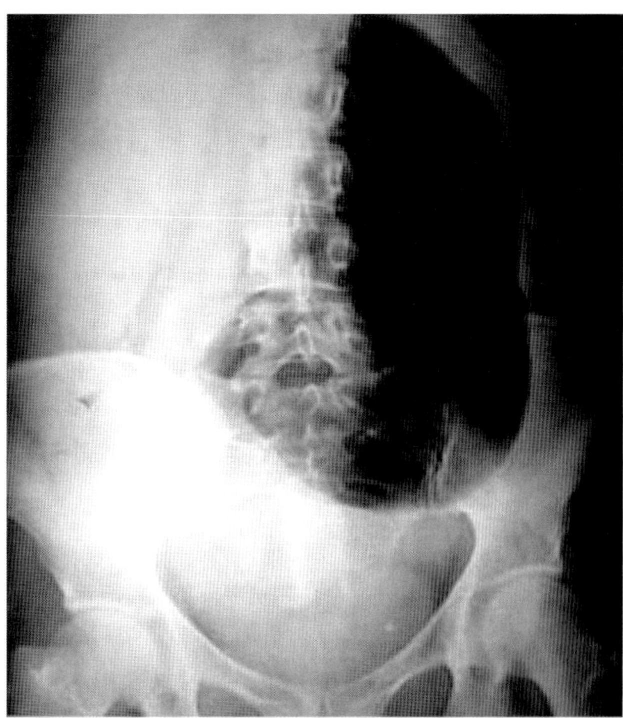

FIGURE 6-8. Plain film of cecal volvulus.

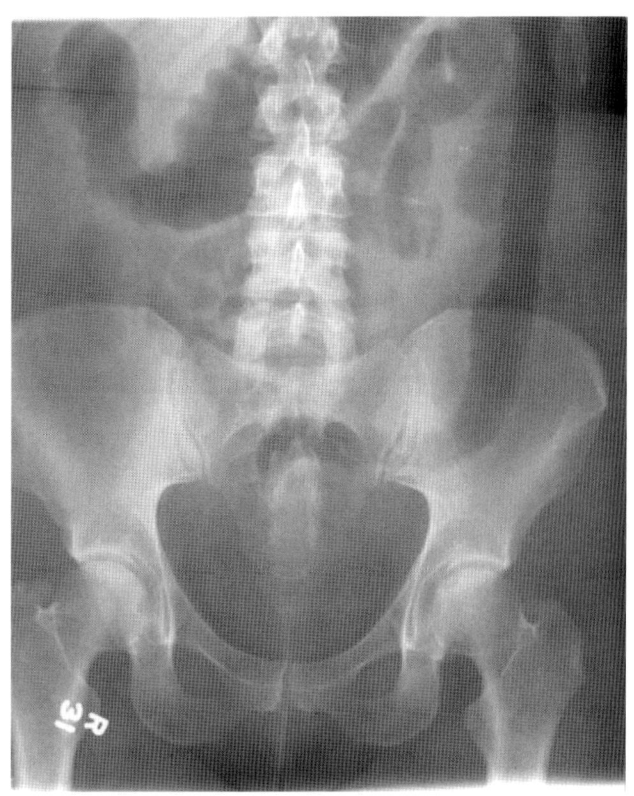

FIGURE 6-9. Plain film of chronic burned out colitis.

Contrast Studies

Contrast Enemas

Contrast enemas can be performed as a single contrast or double contrast enema. The single contrast enema is performed by filling the colon and rectum with barium or a water-soluble agent through a rectal catheter. In double contrast enemas or air contrast enemas, barium is instilled into the colon and rectum until the mid-transverse colon is reached. The colon is then drained of excess barium and air is instilled to allow lumenal distention and prevent mucosal wall apposition. The radiologist can then change the position of the patient and use fluoroscopic guidance to obtain images of the colonic and rectal mucosa throughout its length and in multiple projections without overlap. The double contrast provides mucosal coating and detail that cannot be seen in single contrast studies. Careful technique with mucosal coating, adequate distention, and numerous projections allow discrimination of mucosal abnormalities with the double contrast enema.[16]

The limitations of a contrast enema need to be considered prior to subjecting the patient to this study. In order to visualize the mucosa, the patient must undergo a complete bowel preparation. If a patient does not have mobility to change position on the fluoroscopy table or does not have enough rectal tone to hold the contrast enema, the mucosal coating and projections obtained will be of limited diagnostic value. An incompetent ileocecal valve may allow reflux of contrast into the small bowel and further obscure colonic findings. The rectal catheter may obscure the distal rectum so that internal hemorrhoids or a distal rectal cancer cannot be appropriately discriminated.[17] Finally, there is a risk of perforation as a result of this study. Because barium causes an intense inflammatory response within the peritoneal cavity, in clinical situations for which intestinal continuity is in question or when the bowel wall may be weakened, a water-soluble contrast agent should be used. These scenarios include question of anastomotic integrity, evaluation of a large bowel obstruction, acute colitis, recent snare or forceps biopsy of the colon wall, and suspicion of colonic fistulas.[18] In comparison to barium studies, water-soluble enemas do not coat the mucosa and do not discriminate mucosal changes.

The double contrast technique can be used to detect mucosal disease in an elective setting. This includes the evaluation of colonic polyps and cancer, inflammatory bowel disease, diverticulosis and other mural abnormalities like lipomas, lymphoma, and endometriosis.

The most common reason for a double contrast enema is for colon and rectal cancer screening. Sensitivity of the study depends on the size of the lesion in addition to the coating, distention, and projection of the colon mucosa mentioned earlier. Polyps may be seen as a filling defect if imaged in a puddle of barium or may be outlined as sessile or pedunculated projections into the colon lumen (Figure 6-10). The double contrast enema has a sensitivity of 50% for polyps and cancer

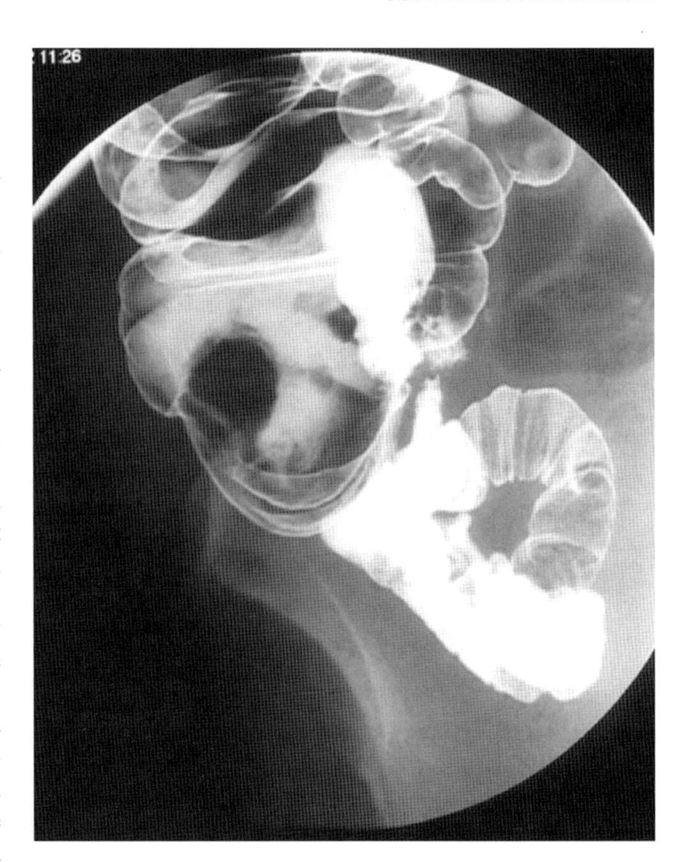

FIGURE 6-10. ACE of polyp or early cancer.

less than 1 cm in size, and 90% sensitivity for those greater than 1 cm.[19,20] Increasing size, ulceration, and circumferential involvement increase the possibility that a polyp has an underlying malignancy. Semiannular lesions, which are seen on contrast enema with abrupt transition from normal to irregular mucosal patterns, shelf-like overhanging borders, and circumferential bowel narrowing, are characteristic of an apple core lesion and are diagnostic of cancer (Figure 6-11). In comparison, benign strictures from ischemic, infectious, or inflammatory etiologies have smooth tapering borders.[21] Overall, double contrast barium enema has a positive predictive value of 96% for a malignant stricture and 84–88% for a benign stricture.[22] Double contrast barium enema has been recommended as one screening modality for patients greater than 50 years of age at average risk of colon and rectal cancer.

Double contrast barium enema can also be diagnostic in the setting of inflammatory bowel disease. It can be used to differentiate Crohn's disease from ulcerative colitis, define the extent and severity of disease burden as well as visualize complications of the disease. In acute ulcerative colitis the mucosa appears stippled with shallow punctuate ulceration (Figure 6-12A). As the inflammation progresses the ulcers enlarge as crypt abscess rupture and expose the submucosa leading to pseudopolyps, which appear as irregular mucosal projections on the contrast enema (Figure 6-12B). Eventually, there is loss of mucosal detail and haustral folds which cause

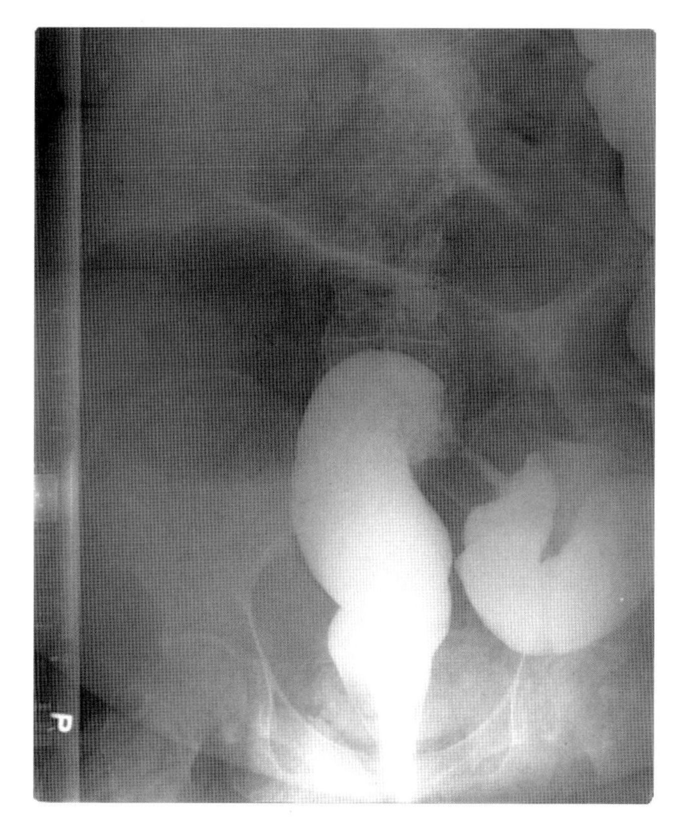

FIGURE 6-11. ACE of annular cancer and "apple core sign."

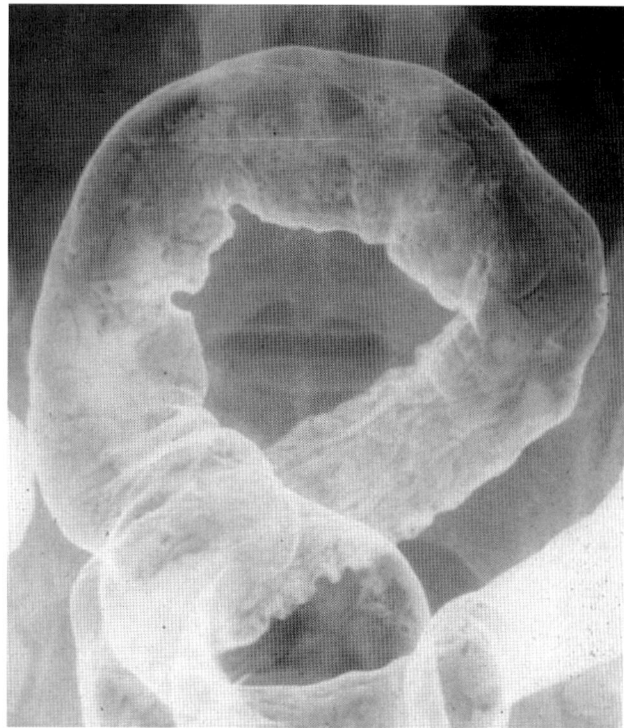

A

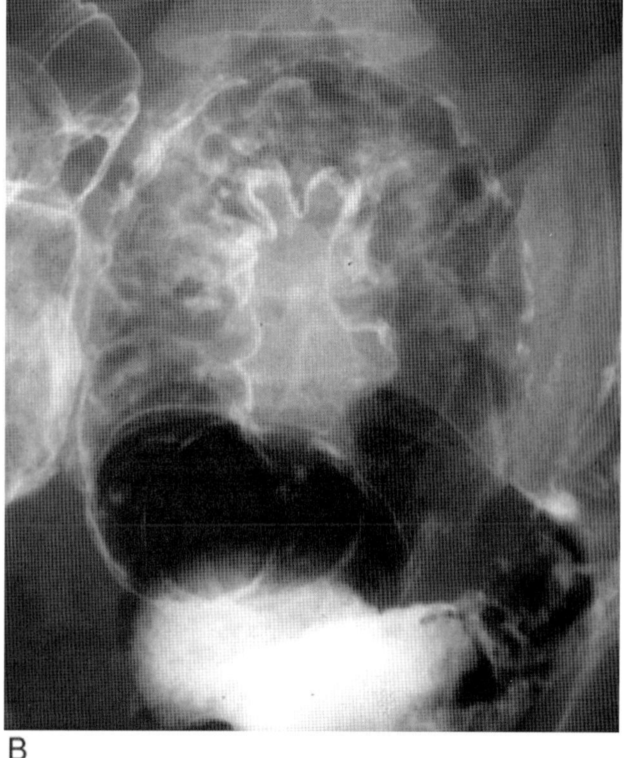

B

FIGURE 6-12. **A** Contrast enema of ulcerative colitis showing stippling ulcers or early colitis. **B** Contrast enema of ulcerative colitis with pseudopolyps.

a tubular or lead pipe appearance of the colon (Figure 6-13). Strictures from ulcerative colitis appear as smooth, symmetric, and circumferential colonic narrowing.[23] In Crohn's disease, the mucosal changes are not continuous and are deeper than the changes seen in ulcerative colitis. Early aphthous ulcers appear as shallow depressions with a radiolucent halo (Figure 6-14A). As Crohn's disease progresses the ulcers widen and coalesce as the muscle in the bowel wall is penetrated. This leads to cobblestoning which appears as irregular white stripes within the colon wall on contrast enema (Figure 6-14B). Deep linear ulceration along the mesenteric border causes "rake" or "bear claw" ulcers that can cause stricturing from transmural fibrosis. Strictures from Crohn's disease appear as noncircumferential, irregular areas of narrowing that are centered at the mesenteric edge (Figure 6-15).[24,25] Complications of Crohn's disease such as strictures and fistulas are well imaged with the double contrast barium technique. In contrast, other complications of inflammatory bowel disease are not easily diagnosed with enema studies. In both ulcerative colitis and Crohn's disease it is difficult to distinguish inflammatory polyps from dysplasia or cancer.[26]

Diverticular disease can also be well characterized with contrast enemas. The size, shape, number, and location of diverticuli are well imaged. In profile, diverticuli appear flask shaped with a neck, which points away from the colonic lumen. En face diverticuli appear as a white spot or meniscus within the colon lumen (Figure 6-16). With acute diverticular inflammation, secondary signs of inflammation such as narrowing of the colon lumen from extrinsic compression and mucosal edema are evident. Complications

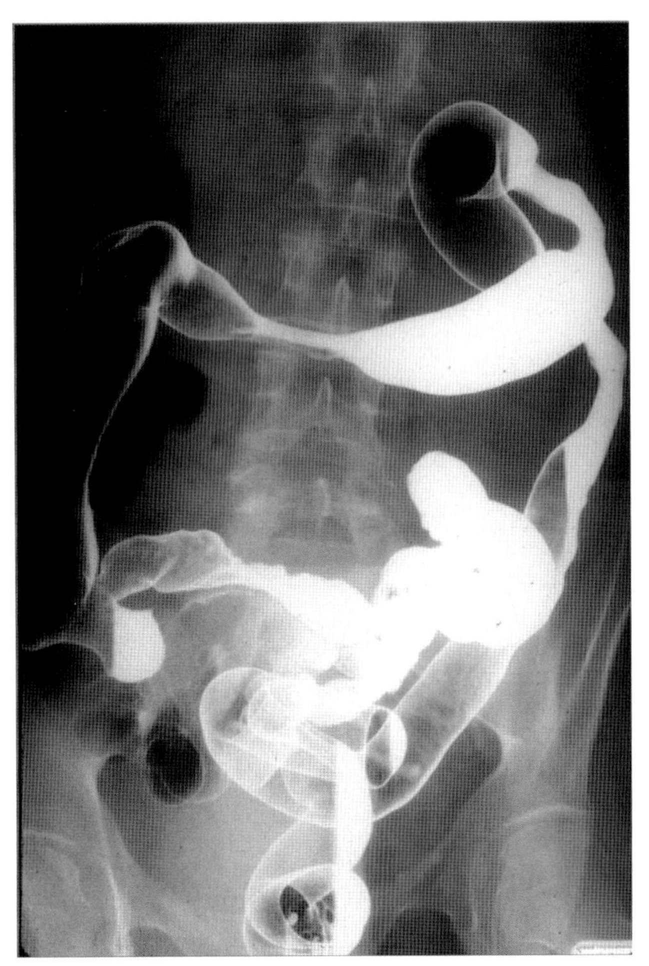

FIGURE 6-13. Contrast enema of chronic ulcerative colitis.

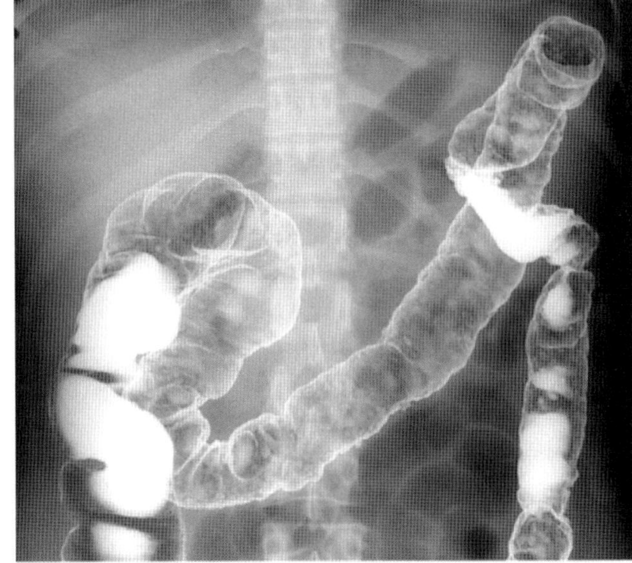

A

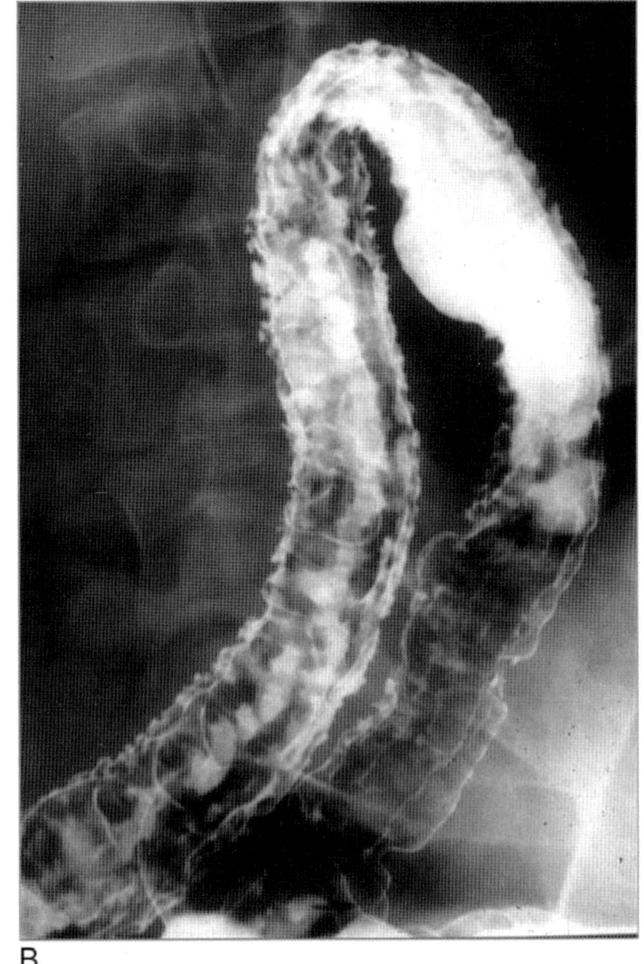

B

FIGURE 6-14. **A** Contrast enema of Crohn's disease showing ulcers. **B** Contrast enema of Crohn's with fissures and long linear ulcers.

of diverticulitis can also be seen. Diverticular perforation results in leaking of extralumenal contrast into the peritoneal cavity, a contained cavity or a blind sinus that drains back into the colon lumen. Strictures appear as smooth transitions in colon caliber with intact mucosa. Abscesses are suggested by a smooth contour defect within the colon lumen which does not distend with additional air or contrast instillation. Fistulae between proximal intestinal loops, the vagina, and bladder may also be seen. Barium contrast enema is safe to perform with active diverticular inflammation in the absence of peritonitis. However, the sensitivity of the contrast enema is low and may not be diagnostic in a patient with complicated diverticulitis.[27]

Double contrast enemas may also reveal colonic lipomas, endometriosis, and lymphoma. Lipomas are seen as a submucosal mass or polypoid lesion with smooth overlying mucosa. The soft pliable nature of the lipoma may be imaged in real time as the barium and air are instilled and show compression of the mass known as the "pillow sign." Endometriosis appears as an extracolonic process with intact but

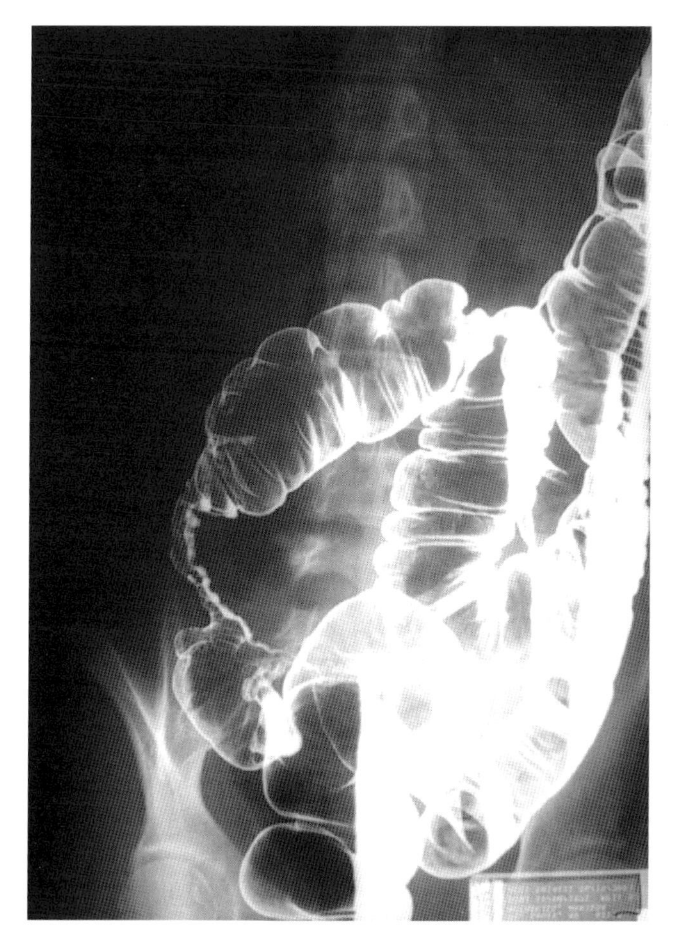

FIGURE 6-15. Contrast enema of Crohn's disease showing a stricture.

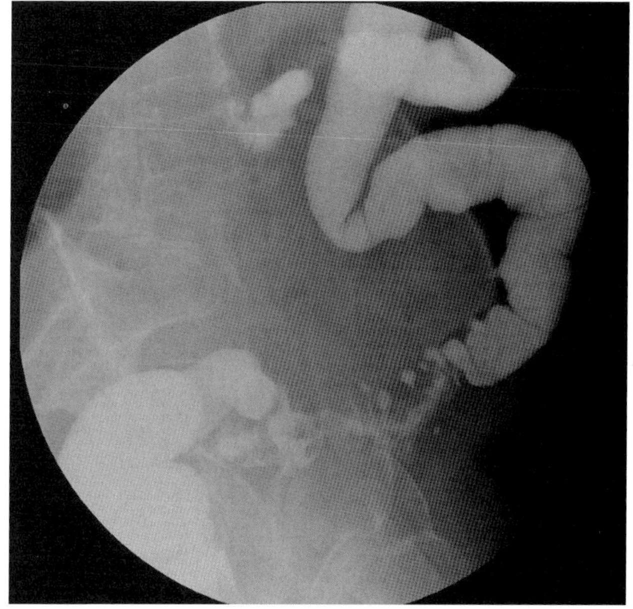

FIGURE 6-16. Barium enema demonstrates a deformed colon wall with diverticular sacs. (From Blanchard TJ, Altmeyer WB, Mathews CC. Limitations of colorectal imaging studies. In: Whitlow CB, Beck DE, Margolin DA, Hicks TC, Timmcke AE, editors. Improved outcomes in colon and rectal surgery. London: Informa Healthcare; 2010. p. 97–131. With permission).

bunched up mucosal folds that result in luminal narrowing and in extreme cases scarring and lumenal contracture (Figure 6-17). Lymphoma appears different from adenocarcinoma on a double contrast enema. In contrast, lymphoma does not narrow the lumen but causes folding and thickening of the mucosa from bowel wall infiltration. The mucosa maintains a smooth appearance (Figure 6-18). All these findings on double contrast enema while suggestive of a specific diagnosis, require correlation with clinical information to be diagnostic of the condition.[28,29]

Water-soluble enemas do not result in the same mucosal coating and colonic distention that can be achieved with double contrast enemas. However, water-soluble contrast is not toxic to the peritoneal lining and can therefore be used in clinical situations in which bowel integrity may be compromised. This includes clinical situations suspicious for colonic obstruction caused by cancer, acute episodes of inflammatory bowel disease, intussusception, volvulus, and fecal impaction. Water-soluble enemas may also be used for evaluation of anastomotic integrity. Colonic intussusception occurs when a portion of proximal colon or ileum telescopes into the lumen of distal colon. A water-soluble contrast

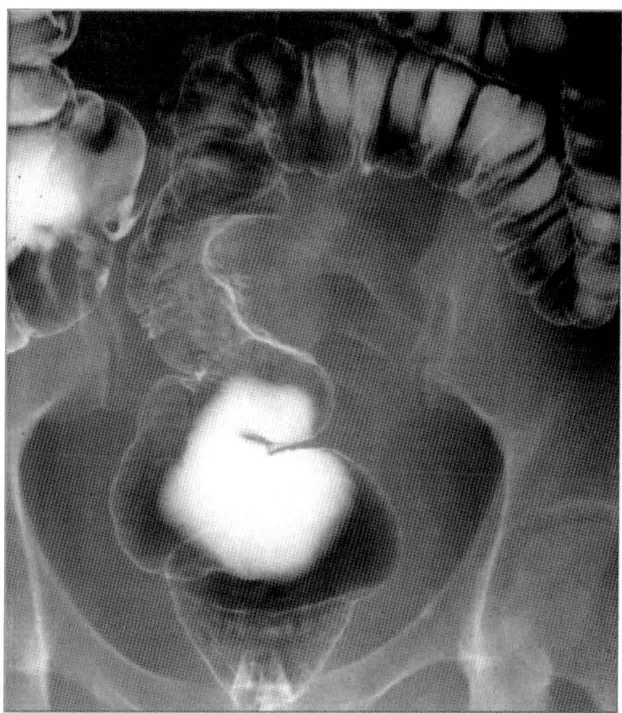

FIGURE 6-17. Contrast enema showing endometriosis.

enema demonstrates a spring coil appearance or crescent sign as contrast gets trapped between the lumens of the two bowel segments and leaves a thin circular line that outlines

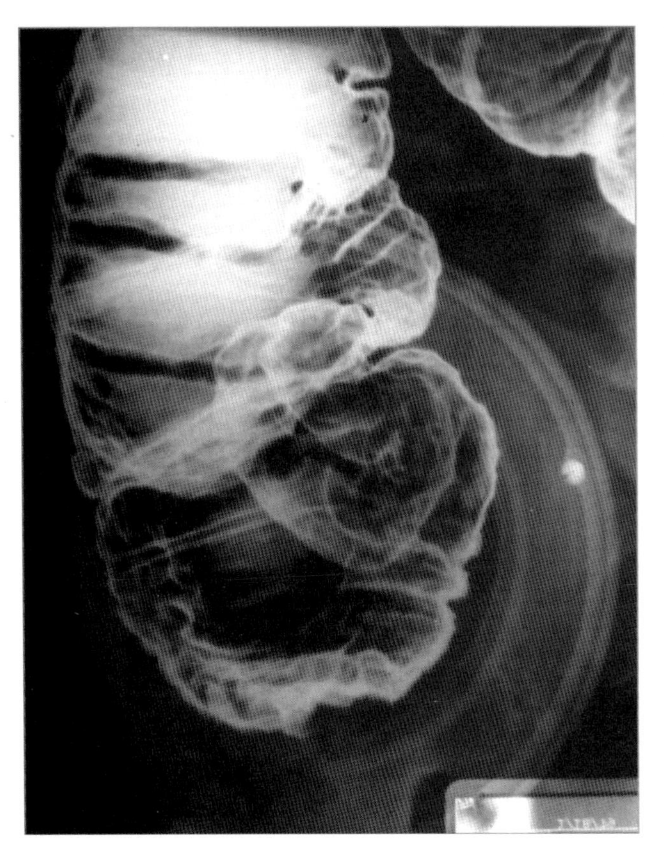

Figure 6-18. Contrast enema showing colonic lymphoma.

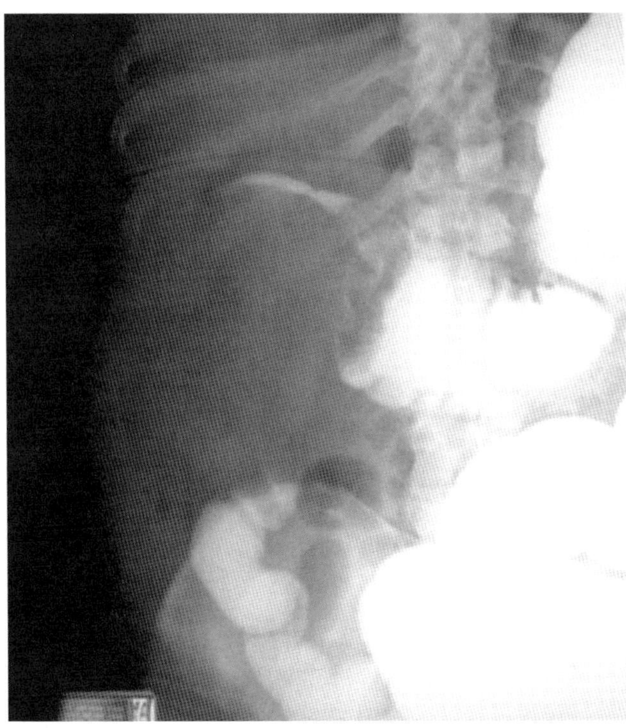

Figure 6-19. Contrast enema showing colonic intussusception.

the proximal bowel in the distal bowel lumen (Figure 6-19). While barium, air, and water-soluble enemas have been used to hydrostatically decompress an intussusception, this is not typically attempted in the older child or adult because the cause is usually a pathologic lead point.[30] Water-soluble enemas can be used to diagnose and occasionally spontaneously decompress a colonic volvulus. Sigmoid volvulus appears as a "bird's beak" as the mucosal folds spiral into the point of obstruction.[31] In cecal volvulus there is abrupt contrast cutoff distal to the torsed colonic segment with a dilated ectopic cecum. This is known as the "column cutoff sign" (Figure 6-20). In the setting of fecal impaction, water-soluble contrast is instilled up to the site of obstruction under fluoroscopic guidance. The high osmolality of the substance allows it to emulsify stool and release impacted stool into smaller pieces that can be passed per anus.[32] Water-soluble enemas are also useful prior to takedown of a diverting stoma, when a colonic stenosis is suspected or in the early postoperative period when a leak is suspected (Figure 6-21A and B). Views of the colon should be obtained in the anteroposterior and lateral views during early luminal filling, full colonic distention and after evacuation of contrast. Multiple colon projections with varying degrees of contrast distention allow for the diagnosis of subtle leaks that may be obscured by full colonic distention with contrast.[16] Overall, water-soluble enemas may not have the same diagnostic sensitivity as a double contrast barium enema but they remain useful in the diagnosis and treatment of colon and rectal disease.

Small Bowel Series and Enteroclysis

The small bowel can be imaged using several methods. To obtain a small bowel series, a patient drinks a large volume of dilute barium and contrast is followed as it advances through the small bowel with fluoroscopy images taken every 15 min. In order to improve visualization of small bowel loops, abdominal pressure and compression can be used to flatten bowel loops and decrease small bowel loop overlap. Transit of contrast through the small bowel normally takes 90–120 min. In comparison, small bowel enteroclysis is a more labor and time intensive method for imaging the small bowel. The patient must undergo colonic cleansing to decrease both the time needed for contrast to reach the terminal ileum as well as the amount of contrast needed to fill the small bowel.[25] With this method, two contrast agents are instilled into the duodenum at separate points in time through a tube inserted through the nose and advanced into the proximal duodenum. The rate of contrast instillation is modified according to the amount of small bowel distention achieved and patient tolerance. Administration of barium in addition to air or methylcellulose allows the barium to act as an interface with the small bowel mucosa for detection of mucosal lesions or subtle mucosal changes. Serial images are obtained with enteroclysis as is done with small bowel series. In comparison to small bowel series, small

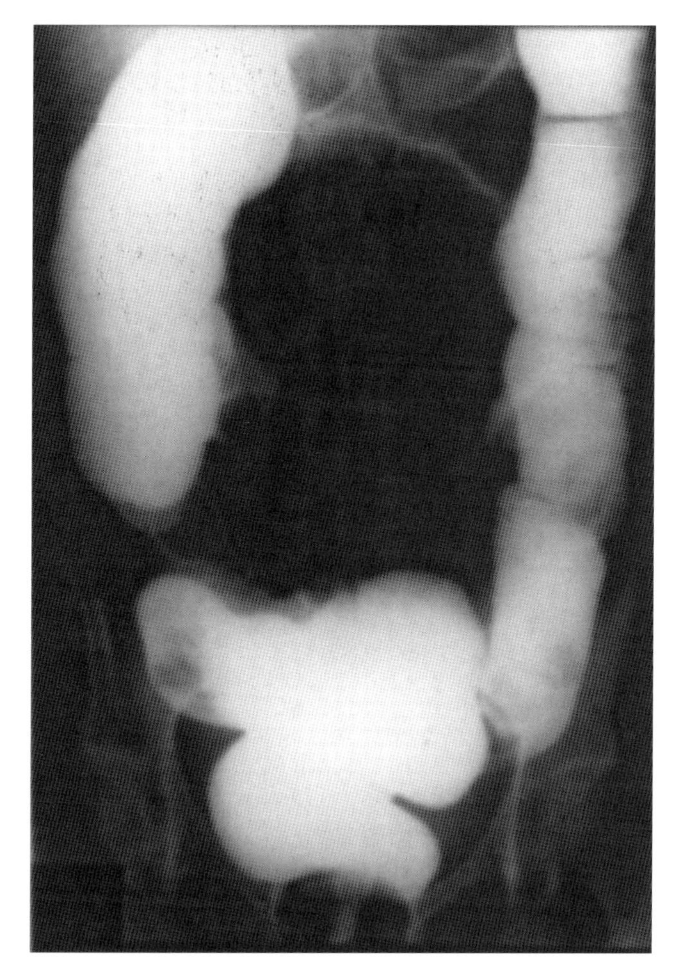

FIGURE 6-20. Water-soluble contrast enema showing cecal volvulus. (From Blanchard TJ, Altmeyer WB, Matthews CC. Limitations of colorectal imaging studies. In: Whitlow CB, Beck DE, Margolin DA, Hicks TC, Timmcke AE, editors. Improved outcomes in colon and rectal surgery. London: Informa Healthcare; 2010. p. 97–131. With permission).

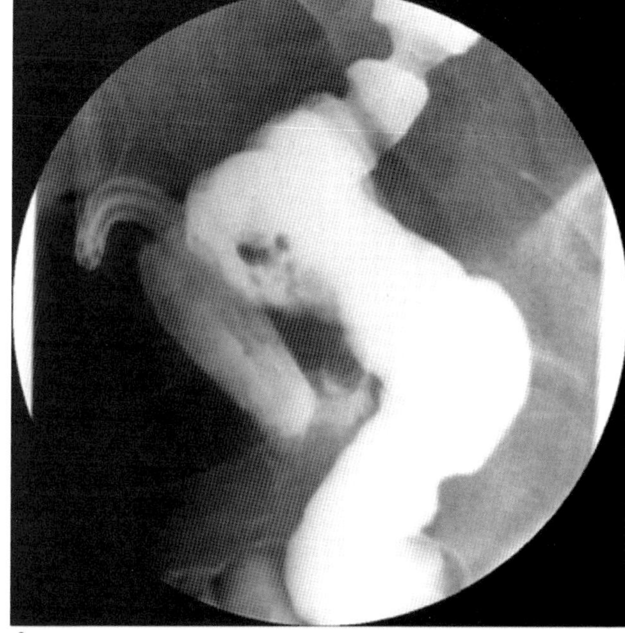

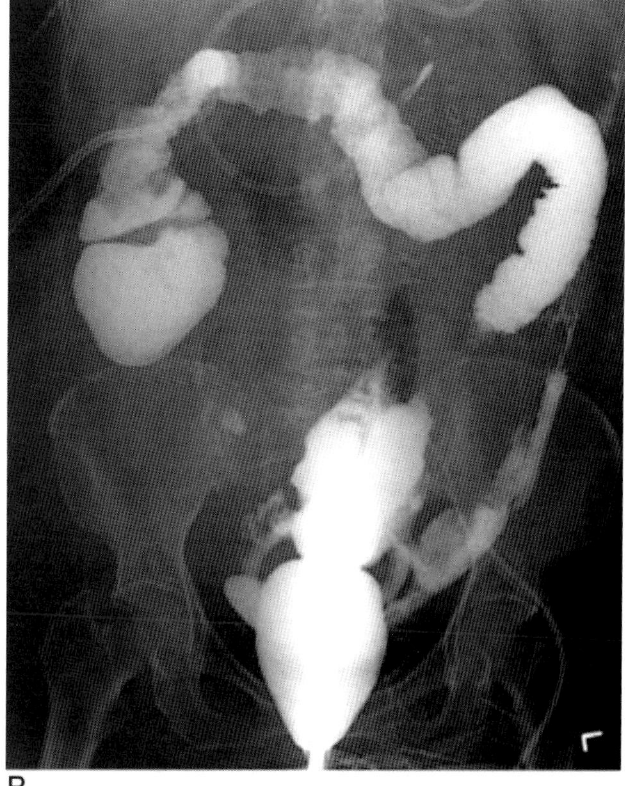

FIGURE 6-21. **A** Contrast enema showing a contained anastomotic leak. **B** Contrast enema showing a free-flowing leak.

bowel enteroclysis requires placement of a nasogastric tube, high radiation doses (up to 21 mSv), and administration of a hyperosmotic contrast agent.[33] Overall, fluoroscopy is a time and labor-intensive method of obtaining radiographic images of the small bowel.

Small bowel imaging is typically useful for patients with unexplained gastrointestinal bleeding, suspected small bowel tumors, Crohn's disease, and partial SBOs. For patients with Crohn's disease, the severity and distribution of disease can be determined (Figure 6-22A and B). In addition, the site of small bowel complications such a fistula and stricture can be located. For patients with suspected SBOs, dilute barium can be used to image the small bowel when there is unclear etiology of the obstruction or when localization of the obstructing point is important. Unlike the colon, barium does not become inspissated in the small bowel while hypertonic water-soluble contrast agents may exacerbate lumenal distention already present in SBO.[34] In all, the small bowel contributes a large amount of mucosal surface and length to be studied. Small bowel radiography should be undertaken only after ruling out other parts of the intestine as the cause of the patient's symptoms or for specific diagnoses that affect the small bowel.

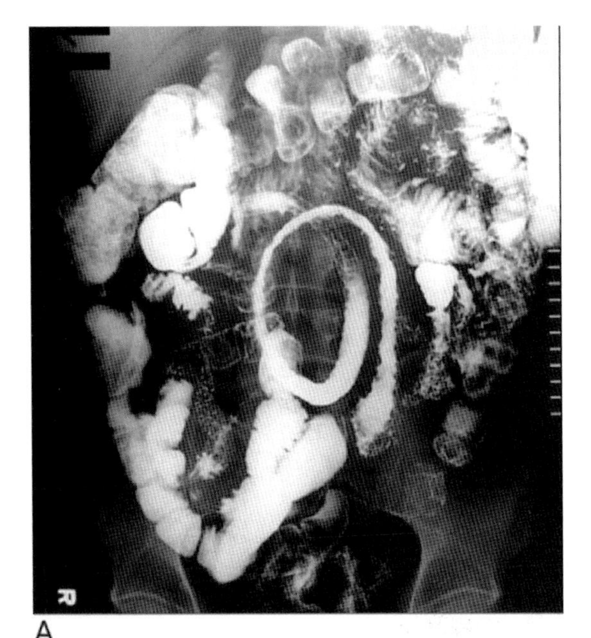

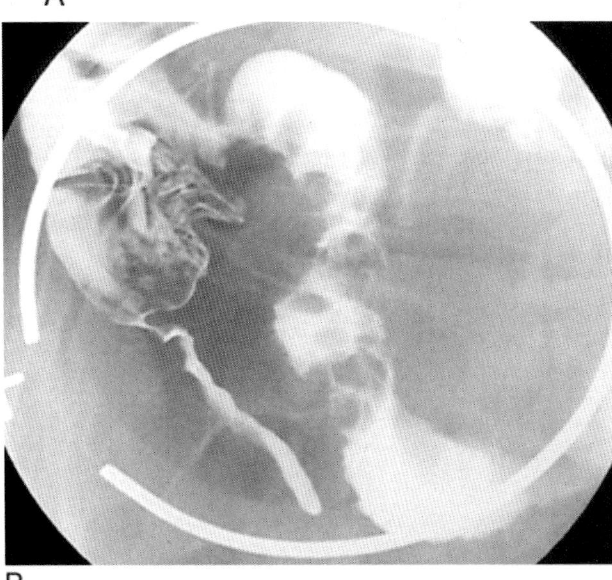

FIGURE 6-22. **A** Small bowel series showing terminal ileum Crohn's disease strictures. **B** Small bowel follow through showing cobblestoning.

Computed Tomography

Computed tomography (CT) has become a routine examination to evaluate a wide range of disease processes, because it is an easy, fast, and accurate test. CT provides detailed and high-resolution cross-sectional images of hollow viscous and solid organs. Accurate interpretation requires optimal opacification of the gastrointestinal tract and vascular structures. The bowel is opacified by administering a water-soluble oral contrast agent. The density of barium interferes with the acquisition of data during the scan and thus should be avoided as a contrast agent. The oral contrast is typically administered 45–60 min before scanning to allow the contrast to opacify as much of the bowel as possible. If pelvic or rectal pathology is being evaluated, the contrast may also be administered per rectum at the time the scan is being performed. Intravenous (IV) contrast agents typically are iodinated so it is important to take a thorough history of allergies. Anaphylactic reaction to the iodinated contrast is a contraindication for administration but simple allergies such as hives can be prevented with steroids and diphenhydramine. Iodinated contrast is administered as a bolus at the time of the examination. The reason for the examination dictates the exact timing between when the contrast is administered and when the CT images are acquired (i.e., venous vs. arterial phase). The CT scan uses ionizing radiation to acquire the images with 5- to 10-mm collimation. Smaller collimation allows for sharper, more detailed images. Radiation exposure to the patient varies depending on protocol design and the type of CT scanner used. However, the average radiation dose for a multidetector CT of the abdomen and pelvis is 13.3 mSv and for a CT of the chest is 6.8.[35] CT is sensitive for the staging of colon and rectal cancer and diagnosis of inflammatory and infectious conditions of the colon, bowel obstruction, and postoperative complications.

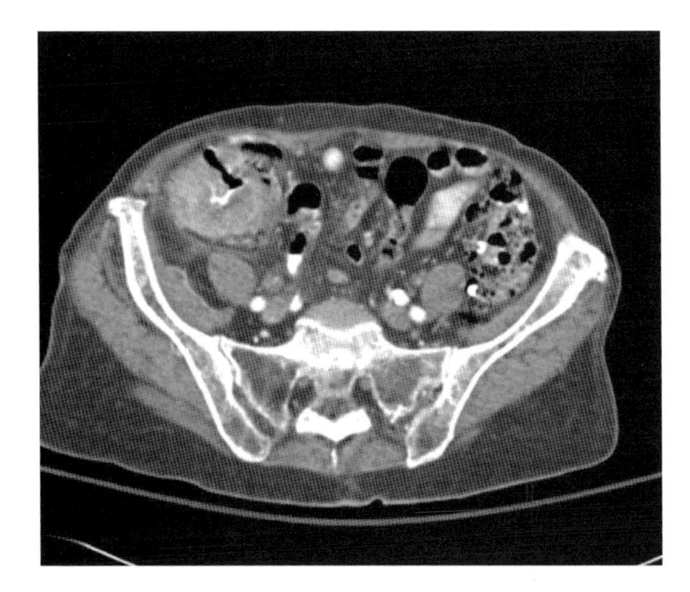

FIGURE 6-23. CT scan showing colon cancer primary lesion and adenopathy.

Colon and Rectal Cancer

CT of the abdomen and pelvis is useful for the initial staging of colon and rectal cancer. CT assists the surgeon in determining the location of the primary tumor, involvement of adjacent organs, enlargement of regional lymph nodes and the presence of distant (liver) metastases. Colon and rectal cancer primary lesions may appear as an exophytic mass within the colon lumen or as an apple core lesion with irregular circumferential bowel wall narrowing (Figure 6-23).[36] CT accuracy for predicting tumoral extension beyond the muscularis propria can be as high as 70–82%[37]; however,

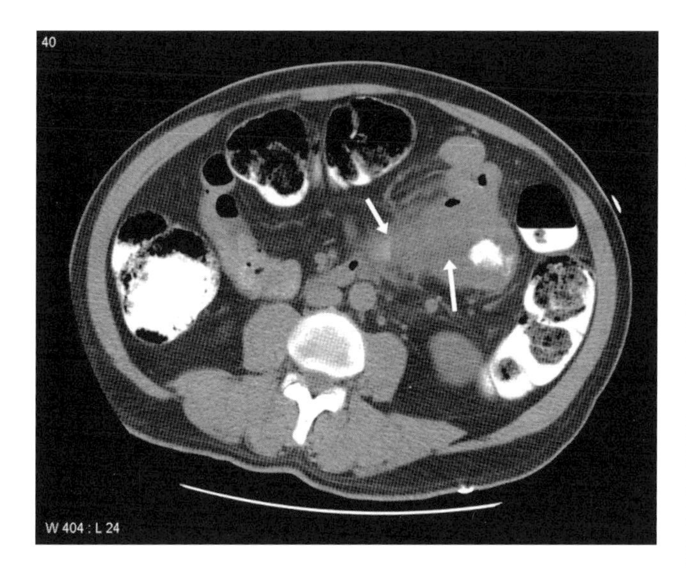

FIGURE 6-24. CT showing a large colonic mass in the descending colon that narrows the lumen. CT cannot differentiate tumor extension through the wall from pericolonic edema or desmoplastic reaction. (From Blanchard TJ, Altmeyer WB, Matthews CC. Limitations of colorectal imaging studies. In: Whitlow CB, Beck DE, Margolin DA, Hicks TC, Timmcke AE, editors. Improved outcomes in colon and rectal surgery. London: Informa Healthcare; 2010. p. 97–131. With permission).

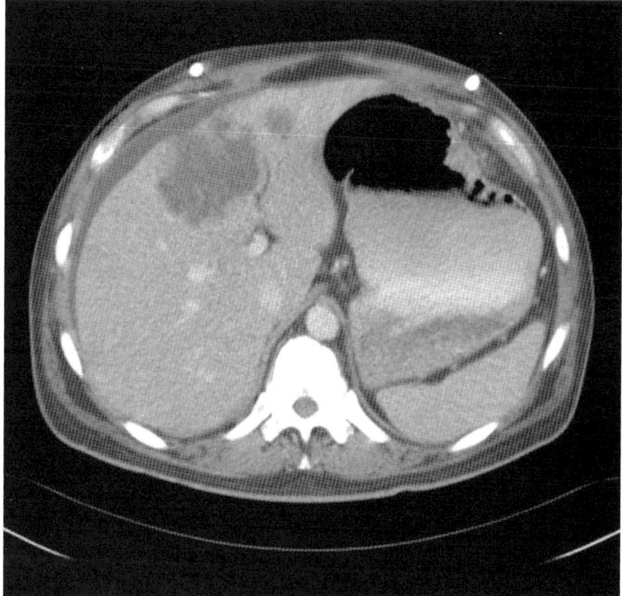

FIGURE 6-25. CT scan showing liver metastasis.

inaccuracies result from the inability to distinguish gross tumor extension from peritumoral desmoplastic reaction (Figure 6-24). CT is also advantageous for determining adjacent organ involvement which will require more extensive en bloc resection of the tumor. Adjacent organ involvement may include the peritoneum, duodenum, stomach, vagina, bladder, and abdominal wall.[38] Lymph nodes are considered pathologic if they are >1 cm in size on CT scan. Accuracy in detecting lymph node involvement can be limited by normal size of tumor bearing nodes and enlargement of lymph nodes in the peritumoral region without nodal metastases.[39,40] Overall, preoperative CT scans can assist the surgeon in determining local tumor extension.

CT scan is an accurate imaging modality for the detection of hepatic metastases as well as hepatic recurrence of colon and rectal cancer. CT images are typically obtained in two phases: the hepatic artery phase (20–25 s after the IV contrast is infused) and the portal venous phase (65–70 s after the IV contrast is infused). Colon and rectal metastases are supplied by the hepatic artery while most of the liver parenchyma is supplied by the portal vein. Therefore, during a portal venous phase CT, colon and rectal liver metastases appear as solid hypodense lesions that do not have dynamic enhancement changes (Figure 6-25).[41] These characteristics allow hepatic metastases to be differentiated from fluid filled hepatic cysts, hemangiomas, and hypervascular liver malignancies. Preoperative CT scan is 85% sensitive for colon and rectal hepatic metastases.[42] Because liver lesions that are <1 cm in size do not demonstrate contrast-enhancing properties, they are labeled as indeterminate lesions. Follow-up studies of patients with colon and rectal cancer and indeterminate liver lesions show that up to 11% of indeterminate lesions on initial CT may progress on subsequent imaging and, therefore, represent early metastases.[43]

CT scan is a recommended part of some surveillance programs for colon and rectal cancer patients in order to detect recurrence. Although surveillance programs have not been shown to improve overall survival, intense follow-up has been shown to improve postrecurrence survival.[44] CT scan, along with carcinoembryonic antigen levels, chest X-ray, and colonoscopy, has been shown to detect asymptomatic recurrence.[45] Recurrence of colon and rectal cancer on CT scan is demonstrated by interval enlargement of soft tissue masses, enlarging lymph nodes, and invasion of adjacent organs (Figure 6-26). New metastases may also be visualized within the liver. Because evidence is lacking that routine CT scan after colon and rectal cancer resection improves overall survival, the ASCRS practice parameters do not recommend routine abdominal imaging as part of a cancer surveillance program.[46]

Other Tumors of the Colon

CT remains the imaging study of choice for detection of benign and malignant tumors of the colon other than adenoma and adenocarcinoma. Metastases to the colon can be seen on contrast-enhanced CT, if they are large enough; but CT cannot differentiate primary tumor from metastasis.[47] One of the most common benign colonic tumors is a lipoma. Lipomas can be easily diagnosed by demonstrating a 2–3 cm, round or ovoid, sharply defined tumor with homogenous fat density.

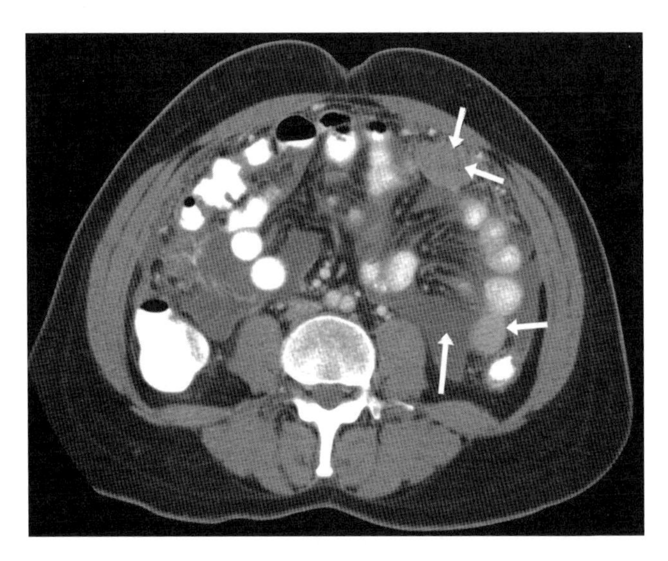

Figure 6-26. CT showing thickening of the peritoneal surfaces, ascites, and two large peritoneal nodules in a patient with colon cancer. (From Blanchard TJ, Altmeyer WB, Matthews CC. Limitations of colorectal imaging studies. In: Whitlow CB, Beck DE, Margolin DA, Hicks TC, Timmcke AE, editors. Improved outcomes in colon and rectal surgery. London: Informa Healthcare; 2010. p. 97–131. With permission).

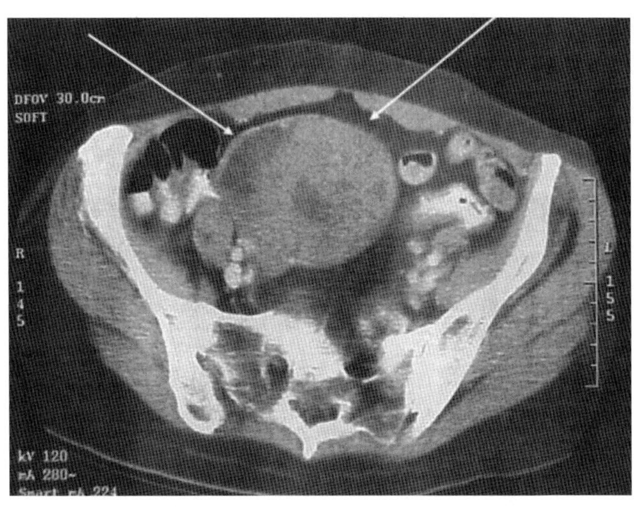

Figure 6-27. CT showing a large heterogenous exophytic mass with cystic degeneration and necrosis that communicates with the lumen of adjacent colon and small bowel. (From Blanchard TJ, Altmeyer WB, Matthews CC. Limitations of colorectal imaging studies. In: Whitlow CB, Beck DE, Margolin DA, Hicks TC, Timmcke AE, editors. Improved outcomes in colon and rectal surgery. London: Informa Healthcare; 2010. p. 97–131. With permission).

Colonic lymphoma usually appears as either a marked thickening of the bowel wall that often exceeds 4 cm, or a homogeneous soft tissue mass without calcification. Lymphoma characteristically causes much larger soft tissue masses than adenocarcinoma. Owing to the softness of the tumor, the lumen is commonly dilated or normal, rather than constricted, and bowel obstruction is uncommon. The absence of desmoplastic reaction and diffuse lymphadenopathy help to differentiate lymphoma from adenocarcinoma.[48,49]

Gastrointestinal stroma tumors (GIST) can be benign or malignant and cannot be differentiated on cross-sectional imaging without distant metastases to the liver or peritoneum.[50] GISTs can appear as an exophytic or intraluminal mass, and size varies from few millimeters to 30 cm (Figure 6-27). Cystic degeneration, hemorrhage, and necrosis are common in large lesions with calcification rarely noted. The tumor cavity may communicate with the colon lumen and contain air or oral contrast. Sarcomas that arise in the bowel, anorectum, or omentum are indistinguishable from malignant GIST.[50] Tissue types include leiomyosarcoma, fibrosarcoma, and liposarcoma.

Diverticulitis

CT scan is the most accurate imaging modality for the diagnosis of diverticulitis and its complications. CT findings of diverticulitis include soft tissue stranding of the pericolonic fat, diverticula, colon wall thickening, and abscess formation.[51] Normally, the colon mesentery and pericolonic tissues are hypodense secondary to the high water content of fatty tissue. This creates sharp boundaries between the colon, colonic mesentery, and adjacent organs. As the inflammatory process develops, the mesentery becomes edematous and hypervascular. The sharp contrast between tissue planes is obscured resulting in so-called dirty fat. When the mesenteric and pericolonic inflammation is associated with colon wall thickening within the sigmoid mesentery, the diagnosis is diverticulitis (Figure 6-28). The inflammatory process can be extensive with an associated phlegmon but no organized abscess. Depending on the size of diverticular perforation, there may be small flecks of extraluminal air within the mesentery or in the upper abdomen above the liver.[52] The identification of diverticula within the colon is not mandatory for the CT diagnosis of diverticulitis. Overall, the CT diagnosis of diverticulitis is based on a thickened short segment of colon with surrounding pericolonic inflammation.

CT scans are also useful for the diagnosis of complicated diverticulitis. Pericolonic abscesses are fluid collections adjacent to the inflamed colon (Figure 6-29). Abscesses are best visualized when surrounding loops of bowel are opacified with oral or rectal contrast and the rim of the abscess is enhanced with intravenous contrast. A colovesicular fistula, an abnormal connection between the colon and bladder, can be diagnosed in several ways. Air within the bladder without previous catheterization is diagnostic (Figure 6-30). In addition, thickening of the bladder wall with adjacent inflamed sigmoid colon can be suggestive of bladder involvement. If the fistula is large enough, enteral contrast may enter the bladder via the intestinal segment.[53] In all, CT is able to diagnose diverticulitis and its complications with a high degree of accuracy.

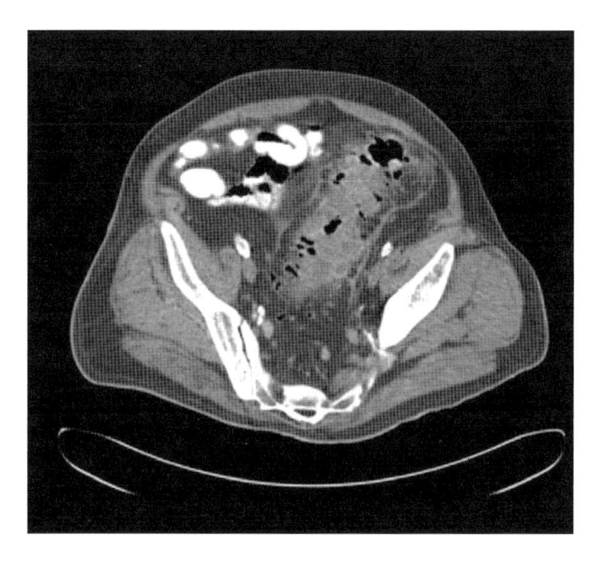

FIGURE 6-28. CT showing uncomplicated diverticulitis.

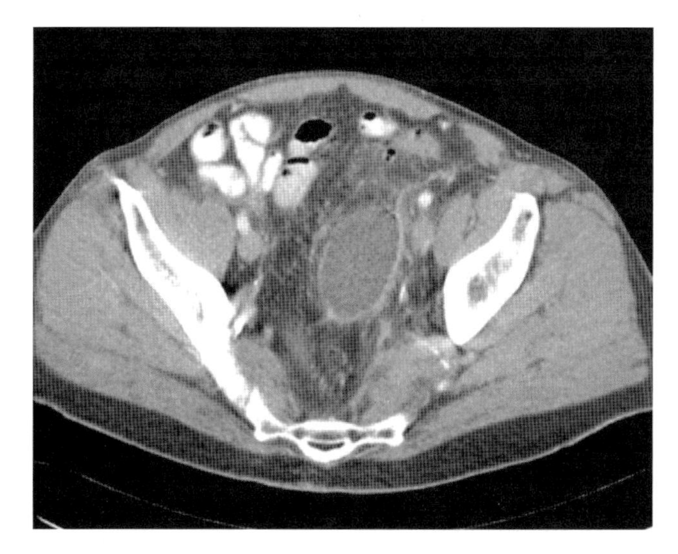

FIGURE 6-29. CT showing a diverticular abscess.

The most important diagnostic determination is to distinguish diverticulitis from colon cancer. Certain CT features may suggest one diagnosis over another. Diverticulitis is more likely to involve a longer colonic segment (>5 cm), cause pericolonic inflammation, perivascular engorgement and fluid at the root of the mesentery.[51] Conversely, colon cancer is more likely to be associated with an intraluminal mass, asymmetric wall thickening, and enlarged lymph nodes.[54] Regardless, a mucosal examination of the affected colon segment should be performed after resolution of the inflammatory changes to make a definitive diagnosis.

Inflammatory Bowel Disease

Crohn's Disease

CT scan is useful for both the diagnosis of Crohn's disease and evaluation of established Crohn's disease. The most common findings associated with Crohn's disease are bowel wall thickening, peri-intestinal inflammation, and regional lymphadenopathy. The bowel wall can reach 11–13 mm in thickness, which can be either symmetric or asymmetric. The halo sign, which is a low-attenuation ring caused by submucosal deposition of fat between the enhancing mucosa and bowel musculature, is a common finding associated with Crohn's disease. The transmural nature of the inflammatory process allows it to extend into the mesentery and adjacent structures so there is often an extensive inflammatory response centered on the affected bowel (Figure 6-31A and B).[55] The presence of creeping fat or fat proliferation within the mesentery separates bowel loops. This can give a characteristic appearance of a predominance of fat and inflammation on one side of the abdomen and a shift of unaffected, healthy bowel on the other side of the abdomen. Complications of Crohn's disease may also be seen on CT scan and include abscesses within mesentery, bowel loops, psoas muscle, pelvis, and abdominal wall (Figure 6-32). Fistulae between bowel loops, the abdominal wall, vagina, and bladder may also be seen on CT. Finally, intestinal strictures with homogenous enhancement from chronic inflammation and fibrosis may also be seen on CT.[56,57] Overall, CT is useful for delineating the extent and severity of Crohn's disease and its complications.

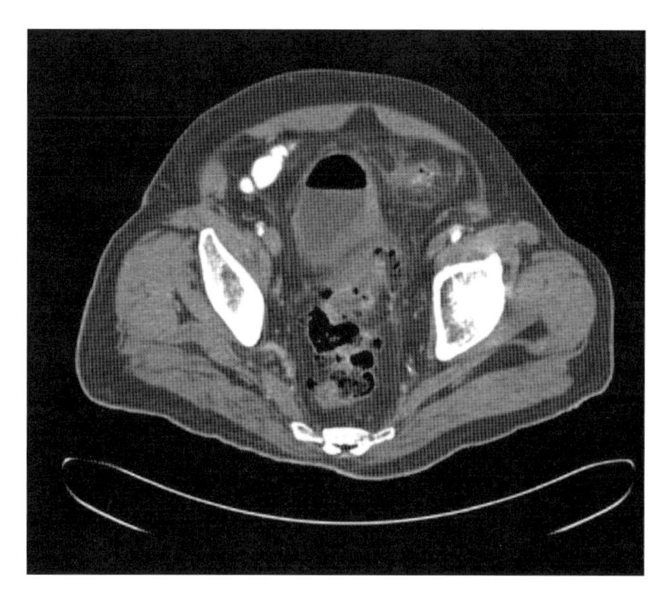

FIGURE 6-30. CT demonstrating a colovesical fistula.

Ulcerative Colitis

Like Crohn's disease, ulcerative colitis is characterized by thickening of the colon wall on CT scan. However, ulcerative colitis is not a transmural disease and, therefore, results in a lesser degree of bowel wall thickening (7–8 mm) in comparison to Crohn's disease (10–20 mm). In addition, bowel wall thickening in ulcerative colitis is circumferential while Crohn's disease may cause eccentric wall thickening.

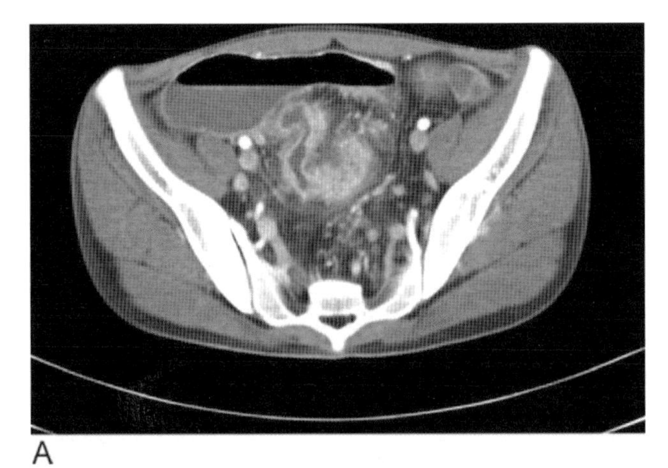

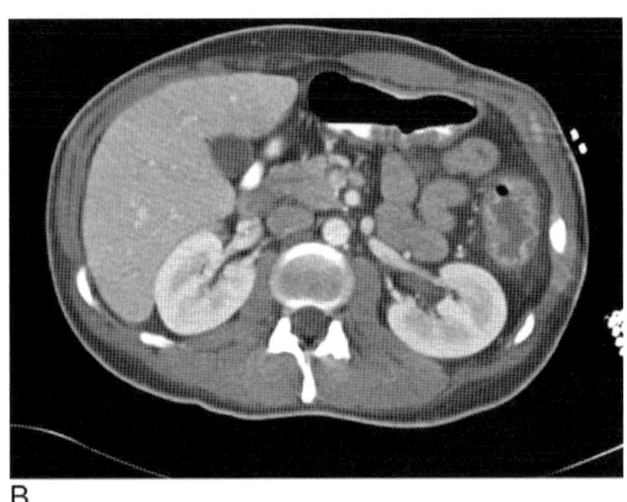

FIGURE 6-31. **A** CT showing terminal ileum Crohn's disease with abscess. **B** CT showing Crohn's colitis.

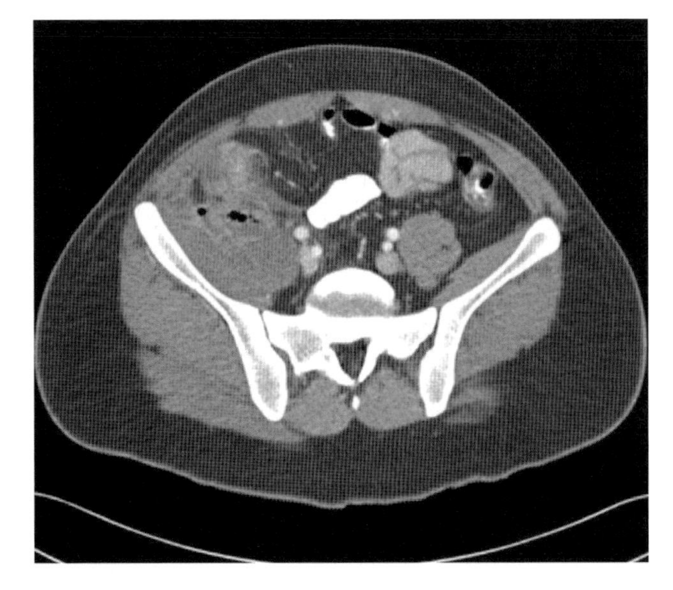

FIGURE 6-32. CT showing a psoas abscess related to Crohn's disease.

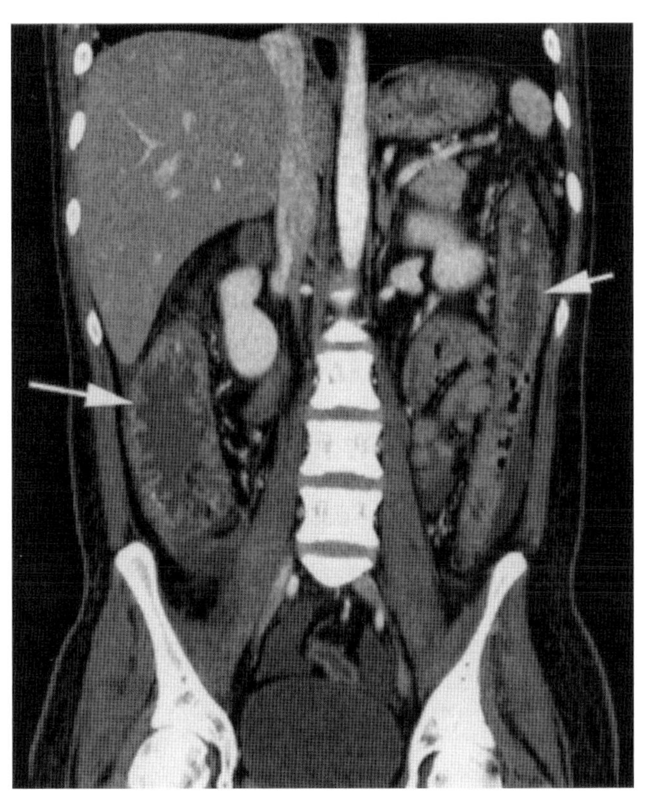

FIGURE 6-33. CT with coronal reformatting showing wall thickening and marked irregularity of the mucosa in the ascending and descending colon consistent with ulcerative colitis. (From Blanchard TJ, Altmeyer WB, Matthews CC. Limitations of colorectal imaging Studies. In: Whitlow CB, Beck DE, Margolin DA, Hicks TC, Timmcke AE, editors. Improved outcomes in colon and rectal surgery. London: Informa Healthcare; 2010. p. 97–131. With permission).

In ulcerative colitis, inflammatory changes extend from the rectum proximally and are continuous (Figure 6-33). Crohn's disease typically affects the terminal ileum and proximal colon, but any area of the intestinal length can be involved with intervening segments of normal bowel (i.e., "skip lesions"). Although ulcerative colitis can cause luminal narrowing of the colon from pseudopolyps, the outer bowel wall tends to remain smooth. In contrast, bowel that is affected by Crohn's disease can be irregular on both the inner and outer bowel wall lining. Finally, ulcerative colitis is not typically associated with abscesses and fistulae. By identifying patterns of bowel involvement, a distinction between Crohn's disease and ulcerative colitis can usually be made with CT scan.[55,58,59]

Other Colitides

Colitis is characterized by colonic wall thickening and may be indicative of an infectious, inflammatory or ischemic process. Colonoscopic evaluation can confirm the underlying disease process as infectious (15%), inflammatory (9%), ischemic (36%), or malignant (7%).[60] However, just as patterns of involvement can differentiate Crohn's disease from ulcerative colitis, they can also be used to differentiate the various causes of bowel wall thickening. In addition, the clinical presentation of various types of colitis differ, so combining the presenting signs and symptoms with the distribution of CT findings will usually lead to the correct diagnosis.

Neutropenic enterocolitis or typhlitis typically occurs in patients who are neutropenic either from cytotoxic chemotherapy or severe immunosuppression. The terminal ileum, cecum, and right colon are most frequently affected. CT is the study of choice for the diagnosis. Circumferential thickening of the terminal ileum, cecum, and variably the right colon are the common CT findings consistent with typhlitis (Figure 6-34). The bowel wall may become so thickened because of edema that a hypodense ring develops between the mucosa and musculature. Complications such as pneumatosis or perforation can also be detected.[61]

Ischemic colitis is the most common vascular abnormality of the colon. Presenting symptoms include abdominal pain associated with bloody diarrhea. The age of the patient and onset of symptoms will help to differentiate between IBD, infectious colitis, and ischemic colitis. Endoscopy is the gold standard for diagnosing ischemic colitis. CT is much more readily available so it is often the first test ordered. The colitis may be segmental or diffuse, typically occurring in the watershed areas of the right colon, splenic flexure, and rectosigmoid. CT findings consist of thickened, edematous colon in these areas (Figure 6-35). The typical "thumbprinting" in the colonic mucosa can be seen on CT scan as well as plain films. There may be a halo sign of either low attenuation caused by edema or high attenuation caused by hemorrhage within the bowel wall. A pericolonic inflammatory response is often present as well. Thrombus within the colonic mesenteric vessels may also be seen. Finally, pneumatosis or portal venous gas may be present indicating bowel infarction.

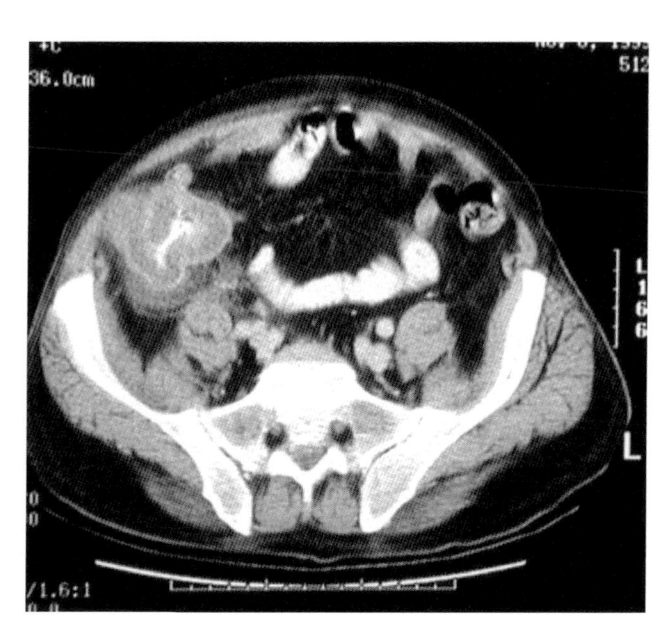

FIGURE 6-34. CT showing neutropenic enterocolitis.

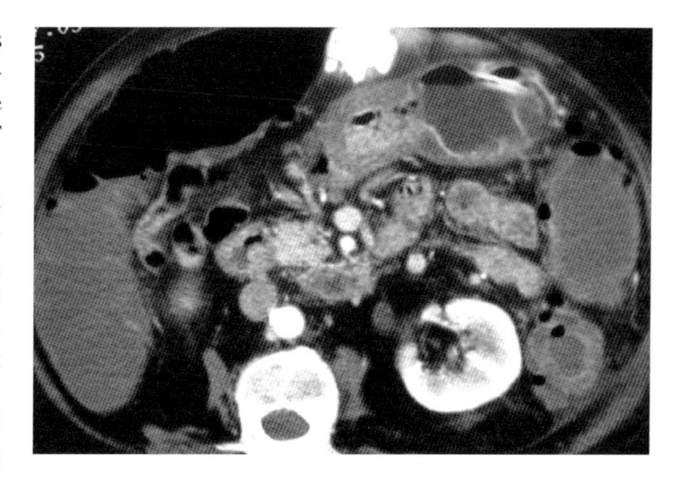

FIGURE 6-35. CT showing of ischemic colitis.

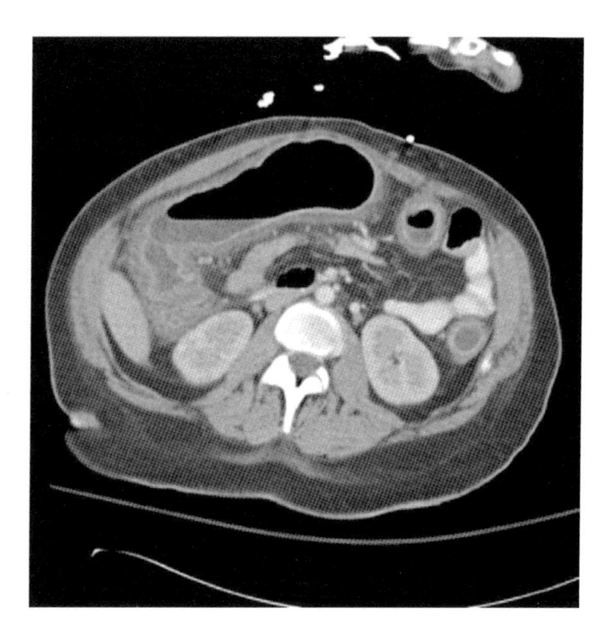

FIGURE 6-36. CT showing pseudomembranous colitis.

Pseudomembranous colitis resulting from the toxins produced by *Clostridium difficile* can cause profound inflammation of the colon. Computed tomographic findings include nonspecific thickening and edema of the colon and pericolonic inflammation. Generally, the edema and thickening of the colon is greater than that seen with infectious colitis or other inflammatory processes. The presence of pancolitis also tends to suggest pseudomembranous colitis vs. other colitides (Figure 6-36). Once again, the CT results must be interpreted in the clinical context of the patient.

Small Bowel Obstruction

SBO is a clinical diagnosis based on the signs, symptoms, and clinical condition of the patient. Radiologic studies are obtained to confirm the clinical diagnosis. The use of CT in the evaluation of an SBO is expanding and in many cases can eliminate delays in diagnosis. CT has the advantages

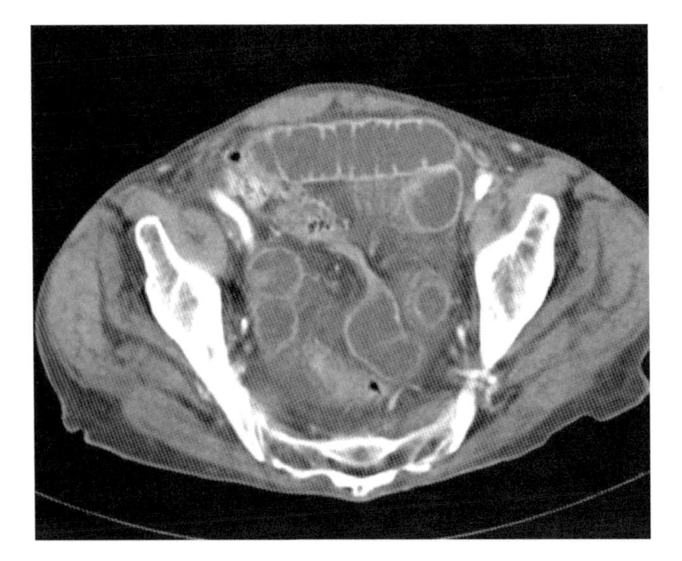

FIGURE 6-37. CT showing a simple small bowel obstruction.

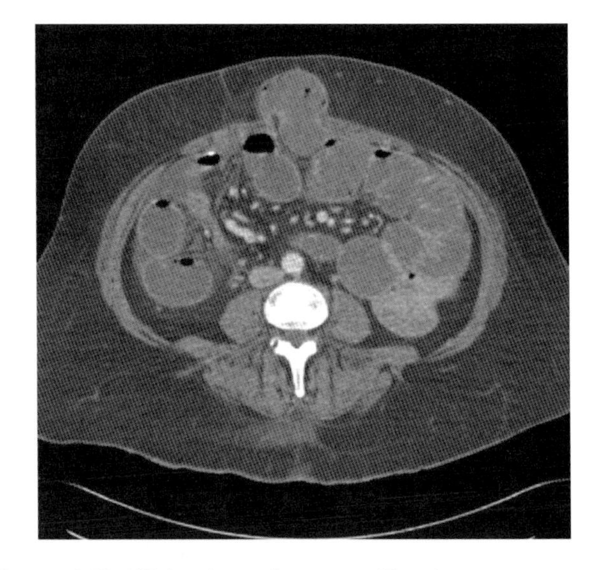

FIGURE 6-38. CT showing an incarcerated hernia.

of being able to identify the site of obstruction, cause of obstruction, and it can provide information regarding vascular compromise of the bowel. Indications when a CT scan is particularly helpful include (1) a patient with no prior surgery, (2) a patient with equivocal plain films and an uncertain diagnosis, and (3) a patient with known intra-abdominal pathology such as Crohn's disease or cancer.[62]

Oral contrast is not always necessary and should be avoided in patients with a high-grade or complete bowel obstruction. The intraluminal fluid often distends the bowel and acts as a natural contrast agent. The low-density intestinal fluid also augments the enhancement of the bowel wall after the administration of IV contrast, which can provide information regarding the flow of blood of the bowel.

The CT diagnostic criteria of a SBO are based on the presence of dilated proximal small bowel (>2.5 cm) and collapsed distal bowel. When a transition between dilated and collapsed bowel is identified, then the diagnosis is confirmed (Figure 6-37). When a transition point is not identified, it is difficult to distinguish between an SBO and adynamic ileus. In such cases, one must search for other clues to differentiate the processes. For example, the presence of "small bowel feces," which are gas bubbles mixed within particulate matter and located in the dilated bowel, is a reliable indicator of a SBO. The presence of other intra-abdominal pathology, particularly inflammatory processes, would generally indicate an adynamic ileus. This is a case in which oral contrast may be particularly helpful because if contrast reaches the colon, a complete SBO is not present.[63,64]

CT can also provide significant information regarding the cause of the obstruction. Once again, the findings must be interpreted in context of the patient's clinical situation. When there is a sharp transition from dilated to decompressed bowel in the absence of other findings, this is highly suggestive of an SBO secondary to adhesions. CT does an excellent job identifying hernias such as inguinal, umbilical, incisional, or other atypical hernias. Often these hernias contain bowel but not all are obstructing. Clues indicating obstruction are dilated bowel going into the hernia and collapsed bowel exiting the hernia, oral contrast proximal to the hernia and no contrast distal to the hernia, and a localized inflammatory process surrounding the hernia, particularly in the subcutaneous tissues (Figure 6-38). Another common extrinsic cause of obstruction is recurrent cancer. A CT scan is often able to demonstrate a mass at the site of obstruction and may also provide evidence of more widespread peritoneal disease. Unexpected causes of obstruction may also be identified such as Crohn's disease, intussusception, or small bowel cancers.[65]

When the affected bowel becomes strangulated, the morbidity and mortality associated with a SBO increase significantly. No test is able to provide definitive proof of strangulated bowel, but CT is able to provide a wealth of information that can indicate concern for vascular compromise. Thickened, congested bowel with increased attenuation at the site of obstruction associated with engorgement of the mesenteric vasculature is concerning for strangulation (Figure 6-39). The mesentery may become hazy or the vasculature may be obliterated as the inflammation progresses, and it becomes filled with fluid or even blood.[66] Other findings of ischemia include lack of enhancement after IV contrast administration or the presence of ascites. The presence of pneumatosis and portal venous gas are the more ominous signs of intestinal ischemia. Finally, a spiral pattern of engorged mesenteric blood vessels may indicate an internal hernia or rotation of small intestine around fixed adhesions.[67]

Postoperative Evaluation

CT has greatly impacted the postoperative evaluation of the surgical patient. It is typically used to evaluate a patient with

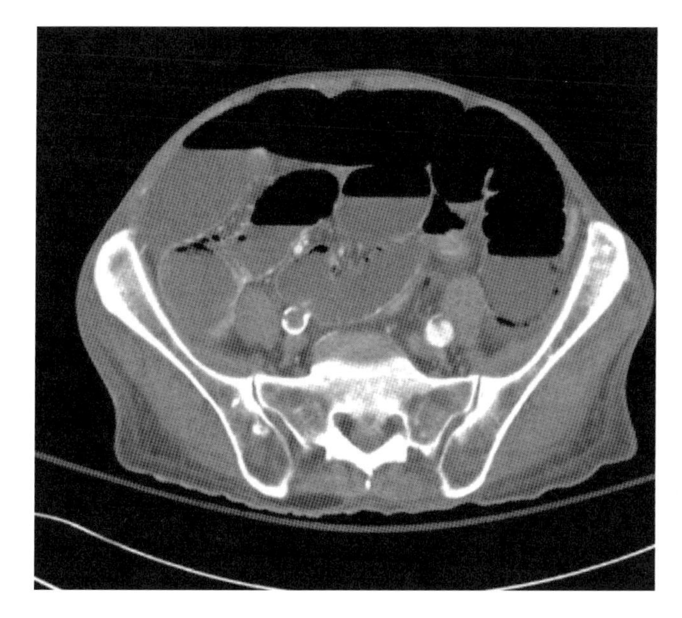

FIGURE 6-39. CT showing a small bowel obstruction with evidence of ischemia.

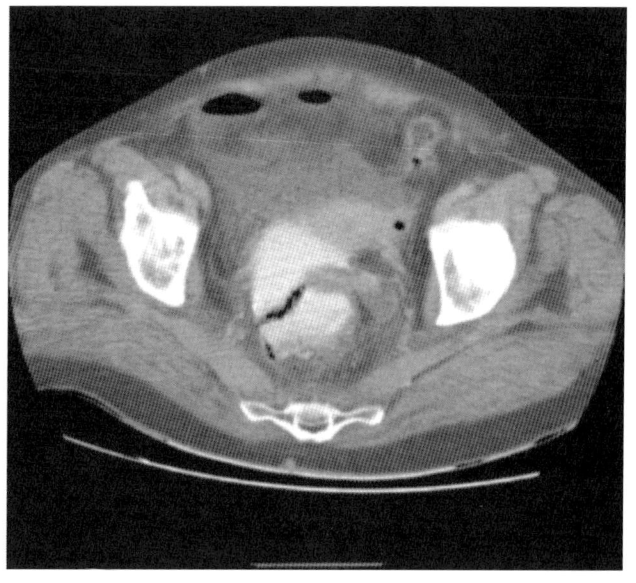

FIGURE 6-40. CT showing a colorectal anastomotic leak.

abdominal pain, fevers, leukocytosis, or persistent ileus in the postoperative period. The yield of a CT scan is greatest when it is obtained 5 days or more after surgery. Before postoperative day 5, it is difficult to differentiate normal postoperative intraperitoneal free air and fluid from air and fluid that represent a leak from a hollow viscus or abscess cavity. It usually takes more than 5 days for an abscess to organize into a walled-off, contained collection.[68] Once again, the findings of the CT scan must be interpreted in the context of the clinical condition of the patient. Therefore, the yield will be greatest when the scan can address a specific question.

Findings highly suggestive of an anastomotic leak include an inappropriate volume of free air or fluid in the abdomen. The presence of extraluminal oral contrast confirms perforation of a hollow viscous. The presence of localized fluid and air around an anastomosis are concerning for a leak but must be taken in context to the postoperative period and the condition of the patient. Water-soluble enemas are more sensitive than CT with rectal contrast for the detection of a colonic anastomotic leak (Figure 6-40). However, a CT is often more easily and readily obtained. An abscess is defined as an organized fluid collection with or without air that has an enhancing rim (Figure 6-41).[69,70] As mentioned above, CT is very good at distinguishing between an ileus and a mechanical bowel obstruction, which is an important distinction in the perioperative period.

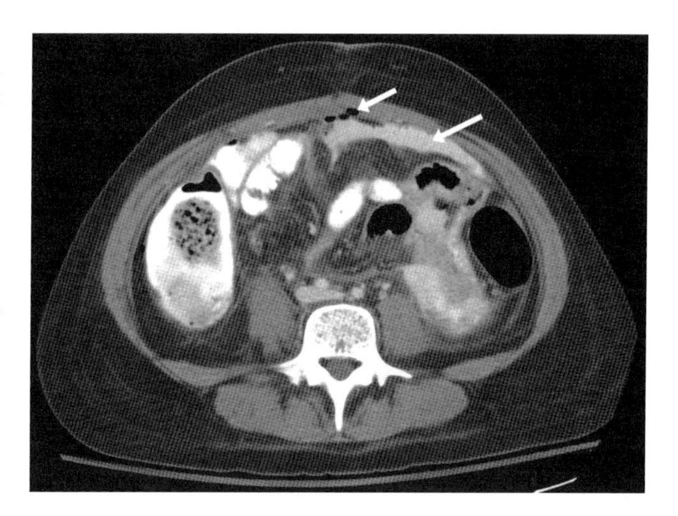

FIGURE 6-41. CT showing an anastomotic leak. *Arrows* point to pneumoperitoneum and high density ascites which represents extravasated oral contrast. (From Blanchard TJ, Altmeyer WB, Matthews CC. Limitations of colorectal imaging studies. In: Whitlow CB, Beck DE, Margolin DA, Hicks TC, Timmcke AE, editors. Improved outcomes in colon and rectal surgery. London: Informa Healthcare; 2010. p. 97–131. With permission).

Computed Tomography Enterography

Computed tomography enterography (CTE) is a technique that uses multidetector row CT to examine the small bowel in a continuous fashion. The volume of information produced can be reconstructed in any plane to produce high-resolution scans with superb image quality.[71] For high quality images the patient must ingest over a liter of oral contrast in a rapid fashion (<1 h) and intravenous contrast is administered for enhancement. Advantages of CTE include the ready availability of CT scanners, a straightforward technique, the speed of the exam (10–15 min), and the potential for less radiation than a standard small bowel follow through. Intestinal and extraintestinal findings of Crohn's disease can be seen on CTE.[72] Intestinal findings include wall hyperenhancement, wall thickening (generally >3 mm), and luminal narrowing (Figures 6-42 and 6-43). Extraintestinal findings include

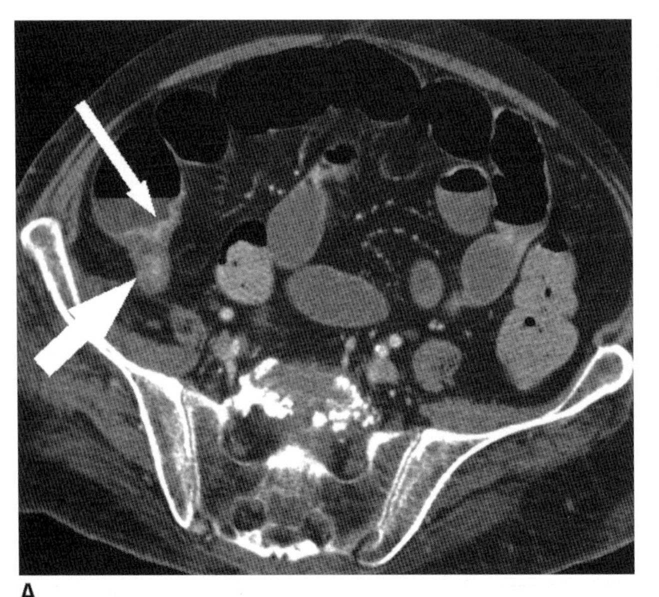

A

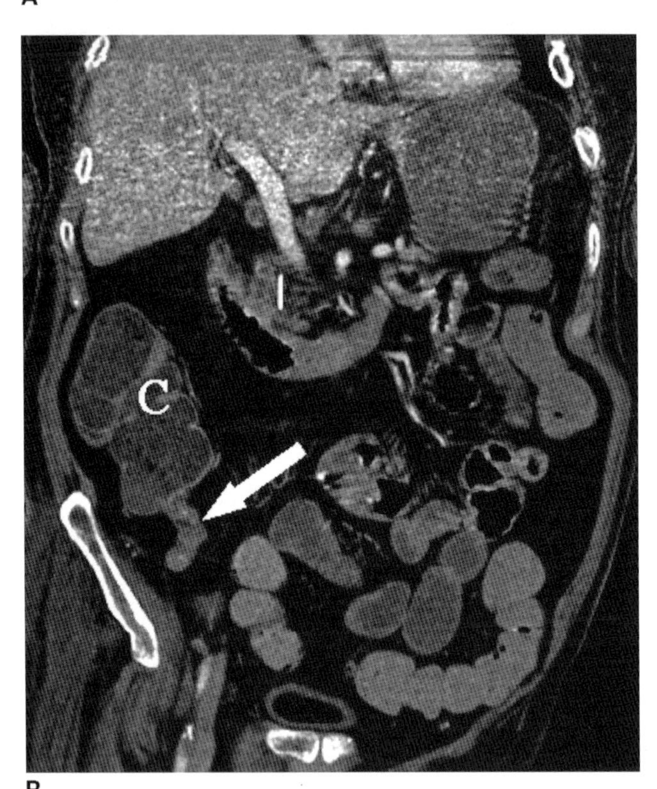

B

FIGURE 6-42. **A** CT enterography of strictured ileal Crohn's disease. Axial scan through the pelvis shows narrowed, strictured neo-terminal ileum (*large arrow*). Note the thin, inner wall hyperenhancement and the peripheral wall hypoenhancement giving a target appearance or mural stratification. Additionally, the inner portion of the wall of the immediate upstream ileum (*long small arrow*) also hyper enhances. The stricture causes significant upstream obstruction. **B** CT enterography of strictured ileal Crohn's disease. Coronal, thin MIP scan through the pelvis shows narrowed, strictured neo-terminal ileum (*arrow*) just proximal to the cecum (C). (From Baker ME, Veniero JC, Kiran RP. Computed tomography enterography and magnetic resonance enterography: the future of small bowel imaging. Clin Colon Rectal Surg. 2008;21:213–19. With permission).

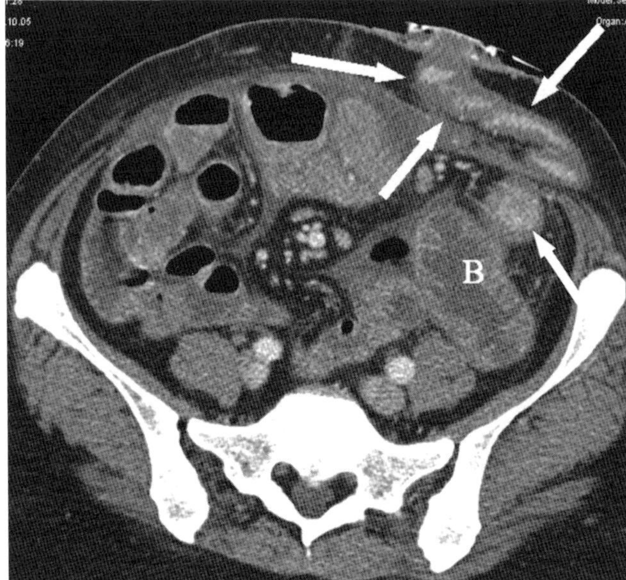

A

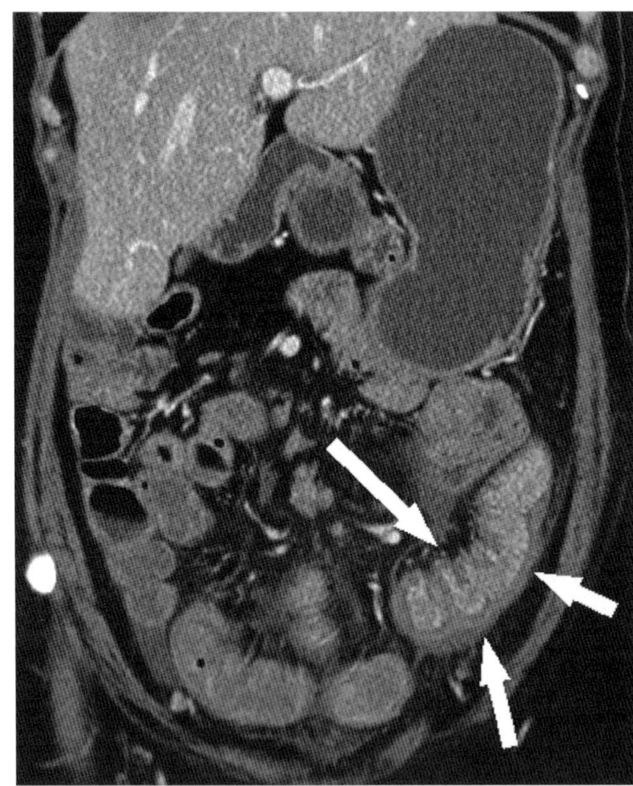

B

FIGURE 6-43. **A** CT enterography of distal ileal Crohn's disease. Axial scan through the pelvis shows a long segment of disease proximal to an end ileostomy (*arrows*). There is mild-to-moderate upstream small bowel (B) dilation. Interestingly, the endoscopy was normal, but the pathology was positive for active disease. **B** CT enterography of distal ileal Crohn's disease. Coronal thin MIP reconstruction through the pelvis shows a long segment of disease proximal to an end ileostomy (*arrows*). (From Baker ME, Veniero JC, Kiran RP. Computed tomography enterography and magnetic resonance enterography: the future of small bowel imaging. Clin Colon Rectal Surg. 2008;21:213–19. With permission).

peribowel vascular engorgement, peribowel fat proliferation, strictures, fistulae, and abscesses. In many centers, CTE is replacing the traditional small bowel follow through.

CT Colonography

CT colonography or virtual colonoscopy is a method for imaging the colon and screening for advanced polyps and colorectal cancers. This technique requires cleansing of the colon to allow differentiation of polyps and haustral folds from fecal material. A newer method of stool tagging which involves patient ingestion of low-density barium and water-soluble contrast the night before the study along with the colon preparation, increases the sensitivity of the exam. The colon is distended during the study through the manual or automated instillation of air or carbon dioxide. The colon is then imaged in two patient positions (supine and prone) using multidetector row CT with thin collimation. The images are then viewed in two- and three-dimensional views for interpretation by a computer and the radiologist. Computer-aided detection identifies suspicious areas and increases the diagnostic accuracy of the reading radiologist. Advances in this technique which include stool tagging, automated colon distention, and multiplanar views of the colon have increased the utility of this technique for colon polyp and cancer screening. In addition, the short amount of time required to obtain images (<15 min), the absence of conscious sedation, and a low perforation rate make CT colonography a promising alternative to optical colonoscopy for colon cancer screening.[73]

CT colonography allows detection of polyps based on size. Polyps which are >10 mm in size are considered high risk and the patient is referred for same day colonoscopy. Polyps between 6 and 10 mm in size are detected and reported but current treatment protocols call for variable management of these polyps. Some patients may be offered CT surveillance and others optical colonoscopy (Figures 6-44 and 6-45). Although polyps which are 5 mm or less in size may be seen on CT colonography, they are not reported in the radiologist's interpretation of the study. This approach has been shown to decrease the number of referrals for optical colonoscopy without sacrificing early treatment of high risk polyps.[74] CT colonography has been shown to have similar sensitivity to optical colonoscopy for the detection of middle and large size polyps in average risk individuals.[75]

Despite advances in sensitivity with CT colonography, this technique still has limitations that must be overcome before its widespread use in screening protocols. For example, CT colonography has a poor sensitivity for flat lesions and may miss up to 66% of flat lesions over 5 mm.[76] In addition, CT colonography is a diagnostic not therapeutic procedure. Up to one in five patients undergoing CT colonography may be referred to optical colonoscopy. CT colonography may also reveal extracolonic findings. While extracolonic cancers have been diagnosed using this technique, between 5 and 16% of patients will be referred for additional imaging and diagnostic procedures when CT colonography findings have no clinical significance.[77] Finally, insurance coverage for this screening technique is limited. For these reasons, CT colonography is recommended for patients who are unable to have a complete colonoscopy, for those who have significant medical problems that put them at increased risk for optical colonoscopy complications (significant pulmonary disease or anticoagulation), and to identify synchronous cancers or polyps in patients with

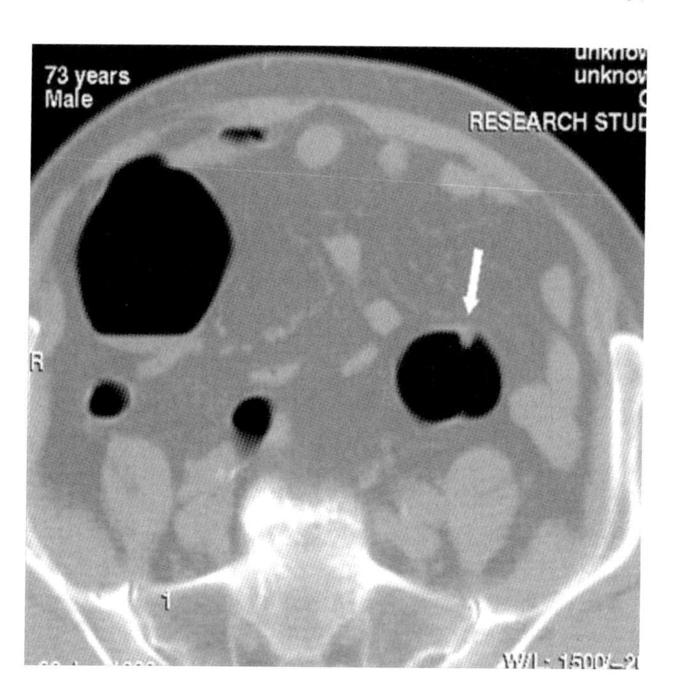

FIGURE 6-44. Axial two-dimensional image from a CT colon study shows a well-defined 6-mm polyp in the sigmoid colon.

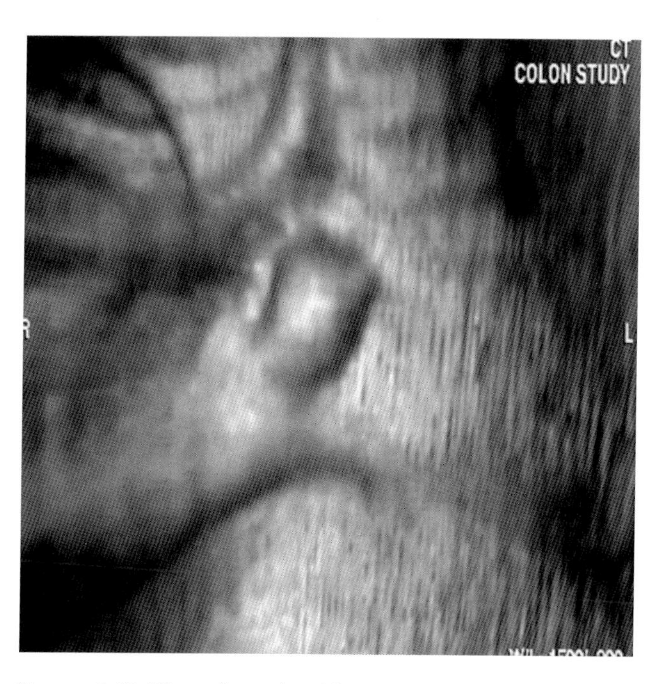

FIGURE 6-45. Three-dimensional image confirms the presence of the polyp in Figure 6-4.

obstructing lesions. CT colonography is contraindicated in patients who are at high risk for colon and rectal cancer such as inflammatory bowel disease patients or those with known genetic syndromes for colon or rectal cancer.[73]

Magnetic Resonance Imaging

Magnetic resonance imaging (MRI) is an imaging technique that measures proton behavior after excitation by a radiofrequency pulse in a magnetic field. Protons within water dense or fat dense tissue can be selectively displayed so that adjacent tissues demonstrate different levels of intensity. Advantages of this technique include the avoidance of ionizing radiation as well as iodinated contrast agents.[78] However, MRI requires expensive equipment and radiologist expertise for interpretation and, therefore, may not be widely available. In addition, image resolution may be degraded by respiratory motion or peristalsis of the bowel. Newer advances enhance image quality despite challenges with motion artifact. Integration of a pelvic phased array coil with the endorectal coil (Figure 6-46) or an external phased array coil used independently results in high-resolution images with a large field of view.[79,80] MRI cannot be performed in patients with implanted devices which may malfunction in a strong magnetic field (cardiac pacemakers, cerebral aneurysm clips, cochlear implants). In addition, patients with chronic renal insufficiency who will require gadolinium for MRI image acquisition are at risk for nephrogenic systemic fibrosis, a progressive fibrotic syndrome which affects the skin and other organs.[81] Despite the utility of MRI in imaging rectal and anal disease with respect to the entire pelvis, not all patients will be candidates for MRI imaging.

MRI can be used for staging rectal cancer. Pretreatment staging of rectal cancer has been shown to have similar accuracy for detection of tumor depth and nodal involvement as endorectal ultrasound.[82] Tumor depth can be determined secondary to the low signal intensity of the muscularis propria which sits between the high intensity layers of the submucosa and perirectal fat (Figure 6-47). Lymph node involvement is not judged solely by size but also by irregular borders and heterogenous signal intensity. Agreement between MRI and pathology staging is 94% for tumor depth, 85% for nodal involvement and 92% for circumferential margin involvement.[83] Advantages of MRI for initial rectal cancer staging include accuracy that does not vary with the height of the rectal lesion and visualization of the entire pelvis This allows surgeons to assess of the radial margin and pelvic sidewall prior to surgery.

Studies have been performed to test the utility of MRI in restaging of rectal cancer after neoadjuvant chemoradiation and after rectal cancer recurrence. The difficulty is in distinguishing inflammation from tumor deposits. Tumor has a high signal intensity and rapid enhancement on T2 images. Granulation tissue, hematoma and radiation-induced inflammation also have a high signal intensity.[82] Therefore, MRI images have a low sensitivity for diagnosing tumor persistence after chemoradiation therapy.[84] Even as inflammation matures over time into fibrosis which appears as an area of low intensity and slow enhancement, the specificity of MRI remains low (29–86%) and can lead to a diagnosis of recurrence when there is not.[84] Overall, utility of MRI in restaging rectal cancer after neoadjuvant treatment and in detecting rectal cancer recurrence remains low.

MRI is now increasingly used for the imaging of complex fistula in ano and fecal incontinence. Fistula in ano is often diagnosed and treated with an exam under anesthesia. However, MRI images may assist the surgeon in identifying primary and secondary fistula tracts and the internal anal

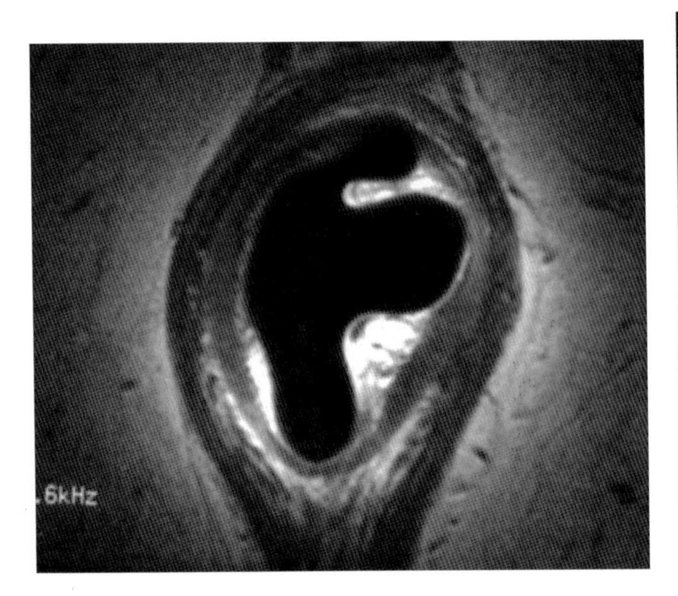

FIGURE 6-46. Endoanal MRI demonstrates a nondisrupted (normal) signal of the internal and external sphincter.

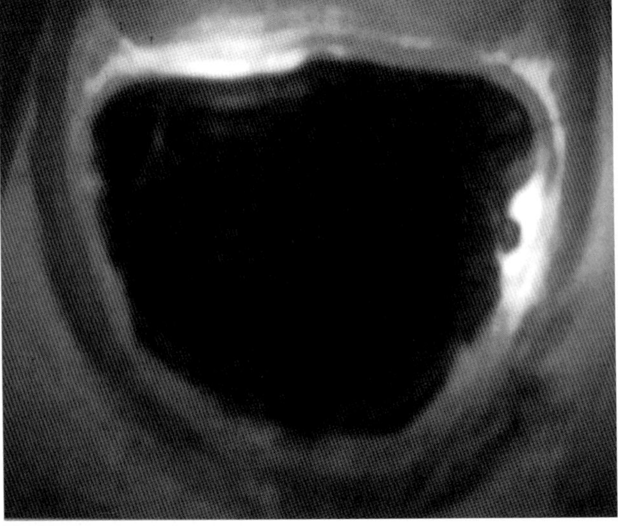

FIGURE 6-47. Endorectal MRI examination shows an ulcerated plaque-like cancer arising from the mucosa and extending to the first muscular layer of the muscularis propria.

canal opening with respect to the sphincter complex prior to definitive surgery. Unlike endoanal ultrasound (EAUS) which may also assist the surgeon, the MRI allows for a large field of view which includes the pelvis, ischiorectal fossa, and gluteal regions that are outside the scope of EAUS images but may be involved if fistulous disease is extensive. In addition, patients with active proctitis or anal stenosis may be more comfortable with an external phased array coil rather than an endoanal coil or ultrasound probe.[85] MRI may also be used for patients with fecal incontinence. While MRI demonstrates defects in the external and internal anal sphincters just as EAUS, MRI may better for imaging external anal sphincter atrophy and other defects in pelvic musculature (puborectalis and levator ani).[86] In all, MRI is an alternative to EAUS for image acquisition in patients with fistula in ano or fecal incontinence and it offers some advantages over the ultrasound technique.

Radionuclide Imaging

Radionuclide images are acquired based on physiologic rather than anatomic differences between tissues. These images have a wide spectrum of use in clinical medicine. Radiopharmaceuticals and gamma cameras are the mainstay of radionuclide imaging. Specific radionuclides are chosen based on their affinity for a particular organ system or ongoing physiologic process (i.e., glucose metabolism or GI bleeding). The image quality depends on the sensitivity of the radionuclide for the target organ or physiologic process. Gamma cameras then generate images based on the summed location and intensity of gamma photons emitted by the radionuclide substance.[87]

Positron Emission Topography

Positron emission topography (PET) is an imaging modality which relies on the physiologic differences in glucose metabolism that exists between tissue types.[88] Cells which have a higher baseline metabolic rate or increased mitotic activity will absorb glucose at a high rate. PET takes advantage of this difference as metabolically active cells will absorb a radioactive analog of glucose, 18-F-2-fluoro-2-deoxy-D-glucose (FDG) at a high concentration. However, structural changes in the FDG molecule prohibit further metabolic degradation and FDG accumulates in the intracellular space of metabolically active tissues.[89] Images are then generated based on differential FDG uptake.

PET image acquisition depends on differential glucose utilization by tissues. In order to maximize tissue differences, prior to the study patients should avoid carbohydrates, fast for 4–6 h immediately before and control serum glucose (<200 mg/dl).[90] Tissues that display increased FDG uptake include the urinary and gastrointestinal tracts, tissue with active inflammation secondary to leukocyte and macrophage activity and malignant tissue.[88] Because of increased FDG avidity of malignant cells, PET scans have become an invaluable tool for the staging of primary and recurrent cancers.

PET is currently approved for use in patients with colon and rectal cancer. While colon and rectal cancer is usually diagnosed with colonoscopy and an initial staging CT, PET obtained for other reasons may be diagnostic of high-grade colon or rectal lesions in 3.3% of patients.[91] However, PET is not recommended for primary staging of colon or rectal cancer where the likelihood of a change in surgical management is low.[92] If there is a question of resectability at initial diagnosis, especially in regard to liver metastases, PET is more accurate in detecting extrahepatic disease and characterizing liver metastases than CT (Figure 6-48A–C). Therefore, PET may be used to determine treatment course in patients with indeterminate initial staging. PET is also useful for the detection of recurrent disease and acts as a complement to CT, CEA, and colonoscopy surveillance.[93] PET is also more sensitive than these other surveillance tests for determining extent of recurrence so a change in CT imaging or CEA level which suggests recurrence can be confirmed by PET imaging (Figure 6-49A and B).[94] Clinical situations in which PET has been studied for use but is not currently approved include monitoring response to chemotherapy and monitoring response after ablation of liver metastases. PET has not been found to be useful in restaging rectal cancer after neoadjuvant chemoradiation since radiation therapy results in inflammation within the tumor bed that causes difficult to interpret changes in FDG avidity. PET has also been investigated for use in anal squamous cell cancer. PET may aid in the initial staging of anal cancer by detecting inguinal lymph node involvement. However, the specificity of inguinal lymph node involvement is low and inguinal nodes may display FDG avidity with benign inflammation.[95] Overall, PET is useful for staging and treatment planning in colon and rectal cancer recurrence or metastatic disease which has been treated medically and is being evaluated for surgical resection.

PET imaging has certain limitations. For example, traditional PET imaging has low spatial resolution. New techniques allow fusion of PET and CT images taken in one imaging session to allow localization of FDG avid structures in relation to specific organ structures. PET also has low specificity resulting in false-positive and -negative studies secondary to inflammation, normal gastrointestinal physiologic uptake, and cancers with low cellular or metabolic density (i.e., mucinous adenocarcinoma or carcinoid).[90] PET/CT allows correlation of FDG avid areas with specific organs found on CT. Therefore, PET/CT not only improves localization of FDG avid lesions but also enhances the certainty in interpreting lesions as normal or abnormal.[96] Overall, PET/CT is proving to be a more accurate test than either of its individual components or the sum of its components viewed side by side in regard to colon and rectal cancer staging.[97] Further studies are required to determine the clinical scenarios in which PET/CT is most appropriate.

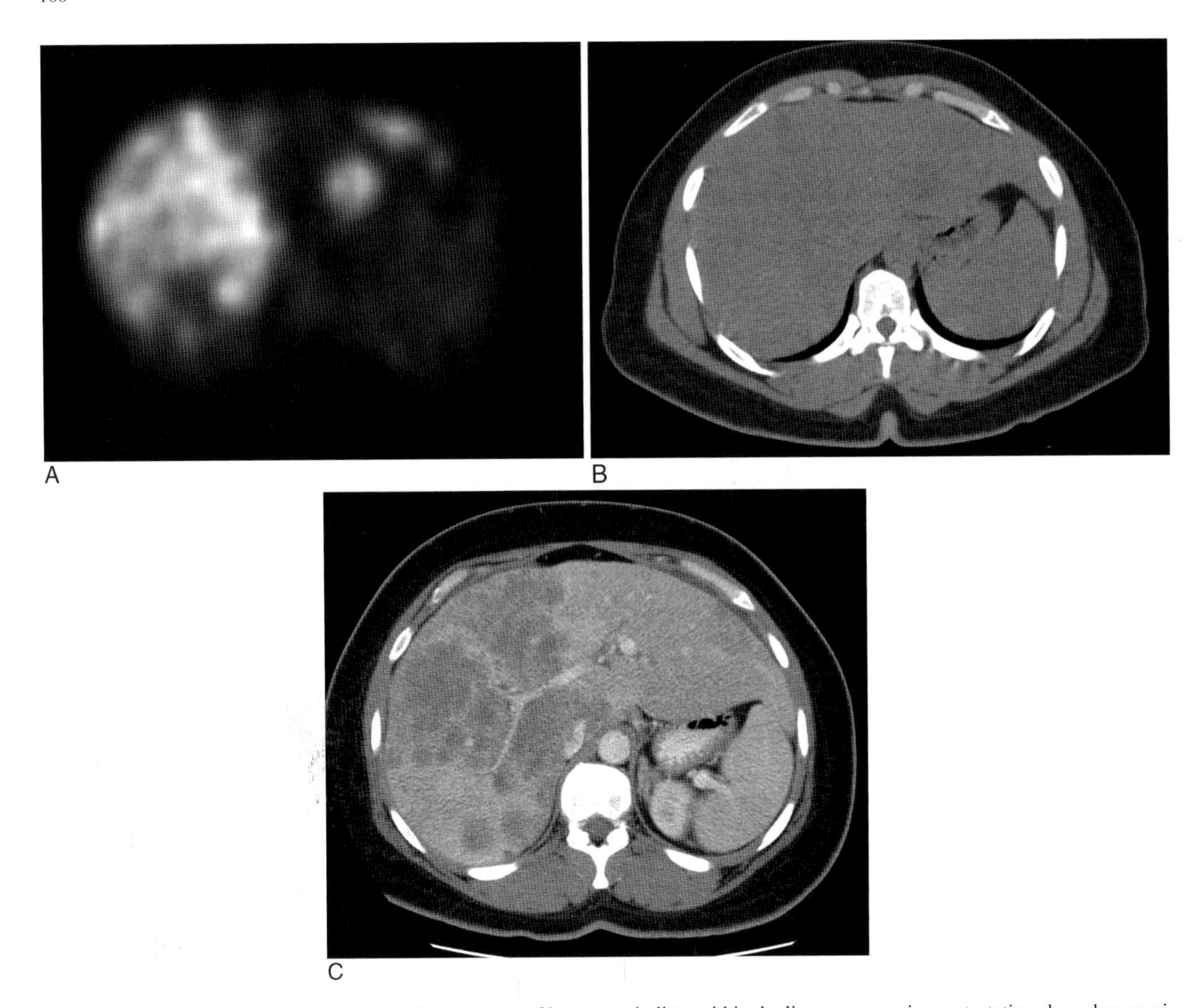

FIGURE 6-48. **A** PET scan showing multiple discrete areas of hypermetabolism within the liver, representing metastatic colon adenocarcinoma. **B** A noncontrast CT of the same patient. The multiple metastatic foci are nearly impossible to detect without contrast. **C** Iodinated contrast helps to delineate between normal hepatic tissue and hypodense metastatic disease (From Blanchard TJ, Altmeyer WB, Matthews CC. Limitations of colorectal imaging studies. In: Whitlow CB, Beck DE, Margolin DA, Hicks TC, Timmcke AE, editors. Improved outcomes in colon and rectal surgery. London: Informa Healthcare; 2010. p. 97–131. With permission).

RBC Scintigraphy

Radionuclide imaging studies are widely used in the diagnosis of lower gastrointestinal bleeding. The principle is that the intravascular tracer will be extravasated into the bowel lumen during active bleeding. Concentration of the radioactive tracer on the acquired images allows for identification of the bleeding site. Technetium 99mTc is the radionuclide used in bleeding scans. This radiopharmaceutical can be used to label colloid or patient red blood cells (RBCs). Radiolabeled colloid is readily available and requires less preparation time. However, the colloid is rapidly metabolized resulting in a lower sensitivity for the detection of gastrointestinal bleeding.[98] RBCs take longer to label but they are metabolized slower and can remain active up to 24 h after injection. Therefore, the use of labeled RBCs is preferred as multiple scans can be obtained in patients with intermittent bleeding episodes. Tagged RBC scans are considered positive if the tracer pattern conforms to bowel anatomy, uptake increases in intensity over time and the tracer propagates in an antegrade or retrograde fashion (Figure 6-50).[99] These criteria help to distinguish true gastrointestinal bleeding from other lesions within the intestine with a high blood density (hepatic hemangioma, colonic angiodysplasia). Tagged RBC scans are sensitive for bleeding but may result in a false negative if the rate of bleeding is below 0.2 cm^3/min or the bleed is episodic. [100] Similar to PET, tagged RBC scans have a low spatial resolution and locate only the vascular territory of the bleed. In addition, the time for radionuclide appearance on bleeding scans may have prognostic significance. Patients who have an early

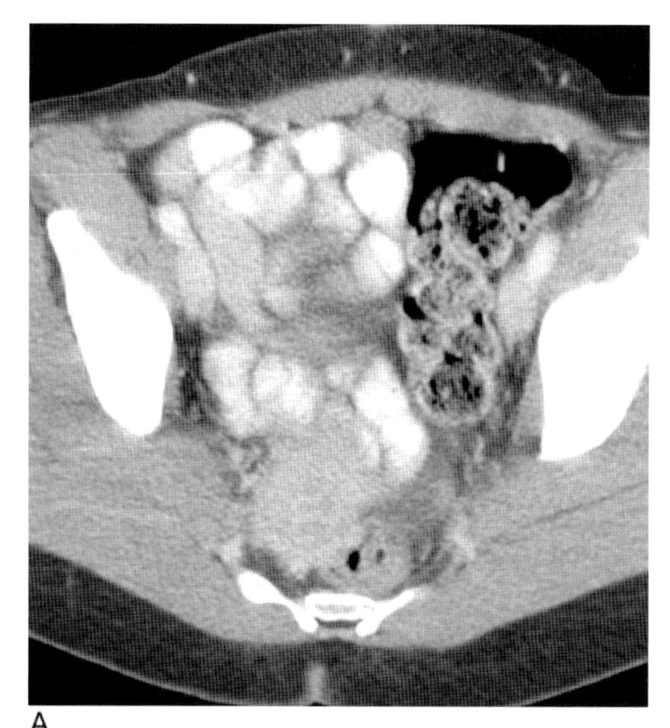

A

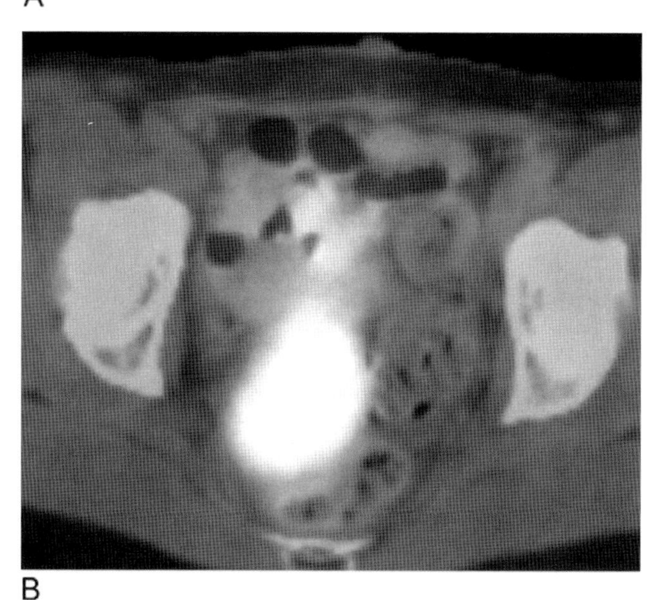

B

FIGURE 6-49. **A** CT in a patient who had prior rectal resection for carcinoma shows soft tissue mass in the surgical bed of the perirectal fat. **B** Follow-up PET examination shows intense FDG uptake within this soft tissue mass consistent with recurrence.

positive scan (<2 min) are more likely to have a blush on arteriogram that can be treated compared to patients with a late positive scan who are more likely to benefit from resuscitation and colonoscopy if necessary.[101] RBC scintigraphy is useful for the stratification of patients with active large volume gastrointestinal bleeding who will benefit from subsequent angiography and those who can be managed with less invasive techniques.

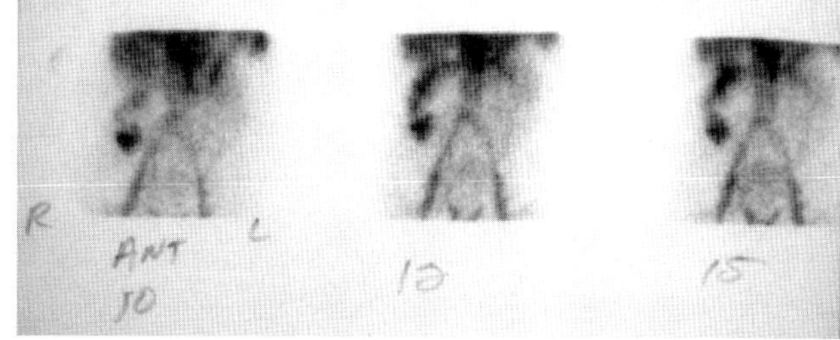

FIGURE 6-50. 99mTc-tagged red blood cell study shows early blood pool activity within the ascending colon in this patient with bleeding after a recent polypectomy.

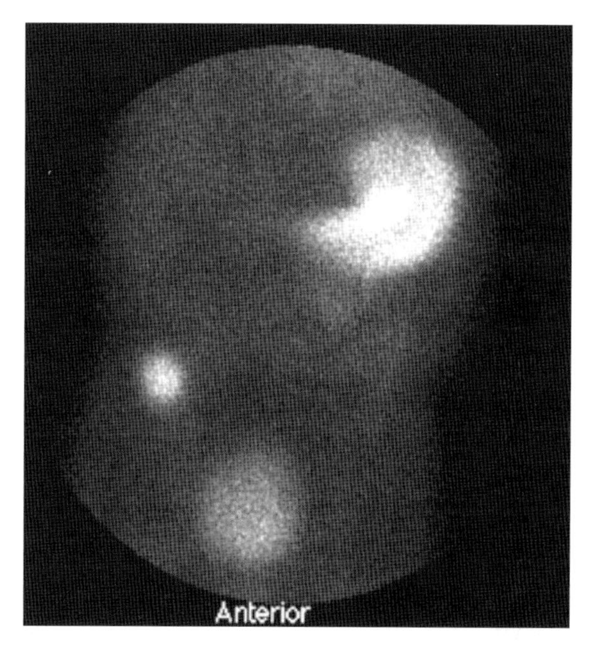

FIGURE 6-51. 99mTc-pertechnetate scan (Meckel's) shows a discrete focus of increased uptake in the right lower quadrant, with approximately the same intensity as the stomach indicating gastric mucosa is present within this Meckel's diverticulum.

Meckel's Scintigraphy

A Meckel's scan, although not used as often as the tagged RBC scan, can be useful in the evaluation of young patients with occult gastrointestinal bleeding with no identifiable colonic source. Meckel's diverticulum causes abnormal bleeding as a result of aberrant gastric mucosa that lines the diverticulum. 99Tc pertechnetate is a radionuclide which is actively concentrated and then excreted by mucous-secreting cells in gastric mucosa.[102] Native as well as ectopic gastric mucosa will concentrate the radionuclide and be visualized within 30–60 min after injection (Figure 6-51). Delayed images will obscure ectopic foci of uptake, secondary to rapid transit of the radiotracer through the gastrointestinal tract. The sensitivity of the Meckel's scan is 85% and the specificity is 95%.[103]

Arteriography

Arteriography is an invasive procedure performed by specialty trained physicians and is used in the diagnosis and treatment of a variety of colorectal diseases. The arteriogram is performed through a percutaneous approach under sterile conditions. The femoral artery is a preferred puncture sight although axillary and brachial arteries may be used. A guidewire is introduced through the needle and a catheter is introduced over the guidewire. Various catheters and guide wires allow the interventional radiologist to access the vessels in question. Arteriography is an invasive procedure with an overall mortality of 1 in 40,000.[104] Complications from the performance of the procedure and manipulation of the wires and catheters are more common than reactions to the contrast itself.[105] The most common complications are related to hematomas or pseudoaneurysms at the puncture sight, dissection or embolization secondary to catheter manipulation. Contrast reactions and contrast toxicity (renal failure) occur in <1% of studies done. Experience and technique can minimize many of the complications. Hydration and IV mannitol can reduce the nephrotoxicity. If the patient has allergies to iodine or has had a prior contrast reaction, premedication with methyl prednisolone is done 12 and 2 hours before arteriography.

The arteriogram is a useful diagnostic and therapeutic modality in the treatment of active lower GI bleeding. If a radionuclide scan is performed and localizes the site of bleeding, a selective angiogram can then be performed. For bleeding localized to the left colon on tagged RBC study, the inferior mesenteric artery is selected first. The superior mesenteric artery is selected first for those bleeds that occur in the right colon. If the bleeding site is not identified after injection of both the superior and inferior mesenteric arteries, a celiac run is performed looking for an upper intestinal bleeding source. Active bleeding can be diagnosed by the accumulation of contrast in the arterial phase that persists through the venous phase (Figure 6-52). Bleeding needs to occur at a higher rate for a positive angiogram (0.5 ml/min) than for nuclear imaging (0.1–0.2 ml/min). Because lower GI bleeding can be intermittent, the bleeding site is sometimes not identified at the time of the angiogram.

Diverticulosis and vascular ectasias are presumed to be the leading cause of lower GI bleeding in most patients. Diverticular bleeds appear as a blush of contrast contained within a diverticulum. Vascular ectasias often occur in the right colon and appear as small vascular clusters, a blush in the wall of the colon, and early opacification of a draining vein.[106] Arteriovenous malformations are developmental in origin and are often seen in the small bowel. They appear as tortuous, dilated arteries and early prominent veins. Capillary telangiectasias (common in Osler Weber Rendu syndrome) appear as multiple, tiny areas of blush and no arteriovenous shunting. Postpolypectomy bleeding has been diagnosed and treated with angiography. A rapid blush of dye occurs at the site of bleeding and often stops with direct infusion of vasopressin or embolization (Figure 6-53A and B).

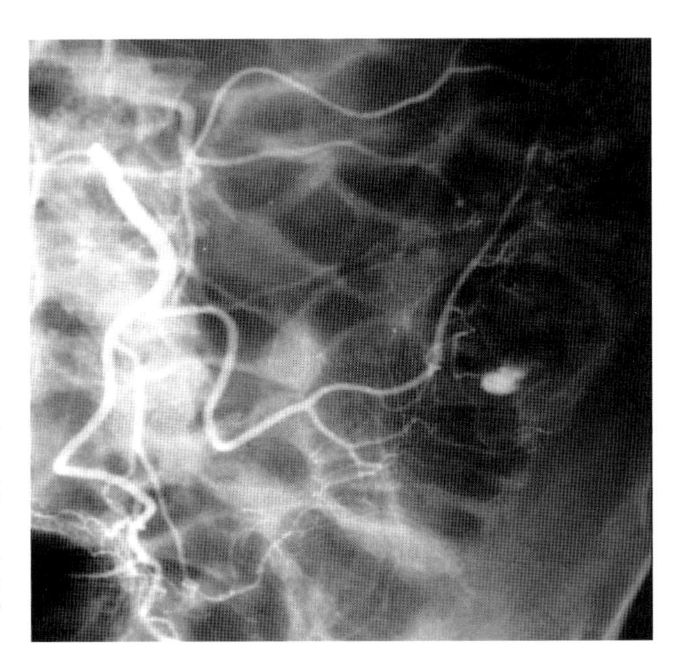

FIGURE 6-52. Mesenteric angiogram shows pooling of contrast in the sigmoid colon in this patient with surgically proven diverticular bleeding.

Acute mesenteric ischemia is one of the most common intestinal disease processes for which arteriography is used for diagnosis and treatment. Acute mesenteric ischemia can be either nonocclusive or occlusive. Nonocclusive mesenteric ischemia arises from a "low flow" state typically secondary to reduction in mesenteric blood flow from cardiac failure or hypotensive shock. This diagnosis can frequently be made with clinical symptoms and computer tomography images. The typical early angiographic images show diffuse vasoconstriction of mesenteric arterial branches and decreased parenchymal vascularity (Figure 6-54). In the late stage there is increased accumulation of contrast in the bowel wall. Treatment includes volume resuscitation and cardiac support. The diagnostic percutaneous catheter can be used to treat the mesenteric phase of constriction with IV glucagon or intra-arterial infusion of the papaverine in an intensive care unit setting.

Occlusive acute mesenteric ischemia is a medical emergency, thus early diagnosis and treatment may prevent bowel necrosis and perforation. These patients typically have severe abdominal pain with nonspecific physical findings.[107] An arteriogram is the most useful diagnostic examination for patients in whom one has a high clinical suspicion of acute occlusive mesenteric ischemia.[47] A catheter is inserted into the aorta and an aortogram is obtained. The celiac and superior mesenteric arteries are catheterized and injected with contrast in order to identify the level of occlusion and document collateral circulation. A superior mesenteric artery embolus typically lodges just proximal or distal to the take off of the middle colic artery and is seen as a meniscus at the site of occlusion and blockage of contrast (Figure 6-55). Atherosclerotic occlusion will often involve the origin of the

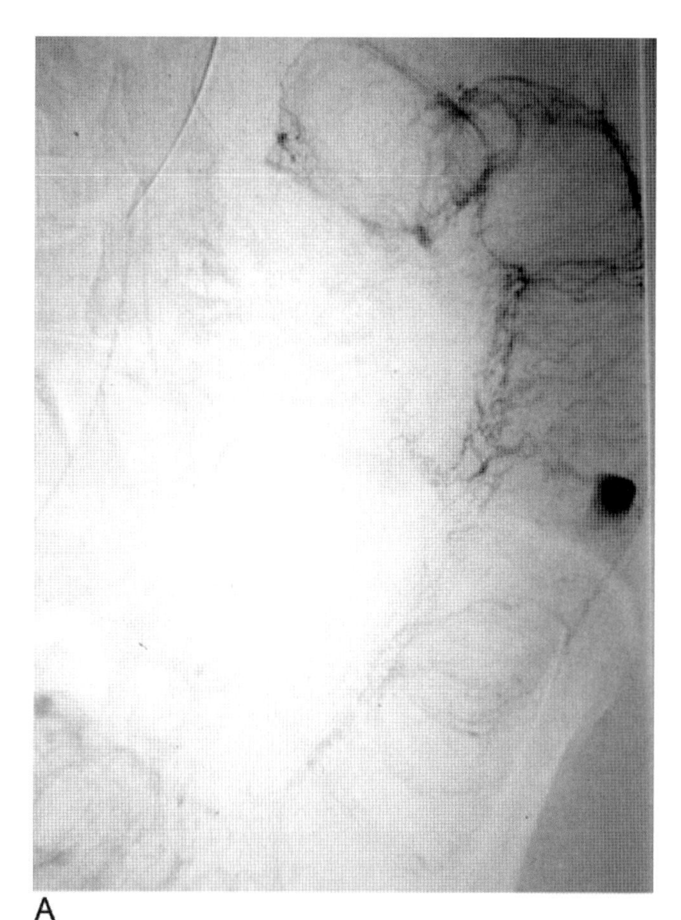

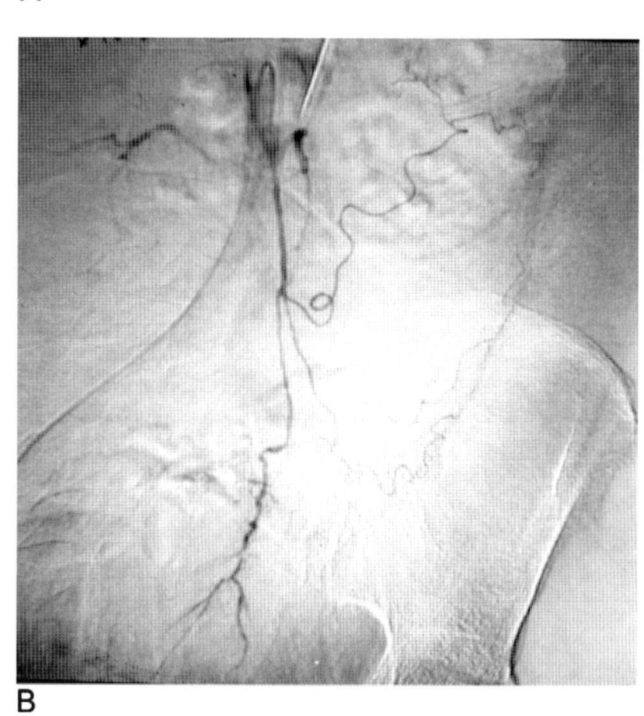

FIGURE 6-53. **A** Mesenteric angiogram shows extravasation of contrast indicating an acute bleed. **B** Acute gastrointestinal bleed that was successfully treated after infusion of pitressin.

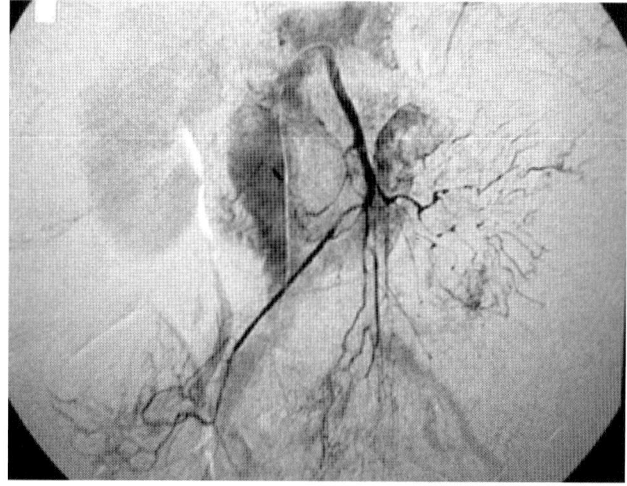

FIGURE 6-54. Mesenteric angiogram shows vasoconstriction and pruning of the superior mesenteric artery and its branches in this patient who presented with mesenteric ischemia secondary to severe hypotension.

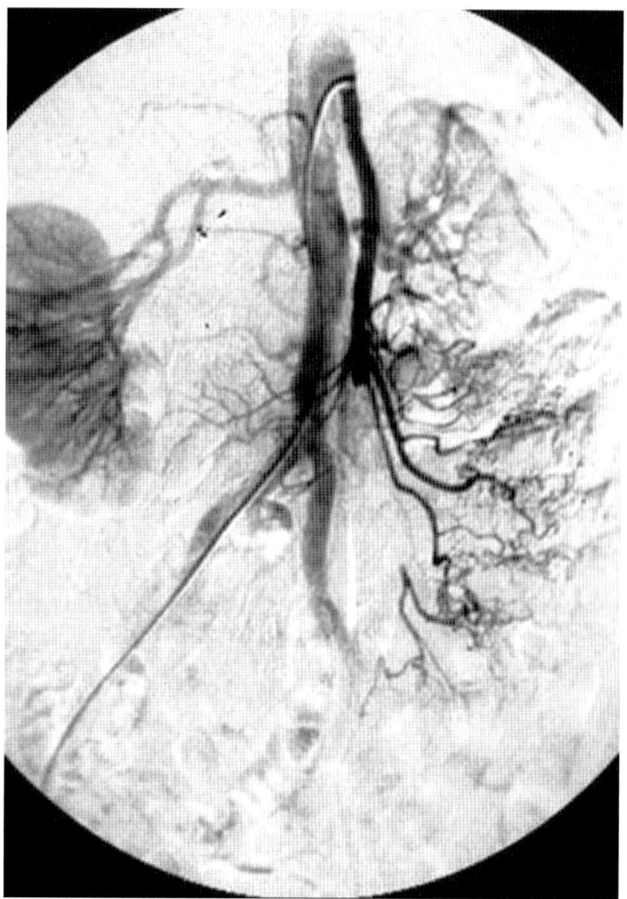

FIGURE 6-55. Mesenteric angiogram shows a large filling defect within the proximal superior mesenteric artery consistent with an embolism in this patient with ischemic bowel.

superior mesenteric artery seen as stenosis or plaque with a trickle of glow beyond. Collaterals will develop from the inferior mesenteric artery through the marginal artery. If the inferior mesenteric artery is occluded or absent, the collaterals will develop from the middle or inferior hemorrhoidal arterial branches of the internal iliac artery.[108,109]

Acknowledgments. This chapter was written by Matthew G. Mutch, Elisa H. Birnbaum, and Christine O. Menias in the first edition of this textbook.

References

1. Novelline RA. Squire's fundamentals of radiology. 5th ed. Cambridge, MA: Harvard University Press; 1997. p. 244–59.
2. Mirvus SE, Young JWR, Keramati B, et al. Plain film evaluation of patient with abdominal pain: are three radiographs really necessary? AJR Am J Roentgenol. 1986;147:501–3.
3. ACR Practice guideline for the performance of abdominal radiography. In: Practice guidelines and technical standards. Reston, VA: American College of Radiology; 2005. p. 1–5.
4. Roszler MH. Plain film radiologic examination of the abdomen. Crit Care Clin. 1994;10(2):277–96.
5. Almer S, Bodemar G, Frazen L, et al. Plain X-ray films and air enema films reflect severe mucosal inflammation in acute ulcerative colitis. Digestion. 1995;56:528–33.
6. Hicks TC, Opelka FG. The hazards of anal sexual eroticism. Perspect Colon Rectal Surg. 1994;7(1):37–57.
7. Miller RE, Nelson SW. The roentgenological demonstration of tiny amounts of free intraperitoneal gas: experimental and clinical studies. AJR Am J Roentgenol. 1971;112:487–90.
8. Miller RE, Becker GJ, Slabough RD. Detection of pneumoperitoneum: optimum body position and respiratory phase. AJR Am J Roentgenol. 1980;135:487–90.
9. Cook C, Campbell-Smith TA, Hopkins R. The abdominal radiograph: a pictorial view. Hosp Med. 2002;63(12): 726–31.
10. Levine MS, Scheiner JD, Rubesin SE, et al. Diagnosis of pneumoperitoneum on supine abdominal radiographs. AJR Am J Roentgenol. 1991;156:731–5.
11. Harvey CJ, Allen S, O'Regan D. Interpretation of the abdominal radiograph. Br J Hosp Med. 2005;66(11):M66–9.
12. Maglinte DD, Kelvin FM, Sandrasegaran K, et al. Radiology of small bowel obstruction: contemporary approach and controversies. Abdom Imaging. 2005;30:160–78.
13. Maglinte D, Heitkamp D, Howard T, et al. Current concepts in imaging of small bowel obstruction. Radiol Clin North Am. 2003;41:263–83.
14. Brant WE, Helms CA. Fundamentals of diagnostic radiology, vol. III. 3rd ed. New York: Lippincott Williams & Wilkins; 2006.
15. Burrell HC, Baker DM, Wardrop P, et al. Significant plain film findings in sigmoid volvulus. Clin Radiol. 1994;49:317–9.
16. Rubesin SE, Maglinte DDT. Double contrast barium enema technique. Radiol Clin North Am. 2003;41:365–76.
17. Levine MS, Kam LW, Rubesin SE, Ekberg O. Internal hemorrhoids: diagnosis with double-contrast barium enema examinations. Radiology. 1990;177:141–4.
18. Maglinte DDT, Strong RC, Strate RW, et al. Barium enema after colorectal biopsies: experimental data. AJR Am J Roentgenol. 1982;139:693–7.
19. Klabunde CN, Jones E, Brown ML, et al. Colorectal cancer screening with double contrast barium enema: a national survey of diagnostic radiologists. AJR Am J Roentgenol. 2002;179:1419–27.
20. Winawer SJ, Stewart ET, Zauber AG, et al. A comparison of colonoscopy and double contrast barium enema from surveillance after polypectomy. N Engl J Med. 2000;342:1766–72.
21. McCarthy PA, Rubesin SE, Levine MS, et al. Colon cancer: morphology detected with barium enema versus histologic stage. Radiology. 1995;197:683–7.
22. Blakeborough A, Chapman AH, AH SS, et al. Strictures of the sigmoid colon: barium enema evaluation. Radiology. 2001;220:343.
23. Almer S, Bodemar G, Franzen L, et al. Use of air enema radiology to assess depth of ulceration during acute attacks of ulcerative colitis. Lancet. 1996;347:1731–5.
24. Hizawa K, Iida M, Kohrogi N, et al. Crohn's disease: early recognition and progress of aphthous lesions. Radiology. 1994;190:451–4.
25. Nolan DJ, Traill ZC. The current role of barium examinations of the small intestine. Clin Radiol. 1997;52:809–20.
26. Giardiello FM, Bayless TM. Colorectal cancer and ulcerative colitis. Radiology. 1996;199:28–30.
27. Najjar SF, Jamal MK, Savas JF, et al. The spectrum of colovesical fistula and diagnostic paradigm. Am J Surg. 2004; 188:617–21.
28. Szucs RA, Turner MA. Gastrointestinal tract involvement by gynecologic disease. Radiographics. 1996;16:1251–70.
29. Thompson WM. Imaging and findings of lipomas of the gastrointestinal tract. AJR Am J Roentgenol. 2005;184:1163–71.
30. Simanovsky N, Hiller N, Koplewitz BZ, et al. Is non-operative intussusception reduction effective in older children? Ten-year experience in a university affiliated medical center. Pediatr Surg Int. 2007;23:261–4.
31. Friedman JD, Odland MD, Bubrick MP. Experience with colonic volvulus. Dis Colon Rectum. 1989;32:409–16.
32. Wood BP, Katzberg RW. Tween 80/diatrizoate enemas in bowel obstruction. AJR Am J Roentgenol. 1978;130(4):747–50.
33. Maglinte DDT, Lappas JC, Heitkamp DE, et al. Technical refinements in enteroclysis. Radiol Clin North Am. 2003;41:213–29.
34. Maglinte DDT, Kelvin FM, O'Connor K, et al. Current status of small bowel radiology. Abdom Imaging. 1996;21:247–57.
35. Jaffe TA, Yoshizumi TT, Toncheva G, et al. Radiation dose for body CT protocols: variability of scanners at one institution. AJR Am J Roentgenol. 2009;193:1141–7.
36. Horton KM, Abrams RA, Fishman EK. Spiral CT of colon cancer: imaging features and role in management. Radiographics. 2000;20:419–30.
37. Burtin S, Brown G, Bees N, et al. Accuracy of CT prediction of poor prognostic features in colonic cancer. Br J Radiol. 2008;81:10–9.
38. Zerhouni EA, Rutter C, Hamilton SR, et al. CT and MR imaging in the staging of colorectal carcinoma: report of the Radiology Diagnostic Oncology Group II. Radiology. 1996;200:443–51.
39. Freeny PC, Marks WM, Ryan JA, Bolen JW. Colorectal carcinoma evaluation with CT: preoperative staging and detection of postoperative recurrence. Radiology. 1986;158:347–53.

40. Acunas B, Rozanes I, Acunas G, Celik L, Sayi I, Gokmen E. Preoperative CT staging of colon carcinoma (excluding the rectosigmoid region). Eur J Radiol. 1990;11:150–3.
41. Scott DJ, Guthrie JA, Arnold P, et al. Dual phase helical CT versus portal venous phase CT for the detection of colorectal liver metastases: correlation with intra-operative sonography, surgical and pathological findings. Clin Radiol. 2001;56:235–42.
42. Bhattacharjya S, Bhattacharjya T, Bader S, et al. Prospective study of contrast-enhanced computed tomography, computed tomography during arterioportography, and magnetic resonance imaging for staging colorectal liver metastasis for liver resection. Br J Surg. 2004;91:1361–9.
43. Lim GH, Chi-Song D, Cheong WK, et al. Natural history of small "indeterminate" hepatic lesions in patients with colorectal cancer. Dis Colon Rectum. 2009;52:1487–91.
44. Jeffrey M, Hickey BE, Hider PN. Follow-up strategies for patients treated for non-metastatic colorectal cancer. Cochrane Database Syst Rev. 2007;(1):CD002200.
45. Tsikitis VL, Nakireddy K, Green EA, et al. Postoperative surveillance recommendations for early stage colon cancer based on results from the clinical outcomes of surgical therapy trial. J Clin Oncol. 2009;27:3671–6.
46. Anthony T, Simmang C, Hyman N, et al. Practice parameters for the surveillance and follow-up of patients with colon and rectal cancer. Dis Colon Rectum. 2004;47:807–17.
47. McDermott VG, Low VH, Keogan MT, et al. Malignant melanoma metastatic to the gastrointestinal tract. AJR Am J Roentgenol. 1996;166(4):809–13.
48. Byun JH, Ha HK, Kim AY, et al. CT findings in peripheral T-cell lymphoma involving the gastrointestinal tract. Radiology. 2003;227:59–67.
49. Tamm EP, Fishman EK. CT appearance of acute abdomen as initial presentation in lymphoma of the large and small bowel. Clin Imaging. 1996;20:21–5.
50. Levy AD, Remotti HE, Thompson WM, et al. Gastrointestinal stromal tumor: radiologic features with pathologic correlation. Radiographics. 2003;23:283–304.
51. Hulnick DH, Megibow AJ, Balthazar EJ, et al. Computed tomography in the evaluation of diverticulitis. Radiology. 1984;152:491–5.
52. Larimore T, Rhea J. Computed tomography evaluation of diverticulitis. J Intensive Care Med. 2004;19:194–204.
53. Jarrett TW, Vaughan Jr ED. Accuracy of computerized tomography in the diagnosis of colovesical fistula secondary to diverticular disease. J Urol. 1995;153:44–6.
54. Chintapalli KN, Chopra S, Ghiatas AA, Esola CC, Fields SF, Dodd GD. Diverticulitis versus colon cancer: differentiation with helical CT findings. Radiology. 1999;210:429–35.
55. Gore RM. CT of inflammatory bowel disease. Radiol Clin North Am. 1989;27:717–30.
56. Gore RM, Cohen MI, Vogelzang RL, et al. Value of computed tomography in the detection of complications of Crohn's disease. Dig Dis Sci. 1985;30:701–9.
57. Kerber GW, Greenberg M, Rubin JM. Computed tomography evaluation of local and intestinal complications in Crohn's disease. Gastrointest Radiol. 1984;9:143–8.
58. Gore RM, Balthazar EJ, Ghahremani GG, Miller FH. CT features of ulcerative colitis and Crohn's disease. AJR Am J Roentgenol. 1996;167:3–15.
59. Horton KM, Corl FM, Fishman EK. CT evaluation of the colon: inflammatory disease. Radiographics. 2000;20:399–418.
60. Wolff JH, Rubin A, Potter JD, et al. Clinical significance of colonoscopic findings associated with colonic thickening on computed tomography: is colonoscopy warranted when thickening is detected? J Clin Gastroenterol. 2008;42(5):472–5.
61. Yu J, Fulcher AS, Turner MA, Halvorsen RA. Helical CT evaluation of acute right lower quadrant pain. II. Uncommon mimics of appendicitis. AJR Am J Roentgenol. 2005;184:1143–9.
62. Furukawa A, Yamasaki M, Takahashi M, et al. CT diagnosis of small bowel obstruction: scanning technique, interpretation and role in the diagnosis. Semin Ultrasound CT MR. 2003;24:336–52.
63. Balthazar EJ. CT of small-bowel obstruction. AJR Am J Roentgenol. 1994;162:255–61.
64. Gazelle GS, Goldberg MA, Wittenberg J, Halpern EF, Pinkney L, Mueller PR. Efficacy of CT in distinguishing small-bowel obstruction from other causes of small-bowel dilatation. AJR Am J Roentgenol. 1994;162:43–7.
65. Frager D, Medwid SW, Baer JW, Mollinelli B, Friedman M. CT of small-bowel obstruction: value in establishing the diagnosis and determining the degree and cause. AJR Am J Roentgenol. 1994;162:37–41.
66. Zalcman M, Sy M, Donckier V, Closset J, Gansbeke DV. Helical CT signs in the diagnosis of intestinal ischemia in small-bowel obstruction. AJR Am J Roentgenol. 2000;175:1601–7.
67. Ha HK, Kim JS, Lee MS, et al. Differentiation of simple and strangulated small-bowel obstructions: usefulness of known CT criteria. Radiology. 1997;204:507–12.
68. Dobrin PB, Gully PH, Greenlee HB, et al. Radiologic diagnosis of an intra-abdominal abscess. Do multiple tests help? Arch Surg. 1986;121:41–6.
69. Aronberg DJ, Stanley RJ, Levitt RG, et al. Evaluation of abdominal abscess with computed tomography. J Comput Assist Tomogr. 1978;2:384–7.
70. Callen PW. Computed tomographic evaluation of abdominal and pelvic abscesses. Radiology. 1997;131:171–5.
71. Baker ME, Einstein DM, Veniero JC. Computed tomography enterography and magnetic resonance enterography: the future of small bowel imaging. Clin Colon Rectal Surg. 2008;21:193–2212.
72. Paulson SR, Hupprich JE, Hara AK. CT enterography: noninvasive evaluation of Crohn's disease and obscure gastrointestinal bleeding. Radiol Clin North Am. 2007;45:303–15.
73. McFarland EG, Fletcher JG, Pickhardt P, et al. ACR Colon Cancer Committee White Paper: status of CT colonography 2009. J Am Coll Radiol. 2009;6:756–72.
74. Pickhardt PJ, Hassan C, Laghi A, Zullo A, Kim DH, Morini S. Cost-effectiveness of colorectal cancer screening with computed tomographic colonography: the impact of not reporting diminutive lesions. Cancer. 2007;109:2213–21.
75. Pickhardt PJ, Choi JR, Hwang I, et al. Computed tomographic virtual colonoscopy to screen for colorectal neoplasia in asymptomatic adults. N Engl J Med. 2003;349:2191–200.
76. Matuchansky C. Computed tomographic colonography for detecting advanced neoplasia. JAMA. 2009;302(14):1527.
77. Johnson CD. CT colonography: coming of age. AJR Am J Roentgenol. 2009;193:1239–42.
78. Yamada T et al. Textbook of gastroenterology. 4th ed. Philadelphia, PA: Lippincott Williams & Wilkins; 2003. p. 3139–55. 3184–97.
79. Sun MRM, Smith MP, Kane RA. Current imaging techniques in imaging of fistula in ano: three dimensional endoanal ultrasound

and magnetic resonance imaging. Semin Ultrasound CT MR. 2008;29:454–71.
80. Raghunathan G, Mortele KJ. Magnetic resonance imaging of anorectal neoplasms. Clin Gastroenterol Hepatol. 2009; 7(4):379–88.
81. Yamada T et al. Textbook of gastroenterology. 4th ed. Philadelphia, PA: Lippincott Williams & Wilkins; 2003. p. 3184–98.
82. Taylor FGM, Swift RI, Blomqvist L, et al. A systematic approach to the interpretation of preoperative staging MRI for rectal cancer. AJR Am J Roentgenol. 2008;191:1827–35.
83. Brown G, Radcliffe AG, Newcombe RG, et al. Preoperative assessment of prognostic factors in rectal cancer using high-resolution magnetic resonance imaging. Br J Surg. 2003;90:355–64.
84. Messiou C, Chalmers A, Boyle PS. Surgery for recurrent rectal carcinoma: the role of preoperative magnetic resonance imaging. Clin Radiol. 2006;61:250–8.
85. Kulkarni T, Gollins S, Maw A, et al. Magnetic resonance imaging in rectal cancer downstaged using neoadjuvant chemoradiation: accuracy of prediction of tumour stage and circumferential resection margin status. Colorectal Dis. 2008;10:479–89.
86. Stoker J. Magnetic resonance imaging in fecal incontinence. Semin Ultrasound CT MR. 2008;29:409–13.
87. Sorenson JA, Phelps ME. Physics in nuclear medicine. 2nd ed. Orlando, FL: Grune & Stratton; 1987.
88. Podoloff DA, Advani RH, Alfred C, et al. NCCN task force report: positron emission tomography (PET)/computed tomography (CT) scanning in cancer. J Natl Compr Canc Netw. 2007;5(1):S1–22.
89. Pauwels E, McCready VR, Stoot JH, et al. The mechanism of accumulation of turnover localizing radiopharmaceuticals. Am J Nucl Med. 1998;25:277.
90. Ziessman HA et al. Nuclear medicine: the requisites. Philadelphia, PA: Mosby; 2006. p. 302–45.
91. Yasuda S, Fujii H, Nakahara T, et al. 18F-FDG PET detection of colonic adenomas. J Nucl Med. 2001;42:989–92.
92. Geus-Oei LF, Vriens D, van Laarhoven HWM, et al. Monitoring and predicting response to therapy with 18F-FDG PET in colorectal cancer: a systematic review. J Nucl Med. 2009;50:43S–54.
93. Desch CE, Benson III AB, Somerfield ME, et al. Colorectal cancer surveillance: 2005 update of an American Society of Clinical Oncology practice guideline. J Clin Oncol. 2005;23:8512–9. Earratum in J Clin Oncol 2006; 24:1224.
94. Huebner RH, Park KC, Shepherd JE, et al. A meta-analysis of the literature for whole body FDG PET detection of recurrent colorectal cancer. J Nucl Med. 2000;41:1177–89.
95. Iagaru A, Kundu R, Jadvar H, et al. Evaluation by 18F-FDG-PET of patients with anal squamous cell carcinoma. Hell J Nucl Med. 2009;12(1):26–9.
96. Cohade C, Osman M, Leal J, et al. Direct comparison of (18) F-FDG PET and PET/CT in patients with colorectal carcinoma. J Nucl Med. 2003;44:1797–803.
97. Hicks RJ, Ware RE, Lau EW. PET/CT: will it change the way that we use CT in cancer imaging? Cancer Imaging. 2006;6:S52–62.
98. Winzelberg GG, McKusick KA, Froelich JW, et al. Detection of gastrointestinal bleeding with Tc 99m-labeled red blood cells. Semin Nucl Med. 1982;12:139–46.
99. Gore RM, Levine MS. Textbook of gastrointestinal radiology. 2nd ed. Philadelphia, PA: W.B. Saunders Company; 2000. p. 1033–4.
100. Mettler FA, Guiberteau MJ. Essentials of nuclear medicine imaging. Philadelphia, PA: Saunders Elsevier; 2006. p. 215–9. 322.
101. Ng DA, Opelka FA, Beck DF, et al. Predictive value of technetium Tc 99m-labeled red blood cell scintigraphy for positive angiogram in massive lower gastrointestinal bleeding. Dis Colon Rectum. 1997;40:471–7.
102. Sfakianakis GN, Conway JJ. Detection of ectopia gastric mucosa in Meckel's diverticulum and in other aberrations by scintigraphy. I. Pathophysiology and 10 year clinical experience. J Nucl Med. 1981;22:647–54.
103. Sfakianakis GN, Conway JJ. Detection of ectopia gastric mucosa in Meckel's diverticulum and in other aberrations by scintigraphy. II. Indications and methods – a 10-year experience. J Nucl Med. 1981;22:732–8.
104. Witten DM, Hirsch FD, Hartman GW. Acute reaction to urographic contrast medium: incidence, clinical characteristics and relationship to history of hypersensitivity states. AJR Am J Roentgenol. 1973;119:832–40.
105. Hessel SJ, Adams DF, Abrams HL. Complications of angiography. Radiology. 1981;138:273.
106. Baum S, Athanasoulis CA, Waltman AC, et al. Angiodysplasia of the right colon: a cause of gastrointestinal bleeding. AJR Am J Roentgenol. 1977;129:789.
107. Tomchik FS, Wittenberg J, Ottinger LW. The roentgenographic spectrum of bowel infarction. Radiology. 1970;96:249.
108. Flickinger EG, Johnsrude IS, Ogburn NL, Weaver MD, Pories WJ. Local streptokinase infusion for SMA thromboembolism. AJR Am J Roentgenol. 1983;140:771–2.
109. Odurny A, Sniderman KW, Colapinto RF. Intestinal angina: percutaneous transluminal angioplasty of the celiac and SMA arteries. Radiology. 1988;167:59.

7 Endoluminal Ultrasound

Donald G. Kim and W. Douglas Wong[†]

Evaluation of the anal canal and rectum has traditionally relied on digital examination, anoscopy, and rigid or flexible proctosigmoidoscopy. The introduction of imaging methods, particularly endoluminal ultrasonography, has brought a greater degree of objectivity to the evaluation of the anorectum.

Endoluminal ultrasound has become the diagnostic procedure of choice in the evaluation of many anorectal disorders. Endorectal ultrasound (ERUS) has evolved into the best imaging modality for accurate staging of rectal neoplasms. The accurate determination of tumor penetration depth and regional lymph node status has become critical to guiding subsequent treatment of rectal malignancies. In addition, endoanal ultrasound (EAUS) has become invaluable in the diagnostic workup of fecal incontinence and anorectal suppurative conditions. This chapter will focus on the use of endoluminal ultrasound in the evaluation of patients with benign and malignant conditions of the anorectum.

History

Endoluminal ultrasound of the rectum was first introduced by Wild and Reid in 1952.[1] They were the first to develop an "echoendo probe," but it was never used clinically. Because of limitations in technology, it was not until 1983 that this type of imaging was introduced into clinical practice by Dragsted and Gammelgaard.[2] They used a Bruel and Kjaer (Type 8901) ultrasound probe with a rigid rotating endosonic probe with 4.5-MHz transducer initially designed for prostatic ultrasound. Thirteen primary rectal cancers were evaluated and invasion was correctly predicted in 11 cases when compared with the final histopathology. Two patients could not be adequately imaged because of stricture. Although successful, they did not define their reporting criteria. In 1985, Hildebrandt and Feifel[3] found that ultrasonography correlated with pathologic finding in 23 of 25 rectal cancers. They proposed a modification of the tumor-node-metastasis (TNM) classification[4] for ultrasound tumor staging (uTNM).[3] The prefix "u" indicated ultrasound staging as opposed to the prefix "p" representing pathologic staging. Similar to Dragsted and Gammelgaard, they also made no reference to the reporting criteria used for degree of invasion. Further refinements of the technique and improvement in the ultrasound equipment have made endoluminal ultrasound routine in the evaluation of patients with anorectal disorders.

Endorectal Ultrasound

As the treatment for rectal cancer has evolved, the importance of accurate preoperative staging of the lesion has become paramount in determining the patient's treatment regimen. Radical surgery, either low anterior or abdominoperineal resection is not always the initial or only therapy available for patients diagnosed with rectal carcinoma. With the development of preoperative neoadjuvant therapies for rectal cancer, accurate staging of these patients' lesions has become increasingly important. In addition, local excision has become an option in highly selected early-stage rectal cancers necessitating accurate preoperative staging.

The goal of preoperatively staging the rectal lesion is an accurate evaluation of the primary tumor, which includes the depth of tumor penetration and an evaluation of regional lymph node disease. ERUS accomplishes these goals using an intraluminal high-frequency sonographic transducer via a handheld rotating probe to accurately image the rectal wall and adjacent structures. For this reason, ERUS has become the preferred method used to stage the patient with rectal cancer.

Equipment and Technique

Equipment used for endoluminal ultrasonography includes a handheld endocavitary probe with rotating transducer which acquires a 360° image. Most investigators use a B-K Medical

[†]Deceased

D.E. Beck et al. (eds.), *The ASCRS Textbook of Colon and Rectal Surgery: Second Edition*,
DOI 10.1007/978-1-4419-1584-9_7,

scanner with a rigid handheld Type 1850 rotating probe and a 7- or 10-MHz transducer (B-K Medical, Wilmington, MA). Transducers of 7 and 10 MHz provide a focal length of 2–5 and 1–4 cm, respectively, rotating in a 90° scanning plane at four to six cycles per second to obtain a 360° radial scan of the rectal wall and surrounding structures. Because of its superior near-image clarity, the 10-MHz transducer is preferred. Rectal imaging requires a latex balloon covering the transducer for acoustic contact. The balloon is instilled with water allowing the ultrasound signals to easily pass through the water to image the rectum. The water instilled distends the rectum allowing the balloon to maintain contact with the rectal wall without separation, preventing any distortion of the image by the interposition of nonconductive air between the probe and the rectal wall.

Patients receive one or two phosphosoda enemas to cleanse the rectum before examination. The procedure is performed with the patient in the left lateral decubitus position without sedation. A digital rectal and proctoscopic examination is performed to assess the tumor size, appearance, location, and distance from the anal verge. Any residual stool or enema effluent that might interfere with the ultrasound is removed. A wide-bore ESI proctoscope (Electrosurgical Instrument Company, Rochester, NY) is inserted into the rectum to examine the rectum and lesion of interest. Optimally, the proctoscope is advanced proximal to the lesion to facilitate complete examination of the tumor by the transducer. The wide-bore ESI proctoscope permits passage of the ultrasound probe through the proctoscope to facilitate positioning of the probe above the lesion. This facilitates complete imaging of the lesion from its most proximal to distal extent as well as the proximal mesorectum, which may harbor involved lymph nodes. This approach is preferred to blind insertion of the ultrasound probe into the rectum. With blind insertion, distortion of the image can occur and the proximal areas of a lesion as well as the adjacent mesorectum will often be missed.

After correct positioning of the wide-bore ESI proctoscope, the ultrasound probe with latex balloon is lubricated and passed through the proctoscope to its full extent. The ultrasound probe is oriented with the stopcock and syringe positioned upright to the patient's right. The proctoscope is slightly withdrawn keeping the ultrasound probe in place to expose the transducer protruding beyond the end of the proctoscope, above the rectal lesion. The latex balloon is filled with 30–60 ml of water providing an optimal acoustic environment surrounding the rotating transducer. Initial preparation of the ultrasound probe includes careful removal of all air bubbles within the latex balloon to minimize acoustic interference. The probe and attached proctoscope are slowly withdrawn together carefully scanning the rectum from proximal to distal. The ultrasonographer observes for alterations of the rectal wall and perirectal tissues to assess depth of invasion and perirectal lymph node involvement. Optimal evaluation often requires several passes back and forth across a lesion. The evaluation of the lesion occurs on the basis of real-time imaging intermittently capturing still images that are representative of the lesion being studied. With the patient and ultrasound probe positioned as above, the images obtained are oriented radially similar to a computed tomography scan, looking up from the patient's feet. The patient's right side is oriented to the left of the image, anterior is up, and posterior is down. The studies can also be videotaped for further review.

Image Interpretation

Most ERUS images display a series of five distinct layers can be identified in the rectal wall. They consist of three hyperechoic (white) layers separated by two hypoechoic (black) layers. Beynon and colleagues[5] proposed a five-layer model based on an anatomic study, demonstrating that the five basic layers seen on an ultrasonographic scan of the rectal wall correspond directly to the anatomic layers present in the rectal wall. It is this five-layer model that we continue to use today (Figure 7-1). The five layers from the center to the periphery consist of the following:

First hyperechoic layer: Interface between the balloon and the rectal mucosal surface
Second hypoechoic layer: Mucosa and muscularis mucosa
Third hyperechoic layer: Submucosa
Fourth hypoechoic layer: Muscularis propria
Fifth hyperechoic layer: Interface between the muscularis propria and perirectal fat

Occasionally, a seven-ring model may be visualized when the muscularis propria is observed as two black rings separated by a white ring (Figure 7-2). This model represents the inner circular and outer longitudinal muscle layers as hyperechoic (black) rings separated by a hypoechoic (white) interface.

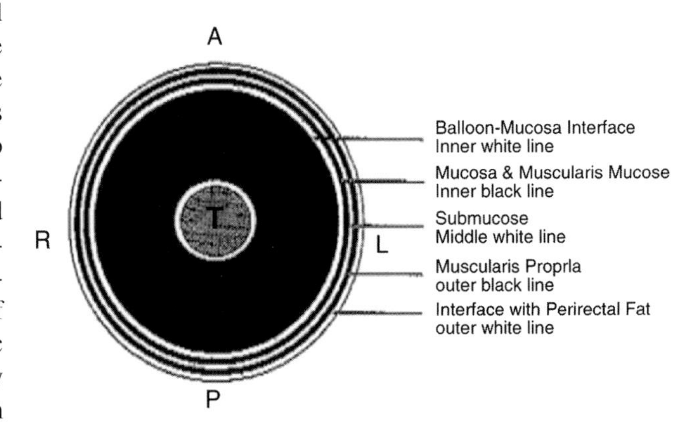

FIGURE 7-1. Five-layer anatomic model of an ERUS scan. Three hyperechoic (*white*) layers and two hypoechoic (*black*) layers are visualized. *A* anterior, *L* left, *P* posterior, *R* right, *T* transducer.

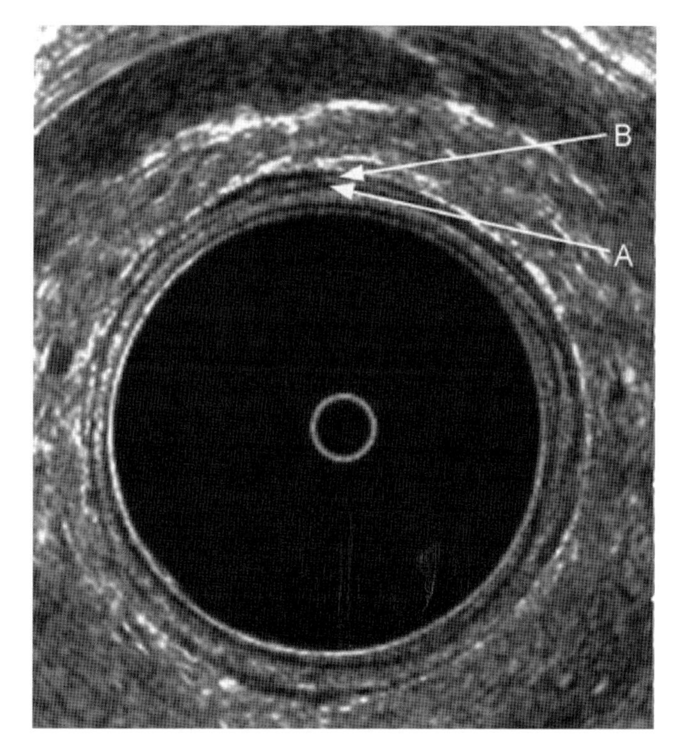

FIGURE 7-2. The typical five layers of the rectal wall. Seven layers are depicted anteriorly, where an interface can be seen between the *inner circular* **A** and outer longitudinal **B** muscle layers of the muscularis propria.

TABLE 7-1. Ultrasound staging classification (uTNM) for rectal cancer

uT0	Noninvasive lesion confined to the mucosa
uT1	Tumor confined to the mucosa and submucosa
uT2	Tumor penetrates into but not through the muscularis propria
uT3	Tumor extends into the perirectal fat
uT4	Tumor involves an adjacent organ
uN0	No evidence of lymph node metastasis
uN1	Evidence of lymph node metastasis

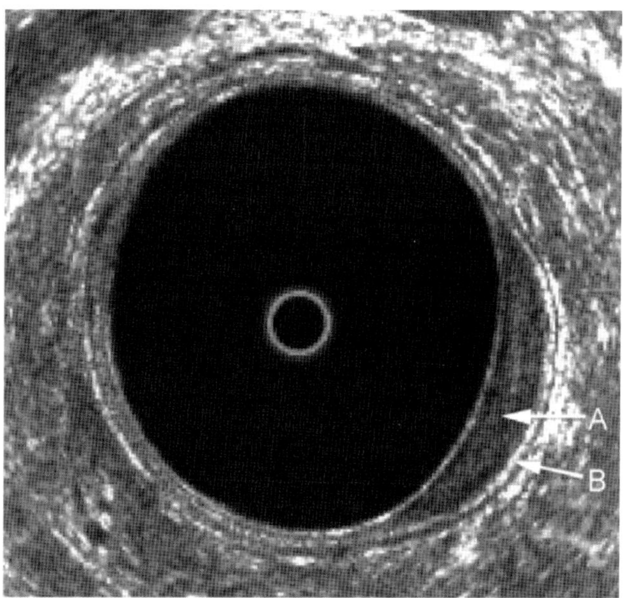

FIGURE 7-3. A benign uT0 lesion in the left posterolateral aspect of the rectum. There is an expansion of the *inner black line* that represents the mucosa **A**, but the submucosa **B** is seen to be completely intact.

Assessment of Rectal Neoplasms

Depth of Invasion

As discussed above, ultrasound classification of rectal tumor stage was initially proposed by Hildebrandt and Feifel[3] as a modification of the TNM classification. Ultrasound staging classification (uTNM) is presented in Table 7-1. The depth of invasion is classified as follows: uT0 lesions are benign, noninvasive lesions confined to the mucosa; uT1 lesions indicate an invasive lesion confined to the mucosa and submucosa; uT2 lesions penetrate but are confined to the muscularis propria; uT3 lesions penetrate the entire bowel wall and invade the perirectal fat; and a uT4 lesions penetrate a contiguous organ (i.e., uterus, vagina, cervix, bladder, prostate, seminal vesicles) or the pelvic sidewall or sacrum.

uT0 Lesions

uT0 lesions are benign, noninvasive lesions confined to the rectal mucosa. Sonographically, the mucosal layer (inner black band) is expanded with an intact submucosa (middle white, hyperechoic line) (Figure 7-3). Benign rectal villous adenomas are classified as uT0 lesions and may be treated with local excision with excellent results. Important in this decision is to accurately exclude any focus of invasion. The accuracy of ERUS is probably highest for T0 lesions. In an initial study by Deen et al.[6] from the University of Minnesota, 47 of 53 lesions (89%) were correctly staged preoperatively. A more recent update reported 129 of 148 patients (87%) were correctly staged preoperatively from that same institution.[7] Pikarsky et al.[8] reported that 25 of 27 patients (96%) were accurately staged a benign lesion when compared with pathologic results. Rectal adenomas excised transanally are frequently misdiagnosed on initial biopsy with the subsequent finding of an invasive cancer in the final pathologic specimen. For this reason, Worrell et al.[9] conducted a systematic literature review to assess the utility of ERUS in the assessment of rectal villous adenomas. He compared the diagnosis by biopsy alone with diagnosis by a combination of biopsy and ERUS. This meta-analysis revealed that, of 258 biopsy-negative rectal adenomas, 24% had focal carcinoma on final histopathology and that ERUS correctly detected the cancer in 81%.

uT1 Lesions

uT1 lesions are early invasive cancers. uT1 lesions have invaded the mucosa and submucosa without penetrating into the muscularis propria. Sonographically this is characterized by an irregular middle white line (submucosa) without alteration of the outer black line (muscularis propria) (Figure 7-4). Irregularities are indicated by a thickening or stippling of the submucosal layer but there must not be a distinct break in the submucosal layer. A distinct break in the submucosal (middle white line) layer indicates invasion of the muscularis propria, hence a T2 lesion.

Local transanal excision is an acceptable treatment method for selected T1 lesions highlighting the need for accurate staging of these cancers. Criteria for the use of local therapies to treat early rectal cancers have been described[10] and include tumor size less than 4 cm, involvement less than one-third of the rectal circumference, location less than 8 cm from the anal verge, well- to moderately well-differentiated histology, absence of lymphatic or vascular invasion, and no involvement of perirectal lymph nodes.

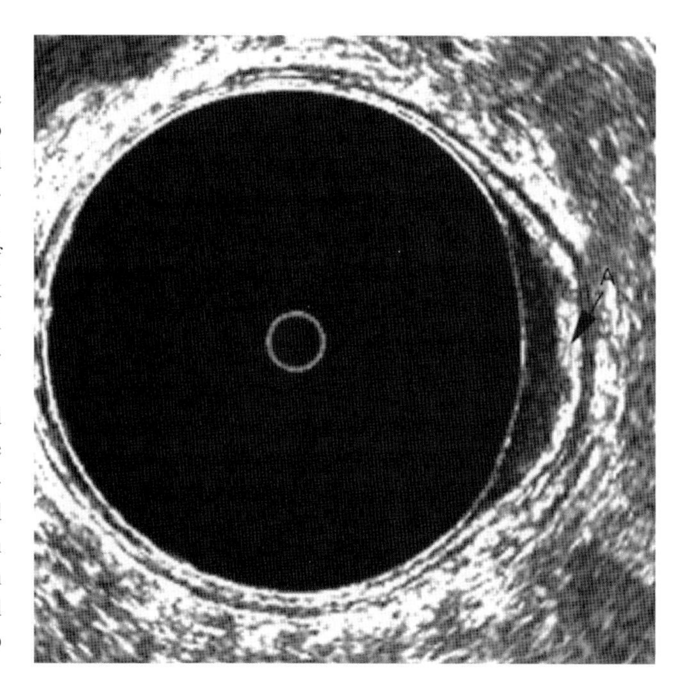

FIGURE 7-4. A uT1 cancer in the left lateral wall of the rectum. The *middle white line* or submucosa is irregular and somewhat thickened **A** but not completely disrupted.

uT2 Lesions

uT2 lesions penetrate into the muscularis propria (second hypoechoic, black line) but are confined to the rectal wall. Sonographically the hallmark finding is a distinct break in the submucosal layer. Characteristically, there is an expansion of the muscularis propria (outer black line) but the interface between the muscularis propria and the perirectal fat (the outermost white line) remains intact. The expansion of the muscularis propria may be variable depending on the degree of invasion. "Early" uT2 lesions may just invade the muscularis propria with minimal expansion of the layer. "Deep" uT2 lesions have significant expansion of the muscularis propria (outer black line) and may appear to scallop the outer aspect of the muscularis propria but preserve the interface with the perirectal fat. An example of a uT2 lesion is illustrated in Figure 7-5.

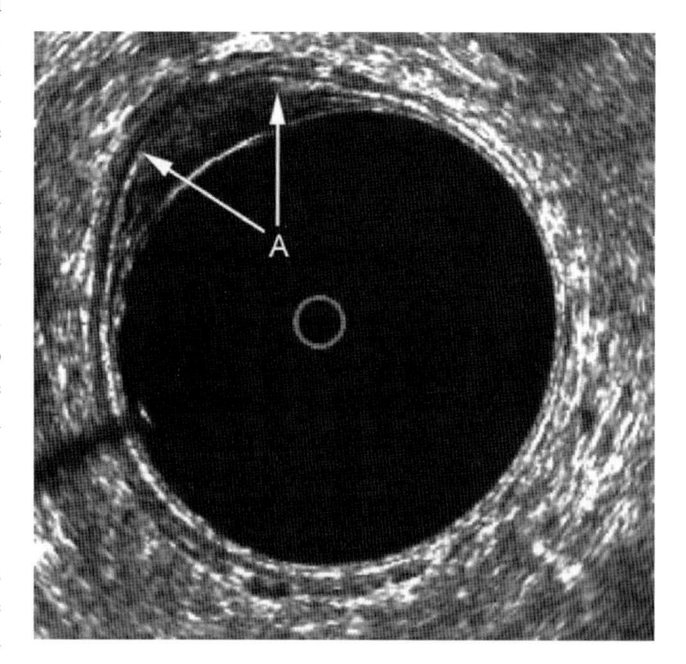

FIGURE 7-5. A uT2 lesion is identified in the right anterior location. The hallmark of a uT2 lesion, as seen on endorectal ultrasonography, is the distinct break **A** in the submucosa (the *middle white line*) as seen in this image.

uT3 Lesions

uT3 lesions penetrate the full thickness of the muscularis propria and into the perirectal fat. Contiguous structures are not involved. The sonographic appearance reveals disruption of the submucosa, thickening of the muscularis propria, and disruption of the outer hyperechoic, white line indicating penetration into the perirectal fat (Figure 7-6). The recognition of perirectal fat invasion is an important determinant in the preoperative evaluation of the rectal cancer patient. Because of the high incidence of lymph node metastases (30–50%), local therapy cannot be recommended for these patients, who are usually candidates for preoperative radiation and chemotherapy followed by surgery. ERUS obviously has an important role in selecting those patients who will undergo preoperative radiation and chemotherapy.

uT4 Lesions

uT4 lesions are locally invasive into contiguous structures such as the uterus, vagina, cervix, bladder, prostate and seminal vesicles, or involve the pelvic sidewall or sacrum. They are clinically fixed and tethered. Sonographically, there is

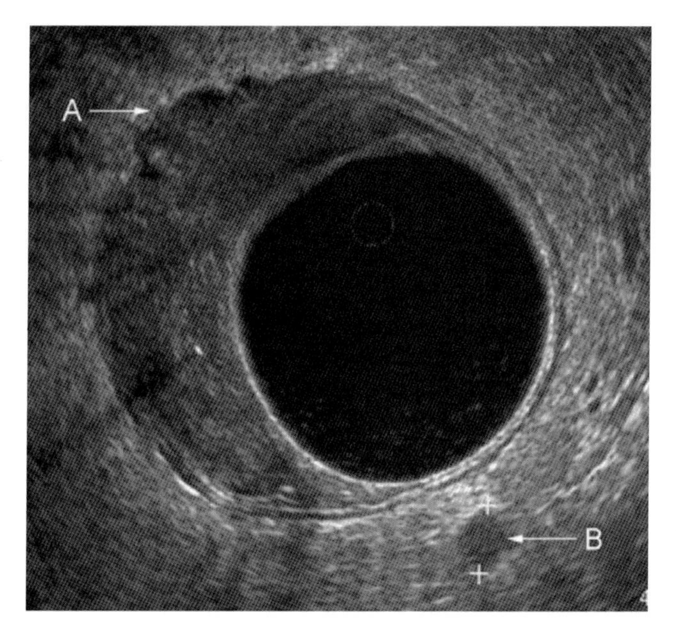

FIGURE 7-6. A uT3N1 lesion. The tumor disrupts all layers of the rectal wall, with extensions evident into the perirectal fat **A**. A lymph node **B** is identified in the left posterior location within the mesorectum.

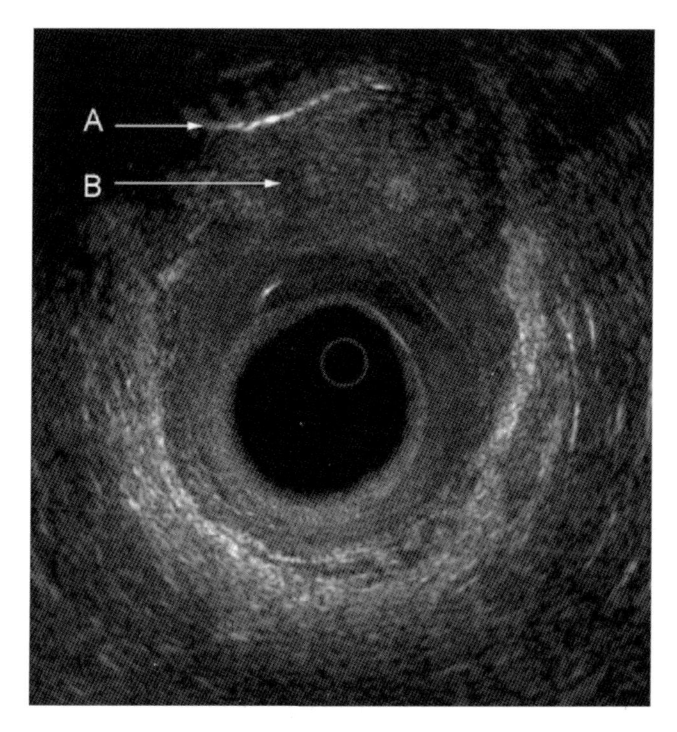

FIGURE 7-7. A T4 lesion in the distal rectum and upper anal canal extending to the vagina. The *curved white line* **A** seen anteriorly represents the examiner's finger in the vagina, and the hypoechoic anterior tumor **B** can be seen to extend into the vagina.

loss of the normal hyperechoic interface between the tumor and adjacent organ (Figure 7-7). Therapy of a T4 lesion usually requires preoperative radiation and chemotherapy followed by surgical resection of the rectal cancer and involved adjacent organ. The overall prognosis is poor, with less than half of patients resected for cure. Preoperative radiation and chemoradiation therapy can shrink the tumor for increased resectability and decreased local recurrence. ERUS provides the means to preoperatively identify those lesions with T4 involvement to adequately plan the patient's treatment.

Nodal Involvement

Lymph node involvement in rectal cancer is associated with decreased survival rates and increased local recurrence rates. ERUS is able to detect metastatic lymph nodes in the mesorectum. Unfortunately, the accuracy of detecting involved lymph nodes is less than the accuracy in determining the depth of invasion. The accuracy of ERUS in detecting lymph node metastases ranges from 50 to 83%.[7,11,12] ERUS determination of metastatic lymph nodes is certainly more accurate than clinical (digital) evaluation[13–15] as well as other imaging modalities including computed tomography (CT)[11,16–18] and conventional magnetic resonance imaging (MRI).[18,19] However, phased array MRI and endorectal coil MRI are comparable to ERUS in lymph node assessment.[20–22]

As indicated in Table 7-1, lymph node staging parallels pathologic TNM staging classifying tumors with (uN1) or without (uN0) lymph node involvement. Undetectable or benign-appearing lymph nodes are classified as uN0. Malignant-appearing lymph nodes are classified as uN1. Normal, nonenlarged lymph nodes are usually not detectable by ERUS. Inflamed, enlarged lymph nodes appear hyperechoic with irregular borders. Lymph nodes suspicious for malignancy include larger, round, hypoechoic lymph nodes with an irregular contour. ERUS findings consistent with metastatic lymph nodes are demonstrated in Figure 7-8. Hypoechoic lymph nodes greater than 5 mm are highly suspicious for metastases. Involved lymph nodes are usually found adjacent to the primary tumor or within the proximal mesorectum.

The echogenic pattern and size of imaged lymph nodes have been suggested to be indicators of metastatic nodal disease. Tio and Tytgat[23] were the first to recognize the hypoechoic pattern of malignant lymph nodes using ERUS. Hildebrandt et al.[24] differentiated two main groups of lymph nodes: hypoechoic and hyperechoic lymph nodes. Compared with pathologic findings, hypoechoic lymph nodes represent metastases, whereas hyperechoic lymph nodes are visualized because of nonspecific inflammation. There is no definitive size threshold to determine if an identified lymph node is malignant. Lymph nodes smaller than 5 mm can harbor metastatic disease.[25–27] In a pathology-based study, Herrera-Ornelas et al.[25] found that two-thirds of metastatic lymph nodes from colorectal cancer were smaller than 5 mm in diameter. Katsura et al.[26] found that 18% of nodes measuring 4 mm or less on ERUS were involved with metastatic disease. Similarly, Akasu et al.[27] found that approximately 50% of cases of lymph nodes measuring 3–5 mm on ERUS harbored metastases. Sunouchi et al.[28] described a "small

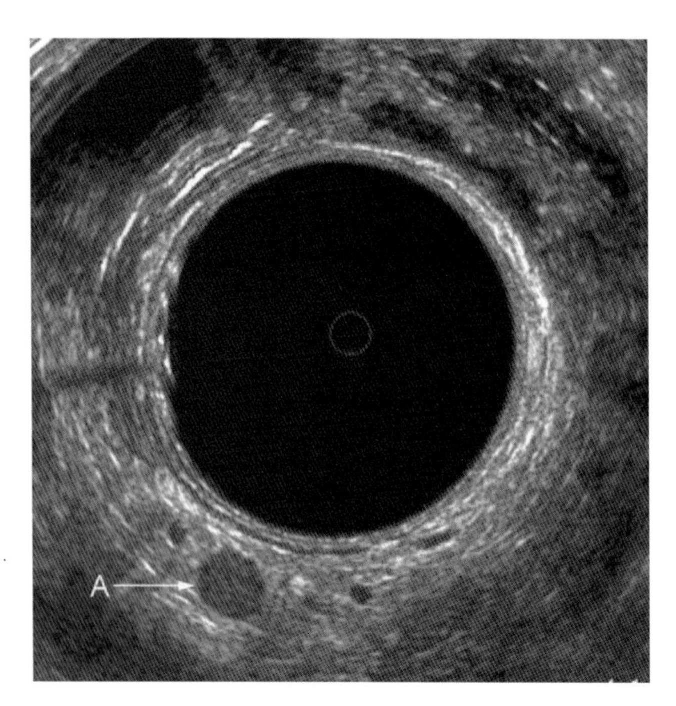

FIGURE 7-8. A typical metastatic lymph node **A**, which is round and hypoechoic.

spot sign" for lesions at the margin of rectal carcinomas on ERUS measuring 1–3 mm in diameter. The small hypoechoic "spots" correlated with massive venous or lymphatic invasion histologically.

Nodes larger than 5 mm harbored metastatic disease 54% of the time. Sunouchi et al.[29] studying hypoechoic lesions larger than 5 mm on ERUS demonstrated that 68% were metastatic lymph nodes and 20% were tumor deposits. Statistically, the incidence of metastatic disease increases as lymph node size increases.

Overall, four nodal patterns are seen with differing probabilities of being involved with metastatic disease. Nonvisible lymph nodes on ultrasound have a low probability of harboring lymph node metastases. Hyperechoic lymph nodes with nonsharply delineated boundaries are more often benign resulting from inflammatory changes. Hypoechoic lymph nodes larger than 5 mm are highly suggestive of lymph node metastases. Mixed echogenic lymph nodes larger than 5 mm are difficult to classify but should be considered malignant.

Accurate lymph node staging of rectal cancers by ERUS relies on the experience of the examiner. False-positive results may occur because of inflammatory lymph nodes or confusing the cross-sectional appearance of perirectal blood vessels for metastatic lymph nodes. Scanning longitudinally will distinguish between blood vessels and lymph nodes because blood vessels will extend longitudinally, change direction, and/or branch. The sonographic continuity of the hypoechoic vessel over a distance greater than the cross-sectional area is the criterion used to distinguish the two. Three-dimensional imaging can help in making this distinction.

False-negative results are also problematic in interpreting nodal involvement on ERUS. Lymph nodes harboring micrometastases are difficult to detect. Grossly malignant lymph nodes may be present outside the range of the ultrasound probe and remain undetectable. This may be the case of lateral pelvic lymph nodes such as the obturator nodes as well as those within the mesorectum beyond the proximal extent of the rigid probe.

Accuracy of Ultrasound in the Diagnosis of Rectal Cancer

The success of any imaging modality is the result of its diagnostic accuracy. Preoperative therapy for rectal cancer depends on the accurate staging of the primary lesion. The determination of the lesion's depth of invasion (T stage) and lymph node involvement (N stage) are important factors dictating the therapeutic options. ERUS has the ability to determine the depth of tumor invasion and lymph node involvement of rectal cancers. ERUS has been found to be accurate in determining the tumor's depth of invasion within the bowel wall, although ERUS is only moderately accurate in the assessment of lymph node involvement.

The accuracy of ERUS for the staging of rectal cancer has been established from studies comparing preoperative ultrasound staging with the pathologic staging from the operative specimens. The accuracy of ERUS for tumor depth of invasion has been reported in the range of 63–93% (Table 7-2). Overstaging has been reported in approximately 11% of patients[16] and is believed to be the result of peritumoral inflammation beyond the leading edge of the tumor. Understaging for depth of wall invasion has been reported to be approximately 5%[16] and is considerably more serious than overstaging because inadequate management may result. With overstaging, potentially more aggressive management is recommended than might be required.

Detection of lymph node metastases with ERUS has been less accurate, ranging from 50 to 83% in reported series (Table 7-2). Solomon and McLeod[41] reviewed the literature and pooled raw data were collected from eight published cross-sectional surveys assessing the degree of tumor penetration in 873 patients and lymph node involvement in 571 patients with primary rectal cancer. As previously noted, ERUS was very accurate in determining tumor penetration (κ=0.85), but only a moderate correlation was found between ERUS and histopathology for detecting lymph node involvement (κ=0.58). Furthermore, the positive predictive value was 74% with a negative predictive value (NPV) of 84%, indicating only moderate accuracy among the included series.

Puli et al.[18] recently conducted a meta-analysis and systematic review to determine the accuracy of ERUS in determining lymph node invasion of rectal cancers. Only ERUS confirmed by surgical histology were selected. Data

TABLE 7-2. Accuracy of ERUS in the staging of rectal cancer

Author	Year	*n*	Accuracy (%) T stage	Accuracy (%) N stage
Hildebrandt and Feifel[3]	1985	25	92	n/a
Saitoh et al.[30]	1986	88	90	75
Holdsworth et al.[31]	1988	36	86	61
Beynon et al.[32]	1989	100	93	83
Rifkin et al.[12]	1989	102	65	50
Glaser et al.[33]	1990	86	88	79
Jochem et al.[34]	1990	50	80	73
Milsom and Graffner[14]	1990	52	83	83
Orrom et al.[35]	1990	77	75	82
Katsura et al.[26]	1992	112	92	n/a
Glaser et al.[36]	1993	154	92	81
Herzog et al.[37]	1993	118	89	80
Deen et al.[6]	1995	209	82	77
Akasu et al.[27]	1997	152	82	76
Adams et al.[38]	1999	70	74	83
Kim et al.[21]	1999	89	81	64
Garcia-Aguilar et al.[7]	2002	545	69	64
Marusch et al.[39]	2002	422	63	n/a
Kauer et al.[40]	2004	458	69	68

were extracted from 35 studies ($N = 2{,}732$) that met the study inclusion criteria. The meta-analysis demonstrated moderate sensitivity and specificity. Pooled sensitivity of ERUS in determining nodal involvement by rectal cancer was 73.2% with a pooled specificity of 75.8%. The positive likelihood ratio of ERUS was 2.84 (95% CI 2.16–3.72) and the negative likelihood ratio was 0.42 (95% CI 0.32–0.52). The positive likelihood ratio of a diagnostic test measures how well the test correctly identifies a disease state. The higher the positive likelihood ratio, the more likely the diagnostic test will correctly identify the true disease state. Contrarily, the negative likelihood ratio of a diagnostic test measures how well the test correctly excludes a disease state. The lower the negative likelihood ratio, the better the diagnostic test's ability to exclude a disease state. ERUS has a low negative likelihood ratio but the positive likelihood ratio is modest. Therefore, based on this meta-analysis, ERUS can better exclude nodal invasion by rectal cancer than confirm nodal invasion. In other words, one would be more confident in a negative (nodal invasion absent) diagnosis than a positive (nodal invasion present) diagnosis.

There is a significant learning curve associated with the performance and interpretation of ERUS. Accuracy rates have been demonstrated to improve significantly with experience.[35] ERUS is highly operator dependent and thus accuracy is dependent on the experience and expertise of the examiner.[7,33]

Several factors can lead to the misinterpretation of ERUS images.[42,43] These factors include a lesion in close proximity to the anal verge, improper balloon inflation with associated balloon-wall separation, a nonperpendicular imaging plane, shadowing artifacts caused by air or stool, reverberation artifacts, refraction artifacts, and a transducer gain setting that is too high.[42] A technically difficult ERUS is likely to give an inconclusive or inaccurate result.[43] Factors causing technical difficulties include stenotic lesions, patient discomfort, poor bowel preparation, and scarring from previous surgery.[43]

Postbiopsy and postsurgical changes, hemorrhage, and bulky or pedunculated tumors can cause changes in the ultrasound image significantly affecting the accuracy of the ERUS interpretation.[44]

The accuracy of ERUS after neoadjuvant therapy is decreased for both depth of penetration and nodal status.[45–50] Radiation therapy can significantly downstage tumors and may in fact leave no residual tumor within the pathologic specimen. In fact, up to 24% of patients treated with preoperative radiation therapy have a complete pathologic response with no evidence of residual tumor.[51] Radiation therapy can cause tissue edema and fibrosis of the rectal lesion making ERUS interpretation difficult. One cannot accurately distinguish radiation-induced changes from residual tumor. In contrast with the disappointing accuracy of ERUS for both T and N staging, the NPV is relatively high (81–82%) in several series.[45,47,48,52] ERUS may allow good prediction of node-negative rectal cancers.[47,48] This may be helpful when local therapy may be considered for a patient after preoperative chemoradiation. Typically, ERUS is felt to be inaccurate and unreliable after radiation therapy, and is not recommended.

Postoperative Follow-Up

Local recurrence continues to be a difficult problem in the treatment of rectal cancer. Overall, local recurrence rates have been reported between 4 and 30% after curative rectal cancer surgery. More than 50% of patients will have local recurrence only at the surgical site without distant metastases.[53,54] Even with newer adjuvant therapies available, surgical resection remains the best chance of cure for the patient with isolated local recurrence. Clearly, early detection of local recurrence is important and follow-up programs should be directed at this goal in order to be successful. ERUS may be used in a variety of settings for surveillance purposes after surgery for rectal cancer. When used in combination with a digital rectal examination and endoscopic surveillance, ERUS may significantly improve the sensitivity of detecting recurrent lesions.[55–57] ERUS may improve the ability to diagnose recurrent neoplasm by as much as 30%.[58] In a series studying ERUS as a means to identify local recurrence, overall local recurrence ranged from 11 to 20% with the proportion of local recurrences diagnosed exclusively by ERUS varying from 18 to 35%.[57–59] These ERUS-only recurrences represent only 3.2–5% of the entire group of patients. The University of Minnesota group presented similar results although the impact on overall survival is unclear.[56]

Although local recurrence can occur within the lumen at the anastomosis, locally recurrent tumors more often extend from extrarectal lesions that invade through the rectum, often at the level of an anastomosis. Extrarectal tumor not involving the mucosa may be undetectable endoscopically but can be identified at an early stage with ERUS. Recurrent tumor appears as a circumscribed hypoechoic lesion in the para-anastomotic tissues with all or a portion of the rectal wall intact on the inner, luminal aspect (Figure 7-9). Early postoperative changes, particularly adjacent to the anastomosis, can make the interpretation of the ERUS difficult. Interpretation is aided if a "baseline" ultrasound is obtained soon (3 months) after surgery and compared with subsequent surveillance images. A baseline examination is useful to document postoperative scarring and to evaluate that area for potential changes on serial examinations. Lesions that increase in size on subsequent examinations are more likely to represent recurrent tumor. Because ERUS cannot establish that a lesion is malignant with absolute certainty, a biopsy of suspicious lesions is recommended to confirm recurrent disease.[60] Biopsies may be performed by ultrasound-guided biopsy or computed tomography scan-guided biopsy.

The optimal interval and length of time for serial follow-up ERUS examinations have not been determined. Because most recurrences present within the first 2 years after surgery, more intensive follow-up is justified during this period. Imaging every 3–4 months for the first 2–3 years may be appropriate with less frequent, every 6-month evaluations until 5 years.

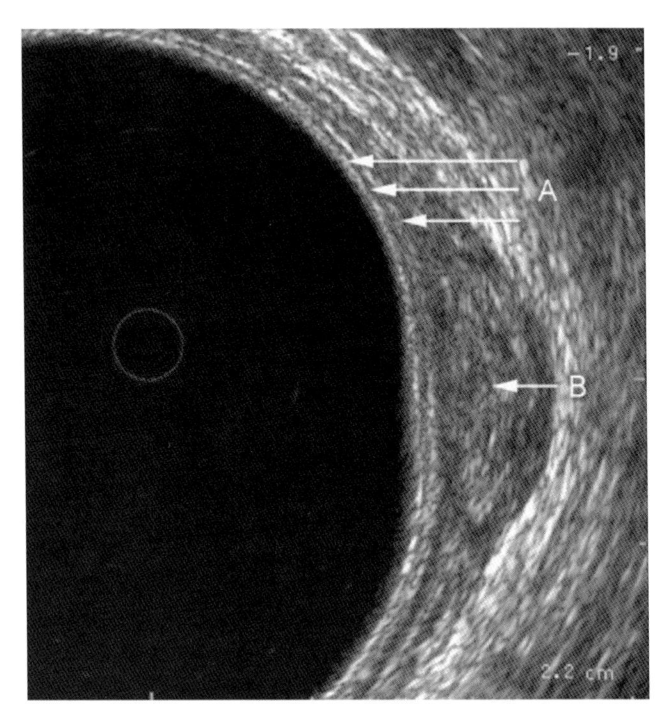

FIGURE 7-9. A recurrent rectal cancer. It is located in the left lateral rectal wall. Note the intact *inner three lines* **A** on the ultrasound image, indicating no involvement of the mucosa or submucosa but an obvious abnormality at the level of the muscularis propria **B**, representing the recurrence.

Comparison of Endorectal Ultrasound, Computed Tomography, and Magnetic Resonance Imaging

In a meta-analysis by Kwok et al.[16] ERUS, CT, and MRI were evaluated as preoperative staging modalities in rectal cancer. In his evaluation of ERUS, Kwok found an overall accuracy rate of 87% (sensitivity, 93%; specificity, 78%) for depth of penetration. Nodal status demonstrated a pooled accuracy rate of 74% (sensitivity, 71%; specificity, 76%). Among those cases staged by TNM classification, 11% were overstaged and 5% were understaged.

In his evaluation of CT, the overall accuracy for depth of penetration was found to be 73% (sensitivity, 78%; specificity, 63%).[16] Nodal status was accurately assessed 66% of the time (sensitivity, 52%; specificity, 78%). Of those staged by TNM classification, 13% were overstaged and 7% were understaged.

With respect to MRI, the accuracy of all MRI modalities for depth of penetration was 82% (sensitivity, 86%; specificity, 77%).[16] Nodal involvement accuracy for MRI was 74% (sensitivity, 65%; specificity 80%). Of those cases staged by TNM classification, 13% were overstaged and 13% understaged. Subgroup analysis found that MRI with an endorectal coil was equivalent to ERUS for depth of penetration with an overall accuracy rate of 84% (sensitivity, 89%; specificity, 79%). Overall accuracy for nodal status was 82% (sensitivity, 82%; specificity; 83%).

In another meta-analysis, Bipat et al.[20] also compared ERUS, CT, and MRI in rectal cancer staging. In this review, duplicate studies were excluded. Studies with the most details or the most patients were included. For muscularis propria invasion, ERUS and MRI had similar sensitivities; specificity of ERUS (86%) was significantly higher than that of MRI (69%) (P=0.02). For perirectal tissue invasion, sensitivity of ERUS (90%) was significantly higher than that of CT (79%) (P<0.001) and MRI (82%) (P=0.003); specificities were comparable. For adjacent organ invasion and lymph node involvement, sensitivities and specificities for ERUS, CT, and MRI were comparable.

In the most recent comparative study, Dinter et al.[22] evaluated ERUS, hydro-CT, and high-resolution endorectal MRI in the preoperative staging of rectal cancer. A total of 23 patients with histologically proven rectal cancer underwent all examinations followed by surgery. All modalities demonstrated correct depth of penetration in 19 of 23 patients (83%). Lymph node staging was correctly determined by ERUS in 19 of 23 patients (83%). Hydro-CT correctly staged lymph nodes in 20 of 23 patients (87%) with endorectal MRI correctly staging 19 of 23 (83%). Only two previous studies have compared ERUS, endorectal MRI, and CT.[21,61] These older studies may have been limited by the available equipment. In the study by Kim et al.[21] CT was performed with a helical single detector scanner with 10-mm slice thickness as compared to a multidetector spiral CT. In Meyenberger's[61] study, only a limited number of patients were evaluated with all methods: 32 patients underwent ERUS, 16 patients underwent CT, 9 MRI, and only 5 endorectal MRI. Overall accuracy of the Dinter et al.[22] study was comparable to that of Kim et al.[21] In lymph node staging, the results were better in all modalities when compared to those of Kim et al.[21] with ERUS accuracy of 83% vs. 63.5%, CT 87% vs. 56.5%, and MRI 83% vs. 78.5%.[22] Although only a limited number of patients were examined, the Dinter et al.[22] study indicates that improved results may be attainable as a result of better technical equipment.

Endoanal Ultrasound

EAUS is useful in the evaluation of the anal canal in both benign and malignant disease. The anal sphincter anatomy can be clearly identified detecting abnormalities in the external and/or internal sphincter. EAUS is routinely used in the evaluation of fecal incontinence and may be particularly useful in the evaluation of complex perianal abscesses and fistulas. EAUS is also useful in the evaluation of anal canal neoplasms accurately staging these lesions.

Equipment and Technique

The equipment used for EAUS is similar to that used for ERUS. The same B-K scanner is used with the 1850 rotating probe and 10-MHz transducer (B-K Medical). In place of the latex balloon, a translucent plastic cap (B-K type WA0453) is placed over the transducer to maintain contact with the anal canal. The plastic cap is again filled with water to provide the acoustic medium. There is a pinhole in the apex of the plastic cap that permits the escape of any air through displacement of the space with water.

The examination technique for EAUS is similar to that of ERUS. Patients are examined in the left lateral decubitus position, again usually without sedation. A careful external examination of the perianal area followed by a digital rectal examination is performed. The probe is lubricated with a water-soluble gel and gently inserted into the anal canal until the plastic cap is no longer visible. This will usually ensure that the transducer is at the level of the upper anal canal. The probe is slowly withdrawn to image the full length of the anal canal. Images are typically obtained in the upper, mid, and distal anal canal. In most instances, patients can be reassured that the examination should cause no more discomfort than a digital rectal examination. Certain instances of complex anorectal sepsis may be painful and require examination under anesthesia to adequately image the patient with EAUS.

Image Interpretation

Normal anal canal anatomy is well visualized with EAUS. As with the rectum, the interpretation of these images must be based on a precise definition of normal endosonographic anatomy of the anal canal that correlates well with anatomy. EAUS of the anal canal and pelvic floor have been correlated with cadaveric anatomic dissections.[62] The ultrasonographic anatomy of the anal canal is generally divided into three levels: the upper, mid, and distal anal canal. Each level has a different appearance on EAUS. The upper anal canal is illustrated in Figure 7-10. The puborectalis is an important

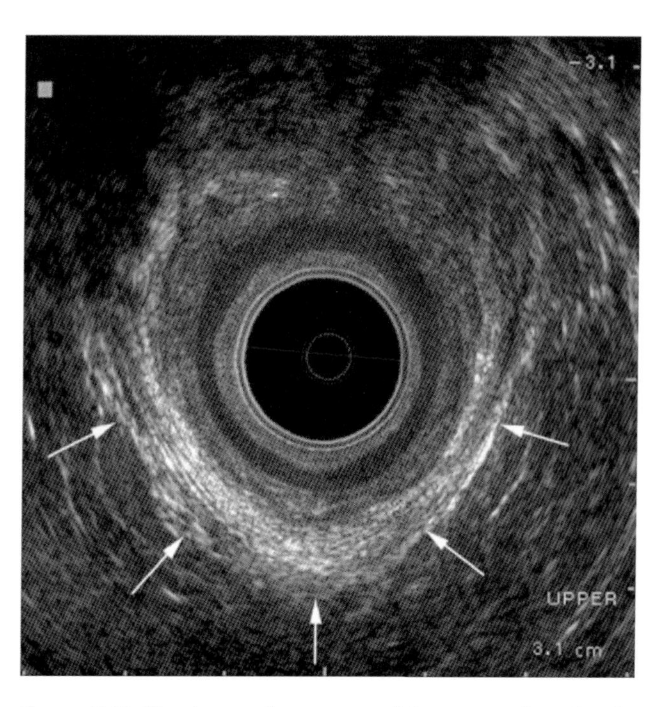

FIGURE 7-10. The ultrasound appearance of the upper anal canal at the level of the puborectalis, which can be seen as the hyperechoic U-shaped structure seen posteriorly and laterally (*arrows*) in this image.

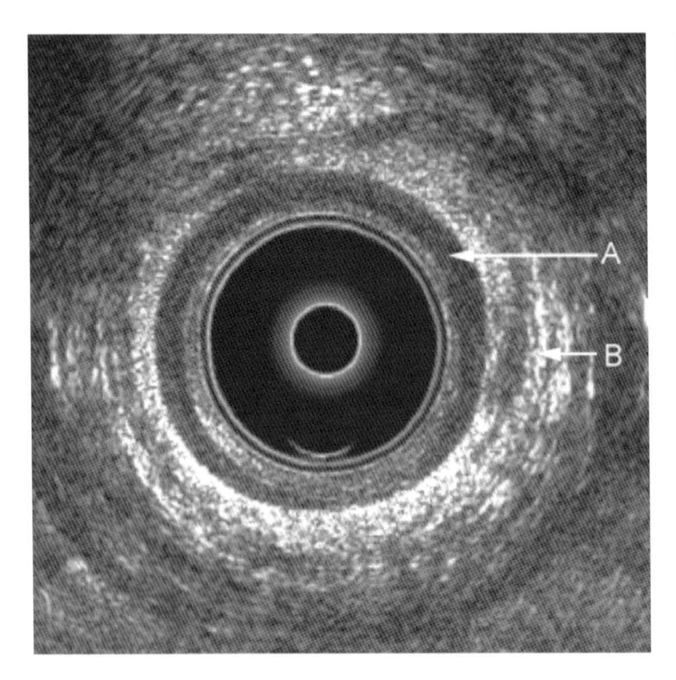

FIGURE 7-11. The characteristic appearance of the mid-anal canal. The circular hypoechoic structure represents the internal anal sphincter **A**, surrounded by the thicker hyperechoic circumferential external anal sphincter **B**.

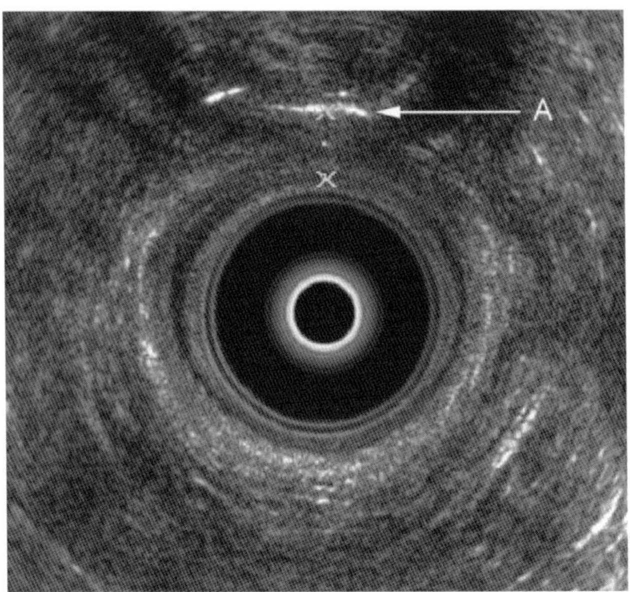

FIGURE 7-12. The technique used to measure the anterior perineal body in a female patient. The examiner's finger is placed in the vagina, and the hyperechoic curvilinear structure **A** seen anteriorly delineates the examiner's finger. The two cross-hatches between the examiner's finger and the transducer measure the thickness of the perineal body in this intact sphincter at the mid-anal canal level.

landmark delineating the upper anal canal. The puborectalis is imaged as a horseshoe-shaped mixed echogenic structure forming the lateral and posterior portion of the upper anal canal.

The mid-anal canal is illustrated in Figure 7-11. Within the mid-anal canal, the internal anal sphincter is represented by a hypoechoic band surrounded by the hyperechoic external anal sphincter. Between the transducer and the internal anal sphincter is an additional hyperechoic ring of variable thickness representing the epithelial, hemorrhoidal, and submucosal tissue. Perineal body measurements can be made at the level of the mid-anal canal (Figure 7-12). With the probe positioned within the mid-anal canal, the right index finger is placed within the vagina against the rectovaginal septum and ultrasound probe. The distance between the hyperechoic ultrasound reflection of the finger and the inner aspect of the internal anal sphincter may be measured and represents the perineal body thickness. Normal measurements for perineal body thickness range from 10 to 15 mm, with a lower limit of normal considered to be approximately 8 mm. This measurement is useful in the evaluation of women with fecal incontinence from anterior sphincter defects. The examining index finger not only better defines the perineal body but may accentuate an anterior sphincter defect that may otherwise appear intact.

The distal anal canal is illustrated in Figure 7-13. The distal anal canal is defined as the point where the internal anal sphincter is no longer seen. Only the hyperechoic external anal sphincter and surrounding soft tissues are visualized.

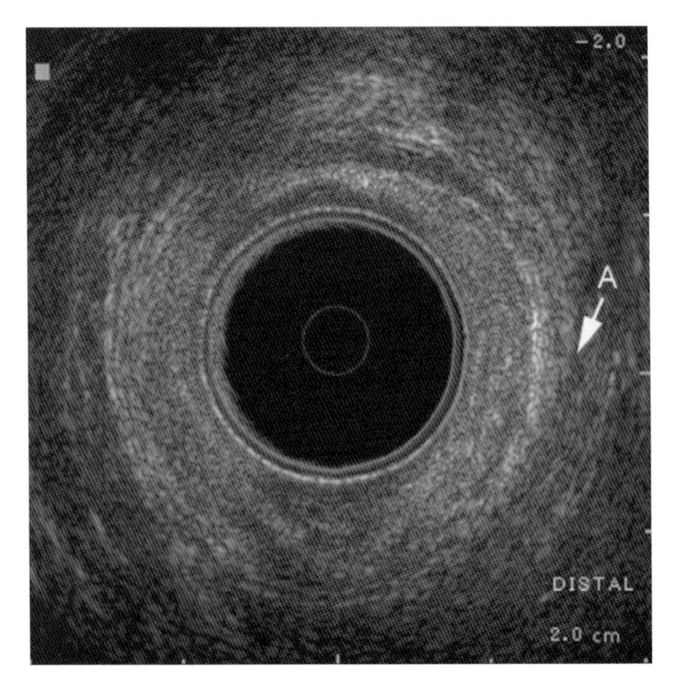

FIGURE 7-13. The distal anal canal below the inferior level of the internal sphincter, where only the hyperechoic circumferential fibers of the superficial external anal sphincter **A** are imaged.

Evaluation of Fecal Incontinence

EAUS has an important role in the evaluation of fecal incontinence, accurately delineating anal sphincter anatomy.[63–65] Causes of anal sphincter defects include obstetric injuries, anorectal surgeries, traumatic injuries, and congenital abnormalities.

Fecal incontinence is eight times more frequent in women,[66] the most common cause being obstetric trauma leading to injury of the anal sphincter muscles or traction neuropathy involving the pudendal nerve.[66–68] Although anal sphincter injury identified during delivery does not lead to significant deterioration in sphincter function immediately, it is suspected to lead to fecal incontinence in approximately 40% of women in long-term follow-up despite primary sphincter repair.[69–71] Anal incontinence is not restricted to patients with recognized third- or fourth-degree obstetric tears. Patients may also develop delayed symptoms of incontinence several years after an unrecognized sphincter injury.[72] The introduction of EAUS has led to the recognition of unsuspected sphincter defects in asymptomatic, continent women thought to have normal perineums.[73–76] Traumatic sphincter disruption can frequently be associated with a subsequent rectovaginal fistula. These patients may be anally continent but have symptoms of fecal incontinence associated with the fistula. Because these patients may have an unrecognized anal sphincter defect, all patients with rectovaginal fistula should undergo preoperative evaluation for occult sphincter defects by EAUS.[77] Local tissues are inadequate for endorectal advancement flap repairs in patients with anal sphincter defects and these patients should be treated by sphincteroplasty with levatoroplasty.[77] EAUS has become an accurate method to image the anal sphincters identifying anal sphincter defects that result in fecal incontinence.[68,78–80]

EAUS has become the best modality to accurately demonstrate the anatomy of the anal canal as well as anal sphincter defects that contribute to fecal incontinence.[65] Defects in the external anal sphincter usually appear hypoechoic, although some may appear hyperechoic or demonstrate mixed echogenicity. Defects of the internal anal sphincter are represented by the lack of segment of the hypoechoic band of internal sphincter muscle. There is usually associated contralateral thickening of the hypoechoic internal anal sphincter. With complete sphincter disruption, EAUS demonstrates the ends of the internal and external anal sphincter widely separated and bridged with intervening scar tissue of variable echogenicity (Figure 7-14). Many times, complete sphincter disruption is not seen, but attenuation of the sphincter mechanism is noted anteriorly, indicating a significant partial sphincter defect. An examining digit[81,82] or vaginal balloon[81] used to measure the perineal body distance in the mid-anal canal can accentuate an anterior sphincter defect, helping to identify a sphincter injury (Figure 7-15).

Other causes of anatomic anal sphincter defects include anorectal trauma or surgery and congenital anomalies.

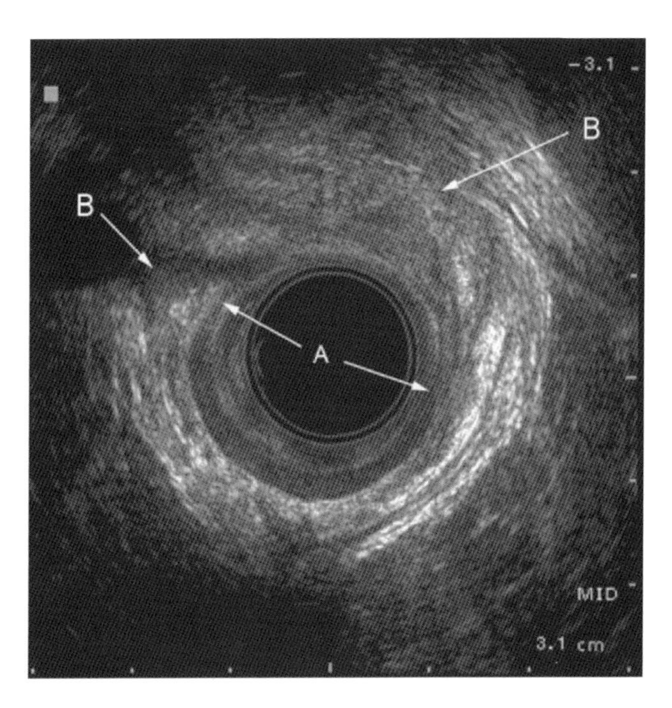

FIGURE 7-14. A complete anterior sphincter disruption in a female patient. The hypoechoic internal anal sphincter can be seen completely disrupted in its anterior location (**A** *arrows*). Similarly, the hyperechoic external anal sphincter is completely disrupted anteriorly (**B** *arrows*).

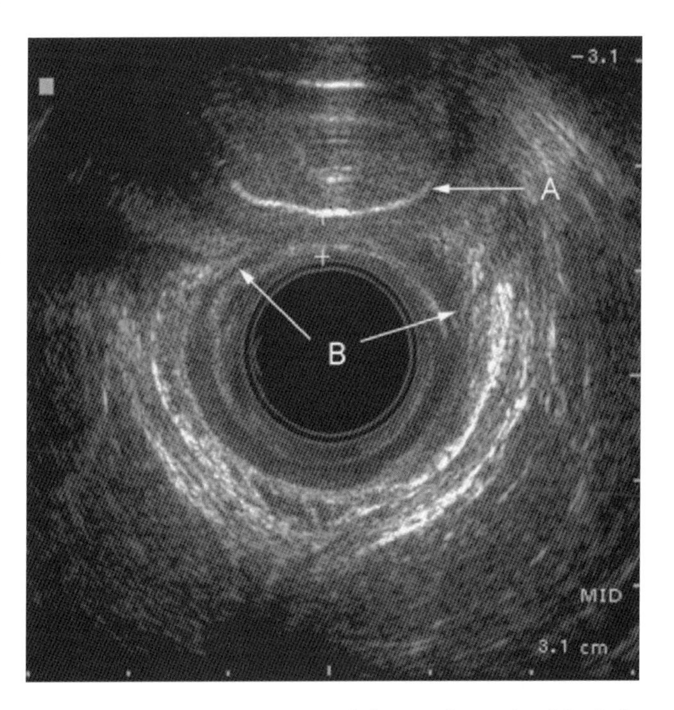

FIGURE 7-15. The measurement of the anterior perineal body in this patient with an anterior sphincter disruption. The curvilinear hyperechoic structure **A** is the examiner's finger in the vagina. This technique can often accentuate the defect **B** seen in the internal anal sphincter and the external anal sphincter, and documents the decreased thickness of the anterior sphincter and perineal body.

Blunt or penetrating trauma to the perineum may involve the sphincter mechanism. Management often includes fecal diversion, and debridement of the associated perineal soft tissues. After the perineal wound has healed, EAUS may be used to assess anal sphincter anatomy to determine if sphincter reconstruction is necessary before colostomy closure.

Patients undergoing anorectal surgery may experience transient minor incontinence in the early postoperative period, which usually resolves spontaneously. Patients who have persistent symptoms of incontinence may warrant evaluation. EAUS provides an objective means to evaluate the anal sphincter mechanism in patients with postoperative fecal incontinence after anorectal surgery such as hemorrhoidectomy, fistulotomy, lateral internal sphincterotomy, or sphincteroplasty.

The surgical correction of congenital anorectal anomalies is based on reconstituting the anatomy of the anorectum. The goal of posterior sagittal anorectoplasty (PSARP) is to place the bowel within the striated muscle complex of the levator ani and external anal sphincter.[83] EAUS has been used to accurately confirm the position of the neo-anus within the anal sphincter complex comparing favorably with MRI.[84] EAUS in fact provided greater detail of the anal muscles than MRI and had better correlation with direct perineal muscle stimulation.[84] Adult patients who present with severe fecal incontinence after previous surgical repair of a congenital anorectal malformation can undergo successful PSARP.[85] Usually, the existing anus is anterior to the sphincteric muscle complex.[85] An EAUS can be performed to help define the relationship of the anus to the sphincteric mechanism. In a recent study, Emblem et al.[86] correlated the endosonographic appearance of the anal sphincter with functional results after operative treatment of anorectal malformations demonstrating EAUS may be used to study the results after different surgical techniques for anorectal malformations.

The identification of localized sphincter defects is important in the evaluation of the incontinent patient, because these defects may be amenable to surgical repair. EAUS can clearly and objectively image the anal sphincter mechanism and has replaced needle electromyography as the procedure of choice for anal sphincter mapping.[65] EAUS is better tolerated and less painful than needle electromyography sphincter mapping. Anorectal manometry and pudendal nerve terminal motor latency testing are complementary but do not definitively correlate with a surgically correctable defect.[68,75,76,87,88] EAUS remains the definitive test that can identify a surgically correctable defect in a symptomatic patient with fecal incontinence.

Evaluation of Perianal Sepsis and Fistula-In-Ano

Typically, the diagnosis of a perianal or perirectal abscess is quite apparent on physical examination and only requires proper identification and prompt drainage. Occasionally, an abscess is strongly suspected on clinical grounds but is not readily identified on physical examination. In these situations, an EAUS may be useful in the evaluation of perianal or perirectal abscesses. EAUS can be helpful to localize an obscure abscess to plan the appropriate surgical intervention.

Often, clinical examination of perianal or perirectal abscesses is quite painful and examination under anesthesia is required. Because the ultrasound equipment is portable, the EAUS examination can be performed in the operating room while the patient is anesthetized. Abscesses appear as hypoechoic areas often surrounded by a hyperechoic border. In patients with perianal Crohn's disease, EAUS may be useful in distinguishing discrete abscesses that require surgical drainage from inflammation that requires medical treatment. The use of EAUS has also been evaluated in patients with ileoanal pouch anastomosis and can be helpful in demonstrating pouch pathology including inflammation, abscesses, and fistulas.[89]

The natural history of a drained perianal/rectal abscess is either complete resolution or fistula formation. The majority of fistulas that occur are simple intersphincteric fistulas that are easily identified and treated by simple unroofing. However, occasionally fistula tracts develop that are extensive and highly complex. These complex fistulas present a diagnostic challenge to even the most experienced colon and rectal surgeon. Use of EAUS can be helpful in identification of fistulous communications in patients with complex and recurrent fistula-in-ano.[90–92] Fistula tracts are generally hypoechoic defects that can be followed to identify direction and extent. The anatomic details of the fistula tract can be delineated in relation to the anal sphincter. The EAUS examination should include the anal canal and distal rectum to search for the presence of high blind tracts. Hydrogen peroxide has been used to enhance the imaging of complex fistula.[93–96] Hydrogen peroxide causes a release of oxygen, accentuating the fistula and appears as a brightly hyperechoic image on the ultrasound image. With the instillation of hydrogen peroxide the internal opening is identified in 62.5–94% of patients.[93,96–99] Lack of the use of hydrogen peroxide result in suboptimal results as is reflected in a recent meta-analysis.[100] An example of a fistula-in-ano with hydrogen peroxide enhancement is demonstrated in Figure 7-16. When evaluating an anal fistula with ERUS, it is important to use both the balloon-covered transducer to evaluate the perirectal region to assess for any supralevator extension as well as the plastic cap for evaluation of the anus and surrounding anatomy.

Anal Canal Neoplasms

Endoanal ultrasonography images the normal anal canal and associated pathologies quite well. EAUS can have an important role in the evaluation of benign and malignant anal canal neoplasms. The normal anatomic structures are clearly defined and any changes in the normal anatomy and their

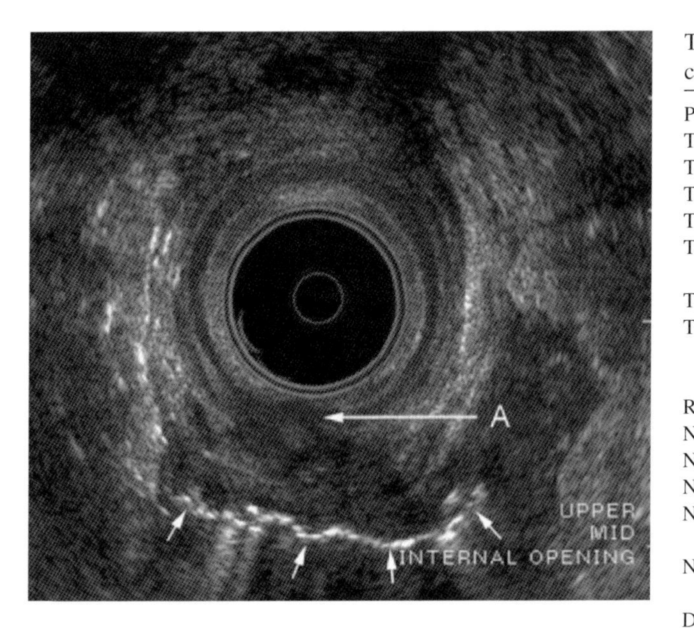

FIGURE 7-16. A fistula-in-ano that has been enhanced by the introduction of hydrogen peroxide. The hyperechoic features posteriorly represent the hydrogen peroxide within the fistula tract (*short arrows*). There is an obvious hypoechoic defect in the internal anal sphincter in the midline posteriorly **A**, representing the internal fistula opening. The hypoechoic horseshoe tract can be seen extending toward the patient's left.

relationships with specific anatomic structures are clearly defined. Benign neoplasms such as lipomas and leiomyomas can be demonstrated along with their relationship to adjacent anal canal structures. Lesions within the anal canal appear as hypoechoic areas. Tissue diagnosis may be obtained with ultrasound-directed needle biopsies when desired.

Anal canal malignancies are an uncommon cancer in the gastrointestinal tract. Diagnosis requires appropriate clinical evaluation and histologic confirmation by tissue biopsy. Anal canal malignancies evaluated by EAUS include leiomyosarcomas, malignant melanomas, anal canal adenocarcinomas, and squamous cell carcinomas. Squamous cell or epidermoid carcinomas of the anal canal are the most common anal canal malignancy. EAUS can be used in the initial evaluation to stage the lesion as well as in follow-up for patients with squamous cell carcinoma of the anal canal.[101–104] Because squamous cell carcinomas of the anus are primarily treated nonoperatively with combined chemoradiation therapy; it is desirable to have an accurate method of staging to assess response to multimodality therapy. EAUS accurately stages the initial tumor and can be used in follow-up to detect residual tumors as well as early recurrences after treatment. Surgical treatment in the form of abdominoperineal resection is reserved as salvage surgery for those patients who fail standard chemoradiation therapy.

Although clinical (digital) examination is important in the assessment of squamous cell carcinoma of the anus, EAUS is more precise in accurately measuring the actual size and

TABLE 7-3. Ultrasound staging classification (uTNM) for anal canal cancer

Primary tumor (T)	
Tx	Primary tumor cannot be assessed
T0	No evidence of primary tumor
Tis	Carcinoma in situ
T1	Tumor 2 cm or less in greatest dimension
T2	Tumor more than 2 cm but no more than 5 cm in greatest dimension
T3	Tumor more than 5 cm in greatest dimension
T4	Tumor of any size that invades an adjacent organ(s), e.g., vagina, urethra, bladder (involvement of the sphincter muscle(s) alone is not classified as T4)
Regional lymph nodes (N)	
Nx	Regional lymph nodes cannot be assessed
N0	No regional lymph node metastasis
N1	Metastasis in perirectal lymph node(s)
N2	Metastasis in unilateral internal iliac and/or inguinal lymph node(s)
N3	Metastasis in perirectal and inguinal lymph nodes and/or bilateral internal iliac and/or inguinal lymph nodes
Distant metastasis	
Mx	Distant metastasis cannot be assessed
M0	No distant metastasis
M1	Distant metastasis

TABLE 7-4. Ultrasound staging classification by depth of invasion (uTNM) for anal canal cancer

uT1	Tumor confined to the submucosa
uT2a	Tumor invades only the internal anal sphincter
uT2b	Tumor penetrates into the external anal sphincter
uT3	Tumor invades through the sphincter complex and into the perianal tissues
uT4	Tumor invades adjacent structures

circumferential involvement of the lesion. EAUS staging (uTNM) of anal cancers corresponds to the TNM [UICC (International Union Against Cancer)] staging (Table 7-3).[105] Tumor staging for anal cancer depends primarily on the maximal tumor diameter, which is accurately measured by EAUS. Additionally, the depth of invasion of the lesion can be measured in relationship to the sphincter mechanism. The extent of sphincter involvement can be determined and other staging systems stage these lesions based on depth of invasion.[104,106] One such staging system is depicted in Table 7-4.[106] The evaluation of squamous cell carcinomas of the anus should include an evaluation of the rectum with ERUS to determine the presence of metastatic lymph nodes within the mesorectum. The mesorectum as well as the anal canal can also be evaluated in follow-up after treatment. Any suspicious areas detected during follow-up may be biopsied if necessary.

Three-Dimensional Ultrasound

Three-dimensional ultrasound allows for multiplanar imaging of both the rectum and the anal canal. This new technology is currently being evaluated to compare its efficacy

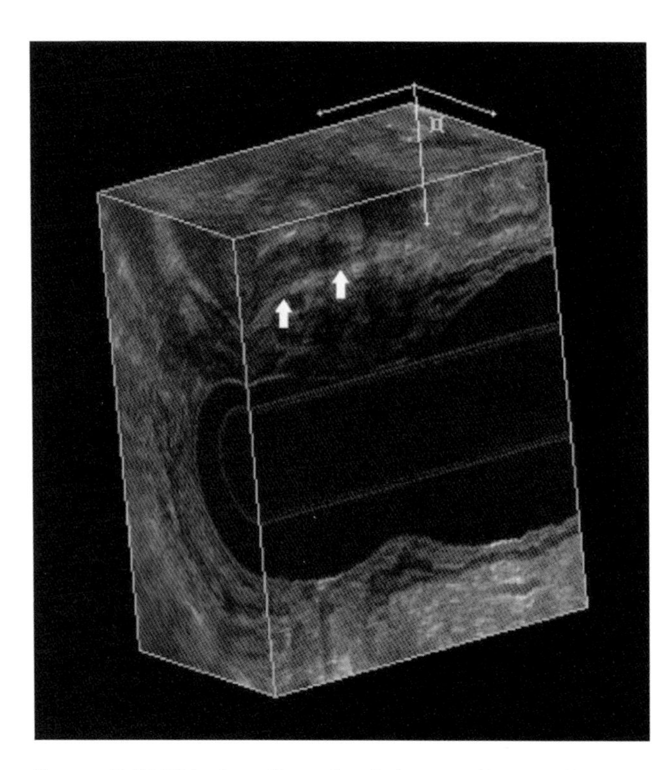

FIGURE 7-17. This three-dimensional ultrasound image of an anteriorly based rectal cancer that extends full thickness through the rectal wall (uT3). However, a clear hyperechoic plane can be seen between the prostate gland and the rectal tumor, as depicted by the *arrows*.

relative to conventional two-dimensional ultrasound as well as to other modalities such as MRI. Three-dimensional ultrasound can be used to assess anal fistulous tracts, to evaluate anal sphincter injury, as well as to stage both rectal and anal tumors. An example of a three-dimensional ERUS image (3D-ERUS) of a rectal cancer is shown in Figure 7-17.

Hunerbein et al.[107] compared standard two-dimensional ultrasound with 3D-ERUS and endorectal MRI and reported accuracy rates for depth of penetration by rectal cancer of 84, 88, and 91%, respectively. Because of the small sample size, these differences were not statistically significant. However, they believed that the additional scan planes improved the understanding of three-dimensional imaging and facilitated interpretation of the findings. In a recent study, Kim et al.[108] reported that 3D ERUS showed greater accuracy than 2D ERUS or CT in rectal cancer staging and lymph node metastases. The accuracy for T-staging was 78% for 3D ERUS vs. 69% for 2D ERUS and 57% for CT ($P<0.001$–0.002). Accuracy for lymph node metastases was 65, 56, and 53%, respectively ($P<0.0001$–0.006).

Three-dimensional EAUS has also been applied to benign anal disorders such as anal sphincter injury and anal fistula assessment. Several comparative studies have been reported evaluating its efficacy and comparing 3D-EAUS with MRI. West et al.[109] reported that 3D-EAUS and endoanal MRI were comparable for detecting external sphincter defects. Gold et al.[110] determined that 3D-EAUS revealed a direct relationship between the length of a sphincter tear and its radial extent. In addition, they demonstrated marked gender differences in anal sphincter configuration using three-dimensional ultrasound imaging. In the evaluation of anal fistula tracts, West et al.[111] reported equivalency between 3D-EAUS and endoanal MRI for the evaluation of anal fistula tracts. In a study by Buchanan et al.[112] 3D-EAUS was found to be very accurate in the assessment of both the internal opening and the primary tract of an anal fistula. They reported an accuracy of 90% in identifying the internal opening and an accuracy of 81% in delineating the primary tract. Three-dimensional EAUS was less accurate (68%) in identifying secondary tracts or extensions. In their study, the use of hydrogen peroxide did not increase the accuracy but in some instances it did make the tract and internal opening more conspicuous.

Summary

Endoluminal ultrasound has been shown to be extremely useful in the evaluation and management of many benign and malignant anorectal conditions. ERUS has become the best imaging technique to accurately stage rectal cancers and anal canal tumors preoperatively. Moreover, ERUS can have a role in the follow-up evaluation of these patients. EAUS is the diagnostic test of choice in the evaluation of fecal incontinence and is used routinely. The EAUS has also been used to help define complex anal fistulas to facilitate their management. The accuracy of diagnosis is operator dependent and improves with experience. Endoluminal ultrasound has made a major contribution to the understanding and management of many anorectal conditions. Three-dimensional ultrasound may prove to be advantageous but requires further study.

References

1. Wild JJ, Reid JM. Diagnostic use of ultrasound. Br J Phys Med. 1956;19(11):248–57.
2. Dragsted J, Gammelgaard J. Endoluminal ultrasonic scanning in the evaluation of rectal cancer: a preliminary report of 13 cases. Gastrointest Radiol. 1983;8(4):367–9.
3. Hildebrandt U, Feifel G. Preoperative staging of rectal cancer by intrarectal ultrasound. Dis Colon Rectum. 1985;28(1):42–6.
4. Edge SB, Byrd DR, Compton CC, Fritz AG, Greene FL, Trotti A. Colon and rectum. AJCC cancer staging manual. 7th ed. New York: Springer; 2009.
5. Beynon J, Foy DM, Temple LN, Channer JL, Virjee J, Mortensen NJ. The endosonic appearances of normal colon and rectum. Dis Colon Rectum. 1986;29(12):810–3.
6. Deen KI, Madoff RD, Wong WD. Preoperative staging of rectal neoplasms with endorectal ultrasonography. Semin Colon Rectal Surg. 1995;6:78–85.
7. Garcia-Aguilar J, Pollack J, Lee S-H, et al. Accuracy of endorectal ultrasonography in preoperative staging of rectal tumors. Dis Colon Rectum. 2002;45(1):10–5.

8. Pikarsky A, Wexner S, Lebensart P, et al. The use of rectal ultrasound for the correct diagnosis and treatment of rectal villous tumors. Am J Surg. 2000;179(4):261–5.
9. Worrell S, Horvath K, Blakemore T, Flum D. Endorectal ultrasound detection of focal carcinoma within rectal adenomas. Am J Surg. 2004;187(5):625–9. discussion 629.
10. Kim DG, Madoff RD. Transanal treatment of rectal cancer: ablative methods and open resection. Semin Surg Oncol. 1998;15(2):101–13.
11. Beynon J, Mortensen NJ, Foy DM, Channer JL, Rigby H, Virjee J. Preoperative assessment of mesorectal lymph node involvement in rectal cancer. Br J Surg. 1989;76(3):276–9.
12. Rifkin MD, Ehrlich SM, Marks G. Staging of rectal carcinoma: prospective comparison of endorectal US and CT. Radiology. 1989;170(2):319–22.
13. Starck M, Bohe M, Fork FT, Lindstrom C, Sjoberg S. Endoluminal ultrasound and low-field magnetic resonance imaging are superior to clinical examination in the preoperative staging of rectal cancer. Eur J Surg. 1995;161(11):841–5.
14. Milsom JW, Graffner H. Intrarectal ultrasonography in rectal cancer staging and in the evaluation of pelvic disease. Clinical uses of intrarectal ultrasound. Ann Surg. 1990;212(5):602–6.
15. Rafaelsen SR, Kronborg O, Fenger C. Digital rectal examination and transrectal ultrasonography in staging of rectal cancer. A prospective, blind study. Acta Radiol. 1994;35(3):300–4.
16. Kwok H, Bissett IP, Hill GL. Preoperative staging of rectal cancer. Int J Colorectal Dis. 2000;15(1):9–20.
17. Pappalardo G, Reggio D, Frattaroli FM, et al. The value of endoluminal ultrasonography and computed tomography in the staging of rectal cancer: a preliminary study. J Surg Oncol. 1990;43(4):219–22.
18. Puli SR, Reddy JB, Bechtold ML, Choudhary A, Antillon MR, Brugge WR. Accuracy of endoscopic ultrasound to diagnose nodal invasion by rectal cancers: a meta-analysis and systematic review. Ann Surg Oncol. 2009;16(5):1255–65.
19. Thaler W, Watzka S, Martin F, et al. Preoperative staging of rectal cancer by endoluminal ultrasound vs. magnetic resonance imaging. Preliminary results of a prospective, comparative study. Dis Colon Rectum. 1994;37(12):1189–93.
20. Bipat S, Glas AS, Slors FJM, Zwinderman AH, Bossuyt PMM, Stoker J. Rectal cancer: local staging and assessment of lymph node involvement with endoluminal US, CT, and MR imaging – a meta-analysis. Radiology. 2004;232(3):773–83.
21. Kim NK, Kim MJ, Yun SH, Sohn SK, Min JS. Comparative study of transrectal ultrasonography, pelvic computerized tomography, and magnetic resonance imaging in preoperative staging of rectal cancer. Dis Colon Rectum. 1999;42(6):770–5.
22. Dinter DJ, Hofheinz R-D, Hartel M, Kaehler GFAB, Neff W, Diehl SJ. Preoperative staging of rectal tumors: comparison of endorectal ultrasound, hydro-CT, and high-resolution endorectal MRI. Onkologie. 2008;31(5):230–5.
23. Tio TL, Tytgat GN. Endoscopic ultrasonography in analysing peri-intestinal lymph node abnormality. Preliminary results of studies in vitro and in vivo. Scand J Gastroenterol Suppl. 1986;123:158–63.
24. Hildebrandt U, Klein T, Feifel G, Schwarz HP, Koch B, Schmitt RM. Endosonography of pararectal lymph nodes. In vitro and in vivo evaluation. Dis Colon Rectum. 1990;33(10):863–8.
25. Herrera-Ornelas L, Justiniano J, Castillo N, Petrelli NJ, Stulc JP, Mittelman A. Metastases in small lymph nodes from colon cancer. Arch Surg. 1987;122(11):1253–6.
26. Katsura Y, Yamada K, Ishizawa T, Yoshinaka H, Shimazu H. Endorectal ultrasonography for the assessment of wall invasion and lymph node metastasis in rectal cancer. Dis Colon Rectum. 1992;35(4):362–8.
27. Akasu T, Sugihara K, Moriya Y, Fujita S. Limitations and pitfalls of transrectal ultrasonography for staging of rectal cancer. Dis Colon Rectum. 1997;40 Suppl 10:S10–5.
28. Sunouchi K, Sakaguchi M, Higuchi Y, Namiki K, Muto T. Small spot sign of rectal carcinoma by endorectal ultrasonography: histologic relation and clinical impact on postoperative recurrence. Dis Colon Rectum. 1998;41(5):649–53.
29. Sunouchi K, Sakaguchi M, Higuchi Y, Namiki K, Muto T. Limitation of endorectal ultrasonography: what does a low lesion more than 5 mm in size correspond to histologically? Dis Colon Rectum. 1998;41(6):761–4.
30. Saitoh N, Okui K, Sarashina H, Suzuki M, Arai T, Nunomura M. Evaluation of echographic diagnosis of rectal cancer using intrarectal ultrasonic examination. Dis Colon Rectum. 1986;29(4):234–42.
31. Holdsworth PJ, Johnston D, Chalmers AG, et al. Endoluminal ultrasound and computed tomography in the staging of rectal cancer. Br J Surg. 1988;75(10):1019–22.
32. Beynon J. An evaluation of the role of rectal endosonography in rectal cancer. Ann R Coll Surg Engl. 1989;71(2):131–9.
33. Glaser F, Schlag P, Herfarth C. Endorectal ultrasonography for the assessment of invasion of rectal tumours and lymph node involvement. Br J Surg. 1990;77(8):883–7.
34. Jochem RJ, Reading CC, Dozois RR, Carpenter HA, Wolff BG, Charboneau JW. Endorectal ultrasonographic staging of rectal carcinoma. Mayo Clin Proc. 1990;65(12):1571–7.
35. Orrom WJ, Wong WD, Rothenberger DA, Jensen LL, Goldberg SM. Endorectal ultrasound in the preoperative staging of rectal tumors. A learning experience. Dis Colon Rectum. 1990;33(8):654–9.
36. Glaser F, Kuntz C, Schlag P, Herfarth C. Endorectal ultrasound for control of preoperative radiotherapy of rectal cancer. Ann Surg. 1993;217(1):64–71.
37. Herzog U, von Flue M, Tondelli P, Schuppisser JP. How accurate is endorectal ultrasound in the preoperative staging of rectal cancer? Dis Colon Rectum. 1993;36(2):127–34.
38. Adams DR, Blatchford GJ, Lin KM, Ternent CA, Thorson AG, Christensen MA. Use of preoperative ultrasound staging for treatment of rectal cancer. Dis Colon Rectum. 1999;42(2):159–66.
39. Marusch F, Koch A, Schmidt U, et al. Routine use of transrectal ultrasound in rectal carcinoma: results of a prospective multicenter study. Endoscopy. 2002;34(5):385–90.
40. Kauer WKH, Prantl L, Dittler HJ, Siewert JR. The value of endosonographic rectal carcinoma staging in routine diagnostics: a 10-year analysis. Surg Endosc. 2004;18(7):1075–8.
41. Solomon MJ, McLeod RS. Endoluminal transrectal ultrasonography: accuracy, reliability, and validity. Dis Colon Rectum. 1993;36(2):200–5.
42. Kruskal JB, Kane RA, Sentovich SM, Longmaid HE. Pitfalls and sources of error in staging rectal cancer with endorectal us. Radiographics. 1997;17(3):609–26.
43. Zammit M, Jenkins JT, Urie A, O'Dwyer PJ, Molloy RG. A technically difficult endorectal ultrasound is more likely to be inaccurate. Colorectal Dis. 2005;7(5):486–91.

44. Goertz RS, Fein M, Sailer M. Impact of biopsy on the accuracy of endorectal ultrasound staging of rectal tumors. Dis Colon Rectum. 2008;51(7):1125–9.
45. Bernini A, Deen KI, Madoff RD, Wong WD. Preoperative adjuvant radiation with chemotherapy for rectal cancer: its impact on stage of disease and the role of endorectal ultrasound. Ann Surg Oncol. 1996;3(2):131–5.
46. Fleshman JW, Myerson RJ, Fry RD, Kodner IJ. Accuracy of transrectal ultrasound in predicting pathologic stage of rectal cancer before and after preoperative radiation therapy. Dis Colon Rectum. 1992;35(9):823–9.
47. Huh JW, Park YA, Jung EJ, Lee KY, Sohn S-K. Accuracy of endorectal ultrasonography and computed tomography for restaging rectal cancer after preoperative chemoradiation. J Am Coll Surg. 2008;207(1):7–12.
48. Maretto I, Pomerri F, Pucciarelli S, et al. The potential of restaging in the prediction of pathologic response after preoperative chemoradiotherapy for rectal cancer. Ann Surg Oncol. 2007;14(2):455–61.
49. Rau B, Hunerbein M, Barth C, et al. Accuracy of endorectal ultrasound after preoperative radiochemotherapy in locally advanced rectal cancer. Surg Endosc. 1999;13(10):980–4.
50. Williamson PR, Hellinger MD, Larach SW, Ferrara A. Endorectal ultrasound of T3 and T4 rectal cancers after preoperative chemoradiation. Dis Colon Rectum. 1996;39(1):45–9.
51. Brown CL, Ternent CA, Thorson AG, et al. Response to preoperative chemoradiation in stage II and III rectal cancer. Dis Colon Rectum. 2003;46(9):1189–93.
52. Radovanovic Z, Breberina M, Petrovic T, Golubovic A, Radovanovic D. Accuracy of endorectal ultrasonography in staging locally advanced rectal cancer after preoperative chemoradiation. Surg Endosc. 2008;22(11):2412–5.
53. Sagar PM, Pemberton JH. Surgical management of locally recurrent rectal cancer. Br J Surg. 1996;83(3):293–304.
54. Michelassi F, Vannucci L, Ayala JJ, Chappel R, Goldberg R, Block GE. Local recurrence after curative resection of colorectal adenocarcinoma. Surgery. 1990;108(4):787–92. discussion 792–783.
55. Beynon J, Mortensen NJ, Foy DM, Channer JL, Rigby H, Virjee J. The detection and evaluation of locally recurrent rectal cancer with rectal endosonography. Dis Colon Rectum. 1989;32(6):509–17.
56. de Anda EH, Lee S-H, Finne CO, Rothenberger DA, Madoff RD, Garcia-Aguilar J. Endorectal ultrasound in the follow-up of rectal cancer patients treated by local excision or radical surgery. Dis Colon Rectum. 2004;47(6):818–24.
57. Mascagni D, Corbellini L, Urciuoli P, Di Matteo G. Endoluminal ultrasound for early detection of local recurrence of rectal cancer. Br J Surg. 1989;76(11):1176–80.
58. Ramirez JM, Mortensen NJ, Takeuchi N, Humphreys MM. Endoluminal ultrasonography in the follow-up of patients with rectal cancer. Br J Surg. 1994;81(5):692–4.
59. Rotondano G, Esposito P, Pellecchia L, Novi A, Romano G. Early detection of locally recurrent rectal cancer by endosonography. Br J Radiol. 1997;70(834):567–71.
60. Morken JJ, Baxter NN, Madoff RD, Finne III CO. Endorectal ultrasound-directed biopsy: a useful technique to detect local recurrence of rectal cancer. Int J Colorectal Dis. 2006;21(3):258–64.
61. Meyenberger C, Wildi S, Kulling D, et al. Tumor staging and follow-up care in rectosigmoid carcinoma: colonoscopic endosonography compared to CT, MRI and endorectal MRI. Praxis (Bern 1994). 1996;85(19):622–31.
62. Tjandra JJ, Milsom JW, Stolfi VM, et al. Endoluminal ultrasound defines anatomy of the anal canal and pelvic floor. Dis Colon Rectum. 1992;35(5):465–70.
63. Rieger N, Tjandra J, Solomon M. Endoanal and endorectal ultrasound: applications in colorectal surgery. ANZ J Surg. 2004;74(8):671–5.
64. Sentovich SM, Wong WD, Blatchford GJ. Accuracy and reliability of transanal ultrasound for anterior anal sphincter injury. Dis Colon Rectum. 1998;41(8):1000–4.
65. Tjandra JJ, Milsom JW, Schroeder T, Fazio VW. Endoluminal ultrasound is preferable to electromyography in mapping anal sphincteric defects. Dis Colon Rectum. 1993;36(7):689–92.
66. Mellgren A, Jensen LL, Zetterstrom JP, Wong WD, Hofmeister JH, Lowry AC. Long-term cost of fecal incontinence secondary to obstetric injuries. Dis Colon Rectum. 1999;42(7):857–65. discussion 865–857.
67. Allen RE, Hosker GL, Smith AR, Warrell DW. Pelvic floor damage and childbirth: a neurophysiological study. Br J Obstet Gynaecol. 1990;97(9):770–9.
68. Sultan AH, Kamm MA, Hudson CN, Thomas JM, Bartram CI. Anal-sphincter disruption during vaginal delivery. N Engl J Med. 1993;329(26):1905–11.
69. Poen AC, Felt-Bersma RJ, Strijers RL, Dekker GA, Cuesta MA, Meuwissen SG. Third-degree obstetric perineal tear: long-term clinical and functional results after primary repair. Br J Surg. 1998;85(10):1433–8.
70. Sorensen M, Tetzschner T, Rasmussen OO, Bjarnesen J, Christiansen J. Sphincter rupture in childbirth. Br J Surg. 1993;80(3):392–4.
71. Tetzschner T, Sorensen M, Lose G, Christiansen J. Anal and urinary incontinence in women with obstetric anal sphincter rupture. Br J Obstet Gynaecol. 1996;103(10):1034–40.
72. Burnett SJ, Spence-Jones C, Speakman CT, Kamm MA, Hudson CN, Bartram CI. Unsuspected sphincter damage following childbirth revealed by anal endosonography. Br J Radiol. 1991;64(759):225–7.
73. Sultan AH, Kamm MA, Hudson CN, Bartram CI. Effect of pregnancy on anal sphincter morphology and function. Int J Colorectal Dis. 1993;8(4):206–9.
74. Varma A, Gunn J, Gardiner A, Lindow SW, Duthie GS. Obstetric anal sphincter injury: prospective evaluation of incidence. Dis Colon Rectum. 1999;42(12):1537–43.
75. Willis S, Faridi A, Schelzig S, et al. Childbirth and incontinence: a prospective study on anal sphincter morphology and function before and early after vaginal delivery. Langenbecks Arch Surg. 2002;387(2):101–7.
76. Zetterstrom J, Mellgren A, Jensen LL, et al. Effect of delivery on anal sphincter morphology and function. Dis Colon Rectum. 1999;42(10):1253–60.
77. Tsang CB, Madoff RD, Wong WD, et al. Anal sphincter integrity and function influences outcome in rectovaginal fistula repair. Dis Colon Rectum. 1998;41(9):1141–6.
78. Deen KI, Kumar D, Williams JG, Olliff J, Keighley MR. Anal sphincter defects. Correlation between endoanal ultrasound and surgery. Ann Surg. 1993;218(2):201–5.

79. Falk PM, Blatchford GJ, Cali RL, Christensen MA, Thorson AG. Transanal ultrasound and manometry in the evaluation of fecal incontinence. Dis Colon Rectum. 1994;37(5):468–72.
80. Farouk R, Bartolo DC. The use of endoluminal ultrasound in the assessment of patients with faecal incontinence. J R Coll Surg Edinb. 1994;39(5):312–8.
81. Titi MA, Jenkins JT, Urie A, Molloy RG. Perineum compression during EAUS enhances visualization of anterior anal sphincter defects. Colorectal Dis. 2009;11(6):625–30.
82. Zetterstrom JP, Mellgren A, Madoff RD, Kim DG, Wong WD. Perineal body measurement improves evaluation of anterior sphincter lesions during endoanal ultrasonography. Dis Colon Rectum. 1998;41(6):705–13.
83. deVries PA, Pena A. Posterior sagittal anorectoplasty. J Pediatr Surg. 1982;17(5):638–43.
84. Jones NM, Humphreys MS, Goodman TR, Sullivan PB, Grant HW. The value of anal endosonography compared with magnetic resonance imaging following the repair of anorectal malformations. Pediatr Radiol. 2003;33(3):183–5.
85. Simmang CL, Huber Jr PJ, Guzzetta P, Crockett J, Martinez R. Posterior sagittal anorectoplasty in adults: secondary repair for persistent incontinence in patients with anorectal malformations. Dis Colon Rectum. 1999;42(8):1022–7.
86. Emblem R, Morkrid L, Bjornland K. Anal endosonography is useful for postoperative assessment of anorectal malformations. J Pediatr Surg. 2007;42(9):1549–54.
87. Gilliland R, Altomare DF, Moreira Jr H, Oliveira L, Gilliland JE, Wexner SD. Pudendal neuropathy is predictive of failure following anterior overlapping sphincteroplasty. Dis Colon Rectum. 1998;41(12):1516–22.
88. Donnelly V, Fynes M, Campbell D, Johnson H, O'Connell PR, O'Herlihy C. Obstetric events leading to anal sphincter damage. Obstet Gynecol. 1998;92(6):955–61.
89. Solomon MJ, McLeod RS, O'Connor BI, Cohen Z. Assessment of peripouch inflammation after ileoanal anastomosis using endoluminal ultrasonography. Dis Colon Rectum. 1995;38(2):182–7.
90. Cataldo PA, Senagore A, Luchtefeld MA. Intrarectal ultrasound in the evaluation of perirectal abscesses. Dis Colon Rectum. 1993;36(6):554–8.
91. Deen KI, Williams JG, Hutchinson R, Keighley MR, Kumar D. Fistulas in ano: endoanal ultrasonographic assessment assists decision making for surgery. Gut. 1994;35(3):391–4.
92. Law PJ, Talbot RW, Bartram CI, Northover JM. Anal endosonography in the evaluation of perianal sepsis and fistula in ano. Br J Surg. 1989;76(7):752–5.
93. Lengyel AJ, Hurst NG, Williams JG. Pre-operative assessment of anal fistulas using endoanal ultrasound. Colorectal Dis. 2002;4(6):436–40.
94. Cheong DM, Nogueras JJ, Wexner SD, Jagelman DG. Anal endosonography for recurrent anal fistulas: image enhancement with hydrogen peroxide. Dis Colon Rectum. 1993;36(12):1158–60.
95. Poen AC, Felt-Bersma RJ, Eijsbouts QA, Cuesta MA, Meuwissen SG. Hydrogen peroxide-enhanced transanal ultrasound in the assessment of fistula-in-ano. Dis Colon Rectum. 1998;41(9):1147–52.
96. Navarro-Luna A, Garcia-Domingo MI, Rius-Macias J, Marco-Molina C. Ultrasound study of anal fistulas with hydrogen peroxide enhancement. Dis Colon Rectum. 2004;47(1):108–14.
97. Cho DY. Endosonographic criteria for an internal opening of fistula-in-ano. Dis Colon Rectum. 1999;42(4):515–8.
98. Ortiz H, Marzo J, Jimenez G, DeMiguel M. Accuracy of hydrogen peroxide-enhanced ultrasound in the identification of internal openings of anal fistulas. Colorectal Dis. 2002;4(4):280–3.
99. Toyonaga T, Tanaka Y, Song JF, et al. Comparison of accuracy of physical examination and endoanal ultrasonography for preoperative assessment in patients with acute and chronic anal fistula. Tech Coloproctol. 2008;12(3):217–23.
100. Sahni VA, Ahmad R, Burling D. Which method is best for imaging of perianal fistula? Abdom Imaging. 2008;33(1):26–30.
101. Goldman S, Norming U, Svensson C, Glimelius B. Transanorectal ultrasonography in the staging of anal epidermoid carcinoma. Int J Colorectal Dis. 1991;6(3):152–7.
102. Herzog U, Boss M, Spichtin HP. Endoanal ultrasonography in the follow-up of anal carcinoma. Surg Endosc. 1994;8(10):1186–9.
103. Roseau G, Palazzo L, Colardelle P, Chaussade S, Couturier D, Paolaggi JA. Endoscopic ultrasonography in the staging and follow-up of epidermoid carcinoma of the anal canal. Gastrointest Endosc. 1994;40(4):447–50.
104. Giovannini M, Bardou VJ, Barclay R, et al. Anal carcinoma: prognostic value of endorectal ultrasound (ERUS). Results of a prospective multicenter study. Endoscopy. 2001;33(3):231–6.
105. Edge SB, Byrd DR, Compton CC, Fritz AG, Greene FL, Trotti A. AJCC cancer staging manual. 7th ed. New York: Springer; 2009. p. 165–74.
106. Tarantino D, Bernstein MA. Endoanal ultrasound in the staging and management of squamous-cell carcinoma of the anal canal: potential implications of a new ultrasound staging system. Dis Colon Rectum. 2002;45(1):16–22.
107. Hunerbein M, Pegios W, Rau B, Vogl TJ, Felix R, Schlag PM. Prospective comparison of endorectal ultrasound, three-dimensional endorectal ultrasound, and endorectal MRI in the preoperative evaluation of rectal tumors. Preliminary results. Surg Endosc. 2000;14(11):1005–9.
108. Kim JC, Kim HC, Yu CS, et al. Efficacy of 3-dimensional endorectal ultrasonography compared with conventional ultrasonography and computed tomography in preoperative rectal cancer staging. Am J Surg. 2006;192(1):89–97.
109. West RL, Dwarkasing S, Briel JW, et al. Can three-dimensional endoanal ultrasonography detect external anal sphincter atrophy? A comparison with endoanal magnetic resonance imaging. Int J Colorectal Dis. 2005;20(4):328–33.
110. Gold DM, Bartram CI, Halligan S, Humphries KN, Kamm MA, Kmiot WA. Three-dimensional endoanal sonography in assessing anal canal injury. Br J Surg. 1999;86(3):365–70.
111. West RL, Dwarkasing S, Felt-Bersma RJ, et al. Hydrogen peroxide-enhanced three-dimensional endoanal ultrasonography and endoanal magnetic resonance imaging in evaluating perianal fistulas: agreement and patient preference. Eur J Gastroenterol Hepatol. 2004;16(12):1319–24.
112. Buchanan GN, Bartram CI, Williams AB, Halligan S, Cohen CRG. Value of hydrogen peroxide enhancement of three-dimensional endoanal ultrasound in fistula-in-ano. Dis Colon Rectum. 2005;48(1):141–7.

8 Preoperative Management

Janice F. Rafferty

Risk Assessment and Management

Preoperative management of a patient who requires surgery of the colon, rectum, or anus mandates thoughtful consideration of associated conditions that may result in perioperative morbidity and mortality. Understanding risks associated with certain comorbid conditions and disease processes allows the surgeon to stratify patients into risk categories, manage them appropriately, and improve short- and long-term outcomes.

Ambulatory Surgery

"Ambulatory surgery" is defined as surgical procedures requiring at least local anesthesia, which are more complex than office-based procedures but less complex than operations requiring at least an overnight stay.[1] Approximately 90% of anorectal surgery to treat fissures, condyloma, fistulas, certain early tumors, hemorrhoids, and pilonidal disease may be suitable for the ambulatory setting.[2,3] The Standards Committee of the American Society of Colon and Rectal Surgeons (ASCRS) has developed a Clinical Practice Guideline about Ambulatory Anorectal Surgery, for practitioners and health care workers, to provide current information from the literature upon which decisions can be made.[4] Data from many nonrandomized trials suggest that most patients with American Society of Anesthesiology (ASA) Classifications I and II, and some Class III are suitable for ambulatory surgery from an anesthesia risk standpoint. However, multiple factors must be considered to determine whether this is appropriate,[5] including the estimation of the magnitude of the operation, type of anesthesia, patient compliance, distance of the patient's home from the surgical center, and availability of support once home.[4]

- In general, the need for bloodwork, electrocardiogram (EKG), and other investigations of the ambulatory surgery patient can be predicted by information obtained with a thorough history and physical exam.[6] In fact routine preoperative testing is rarely helpful except in monitoring of established patient diseases. One study described 5,003 preoperative screening tests that revealed only 225 abnormal results. Slightly more than 100 tests were of potential importance and the plan for surgery was changed in only 17 cases. The authors concluded that only four patients derived true benefit from preoperative screening tests.[7] From studies such as this and others, [8,9] we can conclude that screening tests should be replaced by directed testing, and a thoughtful and thorough history and exam are the most important tools available to the surgeon in determining a patient's risk for outpatient surgery.

Inpatient Surgery

Objective assessment of patient risk for inpatient colorectal surgery is necessary for informed consent and favorable surgical outcome. Scoring systems have been developed to help differentiate those who are at high risk for perioperative complication from those who are not. Scoring systems can be classified as preoperative or physiologic (Table 8-1).[10] Some are specific to colon and rectal surgery.[11–13]

Cardiac Risk

The Goldman risk model determines cardiac risk for surgery.[14] Point scores are assigned to each of nine clinical factors; patients are divided into four risk classes based on the total point score (Table 8-2). Although the system is easy to use and utilizes relative weighting of risk factors, it was designed in the 1970s and has not been updated for modern practice in anesthesia, medicine, or surgery.

Respiratory Risk

The risk for perioperative respiratory complications can be gauged by combining findings on chest examination, chest X-ray, Goldman's cardiac risk index, and the Charlson comorbidity index.[15] Risk reduction strategies initiated preoperatively,

D.E. Beck et al. (eds.), *The ASCRS Textbook of Colon and Rectal Surgery: Second Edition*,
DOI 10.1007/978-1-4419-1584-9_8, © Springer Science+Business Media, LLC 2011

TABLE 8-1. Operative scoring system

Preoperative	Physiologic
ASA grade	APACHE (I and II)
Goldman cardiac risk index	SAPS
Pulmonary complication risk	Sickness score
Prognostic nutritional index	POSSUM
Hospital prognostic index	P-POSSUM
	Sepsis score
	Therapeutic intervention score

APACHE acute physiology and chronic health evaluation, *POSSUM* physiological and operative severity score for enumeration of mortality and morbidity, *SAPS* simplified acute physiology score, and *ASA* American Society of Anesthesia.

Adapted from Kiran RP, Delaney CP, Senagore AJ. Perioperative management. In: Beck DE, editor. Clinics in colon and rectal surgery. 2003;16(2): 75–84.

TABLE 8-2. Goldman cardiac risk index

Cardiac risk event	Points
Myocardial infarction within 6 months	10
Age >70 years	5
S3 gallop or jugular venous distension	11
Important aortic valve stenosis	3
Rhythm other than sinus, or sinus rhythm and atrial premature contractions on last preoperative electrocardiogram	7
More than five premature ventricular contractions per minute anytime before surgery	7
Poor general medical status	3
Intraperitoneal, intrathoracic, or aortic operation	3
Emergency operation	4

Class	Points	Life-threatening complication risk (%)	Cardiac death risk (%)
I	0–5	0.7	0.2
II	6–12	5	2
III	3–25	11	2
IV	≥26	22	56

such as smoking cessation, lung expansion teaching, chronic obstructive pulmonary disease (COPD) treatments, and asthmatic treatments may positively influence outcome after surgery.[16]

American Society of Anesthesiologists Classification

The American Society of Anesthesiologists (ASA) classification system (Table 8-3) was initially developed to alert anesthesiologists to preexisting diseases. It has also been used to estimate operative risk,[17] and correlates directly with perioperative mortality and morbidity. This classification scheme also correlates with perioperative variables such as intraoperative blood loss, duration of postoperative ventilation, and duration of intensive care unit (ICU) stay.[18] The disadvantages to using the ASA score are that it depends on the subjective opinion of the attending anesthesiologist, and because of small numbers of groups available there can be little meaningful comparison between different surgeons or institutions.

TABLE 8-3. American Society of Anesthesia classification

I	Normal healthy patient
II	Mild systemic disease
III	Severe, noncapacitating systemic disease
IV	Incapacitating systemic disease, threatening life
V	Moribund, not expected to survive 24 h
E	Emergency

Nutritional Assessment

Abdominal surgery induces a catabolic response with stress hormone release and insulin resistance; therefore, nutritional parameters should be evaluated in certain chronically ill patients before surgery. Protein catabolism may be accentuated by prolonged fasting and bowel preparation. Increased nutritional risk can influence postoperative morbidity and mortality[19,20] and anastomotic leak rates.[21] The prognostic nutritional index (PNI) was devised in the 1970s to predict complications such as sepsis and death after surgery.[22] The PNI evaluates four factors to predict complications (serum albumin, transferrin, triceps skinfold thickness, and cutaneous delayed-type hypersensitivity), but only albumin, transferrin, and delayed hypersensitivity are accurate predictors of postoperative morbidity and mortality. This index can theoretically be used to identify patients who may benefit from nutritional support in the perioperative period.

Acute Physiology and Chronic Health Evaluation Scoring Systems

The Acute Physiology and Chronic Health Evaluation (APACHE) scoring system was initially designed to assess risk for ICU patients, but has been extended to assess patients with severe trauma, abdominal sepsis, postoperative enterocutaneous fistulas, and acute pancreatitis and to predict postoperative outcome.[23] Scoring for emergency patients being admitted to the ICU is best performed before surgical intervention.[24] This index does not take into consideration the nutritional status of the patient, extent of surgery, or cardiovascular findings that add to operative risk. Several simpler scoring systems have been developed from the APACHE system, including simplified acute physiology score (SAPS), which uses 14 of the 34 variables, and SAPS II, which also takes into consideration the urgency of the procedure and any associated chronic medical illness.[25]

Physiological and Operative Severity Score for Enumeration of Mortality and Mortality

The Physiological and Operative Severity Score for enUmeration of Mortality and morbidity (POSSUM) calculates expected death and expected morbidity rates based on

TABLE 8-4. Parameters for the calculation of the physiological and operative severity score for enumeration of morbidity and mortality (POSSUM) score

Physiologic parameters	Operative parameters
Age (years)	Operative severity
Cardiac signs/chest X-ray	Multiple procedures
Respiratory signs/chest X-ray	Total blood loss (mL)
Pulse rate	Peritoneal soiling
Systolic blood pressure (mmHg)	Presence of malignancy
Glasgow coma score	Mode of surgery
Hemoglobin (g/dL)	
White cell count ($\times 10^{12}$/L)	
Urea concentration (mmol/L)	
Na^+ and K^+ levels (mmol/L)	
Electrocardiogram	

12 physiologic variables and 6 operative variables (Table 8-4). The advantage of POSSUM is that it predicts both morbidity and mortality and can be used to compare performance among surgical units, hospitals, and countries.[26] It does not, however, take into account primary diagnosis, differences among surgeons, anesthetists, and operating time, all of which may influence outcome. Nevertheless, it has been shown that POSSUM is superior to APACHE in predicting mortality in patients after general surgery.[27] P-POSSUM may be a better predictor of mortality and morbidity for gastrointestinal and laparoscopic colorectal surgery.[28,29] Another modification of this index, the CR-POSSUM score, is advocated to assess the risk for patients undergoing major colorectal cancer surgery.[11,12]

Preoperative Assessment Specific to Colorectal Procedures

Assessment of specific organ systems may be necessary and should be done for patients with identified preexisting dysfunction.[30] In general, age, history of chronic heart disease, renal disease, emergency surgery, and type of operation are predictors of the risk of mortality.[31] Fit, young patients undergoing minor and intermediate procedures do not need routine preoperative investigation and, in the pediatric age group, a thorough clinical examination has been found to be of greater value than routine laboratory screening. A good history and physical examination are more important than laboratory data in the development of a treatment plan for anesthesia. For patients undergoing colorectal surgery, a previous major laparotomy may preclude laparoscopic surgery or indicate an increased risk of conversion to open surgery. Body habitus of the patient, mental status, visual acuity, and the presence of other disorders such as arthritis may determine the decision on whether a stoma is formed and its placement. Assessment of patients' attitudes toward surgery, addressing their concerns, and counseling them regarding what to expect during hospitalization is integral part of the preoperative evaluation.

Current Recommendations

Preoperative tests serve to complement the history and physical exam. They have been used to assess levels of known disease, detect unsuspected but modifiable conditions that may be treated to reduce risk before surgery or detect unsuspected conditions that may not be possible to treat, and therefore simply be baseline results before surgery. Many patients undergoing minor surgery need minimal investigation, even if they have chronic medical conditions. Review of current evidence indicates that routine laboratory tests are rarely helpful except in the monitoring of known disease states. New guidelines have a significant impact on reducing preoperative testing and have not caused an increase in untoward perioperative events.[32,33]

Tests that need to be performed prior to major colorectal surgical procedures include hemoglobin for evidence of anemia and as a baseline level for postoperative management. Renal and liver function tests are not routinely carried out. Preoperative blood glucose determination is obtained in patients 45 years of age or older because current recommendations suggest screening of all over that age. In addition, impaired glucose control increases perioperative risks. A urine pregnancy test should be considered for all women of childbearing age. Coagulation tests are only indicated in patients on anticoagulation, with a family or personal history of bleeding disorder, or those with liver disease. Patients undergoing major surgery with a potential for blood loss should have a type and screen, even if transfusion is not expected. This may help to minimize the risk of later transfusion reaction.

EKG is indicated in male patients older than 40 years, and females older than 50 years. Those with a history suggestive of cardiac disorders, myocardial abnormalities, valvular disorders, conduction disorders, and hypertension may benefit from more intensive investigation prior to elective colorectal surgery.[34] Chest X-rays are performed on the basis of findings from the medical history or physical examination. As part of preoperative risk assessment, patients found to have medical conditions requiring further specific therapy before surgery should also be considered for more intensive medical supervision. This is important while in the hospital for their surgery and also as part of their postdischarge follow-up.

Bowel Preparation

Bowel preparation for colon and rectal surgery has traditionally involved two components: mechanical cleansing and antibiotics. Mechanical bowel preparation (MBP) before elective colorectal surgery has its roots in history and has long been a cornerstone of surgical practice. Today, however, there remains little evidence that it is necessary.

Bacteria represent a third of the dry weight of stool[35]; uncontrolled leak of intestinal contents into the abdominal cavity can, therefore, be life threatening. The accepted rationale for MBP includes the evacuation of stool to allow visualization of the luminal surfaces as well as to reduce the fecal flora, which is believed to translate into lower risk of infectious and anastomotic complications at surgery. While the removal of stool permitting mucosal inspection at colonoscopy is well established and not controversial, the latter rationale – the reduction of infectious and anastomotic complications by MBP – has not been supported by evidence and has recently been challenged in the medical literature. In the trauma setting (see Chap. 26), repair of the injured colon and anastomosis has been shown to be safe and less complicated than diversion of the fecal stream,[36,37] unless there is severe fecal contamination, or the need for transfusion of more than four units of blood.[38] These reports led to the question that if primary anastomosis was acceptable in the trauma setting, could its success and safety be translated to elective surgery performed under optimal conditions? Subsequent multiple animal studies failed to strongly support or refute the role of MBP.[39]

To better understand the debate and controversy surrounding the role of MBP in colorectal surgery, it is worthwhile first to review the various regimens currently in use today as well as their mechanisms, effectiveness, and potential side effects.[40] Dietary restriction (5 days of clear liquids), cathartics, and enemas formed the original framework of colon preparation. However, patient discomfort, electrolyte problems, and inadequate caloric intake proved cumbersome as well as costly.[41] Transition to a large volume (8–10 L) orthograde gut lavage with saline solutions was then tried.[42,43] The need of a nasogastric tube, requirement for hospitalization, and large fluid shifts with potential for electrolyte instability led to the search for alternatives.

Mannitol was found to be an excellent cathartic with minimal effects compared with saline lavage. A major detriment was the fermentation by colonic bacteria which generated combustible gases (methane and hydrogen). Multiple case reports described explosions occurring during colonoscopy after mannitol preps. These case reports along with the fear of explosion with the addition of electrocautery during surgery prevented universal acceptance.[44–48]

Polyethylene glycol (PEG) lavage solution was first introduced in 1980.[49] PEG solutions are iso-osmotic nonabsorbable electrolyte lavage solutions that cause little to no fluid shifts or electrolyte disturbances. Colyte™ (Schwarz Pharma, Inc., Milwaukee, WI) and GoLYTELY™ (Braintree Laboratories, Inc., Braintree, MA) are the most familiar commercial examples in practice. Multiple studies have proven these lavage solutions to be safe, effective, and well tolerated when compared with traditional bowel preparative regimens.[50–52]

PEG solutions require ingestion of 3–4 L solution. The salty taste and high volume reduce patient compliance. Addition of bisacodyl, senna, or magnesium citrate to traditional 4 L PEG regimens has been shown to improve colonic cleansing for colonoscopy.[53–55] Addition of these adjuncts has also allowed for lower-volume (2 L) PEG solutions to be administered with equivalent or increased efficacy and improved patient tolerability.[56–58] Prokinetic agents and enemas when combined with oral lavage have not been shown to improve efficacy or decrease patient symptoms.[59,60] PEG solutions are contraindicated in patients with any sensitivity to the components of the solution, gastrointestinal obstruction, gastric retention, bowel perforation, toxic colitis, toxic megacolon, or ileus. PEG solutions are considered Category C drugs in pregnancy and have not been well studied in this patient population.[61]

In 1990, sodium phosphate (NaP), a saline laxative, was introduced as a safe, more efficacious, and less costly form of bowel preparation when compared with PEG in initial and subsequent studies.[52,62] NaP solutions (Fleet Phospho-soda™, Fleet laboratories, Lynchburg, VA) are concentrated, low-volume hyperosmotic solutions that exert an osmotic effect to draw fluid into the bowel lumen to assist in transit of contents.[63] These solutions were administered as two 4.5 oz. dispensations that are diluted and ingested by the patient at preset times, the day prior to elective colorectal surgery. Electrolyte alterations that may occur include hyperphosphatemia, hypocalcemia, hypernatremia, and hypokalemia, which in most patients were minimal and/or transient in nature.

A tablet form of NaP was developed in 2000 showing equal or improved efficacy and/or improved tolerance when compared with both liquid NaP, PEG, and PEG plus bisacodyl regimens.[64–66] These tablet preparations (OsmoPrep™ and Visicol™, both Salix Pharmaceuticals, Morrisville, NC) offer an alternative to the solution-type NaP formulation. The tablet preparation regimen consists of 28–40 tablets given the day prior to the elective procedure or in a split dose manner, similar to the fluid formulation.

Patients with impaired renal function, dehydration, hypercalcemia, hyperphosphatemia, congestive heart failure, or advanced liver disease could experience severe complications with NaP administration including phosphate nephropathy.[67,68] This is especially true in hypertensive patients taking certain medications, namely angiotensin-converting enzyme inhibitors or angiotensin receptor blockers. This led the Federal Drug Administration to issue a Black Box warning for the over-the-counter version of this preparation and the manufacturer to voluntarily remove the preparation from the market. As this preparation is hypertonic, significant fluid and electrolyte shifts can occur and it is necessary to maintain adequate hydration while undergoing the preparation.[69,70] Absolute contraindications to any bowel preparation include obstruction, ileus, perforation, diverticulitis, severe colitis, toxic megacolon, gastric retention, and gastric paresis.

Summary of Trials and Meta-Analyses

Over the past few years and as recent as mid-2008, numerous clinical trials and meta-analyses have been performed in an attempt to understand the role of MBP in elective colorectal

TABLE 8-5. Randomized controlled trials and Cochrane report relating to preoperative mechanical bowel preparation[a]

Author/year	No. of patients	Mechanical bowel preparation agent	Anastomotic leaks	Wound infections	Mortality
Brownson (1992)[70]	179	PEG	11.9 vs. 1.5[b]	5.8 vs. 7.5	0.0 vs. 0.0
Santos (1994)[71]	149	Mineral oil, agar, and phenolphthalein; enema; mannitol (3-day regimen)	10.4 vs. 5.3	23.6 vs. 11.7	0.0 vs. 0.0
Burke (1994)[72]	169	Sodium picosulfate	3.8 vs. 4.6	4.9 vs. 3.4	2.4 vs. 0.0
Fillman (1995)[73]	60	Mannitol	8.7 vs. 4.3	3.3 vs. 6.7	
Miettinen (2000)[74]	267	PEG	4.0 vs. 2.0	4.0 vs. 2.0	0.0 vs. 0.0
Tabusso (2002)[75]	47	Mannitol or PEG	20.8 vs. 0[b]	8.3 vs. 0	
Bucher (2005)[76]	153	PEG	6.4 vs. 1.3	12.8 vs. 4	
Ram (2005)[77]	329	NaP	0.6 vs. 1.3	9.8 vs. 6.1	
Fa-Si-Oen (2005)[78]	250	PEG	5.6 vs. 4.8	7.2 vs. 5.6	
Zmora (2006)[79]	249	PEG	4.2 vs. 2.3	6.7 vs. 10.1	1.7 vs. 0.8
Pena-Soria (2007)[80]	97	PEG	8.3 vs. 4.1	12.5 vs. 12.2	
Jung (2007)[81]	1,343	PEG, NaP, enema	1.9 vs. 2.6	7.9 vs. 6.4	
Contant (2007)[82]	1,354	PEG + Bisacodyl or NaP	4.8 vs. 5.4	13.4 vs. 14.0	

[a] All results as mechanical bowel preparation (MBP) vs. no MBP, %; PEG polyethylene glycol, NaP sodium phosphate.
[b] Significant result.

surgery.[41] These studies are summarized in Table 8-5.[70–82] This issue of MBP vs. no MBP was reviewed in a Cochrane Database review published in 2005.[83] This comprehensive meta-analysis included nine clinical trials and a total of 1,592 patients. The authors reiterated a belief that was raised in other studies, wherein the use of MBP frequently resulted in a "semi prepared" colon full of liquid feces that was difficult to control, often leading to spillage and peritoneal contamination and thus explaining the higher rates of complications found in the MBP group.

The most thorough and current meta-analysis on the subject was recently published by Pineda and colleagues, who completed a systematic review of the literature through early 2008 and found 13 prospective trials available with a total of 4,601 patients, the greatest number of patients available to date.[84] In this meta-analysis, the authors analyzed two primary outcomes – anastomotic leaks and wound infections. They found no statistically significant difference between 2,304 patients receiving MBP compared with 2,297 patients receiving no MBP in either outcome. Anastomotic leaks were reported in 97 patients (4.2%) with MBP and 81 patients (3.5%) without MBP ($p = 0.206$). Wound infections occurred in 9.9 vs. 8.8% ($p = 0.155$). This lack of any statistically significant difference between the two arms in the largest meta-analysis yet performed prompted the authors to conclude that MBP is of no benefit to patients undergoing elective colorectal resection. Though the authors acknowledge certain scenarios when the use of MBP is warranted, such as the anticipated need for intraoperative colonoscopy, they propose that routine MBP need not be considered a "prerequisite of safe colorectal surgery." Despite these data, a 2003 survey of practicing colorectal surgeons revealed that 99% of respondents continue to employ MBP, though 10% did question its role in elective surgery.[85]

Antibiotics

The use of antibiotic prophylaxis in elective colon surgery is mandatory to minimize infection complications.[86] Unfortunately, the choice of antibiotic and route of administration are less clear. The first principle in prophylactic use of antibiotic administration is to provide coverage for the normal bowel flora [aerobic bacteria (*E. coli*) and anaerobic species (*Bacteroides sp.*)]. Oral antibiotics as used in the traditional Nichols–Condon antibiotic preparation have been shown to reduce intraluminal and mucosal bacterial count, while parenteral antibiotics have been shown to reduce systemic bacterial counts at the tissue level.

Colorectal surgery performed prior to 1970 was fraught with infectious complications which occurred in more than 30–50% of all operations. With a better understanding of bacteriology and the availability of an increasing number of antibiotics, surgeons attempted to improve their outcomes with regards to infections.[87–90] In a 1977 VA cooperative study, Nichols and Condon showed that oral neomycin sulfate and erythromycin base decrease the wound infection rate of elective colon resections from 35 to 9%.[91] They also showed that this regimen led to significant decrease in all septic complications (wound infection, anastomotic leak, and abscess) from 43 to 9%.[91–93] The dosing of 1 g of oral neomycin sulfate and erythromycin base at 2 p.m., 3 p.m., and 10 p.m. for an 8 a.m. case became and remains a standard oral antibiotic regime for elective surgery. Unfortunately, the Nichols prep has its drawbacks. While this antibiotic combination is efficacious, it can cause significant gastrointestinal discomfort severely limiting patient compliance with the remainder of the antibiotic preparation and completion of their mechanical preparation.

These limitations, along with the significant increase in number and spectrum of parenteral antibiotics, led many investigators to utilize various IV antibiotic combinations to minimize infectious complications.[86–93] In 1998, Song and colleagues codified modern practice and confirmed that parenteral antibiotics alone decrease the rate of wound infection and that no single regimen is superior as long as the antibiotics chosen cover both aerobic and anaerobic bacteria and are given before incision.[94] In 2003, the Surgical Infection Prevention Guideline Writers Workgroup (SIPGWW), a project endorsed by both the American College of Surgeons (ACS) and the ASCRS, submitted consensus positions for surgical antimicrobial prophylaxis.[95] The standard for parenteral antibiotic prophylaxis in elective colon resections should include:

1. *Timing*: Infusion of the first antimicrobial dose should begin within 60 min prior to surgical incision.
2. *Duration*: Prophylactic antimicrobials should be discontinued within 24 h following surgery.
3. *Dosing*: The initial dose should be adequate based on weight, adjusted dosing weight or BMI. An additional dose should be administered, if the operation continues over two half-lives after the initial dose.
4. *Selection (colon surgery)*: Cefotetan, cefoxitin, cefazolin/metronidazole, and ampicillin/sulbactam.
   - Options for β-lactam allergic patients: clindamycin + gentamicin, ciprofloxacin, or aztreonam.
   - Metronidazole + gentamycin or ciprofloxacin.

Deep Venous Thrombosis Prophylaxis

Deep venous thrombosis (DVT) and its embolic corollary, pulmonary embolism (PE) are a significant source of morbidity and mortality in the perioperative period. Due to the predominance of abdominal and pelvic surgery, colorectal surgery confers a higher risk of these postoperative complications than other general surgical procedures.[96] Yet despite so much emphasis, DVT and PE continue to be the most common cause of preventable deaths during in-hospital admission, accounting for one out of every four hospitalized patients' deaths.[97,98] More concerning, over 50% of all DVTs are asymptomatic, while the vast majority of PEs are detected only after death.[99] Since Virchow's original description of stasis, hypercoaguability and endothelial damage as risk factors, large epidemiological studies have found an increase in the development of symptomatic venous thromboembolism in the perioperative period associated with male gender, malignancy, trauma, immobility, COPD, sepsis, low hematocrit, low albumin, and major surgery.[100]

Prophylaxis of venous thrombotic events centers on both mechanical and medical means. Mechanical methods include intermittent pneumatic compression stockings, while the current mainstays for chemical thromboprophylaxis are unfractionated and low-molecular-weight heparin. Unfractionated heparin works through antithrombin III to inactivate thrombin and other factors in the clotting cascade. Concerns about its increased bleeding events as well as its dose–effect relationship have led many to be wary of its use. Low-molecular-weight heparin has enhanced antifactor Xa activity and more predictable dose–effect relationships.[101] A recent Cochrane review concluded that the combined use of mechanical graduated stockings with either unfractionated or low molecular heparin was the optimal prophylaxis to prevent thromboembolic complications.[102] Only three studies meeting the inclusion criteria, in this review, focused specifically on colon and rectal surgery. Two years later, the group evaluated 558 studies, of which 19 met the inclusion criteria, and again found that unfractionated and fractionated heparin were equally effective, and the addition of either to compression stockings was superior to either alone.[102]

Risk stratification is the mainstay for DVT prophylaxis recommendation. Young healthy patients undergoing routine anorectal surgery with minimal patient-specific risk factors do not require any additional therapy other than mechanical means via graduated compression stockings and/or intermittent pneumatic compression boots and early ambulation. Those patients with multiple risk factors and undergoing high-risk surgery such as pelvic operations warrant more aggressive means such as unfractionated or low-molecular-weight heparin in addition to the mechanical devices. Timing has been somewhat controversial with some studies demonstrating higher bleeding without undue increase in thrombotic events when given after the surgery and others stating that dosing should begin preoperatively. Although this question has yet to be definitively answered based on current literature, it is well accepted that some form of perioperative including intraoperative means has become the standard of care. The risk of bleeding with thromboprophylaxis dosing is small, with the majority revolving around injection site ecchymoses or hematoma in up to 7% of cases.[103] More clinically significant bleeding, such as gastrointestinal or intraabdominal bleeding, occurs in <0.5% and is rarely the cause for secession of therapy.

A concern in colorectal surgery is how to manage anticoagulated patients who require colonoscopy. Recent guidelines suggest that aspirin and other nonsteroidal anti-inflammatory drugs (NSAIDs) do not need to be withheld, with the rate of postpolypectomy bleeding around 2%.[104] Coumadin and other more potent antiplatelet medications (i.e., clopidogrel) are commonly held for 5–7 days prior to the procedure, especially when it is known that a polypectomy or other procedures are likely. There is some evidence that the application of endoclips or detachable loops with polypectomy in anticoagulated patients is safe; however, small sample sizes hinder ability to make broad recommendations.[105] Current recommendations are provided in the

ASCRS Practice Parameters for the prevention of venous thromboembolism (www.fascrs.org).[106]

Beta Blockade

Perioperative treatment with beta-blockers titrated to a heart rate of less than 70 bpm to reduce cardiac risk has been studied in multiple clinical trials.[107] Although some more recent trials have not demonstrated the pronounced benefit of earlier trials on the subject, the aggregate conclusion of the multiple studies suggests benefit with small risk. Preoperative beta blockade is indicated in patients having intermediate risk surgery with one or more clinical risk factors or any patient having vascular surgery. It is not indicated in patients for low risk surgery or intermediate risk surgery without clinical risk factors. Some authors argue that effective beta blockade obviates the need for additional cardiac testing in certain intermediate risk patients.[108] Institution of statin-class medication for patients with one or more clinical risk factors undergoing intermediate risk surgery should be considered.[109]

Transfusion: and Hematologic Evaluation

Most patients with anemia tolerate operations well unless they have associated disease, and therefore anemia rarely changes management unless operative blood losses are expected to be great.[106] Risk of thromboembolism and bleeding disorders can be assessed by a detailed history and by tests that measure coagulation factors (prothrombin and partial thromboplastin time) and that assess platelet count and function (bleeding time). Measures to reduce the risk of thromboembolism have been well documented and are part of the practice parameters available from the ASCRS.[100,101,106]

Blood grouping and cross-matching are obviously critical when planning major surgery in which significant blood losses may occur. An important consideration is to have a routine sample for blood type on file for patients undergoing major surgery, even if transfusion is not expected, and cross-matching would not usually take place. This allows a double level of security when urgent samples are sent if bleeding occurs during surgery. This may help to avoid the risk of transfusion reaction, if there is concern about errors with sample labeling or source at any time.

Anemic patients who are scheduled for elective surgery may be treated preoperatively by allogenic transfusion, but consideration is also given to autologous donation, erythropoietin, intraoperative hemodilution with autotransfusion or consideration of cell salvage techniques which are still being evaluated in colorectal surgery. Preoperative autologous donation (PAD) has been criticized recently because of cost-ineffectiveness, large wastage of PAD units, and the potential for leaving patients more anemic after surgery than without PAD.[102] Techniques including acute normovolemic hemodilution and cell salvage may be more efficient; however, investigations still continue into their use.[103]

Communication with the Patient and Establishing the Expectations for Postoperative Recovery

No preoperative visit is complete without providing information on expected postoperative outcomes. This discussion helps the patient to build confidence and trust in the surgeon. Such discussion is likely to be an important component of any postoperative care pathway, and this may help lead to significant reduction in postoperative stay.

Patients can be advised of the surgery they will undergo, their expected milestones in recovery, and possible complications, including issues such as readmission, which may occur in 10% or more of these patients undergoing major abdominal surgery.

Prophylaxis for Endocarditis and Prosthesis

Patients undergoing invasive colorectal procedures are at varying risk for endocarditis and infection of prosthesis. The ASCRS has published practice parameters to guide surgeons on selecting appropriate measures for at risk patients.[110]

Conclusion

Assessment of the patient undergoing surgery is of extreme importance in providing patients with a safe recovery from their operation. This permits stratification of patients into groups that require intensive, moderate or minimal investigation, or treatment prior to anesthesia. Tests to investigate patients should be used selectively based on increasingly accepted guidelines. Patients who need such evaluation and treatment prior to surgery should also be seen by the relevant medical specialty when in hospital and receive any necessary instructions for appropriate medical follow-up after their surgery.

MBP continues to be used by the majority of colorectal surgeons based on traditional practice patterns. Several randomized controlled trials now suggest that this practice may be unnecessary. Patients undergoing bowel resection should be given antibiotic prophylaxis using one dose of parenteral broad-spectrum agents at the time of induction of anesthesia.

Acknowledgments. This chapter was written by Conor P. Delaney and John M. MacKeigan in the first edition of this textbook.

References

1. Detmer DE. Ambulatory surgery. N Engl J Med. 1981;305: 1406–9.
2. Smith LE. Ambulatory surgery for anorectal diseases: an update. South Med J. 1986;79:163–6.
3. Ferrara A, Gallagher J. The physician-owned ambulatory surgery center for colon and rectal surgery. In: Bailey HR, Snyder MJ, editors. Ambulatory anorectal surgery. New York: Springer; 1999. p. 13–6.
4. Place R, Hyman N, et al. Practice parameters for ambulatory anorectal surgery. Dis Colon Rectum. 2003;46(5):573–6.
5. Snyder MJ. Selection, preoperative assessment and education of the patient for ambulatory surgery. In: Bailey HR, Snyder MJ, editors. Ambulatory anorectal surgery. New York: Springer; 1999. p. 37–45.
6. Kaplan EB, Sheiner LB, Brockmann AJ, et al. The usefulness of preoperative laboratory screening. JAMA. 1985;253:3576–81.
7. Turnbull JM, Buck C. The value of preoperative screening in investigators in otherwise healthy individuals. Arch Intern Med. 1987;147:1101–5.
8. Suchman AL, Mushlin AI. How well does the activated partial thromboplastin time predict postoperative hemorrhage? JAMA. 1986;256:750–3.
9. Freeman WK, Gibbons RJ, Shub C. Preoperative assessment of cardiac patients undergoing noncardiac surgical procedures. Mayo Clin Proc. 1989;64:1105–17.
10. Kiran RP, Delaney CP, Senagore AJ. In Beck DE, Ed. Clinics in Colon and Rectal Surgery: Perioperative Management. 2003;16(2):75–84.
11. Bromage SJ, Cunliffe WJ. Validation of the CR-POSSUM risk adjusted scoring system for major colorectal cancer surgery in a single center. Dis Colon Rectum. 2007;50:192–6.
12. Tekkis PP, Prytherch DR, Kocher HM, et al. Development of a dedicated risk-adjustment scoring system for colorectal surgery (colorectal POSSUM). Br J Surg. 2004;91:1174–82.
13. Fazio VW, Tekkis PP, Remzi F, Lavery IC. Assessment of operative risk in colorectal cancer surgery: the Cleveland Clinic Foundation colorectal cancer model. Dis Colon Rectum. 2004;47:2015–24.
14. Goldman L, Caldera DL, Nussbaum SR, et al. Multifactorial index of cardiac risk in noncardiac surgical procedures. N Engl J Med. 1977;297:845.
15. Lawrence VA, Dhanda R, Hilsenbeck SG, et al. Risk of pulmonary complications after elective abdominal surgery. Chest. 1996;110(3):744–50.
16. Sweitzer BJ, Smetana GW. Identification and evaluation of the patient with lung disease. Anesthesiol Clin. 2009 Dec;27(4):673–86.
17. Menke H, Klein A, John KD, et al. Predictive value of ASA classification for the assessment of perioperative risk. Int Surg. 1993;78:266–70.
18. Wolters U, Wolf T, Stutzer H, et al. ASA classification and perioperative variables as predictors of postoperative outcome. Br J Anaesth. 1996;77(2):217–22.
19. Schweiger I, von Holzen A, Gutzwiller JP, et al. Nutritional risk is a clinical predictor of post-operative mortality and morbidity in surgery for colorectal cancer. Br J Surg. 2010;97(1):92–7.
20. Noblett SE, Watson DS, Huong H, et al. Pre-operative oral carbohydrate loading in colorectal surgery: a randomized controlled trial. Colorectal Dis. 2006;8(7):563–9.
21. Taflampas P, Christodoulakis M, Tsiftsis DD. Anastomotic leakage after low anterior resection for rectal cancer: facts, obscurity, and fiction. Surg Today. 2009;39(3):183–8.
22. Mullen JL, Gertner MH, Buzby GP, et al. Implications of malnutrition in the surgical patient. Arch Surg. 1979;114:121–5.
23. Goffi L, Saba V, Ghiselli R, et al. Preoperative APACHE II and ASA scores in patients having major general surgical operations: prognostic value and potential clinical applications. Eur J Surg. 1999;165:730–5.
24. Koperna T, Semmler D, Marian F. Risk stratification in emergency surgical patients: is the APACHE II score a reliable marker of physiological impairment? Arch Surg. 2001;136(1):55–9.
25. Le Gall JR, Loirat P, Alperovitch A, et al. A simplified acute physiology score for ICU patients. Crit Care Med. 1984;12:975–7.
26. Bennett-Guerrero E, Hyam JA, Shaefi S, et al. Comparison of P-POSSUM risk-adjusted mortality rates after surgery between patients in the USA and UK. Br J Surg. 2003;90:1593–8.
27. Jones DR, Copeland GP, de Cossart L. Comparison of POSSUM with APACHE II for prediction of outcome from a surgical high-dependency unit. Br J Surg. 1992;79:1293–6.
28. Tekkis PP, Kocher HM, Bentley AJ, et al. Operative mortality rates among surgeons: comparison of POSSUM and p-POSSUM scoring systems in gastrointestinal surgery. Dis Colon Rectum. 2000;43(11):1528–32.
29. Senagore AJ, Delaney CP, Duepree HJ, Brady K, Fazio VW. An evaluation of POSSUM and p-POSSUM scoring systems in assessing outcomes with laparoscopic colectomy. Br J Surg. 2003;90:1280–4.
30. Delaney CP, Mackeigan JM. Preoperative management – risk assessment, medical evaluation, and bowel preparation. In: Wolff BG, Fleshman JW, Beck DE, Pemberton JH, Wexner SD, editors. ASCRS textbook of colorectal surgery. New York: Springer; 2007. p. 116–29.
31. Pedersen T, Eliasen K, Henriksen E. A prospective study of mortality associated with anesthesia and surgery: risk indicators of mortality in hospital. Acta Anaesthesiol Scand. 1990;34(3):176–82.
32. Mancuso CA. Impact of new guidelines on physicians' ordering of preoperative tests. J Gen Intern Med. 1999;14(3):166–72.
33. Greer AE, Irwin MG. Implementation and evaluation of guidelines for preoperative testing in a tertiary hospital. Anaesth Intensive Care. 2000;30:326–30.
34. Eagle KA, Berger PB, Calkins H, et al. ACC/AHA guideline update for perioperative cardiovascular evaluation of noncardiac surgery – executive summary: a report of the ACC/AHA task force on practice guidelines (committee to update the 1996 Guidelines on Perioperative Cardiovascular Evaluation for Noncardiac Surgery). J Am Coll Cardiol. 2002;39:542.
35. Arnspiger RC, Helling TS. AN evaluation of results of colon anastomosis in prepared and unprepared bowel. J Clin Gastroenterol. 1988;10:638–41.

36. Stone HH, Fabian TC. Management of perforating colon trauma: randomization between primary closure and exteriorization. Ann Surg. 1979;190:430–6.
37. Sasaki LS, Allaben RD, Golwala R, Mittal VK. Primary repair of colon injuries: a prospective randomized study. J Trauma. 1995;39:895–901.
38. Demetriades D, Murray JA, Chan L, et al. Penetrating colon injuries requiring resection: diversion or primary anastomosis? An AAST prospective multicenter study. J Trauma. 2001;50:765–75.
39. Katz JA, Orkin BA. Bowel preparation for elective colon and rectal surgery. In Clinics in Colon and rectal Surgery. Beck DA, Ed. 2003;16(2):119–130.
40. Duncan JE, Quietmeyer CM. Bowel preparation: current status. Clin Colon Rectal Surg. 2009;22:14–20.
41. Beck DE, Harford FJ, DiPalma JA. Comparison of cleansing methods in preparation for colonic surgery. Dis Colon Rectum. 1985;28:491–5.
42. Bigard MA, Gaucher P, Lassalle C. Fatal colonic explosion during colonoscopic polypectomy. Gastroenterology. 1979;77:1307–10.
43. Taylor EW, Bentley S, Young D, et al. Bowel preparation and the safety of colonoscopic polypectomy. Gastroenterology. 1981;81:1–4.
44. Raillat A, de Saint-Julien J, Abgrall J. Colonic explosion during an endoscopic electrocoagulation after preparation with mannitol. Gastroenterol Clin Biol. 1982;6(3):301–2.
45. Zanoni CE, Bergamini C, Bertoncini M, Bertoncini L, Garbini A. Whole-gut lavage for surgery. A case of intraoperative colonic explosion after administration of mannitol. Dis Colon Rectum. 1982;25(6):580–1.
46. Gross E, Jurim O, Krausz M. Diathermy-induced gas explosion in the intestinal tract. Harefuah. 1992;123(1–2):12–3. 72, 71.
47. Beck DE, Fazio VW, Jagelman DG. Comparison of lavage methods for preoperative colonic cleansing. Dis Colon Rectum. 1986;29:699–703.
48. Davis GR, Santa Ana CA, Morawski SG, et al. Development of a lavage solution associated with minimum water and electrolyte absorption or secretion. Gastroenterology. 1980;78:991–5.
49. Shawki S, Wexner S. Oral colorectal cleansing preparations in adults. Drugs. 2008;68(4):417–37.
50. Beck DE, Harford FJ, DiPalma JA, Brady CE. Colon cleansing with Golytely. South Med J. 1985;78:1414–8.
51. Ziegenhagen DJ, Zehnter E, Tacke W, Kruis W. Addition of senna improves colonoscopy preparation with lavage: a prospective randomized trial. Gastrointest Endosc. 1991;37(5):547–9.
52. Oliveira L, Wexner SD, Daniel N, et al. Mechanical bowel preparation for elective colorectal surgery. A prospective, randomized, surgeon-blinded trial comparing sodium phosphate and polyethylene glycol-based oral lavage solutions. Dis Colon Rectum. 1997;40(5):585–91.
53. Clarkston WK, Smith OJ. The use of GoLYTELY and Dulcolax in combination in outpatient colonoscopy. J Clin Gastroenterol. 1993;17:146–8.
54. Sharma VK, Chockalingham SK, Ugheoke EA, et al. Prospective, randomized, controlled comparison of the use of polyethylene glycol electrolyte lavage solution in four-liter versus two-liter volumes and pretreatment with either magnesium citrate or bisacodyl for colonoscopy preparation. Gastrointest Endosc. 1998;47(2):167–71.
55. Adams WJ, Meagher AP, Lubowski DZ, King DW. Bisacodyl reduces the volume of polyethylene glycol solution required for bowel preparation. Dis Colon Rectum. 1994;37(3):229–33. discussion 233–4.
56. Sharma VK, Steinberg EN, Vasudeva R, Howden CW. Randomized, controlled study of pretreatment with magnesium citrate on the quality of colonoscopy preparation with polyethylene glycol electrolyte lavage solution. Gastrointest Endosc. 1997;46:541–2.
57. Ker TS. Comparison of reduced volume versus four-liter electrolyte lavage solutions for colon cleansing. Am Surg. 2006;72(10):909–11.
58. Brady CE, DiPalma JA, Pierson WP. Golytely lavage – is metoclopramide necessary? Am J Gastroenterol. 1985;80(3):180–4.
59. Lever EL, Walter MH, Condon SC, et al. Addition of enemas to oral lavage preparation for colonoscopy is not necessary. Gastrointest Endosc. 1992;38(3):369–72.
60. Braintree Laboratories, Inc. Full prescribing information (PDF). http://www.nulytely.com/pdf/Golytely_Pres_Info.pdf 2001.
61. Vanner SJ, MacDonald PH, Paterson WG, Prentice RS, Da Costa LR, Beck IT. Randomized prospective trial comparing oral sodium phosphate with standard polyethylene glycol-based lavage solution (Golytely) in the preparation of patients for colonoscopy. Am J Gastroenterol. 1990;85(4):422–7.
62. Lieberman DA, Ghormley J, Flora K. Effect of oral sodium phosphate colon preparation on serum electrolytes in patients with normal serum creatinine. Gastrointest Endosc. 1996;43(5):467–9.
63. Aronchik CA, Lipshutz WH, Wright SH, et al. A novel tableted purgative for colonoscopy: efficacy and safety comparisons with Colyte and Fleet Phospho-Soda. Gastrointest Endosc. 2000;52:346–52.
64. Lichtenstein GR, Grandhi N, Schmalz M, et al. Clinical trial: sodium phosphate tablets are preferred and better tolerated by patients compared to polyethylene glycol solution plus bisacodyl tablets for bowel preparation. Aliment Pharmacol Ther. 2007;26(10):1361–70.
65. Johanson JF, Popp JW, Cohen LB, et al. Randomized, multicenter study comparing the safety and efficacy of sodium phosphate tablets with 2L polyethylene glycol solution plus bisacodyl tablets for colon cleansing. Am J Gastroenterol. 2007;102(10):2238–46.
66. Markowitz GS, Stokes MB, Radhakrishnan J, D'Agati VD. Acute phosphate nephropathy following oral sodium phosphate bowel purgative: an underrecognized cause of chronic renal failure. J Am Soc Nephrol. 2005;16(11):3389–96.
67. Carl DE, Sica DA. Acute phosphate nephropathy following colonoscopy preparation. Am J Med Sci. 2007;334(3):151–4.
68. Bucher P, Gervaz P, Egger JF, Soravia C, Morel P. Morphologic alterations associated with mechanical bowel preparation before elective colorectal surgery: a randomized trial. Dis Colon Rectum. 2006;49(1):109–12.
69. Beloosesky Y, Grinblat J, Weiss A, Grosman B, Gafter U, Chagnac A. Electrolyte disorders following oral sodium phosphate administration for bowel cleansing in elderly patients. Arch Intern Med. 2003;63(7):803–8.
70. Brownson P, Jenkins SA, Nott D, Ellenbogen S. Mechanical bowel preparation before colorectal surgery: results of a prospective randomized trial. Br J Surg. 1992;79:461–2.

71. Santos Jr JC, Batista J, Sirimarco MT, Guimaraes AS, Levy CE. Prospective randomized trial of mechanical bowel preparation in patients undergoing elective colorectal surgery. Br J Surg. 1994;81:1673–6.
72. Burke P, Mealy K, Gillen P, Joyce W, Traynor O, Hyland J. Requirement for bowel preparation in colorectal surgery. Br J Surg. 1994;81:907–10.
73. Fillman EEP, Fillmann HS, Fillmann LS. Elective colorectal surgery without prepare [Cirurgia colorretal eletiva sem prepare]. Rev Bras Coloproctologia. 1995;15:70–1.
74. Miettinen RP, Laitinen ST, Makela JT, Paakkonen ME. Bowel preparation is unnecessary in elective open colorectal surgery. A prospective, randomized study. Dis Colon Rectum. 2000;43:669–75.
75. Tabusso FY, Zapata JC, Espinoza FB, Meza EP, Figueroa ER. Mechanical preparation in elective colorectal surgery, a useful practice or need? Rev Gastroenterol Peru. 2002;22:152–8.
76. Bucher P, Gervaz P, Soravia C, Mermillod B, Erne M, Morel P. Randomized clinical trial of mechanical bowel preparation versus no preparation before elective left-sided colorectal surgery. Br J Surg. 2005;92:409–14.
77. Ram E, Sherman Y, Weil R, Vishne T, Kravarusic D, Dreznik Z. Is mechanical bowel preparation mandatory for elective colon surgery? A prospective randomized study. Arch Surg. 2005;140:285–8.
78. Fa-Si-Oen P, Roumen R, Buitenweg J, van de Velde C, van Geldere D, Putter H, et al. Mechanical bowel preparation or not? Outcome of a multicenter, randomized trial in elective colon surgery. Dis Colon Rectum. 2005;48:1509–16.
79. Zmora O, Mahajna A, Bar-Zakai B, Hershko D, Shabtai M, Krausz MM, et al. Is mechanical bowel preparation mandatory for left-sided colonic anastomosis? Results of a prospective randomized trial. Tech Coloproctol. 2006;10:131–5.
80. Pena-Soria MJ, Mayo JM, Annual-Fernandez R, Arbeo-Escolar A, Fernandez-Represa JA. Mechanical bowel preparation for elective colorectal surgery with primary intraperitoneal anastomosis by a single surgeon: interim analysis of a prospective single-blinded randomized trial. J Gastrointest Surg. 2007;11:562–7.
81. Jung B, Pahlman L, Nystrom PO, Nilsson E. Multicentre randomized clinical trial of mechanical bowel preparation in elective colonic resection. Br J Surg. 2007;94:689–95.
82. Contant CM, Hop WC, van't Sant HP. Mechanical bowel preparation for elective colorectal surgery: a multicentre randomised trial. Lancet. 2007;370:2112–7.
83. Guenega KF, Matos D, Castro AA, Atallah AN, Wille-Jorgensen P. Mechanical bowel preparation for elective colorectal surgery. Cochrane Database Syst Rev. 2005:CD001544.
84. Pineda CE, Shelton AA, Hernandez-Boussard T, Morton JM, Welton ML. Mechanical bowel preparation in intestinal surgery: a meta-analysis and review of the literature. J Gastrointest Surg. 2008;12:2037–44.
85. Zmora O, Wexner SD, Hajjar L, et al. Trends in preparation for colorectal surgery: survey of members of the American Society of Colon and Rectal Surgeons. Am Surg. 2003;69:150–4.
86. Margolin DA, Mayfield S. Preoperative bowel preparation. In: Whitlow CB, Beck DE, Margolin DA, Hicks TC, Timmcke AE, editors. Improved outcomes in colon and rectal surgery. New York: Informa Healthcare; 2009. p. 14–8.
87. Garlock JH, Seley GP. The use of sulfanilamide in surgery of the colon and rectum. Preliminary report. Surgery. 1939;5:787–90.
88. Dearing WH, Needham GM. The effect of terramycin on the intestinal bacterial flora of patients being prepared for intestinal surgery. Proc Staff Meet Mayo Clin. 1951;26(3):49–52.
89. Poth EJ. The role of intestinal antisepsis in the preoperative preparation of the colon. Surgery. 1960;47:1018–28.
90. Clarke JS, Condon RE, Bartlett JG, et al. Preoperative oral antibiotics reduce septic complications of colon operations: results of prospective, randomized, double-blind clinical study. Ann Surg. 1977;186:151.
91. Bartlett JG, Condon RE, Gorbach SL. Veterans Administration Cooperative Study on Bowel Preparation for Elective Colorectal Operations: impact of oral antibiotic regimen on colonic flora, wound irrigation cultures and bacteriology of septic complications. Ann Surg. 1978;188(2):249–54.
92. Condon RE, Bartlett JG, Nichols RL, et al. Preoperative prophylactic cephalothin fails to control septic complications of colorectal operations: results of controlled clinical trial. A Veterans Administration cooperative study. Am J Surg. 1979;137:68.
93. Polk HC, Zeppa R, Warren WD. Surgical significance of differentiation between acute and chronic pancreatic collections. Ann Surg. 1969;169(3):444–6.
94. Song F, Glenny A. Antimicrobial prophylaxis in colorectal surgery: a systematic review of randomized controlled trials. Br J Surg. 1998;85:1232–41.
95. Bratzler DW et al. Antimicrobial prophylaxis for surgery: an advisory statement from the National Surgical Infection Prevention Project. Clin Infect Dis. 2004;38:1706–15.
96. Steele SR, Simmang CL. General postoperative complications. In: Whitlow CB, Beck DE, Margolin DA, Hicks TC, Timmcke AE, editors. Improved outcomes in colon and rectal surgery. New York: Informa Healthcare; 2009. p. 67–78.
97. Nutescu EA. Assessing, preventing, and treating venous thromboembolism: evidence-based approaches. Am J Health Syst Pharm. 2007;64(11 Suppl 7):S5–13.
98. Anaya DA, Nathens AB. Thrombosis and coagulation: deep vein thrombosis and pulmonary embolism prophylaxis. Surg Clin North Am. 2005;85(6):1163–77.
99. Gangireddy C, Rectenwald JR, Upchurch GR, Wakefield TW, Khuri S, Henderson WG, et al. Risk factors and the clinical impact of postoperative symptomatic venous thromboembolism. J Vasc Surg. 2007;45(2):335–41.
100. Buller HR, Agnelli G, Hull RD, Hyers TM, Prins MH, Raskob GE. Antithrombotic therapy for venous thromboembolic disease. Chest. 2004;126(3 Suppl):401S–428.
101. Wille-Jorgensen P, Rasmussen MS, Andersen BR, Borly L. Heparins and mechanical methods for thromboprophylaxis in colorectal surgery. Cochrane Database Syst Rev. 2003;(4):CD001217.
102. Borly L, Wille-Jorgensen P, Rasmussen MS. Systematic review of thromboprophylaxis in colorectal surgery – an update. Colorectal Dis. 2005;7(2):122–7.
103. Leonardi MJ, McGory ML, Ko CY. The rate of bleeding complications after pharmacologic deep venous thrombosis prophylaxis: a systematic review of 33 randomized controlled trials. Arch Surg. 2006;141(8):790–7.

104. Hui AJ, Wong RM, Ching JY, Hung LC, Chung SC, Sung JJ. Risk of colonoscopic polypectomy bleeding with anticoagulants and antiplatelet agents: analysis of 1657 cases. Gastrointest Endosc. 2004;59(1):44–8.
105. Friedland S, Soetikno R. Colonoscopy with polypectomy in anticoagulated patients. Gastrointest Endosc. 2006;64(1): 98–100.
106. Practice parameters for the prevention of venous thromboembolism. Task Force of the American Society of Colon and Rectal Surgeons. Dis Colon Rectum. 2000;43(8): 1037–47.
107. Mardenstein EL, Neragi-Miandoab S, Delaney CP. Preexisting conditions. In: Whitlow CB, Beck DE, Margolin DA, Hicks TC, Timmcke AE, editors. Improved outcomes in colon and rectal surgery. New York: Informa; 2009. p. 1–13.
108. Poldermans D, Bax JJ, Schouten O, et al. Should major vascular surgery be delayed because of preoperative cardiac testing in intermediate-risk patients receiving beta-blocker therapy with tight heart rate control? J Am Coll Cardiol. 2006;48:964–9.
109. Hindler K, Shaw AD, Samuels J, Flton S, Collard CD, Reidel B. Improved postoperative outcomes associated with preoperative statin therapy. Anesthesiology. 2006;105:1260–72.
110. Practice parameters for antibiotic prophylaxis to prevent endocarditis or infected prosthesis during colon and rectal endoscopy. The American Society of Colon and Rectal Surgeons. Dis Colon Rectum. 1992;35(3):227.

9 Postoperative Management

Sharon L. Stein and Conor P. Delaney

Postoperative care of the colorectal patient is focused on decreasing morbidity, mortality, and health-care costs. An estimated 161,000 Medicare patients undergo major intestinal surgery in the USA annually at a cost of 1.75 billion dollars.[1] The average patient remains in the hospital 10.3 days after colorectal surgery, costing approximately $1,055 per day.[2]

Advances and standardization of postoperative care have reduced perioperative morbidity and mortality. Estimates of overall morbidity are 24.3% following colorectal surgery, with the incidence of serious morbidity including organ space surgical site infection, pulmonary embolism, and septic shock at up to 11.4%.[3] Recent NSQIP data estimates mortality at 1.4% for elective procedures and 15.8% for emergency colon and rectal surgery.[4] Although some costs and complications are unavoidable in postoperative care, a substantial percentage result from prolonged hospitalization, complications including surgical site infections, postoperative ileus, and venous thromboembolic events.

Numerous studies demonstrate that most patients can safely leave the hospital within 3–5 days following colon and rectal surgery without increasing rates of complications or readmission.[5–7] By decreasing the length of hospital stay, postoperative complications, and postoperative ileus, clinicians have the potential to save millions of health-care dollars annually, as well as accelerate the recovery of patients after major surgery. An expanding field of literature focuses on optimizing postoperative care and reducing length of stay. Comprehensive enhanced recovery or fast track protocols include several important elements to ensure success: appropriate antibiotic dosing, perioperative fluid optimization, early enteric nutrition, prevention of ileus, early ambulation, venous thromboembolic prophylaxis, and optimized postoperative analgesia.[8] Research has focused on evaluating available treatments and creating a comprehensive postoperative care plan to expedite hospital stay.

This chapter will review the available data for comprehensive enhanced recovery pathways and individual aspects of perioperative care including recommendations for prevention of postoperative complications and optimal treatment of colon and rectal surgery patients.

Standardized Fast Track Protocols or Enhanced Recovery Pathways

Standardized fast track or enhanced recovery protocols have the ability to substantially reduce length of stay. Generally, patients with stable vital signs are deemed ready for discharge when ambulating, tolerating enteric nutrition, and pain is well controlled with oral analgesia, and adequate discharge care (home or transitional facility) is available. In 2005, average length of stay following colectomy was 10.6 days.[1] Using multimodal, enhanced recovery, or fast track protocols, length of stay has dropped to a mean of 4–5 days in many series and as short as 2.5 days in the hands of some authors.[7,9] A truly efficacious postoperative care protocol combines many elements including regulation of postoperative fluids, early ambulation, early feeding and gastric stimulation, postoperative pain control, and pharmacologic treatment of ileus. Multiples studies have demonstrated the feasibility, safety, and success of enhanced recovery protocols.

Initial data on two small series of multimodal recovery protocols incorporated 48 h of epidural analgesia, immediate postoperative ambulation, and early postoperative feeding. Median length of stay after open sigmoid colectomy was 2 days, with a mean of approximately 4.4 days.[9,10] Simultaneously, Bradshaw et al. randomized 72 patients to early removal of nasogastric tubes, oral diet, and early ambulation and found protocol patients had earlier return of bowel function and were discharged on average 1 day prior to controls.[11] In 2001, Delaney et al. applied these premises to 58 patients undergoing reoperative or complex pelvic and rectal surgery.[5] Ambulation, early oral intake, and pain control were important elements of the protocol. Prompt removal of tubes and drains and enterostomal teaching prepared patients for earlier discharge. Patients without significant comorbidities

D.E. Beck et al. (eds.), *The ASCRS Textbook of Colon and Rectal Surgery: Second Edition*,
DOI 10.1007/978-1-4419-1584-9_9, © Springer Science+Business Media, LLC 2011

(DRG 149) left the hospital at 3.5 days, compared with 5.1 days for complicated patients. Eight patients (14%), who were poorly compliant with the protocol, had a mean length of stay of 5.1 days. Readmissions occurred in four patients (7%). A second study on 118 patients undergoing laparoscopic colectomy with standardized postoperative and discharge protocols, found median stay of 3 days.[7] Seventy percent of patients were discharged within 72 h of surgery, with a readmission rate of 8.5%. Patients discharged on days 1–3 were slightly less likely to have complications, but this did not reach statistical significance.

A systematic review of perioperative clinical care pathways found 13 articles incorporating standardized protocols after gastrointestinal surgery.[12] Articles include preoperative (11), intraoperative (7), and postoperative (13) interventions. Postoperative inventions included nutritional management, pain management, early mobilization, education of family and patient, and discharge planning. Overall, 11 of 13 programs demonstrated a significant decrease in length of stay when compared to conventional care; three also found a decrease in complication rates. None of the studies documented an increased risk of negative outcomes in the clinical pathway group when compared to standardized protocol patients. This was supported by several other meta-analyses in which length of stay was significantly decreased in fast track protocols (1.56–2.35 days shorter), and overall morbidity rates favored fast track protocols.[13,14]

Concern over increased readmission rates after early discharge appears to be unfounded. Three individual studies had notably high readmission rates from 22 to 27%[15–17] but meta-analysis has failed to show a significantly higher rate of readmission for fast track protocols (RR=1.17, 95% CI 0.73–1.86).[16] In addition, total hospital stay was analyzed including readmission in several studies and was still found to be approximately 2.5 days shorter than patients on conventional protocols.[14,16,17]

Data on increased use of posthospital services at time of discharge is scant. None of the meta-analyses of enhanced recovery protocols analyzed use of services, and few individual papers have described the use of home nursing or skilled nursing facilities.[15–17] Patients discharged within 1–2 days after surgery were less likely to require postdischarge services.[7,18] Need for posthospital services should be an individualized decision. Patients with new ostomies may require visiting nurse care following discharge for continued education and emotion adjustment.[19] Deconditioned or nonambulatory patients may require evaluation by physical therapy for in-patient or home services. A number of papers have demonstrated the importance of predischarge planning to ensure patient and caregiver comfort and satisfaction after discharge from hospital.[20,21] Laparoscopic surgery tends to be associated with less use of postdischarge care facilities than open surgery.[7]

Implementing a fast track protocol is not simple. Most fast track protocols incorporate 8–12 elements, with ranges varying from 4 to 20 elements.[12,14,16] An example of the University Hospital, Case Medical Center standardized protocol is listed in Table 9-1. Virtually all studies incorporate accelerated mobilization and early postoperative feeding. Other elements include preoperative bowel preparation, prevention of intraoperative hypothermia, early removal of lines and tubes, perioperative fluid management, opioid sparing techniques and pharmacologic treatment of ileus.[22] A key to the success in implementing a fast track program is the involvement of a multidisciplinary team. The team should consist of anesthetists, nurses, physical therapists, social workers and enterostomal therapists all trained, experienced, and committed to the success of the program.

Some studies have looked at the difficulties implementing a fast track protocol. Ionescu et al. randomized 96 patients to standardized protocol versus fast track implemented for

Table 9-1. University Hospital–Case Medical Center enhanced recovery protocol guidelines

Day before surgery
1. Protein/glucose drink
2. Bowel prep as directed
3. Diclofenac 100 mg po
Preoperative holding area
1. Gabapentin 600 mg po 1–2 h prior to induction
2. Alvimopam 12 mg po 1–2 h prior to induction
3. Thromboprophylaxis low-dose unfractionated heparin 5,000 U SC
4. Antibiotics prior to induction 30–60 min prior to induction
Postanesthesia recovery unit
1. Morphine PCA for all patients
2. DC antibiotics unless therapeutic indication
Nursing floor – General orders
1. CBC, BMP POD #1, 3 unless otherwise indicated
2. Ambulate in hallway 5 times per day
3. Sit out of bed 4–6 h per day
4. Foley removed POD#1 if laparoscopic, POD#2 if open
5. Heplock IVF POD#1 if laparoscopic, POD#2 if open
Nursing floor – Dietary orders
1. Clear liquids as tolerated
2. Protein/glucose drink 1 can BID
3. Soft diet POD#1 if laparoscopic, POD#2 if open
4. Chewing gum 1 stick TID × 60 min
Nursing floor medication orders
1. Gabapentin 300 mg po TID while in hospital
2. Alvimopam 12 mg po BID × 7 days while in hospital
3. Ketoroloac 15 mg IV Q6 h × 72 h while in hospital
4. Diclofenac 50 mg TID while in hospital
5. Heparin 5,000 U SC TID while in hospital *may be continued following discharge in high risk patients
6. Lactulose 10 mL po BID
Nursing floor – Oral analgesia
1. Transition to oral analgesia – POD#1 if laparoscopic, POD#2 if open
a. DC PCA
b. Acetaminophen #3 1–2 pills po q4–6 h, first dose 30 min prior to stopping PCA
c. Hold morphine except break through pain

The above guidelines should be modified as clinically appropriate and do not replace clinical evaluation and experience.
POD postoperative day, *PCA* patient controlled analgesia.

the first time at a single institution.[23] The average length of stay was reduced to 6.43 from 9.16 days. Difficulties faced in implementation included maintaining patients in a higher acuity unit to incorporate all elements of the protocol and convincing patients of the safety of accelerated hospital stay. Although patients tolerated oral diet at a mean of 42 h, mean length of stay was 6.43 days ($p<0.001$). Maessen et al. also found that implementation of postoperative care plan and discharge criteria were not sufficient to significantly reduce hospital stay in a multicenter European trial.[24] Although the majority of patients met discharge criteria at 3 days, the median time to discharge was 5 days after surgery. In a study center familiar with the fast track protocol, the percentage of patients discharged upon meeting criteria was 66% versus less familiar centers where only 26% of patients were immediately discharged ($p<0.001$).

Provider hesitancy may also play a role in the slow implementation of fast track programs. Kehlet and colleagues performed a survey in the USA and Europe of 295 hospitals and 1,082 colon surgery patients.[25] Despite evidence demonstrating a lack of efficacy,[26–28] they found that nasogastric tubes were left in situ for an average of 3 days in 40% of US patients and 66% of European patients. After surgery, 50% of patients tolerated their first liquids at 3–4 days and first meals at 4–5 days. However, patients remained in the hospital for a mean length of stay of 7 days in the USA and over 10 days in Europe. Polle et al. compared 55 fast track and 52 conventional patients on two gastrointestinal units at a single hospital using 13 fast track elements.[18] On average only 7.4 elements were applied per patient within the fast track group. Despite this, length of stay was reduced from 8 to 4.5 days for patients undergoing open colorectal surgery ($p=0.02$) but no reduction was noted in laparoscopic patients. Although readmission rates were higher in the fast track group (6% vs. 3%), overall total hospital stay was still decreased by 2.5 days on average ($p=0.03$). Patient satisfaction was not significantly different between the two groups.

Many studies have now analyzed the cost effectiveness of fast track protocols. Pritts et al. used pre-fast track historic and concurrent standard protocol patients to evaluate cost savings of an enhanced recovery protocol.[29] The mean cost per hospital stay was \$19,997.35 ± \$1,244.61 for patients in the historical control group, \$20,835.28 ± \$2,286.26 for those in the simultaneous control group, and \$13,908.53 ± \$1,113.01 for those in the enhanced recovery group ($p<0.05$ vs. other groups). Length of stay was reduced by approximately 2 days when compared to historical and nonpathway groups ($p<0.05$ vs. other groups). Stephen and Berger compared pre- and post-fast track implementation costs and length of stay.[30] After implementation of a fast track protocol, length of stay was reduced from 6.6 to 3.7 days ($p<0.001$) and costs were reduced from \$9,310 ± \$5,170 to \$7,070 ± \$3,670 ($p=0.002$). Kariv et al. looked exclusively at patients undergoing ileal pouch anal anastomosis and found shorter hospital stays (4 days vs. 5 days) ($p=0.012$) and lower direct 30-day costs reduced from \$6,672 to \$5,692 ($p=0.001$).[31]

Clearly, development of an enhanced recovery protocol has potential benefits, including the potential for substantial financial savings. Risk of readmission and complications do not appear to be increased in accelerated patient pathways. Provider and patient comfort is an important element to success and is benefitted by a team committed to a comprehensive protocol.

Fluid Management

Postoperative fluid management is complicated by perioperative changes in homeostasis and appropriate fluid management is essential to optimizing postoperative care. Basic fluid requirements are approximately 2,500 cc/day in a 70 kg adult. This allows for both insensible losses from respiration, perspiration, and feces as well as the 1,500 cc of urine necessary to excrete waste products including urea, potassium, and sodium. A basic formula for calculating fluid needs is 1,500 cc for the first 20 kg and 20 cc/kg for the rest of the weight.

After surgical stress, there is an increase in renin, aldosterone, and antidiuretic hormone release and activation of the sympathetic system resulting in sequestration of fluid (third spacing) and increased volume requirements. Additional losses may occur from evaporation from exposed abdominal cavity, blood loss, diarrhea, nasogastric tubes, and abdominal drains; each of these must be accounted for. In recovering patients, fluid retention begins to resolve with a return of the hormones and sympathetic nervous system toward normal in approximately 72 h.

Data have shown that insufficient perioperative fluid resuscitation increases the risk of hypotension, inadequate tissue perfusion, and renal failure.[32,33] Shires historically advocated aggressive fluid resuscitation in trauma patients to compensate for perioperative third spacing, and the concept was quickly applied to elective surgery.[34] In this regimen, patients were resuscitated in excess of expected or actual intraoperative fluid losses, receiving between 3.5 and 7 L of fluid on the day of surgery. Following surgery, patients might receive 3 L per day for 48 h with weight gains of 3–6 kg postoperatively rendering them hypervolemic.[35,36] However, over-resuscitation is associated with hypoalbuminemia, delayed gastrointestinal recovery, pulmonary complications, and increased cardiac demand.[37,38]

Initial attempts to moderate resuscitation fluids were compared with standard resuscitation. Lobo et al. restricted fluids in ten patients to 2 L per day and noted reductions in complication rates ($p=0.01$), earlier return of gastrointestinal function (4.0 vs. 3.0, $p=0.001$) and reduced length of stay (9.0 vs. 6.0, $p=0.001$).[35] These findings were supported by some studies;[39–41] others failed to show decreases in wound infection rates (11.3% vs. 5.5%, NS)[42] or length of stay (7.2 days vs. 7.2 days).[43] A meta-analysis of seven trials not only demonstrated no evidence of increased rates of serious complications such as anastomotic leaks but also failed to reach definitive recommendations.[44] This body of literature has been criticized for including a heterogeneous mix of resuscitation patterns, definitions, and goals. Postoperative care regimens, time to oral intake, use of colloid supplements, and anesthetic regiments varied greatly between studies. "Restricted" resuscitation rates ranged from 998 to 2,740 mL, and overlapped with liberal fluid resuscitation in other studies. Varied analgesia regimens led to changes in resuscitation; patients with epidural catheters had hypotension associated with sympathetic blockade and vasodilation and required additional fluids.[39] In addition, many studies excluded high-risk patients, who might benefit most from restrictive or goal-directed therapies.[44] Further studies with standardized definitions, perioperative protocols, and more rigorous outcomes are necessary to define optimal management.

More recently, transesophageal Doppler monitoring has been used to guide resuscitation. Monitoring of ejection fraction and stroke volume aid in assessing oxygen tissue delivery.[45,46] Optimization of stroke volume as determined by Doppler is compared with typical postoperative hemodynamic parameters such as urine output, heart rate, and blood pressure. Several studies have shown reduced postoperative gastrointestinal and overall complications[47–50] and earlier return of bowel function.[50] Resuscitation with colloid versus crystalloid did not further improve length of stay.[51] The rate of anastomotic leaks was not increased in the study groups.[52,53] Three studies demonstrated a statistically reduced postoperative length of stay by 1.5 to 2 days[49,50] confirmed in two separate meta-analysis in favor of Doppler-guided resuscitation.[52]

While general trends support restricted perioperative fluids[44,52,53] the ideal resuscitation goals are still being debated. Doppler guidance is available only intraoperatively, and although this can reduce early over resuscitation, postoperative fluids are still based on a variety of subjective hemodynamic parameters. Further studies in the setting of standardized perioperative care module will be helpful in determining best goals for postoperative intravenous fluid administration. In addition, as trends toward earlier enteric intake continue, reducing intravenous fluids in exchange for oral fluids may further change practice parameters.

Postoperative Gastrointestinal Recovery: Nausea, Vomiting, Feeding, Gum Chewing, and Ileus

Postoperative Nausea and Vomiting

Postoperative nausea and vomiting (PONV) is a common early complication after gastrointestinal surgery. Approximately 25% of patients experience PONV within 24 h. Among high-risk patients, the incidence may be as high as 70–80%.[54,55] PONV delays recovery of patients after in-patient surgery and accounts for a significant proportion of unanticipated hospitalizations following ambulatory surgery. PONV leads to patient discomfort and satisfaction but is largely avoidable when properly addressed.

Table 9-2. Risk factors for postoperative nausea and vomiting

Patient-specific risk factors
1. Female sex
2. Nonsmoking status
3. History of PONV/motion sickness

Anesthetic risk factors
1. Use of volatile anesthetics
2. Nitrous oxide
3. Use of intraoperative or postoperative narcotics

Surgical risk factors
1. Duration of surgery
2. Type of surgery

Adapted from Gan TJ. Risk factors for postoperative nausea and vomiting. Anesth Analg. 2006;102:1884–98.[79]
PONV postoperative nausea and vomiting.

Table 9-3. Koivuranta score II for evaluation of postoperative nausea and vomiting

SCORING: Patient risk is calculated based on cumulative number of risk factors:
Risk factors:
Female gender
Previous PONV
Duration of surgery over 60 min
History of motion sickness
Nonsmoker

# of risk factors	Risk of nausea (%)	Risk of vomiting (%)
0-1 factor:	17–18	7
2 factors:	42	17
3 factors:	54	25
4 factors:	74	38
5 factors:	87	61

Adapted from Koivuranta M, Laara E, Snare L, Alahuhta S. A survey of postoperative nausea and vomiting. Anaesthesia. 1997;52:443–9.[59]
PONV postoperative nausea and vomiting.

Risk factors and risk assessment for postoperative nausea have been well studied. Consensus guidelines for managing PONV highlight patient, anesthetic, and surgical risk factors as listed in Table 9-2.[56] Instruments that predict PONV have been validated with a high level of correlation to patient outcome.[57,58] Among the simplest is the Koivuranta score (Table 9-3) which uses only the five strongest risk factors – female gender, previous PONV, duration of surgery, history of motion sickness, and nonsmoking status – as predictors of PONV.[59]

Prevention of PONV is centered on reducing anesthetic and surgical risks, while appropriately adding pharmacologic prophylaxis. Use of regional anesthesia, minimization of narcotics, and avoidance of nitrous oxide and volatile anesthetics have efficacy in reducing PONV.[51,60,61] Propofol induction, increasing hydration, and use of supplemental oxygen are associated with reduction in risk in patients undergoing colorectal surgery.[62]

Many pharmacologic therapies for PONV are familiar to the colorectal surgeon. 5-HT$_3$A agents such as ondansetron, granisetron, and tropisetron are often chosen as first line treatment. They are generally effective (NNT 5–7) with a favorable side effect profile which includes headaches, increased liver enzymes, and constipation.[63,64] Typical dose of ondansetron is 4 mg IV every 8 h, but this may be doubled for increased efficacy. Steroids have also been shown to be effective, particularly if administered prior to induction.[65] Dexamethasone is generally administered as a single dose intravenous of 8–10 mg, although doses as low as 2.5 have been found to be effective (NNT=4).[66] Side effect profile is more concerning to surgeons and includes wound infection and adrenal suppression, but these effects have not been reported after a single bolus dose. Droperidol was commonly administered at the end of surgery in doses of 1 mg IV with good effect (NNT=5) but a FDA "black box" warning recently issued has diminished enthusiasm for this antiemetic.[67] Reports of prolonged QTc intervals, arrhythmias and cardiac death, have been reported after use of droperidol but not following a single prophylactic dose.[68]

Other medications are used less frequently secondary to side effect profiles or questionable efficacy. Promethazine, a phenothiazine, has been shown in a single study to be more effective than ondansetron in preventing nausea (OR=3.4, 95% CI 1.2–9.4) but was not equally effective in preventing vomiting.[69] Additionally, the study was criticized for having a higher proportion of high-risk patients in the ondansetron arm (40% vs. 27%). Phenothiazines are also limited by their significant side effect profile, which include extrapyramidal symptoms, dystonia, tardive dyskinesia and akathisia. Scopalamine is a transdermal anticholinergic agent effective in preventing PONV in a single study (NNR 3.8).[70] However, use of scopolamine is limited by 2–4 h delay in onset of action as well as uncommon hallucinations, disorientation, and memory disturbances. Metoclopramide is a relatively cost effective treatment, which has mixed results in over 54 studies.[71] In a meta-analysis, metoclopramide had higher efficacy than ondansetron for nausea (59% vs. 48%, NS) but was less efficacious at preventing vomiting (35% vs. 50%, $p<0.001$).[72] In addition, side effects affect in up to 20% of patients include somnolence, reduced mental acuity, anxiety, and depression.[73] Despite FDA approval for PONV, metoclopramide is not routinely recommended.[56]

Unconventional treatments may also reduce the incidence of PONV. Acupuncture has been demonstrated to reduce the incidence of PONV when compared to placebo (23% vs. 41%, $p=0.0058$).[74] White et al. found that acupuncture and ondansetron were better than ondanestron alone for both nausea (40% vs. 70%, $p=0.006$) and vomiting (22.5% vs. 50% $p=0.070$).[75] Ernst et al. found that the use of 1 g of ginger was equivalent to the use of metoclopramide in preventing PONV.[76] Other studies demonstrated that ginger was no better than placebo in preventing PONV in women undergoing gynecologic surgery.[77] Aromatherapy including peppermint oil, isopropyl alcohol, or placebo decreased nausea from baseline, but there was no difference between scents in a single study.[78]

Economic and emotional costs of nausea and vomiting are often weighed against the cost of therapy. PONV prophylaxis was not found to be cost effective in patients whose risk of nausea or vomiting are less than 20%.[79] Hill found that prophylactic therapy was cost effective only in higher risk groups when compared to placebo.[80] In high-risk patients, two antiemetic agents were more cost effective than no prophylaxis and rescue therapy.[81] Treating vomiting is typically three times more expensive than treating nausea.[82]

Algorithms for management of PONV are well established.[56,71] Patients should be assessed preoperatively for risk of PONV and if found to be low risk, no prophylactic dosage is generally given. A rescue dose of 5-HT$_3$A, such as ondansetron, may be given if the patient experiences PONV after emersion. Patients are deemed to be at moderate to high risk of PONV are generally treated empirically. Monotherapy agents such as use of dexamethasone, droperidol, or ondansetron may be used or combination therapy of multiple agents can be employed when deemed appropriate.

Early Refeeding and Use of Nasogastric Tubes

Historically, patients were advised to refrain from postoperative nutrition for several days and nasogastric tubes were left in place to protect patients from nausea and vomiting following abdominal surgery.[83,84] Although nasogastric tubes relieved some symptoms of postoperative ileus, there is no evidence that they decreased duration of ileus or PONV.[26,85,86] In 1995, a meta-analysis determined that nasogastric tubes are associated with increased atelectasis and pneumonia.[87] Other studies demonstrated increased gastroesophageal reflux with nasogastric intubation,[28] and a recent meta-analysis demonstrated earlier return of bowel function after colonic surgery without a routine use of nasogastric tube.[26]

Early refeeding is believed to stimulate propulsive activity, decrease intestinal gut mucosal permeability, and induce secretions of gastrointestinal hormones to promote bowel motility. Early feeding was first proposed with laparoscopic surgery and early studies demonstrated that 80–90% of patients tolerated liquids within 24 h of surgery.[88,89] After success in laparoscopic surgery, studies expanded to patients undergoing open surgery.[90,91] A meta-analysis found feeding patients promptly after surgery is associated with decreased rate of infections (RR=0.72, $p=0.036$), and shorter length of stay (RR=0.84, $p=0.001$), but an increased risk of vomiting after surgery (RR=1.27, $p=0.046$).[92] A 2009 Cochrane data review suggested that earlier refeeding was safe and may reduce the risk of postoperative complications but data failed to reach statistical significance.[93]

Accelerated recovery programs uniformly include early refeeding for patients undergoing both open and laparoscopic surgery.[7,13,14] Approximately 5–15% of patients will develop substantial postoperative ileus requiring return to NPO status or nasogastric decompression, but most patients tolerate early feeding without complications.[5,90] Additionally, for the majority of patients who tolerate early refeeding, decreased complications, earlier discharge, and patient comfort are significant benefits.

Preoperative fasting has also been questioned as a routine part of clinical care. Postoperative hyperglycemia and insulin resistance have been proposed as independent factors increasing hospital stay.[94] Preoperative fasting of 8–12 h can deplete available carbohydrate reserves and promote a fasting metabolism. Data have demonstrated administration of a preoperative carbohydrate drink does not increase risk of aspiration or complications on induction.[95,96] A carbohydrate rich drink, given the evening before surgery and 2–3 h prior to surgery, has been shown to significantly reduce patient thirst, hunger, and improve well-being,[97] while also decreasing the loss of muscle mass postoperatively[98] and significantly reducing length of stay by 1.2 days ($p<0.02$).[99,100]

Treatment and Prevention of Ileus

Postoperative ileus is defined as the "transient cessation of coordinated bowel motility after surgical intervention, which prevents effective transit of intestinal contents and/or tolerance of oral intake."[101] The average time until recovery of bowel function after major abdominal surgery is less than 24 h for the small intestine, 24–48 h for the stomach and 48–120 h for the colon.[102,103] In general, ileus should resolve within the fifth postoperative day after open surgery and by the third postoperative day after laparoscopic surgery. Failure to resume gastrointestinal function has many adverse effects including increased postoperative pain, nausea and vomiting, poor wound healing, delay in postoperative mobilization, increase in deconditioning, pulmonary complications and nosocomial infections, prolonged hospitalization, decreased patient satisfaction, and increased health-care costs.

Health Care Financing Administration data estimates that postoperative ileus occurs in approximately 14.9% of patients following large bowel resection and up to 19.2% after small bowel resection.[1] It is estimated that the total health-care cost of postoperative ileus are approximately $1.14 billion dollars annually, or 6.24% of all health-care costs in the USA. The average length of stay of patients with postoperative ileus is almost doubled to 11.5 from 6.5 days for patients without postoperative ileus.[104]

To reduce the incidence and duration of postoperative ileus, multiple pharmacologic interventions have been attempted.[105,106] Beta blockade of adrenergic receptors in the gut might be expected to decrease the incidence of postoperative ileus. A single small study of propanolol in 1983 demonstrated promising results with decreased time to bowel movement of 18 h ($p\leq0.01$), but patients experienced a significant decrease in blood pressure and heart rate.[107] Further studies on propanolol failed to validate results or utility.[108] Neostigamine is an acetylcholinesterase inhibitor, which increases parasympathetic activity in the gut wall and has been used extensively in the treatment of acute colonic obstruction. However, its usefulness in postoperative ileus is limited by side effects which includes abdominal cramps, vomiting, and profound bradycardia.[109] Cisapride is a serotonin receptor antagonist that promotes acetylcholine receptor release from peripheral nerve endings and was demonstrated to have significant utility in decreasing postoperative ileus. However, cardiovascular events resulted in the drug's withdrawal from the market in 2000.[110] Metoclopramide is believed to increase gastrointestinal motility through stimulation of smooth muscle contractions. Although some studies demonstrated decreased nausea and vomiting with its routine use, there are no convincing data establishing a reduction in postoperative ileus.[111–115]

Newer drugs have been designed to selectively block peripheral (mu) μ-opioid receptors that contribute to postoperative ileus (POI). The ideal POI treatment is a peripheral opioid receptor antagonist that reverses GI side effects without crossing the blood–brain barrier, and therefore is unable to compromise postoperative analgesia. Two novel peripheral (mu) μ-opioid receptor antagonists have been studied in patients undergoing abdominal and pelvic surgery.

Methylnaltrexone is a quaternary derivative of naltrexone, which acts selectively on peripheral opioid receptors as a competitive antagonist. Because methylnaltrexone does not cross the blood–brain barrier it does not reverse analgesia or precipitate opioid withdrawal.[101,116] Methylnatrexone was approved in 2008 for treatment of opioid-induced constipation and significantly improved postoperative ileus in a Phase 2 study.[117] A randomized double-blind placebo-controlled trial of 0.3 mg/kg of intravenous methylnaltrexone demonstrated reduced time to first bowel movement (97 h vs. 120 h, $p=0.01$) and time to discharge eligibility (119 h vs. 149 h, $p=0.03$). Side effects included abdominal cramps and flatulence, as well as transient orthostatic hypotension when administered intravenously. Data from Phase III trials failed to show clinical improvement in postoperative ileus, and methylnaltrexone is currently approved only for opioid-induced constipation.

Alvimopan is also a peripherally active (mu) μ-opioid antagonist, but has higher affinity for human (mu) μ-opioid receptors and an active metabolite that appears to be absorbed systemically. Taguchi published the first results on postoperative use of alvimopan in 78 patients showing a dose-related response with significantly decreased time to passage of first flatus (70 h vs. 49 h) first bowel movement (111 h vs. 70 h and ready for discharge (91 h vs. 68 h).[118] Results were validated in a randomized double-blind multicenter trial demonstrating reduced time to GI-3 recovery consisting of two of the following: time to tolerating solid food, time to first flatus, or time to bowel movement. GI-3 recovery was reduced by 86.2 h versus 100.3 h in placebo.[119] Of note, patients undergoing hysterectomy did not have significant decrease in GI recovery time. A second multicenter trial demonstrated a GI-3, dose–response curve to alvimopan with recovery 15 h faster for 6 mg of alvimopan and 22 h faster for 12 mg of alvimopan when compared with placebo.[120] Buchler et al. published a RCT double-blind study in Europe; however, this study varied from the other studies by having much lower use of opioids and some patients who did not receive any opioids.[121] GI-3 bowel function was reduced by 8.5 h in the 6 mg group and 4.8 h in the 12 mg group, but this was not statistically significant. Pooled data analysis of the three US trials showed that alvimopan speeded overall GI-2 (tolerance of solid food and first bowel movement) recovery by 12 h and accelerated time to discharge order (HR = 1.35, $p<0.01$).[122,123] A second meta-analysis of five studies demonstrated similar findings.[124,125] In these studies, alvimopan has not been shown to have an increase in adverse event rates or complications.[104,123,124]

Alvimopan (Entereg®; Adolor and GlaxoSmithKline, Exton, PA) is currently approved for perioperative use only for hospitalized patients in the setting of Entereg Access Support and Education Programs (EASE). The first dose of 12 mg should be given orally prior to surgery, and continued 12 mg BID for 7 days, or until discharge. Alvimopan is contraindicated for patients on chronic opioids, with bowel obstruction, or severe hepatic or renal disease.[126] A cost analysis of alvimopan from the North American studies found mean hospital length of stay to be 1 full day shorter with a mean savings of $879–977 per patient, given an estimated cost of $558 dollars (8.9 × 12 mg doses).[127] Further analysis of the benefits of alvimopan on patients receiving laparoscopic surgery is ongoing, as all of the trials to date have been in patients undergoing open surgery.

Use of Gum Chewing

Gum chewing has also been proposed to decrease the incidence of postoperative ileus. Chewing stimulates the cephalic phase of digestion and serves as a form of sham feeding stimulating neural and hormonal pathways.[128] Mastication and salivation increase vagal cholinergic stimulation and promote the release of gastrointestinal hormones such as gastrin, neurotensin, and pancreatic polypeptide.[129] Cephalic stimulation is accomplished without oral intake, thereby theoretically avoiding complications of food intolerance, which may occur in up to 20% of patients after early oral intake.[130]

Asao et al. first proposed gum chewing to enhance recovery after colectomy in 2002.[131] Nineteen patients randomized to chewing gum three times daily following laparoscopic colectomy were noted to have earlier return of flatus (1.1 days, $p<0.01$), time to defecation (2.7 days, $p<0.01$) and time to discharge (1 days, NS). This data was supported by a multicenter trial by McCormick et al.[132] Patients who chewed gum four times daily after laparoscopic surgery had shorter duration of postoperative ileus (2.6 days vs. 3.3 days, $p=0.0047$) and hospital stay (4.0 days vs. 5.3 days, $p=0.029$).

Data is less compelling on the efficacy of gum chewing following open colectomy. Schuster et al. randomized 34 patients undergoing sigmoid colectomy to gum chewing and noted statistically decreased time to flatus (65.4 h vs. 80.2 h, $p=0.05$), defecation (63.2 h vs. 89.4 h, $p=0.04$), and length of stay (4.3 h vs. 6.8 day, $p=0.01$).[133] But other studies demonstrated no significant difference between groups undergoing open colectomy.[134,135] In a study of 38 open colectomy patients, Quah et al.[134] found slight reductions in passage of flatus (2.7 days vs. 2.4 days), time to defecation (3.9 days vs. 3.2 days), and length of stay (11.1 days vs. 9.4 days), none of which were significant. Matros et al. randomized 66 patients to gum chewing, acupressure wrist bracelets and control groups and demonstrated no significant differences in time to flatus, bowel movement, or discharge.[135] McCormick also found no reduction in time to bowel recovery (3.6 days vs. 3.9 days, $p=0.50$) or discharge (5.6 days vs. 5.3 days, $p=0.5$) in the open arm of their study.[132]

At least five meta-analyses on gum chewing exist in the literature, all of which demonstrate a statistically significant reduction in time to flatus and defecation.[136–140] Cumulative time to flatus and defecation were reduced by as much as 20 and 29 h, respectively.[136] Only Noble et al. demonstrated a significant reduction in length of stay (1.1 days, $p=0.0016$), after including a study of nonrandomized patients undergoing cystectomy.[138,141] Meta-analyses highlight the heterogenicity of trials including frequency and duration of gum chewing, which varied from TID to QID and 5–30 min in duration. Use of epidural anesthesia was varied in open trials; epidurals were used in over 85% of patients in trials by Matros and Quah[134,135] but less than half in the trial by Schuster et al.[133] Thoracic epidural analgesia provides a sympathetic blockade that may negate the parasympathetic stimulation of gum chewing. Most trials were small, and blinding was difficult to perform.

The economic and social costs of gum chewing are minimal. Schuster et al. estimated a cost of gum at $.04 per stick three times daily for 5 days per patients.[133] With over 350,000 colectomies performed annually in the USA, the cost would be under $50,000 per year. An average hospital room was estimated at $1,500 per day, and the cost of ileus is over $750,000,000 annually.[1] In addition, although theoretical complications such as aspiration or small bowel obstruction after gum chewing may exist, no significant complications were reported in any of the trials. Gum chewing appeared well tolerated and probably is a low-risk intervention for patients undergoing colectomy.

Early Ambulation

Early ambulation following abdominal surgery was proposed by Ephraim McDowell as early as 1817, but most surgeons including Sir William Halstead were more cautious, keeping patients immobilized for up to 21 days following laparotomy.[142,143] In 1941, Leithauser popularized early ambulation, listing decreases in pulmonary, circulatory and digestive system complications as benefits.[144,145]

Direct benefits of ambulation on postoperative gastrointestinal recovery are inconclusive. In 1990, Waldenhausen and Schirmer studied myoelectrical recovery of the gastrointestinal tract following surgery and found no difference in recovery times for patients who ambulated on postoperative day 1 versus day 4.[146] Maessen et al. noted ambulating within 24 h of surgery was associated with early discharge, but not reduction in time to flatus or bowel movement.[147] Lin et al. correlated increased length of ambulation with 36.6% earlier discharge following laparoscopic surgery.[148] However Zutshi et al. found no added benefit for early ambulation in patients who participated in comprehensive enhanced recovery protocols.[149]

Early ambulation appears to be correlated with reduced postoperative respiratory and hematologic complications but may not have a direct effect on recovery of bowel function. Additional benefits include preservation of strength and conditioning.[150] As there are virtually no disadvantages to early ambulation, early ambulation is an established component of virtually all accelerated recovery programs. Ideally, patients ambulate on the evening of surgery. To accommodate early ambulation, lines and tubes are minimized after surgery. Foley catheters are removed by postoperative day 1 for laparoscopic surgery or day 2 after open surgery. Drainage catheters are not routinely left in place after surgery.[151,152] By postoperative day 1, patients are encouraged to walk a minimum of 60 m and spend 5 or more hours out of bed.[153]

Prevention of Pulmonary Complications

Pulmonary complications are well established after surgery. Churchill described reductions of up to 80% of vital lung capacity following surgery in 1928; lung volumes are diminished after both general anesthesia and abdominal surgery.[154,155] Interventions including early ambulation, minimally invasive surgery, and smoking cessation have been evaluated to reduce risk of postoperative pulmonary complications.

Delayed ambulation has been directly correlated with worsening pulmonary function. Pain appears to be a factor in both ability to ambulate and pulmonary toilet. Kanat et al. demonstrated increased respiratory complications in patients who failed to ambulate within 48 h.[156] Appropriate pain control can be essential in moderating diminished lung capacity.[157]

Earlier return of forced expiratory volumes was one of the first benefits demonstrated from laparoscopic surgery.[158,159] Several studies have demonstrated early recovery of pulmonary function as evidenced by incentive spirometry.[160] Vignali et al. demonstrated nonsignificant but lower rates of pneumonia in patients undergoing laparoscopy.[161] A retrospective review by Guller found a decreased incidence of postoperative respiratory complications in laparoscopic patients (2.5% vs. 6%, $p<0.001$).[162] A meta-analysis performed by Abraham et al. demonstrated achieving 80% preoperative peak expiratory flow was delayed in 44.3% patients having open surgery, but FEV1 and FVC were not significantly different when compared to laparoscopic groups.[163] These studies have been criticized for a lack of prospective data, disparities between groups, and more importantly the relevance of clinical end points, such as spirometry parameters and radiographic atelectasis.[164]

Although all patients are at risk for pulmonary complications, there appear to be groups who are particularly susceptible. A 2006 review evaluated risk factors and interventions in an attempt to reduce postoperative pulmonary complications.[165] Qaseem et al. determined that patients at high risk included patients with chronic obstructive pulmonary disease, age greater than 60, American Society of Anesthesiologist (ASA) class II or greater, and cardiac failure. Emergency surgery, general anesthesia, abdominal surgery, and procedures longer than 3 h in length all further increase risk. Patients deemed high risk of complications benefit from deep breathing exercises or incentive spirometry, and the selective use of nasogastric tubes, though no single intervention was statistically superior.[165]

Preoperative smoking cessation may not be advantageous. Data regarding postoperative benefits of preoperative smoking cessation is generally inconclusive[166] but appears to be most beneficial for patients who quit 4–6 weeks before surgery.[157] Patients who quit smoking within 2 months of surgery may have a paradoxical increased risk of postoperative pulmonary complications, possibly from increased mucous production.[167]

Prevention of Venous Thromboembolism

Colon and rectal surgery patients are at risk for deep venous thrombosis (DVT) and pulmonary embolism (PE). Estimates are that between 20 and 40% of patients undergoing abdominal surgery will experience DVT and 2–4% will develop a pulmonary embolism.[168] Fatal pulmonary embolism occurs in up to 1.0% of hospitalized patients, and accounts for 10% of hospital deaths, making it the most common preventable cause of hospital death in the USA.[169,170] Colon and rectal surgery patients often have multiple risk factors for venous thromboembolism (VTE), listed in Table 9-4, including diagnoses such as cancer or inflammatory bowel disease, advanced age, and prolonged surgical procedures.[171]

The rationale for thromboprophylaxis in colorectal patients is simple and scientific.[172,173] Many of these events are clinically silent and screening is neither clinically nor economically effective. Prophylaxis for VTE should be a standard element in the care of the postoperative colorectal surgery patients. There are many highly efficacious methods of preventing VTE. Patient risk should be stratified preoperatively

TABLE 9-4. Risk factors for venous thromboembolism

Surgery
Trauma (major or lower extremity)
Malignancy
Cancer therapy (hormonal, chemotherapy, radiotherapy)
Previous venous thromboembolism
Increasing age
Pregnancy/postpartum
Estrogen containing oral contraceptive/hormone therapy/modulation
Acute medical illness
Heart/Respiratory failure
Inflammatory bowel disease
Nephrotic syndrome
Obesity
Smoking
Varicose veins
Central venous catheterization

Modified from Geerts WH, Bergqvist D, Pineo GF, et al. Prevention of venous thromboembolism. Chest 2008;133:381S–453S.[171]

TABLE 9-5. Risk classification of deep venous thrombosis and recommended options for prophylaxis for patients undergoing surgery

Level of risk	Approximate risk of DVT without thromboprophylaxis (%)	Suggested options
Low risk (minor surgery in mobile patients)	<10	Early ambulation
Moderate risk (most general surgery patients)	10–40	Low molecular weight heparin Low dose unfractionated heparin Fondaparinux
High risk	40–80	Low molecular weight heparin Fondaparinux Oral vitamin K antagonist to INR (2–3)

Modified from Geerts WH, Bergqvist D, Pineo GF, et al. Prevention of venous thromboembolism. Chest. 2008;133:381S–453S.[171]
DVT deep vein thrombosis.

and use of prophylactic regiments including elastic stockings, mechanical sequential compression devices (SCDs), and pharmacologic agents should be employed. Risk classification of patients and general guidelines is included in Table 9-5. The American Society of Colon and Rectal Surgeons (ASCRS) has provided practice parameters for the prevention of venous thromoboemoblism.[174]

Elastic Stockings and Sequential Compression Devices

Elastic stockings and SCDs are mechanical methods of increasing venous outflow and reducing stasis in leg veins to decrease the risk of DVT. Graduated compression stockings function purely on a mechanical level to encourage venous return. SCDs are also believed to systemically increase the fibrinolytic activity by reducing plasminogen activator.[175] For maximal benefit in patients undergoing surgery, elastic stockings or SCDs should be placed before the induction of anesthesia and function throughout the operation.

Data on the effectiveness of elastic stockings and SCDs is limited. Both methods have demonstrated efficacy in reducing the risk of DVT, but neither have been shown to decrease the incidence of PE.[176–178] Several factors limit the effectiveness of SCDs and elastic stockings including poor compliance, poor fit, and arterial insufficiency.[179] In an observational study of patient compliance, Cornwell et al. observed that only 19% of patients were fully compliant with use of SCDs and patients were using SCDs at the time of only 53% of observations in this study.[180] If not fitted properly, elastic stockings may actually be constrictive and paradoxically increase venous pressure below the knees.[181] Compression stockings are not recommended for patients with arterial insufficiency or current DVT.[182]

As sole prophylaxis, compressive stockings and SCDs should be reserved for the low-risk patient or patients at high risk of bleeding who cannot tolerate prophylaxis pharmacotherapy.[171] SCDs and elastic stockings may be used in conjunction with pharmacologic prophylaxis.[183,184] Care should be taken to ensure that devices are applied regularly, fit appropriately, and do not limit ambulation postoperatively.

Aspirin

Although aspirin has significant antiplatelet activities and has been used to prevent major vascular events, current recommendations are that aspirin should not be used as primary treatment to prevent VTE.[171] A number of trials demonstrated no significant benefit from aspirin therapy alone.[185,186]

Low-Dose Unfractionated Heparin

Unfractionated heparin has been used as a form of DVT prophylaxis since the 1970s and has been shown to be safe in the majority of surgical patients. It binds to antithrombin (ATIII) and accelerates the inhibition of thrombin and other coagulation factors, particularly factor X. Typically, pTT will be unchanged despite use of unfractionated mini-dose heparin. Heparin can be reversed with use of protamine. Recommendations are that the initial dose of low-dose unfractionated heparin (LDUH) be given 1–2 h preoperatively. Although the standard dosing regimen is 5,000 U subcutaneously every 8–12 h postoperatively, no study has compared dosing regimens directly.

A meta-analysis of LDUH compared 46 randomized clinical trials of LDUH, no thromboprophylaxis or placebo.[187] The rate of DVT, PE, and fatal PE were each significantly reduced (22% vs. 9%, 2.0% vs. 1.3%, and 0.8% vs. 0.3%). Risks of use of LDUH include the risk of postoperative bleeding and heparin-induced thrombocytopenia (HIT). LDUH is associated with an increased rate of bleeding events (5.9% vs. 3.5%), but subsequent analysis demonstrated bleeding was generally associated with wound hematomas and not major bleeding.[188] HIT may occur in 5–15% of patients but is less common than in patients on full anticoagulation. HIT may cause a paradoxical hypercoagulable state with arterial and venous thrombosis. The platelet count typically reduces to less than 50% of baseline levels and should be followed in patients receiving routine heparin and discontinued immediately if diminishing significantly.

Low Molecular Weight Heparin

Low molecular weight heparin (LMWH) consists of heparin molecules in a smaller range and size than LDUH. The mechanism is similar to LDUH in accelerating ATIII inactivation of Xa, but LMWH does not inactivate thrombin or bind as strongly to plasma moieties. LMWH has greater bioavailability, longer half-life, and more predictable plasma levels than LDUH. Because of this, partial thromboplastin time is not affected and does not need to be monitored.[189] Over time, accumulation of antifactor Xa activity and fibrinolysis may accumulate in patients on LMWH, especially in patients with renal failure. Compared to LDUH, LMWH has a longer half-life and may not be reversed with protamine infusion. The incidence of HIT is also lower than LDUH (2.7% vs. 0%).[190,191] Dosing regiments for LMWH are varied. In Europe, LMWH (enoxaparin) is typically dosed 20–40 mg daily. Americans tend to prefer a 30 mg BID dosing.

LMWH is at least as effective as LDUH in preventing DVT in postoperative general surgery and colorectal surgery patients. A large European trial randomized 1,351 patients undergoing abdominal surgery to LDUH or LMWH.[192] The incidence of thromboembolic complications was equal (4.7% vs. 4.3%), but patients in the LMWH group experienced fewer bleeding complications (8.3% vs. 11.8%, $p=0.03$). A meta-analysis of prospective randomized trials including over 5,000 patients confirmed these results.

Despite equal incidence of VTE, cost currently limits the use of LMWH. The Canadian Multicentre Colorectal Deep Vein Thrombosis Prophylaxis Trial attempted a cost analysis in both Canadian and US dollars for the use of LDUH and LMWH in a randomized prospective trial of 936 colorectal surgery patients.[193] Based on their findings of equal efficacy, and a trend toward more bleeding in the LMWH group, they concluded that LDUH was more cost effective. LMWH was twice as expensive as LDUH therapy. This was further supported by the National Institute of Health and Clinical Excellence who failed to note economic benefits of LMWH when compared to LDUH.[194]

Fondaparinux

Fondaparinux is a selective Factor Xa inhibitor that has been successfully used for thromboprophylaxis. A randomized controlled study comparing LMWH and fondaparinux 2.5 mg SC QD demonstrated equivalent rates of VTE, major bleeding, and death.[195] A second trial compared fondaparinux to placebo and SCD's and found that rates of VTE and DVT were significantly lower when using fondaparinux (1.7% vs. 5.3%, $p=0.004$).[196] Fondaparinux has a longer half-life than LMWH and may result in bioaccumulation in patients with altered creatinine clearance. Because of daily dosing, fondaparinux has been noted to be cost effective when compared to LMWH.[197]

VTE Prophylaxis and the Use of Epidural Analgesia

A rare but potential complication of spinal or epidural analgesia is the risk of bleeding into the spinal canal or epidural space. This may result in spinal cord ischemia and paraplegia in patients. Risk factors for the development of hematoma include high level of anticoagulation and continuous use of epidural.[198] Tryba et al.[199] estimated the overall incidence of spinal hematoma to be approximately 1:150,000 after epidural anesthesia and, in the presence of anticoagulation, it is estimated to increase to approximately 1:1,000 to 1:32,500 patients.[200,257]

Initial data in patients receiving neuroaxial anesthesia while receiving prophylactic doses of unfractionated heparin failed to show an increase in the incidence of complications in 5,528 patients.[201] However, the use of LMWH has been correlated with an increase in incidence of hematoma.[202,203] In 1998, after 40 cases of spinal hematoma were reported in 5 years, the Food and Drug Administration (FDA) released a public health advisory that anticoagulation with LMWH or heparinoids for thromboprophylaxis increases risk of developing spinal hematomas.[204] Interestingly, the increased incidence of spinal complications is noted in US patients, but not in European patients. In Europe, patients typically receive a dose of enoxaparin of 20–40 mg once per day, as opposed to US dosing of 30 mg twice per day.[205]

Current recommendations are that LDUH or LMWH and neuroaxial anesthesia can be used concurrently with appropriate caution.[171,206] Dosing guidelines, consideration and precautions are listed in Table 9-6. Currently, the American Society of Regional Anesthesia and Pain Medicine RA do not recommend dosing of fondaparinux with neuraxial anesthesia.

Duration

Although thromoboprophylaxis is traditionally terminated at the time of discharge from the hospital, the risk of DVT and PE continues. Several studies have shown a significant rate of DVT 4–6 weeks after surgery.[207,208] White et al. noted up to 66% of thrombotic events occurred following discharge[209] and Agnelli et al. found that 40% of DVT/PE events occurred more than 21 days after surgery.[210] Bergqvist demonstrated prolonged administration of LMWH significantly reduced the

Table 9-6. Anticoagulation and epidural analgesia

Low dose unfractionated heparin
1. Avoid in patients with underlying intrinsic or acquired coagulopathy
2. Heparin administration should be delayed for 1 h following needle/catheter placement
3. Indwelling catheters should be removed 2–4 h after last heparin dose and after evaluation of coagulation status
4. Resumption of heparin should be delayed 1 h after catheter removal
5. Monitoring of patient postoperatively for early detection of motor block

Additional recommendations for patients treated with low molecular weight heparin
1. Patients on LMWH preoperatively should wait 10–12 h from last dose before needle/catheter insertion
2. Presence of blood during needle or catheter placement does not necessitate postponement of surgery, but LMWH should be delayed for 24 h postoperatively
3. For patients on twice-daily dosing of LMWH, in-dwelling catheter should be removed prior to first dose of LMWH. First dose may be administered 2 h after catheter removal
4. For patients on once daily dosing of LMWH, first dose of LMWH may be administered 6–8 h postoperatively. The catheter should be removed 10–12 h after a dose of LMWH and subsequent dosing should occur minimum of 2 h after removal

Horlocker TT, Wedel DJ, Benzon H, et al. Regional anesthesia in the anticoagulated patient: defining the risks (the second ASRA Consensus Conference on Neuraxial Anesthesia and Anticoagulation). Reg Anesthesia Pain Med. 2003;28:172–197.
LMWH low molecular weight heparin.

Table 9-7. Consensus recommendations of the surgical infection prevention guidelines for colorectal surgery

1. Antibiotic should be received within 1 h of surgical incision
2. Prophylaxis antibiotic should be discontinued within 24 h of surgical completion
3. Proper hair control (no clippers or hair removal)
4. Maintenance of normothermia in colorectal surgery patients

Oral antimicrobial prophylaxis
- Neomycin + erythromycin
- Neomycin + metronidazole

Parental antimicrobial prophylaxis
- Cefotetan, cefoxitan,
- Ampicillin-sulbactam
- Ertapenem
- Or Cefazolin/cefuroxime + metronidazole

Parental antimicrobial prophylaxis with B lactam allergy
- Clindamycin + aminoglycoside
- Clindamycin + quinolone
- Clindamycin + azotrenam
- Or Metronidazole + aminoglycoside
- Metronidazole + fluoroquinolone

Adapted from material prepared by Stratis Health and the Oklahoma Foundation for Medical Quality, the Quality Improvement Organization Support Center for Patient Safety, under contract with the Centers for Medicare & Medicaid Services an agency of the US Department of Health and Human Services. 9SOW-QIOSC-6.2-09-36.

incidence of DVT at 3 weeks and 3 months (12.0 vs. 4.8, $p=0.02$ and 13.8% vs. 5.5% $p=0.01$).[211] A 2009 Cochrane review of four eligible studies noted a decrease in VTE from 1.7 to 0.2% in patients receiving prolonged thromboprophylaxis; the incidence of bleeding complications was slightly but not significantly higher in the treatment groups (3.7 vs. 4.1, $p=0.73$).[212] Based on this data, reviewers concluded that patients should undergo extended thromboprophylaxis for 1 month following surgery. Determination of which patients should receive prolonged therapy and duration of therapy will require further evaluation.

Prophylactic Perioperative Antibiotics

Significant literature has focused on the use of perioperative antibiotics for colorectal surgery. Surgical site infections account for 14–16% of all hospital acquired infection.[213] Although all antibiotics should be based on the presence of infection, culture data, and patient disease, recommendations for type and duration of antibiotics for prophylaxis of infections can now be made.

Prophylaxis is centered on the prevention of surgical wound infections. A 2009 Cochrane review evaluated 50 antibiotics used in over 180 trials and 30,000 patients.[214] Although patients who received antibiotics were less likely to develop surgical wound infections when compared to placebo (RR = 0.30, 95% CI 0.22–0.41), there was no difference for short term versus long term prophylaxis (RR = 1.06, 95% CI 0.89–1.27) or single versus multiple doses (1.17%, 95% CI 0.67–2.05). Additional aerobic and anaerobic coverage reduced the risk of surgical wound infections (RR 0.41 and 0.55) and the use of both oral and intravenous antibiotics was superior to intravenous or oral antibiotics alone. Using these parameters, there was a 75% reduction in surgical wound infections. Further trials to establish timing and dosing were recommended.

Guidelines for perioperative antibiotics have been formalized by the Surgical Care Improvement Project, a partnership of organizations including the Centers of Medicare and Medicaid services (CMS) and US Centers for Disease Control.[215,216] Currently, there are five recommendations relevant to prevention of surgical site infections in colorectal patients (see Table 9-7).[215,216] Antibiotics should be given within a 60 min window of incision and within 2 h when using vancomycin or fluoroquinoles. Ideally, this ensures that antibiotics will be in adequate tissue concentration at the time of incision. Antibiotics given too soon may be eliminated, whereas those given too late will not be therapeutic at time of incision. An increase in preoperative timing intervals was allowed for vancomycin and fluroroquinoles secondary to longer infusion times. Prophylactic antibiotics should be discontinued within 24 h of surgery. Prolongation is costly, promotes bacterial resistance, and is without evidence of benefit to patients. Patients with documented preoperative infections should be treated appropriately and do not fall under these recommendations.

Antibiotic recommendations have been standardized and are listed in Table 9-7. Additional measures to prevent postoperative surgical site infections include appropriate preoperative hair removal, prompt removal of urinary catheters, and immediate postoperative maintenance of normothermia (greater than 96.8°F/36°C) for colorectal patients.[217]

Postoperative Treatment of Adrenal Insufficiency

Glucocorticoids and mineralocorticoids are important in the control of hemostasis including maintenance of blood volume and normal cardiovascular function. In addition to hemodynamic changes, use of chronic steroids may have other perioperative side such as water retention, delayed wound healing, and diabetes.[218] After stress of trauma or surgery, endogenous steroids are increased up to six times from baseline to over 150 mg daily.[219] Patients with adrenal suppression or insufficiency are unable to secrete sufficient corticosteroids.

There are many causes of adrenal insufficiency including primary causes: Addison's disease, tuberculosis, and HIV; or secondary causes such as chronic exogenous administration. In addition to underlying medical illness, patients undergoing colorectal surgery may use steroids chronically as a component of treatment for their primary colorectal disorder; patients with inflammatory bowel disease are often treated acutely with steroids and steroids may be a component of oncologic treatment as well. Patients treated with steroids chronically or with primary steroid deficiencies may suffer from adrenal insufficiency during times of stress, such as surgical intervention. Any patient on doses of 5 mg prednisone for any prolonged period up to 1 year prior to surgery have traditionally been believed to be at risk of postoperative adrenal insufficiency.

In actuality, the occurrence of adrenal insufficiency in the surgical population is quite rare. Current postoperative repletion is based on two anecdotal reports in 1952 and 1953 that led to recommendations that became the standard of care.[220,221] World literature reviews by Salem and Kehlet revealed only three cases of death or hypotension attributable to perioperative adrenal crisis.[222,223] Only two randomized controlled trials, each with small numbers of patients, have results reported. Glowniak and Loriax performed a randomized control trial of 100 mg hydrocortisone versus normal daily dose of glucocorticoids plus placebo in 18 patients with an average baseline daily dose of 7.5 mg of hydrocortisone.[224] One patient in each group experienced hypotension treated with fluid resuscitation. The authors concluded that there were no significant differences between the groups and basal glucorticoid levels were sufficient to counterbalance perioperative stress. The second trial was a randomized crossover study of 20 patients undergoing dental surgery.[225] Patients were randomized to regular dose versus 100 mg hydrocortisone and the authors found no difference in hemodynamic parameters. However, both trials were criticized for limited power and sample size, and the second study was questioned in terms of stress impact of dental surgery in terms of severity of physiologic stress.

Recent systematic reviews of the literature including a 2009 Cochrane review failed to find definitive evidence that preemptive perioperative supraphysiologic dosing of steroids is necessary.[226] The Cochrane review evaluated 37 patients in the two randomized clinical trials and concluded that studies were insufficiently powered to determine whether supplemental steroids were needed. deLange and Kars determined that current perioperative steroids supplementation is not validated by review of the medical literature and recommended continuation of baseline steroids without supplementation until further trials establish further evidence.[227] Marik and Varon concluded that while most patients on exogenous steroids do not require supplementation, there was sufficient evidence to supplement patients with primary hypothalamic pituitary adrenocortical axis failure such as Addison's disease and congenital adrenal hyperplasia.[228] These patients cannot increase steroid hormone production and require 48–72 h of treatment postoperatively following major surgery.

It is important to recognize the signs of adrenal insufficiency because they may occur both in the immediate postoperative period and beyond in the event of a complication. Symptoms may include hypoglycemia, cardiovascular collapse, fatigue, abdominal pain, nausea, and vomiting. In the postoperative patient presenting with a change in intestinal function, steroid withdrawal should be considered in the at-risk population. Stelzer et al. reviewed their 60 steroid-dependent patients who underwent pouch surgery and developed signs and symptoms of a bowel obstruction.[229] They found that 43 had no objective signs of mechanical obstruction and promptly resolved their symptoms within 4 h of steroid administration. At the other extreme of intestinal function, Rai and Hemingway reported on a patient presenting with high ileostomy output responsive to steroids.[230]

Postoperative Analgesia

Analgesia following colon and rectal surgery is of paramount importance in improving patient satisfaction, early ambulation and minimizing sympathetic inhibition postoperatively. Narcotics are used to decrease pain after surgery by crossing the blood–brain barrier and binding to (mu) μ-opioid receptors within the central nervous system. However, a secondary effect of narcotics is stimulation of (mu) μ receptors in the gastrointestinal tract that contribute to inhibition of bowel function postoperatively. Narcotics have been shown to decrease peristaltic activity, delay gastric emptying and play an important role in prolonging postoperative ileus.[231] Cali et al. demonstrated a positive correlation between the amount of morphine used postoperatively and prolonged return of bowel sounds ($r=0.74$, $p=0.001$), time to flatus ($r=0.47$, $p=0.003$) and time to bowel movement ($r=0.48$, $p=0.002$).[232]

The use of epidural analgesia was proposed to minimize systemic narcotics, decrease inflammation, and create sympathetic blockade leading to earlier return of bowel function and decreasing need for narcotics. A randomized trial of epidural analgesia by Liu et al. initially demonstrated that patients receiving local anesthetic plus opioid postoperatively had the best balance of analgesia and return of gastrointestinal function.[233] In 2000, a Cochrane review of eight studies comparing local epidural versus opioid-based regiments concluded patients receiving local anesthetic without narcotic accelerated return of gastrointestinal function with comparable postoperative pain.[234]

More recent data demonstrates equivalency in length of stay and gastrointestinal recovery for patients receiving thoracic epidural analgesia versus intravenous patient controlled analgesia (PCA). A 2001 large multicenter VA study of 1,021 patients demonstrated reduced postoperative pain scores ($p>0.01$) with thoracic epidural but no reduction in length of stay or complications rates.[235] Senagore performed a randomized trial of epidural versus PCA, using identical dietary regimens, and demonstrated similar hospital stays in both groups, 2.3 versus 2.4 days in laparoscopic cases.[236] A 2005 Cochrane review concluded pain scale ratings were higher in the PCA groups, but there was no difference in return of bowel function or length of stay.[237] This is further supported by a recent meta-analysis of 16 studies demonstrating reduced pain scores in the epidural group, slightly decreased time to return of bowel function (weighted mean difference – 1.55 days) but no change in the length of stay.[238]

Notwithstanding the lack of evidence supporting use of epidurals, many centers still use them, particularly in European enhanced recovery pathways. Zutshi noted improved epidural pain scores were not durable; pain scores were reduced at 48 h, but equivocal at discharge.[239] Patients with thoracic epidurals were more likely to experience urinary retention, pruritis, and arterial hypotension postoperatively.[238] Although costs may be lower in patients with thoracic epidurals,[239] difficulty inserting epidurals has been reported in up to 40% of patients.[240] Postoperative reduction of ileus and earlier return of bowel function are effective only with thoracic epidurals using local anesthetic alone without fentanyl,[241,242] and several studies have demonstrated that epidurals should remain in place for 48 h to maximize benefits.[233,243,244] In these cases, continuation of the epidural may prolong hospitalization, especially after laparoscopic resection.[240]

Multiple studies have investigated the use of alternative analgesic regiments to avoid the use of narcotics including ketorolac, diclofenac, and gabapentin. Nonsteroidal anti-inflammatory drugs (NSAIDs) have been shown to reduce interruption of gut motility postoperatively.[245] Ketorolac, at doses of 15–30 mg, has been demonstrated to decrease postoperative pain, the need for narcotics and time to recovery of bowel function after abdominal surgery.[246–248] Schlachta et al. performed a randomized study of patients receiving PCA versus PCA with ketorolac and found patients receiving ketorolac used less narcotics (33 mg vs. 66 mg, $p=0.011$) with improved pain control and were more likely to ambulate, and have earlier return bowel function (2.0 days vs. 3.0 days, $p<0.001$).[249] However, these improvements did not translate into a shorter postoperative length of stay. Chen et al. demonstrated similar improvements in time to bowel movement (1.8 days vs. 2.4 days, $p=0.001$), and patients receiving ketorolac were 5.25 times less likely to have postoperative ileus.[250] Cyclooxygenase-2 inhibitors have been used in postoperative pain management and to promote earlier return of bowel function but cardiac and safety concerns have limited their use in the USA.[251,253] Patients receiving a nonspecific NSAID, diclofenac, have also been shown to have lower use of narcotics postoperatively and may have earlier return of bowel function.[254] Gabapentin is an antiepileptic drug with efficacy in neuropathy, neuralgia, and neuropathic pain has been studied in multiple randomized trials. Although evidence is limited in gastrointestinal surgery, patients undergoing abdominal hysterectomy and mini cholecystectomy had reduced pain scores, opioid consumption, and incidence of nausea after receiving 600 mg of gabapentin 2 h preoperatively.[254–256]

Reducing the use of postoperative narcotics has a role in recovery of bowel function, avoiding postoperative ileus, and reduced length of stay. The use of thoracic epidural appears to reduce postoperative pain but not length of stay. Use of narcotic sparing analgesia such as ketorolac and gabapentin may help improve pain control and reduce the incidence of postoperative ileus.

Conclusion

The care of the postoperative colon and rectal surgery patient has undergone significant changes over the past 20 years. Optimization of perioperative fluids, early ambulation, timing of oral nutrition and gastric stimulation, prophylaxis for VTE, minimization of narcotics, and avoidance of postoperative ileus have led to substantial reductions in length of postoperative stay and improvements in postoperative care. A significant body of literature evaluating and testing various care options is now available. By combining care elements into standardized fast track or enhanced recovery protocols, average length of stay can be reduced without compromising complication or readmission rates. Implementing a fast track protocol requires multidisciplinary teams, with patient and provider education to be truly successful. However, patient care benefits as well as health cost savings may be substantial.[252]

Acknowledgment. This chapter was written by Tracey D. Arnell and Robert W. Beart Jr. in the first edition of this textbook.

References

1. Health Care Financing Administration, Federal Register. http://www.gpoaccess.gov/fr/ (2005). Accessed April 2006.
2. Health Care Financing Administration, Federal Register. http://www.gpoaccess.gov/fr/ (1999–2000). Accessed April 2006
3. Cohen ME, Bilimoria KY, Ko CY, et al. Development of an American College of Surgeons National Surgery Quality Improvement Program: morbidity and mortality risk calculator for colorectal surgery. J Am Coll Surg. 2009;208:1009–16.
4. Visser B, Keegan H, Martin M, et al. Death after colectomy: it's later than we think. Arch Surg. 2009;144:1021–7.
5. Delaney CP, Fazio VW, Senagore AJ, et al. 'Fast track' postoperative management protocol for patients with high comorbidity undergoing complex abdominal and pelvic colorectal surgery. Br J Surg. 2001;88:1533–8.
6. Kehlet H, Wilmore DW. Multimodal strategies to improve surgical outcome. Am J Surg. 2002;183:630–41.
7. Delaney CP. Outcome of discharge within 24 to 72 hours after laparoscopic colorectal surgery. Dis Colon Rectum. 2007;51:181–5.
8. Lassen K, Soop M, Nygen J, et al. Consensus review of optimal perioperative care in colorectal surgery. Arch Surg. 2009;144:961–9.
9. Kehlet H, Morgensen T. Hospital stay of 2 days after open sigmoidectomy with multimodal rehabilitation programme. Br J Surg. 1999;86:227–30.
10. Bardram L, Funch-Jensen P, Jensen P, et al. Recovery after laparoscopic colonic surgery with epidural analagesia, and early oral nutrition and mobilization. Lancet. 1995;345: 763–4.
11. Bradshaw BGG, Liu SS, Thilby RC. Standardized perioperative care protocols and reduced length of stay after colon surgery. J Am Coll Surg. 1998;186:501–6.
12. Lemmens L, van Zelm R, Inkes IB, et al. Clinical and organizational content of clinical pathways for digestive surgery: a systematic review. Dig Surg. 2009;26:91–9.
13. Gouvas N, Tan E, Windsor A, et al. Fast-track vs standard care in colorectal surgery: A meta-analysis update. Int J Colorectal Dis. 2009;24:1119–31.
14. Wind J, Polle SW, Fun Kon Jin PHP, et al. Systematic review of enhanced recovery programs after colonic surgery. Br J Surg. 2006;93:800–9.
15. Basse L, Thorbol JE, Lossl K, Kehlet H. Colonic surgery with accelerated rehabilitation or conventional care. Dis Colon Rectum. 2004;47:271–7.
16. Nygren J, Hausel J, Kehlet H, et al. A comparison of five European Centres of case mix, clinical management and outcomes following either conventional or fast track perioperative care in colorectal surgery. Clin Nutr. 2005;24:455–61.
17. Scattizi M, Kroning KC, Boddi V, et al. Fast track surgery after laparoscopic colorectal surgery; is it feasible in a general surgery unit? Surgery. 2010;147(2):219–26.
18. Polle SW, Wind J, Fuhring JW, et al. Implementation of a fast-track perioperative care program: What are the difficulties? Dig Surg. 2007;24:441–9.
19. Black P. Stoma care nursing management: cost implications in community care. Br J Community Nurs. 2009;14:352–5.
20. Driscoll A. Managing post-discharge care at home: an analysis of patients' and their carer's perceptions of information received during their stay in the hospital. J Adv Nurs. 2000; 31:1165–73.
21. Boughton M, Halliday L. Home alone: patient and carer uncertainty surrounding discharge with continuing clinical needs. Contemp Nurse. 2009;33:30–40.
22. Kehlet H, Wilmore DW. Evidence-based surgical care and the evolution of fast-track surgery. Ann Surg. 2008; 248:189–98.
23. Ionescu D, Iancu C, Ion D, et al. Implementing fast-track protocol for colorectal surgery: a randomized prospective clinical trial. World J Surg. 2009;33:2433–8.
24. Maessen J, Dejong CHC, Hausel J, et al. A protocol is not enough to implement an enhanced recovery programme for colorectal resection. Br J Surg. 2007;94:224–31.
25. Kehlet H, Buchler MW, Beart Jr RW, et al. Care after colonic operation: is it evidence-based? Results from a multinational survey in Europe and the United States. J Am Coll Surg. 2006;202:45–54.
26. Nelson R, Tse B, Edwards S. Systematic review of prophylactic nasogastric decompression after abdominal operations. Br J Surg. 2005;92:673–80.
27. Cheatham ML, Chapman WC, Key SP, et al. A meta-analysis of selective vs routine nasogastric tube decompression after elective laparotomy. Ann Surg. 1995;221:469–71.
28. Manning BJ, Winter DC, McGreal G, et al. Nasogastric intubation causes gastroesophageal reflux in patients undergoing elective laparotomy. Surgery. 2001;130:788–91.
29. Pritts TA, Nussbaum MS, Flesch LV, et al. Implementation of a clinical pathway decreases length of stay and cost for bowel resection. Ann Surg. 1999;230:728–33.
30. Stephen AE, Berger DL. Shortened length of stay and hospital cost reduction with implementation of an accelerated clinical care pathway after elective colon resection. Surgery. 2003;133:277–82.
31. Kariv Y, Delaney CP, Senagore AJ, et al. Clinical outcomes and cost analysis of a 'fast track' postoperative care pathway for ileal pouch-anal anastomosis: a case-control study. Dis Colon Rectum. 2007;50:137–46.
32. Arkilic CF, Taguchi A, Sharma N, et al. Supplemental perioperative fluid administration increases tissue oxygen pressure. Surgery. 2003;133:49–55.
33. Rosenthal MH. Intraoperative fluid management – what and how much? Chest. 1999;115:1065–125.
34. Shires T, Williams J, Brown F. Acute change in extracellular fluids associated with major surgical Procedures. Ann Surg. 1961;154:803–10.
35. Lobo DN, Bostock KA, Neal KR, et al. Effect of salt and water balance on recovery of gastrointestinal function after elective colonic resection: a randomized control trial. Lancet. 2002;359:1812–8.
36. Hannemann P, Lassen K, Hausel J, et al. Patterns in current anaesthesiological peri-operative practice for colonic resections: a survey in five northern European countries. Acta Anaesthesiol Scand. 2006;50:1152–60.
37. Mecray PM, Barden RP, Ravdin IS. Nutritional edema its effect on the gastric emptying time before and after gastric operations. Surgery. 1937;1:53–64.
38. Barden RP, Thompson WD, Ravdin IS, et al. The influence of serum protein on the motility of the small intestine. Surg Gynecol Obstet. 1938;66:819–21.

39. Holte K, Foss NB, Svensen C, et al. Epidural anesthesia, hypotension, and changes in intravascular volume. Anesthesiology. 2004;100:281–6.
40. Brandstrup B, Tonnesen H, Beier-Holgersen R, et al. Effects of intravenous fluid restriction on postoperative complications: Comparison of two perioperative fluid regimens: a randomized assessor-blinded multicenter trial. Ann Surg. 2003;238:641–8.
41. Nisanevich V, Felsenstein I, Almogy G, et al. Effect of intraoperative fluid management on outcome after intraabdominal surgery. Anesthesiology. 2005;103:25–32.
42. Kabon B, Akca O, Taguchi A, et al. Supplemental intravenous crystalloid administration does not reduce the risk of surgical wound infection. Anesth Analg. 2005;101:1546–53.
43. MacKay G, Fearon K, McConnachie A. Randomized clinical trial of the effect of postoperative intravenous fluid resuscitation on recovery after colorectal surgery. Br J Surg. 2006;93:1469–74.
44. Bungaard-Nielsen M, Scher NH, Kehlet H. 'Liberal' vs 'Restrictive perioperative fluid therapy – a critical assessment of the literature. Acta Anaethsiol Scand. 2009;53:843–51.
45. Rivers E, Nguyen B, Havstad S, et al. Early goal-directed therapy in the treatment of severe sepsis and septic shock. N Engl J Med. 2001;345:1368–77.
46. Connors AF, Speroff T, Dawson NV, et al. The effectiveness of right heart catherization in the initial care of critically ill patients. JAMA. 1996;276:889–97.
47. Conway DH, Mayall R, Abdul-Latif MS, et al. Randomized controlled trial investigating the influence of intravenous fluid titration using oesophageal monitoring during bowel surgery. Anaesthesia. 2002;57:845–9.
48. Gan TJ, Soppitt A, Maroof M, et al. Goal-directed intraoperative fluid administration reduces length of hospital stay after major surgery. Anaesthesiology. 2002;97:820–6.
49. Noblett SE, Snowden CP, Shenton BK, et al. Randomized clinical trial assessing the effect of Doppler-optimized fluid management on outcome for elective colorectal resection. Br J Surg. 2006;93:1069–76.
50. Wakeling HG, McFall MR, Jenkins CS, et al. Intraoperative oesophageal Doppler guided fluid management shortens postoperative hospital stay after major bowel surgery. Br J Anaesth. 2005;95:634–42.
51. Senagore AJ, Emery T, Luchtefeld M, et al. Fluid management for laparoscopic colectomy: a prospective randomized assessment of goal-directed administration of balanced salt solution or hetastarch coupled with enhanced recovery program. Dis Colon Rectum. 2009;52:1935–40.
52. Abbas SM, Hill AG. Systematic review of the literature for the use of oesophageal Doppler monitor for fluid replacement in major abdominal surgery. Anaesthesia. 2008;63:44–51.
53. Rahbari NN, Zimermann JB, Schmidt T, et al. Meta-analysis of standard, restrictive and supplemental fluid administration in colorectal surgery. Br J Surg. 2009;96:331–41.
54. Lerman J. Surgical and patient factors involved in postoperative nausea and vomiting. Br J Anaesth. 1992;69 Suppl 1:S24–32.
55. Apfel CC, Laara E, Koivuranta M, et al. A simplified risk score for predicting postoperative nausea and vomiting. Anesthesiology. 1999;91:693–700.
56. Gan TJ, Meyer T, Apfel CC, et al. Consensus guidelines for managing postoperative nausea and vomiting. Anesth Analg. 2003;97:62–71.
57. Eberhart LHJ, Hogel J, Seeling W, et al. Evaluation of three risk scores to predict postoperative nausea and vomiting. Acta Anesthesiol Scand. 2000;44:480–8.
58. Apfel CC, Kranke P, Eberhart LH, et al. Comparison of predictive models of postoperative nausea and vomiting. Br J Anaesth. 2002;88:234–40.
59. Koivuranta M, Laara E, Snare L, Alahuhta S. A survey of postoperative nausea and vomiting. Anaesthesia. 1997;52:443–9.
60. Tramer M, Moore A, McQuay H. Metaanalytic comparison of prophylactic antiemetic efficacy for postoperative nausea and vomiting: propofol anaesthesia vs. omitting nitrous oxide vs total IV anaesthesia with propofol. Br J Anaesth. 1997;78:256–9.
61. Apfel CC, Katz MH, Kranke P, et al. Volatile anaesthetics may be the main cause of early but not delayed postoperative vomiting: a randomized controlled trial of factorial design. B J Anesth. 2002;88:659–68.
62. Greif R, Laciny S, Rapf B, et al. Supplemental oxygen reduces the incidence of postoperative nausea and vomiting. Anesthesiology. 1999;91:1246–52.
63. Tramer MR, Reynolds DJM, Moore RA, McQuay HJ. Efficacy, dose-response, and safety of ondansetron in prevention of postoperative nausea and vomiting: a qualitative systematic review of randomized placebo-controlled trials. Anesthesiology. 1997;87:1277–89.
64. Graczyk SG, McKenzie R, Kallar S, et al. Intravenous dolasetron for the prevention of postoperative nausea and vomiting after outpatient laparoscopic gynecologic surgery. Anesth Analg. 1997;84:325–30.
65. Wang JJ, Ho ST, Tzeng JI, Tang CS. The effect of timing of dexamethasone administration on its efficacy as a prophylactic antiemetic for postoperative nausea and vomiting. Anesth Analg. 2000;91:136–9.
66. Henzi I, Walder B, Tramer MR. Dexamethasome for the prevention of postoperative nausea and vomiting: a quantitative systemic review. Anesth Analg. 1997;85:652–6.
67. Tramer M. A rational approach to the control of postoperative nausea and vomiting: evidence from systemic reviews. II Recommendations for prevention and treatment and research agenda. Acta Anaesthesiol Scand. 2001;45:14–9.
68. FDA strengthens warnings for droperidol. http://www.fda.gov/bbs/topics/ANSWERS/2001/ANS01123.html (2009). Accessed December 2009.
69. Chen JJ, Frame DG, White TJ. Efficacy of ondansetron and prochlorperazine for the prevention of postoperative nausea and vomiting after total hip replacement or total knee replacement procedures. Arch Intern Med. 1998;158:2124–8.
70. Kranke P, Morin AM, Roewer N, et al. The efficacy and safety of transdermal scopolamine for the prevention of postoperative nausea and vomiting: a quantitative systematic review. Anesth Analg. 2002;95:133–43.
71. Wilhelm SM, Dehoorne-Smith ML, Kale-Pradhan PB. Prevention of postoperative nausea and vomiting. Ann Pharmacother. 2006;40:66–78.
72. Domino KB, Anderson EA, Polissar NL, Posner KL. Comparative efficacy and safety of ondansetron, droperidol, and metoclopramide for preventing postoperative nausea and vomiting: a meta-analysis. Anesth Analg. 1999;88:1370–9.
73. Patterson D, Abell T, Rothstein R, et al. A double-blind multicenter comparison of droperidol and metoclopramide in the

treatment of diabetic patients with symptoms of gastroparesis. Am J Gastroenterol. 1999;94:1230–4.

74. Fan C, Tanhui E, Joshi S, et al. Acupressure treatment for prevention of postoperative nausea and vomiting. Anesth Analg. 1997;84:821–5.
75. White PF, Issioui T, Hu J, et al. Comparative efficacy of acustimulation (Relief Band) versus ondansetron (Zofran) in combination with droperidol for preventing nausea and vomiting. Anesthesiology. 2002;97:1075–81.
76. Ernst E, Pittler MH. Efficacy of ginger for nausea and vomiting: a systematic review of randomized clinical trials. Br J Anaesth. 2000;84:367–71.
77. Eberhart LH, Mayer R, Betz O, et al. Ginger does not prevent postoperative nausea and vomiting after laparoscopic surgery. Anesth Analg. 2003;96:995–8.
78. Anderson LA, Gross JB. Aromatherapy with peppermint, isopropyl alcohol, or placebo is equally effective in relieving postoperative nausea. J Perianesth Nurs. 2004;19:29–35.
79. Gan TJ. Risk factors for postoperative nausea and vomiting. Anesth Analg. 2006;102:1884–98.
80. Hill RP, Lubarsky DA, Phillips-Bute B, et al. Cost-effectiveness of prophylactic antiemetic therapy with ondansetron, droperidol, or placebo. Anesthesiology. 2000;92:958–67.
81. Frighetto L, Loewen PS, Dolman J, Marra CA. Cost-effectiveness of prophylactic dolasetron or droperidol vs. rescue therapy in the prevention of PONV in ambulatory gynecologic surgery. Can J Anaesth. 1999;46:536–43.
82. Watcha MF, Smith I. Cost-effectiveness analysis of antiemetic therapy for ambulatory surgery. J Clin Anesth. 1994;6:370–7.
83. Levine M. A new gastroduodenal catheter. JAMA. 1921; 76:1007.
84. Tinkler L. Nasogastric tube management. Br J Surg. 1972;59:637–41.
85. Nathan BN, Pain JA. Nasogastric suction after elective abdominal surgery: a randomized study. Ann R Coll Surg Engl. 1991;73:291–4.
86. Wolff BG, Pemberton JH, Van Heerden JA, et al. Elective colon and rectal surgery without nasogastric decompression. Ann Surg. 1987;154:640–2.
87. Cheatham ML, Chapman WC, Sp K, et al. A meta-analysis of selective vs routine nasogastric tube decompression after elective laparotomy. Ann Surg. 1995;221:469–71.
88. Phillips EH, Franklin M, Carroll BJ, et al. Laparoscopic colectomy. Ann Surg. 1992;216:703–7.
89. Jacobs M, Verdeja GD, Goldstein DS. Minimally invasive colon resection (laparoscopic colectomy). Surg Laparosc Endosc. 1991;1:144–50.
90. Resissman P, Teoh TA, Cohen SM, et al. Is early oral feeding safe after elective colorectal surgery? Ann Surg. 1995;222:73–7.
91. Carr CS, Ling KDE, Boulos P, et al. Randomized trial of safety and efficacy of immediate postoperative enteral feeding in patients undergoing gastrointestinal resection. Br Med J. 1996;312:869–71.
92. Lewis SJ, Egger M, Sylvester PA. Early enteric feeding versus nil by mouth after gastrointestinal surgery; systematic review and meta-analysis of controlled trials. Br Med J. 2001;323:1–5.
93. Andersen HK, Lewis SJ, Thomas S. Early enteral nutrition within 24h of colorectal surgery versus later commencement of feeding for postoperative complications. Cochrane Database Syst Rev 2009;CD004080.
94. Thorell A, Hygren J, Lungquist O. Insulin resistance – a marker of surgical stress. Curr Opin Clin Nutr Metab Care. 1999;2:69–78.
95. Maltby JR, Sutherland AD, Sale JP, Shaffer EA. Preoperative oral fluids: is a five-hour fast justified prior to elective surgery? Anaesth Analg. 1986;65:1112–6.
96. Splinter WM, Schaeffer JD. Unlimited clear fluid ingestion two hours before surgery in children does not affect volume or pH of stomach contents. Anaesth Intensive Care. 1990;18:522–6.
97. Nygren J, Thorell A, Lagerkranser M, et al. Safety and patient well-being after preoperative intake of carbohydrate rich beverage. Clin Nutr. 1996;15S:30.
98. Yuill K, Richardson R, Davidson I, et al. Oral administration of carbohydrate fluids prior to major elective surgery. Br J Surg. 2002;89:92.
99. Ljungqvist O, Nygren J, Thorell A, et al. Preoperative nutrition – elective surgery in the fed or the overnight fasted state. Clin Nutr. 2001;20S:167–71.
100. Hofman Z, van Drunen J, Yuill K, et al. Tolerance and efficacy of immediate pre-operative carbohydrate feeding in uncomplicated elective surgery patients. Clin Nutr. 2001;20S:21.
101. Delaney CP, Kehlet H, Senagore AJ, et al. Clinical consensus update: postoperative ileus: profiles, risk factors and definitions – a framework for optimizing surgical outcomes inpatients undergoing major abdominal and colorectal surgery. Pharmatecture, LLC. http://www.clinicalwebcasts.com/pdfs/GenSurg_WEB.pdf (2006). Accessed 2006.
102. Luckey A, Livingston E, Taché Y. Mechanisms and treatment of postoperative ileus. Arch Surg. 2003;138:206–14.
103. Livingston EH, Passaro Jr EP. Postoperative Ileus. Dig Dis Sci. 1990;35:121–32.
104. Delaney CP, Senagore AJ, Viscusi ER, et al. Postoperative upper and lower gastrointestinal recovery and gastrointestinal morbidity in patients undergoing bowel resection: pooled analysis of placebo data from 3 randomized controlled trials. Am J Surg. 2006;191:315–9.
105. Yeh YC, Klinger EV, Reddy P. Pharmacologic options to prevent postoperative ileus. Ann Pharmacother. 2009;43:1474–85.
106. Zeinali F, Stulbeg JJ, Delaney CP. Pharmacological management of postoperative ileus. Can J Surg. 2009;52:153–7.
107. Abrahamsson H, Lyrenas E, Dotevall G. Effects of beta-adrenoreceptor blocking drugs on human sigmoid colon motility. Dig Dis Sci. 1983;28:590–4.
108. Ferrazz AA, Wanderly GJ, Santos MA, et al. Effects of propranolol on human postoperative ileus. Dig Surg. 2001;18:305–10.
109. Holte K, Kehlet H. Postoperative ileus: progress towards effective management. Drugs. 2002;62:2603–15.
110. Food and Drug Administration. Withdrawal of troglitazone and cisapride. JAMA. 2000;283:2228.
111. Breivik H, Lind B. Anti-emetic and propulsive peristaltic properties of metoclopramide. Br J Anesth. 1971;43:400–3.
112. Kivalo I, Miettienen K. The effects of metoclopramide on postoperative nausea and bowel function. Ann Chirug Gynaecol Fenn. 1970;59:155–8.
113. Tollesson PO, Cassuto J, Faxen A, et al. Lack of effect of metoclopramide on colonic motility after cholecystectomy. Eur J Surg. 1991;157:355–8.
114. Jepsen S, Klaerke A, Nielsen PH, et al. Negative effect of metoclopramide in postoperative adynamic ileus. Br J Surg. 1986;73:290–1.

115. Cheape JD, Wexner SD, James K, et al. Does metoclopramide reduce the length of ileus after colorectal surgery? A prospective randomized trial. Dis Colon Rectum. 1991;34:437–41.
116. Yuan CS, Foss JF, O'Conno M, et al. Methylnaltrexone for reversal of constipation due to chronic methadone use: a randomized controlled trial. JAMA. 2000;283:367–72.
117. Vicusi E, Rathmell J, Fichera A, et al. A double-blind randomized, placebo controlled trial of methylnaltrexone for postoperative bowel dysfunction in segmental colectomy. Proc Am Soc Anesth. 2005;103:A893 (Abstract).
118. Taguchi A, Sharma N, Saleem RM, et al. Selective postoperative inhibition of gastrointestinal opioid receptors. N Engl J Med. 2001;345:935–40.
119. Delaney CP, Weese JL, Hyman NH, et al. Phase III trial of alvimopan: a novel peripherally acting, mu opioid antagonist, for postoperative ileus after major abdominal surgery. Dis Colon Rectum. 2005;48:1114–29.
120. Wolff BG, Michelassi F, Gerkin TM, et al. Alvimopan, a novel peripherally acting mu opioid antagonist. Ann Surg. 2004;240:728–35.
121. Buchler MW, Seilte CM, Monson JRT, et al. Clinical trial: Alvimopan for the management of post-operative ileus after abdominal surgery: results of an international randomized, double-blind, multicenter, placebo-controlled clinical study. Aliment Pharmacol Ther. 2008;28:312–25.
122. Delaney CP, Wolff B, Viscusi E, et al. Alvimopan, for postoperative ileus following bowel resection: a pooled analysis of phase III studies. Ann Surg. 2007;245:355–63.
123. Senagore A, Bauer J, Du W, et al. Alvimopan accelerates gastrointestinal recovery after bowel resection regardless of age, gender, race or concommitant medication use. Surgery. 2007;142:478–86.
124. Tan EK, Cornish J, Darzi AW, et al. Meta-analysis: Alvimopan vs. placebo in the treatment of postoperative ileus. Aliment Pharmacol Ther. 2006;25:47–57.
125. Herzog T, Coleman R, Guerrieri J, et al. A double blind randomized placebo-controlled phase III study of the safety of alvimopan in patients who undergo simple total abdominal hysterectomy. Am J Obstet Gynecol. 2006;195:445–53.
126. Marderstein EL, Delaney CP. Management of postoperative ileus: focus on alvimopan. Ther Clin Risk Manag. 2008;4:965–73.
127. Bell TJ, Poston SA, Kraft MD, et al. Economic analysis of alvimopan in North American phase III efficacy trials. Am J Health Syst Pharm. 2009;66:1362–8.
128. Soffer EE, Adrian TE. Effect of meal composition and sham feeding on duodenojejunal motility in humans. Dig Dis Sci. 1992;37:1009–14.
129. Stern RM, Crawford HE, Steward WR, et al. Sham feeding. Cephalic-vagal influences on gastric myoelectric activit. Dig Dis Sci. 1989;34:521–7.
130. Stewart BT, Woods RJ, Collopy NT. Early feeding after elective open colorectal resections: a prospective randomized trial. Aust N Z J Surg. 1998;68:125–8.
131. Asao T, Kuwano H, Nakamura J, et al. Gum chewing enhances early recovery from postoperative ileus after laparoscopic colectomy. J Am Coll Surg. 2002;195:30–2.
132. McCormick JT, Garvin R, Cuashaj P, et al. The effects of gum-chewing in bowel function and hospital stay after laparoscopic vs open colectomy: a multi-institutional prospective randomized trial. J Am Coll Surg. 2005;201:s66–7.
133. Schuster R, Grewal N, Greaney GC, et al. Gum chewing reduces ileus after elective open sigmoid colectomy. Arch Surg. 2006;141:174–9.
134. Quah HM, Samad A, Neathey AJ, et al. Does gum chewing reduce postoperative ileus following open colectomy for left-sided colon and rectal cancer? – a prospective randomized controlled trial. Colorectal Dis. 2006;8:64–70.
135. Matros E, Rocha F, Zinner M, et al. Does gum chewing ameiliorate postoperative ileus? Results of a prospective randomized placebo controlled trial. J Am Coll Surg. 2006;202:773–8.
136. De Castro SMM, van der Esschert JW, van Heek NT, et al. A Systematic review of the efficacy of gum chewing for the amelioration of postoperative ileus. Dig Surg. 2008;25:39–45.
137. Purkayastha S, Tileny HS, Darzi AW, et al. Meta-analysis of randomized studies evaluating chewing gum to enhance postoperative recovery following colectomy. Arch Surg. 2008;143:788–93.
138. Noble EJ, Harris R, Hoise KB, et al. Gum chewing reduces postoperative ileus? A systematic review and meta-analysis. Int J Surg. 2009;7:100–5.
139. Vasquez W, Hernandez AV, Garcia-Sabrido J. Is gum chewing useful for ileus after elective colorectal surgery? A systematic review and meta-analysis of randomized clinical trials. J Gastrointest Surg. 2009;13:649–56.
140. Fitzgerald JEF, Ahmed I. Systematic review and meta-analysis of chewing gum therapy in the reduction of post-operative paralytic ileus following gastrointestinal surgery. World J Surg. 2009;33(21):2557–66.
141. Kouba EJ, Wallen EM, Pruthi RS. Gum chewing stimulates bowel motility in patients undergoing radical cystectomy with urinary diversion. Urology. 2007;70:1053–6.
142. McDowell E. Three cases of extirpation of diseased ovaria. Eclectic Repertory Anal Rev. 1817;7:242–4.
143. Brieger GH. Early ambulation: a study in the history of surgery. Ann Surg. 1983;197:443–9.
144. Leithauser DJ, Bergo HL. Early rising and ambulatory activity after operation. Arch Surg. 1941;42:108–1093.
145. Leithauser DJ. Early ambulation. Am J Nurs. 1950;50:203–6.
146. Waldenhausen JHT, Schirmer BD. Effect of ambulation of recovery from postoperative ileus. Ann Surg. 2009; 212:671–7.
147. Maessen J, Dejong CHC, Hausel J, et al. A protocol is not enough to implement an enhanced recovery programme for colorectal resection. Br J Surg. 2006;94:224–31.
148. Lin JH, Whelan RL, Sakellarios NE, et al. Prospective study of ambulation after open and laparoscopic colorectal resection. Surg Innov. 2009;16:16–20.
149. Zutshi M, Delaney CP, Senagore AJ, et al. Shorter hospital stay associated with fast track postoperative care pathways and laparoscopic intestinal resection are not associated with increased physical activity. Colorect Dis. 2004;6:477–80.
150. Bauer AJ, Boeckxstaens GE. Mechanisms of postoperative ileus. Neurogastroenterol Motil. 2004;16 Suppl 2:54–60.
151. Jesus EC, Karliczek A, Matos D, et al. Prophylactic anastomotic drainage for colorectal surgery. Cochrane Database Syst Rev 2004;CD0021000.
152. Yeh CY, Changchien C, Wang JY, et al. Pelvic drainage and other risk factors for leakage after elective anterior resection in rectal cancer patients: a prospective study of 978 patients. Ann Surg. 2005;241:9–13.

153. Bardam L, Funch-Jensen P, Jensen P, et al. Recovery after laparoscopic colonic surgery with epidural analgesia, and early oral nutrition and mobilization. Lancet. 1995;345:763–4.
154. Churchill ED, McNeill D. The reduction in vital capacity following operation. Surg Gynecol Obstet. 1927;44:483–8.
155. Von Ungern-Sternberg BS, Regli A, Reber A, et al. Comparison of perioperative spirometric data following spinal or general anaesthesia in normal-weight and overweight gynaecological patients. Acta Anaesthesiol Scand. 2005;49:940–8.
156. Kanat F, Golcuk A, Teke T, et al. Risk factors for postoperative pulmonary complications in upper abdominal surgery. ANZ J Surg. 2007;77:135–41.
157. Canet J, Mazo V. Postoperative pulmonary complications. Minerva Anestesiol. 2009;75:1–5.
158. Milsom JW, Bohm B, Hammerhofer KA, et al. A prospective, randomized trial comparing laparoscopic versus conventional in colorectal cancer surgery: a preliminary report. J Am Coll Surg. 1998;187:46–54.
159. Schwenk W, Bohm C, Witt C. Pulmonary function following laparoscopic or conventional colorectal resection a randomized controlled evaluation. Arch Surg. 1999;134:6–12.
160. Stage JG, Schulze S, Moller P, Overgaard H, Anderson M, Rebsdorf-Pedersen VB, et al. Prospective randomized study of laparoscopic versus open colonic resection for adenocarcinoma. Br J Surg. 1997;84:391–6.
161. Vignali A, Braga M, Zuliana W, et al. Laparoscopic colorectal surgery modifies risk factors for postoperative morbidity. Dis Colon Rectum. 2004;47:1686–93.
162. Guller U, Jain N, Hevey S, et al. Laparoscopic vs open colectomy: outcomes comparison based on large nationwide databases. Arch Surg. 2003;138:1179–86.
163. Young ANS, JM SMJ. Meta-analysis of short-term outcomes after laparoscopic resection for colorectal surgery. Br J Surg. 2004;91:1111–24.
164. Lawrence VA, Cornell JE, Smetana GW. Strategies to reduce postoperative pulmonary complications after noncardiothoracic surgery: systematic review of the American College of Physicians. Ann Intern Med. 2006;144:596–608.
165. Qaseem A, Snow V, Fitterman N, et al. Risk Assessment for Strategies to reduce perioperative pulmonary complications for patients undergoing noncardiothoracic surgery: a guideline from the American College of Physicians. Ann Intern Med. 2006;144:575–80.
166. Moller AM, Villebro N, Pedersen T, et al. Effect of postoperative smoking intervention on postoperative complications: a randomized clinical trial. Lancet. 2002;359:114–7.
167. Bluman LG, Mosca L, Newman N, et al. Preoperative Smoking habits and postoperative pulmonary complications. Chest. 1998;113:883–9.
168. Geerts WH, Heit JA, Clagett GP, et al. Prevention of venous thromboembolism. Chest. 2001;119:132S–75.
169. Lindblad B, Eriksson A, Bergqvist D. Autopsy-verified pulmonary embolism in a surgical department: analysis of the period from 1951 to 1968. Br J Surg. 1991;78:849–52.
170. Sandler DA, Martin JF. Autopsy proven pulmonary embolism in hospital patients: are we detecting enough deep vein thrombosis? J R Soc Med. 1989;82:203–5.
171. Geerts WH, Bergqvist D, Pineo GF, et al. Prevention of venous thromboembolism. Chest. 2008;133:381S–453.
172. Second Thromboembolic Risk Factors (THRiFT II) Consensus Group. Risk of and prophylaxis for venous thromboembolism in hospital patients. Phlebology. 1998;13:87–97.
173. Sullivan SD, Kahn SR, Davidson BL, et al. Measuring the outcomes and pharmacoeconomic consequences of venous thromboembolism prophylaxis in major orthopaedic surgery. Pharmacoeconomics. 2003;21:477–96.
174. Camerota AJ, Chouhan V, Harada RN, et al. The fibrinolytic effects of intermittent pneumatic compression: mechanism of enhanced fibrinolysis. Ann Surg. 1997;226:306–13.
175. Practice parameters for the prevention of venous thromboembolism. The standards task force of the american society of colon and rectal surgeons. Dis Colon Rectum. 2000;43(8):1037–47.
176. Coe NP, Collins RE, Klein LA, et al. Prevention of deep vein thrombosis in urological patients: a controlled, randomized trial of low-dose heparin and external pneumatic compression boots. Surgery. 1978;83:230–4.
177. Agu O, Hamilton G, Baker D. Graduated compression stockings in the prevention of venous thromboembolism. Br J Surg. 1999;86:992–1004.
178. Amarigiri SV, Lees TA. Elastic compression stockings for prevention of deep vein thrombosis. Cochrane Database Syst Rev 2000;(3):CD001484
179. Haddad FS, Kerry RM, McEwen JA, et al. Unanticipated variations between expected and delivered pneumatic compression therapy after elective hip surgery: a possible source of variation in reported patient outcomes. J Arthroplasty. 2001;16:37–46.
180. Cornwell EE, Chang D, Velmahos G, et al. Compliance with sequential compression device prophylaxis in at-risk trauma patients: a prospective analysis. Am Surg. 2002;68:470–3.
181. Best AJ, Williams S, Crozier A, Bhatt R, Gregg PJ, Hui AC. Graded compression stockings in elective orthopedic surgery. An assessment of the in vivo performance of commercially available stockings in patients having hip and knee arthroplasty. J Bone Joint Surg Br. 2000;82:116–8.
182. Heath DI, Kent SJ, Johns DL, et al. Arterial thrombosis associated with graduated pressure antiembolic stockings. BMJ. 1987;295:580.
183. Merrett ND, Hanel KC. Ischaemic complications of graduated compression stockings in the treatment of deep venous thrombosis. Postgrad Med J. 1993;69:232–4.
184. Wille-Jorgensen P. Prophylaxis of postoperative thromboembolism with a combination of heparin and graduated compression stockings. Int Angiol. 1996;15(suppl):15–20.
185. Butterfield WJ, Hicks BH, Ambler AR, et al. Effect of aspirin on postoperative venous thrombosis. Lancet. 1972;2:441–5.
186. Gent M, Hirsh J, Ginsberg JS, et al. Low-molecular-weight heparin is more effective than aspirin in the prevention of venous thromboembolism after surgery for hip fracture. Circulation. 1996;93:80–4.
187. Collins R, Scrimgeour A, Yusuf S. Reduction in fatal pulmonary embolism and venous thrombosis by perioperative administration of subcutaneous heparin: overview of results of randomized trials in general, orthopedic, and urologic surgery. N Engl J Med. 1988;318:1162–73.
188. Clagett GP, Reisch JS. Prevention of venous thromboembolism in general surgical patients: results of meta-analysis. Ann Surg. 1988;208:227–40.

189. Simmons ED. Antithrombotic therapy. In: Bongard FS, Sue DY, editors. Current critical care diagnosis and treatment. 2nd ed. New York: McGraw Hill; 2002. p. 905–24.
190. Warkentin TE, Levine MN, Hirsh J, et al. Heparin-induced thrombocytopenia in patients treated with low-molecular weight heparin or unfractionated heparin. N Engl J Med. 1995;332:1330–5.
191. Mismetti P, Laporte S, Darmon JY, Buchmuller A, Decousus H. Meta-analysis of low molecular weight heparin in the prevention of venous thromboembolism in general surgery. Br J Surg. 2001;88:913–30.
192. Kakkar VV, Boeckl O, Boneu B, et al. Efficacy and safety of a low-molecular-weight heparin and standard unfractionated heparin for prophylaxis of postoperative venous thromboembolism. European multicenter trial. World J Surg. 1997;2:2–8.
193. McLeod RS, Geerts WH, Sniderman KW, et al. Subcutaneous heparin versus low-molecular-weight heparin as thromboprophylaxis in patients undergoing colorectal surgery: results of the Canadian colorectal DVT prophylaxis trial: a randomized, double-blind trial. Ann Surg. 2001;233:438–44.
194. National Institute for Health and Clinical Excellence. Reducing the risk of venous thromboembolism (deep vein thrombosis and pulmonary embolism) in inpatients undergoing surgery. NICE clinical guideline No. 46:1–160. http://www.nice.org.uk/CG046 (2008). Accessed March 31, 2008.
195. Agnelli G, Bergqvist D, Cohen AT, et al. Randomized clinical trial of postoperative fondaparinux versus perioperative dalteparin for prevention of venous thromboembolism in high-risk abdominal surgery. Br J Surg. 2005;92:1212–20.
196. Turpie AG, Bauer KA, Caprini JA, et al. Fondaparinux combined with intermittent pneumatic compression versus intermittent pneumatic compression alone for prevention of venous thromboembolism after abdominal surgery: a randomized, double-blind comparison. J Thromb Haemost. 2007;5:1854–61.
197. Bergqvist D. Review of fondaparinux sodium injection for the prevention of venous thromboembolism. Vasc Health Risk Manag. 2006;2:365–70.
198. Vandermeulen E. Is anticoagulation and central neural blockade a safe combination? Curr Opin Anaesthesiol. 1999;69: 407–11.
199. Tryba M. Epidural regional anesthesia and low molecular heparin. Anästhesiol Intensivmed Notfallmed Schmerzther. 1993;28:179–81.
200. Stafford-Smith M. Impaired haemostasis and regional anaesthesia. Can J Anaesth. 1996;43:R129–41.
201. Schwander D, Bachmann F. Heparin and spinal or epidural anaesthesia: clinical decision making. Ann Fr Anesth Rèanim. 1991;10:284–96.
202. Horlocker TT, Heit JA. Low molecular weight heparin: biochemistry, pharmacology, perioperative prophylaxis regimens, and guidelines for regional anesthetic management. Anesth Analg. 1997;85:874–88.
203. Tryba M, Wedel DJ. Central neuraxial block and low molecular weight heparin (enoxaparin) – lessons learned from different dosage regimens in two continents. Acta Anaesthesiol Scand. 1997;42:99–103.
204. www.accessdata.fda.gov/drugsatfda_docs/label/2009/020164s083lbl.pdf. 2009. Accessed December 2009.
205. Checketts MR, Wildsmith JAW. Editorial II. Central nerve block and thromboprophylaxis – is there a problem? Br J Anaesth. 1999;82:164–7.
206. American Society of Regional Anesthesia and Pain Medicine Second Consensus Conference of Neuraxial Anesthesia and Anticoagulation. http://www.asra.com/consensus-statements/2.html (2002). Accessed December 2009.
207. Scurr JH, Colerigde-Smith PD, Hasty JH. Deep venous thrombosis: a continuing problem. Br Med J. 1998;297:28.
208. Clarke-Pearson DL, Sunan IS, Hinshaw WM, et al. Prevention of postoperative venous thromboembolism by external pneumatic calf compression in patients with gynecologic malignancy. Obstet Gynecol. 1984;63:92–8.
209. White RH, Romano PS, Zhou H. A population-based comparison of the 3 month incidence of thromboembolism after major elective/urgent surgery. Thromb Haemost. 2001;86:2255.
210. Agnelli G, Boli G, Capussotti L, et al. A clinical outcome based prospective study on venous thromboembolism after cancer surgery. Ann Surg. 2006;243:89–95.
211. Bergqvist D, Agnelli G, Cohen AT, et al. Duration of prophylaxis against venous thromboembolism with enoxaparin after surgery for cancer. N Engl J Med. 2002;346:975–80.
212. Rasmussen MS, Jorgensen LN, Wille-Jorgensen P. Prolonged thromboprophylaxis with low molecular weight heparin for abdominal or pelvic surgery. Cochrane Database Syst Rev 2009;1:CD004318.
213. 2009. http://www.qualitynet.org/dcs. Accessed December 2009.
214. Nelson RL, Glenny AM, Song F. Antimicrobial prophylaxis for colorectal surgery. Cochrane Database Syst Rev 2009;CD001181.
215. Bratzler DW, Hunt DR. The Surgical infection prevention and surgical care improvement projects: National initiatives to improve outcomes for patients having surgery. Clin Infect Dis. 2006;43:322–30.
216. Fry DE. Surgical site infections and the surgical care improvement project (SCIP): evolution of national quality measures. Surg Infect. 2008;9:579–84.
217. Specifications Manual for National Hospital Inpatient Quality Measures Discharges 04-01-10 (2Q10) through 09-30-10 (3Q10). Accessed December 2009.
218. Schalghecke R, Kornely E, Satern R, et al. The effect of long-term glucocorticoid therapy on pituitary-adrenal responses to exogenous corticotrophin-releasing hormone. N Engl J Med. 1992;326:226–30.
219. Cooper MS, Stewart PM. Corticosteroid insufficiency in acutely ill patients. N Engl J Med. 2003;348:727–34.
220. Frasier CG, Preuss FS, Bigford WD. Adrenal atrophy and irreversible shock associated with cortisone therapy. J Am Med Assoc. 1952;149:1542–3.
221. Lewis L, Robinson RF, Yee J, et al. Patal adrenal cortical insufficiency precipitated by surgery during prolonged continuous cortisone treatment. Ann Intern Med. 1953;39:116–26.
222. Salem M, Trainish Jr RE, Bomber J, et al. Perioperative glucocorticoid coverage: a reassessment 42 years after emergence of a problem. Ann Surg. 1994;219:416–25.
223. Kehlet H. Clinical course and hypothalamic-pituitary-adrenocortical function in glucocorticoid treated surgical patients. Copenhagen, Denmark: FACL Forlag; 1976.

224. Glowniak JV, Loriaux DL. A double-blind study of perioperative steroid requirements in secondary adrenal insufficiency. Surgery. 1997;121:123–9.
225. Thomason JM, Girdler NM, Kendall-Taylor P, et al. An investigation into the need for supplementary steroids in organ transplant patients undergoing gingival surgery. A double blind, split mouth, cross over study. J Clin Periodontol. 1999;25:577–82.
226. Yong SL, Marik P, Esposito M, et al. Supplemental perioperative steroids for surgical patients with adrenal insufficiency. Cochrane Database Syst Rev 2009;CD005367.
227. de Lange DW, Mars M. Perioperative glucocorticosteroid supplementation is not supported by evidence. Eur J Intern Med. 2008;19:461–7.
228. Marik PE, Varon J. Requirement of perioperative stress doses of corticosteroids: a systematic review of the literature. Arch Surg. 2008;143:1222–6.
229. Stelzer M, Phillips JD, Fonkalsrud EW. Acute ileus from steroid withdrawal simulating intestinal obstruction after surgery for ulcerative colitis. Arch Surg. 1990;125:914–7.
230. Rai S, Hemingway D. Acute adrenal insufficiency presenting as high output ileostomy. Ann R Coll Surg Engl. 2003;85:105–6.
231. Prasad M, Matthews JB. Deflating postoperative ileus. Gastroenterology. 1999;117:489–92.
232. Cali RL, Meade PG, Swanson MS, et al. Effect of morphine and incision length on bowel function after colectomy. Dis Colon Rectum. 2000;43:163–8.
233. Liu SS, Carpenter RL, Mackey DC, et al. Effects of perioperative analgesic technique on recovery after colon surgery. Anesthesiology. 1995;83:757–65.
234. Jorgensen H, Wetterslev J, Moiniche S, et al. Epidural local anaesthetics versus opioid-based analgesic regimens on postoperative gastrointestinal paralysis, PONV and pain after abdominal surgery. Cochrane Database Syst Rev 2000;CD001893.
235. Park WY, Thompson JS, Lee KK. Effect of epidural anesthesia and analgesia on perioperative outcome: a randomized controlled Veterans Affairs cooperative study. Ann Surg. 2001;234:560–9.
236. Senagore AJ, Delaney CP, Mekhail N. Randomized clinical trial comparing epidural anaesthesia and patient-controlled analagesia after laparoscopic segmental colectomy. Br J Surg. 2003;90:1195–9.
237. Werawatganon T, Charuluanun S. Patient controlled intravenous opioid analgesia versus continuous epidural analgesia for pain after intra-abdominal surgery. Cochrane Database Syst Rev 2005;CD004088.
238. Marret E, Remy C, Bonnet F, et al. Meta-analysis of epidural analgesia versus parental opioid analgesia after colorectal surgery. Br J Surg. 2007;94:665–73.
239. Zutshi M, Delaney CP, Senagore AJ, et al. Randomized controlled trial comparing the controlled rehabilitation with early ambulation and diet pathway versus the controlled rehabilitation with early ambulation and diet with preemptive epidural anesthesia/analgesia after laparotomy and intestinal resection. Am J Surg. 2005;189:268–72.
240. Levy BF, Tilney HS, Dowson HMP, et al. A systematic review of post-operative analgesia following laparoscopic colorectal surgery. Colorectal Dis. 2010;12:5–15.
241. Paulsen EK, Porter MG, Helner SD, et al. Thoracic epidural versus patient-controlled analgesia in elective bowel resections. Am J Surg. 2001;182:570–7.
242. Neudecker J, Schwenk W, Junghans T, et al. Randomised controlled trial to examine the influence of thoracic epidural analgesia on postoperative ileus after laparoscopic sigmoid resection. Br J Surg. 1999;86:1292–5.
243. Holte K, Kehlet H. Postoperative ileus: a preventable event. Br J Surg. 2000;87:1480–93.
244. Carli F, Trudel JL, Belliveau P. The effect of intraoperative thoracic epidural anesthesia and postoperative analgesia on bowel function after colorectal surgery: a prospective, randomized trial. Dis Colon Rectum. 2001;44:1083–9.
245. Kalff JC, Turler A, Schwarz NT, et al. Intra-abdominal activation of a local inflammatory response within the human muscularis externa during laparotomy. Ann Surg. 2003;237:301–15.
246. Brown CR, Mazzulla JP, Mok MS, et al. Comparison of repeat doses of intramuscular ketorolac tromethamine and morphine sulfate for analgesia after major surgery. Pharmacotherapy. 1990;10:45S–50.
247. Cataldo PA, Senagore AJ, Kilbride MJ. Ketorolac and patient controlled analgesia in the treatment of postoperative pain. Surg Gynecol Obstet. 1993;176:435–8.
248. Ferraz AAB, Cowles VE. Nonopioid analgesics shorten the duration of postoperative ileus. Am Surg. 1995;61:1079–84.
249. Schlachta CM, Burpee SE, Fernandez C, et al. Optimizing recovery after laparoscopic colon surgery. Surg Endosc. 2007;21:2212–9.
250. Chen JY, Ko TL, Wen YR, et al. Opioid-sparing effects of ketorolac and its correlation with the recovery of postoperative bowel function in colorectal surgery patients: a prospective randomized double-blinded study. Clin J Pain. 2009; 25:485–9.
251. Lacy AM, Garcia-Valdecasas JC, Delgado S, et al. Laparoscopy-assisted colectomy versus open colectomy for treatment of non-metastatic colon cancer: a randomised trial. Lancet. 2002;359:2224–9.
252. Fearon KC, Ljungqvist O, Von Meyenfeldt M, et al. Enhanced recovery after surgery: a consensus review of clinical care for patients undergoing colonic resection. Clin Nutr. 2005; 24:466–7.
253. Wattchow DA, Fontgalland DD, Bampton PA, et al. Clinical trial: the impact of cyclooxygenase inhibitos on gastrointestinal recovery after major surgery – a randomized double blind controlled trial of celecoxib or diclofenac vs placebo. Aliment Pharmacol Ther. 2009;30:987–98.
254. Mathiesen O, Moiniche S, Dahl JB. Gabapentin and postoperative pain: a qualitative and quantitative systemic review, with focus on procedure. BMC Anesthesiol. 2007;7:6.
255. Srivastava U, Kumar A, Saxena S, et al. Effect of preoperative gabapentin on postoperative pain and tramadol consumption after mini open cholecystectomy: a randomized double blind placebo controlled trial. Eur J Anaesthesiol. 2010; 27(4):331–5.
256. Pandey CK, Priye S, Ambesh SP, et al. Prophylactic gabapentin for prevention of postoperative nausea nd vomiting in patients undergoing laparoscopic cholecystectomy: a randomized, double blind, placebo controlled study. J Postgrad Med. 2006;52:97–100.
257. Horlocker T, Wedel DJ. Neuraxial block and low-molecular weight heparin: balancing perioperative analgesia and thromboprophylaxis. Reg Anesth Pain Med. 1998;23 Suppl 2: 164–77.

10 Postoperative Complications

David W. Dietz

Whether practicing in a small rural hospital or a large tertiary referral center, colorectal surgeons will encounter a variety of postoperative complications. The ability to minimize, recognize, and effectively treat these problems is paramount to achieving quality outcomes for our patients. This chapter focuses on those surgical complications most often encountered by colorectal surgeons: injuries to the bowel and genitourinary structures, pelvic hemorrhage, small bowel obstruction, wound infections, abscesses, and anastomotic leaks, strictures, and bleeding.

Unrecognized Enterotomies and Enterocutaneous Fistulae

Patients undergoing extensive adhesiolysis are at the highest risk for enterotomies. An enterotomy, while a complication, can be easily and promptly managed. In cases in which any significant degree of adhesiolysis is performed, the entire bowel should be carefully inspected at the end of the procedure. Although the natural history of serosal tears is unknown, they should be repaired when recognized with imbricating seromuscular sutures. Full-thickness enterotomies can be repaired using a number of different and equally effective techniques: one common method is a two-layer closure using an inner layer of absorbable seromuscular sutures and an outer layer of permanent Lembert sutures. In cases in which multiple enterotomies have occurred within a short segment of bowel, resection of the involved segment with primary anastomosis is performed. If the mesentery has also been injured during the course of adhesiolysis, the viability of the bowel ends should be confirmed before anastomosis. Imbrication of excessive amounts of mucosa and submucosa may cause excessive luminal narrowing with subsequent obstructive symptoms. Thus, long longitudinal seromyotomies may be treated by converting them to full-thickness lacerations and closing them in a strictureplasty fashion.

Failure to recognize an enterotomy at the time of surgery will lead to one of several postoperative complications. The patient may develop peritonitis within the first 24–48 h after surgery. This problem may be difficult to detect in the background of narcotic analgesia and the surgeon and patient's expectation of postoperative incisional pain. The diagnosis is purely based on patient's appearance and examination. The usual markers of bowel perforation (leukocytosis, fever, and pneumoperitoneum) are not reliable, because they are normal findings in the early postoperative patient. A high index of suspicion should be maintained with a low threshold for reexploration. Reoperation within the first several days is usually not difficult because significant adhesions have not yet formed. Most enterotomies found in this situation can be primarily repaired, provided that the bowel edges are viable. If conditions are not favorable for primary repair, a diverting stoma should be created proximal to the repair. An especially difficult situation is that in which bilious fluid is encountered at reexploration but no enterotomy can be found. After running both the small and large bowel at least twice and excluding a duodenal, gastric, or gallbladder injury, the only remaining option may be to place drains in both paracolic gutters and the pelvis in hopes of creating a controlled enterocutaneous fistula. Insufflation of the small bowel with carbon dioxide gas through a nasogastric tube has also been described as a method for localizing small enterotomies. Gas bubbles may be seen emanating from the site of injury after the abdomen has been filled with saline.

An unrecognized enterotomy may also present as an enterocutaneous fistula, with enteric drainage emanating from the incision or wound later in the postoperative course. If there are no signs of sepsis, a nonoperative approach may be considered, especially if the patient is more than 1 week removed from surgery. Laparotomy after the first postoperative week is often extremely difficult. Dense, vascular adhesions may be encountered and there is significant risk of making the situation worse with further enterotomies or

D.E. Beck et al. (eds.), *The ASCRS Textbook of Colon and Rectal Surgery: Second Edition*,
DOI 10.1007/978-1-4419-1584-9_10, © Springer Science+Business Media, LLC 2011

mesenteric vascular injury. Instead, the patient is placed on complete bowel rest, a nasogastric tube is inserted, broad-spectrum antibiotic coverage is initiated, and a computed tomography (CT) scan is obtained to assess for an associated abscess or fluid collection. If a fluid collection greater than 4 cm in diameter is present, percutaneous, radiologically guided drainage should be used. If available, an enterostomal therapist should be involved to assist with pouching the fistula in order to protect the skin from irritating enteric contents. In most cases, parenteral nutrition will be started to meet the patient's caloric and protein requirements in anticipation of a prolonged period of fasting. H2 antagonists should be added to decrease gastric secretions. Somatostatin analogs may also be used to decrease the volume of fistula output, although they do not seem to increase the rate of spontaneous fistula closure.[1] The rate of spontaneous small bowel fistula closure varies but is typically less than 50%. Chances of spontaneous closure are thought to be reduced by high output because of proximal location, distal obstruction, local sepsis, radiation exposure, a short or epithelialized tract, malignancy, a foreign body in the tract such as mesh and/or sutures, Crohn's disease, and malnutrition.[2,3]

Most enterocutaneous fistulas that spontaneously close will do so within the first month. If the fistula persists, fibrin glue injection can be attempted. Several reports have been published describing this technique and successful closure has been achieved in some cases.[4–6] Although no large series exists to define the success rate, little progress is lost in making the attempt. Surgical intervention should be delayed until all sepsis has resolved, adequate nutrition has been restored, and intraabdominal adhesions have softened to the point of allowing safe reoperation. Most authors recommend a delay of at least 6 weeks since the last laparotomy, but 3–6 months may be more appropriate.[7,8] Experience has dictated that the longer one can wait until reoperation, the better. This must, of course, be balanced against the patient's medical and social condition, and their degree of patience. Appropriate management of the often highly caustic effluent including pouching by an enterostomal therapist is a very important measure.

The outcome from our department regarding the surgical management of over 200 patients with small bowel enterocutaneous fistulas was recently reported. Following the principles outlined above, the ultimate healing rate was approximately 80% with a median follow-up of 9.5 months. Most fistulas that recurred did so within the first 3 months. The only statistically significant predictor of recurrence identified was surgical technique. Fistulas that were primarily repaired recurred in 36% of cases, whereas the recurrence rate in those treated with segmental bowel resection was only 16%. There was a trend toward better outcomes with a longer interval between the index surgery and the operation for fistula repair (<3 months, recurrence rate 28%; 3–6 months, recurrence rate 15%; >6 months, recurrence rate 10%). Ninety-day operative mortality was 3.5%.[8]

Anastomotic Complications

Anastomotic complications are among the most feared in colorectal surgery. They can lead to emergent reoperation and/or a prolonged, complicated, and costly postoperative hospitalization. If the patient recovers from the acute event, chronic sequelae may develop because of stricture or pelvic fibrosis leading to poor bowel function and the possibility of further revisionary surgery or permanent fecal diversion.

Anastomotic complications are usually related to technical factors such as ischemia, tension, poor technique, stapler malfunction, or preexisting conditions such as local sepsis, poor nutrition, immunosuppression, morbid obesity, and radiation exposure. The contribution of the former set of variables may be minimized by a careful, methodical approach to construction of the anastomosis (Table 10-1). For colorectal anastomoses, a tension-free anastomosis may be achieved by full division of the lateral attachments of the descending colon, complete mobilization of the splenic flexure, high ligation of the inferior mesenteric artery (IMA), separation of the omentum from the distal transverse colon and mesocolon, and division of the inferior mesenteric vein (IMV) at the lower edge of the pancreas. Adequate blood supply should be confirmed by cutting across the marginal artery or bowel wall with anything less than pulsatile bleeding considered unacceptable. Further colon resection should be performed until adequate bleeding is encountered. If necessary, anastomoses between the hepatic flexure or distal ascending colon and rectum are easily achieved by passing the colon through a window in the mesentery of the terminal ileum.

Nutritional status, degree of immunosuppression, and general medical condition should be considered when deciding whether or not to perform a primary anastomosis. If severe malnutrition (albumin <2.0 or weight loss >15%) or significant immunosuppression (chemotherapy, high-dose steroids, antitumor necrosis factor drugs) are present, either an end-colostomy and Hartmann stump or a proximal loop ileostomy will minimize the risk of complications. Stoma takedown can then be performed if and when these factors have been corrected. A 3-month waiting period is advised for closure of a

TABLE 10-1. Steps to minimize risk of leak from colorectal or coloanal anastomoses

1. Ensure good blood supply (pulsatile bleeding from marginal artery at level of anastomosis)
2. Ensure tension-free anastomosis by complete mobilization of splenic flexure (includes high ligation of inferior mesenteric artery and ligation of inferior mesenteric vein at lower border of pancreas)
3. Avoid use of sigmoid colon in creation of anastomoses
4. Inspection of anastomotic donuts for completeness after circular stapled anastomoses
5. Air or fluid insufflation test to rule out anastomotic leak immediately after construction in the operating room

loop ileostomy. Laparotomy for takedown of an end stoma is generally deferred for 6 months. Preoperative weight loss, if able to be accomplished by the morbidly obese patient, will make the construction of deep pelvic anastomoses easier. When operating in the radiated pelvis, one end of the bowel used to construct the anastomosis should come from outside the field of radiation.[9] The double-stapled technique and other intersecting staple lines may have a higher predisposition to leak than a single stapled or hand sutured anastomosis.

Bleeding

Anastomotic bleeding is common and varies greatly in severity. In most cases, bleeding is minor and is manifested by the passage of dark blood with the patient's first bowel movements after surgery. In rare instances, bleeding can be significant and require transfusion and active intervention.

Bleeding can occur after either stapled or hand-sewn anastomoses, but is probably more common with the former. This complication can be reduced by careful inspection of the staple line, particularly in the case of side-to-side/functional end-to-end anastomoses. Before closing the enterotomy through which the stapler was introduced, the linear staple line can be everted and inspected. Routine intraoperative endoscopy after the construction of coloanal or colorectal anastomoses may allow intraoperative rather than postoperative control of bleeding.[10] Bleeding points should be controlled with sutures rather than cautery to prevent a deep burn injury which may lead to delayed leak. The incidence of bleeding from the linear staple line can be minimized by using the antimesenteric borders of each limb to construct the anastomosis, thus avoiding inclusion of the mesentery in the staple line. Alternatively, full-thickness staple line reinforcement may be undertaken with interrupted sutures to ensure optimal hemostasis.

Bleeding from circular stapled anastomoses or from the staple lines of ileal or colonic J pouches is usually not diagnosed until after the patient has left the operating room. After performing proctoscopy to evacuate clot from the rectum or neorectum, a rectal tube is inserted and a 1:100,000 solution of saline and epinephrine is instilled. The tube is then clamped for 15 min. If bleeding persists after the solution is allowed to drain, the procedure may be repeated. If bleeding continues or hypotension develops, the patient should be returned to the operating room for transanal examination of the anastomosis or pouch under anesthesia. Bleeding from anastomoses that are not accessible using these techniques, such as ileocolic or enteroenteric, may be managed with supportive care and correction of any underlying coagulopathy. If bleeding is severe, angiography may be required to localize the site and allow selective infusion of vasopressin. Alternatively, colonoscopy may be used. If the anastomosis can be visualized, the bleeding site can be treated with either cautery, injection of epinephrine, or endoscopic clips. In rare cases, reoperation with oversewing or resection of the bleeding anastomosis may be required.

Leaks

The incidence of anastomotic leak varies widely and is related to the factors listed above as well as the type of anastomosis. The lowest leak rates are seen after small bowel or ileocolic anastomosis (1–3%), whereas the highest occur after coloanal anastomosis (10–20%). Vignali et al. reported on 1,014 colorectal anastomoses.[11] The overall clinical leak rate was 2.9%. The incidence of leak was strongly associated with the distance of the anastomosis from the anal verge. Eight percent of low anastomoses (<7 cm from anal verge) leaked compared with only 1% of high anastomoses (>7 cm from anal verge). Although diabetes mellitus, use of a pelvic drain, and duration of surgery were each related to anastomotic leak in the univariate analysis, only low anastomosis was predictive in the multivariate model. Again, this higher leak rate may be related to the double stapling technique.

Another high-risk anastomosis is the ileal pouch-anal anastomosis. Leak rates of 5–10% have been reported.[12–14] Data from series of ileal pouch-anal anastomosis in patients with ulcerative colitis identify immunosuppressive drug therapy as a significant risk factor. Prednisone >40 mg/day and antitumor necrosis factor alpha agents have both been shown to increase the risk of ileal pouch-anal anastomotic leaks and pelvic sepsis in some studies.[15,16]

Role of Fecal Diversion

The creation of a proximal diverting stoma minimizes the severe consequences of an anastomotic leak but it does not reduce the incidence of leak itself.[17–19] A diverting stoma should be considered for any high-risk anastomosis [coloanal, low colorectal (<6 cm from anal verge), ileoanal]. In addition, patient factors such as severe malnutrition, significant immunosuppression, hemodynamic instability, excessive intraoperative blood loss, and purulent peritonitis or pelvic sepsis should be considered as indications for diversion (Table 10-2). Consideration should also be given to the patient's comorbidities and general condition; in cases in which the "physiologic reserve" necessary to tolerate an anastomotic leak does not exist, the use of a proximal stoma should be strongly entertained even if other risk factors are not present. Neoadjuvant radiation therapy does not seem to increase the incidence of anastomotic leak in patients undergoing restorative proctectomy for rectal cancer[20,21] but this may be because of the tendency for surgeons to cover these anastomoses with a proximal stoma, thus reducing the clinical manifestations of a leak. In fact, recent data from a large randomized trial assessing the efficacy of short-course neoadjuvant radiation therapy in rectal cancer found that a protecting stoma reduces the need for surgical intervention

TABLE 10-2. Indications for a diverting loop ileostomy

1. Coloanal or low colorectal anastomosis (<6 cm from anal verge)
2. Ileoanal anastomosis
3. Severe malnutrition
4. Significant immunosuppression (i.e., prednisone >40 mg/day, anti-TNF agents)
5. Hemodynamic instability
6. Excessive intraoperative blood loss
7. Purulent peritonitis
8. Pelvic sepsis
9. Neoadjuvant therapy

should an anastomotic leak occur.[22] When in doubt it is definitely safer to divert than to avoid diversion.

Role of Pelvic Drains

The use of pelvic drains is controversial. Whereas surgeons have long believed that preventing the collection of fluid or hematoma in the pelvis minimizes the risk of anastomotic leak, the use of drains has not been shown to be of benefit or harm in a recent, large randomized study[23] and in a metaanalysis.[24] However, examination of the data from the Dutch TME trial showed that the use of pelvic drains reduced the incidence of clinical anastomotic leak after short-course neoadjuvant radiation therapy from 23 to 9%. In the absence of data suggesting harm, the author routinely drains low colorectal or coloanal anastomoses, especially after neoadjuvant therapy.

Diagnosis and Management of Anastomotic Leak

Anastomotic leaks can be divided into "free" and "contained" varieties. Free leaks are those in which fecal contents leak from the anastomosis and spread throughout the abdominal cavity. Patients usually present with fever, tachycardia, leukocytosis, and diffuse peritonitis. Feculent fluid may present itself through the surgical incision or via the pelvic drains. Hypotension and other signs of systemic sepsis may ensue. If the patient is stable, radiologic investigation may be helpful to localize the leak and to determine its size and severity, although this is usually readily apparent at laparotomy. Radiographic studies, however, should not be allowed to delay reoperation.

Patients with "free" leaks should be taken to the operating room after fluid resuscitation and administration of broad-spectrum intravenous antibiotics. Surgical treatment will be dictated by the findings at operation. Most leaking colorectal anastomoses will require abdominal washout and takedown of the anastomosis with creation of an end-colostomy and Hartmann stump. If the stump cannot be stapled or sutured closed because of the friability of the tissues, transabdominal pelvic and per-anal drains should be placed. However, leaking ileocolic or small bowel to small bowel anastomoses can occasionally be repaired primarily in carefully selected circumstances, i.e., small defect with viable edges. However, resection of the anastomosis with either reconstruction or creation of a stoma is the most conservative option. Placing the repaired anastomosis directly under the midline incision will usually result in an enterocutaneous fistula rather than a second bout of peritonitis should the repair fail. If the viability of the bowel ends is questionable, takedown of the anastomosis and creation of a stoma is mandatory. Small defects in colorectal anastomoses may also, under ideal circumstances, be repaired primarily and covered with a proximal ileostomy. This is contraindicated, however, if there is a significant fecal load present between the ileostomy and the site of repair. Despite recent trends, mechanical bowel preparation for left-sided colorectal resections may still be wise for this reason alone.

Creating a stoma in the setting of an anastomotic leak can be particularly challenging. Severe peritonitis with a thickened and rigid mesentery may make it difficult to create an end-colostomy in the conventional manner. If a stoma does not reach skin level through an aperture away from the midline incision, two options exist. The first is to create a "loop-end" stoma. This often provides extra mesenteric length and also has better blood supply than a traditional end stoma. The second option is to bring the stoma up to the skin through the upper aspect of the midline wound. While this may present pouching difficulties for the patient, it is sometimes the only alternative in cases of intraabdominal catastrophe. Simply wrapping the exteriorized bowel with gauze and then performing delayed maturation of the stoma in 5–7 days will ensure viability of the stoma and insure against complete mucocutaneous separation and retraction.

"Contained" leaks are those in which the extravasation of contrast material is limited to the pelvis and usually result in the development of a pelvic abscess (Figure 10-1). If the abscess cavity is small and contrast flows freely back into the bowel, the patient may be treated with intravenous antibiotics, bowel rest, and observation. If the abscess is larger or somewhat removed from the site of the anastomosis, then percutaneous abscess drainage using CT or ultrasound guidance may avoid laparotomy. Such leaks rarely require immediate operation for fecal diversion, but surgery may eventually be required if the patient is left with a cutaneous fistula, anastomotic stricture, or chronic presacral cavity as a consequence.

Fistulae

Anastomotic leaks may also result in fistulae to the skin, vagina, male genitourinary system, or chronic presacral abscess (presacral sinus). Colocutaneous fistulae will frequently close with conservative management consisting of either bowel rest with total parenteral nutrition or a low residue diet and pouching

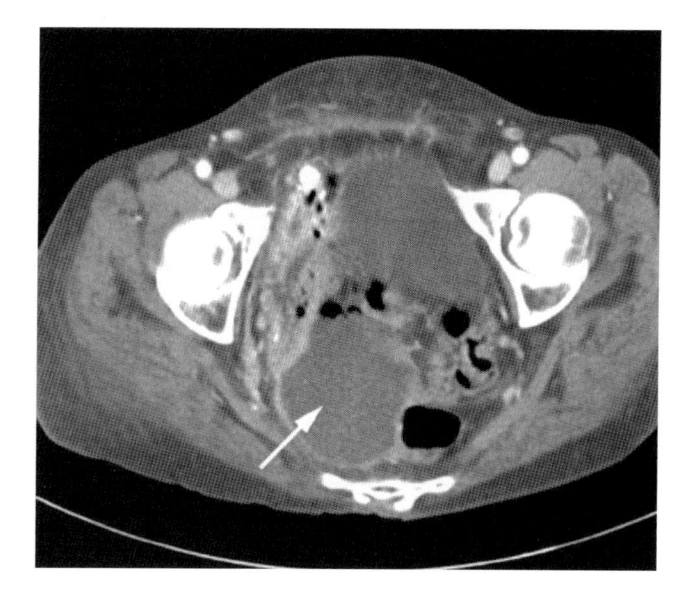

FIGURE 10-1. Pelvic abscess resulting from ileocolic anastomotic leak (*white arrow*). Extravasated enteric contrast can be seen in the right pelvis tracking down toward the abscess.

of the fistula to protect the surrounding skin. If drainage persists, reoperation for fistula takedown and reconstruction of the anastomosis can be performed after a delay of 3–6 months. Patients can usually eat a normal diet during this time period to maintain nutritional status. Fibrin glue injection has been reported as a successful alternative to surgery.[6]

Colovaginal fistulae are usually the consequence of either an anastomotic leak necessitating through the vaginal cuff in a patient who has undergone a prior hysterectomy or the inadvertent inclusion of the vagina during creation of a stapled anastomosis. In either case, spontaneous closure is rare. If the vaginal drainage is copious and intolerable to the patient, proximal fecal diversion may be necessary. An alternative measure to avoid a stoma during the period of fistula maturation is to use a large-volume daily enema to evacuate the colonic contents at a predictable time each day. After a waiting period of 3–6 months, reoperation may be performed. Options include attempts at local repair using advancement flaps (colonic or vaginal)/sleeve advancements, tissue interposition (labus majorum or gracilis), or laparotomy with redo coloanal anastomosis.

Chronic presacral abscess or sinus may result from a posterior leak from a coloanal or ileal pouch-anal anastomosis. Patients may have an occult presentation consisting of vague pelvic pain, fevers, frequency of stool, urgency, and bleeding. A pelvic CT scan usually shows presacral inflammatory changes and a contrast enema confirms the presence of a sinus tract originating from the posterior midline of the anastomosis and extending cephalad into the presacral space (Figure 10-2). Examination under anesthesia can then be performed with careful inspection of the anastomosis. A probe or clamp is placed through the anastomotic defect and the chronic presacral cavity is simply lain open using

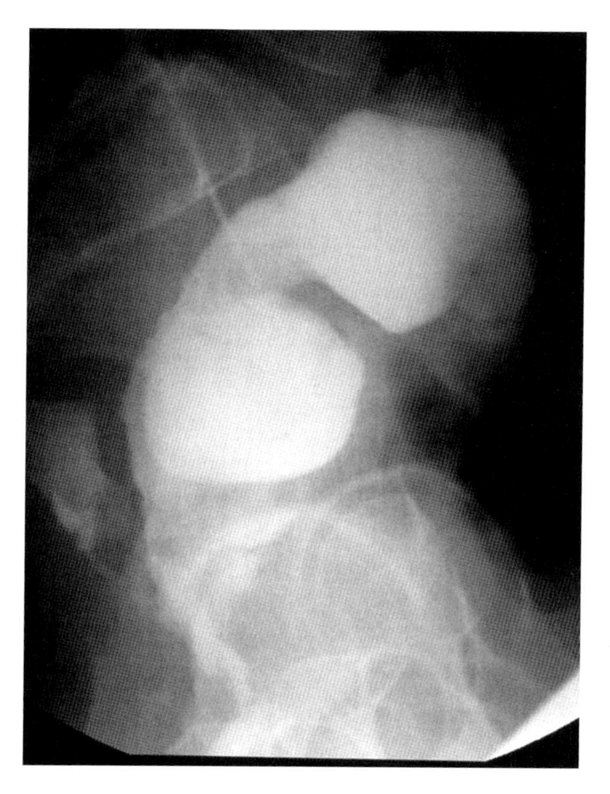

FIGURE 10-2. Gastrografin enema demonstrating chronic presacral sinus in a patient after ileal pouch-anal anastomotic leak.

cautery and gently curetted of granulation tissue. An alternative to using cautery is to open the sinus with a laparoscopic linear cutting stapler to divide the luminal-cavity septum. Either method allows free drainage of the presacral abscess and healing by secondary intention. This may result in a chronic posterior sinus or "pseudo-diverticulum." Successful management of an anastomotic sinus or chronic cavity has been described in Europe with an endoscopically placed vacuum-sponge device. A Dutch multicenter experience included 16 patients with early and late sinuses.[25] Closure was obtained in 11 of the 16 patients at a mean of 40 days and a median of 13 sponge replacements. If these approaches fail, then a redo coloanal anastomosis may be considered.

An especially useful, but not widely known, operation that can be employed in these situations is the "Turnbull–Cutait" abdominoperineal pull-through procedure. This operation was devised and reported on by Turnbull, Cutait, and Bacon, among others.[26–28] The technique involves two stages. In the first stage, after the failed coloanal anastomosis has been resected and pelvic sepsis debrided, the mobilized descending colon is brought through the anal canal and exteriorized to the extent that it can be wrapped with gauze to secure it in place. Five to ten days later, the patient is returned to the operating room for the second phase where the exteriorized portion of colon is excised and the delayed coloanal anastomosis is performed by a perineal approach (Figure 10-3A–D). Remzi et al.[29] have recently reported our experience with this procedure in 67 patients, mostly for salvage of pelvic anastomotic

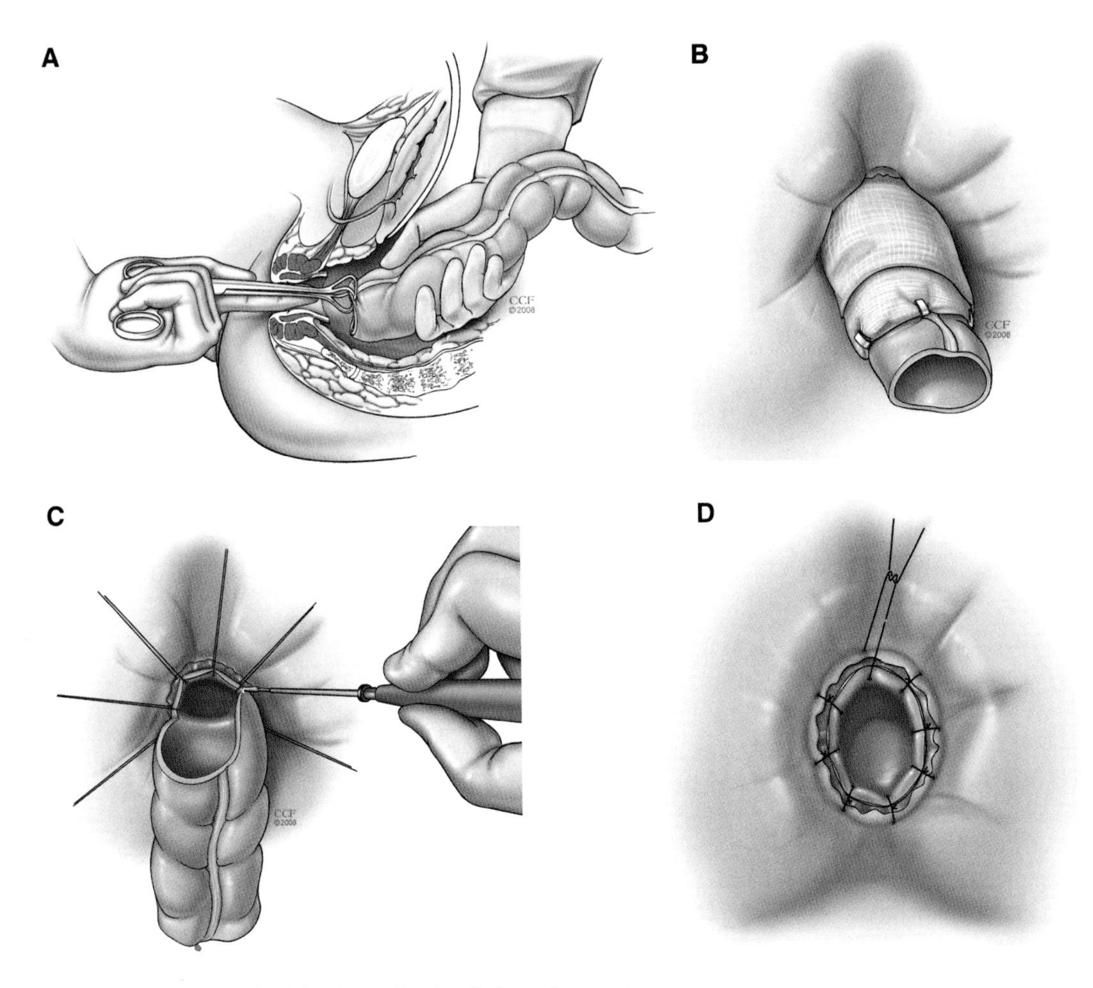

FIGURE 10-3. **A–D** Turnbull–Cutait abdominoperineal pull-through procedure.

complications (recto-vaginal and -urethral fistulas, strictures, presacral abscess, etc.). The procedure was successful in 75% of patients. Bowel function was felt to be satisfactory by most patients and was comparable to a matched group undergoing primary coloanal anastomosis for rectal cancer.

Stricture

Anastomotic stricture may be the end result of anastomotic leak or ischemia. It typically presents 2–12 months after surgery with increasing constipation and difficulty evacuating. If the initial resection was done for malignancy, recurrence as a cause of the stricture must be excluded with a combination of CT scan and fluorodeoxyglucose–positron emission tomography (PET) scan. Biopsy is mandated if a mass or abnormality is identified. Low colorectal, coloanal, or ileal pouch-anal anastomotic strictures may be successfully treated with repeated dilatations using an examining finger or rubber dilators. Dilatation is more successful if initiated within the first few weeks after surgery. In fact, almost all coloanal or ileoanal anastomoses stricture to some degree during the early postoperative period, especially if a diverting stoma is present. All such anastomoses should undergo digital examination at 4–6 weeks after surgery and just before stoma closure (usually at 2–3 months). Strictures are usually soft and easily dilated during these examinations. Higher colorectal, colocolic, or ileocolic strictures may be approached using endoscopic balloon dilatation (Figure 10-4). If these measures fail, or if the stricture is extremely tight or long, revisionary surgery may be required. These are difficult operations, however, because of the pelvic fibrosis that develops after anastomotic leak and complications are common. In some cases, permanent fecal diversion is the only option.[30,31]

Genitourinary Complications

Ureteral Injuries

Injury to the ureters typically occurs at one of four specific points during pelvic intestinal surgery. The first is during high ligation of the IMA where the junction between the upper and middle thirds of the left ureter lies in close

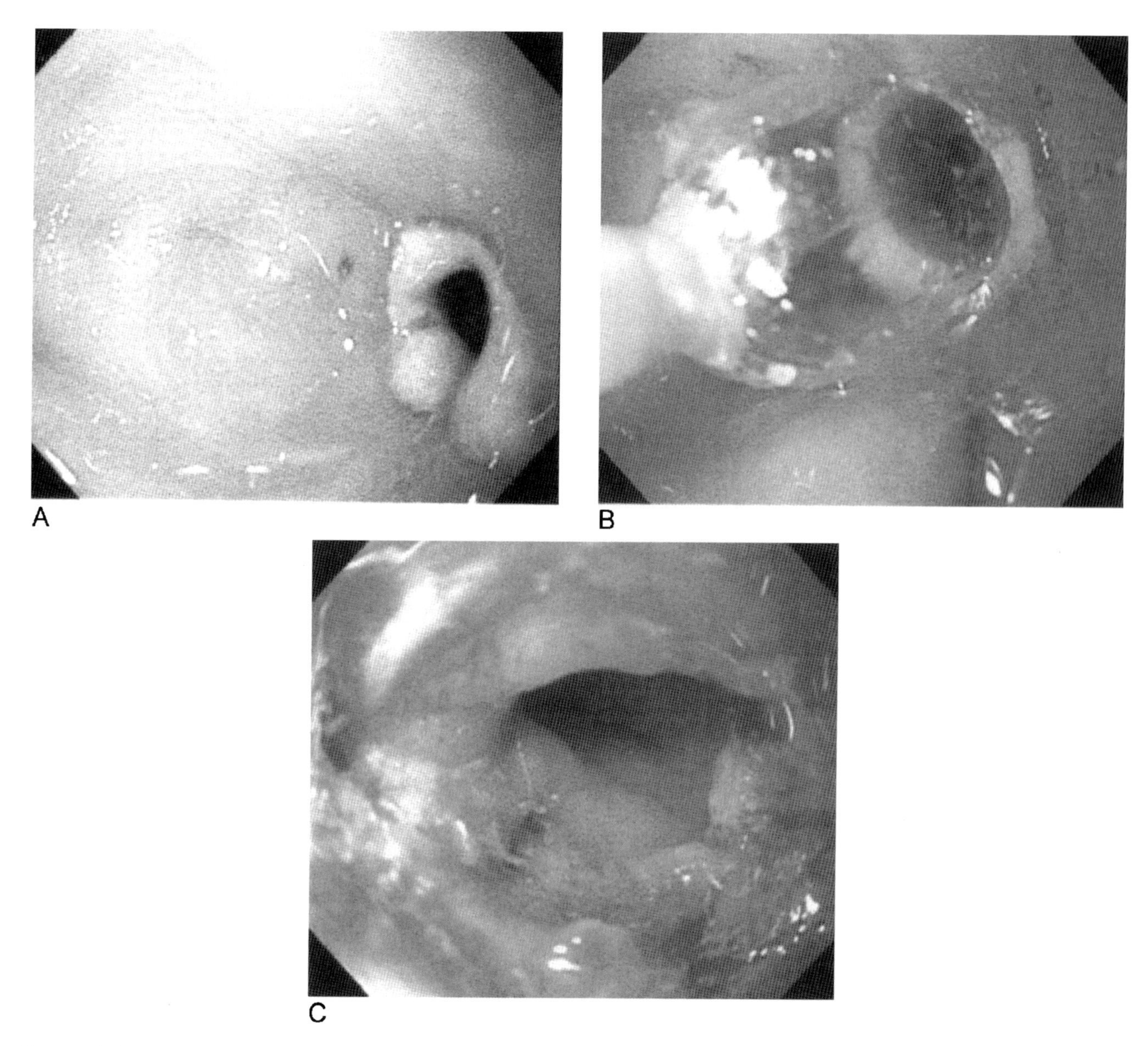

FIGURE 10-4. Endoscopic balloon dilatation of a colorectal anastomotic stricture: **A** 5-mm colorectal anastomotic stricture, **B** balloon dilator inflated, **C** result.

proximity to the vessels. Failure to mobilize the ureter laterally before ligation of the IMA may result in its inclusion with the vascular pedicle when clamped and subsequent division. It is good practice to always confirm the position of the left ureter before and after applying clamps to the IMA and before division of the vessel. Injury at this level is usually limited to transection and can be repaired primarily using an end-to-end, spatulated anastomosis performed over a stent. The second point of danger is during mobilization of the upper mesorectum near the level of the sacral promontory. It is at this point that the ureters cross over the bifurcation of the iliac artery and course medially as they enter the pelvis. The left ureter may be closely associated with the sigmoid colon and can even be adherent secondary to prior inflammatory processes. The injury may be tangential and not readily recognized in the setting of a phlegmon or abscess. Ureteral stents in this setting are most beneficial in identifying the injury rather than preventing it. Injury at this level is usually managed by either primary repair or ligation of the distal stump and creation of a ureteroneocystostomy with a Boari flap or psoas hitch repair.

The third point of risk is during the deepest portion of the abdominal phase of the operation. Anterolateral dissection in the plane between the lower rectum, pelvic sidewall, and bladder base can result in ureter injury at the ureterovesical junction. The ureter may also be injured at this level during division of the lateral stalks. The final area of risk is during the most cephalad portion of the perineal phase of the operation. If exposure is limited (obese patient, android pelvis), the ureter may be unknowingly divided near the ureterovesical junction. In either of these circumstances, the injury can be managed by creating a ureteroneocystostomy. The ureter is reimplanted into the bladder by tunneling the ureter through the bladder wall and creating a mucosa to mucosa anastomosis.

Should ureteral injury occur, the key to minimizing its consequence is immediate (intraoperative) recognition and repair of the injury. In cases in which a difficult pelvic dissection is anticipated, because of prior pelvic surgery, inflammation, or a locally advanced tumor, the preoperative placement of ureteral stents can be invaluable. Although the literature does not demonstrate that stents prevent ureteral injuries, palpation of the stents can aid in localization of the ureters and can also facilitate identification and repair should injury occur. In cases in which the surgeon is suspicious of occult injury, indigo carmine can be administered intravenously. After several minutes, the urine turns blue-green and the operative field can then be inspected for staining. Unfortunately, the literature suggests that less than 50% of ureteral injuries are identified intraoperatively, usually because the injury is not suspected. Ureteral stents should be used selectively, however, because their use can lead to complications such as obstruction secondary to hematoma, perforation, or acute renal failure. As is the case with all complications, it is far better to avoid them than to treat them; Specifically in this instance, if there is a premonition of significant anatomic distortion at one or more of the points of potential ureteric injury then intraoperative ureteric catheterization should be undertaken. These settings typically include patients with recurrent Crohn's disease, chronic diverticulitis, leaked pelvic anastomoses, and pelvic irradiation.

Urethral Injuries

Iatrogenic injury to the urethra occur during abdomino-perineal resection (APR) or total proctocolectomy. The injury typically occurs during the perineal portion of the procedure and usually involves the membranous or prostatic portion. Intraoperatively, urethral injury may be recognized by visualization of the bladder catheter through the defect. These injuries may be difficult to avoid in the presence of a large, deeply penetrating anterior tumor in which the involvement of the prostate gland can occur. Desmoplastic reaction to the tumor or edema from neoadjuvant radiation therapy may also obscure anatomic planes. Small injuries can be repaired at the time of surgery using 5-0 chromic sutures with the Foley catheter left in place to stent the repair for 2–4 weeks. Larger injuries or those not presenting until the postoperative period (urine draining from the perineal wound) require proximal urinary diversion via suprapubic catheter and delayed repair. This should be performed by a skilled urologist with experience in urethral reconstruction and typically utilizes a gracilis muscle flap. If the patient is deemed at high risk for a urethral injury the intraoperative placement of a large diameter bladder catheter may be useful to avoid the injury.

Bladder Injury

Bladder injuries are relatively frequent and are, in most cases, related to resection of an adherent rectosigmoid tumor or diverticular phlegmon. When created purposefully or recognized immediately, defects in the bladder dome are easily repaired in two layers with a Foley catheter then left in place for 7–10 days postoperatively. Before removal, a cystogram may be obtained to confirm healing. Injuries to the base of the bladder are more problematic. The major risk of repair in this situation is occlusion of the ureteral orifice at the trigone. Most urologists advocate opening of the bladder dome to gain access to the bladder lumen with subsequent repair of the trigone injury under direct vision from the interior. Ureteral patency is confirmed at the conclusion of the repair before closing the cystotomy. Injuries not recognized at the time of surgery will present in the postoperative period with urine in the abdominal cavity, pneumaturia, or fecaluria. Initially, fecal and urinary diversion may be necessary to temporize the situation until reoperation can be safely performed. At that time, takedown of the colovesical fistula can be performed with primary repair of the bladder. If available, omentum may be interposed between the bladder repair and any bowel anastomosis. Regardless of whether or not a repair was undertaken, catheter drainage of the bladder is maintained for 1–2 weeks after which a cystogram is performed to confirm integrity of the repair prior to catheter removal.

Urinary Dysfunction

Urinary dysfunction is one of the most common urinary complications of APR.[32] Some degree of voiding difficulty occurs in up to 70% of patients after APR, but it is usually confined to the early postoperative period. In most instances, urinary retention is the result of denervation of the detrusor muscle causing partial paralysis. Bladder contractility is under parasympathetic control via pelvic nerve branches originating from the inferior hypogastric plexus. These nerves can be injured if the endopelvic fascia is breached, especially during blunt dissection of the rectum. Temporary dysfunction of these nerves is nearly universal after APR, even when a meticulous sharp dissection is used. Most patients, however, only require maintenance of a bladder catheter for 5–7 days postoperatively. In a small percentage of patients, the problem persists beyond several months and urologic consultation is required. A small percentage of these patients may require prostatectomy or even intermittent self-catheterization on a long-term basis.

Sexual Dysfunction

Recent series report an incidence of sexual dysfunction of 15–50% in male patients undergoing APR for rectal cancer.[33–35]

This wide range is likely attributable to several factors such as patient age, preoperative libido, use of adjuvant radiation therapy, varying definitions of dysfunction, time point of follow-up, and social barriers preventing a frank discussion of the problem. The type of dysfunction is dependent on the pattern of nerve injury. Damage to the superior hypogastric (sympathetic) plexus during high ligation of the IMA or to the hypogastric nerves at the sacral promontory during mobilization of the upper mesorectum results in ejaculatory problems such as retrograde ejaculation. This is the most common type of sexual dysfunction seen in male patients after APR and is also the type most likely to resolve with time (6–12 months). Damage to the pelvic plexus during the lateral dissection or to the nervi erigentes or cavernous nerves while dissecting the anterior plane (abdominal or perineal phase) may result in erectile dysfunction. The cavernous nerves arise from branches of the pelvic plexus and course anterior to Denonvillier's fascia at the lateral border of the seminal vesicles. Parasympathetic innervation from these routes controls the inflow to and retention of blood within the corpora cavernosa. The important anatomic relations of the pelvic nerves are illustrated in Figure 10-5.

Risk of injury to these nerves may be reduced by tailoring the anterior dissection based on the location of the tumor. The highest risk of parasympathetic nerve injury occurs when dissection is performed in the plane anterior to Denonvillier's fascia and flush with the posterior aspect of the seminal vesicles and prostate. Whereas some believe that this plane is a vital part of total mesorectal excision for any low rectal cancer, others will only include Denonvillier's fascia in the resection specimen for an anterior tumor where it may help obtain a clear radial margin.[36] For posterior tumors, Denonvillier's fascia is preserved by dissecting between it and the fascia propria of the rectum in order to protect the small cavernous nerves. Using a "nerve sparing" approach to total mesorectal excision, several authors have reported an incidence of erectile dysfunction of 5–15% after proctectomy for rectal cancer. Factors shown to increase risk are older age, poor preoperative libido, and low rectal tumor requiring APR (two- to threefold increase compared with low anterior resection).

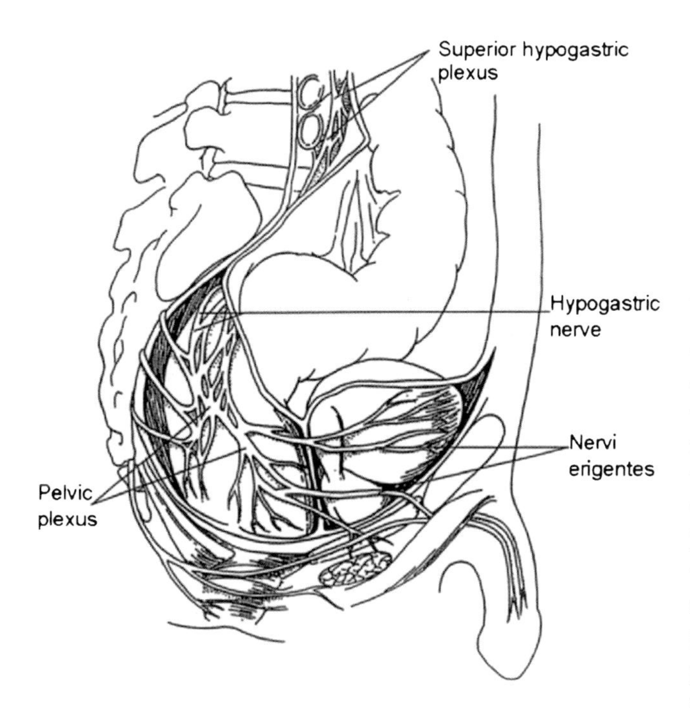

FIGURE 10-5. Anatomic relations of the pelvic nerves. Damage to the superior hypogastric plexus during high ligation of the inferior mesenteric artery (IMA) or to the hypogastric nerves at the sacral promontory during mobilization of the upper mesorectum results in retrograde ejaculation. Damage to the pelvic plexus during the lateral dissection or to the nervi erigentes or cavernous nerves while dissecting the anterior plane may result in erectile dysfunction.

Sildenafil has been shown to be an effective treatment for male patients suffering from erectile dysfunction after proctectomy. A randomized, double-blind, placebo-controlled trial by Lindsey and Mortensen[37] found that the treatment with sildenafil completely reversed or satisfactorily improved erectile dysfunction in 79% of patients, compared with 17% in the placebo group. Side effects were mild and well tolerated.

Although harder to quantify, sexual dysfunction also occurs in women after proctectomy. It is characterized by dyspareunia and inability to produce vaginal lubricant and achieve orgasm. The incidence is lower than that seen in males and varies between 10 and 20%.[35,38,39]

Female Infertility

Several recent studies have documented decreased fertility in women who have undergone restorative proctocolectomy for ulcerative colitis or familial adenomatous polyposis.[40,41] The postoperative infertility rate exceeds 50% in this group when defined as "one year of unprotected intercourse without conception." This has important implications in both preoperative patient counseling and in the modification of operative technique to minimize the effect of pelvic adhesions on fertility. Women of childbearing age should be informed of this potential complication before elective restorative proctocolectomy because it may influence the timing of surgery. In addition, because pelvic adhesions are thought to interfere with egg transit from the ovary to the fallopian tube, measures to minimize their occurrence may be of benefit. Tacking the ovaries to the anterior abdominal wall outside of the pelvis and wrapping the adnexa with an antiadhesion barrier sheet are frequently used techniques but there are no data to support their efficacy.

Trapped Ovary Syndrome

Trapped ovary syndrome is a fairly common complication after restorative proctocolectomy in young women (Figure 10-6).

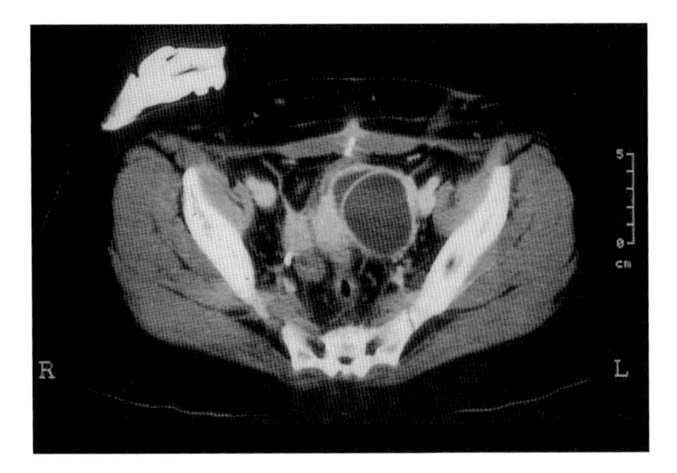

FIGURE 10-6. CT scan demonstrating "trapped" ovary in the right pelvis.

The adhesions that form after ileal pouch-anal anastomosis trap the ovaries in the pelvis and cover the fallopian tubes. With each ovulatory cycle, there is release of fluid into the pelvic cavity defined by these adhesions. As fluid accumulates and the cavity expands, patients will complain of pelvic or lower abdominal pain relevant to the side of the trapped ovary. A CT scan or ultrasound reveals a cystic lesion in the pelvis containing no air and with no surrounding inflammatory reaction. Operative findings are a cyst containing clear or tan fluid, surrounded by adhesions and with the ovary attached. Treatment consists of unroofing and evacuation of the cyst, pelvic adhesiolysis, and suspension of the ovary to the pelvic brim or iliac fossa with sutures. Trapped ovary syndrome may be prevented by suspending the ovaries at the time of restorative proctocolectomy and by placing an adhesion barrier film in the pelvis.

Small Bowel Obstruction

Perhaps the most critical components in the management of patients with bowel obstruction are the recognition and prevention of the disastrous effects of bowel ischemia. Timely surgical intervention, before the development of transmural necrosis, will limit complications and improve outcome. In one recently published series of more than 1,000 patients undergoing surgery for small bowel obstruction, nonviable strangulated bowel was present at laparotomy in only 16% of cases but the risk of death in this group was increased fourfold.[42] It is also important to distinguish between early (<30 days) and late postoperative small bowel obstruction.

Presentation and Diagnosis

Nausea and vomiting, colicky pain, abdominal bloating, and obstipation are the hallmark signs of small bowel obstruction. The degree to which each of these contributes to the clinical picture will depend on the location, degree, and duration of the obstruction.

The commonly regarded hallmarks of strangulated bowel are fever, tachycardia, leukocytosis, sepsis, peritoneal signs, and the presence of continuous as opposed to intermittent pain. If any of these are found, the suspicion of ischemia should be high. These signs may also be found in patients without strangulation and are, therefore, nonpathognomonic. In many cases, however, this determination is not made until laparotomy, and timely surgical intervention in symptomatic patients may be the best means of avoiding the progression to bowel ischemia. This fact is underscored by a report from Sarr et al.[43] who found that the traditional clinical parameters frequently used to predict strangulation were neither sensitive nor specific. Nearly one-third of patients with strangulation were not diagnosed until the time of surgery.

Radiographic Studies

Plain Radiographs

An acute abdominal series is the initial imaging study performed in most patients suspected of having small bowel obstruction and consists of both upright and supine abdominal films and an upright chest X-ray. Typical findings include dilated, air-filled loops of small bowel, air-fluid levels, and an absence or paucity of colonic air. These findings may be absent, however, when the obstruction is proximal or the dilated bowel loops are mostly fluid filled. The sensitivity of plain radiographs in detecting small bowel obstruction is approximately 60%. The findings of pneumatosis intestinalis or portal vein gas are worrisome for advanced bowel ischemia.

CT Scan

Abdominopelvic CT scanning is increasingly used as a primary imaging modality in patients suspected of having small bowel obstruction. In addition to establishing the diagnosis, CT may also be able to precisely define a transition point and reveal secondary causes of obstruction such as tumor, hernia, intussusception, volvulus, or inflammatory conditions such as Crohn's disease and radiation enteritis. CT may also reveal closed loop obstructions or signs of progressing ischemia such as bowel wall thickening, pneumatosis, or portal vein gas. Several studies have shown that the sensitivity of CT in diagnosing small bowel obstruction approaches 90–100%.

Contrast Studies

Contrast studies using water-soluble agents are frequently used in patients with acute small bowel obstruction. In patients with distal small bowel obstruction, a contrast enema is an efficient means by which colonic obstruction can be excluded. Antegrade studies of the small bowel can help to differentiate partial from complete obstruction, and may therefore predict the need for surgical intervention. In fact, some authors have used small bowel contrast studies as a "screening test" for patients presenting with adhesive obstructions. Failure of contrast material to reach the colon by 24 h is used as an indication for prompt surgical exploration. Several studies have also shown that the antegrade administration of contrast agents may speed the resolution of partial small bowel obstruction, presumably through an osmotic effect. However, conflicting data also exist and the therapeutic effects of the small bowel contrast study remain to be defined.

Initial Therapy and Nonoperative Management

Once the diagnosis of small bowel obstruction is made, the patient is admitted to the hospital. Those with peritonitis, perforation, or signs of ischemic bowel are immediately prepared for laparotomy with expeditious correction of fluid and electrolyte deficits. A urinary catheter is inserted to guide resuscitation with the end points being resolution of tachycardia and hypotension and/or achieving a urine output of at least 0.5 cm^3/kg/h. Broad-spectrum antibiotics are initiated. A nasogastric tube is inserted preoperatively to decompress the stomach, because these patients are at risk for aspiration on induction of general anesthesia.

If signs of perforation or ischemia are not present, a trial of expectant management may be undertaken. Patients with partial small bowel obstructions secondary to adhesions will resolve with a nonoperative approach in 80% of cases.[44–46] The success rate for patients initially presenting with complete obstruction is significantly lower. The nonoperative management of small bowel obstruction consists of fluid and electrolyte replacement, bowel rest, and tube decompression. The debate between standard nasogastric tube vs. long nasoenteric tube decompression has mostly settled in favor of the nasogastric tube. This is in part attributable to the fact that long tubes with mercury-weighted tips (Miller-Abbott) are no longer available for use (because of concern about the elemental Mercury) and have been replaced with a balloon-tipped tube (Gowen tube) that requires endoscopic placement. Long tubes are more difficult to place, requiring special expertise, serial radiographic studies, or endoscopy to guide insertion. There has been some recent resurgence in interest in the use of nasoenteric tubes, mostly among radiologists. Indications for long tube management of small bowel obstruction include early postoperative obstruction and recurrent partial obstruction where the transition point is difficult to identify on contrast studies.

Narcotic analgesics may be administered to comfort the patient, but not to the point of diminishing mental status. The practice of withholding pain medication to avoid masking the signs of perforation or ischemia is probably unnecessary. Serial abdominal examinations (ideally just before the next dose of analgesics) should be performed to assess for increasing tenderness or the presence of peritoneal signs. Any change in the patient's condition that suggests developing bowel ischemia mandates exploratory laparotomy. In general, a nonoperative course may be followed for 24–48 h. If the obstruction has not resolved within that time period, it is unlikely to do so and laparotomy is advised.

Decision to Operate

Several studies have attempted to define certain criteria that would reliably predict the presence or absence of strangulated bowel. Unfortunately, none have been shown to be particularly accurate and the best tool remains sound clinical judgment. Certainly, patients with fever, peritonitis, pneumoperitoneum, or overt sepsis should undergo emergent laparotomy because these are hard signs of transmural bowel necrosis. The presence of early ischemia, however, is much more difficult to discern. It is not uncommon for patients with small bowel obstruction to present with tachycardia, relative hypotension, mild acidosis, and leukocytosis, all of which may be secondary to dehydration. These patients should be aggressively rehydrated with isotonic intravenous fluids and the above parameters should be reassessed. Persistence of any of these signs after fluid resuscitation should prompt immediate laparotomy. Adherence to this simple algorithm should minimize the progression to strangulation while limiting the number of unnecessary laparotomies.

Distinguishing between partial and complete obstruction is also a key element in deciding which patients should be taken for early operation. As stated above, the likelihood of resolution of a complete obstruction with expectant management is low (20%). Delaying operative therapy until after a nonviable strangulation or perforation has occurred will substantially increase the mortality rate. Although this distinction may be difficult to make clinically, there are some useful caveats. The passage of stool or flatus cannot be relied on as an accurate predictor because patients with complete obstruction may continue to pass stool and flatus until the bowel distal to the site of obstruction is evacuated. However, if bowel function continues for more than 12 h after the onset of obstructive symptoms, the likelihood of complete obstruction is diminished. The passage of large volumes of nonbloody, watery stool along with vomiting and distension is pathognomonic for partial small bowel obstruction. The onset of flatus, however, usually signals the beginning of resolution of the obstruction because flatus is produced from swallowed air.

Surgical Technique

After the adequacy of resuscitation is confirmed and broad-spectrum antibiotics active against enteric pathogens are administered, the peritoneal cavity is entered through a midline incision. This is a point in the operation where the risk of inadvertent enterotomy is very high because bowel loops are distended and often adherent to the undersurface of the abdominal wall. Once the fascia is encountered, the application of gentle pressure with the bevel of the scalpel blade, rather than a cutting stroke, is used to breach the peritoneal cavity. Using this technique, it is usually possible to recognize an adherent bowel loop before enterotomy occurs.

In the most favorable scenario, a single constricting band will be encountered that can be sharply divided to relieve the obstruction. In the worst cases, the peritoneal cavity will be totally obliterated by scar tissue. An orderly and systematic approach to adhesiolysis is advised in these instances. First, the underside of the midline scar is cleared so that the entire length of the incision can be opened if necessary. Next, adhesions to the abdominal wall are dissected laterally until both paracolic gutters are reached. This allows the placement of a self-retaining retractor to facilitate exposure. In cases in which bowel distension is severe, needle decompression may be used to gain additional working space. Particularly severe adhesions that defy identification of the bowel and peritoneal surfaces ("frozen abdomen") may be injected with saline through a fine-gage needle to separate the surfaces and thus facilitate adhesiolysis. Attention is then turned to the pelvis where the most difficult adhesions are often encountered. Rather than separating individual bowel loops at this stage, the small bowel residing in the pelvis should be mobilized "en-masse" by lysing adhesions to the pelvic structures in an anterior to posterior manner in order to roll the mass of intestine up and out of the pelvis. The final portion of this stage of the operation involves mobilizing the plane between the small bowel mesentery and the retroperitoneum until the duodenum is encountered. Only at this point are all adhesions between individual bowel loops lysed in order to free the entire length of the small intestine. The bowel is then inspected for any coexisting pathology and for enterotomies or serosal tears created in the course of mobilization.

Assessment of bowel viability is usually possible by using the triad of color, peristalsis, and mesenteric pulsations. In cases in which these signs are questionable, the ischemic segment should be wrapped in warm, wet packs and viability reassessed after 15 min. If viability is still in doubt, use of the Doppler probe or systemic injection of fluorescein dye followed by inspection of the bowel under a Wood's lamp may aid in decision making. If the area in question is a short segment, it may be best to proceed with resection. If an extensive segment of questionable viability is present, then a second-look operation 24 h later should be planned before committing the patient to a massive small bowel resection.

There is some debate as to the need for complete adhesiolysis when the point of obstruction is encountered early in the operation. It is our policy to divide the majority of adhesions if this can be done safely. This facilitates the inspection of the entire length of the small bowel and allows for the placement of anti-adhesion barriers if desired (see below).

Special Situations

Early Postoperative Bowel Obstruction

Early postoperative bowel obstruction is generally defined as mechanical obstruction occurring within 1 month of abdominal or pelvic surgery. This condition is special in that attempts at relaparotomy in the early postoperative period frequently result in disastrous complications. The mantra of "never let the sun rise or set on a patient with bowel obstruction" should not be broadly applied in this group. An intense inflammatory response usually begins within the abdomen at 7–10 days postoperatively and persists for at least 6 weeks. If forced to operate during this period of time, the surgeon is likely to encounter dense hypervascular adhesions that may obliterate the peritoneal cavity. The risk of enterotomy and subsequent fistulization is extremely high. In addition, vascular or extensive serosal injury of the bowel may lead to massive resections. Therefore, immediate reoperation for early postoperative bowel obstruction is not advised, especially considering the fact that the development of strangulation in this setting is extremely rare. These patients should be managed conservatively with nasogastric or long tube suction and intravenous fluids. If resolution does not occur within the first 5–7 days, a percutaneous gastrostomy tube may be placed for long-term decompression, and the patient is started on hyperalimentation. Patients may be discharged from the hospital on this regimen and laparotomy performed in 6–12 weeks if the obstruction has not resolved. However, if peritonitis or signs of sepsis are present initially or develop during the course of nonoperative therapy, a CT scan should be performed immediately. Any abscess or fluid collection caused by an enteric leak can be percutaneously drained and a controlled enterocutaneous fistula established. Exploration is usually only required in cases of ischemic or necrotic bowel. There is a place for very early exploration within the first 10 days postoperatively if obstruction is recognized promptly. The adhesions encountered during this time period have not usually become severe and can be dealt with safely. There is also a role for laparoscopic enterolysis in the selected settings when performed by appropriately trained skilled surgeons.[34]

Anastomotic "Overhealing"

Anastomotic overhealing is a rare cause of postoperative small bowel obstruction. It is most often attributable to early adhesion and healing of the staple lines of the linear cutter between the limbs of a functional end-to-end/side-to-side anastomosis. This is best prevented by maximally distracting the two staple lines as the transverse staple line is placed to close the enterotomy made to introduce the side-to-side stapler. When this occurs in the early postoperative period, it will be easily diagnosed with a water-soluble contrast study, especially if administered via a long tube near the point of obstruction. The treatment should be conservative initially and may include long tube decompression. In some cases, the balloon-tipped catheter itself has broken through the healing web and relieved the obstruction. In the case of an obstructed ileocolic anastomosis, colonoscopic balloon dilatation may be carefully used. Operative intervention should be a last resort and usually requires resection and reanastomosis.

Prevention of Adhesions

More than 90% of patients undergoing abdominal surgery will develop some degree of intraabdominal adhesions.

Adhesion formation can occur wherever the visceral or parietal peritoneum has been disturbed. Once an area of injury is established, fibrin is deposited and then organizes to form a matrix for collagen deposition. Bowel motility and endogenous lubricants attempt to counteract this process, but in most cases, adhesions will eventually result as the deposited collagen matures. As discussed earlier, the progression from early to mature adhesions usually takes approximately 6 weeks.

Several strategies have been developed to minimize, prevent, or influence adhesion formation. Gentle handling of tissues, avoiding the deposition of talc by wearing powder-free gloves, and copious lavage of the peritoneal cavity at the conclusion of the operative procedure are simple means that should be used in all cases. In instances in which particularly severe adhesion formation can be anticipated, for instance patients with multiple recurrences of small bowel obstruction, the use of long intestinal tubes placed at the conclusion of surgery to "splint" the bowel open during adhesion formation has been advocated. This is usually accomplished by inserting a Baker tube via a proximal jejunostomy.

Recently, several chemoprophylactic agents have been developed in an attempt to reduce or eliminate adhesions through a barrier mechanism. The best studied of these is a bioresorbable membrane of modified sodium hyaluronate and carboxymethylcellulose. A large multicenter study by Becker et al.[47] has shown that this material substantially reduces the extent, incidence, and severity of adhesion formation. Its efficacy in reducing the incidence of adhesive bowel obstruction has recently been reported.[48] However, the decrease in incidence of bowel obstruction requiring reoperation from 3.4% in the control group to 1.8% in the treatment group is of uncertain clinical significance. The use of adhesion barriers in patients at high risk for subsequent reoperation because of disease or previous adhesions may be justified by the likely improvement in the ease and safety of the subsequent abdominal reentry and explorations. One of the problems with the barrier material is that it only prevents adhesions between the surfaces where it is applied.

Pelvic Bleeding

Serious pelvic bleeding may be encountered during proctectomy and is usually caused by injury to the presacral venous plexus or the internal iliac vessels or their branches. Although rare, pelvic bleeding can be a devastating event and is a significant cause of operative mortality. If bleeding is moderate, the best course of action is to complete the proctectomy. Bleeding will often stop, or at least slow significantly, once the rectum has been removed. Presacral venous hemorrhage is especially challenging because the anatomy and fragility of the presacral venous plexus make control of bleeding difficult. Attempts at electrocoagulation or suture ligation of these vessels usually results in an increase in bleeding and is not advised. Direct finger pressure should be used to gain temporary control of bleeding while allowing the anesthesia team to "catch up" with the resuscitation. Finger pressure can then be replaced with pressure applied by a cotton pledget on a long clamp. This will improve exposure and visualization for the attempt at repair. Once the patient is stabilized, several methods exist for permanent hemostasis. The most common of these is the use of sterile thumbtacks or specially designed "occluder pins" that are driven into the sacrum at right angles and directly over the site of bleeding.[49,50] If this maneuver is unsuccessful, a rectus abdominus muscle flap may be rotated down into the pelvis based on the inferior epigastric pedicle. Heavy sutures are then placed on either side of the sacrum and tied down to compress the rectus flap against the sacrum to tamponade the bleeding.[51] Other methods to control presacral bleeding have also been described,[51–54] such as removing a 2×2 cm square of rectus muscle and tacking this to the sacrum with absorbable sutures placed on either side of the bleeding site and tied tightly to secure the muscle patch. Application of electrocautery to the muscle then produces a secure coagulum on the surface of the bleeding venous plexus. If these measures fail, pelvic bleeding may be controlled by packing several laparotomy sponges tightly into the pelvis with the ends being brought out through the lower portion of the abdominal wound. The abdomen is then closed and the patient is taken to the intensive care unit for blood transfusion, fluid resuscitation, correction of coagulopathy, and general support. After 24–48 h, the patient is returned to the operating room for removal of the packs.[55]

Wound Infection and Intraabdominal Abscess

Wound Infection

Because of the large bacterial content of the colon (10^{10} anaerobes and 10^{8} aerobes/g of stool), wound infection rates are high after colorectal surgical procedures.[51,54,62] The introduction of an oral antibiotic preparation before surgery by Nichols and Condon reduced wound infection rates from 40% historically to the present day level of 5–10%. In many centers, a single parenteral dose of antibiotics at induction has replaced the more complicated "Nichol's prep." Several single-agent or combination choices exist, each with adequate gram-negative and anaerobic coverage. Risk factors for wound infection have been identified and include malnutrition, diabetes mellitus, immunosuppression, age >60 years, American Society of Anesthesia score >2, fecal contamination, length of hospitalization before surgery, and extensive surgery.[8,55] Recently, there is a growing body of literature that shows that mechanical bowel preparation does not decrease the incidence of wound infection. Several metaanalyses have examined this question and are in agreement.[56,57] The largest and most recent also found that the risk of anastomotic leak was actually increased in patients receiving a bowel preparation (odds ratio 1.75).[58]

Wound infections typically present on or around the fifth postoperative day and are characterized by erythema, warmth, tenderness, fever, and purulent drainage. Initial treatment consists of opening a portion of the skin incision over the area of maximal change to allow drainage. Antibiotics are not prescribed unless there is cellulitis present. If a significant amount of necrotic tissue is present, it should be debrided. Once the wound is adequately drained, a packing regimen is begun and the wound is allowed to heal by secondary intention. Large wounds may be treated with the application of a vacuum-assisted wound closure device. After the wound has been debrided by several days of wet to dry dressing changes, the vacuum-assisted closure device is applied (V.A.C.; KCI Therapeutic Services, San Antonio, TX). The advantages of this system are simplification of wound care and quicker closure. The dressing only needs to be changed every 4–5 days and wounds typically close within several weeks.

Several situations require more aggressive treatment. Deep infection involving the rectus muscle and fascia may occur and result in dehiscence. These patients should be taken back to the operating room for debridement of the necrotic fascial edges and repair of the dehiscence. Invasive wound infections with either clostridium perfringens or beta-hemolytic streptococcus is a potentially life-threatening complication. These infections may have an atypical presentation in that they can occur within the first 1–2 days after surgery and may be associated with minimal skin changes. The combination of fever and unusually severe wound pain early in the postoperative course should prompt opening of the skin incision. A necrotizing infection is suggested by the drainage of thin gray fluid. The key to timely diagnosis and treatment of these severe infections is a high level of suspicion. The patient should be taken to the operating room for a thorough wound exploration. All devitalized tissue should be removed and the fascia excised back to healthy, bleeding edges. Broad-spectrum antibiotic coverage should include high-dose penicillin.

Intraabdominal Abscess

Intraabdominal abscesses can result from anastomotic leaks, enterotomies, or spillage of bowel contents at the time of surgery. Patients will usually present with fever, leukocytosis, and abdominal or pelvic pain 5–7 days after surgery. The diagnostic modality of choice is a CT scan of the abdomen and pelvis performed with intravenous and oral contrast (and rectal contrast in the patient with a colorectal anastomosis). The finding of a fluid collection with a thickened, enhancing rim and surrounding inflammatory stranding is diagnostic. Air bubbles may also be present in the collection. Proximity to a staple line and the presence of contrast material in the abscess suggest an anastomotic leak as its cause.

Most intraabdominal or pelvic abscesses can be successfully treated with percutaneous catheter drainage performed under ultrasound or CT guidance. Intravenous antibiotics should also be administered. The CT scan is repeated 48 h after drainage to assess its efficacy. Further follow-up is usually performed by contrast studies obtained by injecting the drainage catheter. Once the abscess cavity has collapsed and no fistula to the bowel is identified, the catheter can be safely removed. Some abscesses cannot be drained percutaneously because of their location and lack of a safe "radiographic window" for drainage. Reported success rates for percutaneous drainage of intraabdominal abscesses range from 65 to 90% and depend on size, complexity, etiology, and microbial flora.[58–61]

Perineal Wound Infection

Perineal wound infection and delayed healing are major causes of morbidity after APR with the incidence ranging from 11 to 50%.[62–65] The rigidity of the lower pelvis combined with wide resection of the perineal soft tissues and levator muscles is mostly to blame, because this results in dead space cephalad to the skin closure which is easily infected.[66] Technical modifications that may help reduce the incidence of perineal wound problems include reapproximation of the subcutaneous tissues, suction drainage of the pelvis (with or without irrigation) to prevent hematoma formation and resultant fibrosis,[67] and filling of the dead space with an omental pedicle graft.[68–72] The area of raw surface deep in the pelvis also frequently fills with small bowel and may lead to small bowel obstruction. The bowel can be excluded from the pelvis by closing the pelvic peritoneum when possible, posteriorly retroverting the uterus to close the defect, or by rotating the cecum into the pelvis. The use of absorbable mesh has also been described, but this has been associated with multiple reports of obstruction and fistulization. In benign disease, a cuff of levator muscle can be left by incising the pelvic floor just outside of the external sphincter muscle. This method should always be possible for small rectal cancers. This technique allows closure of the levator muscles in the midline and prevents dead space formation and perineal hernia. Several risk factors for perineal wound complications have been identified. Foremost among these is the use of neoadjuvant radiation therapy. In one study, the incidence of perineal wound infection increased from 13 to 34% with the addition of preoperative radiation, whereas the rate of nonhealing at 30 days increased from 19 to 51%. Rates of perineal wound complications were even higher if intraoperative radiation was used.[73] Other factors are long operative time (>300 min), intraoperative hypothermia, and fecal contamination during the perineal dissection.[68,74–77] Patients with anorectal Crohn's disease are also at increased risk when undergoing APR for rectal cancer. However, an intersphincteric dissection in patients with inflammatory bowel disease allows closure of the external sphincter and may improve wound healing (Figure 10-7A–C).

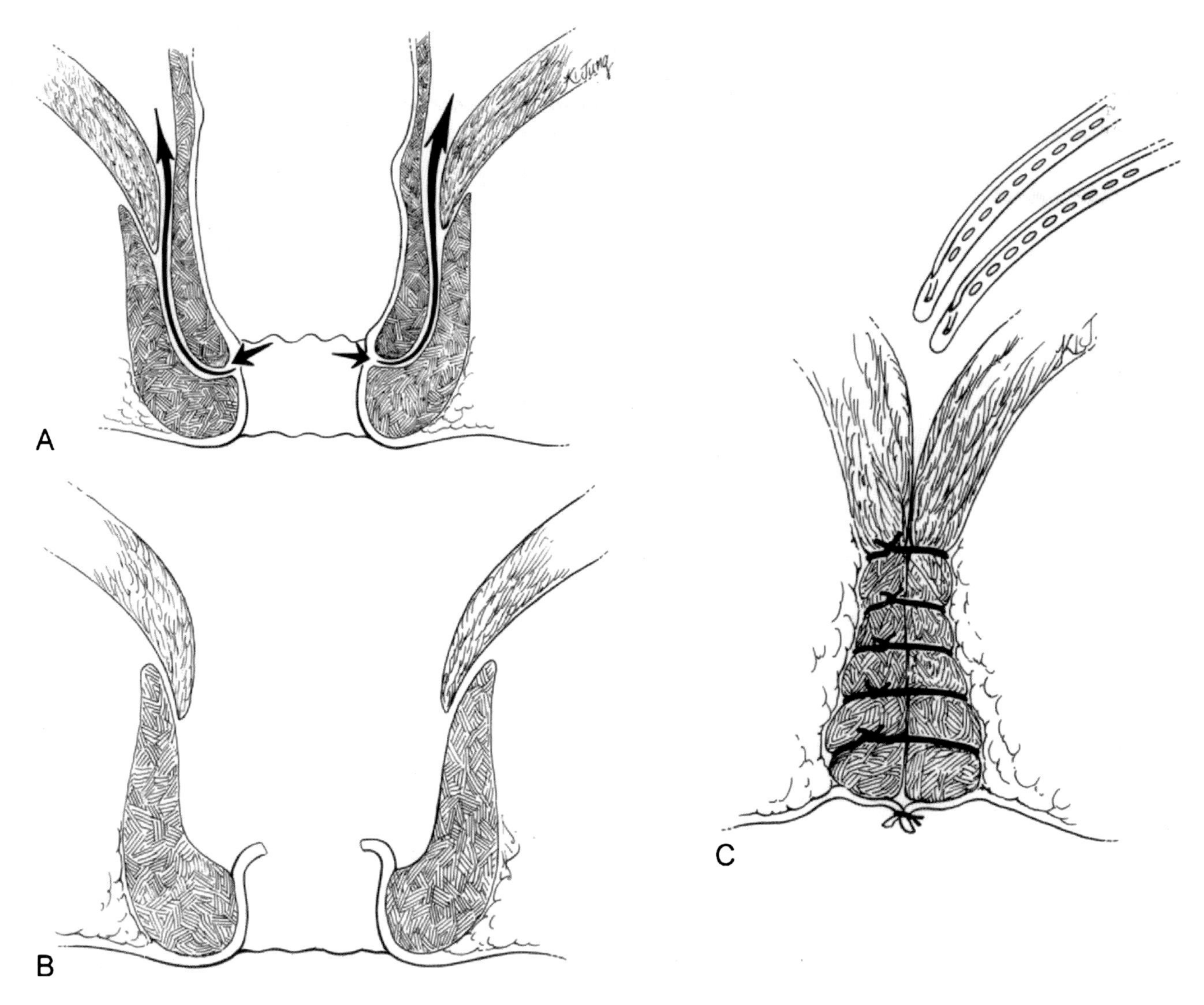

FIGURE 10-7. **A** Technique of intersphincteric proctectomy, **B** the mucosa overlying the intersphincteric groove is incised near the dentate line and the dissection is carried cephalad between the internal and external sphincters, **C** this results in retention of the external sphincters and levators which are then able to be closed in the midline.

If infection does occur, the skin should be opened to allow drainage and a program of wet to dry packing begun. A vacuum-assisted closure device can then be placed, as described above. In cases in which a chronic perineal sinus develops, closure of the defect may require wound debridement and myocutaneous flap reconstruction with gracilis, inferior gluteus, or rectus abdominus muscle.

References

1. Sancho JJ, di Costanzo J, Nubiola P, et al. Randomized double-blind placebo-controlled trial of early octreotide in patients with postoperative enterocutaneous fistula. Br J Surg. 1995;82(5):638–41.
2. Berry SM, Fischer JE. Enterocutaneous fistulas. Curr Probl Surg. 1994;31(6):469–566.
3. Joyce MR, Dietz DW. Management of complicated gastrointestinal fistulas. Curr Probl Surg. 2008;46(5):373–432.
4. Huang CS, Hess DT, Lichtenstein DR. Successful endoscopic management of postoperative GI fistula with fibrin glue injection: report of two cases. Gastrointest Endosc. 2004;60(3):460–3.
5. Okamoto K, Watanabe Y, Nakachi T, et al. The use of autologous fibrin glue for the treatment of postoperative fecal fistula following an appendectomy: report of a case. Surg Today. 2003;33(7):550–2.
6. Lamont JP, Hooker G, Espenschied JR, Lichliter WE, Franko E. Closure of proximal colorectal fistulas using fibrin sealant. Am Surg. 2002;68(7):615–8.
7. Fazio VW, Coutsoftides T, Steiger E. Factors influencing the outcome of treatment of small bowel cutaneous fistula. World J Surg. 1983;7(4):481–8.
8. Hollington P, Mawdsley J, Lim W, Gabe SM, Forbes A, Windsor AJ. An 11-year experience of enterocutaneous fistula. Br J Surg. 2004;91(12):1646–51.
9. Galland RB, Spencer J. Natural history and surgical management of radiation enteritis. Br J Surg. 1987;74(8):742–7.

10. Li VKM, Wexner SD, Pulido N, Wang H, Jin HY, Weiss EG, et al. Use of routine intraoperative endoscopy in elective laparoscopic colorectal surgery: can it further avoid anastomotic failure? Surg Endosc. 2009;23(11):2459–65.
11. Vignali A, Fazio VW, Lavery IC, Milsom JW, Church JM, Hull TL, et al. Factors associated with the occurrence of leaks in stapled rectal anastomoses: a review of 1,014 patients. J Am Coll Surg. 1997;185(2):105–13.
12. Fazio VW, Ziv Y, Church JM, et al. Ileal pouch-anal anastomoses complications and function in 1005 patients. Ann Surg. 1995;222(2):120–7.
13. Dayton MT, Larsen KR, Christiansen DD. Similar functional results and complications after ileal pouch-anal anastomosis in patients with indeterminate vs. ulcerative colitis. Arch Surg. 2002;137(6):690–4.
14. Sugerman HJ, Sugerman EL, Meador JG, Newsome Jr HH, Kellum Jr JM, DeMaria EJ. Ileal pouch anal anastomosis without ileal diversion. Ann Surg. 2000;232(4):530–41.
15. Heuschen UA, Hinz U, Allemeyer EH, et al. Risk factors for ileoanal J pouch-related septic complications in ulcerative colitis and familial adenomatous polyposis. Ann Surg. 2002;235(2):207–16.
16. Selvasekar CR, Cima RR, Larson DW, et al. Effect of infliximab on short-term complications in patients undergoing operation for chronic ulcerative colitis. J Am Coll Surg. 2007;204(5):956–62.
17. Marusch F, Koch A, Schmidt U, et al. Value of a protective stoma in low anterior resections for rectal cancer. Dis Colon Rectum. 2002;45(9):1164–71.
18. Pakkastie TE, Ovaska JT, Pekkala ES, Luukkonen PE, Jarvinen HJ. A randomised study of colostomies in low colorectal anastomoses. Eur J Surg. 1997;163(12):929–33.
19. Dehni N, Schlegel RD, Cunningham C, Guiguet M, Tiret E, Parc R. Influence of a defunctioning stoma on leakage rates after low colorectal anastomosis and colonic J pouch-anal anastomosis. Br J Surg. 1998;85(8):1114–7.
20. Enker WE, Merchant N, Cohen AM, et al. Safety and efficacy of low anterior resection for rectal cancer: 681 consecutive cases from a specialty service. Ann Surg. 1999;230(4):544–52.
21. Kapiteijn E, Marijnen CA, Nagtegaal ID, et al. Preoperative radiotherapy combined with total mesorectal excision for resectable rectal cancer. N Engl J Med. 2001;345(9):638–46.
22. Peeters KC, Tollenaar RA, Marijnen CA, et al. Risk factors for anastomotic failure after total mesorectal excision of rectal cancer. Br J Surg. 2004;92(2):211–6.
23. Merad F, Hay JM, Fingerhut A, et al. Is prophylactic pelvic drainage useful after elective rectal or anal anastomosis? A multicenter controlled randomized trial. French Association for Surgical Research. Surgery. 1999;125(5):529–35.
24. Urbach DR, Kennedy ED, Cohen MM. Colon and rectal anastomoses do not require routine drainage: a systematic review and meta-analysis. Ann Surg. 1999;229(2):174–80.
25. van Koperen PJ, van Berge Henegouwen MI, Rosman C, Bakker CM, Heres P, Slors JFM, et al. The Dutch multicenter experience of the Endo-Sponge treatment foe anastomotic leakage after colorectal surgery. Surg Endosc. 2009;23:1379–83.
26. Turnbull Jr RB. Pull-through resection of the rectum, with delayed anastomosis, for cancer or Hirschsprung's disease. Surgery. 1966;59:498–502.
27. Cutait DE, Cutait R, Ioshimoto M, et al. Abdominoperineal endoanal pull-through resection. A comparative study between immediate and delayed colorectal anastomosis. Dis Colon Rectum. 1985;28:294–9.
28. Bacon HE. Present status of the pull-through sphincter-preserving procedure. Cancer. 1971;28:196–203.
29. Remzi FH, El Gazzaz G, Kiran RP, et al. Outcomes following Turnbull–Cutait abdominoperineal pull-through compared with coloanal anastomosis. Br J Surg. 2009;96:424–9.
30. Di Giorgio P, De Luca L, Rivellini G, Sorrentino E, D'amore E, De Luca B. Endoscopic dilation of benign colorectal anastomotic stricture after low anterior resection: a prospective comparison study of two balloon types. Gastrointest Endosc. 2004;60(3):347–50.
31. Suchan KL, Muldner A, Manegold BC. Endoscopic treatment of postoperative colorectal anastomotic strictures. Surg Endosc. 2003;17(7):1110–3.
32. Hollabaugh Jr RS, Steiner MS, Sellers KD, Samm BJ, Dmochowski RR. Neuroanatomy of the pelvis: implications for colonic and rectal resection. Dis Colon Rectum. 2000;43(10):1390–7.
33. Walsh PC, Schlegel PN. Radical pelvic surgery with preservation of sexual function. Ann Surg. 1988;208(4):391–400.
34. Cirocchi R, Abraha I, Farinella E, Montedori A, Sciannameo F. Laparoscopic versus open surgery in small bowel obstruction. Cochrane Database Syst Rev. 2010;(2):CD007511.
35. Havenga K, Enker WE, McDermott K, Cohen AM, Minsky BD, Guillem J. Male and female sexual and urinary function after total mesorectal excision with autonomic nerve preservation for carcinoma of the rectum. J Am Coll Surg. 1996;182(6):495–502.
36. Masui H, Ike H, Yamaguchi S, Oki S, Shimada H. Male sexual function after autonomic nerve-preserving operation for rectal cancer. Dis Colon Rectum. 1996;39(10):1140–5.
37. Lindsey I, Mortensen NJ. Iatrogenic impotence and rectal dissection. Br J Surg. 2002;89(12):1493–4.
38. Lindsey I, George B, Kettlewell M, et al. Randomized, double-blind, placebo-controlled trial of sildenafil (Viagra) for erectile dysfunction after rectal excision for cancer and inflammatory bowel disease. Dis Colon Rectum. 2002;45(6):727–32.
39. daSilva GM, Hull T, Roberts PL, Ruiz DE, Wexner SD, Weiss EG, et al. The effect of colorectal surgery in female sexual function, body image, self esteem and general health: a prospective study. Ann Surg. 2008;248(2):266–72.
40. Gorgun E, Remzi FH, Goldberg JM, et al. Fertility is reduced after restorative proctocolectomy with ileal pouch anal anastomosis: a study of 300 patients. Surgery. 2004;136(4):795–803.
41. Olsen KO, Joelsson M, Laurberg S, Oresland T. Fertility after ileal pouch-anal anastomosis in women with ulcerative colitis. Br J Surg. 1999;86(4):493–5.
42. Fevang BT, Fevang J, Stangeland L, Soreide O, Svanes K, Viste A. Complications and death after surgical treatment of small bowel obstruction: a 35-year institutional experience. Ann Surg. 2000;231(4):529–37.
43. Sarr MG, Bulkley GB, Zuidema GD. Preoperative recognition of intestinal strangulation obstruction. Prospective evaluation of diagnostic capability. Am J Surg. 1983;145(1):176–82.
44. Biondo S, Pares D, Mora L, Marti RJ, Kreisler E, Jaurrieta E. Randomized clinical study of gastrografin administration in patients with adhesive small bowel obstruction. Br J Surg. 2003;90(5):542–6.

45. Choi HK, Chu KW, Law WL. Therapeutic value of gastrografin in adhesive small bowel obstruction after unsuccessful conservative treatment: a prospective randomized trial. Ann Surg. 2002;236(1):1–6.
46. Chen SC, Lin FY, Lee PH, Yu SC, Wang SM, Chang KJ. Water-soluble contrast study predicts the need for early surgery in adhesive small bowel obstruction. Br J Surg. 1998;85(12):1692–4.
47. Becker JM, Dayton MT, Fazio VW, et al. Prevention of postoperative abdominal adhesions by a sodium hyaluronate-based bioresorbable membrane: a prospective, randomized, double-blind multicenter study. J Am Coll Surg. 1996;183(4):297–306.
48. Fazio VW, Cohen Z, Fleshman JW, et al. Adhesion Study Group. Reduction in adhesive small bowel obstruction by Seprafilm® adhesion barrier after intestinal resection. Dis Colon Rectum. 2006;48:1–9.
49. Nivatvongs S, Fang DT. The use of thumbtacks to stop massive presacral hemorrhage. Dis Colon Rectum. 1986;29(9):589–90.
50. Stolfi VM, Milsom JW, Lavery IC, Oakley JR, Church JM, Fazio VW. Newly designed occluder pin for presacral hemorrhage. Dis Colon Rectum. 1992;35(2):166–9.
51. Remzi FH, Oncel M, Fazio VW. Muscle tamponade to control presacral venous bleeding: report of two cases. Dis Colon Rectum. 2002;45(8):1109–11.
52. Cosman BC, Lackides GA, Fisher DP, Eskenazi LB. Use of tissue expander for tamponade of presacral hemorrhage. Report of a case. Dis Colon Rectum. 1994;37(7):723–6.
53. Losanoff JE, Richman BW, Jones JW. Cyanoacrylate adhesive in management of severe presacral bleeding. Dis Colon Rectum. 2002;45(8):1118–9.
54. Xu J, Lin J. Control of presacral hemorrhage with electrocautery through a muscle fragment pressed on the bleeding vein. J Am Coll Surg. 1994;179(3):351–2.
55. Metzger PP. Modified packing technique for control of presacral pelvic bleeding. Dis Colon Rectum. 1988;31(12):981–2.
56. Rau HG, Mittelkotter U, Zimmermann A, Lachmann A, Kohler L, Kullmann KH. Perioperative infection prophylaxis and risk factor impact in colon surgery. Chemotherapy. 2000;46(5):353–63.
57. Platell C, Hall JC. The prevention of wound infection in patients undergoing colorectal surgery. J Hosp Infect. 2001;49(4):233–8.
58. Slim K, Vicaut E, Panis Y, Chipponi J. Meta-analysis of randomized clinical trials of colorectal surgery with or without mechanical bowel preparation. Br J Surg. 2004;91(9):1125–30.
59. Platell C, Hall J. What is the role of mechanical bowel preparation in patients undergoing colorectal surgery? Dis Colon Rectum. 1998;41(7):875–82.
60. Guenaga KF, Matos D, Castro AA, Atallah AN, Wille-Jorgensen P. Mechanical bowel preparation for elective colorectal surgery. Cochrane Database Syst Rev. 2003;(2):CD001544.
61. Khurrum BM, Hua ZR, Batista O, et al. Percutaneous postoperative intra-abdominal abscess drainage after elective colorectal surgery. Tech Coloproctol. 2002;6(3):159–64.
62. Schechter S, Eisenstat TE, Oliver GC, Rubin RJ, Salvati EP. Computerized tomographic scan-guided drainage of intra-abdominal abscesses. Preoperative and postoperative modalities in colon and rectal surgery. Dis Colon Rectum. 1994;37(10):984–8.
63. Benoist S, Panis Y, Pannegeon V, et al. Can failure of percutaneous drainage of postoperative abdominal abscesses be predicted? Am J Surg. 2002;184(2):148–53.
64. Cinat ME, Wilson SE, Din AM. Determinants for successful percutaneous image-guided drainage of intra-abdominal abscess. Arch Surg. 2002;137(7):845–9.
65. Pollard CW, Nivatvongs S, Rojanasakul A, Ilstrup DM. Carcinoma of the rectum. Profiles of intraoperative and early post-operative complications. Dis Colon Rectum. 1994;37(9):866–74.
66. Rosen L, Veidenheimer MC, Coller JA, Corman ML. Mortality, morbidity, and patterns of recurrence after abdominoperineal resection for cancer of the rectum. Dis Colon Rectum. 1982;25(3):202–8.
67. Rothenberger DA, Wong WD. Abdominoperineal resection for adenocarcinoma of the low rectum. World J Surg. 1992;16(3):478–85.
68. Nissan A, Guillem JG, Paty PB, et al. Abdominoperineal resection for rectal cancer at a specialty center. Dis Colon Rectum. 2001;44(1):27–35.
69. Silen W, Glotzer DJ. The prevention and treatment of the persistent perineal sinus. Surgery. 1974;75(4):535–42.
70. Wang JY, Huang CJ, Hsieh JS, Huang YS, Juang YF, Huang TJ. Management of the perineal wounds following excision of the rectum for malignancy. Gaoxiong Yi Xue Ke Xue Za Zhi. 1994;10(4):177–81.
71. Hay JM, Fingerhut A, Paquet JC, Flamant Y. Management of the pelvic space with or without omentoplasty after abdominoperineal resection for carcinoma of the rectum: a prospective multicenter study. The French Association for Surgical Research. Eur J Surg. 1997;163(3):199–206.
72. Rice ML, Hay AM, Hurlow RH. Omentoplasty in abdominoperineal resection of the rectum. Aust N Z J Surg. 1992;62(2):147–9.
73. Ferguson CM. Use of omental pedicle grafts in abdominoperineal resection. Am Surg. 1990;56(5):310–2.
74. Smith SR, Swift I, Gompertz H, Baker WN. Abdominoperineal and anterior resection of the rectum with retrocolic omentoplasty and no drainage. Br J Surg. 1988;75(10):1012–5.
75. Moreaux J, Horiot A, Barrat F, Mabille J. Obliteration of the pelvic space with pedicled omentum after excision of the rectum for cancer. Am J Surg. 1984;148(5):640–4.
76. Baudot P, Keighley MR, Alexander-Williams J. Perineal wound healing after proctectomy for carcinoma and inflammatory disease. Br J Surg. 1980;67(4):275–6.
77. Irvin TT, Goligher JC. A controlled clinical trial of three different methods of perineal wound management following excision of the rectum. Br J Surg. 1975;62(4):287–91.

11 Hemorrhoids

Marc Singer

Anatomy

Hemorrhoids are a normal component of anorectal anatomy. The terms "hemorrhoids" – as used by patients – or "hemorrhoidal disease" refer to the state of symptoms attributed to the vascular cushions present in the anal canal. It is critical for both surgeons and patients alike to consider this fact when evaluating and managing hemorrhoidal symptoms, as patients may desire removal of hemorrhoids, whereas control of symptoms should be the primary treatment goal.

Thomson's classic description introduced the concept of hemorrhoids as anatomically distinct vascular cushions in 1975.[1] The internal hemorrhoids are not merely a thickening of the mucosa or submucosa within the anal canal, rather, discrete specialized structures with specific physiologic functions. Hemorrhoids, also known as piles, are vascular cushions contained within the submucosal space of the anal canal. These cushions are a normal anatomic component of the anus, and serve to maintain closure of the anal canal, thus contributing toward fecal continence. The hemorrhoids are composed of blood vessels, connective tissue, smooth muscle, and elastic tissue. The smooth muscle contained within the submucosal space, and therefore within the hemorrhoids, known as Trietz's muscle, originates from the conjoined longitudinal muscle and the internal sphincter. These fibers support the hemorrhoid, keeping it adherent to the internal sphincter. Hemorrhoids typically exist at three locations: the left lateral, right anterior, and right posterior positions of the anal canal.[1] These positions are often referred by the misnomer "quadrants." Hemorrhoidal tissue is not necessarily limited to these locations, and there is frequently additional hemorrhoidal tissue in between these three specific locations. In fact, less than 20% of cadavers were found to have the specific configuration of hemorrhoids at the three standard positions.[1] Gross inspection of the hemorrhoids reveals a blue hue, which may suggest similarity to veins. However, histologic analysis of hemorrhoids reveals an absent muscular wall, characterizing the cushions as sinusoids, technically not veins or arteries. Furthermore, hemorrhoidal bleeding is typically described as "bright red," suggestive of well-oxygenated arterial blood. A pH analysis of hemorrhoidal blood is most consistent with arterial blood.[2]

The arterial inflow supplying hemorrhoids consists of the terminal blanches of the superior hemorrhoidal artery, with some contribution by the branches of middle hemorrhoidal arteries. The more distal aspects also receive inflow from the inferior hemorrhoidal arteries.[3] The specific locations of the terminal branches of the superior hemorrhoidal artery do not relate to the three common locations of hemorrhoids (left lateral, right anterior, and right posterior). A renewed interest in the anatomy and the number of terminal branches of the arterial inflow has occurred, as directed ligation of these branches has become a popular treatment option. The venous drainage of the hemorrhoidal plexus distal to the dentate line (external hemorrhoids) includes the inferior hemorrhoidal veins, which flow into the pudendal veins, and ultimately the internal iliac veins. The middle hemorrhoidal veins contribute toward venous outflow from the internal hemorrhoids, located proximal to the dentate line, and also drain into the iliac veins.[4]

The anal canal, proximal to the dentate line, is innervated by sympathetic and parasympathetic nerves, as well as noncholinergic/nonadrenergic mediators. The anal canal distal to the dentate line, as well as the anoderm, is innervated by somatic nerves. For this reason, the distal anal canal and the associated external hemorrhoids are sensitive to touch, pain, temperature, and stretch.

There are multiple theories regarding the function of hemorrhoids. The most commonly believed hypothesis is that the hemorrhoids contribute toward maintaining fecal continence. Closure of the sphincter complex does not completely close the anal canal, and the bulkiness of the hemorrhoidal tissue provides closure of the central aspect of the anus. As one strains, sneezes, or exerts themselves, the vascular cushions engorge and distend, which completely closes the anus while at highest risk of fecal leakage. It has been theorized that hemorrhoids contribute up to 20% of the resting pressure of the anus.[5] The anal canal, including the hemorrhoids, is highly sensitive toward the discrimination of an

D.E. Beck et al. (eds.), *The ASCRS Textbook of Colon and Rectal Surgery: Second Edition*,
DOI 10.1007/978-1-4419-1584-9_11, © Springer Science+Business Media, LLC 2011

empty rectum, gas, liquid, or solid stool. The loss of bulk and sensation within the anal canal may put patients with marginal continence at high risk for postoperative incontinence after hemorrhoidectomy. Besides aiding continence, the soft and pliable hemorrhoid tissue may protect the sphincters from trauma related to passing stool.

Internal hemorrhoids are lined by columnar epithelium. Near the dentate line, there may be transitional epithelium. This mucosa is viscerally innervated, which means patients will report sensations such as vague fullness and pressure, but do not perceive touch, pain, stretch, or temperature such as on the skin. This makes office-based treatments possible without anesthesia.

The anoderm is specialized squamous epithelium that lacks skin structures such as hair follicles or sweat glands. The distal most aspects are lined by normal skin, including the appendages. The anoderm and perianal skin are somatically innervated, which means external hemorrhoids are very sensitive to touch, requiring anesthesia for procedures.

Etiology

A long list of conditions, diagnoses, behaviors, and comorbidities have been suggested as possible causes of symptomatic hemorrhoids. Conditions that impair venous drainage, promote prolapse of the vascular cushions, dietary patterns, behavioral factors, and sphincter function are among the features commonly believed to contribute toward the exacerbation of hemorrhoid symptoms.

Venous congestion with subsequent hypertrophy of the internal hemorrhoids is the most common event leading to symptomatic hemorrhoids. During normal straining and defecation, hemorrhoids engorge and then return to normal. If patients strain for prolonged periods, as with chronic constipation, the internal hemorrhoids become congested but do not rapidly decompress because the increased abdominal pressure impairs venous return. This process occurs as a result of constipation as well as pregnancy, chronic cough, pelvic mass, pelvic floor dysfunction, or ascites.

The internal hemorrhoids are normally supported by the fibers of Trietz's muscle and the elastic tissues in the submucosa. These supportive tissues can become attenuated, and therefore the hemorrhoids become progressively more mobile and begin to prolapse. As they prolapse, the venous return becomes obstructed, and the hemorrhoids will become more engorged. The bulk of the hemorrhoid will lead to further weakening of the supporting structures. Thompson described this cycle of progressive prolapse and engorgement as the sliding anal cushion theory.[1] If the prolapse is outside the sphincter, then the pressure of the sphincter further impairs blood return and the hemorrhoids become further congested.

Dietary and behavioral features contribute to symptomatic hemorrhoids. The low fiber diet of Western society creates hard dry stools. Constipation causes excessive straining, which exacerbates the hemorrhoids. The hard stool will also cause local tissue trauma, thus inducing bleeding. Toileting behavior and defecation habits are widely believed to contribute toward the development of hemorrhoid symptoms, but objective evidence is limited. This may be an indirect reflection of constipation. Some patients may spend prolonged time periods sitting on the commode because they are determined to have a bowel movement at a selected time or to move the bowels daily, even if not necessary. Some patients may read while on the toilet, which may subconsciously lead to prolonged straining.

Although constipation is well known to exacerbate hemorrhoid symptoms, diarrhea or frequent bowel movements can have the same effect. Advancing age is a known risk factor, independent of the other comorbidities. There is histologic evidence suggesting that the supporting soft tissues of the hemorrhoids, including Trietz's muscles, become less supportive with age, which leads to prolapse.[6] It has also been suggested that erect posture contributes to hemorrhoids due to the gravitational effects and venous pooling.

Hemorrhoids are not typically due to mucosal abnormalities, such as inflammation or dysplastic changes, or intrinsic sphincter abnormalities. However, there is objective evidence that patients with hemorrhoid symptoms demonstrate elevated manometric sphincter pressures compared to controls.[6–12] It may be possible that elevated sphincter pressures impair venous drainage of the hemorrhoids in some patients. Excisional hemorrhoidectomy has been documented to reverse this finding.[9]

There is sparse objective evidence for any of the purported hypotheses. It is likely that the development of symptoms is multifactorial, including a number of patient-specific anatomic, behavioral, dietary, and possibly genetic influences.

Epidemiology

The true incidence of hemorrhoids is difficult to accurately assess. Many patients do not seek medical attention for their symptoms.[7,10] Patients often self-medicate with any number of the large variety of over-the-counter products that are available. Statistics such as operative procedures may be straightforward to monitor; however, a very small proportion of patients with symptoms actually require operative therapy. In addition, patients seek care from a large number of different specialists including surgeons, gastroenterologists, internists, family practitioners, pediatricians, gynecologists, and practitioners of alternative medicine. Finally, patients self-diagnose many other anorectal diseases as "hemorrhoids."

The prevalence of hemorrhoids in the USA has been estimated at 4.4%[10] or 8.5 million patients.[11] It may be as high as 36% of patients seeking care in a general medical practice.[12] Fortunately, the number of deaths attributed to hemorrhoids is exceedingly small.[13] The prevalence is highest in Caucasian patients between 45 and 65 years of age and of elevated socioeconomic status. This may represent selection bias and access to care, as this cohort typically would have the greatest access. Johanson and Sonnenberg[14] suggest that the incidence of hemorrhoidal symptoms has decreased in the last 50 years based on self-reporting of patients in the USA and UK. By any measure, this represents a common problem with between 1.9 and 3.5 million physician visits[15,16] and 168,000 hospitalizations, annually.[17] There are nearly two million prescriptions written annually for hemorrhoid therapies,[18] accounting for over $43,000,000. This is independent of over-the-counter, herbal, and homeopathic remedies.[19]

Classification

Hemorrhoids are generally divided into two categories: internal and external. Internal hemorrhoids originate proximal to the dentate line. This can be a source of confusion in the setting of prolapse completely through the anus. Patients perceive the hemorrhoids to be outside of the anorectum, but in fact, the hemorrhoids originate proximal to the dentate line. Internal hemorrhoids are lined by columnar epithelium. External hemorrhoids are located distal to the dentate line, and are lined by anoderm and skin at the distal most aspect. A mixed, or combined, hemorrhoid is a condition in which both internal and external hemorrhoids are present.

In 1985, Banow et al.[20] described a classification system based on clinical prolapse (Table 11-1). This system has become popular among surgeons because it describes the symptoms of prolapse, which is one of the main factors driving treatment decisions. Unfortunately, it does not incorporate size, discomfort, or bleeding, which also commonly direct therapeutic decisions.

Clinical Presentation

Patients with essentially any anorectal pathology may present with the complaint of "hemorrhoids." Patients and physicians unfamiliar with specific anorectal pathology commonly use this label. A number of patients may suffer from other benign anorectal conditions such as fissures, fistulas, pruritis, abscesses, and condylomata. These are pathologies also addressed by a colon and rectal surgeon, making a referral appropriate under any circumstance. More importantly, patients with warning signs, like bleeding, should not be overlooked as colon, rectal, or anal cancer can present with such symptoms.

TABLE 11-1. Classification of hemorrhoids

Grade I – Internal hemorrhoids bulge into the anus without prolapse
Grade II – Internal hemorrhoids prolapse during defecation, spontaneously reduce
Grade III – Internal hemorrhoids prolapse, requiring manual reduction
Grade IV – Hemorrhoids prolapsed and irreducible

Internal Hemorrhoid Symptoms

Patients with symptomatic internal hemorrhoids may complain of bleeding, itching, burning, pain, prolapse, swelling, mucus discharge, and difficulty with perineal hygiene. The edematous hemorrhoids may cause the patient to feel as if they are sitting on a foreign object. Patients with prolapsing hemorrhoids may not always recognize the prolapsing nature of the hemorrhoids, but may report wetness, itching, and soiling of the undergarments. Traditionally, it has been suggested that internal hemorrhoids do not cause somatic pain because they originate proximal to the dentate line. However, patients commonly complain of anal or rectal pain. It may be that patients use the word "pain" as a surrogate for itching, burning, or an overall sense of discomfort or unpleasantness. When patients are specifically queried, patients do report hemorrhoidal pain, even if afforded the opportunity to differentiate pain from burning, wetness, or other symptoms.[21] Although the anatomic location suggests that internal hemorrhoids should not cause pain, such objective evidence should not be entirely discounted, and patient complaints of pain should be addressed. It remains critical to identify and treat alternative causes of pain such as associated fissures or perianal excoriation. A subtle volume of mucus may be discharged at the time of hemorrhoid prolapse, which can cause significant perianal irritation. Severe pain may be indicative of thrombosed or strangulated internal hemorrhoids.

The specific details of the rectal bleeding should be elicited. The classic hemorrhoidal bleeding is bright red blood at the time of bowel movements. Patients may report blood on the toilet paper, blood dripping into the toilet, or even blood squirting into the toilet. Hemorrhoidal bleeding will typically occur at the end of the bowel movement, presumably because the stool itself causes trauma to the engorged hemorrhoids. An attempt should be made to differentiate this from blood mixing into the stool, or melena, which suggests a colorectal malignancy. Patients may not be able to reliably distinguish these patterns, and for that reason, bleeding must be carefully considered and worked up in the appropriate patients. Age, personal history, family history, or other risk factors must weigh into the decision regarding further workup of bleeding. It is not always necessary to complete this workup at the onset of treatment. A mechanical bowel preparation and colonoscopy may exacerbate hemorrhoid symptoms. Deferral until after hemorrhoids have been treated is appropriate, but it must not be postponed indefinitely. Bleeding may occur in microscopic quantities only, resulting in a positive guaiac test. Anemia due to hemorrhoidal bleeding is sufficiently rare that it warrants a full assessment of the gastrointestinal tract.

The internal hemorrhoids may be prolapsing internally, which can cause a sensation of fullness, the urge to defecate, or the sensation of incomplete evacuation after bowel movements. If hemorrhoids prolapse completely through the anus, then patients will perceive a mass or lump, but can also cause wetness or soiling. As the mucosa prolapses, it carries mucus, blood, or stool from inside the anal canal out to the perineum. This can make hygiene difficult after a bowel movement. Patients may complain that excessive wiping is required, or shortly after a bowel movement they find their undergarments to be soiled. Patients should be asked about spontaneous or manual reduction of prolapsing hemorrhoids. Finally, lifestyle questions should be directed toward uncovering additional precipitating factors such as constant straining due to heavy lifting, chronic coughing due to chronic obstructive pulmonary disease (COPD), and limited bathroom access leading to hard dry stools.

External Hemorrhoid Symptoms

External hemorrhoids may present with redundant tissue around the anus, bleeding, or difficulty in maintaining hygiene after bowel movements. In addition, they may become inflamed. Symptoms are typically less severe than those of internal hemorrhoids, with the exception of acute thrombosis of an external hemorrhoid. Patients will experience the acute onset of mild to excruciating anal pain. This may be precipitated by an episode of diarrhea or constipation, but many times there is no identifiable inciting factor. Patients will also complain of a firm lump at the anus. Patients sometimes undertake unusual maneuvers in order to visualize their own anus, and may report a blue or purple color to the lump. This will be at the level or distal to the dentate line. Bleeding will not usually occur immediately following the onset of pain; however, when the pressure of the thrombus erodes through the skin, then the clot will spontaneously drain. The necrotic skin may become gangrenous and rarely cause surrounding cellulitis. After the external hemorrhoid thrombus drains spontaneously or is surgically evacuated, the expanded external hemorrhoid will reduce in size; however, patients are often left with resultant skin tags. These tags may reduce in size over time, but typically do not completely regress. Tags may cause symptoms in the future, such as itching and difficulty with hygiene, even after the hemorrhoid symptoms have long resolved. Such tags may also be embarrassing for patients. The differential diagnosis of common hemorrhoidal problems based on anorectal symptoms is presented in Table 11-2.

TABLE 11-2. Differential diagnosis based on anal symptoms

Symptom	Differential diagnoses
Pain	Thrombosed hemorrhoids, fissure, abscess, fistula, pruritis, anorectal Crohn's disease, anismus, abscess
Bleeding	Internal or external hemorrhoids, fissure, fistula, hypertrophic papilla, polyps, anal or colorectal cancer, ulcerative colitis, Crohn's disease, infectious colitis, draining thrombosed hemorrhoids, rectal prolapse
Pruritis	Prolapsing hemorrhoids, fistula, incontinence, anal condylomata, rectal prolapse, pruritis ani, anal papilla, dermatitis, dietary causes
Mass	Thrombosed or prolapsed hemorrhoids, abscess, anal cancer, prolapsing polyp or papilla, skin tags, prolapsing tumor, rectal prolapse, condylomata

Evaluation

History

The goal of management of hemorrhoids is control of the symptoms, but not necessarily to extirpate all hemorrhoid tissue. For this reason, a careful ascertainment of specific symptoms is critical toward guiding the evaluation and directing the therapeutic options.

A detailed history, including a complete discussion of the patient's bowel habits, is the starting point in the workup of symptomatic hemorrhoids. Symptoms are intimately related to bowel habits. Constipation, diarrhea, urgency, frequency, and changes in the bowel habit must be documented. For selected patients, a prospectively maintained bowel diary including standardized instruments, such as the Bristol Stool Scale which specifically describes stool types (texture and shape), and includes visuals (see Chap. 32) may be helpful to accurately characterize bowel movements over time.[22]

This bowel history is also useful in eliciting "red flag" symptoms, such as bleeding or changes in bowel habit, which may be indicative of malignancies. Furthermore, the history can help to differentiate hemorrhoids from other benign anorectal pathology. Chronic diarrhea with anal pain may suggest Crohn's disease. A lump that drains pus suggests an abscess or fistula. Chronic itching without bleeding or prolapse suggests pruritis. Extreme pain with bowel movements suggests a fissure.

A dietary history, and the effects on the bowel habit, is also critical toward management of hemorrhoid symptoms. Specific foods or eating patterns that worsen constipation of diarrhea must be addressed at the beginning of the management plan. A common cause of constipation in Western countries is in adequate dietary fiber and/or fluid intake. Although it can be difficult to estimate fiber intake, patients committed to dietary and medical management of hemorrhoid symptoms may benefit from a diet journal. Special attention should be paid to foods that commonly cause diarrhea (fats, caffeine, or alcohol) or constipation (cheese, beef, or bananas). Recent changes in diet or bowel habit due to acute illness or travel should be noted.

Physical Examination

A generalized physical examination may reveal relevant physical signs of liver disease, COPD, or coagulopathy. The abdominal examination should be directed toward the signs of constipation, such as abdominal distension or a palpable fecal impaction in the left colon. Finally, the examination should be directed toward the anorectum. The anorectal examination can be embarrassing for many patients. This may be especially true of younger patients who have never undergone an anorectal examination by their primary care physician or gynecologist. The patient should be reassured that the examination will be brief and, although uncomfortable, will not be painful. Patients should be offered to have a same-gender chaperone in the room during the examination, if feasible. These steps will relax the patient and facilitate a more complete and thorough examination. If the patient is uncomfortable or uncooperative, then the clinician may inadvertently abbreviate the examination or be reluctant to complete some aspects of the evaluation such as a proctoscopy.

The prone jackknife position on a proctologic table allows for maximal exposure of the perineum and anus. This can be particularly true for obese patients, in whom retraction of the buttocks can be difficult. In addition, if examining the patient without the aid of an assistant, the prone position does not mandate retraction of the buttocks. If a proctologic table is unavailable or impractical because the patient is too obese, pregnant, or orthopedic issues preclude the prone position, then the lateral position (Sims) or lithotomy positions will suffice. Regardless of the position in which the patient is examined, the anatomy and pathology should be described in anatomical terms (left, right, anterior, or posterior), but *not* the positions of a clock. The convention of clock positions can be confusing as different practitioners may examine patients in different positions. Furthermore, vague terms such as above or below should not be used to describe proximal or distal to the dentate line or anal verge.

The examining surgeon gently spreads the buttocks and inspects the perineum, anoderm, and sacrococcygeal regions. The surgeon then identifies external hemorrhoids, skin tags, prolapsing internal hemorrhoids, rectal prolapse, excoriated skin, fissures, fistulas, abscesses, anal cancers, thrombosed external hemorrhoids, rashes, or dermatitites. Careful palpation should also be performed in order to assess for induration, tenderness, masses, or thrombus in the external hemorrhoids. Next, a digital examination of the anal canal should be performed to assess sphincter tone, identify masses, abscesses, and localize pain. Weak resting sphincter tone should be further interrogated by asking the patient to voluntarily squeeze on the examiner's finger in order to grossly assess squeeze pressures.

At a minimum, anoscopy is required to thoroughly assess hemorrhoids. Several types of anoscopes are available (Figure 11-1A and B). A slotted or side viewing anoscope is best for assessing internal hemorrhoids. The slot allows the internal hemorrhoids to prolapse into the scope, giving the examiner a sense of the bulk of the hemorrhoids. Translucent plastic anoscopes are available, which are conveniently disposable. Also, the clear plastic allows for simultaneous visualization of the entire anal canal, especially the relationship between the hemorrhoids and the dentate lane. However, the lack of a slot on some plastic anoscopes can impair rubber band ligation (RBL). Some anoscopes contain multiple slots, which may facilitate RBL of multiple quadrants in a single setting.[23]

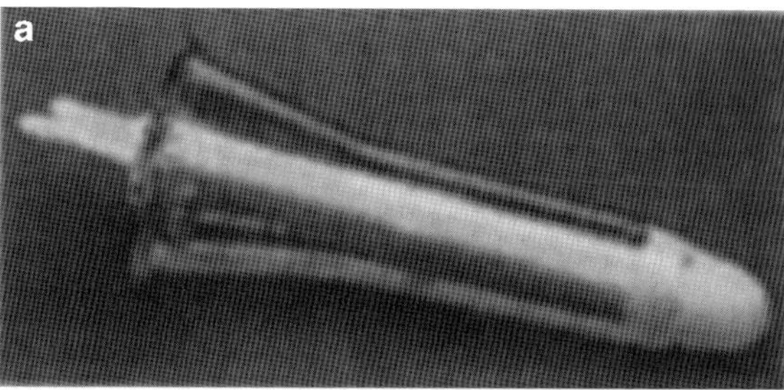

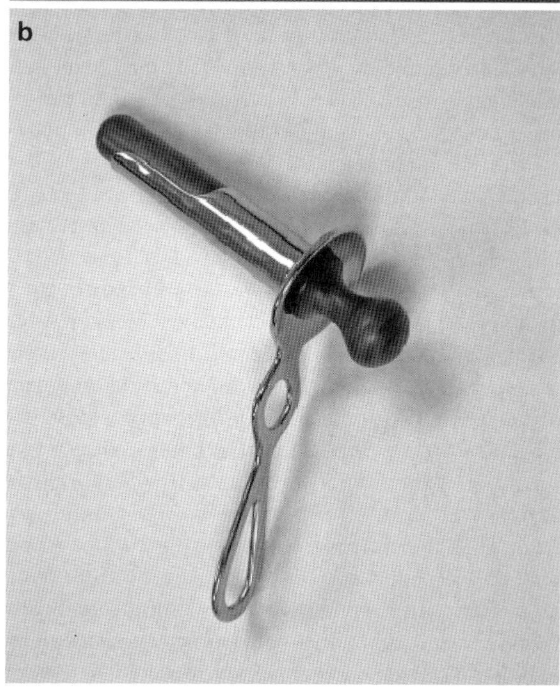

FIGURE 11-1. **a** Ives Fansler Anoscope and **b** a clear plastic anoscope.

The degree of prolapse should be assessed by asking the patient to strain or simulate a bowel movement. This may be underestimated in the prone jackknife position. If the degree of prolapse is questionable, then the patient should be moved to a commode or onto a toilet. The examiner should request the patient to push or strain, and then carefully inspect the anus while the patient is in this more physiologic situation.

Patients should also undergo rigid or flexible proctoscopy. The rectum should be evaluated for inflammatory conditions, polyps, or tumors. This is certainly true in patients with red flag symptoms of bleeding, weight loss, anemia, or change in bowel habits. At least at the initial evaluation of a new patient, an effort should be made to understand the status of the rectum. Hemorrhoids in the setting of rectal inflammation may be treated differently than hemorrhoids in a patient with a normal rectum.

The patient should be considered for formal evaluation of the entire colon with either colonoscopy or double contrast enema. Clinical factors such as red flag symptoms, age, personal and family history of colorectal pathology, duration of symptoms, or the nature of bleeding can be used to determine which patients should undergo additional evaluation. In suitable patients, it is appropriate to treat hemorrhoids first and defer formal evaluation of the colon until a later date. There is reluctance to administer a full cathartic bowel preparation in a patient experiencing significant symptoms already. It would be reasonable to defer evaluation for several weeks to months to allow treatments of the hemorrhoids. The ability of the patient to accurately characterize the blood per rectum may not be reliable enough to sufficiently differentiate benign versus malignant causes of bleeding in many cases. Therefore, the entire clinical scenario must be considered in the decision to evaluate the colon entirely for bleeding.[24–28] Patients fulfilling specific criteria (such as those proposed by the Multi-Society Task Force on Colorectal Cancers) should be considered for additional workup.[26,27]

In addition, patients with risk factors, such as being part of an HNPCC family or those with atypical bleeding, should also undergo colonoscopy.[29,30] Hemorrhoids often present in younger patients, in whom the risk of colorectal malignancy is relatively low. This often raises the question of total colon examination. Simple hemorrhoidal bleeding does not require total colon evaluation in a young patient without other risk factors (family history); however, hemorrhoids rarely cause anemia. Thus, hemorrhoids with anemia warrant colonoscopy or contrast enema.[31,32]

As a general rule, younger patients (<40 years old) with hemorrhoids and symptoms compatible with their disease may undergo office anoscopy and proctoscopy. If treatment immediately ceases bleeding, then no future evaluation is indicated. Patients >40 years of age with a family history or symptoms that seem out of proportion to their exam should undergo total colon evaluations.

Table 11-3. Amount of fiber in common foods

Foods	Serving size	Total fiber (g)
Navy beans, cooked	1 Cup	19.1
Lentils, cooked	1 Cup	15.6
Pinto beans, cooked	1 Cup	15.4
Black beans, cooked	1 Cup	15.0
Artichokes, cooked	1 Cup	14.4
Lima beans, cooked	1 Cup	13.2
Garbanzo beans	1 Cup	12.5
Baked beans, cooked	1 Cup	10.4
Soybeans, boiled	1 Cup	10.3
Peas, cooked	1 Cup	8.8
Raspberries	1 Cup	8.0
Blackberries	1 Cup	7.6
Spinach, frozen, cooked	1 Cup	7.0
Lettuce, iceberg	1 Head	6.5
Pear, with skin	1 Medium	5.5
Bran flakes	3/4 Cup	5.3
Oat bran muffin	1 Medium	5.2
Broccoli, boiled	1 Cup	5.1
Apple, with skin	1 Medium	4.4
White Rice, cooked	1 Cup	4.1
Brussels sprouts, cooked	1 Cup	4.1
Oatmeal, cooked	1 Cup	4.0
Strawberries	1.25 Cup	3.8
Brown rice, cooked	1 Cup	3.5
Almonds	1 Oz	3.5
Strawberries	1 Cup	3.3
Orange	1 Medium	3.1
Banana	1 Medium	3.1
Potato, with skin, baked	1 Medium	2.9
Cucumber, peeled, raw	1 Large	2.0
Bread, whole-wheat	1 Slice	1.9
Corn, sweet	1 Ear	1.8
Carrot	1 Medium	1.7
Raisins	2 Tablespoons	1.0
Bread, wheat	1 Slice	0.9
Bread, white	1 Slice	0.6
Grapes, red or green	10 Grapes	0.5

Adapted from: United States Department of Agriculture (USDA) National Nutrient Database for Standard Reference, Release 22; www.ars.usda.gov.

Treatment

The treatment of symptomatic hemorrhoids is directed by the symptoms themselves. Patients should be reassured that hemorrhoids are normal components of human anatomy and that it is not necessary to remove all hemorrhoidal tissue. Treatments can be broadly categorized into three groups: (1) medical management, including dietary and behavioral therapies, (2) office-based procedures, and (3) operative therapies.

Dietary and Lifestyle Modification

Hemorrhoid symptoms are frequently related to alteration of the bowel habit. Therefore, initial therapy should be directed at modifying the stool. Constipation is most commonly related to a relative lack of dietary fiber and fluid intake. The recommendation of 25 g/day for women and 38 g/day for men is rarely achieved. The United States Department of Agriculture (USDA) estimates that mean fiber intake for Americans is merely 15 g/day.[33] A high fiber diet (Table 11-3) and 64 oz of water daily should be the initial recommendations. Also, behavioral modifications such as a regular sleep/wake cycle and exercise schedule can be helpful to maintain a regular bowel habit, and therefore reduce hemorrhoid symptoms.

It can be difficult to ingest 25–35 g/day of dietary fiber, making the fiber supplement a necessary option (Table 11-4). Bulk-forming agents such as psyllium are generally well tolerated and cost-effective. The objective data regarding fiber supplements is somewhat conflicting, but available publications do support the use of bulk-forming agents to treat hemorrhoid symptoms. Moesgaard et al.[34] have

Table 11-4. Fiber supplements

Fiber supplement	Brand name products
Psyllium	Metamucil, Konsyl Fiberall, Hydrocil, Perdiem, Serutan
Methylcellulose	Citrucel
Calcium Polycarbophil	FiberCon, Fiber-lax, Equalactin, Mitrolan
Wheat Dextrin	Benefiber
Inulin	FiberChoice

demonstrated that a high fiber diet can reduce bleeding and pain as related to hemorrhoids; however, other authors have not been able to document such benefits.[35–37] Alonso-Coello et al.[38] conducted a systematic review of trials examining fiber for the treatment of hemorrhoids. He examined seven trials with nearly 400 patients comparing fiber to a control group. Fiber showed a consistent benefit for the reduction of bleeding and other symptoms.

Bulk-forming agents treat hemorrhoids by modifying the quality of the stool. They work in combination with oral fluids to add moisture and soften the stool. For this reason, supplements are best administered in the morning, so that fluid can be consumed throughout the day. If ingested at bedtime, as some patients prefer to take their other medications, the fiber will remain in the intestinal track overnight, without additional fluid, and may, in fact, dehydrate the stool and worsen constipation. Divided dosing throughout the day is appropriate, but it is imperative that patients drink fluids with the dose and then throughout the day.

The addition of stool softeners (docusate) or lubricants (mineral oil) can be helpful toward treating constipation. Hyperosmolar (plyethylene glycol), saline (magnesium citrate), or stimulate laxatives (senna and bisacodyl) are safe and effective. There is no creditable evidence that long-term use is harmful. Patients may require such laxatives to break a fecal impaction, but should be transitioned to a regimen of fiber and stool softeners as quickly as possible. The goal of the fiber supplement, stool softeners, and increased fluid consumption is create bulky, but soft stools that move regularly. The goal of this therapy, in terms of the quantity and frequency of bowel movements, is determined by the comfort and symptoms of a patient.

Patients with diarrhea may require additional assessment. Patients with loose stools related to a diet, which is low in fiber and high in fats, need only dietary modification. This is often exacerbated by caffeine, alcohol, and an irregular sleep/wake cycle. Profound or bloody diarrhea may require stool cultures, fecal fat analysis, or endoscopy, among others. Loose stools can be treated initially with fiber supplementation. Although 25–35 g/day is the recommended target, patients will require titration of the dose.

Typically, the high fiber diet and fiber supplements and stool softeners should be trialed for 4–6 weeks. Reevaluation should focus on symptom management. The appearance of internal hemorrhoids during anoscopy may be unchanged, but if symptoms are well controlled, this should be considered a successful outcome. Long-term compliance with these measures can be problematic, as many patients will not commit to indefinite treatment. In addition, many fiber supplements carry significant noncompliance due to poor palatability or side effects such as abdominal bloating, excessive flatus, or crampy abdominal pain. Patients should be started on a low dose and titrated up to the desired effect in order to minimize the side effects.

Toileting Behavior

Patients with hemorrhoids commonly exhibit dysfunctional toileting behaviors. It is not clear that this is a result of hemorrhoidal symptoms or a contributing factor toward symptoms. Common issues include excessive straining, pushing, Valsalva maneuver, and prolonged time on the toilet. Patients should be encouraged to spend 3–5 min on the toilet as a general guideline. Patients should refrain from the common practice of reading on the toilet, as this may lead to prolonged periods of straining. Patients requiring excessive time on the toilet (>30 min) or those with multiple unsuccessful attempts should be considered for evaluation of a pelvic floor disorder. In addition, perianal hygiene routines should be addressed. Patient with soft or pasty stool commonly complain of excessive wiping. Some patients become compulsive with cleaning rituals. Patients should be encouraged to wipe only until clean. Excessive wiping can cause local trauma, contributing to inflammation of prolapsing internal hemorrhoids, bleeding of external hemorrhoids, and worsening pruritis. The use of premoistened wipes (baby wipes and witch hazel wipes) is safe and often less traumatic. Patients should be cautioned to dry the perineum afterwards because a wet perineum will lead to further skin maceration and symptoms.

Sitz Baths

Sitz baths are commonly recommended as part of the initial treatment plan and can aid with hygiene, particularly after bowel movements. They often provide symptomatic relief of pain, itching, burning, and may facilitate the manual reduction of prolapsed hemorrhoids. Sitz baths may alleviate sphincter and pelvic floor spasm, which contribute to the discomfort in some patients.

Sitz baths should be warm, as if a patient were taking a normal bath (approximately 40°C) but not scalding hot. In attempt to maximize the therapeutic benefits of sitz baths, patients have been known to scald their perineal skin. Sitz baths are best accomplished in a traditional bathtub, however, older patients may not be able to get in/out of a bathtub due to orthopedic issues and some patients may not have access to a bathtub. In such cases, portable sitz baths are available (Figure 11-2). These are placed on top of the

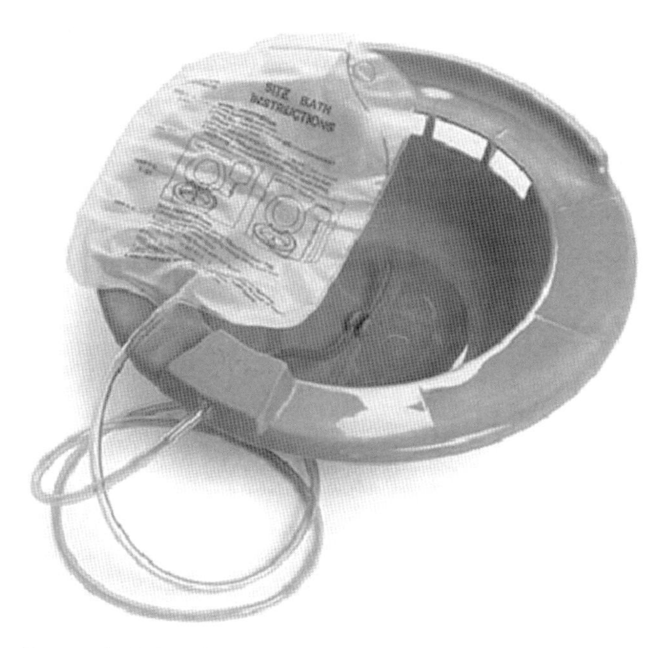

FIGURE 11-2. Portable Sitz bath.

toilet and allow patients to soak the perineum only. Soaking time should be limited to approximately 15 min. Prolonged soaking in water may contribute to edema. Patients should be discouraged from adding salts, oils, or lotions to the water. These products may cause further inflammation of prolapsing hemorrhoids.

There is a dearth of objective evidence supporting the use of sitz baths for hemorrhoids or other anorectal disorders.[39] However, many patients subjectively report relief from this practice. Considering the low cost and low risk, it is appropriate to continue to recommend sitz baths.

For a large number of patients, increasing fiber and water, sitz baths, and simple behavioral modifications are adequate to completely treat hemorrhoid symptoms. If dietary and behavioral modifications are unsuccessful, then additional treatment options should be considered.

Medical Therapy

A large number of topical medications, suppositories, and wipes are available to patients. Patients will frequently attempt self-medication with over-the-counter products before seeking treatment from a physician. Objective evidence regarding the effectiveness of these products is sparse. Most available data does not rigorously examine products compared to controls or placebo, or make use of standardized definitions and survey instruments. It is therefore inappropriate to make firm recommendations in support of any of the products. The use of these products is so common that surgeons should be familiar with them so that appropriate discussion can be entertained with patients.

Common over-the-counter products include ointments, creams, gels, suppositories, foams, and wipes. Most products contain a combination of agents including a barrier protectant and another active ingredient. Local anesthetics applied topically may provide temporary relief of pain, itching, and burning. The delivery vehicles may cause local irritation to the anoderm. The active ingredients include benzocaine, benzyl alcohol, dibucaine, dyclonine, lidcaine, pramoxine, and tetracain. Vasoconstricting agents can be used in an effort to reduce swelling and engorgement of hemorrhoids. Available drugs include ephedrine, epinephrine, and phenylephrine. Barrier protectants aim to prevent skin irritation by keeping mucus, stool, or mucosa from directly contacting the perianal skin. Common products include aluminum hydroxide gel, cocoa butter, glycerin, kaolin, lanolin, mineral oil, petrolatum, starch, and zinc oxide. Astringents can be used to clean and dry the perineum. These products include calamine, zinc oxide, and witch hazel. Analgesics aim to sooth the anus. These include camphor, juniper tar, and menthol. Corticosteroids are anti-inflammatory drugs. These serve to reduce perianal inflammation, itching, and pain. Prolonged use may cause thinning of the skin and therefore should not be used for longer than a few weeks.

Patients commonly attempt symptomatic relief with suppositories. Suppositories do not typically remain localized within the anal canal. They are often expelled immediately after insertion, in which case they cannot deliver a sustained dose of medication. Alternatively, they may migrate proximally into the rectum, where the medication will be delivered. However, as these medications are meant to act topically within the anus, they are not affecting the appropriate mucosa. Suppositories may provide indirect benefit by either mechanically stimulating the rectum to evacuate or they may deliver lubrication to the anal canal and rectum, which can provide some benefit by lubricating the anus, and thus mitigating the effects of stool trauma on the hemorrhoids. A variety of soothing creams and ointments are contained within the suppositories. Frequently, steroids and/or local anesthetics will be combined with these agents.

Phlebotonics

Phlebotonics are a heterogeneous collection of substances that are used to treat venous insufficiency, lymphedema, venous stasis ulcers, and certain bleeding conditions, but also to treat hemorrhoids. Some of these products are plant extracts (flavonoids and saponosedes), and some are synthetic compounds (calcium dobesilate and naftazone). These compounds are purported to improve venous blood flow, which may ameliorate conditions such as lower extremity venous insufficiency or engorged hemorrhoids. The specific mechanisms of action are largely unknown, but they are believed to improve venous tone, stabilize capillary permeability, and increase lymphatic drainage.[40–42] Documented benefits are largely unknown due to the lack of controlled studies. Some compounds have specific safety concerns, such as the flavonoids which can cause GI side effects or calcium dobesilate which can cause agranulocytosis.[43]

The citrus bioflavoinoids, which create pigmentation in fruits, are most often used in Europe. There are multiple alleged health benefits, but most are not substantially documented. The most common compounds include diosmin, hesperidin, rutin, naringin, tangeretin, diosmetin, narirutin, neohesperidin, nobiletin, and quercetin. A commercially available diosmin product has been shown to be effective for the treatment of hemorrhoids, but such products are not available in pharmaceutical grade in the USA.[44–48] They are available as nutritional supplements (Daflon 500® Les Laboratories, Servier, France) and with the increasing incidence of patients ordering international products through the internet, it is critical to be familiar with this and related supplements. Other naturally occurring compounds include "flavonoids," Rutosides,[49,50] buckwheat herb, ruscus aculeastus (butcher's broom), hidrosmin, gingko biloba, saponsides, escin (horse chestnut seed), and Hamamelis Virginiana (Witch Hazel).

Synthetic products include calcium dobesilate, naftazone, aminaftone, chromocarbe, iquinosa, flunarizine, and sulfomucopolysaccharide. Of this group, calcium dobesilate may be the most widely examined. Its function stems from the capacity to stabilize capillary permeability, decrease platelet aggregation, and improve lymphatic transport. Metes et al.[51] sought to determine the clinical efficacy of calcium dobesiliate for hemorrhoids by conducting a randomized clinical trial comparing effects to fiber supplementation alone. Patient symptoms significantly improved after only 2 weeks of treatments.[51]

A recent meta-analysis examining the utility of flavonoids to treat hemorrhoids reviewed 14 trials.[52] There was significant heterogeneity between trials, but there did appear to be a beneficial effect. Patients enjoyed decreased bleeding, pain, and itching. The doses and formulations of the investigated compounds were highly variable.

Office Treatments

A variety of office-based treatments are available as options for patients including RBL, infrared coagulation, bipolar diathermy, direct-current electrotherapy, injection sclerotherapy, dilation, and cryotherapy. The choice of therapies depends on surgeon experience, patient preference, availability of equipment, and medical status of the patient. It should be emphasized that all of these techniques are directed toward treatment of internal hemorrhoids. The lack of somatic innervations proximal to the dentate line permits such treatments, but excludes office-based directed treatments directed specifically toward external hemorrhoids.

Rubber Band Ligation

RBL is one of the most commonly performed office procedures to treat hemorrhoids. It has been widely adopted due to its efficacy, safety, and cost effectiveness. RBL is a technique of internal hemorrhoid fixation. A small rubber band is applied at the apex of the internal hemorrhoid, which creates an inflammatory response. The fibrotic reaction creates fixation of the hemorrhoid high in the anal canal at the normal anatomic position. By correcting the prolapse, the venous drainage improves and the hemorrhoids shrink in size.

Mechanical bowel preparation is not required, although an enema shortly before the procedure can improve visualization. Patients are ideally positioned in the prone jackknife position on a proctology table. The next best option is the left lateral decubitus position. The patient must be able to tolerate a complete anoscopic exam. If the patient cannot tolerate this examination, then this procedure may require sedation in a monitored setting. Fortunately, discomfort is quite rare.

After a formal anoscopic examination, the grasping instrument is used to bring the redundant mucosa at the proximal aspect of the internal hemorrhoids into the barrel of the banding instrument. The grasper is used to gently bring as much tissue as possible into the barrel (Figure 11-3). The band is

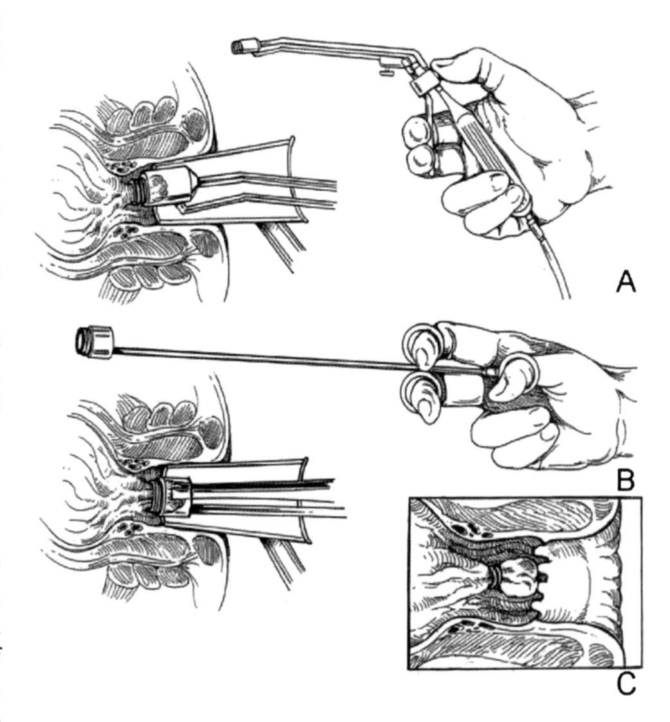

FIGURE 11-3. Rubber banding an internal hemorrhoid. **A** The internal hemorrhoid is teased into the barrel of the ligating gun with a McGown suction ligator or **B** a McGivney type ligator. **C** The apex of the banded hemorrhoid is well above the dentate line in order to minimize pain. (Reprinted from Beck D, Wexner S. Fundamentals of Anorectal surgery, 2nd ed. Copyright 1998, with permission from David Beck, MD).

then applied to this redundant mucosa, allowing reduction of the prolapse and fixation of the hemorrhoid. It is critical to place the band proximal to the dentate line (approximately 2 cm proximal). If the band is applied less than 2 cm proximal from the dentate line, the patient may feel significant pain. The band causes relative ischemia to the tissue contained within, which will then slough in 5–7 days. This creates an ulcer at the site, with an inflammatory response surrounding it. As the ulcer develops and subsequently heals, the accompanying fibrosis will secure the internal rectal mucosa to the underlining sphincter. A common misperception is that the rubber band strangulates the entire internal hemorrhoid. It is the ulcer, and subsequent scarring that causes fixation. By returning the internal hemorrhoid to its normal anatomic position, the hemorrhoid will no longer prolapse outside the anus, venous return will improve, and the hemorrhoid will shrink.

There are a variety of banding instruments available for RBL, but all make use of the same basic principles. The categories include variations of the McGivney type of ligators, McGown suction-type ligators, endoscopic, and disposable instruments. The McGivney ligators come in several styles and require the use of an atraumatic Allis-type grasper. A trigger is activated to deploy the rubber band. This requires two hands to operate and typically an assistant to hold the anoscope in place.

The second type of banding instrument is the McGown type suction ligator. (McGown, Pembroke Pines, FL). This instrument makes use of suction to draw the hemorrhoid into the barrel. It is positioned and activated with the same hand, which leaves the other hand free to position the anoscope. This may allow the surgeon to perform the procedure independently.[53] The barrel of the suction ligator is smaller than the more traditional devices, therefore less tissue is banded.

RBL can be safely and effectively performed with an endoscopic variceal ligator in conjunction with a flexible endoscope.[54–56] Gastroenterologists commonly perform banding of esophageal varices with this instrument. The cost and risks of performing flexible endoscopy may not be justified in all patients, but if diagnostic endoscopy is indicated, then combining banding with the procedure may be appropriate.

Finally, two varieties of disposable instrumentation have been developed for banding. The first is a disposable suction ligator (ShortShot® Saeed Hemorrhoidal Multi-Band Ligator, Cook Medical) (Figure 11-4), with four preloaded rubber bands. The device is placed over the site of ligation, a thumb hole is occluded to activate the suction, and a dial rotated to deploy a band. This is similar to the McGown ligators, in that it makes use of suction, and may eliminate the need for an assistant.[57,58]

The second type of disposable ligator (O'Reagan Ligating System) (Figure 11-5A–C) makes use of a syringe type of device. The surgeon can also perform this procedure alone.

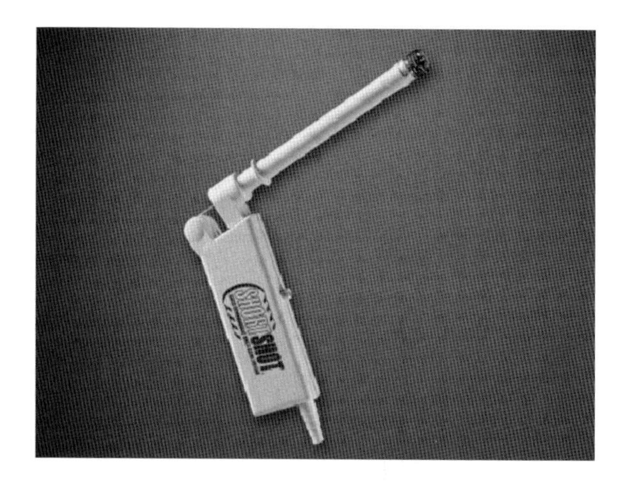

FIGURE 11-4. A ShortShot®Saeed Hemorrhoidal Multi-Band Ligator (Cook Medical).

As depicted in the illustration, the ligator is placed at the site, the syringe withdrawn, thus creating negative pressure and drawing tissue into the device, and the band deployed with a thumb trigger. This device has been reported to be safe and effective similar to other devices.[58]

Regardless of the type of banding instrumentation, an anoscope, a bright light, and possibly an assistant are the only requirements for this procedure. It is appropriate for first-, second-, and third-degree hemorrhoids. However, patients with very large and bulky hemorrhoids may require multiple treatments. Typically, the largest or most symptomatic hemorrhoid should be banded first. If the patient experiences a complication or pain and the procedure must be aborted, then the most symptomatic quadrant was already addressed. Some surgeons prefer to place two bands at the hemorrhoidal bundle (by loading two bands onto the ligator) in case one band slips or sloughs early.

Patients should be instructed to resume normal activities immediately after the procedure. The band and some of the internal hemorrhoid will slough approximately 5–7 days after the procedure. Patients may experience blood per rectum and should be informed of this ahead of time to ease anxieties. More importantly, patients should specifically be instructed, if medically possible, to refrain from anticoagulation [including aspirin and nonsteroidal anti-inflammatory drugs (NSAIDs)] for 10 days. There is no evidence supporting this strategy; however, it seems reasonable to avoid anticoagulation in anticipation of a known bleeding event. RBL is relatively contraindicated in patients on systemic anticoagulation with warfarin, antiplatelet therapy, heparin, or low molecular-weight heparin. The procedure itself can usually be performed bloodless fashion, but the bleeding that occurs 1 week after the procedure occurs in an uncontrolled setting and may potentially lead to a massive bleeding episode. Patients should be maintained on the bowel regimen started previously or at that time.

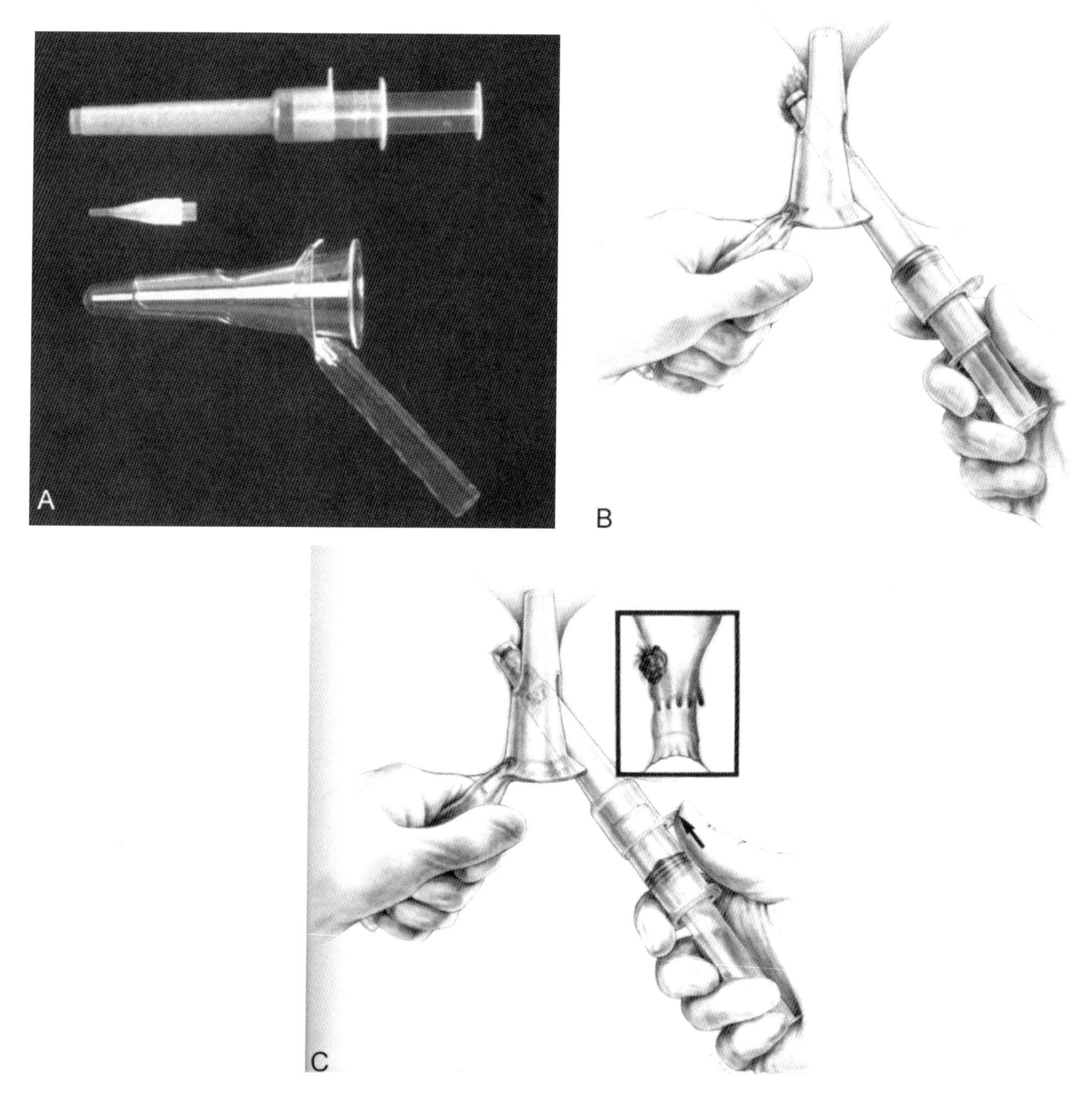

FIGURE 11-5. **A** O'Regan disposable banding system (Medsurge Medical Products Corp., Vancouver, Canada). **B**, **C** Technique of internal hemorrhoidal ligation using the O'Regan ligating system.

Constipation has been specifically correlated with less successful outcomes after banding.[59]

It has been demonstrated that banding multiple hemorrhoids in the same setting is safe and that there are no significant increases in complications.[20,60–64] Although the majority of patients tolerate banding of multiple sites with minimal discomfort or complications, there is data suggesting greater pain (29 vs. 4.5%), vasovagal symptoms (5 vs. 2%), and urinary retention (12 vs. 0%) if multiple hemorrhoids are banded.[63] For this reason, some surgeons will choose to apply one band at the first setting, and depending on the patient response and outcome, apply additional bands at subsequent visits if necessary.

Complications after RBL fortunately are rare and usually minor. The most common complications are pain, thrombosis, bleeding, and urinary hesitation or retention. The most common complication after banding is pain. Because the bands are placed proximal to the dentate line, patients typically experience vague pressure or fullness more commonly than somatic pain. It may also be common to experience the urgency to evacuate the rectum or the sensation of incomplete evacuation. These sensations typically subside in 24–48 h. Patients may resume sitz baths if their symptoms dictate, and this may relieve the pressure and/or fullness. Pain has been reported some series as low as 5%, but also as high at 60%.[27,58,65–67] Severe pain is rare, and usually due to one of the several clinical situations. Pain immediately after the procedure is related to a band misplaced too close to the dentate line. If the pain becomes unbearable, and the patient can no longer tolerate the anoscopy, then the surgeon can attempt a local anal block in the office setting to facilitate band removal, or even proceed to the operating room where anesthesia providers and sedation are more readily available. The delayed onset of pain may signify the complications of thrombosed internal and/or external hemorrhoids. This is typically treated with analgesics, sitz baths, and observation. If the pain is severe enough, then hemorrhoidectomy may rarely be indicated.

Other complications such as abscess, early band slippage, and urinary dysfunction are reported but rare.[68] The most concerning complication of RBL is pelvic sepsis. This is an extremely rare, but potentially fatal complication. There have been several documented case reports of this situation.[69–72] The clinical picture of worsening pain, fever, and urinary retention mandates immediate attention, including examination under anesthesia if necessary, as this may suggest the diagnosis of pelvic sepsis.[72] CT scan of the pelvis may demonstrate extrarectal air and/or inflammation, which may require exploratory laparotomy and pelvic drainage and/or fecal diversion. This potentially devastating complication may be increasing as the number of immunocompromised patients grows.[73]

Finally, it should be noted that most rubber bands are made with latex. Latex-free bands are available. Patients with true latex hypersensitivity should be advised not to undergo the procedure. Anaphylaxis from this application has not been reported, but a known fatal side effect should be avoided for a minor outpatient procedure.

The large majority of patients will respond to treatment of first- or second-degree hemorrhoids.[54,74,75] It may be common that patients require multiple treatment sessions. Savioz et al.[75] followed a small cohort of patients over 10 years. Thirty-two percent required repeat banding by 10 years. Bayer et al.[76] followed nearly 3,000 patients over 12 years. Eighteen percent required repeat banding and 2% required formal hemorrhoidectomy. This is a fairly durable procedure and can be easily and safely repeated if necessary. Many patients would find banding, and even repeat banding, preferable to the significantly more painful hemorrhoidectomy.

Infrared Photocoagulation, Bipolar Diathermy, and Direct-Current Electrotherapy

Surgeons utilize infrared photocoagulation, bipolar diathermy, and direct-current electrotherapy much less commonly as compared to RBL. These procedures are similar to RBL in that all are techniques of fixation. The difference is only in the method of fixation. The management issues such as patient preparation, positioning, and anticoagulation are similar to RBL.

Infrared photocoagulation employs infrared radiation to generate heat, which coagulates proteins and creates an inflammatory bed (Figure 11-6). The subsequent eschar formation and scarring at the site of application create the point of fixation for the internal hemorrhoid during the 2 weeks following the procedure.[77] A tungsten halogen lamp is used to generate the infrared radiation (Redfield Corp, Montvale, NJ) (Figure 11-7). The applicator tip is placed at the apex of the internal hemorrhoid for a 1.0–1.5 pulse of energy. Typically three or four applications at each hemorrhoid are performed. Up to three internal hemorrhoids may be treated at a single visit.[57] The application of this device will yield a 4 mm^2 focus of coagulation with a 2.5 mm deep ulcer. Complications are minor and rare. If the radiation is applied too close to the dentate line, then postprocedural pain may occur as the tissue ulcerates. Bleeding may be caused by excessive application of the energy. Infrared coagulation is best applied to small first- and second-degree hemorrhoids. There is some evidence that it may be less painful than banding.[78] At least three prospective randomized clinical trials have suggested that infrared coagulation controls bleeding in the majority of patients with first- or second-degree hemorrhoids.[57,71,72] One drawback of this technique is the expense of the device, which is clearly more costly than a rubber band ligator.

Bipolar diathermy is an alternative technique of fixation. Rather than a rubber band or an infrared-induced ulcer creating the point of fixation, bipolar radiofrequency energy is applied to the apex of the hemorrhoid. Bipolar energy does

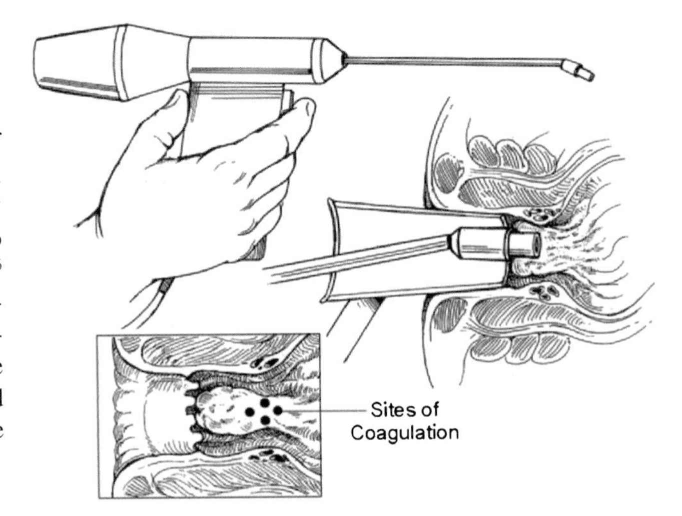

FIGURE 11-6. **A** Infrared photocoagulation. The infrared photocoagulator creates a small thermal injury. Thus, several applications are required for each hemorrhoidal column. (Reprinted from Beck D. Hemorrhoids. Handbook of Colorectal Surgery. 2nd ed. Copyright 2003 by Taylor & Francis Group LLC).

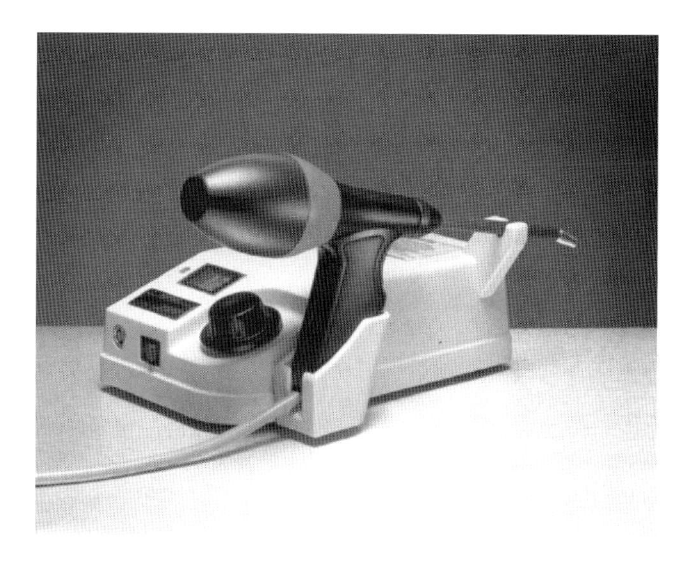

FIGURE 11-7. Infrared coagulation IRC2100™ (Redfield Corporation, Rochelle Park, NJ).

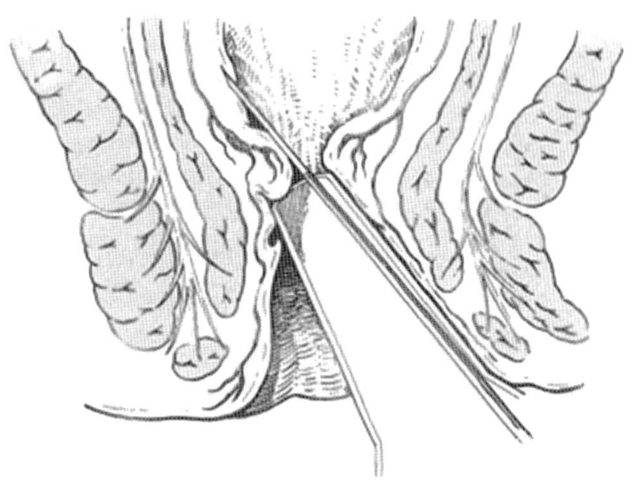

FIGURE 11-8. Injection Sclerotherapy. The needle is placed proximal to the apex of the internal hemorrhoids into the submucosal space.

not penetrate as deeply as monopolar electrocautery. The energy is applied in a pulsatile fashion until the tissue coagulates. The depth of coagulation is 2.2 mm. Success rates of treatment have been reported from 88 to 100%, however, up to 20% of patients may ultimately require excisional hemorrhoidectomy for prolapse.[79–81]

Direct-current electrotherapy is an additional method of applying energy to the site, with the intent of creating a scar, and thus securing the internal hemorrhoid in place. An applicator is directed to the apex of the internal hemorrhoids, and a 110-V direct current is delivered at increasing amperage up to the maximum tolerable level, which is approximately 16 mA. The energy is then delivered for 10 min. Patients frequently require multiple treatments at the same hemorrhoid. This technique has not gained popularity, primarily because of the time course required to treat each site and inability to treat larger grade III hemorrhoids.[82–84]

Sclerotherapy

Sclerotherapy is also a technique of internal hemorrhoidal fixation. Unlike the previously described techniques which rely on energy delivery to the site, this office technique employs chemical agents to create fibrosis and fixation of the hemorrhoids. The sclerosing agent obliterates the vascularity of the internal hemorrhoid, reduces the hemorrhoid in size, and secures it at the anatomic position. This is also performed in the office in a manner similar to RBL. A variety of sclerosing agents are available, but commonly used solutions include 5% phenol in an oil base, 5% quinine and urea, or a hypertonic saline solution. A spinal needle can be convenient to prevent the surgeon's hands and syringe from obstructing the anoscopic view. A 25 gauge (or smaller) needle should be used to minimize bleeding; 2–3 ml of the sclerosant is injected 1–2 cm proximal to the dentate line at or near the base of the internal hemorrhoid (Figure 11-8). The injection should go into the submucosal space, and the surgeon should take caution to avoid injection into the mucosa or intramuscular spaces, which may cause either mucosal sloughing with a large ulcer or significant pain.

Sclerotherapy can be safely used in patients on systemic anticoagulation since it does not induce sloughing, but rather a fibrotic reaction. Multiple repeated attempts at sclerotherapy should be avoided due to the potential complication of stricture. Complications are generally related to injection of the sclerosant into an unintended anatomical space.[85] On rare occasion, the sclerosant or the oil vehicle may cause a significant inflammatory reaction with subsequent abscess, urinary retention, or even impotence.[86] Sclerotherapy is best indicated for first- or second-degree internal hemorrhoids. Success rates are generally reported to be high. A prospective randomized trial comparing single versus multiple injections of phenol yielded similar results, with symptom control in nearly 90% of patients.[87] However, not all data are as impressive, with some series reporting 30% recurrence of symptoms 4 years after injection.[66] One trial even suggests that sclerotherapy plus fiber yields similar bleeding control rates as fiber alone.[88]

In many practices, RBL or infrared coagulation have become the preferred office-based procedures, except in anticoagulated patients, in whom injection sclerotherapy is the safest option.

Anal Dilation

Anal dilation – also known as Lord's procedure – was originally described as dilation to accommodate four fingers of both hands.[89] This essentially creates an uncontrolled stretch injury to the sphincter. Ultrasonographic evidence and postoperative incontinence have precluded this treatment from gaining acceptance in the USA.[90–92]

Cryotherapy

Cryotherapy is an alternative method of fixation of the internal hemorrhoids. This technique makes use of freezing as a method of local tissue destruction. A specialized probe is cooled by nitrous oxide (−70°C) or liquid nitrogen (−196°C). The probe is then applied to the desired location at the apex of the internal hemorrhoids. The procedure can be time-consuming, and the patients can experience pain and a foul smelling discharge per rectum afterwards.[93–95] In addition, the probe is not widely available, and inappropriate applications can lead to anal stenosis, sphincter damage, or even fecal incontinence. This technique is rarely offered and should likely be abandoned.

Operative Hemorrhoidectomy

In broad terms, operative hemorrhoidectomy is indicated for patients who fail nonoperative management techniques, have advanced disease unlikely to be amenable to nonoperative techniques, or significant external hemorrhoids requiring excision. In addition, patients with other anorectal pathology, such as fissures, fistulas, or abscesses requiring operative intervention may elect for concomitant hemorrhoidectomy. Patients unable to tolerate office procedures or coagulopathic patients requiring definitive control of bleeding are also suitable candidates for operative therapies.

A relatively small number of patients, 5–10%,[96,97] require operative hemorrhoidectomy compared to the very large number of patients experiencing hemorrhoidal symptoms. Surgical treatment falls into three categories: excisional hemorrhoidectomy, stapled hemorrhoidopexy, and a relatively newer technique of Doppler-guided transanal devascularization.

Excisional hemorrhoidectomy remains the gold standard treatment to which other operations must be compared. Its safety and efficacy have withstood the test of time for decades. The obvious drawback to this operative approach is the notorious postoperative pain. There are three variations of excisional hemorrhoidectomy: the open technique, the closed technique, and the circumferential (Whitehead) technique.

Closed Hemorrhoidectomy (Ferguson Hemorrhoidectomy)

Described by Ferguson some 40 years ago, the closed hemorrhoidectomy or Ferguson hemorrhoidectomy remains the most common operation for hemorrhoids in the USA.[98]

Patients do not require a formal mechanical bowel preparation or perioperative antibiotics. Enemas prior to surgery are sufficient for evacuation of the rectum. Prone jackknife position with the buttocks taped widely apart allows maximum exposure. Some surgeons prefer the lateral decubitus position. This operation can be performed under general, regional, or local anesthesia with intravenous sedation. Sedation with local anesthesia is safe and can facilitate an expeditious recovery and discharge.[99]

The operation begins with a formal anoscopic examination and a proctoscopic examination if indicated. A deep anchoring suture is placed at the apex of the internal hemorrhoid using absorbable suture material. The ligature should be deep to the submucosa, so as to incorporate the feeding artery and devascularize the pedicle. A diamond-shaped incision is made to plan the dissection, with either scalpel or a cautery device. The incision should begin immediately distal to the anchoring suture, incorporate the bulk of the internal/external hemorrhoid, and extend widely onto the perineum. A long incision will give a smooth contour when the wound is closed. Next, starting at the distal aspect of the diamond-shaped incision, the hemorrhoidectomy is initiated. A hemostatic clamp can be applied to the external hemorrhoids in order to facilitate traction of the specimen; however, the surgeon must be confident that there is not a significant amount of sphincter within the clamp. The skin and subcutaneous tissues are dissected with scalpel, scissors, or cautery. The dissection proceeds to remove the external hemorrhoid, and the base of the wound will now expose the external sphincter. Care should be taken to dissect the mucosa and submucosal away from the underlying sphincter fibers. As long as the submucosal plane is not traversed, the muscle fibers can usually be easily swept downward, away from the hemorrhoid tissue. The dissection proceeds proximally, separating the internal hemorrhoids from the external and finally the internal sphincter. This portion of the dissection, with good visualization of the sphincter, is the critical aspect in preventing injury to the sphincter. The use of cautery, scalpel, scissors, or even an advanced energy device does not change this critical element. The specimen is amputated just distal to the anchoring stitch. The wound is inspected for hemostasis. The suture at the apex stitch is retrieved and used to close the wound. If the mucosal edges are bleeding, a running locked suture can aid hemostasis. If there is significant dead space deep to the closure, then a three-point stitch, incorporating a small amount of sphincter, will obliterate this space.

Another variation of the techniques uses an hourglass-shaped incision around the hemorrhoid bundle. The bundle is dissected carefully off the muscle until the proximal vascular bundle is encountered. This structure is clamped and the hemorrhoidal bundle is excised. The vascular pedical is suture ligated and the stitch is used to approximate the mucosa as described above. This variation ensures that maximal anoderm is retained and there is no suture to obstruct the dissection (Figure 11-9).

Care should be taken with both techniques to match up the anal verge from both sides of the wound. The distal most aspect of the wound (5 mm) should be left open to drain. The wound should be dressed with a nonadherent dressing, or antibiotic ointment and gauze, and mesh panties. Tape on the buttocks should be avoided so as to prevent the painful removal and avoid putting tension on the new suture lines.

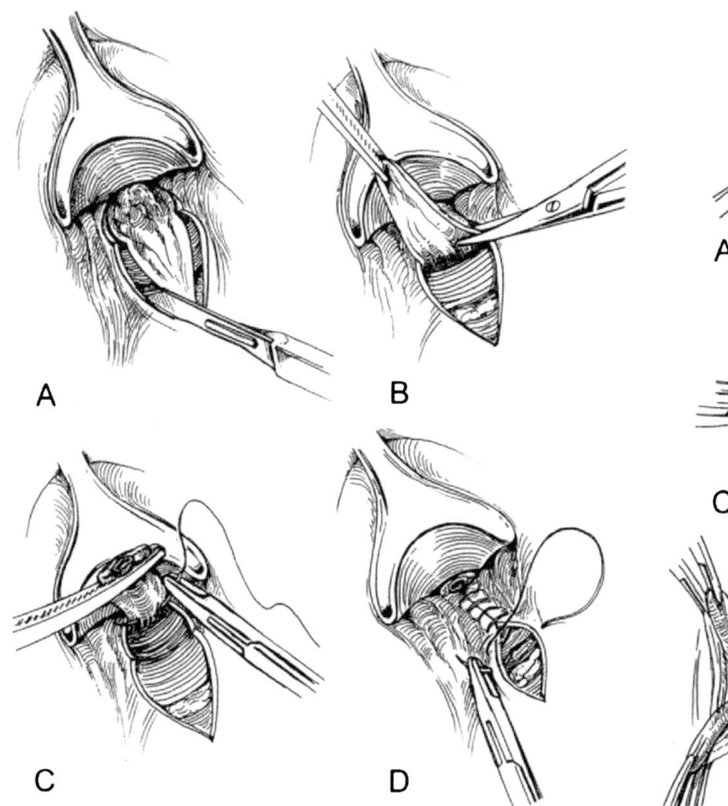

FIGURE 11-9. Ferguson closed hemorrhoidectomy. **A** An incision is made in the mucosa and anoderm around the hemorrhoid bundle. **B** The hemorrhoid dissection is carefully continued cephalad by dissecting the sphincter away from the hemorrhoid. **C** After dissection of the hemorrhoid to its pedicle, it is clamped, secured, or excised. The pedicle is suture ligated. **D** The wound is closed with a running stitch. Excessive traction on the suture is avoided to prevent forming dog-ears or displacing the anoderm caudally.

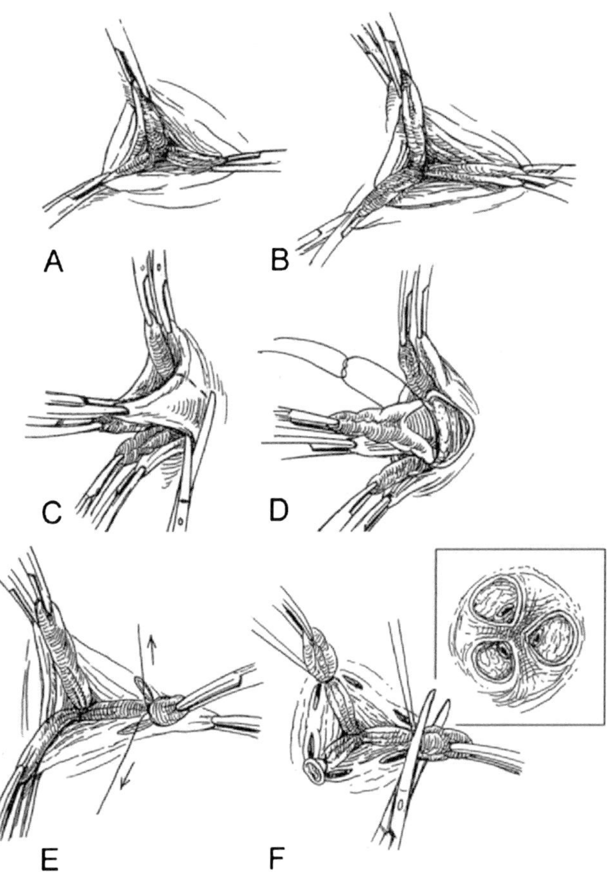

FIGURE 11-10. Open (Milligan–Morgan) hemorrhoidectomy. **A** External hemorrhoids grasped with forceps and retracted outward. **B** Internal hemorrhoids grasped with forceps and retracted outward with external hemorrhoids. **C** External skin and hemorrhoid excised with scissors. **D** Suture placed through proximal internal hemorrhoid and vascular bundle. **E** Ligature tied. **F** Tissue distal to ligature is excised. Inset depicts completed three-bundle hemorrhoidectomy.

Patients can be discharged home in most cases. One, two, or three quadrants may be excised at a single operation. Maintaining bridges of viable skin and mucosa in between each excision will prevent anal stenosis.

The operative specimen does not require routine pathologic examination as the incidence of significant pathology as a clinically normal exam is not justified.

Open Hemorrhoidectomy (Milligan–Morgan)

The open technique, or Milligan–Morgan, is more commonly used in the UK and follows the technique described by Milligan and Morgan.[100] Perioperative management is identical to Ferguson hemorrhoidectomy.

The external hemorrhoids are grasped with a hemostat and retracted in the caudal direction. This exposes the internal hemorrhoids, which are also grasped with hemostats. Traction on the three internal/external bundles exposes the apex of each group. A V-shaped incision is made on the anoderm extending to the mucocutaneous junction. The sphincter fibers are exposed and gently dissected away from the hemorrhoid with sharp and blunt dissection. As with open hemorrhoidectomy, care is taken to separate the sphincter fibers from the hemorrhoid bundle. The apex of the pedicle is then suture ligated, and the hemorrhoid amputated (Figure 11-10). One, two, or three columns can be excised.[101] The wounds are left open to granulate.

Circumferential Technique (Whitehead Hemorrhoidectomy)

The Whitehead hemorrhoidectomy involves a circumferential excision of the internal hemorrhoids and redundant mucosa just proximal to the dentate line.[102–105] The technique describes total excision of the hemorrhoids and mucosa from the dentate line and progressing proximally (Figure 11-11). It had been used more commonly in the UK, but became much less popular. It was never widely adopted in the USA. Many surgeons would suture the proximal rectal mucosa to the anal

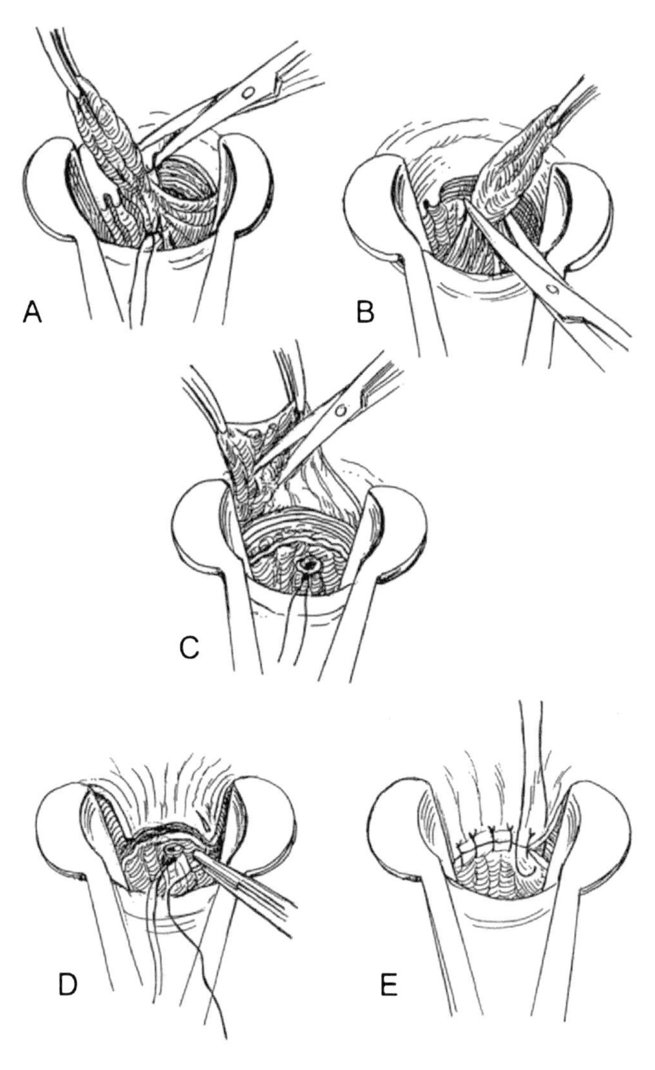

FIGURE 11-11. Whitehead hemorrhoidectomy. **A** Suture placed through proximal internal hemorrhoid for orientation. Excision started at dentate line and continued to proximal bundle. **B** Internal hemorrhoidal tissue excised above ligated bundle. **C** Vascular tissue excised from underside of elevated anoderm. **D** End of anoderm reapproximated with sutures to original location of dentate line. **E** Completed procedure.

skin, which resulted in a significant mucosal ectropion, the so-called Whitehead's deformity. In addition, high rates of stenosis and incontinence have lead to abandonment of this technique at most centers.

Results of Hemorrhoidectomy

The long-term results of excisional hemorrhoidectomy are excellent. There are however, relatively few studies with long-term follow-up on a large number of patients. MacRae et al.[106] reviewed available data and found that the recurrence of symptoms or need for subsequent treatment is low.

The debate regarding open or closed hemorrhoidectomy is longstanding. Multiple clinical trials have examined the relative merits of each technique. In recent years, there have been at least four randomized comparative trials examining open versus closed hemorrhoidectomy.[107–110] These trials revealed similar postoperative pain, analgesic requirement, length of stay, and complications. Some authors suggest complete wound healing was superior in open hemorrhoidectomy,[110] similar between groups,[93,94] or closed hemorrhoidectomy.[108,109]

Ho and Buettner[111] performed a meta-analysis comparing open and closed techniques. Six trials including nearly 700 patients were included. There were no significant differences in cure rates, length of stay, maximum pain score, or complications rates. Open hemorrhoidectomy was faster to perform, but closed hemorrhoidectomy wounds did heal faster. In summary, there were no clear differences between the two techniques. As with any operations in which equivalent results have been documented, the surgeon should offer whichever operation he/she is most comfortable performing.

The greatest patient concern regarding hemorrhoidectomy is postoperative pain. This experience has become a significant deterrent to many patients and often causes delay in seeking surgical care for hemorrhoids. Even relatively recent trials, which incorporate the most modern anesthesia and postoperative analgesic practices, demonstrate the frequent need for narcotic pain medication and the prolonged delay in returning to normal activities for up to a month.[112–115]

Due to the significant postoperative pain, several methods have been examined in an effort to minimize postoperative pain. Alternative methods of tissue dissection have been investigated. The LigaSure™ bipolar energy device (Valleylab, Boulder, CO) as well as the Harmonic® Ultrasonic Device (Ethicon Endosurgery, Cincinnati, OH) have been examined for hemorrhoidectomy. The supposition is that the advanced energy devices may create less thermal injury, less tissue destruction, and therefore less postoperative pain. Multiple randomized trials have examined these devices as compared to diathermy hemorrhoidectomy.[111,116–129]

These trials were all modest size (30–86 patients). The data suggests that advanced energy devices may save operating time, with a lower blood loss. The clinical significance of the difference in blood loss was questionable in most cases (<25 mL). The postoperative pain was similar or less than diathermy in the Ligasure™ and Harmonic® studies. Unfortunately, there is little long-term data regarding the safety and durability of these devices for this application. Furthermore, the cost of these devices is clearly in excess of the traditional instrumentation required for excisional hemorrhoidectomy. The potentially shorter operative time may not offset this cost. A recent Cochrane review of Ligasure™ hemorrhoidectomy compared to excisional hemorrhoidectomy was performed.[111] This review included 12 trials with over 1,100 patients. Ligasure patients experienced less pain on the first postoperative day, and most studies suggested less analgesic requirements. This benefit disappeared by postoperative day 14. Excisional hemorrhoidectomy required nine additional minutes to perform. There were no differences in complications, recurrent bleeding, or incontinence. Ligasure™ patients returned to work 5 days sooner than control patients.

Both Harmonic® and Ligasure™ hemorrhoidectomy appear to offer patients reduced postoperative pain, but the lack of long-term follow-up precludes a firm recommendation at this time. If the seemingly low rate of recurrence and functional results are sustained during longer-term follow-up, these techniques will likely grow in popularity. The issue will be comparative effectiveness to address the relative cost efficiency of these techniques compared to standard hemorrhoidectomy.

Several trials have examined diathermy versus scissor hemorrhoidectomy. There are not significant differences between the two techniques and this should remain surgeon preference.[130–132] Laser hemorrhoidectomy with NdYAG laser has been evaluated as an alternative technique of excisional hemorrhoidectomy. There were not significant improvements in clinical outcome compare to excisional hemorrhoidectomy.[133–135] This technique suffers from a large cost and may also create compromised wound healing.[135]

Additional techniques or adjuncts to hemorrhoidectomy have been examined in an effort to decrease postoperative pain. Ui[136] proposed hemorrhoidectomy with limited incisions, and Patel and O'Connor[137] described suture ligation of the vascular pedicle alone. Concomitant lateral internal sphincterotomy has been demonstrated to reduce postoperative pain.[138] It may be that sphincterotomy mitigates the painful sphincter spasm experienced after hemorrhoidectomy. The uses of postoperative oral[139] as well as 10% topical metronidazole[140] have been demonstrated to reduce pain. It is unclear whether this represents an anti-inflammatory or an antibacterial effect of the drug. Nitroglycerin ointment, a known smooth muscle relaxant, commonly used to treat spasm associated with fissures has been examined for postoperative pain as well.[141,142] Additional agents, such as local anesthetics, anxiolytics, parasympathomimetics, and other sphincter relaxants have been employed, but none have definitively reduced pain and warrant routine use.[143–147] Routine pathologic examination of hemorrhoidectomy specimens may not be necessary. A recent review suggests that 1.4% of 914 patients contained histologic abnormalities.[100] During a 20-year period at Ferguson Hospital, only 1 of 21,257 specimens made was found to contain carcinoma.[148]

Complications of Hemorrhoidectomy

Bleeding is one of the more common complications after hemorrhoidectomy, although delayed severe hemorrhage occurs less than 5% of cases.[149,150] This may be related to infections at the vascular pedicle, however, it may be more related to technical factors. One large prospective trial documents that male patients (narrow anal canal) and surgeon as independent risks. This suggests technical issues are the cause of bleeding.[151] If patients present with massive postoperative bleeding, then immediate packing of the anal canal or inflation of a balloon-tipped catheter will adequately tamponade bleeding. If unsuccessful, then proceeding to the operating room for surgical control is appropriate. Patients may accumulate large quantities of old clot within the rectosigmoid, which should be differentiated from ongoing bleeding. Rectal irrigation can help to distinguish these so that selection for operative management can be made.[152]

Other common complications after hemorrhoidectomy include: urinary retention (0.2–36%), infection (0.2–6%), fecal incontinence (2–12%), fecal impaction (0.4%), and anal stenosis (0–6%).[153–158]

Stapled Hemorrhoidopexy

An alternative to excisional hemorrhoidectomy is the stapled hemorrhoidopexy, which was first described, and subsequently modified, by Italian surgeons.[159,160] This operation makes use of modified circular stapler, traditionally used for creating circular end-to-end intestinal anastomoses (Ethicon Endosurgery). The operation is primarily a hemorrhoidopexy, an operative form of hemorrhoid fixation. The transanal stapler circumferentially excises mucosa and submucosa, well proximal to the dentate line. A stapled anastomosis is created, thus lifting and securing the redundant mucosa and internal hemorrhoids in the normal anatomic position, which improves venous outflow. Also, the staple line may divide the arterial inflow contained in the submucosal space, thus devascularizing the hemorrhoids. This procedure offers the convenience of single setting treatment without the painful incisions in the highly sensitive anoderm.

This procedure combines elements of several other procedures. It is an operative technique, like excisional hemorrhoidectomy. It excises a circumferential ring of mucosa, like Whitehead hemorrhoidectomy. It is a technique of fixation, like RBL or sclerotherapy. It also devascularizes the hemorrhoids, like transanal hemorrhoidal devascularization (described below). The main benefit of this procedure as compared to excisional techniques is reduced pain. As all the staples are within the anal canal, proximal to the dentate line, there are no incisions on the highly sensitive anoderm, and therefore does not create the same degree of somatic pain as excisional hemorrhoidectomy.

The procedure has been cited by several names. Stapled hemorrhoidopexy most accurately reflects the nature of this operation as a technique of fixation. It is not a hemorrhoidectomy in that excision of hemorrhoid tissue is only a minor component. Authors have also referred to it as stapled anopexy, stapled prolapsectomy, and stapled mucosectomy. Procedure for prolapse and hemorrhoids (PPH) is a proprietary name coined by the manufacturer (Ethicon Endosurgery).

Stapled hemorrhoidopexy is best considered an alternative to excisional hemorrhoidectomy; therefore, the indications are similar. Indications include second- and third-degree hemorrhoids that either fail nonoperative methods or in patients who desire single setting treatment rather than multiple RBL.

Some exceptions include patients with thrombosed internal or external hemorrhoids, who should undergo excisional hemorrhoidectomy. Fourth-degree hemorrhoids also require excision, as reduction of the hemorrhoids is necessary for the conduct of the procedure. Some limited data does support the use in irreducible fourth-degree hemorrhoids if they can be reduced in the operating room.[114]

Patent preparation, anesthesia, positioning, and management are identical to excisional hemorrhoidectomy. The anal canal is examined per routine. The included disposable circular anoscope inserted. This anoscope is translucent to allow visualization of the dentate line during the procedure. A purse string suture anoscope is placed through the circular anoscope to facilitate the placement of a circumferential pursestring suture (2-0 polypropelene) into the submucosa 2 cm proximal to the apex of the hemorrhoids. The stapler is inserted through the anoscope with the head maximally opened. The head is passed through the pursestring, and the suture is tightened. Gentle traction on the pursestring suture then draws the redundant tissue into the stapler. The stapler is closed and fired, thus creating a circular partial thickness anastomoses proximal to the dentate line, while excising a ring of mucosa/submucosa approximately 1–3 cm wide (Figure 11-12). The staple line should be carefully inspected for bleeding and oversewn, as necessary.

The purse string suture is a critical element as it drives the operation. It determines the height of the staple line relative to the dentate line. If too proximal, inadequate retraction of the hemorrhoids may result in recurrent prolapse. If too distal, the staple line will be near the dentate line and cause pain. If too deep, the patient may experience full thickness anastomoses, which can pose a risk of pelvic abscess, fistula, or stapled rectovaginal fistula. Multiple examinations of the vagina during placement of the suture and before firing the stapler may prevent this complication.

The external hemorrhoids are indirectly treated to a limited extent. They are drawn into the anal canal, and the devascularization does create some resolution of the external hemorrhoids. Significant tags or thrombosed external hemorrhoids can be treated concomitantly if symptomatic or in a deferred fashion as needed. The large majority of patients will not require further treatment of these after stapled hemorrhoidopexy.[146]

A large number of randomized controlled trials have been conducted in the last 10 years. The large majority of these trials demonstrated significantly less postoperative pain compared to excisional hemorrhoidectomy.[21,111,113,114,161–180] In order to help understand this rapid influx of data, there have been several meta-analyses of the results of stapled hemorrhoidopexy.

In 2004, Nisar et al.[181] performed a formal systematic review of 15 randomized trials examining the safety and efficacy compared to excisional techniques. The review suggested that there were no difference in total complications and less frequent immediate postoperative bleeding in PPH. There was a shorter hospital stay and return to normal activity. Pain was significantly improved with PPH at 24 h postoperative. Recurrent prolapse at 6 months was higher in PPH, but this was obviously a short follow-up.

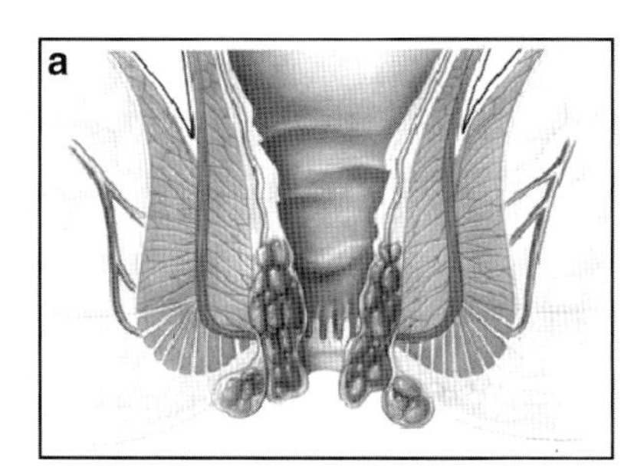

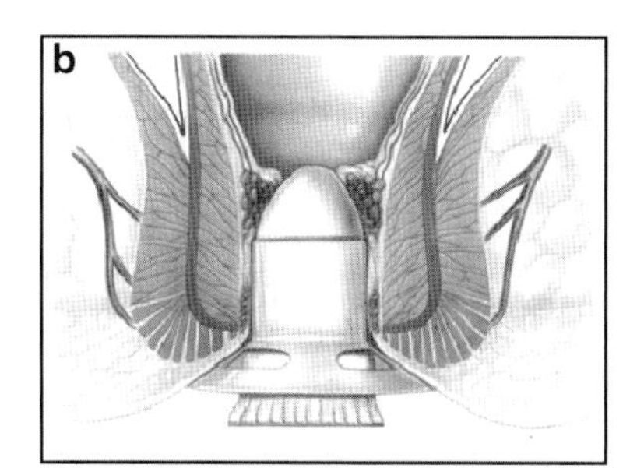

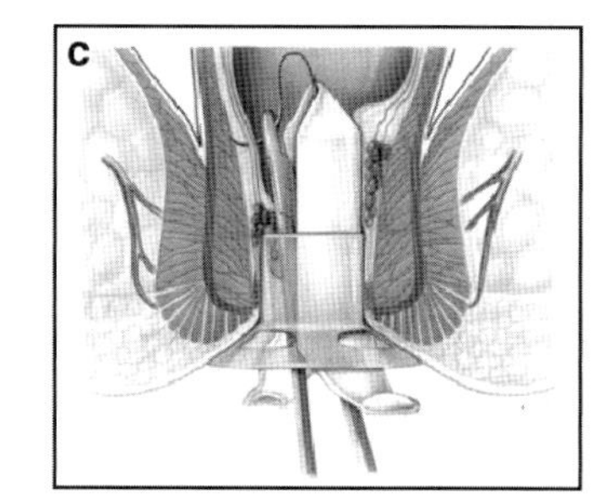

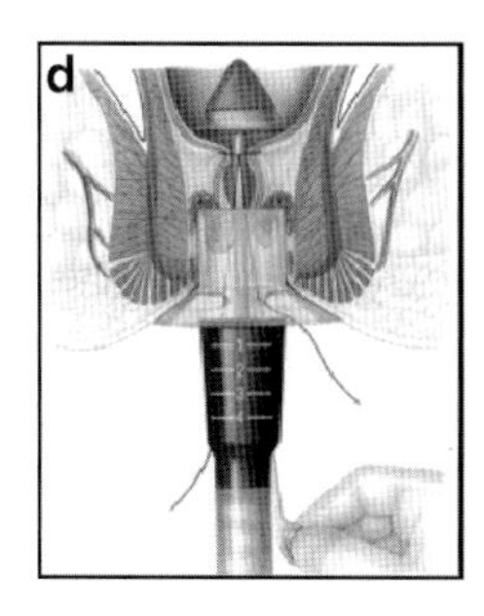

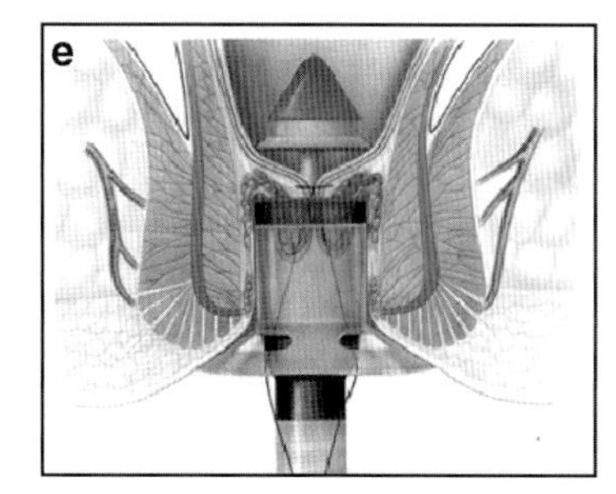

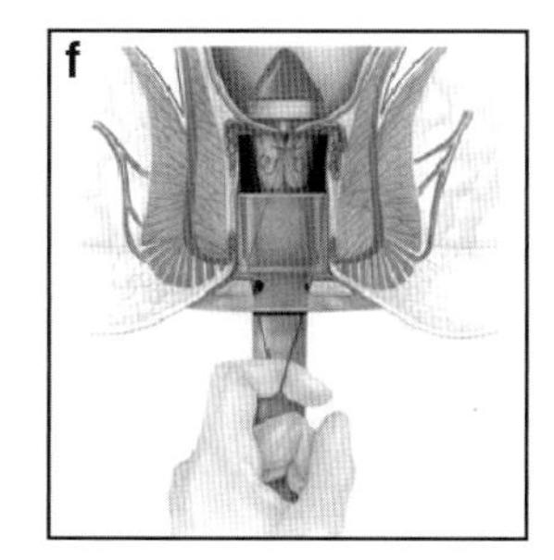

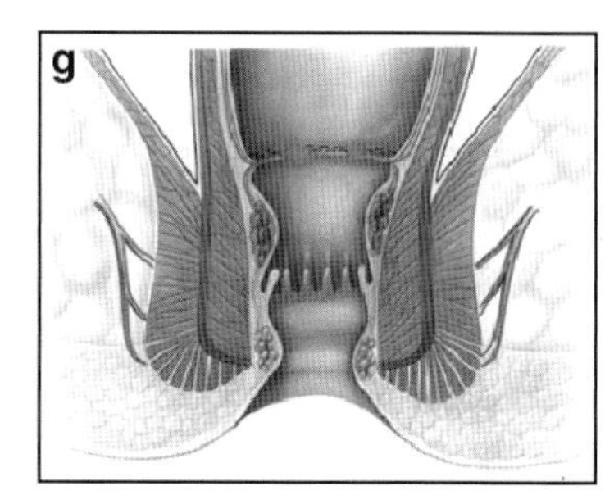

FIGURE 11-12. Stapled hemorrhoidopexy. **a** Prolapsing internal hemorrhoids and external hemorrhoids. **b** Circular anoscope is inserted. **c** Purse string anoscope is inserted and circumferential purse string suture is placed proximal to hemorrhoids. **d** The purse strings are drawn through the stapler. **e** Traction on the purse string draws the redundant mucosa into the head of the stapler. **f** The stapler is closed onto the mucosa and fired. **g** The final staple line draws the hemorrhoids into the anatomic positions.

Next, Lan et al.[182] performed a systematic review in 2006. This review included ten prospective RCT comparing PPH to Milligan–Morgan for grades III and IV hemorrhoids. Safety and bleeding was similar up to 3 months postoperative. Complications were similar. Postoperative pain, operative time, length of stay, and patient satisfaction favored stapled hemorrhoidopexy. Postoperative skin tags and recurrent prolapse were more frequent in PPH patients.

A more recent systematic review[183] evaluated PPH compared to excisional techniques for short- and long-term outcomes. Twenty-nine trials were examined including 2,056 patients (20–200 per study). The rate of overall complications was similar between groups. There was a higher rate of bleeding requiring reintervention after PPH. There were similar rates of external thrombosis and urinary retention. PPH caused fewer fecal impactions, required less operating room time, a shorter length of stay, and faster return to normal activities. Postoperative pain was significantly lower in the PPH patients at 24 h postoperative, at the time of first bowel movement, and 1–2 weeks postoperative. Recurrent prolapse was more common after PPH, but the requirement for further operative intervention was similar.

Although the meta-analyses conclude that stapled hemorrhoidopexy is a safe operation with shorter operative time, less postoperative pain, and shorter recovery than excisional hemorhriodectomy,[181–183] there are several complications important to specifically note. Rectal obstruction, rectal perforation, retroperitoneal sepsis, and pelvic sepsis have all been documented as a result of stapled hemorrhoidopexy.[184–188] There is potential for sphincter injury if the muscle is incorporated into the stapler. Histologic analysis of the resection tissue reveals sphincter muscles fibers.[189,190] The rate of incontinence is not alarming, however, this finding highlights the potential for injury. In addition, rectovaginal fistula has been reported.[167,191,192] This complication is exceedingly rare in excisional hemorrhoidectomy, but is a significant concern in PPH. The actual incidence is very low, however, the nature of the operation puts women at risk due to the demands of precise placement of the purse string suture.

The large majority of data confirms that stapled hemorrhoidopexy is at least as safe at excisional hemorrhoidectomy, with significantly less postoperative pain and faster return to normal activities compared to excisional techniques.

Transanal Hemorrhoidal Dearterialization

The newest addition to surgical armamentarium is Doppler-guided arterial ligation with hemorrhoidopexy. In 1995, Morinaga et al.[193] described a novel surgical treatment for hemorrhoids [Hemorrhoidal Artery Ligation (HAL)]. The specific techniques and commercially available instrumentation have evolved since that time, but the principle remains. The HAL is a nonexcisional operative technique that employs Doppler-guided ligation of the arterial inflow to the hemorrhoids. Some years later, suture rectopexy was added to the ligation.

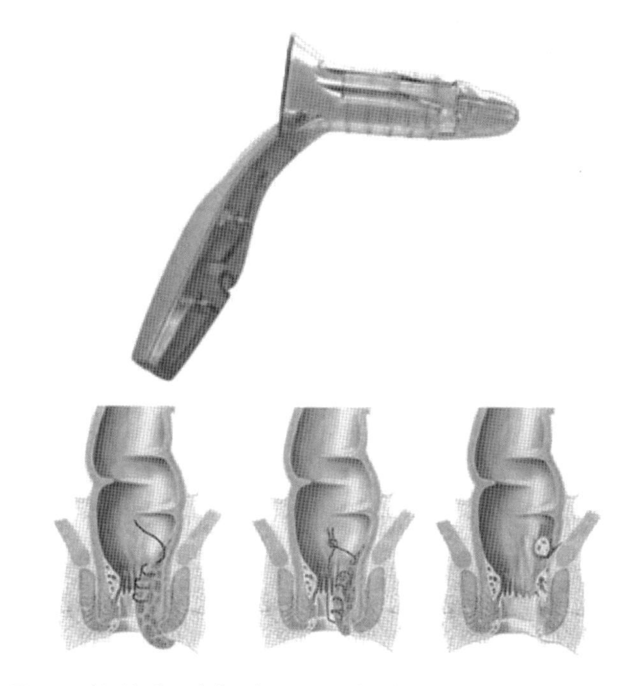

Figure 11-13. Specialized anoscope for the transanal hemorrhoidal dearterialization (AMI Surgical).

This combined technique was introduced into the USA in 2008. There are currently two available products in the USA: transanal hemorrhoidal dearterialization (THD; America, Ankeny IA) and hemorrhoidal artery ligation and recto anal repair (HAL/RAR; A.M.I. Inc, Natck MA).

This nonexcisional technique relies upon detection of the hemorrhoidal arterial inflow by Doppler-guided identification and ligation of the branches of the superior hemorrhoidal arteries.[193] This reduced inflow facilitates reduction in size of the hemorrhoids. Suturing is well proximal to the dentate line, so as to avoid the highly sensitive anoderm. The suture hemorrhoidopexy addresses the redundant and prolapsing mucosal and internal hemorrhoid.

The procedure is performed in the operating room and requires anesthesia as a hemorrhoidectomy. A specialized anoscope is inserted into the anal canal (Figure 11-13). The anoscope contains within it a removable Doppler ultrasound probe. The anoscope is axially rotated until one of the feeding arteries is precisely identified. At this point, the artery is ligated. A slot in the anoscope that allows for placement of a suture immediately proximal to the ultrasound probe. A "figure of eight" suture ligation of the artery is performed. The adequacy of the ligation may be immediately confirmed by assessing the change in Doppler signal. The anoscope is then rotated axially so as to identify the next artery. Most often, 4–6 arteries are identified and ligated, but this varies depending upon each patient's unique anatomy. Once the ligation is completed, a hemorrhoidopexy or mucopexy is performed. This may be accomplished immediately following the arterial ligation, using the same suture, or each of the ligations may be performed first, followed by the mucopexies. Although the same specialized anoscope is used, the Doppler feature is not important for this part of the operation. The suture is anchored at the apex of the internal hemorrhoid, and a running suture is then performed from proximal toward distal. With each successive purchase, tension is applied to the suture so as to progressively draw more of the hemorrhoid and redundant into the anoscope, and thus become incorporated into the running suture. This suture line is terminated proximal to the dentate line, so as to minimize pain. The distal tail of the suture is then tied to the proximal tail, which lifts the hemorrhoid and fixes it high within the anal canal. This hemorrhoidopexy may be repeated in association with each artery ligation, or only at locations of redundant and/or prolapsing mucosa. Typically, the procedure is performed 2–4 times.

The operation requires a relatively short operative time. It purports to accomplish the same goals as stapled hemorrhoidopexy in that it devascularizes the hemorrhoids by ligation of the arterial inflow and also creates a hemorrhoidopexy by securing the redundant mucosa high within the anal canal. The benefits of this operation are similar to PPH in that the sutures are proximal to the dentate line, offering patients reduced postoperative pain compared to excisional techniques. This does, however, represent an operative procedure, which includes the anesthesia risks, operating room expense, and usual surgical risks of bleeding, infection, urinary retention, and postoperative pain.

The specialized anoscope and Doppler ultrasound probe are disposable; therefore, add a significant cost when compared with excisional hemorrhoidectomy, but less expensive than a stapled procedure.

Long-term data are lacking, but these procedures are gaining in popularity, and therefore future cost–benefit analyses and long-term follow-up on durability of the repair and need for future treatments are anticipated.

A retrospective review of 330 patients with grades II and III hemorrhoids reported a 7% complication rate. The mean postoperative pain score was 1.32. A total of 219 patients were followed for a mean 43 months; of these 93% experienced complete resolution of symptoms.[194] There are a variety of additional publications documenting the safety of this technique.[195–203]

In order to better understand the limited available data, Giordano et al.[203] performed a systematic review. Seventeen trials were analyzed, but only one was a RCT, which included 1996 patients. A combination of instruments were used [HAL-Doppler instrument, KM-25 device (VaiDan Medical Corp), KM025 Moricorn (Hayashi Denki Co), and the THD Instrument]. The number of arteries ligated were 4–6 in most patients. Early postoperative results were: pain on day 1 in 19%, residual prolapse in 13%, bleeding in 4%, and urinary retention in 0.7%. Normal activities resumed 2–3 days postoperative. Twenty-seven percent required a second THD for persistence prolapse. At 1 year, prolapsed was reported in 11%, bleeding in 10%, and pain in 9%. The addition of mucosopexy alone reduced recurrence to 11%.[194]

TDH is safe and effective for grades II and III hemorrhoids with reduced pain and short recovery, but quality and quantity of data is very limited at this time. It offers surgeons and patients another reliable option.

External Hemorrhoids

Due to the fact that external hemorrhoids are distal to the dentate line, and therefore innervated by somatic nerves, office-based procedures are generally not applicable. Patients requiring specific treatment of the external hemorrhoids are usually treated in two settings, either elective hemorrhoidectomy or the treatment of thrombosed external hemorrhoids.

Acute Thrombosis of External Hemorrhoid

Patients with acute thrombosis will complain of acute onset of severe anal pain. This may be precipitated by an episode of constipation, diarrhea, excessive straining (weightlifting), coughing (COPD exacerbation), or there may not be any precipitating features at all. A firm or hard lump at the anus typically accompanies the pain. The pain rapidly progresses, and the peak of the pain cycle will occur at approximately 48 h and then diminishes by the fourth day. The skin overlying the thrombus may succumb to pressure necrosis and ulcerate. The thrombus will necessitate at this time, resulting in evacuation of thrombus or liquefied hematoma. This may provide relief as a result of the decrease in pressure.

Management of this clinical scenario is directed at pain control. For this reason, the timing of the presentation is critical. If the patient presents in the first 3 or 4 days since the onset of pain, and pain is severe, then excision of the thrombus is warranted. It should be emphasized that this decision is made based not only on timing, but also pain intensity. Some patients may have a large thrombus that does not cause significant pain. This may be safely treated with medical management. Conversely, a small thrombus causing severe pain should sway the surgeon toward operative management (Figure 11-14).

The operative treatment of a thrombosed external hemorrhoid is excision of the thrombus. This procedure can be safely performed in the office setting or the operating room. Local anesthesia, a mixture of 0.5% lidocaine and 0.25% bupivicaine with 1:200,000 epinephrine, should be infiltrated to create a field block at the level of the thrombosed external hemorrhoid. The skin overlying the thrombus is then incised in an elliptical fashion. The entirety of the thrombus should be removed. Bleeding can be controlled with pressure, ferric subsulfate (Monsel's solution), silver nitrate, or topical hemostatic agents such as thrombin or epinephrine soaked gauze. The skin edges may be left open to maximize drainage of residual thrombus and prevent new thrombus from creating pressure. Alternatively, the skin edges may

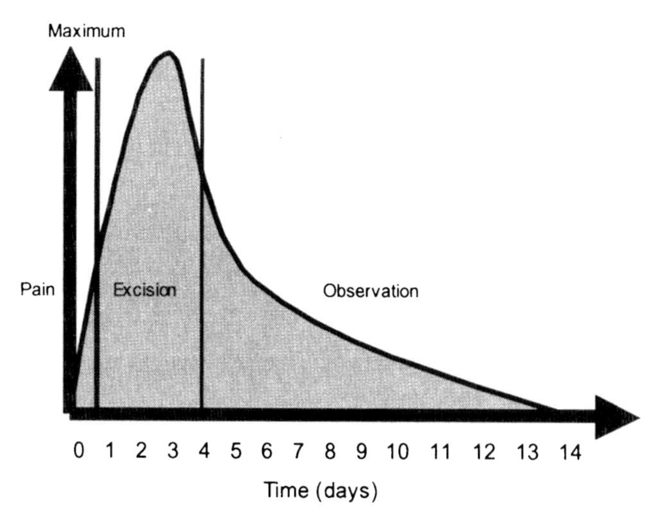

FIGURE 11-14. Thrombosed hemorrhoid management. Timing of excision of a thrombosed external hemorrhoid.

be sutured closed. Closure provides additional hemostasis and leaves a cosmetically improved wound. After excision, patients should be offered analgesics, and instructed to take frequent sitz baths, and placed on a bowel regimen of bulk-forming agents (psyllium) and a stool softener or lubricant (mineral oil).

If the patient presents in a delayed fashion (>4 days) or has minimal pain, then nonoperative management is appropriate. This includes fiber, a stool softener, analgesics, and sitz baths. Anoscopy should be deferred until pain is controlled, but the anus and rectum should be evaluated at some point. The reason for avoiding excision of thrombus at that time is that the procedure is likely to cause as much discomfort as the patient is already experiencing. The injection of local anesthetic does in fact cause some pain. Therefore, the clinician and patient must decide together which option to choose.

Special Clinical Scenarios

Strangulated Hemorrhoids

Strangulated hemorrhoids are prolapsed internal hemorrhoids that become incarcerated. Patients will present with a history of prolapsing hemorrhoids that became acutely painful and may also experience urinary retention. Physical examination will reveal bulky external hemorrhoids with significant thrombosis and edema. The internal hemorrhoids will be prolapsed, incarcerated, and edematous. The patient will be exquisitely tender and cannot tolerate anoscopy. Depending on the time course, ulceration, necrosis, and gangrene may occur.

Such patients must be urgently treated with excisional hemorrhoidectomy in the operating room. Incisions or excision of thrombus alone is not appropriate for this clinical scenario. A Ferguson or Milligan–Morgan technique can be used, depending on surgeon preference; however, if devitalized tissue and/or abscess are present, then wounds should be left open to prevent postoperative abscess. This operation is generally safe if all devitalized tissue is debrided.[155] Other than hemorrhoidectomy, or if the operating room is not available, then anther treatment option is to infiltrate a local perianal block, gently reducing internal hemorrhoids, placing multiple RBLs, and performing thrombectomies on the external hemorrhoids. Patients will not typically require future hemorrhoidectomy.[204] Patients must be highly motivated for this technique. A randomized trial suggested both excisional hemorrhoidectomy and this technique were safe options.

Hemorrhoids, Varices, and Portal Hypertension

It should be made clear that rectal varices are a distinct entity from hemorrhoids although often confused. Internal hemorrhoids drain into the middle rectal veins, subsequently the iliac veins and finally the systemic circulation. External hemorrhoids drain into the inferior rectal veins, the internal lilac veins, and the systemic circulation. Rectal varices are a distinct anatomic structure, which provide collateral circulation from the portal system into the systemic venous system.[205] This collateral circulation would seem to exacerbate hemorrhoid symptoms in patients with portal hypertension; however, the incidence of hemorrhoid symptoms is similar in this population to the general populations.[206–208] Rectal varies are very common in patients with portal hypertension (59 and 78%).[207,209] Fortunately, in contrast to esophageal varices, these varies rarely bleed.[210] Treatment of bleeding from rectal varices in this setting ranges widely from medical management of portal pressures, sclerotherapy,[205,211] to suture ligation,[211] stapled anopexy,[212] all the way to TIPS and portosystemic shunts.[213–216]

Hemorrhoids in Pregnancy

Hemorrhoids are not uncommon during pregnancy, likely due to increased circulating blood volume, impaired venous return, straining secondary to constipation, and the prolonged staring associated with labor. While pregnant, most women can be satisfactorily treated with conventional medical and behavioral treatments. If hemorrhoids become severe, or intensify during labor, the large majority will spontaneously resolve in the postpartum period. Like many surgical therapies, operative therapy for pregnancy would be reserved only for severe cases including strangulated hemorrhoids and acute external thrombosis. Operations under local anesthesia while in the left lateral position are preferred. Fortunately, only 0.2% of pregnancy women require emergent hemorrhoidectomy for grave IV hemorrhoids.[217]

Hemorrhoids and Crohn's Disease

Patients with Crohn's disease may be prone to hemorrhoid symptoms, likely related to exacerbations with diarrhea.

Hemorrhoids per say are not part of the anorectal Crohn's picture, but are common, perhaps due to engorgement related to local inflammation. As with other anorectal pathologies such as fissure, skins tags, etc., caution should be exercised with Crohn's patients. Prolonged wound healing and ulceration should be considered when discussing surgical options for hemorrhoids. If anorectal disease is well controlled, and there is little active inflammation, then Crohn's disease is not an absolute contraindication to operative therapy. Jeffery et al.[218] documented a very high complication rate for patients treated for hemorrhoids, with 30% subsequently requiring proctectomy. This was however prior to many of the currently available medical therapies for Crohn's disease. More recently, Wolkomir and Luchtefeld[219] document nearly 90% healing rate in selected patients in whom ileocolic disease was well managed. These results are encouraging for patients in whom hemorrhoidectomy is necessary. However, extreme caution should be exercise in all patient with Crohn's disease.

Hemorrhoids and the Immunocompromised Patient

As the incidence of immunocompromised patients increases due to the long survival of HIV patients, the number of patients treated with immunosuppressants, steroids, and chemotherapy grows, the issues of anorectal surgery in this population become more significant. Commonly, this population has many difficulties healing anorectal surgical wounds and is at increased risk for infectious complications. Similar to Crohn's disease, great caution should be exercised when considering surgical therapies in this population. Neutropenic patients do not suffer a higher rate of mortality due to operative therapy.[220] Nevertheless, nonoperative methods should be exhausted first. Morandi et al.[221] suggested that patients with HIV do suffer a greater degree of complications after hemorrhoidectomy.

As a general rule, all patients in these categories should have their medical conditions optimized, medical and topical therapies exhausted, and hemorrhoidectomy reserved only as needed. Patients with thrombocytopenia should likely have hemorrhoidectomy to provide most definitive control rather than delayed bleeding like in RBL.

Acknowledgment. This chapter was written by Jose R. Citron and Herand Abcarian in the first edition of this textbook.

References

1. Thomson WH. The nature of haemorrhoids. Br J Surg. 1975;62(7):542–52.
2. Thulesius O, Gores JE. Arterio-venous anastomoses in the anal region with reference to the pathogenesis and treatment of haemorrhoids. Acta Chir Scand. 1973;139(5):476–8.
3. Parnaud E, Guntz M, Bernard A, et al. Anatomie normale macroscopique et microscopique du reseau vasculaire hemorrhoidal. Arch Fr Mal Appar Dig. 1976;65:501.
4. Hansen HH. Pathomorphologieund therapie des hamorrhoidalleidens. Hautartzt. 1977;28:364.
5. Lestar B, Penninck F, Kerremans R. The composition of anal basal pressure. An in vivo and in vitro study in man. Int J Colorectal Dis. 1989;4(2):118–22.
6. Haas PA, Fox TA, Hass GP. The pathogenesis of hemorrhoids. Dis Colon Rectum. 1984;27(7):442–50.
7. Galizia G, Lieto E, Castellano P, Pelosio L, Imperator V, Pigantelli C. Lateral internal sphincterotomy together with haemorhroidectomy for treatment for haemorrhoids: a randomized prospective study. Eur J Surg. 2000;166:223–8.
8. Farouk R, Duthie GS, MacGregor AB, Bartolo DC. Sustained internal sphincter hypertonia in patients with chronic anal fissure. Dis Colon Rectum. 1994;37:424–9.
9. Loder PB, Kamm MA, Nicholls RJ, Phillips RK. Haemorrhoids: pathology, pathophysiology, and aetiology. Br J Surg. 1994;81(7):946–54.
10. Johanson JF, Sonnenberg A. The prevalence of hemorrhoids and chronic constipation. An epidemiologic study. Gastroenterology. 1990;98(2):380–6.
11. Adams PF, Hendershot GE, Marano MA. Current estimates from the National Health Interview Survey, 1996. Natl Center Health Stat Vital Health Stat. 1999;10(200):1–203.
12. Abramowitz L, Godeberge P, Staumont G, Soudan D. Clinical practice guidelines for the treatment of hemorrhoid disease. Gastroenterol Clin Biol. 2001;25(6–7):674–702.
13. National Center for Health Statistics. (Technical Appendix from Vital Statistics of the United States: Mortality). 2002. Hyattsville, Maryland: 2004.
14. Johanson JF, Sonnenberg A. Temporal changes in the occurrence of hemoohids in the United States and England. Dis Colon Rectum. 1991;34(7):585–91.
15. Burt CW, Schappert SM. Ambulatory care visits to physician offices, hospital outpatient departments, and emergency departments: United States, 1999–2000. Natl Center Health Stat Vital Health Stat. 2004;13(157):1–70.
16. Helmick CG, Griffin PM, Addiss DG, Tauxe RV, and Juranek DD. Chapter 3 in Everhart, James. E. (ed.), *Digestive Diseases in the United States: Epidemiology and Impact*. U.S. Dept. of Health and Human Services, Public Health Service, National Institutes of Health, National Institute of Diabetes and Digestive and Kidney Diseases: U.S. Government Printing Office, May 1994, NIH Pub. No. 94-1447, pp. 85–123
17. Kozak LJ, Owings MF, Hall MJ. National Hospital Discharge Survey: 2002 annual summary with detailed diagnosis and procedure data. Natl Center Health Stat Vital Health Stat. 2005;13(158):1–199.
18. Johanson JF. Hemorrhoids. In: Everhart JE, editor. Digestive diseases in the United States: epidemiology and impact. US Department of Health and Human Services, Public Health Service, National Institutes of Health, National Institute of Diabetes and Digestive and Kidney Diseases. Washington, DC: US Government Printing Office, 1994; NIH Publication No. 94-1447 pp. 271–298.
19. Everhart JE, ed. The burden of digestive diseases in the United States. US Department of Health and Human Services, Public Health Service, National Institutes of Health, National Institute

of Diabetes and Digestive and Kidney Diseases. Washington, DC: US Government Printing Office, 2008; NIH Publication No. 09-6443.
20. Banov Jr J, Kneopp Jr JF, Erdman JH, Alia RT. Management of hemorrhoidal disease. J S C Med Assoc. 1985;81(7):398–401.
21. Senagore AJ, Singer M, Abcarian H, et al. A prospective, randomized, controlled, multicenter trial comparing stapled hemorrhoidopexy and Ferguson hemorrhoidectomy: peripoperative and one year result. Dis Colon Rectum. 2004;47(11):824–36.
22. O'Donnell LJD, Heaton KW. Pseudo-diarrhea in the irritable bowel syndrome: patients' records of stool form reflect transit time while stool frequency does not. Gut. 1988;29:A1455.
23. Armstrong DN. Multiple hemorrhoidal ligation: a prospective, randomized trial evaluating a new technique. Dis Colon Rectum. 2003;46(2):179–86.
24. Segal WN, Greenberg PD, Rockey DC, Cello JP, McQuaid KR. The outpatient evaluation for hematochezia. Am J Gastroenterol. 1998;93(2):179–82.
25. Church JM. Analysis of the colonoscopic findings in patients with rectal bleeding according to the pattern of their presenting symptoms. Dis Colon Rectum. 1991;34:391–5.
26. Rex DK, Bond JH, Winawer S, et al. Quality in the technical performance of colonoscopy and the continuous quality improvement process for colonoscopy: recommendations of the U.S. Multi-Society Task Force on colorectal cancer. Am J Gastroenterol. 2002;97:1296–308.
27. Cataldo P, Ellis N, Gregorcyk S, et al. Practice parameters for the management of hemorrhoids (Revised). Dis Colon Rectum. 2005;48:189–94.
28. Clinical Practice Committee, American Gatroenterological Association. American Gastroenterological Association medical position statement; diagnosis and treatment of hemorrhoids. Gastroenterology 2004; 126(5); 1461–1462.
29. Korkis AM, McDougall CJ. Rectal bleeding in patients less than 50 years of age. Dig Dis Sci. 1995;40(7):1520–3.
30. Nakama H, Kamijo N, Fujimori K, Horiuchi A, Abdul Fattah S, Zhang B. Immunochemical fecal occult blood test is not suitable for diagnosis of hemorrhoids. Am J Med. 1997;102(6):551–4.
31. Madoff RD, Fleshman JW. American Gastroenterological Association technical review on the diagnosis and treatment of hemorrhoids. Gastroenterology. 2004;126(5):1463–73.
32. Kluiber RM, Wolff BG. Evaluation of anesmia caused by hemorrhoidal bleeding. Dis Colon Rectum. 1994;37(10):1006–7.
33. USDA, Agricultural research service. Dietary Intake Data from the Third National Health and Nutrition Examination Survey (NHANES III) 1988.
34. Moesgaard F, Nielsen ML, Hansen JB, Knudse JT. High fiber diet resuces bleeding and pain in patients with hemorrhoids: a double-blind trial of Vi-Siblin. Dis Colon Rectum. 1982;25(2):454–6.
35. Broader JH, Gunn IF, Alexander-Williams J. Evaluation of a bulk-forming evacuant in the management of haemorrhoids. Br J Surg. 1974;61(2):142–4.
36. Webster DJ, Gough DC, Craven JL. The use of bulk evacuant in patients with haemorrhoids. Br J Surg. 1978;65(4):291–2.
37. Perez-Miranda M, Gomez-Cedenilla A, Leon-Colombo T, Pajares J, Mate-Jimenez J. Effect of fiber supplements on internal bleeding hemorrhoids. Hepatogastroenterology. 1996;43(12):1504–7.
38. Alonso-Coello P, Mills E, Heels-Ansdell D, López-Yarto M, Zhou Q, Johanson JF, et al. Fiber for the treatment of hemorrhoids complications: a systematic review and meta-analysis. Am J Gastroenterol. 2006;101(1):181–8.
39. Tejirian T, Abbas MA. Sitz bath: where is the evidence? Scientific basis for a common practice. Dis Colon Rectum. 2005;48(12):2336–40.
40. Smith PD. Neutrophil activation and mediators of inflammation in chronic venous insufficiency. J Vasc Res. 1999;36:24–36.
41. Shoab SS, Porter J, Scurr JH, Coleridge-Smith PD. Endothelial activation response to oral micronised flavonoid therapy in patients with chronic venous disease – a prospective study. Eur J Vasc Endovasc Surg. 1999;17:313–8.
42. Struckmann JR. Clinical efficacy of micronized purified flavonoid fraction: an overview. J Vasc Res. 1999;36:37–41.
43. Ibañez L, Ballarín E, Vidal X, Laporte JR. Agranulocytosis associated with calcium dobesilate. Clinical course and risk estimation with the case-control and the case-population approaches. Eur J Clin Pharmacol. 2000;56:763–7.
44. Godeberge P. Daflon 500 mg in the treatment of hemorrhoidal disease: a demonstrated efficacy in comparison with placebo. Angiology. 1994;45:574–8.
45. Cospite M. Double-blind, placebo-controlled evaluation of clinical activity and safety of Daflon 500 mg in the treatment of acute hemorrhoids. Angiology. 1994;45:566–73.
46. Thanapongsathorn W, Vajrabukka T. Clinical trial of oral disomin (Daflon) in the treatment of hemorrhoids. Dis Colon Rectum. 1992;35(11):1085–8.
47. Misra MC, Parshad R. Randomized clinical trial of micronized flavonoids in the early control of bleeding from acute internal haemorrhoids (comment). Br J Surg. 2000;87(7):868–72.
48. Ho YH, Foo CL, Seow-Choen F, Goh HS. Prospective randomized controlled trial of a micronized flavonidic fraction to reduce bleeding after haemorrhoidectomy. Br J Surg. 1995;82(8):1034–5.
49. Wijayanegara H, Mose JC, Achmad L, Sobarna R, Permadi W. A clinical trial of hydroxyethylrutoside in the treatment of haemorrhoids of pregnancy. J Int Med Res. 1992;20(1):54–60.
50. Squadrito F, Altavilla D, Oliaro Bosso S. Double blind, randomized clinical trial of troxerutin-carbazochrome in patients with hemorrhoids. Eur Rev Med Pharmacol Sci. 2000;4(1–2):21–4.
51. Mentes BB, Gorgul A, Tatlicioglu E, Ayoglu F, Unal S. Efficacy of calcium dobesilate in treating acute attacks of hemorrhoidal disease. Dis Colon Rectum. 2001;4(10):1489–95.
52. Alonso-Coello P, Zhou Q, Martinez-Zapata MJ, Heels-Ansdell D, Johanson JF, Guyatt G. Meta-analysis of flavonoids for the treatment of haemorrhoids. Br J Surg. 2006;93:909–20.
53. Budding J. Solo operated haemorrhoid ligator rectoscope. A report on 200 consecutive bandings. Int J Colorectal Dis. 1997;12(1):42–4.
54. Berkelhammer C, Moosvi SB. Retroflexed endoscopic band ligation of bleeding internal hemorrhoids. Gastroinest Endosc. 2002;55(4):532–7.
55. Su MY, Chiu CT, Wu CS, et al. Endoscopic hemorrhoidal ligation of symptomatic internal hemorrhoids. Gastrointest Endosc. 2003;58(6):871–4.
56. Ramzisham AR, Sagap I, Nadeson S, Ali IM, Hasni MJ. Prospective randomized clinical trial on suction elastic band ligator versus forceps ligator in the treatment of haemorrhoids. Asian J Surg. 2005;28(4):241–5.

57. Khaliq T, Shah SA, Mehboob A. Outcome of rubber band ligation of haemorrhoids using suction ligator. J Ayub Med Coll Abbottabad. 2004;16(4):34–7.
58. O'Regan PH. Disposable device and a minimally invasive technique for rubber band ligation of haemorrhoids. Dis Colon Rectum. 1999;42(5):683–5.
59. Mattana C, Maria G, Pescatori M. Rubber band ligation of hemorrhoids and rectal mucosal prolapse in constipated patients. Dis Colon Rectum. 1989;32(5):372–5.
60. Lau WY, Chow HP, Poon GP, Wong SH. Rubber band ligation of three primary hemorrhoids in a single session. A safe an effective procedure. Dis Colon Rectum. 1982;25(4):336–9.
61. Khubchandani IT. A randomized comparison of single and multiple rubber band ligations. Dis Colon Rectum. 1983;26(11):705–8.
62. Poon GP, Chu KW, Lau WY. Conventional vs. triple rubber band ligation for hemorrhoids. A prospective, randomized trial. Dis Colon Rectum. 1986;29(12):836–8.
63. Lee HH, Spencer RJ, Beart Jr RW. Multiple hemorrhoidal bandings in a single session. Dis Colon Rectum. 1994;37(1):37–41.
64. Law WL, Chu KW. Triple rubber band ligation for hemorrhoids: prospective, randomized trial of use of local anesthetic injection. Dis Colon Rectum. 1999;42(3):363–6.
65. Ambrose NS, Hares MM, Alexander Williams J, Keighley MR. Prospective randomized comparison of photocoagulation and rubber band ligation in treatment of haemorrhoids. Br Med J (Clin Res Ed). 1983;286(6375):1389–91.
66. Templeton JL, Spence RA, Kennedy TL, Parks TG, Mackenzie G, Hanna WA. Comparison of infrared coagulation and rubber band ligation for first and second degree haemorrhoids: a randomised prospective clinical trial. Br Med J (Clin Red Ed). 1983;286(6375):1387–9.
67. Walker AJ, Leiceste RJ, Nicholls RJ, Mann CV. A prospective study of infrared coagulation injection and rubber band ligation in the treatment of haemorrhoids. Int J Colorectal Dis. 1990;5(2):113–6.
68. Bat L, Melzer E, Koler M, Dreznick Z, Shemesh E. Complications of rubber band ligation of symptomatic internal hemorrhoids. Dis Colon Rectum. 1993;36(3):287–90.
69. O'Hara VS. Fatal clostridial infection following hemorrhoidal banding. Dis Colon Rectum. 1980;23(8):570–1.
70. Russell TR, Donohue JH. Hemorrhoidal banding. A warning. Dis Colon Rectum. 1985;25(5):291–3.
71. Scarpa FJ, Hillis W, Sabetta JR. Pelvic cellulitis: a life threatening complication of hemorrhoidal banding. Surgery. 1988;103(3):383–5.
72. Quevedo-Bonilla G, Farkas AM, Abcarian H, Hambrick E, Orsay CP. Septic complications of hemorrhoidal banding. Arch Surg. 1988;123(5):650–1.
73. Shemesh EI, Kodner IJ, Fry RD, Neufeld DM. Sever complications of rubber band ligation of internal hemorrhoids. Dis Colon Rectum. 1987;30(3):199–200.
74. Wrobleski DE, Corman ML, Veidenheimer MC, Coller JA. Long-term evaluation of rubber ring ligation in hemorrhoidal disease. Dis Colon Rectum. 1980;23(7):478–82.
75. Savioz D, Roche B, Glauser T, Dobrinov A, Ludwig C, Marti MC. Rubber band ligation of hemorrhoids: relapse as a function of time. Int J Colorectal Dis. 1998;12(4):154–6.
76. Bayer I, Myslovaty B, Picovsky BM. Rubber band ligation of hemorrhoids. Convenient and economic treatment. J Clin Gastroenterol. 1996;23(1):50–2.
77. Dennison A, Whiston RJ, Rooney S, Chadderton RD, Wherry DC, Morris DL. A randomized comparison of infrared photocoagulation with bipolar diathermy for the outpatient treatment of hemorrhoids. Dis Colon Rectum. 1990;33(1):32–4.
78. Peon AC, Felt-Bersma RJ, Cuesta MA, Deville W, Meuwissen SG. A randomized controlled trial of rubber band ligation versus infra-red coagulation in the treatment of internal haemorrhoids. Eur J Gastroenterol Hepatol. 2000;12(5):535–9.
79. Hinton CP, Morris DL. A randomized trial comparing direct current therapy and bipolar diathermy in the outpatient treatment of third-degree hemorrhoids. Dis Colon Rectum. 1990;33(11):931–2.
80. Randall GM, Jensen DM, Machicado GA, et al. Prospective randomized comparative study of bipolar versus direct current electrocoagulation for treatment of bleeding internal hemorrhoids. Gastrointest Endosc. 1994;40(4):403–10.
81. Jensen DM, Jutabha R, Machicado GA, et al. Prospective randomized comparative study of bipolar electrocoagulation versus hater probe for treatment of chronically bleeding internal hemorrhoids. Gastrointest Endosc. 1997;46(5):435–43.
82. Norman DA, Newton R, Nicholas GV. Direct current electrotherapy of internal hemorrhoids: an effective, safe, and painless outpatient approach. Am J Gastroenterol. 1989;84(5):482–7.
83. Zinberg SS, Stern DH, Furman DS, Wittles JM. A personal experience in comparing three nonoperative techniques for treating internal hemorrhoids. Am J Gastroenterol. 1989;84(5):488–92.
84. Varma JS, Chung SC, Li AK. Propsective randomized comparison of current coagulation and infection sclerotherapy for the outpatient treatment of haemorrhoids. Int J Colorectal Dis. 1991;6(1):42–5.
85. Sim AJ, Murie JA, Mackenzie I. Three year follow up study on the treatment of first and second degree hemorrhoids by sclerosant injection or rubber band ligation. Surg Gynecol Obstet. 1983;157(6):534–6.
86. Bullock N. Importance after sclerotherapy of haemorrhoids: case reports. BMJ. 1997;314(7078):419.
87. Khoury GA, Lake SP, Lewis MC, Lewis AA. A randomized trial to compare single with multiple phenol injection treatment for haemorrhoids. Br J Surg. 1985;72(9):741–2.
88. Senapati A, Nicholls RJ. A randomized trial to compare the results of injection sclerotherapy with a bulk laxative alone in the treatment of bleeding haemorrhoids. Int J Colorectal Dis. 1988;3(2):124–6.
89. Lord PH. A new regime for the treatment of haemorrhoids. Proc R Soc Med. 1968;61(9):935–6.
90. Speakman CT, Burnett SJ, Kamm MA, Bartram CI. Sphincter injury after anal dilatation demonstrated by anal endosonography. Br J Surg. 1991;78(12):1429–30.
91. MacDonald A, Smith A, McNeill AD, Finlay I. Manual dilatation of the anus. Br J Surg. 1992;79(12):1381–2.
92. Konsten J, Baeten CG. Hemorrhoidectomy vs Lord's method: 17-year follow up of a prospective, randomized trial. Dis Colon Rectum. 2000;43(4):503–6.
93. Goligher JC. Cryosurgery for hemorrhoids. Dis Colon Rectum. 1976;19(3):213–8.
94. Smith LE, Goodreau JJ, Fouty WJ. Operative hemorrhoidectomy versus cryodestruction. Dis Colon Rectum. 1979;22(1):10–6.
95. O'Callaghan JD, Matheson TS, Hall R. Inpatient treatment of prolapsing piles:cryosurgery versus Milligan-Morgan haemorrhoidectomy. Br J Surg. 1982;69(3):157–9.

96. Dennison AR, Whiston RJ, Rooney S, Morris DL. The management of hemorrhoids. Am J Gastroenterol. 1989;84(5): 475–81.
97. Bleday R, Pena JP, Rothenberger DA, Goldberg SM, Buls JG. Symptomatic hemorrhoids: current incidence and complications of operative therapy. Dis Colon Rectum. 1992;35(5): 477–81.
98. Ferguson JA, Mazier WP, Ganchrow MI, Friend WG. The closed technique of hemorrhoidectomy. Surgery. 1971;70(3):480–4.
99. Read TE, Henry SE, Hovis RM, Fleshman JW, Birnbaum EH, Caushaj PF, et al. Prospective evaluation of anesthetic technique for anorectal surgery. Dis Colon Rectum. 2002;45(11):1553–8.
100. Lohsiriwat V, Vongjirad A, Lohsiriwat D. Value of routine histopathologic examination of three common surgical specimens: appendix, gallbladder, and hemorrhoid. World J Surg. 2009;33(10):2189–93.
101. Milligan ET, Morgan CN, Jones LE. Surgical anatomy of the anal canal and the operative treatment of hemorrhoids. Lancet. 1937;2:119–24.
102. Whitehead W. The surgical treatment of hemorrhoids. Br Med J. 1882;1:148–50.
103. Wolff BG, Culp CE. The Whitehead hemorrhoidectomy. An unjustly maligned procedure. Dis Colon Rectum. 1988;31(8):587–90.
104. Devien CV, Pujol JP. Total circular hemorrhoidectomy. Int Surg. 1989;74(3):154–7.
105. Boccasanta P, Venturi M, Orio A, et al. Circular hemorrhoidectomy in advanced hemorrhoidal disease. Hepatogastroenterology. 1998;45(22):969–72.
106. MacRae HM, Temple LK, McLeod RS. A meta-analysis for hemorrhoidal treatments. Semin C R Surg. 2002;13:77–83.
107. Ho YH, Seow-Choen F, Tan M, Leong AF. Randomized controlled trial of open and closed haemorrhoidectomy. Br J Surg. 1997;84(12):1729–30.
108. Carapeti EA, Kamm MA, McDonald PH, Chadwick SJ, Phillips RK. Randomized trial of pen versus closed day-case haemorrhoidectomy. Br J Surg. 1999;86(5):612–3.
109. Arbman G, Krook H, Haapaniemi S. Closed vs. open hemorrhoidectomy – is there any difference? Dis Colon Rectum. 2000;43(1):31–4.
110. Gencosmanoglu R, Sad O, Koc D, Inceoglu R. Hemorrhoidectomy: open or closed technique? A prospective randomized clinical trial. Dis Colon Rectum. 2002;45(1):70–5.
111. Ho YH, Buettner PG. Open compared with closed haemorrhoidectomy: meta-analysis of randomized controlled trials. Tech Coloproctol. 2007;11(2):135–43.
112. Mehigan BJ, Monson JR, Hartley JE. Stapling procedure of haemorrhoids versus Milligan-Morgan haemorrhoidectomy: randomized controlled trial. Lancet. 2000;355(9206): 782–5.
113. Shalaby R, Desoky A. Randomized clinical trial of stapled versus Milligan-Morgan haemorrhoidectomy. Br J Surg. 2001;88(8):1049–53.
114. Boccasanta P, Capretti PG, Venturi M, et al. Randomised controlled trial between stapled circumferential mucosectomy and conventional circular hemorrhoidectomy in advanced hemorrhoids with external mucosal prolapse. Am J Surg. 2001;182(1):64–8.
115. Hetzer FH, Demartines N, Handschin AE, Clavien PA. Stapled vs excision hemorrhoidectomy: long term-results of a prospective randomized trial. Arch Surg. 2002;127(3):337–40.
116. Khan S, Pawlak SE, Eggenberger JC, et al. Surgical treatment of hemorrhoids: prospective, randomized trial comparing closed excisional hemorrhoidectomy and the Harmonic Scalpel technique for excisional hemorrhoidectomy. Dis Colon Rectum. 2001;44(6):845–9.
117. Armstrong DN, Ambroze WL, Schertzer ME, Orangio GR. Harmonic scalpel vs electrocautery hemorrhoidectomy: a prospective evaluation. Dis Colon Rectum. 2001;44(4):558–64.
118. Tan JJ, Seow-Choen F. Prospective, randomized trial comparing diathermy and Harmonic Scalpel hemorrhoidectomy. Dis Colon Rectum. 2001;44(5):677–9.
119. Franklin EJ, Seetharam S, Lowney J, Horgan PG. Randomized clinical trial of Ligasure vs conventional diathermy in hemorrhoidectomy. Dis Colon Rectum. 2003;46(10):1380–3.
120. Chung YC, Wu HJ. Clinical experience of sutureless closed hemorrhoidectomy with LigaSure. Dis Colon Rectum. 2003;4(1):87–92.
121. Chung CC, Ha JP, Tai YP, Tsang WW, Li MK. Double blind randomized trial comparing Harmonic Scalpel hemorrhoidectomy, bipolar scissors hemorrhoidectomy, and scissor excision: ligation technique. Dis Colon Rectum. 2002;45(6):789–94.
122. Jayne DG, Botterill I, Ambrose NS, Brennan TG, Guilou PH, O'Riordain DS. Randomized clinical trial of Ligasure versus conventional diathermy for day case haemorrhoidectomy. Dr J Surg. 2002;89(4):428–32.
123. Palazzo FF, Francis DL, Cligton MA. Randomized clinical trial of Ligasure versus open haemorrhoidectomy. Br J Surg. 2002;89(2):154–7.
124. Abo-hashem AA, Sarhan A, Aly AM. Harmonic Scalpel compared with bipolar electro-cautery hemorrhoidectomy: a randomized controlled trial. Int J Surg. 2010;8(3):243–7.
125. Sohn VY, Martin MJ, Mullenix PS, Cuadrado DG, Place RJ, Steele SR. A comparison of open versus closed techniques using the Harmonic Scalpel in outpatient hemorrhoid surgery. Mil Med. 2008;173(7):689–92.
126. Fareed M, El-Awady S, Abd-El monaem H, Aly A. Randomized trial comparing LigaSure to closed Ferguson hemorrhoidectomy. Tech Coloproctol. 2009;13(3):243–6.
127. Castellí J, Sueiras A, Espinosa J, Vallet J, Gil V, Pi F. Ligasure versus diathermy hemorrhoidectomy under spinal anesthesia or pudendal block with ropivacaine: a randomized prospective clinical study with 1-year follow-up. Int J Colorectal Dis. 2009;24(9):1011–8.
128. Tan KY, Zin T, Sim HL, Poon PL, Cheng A, Mak K. Randomized clinical trial comparing LigaSure haemorrhoidectomy with open diathermy haemorrhoidectomy. Tech Coloproctol. 2008;12(2):93–7.
129. Muzi MG, Milito G, Nigro C, Cadeddu F, Andreoli F, Amabile D, et al. Randomized clinical trial of LigaSure and conventional diathermy haemorrhoidectomy. Br J Surg. 2007;94(8):937–42.
130. Seow-Choen F, Ho YH, Ang HG, Goh HS. Prospective randomized trial comparing pain and clinical function after conventional scissors excision/ligation vs. diathermy excision without ligation for symptomatic prolapsed hemorhoides. Dis Colon Rectum. 1992;35(12):1165–9.

131. Andrews BT, Layer GT, Jackson BT, Nicholls RJ. Randomized trial comparing diathermy hemorrhoictomy with the scissor dissection in Milligan-Morgan operation. Dis Colon Rectum. 1993;36(6):580–3.
132. Ibrahim S, Tsang C, Lee YL, Eu KW, Seow-Choen F. Prospective, randomized trial comparing pain and complications between diathermy and scissors for closed hemorrhoidectomy. Dis Colon Rectum. 1998;41(11):1418–20.
133. Wang JY, Chang-Chien CR, Chen JS, Lai CR, Tang RP. The role of lasers in hemorrhoidectomy. Dis Colon Rectum. 1991;34(1):78–82.
134. Iwagaki H, Higuchi Y, Fuchimoto S, Ortia K. The laser treatment of hemorrhoids: results of a study on 1816 patients. Jpn J Surg. 1989;19(6):658–61.
135. Senagore A, Mazier WP, Luchtefeld MA, MacKeigan JM, Wengert T. Treatment of advanced hemorrhoidal disease: a prospective, randomized comparison of cold scalper vs contact ND:YAG laser. Dis Colon Rectum. 1993;36(11):1042–9.
136. Ui Y. Anoderm-preserving, completely closed hemorrhoidectomy with no mucosal incision. Dis Colon Rectum. 1997;40(10):S99–S101.
137. Patel N, O'Connor T. Suture haemorrhoidectomy: a day-only alternative. Aust N Z J Surg. 1996;66(12):830–1.
138. Mathai V, Ong BC, Ho YH. Randomized controlled trial of lateral internal sphincterotomy with haemorrhoidectomy. Br J Surg. 1996;83(3):380–2.
139. Carapeti EA, Kamm MA, McDonald PJ, Phillips RK. Double-blind randomized controlled trial of effect of metronidazole on pain after day-case haemorrhoidectomy. Lancet. 1998;351(9097):169–72.
140. Nicholson TJ, Armstron D. Topical metronidazole (10 percent) decreases posthemorrhoidectomy pain and improves healing. Dis Colon Rectum. 2004;47:711–6.
141. Wasvary HJ, Hain J, Mosed-Vogel M, Bendick P, Varkel DC, Klein SN. Randomized, prospective, double-blind, placebo controlled trial of effect of nitroglycerin ointment on pain after hemorrhoidectomy. Dis Colon Rectum. 2001;44(8):1069–73.
142. Karanlik H, Akturk R, Camlica H, Asoglu O. The effect of glyceryl trinitrate ointment on posthemorrhoidectomy pain and wound healing: results of a randomized, double-blind, placebo-controlled study. Dis Colon Rectum. 2009;52(2):280–5.
143. Hussein MK, Taha AM, Haddad FF, Bassim YR. Bupivacaine local injection in anorectal surgery. Int Surg. 1009;83(1):56–7.
144. Pryn SJ, Crosse MM, Murison MS, McGinn FP. Postoperative analgesia for haemorrhoidectomy. A comparison between caudal and local infiltration. Anaesthesia. 1989;44(12):964–6.
145. Chester JF, Standford BJ, Gazet JC. Analgesia benefit of locally injected bupivacaine after hemorrhoidectomy. Dis Colon Rectum. 1990;33(6):487–9.
146. Ho YH, Seow-Choen F, Low JY, Tn M, Leong AP. Randomized controlled trial of trimebutine (anal sphincter relaxant) for pain after haemorrhoidectomy. Br J Surg. 1997;84(3):377–9.
147. Gottesman L, Milsom JW, Mazier WP. The use of anxiolytic and parasympathomimetic agents in the treatment of postoperative urinary retention following anorectal surgery. A prospective, randomized, double-blind study. Dis Colon Rectum. 1989;32(10):687–870.
148. Cataldo PA, MacKeigan JM. The necessity of routine pathologic evaluation of hemorrhoidectomy specimens. Surg Gynecol Obstet. 1992;174(4):302–4.
149. Rosen L, Sipe P, Stasik JJ, et al. Outcome of delayed hemorrhage following surgical hemorrhoidectomy (letter). Dis Colon Rectum. 1994;37:288–9.
150. Basso L, Pescatroi M. Outcome of delayed hemorrhoids following surgical hemorrhoidectomy (letter). Dis Colon Rectum. 1994;37:288–9.
151. Chen HH, Wang JY, Changchien RC, et al. Risk factors associated with post-hemorrhoidectomy secondary hemorrhoidage. A single institution prospective study of 4880 consecutive hemorrhoidectomies. Dis Colon Rectum. 2003;45:1096–9.
152. Chen HH, Wang J, Changchien CR, Yeh CY, Tsai WS, Tang R. Effective management of posthemorrhoidectomy secondary hemorrhage using rectal irrigation. Dis Colon Rectum. 2002;45:234–8.
153. Tajana A. Hemorrhoidectomy according to Milligan-Morgan: ligature and excision technique. Int Surg. 1989;74(3):158–61.
154. Johnstone CS, Isbisteer WH. Inpatient management of pile: a surgical audit. Aust N Z J Surg. 1992;62(9):720–4.
155. Eu KW, Seow-Choen F, Goh HS. Comparison of emergency and elective haemorrhoidectomy. Br J Surg. 1994;81(2):308–10.
156. Ganchrow MI, Mazier WP, Friend WG, Ferguson JA. Hemorrhoidectomy revisited: a computer analysis of 2038 cases. Dis Colon Rectum. 1971;14:128–33.
157. Goldberg SM, Gordon PH, Nivatvongs S. Hemorrhoids. In: Essentials of Anorectal Surgery. Philadelphia: Lippincott, 1980.
158. McConnell JC, Khubchandani IT. Long term follow up of closed haemorrhoidectomy. Dis Colon Rectum. 1983;26:797–9.
159. Pescatori M, Favetta U, Dedola S, Orsini S. Transanal stapled excision for rectal mucosal prolapse. Tech Coloproctol. 1997;1:96–8.
160. Longo A. Treatment of hemorrhoidal disease by reduction for mucosa and haemorrhoidal prolapse with a circular stapling device: a new procedure – 6th World Congress of Endoscopic Surgery. Mundozzi Editore 1998; 777–84.
161. Ho YH, Cheong WK, Tsang C, et al. Stapled hemorrhoidectomy cost and effectiveness. Randomized, controlled trial including incontinence scoring, anorectal manometry, and endoanal ultrasound assessments at up to three months. Dis Colon Rectum. 2000;43(12):1666–75.
162. Brown SR, Ballan K, Ho E, et al. Stapled mucosectomy for acute thrombosed circumferentially prolapsed piles: a prospective randomized comparison with conventional haemorrhoidectomy. Colorectal Dis. 2001;3(3):175–8.
163. Hetzer FH, Demartines N, Handschin AE, et al. Stapled vs excision hemorrhoidectomy: long-term results of a prospective randomized trial. Arch Surg. 2002;137(3):337–40.
164. Ortiz H, Marzo J, Armendariz P. Randomized clinical trial of stapled haemorrhoidopexy versus conventional diathermy haemorrhoidectomy. Br J Surg. 2002;89(11):1376–81.
165. Pavlidis T, Papaziogas B, Souparis A, et al. Modern stapled Longo procedure vs. conventional Milligan-Morgan hemorrhoidectomy: a randomized controlled trial. Int J Colorectal Dis. 2002;17(1):50–3.
166. Palimento D, Picchio M, Attanasio U, et al. Stapled and open hemorrhoidectomy: randomized controlled trial of early results. World J Surg. 2003;27(2):203–7.

167. Kraemer M, Parulava T, Roblick M, et al. Prospective, randomized study: proximate PPH stapler vs. LigaSure for hemorrhoidal surgery. Dis Colon Rectum. 2005;48(8): 1517–22.
168. Correa-Rovelo JM, Tellez O, Obregon L, et al. Stapled rectal mucosectomy vs. closed hemorrhoidectomy: a randomized clinical trial. Dis Colon Rectum. 2002;45(10):1367–74 [discussion:1374–5].
169. Wilson MS, Pope V, Doran HE, et al. Objective comparison of stapled anopexy and open hemorrhoidectomy: a randomized, controlled trial. Dis Colon Rectum. 2002;45(11):1437–44.
170. Rowsell M, Bello M, Hemingway DM. Circumferential mucosectomy (stapled haemorrhoidectomy) versus conventional haemorrhoidectomy: randomised controlled trial. Lancet. 2000;355(9206):779–81.
171. Cheetham MJ, Cohen CR, Kamm MA, et al. A randomized controlled trial of diathermy hemorrhoidectomy vs. stapled hemorrhoidectomy in an intended day-care setting with longer-term follow-up. Dis Colon Rectum. 2003;46(4):491–7.
172. Bikhchandani J, Agarwal PN, Kant R, et al. Randomized controlled trial to compare the early and mid-term results of stapled versus open hemorrhoidectomy. Am J Surg. 2005;189(1):56–60.
173. Kairaluoma M, Nuorva K, Kellokumpu I. Day-case stapled (circular) vs. diathermy hemorrhoidectomy: a randomized, controlled trial evaluating surgical and functional outcome. Dis Colon Rectum. 2003;46(1):93–9.
174. Gravie JF, Lehur PA, Huten N, et al. Stapled hemorrhoidopexy versus Milligan-Morgan hemorrhoidectomy: a prospective, randomized, multicenter trial with 2-year postoperative follow up. Ann Surg. 2005;242(1):29–35.
175. Chung CC, Cheung HY, Chan ES, et al. Stapled hemorrhoidopexy vs. Harmonic Scalpel hemorrhoidectomy: a randomized trial. Dis Colon Rectum. 2005;48(6):1213–9.
176. Ortiz H, Marzo J, Armendariz P, et al. Stapled hemorrhoidopexy vs. diathermy excision for fourth-degree hemorrhoids: a randomized, clinical trial and review of the literature. Dis Colon Rectum. 2005;48(4):809–15.
177. Ganio E, Altomare DF, Gabrielli F, et al. Prospective randomized multicentre trial comparing stapled with open haemorrhoidectomy. Br J Surg. 2001;88(5):669–74.
178. Smyth EF, Baker RP, Wilken BJ, et al. Stapled versus excision haemorrhoidectomy: long term follow up of a randomised controlled trial. Lancet. 2003;361(9367):1437–8.
179. Racalbuto A, Aliotta I, Corsaro G, et al. Hemorrhoidal stapler prolapsectomy vs. Milligan-Morgan hemorrhoidectomy: a long-term randomized trial. Int J Colorectal Dis. 2004;19(3): 239–44.
180. Krska Z, Kvasnieka J, Faltyn J, et al. Surgical treatment of haemorrhoids according to Longo and Milligan Morgan: an evaluation of postoperative tissue response. Colorectal Dis. 2003;5(6):573–6.
181. Nisar PJ, Acheson AG, Neal KR, et al. Stapled hemorrhoidopexy compared with conventional hemorrhoidectomy: systematic review of randomized, controlled trials. Dis Colon Rectum. 2004;47(11):1837–45.
182. Lan P, Wu X, Zhou X, et al. The safety and efficacy of stapled hemorrhoidectomy in the treatment of hemorrhoids: a systematic review and meta-analysis of ten randomized control trials. Int J Colorectal Dis. 2006;21(2):172–8.
183. Shao WJ, Li GCH, Zhang ZHK, Yang BL, Sun GD, Chen YQ. Systematic review and meta-analysis of randomized controlled trials comparing stapled haemorrhoideopexy with conventional haemorrhoidectomy. Br J Surg. 2008;95: 147–60.
184. Cipriani S, Pescatori M. Acute rectal obstruction after PPH stapled haemorrhoidectomy. Colorectal Dis. 2002;4(5): 367–70.
185. Wong LY, Jiang JK, Chang SC, et al. Rectal perforation: a life-threatening complication of stapled hemorrhoidectomy: report of a case. Dis Colon Rectum. 2003;46(1):116–7.
186. Maw A, Eu KW, Seow-Choen F. Retroperitoneal sepsis complicating stapled hemorrhoidectomy: report of a case and review of the literature. Dis Colon Rectum. 2002;45(6): 826–8.
187. Molloy RG, Kingsmore D. Life threatening pelvic sepsis after stapled haemorrhoidectomy. Lancet. 2000;355(9206):810.
188. Ripetti V, Caricato M, Arullani A. Rectal perforation, retropneumoperitoneum, and pneumomediastinum after stapling procedure for prolapsed hemorrhoids: report of a case and subsequent considerations. Dis Colon Rectum. 2002;45(2): 268–70.
189. Ho YH, Seow-Cheen F, Tsang C, Eu KW. Randomized trial assessing anal sphincter injuries after stapled haemorrhoidectomy. Br J Surg. 2001;88(11):1449–55.
190. George BD, Shetty D, Lindsey I, Mortensen NJ, Warren BF. Histopathology of stapled haemorrhoidectomy specimens: a cautionary note. Colorectal Dis. 2002;4(6):473–6.
191. Roos P. Haemorrhoid surgery revised. Lancet. 2000;355(9215): 1648.
192. Pescatori M. Prospective randomized multicentre trial comparing stapled with open haemorrhoidectomy. Br J Surg. 2002;89(1):122.
193. Morinaga K, Hasuda K, Ikeda T. A novel therapy for internal hemorrhoids: ligation of the hemorrhoidal artery with a newly devised instrument (Moricorn) in conjunction with a Doppler flowmeter. Am J Gastroenterol. 1995;90(4):610–3.
194. Dal Monte PP, Tagariello C, Giordano P, Cudazzo E, Shafi A, Sarago M, Franzini M. Transanal haemorrhoidal dearterialisation:nonexcisional surgery for heat treatment of haemorrhoidal disease. Tech Coloproctol 2007;11(4):333–9.
195. Charua Guindic L, Fonseca Munoz E, García Perez NJ, et al. Hemorrhoidal dearterialization guided by Doppler. A surgical alternative in hemorrhoidal disease management. Rev Gastroenterol Méx. 2004;69:83–7.
196. Bursics A, Morvay K, Kupcsulik P, Flautner L. Comparison of early and 1-year follow-up results of conventional hemorrhoidectomy and hemorrhoid artery ligation: a randomized study. Int J Colorectal Dis. 2004;19:176–80.
197. Ramirez JM, Gracia JA, Aguilella V, Elia M, Casamayor MC, Martinez M. Surgical management of symptomatic haemorrhoids: to cut, to hang or to strangle? A prospective randomized controlled trial. Colorectal Dis. 2005;7:52.
198. Ramirez JM, Aguilella V, Elía M, Gracia JA, Martínez M. Doppler-guided hemorrhoidal artery ligation in the management of symptomatic hemorrhoids. Rev Esp Enferm Dig. 2005;97:97–103.
199. Felice G, Privitera A, Ellul E, Klaumann M. Doppler-guided hemorrhoidal artery ligation: an alternative to hemorrhoidectomy. Dis Colon Rectum. 2005;48:2090–3.

200. Greenberg R, Karin E, Avital S, Skornick Y, Werbin N. First 100 cases with Doppler-guided hemorrhoidal artery ligation. Dis Colon Rectum. 2006;49:485–9.
201. de Vries BM Wallis, van der Beek ES, de Wijkerslooth LR, et al. Treatment of grade 2 and 3 hemorrhoids with Doppler-guided hemorrhoidal artery ligation. Dig Surg. 2007;24:436–40.
202. Abdeldaim Y, Mabadeje O, Muhammad KM, Mc Avinchey D. Doppler-guided haemorrhoidal arteries ligation: preliminary clinical experience. Ir Med J. 2007;100:535–7.
203. Giordano P, Overton J, Madeddu F, Zaman S, Gravante G. Transanal hemorrhoidal de-arterialization: A systematic review. Dis Colon Rectum. 2009;52:1665–71.
204. Rasmussen OO, Larsen KG, Naver L, Christiansen J. Emergency haemorrhoidectomy compared with incision and banding for the treatment of acute strangulated haemorrhoids. A prospective randomised study. Eur J Surg. 1991;157(10):613–4.
205. McCormack TT, Bailey HR, Simms JM, Johnson AG. Rectal varices are not piles. Br J Surg. 1984;71:163.
206. Bernstein WC. What are hemorrhoids and what is their relationship to the portal venous system? Dis Colon Rectum. 1983;23(12):829–34.
207. Hosking SW, Smart HL, Johnson AG, Triger DR. Anorectal varices, haemorrhoids, and portal hypertension. Lancet. 1989;1(8624):349–52.
208. Goenka MK, Kochhar R, Nagi B, Mehta SK. Rectosigmoid varices and other mucosal changes in patients with portal hypertension. Am J Gastroenterol. 1991;86(9):1185–9.
209. Chawla Y, Dilawari JB. Anorectal varices – their frequency in cirrhotic and non-cirrhotic portal hypertension. Gut. 1991;32(3):309–11.
210. Johansen K, Bardin J, Orloff MJ. Massive bleeding from hemorrhoidal varices in portal hypertension. JAMA. 1980;244(18):2084–5.
211. Hosking SW, Johnson AG. Bleeding anorectal varices – a misunderstood condition. Surgery. 1988;104(1):70–3.
212. George BS, ML LAJ. Stapled anopexy in the treatment of anal varices: report of a case. Dis Colon Rectum. 2003;46(9):1284–5.
213. Shibata D, Brophy DP, Gordon FD, Anastopoulos HT, Sentovich SM, Bleday R. Transjugular intrahepatic portosystemic shunt for treatment of bleeding ectopic varices with portoal hypertension. Dis Colon Rectum. 1999;42(12):1581–5.
214. Fantin AC, Zala G, Risti B, Debatin JF, Schopke W, Meyenberger C. Bleeding anorectal varices: successful treatment with transjugular intrahepatic portosystemic shuntin (TIPS). Gut. 1996;38(6):932–5.
215. Montemurro S, Polignano FM, Caliandro C, Rucci A, Ruggieri E, Sciscio V. Inferior mesocaval shunt for bleeding anorectal varices and portal vein thrombosis. Hepatogastroenterology. 2001;48(40):980–3.
216. Rahmani O, Wolpert LM, Drezner AD. Distal inferior mesenteric veins to renal vein shunt for treatment of bleeding anorectal varices: case report and review of literature. J Vasc Surg. 2002;36(6):1264–6.
217. Saleeby Jr RG, Rosen L, Stasik JJ, Tiether Rd, Sheets J, Khubchandani IT. Hemorrhoidectomy during pregnancy: risk or relief? Dis Colon Rectum. 1991;34(3):260–1.
218. Jeffery PJ, Parks AG, Ritchie JK. Treatment of haemorrhoids in patients with inflammatory bowel disease. Lancet. 1977;1(8021):1084–5.
219. Wolkomir AF, Luchtefeld MA. Surgery for symptomatic hemorrhoids and anal fissures in Crohn's disease. Dis Colon Rectum. 1993;36(6):545–7.
220. Grewal H, Guillem JG, Quan SH, Enker WE, Cohen AM. Anorectal disease in neutropenic leukemic patients. Operative vs nonoperative management. Dis Colon Rectum. 1994;37(11):1095–9.
221. Morandi E, Merlini D, Salvaggio A, Foschi D, Trabucci E. Prospective study of healing time after hemorrhoidectomy: influence of HIV infection, acquired immunodeficiency syndrome, and anal wound infection. Dis Colon Rectum. 1999;42(9):1140–4.

12
Anal Fissure

Rocco Ricciardi, Sharon L. Dykes, and Robert D. Madoff

Introduction

An anal fissure, or fissure-in-ano, is a linear or an oval-shaped tear distal to the dentate line in the anal canal. Patients afflicted with this disorder most commonly complain of severe pain with bowel movements as well as bright red blood per rectum. Anal fissures are assumed to be very common although it is difficult to estimate disease prevalence since diagnosis of anorectal disorders is generally inaccurate. In addition, it is likely that a large proportion of patients with anal fissures never seek medical care and thus the condition is much more prevalent in the general population as compared to what is seen in clinical practice. In one survey, 80% of participants with symptoms attributed to the anorectum did not consult a physician.[1]

Large case series have provided much of the background information regarding fissure epidemiology. Data from these studies should be viewed with the understanding that there may be particular groups of patients who never seek medical counsel. Given this information, it appears that anal fissures occur equally in men and women and tend to occur in younger age groups with a mean age of 39.9 in one large study from Montreal Canada.[2] In almost 75% of cases, fissures are identified in the posterior midline but can be seen in the anterior midline in up to 25% of affected women and 8% of affected men.[2] An additional 3% of patients have both anterior and posterior fissures. When fissures occur in atypical locations or multiple fissures are identified, the clinician should investigate for other potentially complicated disease processes, such as Crohn's disease, trauma, tuberculosis, syphilis, HIV/AIDS, or anal carcinoma (Figure 12-1).

Early, or acute, fissures have the appearance of a simple tear in the anoderm. When symptoms last longer than 8–12 weeks, the fissure generally takes on chronic features, demonstrating evidence of edema and fibrosis. Inflammatory manifestations of chronic fissures include sentinel piles, or skin tags, at the distal fissure margin and a hypertrophied anal papilla proximal to the fissure in the anal canal. In addition to these changes, fibers of the internal anal sphincter (IAS) are often visible at the fissure base with chronicity.

Etiology

There has been considerable debate regarding the etiology of anal fissures. Most patients report some element of trauma to the anal canal, often after the passage of either hard or loose stool. Yet, many patients pass hard bowel movements or experience episodes of diarrhea without ever developing a fissure; thus, the trauma hypothesis may explain some element of cause, but it is not the complete story. The potential role of constipation has also been debated, but a history of constipation is not universally obtained and as stated, some patients report diarrhea prior to the onset of symptoms.

It is likely that many patients develop fissures but most heal within a very short period. However, others develop fissure persistence which is associated with increased resting anal pressure – an observation first reported in the mid-1970s.[3,4] Physiologic studies using ambulatory manometry have confirmed the presence of sustained resting hypertonia in fissure patients.[5] Further observational data have delineated an inverse relationship between anal canal pressure and perfusion of the anoderm. The ischemia hypothesis was initially proposed as an instigator of fissure persistence by Gibbons and Read[6] in 1986. Later support was provided by angiographic studies of the inferior rectal artery in cadavers, which demonstrated a paucity of blood vessels in the posterior midline of the anal canal in 85% of those examined.[7] Schouten et al.[8] measured anodermal blood flow in healthy individuals using Doppler laser flowmetry and found that the posterior midline had the lowest perfusion when compared to the other quadrants. In addition, there was a significant inverse correlation between posterior midline anodermal blood flow and maximum resting anal pressure in a large cohort of patients that included normal controls as well as fissure patients. Those patients with fissures demonstrated the

D.E. Beck et al. (eds.), *The ASCRS Textbook of Colon and Rectal Surgery: Second Edition*,
DOI 10.1007/978-1-4419-1584-9_12, © Springer Science+Business Media, LLC 2011

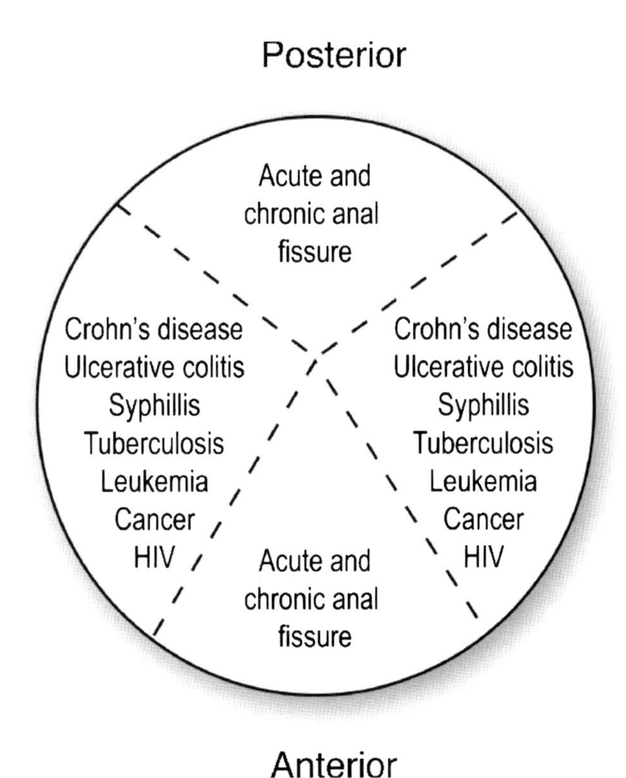

FIGURE 12-1. The location of anal fissure suggests etiology.

highest resting anal pressures and the lowest posterior blood flow of any group. In addition to these data, improvement in posterior midline blood flow was noted to occur after reduction of anal pressure with anesthesia. These same authors were able to demonstrate normalization of sphincter hypertonia and anodermal blood flow after lateral internal sphincterotomy (LIS) in patients with anal fissures.[8]

Symptoms

The clinical hallmark of an anal fissure is pain during, and particularly after, defecation. In acute fissures, pain may be short-lived, but it can last several hours or even all day in the presence of a chronic fissure. Patients often describe the pain as a sensation of "passing razor blades or glass" from their rectum. Understandably, patients with anal fissures describe fear of having a bowel movement. In addition, a large subset of patients will describe rectal bleeding, which is generally limited to minimal bright red blood seen on the toilet tissue.

Diagnosis

Diagnosis is suggested by the characteristic description of pain with bowel movements and is generally easily confirmed by physical examination. Most fissures are readily identified by simply spreading the buttocks with opposing traction of the thumbs and a quick look at the anterior or posterior midline (Figure 12-2). Although some clinicians use a cotton swab to depress the fissure and identify pain with contact, the authors find this approach to be unnecessary. Once the presence of a fissure is verified, further attempt to examine the anal canal with insertion of a finger or endoscopic instrumentation (anoscope, proctoscope or sigmoidoscope) is of little value. Since most patients are far too uncomfortable to justify such invasive anoscopic evaluation, further investigation is delayed until after symptoms have resolved.

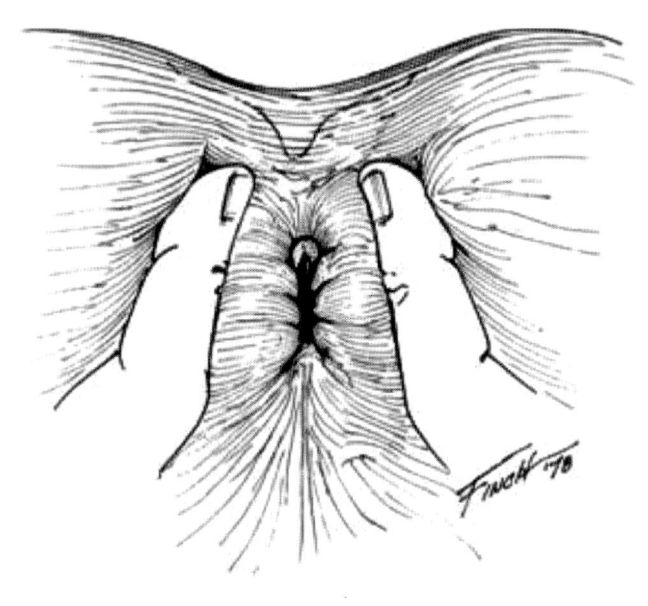

FIGURE 12-2. Examination revealing an anal fissure.

Fissures are often self-diagnosed as hemorrhoids. Similarly, patients may have seen their primary care provider and diagnosed with hemorrhoids. These patients are often troubled by the fact that they have different diagnosis on further examination but can be redirected with a simple understanding of the normalcy of hemorrhoids. The practicing clinician also should be alert for the potential concomitant presence of perianal abscess, anal fistula, inflammatory bowel disease, sexually transmitted disease, and anal carcinoma when the patient complains of anal pain. In addition, atypical fissures such as those occurring off the midline and multiple, painless, and nonhealing fissures, warrant further evaluation via examination under anesthesia and possible biopsy and cultures.

Management

It is estimated that half of all patients diagnosed with an acute fissure will heal with nonoperative measures, such as sitz baths and psyllium fiber supplementation, with or without the addition of topical anesthetics or anti-inflammatory ointments. In a retrospective review by Shub et al.[9] healing occurred in 44% of fissure patients using psyllium fiber, sitz baths, and emollient suppositories. During a 5-year follow-up period, there were treatment failures or recurrences in 27% of patients initially considered healed. A second retrospective review almost 20 years later demonstrated similar findings. Hananel and Gordon[2] reported initial healing in 44% and recurrence in 18.6% of their fissure patients with bulking agents and sitz baths.

Jensen[10] conducted two randomized controlled trials examining the effects of unprocessed bran in both initial treatment and maintenance therapy of acute fissures. In the first study, 103 patients with acute posterior anal fissures were randomized to receive either lignocaine ointment, hydrocortisone ointment, or sitz baths with unprocessed bran for 3 weeks. After weeks 1 and 2, patients treated with sitz baths and bran were found to have significant evidence of symptomatic relief as compared with the other two groups. By the 3-week end point, however, there were no differences among the three groups. At 1 year, fissure recurrence was 16% in patients receiving 15 g of unprocessed bran daily as compared to 60% of patients receiving 7.5 g of bran daily or 68% of patients receiving placebo.[11]

Sphincter Relaxants

Given the theory of increased sphincter tone in patients with anal fissure, a number of topical, oral, and injectable drugs have been tested with the aim of reducing mean maximum resting anal pressure. Preparations include (1) various nitrate formulations such as nitroglycerin ointment (NTG), glyceryl trinitrate (GTN), and isosorbide dinitrate; (2) oral and topical calcium channel blockers, including nifedipine and diltiazem (DTZ); (3) adrenergic antagonists; (4) topical muscarinic agonists, i.e., bethanechol; (5) phosphodiesterase inhibitors; and (6) botulinum toxin. Given the vast number of agents available, the reader might assume that none of the agents are "ideal." As suggested, the comparative data in this area are quite controversial as one recent review concluded "first-line use of medical therapy cures most chronic fissures cheaply and conveniently,"[12] while a second review concluded that "medical therapy for chronic anal fissure … may be applied with a chance of cure that is only marginally better than placebo… [and] far less effective than surgery."[13] These reviews will be considered in more detail with the other published literature in the following paragraphs.

Topical Nitrates

The IAS is a smooth muscle whose tone is affected by both intrinsic myogenic properties and extrinsic neural influences. Nitric oxide is the predominant nonadrenergic, noncholinergic neurotransmitter in the IAS. Release of nitric oxide results in IAS relaxation, which theoretically improves blood flow to the fissure and promotes healing. Exogenous nitrates release nitric oxide in vivo and have been used as nitric oxide donors to treat patients with anal fissures as well as other conditions.

Studies by Loder et al.[14] and Guillemot et al.[15] demonstrated decreased resting anal pressure with application of 0.2% topical GTN. This led to a series of retrospective and prospective reports, as well as randomized trials supporting the use of various nitrate preparations in the treatment of anal fissures (Table 12-1). One early clinical trial by Bacher et al.[18] randomized 35 patients with acute and chronic anal fissures to receive either topical 0.2% NTG ointment or 2% lidocaine gel for 4 weeks. After 1 month, the healing rate was 80% for patients receiving NTG, which was significantly higher than the 40% healing rate reported for patients receiving topical lidocaine. Manometric data on the 28th day of treatment also revealed a decrease in overall maximum resting anal pressure from a mean of 110 to 87 cm H_2O in the NTG group but not in patients receiving lidocaine ointment. The authors postulated that the persistence and recurrence of chronic fissures was due to lack of sphincter tone reduction.[18]

Subsequent randomized placebo-controlled trials have attempted to determine whether higher doses of NTG ointment promote healing and lessen recurrence in chronic anal fissures. Carapeti et al.[20] found no difference in chronic fissure healing between patients randomized to receive an 8-week treatment of either 0.2% topical GTN three times daily or 0.2% GTN titrated in 0.1% increments to a maximum of 0.6%. The authors found that by escalating GTN dose, healing was not accelerated. Thus, 67% of patients treated with either dose of GTN preparation healed as compared to 32% of placebo patients. Bailey et al.[27] and Scholefield et al.[28] reported similar findings when patients with chronic anal fissures were either randomized to receive placebo, 0.1%, 0.2%, or 0.4% GTN ointment twice or three times daily. In both studies, there were no significant differences in fissure healing among treatment groups as healing occurred in approximately 50% of all patients.

Additional randomized placebo-controlled trials have demonstrated comparable healing rates of 46–70% in patients with chronic anal fissures after application of 0.2% GTN ointment two to three times daily for 4–8 weeks (Table 12-1). Supportive data demonstrate statistically significant decreases in pain scores and maximal anal resting pressures in patients treated with GTN as compared to placebo. However, in a study by Altomare et al.[21], 132 patients with chronic fissures were randomized to receive 0.2% topical GTN or placebo for 4 weeks. He confirmed the effects of GTN on anodermal blood flow and sphincter pressure, but unlike similarly designed trials, they demonstrated no significant difference in healing rates between GTN and placebo (49.2% vs. 51.7%).

A series of randomized trials have also sought to compare 0.2% GTN with surgery, i.e., LIS. While initial healing rates during 4–8-week evaluation periods were similar to those in placebo-based trials (and up to 83.3% in a study by Oettle et al.),[17] healing rates were far superior for LIS (91.7–100%). In one clinical trial, Evans et al. demonstrated healing in 60.6% of patients treated with GTN as compared

TABLE 12-1. Randomized trials of nitroglycerine therapy

Year	Author	*n*	Treatment	Follow-up	Success (%)
1997	Lund and Scholefield[16]	80	0.2% GTN bid	8 weeks	68
			placebo		39[b]
1997	Oettle[17]	24	0.2% GTN tid	4 weeks	83.3
			LIS		100[a]
1997	Bacher et al.[18]	35	0.2% GTN	4 weeks	80
			2% lidocaine		40[b]
1999	Kennedy et al.[19]	43	0.2% GTN	4 weeks	46
			placebo		16[b]
1999	Carapeti et al.[20]	70	0.2% GTN tid	8 weeks	67
			0.2% GTN tid (titrated to 0.6%)		
			placebo		32[b]
2000	Altomare et al.[21]	132	0.2% GTN bid	4 weeks	49.2
			placebo		51.7[a]
2000	Zuberi et al.[22]	42	0.2% GTN	8 weeks	66.7
			10 mg NTG patch		63.2
			LIS		91.7[a]
2000	Richard et al.[23]	82	0.2% GTN	6 months	27.2
			LIS		92.1[b]
2001	Evans et al.[24]	65	0.2% GTN tid	8 weeks	60.6
			LIS		97[b]
2001	Chaudhuri et al.[25]	19	0.2% GTN bid	6 weeks	70
			placebo		22.2[b]
2002	Libertiny et al.[26]	70	0.2% GTN	2 years	45.7
			LIS		97.1[b]
2002	Bailey et al.[27]	304	0.1%, 0.2%, and 0.4% GTN bid/tid	8 weeks	50% across board[a]
			placebo		
2003	Scholefield et al.[28]	200	0.1%, 0.2%, and 0.4% GTN bid/tid	8 weeks	46.9, 40.4, 54.1
			placebo		37.5[a]
2005	Mishra et al.[29]	40	0.2% GTN	6 weeks	90
			LIS		85[a]

GTN glyceryl trinitrate, *NTG* nitroglycerin, *LIS* lateral internal sphincterotomy, *bid* twice daily, *tid* three times daily.
[a] Not statistically significant comparison.
[b] Statistically significant comparison.

to 97% of patients treated with sphincterotomy.[24] In addition, of the 33 patients initially treated with GTN, 12 eventually underwent sphincterotomy for persistent fissures. Despite early healing with GTN, 50% of those whose fissures healed with GTN treatment developed recurrences.[24] Similarly, in a randomized, controlled trial by the Canadian Colorectal Surgical Trials Group of LIS compared to topical NTG, 89.5% of patients in the LIS group compared to 29.5% in the NTG group had complete healing of fissures.[23] In addition, side effects were observed more frequently in patients treated with NTG (84%) compared to LIS (28.9%).[23] Follow-up was performed 6 years later and revealed a more durable treatment result for LIS-treated patients as compared to patients treated with topical nitroglycerin therapy.[30]

Other randomized, controlled trials drew different conclusion following GTN treatment. Libertiny et al.[26] randomized 70 patients with chronic anal fissure to receive 0.2% GTN or LIS. Only 16 of 35 patients initially treated with GTN healed without recurrence during a 24-month follow-up, in contrast to operative cure in 34 of 35 patients treated with LIS. Despite the superiority in healing for LIS patients, the authors concluded that chemical sphincterotomy with GTN should be the initial treatment in patients with chronic anal fissure and LIS should be reserved for treatment failures.[26] Zuberi et al.[22] similarly concluded that GTN ointment and NTG patch were effective treatment options in patients with anal fissures. In their prospective trial of 42 patients, healing rates were 66.7% in patients receiving 0.2% GTN, 63.2% for those receiving a 10-mg NTG patch applied at a distance from the fissure, and 91.7% in patients who underwent LIS. Their findings support the use of GTN as a first-line agent in chronic anal fissures, as the difference in healing rates was not statistically significant between groups.[22]

In addition to GTN and NTG, other nitrate preparations have also been used to treat anal fissures. A prospective, uncontrolled study by Schouten et al.[31] demonstrated reduction in anal pressure and improvement in anodermal blood flow in patients with chronic anal fissures treated with isosorbide dintirate. Topical use of isosorbide dintirate led to fissure healing in 88% after 12 weeks. Two randomized, placebo-controlled trials confirmed these findings.[32,33] In a study by Were et al.[32], healing was noted in 85% of patients with chronic anal fissure treated with isosorbide dintirate for 5 weeks as compared to 35% of patients who received placebo. Tankova et al.[33] subsequently reported fissure healing in 80% of patients actively treated with mononitrate. In a dose-finding study, Lysy et al.[34] found that 2.5 mg of topically applied isosorbide dintirate three times daily resulted in a greater reduction in maximum anal resting pressure than 1.25 mg and excellent fissure healing rates. In a prospective randomized trial, isosorbide dinitrate had comparable levels of fissure healing as compared to surgical sphincterotomy. The authors concluded that isosorbide dinitrate ointment must be considered as the first choice of treatment in patients with chronic anal fissure.[35]

Endogenous nitric oxide donors, such as L-arginine, are also effective in producing relaxation of the anal sphincter. Preliminary in vivo studies in rats have demonstrated a decline in sphincter pressure with administration of 10 mg L-arginine rectally. This effect was reversed with the use of L-arginine antagonists.[36] In a placebo-controlled trial, 46% reduction in resting anal pressure was observed 5 min after topical application of L-arginine, and maintained for 2 h.[37] In a clinical trial of 15 patients, topical application of L-arginine promoted fissure healing without headache in 62% of patients.[38]

Despite encouraging results regarding initial healing rates with topical nitrates, concerns about long-term outcomes and adverse reactions have limited their use. Recurrence rates of 35% have been documented as well as lack of compliance with only 67% completing treatment in one study.[39] In a non-randomized, prospective trial, Graziano et al.[40] demonstrated a 67% recurrence rate for chronic fissures during a 9-month follow-up period while 77% reported headaches. Mild headaches were also described by Bacher et al.[18] in 20% of patients receiving 0.2% topical GTN. Altomare et al.[21] reported that 34% of chronic fissure patients treated with GTN had headaches and nearly 6% of patients had orthostatic hypotension. Carapeti et al.[20] noted headaches in 72% of patients receiving GTN vs. 27% of controls receiving placebo.

Calcium Channel Blockers

The effect of nifedipine on the anal sphincter was first evaluated by Chrysos et al.[41] in a prospective trial in 1996. Anorectal manometry was performed on ten patients with hemorrhoids and/or anal fissure and ten controls, before and 30 min after receiving 20 mg of sublingual nifedipine. Anal resting pressure was reduced by almost 30% in both groups.[41] This study set the stage for further prospective clinical trials examining the efficacy of nifedipine and other calcium channel blockers in treating anal fissures. In addition to nifedipine, others have used topical DTZ to treat anal fissures.[42] In one initial trial of 2% DTZ gel in ten patients, 67% of fissures healed while no patient reported a headache or any other side effect.

Further prospective trials have substantiated the findings of these early studies. Knight et al.[43] evaluated the effects of 2% DTZ gel in 71 patients and was able to achieve healing in 75%. Side effects were reported in five patients overall: four experienced perianal dermatitis and one patient, headache. Agaoglu et al.[44] described healing in 60% of patients treated with 20 mg oral nifedipine twice daily, while headaches were reported in only one patient. Ansaloni et al.[45] also reported encouraging results regarding efficacy of 6 mg oral lacidipine, a calcium channel blocker with long duration of action and a particular affinity for blood vessels. Although 90.4% of treated patients' fissures had healed at 2 months follow-up, 33% of patients had side effects.

Randomized, controlled trials comparing topical nifedipine gel with a combination of topical lidocaine and hydrocortisone gels have also demonstrated superiority of nifedipine in the treatment of anal fissures. Antropoli et al.[46] randomized 283 patients to either receive 0.2% nifedipine gel every 12 h or lidocaine/hydrocortisone gel. Complete healing occurred in 95% of patients receiving nifedipine as compared to 50% of controls. Perrotti et al.[47] similarly randomized 110 patients with anal fissure to receive 0.3% nifedipine gel with 1.5% lidocaine or a lidocaine/hydrocortisone mixture twice daily. In the nifedipine group, 94.5% of patients healed completely as compared to 16.4% of controls.

Calcium channel blockers can be administered in either oral form or topically to treat anal fissures. Jonas et al.[48] performed a randomized, controlled trial to ascertain whether different routes of DTZ administration had similar healing rates. The authors identified fissure healing in 38% of those individuals receiving oral DTZ and 65% of patients on topical treatment. In addition, oral DTZ caused far more side effects while no side effects were identified in those receiving topical therapy. At this time, the number of patients evaluated in trials of oral vs. topical therapy has been too small to allow for definitive conclusions.

Although long-term follow-up studies are lacking, several randomized controlled trials comparing calcium channel blockers and nitrates have been performed. Kocher et al.[49] randomized 61 patients with chronic anal fissures to receive 0.2% GTN or 2% DTZ. After 6–8 weeks of treatment, therapeutic efficacy was similar between both groups but patients in the GTN group experienced far more side effects. Bielecki and Kolodziejczak[50] also found equal healing rates between topical 0.2% GTN and 2% DTZ, as well as fewer headaches with 2% DTZ. Yet in another randomized trial, side effects of GTN and DTZ were comparable.[51] Ezri and Susmallian[52] noted improved healing with nifedipine (89%) as compared to GTN (58%) with far more side effects in the GTN (40%) group as compared to nifedipine (5%) and no differences in recurrence. Given these results, many authors have concluded that calcium channel blockers should be considered the preferred first-line treatment because of fewer side effects as compared to GTN.[49,53]

Topical calcium channel blockers have also been compared to surgical sphincterotomy. In one randomized trial, no significant difference in fissure healing was noted in patients treated with topical nifedipine (97%) as compared to LIS

(100%).[54] More side effects and relapses were identified in the nifedipine group, whereas no one in the sphincterotomy group relapsed.[54] In a similar study from Singapore, less convincing results for topical nifedipine were described. Ho found improvements in pain relief, patient satisfaction, and healing rates in patients randomized to internal sphincterotomy as compared to topical nifedipine.[55] In addition, the investigators indicated that there were substantial problems with compliance in the nifedipine group related to side effects and slow healing.[55]

It has become clear to this author that the use of pharmaceutical adjuncts is often based on preferences, but it should be remembered that many of the topical preparations are only available through compounding pharmacies. For this reason, a clinician should become familiar with the pharmaceutical resources available prior to becoming dependent on one medical treatment or another.

Adrenergic Antagonists

The effect of alpha-1 adrenergic blockade on anal sphincter pressure has been studied in two prospective trials. Pitt et al.[56,57] administered 20 mg of indoramin, an alpha-1 blocker, to seven patients with chronic anal fissure and six healthy controls. Reduction in anal pressure was observed in both groups: 35.8% in patients with fissure and 39.9% in those without. In a placebo-controlled trial, 23 patients with chronic anal fissure were randomized to receive 20 mg indoramin or placebo twice daily.[57] Although a 29.8% reduction in maximum anal resting pressure was observed 1 h after active treatment, healing occurred in only one patient (7%), despite 6 weeks of therapy. In the placebo group, 22% of patients achieved healing, although no significant change in anal pressure was observed, the trial was not completed due to lack of efficacy.

Cholinergic Agonists

Carapeti et al.[58] documented reduced anal sphincter pressure using bethanechol in a dose-finding study. The authors demonstrated a 24% reduction in maximal anal resting pressure with a dose of 0.1% of bethanechol. In a subsequent study, they reported fissure healing in 9 of 15 patients treated with 0.1% bethanechol gel three times daily.[42] Maximum resting sphincter pressure was significantly lower after treatment compared with pretreatment values with no side effects.

Phosphodiesterase Inhibitors

Early work by Jones et al.[59] has demonstrated an in vitro effect of increasing concentrations of various phosphodiesterase inhibitors on internal sphincter tone. In a study of 19 consecutive patients with anal fissures, topical administration of a phosphodiesterase-5 inhibitor (sildenafil) significantly reduced anal sphincter pressure in patients with chronic anal fissure. The beneficial effect of sildenafil may not have derived solely from the nitric oxide donor but rather the phosphodiesterase-5 inhibitor. This agent may spark future clinical trials in the treatment of anal fissure.[60]

Botulinum Toxin

Botulinum toxin (BT) is an exotoxin produced by the bacterium *Clostridium botulinum*. When injected locally, BT binds to the presynaptic nerve terminal at the neuromuscular junction, thereby preventing release of acetylcholine and resulting in temporary muscle paralysis. Its mechanism of action on the IAS has been extensively studied in animal studies. In a series of experiments, Jones et al.[61] injected BT into porcine anal sphincters, which responded with decreased mean anal resting pressure following manometric analyses. Strips of sphincter muscle were then isolated and examined in vitro. Application of electrical field stimulation and nicotinic agonists resulted in increased myogenic tone, which was blocked by guanethidine and attenuated by BT injection. These findings suggested that the predominant effect of BT on the IAS is sympathetic blockade.

BT injections can be given easily, on an outpatient basis, and are well tolerated. The commercial availability of BT has prompted several prospective trials examining its efficacy in the treatment of anal fissure (Table 12-2). One placebo-controlled trial randomized 30 patients to receive either two injections of 20 U BT or saline.[62] After 2 months, complete healing occurred in 73% of patients receiving BT and 13% of patients receiving placebo; no recurrences were observed during initial follow-up. In another clinical trial comparing BT with lidocaine in the treatment of anal fissure, Colak et al.[64] demonstrated superiority of BT, with complete fissure epithelialization in 71% of patients in the BT group vs. 21% in the lidocaine group.

The dosing and injection site for BT has also been examined in several trials. In a randomized, double-blind trial of chronic anal fissure treatment, Siproudhis et al.[66] reported that a single 20 U injection of BT was not superior to that of placebo. In a dose-finding study, Brisinda et al.[65] randomized 150 patients to initial treatment with 20 U BT followed by 30 U BT for fissure persistence, or initial treatment with 30 U BT followed by 50 U BT for persistence. One month after BT injections, greater success was noted with higher doses, with little increase in complications or side effects, which is probably related to the diffusion of the toxin to the external sphincter.[65] In addition to dosing, injection site has also been studied. Injection on each side of the anterior midline lowered resting anal pressure to a greater degree and produced an earlier healing scar than compared to BT injection on each side of the posterior midline.[73] The use of BT injections for GTN treatment failures has also been evaluated in prospective trials by Madalinski et al.[74] and Lindsey et al.[75] Both studies concluded that BT injection is an excellent second-line agent in the treatment of chronic anal fissures. Given these data, it

TABLE 12-2. Prospective botulinum toxin trials

Year	Author	*n*	Treatment	Follow-up	Success (%)	Side effects
1998	Maria et al.[62]	30	BT 20 U (2 doses)	2 months	73.3	
			Saline		13.3[a]	
1999	Brisinda et al.[63]	50	BT 20 U (2 doses)	2 months	96	20% headaches
			0.2% NTG		60[a]	
2002	Colak et al.[64]	62	BT	2 months	70.6	
			Lidocaine		21.4[a]	
2002	Brisinda et al.[65]	150	BT 20 U, 30 U	2 months	89	
			BT 30 U, 50 U		96 (NC)	
2003	Siproudhis et al.[66]	44	BT 20 U (1 dose)	4 weeks	22.7	
			Saline		22.7[b]	
2003	Mentes et al.[67]	101	BT 0.3 U/kg	12 months	75.4	16% incontinence
			LIS		94[a]	
2005	Arroyo et al.[68]	80	BT 25 U	12 months	45	5% incontinence
			LIS		92.5[a]	
2005	Iswariah et al.[69]	38	BT 20 U (2 doses)	26 weeks	41	
			LIS		91[a]	
2006	De Nardi et al.[70]	30	BT 30 U	36 months	40	20% headaches
			0.2% GTN		33.3[b]	
2006	Fruehauf et al.[71]	50	BT 30 U	2 weeks	24	48% headaches
			0.2% NTG		52[a]	
2007	Brisinda et al.[72]	100	0.2% GTN	2 months	70	34% headaches
			BT 30 U		92[a]	6% incontinence

BT botulinum toxin, *U* units, *LIS* lateral internal sphincterotomy, *NC* no comparison performed.
[a] Statistically significant comparison.
[b] Not statistically significant comparison.

is the authors practice to inject 20 U of BT on either side of the anterior midline in the intersphincteric groove.

The efficacy of a single injection of BT has been directly compared to topical agents. In a prospective, randomized trial, Brisinda et al.[63] directly compared BT injection and topical NTG as first-line agents in the treatment of chronic anal fissure. BT injections (20 U) were given on each side of the IAS and 0.2% NTG ointment was applied twice daily. Fissures healed in 96% of the patients in the BT group and 60% of the patients in the NTG group with more side effects in the NTG group.[63] A follow-up to this study by the same authors revealed similar findings.[72] Others have used a single dose of 30 U BT and compared it to topical 0.2% NTG twice a day and found nitroglycerin ointment to be superior to the more expensive and invasive botulinum toxin injections for initial healing of chronic fissures.[71] De Nardi et al.[70] performed a similar analysis but used 20 U BT on either side of the anterior midline with dismal healing results for both BT and NTG, 40 and 33%, respectively.

There have been several prospective, randomized trials comparing BT to LIS in the treatment of chronic anal fissures. Mentes et al.[67] reported the results of 61 patients receiving a total of 0.3 U/kg BT in two divided doses and 50 patients who underwent sphincterotomy. By 2 months, healing rates were 74% in the BT group and 98% in the LIS group. By 12 months, however, fissures recurred in seven patients in the BT group leading to an overall healing rate of 75% which was significantly lower than the LIS group. Anal incontinence, predominantly to flatus, was reported in 16% of patients in the LIS group while no side effects were observed with BT. Similarly, Iswariah et al.[69] randomized 38 patients with anal fissures to either BT or sphincterotomy and found significantly higher 2-week pain scores, reoperation rates, and poorer healing in the BT group. In another randomized trial, Arroyo et al.[68] concluded that surgical sphincterotomy should be the first therapeutic approach for anal fissure as compared to BT.

Late recurrence rates 42 months after BT treatment of chronic anal fissures have been reported in a prospective trial by Minguez et al.[76] Patients with complete healing at 6 months after BT were reassessed at 6 month intervals with fissure recurrence demonstrated in 41.5% of patients. Stratification by various clinical parameters revealed that higher risk of recurrence was associated with anterior location, chronicity of disease (longer than 12 months), and multiple injections. They comment that lack of recurrences cited in earlier reports by Maria et al.[62] and Brisinda et al.[63] may be due to strict exclusion criteria.

Many of the studies of BT therapy for anal fissure have focused solely on short-term outcomes such as acute fissure healing. However, as stated above, recurrences are likely common. Some investigators believe that patients with fissure recurrence after one BT injection may experience some improvement in their symptoms with repeated BT injections. In the study by Maria et al.[62], repeated BT injections in four patients with recurrent fissures using 25 U of BT led to healing in all patients. In addition to high recurrence rates with BT, associated complications have been historically minimal. Injections of BT have led to perianal hematomas in 20% of patients treated by Tilney et al.[77] and rare cases of perianal thrombosis in a study by Jost et al.[78] although thrombosis was not reported in a later study by this same author.[79] Most recently, the US Food and Drug Administration (FDA) issued a warning regarding a small number of adverse reactions to BT injections, including respiratory failure and death.[80] In early communications, the agency indicated that these serious reactions to BT injections may have been related to overdosing.[80]

Operative Treatment

The primary goal in the treatment of a nonhealing anal fissure is to decrease abnormally elevated resting anal tone. Operative procedures, such as manual anal dilatation or internal sphincterotomy, have been described as initial modes of treatment because they produce permanent reductions in maximum resting anal pressures.

Anal Dilatation

Manual dilatation of the anus for anal fissure was first reported in 1964.[81] A variety of means to enlarge the anal canal have been described including the use of four fingers and an assortment of dilation instruments. Inconsistencies with regard to technique, specifically extent and duration of sphincter stretch, have cast some doubt about true success rates of dilatation procedures. Yet, reports of anal dilatation continue to surface and recommend its use as the "first management choice in the treatment of anal fissure."[82–85] Given the controversy regarding standardization of the technique, Sohn et al.[86] standardized the anal dilatation procedure with either a Parks' retractor opened to 4.8 cm or a pneumatic balloon inflated to 40 mm and found fissure healing in up to 94%. A more recent study used pneumatic balloon dilatation in the management of chronic anal fissure and found this technique to be effective and safe without producing endosonographically detectable sphincter damage.[87]

Despite few studies describing the benefits of anal dilatation on anal fissure, long-term outcomes of anal dilatation are rare. Additional widespread criticism of the technique stems from reported complications of incontinence, secondary to diffuse sphincter damage. In a retrospective analysis of anal dilatation for anal fissure by MacDonald et al.,[84] not only was dilatation unsuccessful in 56% of patients but incontinence occurred in 27% of patients overall. Speakman et al.[88] performed endoanal ultrasound and anorectal physiology studies on 12 men with fecal incontinence after anal dilatation and found internal and external anal sphincter defects in 11 and 3 patients, respectively. Sphincter defects after anal dilatation were also recognized by Nielsen et al.[89], who reported minor incontinence in 12.5% of patients overall.

Comparisons between sphincterotomy and medical measures, combined with anal dilatation, have also been reported. In one retrospective review, questionnaires were sent to 160 patients who underwent either anal dilatation or LIS. Fewer fissure recurrences or reports of incontinence were reported in patients treated by sphincterotomy.[90] Other prospective, randomized trials did not support these findings.[91–94] In some studies, recurrence and incontinence rates were equal between groups[91,93,94]; in another, significantly worse after LIS.[92] Four months after randomization in a trial by Marby et al.[92], symptomatic improvement was reported in 93% after dilatation vs. 78% after sphincterotomy. During the same time period, recurrence rates were 10% after dilatation and 29% following sphincterotomy. Most recently, randomized trials have demonstrated superior functional results, in terms of incontinence, after LIS.[95] While recurrence rates were 3.5–10% up to 1 year after LIS, higher rates of 26–30% were observed after anal dilatation.[93,96] Although anal dilatation is still performed by some centers, clinical practices across North America no longer commonly use this technique as a primary treatment for anal fissure.

Fissurectomy

Excision of the fissure with or without sphincterotomy has been proposed as a good therapeutic approach to anal fissure. Given that the etiology of anal fissures is thought to be secondary to inadequate blood flow and spasm, one would venture to guess that this approach is unlikely to be useful. In one clinical trial by Mousavi et al.[97], fissurectomy was considered inferior to LIS, which was associated with fewer complications.

Lateral Internal Sphincterotomy

The American Society of Colon and Rectal Surgeons (ASCRS) practice parameters for the management of anal fissures recommends LIS as the surgical treatment of choice for refractory anal fissures.[98] Internal sphincterotomy was first introduced by Eisenhammer[99] in the early 1950s, but his initial approach through the bed of the fissure in the posterior midline often resulted in a scarred groove, or "keyhole deformity." The functional impairment which evolved included gas and/or stool incontinence. Subsequently, LIS emerged as an alternative and was believed to be associated with less functional impairment.[100]

LIS can be performed with an open or closed technique (Figures 12-3 and 12-4). The open technique is performed with a small incision over the intersphincteric groove and direct division of the internal sphincter with electrocautery or other instrument. The closed technique is performed by placing a small scalpel such as a beaver blade into the intersphincteric groove and carefully dividing the internal sphincter. Although the blade can be placed into the submucosal space and then rotated toward the internal sphincter, most

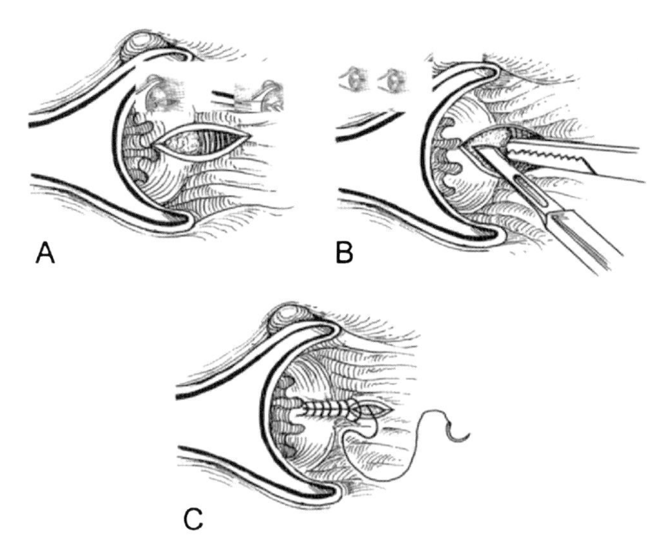

FIGURE 12-3. Open lateral internal sphincterotomy. **A** Radial skin incision distal to the dentate line exposing the intersphincteric groove. **B** Elevation and division of the internal sphincter. **C** Primary wound closure.

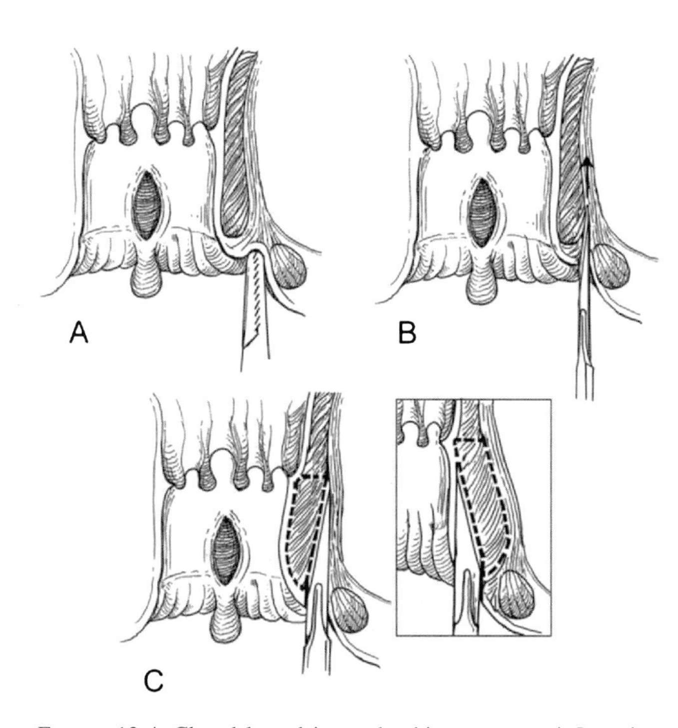

FIGURE 12-4. Closed lateral internal sphincterotomy. **A** Location of the intersphincteric groove. **B** Insertion of the knife blade in the intersphincteric plane. **C** Lateral to medial division of the internal anal sphincter (*inset*: medial to lateral division of the muscle).

find that placing the knife in the intersphincteric groove preferable. Several retrospective studies support the use of LIS as the preferred operative method for the treatment of anal fissures, whether open or closed (Table 12-3).[101,104,107,110,115,117,121] Although there was no significant difference in *acute* complications in one randomized study of open vs. closed LIS, long-term persistent complications were more frequent in the open (55%) than the closed (20%) sphincterotomy group.[109] Similarly, the degree of continence following open vs. closed sphincterotomy was assessed by questionnaire and favored closed LIS.[116]

Persistent incontinence to gas and stool has emerged as a major concern following sphincterotomy. Incontinence rates of up to 36% have been reported, but these vary widely among studies.[109,111,112,116,119] Much of this variation can be attributed to differences in definition and assiduousness of follow-up. Reasons for incontinence after LIS have been related to the type and extent of sphincter muscle divided. Sultan et al.[122] prospectively performed endoanal ultrasonography prior to and 2 months after sphincterotomy in 15 patients. The authors found more complete sphincter deficits in women than men due to the lack of appreciation for shorter anal canals in this population and suggested that post sphincterotomy incontinence may be further lessened if external anal sphincter deficits are recognized preoperatively.

Littlejohn and Newstead[118] reported a retrospective review of 287 patients who underwent tailored sphincterotomy, division of the IAS for the length of the fissure, rather than to the dentate line. There were no reports of incontinence to liquid or solid stool in either group. In another study that sought to identify fecal incontinence related to chronic anal fissure before and after LIS and its relationship to the extent of IAS division, Elsebae[123] concluded that a mild degree of fecal incontinence may be related to the underlying pathology rather than the sphincterotomy. In addition, troublesome fecal incontinence after LIS is uncommon but much more common when sphincterotomy is performed up to the dentate line rather than up to the fissure apex. It is the authors' practice to limit the extent of sphincterotomy to include solely the length of the fissure.

In addition to the length of the sphincterotomy, other technical issues should be considered. Excision of hypertrophied anal papillae and fibrous anal polyps has been advocated by Gupta and Kalaskar.[124] In a randomized trial, patient satisfaction was rated as excellent or good after removal of these structures in 84% of patients, compared to 58% of patients whose papillae were left in vivo. In a separate prospective study, earlier wound healing rates were achieved with primary closure after open LIS as compared to healing by secondary intention.[125] Last, in patients who return with fissure recurrence after sphincterotomy, it should be understood that improper division of the IAS significantly alters fissure healing. In a study by Farouk et al.[126], ultrasound evaluations performed in patients with persistent fissures after sphincterotomy demonstrated a lack of internal sphincter division in almost 70% of patients.

Advancement Flaps

Endorectal advancement flaps have also been employed in the treatment of anal fissure. One prospective trial randomized patients with anal fissure to either LIS or advancement flap

Table 12-3. Results of lateral internal sphincterotomy

Year	Author	n	Success (%)	Recurrence (%)	Incontinence (%)[a]	Follow-up (months)
1980	Abcarian[101]	150	100	1.3	0	NS
1981	Keighley et al.[102]	71	100	25	2	12
1982	Ravikumar et al.[103]	60	97	0	5	24
1984	Hsu and MacKeigan[104]	89	100	5.6	0	NS
1984	Jensen et al.[96]	30	100	3	0	18
1985	Walker et al.[105]	306	100	0	15	52
1987	Gingold[106]	86	100	3.5	0	24
1987	Weaver et al.[91]	39	93	5.1	2.5	17
1988	Lewis et al.[107]	350	94	6	6	37
1988	Zinkin[108]	151	94.7	NS	NS	0
1989	Khubchandani and Reed[109]	717	97.7	NS	35.1	52.9
1992	Kortbeek et al.[110]	112	95.5	NS	NS	1.5
1994	Pernikoff et al.[111]	500	99	2	16	78
1994	Romano et al.[112]	44	100	0	9	8
1995	Leong and Seow-Choen[113]	20	100	NS	0	6.5
1995	Prohm and Bonner[114]	177	96	3.3	1.6	1.5
1995	Usatoff and Polglase[115]	98	90	20	18	41
1996	Garcia-Aguilar et al.[116]	864	96	11	37.8	63.5
1997	Hananel and Gordon[117]	312	98.6	1.4[b]	–	NS
1997	Littlejohn and Newstead[118]	352	99.7	1.4	1.4	9
1999	Nyam and Pemberton[119]	585	96	8	15	72
2004	Wiley et al.[120]	76	96	NS	6.8	12
2004	Parellada[35]	27	100	NS	15	2.5
2005	Arroyo et al.[68]	40	92.5	NS	5	36
2005	Iswariah et al.[69]	21	91	NS	NS	6
2007	Brown et al.[30]	24	NS	0	NS	79

NS not stated.
[a] Includes seepage and incontinence to flatus and stool.
[b] Recurrence and persistence combined.

and found no significant difference in healing rates (100% in the sphincterotomy group vs. 85% in the flap group).[113] Incontinence was not observed in either group. The authors concluded that anal advancement flap is an alternative to LIS for chronic anal fissure. The advancement flap procedure may be particularly useful in those patients with low-pressure fissures but more data is needed before it can be recommended in the patient with traditional spasm-related anal fissure.

Summary of Treatment Options

Treatment options for anal fissures are varied and unfortunately the data presented above are difficult to summarize into a cogent management algorithm. In addition to clinical experience, the clinician can utilize the findings of systematic reviews in making decisions regarding care. In the most recent systematic review of medical options and surgical sphincterotomy, Nelson[127] found that GTN was significantly better than placebo in healing anal fissures but late recurrences were common. Botulinum toxin and calcium channel blockers were equivalent to GTN in efficacy with fewer adverse events. Nelson[127] concluded that no medical therapy came close to the efficacy of surgical sphincterotomy, although a low risk of incontinence must be considered with surgery. Nelson[128] also reviewed the results for all surgical procedures used to treat anal fissures and concluded that anal stretch and posterior midline internal sphincterotomy should probably be abandoned, while open and closed partial LIS appear to be equally efficacious. Given these data, it is our practice to step up treatment from topical agents to injectables or surgical sphincterotomy depending on the patients' potential risk for future incontinence. In women who have had children or are planning on having children, it is the authors' preference to maximize nonsurgical options prior to resorting to surgical sphincterotomy.

Atypical Fissures

The majority of anal fissures have classic signs and symptoms and respond well to LIS. However, there are groups of patients who have fissures identified at the time of anorectal examination for rectal bleeding but deny pain or complain of incontinence yet have obvious signs of anal fissure. Incontinent patients with evidence of anal fissure are generally identified as having low-pressure fissures and they are often postpartum.[129] In a prospective study of 209 primigravid women who underwent anal manometry both pre and postpartum, 9% went on to develop fissures after birth.[130] Interestingly, in those patients who developed fissures, manometric measurements were similar both before and after birth. The authors concluded that, "surgical interference with the anal sphincter mechanism should be avoided," in patients with low-pressure fissures.[130]

It remains unclear as to optimal therapy for low-pressure fissures. A trial of conservative management should be initiated. If unsuccessful, some have advocated the advancement of healthy tissue over the fissure in the form of an island flap or a sliding endoanal advancement flap. In one study, island flaps were advanced into the anal canal leading to fissure healing in all patients and no postoperative incontinence.[131] The authors concluded that island advancement flaps may prove particularly useful for low-pressure fissures or in those patients who may be poor candidates for sphincterotomy. In addition, there are advocates of silver nitrate application to the low-pressure fissure bed, but little evidence exists to substantiate this approach.

Crohn's Disease

Patients with Crohn's disease often present with anorectal manifestations of their disease including asymptomatic or bleeding, deep, anal fissures among other disease pathology. Anal fissures complicating Crohn's most commonly follow the same pathophysiology of benign idiopathic fissures, but persistent nonhealing fissures can evolve into fistulae or perianal abscess.[132] Findings of multiple fissures, nonhealing fissures, and asymptomatic fissures should raise the index of suspicion for Crohn's disease. Large edematous and tender skin tags are also very common in Crohn's disease. In those patients in whom Crohn's disease is suspected based on anorectal examination, thorough evaluation with endoscopy and imaging is recommended.

In a review of 306 patients with Crohn's disease, anal pathology leading to symptoms was identified in 42.4% of patients.[133] The commonest presentations were perianal abscess (29.5%), anal fissure (27.6%), and low anal fistula (26.7%).[133] In another analysis of Crohn's patients treated surgically for perianal complaints, 31.8% had evidence of anal fissure.[134] In a study from the Lahey Clinic, 84% of patients with Crohn's fissures were found to be symptomatic while one-third had multiple fissures.[132] This series documented that unhealed fissures frequently progress to more ominous anal pathology, yet this finding may be related to more virulent disease in this patient population.[132]

As indicated, anorectal surgery has traditionally been contraindicated in patients with Crohn's disease. Concerns of postoperative incontinence, nonhealing wounds, and eventual proctectomy led many to avoid surgery in patients with Crohn's disease. Thus, most clinicians have advocated medical management of Crohn's fissures with a focus on reducing diarrhea, bulking the stool, and comfort measures. This regimen led to healing in 61% of patients treated medically for Crohn's fissures.[135] However, if medical management fails, an exam under anesthesia is indicated to rule out the presence of other pathology. Although, data to support the use of BT for Crohn's fissures is not available, the authors have had limited success with this approach.

Surgical outcomes following sphincterotomy for Crohn's fissures are limited to case series. Surgery for Crohn's fissures was successful in a small study published by Wolkomir et al.[136] as very few patients went on to require proctectomy. At the Lahey Clinic, patients with Crohn's fissures were more likely to report successful healing after partial internal sphincterotomy as compared to medical treatment.[132] Others have reported limited success with anal dilatation for Crohn's fissures,[82] while Allan and Keighley[137] reported the development of incontinence in one patient treated with dilatation. The authors' approach in the patient with a Crohn's fissure has been to try to control the underlying disease with medical management prior to resorting to permanent surgical therapy with LIS.

Human Immunodeficiency Virus

The patient with HIV and anorectal pain often presents with challenging pathology leading to a long differential diagnosis. However, the presence of severe pain should alert the clinician to the potential for fissures or ulcers of the anal canal. Often these findings are mistakenly interchanged, but it is important to understand the distinction between HIV-associated fissures as compared to ulcerating diseases of the anus. Classic anal fissures are common in the HIV patient as in non-HIV patients and are readily identifiable by the typical fissure appearance. Conversely, anorectal ulcers in the HIV patient are deep and boring with a broad base which may be located anywhere in the anus.[138,139] Patients with HIV and classic fissures can be treated with the same modalities that are used in non-HIV patients. In fact, early case reports of wound complications and incontinence after surgical sphincterotomy for fissures likely included a heterogeneous patient population that included patients with HIV-associated anorectal ulcers.[139] In one case series of HIV-associated anal fissures, symptomatic improvement was noted in 92% of patients treated with surgical sphincterotomy.[138] In addition, although theoretically safe, there is little data regarding the risks and benefits of BT on HIV-associated fissures. The introduction of highly active antiretroviral therapy has led some to speculate that the prevalence and distribution of HIV-associated anorectal pathology has changed considerably; however, this theory was not proven in a review at the University of Southern California HIV clinic.[140]

Conclusions

The astute clinician can often make the diagnosis of anal fissure based on a simple history and classic appearance of fissure without inflicting unnecessary pain from examination. Trauma is thought to predispose the development of anal fissures, but elevated sphincter pressure and reduced blood flow are likely to play a role in the pathogenesis. Traditionally, the standard therapeutic approach to anal fissures included oral fiber, sitz baths, and analgesics. At this time, a number of medical treatment options are available including nonoperative care, topical nitrates, topical or oral calcium channel blockers, and injections of BT. Unfortunately, medical care has had pedestrian results as the most recent Cochrane review concluded that medical therapy for anal fissures is only marginally better than placebo and for chronic fissures far less effective than surgery.[127] Despite the mixed results with medical therapy, it is our practice to trial these medical measures unless the patient is extremely uncomfortable.

References

1. Nelson RL, Abcarian H, Davis FG, Persky V. Prevalence of benign anorectal disease in a randomly selected population. Dis Colon Rectum. 1995;38(4):341–4.
2. Hananel N, Gordon PH. Re-examination of clinical manifestations and response to therapy of fissure-in-ano. Dis Colon Rectum. 1997;4:229–33.
3. Hancock BD. The internal sphincter and anal fissure. Br J Surg. 1977;64(2):92–5.
4. Nothmann BJ, Schuster MM. Internal anal sphincter derangement with anal fissures. Gastroenterology. 1974;67(2):216–20.
5. Farouk R, Duthie GS, MacGregor AB, Bartolo DC. Sustained internal sphincter hypertonia in patients with chronic anal fissure. Dis Colon Rectum. 1994;37(5):424–9.
6. Gibbons CP, Read NW. Anal hypertonia in fissures: cause or effect? Br J Surg. 1986;73:443–5.
7. Klosterhalfen B, Vogel P, Rixen H, Mittermayer C. Topography of the inferior rectal artery: a possible cause of chronic, primary anal fissure. Dis Colon Rectum. 1989;32(1): 43–52.
8. Schouten WR, Briel JW, Auwerda JJ, De Graaf EJ. Ischaemic nature of anal fissure. Br J Surg. 1996;83(1):63–5.
9. Shub HA, Salvati EP, Rubin RJ. Conservative treatment of anal fissure: an unselected, retrospective and continuous study. Dis Colon Rectum. 1978;21:582–3.
10. Jensen SL. Treatment of first episodes of acute anal fissure: prospective randomised study of lignocaine ointment versus hydrocortisone ointment or warm sitz baths plus bran. Br Med J (Clin Res Ed). 1986;292(6529):1167–9.
11. Jensen SL. Maintenance therapy with unprocessed bran in the prevention of acute anal fissure recurrence. J R Soc Med. 1987;80(5):296–8.
12. Lindsey I, Jones OM, Cunningham C, Mortensen NJ. Chronic anal fissure. Br J Surg. 2004;91(3):270–9.
13. Nelson R. A systematic review of medical therapy for anal fissure. Dis Colon Rectum. 2004;47(4):422–31.
14. Loder PB, Kamm MA, Nicholls RJ, Phillips RK. "Reversible chemical sphincterotomy" by local application of glyceryl trinitrate. Br J Surg. 1994;81:1386–9.
15. Guillemot F, Leroi H, Lone YC, Rousseau CG, Lamblin MD, Cortot A. Action of in situ nitroglycerin on upper anal canal pressure of patients with terminal gconstipation. A pilot study. Dis Colon Rectum. 1993;36:372–6.
16. Lund JN, Scholefield JH. A randomised, prospective, double-blind, placebo-controlled trial of glyceryl trinitrate ointment in treatment of anal fissure [see comments]. Lancet. 1997;349(9044):11–4 [published erratum appears in Lancet 1997 Mar 1;349(9052):656].
17. Oettle GJ. Glyceryl trinitrate vs. sphincterotomy for treatment of chronic fissure-in-ano: a randomized, controlled trial. Dis Colon Rectum. 1997;40:1318–20.
18. Bacher H, Mischinger HJ, Werkgartner G, et al. Local nitroglycerin for treatment of anal fissures: an alternative to lateral sphincterotomy? Dis Colon Rectum. 1997;40(7):840–5.
19. Kennedy ML, Sowter S, Nguyen H, Lubowski DZ. Glyceryl trinitrate ointment for the treatment of chronic anal fissure: results of a placebo-controlled trial and long-term follow-up. Dis Colon Rectum. 1999;42(8):1000–6.
20. Carapeti EA, Kamm MA, McDonald PJ, Chadwick SJ, Melville D, Phillips RK. Randomised controlled trial shows that glyceryl trinitrate heals anal fissures, higher doses are not more effective, and there is a high recurrence rate. Gut. 1999;44(5):727–30.
21. Altomare DF, Rinaldi M, Milito G, et al. Glyceryl trinitrate for chronic anal fissure – healing or headache? Results of a multicenter, randomized, placebo-controlled, double-blind trial. Dis Colon Rectum. 2000;43(2):174–9.
22. Zuberi BF, Rajput MR, Abro H, Shaikh SA. A randomized trial of glyceryl trinitrate ointment and nitroglycerin patch in healing of anal fissures. Int J Colorectal Dis. 2000;15:243–5.
23. Richard CS, Gregoire R, Plewes EA, et al. Internal sphincterotomy is superior to topical nitroglycerin in the treatment of chronic anal fissure: results of a randomized, controlled trial by the Canadian Colorectal Surgical Trials Group. Dis Colon Rectum. 2000;43(8):1048–57.
24. Evans J, Luck A, Hewett P. Glyceryl trinitrate vs. lateral sphincterotomy for chronic anal fissure: prospective, randomized trial. Dis Colon Rectum. 2001;44:93–7.
25. Chaudhuri S, Pal AK, Acharya A, et al. Treatment of chronic anal fissure with topical glyceryl trinitrate: a double-blind, placebo-controlled trial. Indian J Gastroenterol. 2001;20(3):101–2.
26. Libertiny G, Knight JS, Farouk R. Randomised trial of topical 0.2% glyceryl trinitrate and lateral internal sphincterotomy for the treatment of patients with chronic anal fissure: long-term follow-up. Eur J Surg. 2002;168:418–21.
27. Bailey HR, Beck DE, Billingham RP, et al. A study to determine the nitroglycerin ointment dose and dosing interval that best promote the healing of chronic anal fissures. Dis Colon Rectum. 2002;45:1192–9.
28. Scholefield JH, Bock JU, Marla B, et al. A dose finding study with 0.1%, 0.2%, and 0.4% glyceryl trinitrate ointment in patients with chronic anal fissures. Gut. 2003;52:264–9.
29. Mishra R, Thomas S, Maan MS, Hadke NS. Topical nitroglycerin versus lateral internal sphincterotomy for chronic

anal fissure: prospective, randomized trial. ANZ J Surg. 2005;75(12):1032–5.
30. Brown CJ, Dubreuil D, Santoro L, Liu M, O'Connor BI, McLeod RS. Lateral internal sphincterotomy is superior to topical nitroglycerin for healing chronic anal fissure and does not compromise long-term fecal continence: six-year follow-up of a multicenter, randomized, controlled trial. Dis Colon Rectum. 2007;50(4):442–8.
31. Schouten WR, Briel JW, Boerma MO, Auwerda JJ, Wilms EB, Graatsma BH. Pathophysiological aspects and clinical outcome of intra-anal application of isosorbide dinitrate in patients with chronic anal fissure. Gut. 1996;39:465–9.
32. Werre AJ, Palamba HW, Bilgen EJ, Eggink WF. Isosorbide dinitrate in the treatment of anal fissure: a randomised, prospective, double blind, placebo-controlled trial. Eur J Surg. 2001;167:382–5.
33. Tankova L, Yoncheva K, Muhtarov M, Kadyan H, Draganov V. Topical mononitrate treatment in patients with anal fissure. Aliment Pharmacol Ther. 2002;16:101–3.
34. Lysy J, Israelit-Yatzkan Y, Sestiere-Ittah M, Keret D, Goldin E. Treatment of chronic anal fissure with isosorbide dinitrate: long-term results and dose determination. Dis Colon Rectum. 1998;41:1406–10.
35. Parellada C. Randomized prospective trial comparing 0.2 percent isosorbide dinitrate ointment with sphincterotomy in treatment of chronic anal fissure: a two-year follow-up. Dis Colon Rectum. 2004;47(4):437–43.
36. Hechtman HB, Barlow C. Moderation of anal sphincter tone with nitric oxide agonists and antagonists. Arch Surg. 1996;131(7):775–84.
37. Griffin N, Zimmerman DD, Briel JW, et al. Topical L-arginine gel lowers resting anal pressure: possible treatment for anal fissure. Dis Colon Rectum. 2002;45:1332–6.
38. Gosselink MP, Darby M, Zimmerman DD, Gruss HJ, Schouten WR. Treatment of chronic anal fissure by application of L-arginine gel: a phase II study in 15 patients. Dis Colon Rectum. 2005;48(4):832–7.
39. Dorfman G, Levitt M, Platell C. Treatment of chronic anal fissure with topical glyceryl trinitrate. Dis Colon Rectum. 1999;42:1007–10.
40. Graziano A, Svidler Lopez L, Lencinas S, Masciangioli G, Gualdrini U, Bisisio O. Long-term results of topical nitroglycerin in the treatment of chronic anal fissures are disappointing. Tech Coloproctol. 2001;5:143–7.
41. Chrysos E, Xynos E, Tzovaras G, Zoras OJ, Tsiaoussis J, Vassilakis SJ. Effect of nifedipine on rectoanal motility. Dis Colon Rectum. 1996;39:212–6.
42. Carapeti EA, Kamm MA, Phillips RK. Topical diltiazem and bethanechol decrease anal sphincter pressure and heal anal fissures without side effects. Dis Colon Rectum. 2000;43:1359–62.
43. Knight JS, Birks M, Farouk R. Topical diltiazem ointment in the treatment of chronic anal fissure. Br J Surg. 2001;88:553–6.
44. Agaoglu N, Cengiz S, Arslan MK, Turkyilmaz S. Oral nifedipine in the treatment of chronic anal fissure. Dig Surg. 2003;20:452–6.
45. Ansaloni L, Bernabe A, Ghetti R, Riccardi R, Tranchino RM, Gardini G. Oral lacidipine in the treatment of anal fissure. Tech Coloproctol. 2002;6:79–82.
46. Antropoli C, Perrotti P, Rubino M, et al. Nifedipine for local use in conservative treatment of anal fissures: preliminary results of a multicenter study. Dis Colon Rectum. 1999;42(8):1011–5.
47. Perrotti P, Bove A, Antropoli C, et al. Topical nifedipine with lidocaine ointment vs. active control for treatment of chronic anal fissure: results of a prospective, randomized, double-blind study. Dis Colon Rectum. 2002;45:1468–75.
48. Jonas M, Neal KR, Abercrombie JF, Scholefield JH. A randomized trial of oral vs. topical diltiazem for chronic anal fissures. Dis Colon Rectum. 2001;44:1074–8.
49. Kocher HM, Steward M, Leather AJ, Cullen PT. Randomized clinical trial assessing the side-effects of glyceryl trinitrate and diltiazem hydrochloride in the treatment of chronic anal fissure. Br J Surg. 2002;89:413–7.
50. Bielecki K, Kolodziejczak M. A prospective randomized trial of diltiazem and glyceryltrinitrate ointment in the treatment of chronic anal fissure. Colorectal Dis. 2003;5:256–7.
51. Mustafa NA, Cengiz S, Türkyilmaz S, Yücel Y. Comparison of topical glyceryl trinitrate ointment and oral nifedipine in the treatment of chronic anal fissure. Acta Chir Belg. 2006;106(1):55–8.
52. Ezri T, Susmallian S. Topical nifedipine vs. topical glyceryl trinitrate for treatment of chronic anal fissure. Dis Colon Rectum. 2003;46:805–8.
53. Shrivastava UK, Jain BK, Kumar P, Saifee Y. A comparison of the effects of diltiazem and glyceryl trinitrate ointment in the treatment of chronic anal fissure: a randomized clinical trial. Surg Today. 2007;37(6):482–5.
54. Katsinelos P, Papaziogas B, Koutelidakis I, Paroutoglou G, Dimiropoulos S, Souparis A, et al. Topical 0.5% nifedipine vs. lateral internal sphincterotomy for the treatment of chronic anal fissure: long-term follow-up. Int J Colorectal Dis. 2006;21(2):179–83.
55. Ho KS, Ho YH. Randomized clinical trial comparing oral nifedipine with lateral anal sphincterotomy and tailored sphincterotomy in the treatment of chronic anal fissure. Br J Surg. 2005;92(4):403–8.
56. Pitt J, Dawson PM, Hallan RI, Boulos PB. A double-blind randomized placebo-controlled trial of oral indoramin to treat chronic anal fissure. Colorectal Dis. 2001;3:165–8.
57. Pitt J, Craggs MM, Henry MM, Boulos PB. Alpha-1 adrenoceptor blockade: potential new treatment for anal fissures. Dis Colon Rectum. 2000;43:800–3.
58. Carapeti EA, Kamm MA, Evans BK, Phillips RK. Topical diltiazem and bethanechol decrease anal sphincter pressure without side effects. Gut. 1999;45(5):719–22.
59. Jones OM, Brading AF, Mc CMNJ. Phosphodiesterase inhibitors cause relaxation of the internal anal sphincter in vitro. Dis Colon Rectum. 2002;45:530–6.
60. Torrabadella L, Salgado G, Burns RW, Berman IR. Manometric study of topical sildenafil (Viagra) in patients with chronic anal fissure: sildenafil reduces anal resting tone. Dis Colon Rectum. 2004;47(5):733–8.
61. Jones OM, Moore JA, Brading AF, Mortensen NJ. Botulinum toxin injection inhibits myogenic tone and sympathetic nerve function in the porcine internal anal sphincter. Colorectal Dis. 2003;5:552–7.
62. Maria G, Cassetta E, Gui D, Brisinda G, Bentivoglio AR, Albanese A. A comparison of botulinum toxin and saline for

the treatment of chronic anal fissure [see comments]. N Engl J Med. 1998;338(4):217–20.

63. Brisinda G, Maria G, Bentivoglio AR, Cassetta E, Gui D, Albanese A. A comparison of injections of botulinum toxin and topical nitroglycerin ointment for the treatment of chronic anal fissure [see comments]. N Engl J Med. 1999;341(2):65–9 [published erratum appears in *N Engl J Med.* 1999;341(8):624].
64. Colak T, Ipek T, Kanik A, Aydin S. A randomized trial of botulinum toxin vs lidocain pomade for chronic anal fissure. Acta Gastroenterol Belg. 2002;65:187–90.
65. Brisinda G, Maria G, Sganga G, Bentivoglio AR, Albanese A, Castagneto M. Effectiveness of higher doses of botulinum toxin to induce healing in patients with chronic anal fissures. Surgery. 2002;131:179–84.
66. Siproudhis L, Sebille V, Pigot F, Hemery P, Juguet F, Bellissant E. Lack of effficacy of botulinum toxin in chronic anal fissure. Aliment Pharmacol Ther. 2003;18:515–24.
67. Mentes BB, Irkorucu O, Akin M, Leventoglu S, Tatlicioglu E. Comparison of botulinum toxin injection and lateral internal sphincterotomy for the treatment of chronic anal fissure. Dis Colon Rectum. 2003;46:232–7.
68. Arroyo A, Pérez F, Serrano P, Candela F, Lacueva J, Calpena R. Surgical versus chemical (botulinum toxin) sphincterotomy for chronic anal fissure: long-term results of a prospective randomized clinical and manometric study. Am J Surg. 2005;189(4):429–34.
69. Iswariah H, Stephens J, Rieger N, Rodda D, Hewett P. Randomized prospective controlled trial of lateral internal sphincterotomy versus injection of botulinum toxin for the treatment of idiopathic fissure in ano. ANZ J Surg. 2005;75(7):553–5.
70. De Nardi P, Ortolano E, Radaelli G, Staudacher C. Comparison of glycerine trinitrate and botulinum toxin-a for the treatment of chronic anal fissure: long-term results. Dis Colon Rectum. 2006;49(4):427–32.
71. Fruehauf H, Fried M, Wegmueller B, Bauerfeind P, Thumshirn M. Efficacy and safety of botulinum toxin a injection compared with topical nitroglycerin ointment for the treatment of chronic anal fissure: a prospective randomized study. Am J Gastroenterol. 2006;101(9):2107–12.
72. Brisinda G, Cadeddu F, Brandara F, Marniga G, Maria G. Randomized clinical trial comparing botulinum toxin injections with 0.2 per cent nitroglycerin ointment for chronic anal fissure. Br J Surg. 2007;94(2):162–7.
73. Maria G, Brisinda G, Bentivoglio AR, Cassetta E, Gui D, Albanese A. Influence of botulinum toxin site of injections on healing rate in patients with chronic anal fissure. Am J Surg. 2000;179(1):46–50.
74. Madalinski MH, Slawek J, Zbytek B, et al. Topical nitrates and the higher doses of botulinum toxin for chronic anal fissure. Hepatogastroenterology. 2001;48:977–9.
75. Lindsey I, Jones OM, Cunningham C, George BD, Mortensen NJ. Botulinum toxin as second-line therapy for chronic anal fissure failing 0.2 percent glyceryl trinitrate. Dis Colon Rectum. 2003;46:361–6.
76. Minguez M, Herreros B, Espi A, et al. Long-term follow-up (42 months) of chronic anal fissure after healing with botulinum toxin. Gastroenterology. 2002;123:112–7.
77. Tilney HS, Heriot AG, Cripps NP. Complication of botulinum toxin injections for anal fissure. Dis Colon Rectum. 2001;44:1721–4.
78. Jost WH, Schanne S, Mlitz H, Schimrigk K. Perianal thrombosis following injection therapy into the external anal sphincter using botulin toxin. Dis Colon Rectum. 1995;38:781.
79. Jost WH. Ten years' experience with botulin toxin in anal fissure. Int J Colorectal Dis. 2002;17:298–302.
80. U.S. Food and Drug Administration, Center for Drug Evaluation and Research. Early communication about an ongoing safety review. Botox and Botox Cosmetic (Botulinum toxin type A) and Myobloc (Botulinum toxin type B). Available at www.fda.gov/cder/drug/early_comm/botulinium_toxins.htm. Accessed 22 Oct 2009.
81. Watts JM, Bennett RC, Goligher JC. Stretching of anal sphincters in treatment of fissure-in-ano. Br Med J. 1964;2:342–3.
82. Isbister WH, Prasad J. Fissure in ano. Aust N Z J Surg. 1995;65(2):107–8.
83. O'Connor JJ. Lord procedure for treatment of postpartum hemorrhoids and fissures. Obstet Gynecol. 1980;55(6):747–8.
84. MacDonald A, Smoth A, McNeill AD, Finlay IG. Manual dilatation of the anus. Br J Surg. 1992;79:1381–2.
85. Giebel GD, Horch R. Treatment of anal fissure: a comparison of three different forms of therapy. Nippon Geka Hokan. 1989;58:126–33.
86. Sohn N, Eisenberg MM, Weinstein MA, Lugo RN, Ader J. Precise anorectal sphincter dilatation – its role in the therapy of anal fissures. Dis Colon Rectum. 1992;35:322–7.
87. Renzi A, Brusciano L, Pescatori M, Izzo D, Napolitano V, Rossetti G, et al. Pneumatic balloon dilatation for chronic anal fissure: a prospective, clinical, endosonographic, and manometric study. Dis Colon Rectum. 2005;48(1):121–6.
88. Speakman CT, Burnett SJ, Kamm MA, Bartram CI. Sphincter injury after anal dilatation demonstrated by anal endosonography. Br J Surg. 1991;78:1429–30.
89. Nielsen MB, Rasmussen OO, Pedersen JF, Christiansen J. Risk of sphincter damage and anal incontinence after anal dilatation for fissure-in-ano. An endosonographic study. Dis Colon Rectum. 1993;36(7):677–80.
90. Collopy B, Ryan P. Comparison of lateral subcutaneous sphincterotomy with anal dilatation in the treatment of fissure in ano. Med J Aust. 1979;2:461–7.
91. Weaver RM, Ambrose NS, Alexander-Williams J, Keighley MR. Manual dilatation of the anus vs. lateral subcutaneous sphincterotomy in the treatment of chronic fissure-in-ano. Results of a prospective, randomized, clinical trial. Dis Colon Rectum. 1987;30(6):420–3.
92. Marby M, Alexander-Williams J, Buchmann P, et al. A randomized controlled trial to compare anal dilatation with lateral subcutaneous sphincterotomy for anal fissure. Dis Colon Rectum. 1979;22(5):308–11.
93. Olsen J, Mortensen PE, Krogh Petersen I, Christiansen J. Anal sphincter function after treatment of fissure-in-ano by lateral subcutaneous sphincterotomy versus anal dilatation. A randomized study. Int J Colorectal Dis. 1987;2(3):155–7.
94. Yucel T, Gonullu D, Oncu M, Koksoy FN, Ozkan SG, Aycan O. Comparison of controlled-intermittent anal dilatation and lateral internal sphincterotomy in the treatment of chronic anal fissures: a prospective, randomized study. Int J Surg. 2009;7(3):228–31.
95. Saad AM, Omer A. Surgical treatment of chronic fissure-in-ano: a prospective randomised study. East Afr Med J. 1992; 69:613–5.

96. Jensen SL, Lund F, Nielsen OV, Tange G. Lateral subcutaneous sphincterotomy versus anal dilatation in the treatment of fissure in ano in outpatients: a prospective randomised study. Br Med J (Clin Res Ed). 1984;289(6444):528–30.
97. Mousavi SR, Sharifi M, Mehdikhah Z. A comparison between the results of fissurectomy and lateral internal sphincterotomy in the surgical management of chronic anal fissure. J Gastrointest Surg. 2009;13(7):1279–82.
98. The Standards Practice Task Force. American Society of Colon and Rectal Surgeons. Practice parameters for the management of anal fissures (revisited). Dis Colon Rectum. 2004;47:2003–7.
99. Eisenhammer S. The evaluation of the internal anal sphincterotomy operation with special reference to anal fissure. Surg Gynecol Obstet. 1959;109:583–90.
100. Notaras MJ. Lateral subcutaneous sphincterotomy for anal fissure – a new technique. Proc R Soc Med. 1969;62:713.
101. Abcarian H. Surgical correction of chronic anal fissure: results of lateral internal sphincterotomy vs. fissurectomy – midline sphincterotomy. Dis Colon Rectum. 1980;23(1):31–6.
102. Keighley MR, Greca F, Nevah E, Hares M, Alexander-Williams J. Treatment of anal fissure by lateral subcutaneous sphincterotomy should be under general anaesthesia. Br J Surg. 1981;68(6):400–1.
103. Ravikumar TS, Sridhar S, Rao RN. Subcutaneous lateral internal sphincterotomy for chronic fissure-in-ano. Dis Colon Rectum. 1982;25(8):798–801.
104. Hsu TC, MacKeigan JM. Surgical treatment of chronic anal fissure. A retrospective study of 1753 cases. Dis Colon Rectum. 1984;27(7):475–8.
105. Walker WA, Rothenberger DA, Goldberg SM. Morbidity of internal sphincterotomy for anal fissure and stenosis. Dis Colon Rectum. 1985;28(11):832–5.
106. Gingold BS. Simple in-office sphincterotomy with partial fissurectomy for chronic anal fissure. Surg Gynecol Obstet. 1987;165(1):46–8.
107. Lewis TH, Corman ML, Prager ED, Robertson WG. Long-term results of open and closed sphincterotomy for anal fissure. Dis Colon Rectum. 1988;31(5):368–71.
108. Zinkin L. Left lateral internal sphincterotomy for anal fissure – as an office procedure. N J Med. 1988;85(1):43–5.
109. Khubchandani IT, Reed JF. Sequelae of internal sphincterotomy for chronic fissure in ano. Br J Surg. 1989;76(5):431–4.
110. Kortbeek JB, Langevin JM, Khoo RE, Heine JA. Chronic fissure-in-ano: a randomized study comparing open and subcutaneous lateral internal sphincterotomy. Dis Colon Rectum. 1992;35(9):835–7.
111. Pernikoff BJ, Eisenstat TE, Rubin RJ, Oliver GC, Salvati EP. Reappraisal of partial lateral internal sphincterotomy. Dis Colon Rectum. 1994;37(12):1291–5.
112. Romano G, Rotondano G, Santangelo M, Esercizio L. A critical appraisal of pathogenesis and morbidity of surgical treatment of chronic anal fissure. J Am Coll Surg. 1994;178(6):600–4.
113. Leong AF, Seow-Choen F. Lateral sphincterotomy compared with anal advancement flap for chronic anal fissure. Dis Colon Rectum. 1995;38(1):69–71.
114. Prohm P, Bonner C. Is manometry essential for surgery of chronic fissure-in-ano? Dis Colon Rectum. 1995; 38(7):735–8.
115. Usatoff V, Polglase AL. The longer term results of internal anal sphincterotomy for anal fissure. Aust N Z J Surg. 1995;65(8):576–8.
116. Garcia-Aguilar J, Belmonte C, Wong WD, Lowry AC, Madoff RD. Open vs. closed sphincterotomy for chronic anal fissure: long-term results. Dis Colon Rectum. 1996; 39(4):440–3.
117. Hananel N, Gordon PH. Lateral internal sphincterotomy for fissure-in-ano – revisited. Dis Colon Rectum. 1997;40(5): 597–602.
118. Littlejohn DR, Newstead GL. Tailored lateral sphincterotomy for anal fissure. Dis Colon Rectum. 1997;40(12): 1439–42.
119. Nyam DC, Pemberton JH. Long-term results of lateral internal sphincterotomy for chronic anal fissure with particular reference to incidence of fecal incontinence. Dis Colon Rectum. 1999;42:1306–10.
120. Wiley M, Day P, Rieger N, Stephens J, Moore J. Open vs. closed lateral internal sphincterotomy for idiopathic fissure-in-ano: a prospective, randomized, controlled trial. Dis Colon Rectum. 2004;47(6):847–52.
121. Hyman N. Incontinence after lateral internal sphincterotomy: a prospective study and quality of life assessment. Dis Colon Rectum. 2004;47:35–8.
122. Sultan AH, Kamm MA, Nicholls RJ, Bartram CI. Prospective study of the extent of internal anal sphincter division during lateral sphincterotomy. Dis Colon Rectum. 1994;37(10): 1031–3.
123. Elsebae MM. A study of fecal incontinence in patients with chronic anal fissure: prospective, randomized, controlled trial of the extent of internal anal sphincter division during lateral sphincterotomy. World J Surg. 2007;31(10): 2052–7.
124. Gupta PJ, Kalaskar S. Removal of hypertrophied anal papillae and fibrous anal polyps increases patient satisfaction after anal fissure surgery. Tech Coloproctol. 2003;7:155–8.
125. Aysan E, Aren A, Ayar E. A prospective, randomized, controlled trial of primary wound closure after lateral internal sphincterotomy. Am J Surg. 2004;187:291–4.
126. Farouk R, Monson JR, Duthie GS. Technical failure of lateral sphincterotomy for the treatment of chronic anal fissure: a study using endoanal ultrasonography. Br J Surg. 1997; 84:84–5.
127. Nelson R. Non surgical therapy for anal fissure. Cochrane Database Syst Rev. 2006;18(4):CD003431.
128. Nelson R. Operative procedures for fissure in ano. Cochrane Database Syst Rev. 2005;18(2):CD002199.
129. Jenkins JT, Urie A, Molloy RG. Anterior anal fissures are associated with occult sphincter injury and abnormal sphincter function. Colorectal Dis. 2008;10(3):280–5.
130. Corby H, Donnelly VS, O'Herlihy C, O'Connell PR. Anal canal pressures are low in women with postpartum anal fissure. Br J Surg. 1997;84(1):86–8.
131. Nyam DC, Wilson RG, Stewart KJ, Farouk R, Bartolo DC. Island advancement flaps in the management of anal fissures. Br J Surg. 1995;82:326–8.
132. Fleshner PR, Schoetz Jr DJ, Roberts PL, Murray JJ, Coller JA, Veidenheimer MC. Anal fissure in Crohn's disease: a plea for aggressive management. Dis Colon Rectum. 1995;38(11):1137–43.

133. Platell C, Mackay J, Collopy B, Fink R, Ryan P, Woods R. Anal pathology in patients with Crohn's disease. Aust N Z J Surg. 1996;66(1):5–9.
134. Sangwan YP, Schoetz Jr DJ, Murray JJ, Roberts PL, Coller JA. Perianal Crohn's disease. Results of local surgical treatment. Dis Colon Rectum. 1996;39(5):529–35.
135. Sweeney JL, Ritchie JK, Nicholls RJ. Anal fissure in Crohn's disease. Br J Surg. 1988;75(1):56–7.
136. Wolkomir AF, Luchtefeld MA. Surgery for symptomatic hemorrhoids and anal fissures in Crohn's disease. Dis Colon Rectum. 1993;36(6):545–7.
137. Allan A, Keighley MR. Management of perianal Crohn's disease. World J Surg. 1988;12(2):198–202.
138. Viamonte M, Dailey TH, Gottesman L. Ulcerative disease of the anorectum in the HIV+ patient. Dis Colon Rectum. 1993;36(9):801–5.
139. Weiss EG, Wexner SD. Surgery for anal lesions in HIV-infected patients. Ann Med. 1995;27(4):467–75.
140. Gonzalez-Ruiz C, Heartfield W, Briggs B, Vukasin P, Beart RW. Anorectal pathology in HIV/AIDS-infected patients has not been impacted by highly active antiretroviral therapy. Dis Colon Rectum. 2004;47(9):1483–6.

13
Anorectal Abscess and Fistula

Carol-Ann Vasilevsky

Anorectal abscesses and fistula-in-ano represent different stages along the continuum of a common pathogenic spectrum. The abscess represents the acute inflammatory event while the fistula is representative of the chronic process.

Abscess

Anatomy

Successful eradication of anorectal suppuration and fistula-in-ano requires an in-depth understanding of anorectal anatomy. Essential is an understanding of the existence of potential anorectal spaces (Figure 13-1A).[1] The perianal space is located in the area of the anal verge. It becomes continuous with the ischioanal fat laterally while it extends into the lower portion of the anal canal medially. It is continuous with the intersphincteric space. The ischioanal space extends from the levator ani to the perineum. Anteriorly it is bound by the transverse perineal muscles; the lower border of the gluteus maximus and the sacrotuberous ligament form its posterior border. The medial border is formed by the levator ani and external sphincter muscles; the obturator internus muscle forms the lateral border. The intersphincteric space lies between the internal and external sphincters and is continuous inferiorly with the perianal space and superiorly with the rectal wall. The supralevator space is bounded superiorly by peritoneum, laterally by the pelvic wall, medially by the rectal wall and inferiorly by the levator ani muscle. The deep postanal space is located between the tip of the coccyx posteriorly and lies below the levator ani and above the anococcygeal ligament (Figure 13-1B).

At the level of the dentate line, the ducts of the anal glands empty into the anal crypts.

Some 80% of the anal glands are submucosal in extent, 8% extend to the internal sphincter, 8% to the conjoined longitudinal muscle, 2% to the intersphincteric space, and 1% penetrate the internal sphincter.[2]

Pathophysiology

Etiology

Ninety percent of all anorectal abscesses result from nonspecific cryptoglandular infection while the remainder result from the causes as listed in Table 13-1. According to the cryptoglandular theory championed by Parks,[3] abscesses result from the obstruction of the anal glands and ducts. The obstruction of a duct may result in stasis, infection and formation of an abscess. Persistence of anal gland epithelium in part of the tract between the crypt and the blocked part of the duct results in the formation of a fistula. Predisposing factors include diarrhea and trauma in the form of a hard stool. Associated factors may be anal fissures, infection of a hematoma or Crohn's disease.

Classification

Abscesses are classified according to their location in the aforementioned potential anorectal spaces: perianal, ischioanal, intersphincteric, and supralevator (Figure 13-2). Perianal abscesses are the most common type while supralevator abscesses are the rarest. Pus can also spread circumferentially through the intersphincteric, supralevator or ischioanal spaces, the latter via the deep postanal space, resulting in a horseshoe abscess.

Evaluation

Symptoms

Pain, swelling, and fever are the hallmarks associated with an abscess. The patient with a supralevator abscess may complain of gluteal pain.[4] Rectal bleeding has been reported. Severe rectal pain accompanied by urinary symptoms, such as dysuria, retention, or inability to void may be suggestive of an intersphincteric or supralevator abscess.

D.E. Beck et al. (eds.), *The ASCRS Textbook of Colon and Rectal Surgery: Second Edition*,
DOI 10.1007/978-1-4419-1584-9_13, © Springer Science+Business Media, LLC 2011

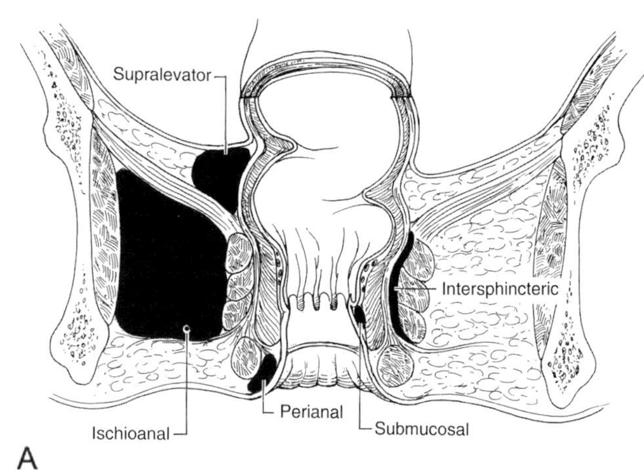

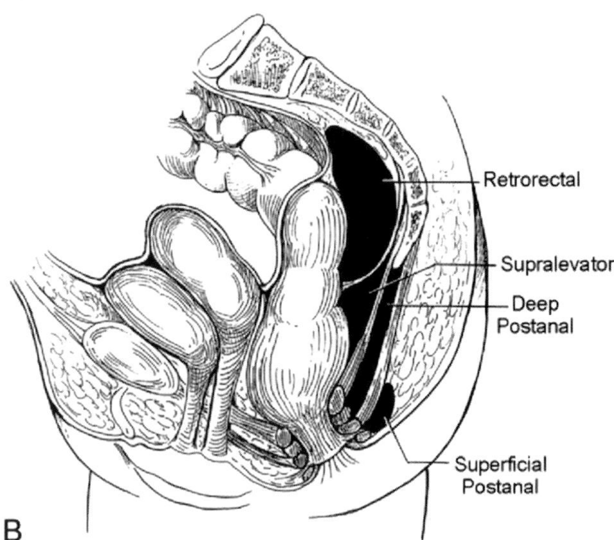

FIGURE 13-1. Anorectal spaces: **A** coronal section, **B** sagital section. (From Vasilevsky CA. Anorectal abscess and fistula-in ano. In Beck DE (ed). Handbook of colorectal surgery. St Louis, Mo: Quality Medical Publishing, 1997. With permission).

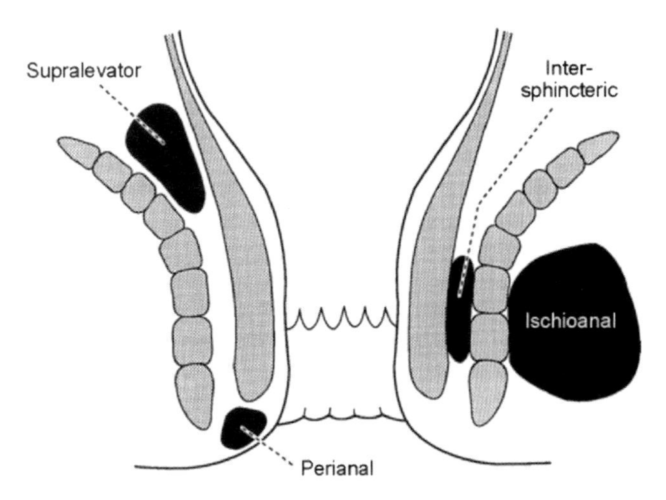

FIGURE 13-2. Classification of anorectal abscess. (From Vasilevsky CA. Fistula-in-Ano and Abscess. In Beck DE, Wexner SD (eds) Fundamentals of Anorectal Surgery. London: WB Saunders, 1998. With permission).

TABLE 13-1. Etiololgy of anorectal abscess

Nonspecific
Cryptoglandular
Specific
Inflammatory bowel disease
Crohn's disease
Ulcerative colitis
Infection
Tuberculosis
Actinomycosis
Lymphogranuloma venereum
Trauma
Impalement
Foreign body
Surgery
Episiotomy
Hemorrhoidectomy
Prostatectomy
Malignancy
Carcinoma
Leukemia
Lymphoma
Radiation

Physical Examination

Inspection reveals erythema, swelling, and possible fluctuation. It is crucial to recognize that no visible external manifestations are present with the intersphincteric or supralevator abscesses despite the patient's complaint of excruciating pain.[1] Although digital examination may not be possible because of extreme tenderness, palpation, if possible, will demonstrate tenderness and a mass. With a supralevator abscess, a tender mass may be palpated on rectal or vaginal examination.[4] Anoscopy and sigmoidoscopy are inappropriate in the acute setting.

Treatment

General Principles

Essentially, the treatment of an anorectal abscess involves incision and drainage. Watchful waiting under the cover of antibiotics is ineffective and may allow the suppurative process to progress resulting in the creation of a more complicated abscess and thus possible injury to the sphincter mechanism. Rarely, delay in diagnosis and management of anorectal abscesses may result in life-threatening necrotizing infection and death.[5] The American Society of Colon and Rectal Surgeons has issued practice parameters for the treatment of perianal abscess and fistula-in-ano.[6]

Operative Management

Incision and Drainage

Perianal abscesses can be effectively drained under local anesthesia.[4,7] After the most tender point has been determined,

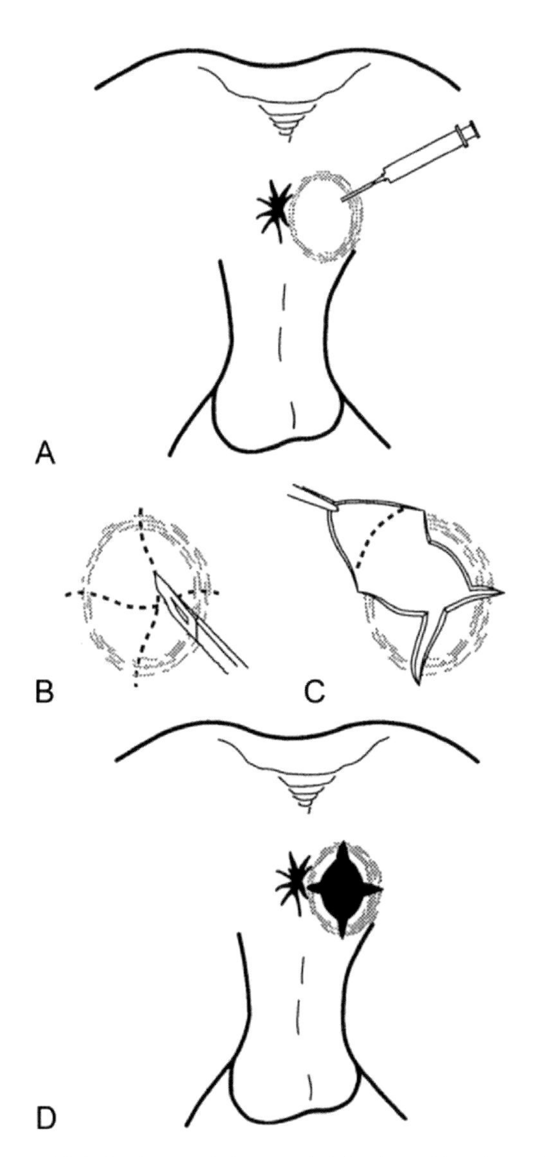

FIGURE 13-3. Drainage of abscess: **A** injection of local anesthesia, **B** cruciate incision, **C** excision of skin, **D** drainage cavity.

the area is infiltrated with 0.5% lidocaine with 1:200,000 epinephrine. A cruciate or elliptical incision is made and the edges are trimmed to prevent coaptation which may result in poor drainage or recurrence (Figure 13-3). No packing is required.

Most ischioanal abscesses can be incised and drained in a similar fashion with the site of incision shifted as close to the anal side of the abscess, minimizing the complexity of a subsequent fistula. Large ischioanal or horseshoe abscesses often require drainage with the patient under a regional or general anesthetic with the patient in the prone jackknife or left lateral (Sim's) position. The location of infection is often in the deep postanal space. Access to this space may be achieved by a midline incision between the coccyx and anus, spreading the superficial external sphincter to enter the space. An opening is made in the posterior midline and the lower half of the internal sphincter is divided to drain the

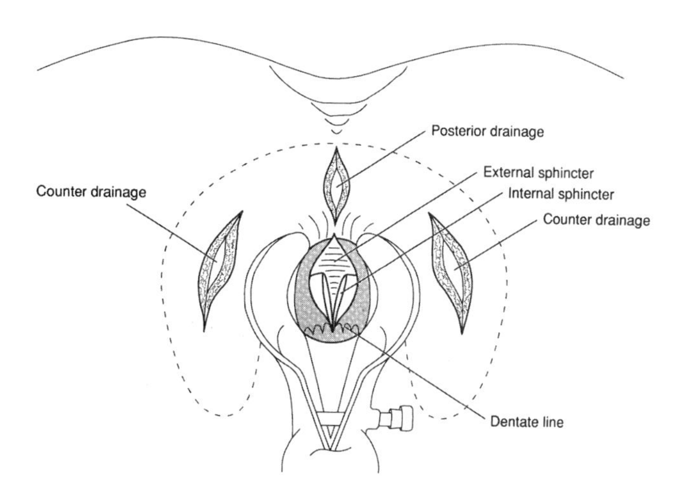

FIGURE 13-4. Drainage of horseshoe abscess.

anal gland in which the infection originated.[4] Counter-incisions are made over each ischioanal fossa to allow drainage of the anterior extensions of the abscess (Hanley procedure) (Figure 13-4).[7]

Since the diagnosis of an intersphincteric abscess is entertained when the patient presents with pain out of proportion to the physical findings, an examination under anesthesia is mandatory to completely assess the cause of the pain. Once the diagnosis is established, either by palpation of a protrusion into the anal canal or by needle aspiration in the intersphincteric plane, treatment consists of dividing the internal sphincter along the length of the abscess cavity. The wound is then marsupialized to allow adequate drainage and quicker healing.

Prior to the treatment of a supralevator abscess, it is essential to determine its origin since it may arise from an upward extension of an intersphincteric or an ischioanal abscess, or downward extension of a pelvic abscess.[1,4] The treatment in each case is different. If the origin is an intersphincteric abscess, it should be drained through the rectum by dividing the internal sphincter and not through the ischioanal fossa, since this will result in the creation of a suprasphincteric fistula. However, if it arises from an ischioanal abscess, it should be drained through the perineal skin and not through the rectum; otherwise an extrasphincteric fistula will occur (Figure 13-5). If the abscess is of pelvic origin, it may be drained through the rectum, ischioanal fossa or abdominal wall via percutaneous drainage depending on the direction to which it is pointing.

Catheter Drainage

An alternative method of treatment for selected patients is catheter drainage. Patients suitable for this technique should not have severe sepsis or any serious systemic illness.[8] The patient is placed in the prone jackknife position or left lateral (Sim's) position. The skin is prepared with a proviodine-iodine solution and the fluctuant point of the abscess is selected. Local anesthesia consisting of 0.5% lidocaine with 1:200,000 epinephrine is injected into a 1 cm area of skin and a stab incision is made to drain the pus.

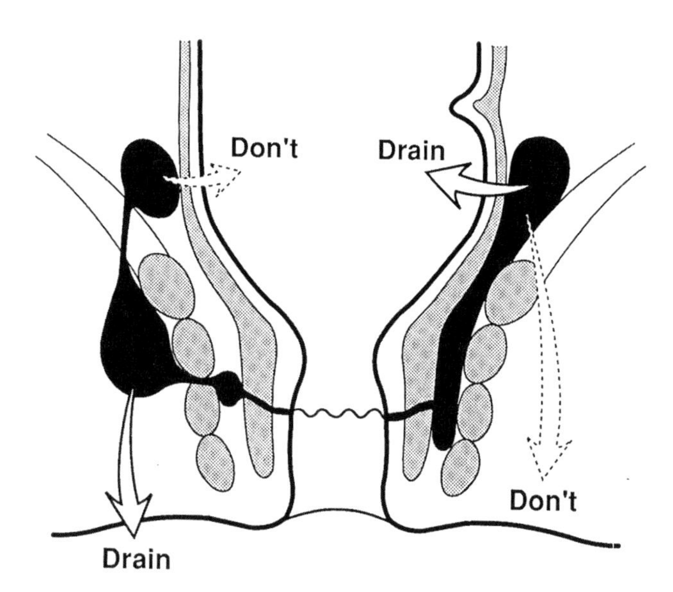

FIGURE 13-5. Drainage of a supralevator abscess.

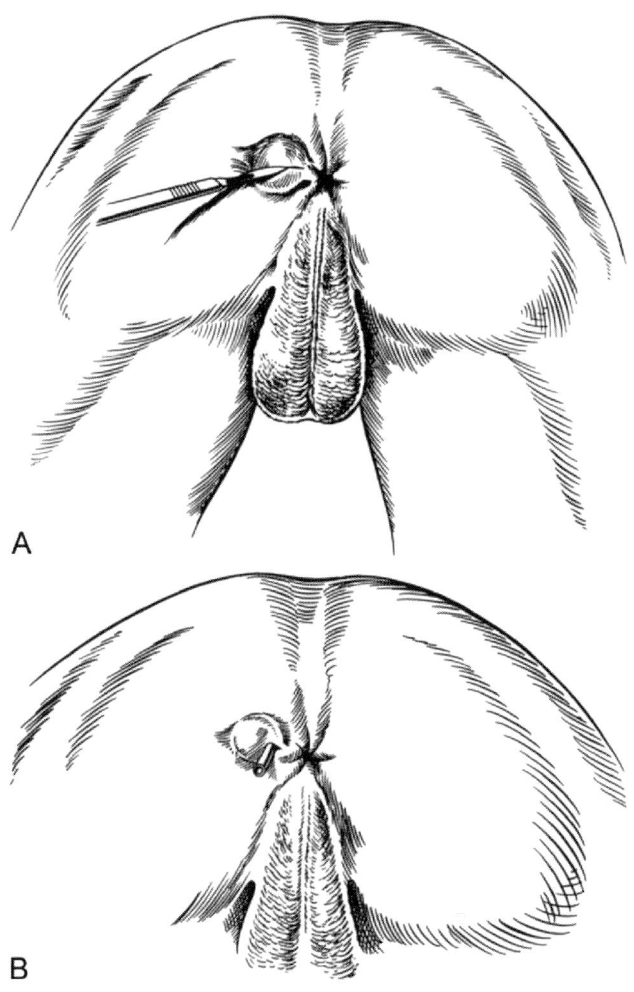

FIGURE 13-6. Catheter drainage of an abscess: **A** stab incision, **B** catheter in abscess cavity.

The lidocaine should be injected into the skin around rather than immediately over the point of maximal fluctuation because the acid environment may otherwise preclude adequate anesthesia (Figure 13-6A). A 10–16 French soft latex mushroom catheter is inserted over a probe into the abscess cavity. When released, the shape of the catheter tip holds the catheter in place, obviating the need for sutures. The external portion of the catheter is shortened to leave 2–3 cm outside the skin with the tip in the depth of the abscess cavity (Figure 13-6B). This reduces the chances of the catheter falling out of or into the abscess cavity. A small bandage is placed over the catheter.

When using this technique, it is important that the stab incision be placed as close as possible to the anus, minimizing the amount of tissue that must be opened if a fistula is found following the resolution of inflammation (Figure 13-6A) and the size and length of the catheter should correspond to the size of the abscess cavity (Figure 13-7A). A catheter that is too small or too short may fall into the wound (Figure 13-7B). The length of time that the catheter should be left in place depends on the size of the original abscess cavity, the amount of granulation tissue around the catheter and the character and amount of drainage. If there is doubt, it is better to leave the catheter in place for a longer period of time.

Primary Fistulotomy

In the recent past, a contentious issue has been whether primary fistulotomy should be performed at the time of initial abscess drainage. With the advent of noninvasive techniques, such as fibrin glue and the anal fistula plug, many of the former proponents of this procedure have since abandoned this approach, electing to await the appearance of a fistula following drainage only to treat it with one of the former less invasive methods so as to avoid cutting any sphincter muscle.

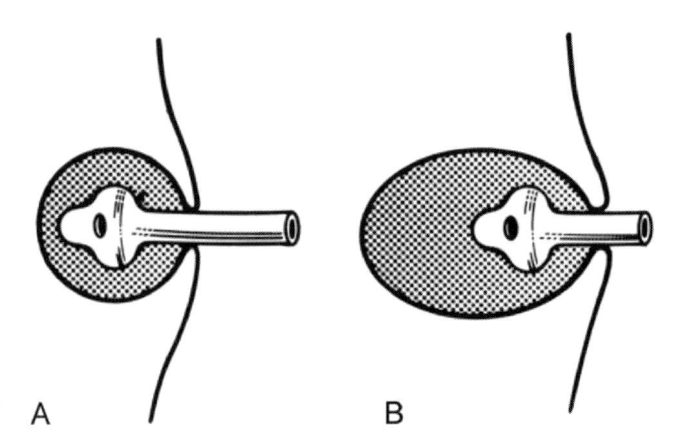

FIGURE 13-7. Catheter in an abscess cavity: **A** correct size and length of catheter, **B** catheter too short.

The argument was based on the feeling that in the acute phase one can better trace the suppurative process because of the presence of pus. Primary fistulotomy, it was believed, eliminated the source of infection and decreased the rate of recurrence, obviating the need for subsequent surgery with the potential to decrease disability and morbidity. A meta-analysis of five randomized controlled trials comparing drainage alone to drainage plus fistulotomy when a fistula was identified showed an 83% decrease in subsequent fistula formation[9] with no increase in incontinence.

Opponents are reluctant to perform primary fistulotomy in the presence of acute inflammation since the search for an internal opening may lead to the creation of false passages resulting in neglect of the main source of infection.[10,11] Failure to identify an internal opening has been reported to occur in as high as 66% of patients.[12] In addition, 34–50% of patients who present with an abscess for the first time will not develop a fistula.[7,12] A recent retrospective cohort study showed that age less than 40 significantly increased the risk of developing a fistula or recurrent abscess after drainage of the initial perianal abscess.[13] Thus, primary fistulotomy in these patients would be unnecessary and may result in needless disturbances of continence. Of those patients whose abscesses are drained, 11% may develop a fistula while 37% may develop a recurrent abscess.[10] This is most often observed in conjunction with ischioanal abscesses.[10] The search for an internal opening converts the operative procedure from one that can be performed under local anesthesia to one that requires regional or general anesthesia. A prospective randomized trial of drainage alone versus drainage and fistulotomy for acute perianal abscesses with proven internal openings revealed that incision and drainage alone demonstrated no statistical significance in recurrence compared with concurrent fistulotomy although there was a tendency to recurrence in the former group.[14] Another prospective study advocated a conservative approach in the treatment of anorectal abscess, reserving fistulotomy as a second-stage procedure, if necessary.[15]

If the internal opening of a low transsphincteric fistula is readily apparent at the time of abscess drainage, primary fistulotomy is feasible with the following exceptions: (1) patients with Crohn's disease, (2) patients with acquired immune deficiency syndrome (AIDS), (3) elderly patients, (4) patients with high transsphincteric fistulas, and (5) women with anterior fistulas and episiotomy scars.

The decision to perform a primary fistulotomy should be individualized but should only be attempted by a surgeon with a sound knowledge of the regional anatomy. Insistence upon finding a fistula may encourage the creation of a false passage and unnecessary division of sphincter muscle.

Antibiotics

There is little if any role for antibiotics in the primary management of anorectal abscesses except as an adjunct in patients with valvular heart disease or prosthetic valves, extensive soft tissue cellulitis, prosthestic devices, diabetes, immunosuppression, or systemic sepsis.

Postoperative Care

Patients are instructed to continue with a regular diet and to take a bulk-forming agent, noncodeine-containing analgesic and sitz baths. Patients are generally seen in follow-up in 2–4 weeks or for intersphincteric or supralevator abscesses, 2 weeks postoperatively. Those patients in whom catheter drainage has been performed are seen within 7–10 days post procedure. If the cavity has closed around the catheter and drainage has ceased, the catheter is removed. If the cavity has not healed, the catheter is left in place or replaced with a smaller one. In all cases, patients are observed until complete healing has occurred.

Complications

Recurrence

Following incision and drainage, ischioanal, and intersphincteric abscesses are associated with the development of recurrent abscesses or fistulas in as many as 89% of patients.[10,15,16] Recurrence is more likely to occur in patients with a history of previous abscess drainage perhaps because the natural barriers to infection have been destroyed.[10,15,16] Reasons for recurrence of anorectal infections include missed infection in adjacent anatomic spaces, the presence of an undiagnosed fistula or abscess at initial abscess drainage, and failure to completely drain the abscess.[5]

If a patient waits too long for follow-up following catheter drainage, the skin may seal and a second incision may be required to retrieve the catheter or redrain a recurrent abscess.

Failure to detect a primary opening at the time of primary fistulotomy and abscess drainage may result in persistence of the infection.

Extra-anal Causes

Extra-anal disease should be considered once the usual causes of recurrence have been ruled out. Hidradentis suppurativa and downward extension of a pilonidal abscess should be considered.[1] A prospective review of recurrent anorectal abscesses by Chrabot et al.[17] reported hidradenitis in one third of patients with recurrent abscesses. In addition, the possibility of Crohn's disease should be suspected as well as tuberculosis, human immunodeficiency virus (HIV) infection, perianal actinomycosis, rectal duplication, lymphogranuloma venereum, trauma, foreign bodies, and a perforated rectal carcinoma.

Incontinence

Incontinence may result after incision and drainage of an abscess either from iatrogenic damage to the sphincter or inappropriate wound care. Continence may be compromised if the superficial external sphincter is inadvertently divided during drainage of a perianal or deep postanal abscess in a patient with preoperative borderline continence. Drainage of a supralevator abscess may lead to incontinence if the puborectalis is inappropriately divided.[18] Prolonged packing of a drained abscess may impair continence by preventing the development of granulation tissue and promoting the formation of excess scar tissue.[19]

Although advocated to decrease recurrence rates, primary fistulotomy may result in unnecessary division of sphincter muscle in acutely inflamed tissue. Schouten and van Vroonhoven[15] reported a 39% rate of continence disturbances in a prospective randomized trial.

Special Considerations

Necrotizing Anorectal Infection

Rarely, anorectal abscesses may result in necrotizing infection and death. Factors thought to be responsible include delay in diagnosis and management, virulence of the organism involved, bacteremia and metastatic infections, or underlying disorders, such as diabetes, blood dyscrasias, heart disease, chronic renal failure, hemorrhoids, and previous abscess or fistula.[5] Obesity and cigarette smoking are thought to be risk factors.

Symptoms and Signs

Spreading soft tissue infection of the perineum can be classified into two groups.[20] The first group includes anorectal sepsis in which the infection extends superficially around the perineum resulting in necrosis of skin, subcutaneous tissue, fascia, or muscle. Perianal crepitation, erythematous, indurated skin, blistering, or gangrene may be present (Figure 13-8). A black spot may appear early and indicates a widespread necrotizing infection.[21] The second group includes sepsis in which the preperitoneal or retroperitoneal spaces have become involved.[20] Subtle signs may be present which include abdominal wall induration, tenderness, or a vague mass. It is important to realize that systemic symptoms, such as fever, tachycardia, and vascular volume depletion may precede the appearance of overt signs of infection.[22] Computed tomography (CT) scan is an excellent diagnostic tool since it demonstrates the origin as well as the extent of infection.[23]

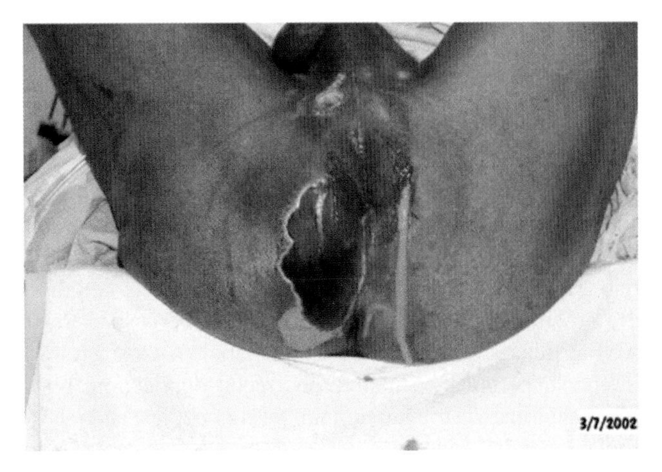

FIGURE 13-8. Necrotizing anorectal infection.

Treatment

Early recognition and aggressive surgical therapy as well as selection of the appropriate antibiotics result in a decrease in mortality.[24] The mean interval from the onset of symptoms to surgical intervention is seen as the most important prognostic factor with a significant impact on outcome.[24]

Treatment consists of vigorous intravenous fluid hydration, restoration of electrolyte balance, and insertion of a Foley catheter. Accompanying coagulopathy, respiratory insufficiency and renal failure must be aggressively treated. Invasive monitoring and ventilatory support may be necessary.[25] Pus or necrotic tissue from the infected region must be cultured for aerobes and anaerobes. A Gram stain can be used to distinguish between the presence of clostridial and nonclostridial organisms.[26] Empiric broad-spectrum antibiotic therapy should be instituted regardless of Gram stain and culture results. The chosen antibiotic regimen should be effective against staphylococci and streptococci, gram-negative coliforms, Pseudomonas, Bacteroides, and Clostridium. For gram-positive rods seen on Gram stain, antibiotics administered should include sodium penicillin G in doses of 24–30 million units per day and an aminoglycoside. Tetanus toxoid should also be administered.[25]

Surgical treatment consists of wide radical debridement until healthy tissue is encountered. The goals of surgical debridement are to remove all nonviable tissue, halt the progression of infection and alleviate the systemic toxicity.[22] It is crucial to realize that the preoperative skin changes may be minimal compared to the operative findings which may include edema, liquefactive necrosis of subcutaneous tissues, watery pus formation, and extensive necrosis of underlying fascia.[25] Re-examination under anesthesia is usually necessary since this is the only manner by which adequate wound examination can be conducted.[25] Vacuum-assisted closure of the resulting wounds may be a useful adjunct in healing of these wounds which may be rather extensive.[27] The need for colostomy is a debatable issue and has been recommended if the sphincter muscle is grossly infected, if there is colonic or rectal perforation, if the rectal wound is large, if the patient is immunocompromised or if incontinence is present.[20,22] While some authors feel that colostomy is seldom necessary,[26] fecal diversion may also be accomplished with the use of a "medical colostomy" consisting of enteral or parenteral nutrition. Controversy also exists with regards to the need for urinary diversion by suprapubic catheterization. It has been suggested that this may be indicated in the presence of known stricture and urinary extravasation with phlegmon.[28]

Although antibiotics and adequate surgical drainage are thought to be sufficient, the use of hyperbaric oxygen (HBO) has been advocated as an adjunct to treatment, particularly in patients with diffuse spreading infections who do not have chronic obstructive pulmonary disease.[29] It is postulated that HBO has a direct antibacterial effect on anaerobic bacteria by diminishing the effect of endotoxins and optimizing leukocyte phagocytic function.[21] HBO may also promote would healing by facilitating fibroblast proliferation.[29] HBO is delivered as 100% oxygen through an oronasal mask or endotracheal tube at 3 ATM for one or two cycles each lasting 2 h. If HBO is to be used as an adjunctive therapy, appropriate surgical intervention with wide debridement cannot be compromised since ischemic tissue cannot be salvaged by HBO.[22]

Despite aggressive surgical and multidisciplinary management of anorectal sepsis, mortality rates ranging from 8 to 67% have been reported.[20,22] This high mortality rate is due in part to the aggressive nature of the infection and to the underlying comorbid diseases that are present in these patients.[22] Mortality rates are two to three times higher in diabetics, in elderly patients and in patients in whom treatment is delayed.[21]

Extent of disease at presentation and metabolic status are of utmost importance in determining prognosis.[30]

Anal Infection and Hematologic Diseases

Acute anorectal suppuration poses an interesting and often life-threatening problem in patients with acute hematologic diseases. In patients with acute leukemia, mortality rates of 45–78% have been reported.[31] There is a definite relationship between the number of circulating granulocytes and the incidence of perianal infection in patients with hematologic diseases. In one study, patients with neutrophil counts below 500 per cubic millimeter had an incidence of anorectal infections of 11%, whereas those with counts greater than 500 per cubic millimeter had an incidence of 0.4%.[32] Glenn et al.[33] reported that 63% of anorectal infectious episodes occurred when fewer than 500 neutrophils were present per cubic millimeter. The risk of developing anorectal infection in this patient population has been found to be related to the severity and duration of the neutropenia.[31] The most important prognostic indicator was the number of days of neutropenia during the infectious episode.[33]

The most common presenting symptoms include fever, which precedes pain, and urinary retention. Point tenderness and poorly demarcated induration constitute the earliest signs[31] while external swelling and fluctuation often appear late in the course of infection.[33]

Controversy surrounds the treatment of acute anorectal infections in patients with hematologic malignancies. Surgery has generally been avoided since what may seem to be simple incision and drainage may produce scant or no pus and may instead cause hemorrhage, poor wound healing or expanding soft tissue infection.[33]

Any patient with perianal pain is assumed to have a perianal complication and is started on precautionary measures which consist of no digital rectal examinations, suppositories, or enemas.[34] Sitz baths, stool softeners, bulk agents, and analgesia are advised. On aspiration of most abscesses in this group, the most common organisms are *Escherichia coli* and group D streptococcus. Consequently, infections are successfully controlled with a third-generation cephalosporin combined with anaerobic coverage or an extended spectrum of penicillin in combination with an aminoglycoside and an antianaerobic antibiotic. This combination has been associated with an 88% success rate.[33]

Barnes et al.[31] recommend an aggressive surgical approach. Through this approach, 13 of 15 patients who were severely neutropenic with neutrophil counts of fewer than 100 per cubic millimeter recovered with incision and drainage. It must be noted that these patients were found to have extensive soft tissue infection. Since appropriate antibiotic coverage has been found to control infection successfully, surgery has generally been recommended only if there is obvious fluctuation, progression of soft tissue infection, or persistent sepsis after a trial of antibiotic therapy.[33]

With severe neutropenia of fewer than 500 neutrophils per cubic millimeter, low dose radiation therapy of 300–400 rad for a period of 1–3 days has been suggested. Spontaneous drainage or subsidence of induration has been found to occur in 3–5 days.[34] A randomized controlled study, however, has failed to confirm the utility of this approach.[35]

Anorectal Sepsis in the HIV-Positive Patient

Patients who are HIV-positive and present with abscesses require drainage either by incision and drainage or the use of catheter drainage. Since these patients are immunosuppressed, adjunctive antibiotics should be used. Efforts should be directed at keeping wounds small since these patients are at risk of poor wound healing.[36] An increased incidence of perianal sepsis may be observed in HIV positive patients.[37] Serious septic complications or uncommon presentations of anorectal sepsis were found in 13% of patients who initially presented with anorectal suppuration in one study.[36] In another study, perianal sepsis was associated with in situ neoplasia.[38]

Fistula-in-ano

Familiarity of the surgeon with the anatomy of the anorectal area and with the pathogenesis and classification of fistulas is essential for their adequate management.

Pathophysiology

Etiology

A fistula is defined as an abnormal communication between any two epithelium-lined surfaces. A fistula-in-ano is an abnormal tract or cavity communicating with the rectum or anal canal by an identifiable internal opening. Most fistulas are thought to arise due to cryptoglandular infection.

Classification

The most helpful yet complicated classification of fistula-in-ano is that described by Parks[39] (Table 13-2). It has been suggested that its use is particularly applicable to the treatment of recurrent fistulas.

Intersphincteric Fistula-in-ano

This fistula is the result of a perianal abscess. The tract passes within the intersphincteric space (Figure 13-9A). This is the most common type of fistula and accounts for approximately 70% of fistulas.[39] A high blind tract passing from the fistula tract to the rectal wall may occur; in addition, the tract may also pass into the lower rectum. The infectious process may pass into the intersphincteric plane and terminate as a blind tract. There is no downward extension to the anal margin, and thus no external opening is present. Infection may also spread in the intersphincteric plane to reach the pelvic cavity to lie above the levator ani muscles. Lastly, an intersphincteric fistula may originate in the pelvis as a pelvic abscess but manifest itself in the perianal area.

TABLE 13-2. Classification of fistula-in-ano

Intersphincteric
Simple low tract
High blind tract
High tract with rectal opening
Rectal opening without perineal opening
Extrarectal extension
Secondary to pelvic disease
Transsphincteric
Uncomplicated
High blind tract
Suprasphincteric
Uncomplicated
High blind tract
Extrasphincteric
Secondary to anal fistula
Secondary to trauma
Secondary to anorectal disease
Secondary to pelvic inflammation

Adapted from Parks[3]

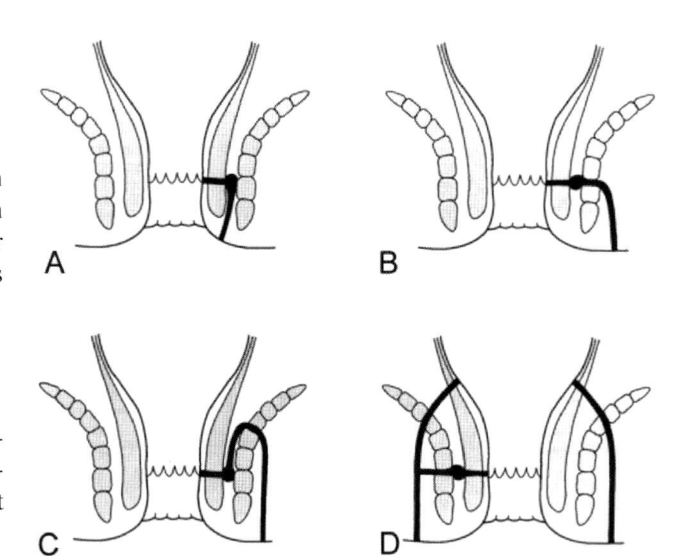

FIGURE 13-9. Classification of fistula-in-ano: **A** intersphincteric, **B** transsphincteric, **C** suprasphincteric, **D** extrasphincteric.

Transsphincteric Fistula-in-ano

In its usual variety, this fistula results from an ischioanal abscess and constitutes approximately 23% of fistulas seen.[39] The tract passes from the internal opening through the internal and external sphincters to the ischioanal fossa (Figure 13-9B). A high blind tract may also occur in this situation in which the upper arm of the tract may pass toward the apex of the ischioanal fossa or may extend through the levator ani muscles and thereby into the pelvis. One form of transsphincteric fistula is the rectovaginal fistula. This is discussed further in Chap. 14.

Suprasphincteric Fistula-in-ano

This fistula results from a supralevator abscess and accounts for approximately 5% of fistulas in some series.[39] The tract passes above the puborectalis after arising as an intersphincteric abscess. The tract curves downward lateral to the external sphincter in the ischioanal space to the perianal skin (Figure 13-9C). A high blind tract may also occur in this variety and result in a horseshoe extension.

Extrasphincteric Fistula-in-ano

This constitutes the rarest type of fistula and accounts for 2% of fistulas.[39] The tract passes from the rectum above the levators and through them to the perianal skin via the ischioanal space (Figure 13-9D). This fistula may result from foreign body penetration of the rectum with drainage through the levators, from penetrating injury to the perineum, or from Crohn's disease or carcinoma or its treatment. However, the most common cause may be iatrogenic secondary to vigorous probing during fistula surgery.[4]

Evaluation and Treatment

Symptoms

A patient with a fistula-in-ano often recounts a history of an abscess that has been drained either surgically or spontaneously. Patients may complain of drainage, pain with defecation, bleeding due to the presence of granulation tissue at the internal opening, swelling or decrease in pain with drainage. Additional bowel symptoms may be present when the fistula is secondary to proctocolitis, Crohn's disease, actinomycosis, or anorectal carcinoma.[40] Systemic diseases such as HIV, carcinoma, and lymphoma should be entertained.[40]

Physical Examination

The external or secondary opening may be seen as an elevation of granulation tissue discharging pus. This may be elicited on digital rectal examination. In most cases, the internal or primary opening is not apparent. The number of external openings and their location may be helpful in identifying the primary opening. According to Goodsall's rule (Figure 13-10), an opening seen posterior to a line drawn transversely across the perineum originates from an internal opening in the posterior midline. An anterior external opening originates in the nearest crypt. Generally, the greater the distance from the anal margin the greater the probability of a complicated upward extension. Cirocco and Reilly[41] found that Goodsall's rule was accurate in describing the course of anal fistulas with a posterior external opening. It was inaccurate in patients with anterior external openings since 71% of these fistulas tracked to a midline anterior primary opening. This was especially true in women in whom fistulas with anterior external openings tracked in a radial fashion in only 31%.[41]

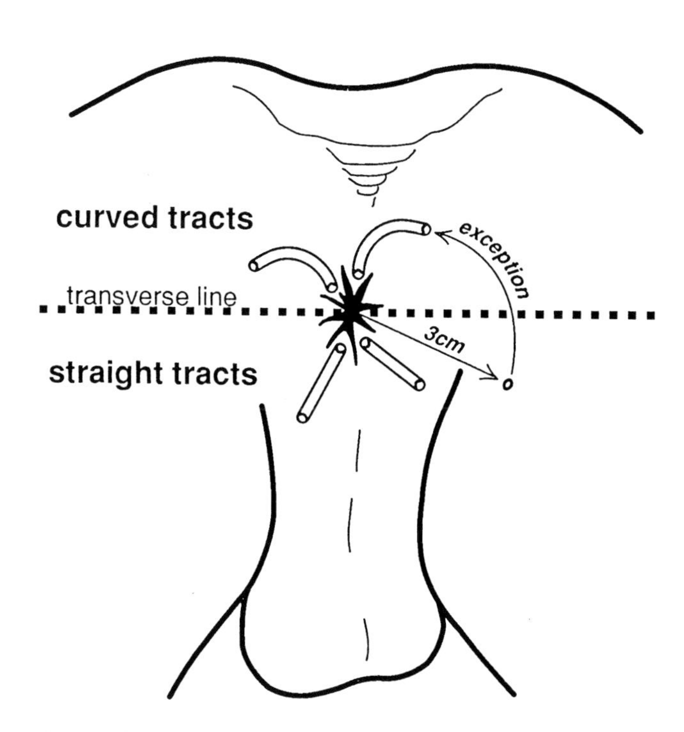

FIGURE 13-10. Goodsall's rule.

Digital rectal examination may reveal an indurated cord-like structure beneath the skin in the direction of the internal opening with asymmetry between right and left sides. Internal openings may be felt as indurated nodules or pits leading to an indurated tract.[41] Posterior or lateral induration may be palpable indicating fistulas deep in the postanal space or horseshoe fistulas.[40,41] Bidigital rectal examination defines the relationship of the tract to the sphincter muscles and provides information as to preoperative sphincter tone, bulk, and voluntary squeeze pressure which need to be assessed preoperatively because of a possible risk of incontinence.[18,40]

Investigations

Anoscopy should be done prior to operation in an attempt to identify the primary opening. Sigmoidoscopy should be performed to locate a proximal internal opening and to exclude underlying pathology, such as proctitis or neoplasia. Colonoscopy or barium enema and a small bowel series are indicated in patients who have symptoms suggestive of inflammatory bowel disease and in patients with multiple or recurrent fistulas. Although anal manometry is not generally required, it may be useful as an adjunct to plan the operative approach in women with previous obstetric trauma, in an elderly patient, a patient with Crohn's disease or AIDS, or in a patient with a recurrent fistula.[42]

The role of preoperative imaging is to demonstrate clinically undetected sepsis, to serve as a guide at the time of the initial surgery, to determine the relationship of the fistula tract to the sphincter mechanism, and to reveal the site of sepsis in a recurrent fistula, all serving to decrease recurrence rates associated with fistula surgery. Imaging may take the form of fistulography, CT scan, endoanal ultrasound, and magnetic resonance imaging (MRI).

Fistulography

Fistulography, which involves cannulation of the external opening with a small feeding tube and injection of water soluble contrast may be useful in the evaluation of recurrent fistulas or in Crohn's disease where previous surgical forays or disease may have altered anorectal anatomy (Figure 13-11).[43] Contrast is introduced at low pressures for fear of tissue disruption. This may not allow secondary tracts to fill with contrast. It is difficult to distinguish between an abscess located high in the ischioanal fossa and one located in the supralevator space. In addition, the level of the internal opening may be difficult to see because of the absence of precise landmarks. Contrast may reflux into the rectum wrongly suggesting an

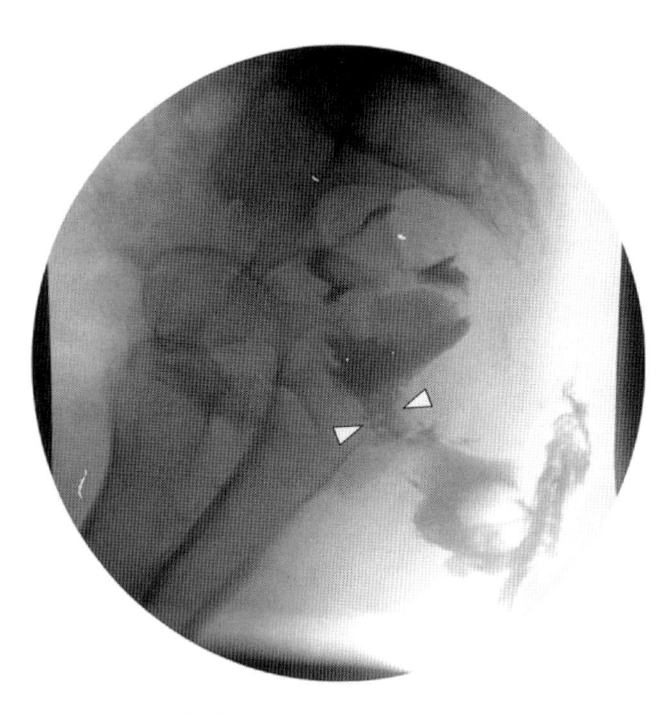

FIGURE 13-11. Fistulogram.

extrasphincteric tract with a rectal opening thus resulting in injudicious probing. Accuracy rates in identifying the internal openings and extensions in one study were found to be 16%, while a subsequent study found fistulography to be useful in 96%.[43,44] Its use resulted in altered surgical management or revealed other surgical pathology in 48%.[43] It was found, for reasons outlined previously, to have a false positive rate of 12%.[44] Fistulography is invasive and potentially may result in the dissemination of sepsis.

Computed Tomography Scan

CT scanning performed with intravenous and rectal contrast is a noninvasive method used to assess the perirectal spaces. Its use may be to distinguish an abscess requiring drainage from perirectal cellultitis. It does not permit visualization of tracts in relation to the levators but may be helpful in assessing the degree of rectal inflammation in patients with inflammatory bowel disease.

Endoanal Ultrasound

The role of endoanal ultrasound is to establish the relation of the primary tract to the anal sphincters, to determine if the fistula is simple or complex with extensions and to determine the location of the primary opening. It may aid in the identification of complex fistulas and may serve as an adjunct in the evaluation of complex suppuration to assess the adequacy of drainage (Figure 13-12A).[45] A prospective study which compared this modality to digital examination found that while endosonography was able to detect a large portion of intersphincteric and transsphincteric tracts, it was unable to detect primary superficial, extrasphincteric, and suprasphincteric tracts or secondary supralevator or infralevator tracts.[46] A study conducted 10 years later using a 10 mHz probe along with injection of hydrogen peroxide into the tract, was able to identify the internal opening in 93%.[47] While this investigative modality is rapid and well tolerated, it is operator dependent and scars or defects caused by previous sepsis, surgery or trauma confuses ultrasonographic interpretation and makes delineation of fistula tracts difficult.[46] The concomitant use of enhancing agents such as hydrogen peroxide (Figure 13-12B) or Levovist™[48] at the time of ultrasound examination has been found to improve its accuracy and it has been suggested that it be used prior to operative treatment since it assists the surgeon by delineating the anatomy of the fistulous tract and provides information that may be of value in planning therapeutic surgery, thereby reducing the risks of incontinence and recurrence.[49,50]

Magnetic Resonance Imaging

MRI in the form of endoanal coil, body coil, and phase array (Figure 13-13) coil may be of value in the assessment of patients with complex fistulas and in those with anatomic distortion resulting from previous surgery. Since MRI can provide multiplanar visualization of the sphincter muscles, differentiation of supralevator from infralevator lesions is easier.[51] MRI has been found to accurately delineate the presence and course of a primary fistulous tract, but also demonstrates the site and presence of any secondary extensions.[52] It also provides the most accurate imaging technique of localizing the site of the internal opening since its location can be inferred from the proximity of the tract in the intersphincteric space.[52] A prospective study which compared the accuracy of MRI in the preoperative assessment of anal fistulas to operative findings, found concordance rates of 88% for the presence and course of the primary tract, 91% for the presence and site of secondary extensions or abscesses, 97% for the presence of horseshoeing, and 80% for the position of the internal openings.[45] In the same study, failure of healing in 9% was found to be related to pathology missed at the time of surgery which had been documented on preoperative MRI.[52] Difficulties in interpretation, however, may occur since neural and vascular structures may be mistaken for fistulas and chemical shift artifacts may simulate a fistula filled with fluid.[52] The use of the endoanal coil has been found to be superior to external MRI for the identification of complex sphincter anatomy especially in the demonstration of the morphology of the internal and external sphincters;[53,54] however, definition may fall off outside the sphincter and may fail to show the tracts that lie beyond its range. It is also painful. A prospective study comparing hydrogen peroxide endoanal ultrasound to endoanal MRI found good agreement for the classification of the primary fistula tract and the location of the internal opening. These results also demonstrated good agreement with the surgical findings enabling both to be reliable for the preoperative evaluation of fistulas.[55]

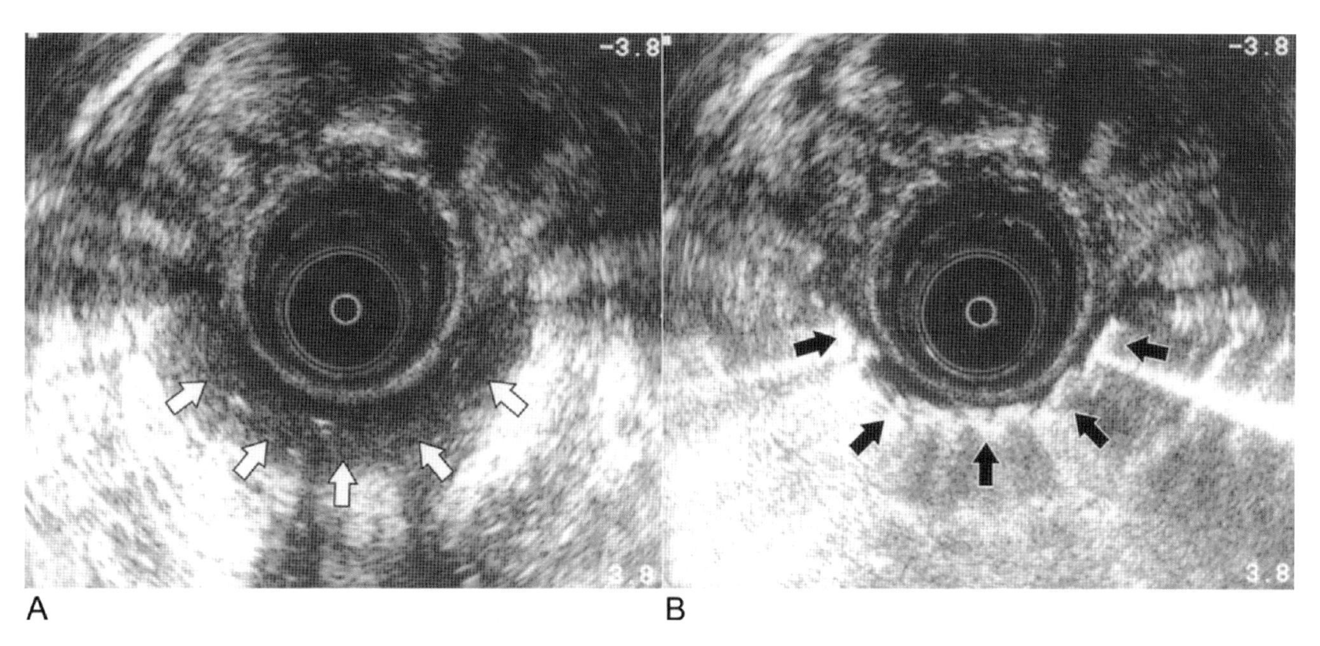

FIGURE 13-12. **A** Anal endosonogram, **B** with hydrogen peroxide. Courtesy Dr. Julio Faria.

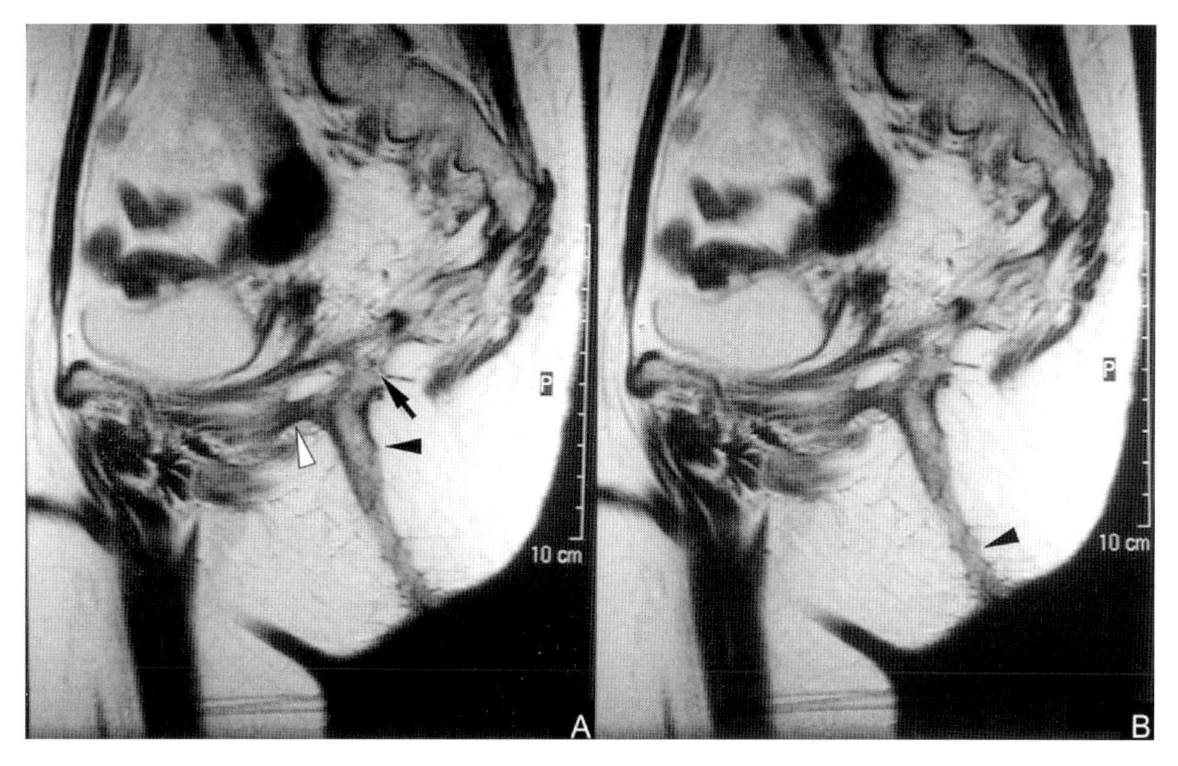

FIGURE 13-13. Phase array MRI.

A prospective trial comparing the use of the endoanal coil to the body coil found that surgical concordance for the endoanal coil was 68% versus 96% for the body coil, presumably due to field of view limitations.[56] This can be overcome with the use of the phase array coil which has a larger field of view and may be useful in Crohn's disease and recurrent fistulas.[57]

In a prospective study to determine the impact of MRI with primary fistulas, Buchanan et al.[58] found that MRI changed the surgical approach in 10%. In another study with respect to recurrent fistulas, recurrence rates were found to be higher for those surgeons who never used MRI.[59] They concluded that MRI-guided surgery can decrease recurrence rates by 75% in surgery for recurrent fistulas.

Treatment

General Principles

The principles of fistula surgery are to eliminate the fistula, prevent recurrence, and preserve sphincter function. Success is usually determined by identification of the primary opening and dividing the least amount of muscle possible. Several methods have been proposed to identify the primary opening in the operating room.[1,4]

1. Passage of a probe or probes from the external opening to the internal opening or vice versa.
2. Injection of a dye such as dilute solution of methylene blue, milk, or hydrogen peroxide and noting their appearance at the dentate line. Although methylene blue may stain surrounding tissues, diluting it with saline or hydrogen peroxide obviates this problem.
3. Following the granulation tissue present in the fistula tract.
4. Noting puckering of an anal crypt when traction is placed on the tract. This may be useful with simple fistulas but is less successful in the more complicated varieties.

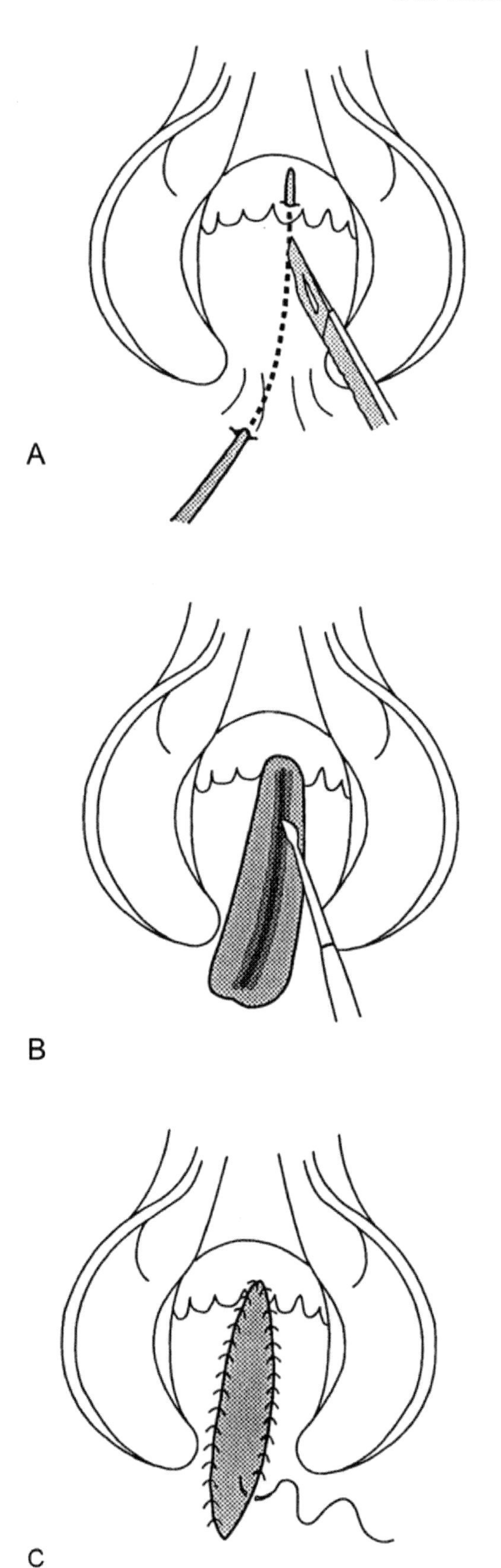

FIGURE 13-14. Technique of laying open: **A** insertion of probe and incision of tissue overlying probe, **B** curettage of granulation tissue, **C** marsupialization of wound edges.

Operative Management

Lay-open Technique

For the treatment of simple intersphincteric and low transsphincteric fistulas, the patient is placed in the prone jackknife position following the induction of a regional anesthetic. Local anesthesia consisting of 0.5% lidocaine or 0.25% bupivacaine hydrochloride with 1:200,000 epinephrine is injected along the fistula tract for hemostasis following the insertion of an anal speculum. Use of bupivacaine provides analgesia of longer duration than most regional anesthetics. A probe is inserted from the external opening along the tract to the internal opening at the dentate line. The tissue overlying the probe is incised and the granulation tissue curetted and sent for pathologic evaluation. A gentle probe is used to identify any high blind tracts or extensions, which are unroofed, if found. If desired, the wound may be marsupialized on either edge by sewing the edges of the incision to the tract with a running locked absorbable suture. There is no need to insert packing if an adequate unroofing has been accomplished (Figure 13-14A–C).

Seton

The problem of preserving anal continence and treating the fistula is more complicated when managing high transsphincteric fistulas. If the tract is seen to cross the sphincter muscle at a high level, the use of the lay-open technique in combination with insertion of a seton is safer. A seton may be any foreign substance which can be inserted into the fistula tract to encircle the sphincter muscles. Materials commonly

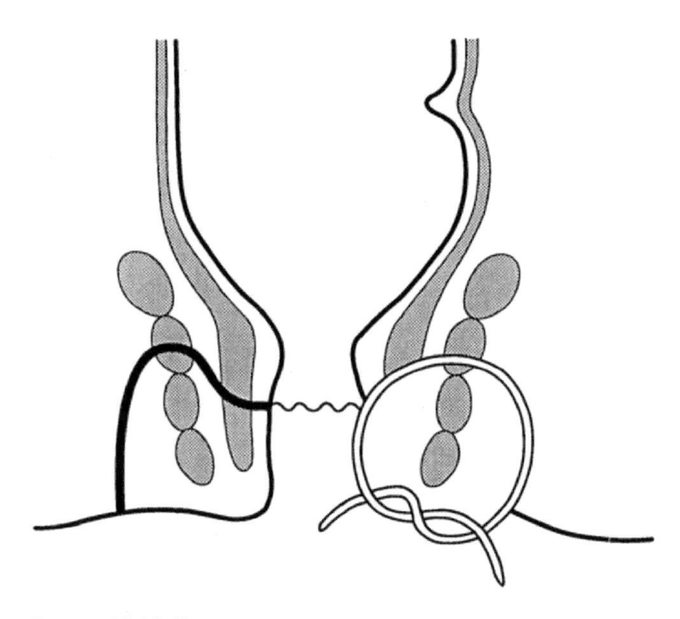

FIGURE 13-15. Seton.

employed include silk or other nonabsorbable suture material, penrose drains, rubber bands, vessel loops, and Silastic catheters.[18] The lower portion of the internal sphincter is divided along with the skin to reach the external opening and a nonabsorbable suture or elastic suture is inserted into the fistulous tract. The ends of the suture or elastic are tied with multiple knots to create a handle for manipulation (Figure 13-15). This form of seton, known as a cutting seton, is tightened at regular intervals to slowly cut through the sphincter. This allows the tract to become more superficial, converting a high fistula into a low one. The proximal fistulotomy subsequently heals by stimulating fibrosis behind it reestablishing continuity of the anorectal ring to prevent separation or retraction of the sphincter muscle at a second stage repair 8 weeks later when the remaining external sphincter is divided. The seton also allows delineation of the amount of remaining muscle thus enabling improved postoperative assessment by outlining the tract. A seton may also be used as a drain which is left loosely in place to facilitate prolonged drainage, thereby referred to as a draining seton. In the past, specific indications for seton use included:[60] (1) To identify and promote fibrosis around a complex anal fistula that encircles most or all of the sphincter mechanism; (2) To mark the site of a transsphincteric fistula in cases of massive anorectal sepsis where the normal anatomic landmarks have been distorted; (3) Anterior, high transsphincteric fistulas in women. Since the puborectalis is absent in this area and the external sphincter is quite tenuous, primary fistulotomy may result in incontinence; (4) The presence of a high transsphincteric fistula in a patient with AIDS in whom healing is known to be poor; (5) To avoid premature skin closure and formation of recurrent abscesses and promote long-term drainage in patients with Crohn's disease. In these patients, a Silastic catheter can be left in place for a prolonged period of time to promote epithelialization of the fistula tract or tracts; (6) When there is suspicion that primary fistulotomy results in incontinence such as in those patients with multiple simultaneous fistulas, patients who have undergone multiple prior sphincter operations, such as fistulotomy or internal sphincterotomy and in elderly patients with weakened sphincter muscles. A recent extensive literature search suggested that the use of cutting setons be abandoned because of high incontinence rates of 12% since ultimately they damage the sphincters.[61] This position was supported by the Association of Coloproctologists of Great Britain and Ireland (ACGBI) who recommended that a cutting seton be used only for low transsphincteric fistula or as the secondary treatment for a low transsphincteric fistula.[62]

Another option available to treat transsphincteric fistulas without division of muscle involves the use of a dermal island flap.[63] Division of muscle was able to be avoided in 90%, however, a 23% failure rate was reported. This was found to be more likely in males, patients who had previous treatment of their fistulas, patients with large fistulas requiring combined flaps and patients who underwent simultaneous fibrin glue injection.

Treatment of suprasphincteric fistulas requires an appreciation that the tract involves the entire external sphincter complex as well as the puborectalis muscle. Laying-open the entire tract would render the patient incontinent. Thus, several methods have been proposed to manage this fistula without the ensuing devastating consequences. The use of a seton has been advocated in combination with division of the internal sphincter and the superficial portion of the external sphincter to the external opening. The seton is placed around the remaining external sphincter as was previously described.[64]

A modification of this approach has been proposed by Kennedy and Zegarra[65] in which an internal sphincterotomy is performed, followed by opening of the tracts outside the external sphincter without division of any portion of the external sphincter which is encircled by a seton to promote fibrosis and assure adequate drainage. Complete healing using the latter approach has been reported in 66% with posterior fistulas and in 88% with anterior fistulas.[65] Parks[64] obtained healing in 63%. Another method that has been proposed to treat this type of fistula is the anorectal advancement flap which is described.

The horseshoe variety of the suprasphincteric fistula also presents the problem of complete sphincter involvement combined with the presence of multiple external openings a great distance from the cryptoglandular source. Treatment consists of identification of the internal opening and proper drainage of the postanal space as was previously described. The horseshoe extensions are enlarged for counter-drainage and the granulation tissue is curetted.

The treatment of an extrasphincteric fistula depends on its etiology. If the fistula arises secondary to an anal fistula, a secondary opening above the puborectalis is thought to be iatrogenic due to extensive probing of a transsphincteric fistula. The lower portion of the internal sphincter is divided and the rectal opening is closed with a nonabsorbable suture. A temporary colostomy may be necessary but a medical colostomy consisting of preoperative mechanical and antibiotic bowel preparation followed by enteral feeding may suffice. If the fistula is the result of entrance of a foreign body, it must be removed, drainage must be established, the internal opening closed and a temporary colostomy constructed to decrease rectal pressure. This type of fistula may also be a manifestation of Crohn's disease. Treatment depends on the nature of the anorectal mucosa and drainage may be assisted by the placement of a seton. Finally, the fistula may be the result of downward tracking of a pelvic abscess which must be drained so that the fistula can heal.

Figure 13-16A–D shows the anorectal advancement flap.

When the traditional laying-open technique may be inappropriate, for example, in anterior fistulas in women, in patients with inflammatory bowel disease, in patients with high transsphincteric and suprasphincteric fistulas as well as in those with previous multiple sphincter operations, multiple and complex fistulas, the use of an anorectal advancement flap has been advocated.[66] Advantages of this technique include a reduction in the duration of healing, reduced associated discomfort, lack of deformity to the anal canal as well as little potential additional damage to the sphincter muscles since no muscle is divided.[18]

Following full mechanical and antibiotic bowel preparation, the patient is placed in the prone jackknife of left lateral position. Under a regional or general anesthetic, following

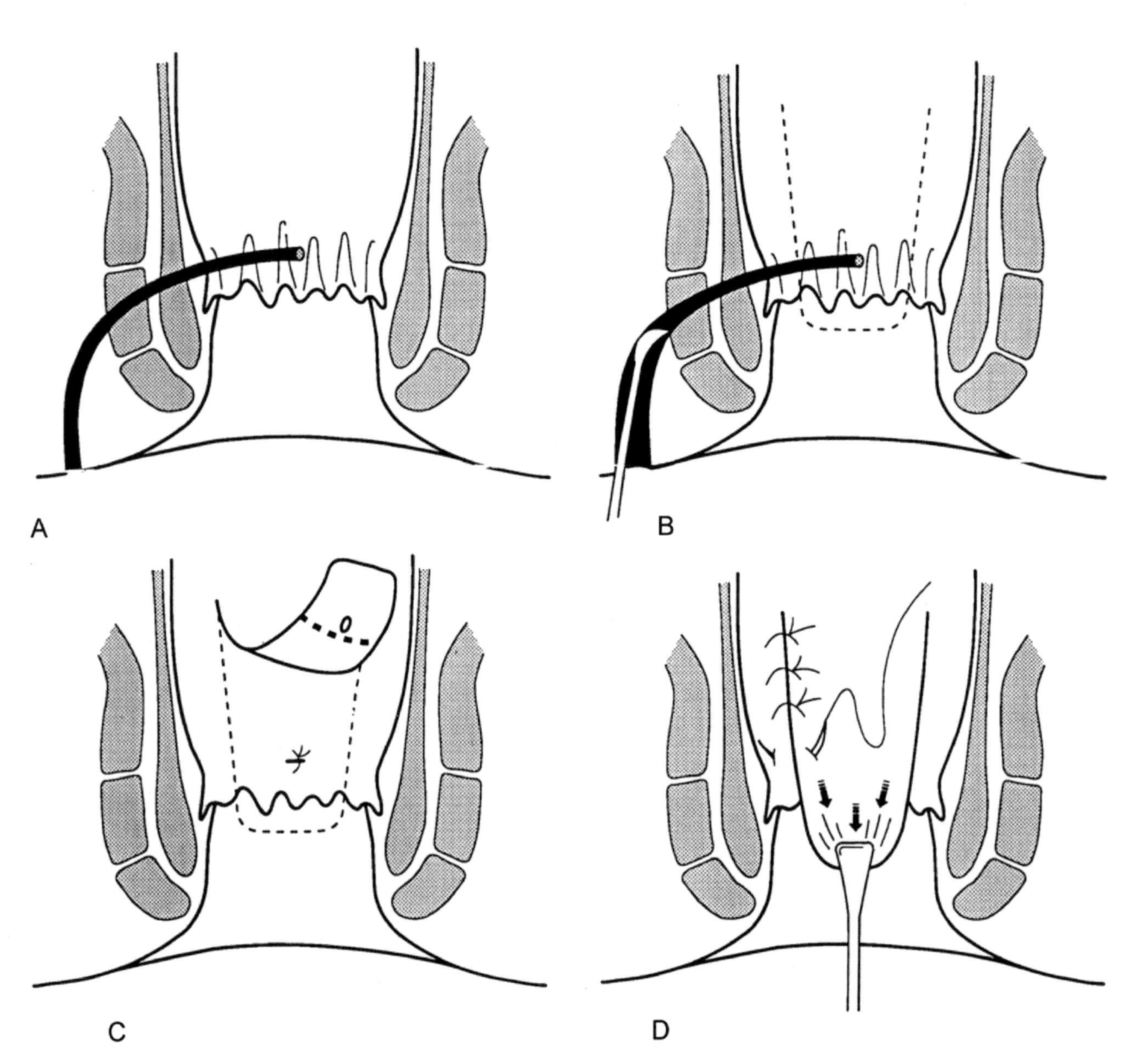

FIGURE 13-16. Anorectal advancement flap: **A** transsphincteric fistula-in-ano, **B** enlargement of external opening and curettage of granulation tissue, **C** mobilization of flap and closure of internal opening, **D** suturing of flap in place covering internal opening.

insertion of a Foley catheter, the fistula tract is identified with a probe and either cored out or curetted. The internal opening is identified and excised. The external opening is enlarged to allow for drainage. A full thickness flap of rectal mucosa, submucosa and part of the internal sphincter is raised. The residual internal opening is closed with absorbable suture. The flap is then advanced 1 cm below the internal opening. The tip of the flap containing the fistulous opening is excised and the flap is sewn into place with absorbable sutures ensuring that the mucosal and muscular suture lines do not overlap. The base of the flap should be twice the width of the apex to maintain good blood supply. Successful results have reported in over 90% of patients.[67] Factors associated with poor outcomes include Crohn's disease and steroids.[68] Cigarette smoking was found to be another significant variable in another study.[69]

Fistulectomy

Although excision of the fistula or fistulectomy was thought to be a satisfactory method of treatment of fistula-in-ano, its use is no longer recommended. Larger wounds are created significantly prolonging wound healing time.[70] A greater separation of muscle ends occurs[1] and there is greater risk of injuring or excising underlying muscle,[66] thereby increasing the risk of incontinence. Schouten and van Vroonhoven[14] have found that fistulectomy, whether primary or secondary, was associated with a clinically significant disturbance in anal function. In recent years, alternative therapies have been developed to avoid division of the sphincters but aimed to obliterate the fistula tract. These include fibrin glue and the anal fistula plug (AFP).

Fibrin Glue

The use of fibrin glue (Tisseel, Baxter Healthcare Corp, Deerfield, IL) as a primary treatment alone or in combination with an advancement flap was appealing since it is a simple, noninvasive approach that avoids the risk of incontinence associated with fistulotomy. In the case of failure, it may be repeated several times without jeopardizing continence. As with fistulotomy, the fistula tract along with its internal and external openings is identified and curetted (with currettes or flexible brushes). Fibrin glue is injected into the fistula tract through a Y connector so that the entire tract is filled and the glue can be seen emerging from the internal opening. The injecting catheter is slowly withdrawn so that the entire tract is filled. Petrolatum jelly gauze may be placed over the external opening.

Enthusiasm generated because of short-term success rates of 70–74%[71,72] has been tempered due to delayed fistula recurrence despite initial apparent healing.[73] With longer follow up, 60% of fistulas were found to have healed in a recent study although patients underwent a two-stage approach consisting of seton placement followed by glue injection at a second stage.[74] Patients who failed underwent

TABLE 13-3. Results with fibrin glue

Authors	Year	*n*	Success rate (%)
Cintron et al.[73]	2000	79	61
Sentovitch[74]	2003	48	70
Buchanan et al.[75]	2003	22	14
Zmora et al.[78]	2005	60	53
Johnson et al.[79]	2006	25	40
Adams et al.[80]	2008	17	94
Yeung et al.[81]	2010	12	42 (simple); 29 (complex)

repeat injection which allowed 69% to heal. The 29% who failed to heal underwent either fistulotomy or advancement flap. Late recurrences (6%) occurred more than 6 months postoperatively and were treated with reinjection. Buchanan et al.[75] found fibrin glue injection to be useful in 14% with complex anal fistulas without extensions.

Although the exact mechanisms responsible for failure have not been entirely appreciated, it has been suggested that curettage may not adequately remove all granulation or epithelialized tissue thus failing to provide the correct environment for the glue to work.[75] Other adverse factors shown to influence healing include the presence of a short tract which may make it easier for the fibrin glue plug to become dislodged as well as the presence of a cavity on endoanal ultrasound.[76] The latter was associated with a complication of perianal abscess since the tract may not have been entirely filled with glue.[77–81] Fibrin glue is associated with a low incontinence rate as well as a disappointing low cure rate. Results using fibrin glue are summarized in Table 13-3.[73–75,78–81]

Anal Fistula Plug

Recently, the use of a bioprosthetic plug made from lyophilized porcine intestinal submucosal has been described for the treatment of complex anal fistulas.[79] The Surgisis AFP™ (Cook Surgical Inc, Bloomington, IN), when implanted, is colonized by host tissue cells and blood vessels and thus provides a scaffold to allow infiltration of the patient's connective tissue. A consensus conference[82] defined the indications for the use of the plug in fistulous disease to include: (1) Transsphincteric fistula; (2) Intersphincteric fistula if conventional fistulotomy posed a risk of incontinence, such as in patients with inflammatory bowel disease; and (3) Extrasphincteric fistula. Contraindications for the use of the plug included: (1) Fistula with persistent abscess cavity; (2) Fistula with infection; (3) Allergy to porcine products; and (4) Inability to identify both the external and internal openings. The latter constitutes an absolute contraindication for the use of the plug. Following full mechanical bowel preparation or the use of a small volume enema along with a single preoperative dose of antibiotics, the patient is placed in the prone jackknife position. The internal and external openings must be clearly delineated. This can be accomplished by irrigation with saline or peroxide. Gentle passage of a probe is essential to confirm the position of the tract and facilitate insertion of the plug. Debridement or curettage of the tract should not be performed. A seton should always be used temporarily only if there is acute inflammation or drainage. The plug should be immersed in sterile saline for 2 min and thus rehydrated. A fistula probe is placed through the tract and a 2-0 suture is placed through the tapered end of the plug and the ends of this suture are attached to the fistula probe at the primary opening. The suture is pulled from the primary opening, through the fistula tract to exit at the secondary opening. For patients with a "horseshoe" fistula, an incision is made over the fistula tract distal to the anal verge to create a secondary opening that the ends of the suture are brought through. With gentle traction on the suture, the porcine plug is pulled into the primary opening of the fistula until "wrinkling" of the superficial layer of the plug is first seen. The plug is not forced tightly. Excess plug is removed by transecting the plug at the level of the primary opening. The plug is secured in the primary opening using a 2-0 absorbable suture placed in a "figure 8" fashion with the suture crossing through the center of the plug and incorporating a generous portion of the sphincter mechanism on both sides. Any plug protruding through the secondary opening is also excised. The distal end of the plug is not sutured to the fistula tract and the distal opening is left open for drainage. Patients are advised to avoid vigorous physical activity for 2 weeks after plug placement to minimize the chance of plug dislodgement. No dietary restrictions are necessary nor are topical antibiotics indicated.

The first prospective study comparing the AFP to fibrin glue in 25 patients with high transsphincteric or deeper fistulas found greater success rates with the plug (87% vs. 40%) at 3 months.[79] The authors concluded that closure of the primary opening of a fistula tract using a suturable biologic AFP is an effective method of treating anorectal fistulas. Although the technique has appeal for its simplicity and avoidance of sphincter injury, more recent reports, however, have tempered enthusiasm with success rates ranging from 13.9 to 87% (Table 13-4).[79,83–92] Dislodgement has been reported in 9 (41%) while sepsis requiring abscess drainage has been reported in 4 (29%) patients.[83–92]

TABLE 13-4. Results with anal Anal Fistula Plug™

Authors	Year	# Healed	% Healed
Johnson et al.[79]	2006	12/15	87
Champagne et al.[83]	2006	38/46	83
Ellis[84]	2007	16/18	88
Schwandner et al.[85]	2007	37/60	62
van Koperen et al.[86]	2007	7/17	41
Lawes et al.[87]	2008	4/17	24
Garg[88]	2008	15/21	71
Thekkinkottil and Botterill[89]	2009	20/45	44
Christoforidis et al.[90]	2008	12/37	32
Safar et al.[91]	2009	5/36	13.9
Ortiz et al.[92]	2009	3/15	20

Ligation of the Intersphincteric Fistula Tract Procedure

Recently, a new sphincter-sparing technique has been introduced [ligation of the intersphincteric fistula tract (LIFT)].[93] The LIFT technique is based on the secure closure of the internal opening and removal of the infected cryptoglandular tissue in the intersphincteric space. The only patients not suitable are those with early fistulous abscess in which the intersphincteric tract is not well formed.

Technique

Patients undergo mechanical bowel preparation and are placed in the prone jackknife position. A Fansler anoscope is inserted into the anal canal and

1. Internal opening is identified.
2. 1.5–2.0 cm curvilinear incision is made at the intersphincteric groove overlying the fistula tract.
3. Cautery is used to dissect into the intersphincteric plane staying close to the external sphincter avoiding cutting through the internal sphincter and breaching anal mucosa.
4. Internal and external sphincters are retracted. The intersphincteric tract is dissected and ligated next to the internal opening with a 3-0 absorbable suture.
5. Tract next to the suture is ligated.
6. Tract excision is confirmed by injection or probing of the external opening.
7. Granulation tissue is curetted.
8. The external opening is sutured through the intersphincteric wound.
9. Incision is closed with 3-0 absorbable suture.

Postoperatively wounds are cleansed with tap water twice a day and following bowel movements. Patients are given 2 weeks of Ciprofloxacillin and Metronidazole.

A pitfall with this technique may be the intersphincteric approach for high tracts especially with horseshoe tracts. Also exposure of the intersphincteric space may damage the internal sphincter.

Although there are only a few reports in the literature, success rates of 58–94% have been reported.[93,94] In addition, time to failure has ranged from 4 to 64 weeks with a median of 19 weeks.[93,94]

New Biologic Injectables

Recently, new options in viable alternative treatments have been promoted experimentally. These include the injection of human acellular dermal matrix, a biologic plug consisting of dermis without cellular components.[95] The graft serves as a scaffold that allows native cellular ingrowth and remodeling. A healing rate at 6 months was 86%, however, failures were observed with longer follow-up of 3–6 months.

Permacol Injection™ (Covidien, Mansfield, MA) is a suspension of cross-linked porcine dermal collagen matrix in saline. It is readily colonized by host tissue cells and blood vessels, minimizing infection. Although initially evaluated in a porcine model, there is one case report documenting its success in fistula healing.[96] It is a liquid injected into the fistula tract and all around the fistula. This may prove to be an effective first-line nonoperative procedure which remains to be evaluated in large trials.

Postoperative Care

Following the lay-open technique, patients are placed on regular diets, bulk agents and noncodeine-containing analgesia. Patients are instructed to take frequent sitz baths to ensure perianal hygiene. Patients are evaluated at 2-week intervals to ensure that healing has occurred from the depths of the tract. Granulation tissue can be cauterized using silver nitrate sticks and cotton-tipped swabs are often used to probe the depths of the incision to ensure that adequate healing is occurring. Following the advancement flap technique, the Foley catheter is removed on the following day. Patients are discharged as soon as they can tolerate a diet.

Complications

Incontinence

Incontinence following fistulotomy depends both on the amount of muscle divided at operation as well as on preexisting sphincter damage and scarring of the anal canal.

Minor disorders of continence following fistulotomy have been reported to range from 18 to 52% while soiling and insufficiency have been reported in as many as 35–45% (Table 13-5).[97,98,100–104] The occurrence of continence disorders has been found to be related to the complexity of the fistula and to the level and location of the internal opening.[97]

Patients with complicated fistulas, high openings, posterior openings, and fistula extensions have been found to be at higher risk.[97] In the treatment of complicated fistulas and those with high openings, more muscle is divided thus decreasing anal pressures while posterior fistula wounds have been associated with higher rates of incontinence because of their more circuitous routes.[97] Drainage of extensions may accidentally damage small nerves and create more scar tissue around the anorectum.[97] If the edges of the fisulotomy wound do not approximate precisely, the anus may be unable to properly close, resulting in intermittent leakage of gas and stool.[61] In addition to these factors, impaired continence was associated with increasing age[97] and female gender.[97,98] The latter is probably the result of partial anal sphincter disruption and/or traction injury to the pudendal nerves sustained during vaginal delivery.[98]

Although excellent results employing a seton have been reported,[105] its use does not protect against the development of impaired continence.[99] Minor continence disorders were reported in 73%,[99] while Williams et al.[106] reported minor disturbances in 54%. Parks and Stitz[64] found that minor incontinence occurred in 39% with the two-stage approach versus 17% when only the first stage was performed and the seton was removed rather than dividing the muscle. Major fecal incontinence was reported in 6.7%[60] after a review of several series (Table 13-6).[60,99,100,105–109] The degree of incontinence is thought to be influenced by the patient's preoperative state of control as well as to how the anal wound heals.[61] Analysis of data compiled in a recent literature search found that a 12% rate of incontinence with the rate increasing as the location of the internal opening moved more proximally.[62] Excellent results with respect to continence have been reported with the use of the advancement flap[69] although recent reports have observed disturbances in continence in 9–35%,[110,111] attributed to over-stretching of the sphincters by self-retaining retractors. Disruption of the internal sphincter also occurs if some internal sphincter fibers are developed with the flap.[112]

As would be expected, continence is unaffected with the use of fibrin glue and the fistula plug. In a study that looked at changes in anorectal morphologic and functional parameters after fistula surgery, it was found that fistulotomy and advancement flaps were most associated with changes in internal anal sphincter defects with decreased resting and squeeze pressure on manometry noted after fistulotomy while rectal advancement flaps were associated with decrease in resting pressure.[113] It therefore behooves the surgeon to recognize preexisting sphincter defects by endoanal ultrasound prior to embarking on fistula surgery.[113]

TABLE 13-5. Results of fistula surgery

Authors	Year	#Patients	% Recurrence	% Incontinence
Marks and Ritchie[97]	1977	793	–	3, 17, 25[a]
Vasilevsky and Gordon[98]	1985	160	6.3	0.7, 2.0, 3.3[b]
Van Tets and Kuijpers[99]	1994	19	–	33.0
Sangwan[98]	1994	461	6.5	2.8
Garcia-Aguilar et al.[100]	1996	293	7.0	42.0
Mylonakis et al.[101]	2001	100	3.0	6.0, 3.0[c]
Malouf et al.[102]	2002	98	4.0	10
Westerterp et al.[103]	2003	60	0	50

[a] 3% solid stool, 17% liquid stool, 25% flatus.
[b] 0.7% solid stool, 2.0% liquid stool, 3.3% flatus.
[c] 0 solid stool, 6.0% soiling, 3,0% gas.

TABLE 13-6. Results of staged fistulotomy using a seton

Authors	Year	Recurrence (%)	Incontinence (%)
Ramanujam et al.[105]	1983	1/45 (2)	1/45 (2)
Fasth et al.[107]	1990	0/7 (0)	0/7 (0)
Williams et al.[106]	1991	2/28 (8)	1/24 (4)
Pearl et al.[60]	1993	3/116 (3)	5/116 (5)
Van Tets and Kuijpers[99]	1994	–	15/29 (54)
Graf et al.[108]	1995	2/25 (8)	11/25 (44)
Garcia-Aguilar et al.[100]	1996	6/63 (9)	39/61(64)
Hasegawa et al.[109]	2000	8/32 (25)	15/32 (4.8)

Recurrence

Recurrence rates following fistulotomy range from 0 to 18%.[97] Causes include failure to identify a primary opening or recognize lateral or upward extensions of a fistula.[98,104] Inability to locate the primary opening may imply a circuitous tract, spontaneous closure of the primary opening or a microscopic opening.[104] The presence of secondary tracts[98] which can be easily missed accounted for early recurrence in 20%.[104] Premature closure of the fistulotomy wound can be obviated by producing an external wound twice the size of the anal wound resulting in proper healing of the internal wound prior to the external wound.[98] Diligent postoperative care can also reduce recurrence rates by avoiding bridging and pocketing of the wound.[114] Epithelialization of the fistula tract from internal or external openings rather than chronic infection of an anal gland has also been suggested as the cause of a persistent anal fistula.[115]

Recurrence rates following staged repairs utilizing a seton range from 0 to 29%.[59]

Although recurrence rates following anorectal advancement flaps were initially reported to be low, with long-term follow-up, recurrence rates of 40% have been reported.[111] Recurrence can be minimized provided that care has been taken to avoid necrosis or retraction of the flap. The use of full-thickness rectal wall has been advocated to prevent ischemic necrosis of the flap.[116]

Early postoperative complications that have been reported following fistula surgery include urinary retention, hemorrhage, fecal impaction, and thrombosed external hemorrhoids which were found to occur in less than 6% of cases.[19] Late complications, such as pain, bleeding, pruritus, and poor wound healing have been reported in 9% of patients.[66] Anal stenosis may occur and is usually the result of loose stools allowing healing of the anal canal by scar contracture.[40] Mucosal prolapse due to extensive division of sphincter muscle may also occur and can be treated by band ligation, sclerosis, or excision.[66] With attention to both operative detail and postoperative follow-up, these complications can be reduced to a minimum.

Special Considerations

Crohn's Disease

Anal fistulas are the most difficult and challenging complication of Crohn's disease to manage. They constitute the most common perianal manifestations, occurring in 6–34% of patients.[117] The location of Crohn's disease in the bowel has an impact on the frequency of fistulas. Patients with colonic Crohn's have a higher incidence with the rate approaching 100% in those with rectal Crohn's.[118]

As discussed previously, patients with Crohn's disease should undergo sigmoidoscopy, colonoscopy, and small bowel follow through to determine the extent of disease. Delineation of the fistulous tract is especially important in Crohn's disease since many fistulas may be complex in nature. In this context, endoanal ultrasound has been found to be as useful as MRI. MRI has been found to detect abscesses that were clinically unsuspected on clinical exam and has been helpful in determining the relationship of the fistulous tract to the sphincter muscles.[119]

Therapeutic goals in managing anorectal fistulas in Crohn's disease remain the alleviation of symptoms and preservation of continence. Surgical treatment of fistulas is associated with poor and delayed wound healing and with the risk of sphincter injury. Alexander-Williams[120] stated that, "Incontinence is likely to be the result of aggressive surgeons, not of aggressive disease." A conservative approach has therefore been advocated, especially since 38% of such fistulas have been reported to heal spontaneously without any surgical intervention. Medications used in the treatment of fistulas include antibiotics such as metronidazole and ciprofloxacin and immunomodulators such as corticosteroids, 6 mercaptopurine (MP), azathioprine, and infliximab. Although several studies have reported spontaneous closure of fistulas in 34–50% of patients treated with metronidazole, improvement is usually seen after 6–8 weeks of treatment with relapses common once the medication is discontinued.[118] A recent placebo-controlled trial comparing a 10-week course of metronidazole, ciprofloxacillin, and placebo in patients with perianal Crohn's disease found a 40% response in the ciprofloxacillin group compared to 14.3% in the metronidazole group and 12.5% in the placebo group. These differences, however, were not significant.[121] In another study, 6MP and azathioprine were found to be efficacious in only one third of patients with fistulizing perianal disease.[122] These effects seemed unrelated to their effects on intestinal disease. The authors concluded that their results did not support the use of these medications solely for the improvement of perianal disease. The use of infliximab has been associated with a 62% reduction in draining fistulas.[123] The combination of infliximab and 6MP may prolong the effect of initial infliximab treatment on fistula closure.[124] Selective seton placement combined with infusion of infliximab and maintenance therapy with azathioprine or methotrexate resulted in complete healing in 67% with Crohn's fistulas in a recently reported retrospective study.[125] Maintenance therapy with infliximab has been reported to result in the absence of draining fistulas in 36% of patients compared to 19% in placebo patients at 54-week follow-up.[126]

Although fistulas may occur in as many as 73% of patients after previous abscess drainage, it is imperative that primary fistulotomy not be performed because of the high risk of creating false passages and injuring the sphincter mechanism.[117] Asymptomatic fistulas require no treatment. Low fistulas with simple tracts can be managed with the standard lay-open method in the absence of active proctitis. Successful outcome as gauged by healing has been reported to occur in 42–100%, mostly in the 70–80% range of procedures.[127]

Fistulotomy has been associated with prolonged healing.[128] Factors associated with delayed healing are rectal involvement;[12,100] anorectal complications, especially strictures;[129] and the presence or absence of an internal opening.[129] Successful healing has occurred in patients with a classic internal opening at the dentate line and in those without rectal involvement[129] although Halme and Sainio[128] found that delayed healing occurred in 80% of patients despite the presence of a normal rectum and Van Dongen and Lubbers[130] found no difference in healing even in the presence of rectal involvement. Nonetheless, initial therapy should be directed at resolving inflammation in the rectum. This can be accomplished with the use of topical steroid or 5-acetylsalycylic enemas or suppositories. In addition, oral medication may be necessary.

Incontinence has been reported in patients with proctitis who have not undergone anal surgery.[130] A patient with severe rectal involvement and even a simple low fistula is not a candidate for fistulotomy. Division of any sphincter muscle in this situation may result in frank incontinence because the noncompliant rectum acts as a conduit rather than as a reservoir. Continence problems have been reported in 25% of patients after simple incision and drainage of abscesses during which the sphincter mechanism has not been touched.[130] Allan and Keighley[131] reported a 50% frequency of major fecal incontinence and minor incontinence has been described in 33% of patients who have undergone only simple drainage or local surgery.[128] It is thought that diarrhea from either associated intestinal involvement or multiple previous small bowel resections is important in control disorders in these patients.[117,128,130] Appropriate medical therapy should be employed to control the diarrhea.

Complex fistulas with high rectal openings might best be managed conservatively because impaired continence may certainly result if the sphincter muscle is divided. Eradication of the fistula in this situation may not be possible because of the complexity of the tracts. Seton placement has been advocated to promote drainage, limit recurrent suppuration, and preserve sphincter function.[132] Rectal advancement flaps have been used in the absence of severe rectal disease.[133] These have been found to succeed in patients without concomitant small bowel Crohn's.[134]

The importance of quiescent intestinal disease for successful outcome of local fistula surgery has been suggested, but not generally accepted and practical. Proximal fecal diversion has also been suggested as an option to ameliorate severe perianal disease since diversion of the fecal stream may reduce perianal inflammation.[135] However, improvement is temporary because fistulas reactivate following restoration of intestinal continuity.[14]

Complicated fistulas are more likely to recur due to the reluctance of the surgeon to divide sphincter muscle. The use of a long-term in-dwelling seton as a drain is therefore recommended.[132] Fistula recurrence may be as high a 39% following the removal of the seton and may necessitate the use of concomitant medical therapy.[117] The use of a rectal advancement flap has been successful; however, breakdown is possible because of sepsis.[133] In patients with mild proctitis, a 20% success rate has been reported.[133] The presence of a protective stoma in this situation does not guarantee success, with failure reported in 55% of patients.[133] A covering stoma may be beneficial in the patient who has undergone multiple unsuccessful repairs.[115]

Disappointing results with standard treatment of anal fistulas has led to the use of noninvasive procedures, such as the fibrin glue and the AFP™ in the armamentarium of treating fistulous Crohn's disease.[136,137] A closure rate of 60% has been reported in one study with the use of fibrin glue. This may also be combined with an endorectal advancement flap in the absence of rectal involvement. Excellent short-term success rates of 77–83% have also been associated with the use of the AFP without alteration in continence.[83,138] Many fistulas may require repeat fistulotomy to achieve complete healing or repeat injections of fibrin glue or repeated use of the plug.[128]

A novel approach reported on recently is the use of mesenchymal adipose stem cells used to stimulate fistula closure.[139] In a randomized controlled trial comparing adipose-derived stem cells and fibrin glue to fibrin glue alone, the fistula closed in 71% in the stem cell group compared to 16% in the fibrin glue group.[138] For severe intractable disease, an intersphincteric proctectomy may ultimately become necessary. The intersphincteric technique reduces the size of the resulting wound and reduces the incidence of unhealed sinuses.

Fistula-in-ano in the HIV Positive Patient

Anal fistulas are prevalent in the anoreceptive HIV positive individual.[140] Disturbed locoregional defenses may allow infection to occur.[141] Although anal fistulas in HIV positive patients arise from the dentate line similar to those in HIV negative patients, they are more likely to have incomplete anal fistulas leading to blind sinus tracts.[142] Concern for wound healing has tempered enthusiasm for operative intervention. However, selective operative management results in a high rate of complete or partial wound healing with symptomatic relief without excessive morbidity or mortality.[142] Severity of illness must be assessed prior to operative intervention since patients with more advanced disease are less likely to heal their wounds. Data are conflicting as to whether preoperative CD4+ lymphocyte counts can be related to poor wound healing,[142] however, Consten[31] found that low CD4+ lymphocyte counts in patients with perianal sepsis were a risk factor for disturbed wound healing. Use of Highly Active Antiviral Therapy (HAART) may reduce the incidence of opportunistic infections and anorectal disease and aid healing.[142]

Asymptomatic fistulas require no treatment. Perioperative antibiotic therapy over a 5-day course has been recommended because of the high risk of infectious complications.[142] Care should be exercised to avoid creation of large wounds and to preserve as much sphincter muscle as possible since these patients may be prone to diarrhea which may overwhelm a partially divided sphincter.[142] In patients who are good operative risks, fistulotomy is appropriate in patients with intersphincteric or low transsphincteric fistulas. For high or complex fistulas as well as for those patients who are poor operative risks, liberal use of draining setons is recommended.[40,142] It is important to realize that cellulitis may be seen with a fistula without concomitant underlying exudates.[142] Metastatic abscesses to other organs, including brain, liver, and mediastinum have been reported with asymptomatic perianal fistulas.[31] Healing has been reported in 55–80% of patients.[36,142]

Mucinous Adenocarcinoma Arising from a Fistula-in-ano

Mucinous adenocarcinoma carcinoma arising from an anal fistula is an extremely rare entity with a handful of cases having been reported in the literature.[143,144] It is associated with a longstanding fistula-in-ano and the chronic inflammatory changes associated with it. Diagnostic criteria include: (1) The fistula should antedate the carcinoma by 10 years; (2) The only tumor present should be secondary to direct extension from the carcinoma into the fistula; (3) The internal opening should be in the anal canal and not into the tumor itself.[145]

Early diagnosis is difficult since the lesion may be obscured within the ischioanal fossa or perineum. Patients do not have bleeding and digital exam may only reveal induration at the site of the fistula. MRI is the most helpful diagnostic tool with several characteristics having been identified. These include pools of extracellular mucin lined by columns of malignant cells, cords, and vessels which produce a mesh-like structure[146] and the presence of a fistula between the mass and the anus.[147] Management has traditionally consisted of abdominoperineal resection; however, more recently improved survival rates have been reported from combined pre- and postoperative chemoradiation or from chemoradiation alone, reserving abdominoperineal resection as a salvage procedure.[147]

Rectourethral Fistulas

Pathophysiology

Rectourethral fistulas are rare but devastating complications that may occur following radical open or laparoscopic prostatectomy, radiation treatment for prostate cancer, trauma, and recurrent perineal abscess of cryptoglandular origin or due to Crohn's disease or following treatment with radiofrequency hyperthermia for benign prostatic hypertrophy. The prostatic urethra is the most common site for fistulization to occur since this portion of the urethra is adjacent to the rectal wall.

Evaluation and Treatment

Symptoms

The most common symptoms include leakage of urine through the rectum during voiding, pneumaturia, and fecaluria. These symptoms tend to occur during the early postoperative period following prostatectomy. In addition, recurrent urinary tract infections resistant to antibiotic treatment following one of the aforementioned causes should suggest this diagnosis.

Investigations

PSA determination should be done to rule out recurrence of carcinoma. Digital rectal examination should always be performed to determine if there is any anorectal pathology that could be the cause. Sigmoidoscopy shows the fistula opening which is located on the anterior rectal wall and in addition rule out rectal pathology as a source. Cystoscopy and retrograde urethral cystography should be performed to determine the presence of a urethral stricture. Assessment of urinary continence should be done prior to any attempt at surgical repair.

Operative Treatment

Operative repair of rectourethral fistulas is challenging due to technical difficulties that are often encountered due to difficult exposure. Multiple repairs have been developed but there is no consensus as to which is best. Traditionally, it has been suggested that the first attempt at repair is the best and that subsequent repairs become more difficult.[148]

Rectal injury during laparoscopic radical prostatectomy may be repaired laparoscopically.[149] Most importantly, they must be recognized at the time of injury. Small fistulas can be managed conservatively with an indwelling foley catheter.[150] Treatment consisting of fecal diversion with either colostomy or ileostomy and urinary diversion with suprapubic catheterization under cover of antibiotics has been described in the management of rectourethral fistulas secondary to radiation when the urethral defect has been found to be too large to repair. This has been associated with bouts of recurrent sepsis and persistent symptoms.[150]

Transabdominal Approach

The transabdominal approach combines the use of abdominoanal pullthrough in combination with omental interposition.

Difficulties with this procedure include limited exposure deep in the male pelvis making closure of the urethral defect very difficult. A fenestrated splinting catheter apposed to the omentum has been used when leaving the prostatic defect open. Complications associated with this approach include impotence and urethral stricture.[151]

Perineal Approach

Perineal approaches using the gracilis muscle, dartos, or Martius flap have all been described. The most popular and easiest involves the use of a rotation flap of the gracilis muscle due to its ease of mobilization and its sufficient length. Several principles important for repair include excision of the fistula, development of layers on the urinary and rectal sides of the fistula and closure of nonoverlapping suture lines with interposition of the levators, when possible. Placement of the gracilis muscle between the rectum and the urethra provides well-vascularized tissue as an interface between these two surfaces allowing healing to occur. Several studies have documented from 97 to 100% success rates with the employment of the gracilis interposition.[152–154] Complications with this procedure include urinary incontinence and stricture as well as complications associated with the muscle harvest.

Anterior Transanorectal Approach

In this approach, a midline perineal incision is deepened by incising all structures superficial to the prostatic capsule which include the superficial perineal fascia, the central tendon of the perineum and the internal and external sphincters.[154] This approach allows better access in the repair of complicated membranoprostatic fistulas with the preservation of continence and erectile function.

Peranal Approach

This approach has the theoretical advantages of minimal scarring and fewer wound infections although it suffers from limited exposure. Initially described by Parks and Motson,[155] it involves the use of a full thickness advancement of anterior rectal wall protected by diverting colosotomy. Success rates of 83% have recently been reported when combined with fecal diversion, urinary diversion, both, or none at all.[155] Success rates have been found to be higher when the flap was done for fistulas secondary to iatrogenic causes or trauma as opposed to Crohn's disease.[155] Advancement flap repair can be achieved with minimal morbidity and good postoperative quality of life without compromise to future interventions if needed.

Kraske Laterosacral Approach

This approach provides excellent exposure without division of the sphincter mechanism. The need to excise two to three sacral segments as well as the nerves, muscles, and ligaments around them pose a disadvantage.[156]

York Mason (Transsphincteric) Approach

This approach affords a rapid, bloodless exposure through fresh territory and allows for complete separation of the urinary and fecal streams. It avoids the neurovascular bundles and pelvic floor structures essential in maintaining continence and sexual function. It may be performed in combination with a diverting colostomy or a so-called medical colostomy consisting of mechanical preparation and postoperative elemental diet.

It has been associated with longer operative times and more postoperative pain than the other procedures mentioned but has a reported 100% success rate.[157]

Transanal Endoscopic Microsurgery

This highly specialized technique allows for a meticulous two-layer closure of the rectal wall and may be combined with transurethral fulguration of the opposite urethral opening of the fistula.[158] There has been no reported morbidity associated with this procedure although experience is very limited.

Cystectomy and Ileal Conduit

Cystectomy and ileal conduit may be considered for those patients with a low probability of success in resolving the fistula or in maintenance of urinary continence.[148]

References

1. Gordon PH. Anorectal abscess and fistula-in-ano. In: Gordon PH, Nivatvongs S, editors. Principles and practice of surgery for the colon, rectum and anus. St. Louis: Quality Medical Publishing; 1999. p. 241–86.
2. Seow-Choen F, Ho JMS. Histoanatomy of anal glands. Dis Colon Rectum. 1994;37:1215–8.
3. Parks AG. Pathogenesis and treatment of fistula-in-ano. Br Med J. 1961;1:463–9.
4. Goldberg SM, Gordon PH, Nivatvongs S. Essentials of anorectal surgery. Philadelphia: JB Lippincott; 1980. p. 100–27.
5. Abcarian H. Surgical management of recurrent anorectal abscess. Contemp Surg. 1982;21:85–91.
6. Whiteford MH, Kilkenny 3rd J, Hyman N, Buie WD, et al. Practice parameters for the treatment of perianal abscess and fistula-in-ano (revised). Dis Colon Rectum. 2005;48(7): 1337–42.
7. Rosen SA, Coloquhoun P, Efron J, et al. Horseshoe abscesses and fistulas: how are we doing? Surg Innov. 2006;13:17–21.
8. Beck DE, Fazio VW, Lavery IC, et al. Catheter drainage of ischiorectal abscesses. South Med J. 1988;81:444–6.
9. Quah HM, Tang CL, Eu KW. Meta-analysis of randomized controlled trials comparing drainage alone vs. drainage and fistulotomy for acute perianal abscesses with proven internal opening. Int J Colorectal Dis. 2005;30:1–8.
10. Vasilevsky CA, Gordon PH. The incidence of recurrent abscesses or fistula-in-ano following anorectal suppuration. Dis Colon Rectum. 1984;27:126–30.
11. Scoma JA, Salvati EP, Rubin RJ. Incidence of fistulas subsequent to anal abscesses. Dis Colon Rectum. 1974;17:357–9.

12. Read DR, Abcarian H. A prospective survey of 474 patients with anorectal abscess. Dis Colon Rectum. 1979;22:566–9.
13. Hamadani A, Haigh PI, Lio IL. Who is at risk for developing chronic anal fistula or recurrent anal sepsis after initial perianal abscess? Dis Colon Rectum. 2009;52:217–21.
14. Tang C-L, Chew S-P, Seow-Choen F. Prospective randomized trial of drainage alone vs. drainage and fistulotomy for acute perianal abscesses with proven internal opening. Dis Colon Rectum. 1996;39:1415–7.
15. Schouten WR, van Vroonhoven TMJV. Treatment of anorectal abscesses with or without primary fistulectomy: results of a prospective randomized trial. Dis Colon Rectum. 1991;34:60–3.
16. Buchan R, Grace RH. Anorectal suppuration: the results of treatment and factors influencing the recurrence rate. Br J Surg. 1973;60:537–40.
17. Chrabot CM, Prasad ML, Abcarian H. Recurrent anorectal abscesses. Dis Colon Rectum. 1984;27:126–30.
18. Seow-Choen F, Nicholls RJ. Anal fistula. Br J Surg. 1992;79:197–205.
19. Mazier WP. The treatment and care of anal fistulas: a study of 1000 patients. Dis Colon Rectum. 1971;14:134–44.
20. Huber Jr P, Kissack AS, Simonton ST. Necrotizing soft tissue infection from rectal abscess. Dis Colon Rectum. 1983;26:507–11.
21. Bubrick MP, Hitchcock CR. Necrotizing anorectal and perineal infections. Surgery. 1979;86:655–62.
22. Laucks SS. Fournier's gangrene in anorectal surgery. Surg Clin North Am. 1994;74:1339–52.
23. Yague-Romeo D, Angulo Hervas E, Bernai L. Fournier's gangrene in a 44 year old woman. CT scan findings. Arch Exp Urol. 2009;62:483–5.
24. Kara E, Muezzinoglu T, Temellas G. Evaluation of risk factors and severity of a life threatening surgical emergency: Fournier's gangrene (a report of 15 cases). Acta Chir Belg. 2009;109:191–7.
25. Kovalcik P, Jones J. Necrotizing perineal infections. Am Surg. 1983;49:163–6.
26. Abcarian H, Eftaiha M. Floating free-standing anus. A complication of massive anorectal infection. Dis Colon Rectum. 1983;26:516–21.
27. Cuccia G, Mucciardi G, Morgia G. Vacuum-assisted closure for treatment of Fournier's gangrene. Urol Int. 2009;82:426–31.
28. Bode WE, Ramos R, Page CP. Invasive necrotizing infection secondary to anorectal abscess. Dis Colon Rectum. 1982;25:416–9.
29. Lucca M, Unger H, Devenny A. Treatment of Fournier's gangrene with adjunctive hyperbaric oxygen therapy. Am J Emerg Med. 1990;8:385–7.
30. Kabay S, Yucel M, Yaylak F. The clinical features of Fournier's gangrene and the predictability of the Fournier's Gangrene Severity Index on the outcomes. Int Urol Nephrol. 2008;40:997–1004.
31. Barnes SG, Sattler FR, Ballard JO. Perirectal infections in acute leukemia. Improved survival after incision and debridement. Ann Intern Med. 1984;100:515–6.
32. Vanheuverzwyn R, Delannoy A, Michaux JL, Dive C. Anal lesions in hematologic diseases. Dis Colon Rectum. 1980;23:310–2.
33. Glenn J, Cotton D, Wesley R, Pizzo P. Anorectal infections in patients with malignant diseases. Rev Infect Dis. 1988;10:42–52.
34. Sehdev MK, Daviing MD, Seal SH, Stearns MW. Perianal and anorectal complications in leukemia. Cancer. 1973;31:149–52.
35. Levi JA, Schempff SC, Slawson RC, Wiernik PH. Evaluation of radiotherapy for localized inflammatory skin and perianal lesion in adult leukemia: a prospectively randomized double-blind study. Cancer Treat Rep. 1977;61:1301–5.
36. Consten CJ, Siors FJM, Noten HJ, et al. Anorectal surgery in human immunodeficiency virus-infected patients. Dis Colon Rectum. 1995;38:1169–75.
37. Sim A. Anorectal infection in HIV infection and AIDS: diagnosis and management. Baillières Clin Gastroenterol. 1992;6:95–103.
38. Miles AJG, Mellor CH, Gazzard B, et al. Surgical management of anorectal disease in HIV-positive homosexuals. Br J Surg. 1990;77:869–71.
39. Parks AG, Gordon PH, Hardcastle JD. A classification of fistula-in-ano. Br J Surg. 1976;63:1–12.
40. Wexner SD, Rosen L, Roberts PL, et al. Practice parameters for treatment of fistula-in-ano-supporting documentation. Dis Colon Rectum. 1996;39:1363–72.
41. Cirocco WC, Reilly JC. Challenging the predictive accuracy of Goodsall's rule for anal fistulas. Dis Colon Rectum. 1992;35:537–42.
42. Sainio P, Husa A. A prospective manometric study of the effect of anal fistula surgery on anorectal function. Acta Chir Scand. 1985;151:279–88.
43. Weisman RI, Orsay CP, Pearl RK, Abcarian H. The role of fistulography in fistula-in-ano. Report of five cases. Dis Colon Rectum. 1991;34:181–4.
44. Kuijpers HC, Schulpen T. Fistulography for fistula-in-ano: is it useful? Dis Colon Rectum. 1985;28:103–4.
45. Cataldo P, Senagore J, Luchtefeld MA, et al. Intrarectal ultrasound in the evaluation of perirectal abscesses. Dis Colon Rectum. 1993;36:554–8.
46. Seow-Choen F, Burnett S, Bartram CI, Nicholls RJ. Comparison between anal endosonography and digital examination in the evaluation of anal fistulas. Br J Surg. 1991;78:445–7.
47. Lengyel AJ, Hurst NG, William JG. Preoperative assessment of anal fistulas using endoanal ultrasound. Colorectal Dis. 2002;4:436–40.
48. Chew SSB, Yang JL, Newstead GL, et al. Anal fistula: Levovist™ – enhanced endoanal ultrasound. A pilot study. Dis Colon Rectum. 2003;46:377–84.
49. Tepes B. The use of different diagnostic modalities in diagnosing fistula-in-ano. Hepatogastroenterology. 2009;54:912–5.
50. Toyonaga TI, Tajaka Y, Sing JF. Comparison of accuracy of physical examination and endoanal endosonography for preoperative assessment in patients with acute and chronic anal fistula. Tech Coloproctol. 2008;12:217–23.
51. Rafal RB, Nicholls JN, Cennerazzo WJ, et al. MRI for evaluation of perianal inflammation. Abdom Imaging. 1995;20:248–52.
52. Barker PG, Lunniss PJ, Armstrong P, et al. Magnetic resonance imaging of fistula-in-ano: technique, interpretation and accuracy. Clin Radiol. 1994;49:7–13.

53. Myhr GE, Myrvold HE, Nilsen G, et al. Perianal fistulas: use of MR imaging for diagnosis. Radiology. 1994;191:545–9.
54. Stoker J, Hussain SM, van Kempen D, et al. Endoanal coil in MR imaging of anal fistulas. AJR Am J Roentgenol. 1996;166:360–2.
55. West RL, Zimmerman DE, Dwarkasing S, et al. Prospective comparison of hydrogen peroxide 3-dimensional endoanal ultrasonography and endoanal magnetic resonance imaging of perianal fistulas. Dis Colon Rectum. 2003;46:1407–15.
56. Halligan S, Bartram CI. MR imaging of fistula-in-ano: are endoanal coils the gold standard? Am J Roentgenol. 1998;171:407–12.
57. Beets-Tan RGH, Beets GL, van de Hoop AG, et al. Preoperative MR imaging of anal fistulas: does it really help the surgeon? Radiology. 2001;218:75–84.
58. Buchanan GN, Halligan S, Williams AB, et al. Magnetic resonance imaging for primary fistula in ano. Br J Surg. 2003;90:877–81.
59. Buchanan G, Halligan A, Cohen CRG, et al. Effect of MRI on clinical outcome of recurrent fistula-in-ano. Lancet. 2002;360:1661–2.
60. Pearl RK, Andrews JR, Orsay CP, et al. Role of the seton in the management of anorectal fistulas. Dis Colon Rectum. 1993;36:573–9.
61. Ritchie RD, Sackier JM, Hode JP. Incontinence rates after cutting seton treatment for anal fistula. Colorectal Dis. 2009;11:564–71.
62. William JG, Farrands PA, Williams AB. The treatment of anal fistula: ACPGBI position statement. Colorectal Dis. 2007;9:18–50.
63. Nelson RL, Cintron J, Abcarian H. Dermal-island flap anoplasty for transsphincteric fistula-in-ano: assessment of treatment failures. Dis Colon Rectum. 2000;43:681–4.
64. Parks AG, Stitz RW. The treatment of high fistula-in-ano. Dis Colon Rectum. 1976;19:487–99.
65. Kennedy HL, Zegarra JP. Fistulotomy without external sphincter division for high anal fistulae. Br J Surg. 1990;77:898–901.
66. Fazio VW. Complex anal fistulae. Gastroenterol Clin North Am. 1987;16:93–114.
67. Kodner IJ, Mazor A, Shemesh GI, et al. Endorectal advancement flap repair of rectovaginal and other complicated anorectal fistulas. Surgery. 1993;114:682–90.
68. Sonoda T, Hull T, Piedmonte MR, Fazio VW. Outcomes of primary repair of anorectal and rectovaginal fistulas using the endorectal advancement flap. Dis Colon Rectum. 2002;45:1622–8.
69. Zimmerman DD, Delemarre JB, Gosselink MP, et al. Smoking affects the outcome of transanal mucosal advancement flap repair of transsphincteric fistulas. Br J Surg. 2003;90:351–4.
70. Kronberg O. To lay open or excise a fistula-in-ano. Br J Surg. 1985;72:970.
71. Cintron JR, Park JJ, Orsay CP, et al. Repair of fistula-in-ano using autologous fibrin tissue adhesive. Dis Colon Rectum. 1999;42:607–13.
72. Patrij L, Kooman B, Mortina CM, et al. Fibrin glue-antibiotic mixture in the treatment of anal fistulae: experience with 69 cases. Dig Surg. 2000;17:77–80.
73. Cintron JR, Park JJ, Orsay CP, et al. Repair of fistulas-in-ano using fibrin adhesive. Long term follow up. Dis Colon Rectum. 2000;43:944–50.
74. Sentovitch SM. Fibrin glue for anal fistulas: long-term results. Dis Colon Rectum. 2003;46:498–502.
75. Buchanan GN, Bartram CI, Phillips RKS, et al. Efficacy of fibrin sealant in the management of complex anal fistulas. A prospective trial. Dis Colon Rectum. 2003;46:1167–74.
76. You SY, Mizrahi N, Zmora O, et al. The role of endoanal ultrasound as a predictive factor in endoanal advancement flap surgery (abstract). Colorectal Dis. 2001;3 Suppl 1:76.
77. Lindsey I, Smilgen-Humphreys MM, Cunningham C, et al. Randomized controlled trial of fibrin glue vs. conventional treatment for anal fistula. Dis Colon Rectum. 2002;45:1608–15.
78. Zmora O, Neufeld D, Ziv Y, et al. Prospective, multienter evaluation of highly concentrated fibrin glue in the treatment of complex cryptogenic perianal fistulas. Dis Colon Rectum. 2005;48:2167–72.
79. Johnson EK, Gaw JU, Armstrong DN. Efficacy of anal fistula plug vs. fibrin glue in closure of anorectal fistulas. Dis Colon Rectum. 2006;49:371–6.
80. Adams T, Yang J, Kondylis LA, Kondylis PD. Long-term outlook after successful fibrin glue ablation of cryptoglandular transsphincteric fistula-in-ano. Dis Colon Rectum. 2008;51:1488–90.
81. Yeung JMC, Simpson JAD, Tang SW, et al. Fibrin glue for the treatment of fistulae-in-ano – a method worth sticking to? Colorectal Dis. 2010;12:363–6.
82. The Surgisis AFP anal fistula plug: report of a consensus conference. Colorectal Dis. 2007;10:17–20.
83. Champagne BJ, O'Connor LM, Ferguson M. Efficacy of anal fistula plug in closure of cryptoglandular fistulas, long term follow up. Dis Colon Rectum. 2006;49:1817–21.
84. Ellis CN. Bioprosthetic plug for complex anal fistulas: an early experience. J Surg Educ. 2007;64:36–40.
85. Schwandner O, Stadler F, Dietl O, et al. Initial experience on efficacy in closure of cryptoglandular and Crohn's transsphincteric fistulas by the use of the anal plug. Int J Colorectal Dis. 2007;64:36–40.
86. van Koperen P, D'Hoore A, Wolthuis AM, et al. Anal fistula plug for closure of difficult anorectal fistula: a prospective study. Dis Colon Rectum. 2007;50:2168–72.
87. Lawes DA, Efron JE, Abbas M, et al. Early experience with bioabsorbable anal fistula plug. World J Surg. 2008;32:1157–9.
88. Garg P. To determine the efficacy of anal fistula plug in the treatment of high fistula-in-ano: an initial experience. Colorectal Dis. 2008;11:588–91.
89. Thekkinkattil D, Botterill I, Ambrose S, et al. Efficacy of the anal fistula plug in complex anorectal fistulae. Colorectal Dis. 2008;11:584–7.
90. Christoforidis D, Eltzioni DA, Goldberg SM, et al. Treatment of complex anal fistulas with the collagen fistula plug. Dis Colon Rectum. 2008;51:1482–7.
91. Safar B, Jobanputra S, Sands D, et al. Anal fistula plug: initial experience and outcomes. Dis Colon Rectum. 2009;52:248–52.
92. Ortiz H, Marzo J, Ciga F, et al. Randomized clinical trial of anal fistula plug versus endorectal advancement flap for the treatment of high crytoglandular fistula in ano. Br J Surg. 2009;96:608–12.

93. Rojanasakul A. LIFT procedure: a simplified technique for fistula-in-ano. Tech Coloproctol. 2009;131:237–40.
94. Moloo H, Goldberg SM. Novel correction of intersphincteric perianal fistulas preserves anal sphincter. Presented at the American College of Surgeons, October 2008, San Francisco.
95. Han JG, Xu HM, Song WL. Histologic analysis of acellular dermal matrix in the treatment of anal fistula in an animal model. J Am Coll Surg. 2009;208:1099.
96. Milito G, Cadeddu F. Conservative treatment for anal fistula: collagen matrix injection. J Am Coll Surg. 2009;209:542–3.
97. Marks CG, Ritchie JK. Anal fistulas at St. Mark's Hospital. Br J Surg. 1977;64:84–91.
98. Vasilevsky CA, Gordon PH. Results of treatment of fistula-in-ano. Dis Colon Rectum. 1985;28:225–31.
99. Van Tets WF, Kuijpers HC. Continence disorders after anal fisulotomy. Dis Colon Rectum. 1994;37:1194–7.
100. Garcia-Aguilar JC, Belmonte C, Wong WD, et al. Surgical treatment of fistula-in-ano. Factors associated with recurrence and incontinence. Dis Colon Rectum. 1996;39:723–9.
101. Mylonakis E, Katsios C, Godevenos D, et al. Quality of life of patients after surgical treatment of anal fistula; the role of anal manometry. Colorectal Dis. 2001;3:417–21.
102. Malouf AJ, Buchanan GN, Carapeti A, et al. A prospective audit of fistula-in-ano at St. Mark's hospital. Colorectal Dis. 2002;4:13–9.
103. Westerterp M, Volkers NA, Poolman RW, van Tets WF. Anal fistulotomy between Skylla and Charybdis. Colorectal Dis. 2003;5:549–55.
104. Sangwan YP, Rosen L, Riether RD, et al. Is simple fistula-in-ano simple? Dis Colon Rectum. 1994;37:885–9.
105. Ramanujam PS, Prasad ML, Abcarian H. The role of seton in fistulotomy of the anus. Surg Gynecol Obstet. 1983;157: 419–22.
106. Williams JG, Macleod CAH, Goldberg SM. Seton treatment of high anal fistula. Br J Surg. 1991;78:1159–61.
107. Fasth SB, Nordgren S, Hulten L. Clinical course and management of suprasphincteric and extrasphincteric fistula-in-ano. Acta Chir Scand. 1990;156:397–402.
108. Graf W, Pahlman L, Egerbald S. Functional results after seton treatment of high transsphincteric anal fistulas. Eur J Surg. 1995;161:289–91.
109. Hasegawa H, Radley S, Keighley MR. Long term results of cutting seton fistulotomy. Acta Chir Iugosi. 2000;47(4 Suppl 1):19–21.
110. Schouten WR, Zimmerman DD, Briel JW, Briel JW. Transanal advancement flap repair of transsphincteric fistulas. Dis Colon Rectum. 1999;42:1419–23.
111. Mizrahi N, Wexner SD, Zmora O, et al. Endorectal advancement flap: are there predictors of failure? Dis Colon Rectum. 2002;45:1616–21.
112. Wang JY, Garcia-Aguilar J, Sternberg JA. Treatment of transsphincteric anal fistulas: are fistula plugs an acceptable alternative? Dis Colon Rectum. 2009;52:692–7.
113. Roig JV, Jordan J, Garcia-Armengol J. Changes in anorectal morphologic and functional parameters after fistula-in-ano surgery. Dis Colon Rectum. 2009;52:1462–9.
114. Seow-Choen F, Phillips RKS. Insights gained from the management of problematical anal fistulae at St. Mark's Hospital, 1984–88. Br J Surg. 1991;78:539–41.
115. Lunniss PJ, Sheffield JP, Talbot IC, et al. Persistence of idiopathic anal fistula may be related to epithelialization. Br J Surg. 1995;82:32–3.
116. Lewis P, Bartolo DCC. Treatment of trans-sphincteric fistulae by full thickness anorectal advancement flaps. Br J Surg. 1990;77:1187–9.
117. Williams JG, Rothenberger DA, Nemer FD, Goldberg SM. Fistula-in-ano in Crohn's disease. Results of aggressive surgical treatment. Dis Colon Rectum. 1991;34:378–84.
118. Schwartz DA, Pemberton JH, Sandborn WJ. Diagnosis and treatment of perianal fistulas in Crohn's disease. Ann Intern Med. 2001;135:906–18.
119. Jenss H, Starlinger M, Skaleij M. Magnetic resonance imaging in perianal Crohn's disease. Lancet. 1992;340:1286.
120. Buchmann P, Keighley MRB, Allan RN, et al. Natural history of perianal Crohn's disease: ten-year follow-up. A plea for conservatism. Am J Surg. 1980;140:642–64.
121. Thia KT, Mahadavan U, Feagen BG. Ciprofloxacin or metronidazole for the treatment of perianal fistulas in patients with Crohn's disease: a randomized double blind placebo-controlled pilot study. Inflamm Bowel Dis. 2009;15: 17–24.
122. Lecomte T, Contou JF, Beaugerie L, et al. Predictive factors of response of perianal Crohn's disease to azathioprine or 6-Mercaptopurine. Dis Colon Rectum. 2003;46:1469–75.
123. Present DH, Rutgeerts P, Targan S, et al. Infliximab for the treatment of fistulas in patients with Crohn's disease. N Engl J Med. 1999;340:1398–405.
124. Ochsonkuhn T, Goke B, Sackman M. Combining infliximab with 6MP for fistula therapy in Crohn's disease. Am J Gastroenterol. 2002;97:2022–5.
125. Topstad D, Panaccione R, Heine JA, et al. Combined seton placement, infliximab infusion and maintenance immunosuppressives improve healing rate in fistulizing anorectal Crohn's disease. A single center experience. Dis Colon Rectum. 2003;46:577–83.
126. Sands BE, Anderson FH, Bernstein CN, et al. Infliximab maintenance therapy for fistulizing Crohn's disease. N Engl J Med. 2004;350:876–85.
127. Nivatvongs S, Gordon PH. Crohn's disease. In: Gordon PH, Nivatvongs S, editors. Principles and practice of surgery for the colon, rectum and anus. St. Louis: Quality Medical Publishing; 1999. p. 952–4.
128. Halme L, Sainio P. Factors related to frequency, type and outcome of anal fistulas in Crohn's disease. Dis Colon Rectum. 1995;38:55–9.
129. Levien DH, Surrell J, Mazier WP. Surgical treatment of anorectal fistula in patients with Crohn's disease. Surg Gynecol Obstet. 1989;169:133–6.
130. Van Dongen LM, Lubbers GJC. Perianal fistulas in Crohn's disease. Arch Surg. 1986;121:1187–90.
131. Allan A, Keighley MRB. Management of perianal Crohn's disease. World J Surg. 1988;12:198–202.
132. White RA, Eisenstat TE, Rubin RJ, Salvati EP. Seton management of complex anorectal fistulas in patients with Crohn's disease. Dis Colon Rectum. 1990;33:587–9.
133. Jones OJ, Fazio VW, Jagelman DG. The use of transanal rectal advancement flaps in the management of fistulas involving the anorectum. Dis Colon Rectum. 1987;30:919–23.

134. Joo JS, Weiss EG, Nogueras JJ, Wexner SD. Endorectal advancement flap in perianal Crohn's disease. Am Surg. 1998; 64:147–50.
135. Wolff BE, Culp CE, Beart RW, et al. Anorectal Crohn's disease: a long term prospective. Dis Colon Rectum. 1985;28: 709–11.
136. McLeod RS. Management of fistula-in-ano: 1990 Roussel lecture. Can J Surg. 1991;34:581–5.
137. Beck DE. Management of anorectal Cohn's fistulas. Clin Colon Rectal Surg. 2001;14:117–28.
138. Schwander O, Fuerst A. Preliminary results on efficacy in closure of transsphincteirc and rectovaginal fistulas associated with Crohn's disease using new materials. Surg Innov. 2009;16:162–8.
139. Garcia-Olmo D, Garcia-Arranz M, Herreros D. Expanded adipose-derived stem cells for the treatment of complex perianal fistula including Crohn's disease. Expert Opin Bio Ther. 2008;8:1417–23.
140. Savafi A, Gottesman L, Dailey TH. Anorectal surgery in the HIV+ patient: update. Dis Colon Rectum. 1991;34: 299–304.
141. Manookian CM, Sokol TP, Hendrick C. Does HIV status influence the anatomy of anal fistulas. Dis Colon Rectum. 1998;41:1529–33.
142. Aleali M, Gottesman L. Anorectal disease in HIV-positive patients. Clin Colon Rectal Surg. 2001;14:265–73.
143. Schaffzin DM, Tj S, Smith LE. Perianal mucinous adenocarcinoma: unusual case presentations and review of the literature. Am Surg. 2003;69:166–9.
144. Sierra EM, Saenz V, Martinez PH. Mucinous adenocarcinoma associated with fistula in ano: report of a case. Tech Coloproctol. 2006;10:51–3.
145. Teixeira CR, Tanaka S, Haruma K. The clinical significance of the histologic subclassification of colorectal carcinoma. Oncology. 2004;50:495–9.
146. Hama Y, Makita K, Yanmana T. Mucinous adenocarcinoma arising from fistula in ano: MRI findings. AJR Am J Roentgenol. 2006;187:517–21.
147. Yang B-L, Shaw WJ, Sun G-D. Perianal mucinous adenocarcinoma arising from chronic anorectal fistulae: a review from single institution. Int J Colorectal Dis. 2009;24:1001–6.
148. Bukowski TP, Chakrabarty A, Powell IJ, et al. Acquired rectourethral fistula: methods of repair. J Urol. 1995;153:730–3.
149. Blumberg JM, Lesser T, Tran VQ. Management of rectal injuries sustained during laparoscopic radical prostatectomy. Urology. 2009;73:163–6.
150. Thompson IM, Marx AC. Conservative therapy of rectourethral fistula: five-year follow up. Urology. 1990;6:533–6.
151. Zmora O, Potenti FM, Wexner SD, et al. Gracilis muscle transposition for iatrogenic rectourethral fistula. Ann Surg. 2003;237:483–7.
152. Zmora O, Tulchinsky H, Gur E, et al. Gracilis muscle transposition for fistulas between the rectum and urethra or vagina. Dis Colon Rectum. 2006;49:1316–21.
153. Gupta G, Kumar S, Kekre N, Gopalakrishnan G. Surgical management of rectourethral fistula. Urology. 2008;71:267–71.
154. Wexner SD, Ruiz DE, Genua J, et al. Gracilis muscle interposition for the treatment of rectourethral, rectovaginal and pouch-vaginal fistula. Results in 53 patients. Ann Surg. 2008;248:39–43.
155. Parks AG, Motson RW. Perianal repair of rectoprostatic fistula. Br J Surg. 1983;70:725–6.
156. Garofalo TE, Delaney CP, Jones SM, et al. Rectal advancement flap repair of rectourethral fistula. A 20-year experience. Dis Colon Rectum. 2003;46:762–9.
157. Prasad ML, Nelson R, Hambrick E, Abcarian H. York Mason procedure for repair of postoperative rectoprostatic urethral fistula. Dis Colon Rectum. 1983;26:716–20.
158. Wilbert DM, Buess G, Bichler K-H. Combined endoscopic closure of rectourethral fistula. J Urol. 1996;155:256–8.

14
Benign Anorectal and Rectovaginal Fistulas

David A. Etzioni and Ann C. Lowry

Introduction

Although infrequently life-threatening, rectovaginal fistulas are an aggravation to both patients and surgeons. Passing flatus or stool through the vagina is understandably distressing to patients; the lack of a uniformly successful repair is frustrating to surgeons.

Etiology

Rectovaginal fistulas arise from a broad range of causes, and may be congenital or acquired. Congenital rectovaginal fistulas are outside the scope of this chapter.

Obstetrical injury is the most frequent cause of acquired rectovaginal fistulas. In general, immediate repair is the treatment of choice after a third or fourth-degree laceration. After an obstetrical injury the fistula may manifest immediately but more commonly appears 7–10 days after delivery. Inadequate repair, breakdown of the repair or infection may result in fistula formation. In developed nations, rectovaginal fistulas occur after 0.06–0.1% of vaginal deliveries.[1–3] In developing countries, the incidence of rectovaginal and vesicovaginal fistula after childbirth is almost three times higher, with more than half of these fistulas being larger than 4 cm in diameter.[4,5] In these countries prolonged labor, causing necrosis of the rectovaginal septum, leads to the formation of a fistula. The resultant social stigma generates significant suffering for these women who have limited access to treatment.[6]

Infectious and inflammatory disease processes may also cause rectovaginal fistulas. The most common infectious cause is cryptoglandular infection with an abscess that spontaneously drains into the vagina. Women with inflammatory bowel disease (IBD) – more commonly Crohn's disease than ulcerative colitis – develop spontaneous rectovaginal fistulas with some frequency. In a population-based study of patients with Crohn's disease in Olmsted County, 8 of 169 patients developed a rectovaginal fistula.[7] In a similar study of patients in St. Mark's Hospital, 90 of the 886 women with Crohn's disease and an intact rectum developed a rectovaginal fistula during a 30-year follow-up.[8]

Operative and nonoperative trauma may also result in a rectovaginal fistula. Complications of rectal or vaginal surgery usually result in fistulas opening low in the rectum. High fistulas are most frequently complications of stapled anastomoses. In one series of 140 patients undergoing low anterior resection for rectal carcinoma four (2.9%) developed a rectovaginal fistula.[9] Rectovaginal fistula is also reported after stapled transanal resection for obstructed defecation syndrome, stapled hemorroidopexy, and in 3–12% of patients undergoing an ileoanal pouch procedure.[10–16] Fistulas have also been documented after dilatation of a radiated vaginal cuff, fecal impaction, viral/bacterial infection in human immunodeficiency virus (HIV) patients, sexual assault, and spontaneously in patients undergoing treatment with antiangiogenic chemotherapeutics.[17–24] Finally, anorectal and gynecologic malignancies may result in fistulas due to local extension of the tumor or secondary to treatment with radiotherapy.

Evaluation

Initial evaluation of a woman with a known or suspected rectovaginal fistula should focus first on confirming the presence of a fistula, and subsequently on evaluating the anatomy of the fistula and the integrity of the surrounding tissues. The specific types of investigations required vary mainly according to the underlying etiology of the fistula.

History

Several important aspects of a woman's history may have a significant impact on a patient's workup and selection of surgical treatment. Any history of anorectal or gynecologic malignancy should prompt a thorough investigation for recurrence, both in the rectovaginal septum and pelvis. Prior treatment

D.E. Beck et al. (eds.), *The ASCRS Textbook of Colon and Rectal Surgery: Second Edition*,
DOI 10.1007/978-1-4419-1584-9_14, © Springer Science+Business Media, LLC 2011

with radiation should be specifically elicited. Issues related to continence should also be documented. If the mechanism of injury is childbirth, the patient with a fistula is at significant risk of a sphincter defect. In a review by the University of Minnesota, 48% of women with rectovaginal fistulas complained of incontinence preoperatively.[25] Bowel function as well as signs/symptoms of IBD should also be targeted as possible areas for workup and preoperative optimization. Evaluation of the intestinal tract by colonoscopy and contrast studies is indicated in patients with known or suspected IBD.

Physical Examination

Information obtained from physical examination is critical to the evaluation and surgical decision-making for women with rectovaginal fistula. During the initial examination, the possibility of local sepsis should be considered. Findings of fluctuance, cellulitis, or any other harbingers of active infection should prompt an exam under anesthesia and drainage with or without placement of seton(s). Any mass lesion discovered on exam should be biopsied to evaluate for malignancy. In patients with a prior history of anorectal or gynecologic malignancy, the threshold for a biopsy should be especially low. In patients with a history of radiation treatment for malignancy an examination under anesthesia with biopsies is often necessary.

The site of rectovaginal fistula can usually be readily identified on digital examination as a palpable dimple in the anterior midline. Multiple perianal fistulas suggest Crohn's disease as the etiology. The rectal opening is frequently visible on anoscopy, but in some women the diagnosis may be elusive. A methylene blue test may confirm the presence of a communication and aid in locating the site. During this test, the patient is placed in prone position and a vaginal tampon is inserted; a 20–30-ml enema colored with methylene blue is then administered. Staining on the tampon is diagnostic of a rectovaginal fistula, assuming no spillage of dye. Alternatively, saline can be instilled in the vagina with the patient in the lithotomy position. The rectum is then insufflated with air and the vagina observed for bubbles.

A patient's sphincter function should also be assessed during the physical examination. Patients with clinically significant sphincter interruption may benefit from a surgical approach which encompasses a sphincter repair.

Radiography

Radiographic tests may help identify an elusive fistula. Vaginography can detect fistulas that are obscure to the maneuvers described above, and gives objective determination of fistula location. It is performed by instilling contrast into the vagina through a Foley catheter with the balloon inflated to occlude the vaginal opening. The technique has a sensitivity of 79–100% for the detection of the fistula tract. Vaginography is most helpful for colovaginal and enterovaginal fistulas; it is less useful for low rectovaginal fistulas.[26,27]

Computed tomography (CT) scans may identify the fistula tract and characterize the surrounding tissue. Contrast material in the vagina after oral or rectal administration is diagnostic of a fistula. Suggestive evidence includes air or fluid in the vagina if there is no history of recent instrumentation. Magnetic resonance imaging (MRI) and endorectal ultrasound are also useful in identifying fistulas; the injection of hydrogen peroxide into fistulas has been shown to increase the yield of ultrasonography.[28] At present there is no clear "best" radiologic test to detect elusive fistulas. Since results are likely highly operator-dependent, local expertise should be considered when selecting a test.

Endoanal ultrasound and MRI also have an important role in assessing the structural integrity of the anal sphincter. One study found that 100% of women presenting with an obstetric rectovaginal fistula had evidence of an anterior sphincter defect.[29] Symptoms of the fistula frequently mask anal incontinence; failure to study the sphincter may lead to a poor choice of repair and persistent incontinence postoperatively.[25,30] Endoanal ultrasound and MRI are reported to be essentially equivalent in detection of a sphincter defect.[31]

MRI, CT, and endosonography also have a role in evaluating for the presence of local sepsis. MRI appears to be more accurate than ultrasound for this purpose, but its superiority to CT has not been demonstrated.[32] Ultrasonography may be a useful tool for intraoperative radiologic guidance for drainage of complex abscesses.[33]

Classification

A variety of classification systems exist for rectovaginal fistulas. Each has importance in terms of generating aspects of the patient's workup and treatment.

Fistula Height

Daniels classified fistulas by their location along the rectovaginal septum as low, middle, or high.[34] With low fistulas, the rectal opening is at the dentate line and the vaginal opening just inside the vaginal fourchette. The vaginal opening is at or near the cervix in high fistulas. Middle fistulas are located between high and low fistulas. In general, high fistulas are more likely to require laparotomy; perineal approaches are appropriate for most low and middle fistulas. Fistulas may also be classified by the location of the rectal opening. Ones opening at the dentate line or above are considered rectovaginal fistulas; fistulas opening below the dentate line as "anovaginal fistulas." The use of this classification is quite inconsistent and has not translated to clear differences in etiology or surgical approach.

Simple vs. Complex Fistulas

Another system classifies fistulas as simple vs. complex.[35] Simple fistulas are small (<2.5 cm), low and secondary to trauma or infection. Complex fistulas are large, high, caused by IBD, radiation or malignancy, or persistent after failed repair(s). This system has some utility in directing surgical decision-making because it reflects the status of the local tissue. Simple fistulas are more amenable to local repairs, whereas complex fistulas are more likely to require resection or interposition. Fecal diversion is a consideration for complex fistulas but rarely, if ever, necessary for simple fistulas.

Surgical Management

In this section, we will catalog the main options for surgical treatment. The following section will discuss the main considerations that should drive decision-making regarding the choice of procedure.

General Considerations

Patients undergo mechanical and antibiotic preparation preoperatively. Most procedures require general anesthesia, although some repairs may be performed under regional anesthesia. A urinary catheter is inserted. Prone jackknife position with taping of the buttocks provides the best exposure for transanal and perineal approaches, while lithotomy position is better for transvaginal repairs. A well-functioning headlight is critical. Depending on the procedure at hand, operative exposure may be greatly facilitated by access to a Lone Star retractor, Pratt bivalve or Fansler anoscope, Wylie renal vein retractors, and narrow Deaver or malleable retractors.

Fistulotomy

Simple fistulotomy is an option for only a very select group of rectovaginal fistulas. Patients who may benefit more than be harmed by this approach have very low fistulas with no (or vanishingly little) sphincter involvement. Fistulotomy should be avoided in other rectovaginal fistulas due to the risk of incontinence.

Fibrin Sealant

A significant body of experience has been accumulated regarding the efficacy of fibrin glue instillation for various types of fistula-in-ano. The technique is straightforward, requiring the gentle curettage of the fistula, followed by injection of an admixture of cryoprecipitate and thrombin. Success rates for fistula-in-ano vary widely, ranging from 31 to 61%.[36,37] An interesting approach – adding fibrin glue to mucosal advancement flap repair was analyzed by Ellis and Clark[38] with similar outcomes.

The accumulated experience in using fibrin glue for rectovaginal fistulas is more limited. Abel et al.[39] reported healing in three of five patients, and Venkatesh and Ramanujam[40] reported success in six of eight patients. These series are too small to yield stable estimates regarding the true effectiveness of fibrin glue for rectovaginal fistulas. Unpublished experience with fibrin sealant has not yet matched the enthusiasm and success rates of these initial reports. The approach has appeal mainly in that the risk (in terms of injury to surrounding tissues) is minimal, and the success rate appears to be greater than zero.

Mucosal Advancement Flaps

Mucosal advancement flaps aim to eradicate rectovaginal fistulas by occluding one side or the other of the tract with healthy epithelial tissue. The approach can be undertaken either transanally or vaginally. The transanal approach is intuitively preferable in that the repair is on the high pressure side of the fistula. With the patient in the prone jackknife position and adequate exposure, a U-shaped flap of mucosa, submucosa, and circular muscle is raised for a distance sufficient to allow a tension-free repair (usually 4–5 cm). Dissection should generate a flap with a base two to three times wider than the apex. The fistula tract is debrided (not excised), and the muscles are approximated over the fistula opening with long-acting absorbable suture in 1–2 layers. Distally, the end of the flap including the fistula site is excised and the flap sutured in place; the vaginal side is left open for drainage (Figure 14-1). Patients typically resume a normal diet with fiber supplements to prevent constipation. Diarrhea must also be controlled as it will affect healing as much as constipation. Postdischarge instructions should include avoiding intercourse and the use of tampons for 6 weeks.

A vaginal approach is performed in similar fashion, with an incision in the posterior vaginal wall near the introitus. A flap of vaginal wall is raised laterally to the ischial tuberosities to provide adequate mobility. The vaginal and rectal defects are closed with absorbable sutures, and the levator ani muscles are approximated in the midline; this portion of the repair is felt to be critical to its success. Absorbable suture are then used to suture the vaginal flap in place.

The success rates of endorectal and vaginal advancement flaps for rectovaginal fistulas have been reported widely in the literature (Table 14-1). Variations in outcomes are likely attributable more to the small size of these series than any underlying patient or technical factor. Differences in length of follow-up are also important, as fistulas may recur more than 4 years postrepair.[58] Importantly, success rates are measured in terms of fistula closure, and measures of continence are rarely included. Studies examining advancement flaps in the treatment of patients with fistula-in-ano document disturbances to continence in 21–40% of patients.[52,53,56] The lack of standardized measures of continence in these reports makes objective comparison challenging, however. Several technical modifications have been attempted with the goal of improving success rates with advancement flaps. One group of investigators added labial fat transposition to endorectal advancement flap but had outcomes no different from an advancement flap alone.[54] At least two early

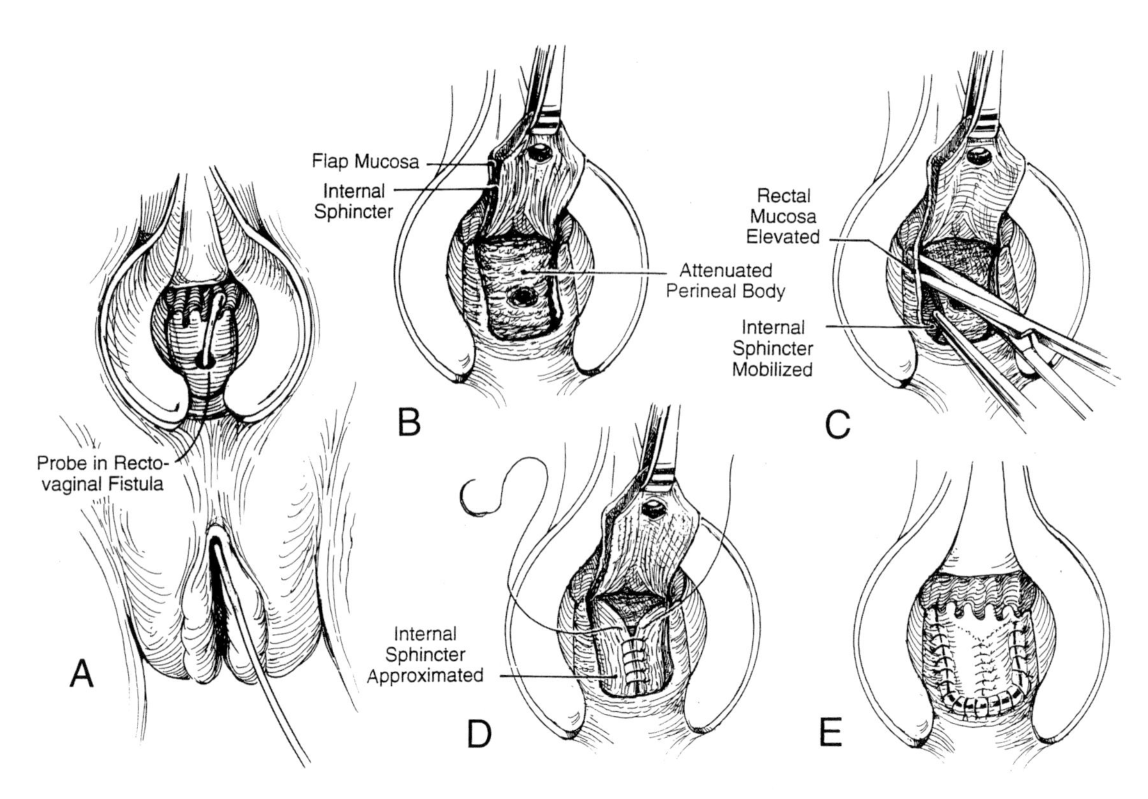

FIGURE 14-1. Endorectal advancement flap.

TABLE 14-1. Results of endorectal advancement flaps

Author	Year	Number of patients	Success (%)	Comments
Greenwald et al.[41]	1978	20	100	Tract excised, layered closure under flap
Hoexter et al.[42]	1985	15	100	Repair as above
Wise et al.[43]	1991	40	85	15 concomitant sphincteroplasty
Lowry et al.[44]	1991	85	78	25 concomitant sphincteroplasty
Kodner et al.[45]	1993	71	93	Unknown # sphincteroplasty
Khanduja et al.[30]	1994	16	100	Patients without incontinence
MacRae et al.[46]	1995	28	29	50% obstetric, previous failed repairs
Mazier et al.[47]	1995	19	95	67% simple
Watson and Phillips[48]	1995	12	58	Ultimate success 83%, 25% stomas
Tsang et al.[25]	1998	27	41	All obstetric
Hyman[49]	1999	12	91	Etiology not reported
Joo et al.[50]	1998	20	75	Ultimate success, all Crohn's
Baig et al.[51]	2000	19	74	7 concomitant sphincteroplasty
Mizrahi et al.[52]	2002	32	56	Mixture of etiologies
Sonoda et al.[53]	2002	37	43	Mixture of etiologies
Zimmerman et al.[54]	2002	21	48	6 concomitant sphincteroplasty 12 labial flap transposition
Casadesus et al.[55]	2006	12	75	Vaginal advancement flap
Uribe et al.[56]	2007	56	93	Endorectal advancement flaps; four failures successfully re-repaired
Abbas et al.[57]	2008	8	50	All were recurrent prior to repair

reports documented the successful use of transanal endoscopic microsurgery (TEM) to facilitate mucosal flap repair for rectovaginal fistula.[59,60] Interestingly, smoking has been linked to failure of endorectal advancement flaps, possibly the result of impairments in mucosal blood flow.[61,62] It is not known whether smoking cessation prior to surgery can increase rates of success.

Retrograde anocutaneous flaps are an option for very low rectovaginal fistulas. A flap of anoderm and perineal skin is raised and advanced into the anal canal. After the fistula is debrided, the flap is sutured into place.[63] A similar approach has also been utilized on the vaginal side in conjunction with an endoanal advancement flap.[64] Only a small number of cases have been reported with either technique.

Fistulectomy with Layered Closure

Another option that can be approached through the rectum, vagina, or perineum is excision of the fistula tract. An elliptical incision is made around the fistula and mucosal flaps are raised for 2–3 cm. The fistula is excised in its entirety. Vaginal mucosa, rectovaginal septum, rectal muscle, and rectal mucosa are closed in succession. Plication of the levator muscles is added by some surgeons. If done through the perineum, a transverse incision is made and extended down to the fistula tract. The fistula is then cored out of the rectal and vaginal walls and a layered closure performed. Using layered closure, successful repair is reported in 88–100% of patients in several small series.[65–68]

Rectal Sleeve Advancement

Rectal sleeve advancement involves the circumferential mobilization of the distal rectum and advancement to cover the anorectal side of a fistula. This technique is reserved for situations where there is a rectovaginal fistula and co-existing diffuse disease in the proximal anal canal and/or distal rectum. Simmang et al.[69] emphasized that this approach is useful for someone with a rectovaginal fistula and an anal stricture, as both problems will be corrected with the procedure.

Technically, the procedure is performed using a circumferential incision at the dentate line which is deepened through the submucosa into the internal sphincter. This plane is continued cephalad, becoming full thickness above the anorectal ring. Mobilization continues until healthy, nonscarred tissue is reached and that tissue can be pulled down to the dentate line without tension. The remaining diseased anorectal mucosa is pulled through the anal canal, and excised; healthy rectum is then sutured to anoderm below the dentate line. In a series of five patients with rectovaginal fistulas and Crohn's disease reported by the Cleveland Clinic, all three of the patients with fecal diversion healed.[70] One patient required two rectal sleeve advancements before healing occurred. Of the two patients without fecal diversion, one healed.

Two variations of the sleeve advancement deserve mention. Schouten and Oom[71] reported using a Kraske approach to sleeve advancement for six women with rectovaginal fistulas after prior failed treatment; they reported success with five. A second variation of the sleeve advancement technique is the modified Noble–Mengert–Fish technique.[72] With this method the full thickness of the anterior rectal wall is mobilized. A curvilinear incision is made at the mucocutaneous junction over the anterior 180° of the anal canal. The dissection continues until the rectovaginal septum is entered. The superior limit is the vault of the vagina; the lateral margin is the full width of the rectovaginal space. There needs to be adequate dissection to ensure that the flap will reach the area of the external sphincter without tension. The flap is then anchored to the external anal sphincter and the perineal skin forming a new mucocutaneous junction. Older reports of this technique documented successful repair of rectovaginal fistulas in 86–100% of patients. Minor incontinence troubled 25% of patients.[73–75] The only recent report combined this repair with sphincter reconstruction or perineal body repair in the majority of patients.[72] The overall anatomic success was 94%; the results for the anterior rectal wall advancement alone were not reported separately.

Sphincteroplasty and Perineo-Proctotomy

Sphincteroplasty and perineo-proctotomy are related techniques in that they both involve converting the rectovaginal fistula to a fourth-degree laceration, with a subsequent layered anatomical repair of mucosa and intervening tissues. A sphincteroplasty procedure is commonly utilized when a defect in the external sphincter is present with the rectovaginal fistula. In that situation, an overlapping sphincteroplasty serves dual purpose, both obliterating the fistula and repairing the sphincter defect. The technical details are described and illustrated in Chap. 46 on incontinence. Successful closure of rectovaginal fistulas with this operation is reported in 65–100% of patients (Table 14-2).[25,29,30,43,44,46,74,77]

The perineo-proctotomy technique differs from the sphincteroplasty primarily in that it is performed in a patient with an intact sphincter complex. This approach begins with the identification of the fistula and division of the bridge of skin, subcutaneous tissue, sphincter muscle, rectal and vaginal walls overlying the fistula. The tract is excised and both the rectal and vaginal walls are dissected away from the muscle. Internal and external sphincter musculature must be adequately mobilized in order to avoid tension when they are reapproximated. After repair of both the rectal and vaginal defects, the sphincter muscles are sutured together. The perineal body is reconstructed and the skin closed (Figure 14-2).

Women with rectovaginal fistula and an accompanying sphincter defect are ideal candidates for sphincteroplasty; the reapproximation of the sphincter may theoretically improve continence, although this has not been proven. The extension of this approach to patients with an intact sphincter (perineo-proctotomy) should not be undertaken lightly. Perineo-proctotomy has a high success rate – success rates for fistula closure range from 87 to 100% in small series.[40,47,68,79] The impact of the procedure on postoperative continence has not been well-studied, but Mazier et al.[47] report that none of 38 women undergoing this repair were incontinent

TABLE 14-2. Results of sphincteroplasty for rectovaginal fistula

Author	Year	Number of patients	Success (%)
Russell and Gallagher[74]	1977	9	96
Lowry et al.[76]	1988	29	93
Wise et al.[43]	1991	15	100
Khanduja et al.[30]	1994	11	100
MacRae[46]	1995	7	86
Tsang et al.[25]	1998	35	80
Yee et al.[29]	1999	22	91
Halverson et al.[77]	2001	14	65
Rahman et al.[78]	2003	8	100

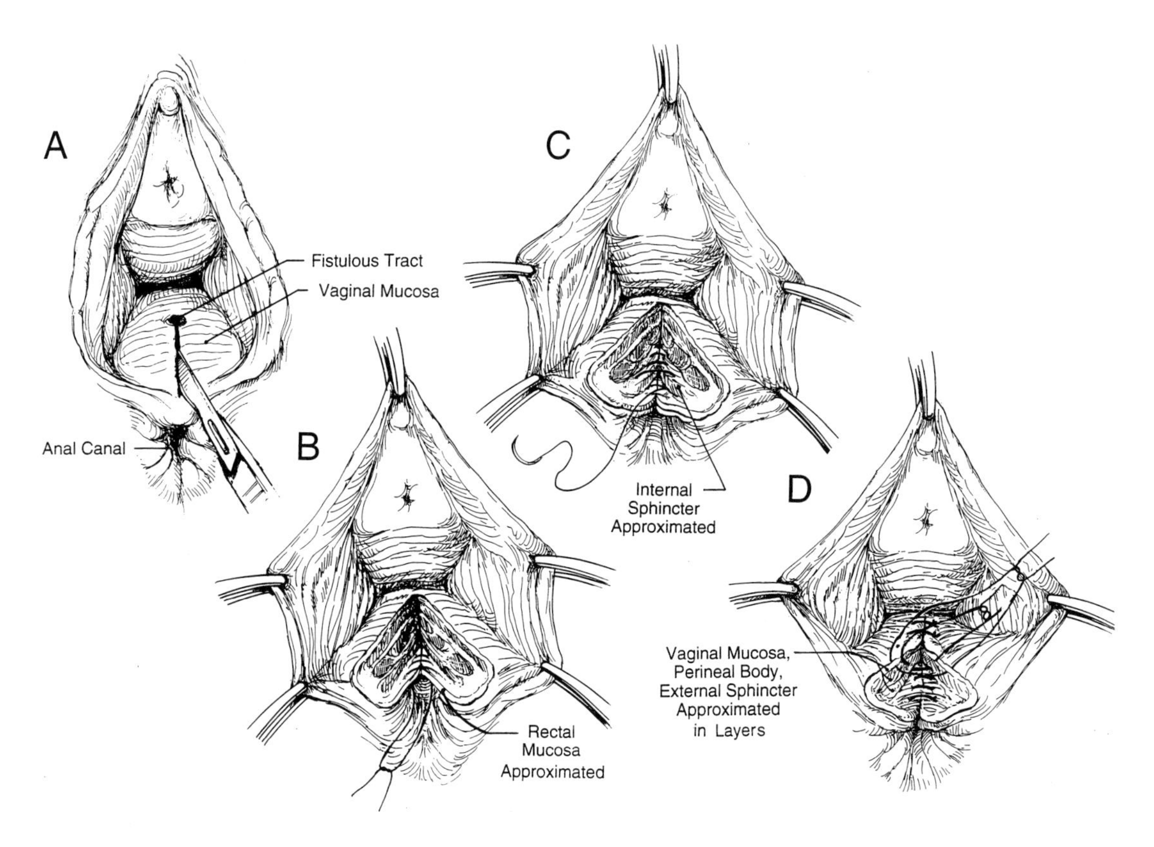

FIGURE 14-2. Perineo-proctotomy.

postoperatively. Despite these results, the potential for significant short- and long-term impairment of continence as a result of injury to an intact sphincter mechanism cannot be ignored. We recommend a dedicated trial of one or more attempts at repairs which do not significantly injure the sphincter mechanism before attempting perineo-proctotomy.

Inversion of Fistula

Inversion of the fistula is a simple technique usually performed through the vagina. The vaginal mucosa is mobilized circumferentially around the fistula, and the tract is excised. A purse-string suture is then used to invert the fistula into the rectum and the vaginal wall is closed over the inversion.[80] One recent series reports a 100% success rate in 39 women with this technique.[78] A similar procedure – ligation of the intersphincteric fistula tract (LIFT) – has generated significant enthusiasm for the treatment of fistula-in-ano.[81,82] With this approach, an intersphincteric dissection is performed to encircle the fistula. The fistula track is divided and suture ligated on both sides; the perineal side is curetted and allowed to drain. While there is only limited experience in using the LIFT procedure for rectovaginal fistulas, the success rates with fistula-in-ano (60–94%) are encouraging.[82,83] There is no intuitive reason why this technique could not be applied to rectovaginal fistulas occurring within the sphincter mechanism. A good candidate for this procedure is a patient with an intact sphincter and a fistula that traverses the sphincter complex. We believe it is unlikely that any repair which depends entirely on anorectal and/or vaginal mucosa has a good chance of success; it is the ability of the intersphincteric plane to heal to itself that is critical to the success of this repair.

Tissue Interposition: General Considerations

The insertion of healthy, well-vascularized tissue between the anorectal and vaginal sides of a rectovaginal fistula is an effective treatment for rectovaginal fistulas. Muscular tissue from a wide range of sources has been used in this capacity, including rectus, bulbocavernous, gracilis, gluteus and sartorius muscles (Table 14-3).[5,84–97] Regardless of which muscle is used, the perineal dissection is similar. The posterior vaginal wall is separated from the anal sphincter and anterior rectal wall until soft, pliable tissue is reached. This dissection is often difficult because of dense scarring. Care must be taken to avoid entering the rectum; injection of saline (with or without epinephrine) may widen this plane and decrease the risk of mucosal injury. Digital manipulation of the rectovaginal septum throughout the dissection is helpful to maintain the appropriate plane. At the site of the fistula, the rectal and vaginal walls are closed with absorbable sutures. It is generally not necessary to trim the vaginal or rectal wall, and doing so often only makes a significantly larger defect. The mobilized

TABLE 14-3. Results of muscle interposition procedures for rectovaginal fistula

Author	Year	Type of interposition	Number of patients	Success (%)
Ulrich et al.[84]	2009	Gracilis	9	Unable to determine
Reisenauer et al.[85]	2009	Martius	2	100
Onishi et al.[86]	2009	Gluteal	1	100
Lefevre et al.[87]	2009	Gracilis	8	75
Cui et al.[88]	2009	Martius	9	100
Wexner et al.[89]	2008	Gracilis	17	53
McNevin et al.[90]	2007	Martius	16	94
Zmora et al.[91]	2006	Gracilis	6	83
Rabau et al.[92]	2006	Gracilis	6	Unable to determine
Onodera et al.[93]	2003	Gluteal	4	100
Tran et al.[94]	1999	Rectus	10	100
Pinedo et al.[95]	1998	Martius	8	75
Margolis et al.[5]	1994	Martius	4	100
Elkins[96]	1994	Martius	35	87
White et al.[97]	1982	Martius	12	92

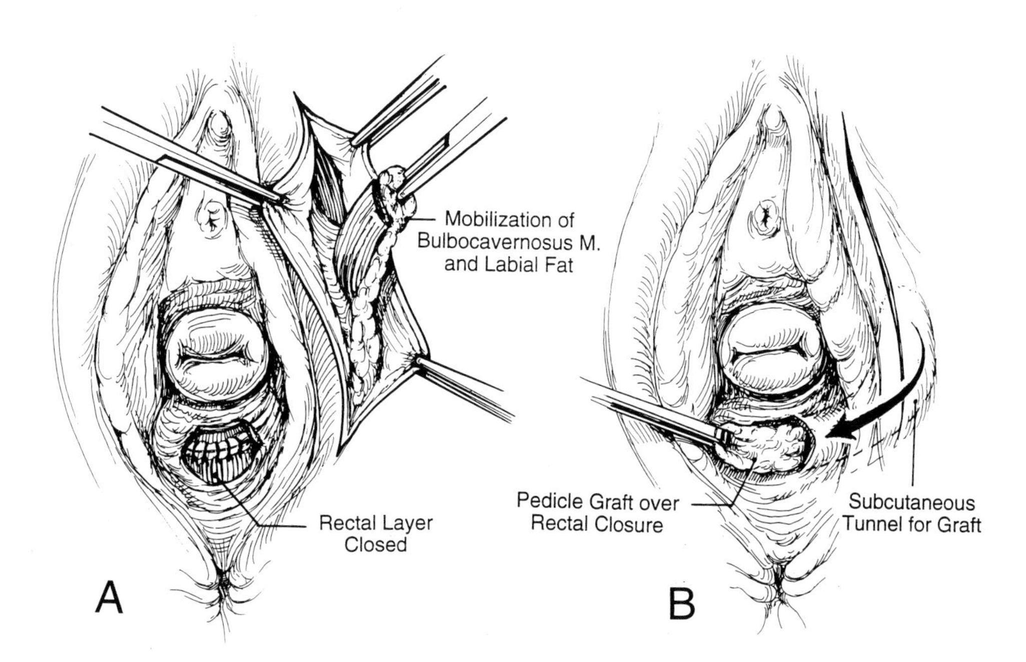

FIGURE 14-3. **A** Martius graft: perineal dissection and mobilization of graft. **B** Martius graft: interposition of labial graft.

muscle is then inserted between the rectum and the vagina and tacked to the posterior vaginal wall, and the incision is closed loosely over a closed suction drain.

Tissue Interposition: Labial Fat Pad or Bulbocavernous Muscle

The labial fat pad (also known as Martius flap) is an excellent source of tissue for transposition into a rectovaginal fistula. This technique is performed with the patient in modified lithotomy position. After a standard perineal dissection is performed, a longitudinal incision is made over the labia majora and skin flaps are raised laterally and medially. There is often a plane similar to Scarpa's fascia for this portion of the dissection. The dissection is continued to the periosteum of the pubis posteriorly and superiorly to the pubic symphysis. Once the entire fat pad with the bulbocavernous muscle is mobilized, the anterior end is divided, preserving the posterior pedicle with the perineal branch of the pudendal artery. A subcutaneous, subvaginal tunnel is created from the base of the pedicle to the perineal incision. The flap is pulled through this tunnel and sutured to the posterior vaginal wall cephalad to the site of the fistula. The labial and perineal incisions are then closed in two layers over drains (Figure 14-3). When vaginal stenosis is a concern, inclusion of an island of skin from the inner thigh with the pedicle is an alternative.[5] Aartsen and Sindram[98] reported 100% initial success in 14 patients with rectovaginal fistulas secondary to radiation damage. Their report has a cautionary note; however, finding that after a 10-year follow-up 8 of the 14 patients required diversion for progressive radiation damage.[98] Others report success in 78–84%.[97,99,100]

Tissue Interposition: Bioprosthetics

The use of bioprosthetic materials to treat rectovaginal fistulas was initially reported in small series in 2004.[101,102] These materials can be interposed trans-perineally between an interrupted rectovaginal fistula or as a "plug" that is inserted into the tract itself. Ellis[103] reported a series of 34 patients treated for rectovaginal fistulas with a bioprosthetic comprised of porcine intestinal submucosa. Of 27 patients who underwent a trans-perineal approach, the success rate was 81%; the seven patients who were treated with a plug had a success rate of 86%.[103] Another series reported by Schwandner et al.[104] reported a 71% primary success rate with a trans-perineal approach in 21 patients. While these reports should be cause for optimism, experience with the plug for fistula-in-ano has been sobering. Initial reports of bioprosthetic quoted success rates of 80–83%.[105,106] Other recent series have been more pessimistic, with healing in 34–43% fistulas.[107,108] In general, the attraction of bioprosthetics in the treatment of rectovaginal fistulas is that the approach is technically straightforward, and there is no injury to the sphincter mechanism. The plug procedure has the additional advantage of avoiding dissection within the perineum, and therefore not impeding future repairs. Likelihood of success is still uncertain, but patients and physicians should expect that these approaches are at least as likely to fail as succeed.

One recent innovation worthy of note is a bioprosthetic plug designed specifically for use in rectovaginal fistulas.[109] The effectiveness of this plug was recently examined in one series of 12 patients.[110] Success was achieved in three of five rectovaginal fistulas and four of seven pouch-vaginal fistulas. A total of 20 plug placements were required, yielding a procedural success rate of 35% and an overall success rate of 58%.

Tissue Interposition: Muscle

Healthy, well-vascularized muscle is an ideal material for interposition and obliteration of a rectovaginal fistula. Several options are available for this approach, but the technique most commonly performed utilizes a gracilis muscle pedicled flap. The outcomes achieved with gracilis interposition are excellent, with successful repairs in 75–83% in recent series.[87,89,91] Healing has been noted to occur less often in patients with Crohn's disease.[89] Rectus, sartorius, and gluteal muscle flaps have also been reported as case reports or small series.[86,94,111,112] Fecal diversion is routinely performed for these procedures.

The major problem with this approach is the morbidity associated with the mobilization of the pedicled muscle flap and the extent of perineal dissection required to accommodate the bulky interposed tissue. Details of mobilization of the rectus, gracilis, and sartorius muscles are beyond the scope of this chapter.

Tissue Interposition: Bowel

Healthy bowel can also be used as an interposition for patients with high rectovaginal fistulas, a procedure described by Bricker and Johnston.[113] Through an abdominal incision the fistula is divided. The sigmoid colon is mobilized and divided; the proximal end is used for a temporary colostomy, and the distal end is sutured in an end to side manner to the debrided edges of the defect in the rectal wall. When healing is confirmed with a contrast study, the proximal sigmoid colon is sutured to the loop of colon utilized in the repair (Figure 14-4). Bricker et al.[114] reported excellent or satisfactory results in 19 of 26 patients.

Resection

An extended low anterior resection may be done with excision of the rectum containing the fistula and creation of an anastomosis below. The vaginal defect is closed and if possible separated from the new anastomosis with omentum. Parks and associates described a sleeve coloanal technique when the fistula is very low.[115] The rectum is mobilized to a level below the fistula and divided. From a perineal approach, a distal rectal mucosectomy is performed and

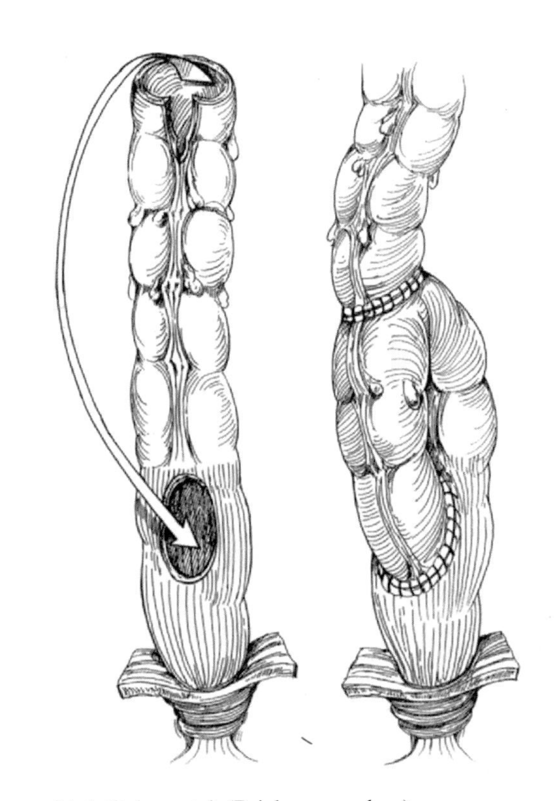

FIGURE 14-4. Onlay patch (Bricker procedure).

the proximal healthy colon is pulled through the muscular sleeve covering the fistula. A hand-sewn coloanal anastomosis is then completed, and proximal diversion is customary. Technical success is reported in 78–100% of patients.[115–117] In a review of functional results after stoma closure, 64% of patients were completely continent at 6 months and 75% at 1 year.[117]

Choice of Treatment

Not all rectovaginal fistulas require surgical treatment. Initial medical management is appropriate for women with small fistulas and minimal symptoms. Obstetric fistulas, in particular have a high rate of spontaneous closure in the 6–9 month postpartum period. Optimizing the patient's bowel function, particularly controlling diarrhea, can only improve the success of any treatment program. Unfortunately, for the majority of women with rectovaginal fistulas the symptoms are intolerable, and many require one (or more) efforts at surgical repair.

Fibrin glue instillation or fistula plug are reasonable initial attempts particularly in low, small fistulas. Their success rates are unproven, but these procedures are well tolerated, carry minimal risk, and do not impede future efforts at repair. Other surgical options should be selected on the basis of factors related to the patient and their disease process.

Rectovaginal Fistulas Secondary to Obstetrical Injury

Rectovaginal fistulas may close spontaneously in the early postpartum period (3–6 months); all others require surgery to close.[78] To facilitate surgical repair and healing, the surrounding tissue must be free of local sepsis before proceeding with surgery; this may involve surgical debridement and draining setons. Once the surrounding tissue is amenable to repair, timing of operation may be chosen by the patient together with her surgeon. Patients with significant symptoms need not wait until their childbearing is complete, although depending upon the choice of repair subsequent children should be delivered by cesarean section.

As mentioned above, an important part of the evaluation of women with rectovaginal fistulas caused by obstetrical injury is assessment of anal sphincter anatomy and function. In multiple studies, the incidence of associated sphincter defect is close to 100% in this subset of patients.[25,29,30] In women with sphincter defects, sphincteroplasty addresses both the fistula and the sphincter defect. The advantage of this technique is the excellent exposure it provides; the disadvantage is the potential risk of incontinence if intact sphincter muscle is divided. For women with intact sphincters and a rectovaginal fistula after childbirth, an advancement flap or layered fistulectomy are recommended as the initial approach. Failure should prompt an attempt with tissue interposition –Martius flap or bioprosthetics are good options. Perineo-proctotomy and sleeve advancement are best reserved for use only after multiple other approaches have failed. Preoperative diversion should be strongly considered as an adjunct in these difficult cases. Despite the many studies performed to date, the literature does not categorically support a single technique as superior; the choice of the repair should be based upon the surgeon's experience.

Rectovaginal Fistulas Secondary to Cryptoglandular Disease

Rectovaginal fistulas secondary to cryptoglandular disease are rare. Evaluation must include evaluation/treatment of associated local sepsis, and endoanal ultrasound to exclude an occult sphincter defect. In the absence of a significant sphincter defect, endorectal/endoanal advancement flap, fibrin glue, and fistula plugs are reasonable alternatives.

Rectovaginal Fistulas Secondary to Crohn's Disease

The treatment of patients with rectovaginal fistulas secondary to Crohn's disease differs from other patients with rectovaginal fistulas in several ways. Given the nature of Crohn's disease, control of symptoms becomes the primary goal as opposed to elimination of the fistula in this subset of patients.

Once any associated sepsis is controlled, medical management with antibiotics and immunosuppressive medication is the initial approach to treatment for virtually all patients with Crohn's disease and rectovaginal fistulas. Recently, infliximab (antitumor necrosis α) has demonstrated efficacy in healing Crohn's rectovaginal fistulas. In 1999, Present et al.[118] reported the results of a randomized trial comparing infliximab to placebo for Crohn's perianal fistulas with closure in 55% for infliximab vs. 13% for placebo. The multicenter trial entitled, A Crohn's disease clinical trial evaluating infliximab in a new long-term treatment regimen in patients with fistulizing Crohn's disease (ACCENT II), investigated the importance of infliximab maintenance on fistula closure; in a subset analysis of patients with rectovaginal fistulas, Sands et al.[119] reported a 44.8% closure rate at 14 weeks in 25 patients. These data are still early, and the true long-term effectiveness of infliximab is unknown, especially given the fact that the radiological healing rate is lower than the clinical healing rate.[120] Results are better when drainage of local sepsis and placement of a seton are done prior to initiating infliximab.[121] If the goal is complete healing, the seton must be removed before the completion of the course of infliximab.

In cases where medical management is able to control Crohn's proctitis, then surgical intervention for fistula repair can be considered. In these patients, the same considerations apply as in the treatment of rectovaginal fistulas in patients without Crohn's. One possible difference is that procedures which involve a significant injury to the sphincter complex (e.g., perineo-proctotomy/sphincteroplasty) should be avoided. The necessity of diversion is controversial, but it is commonly performed in this subset of patients particularly ones requiring immunosuppressive medication to control their intestinal disease. Eradication of the fistula with an endorectal advancement flap is reported in 30–70% of patients.[53,122] Kodner et al.[45] reported an initial healing rate of 71% which increased to 92% with additional procedures. The Cleveland Clinic surgeons tailor the advancement flap according to the height and length of the fistula and the presence of rectal ulceration or inflammation.[70] They report an initial healing rate of 54% and an overall success rate of 68% including repeat repairs. All of these results predate the introduction of infliximab.

For patients with rectovaginal fistulas and medically refractory Crohn's proctitis, surgical options are limited. The inflamed, friable anorectal tissue responds poorly to any intervention. Long-term use of draining setons should be considered in these patients as a bridge to future abatement of disease or progression to definitive treatment (often proctectomy). Patients with anal stricture and active colonic disease appear to be most likely to progress to proctectomy.[123] Of significant concern is the potential for developing a malignancy in the fistula. In one study, Heyen et al.[124] traced the course of 28 women with Crohn's disease and a rectovaginal fistula. Malignancy resulting in death developed in the fistula of two patients.

Rectovaginal Fistulas Secondary to Malignancy

The treatment of rectovaginal fistulas associated with underlying malignancy is dictated primarily by the therapy required for the patient's cancer. For rectal cancer, neoadjuvant chemoradiation therapy followed by surgery (including vaginectomy, with or without reconstruction) is the standard of care for nonmetastatic disease. Fecal diversion prior to initiation of treatment may be necessary for patient comfort. When resection is performed, interposition of tissue (e.g., omentum, rectus muscle) between the colorectal anastomosis and closure of the vagina may prevent a postoperative fistula if a pelvic abscess or anastomotic leak occurs.

For squamous cell carcinoma of the anus, a preexisting fistula or one that develops during chemoradiation often requires diversion for symptom control. If there is complete resolution of the tumor after chemoradiation, repair of the fistula with interposition of the bulbocavernous or gracilis muscle is indicated after a waiting period to allow for resolution of any acute radiation changes. It is unlikely that a local repair would be successful in an irradiated field. If tumor persists after chemoradiation an abdominoperineal resection is necessary. Low rates of perineal wound healing in this situation have led many surgeons to use muscle flaps for wound closure either routinely or selectively.

Rectovaginal Fistulas Secondary to Radiation Therapy

Patients with rectovaginal fistulas resulting from radiation therapy pose a challenging clinical problem. In the diagnostic evaluation of these patients, a thorough examination of the fistula site, preferably under anesthesia should be undertaken, including biopsies of the fistula to exclude recurrent cancer. Fecal diversion should be strongly considered to allow inflammation in the surrounding tissue to resolve.

Decisions regarding surgical intervention center on the patient's overall medical condition, the degree of symptoms caused by the fistula, associated abnormalities, and the risk of a proposed corrective procedure. Not uncommonly, the combination of those factors makes a colostomy alone the most reasonable choice. Permanent diversion is particularly appropriate if the patient is experiencing significant fecal incontinence. However, a variety of surgical options do exist, but these are generally different from those offered to patients who have not been treated with radiation. A guiding principle is that without interposing healthy (nonirradiated) tissue into the fistula tract, the likelihood of success is so small as to render the approach futile.

In cases where the fistula is low and the rectum is relatively normal, tissue interposition (e.g., gracilis muscle, Martius flap) through the perineum is a reasonable choice. If the fistula is high, tissue interposition (e.g., rectus muscle, Bricker procedure) through the abdomen is preferable. Stricture or severe radiation proctitis may require proctectomy, with the introduction of nonirradiated colon as a neorectum. The morbidity of this approach is high, 24% in one series.[125] A Bricker procedure avoids the morbidity of proctectomy and pelvic dissection but leaves a diseased rectum in place. The final option for some patients is an end colostomy, which may provide a quality of life superior to a poorly functioning anorectum. Patient selection and operative choice must be based on clinical experience as comparative studies do not exist.

Iatrogenic Rectovaginal Fistula

The choice of treatment for an iatrogenic rectovaginal fistula is dictated by the factors discussed previously. Fistulas developing after rectal resection almost always arise at the anastomosis and are reported after both hand-sewn and stapled anastomoses.[126,127] An important step toward preventing this complication is to palpate the posterior wall of the vagina while simultaneously rotating the closed EEA stapler during creation of the anastomosis. If dimpling is felt or the vaginal mucosa is felt to be in close apposition to the stapler, the device should be repositioned. Once a fistula occurs, the first goal of therapy is to control local sepsis, which may require temporary diversion and/or drainage procedures. Repair is determined by the level of the fistula. Low fistulas may be amenable to rectal or vaginal advancement flaps; a trans-perineal approach with interposed bioprosthetic material or muscle is also reasonable. High fistulas usually require repeat resection with anastomosis or interposition of omentum or muscle. Large fistulas or those failing initial attempts at repair will usually require tissue interposition.

Persistent Rectovaginal Fistula

There are little data regarding fistulas which persist after an attempted repair. Repeat repairs after one failed attempt appear to have a reasonable success rate, but failure rate after additional procedures increases dramatically so subsequent options should be chosen carefully.[76,77] Work by MacRae et al.[46] highlights the importance of tailoring the surgical approach. They retrospectively reviewed 28 patients who had failed at least one previous attempt at repair. Of 18 patients with simple fistulas, successful repair was accomplished in 13; these successes included 5 advancement flaps, 5 sphincteroplasties, and 3 coloanal anastomoses. In ten patients with complex fistulas, only four patients healed; these involved one sphincteroplasty, one coloanal anastomosis, and two gracilis muscle interpositions. In a report from the Cleveland Clinic, Halverson et al.[77] retrospectively reviewed 33 patients with recurrent rectovaginal fistulas. Advancement flap, sphincteroplasty, rectal sleeve advancement, insertion of fibrin glue, and ileal pouch revision were utilized. Fistula closure was accomplished in 27 of these 33 patients (82%) after a median of two operations. While the overall results are encouraging, the highly heterogenous patient cohort makes it difficult to extract meaningful recommendations for specific patient populations.

Recent studies on bioprosthetic material offer an encouraging alternative to the surgical options described by Halverson et al.[77] and MacRae et al.[46] Ellis[103] reported success in 10 of 14 women (71%) with recurrent rectovaginal fistula using a trans-perineal placement of porcine intestinal submucosal biologic mesh. Similar success has been reported by Schwandner et al.[104] who achieved closure in 15 of 21 women (71%) with recurrent fistulas. Of note, 38% of patients in the Schwandner study had their procedures performed with fecal diversion; no data regarding diversion were reported by Ellis.

From the data available, it appears that a reasonable approach to recurrent rectovaginal fistulas would begin with a period of conservative treatment during which any areas of sepsis are drained and the integrity of the sphincters are evaluated. For low fistulas, the treatment choice depends upon the status of the sphincter and the number of prior repairs. If the sphincter is intact and only one or perhaps two previous repairs have been attempted, an advancement flap or rectal sleeve advancement would be appropriate. Insertion of fibrin glue is a safe alternative but there are little data regarding the expected success rate. If there is a defect in the sphincter muscle, sphincteroplasty or perineo-proctotomy is an appropriate choice. In cases where the sphincter is intact and two or more repairs have failed then an interposition technique should be considered. The choice of technique depends on the expertise of the surgeon; insertion of bulbocavernous muscle is the least morbid transposition method, but there are no good comparative data regarding outcomes of the various interposition methods. Fecal diversion is not absolutely necessary but likely increases the success of repair, especially in patients with Crohn's disease. Recurrent fistulas involving the middle of the vagina almost always require tissue interposition. The choice depends upon the level of the fistula and the body habitus of the patient. Bulbocavernous muscle may not reach if the patient is obese or the fistula is in the upper middle third of the vagina. Gracilis muscle would be a good alternative in those situations. High fistulas require resection or tissue interposition through an abdominal approach.

Conclusion

The literature on rectovaginal fistulas documents a wealth of clinical experience. However, there is a definite lack of uniform terminology, standardized evaluation and comparative studies. Given the multitude of etiologies and the varying nature of the anatomy and condition of surrounding tissue, improving the quality of research will be challenging. However, continued work is necessary to determine appropriate patient selection and optimal surgical repair.

References

1. Homsi R, Daikoku NH, Littlejohn J, Wheeless Jr CR. Episiotomy: risks of dehiscence and rectovaginal fistula. Obstet Gynecol Surv. 1994;49:803–8.
2. Venkatesh KS, Ramanujam PS, Larson DM, Haywood MA. Anorectal complications of vaginal delivery. Dis Colon Rectum. 1989;32:1039–41.
3. Beynon CL. Midline episiotomy as a routine procedure. J Obstet Gynaecol Br Commonw. 1974;81:126–30.
4. Hamlin C, Turnbull GB. The treatment of rectovaginal and vesicovaginal fistulas in women with childbirth injuries in Ethiopia. J Wound Ostomy Continence Nurs. 1997;24:187–9.
5. Margolis T, Elkins TE, Seffah J, Oparo-Addo HS, Fort D. Full-thickness Martius grafts to preserve vaginal depth as an adjunct in the repair of large obstetric fistulas. Obstet Gynecol. 1994;84:148–52.
6. Ahmed S, Genadry R, Stanton C, Lalonde AB. Dead women walking: neglected millions with obstetric fistula. Int J Gynaecol Obstet. 2007;99 Suppl 1:S1–3.

7. Schwartz DA, Loftus Jr EV, Tremaine WJ, et al. The natural history of fistulizing Crohn's disease in Olmsted County, Minnesota. Gastroenterology. 2002;122:875–80.
8. Radcliffe AG, Ritchie JK, Hawley PR, Lennard-Jones JE, Northover JM. Anovaginal and rectovaginal fistulas in Crohn's disease. Dis Colon Rectum. 1988;31:94–9.
9. Nakagoe T, Sawai T, Tuji T, et al. Avoidance of rectovaginal fistula as a complication after low anterior resection for rectal cancer using a double-stapling technique. J Surg Oncol. 1999;71:196–7.
10. Bassi R, Rademacher J, Savoia A. Rectovaginal fistula after STARR procedure complicated by haematoma of the posterior vaginal wall: report of a case. Tech Coloproctol. 2006;10:361–3.
11. Cirocco WC. Life threatening sepsis and mortality following stapled hemorrhoidopexy. Surgery. 2008;143:824–9.
12. Groom JS, Nicholls RJ, Hawley PR, Phillips RK. Pouch-vaginal fistula. Br J Surg. 1993;80:936–40.
13. Jayne DG, Schwandner O, Stuto A. Stapled transanal rectal resection for obstructed defecation syndrome: one-year results of the European STARR Registry. Dis Colon Rectum. 2009;52:1205–12. discussion 12-4.
14. O'Kelly TJ, Merrett M, Mortensen NJ, Dehn TC, Kettlewell M. Pouch-vaginal fistula after restorative proctocolectomy: aetiology and management. Br J Surg. 1994;81:1374–5.
15. Paye F, Penna C, Chiche L, Tiret E, Frileux P, Parc R. Pouch-related fistula following restorative proctocolectomy. Br J Surg. 1996;83:1574–7.
16. Wexner SD, Rothenberger DA, Jensen L, et al. Ileal pouch vaginal fistulas: incidence, etiology, and management. Dis Colon Rectum. 1989;32:460–5.
17. Schwartz J, Rabinowitz H, Rozenfeld V, Leibovitz A, Stelian J, Habot B. Rectovaginal fistula associated with fecal impaction. J Am Geriatr Soc. 1992;40:641.
18. Hoffman MS, Wakeley KE, Cardosi RJ. Risks of rigid dilation for a radiated vaginal cuff: two related rectovaginal fistulas. Obstet Gynecol. 2003;101:1125–6.
19. Sharland M, Peake J, Davies EG. Pseudomonal rectovaginal abscesses in HIV infection. Arch Dis Child. 1995;72:275.
20. Parra JM, Kellogg ND. Repair of a recto-vaginal fistula as a result of sexual assault. Semin Perioper Nurs. 1995;4:140–5.
21. Chereau E, Stefanescu D, Selle F, Rouzier R, Darai E. Spontaneous rectovaginal fistula during bevacizumab therapy for ovarian cancer: a case report. Am J Obstet Gynecol. 2009;200:e15–6.
22. Buyukasik O, Hasdemir OA, Col C. Rectal lumen obliteration from stapled hemorrhoidopexy: can it be prevented? Tech Coloproctol. 2009;19:19.
23. Ijaiya MA, Mai AM, Aboyeji AP, Kumanda V, Abiodun MO, Raji HO. Rectovaginal fistula following sexual intercourse: a case report. Ann Afr Med. 2009;8:59–60.
24. Powers K, Grigorescu B, Lazarou G, Greston WM, Weber T. Neglected pessary causing a rectovaginal fistula: a case report. J Reprod Med. 2008;53:235–7.
25. Tsang CB, Madoff RD, Wong WD, et al. Anal sphincter integrity and function influences outcome in rectovaginal fistula repair. Dis Colon Rectum. 1998;41:1141–6.
26. Bird D, Taylor D, Lee P. Vaginography: the investigation of choice for vaginal fistulas? Aust N Z J Surg. 1993;63:894–6.
27. Giordano P, Drew PJ, Taylor D, Duthie G, Lee PW, Monson JR. Vaginography – investigation of choice for clinically suspected vaginal fistulas. Dis Colon Rectum. 1996;39:568–72.
28. Sudol-Szopinska I, Jakubowski W, Szczepkowski M. Contrast-enhanced endosonography for the diagnosis of anal and anovaginal fistulas. J Clin Ultrasound. 2002;30:145–50.
29. Yee LF, Birnbaum EH, Read TE, Kodner IJ, Fleshman JW. Use of endoanal ultrasound in patients with rectovaginal fistulas. Dis Colon Rectum. 1999;42:1057–64.
30. Khanduja KS, Yamashita HJ, Wise Jr WE, Aguilar PS, Hartmann RF. Delayed repair of obstetric injuries of the anorectum and vagina. A stratified surgical approach. Dis Colon Rectum. 1994;37:344–9.
31. Stoker J, Rociu E, Schouten WR, Lameris JS. Anovaginal and rectovaginal fistulas: endoluminal sonography versus endoluminal MR imaging. AJR Am J Roentgenol. 2002;178:737–41.
32. Maier AG, Funovics MA, Kreuzer SH, et al. Evaluation of perianal sepsis: comparison of anal endosonography and magnetic resonance imaging. J Magn Reson Imaging. 2001;14:254–60.
33. Zbar AP, Armitage NC. Complex perirectal sepsis: clinical classification and imaging. Tech Coloproctol. 2006;10:83–93.
34. Daniels B. Rectovaginal fistula: a clinical and pathological study. Pathology. Minneapolis, MN: University of Minnesota; 1940.
35. Rothenberger DA, Goldberg SM. The management of rectovaginal fistulas. Surg Clin North Am. 1983;63:61–79.
36. Cintron JR, Park JJ, Orsay CP, et al. Repair of fistulas-in-ano using fibrin adhesive: long-term follow-up. Dis Colon Rectum. 2000;43:944–9. discussion 9-50.
37. Loungnarath R, Dietz DW, Mutch MG, Birnbaum EH, Kodner IJ, Fleshman JW. Fibrin glue treatment of complex anal fistulas has low success rate. Dis Colon Rectum. 2004;47:432–6.
38. Ellis CN, Clark S. Fibrin glue as an adjunct to flap repair of anal fistulas: a randomized, controlled study. Dis Colon Rectum. 2006;49:1736–40.
39. Abel ME, Chiu YS, Russell TR, Volpe PA. Autologous fibrin glue in the treatment of rectovaginal and complex fistulas. Dis Colon Rectum. 1993;36:447–9.
40. Venkatesh KS, Ramanujam P. Fibrin glue application in the treatment of recurrent anorectal fistulas. Dis Colon Rectum. 1999;42:1136–9.
41. Greenwald JC, Hoexter B. Repair of rectovaginal fistulas. Surg Gynecol Obstet. 1978;146:443–5.
42. Hoexter B, Labow SB, Moseson MD. Transanal rectovaginal fistula repair. Dis Colon Rectum. 1985;28:572–5.
43. Wise Jr WE, Aguilar PS, Padmanabhan A, Meesig DM, Arnold MW, Stewart WR. Surgical treatment of low rectovaginal fistulas. Dis Colon Rectum. 1991;34:271–4.
44. Lowry AC, Goldberg SM. Simple rectovaginal fistula. In: Cameron J, editor. Current Surgical Therapy. 4th ed. St. Louis, MO: Mosby; 1991.
45. Kodner IJ, Mazor A, Shemesh EI, Fry RD, Fleshman JW, Birnbaum EH. Endorectal advancement flap repair of rectovaginal and other complicated anorectal fistulas. Surgery. 1993;114:682–9. discussion 9-90.
46. MacRae HM, McLeod RS, Cohen Z, Stern H, Reznick R. Treatment of rectovaginal fistulas that has failed previous repair attempts. Dis Colon Rectum. 1995;38:921–5.

47. Mazier WP, Senagore AJ, Schiesel EC. Operative repair of anovaginal and rectovaginal fistulas. Dis Colon Rectum. 1995; 38:4–6.
48. Watson SJ, Phillips RK. Non-inflammatory rectovaginal fistula. Br J Surg. 1995;82:1641–3.
49. Hyman N. Endoanal advancement flap repair for complex anorectal fistulas. Am J Surg. 1999;178:337–40.
50. Joo JS, Latulippe JF, Alabaz O, Weiss EG, Nogueras JJ, Wexner SD. Long-term functional evaluation of straight coloanal anastomosis and colonic J-pouch: is the functional superiority of colonic J-pouch sustained? Dis Colon Rectum. 1998;41:740–6.
51. Baig MK, Zhao RH, Yuen CH, et al. Simple rectovaginal fistulas. Int J Colorectal Dis. 2000;15:323–7.
52. Mizrahi N, Wexner SD, Zmora O, et al. Endorectal advancement flap: are there predictors of failure? Dis Colon Rectum. 2002;45:1616–21.
53. Sonoda T, Hull T, Piedmonte MR, Fazio VW. Outcomes of primary repair of anorectal and rectovaginal fistulas using the endorectal advancement flap. Dis Colon Rectum. 2002;45:1622–8.
54. Zimmerman DD, Gosselink MP, Briel JW, Schouten WR. The outcome of transanal advancement flap repair of rectovaginal fistulas is not improved by an additional labial fat flap transposition. Tech Coloproctol. 2002;6:37–42.
55. Casadesus D, Villasana L, Sanchez IM, Diaz H, Chavez M, Diaz A. Treatment of rectovaginal fistula: a 5-year review. Aust N Z J Obstet Gynaecol. 2006;46:49–51.
56. Uribe N, Millan M, Minguez M, et al. Clinical and manometric results of endorectal advancement flaps for complex anal fistula. Int J Colorectal Dis. 2007;22:259–64.
57. Abbas MA, Lemus-Rangel R, Hamadani A. Long-term outcome of endorectal advancement flap for complex anorectal fistulas. Am Surg. 2008;74:921–4.
58. Ozuner G, Hull TL, Cartmill J, Fazio VW. Long-term analysis of the use of transanal rectal advancement flaps for complicated anorectal/vaginal fistulas. Dis Colon Rectum. 1996;39:10–4.
59. Vavra P, Dostalik J, Vavrova M, et al. Transanal endoscopic microsurgery: a novel technique for the repair of benign rectovaginal fistula. Surgeon. 2009;7:126–7.
60. Darwood RJ, Borley NR. TEMS: an alternative method for the repair of benign recto-vaginal fistulas. Colorectal Dis. 2008;10:619–20.
61. Zimmerman DD, Gosselink MP, Mitalas LE, et al. Smoking impairs rectal mucosal bloodflow – a pilot study: possible implications for transanal advancement flap repair. Dis Colon Rectum. 2005;48:1228–32.
62. Zimmerman DD, Delemarre JB, Gosselink MP, Hop WC, Briel JW, Schouten WR. Smoking affects the outcome of transanal mucosal advancement flap repair of trans-sphincteric fistulas. Br J Surg. 2003;90:351–4.
63. Hesterberg R, Schmidt WU, Muller F, Roher HD. Treatment of anovaginal fistulas with an anocutaneous flap in patients with Crohn's disease. Int J Colorectal Dis. 1993;8:51–4.
64. Haray PN, Stiff G, Foster ME. New option for recurrent rectovaginal fistulas. Dis Colon Rectum. 1996;39:463–4.
65. Hibbard LT. Surgical management of rectovaginal fistulas and complete perineal tears. Am J Obstet Gynecol. 1978;130: 139–41.
66. Lawson J. Rectovaginal fistulas following difficult labour. Proc R Soc Med. 1972;65:283–6.
67. Lescher TC, Pratt JH. Vaginal repair of the simple rectovaginal fistula. Surg Gynecol Obstet. 1967;124:1317–21.
68. Tancer ML, Lasser D, Rosenblum N. Rectovaginal fistula or perineal and anal sphincter disruption, or both, after vaginal delivery. Surg Gynecol Obstet. 1990;171:43–6.
69. Simmang CL, Lacey SW, Huber Jr PJ. Rectal sleeve advancement: repair of rectovaginal fistula associated with anorectal stricture in Crohn's disease. Dis Colon Rectum. 1998;41:787–9.
70. Hull TL, Fazio VW. Surgical approaches to low anovaginal fistula in Crohn's disease. Am J Surg. 1997;173:95–8.
71. Schouten WR, Oom DM. Rectal sleeve advancement for the treatment of persistent rectovaginal fistulas. Tech Coloproctol. 2009;19:19.
72. Veronikis DK, Nichols DH, Spino C. The Noble–Mengert–Fish operation-revisited: a composite approach for persistent rectovaginal fistulas and complex perineal defects. Am J Obstet Gynecol. 1998;179:1411–6. discussion 6-7.
73. Mengert WF, Fish SA. Anterior rectal wall advancement; technic for repair of complete perineal laceration and rectovaginal fistula. Obstet Gynecol. 1955;5:262–7.
74. Russell TR, Gallagher DM. Low rectovaginal fistulas. Approach and treatment. Am J Surg. 1977;134:13–8.
75. Hilsabeck JR. Transanal advancement of the anterior rectal wall for vaginal fistulas involving the lower rectum. Dis Colon Rectum. 1980;23:236–41.
76. Lowry AC, Thorson AG, Rothenberger DA, Goldberg SM. Repair of simple rectovaginal fistulas. Influence of previous repairs. Dis Colon Rectum. 1988;31:676–8.
77. Halverson AL, Hull TL, Fazio VW, Church J, Hammel J, Floruta C. Repair of recurrent rectovaginal fistulas. Surgery. 2001;130:753–7. discussion 7-8.
78. Rahman MS, Al-Suleiman SA, El-Yahia AR, Rahman J. Surgical treatment of rectovaginal fistula of obstetric origin: a review of 15 years' experience in a teaching hospital. J Obstet Gynaecol. 2003;23:607–10.
79. Pepe F, Panella M, Arikian S, Panella P, Pepe G. Low rectovaginal fistulas. Aust N Z J Obstet Gynaecol. 1987;27: 61–3.
80. Hudson CN. Acquired fistulas between the intestine and the vagina. Ann R Coll Surg Engl. 1970;46:20–40.
81. Rojanasakul A. LIFT procedure: a simplified technique for fistula-in-ano. Tech Coloproctol. 2009;13:237–40.
82. Rojanasakul A, Pattanaarun J, Sahakitrungruang C, Tantiphlachiva K. Total anal sphincter saving technique for fistula-in-ano; the ligation of intersphincteric fistula tract. J Med Assoc Thai. 2007;90:581–6.
83. Bleier JI, Moloo H, Goldberg SM. Ligation of the intersphincteric fistula tract: an effective new technique for complex fistulas. Abstract presented at the American Society of Colon and Rectal Surgeons Annual Meeting, May, 2009.
84. Ulrich D, Roos J, Jakse G, Pallua N. Gracilis muscle interposition for the treatment of recto-urethral and rectovaginal fistulas: a retrospective analysis of 35 cases. J Plast Reconstr Aesthet Surg. 2009;62:352–6.
85. Reisenauer C, Huebner M, Wallwiener D. The repair of rectovaginal fistulas using a bulbocavernosus muscle-fat flap. Arch Gynecol Obstet. 2009;279:919–22.

86. Onishi K, Ogino A, Saida Y, Maruyama Y. Repair of a recurrent rectovaginal fistula using gluteal-fold flap: report of a case. Surg Today. 2009;39:615–8.
87. Lefevre JH, Bretagnol F, Maggiori L, Alves A, Ferron M, Panis Y. Operative results and quality of life after gracilis muscle transposition for recurrent rectovaginal fistula. Dis Colon Rectum. 2009;52:1290–5.
88. Cui L, Chen D, Chen W, Jiang H. Interposition of vital bulbocavernosus graft in the treatment of both simple and recurrent rectovaginal fistulas. Int J Colorectal Dis. 2009;24:1255–9.
89. Wexner SD, Ruiz DE, Genua J, Nogueras JJ, Weiss EG, Zmora O. Gracilis muscle interposition for the treatment of rectourethral, rectovaginal, and pouch-vaginal fistulas: results in 53 patients. Ann Surg. 2008;248:39–43.
90. McNevin MS, Lee PY, Bax TW. Martius flap: an adjunct for repair of complex, low rectovaginal fistula. Am J Surg. 2007;193:597–9. discussion 9.
91. Zmora O, Tulchinsky H, Gur E, Goldman G, Klausner JM, Rabau M. Gracilis muscle transposition for fistulas between the rectum and urethra or vagina. Dis Colon Rectum. 2006;49:1316–21.
92. Rabau M, Zmora O, Tulchinsky H, Gur E, Goldman G. Recto-vaginal/urethral fistula: repair with gracilis muscle transposition. Acta Chir Iugosl. 2006;53:81–4.
93. Onodera H, Nagayama S, Kohmoto I, Maetani S, Imamura M. Novel surgical repair with bilateral gluteus muscle patching for intractable rectovaginal fistula. Tech Coloproctol. 2003;7:198–202.
94. Tran KT, Kuijpers HC, van Nieuwenhoven EJ, van Goor H, Spauwen PH. Transposition of the rectus abdominis muscle for complicated pouch and rectal fistulas. Dis Colon Rectum. 1999;42:486–9.
95. Pinedo G, Phillips R. Labial fat pad grafts (modified Martius graft) in complex perianal fistulas. Ann R Coll Surg Engl. 1998;80:410–2.
96. Elkins TE. Surgery for the obstetric vesicovaginal fistula: a review of 100 operations in 82 patients. Am J Obstet Gynecol. 1994;170:1108–18. discussion 18-20.
97. White AJ, Buchsbaum HJ, Blythe JG, Lifshitz S. Use of the bulbocavernosus muscle (Martius procedure) for repair of radiation-induced rectovaginal fistulas. Obstet Gynecol. 1982;60:114–8.
98. Aartsen EJ, Sindram IS. Repair of the radiation induced rectovaginal fistulas without or with interposition of the bulbocavernosus muscle (Martius procedure). Eur J Surg Oncol. 1988;14:171–7.
99. Boronow RC. Repair of the radiation-induced vaginal fistula utilizing the Martius technique. World J Surg. 1986;10:237–48.
100. Zacharin RF. Grafting as a principle in the surgical management of vesicovaginal and rectovaginal fistulas. Aust N Z J Obstet Gynaecol. 1980;20:10–7.
101. Pye PK, Dada T, Duthie G, Phillips K. Surgisistrade mark mesh: a novel approach to repair of a recurrent rectovaginal fistula. Dis Colon Rectum. 2004;47:1554–6.
102. Moore RD, Miklos JR, Kohli N. Rectovaginal fistula repair using a porcine dermal graft. Obstet Gynecol. 2004;104:1165–7.
103. Ellis CN. Outcomes after repair of rectovaginal fistulas using bioprosthetics. Dis Colon Rectum. 2008;51:1084–8.
104. Schwandner O, Fuerst A, Kunstreich K, Scherer R. Innovative technique for the closure of rectovaginal fistula using Surgisis mesh. Tech Coloproctol. 2009;13:135–40.
105. Champagne BJ, O'Connor LM, Ferguson M, Orangio GR, Schertzer ME, Armstrong DN. Efficacy of anal fistula plug in closure of cryptoglandular fistulas: long-term follow-up. Dis Colon Rectum. 2006;49:1817–21.
106. O'Connor L, Champagne BJ, Ferguson MA, Orangio GR, Schertzer ME, Armstrong DN. Efficacy of anal fistula plug in closure of Crohn's anorectal fistulas. Dis Colon Rectum. 2006;49:1569–73.
107. Wang JY, Garcia-Aguilar J, Sternberg JA, Abel ME, Varma MG. Treatment of transsphincteric anal fistulas: are fistula plugs an acceptable alternative? Dis Colon Rectum. 2009;52:692–7.
108. Christoforidis D, Etzioni DA, Goldberg SM, Madoff RD, Mellgren A. Treatment of complex anal fistulas with the collagen fistula plug. Dis Colon Rectum. 2008;51:1482–7.
109. http://www.cookmedical.com/sur/content/mmedia/SUR-BM-RVP-EN-200709.pdf. Accessed 11 Sept 2009.
110. Gonsalves S, Sagar P, Lengyel J, Morrison C, Dunham R. Assessment of the efficacy of the rectovaginal button fistula plug for the treatment of ileal pouch-vaginal and rectovaginal fistulas. Dis Colon Rectum. 2009;52:1887–81.
111. Horch RE, Gitsch G, Schultze-Seemann W. Bilateral pedicled myocutaneous vertical rectus abdominus muscle flaps to close vesicovaginal and pouch-vaginal fistulas with simultaneous vaginal and perineal reconstruction in irradiated pelvic wounds. Urology. 2002;60:502–7.
112. Byron Jr RL, Ostergard DR. Sartorius muscle interposition for the treatment of the radiation-induced vaginal fistula. Am J Obstet Gynecol. 1969;104:104–7.
113. Bricker EM, Johnston WD. Repair of postirradiation rectovaginal fistula and stricture. Surg Gynecol Obstet. 1979;148:499–506.
114. Bricker EM, Kraybill WG, Lopez MJ. Functional results after postirradiation rectal reconstruction. World J Surg. 1986;10:249–58.
115. Parks AG, Allen CL, Frank JD, McPartlin JF. A method of treating post-irradiation rectovaginal fistulas. Br J Surg. 1978;65:417–21.
116. Nowacki MP, Szawlowski AW, Borkowski A. Parks' coloanal sleeve anastomosis for treatment of postirradiation rectovaginal fistula. Dis Colon Rectum. 1986;29:817–20.
117. Cooke SA, de Moor NG. The surgical treatment of the radiation-damaged rectum. Br J Surg. 1981;68:488–92.
118. Present DH, Rutgeerts P, Targan S, et al. Infliximab for the treatment of fistulas in patients with Crohn's disease. N Engl J Med. 1999;340:1398–405.
119. Sands BE, Blank MA, Patel K, van Deventer SJ. Long-term treatment of rectovaginal fistulas in Crohn's disease: response to infliximab in the ACCENT II Study. Clin Gastroenterol Hepatol. 2004;2:912–20.
120. Van Assche G, Vanbeckevoort D, Bielen D, et al. Magnetic resonance imaging of the effects of infliximab on perianal fistulizing Crohn's disease. Am J Gastroenterol. 2003;98:332–9.
121. Topstad DR, Panaccione R, Heine JA, Johnson DR, MacLean AR, Buie WD. Combined seton placement, infliximab infusion, and maintenance immunosuppressives improve healing rate in fistulizing anorectal Crohn's disease: a single center experience. Dis Colon Rectum. 2003;46:577–83.
122. Morrison JG, Gathright Jr JB, Ray JE, Ferrari BT, Hicks TC, Timmcke AE. Results of operation for rectovaginal fistula in Crohn's disease. Dis Colon Rectum. 1989;32:497–9.
123. Galandiuk S, Kimberling J, Al-Mishlab TG, Stromberg AJ. Perianal Crohn disease: predictors of need for permanent diversion. Ann Surg. 2005;241:796–801. discussion-2.

124. Heyen F, Winslet MC, Andrews H, Alexander-Williams J, Keighley MR. Vaginal fistulas in Crohn's disease. Dis Colon Rectum. 1989;32:379–83.
125. Nowacki MP. Ten years of experience with Parks' coloanal sleeve anastomosis for the treatment of post-irradiation rectovaginal fistula. Eur J Surg Oncol. 1991;17:563–6.
126. Rex Jr JC, Khubchandani IT. Rectovaginal fistula: complication of low anterior resection. Dis Colon Rectum. 1992;35:354–6.
127. Sugarbaker PH. Rectovaginal fistula following low circular stapled anastomosis in women with rectal cancer. J Surg Oncol. 1996;61:155–8.

15 Pilonidal Disease and Hidradenitis Suppurativa

Harry T. Papaconstantinou and J. Scott Thomas

Pilonidal Disease

Background and Incidence

Pilonidal disease refers to a subcutaneous infection occurring in the upper half of the gluteal cleft. It may present as an acute pilonidal abscess with pain, erythema, and induration or as a pilonidal sinus, which is an indolent wound that is resistant to spontaneous healing, and can cause significant discomfort and drainage. Pilonidal disease is commonly found in young adults, and typically present in the second decade of life.[1] Men are more frequently affected than women at a ratio of three or four to one, and is more commonly seen in individuals with more body hair.[1] It is not known to be more common in any one racial group; however, certain occupations such as the military, hairdressers, and sheepshearers have been associated with the development of pilonidal disease.[2–4] Other predisposing factors to pilonidal disease have been suggested and include obesity, being a vehicle driver, a sedentary occupation, and having a history of a furuncle at another site on the body.[5,6] Others have implicated anatomic factors such as natal cleft as risk factors for pilonidal disease.[7] In a study of 50 patients with pilonidal disease, the depth of natal cleft was compared to 51 volunteers.[7] The report shows a significantly deeper natal cleft in the pilonidal disease group (27.1 vs. 21.1 mm; $p<0.01$). Although a genetic predisposition has not been determined, family history does seem to play a role in this disease process. A recent report indicates that a family history of pilonidal disease predisposes patients to earlier onset of the disease and higher long-term (25 years) recurrence rate of over 50%.[8]

The incidence of pilonidal disease is not accurately known, but has been reported to affect up to 0.7% of adolescents and young adults[1] and up to 8.8% of recruits in the Turkish army.[5] Others have calculated the incidence of the disease at 26 per 100,000 persons regardless of age.[6]

Pilonidal disease first appeared in the medical literature in 1833 when William Mayo published his first descriptions of this problem.[9,10] In 1880, Hodges[11] introduced the term "pilonidal," which means "hair nest." The term pilonidal "cyst" is a misnomer, because no epithelialized wall exists in the cavities this disease creates. Pilonidal "sinus" or "disease" are the more accurate terms. Pilonidal disease itself, and the surgical and medical treatment related to it, can be a significant source of morbidity and disability. This disease disables patients primarily because of pain and its inconvenient location in the gluteal cleft.

Traditionally, treatment for pilonidal disease was wide local excision; however, in World War II entire hospital wards were filled with soldiers convalescing from these large excisional operations.[12] In fact, nearly 80,000 soldiers were hospitalized for an average of 55 days for wound healing.[13] It became such a problem that the Surgeon General forbade wide local excision as primary therapy. Thus, World War II symbolizes a paradigm shift that occurred in favor of conservative management for pilonidal disease. Much has evolved in the treatment of pilonidal disease and ranges from nonoperative treatments such as shaving and hygiene to operative procedures ranging from excision to flap reconstruction. Each has its role in treating this disease spectrum, and management of pilonidal disease should be tailored to the individual clinical presentation; however, no treatment has proved completely satisfactory. Treatment goals should be maintained and include the complete resolution of the pilonidal disease through methods that have low recurrence and low morbidity.

Pathogenesis

The etiology of pilonidal disease has been controversial, with initial beliefs tied to embryologic origins. Pilonidal disease was considered to be an inborn defect of the skin in the intergluteal region secondary to a remnant of the medullary canal and infolding of the surface epithelium; however, empiric data currently supports this disease as being an acquired condition. First, the disease is not present at birth, but in young adults; second, it is more frequent in hirsute men; and third,

D.E. Beck et al. (eds.), *The ASCRS Textbook of Colon and Rectal Surgery: Second Edition*,
DOI 10.1007/978-1-4419-1584-9_15, © Springer Science+Business Media, LLC 2011

certain occupations predispose people to develop pilonidal disease.[14] Pilonidal disease has been observed in the hands of barbers and sheep shearers, implying that shed hairs may initiate the condition.[3,4]

The acquired theory of pilonidal disease is most popular, but the mechanism varies widely. This disease most likely results from problems that attack the epidermis in the gluteal cleft, rather than from a problem in the deep tissues.[13] Bascom believes that the skin in the natal cleft is normal; however, conditions may exist that predispose a patient to pilonidal disease.[13,15] Bascom[16] believes that hair follicles in the natal cleft become distended with keratin and then infected, forming an abscess that eventually ruptures into the subcutaneous tissue. Vacuum forces and negative suction in the natal cleft draws hair and debris into the midline pits of the hair follicle then into the abscess cavity (pilonidal abscess).[9] Karydakis[17] proposed that hair with chisel-like roots inserts itself into the natal cleft leading to foreign body tissue reaction and infection. Both theories seems plausible as pilonidal lesions have the pathologic characteristics of a foreign body reaction, presumably from burrowed or subcutaneously displaced hair and epithelial debris[1]; however, no published study exist which directly prove or refute the current theories about how pilonidal disease occurs.

Certain anatomic features of pilonidal disease are well established and not associated with any particular theory.[14] They include a midline pit in the natal cleft that is referred to as the primary opening. The pit often extends into a subcutaneous fibrous tract called the pilonidal sinus, which connects to a secondary opening. The secondary opening is located off the midline and is characterized by drainage of purulent or serosanguinous fluid, the presence of granulation tissue, and hypertrophy of the epithelium surrounding the opening. Hair is seen extruding from the primary opening. The pilonidal sinus tract may be single or multiple, short or long, and up to 93% run in the cephalad direction. If the pilonidal sinus runs caudad, the secondary opening may resemble the opening of a fistula-in-ano.

Clinical Presentation and Diagnosis

Pilonidal disease can present acutely as a pilonidal abscess or as a chronically draining sinus tract with intermittent symptoms of pain and drainage followed by long quiescent periods. Diagnosis is indicated by the site and appearance of the disease, and identification of midline pits in the natal cleft skin. Findings can be classified into *acute pilonidal abscess*, *chronic pilonidal sinus*, and *recurrent* or *complex pilonidal sinus*.

Acute pilonidal abscess can be characterized by a tender fluctuant subcutaneous mass with surrounding cellulitis located off midline of the natal cleft. Onset is rapid and pain is severe. *Chronic pilonidal sinus* has a primary pit in the midline natal cleft located 4–5 cm cephalad to the anus. The pit will sometimes have hair extruding from the opening. There may be a secondary opening located cephalad and off midline at a variable distance from the primary opening. Patients with long-standing disease may have *complicated pilonidal sinus* with multiple sinus tracts and partially drained abscess cavities. Uncommonly, this process can be quite destructive with large sinus cavities extending out into the lateral gluteal regions. Occasionally, patients may present with *recurrent pilonidal disease* having had many different surgical procedures performed in the past for their disease. These patients may have a persistent wound from a midline excision or a failed flap procedure.

The differential diagnosis for these patients includes hidradenitis suppurativa and fistula-in-ano, and, less commonly, actinomycosis and syphilitic or tuberculous granulomas. Patients with chronic draining wounds or multiple failed operations for pilonidal disease may have osteomyelitis with draining sinus tracts. In these patients, a bone scan or magnetic resonance imaging (MRI) should be considered.

Treatment

The treatment of pilonidal disease is determined by the initial presentation of the disease. All *acute pilonidal abscesses* must be incised and drained. Most simple *chronic pilonidal sinuses* can be layed open, while *recurrent* and *complex pilonidal sinuses* may require excision with reconstruction. Optimal treatment protocols for each group include the following goals: ease of performance; short or no hospitalization; low recurrence rate; minimal pain and wound care; fast return to normal activity; and cost effectiveness. It is important to remember that no single procedure or treatment meets all these criteria.

Acute Pilonidal Abscess

Drainage of a pilonidal abscess can be performed in the office or emergency room under local anesthesia. The incision is made parallel to the midline and at least 1 cm laterally, to facilitate healing of the wound (Figure 15-1). A small ellipse of skin from the wound is removed to prevent the skin edges from sealing and reforming the abscess. Packing of these wounds is painful and potentially interferes with drainage and healing, and is therefore discouraged. Simply cover the wound with a dressing and have the patient do Sitz baths or use a hand-held shower to clean the wound and remove hair and debris two to three times a day. Antibiotics are only necessary in the patient with diabetes, prosthetic implants, immunocompromized diseases, or significant cellulitis. The patient should return to the office every week or two until the wound heals. Any hair that has grown back within 2 in. of the entire gluteal cleft is shaved during each visit (Figure 15-2). Once the wound has healed, the recurrence rate is 50% and may be in the form of an abscess or chronic pilonidal sinus.[14]

Chronic Pilonidal Sinus

Chronic uncomplicated pilonidal sinus has minimal to no acute inflammation. Primary and secondary openings are

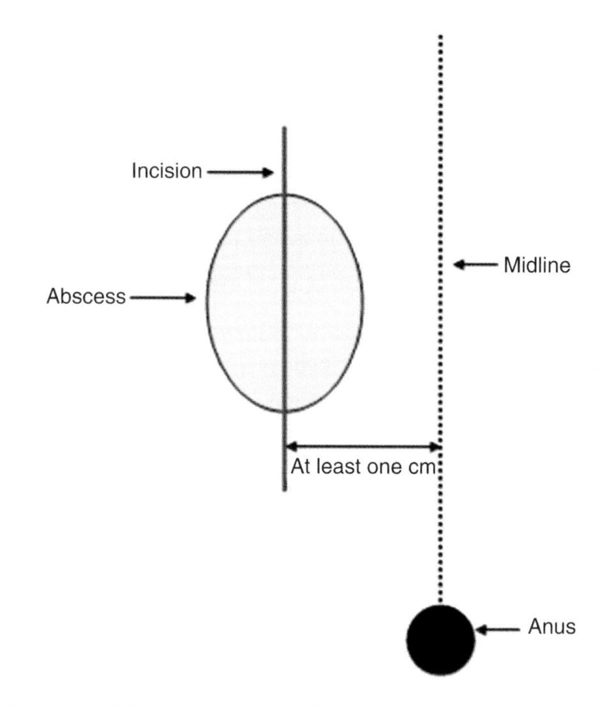

FIGURE 15-1. Incision placement for acute pilonidal abscess.

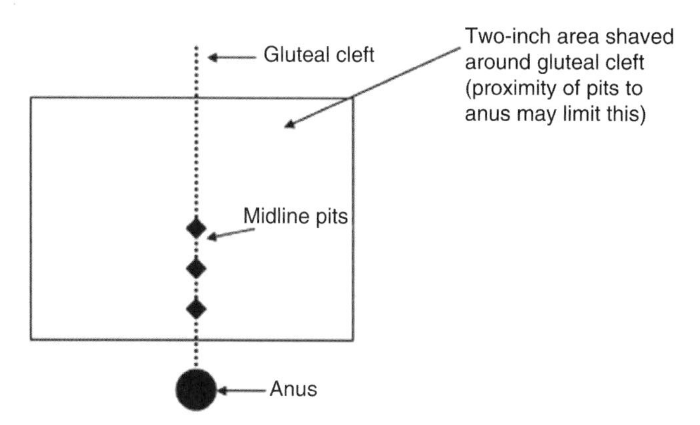

FIGURE 15-2. Shaving technique.

frequently visualized and the sinus tract connecting the two may be palpable. In these patients, treatment can be either nonoperative or operative. The choice of treatment is determined by extent of disease and patient preference.

Nonsurgical Approach

Hair Removal

For the initial treatment of chronic pilonidal sinus, shaving alone has been advocated as the sole alternative to surgery. In 1994, Armstrong and Barcia[15] tested the hypothesis that wide, meticulous shaving was equal or superior to surgical therapy of any kind for patients with chronic pilonidal sinus. The authors performed a pilot nonrandomized cohort study with retrospectively obtained follow-up. One group of patients was treated with weekly strip shaving (5 cm circumferentially around the entire gluteal cleft) until healing occurred and the other group was treated with surgery (any method). They then followed the patients for 3 years, comparing the number of occupied bed days and number of operations required. The authors found a highly statistically significant difference in favor of the group that received only shaving with lower number of occupied bed-days, with only 23 operations required in 101 consecutive cases of conservative management with weekly shaving. Although this study shows significant benefit for shaving alone, it is important to note that the authors did not control for the type of surgery performed in the nonconservative group, or for the severity of disease. Healing and recurrence rates were not reported, which is a major factor to consider when choosing a treatment modality. Furthermore, the data may be flawed in that it is plausible that although conservatively treated patients were not occupying hospital beds, they still could have been suffering from persistence of their disease, or they may have just sought treatment elsewhere. Despite these limitations, this study provides evidence that conservative nonsurgical treatment through shaving can improve pilonidal sinus healing.

Recently, several authors have described laser hair removal as an alternative to shaving.[18–20] In a recent retrospective review on laser depilation of the natal cleft to aid in healing pilonidal sinus, the authors report 14 patients treated over 5 years.[20] Only four patients (29%) had on-going disease requiring further depilation using the Alexandrite laser. All patients subsequently healed without complication. The authors concluded that although laser depilation in the natal cleft is not a cure for pilonidal disease, it does represent an alternative means of hair removal that is long lasting and allows sinuses to heal rapidly.

Collectively, these data suggest that control of hair in the natal cleft by shaving or laser hair removal may be an effective initial therapy in patients with chronic pilonidal sinus without an acute or chronic abscess; however, it is important to note that it is unknown how long one should continue shaving in order to prevent recurrence. Currently, we recommend shaving until complete healing has occurred.

Surgical Approaches

Surgery for pilonidal disease includes incisional procedures and excisional procedures with or without primary closure. As the acquired theory for pilonidal disease has gained wide acceptance, wide excision techniques have fallen out of favor. Minimal surgical techniques for pilonidal disease are now considered as the treatments of choice, and benefit the patient by decreasing hospital stay and minimizing morbidity. For thoroughness, we will describe all surgical options for chronic pilonidal sinus.

Midline Excision

Most chronic pilonidal sinus are located midline, therefore, the most common operation performed is midline excision, with or without primary closure. En block excision is made of the entire pilonidal sinus. It is not necessary to always excise down to presacral fascia. The wound can be packed with moist gauze and dressings are changed daily. Excision without closure is associated with prolonged wound healing times, and it seems logical that excision with primary closure would decrease wound healing time and may afford improved outcomes.

Surprisingly, the literature contains only four randomized, prospective studies comparing open excision to excision and primary closure. In 1985, Kronborg et al.[21] randomized 88 patients to one of three treatment groups: excision, leaving the wound open; excision and wound closure; and excision and closure with postoperative clindamycin coverage. This study is important because it was the first to look at the utility of using antibiotics after pilonidal excision. The authors then looked at recurrence and healing rates. They followed each patient for 3 years. Healing rates between each of the primary closure groups were not statistically significant, and there was no benefit shown from the addition of clindamycin (14 vs. 11 days, $p>0.10$). Healing took a substantially longer amount of time in the open group compared to the primary closure groups (64 vs. 15 days, $p>0.001$). Recurrence rates were not significant in any of the groups ($p>0.40$); however, there was a tendency toward more recurrences in the primary closure group (7 vs. 0 at 3 months and 7 vs. 4 at 3 years).

Fuzun et al.[22] randomized 91 patients to either excision without closure or excision with primary closure. The authors then followed the patients for a minimum of 4 months. They primarily looked at infection and recurrence rates. In the two patients who experienced infection in the closed group, this was treated with simple suture removal and healing by secondary intent without the need for further hospitalization. They used no antibiotics. Patients whose wounds were left open had a lower infection rate (1.8% vs. 3.6%, $p<0.01$) and no instances of recurrence, while the recurrence rate for those undergoing wound closure was 4.4% ($p<0.01$). They did not specify the duration of healing for either group. Patients who had delayed healing were those few who developed a wound infection. Despite the statistically significant differences in favor of open excision, the authors concluded that either method is acceptable.

Sondenaa et al.[23] randomized 153 patients to midline excision and primary closure with or without cefoxitin prophylaxis; 78 patients received preoperative antibiotics and 75 patients did not receive antibiotics. The complication rate (44% vs. 43%) and wound healing at 1 month (69% vs. 64%) was no different between the groups. Based on this data the authors did not recommend cefoxitin antibiotic prophylaxis. In a follow-up study published a year later the same group reported their results of a randomized trial of open excision or excision with primary closure for chronic pilonidal sinus.[24] A total of 120 patients were enrolled with half in the excision and primary closure arm and the remainder in the open excision only arm. The patients were followed for a median of 4.2 years. The authors detected no significant difference between the groups, and therefore, concluded that either method was acceptable.

Collectively, these data suggest that excision with primary closure decreases wound healing time; however, this accelerated wound healing time may come with the price of increased wound complications and recurrence of pilonidal disease. Furthermore, the routine use of prophylactic antibiotics is not necessary.

Unroofing and Secondary Healing

Midline excision without primary closure leaves a large wound that is associated with prolonged healing times. If wound closure is not indicated (i.e. with an associated abscess), a smaller wound with much shorter healing times can be achieved with unroofing or laying open the pilonidal sinus. In fact, unroofing and curettage has been advocated for the treatment of acute pilonidal abscess and chronic pilonidal sinus. In a recent study, 297 consecutive patients presenting with chronic pilonidal sinus, acute abscess, or recurrent disease were treated with unroofing and curettage for removal of hair and granulation tissue.[25] The wound was left open to heal by secondary intention. The investigators found that patients returned to work on average of 3.2 days after the procedure. Mean time for wound healing was 5.4 weeks; however, classification of disease to chronic, recurrent, and abscess revealed a longer wound healing time for abscess group (4.9 vs. 5.0 vs. 7.2 weeks; $p<0.001$, respectively). Six patients (2%) developed recurrence, which were believed to be consequences of poor compliance and follow-up. Postoperative wound care included weekly follow-up with wound debridement and separation of premature skin bridges. Furthermore, the wound area was kept free of hair during wound healing, and the authors stress the importance of hair control to prevent recurrence through the dictum, "No hair, no pilonidal sinus." Others have reported similar good results.[26,27] It is important to keep in mind that open wounds require dressing changes and wound care, but unroofing is associated with half the healing time of wide and deep excision, and marsupialization of the skin edges to the fibrous tract can decrease the wound surface by 50–60%.[21]

Bascom's Chronic Abscess Curettage and Midline Pit Excision (Bascom I)

Bascom bases this procedure on the premise that efforts to treat pilonidal disease should be directed at changing the gluteal cleft conditions rather than excising a large amount of normal tissue associated with the diseased area. In patients who present initially with a chronic abscess, this procedure has given excellent results. He does this by making a generous, vertically oriented incision through the site of the abscess cavity more than 1 cm off the midline (Figure 15-3A) and then removing hair and debris through curettage. The fibrous sinus tract or abscess wall is left in place. The connecting

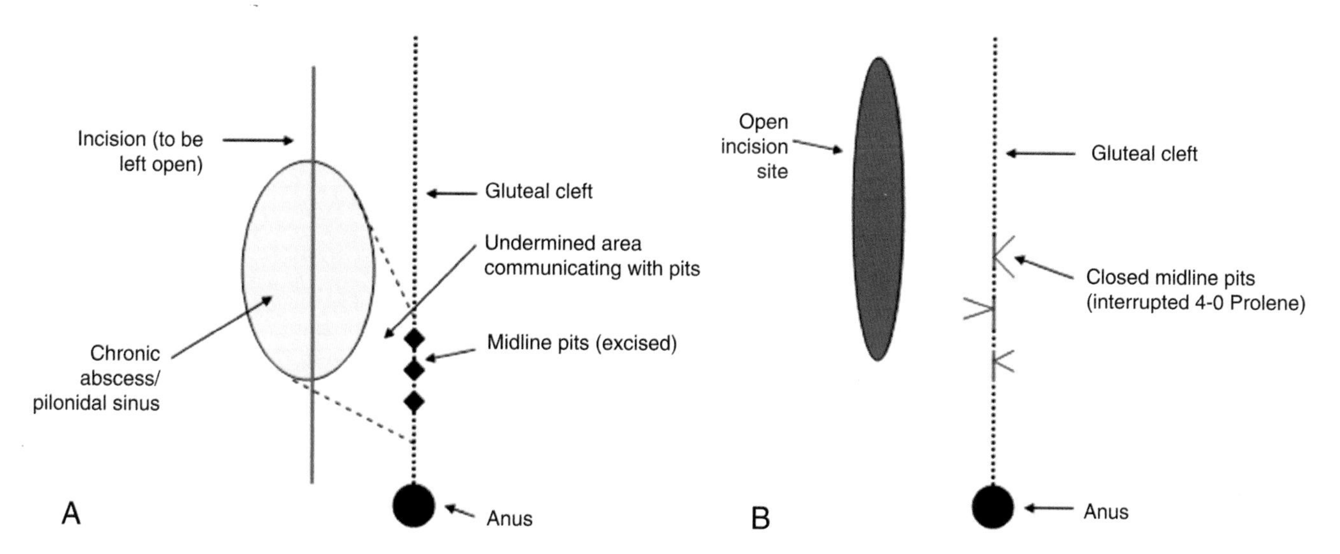

FIGURE 15-3. **A** Bascom procedure. Lateral incision and debridement of cavity. **B** Bascom procedure. Removal of a midline pit with small incisions after lateral debridement, and closure of midline wounds without closure of the lateral incision.

tracts to the midline pits are identified and the overlying skin undermined so that they drain to the site of the incision. The midline pits are then excised utilizing a small diamond-shaped incision to circumferentially remove each of them.[13,16] According to Bascom, the excised pit should be about the size of a grain of rice. The undermined flap of skin, between the incision and drainage site and the excised midline pits, is then tacked down, and the pit excision sites are closed with either subcuticular or vertical mattress, nonabsorbable suture (4-0 or 3-0) (Figure 15-3B). Once this has been accomplished, meticulous shaving of the gluteal cleft should continue at least once a week until the wound has healed. Shaving can be done in the physician's office, or at home by a family member or friend who has been properly instructed.

Senapati et al.[28] published a prospective series of 218 patients treated with Bascom's operation described above. The mean follow-up was 12.1 months (range 1–60), and consisted of phone calls, office visits, and mailed questionnaires. All but one patient healed his or her pit excision sites. The lateral wound in one patient failed to heal and required further excision. All the other wounds healed at an average of 4 weeks (range 1–15 weeks). Eight percent of patients reformed their abscesses when the lateral skin wound healed before the underlying cavity completely healed. This required reopening the lateral wound. Ninety percent of patients healed completely with only 21 patients (10%) ultimately requiring further surgery for recurrent pilonidal disease. Furthermore, patients who failed to heal or recurred were not any worse than when they initially presented. Therefore, the authors recommend the use of this technique. To date, no trials compare Bascom's procedure with another approach to chronic pilonidal sinus and abscess.

Karydakis Procedure (Advancing Flap)

The Karydakis procedure was first performed by Dr. Karydakis in Athens, Greece in 1965. The procedure involves an elliptical incision that is made parallel to the midline at a distance at least 1 cm from the midline. The skin and gluteal fat that contains the pilonidal sinus are then excised down to the sacral fascia (Figure 15-4). Mobilization of the subcutaneous flap is performed on the side closest to the midline to allow advancement to the opposite side. This flap is then sutured down to the sacral fascia, and skin closure should be entirely lateral to the cleft. This procedure achieves two goals: (1) eccentrically excise "vulnerable" tissue in the midline, or laterally displace it, and, (2) laterally displace the surgical wound out of the midline gluteal cleft.

In 1992, Karydakis[17] reported the results of this approach in 7,471 patients over a period of 34 years from 1966 to 1990, and is one of the largest series in the surgical literature. Follow-up was obtained in 95% of cases, and ranged from 2 to 20 years. He reported a recurrence rate of 1% in the first 6,545 cases, finding that new disease occurred from new midline pits. The overall complication rate was 8.5%, mainly from infections and seromas or fluid collections. Antibiotics were not routinely used; however, a drain was always placed at the upper end of the wound for 2–3 days.

Recently, the Karydakis procedure was compared to a midline primary closure in a study conducted by the military hospital in Ardahan, Turkey.[29] This retrospective review reported results on 200 military service members treated for pilonidal disease over a 30-month period. The Karydakis procedure was performed on 78 patients and midline primary closure in 122 patients. The authors reported that the Karydakis procedure group had a significantly lower recurrence rate

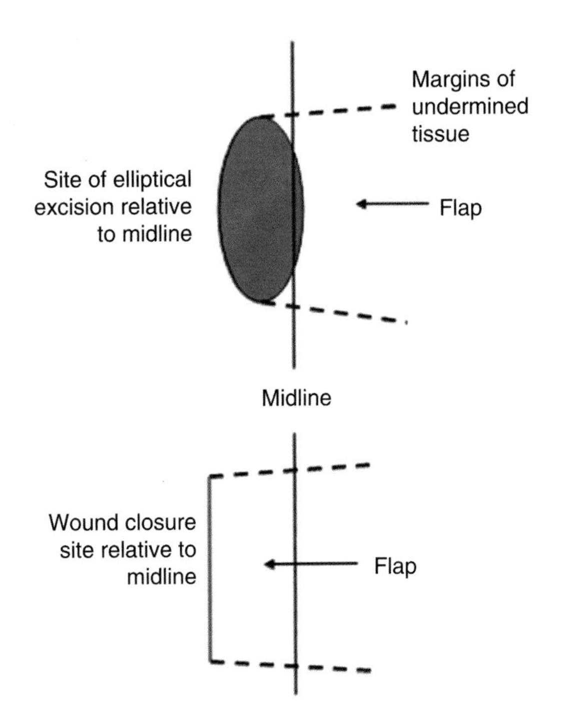

FIGURE 15-4. Karydakis advancing flap operation.

TABLE 15-1. Complex pilonidal procedure results

Procedure	% Healing (mean)	% Complications (mean)	% Recurrence (mean)
Rhomboid flap[31,32]	100	13.5	4.9
Karydakis[17]	–	8.5	1
Bascom cleft lift[13]	100	–	0
V-Y plasty[35]	100	8	0
Z-plasty[36,37]	100	–	0
Myocutaneous flap[38]	100	100	0
Skin graft[39]	96.6	–	1.7

(4.6% vs. 18.4%; $p<0.03$), lower complication rate (8.9% vs. 30.3%; $p<0.02$), and higher degree of patient satisfaction (70.8% vs. 32.6%; $p<0.001$).

These studies indicate that this procedure is highly successful with low complication and recurrence rates; however, comparative series report inpatient hospital stay of over 5 days.[29] This may be due to institution and physician preference as one recent study reported on the successful treatment of chronic pilonidal sinus using the Karydakis flap in a day-surgery setting. These data suggest the Karydakis flap is an effective procedure in the treatment of chronic pilonidal sinus, and should be considered in recurrent or complex cases.

Recurrent or Complex Pilonidal Sinus

Controversy exists over how to manage patients with recurrent and complex pilonidal sinus. Many of these patients have failed standard surgical treatments and conservative measures such as midline excision and hair control and elimination techniques. In these complex patients, excision of the pilonidal sinus is combined with a flap closure and modification of the midline natal cleft. These procedures include rhomboid flaps, Z-plasty, the Karydakis procedure (see above), Bascom's cleft lift procedure, V-Y plasty, gluteus maximus myocutaneous flaps, and skin grafting (Table 15-1). Some level-one evidence exists regarding flap-based or asymmetric closures off the midline for pilonidal disease, but most data comes from patient series and retrospective reports. The major disadvantages with flaps are longer operative times, greater blood loss, potential flap loss, and infection. However, these flap-based procedures offer a quicker time to healing than midline excision, with no increase in infection rate.

Asymmetric wound closure technique is believed to be one advantage in flap procedures used for reconstruction after excision of complex pilonidal disease. This avoids midline closure and obliterates the natal cleft that are both implicated in wound complications following surgery. In a retrospective review of the literature, Petersen et al.[30] reported their findings comparing asymmetric closure techniques to midline excision for pilonidal disease. Asymmetric closure was associated with a significantly decreased incidence of recurrence, and the midline pits recurred less often than the midline excision groups.

Rhomboid Flap

The rhomboid, or Limberg flap, is a cutaneous rotational flap used to fill soft tissue defects. It is ideally suited for pilonidal disease as it brings adjacent healthy tissue to fill the defect after wide excision of sinus tracts and removes the natal cleft from midline (Figure 15-5A–D). In 2009, Darwish and Hassanin[31] reported their experience with superior-based Limberg flap. Over a 3-year period, they treated 25 male patients with pilonidal sinus using this flap technique. Operative time averaged 40 (range 30–45) min, and hospital stay averaged 2 (range 1–6) days. Primary healing was observed in 22 patients, with two patients developing sterile seromas and one patient superficial wound infection. Complete healing of all patients occurred without recurrence during the follow-up period. A larger prospective series used the rhomboid flap on 102 patients regardless of the severity of their disease.[32] Complete healing of the wounds was reportedly 100%; however, time to complete healing was unspecified. They reported a 6% complication rate consisting of three seromas, two partial wound dehiscence, and one wound infection. The recurrence rate was 4.9%, and these patients were successfully treated with a repeat rhomboid flap. Average time to return to normal activity was 7 days. Collectively, these data suggest that the use of the rhomboid flap for reconstruction after excision of chronic pilonidal sinus is reliable, can be quickly performed in the operating room, and is associated with low complication and recurrence rates.

Given these findings, one may ask, "How does the rhomboid flap compare to surgical excision with primary closure?"

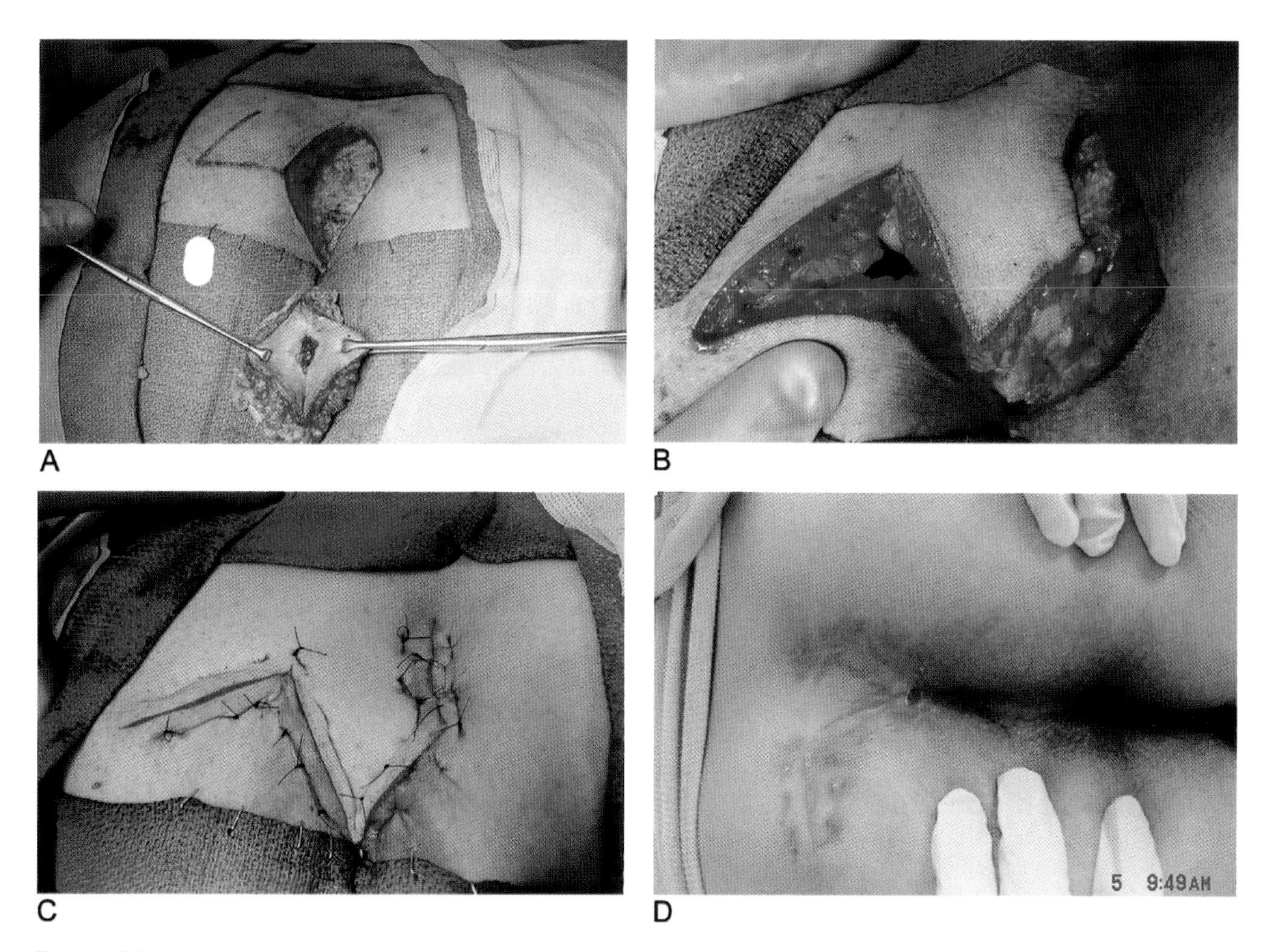

FIGURE 15-5. Rhomboid flap technique for recurrent pilonidal disease. **A** Initial excision of the sinus cavity. Counter incisions are created as shown. **B** Flaps are raised and maneuvered as shown to close defect. **C** Final surgical result. **D** Result at 1 month postoperatively.

Abu Galala et al.[33] randomized 46 patients with chronic pilonidal sinuses either to the rhomboid flap or to midline excision with primary closure. Reported follow-up included postoperative wound healing and recurrence of disease. Wound healing in the rhomboid flap patients was 100% and was significantly higher than the midline excision with primary closure group (77%; $p<0.02$). Furthermore, recurrence rate after 18 months follow-up was higher in the midline excision with primary closure group (9% vs. 0%). These data indicate that rhomboid flap closure after complex pilonidal sinus excision may improve wound healing and decrease recurrence rates.

Flap closure results in the creation of large spaces under the flap tissue. Drains have been used to prevent seroma formation and deep wound space infections in an attempt to improve outcomes. However, recent evidence indicates that drains may not improve outcomes. A recent randomized, prospective trial compared the use of drains after rhomboid flap surgery for chronic pilonidal disease.[34] The authors randomized a total of 40 patients, where drains were used in one-half. The study found no difference in wound healing or recurrence ($p>0.05$), but the drain group did experience a significantly longer hospital stay ($p<0.001$).

Despite the overall good results with use of the rhomboid flap for recalcitrant pilonidal disease, this technique necessitates excision of a large amount of normal tissue and subsequently creates a large scar at the flap site (Figure 15-5). Furthermore, chronic abscesses may be located far lateral and cephalad to the midline pits making the use of this technique more morbid due to the size of the flap required to cover the excised area. However, if the disease is localized close to the midline, the abscess cavity, sinus tracts and midline pits are easily excised. Additionally, this technique should be considered for flap coverage of chronic wounds in the gluteal cleft that have failed to heal over a prolonged period of time.

Bascom Cleft Lift (Bascom II)

This procedure may be the most technically challenging of all the techniques dealing with multiple recurrent and severe pilonidal disease. It also may prove to be the most revolutionary technique to come along since the Karydakis procedure. The key difference between the cleft lift procedure and other flap-based procedures is that normal subcutaneous tissue is not excised in the cleft lift procedure. As described above, the Karydakis procedure does excise normal fat in order to create the flap. The only tissue excised during the cleft lift is a portion of skin. The goal of the cleft lift procedure is to undermine and completely obliterate the gluteal cleft in the diseased area.[13] This procedure detaches the skin of the gluteal cleft from the underlying subcutaneous tissue as a flap. A portion of this flap containing the diseased skin (containing pits) is then excised from the side of the buttocks to which the flap will be sutured (Figure 15-6A). When the flap is pulled across the midline, the gluteal subcutaneous tissue is approximated underneath the flap, thus obliterating the gluteal cleft. Any open chronic wounds or sinus cavities are simply curetted out, but not excised. The raised skin flaps cover these prior wound sites in addition to coapting the normal gluteal fat. The final suture line lies parallel to, but well away from, the midline, and is free from tension (Figure 15-6B). Bascom and Bascom[13] studied 28 consecutive patients with recurrent, festering wounds who received this treatment; 22 patients healed their wounds immediately and had their sutures removed at 1 week. Six patients took longer to heal due to small wound separations. Three patients required operative revision to achieve healing. Finally, one obese patient took 13 months to heal. The median follow-up was 20 months (range 1 month to 15 years) and all patients remained healed. This procedure has enjoyed spectacular results in Dr. Bascom's hands, but these results await duplication.

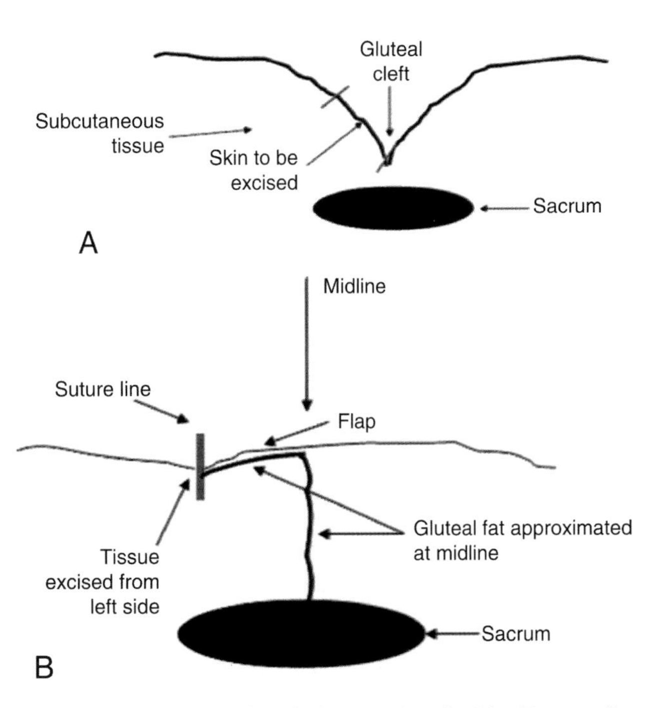

FIGURE 15-6. **A** Cleft lift technique as described by Bascom for nonhealing midline wounds. **B** Final result after flaps are raised and underlying gluteal fat is approximated.

V-Y Flap

Advancement flaps are designed to slide along the flap's long axis, and moves healthy tissue for reconstruction into the excised area. The size of flap, and therefore, the volume of tissue used, is primarily determined by the arterial input (and venous drainage) not length-to-breadth ratios. The V-Y flap maintains blood supply from the fascia, and division of the blood supply and venous drainage should be avoided.

The use of these advancement flaps have been applied to the surgical treatment of pilonidal disease. Schoeller et al.[35] retrospectively investigated their use of the V-Y advancement flap in 24 patients with complex pilonidal sinus. The mean follow-up was 4.5 years. The investigators reported two cases of wound dehiscence, but achieved healing in all cases. There were no recurrences. Overall, they found the method to be satisfactory, but demanding, and recommended a simpler approach. However, it may have applicability in some situations where other flaps have failed, such as the rhomboid flap.

Z-Plasty

Combining excision with Z-plasty for reconstruction is a well-suited treatment option for complex pilonidal sinus. The diseased tissue is excised and the natal cleft is obliterated with a Z-plasty for reconstruction. The limbs of tissue are fashioned 30–45° angles from the wound axis. Full thickness subcutaneous skin flaps are raised and transposed before suturing the skin edges. Early application of this technique showed promise with one study reporting no recurrences in 110 patients with pilonidal sinus disease treated with excision and Z-plasty.[36]

Hodgson and Greenstein[37] reported his results of a randomized, prospective study on complex pilonidal sinus treated with Z-plasty vs. midline excision. The Z-plasty group required no further surgery, but 40% of the open excision group did go on to have repeat operations. In addition to advocating Z-plasty for complex pilonidal sinus excision, this study provides evidence that open excision, while eliminating risk of wound breakdown, does not decrease risk of short-term wound complications.

Myocutaneous Flaps

Myocutaneous flaps are rarely used due to the large nature of the defect and reconstruction created. The procedure may be significantly debilitating as most myocutaneous rotational flaps are harvested from the gluteal area; however, they can be successful for the treatment of pilonidal disease. Rosen and Davidson[38] reported their series of five patients with severe pilonidal disease treated with gluteus myocutaneous flaps. They were all young males and had received an average of six previous procedures. All patients healed with an average follow-up of 40 months and 13 hospital days. Most surgeons reserve this technique for the most severe cases, usually after failure of multiple simpler techniques.

Skin Grafting

Skin grafting is an infrequent procedure used for the treatment of pilonidal disease. Guyuron et al.[39] published their retrospective study of 58 patients with pilonidal disease treated with excision and split-thickness skin grafting. Over 70% of these patients initially presented with recurrent disease. The authors reported a 1.7% recurrence rate and a 3.4% graft failure rate. The authors recommended usc of this method for recurrent or extensive pilonidal disease; however, there have been no further publications on skin grafting for the treatment of pilonidal disease. This can be explained conceptually, as it does not achieve the modern goals of surgical treatment for pilonidal disease. Skin grafting leaves the natal cleft left unchanged, requires prolonged hospital stay for wound care of donor site and graft site, and the graft site, generally the sacrum and/or gluteal area is in zones of high friction. Furthermore, graft success is likely to require significant immobility that prolongs return to normal activity. Taking these factors into account, we cannot recommend skin grafting for the treatment of pilonidal disease.

Summary

Treatment of pilonidal disease is dependent on the disease presentation. Pilonidal abscess, chronic sinus, complex sinus tracts, and chronic recurrent pilonidal abscess and sinus encompass the spectrum of pilonidal disease. Each has specific considerations in the treatment and management of this disease process; however, the cornerstone of all surgical and nonsurgical therapeutic interventions for pilonidal disease should always include wide, meticulous shaving and hygiene. The algorithm in Figure 15-7 outlines a common approach to pilonidal disease based on the evidence presented in this chapter. In patients presenting initially with simple midline pits, or sinus tracts without acute abscess, shaving can be offered as the initial treatment. Meticulous and ritualistic shaving is critical as one single hair protruding from a midline pit will keep it open and result in recurrent or persistent disease. During both the primary and postoperative healing phase, shaving should be continued on a weekly basis until healing is complete.

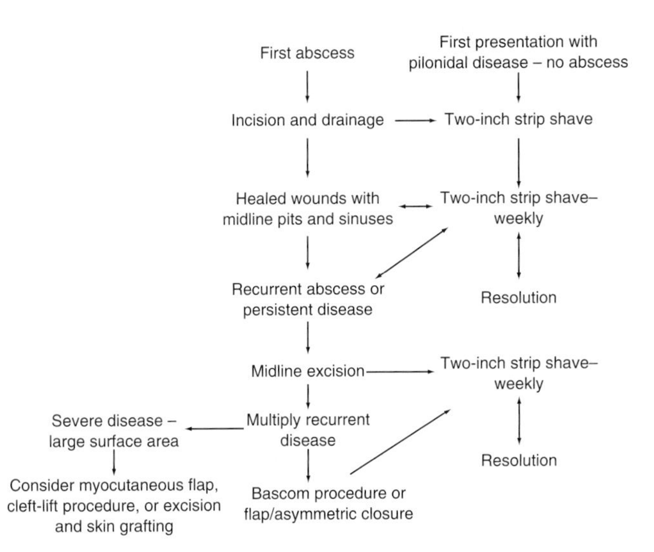

FIGURE 15-7. Pilonidal disease algorithm.

Patients with acute pilonidal abscess require incision and drainage, ideally making the incision lateral to the midline whenever possible. At the same time, one should do a 2-in. strip shave circumferentially around the affected area. Dressing changes, Sitz baths, and shaving are continued until the wound has healed. The majority of acute pilonidal abscess treated in this manner do not recur.

Many patients will present initially with chronic pilonidal sinus. Location of the sinus relative to the midline helps guide the choice of management. In the case where all the disease, sinuses, and pits are located near and in the midline, then a conservative midline excision or unroofing with curettage is a reasonable first line treatment; however, if multiple draining sinuses exist, and they are located far from the midline, then simple midline excision becomes impractical due to the larger wound created. In this case, we recommend the Bascom I procedure or excision with rhomboid flap reconstruction. These procedures are also useful for patients who have failed midline excisions. Patients presenting with multiple recurrent pilonidal disease, or chronic persistent abscess despite conservative management, are more challenging to treat. Continued shaving in this situation is unlikely to succeed, since the abscess cavity and the epithelialized tracts connecting it to the midline pits will contain a great deal of burrowed hair. In this case, we recommend the Bascom I procedure with chronic abscess curettage and midline pit excision. Alternatively, a cutaneous flap procedure with asymmetric closure is also effective.

In the event, a prior operation results in a chronic nonhealing wound, a rotational flap is ideal. These flaps should move the wound closure and natal cleft off the midline. In these circumstances, we suggest the rhomboid flap for this purpose. For extensive recurrence in the midline with abscesses and multiple nonhealing wounds, the Bascom II cleft lift procedure or Z-plasty may be effective. Myocutaneous flaps are reserved for patients with severe complex pilonidal disease or persistent wounds encompassing large surface areas. In these situations, consultation with a plastic surgeon may be advised.

Hidradenitis Suppurativa

Background

Hidradenitis suppurativa is an uncommon cutaneous condition, which primarily affects young individuals and exhibits its chronicity with frequent flare-ups followed by quiescent periods. The severity of this disease is variable. It may present initially as an abscess, but is typically chronic or multiply recurrent in the affected area, and ultimately can lead to severe scarring, contracture, possible malignancy, and disability for the patient. Hidradenitis suppurativa commonly occurs in the perineum, axilla, and groin, but can also be seen in the inguinal and mammary regions as well.[40] These areas contain high concentration of apocrine glands, which may play a role in the disease.

Incidence and Etiology

The exact incidence of hidradenitis suppurativa is not known; however, 1 in every 300 individuals may be affected in some way.[41] African Americans appear to be affected more often than Caucasians, and perianal disease is approximately twice as common in males.[14,40,41] Almost all patients present after puberty in the second and third decades of life, thereby implicating hormones and the development of secondary sexual characteristics as potential causative factors.[41] Harrison et al.[43] demonstrated androgen excess and a decrease in progesterone in patients with hidradenitis. Obesity has been suggested as a predisposing factor through increased shear forces in the affected areas; however, it is more likely an aggravating factor rather than a causative factor.[14,41] Additional predisposing factors include tobacco use, acne, stress, poor skin hygiene, excessive heat, hyperhidrosis, and chemical depilatories. In a series from the Ochsner clinic, 70% of affected patients were smokers, but no causal relationship could be definitively shown.[41] Proposed mechanism of tobacco influence suggests that smoking may alter granulocytes, modify sweat gland activity, and give off toxic metabolites in sweat. Perianal hidradenitis affects males twice as often as females, but hidradenitis in all locations may be more common in females and African–American persons.[41,42] Fortunately, for sufferers of perianal hidradenitis, it appears to recur less often after surgical treatment (<0.5%) than does inguinal–perineal disease (37–74%).[40,42]

Bacteriology

Wound cultures from hidradenitis patients have grown *Staphylococcus epidermidis*, *Escherichia coli*, *Klebsiella*, *Proteus*, *α-Streptococcus*, anaerobic bacteria, and diphtheroids; however, one study reported that wound cultures of early lesions were negative.[44] *S. epidermidis* and *Staphylococcus aureus* are the most frequently isolated organisms from hidradenitis suppurativa lesions.[14,45] *Chlamydia trachomatis*, often associated with lymphogranuloma venereum, and *Bilophila wadsworthia* infection have also been implicated in hidradenitis, but the clinical significance is not known.[41,42]

Pathophysiology

It is believed that hidradenitis suppurativa originates from the occlusion of hair follicles.[46,47] Dilation and rupture of hair follicles into the dermis leads to dermal infiltration by inflammatory cells, giant cells, and formation of sinus tracts, and fibrosis.[48] Involvement is typically in skin that contains apocrine sweat glands, but the inflammation and destruction of these glands seems to be incidental rather than a causative factor.[24] Attanoos et al.[45] examined 118 pathologic hidradenitis specimens and found some degree of keratin plugging in all cases along with an active deep folliculitis. They concluded that plugging of the hair follicle itself led to apocrine inflammation, making the actual apocrine gland destruction of hidradenitis suppurativa a secondary process.[45] These glands secrete a milky, odorless fluid that only becomes malodorous after it interacts with bacteria on the skin. The apocrine glands secrete into the hair follicle as opposed to directly onto the skin like eccrine sweat glands. The function of apocrine secretion is unknown. Nevertheless, obstruction leads to secondary bacterial infection and rupture of the gland into the dermis and subcutaneous tissue, thus causing cellulitis, abscess, and draining sinuses. This process then leads to the characteristic "pit like" scars from chronic fibrosis of the destroyed glandular unit. Over time, this disease can become not only disfiguring, but also debilitating. Microscopically, the pathognomonic serpentine epithelialized sinus tracks with giant cells and granulomas are typically seen.[40,41,49,50]

Clinical Presentation and Diagnosis

Patients with hidradenitis suppurativa typically presents with pain, erythema, and swelling in the affected area. There is frequently a malodorous discharge from the affected skin. Physical examination may reveal a spectrum of indurated subcutaneous nodules, subcutaneous abscess, and/or draining skin sinuses. Sinuses may be simple or complex coalescing to form a network of subcutaneous cavities and tracts with extensive fibrosis.

The diagnosis is based on clinical findings, and diagnostic biopsy is seldom required; however, if the differential diagnosis includes perianal Crohn's disease or cancer, biopsies should be obtained to establish a definitive diagnosis. Differentiating hidradenitis suppurativa from other inflammatory conditions of the perianal region can be difficult, and some of them may coexist. Cutaneous infections such as furuncles, carbuncles, lymphogranuloma venereum, erysipelas, epidermoid or dermoid cysts, and tuberculosis may present in a similar fashion. It is important to distinguish hidradenitis from other fistulizing or sinus-forming processes of the perineum such as Crohn's disease or cryptoglandular perianal abscess. Crohn's disease typically affects the anus and rectum with fistulas arising from the dentate line or higher in the rectum. Fistula-in-ano or perianal abscesses that are cryptoglandular origin will arise from the dentate line and involve the sphincter complex. In contrast, hidradenitis does not affect the rectum or involve the dentate line, because apocrine glands only exist in the lower two-thirds of the anal canal and do not penetrate into the sphincter complex. Thus, patients will not have sinus or fistula tracks to or from the rectum.[40,41] If fistulas are present, then the surgeon should perform anoscopy to rule out the possibility of fistula-in-ano from a cryptoglandular source or consider Crohn's disease as the etiology. Fistulas from hidradenitis should only connect areas of involved skin, and not penetrate the anal sphincters or involve the dentate line. Several case reports have been published describing the association of Crohn's disease and hidradenitis, but no definitive link between the two conditions has ever been proven.[51–55] Nonspecific granulomas (required for a pathologic diagnosis of Crohn's disease) are seen in pathologic specimens in both diseases and may be confused with one another.

In patients with longstanding history of hidradenitis and chronic nonhealing wounds, it is important to rule out malignancy (Figure 15-8). There have been several reports of squamous cell carcinoma arising in chronic hidradenitis wounds.[56–60] A retrospective review of a Swedish database of hospital discharge diagnoses from 1965 to 1997 revealed a 50% increased risk of developing *any* cancer in patients with hidradenitis suppurativa over the general population, but significant increases were specifically found in nonmelanoma skin cancers, buccal cancer, and primary liver cancer.[61] Most patients with cancers had untreated disease for longer than 20 years. In fact, a recent review reports that the mean duration of hidradenitis suppurativa before diagnosis of malignancy is 25 years.[60] One should at least keep a high index of suspicion for this entity in patients with long standing disease and extensive scarring in the affected areas.

Treatment

The clinical presentation of hidradenitis suppurativa encompasses a wide spectrum of severity. Furthermore, the persistent and recurring nature of the disease requires an individualized treatment plan. This may include nonsurgical and surgical techniques for acute and chronic disease. It is imperative to educate the patient about the chronic relapsing nature of the disease, and to reassure the patient that the disease is not contagious or due to poor hygiene.[62]

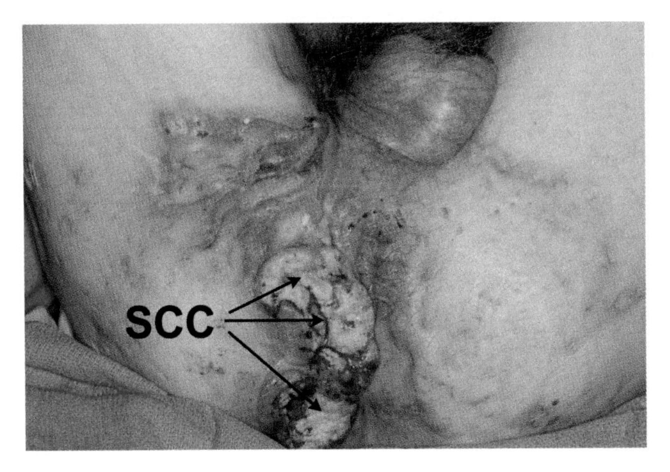

FIGURE 15-8. A large squamous cell cancer (SCC) arising in an area of chronic hidradenitis suppurativa.

Nonsurgical Treatment

Antibiotic therapy is the cornerstone for nonsurgical treatment of hidradenitis. Patients with cellulitis and no definable abscess may be successfully treated with antibiotics for 1–2 weeks. Both topical (clindamycin) and systemic (tetracycline) antibiotics have been advocated, and antimicrobial spectrum must cover skin flora, particularly *Staphylococcus* species. No evidence exists supporting the use of prophylactic antibiotics beyond the initial treatment course, and it is unclear if the natural history or disease process is altered by such therapy.[60]

Other medications have been used for the treatment of hidradenitis suppurativa, and include retinoids, antiandrogen therapy, immunomodulators and anti-inflammatory (etanercept, infliximab, adalimumab) drugs.[60] Most were evaluated through retrospective chart reviews and meaningful conclusions are difficult to draw; however, the potential side effects of these medications are significant and should be considered prior to initiation. Radiotherapy has been used in the past with modest success.[60] These positive results are likely a direct result of hair follicle destruction, but wound healing problems are significant. Others have reported the use of photodynamic therapy, cryosurgery, carbon dioxide laser therapy, and radiofrequency treatments with variable success.

Surgical Treatment

The surgical management of hidradenitis suppurativa can be divided into two categories: (1) surgery to control local infection; and (2) surgery for curative intent. Incision and drainage of abscess and sinus tracts are simple methods that control local infection; however, diseased skin remains and recurrence is highly likely. This is illustrated by a recent report that compared recurrence rates of hidradenitis suppurativa after incision and drainage/limited excision vs. wide excision of disease.[63] After a 3-month follow-up, the study found 100% recurrence after limited excision and 27% recurrence after wide excision of disease. These data suggest that the surgeon must excise the entire involved area, otherwise, the patient will be at risk for recurrence. For this reason, once local inflammation has been controlled with incision and drainage, the patient is offered further surgery for curative intent or initiated on nonsurgical treatment modalities for disease control.

Surgery for curative intent requires complete excision of diseased skin. Excision with primary closure may be performed in selected small wounds if it can be closed without tension. This treatment modality results in decreased morbidity, decreased length of hospitalization and decreased postoperative disability.[64,65] Others have advocated wide excision and healing by secondary intention. All of the grossly involved apocrine bearing skin in the perianal area should be excised full-thickness into the uninvolved gluteal fat. Excision to involve a wide margin has proven to be beneficial. In addition, this method is simple, does not require fecal diversion, and depending on size excised, may be performed as an outpatient procedure. Patients with large areas of involvement may require staged excision. The extent of excision should remain outside the anal verge as long as there is no obvious involvement or history of involvement in the anal canal. If excision near the anal canal is necessary, it should be limited, or staged, in order to prevent anal stricture. Prolonged wound healing of 1 month or longer is a significant disadvantage of this method. These patients require daily wound care and consideration should be given to physical therapy to prevent contracture formation.

Recently, reports on the use of negative pressure dressings have appeared as a way to promote healing and shorten the time to wound closure.[66] The purported benefits of these dressings include increased wound oxygen tension, decreased bacterial counts, better control of fluid produced by the wound, increased granulation tissue formation, and decreased shear forces. Negative pressure dressings have been used successfully on open wounds and on skin grafts[66,67]; however, consideration must be given to cost and technical difficulties inherent to dressings placed in the perianal area. These dressings require an air-tight seal at all times, which can be difficult to achieve near the anal verge and perineum.

Patients with chronic disease, extensive scarring, and sinus tracts rarely respond to conservative measures (Figure 15-9A). The gold standard of care remains wide excision of all hidradenitis involved skin bearing apocrine glands (Figure 15-9B and C). Reconstruction then can follow a number of paths – cutaneous flap closure, myocutaneous flap closure, immediate or delayed split-thickness skin grafting (Figure 15-9D), or excision, and simple healing by secondary intent. Cutaneous or myocutaneous flaps are typically taken from the posterior thigh, gluteus muscle, or lumbosacral region. They are analogous to those used for pilonidal disease. Patients who might benefit from diversion

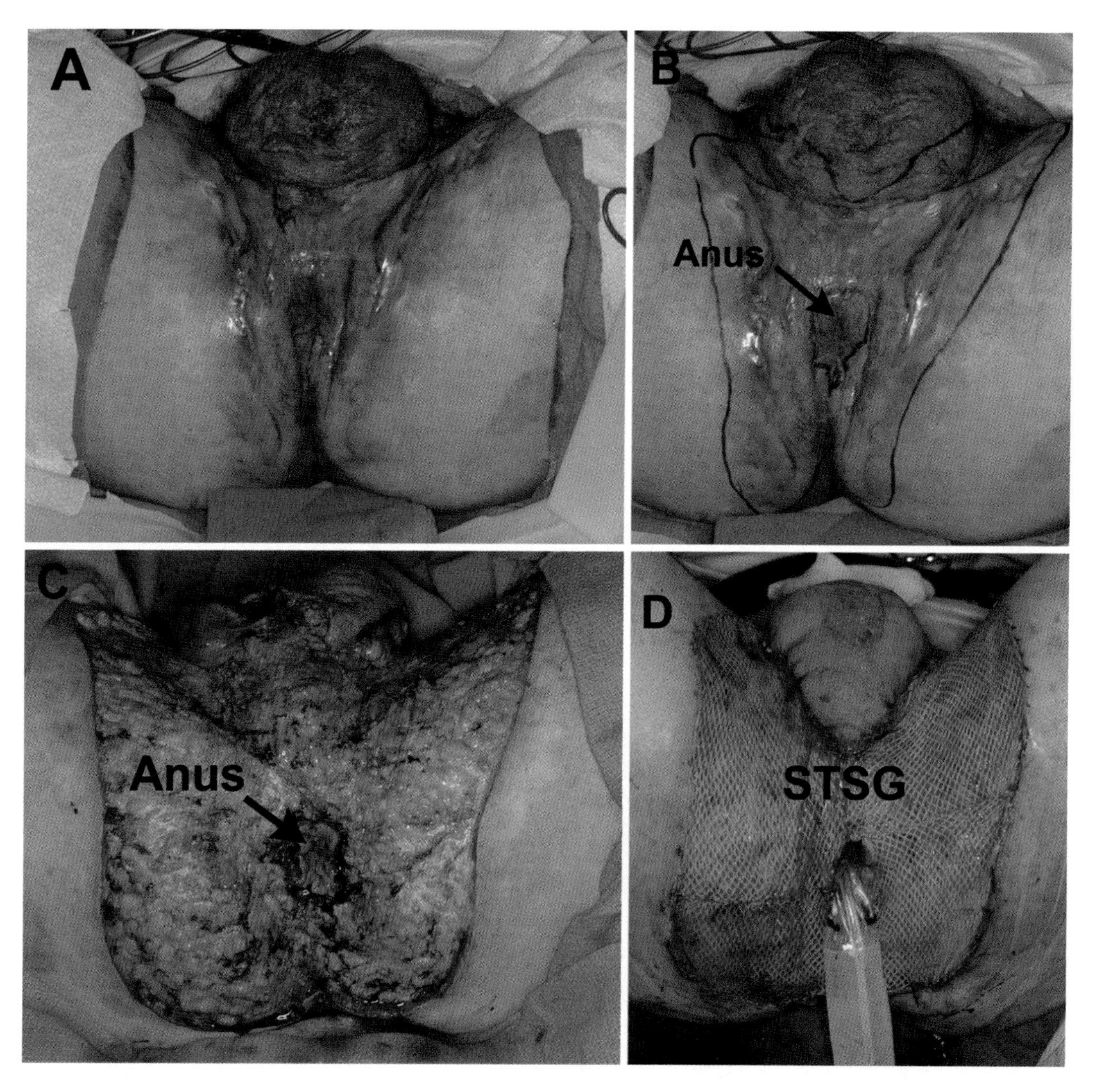

FIGURE 15-9. A male patient with significant perianal and inguinal hidradenitis suppurativa of a chronic nature. **A** Preoperative photo of extent of disease. **B** Planned surgical resection preserving skin at the anal verge. **C** Wide excision of perianal and inguinal hidradenitis suppurativa. **D** Split thickness skin graft (STSG) used for immediate reconstruction.

are those who cannot take care of their wounds long term and those who suffer from both hidradenitis and Crohn's disease, although this is rarely needed.[41,68]

Summary

Hidradenitis suppurativa is a skin disease that typically affects young adults and is characterized by intermittent flares and periods of quiescence. The algorithm in Figure 15-10 outlines one suggested approach to treating patients with perianal hidradenitis suppurativa. Patients who present with acute disease and abscess should have incision and drainage, ideally in an office setting.[69] Antibiotics may be used for excessive cellulitis and to decrease acute inflammation. This process can be repeated, if necessary, and is usually performed for recurrent disease. It is important to rule out other causes of fistulous disease such as Crohn's disease or perirectal abscess from a cryptogladular source. For patients with chronic or recurring disease, definitive excision should be considered. This may include excision with primary closure for small areas of disease, healing by secondary intent for larger areas of disease, or reconstruction with split-thickness skin graft or flap closure for wide excision. Flap procedures are typically reserved for patients with extensive scarring and tissue damage that involves large areas of perianal skin around the anus extending out to the buttocks. By the time a patient reaches the point where they desire surgery, they have usually suffered for many years with recurrent abscesses in the affected area.

Acknowledgments. This chapter was written by Jeffery Nelson and Richard Billingham in the first edition of this textbook.

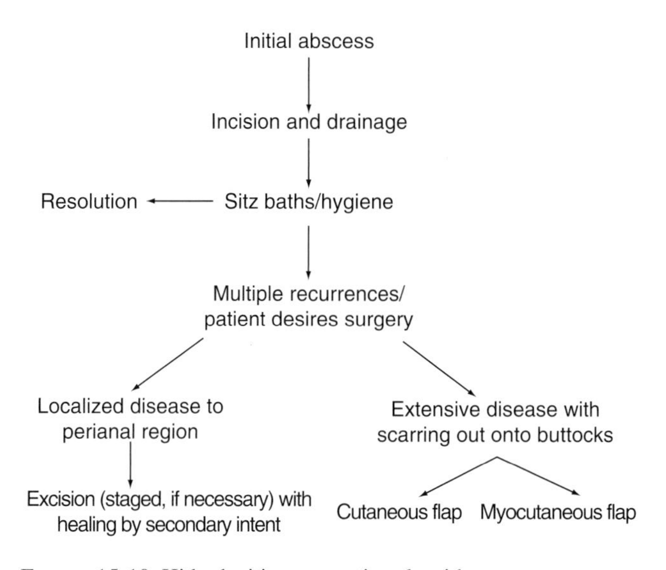

FIGURE 15-10. Hidradenitis suppurativa algorithm.

References

1. da Silva JH. Pilonidal cyst: cause and treatment. Dis Colon Rectum. 2000;43(8):1146–56.
2. Buie LA. Jeep disease (pilonidal disease of mechanized warfare). South Med J. 1944;37:103–9.
3. Patel MR, Bassini L, Nashad R, et al. Barber's interdigital pilonidal sinus of the hand: a foreign body hair granuloma. J Hand Surg. 1990;15A:652–5.
4. Phillips PJ. Web space sinus in a shearer. Med J Aust. 1966;2:1152–3.
5. Akinci OF, Bozer M, Uzunkoy A, Duzgun SA, Coskun A. Incidence and aetiological factors in pilonidal sinus among Turkish soldiers. Eur J Surg. 1999;165(4):339–42.
6. Sondenaa K, Andersen E, Nesvik I, Soreide JA. Patient characteristics and symptoms in chronic pilonidal sinus disease. Int J Colorectal Dis. 1995;10:39–42.
7. Akinci OF, Kurt M, Terzi A, Atak I, Subasi IE, Akbilgic O. Natal cleft deeper in patients with pilonidal sinus: implications for surgical procedure. Dis Colon Rectum. 2009;52:1000–2.
8. Doll D, Matevossian E, Wietelmann K, Evers T, Kriner M, Petersen S. Family history of pilonidal sinus predisposes to earlier onset of disease and 50% long-term recurrence rate. Dis Colon Rectum. 2009;52:1610–5.
9. Hull TL, Wu J. Pilonidal disease. Surg Clin N Am. 2002;82:1169–85.
10. Mayo OH. Observations on injuries and diseases of the rectum. London: Burgess and Hill; 1833. p. 45–6.
11. Hodges RM. Pilonidal sinus. Boston Med Surg J. 1880;103: 485–6.
12. Casberg MA. Infected pilonidal cysts and sinuses. Bull US Army Med Dep. 1949;9:493–6.
13. Bascom J, Bascom T. Failed pilonidal surgery – new paradigm and new operation leading to cures. Arch Surg. 2002;137:1146–50.
14. Velasco AL, Dunlap WW. Pilonidal disease and hidradenitis. Surg Clin N Am. 2009;89:689–701.
15. Armstrong JH, Barcia PJ. Pilonidal sinus disease. The conservative approach. Arch Surg. 1994;129(9):914–9.
16. Bascom JU. Pilonidal sinus. Curr Pract Surg. 1994;6:175–80.
17. Karydakis GE. Easy and successful treatment of pilonidal sinus after explanation of its causative process. Aust N Z J Surg. 1992;62(5):385–9.
18. Lavelle M, Jafri Z, Town G. Recurrent pilonidal sinus treated with epilation using a ruby laser. J Cosmet Laser Ther. 2002;4(2):45–7.
19. Downs AM, Palmer J. Laser hair removal for recurrent pilonidal sinus disease. J Cosmet Laser Ther. 2002;4(3–4):91.
20. Odili J, Gault D. Laser depilation of the natal cleft – an aid to healing the pilonidal sinus. Ann R Coll Surg Engl. 2002;84(1):29–32.
21. Kronborg O, Christensen K, Zimmermann-Nielsen C. Chronic pilonidal disease: a randomized trial with a complete 3-year follow-up. Br J Surg. 1985;72(4):303–4.
22. Fuzun M, Bakir H, Soylu M, et al. Which technique for treatment of pilonidal sinus – open or closed? Dis Colon Rectum. 1994;37(11):1148–50.
23. Sondenaa K, Nesvik I, Gullaksen FP, et al. The role of cefoxitin prophylaxis in chronic pilonidal sinus treated with excision and primary suture. J Am Coll Surg. 1995;180(2):157–60.
24. Sondenaa K, Nesvik I, Anderson E, Soreide JA. Recurrent pilonidal sinus after excision with closed or open treatment: final result of a randomised trial. Eur J Surg. 1996;162(3):237–40.

25. Kepenekci I, Demirkan A, Celasin H, Gecim IE. Unroofing and curettage for the treatment of acute and chronic pilonidal disease. World J Surg. 2010;34(1):153–7.
26. Solla JA, Rothenberger DA. Chronic pilonidal disease: an assessment of 150 cases. Dis Colon Rectum. 1990;33:758–61.
27. Spivak H, Brooks VL, Nussbaum M, Friedman I. Treatment of chronic pilonidal disease. Dis Colon Rectum. 1996;39(10): 1136–9.
28. Senapati A, Cripps NP, Thompson MR. Bascom's operation in the day-surgical management of symptomatic pilonidal sinus. Br J Surg. 2000;87(8):1067–70.
29. Can MF, Sevinc MM, Yilmaz M. Comparison of Karydakis flap reconstruction versus primary midline closure in sacrococcygeal pilonidal disease: results of 200 military service members. Surg Today. 2009;39:580–6.
30. Petersen S, Koch R, Stelzner S, Wendlandt TP, Ludwig K. Primary closure techniques in chronic pilonidal sinus: a survey of the results of different surgical approaches. Dis Colon Rectum. 2002;45(11):1458–67.
31. Darwish AM, Hassanin A. Reconstruction following excision of sacrococcygeal pilonidal sinus with a perforator-based fasciocutaneous limberg flap. J Plast Reconstr Aesthet Surg. 2010;63(7):1176–80.
32. Urhan MK, Kukukel F, Topgul K, Ozer I, Sari S. Rhomboid excision and Limberg flap for managing pilonidal sinus: results of 102 cases. Dis Colon Rectum. 2002;45(5):656–59.
33. Abu Galala KH, Salam IM, Abu Samaan KR, El Ashaal YI, Chandran VP, Sabastian M, et al. Treatment of pilonidal sinus by primary closure with a transposed rhomboid flap compared with deep suturing: a prospective randomised clinical trial. Eur J Surg. 1999;165(5):468–72.
34. Erdem E, Sungurtekin U, Nessar M. Are postoperative drains necessary with the Limberg flap for treatment of pilonidal sinus? Dis Colon Rectum. 1998;41(11):1427–31.
35. Schoeller T, Wechselberger G, Otto A, Papp C. Definite surgical treatment of complicated recurrent pilonidal disease with a modified fasciocutaneous V-Y advancement flap. Surgery. 1997;121(3):258–63.
36. Toubanakis G. Treatment of pilonidal sinus disease with Z-plasty procedure (modified). Am Surg. 1986;52:611–2.
37. Hodgson WJ, Greenstein RJ. A comparative study between Z-plasty and incision and drainage or excision with marsupialization for pilonidal sinus. Surg Gynecol Obstet. 1981;153(6):842–4.
38. Rosen W, Davidson JS. Gluteus maximus musculocutaneous flap for the treatment of recalcitrant pilonidal disease. Ann Plast Surg. 1996;37(3):293–7.
39. Guyuron B, Dinner MI, Dowden RV. Excision and grafting in treatment of recurrent pilonidal sinus disease. Surg Gynecol Obstet. 1983;156(2):201–4.
40. Rubin RJ, Chinn BT. Perianal hidradentitis suppurativa. Surg Clin N Am. 1994;74(6):1317–25.
41. Mitchell KM, Beck DE. Hidradentitis suppurativa. Surg Clin N Am. 2002;82:1187–97.
42. Banerjee AK. Surgical treatment of hidradenitis suppurativa. Br J Surg. 1992;79:863–6.
43. Harrison BJ, Read GF, Hughes LE. Endocrine basis for the clinical presentation of hidradenitis suppurativa. Br J Surg. 1988;75(10):972–5.
44. Jemec GB, Faber M, Gutschick E, Wendelboe P. The bacteriology of hidradenitis suppurativa. Dermatology. 1996;183(3): 203–6.
45. Attanoos RL, Appleton MA, Douglas-Jones AG. The pathogenesis of hidradentitis suppurativa: a closer look at apocrine and apoeccrine glands. Br J Dermatol. 1995;133(2):254–8.
46. Plewig G, Steger M. Acne inverse (alias acne triad, acne tetrad or hidradenitis suppurativa). In: Marks R, Plewig G, editors. Acne and related disorders. London: Martin Dunitz; 1991. p. 345–57.
47. Jansen T, Plewig G. Whats new in acne inverse (alias hidradenitis suppurativa)? J Eur Acad Dermatol Venereol. 2000;14:342–3.
48. Slade DE, Powell BW, Mortimer PS. Hidradenitis suppurativa: pathogenesis and management. Br J Plast Surg. 2003;56: 451–61.
49. Jemec GBE, Hansen U. Histology of hidradenitis suppurativa. J Am Acad Dermatol. 1996;34:994–9.
50. Gilliland R, Wexner SD. Complicated anorectal sepsis. Surg Clin N Am. 1997;77(1):115–48.
51. Burrows NP, Jones RR. Crohn's disease in association with hidradenitis suppurativa – letter to the editor. Br J Dermatol. 1992;126:523–9.
52. Katsanos KH, Christodoulou DK, Tsianos EV. Axillary hidradenitis suppurativa successfully treated with Infliximab in a Crohn's disease patient – letter to the editor. Am J Gastroenterol. 2002;97(8):2155–6.
53. Tsianos EV, Dalekos GN, Tzermias C, Merkouropoulos M, Hatzis J. Hidradenitis suppurativa in Crohn's disease – a further support to this association. J Clin Gastroenterol. 1995;20(2):151–3.
54. Roy MK, Appleton MAC, Delicata RJ, Sharma AK, Williams GT, Carey PD. Probable association between hidradenitis suppurativa and Crohn's disease: significance of epithelioid granuloma. Br J Surg. 1997;84:375–6.
55. Ostlere LS, Langtry JAA, Mortimer PS, Staughton RCD. Hidradenitis suppurativa in Crohn's disease. Br J Dermatol. 1991;125:384–6.
56. Anstey AV, Wilkinson JD, Lord P. Squamous cell carcinoma complicating hidradentis suppurativa. Br J Dermatol. 1990;123:527–31.
57. Gur E, Neligan PC, Shafir R, Reznick R, Cohen M, Shpitzer T. Squamous cell carcinoma in perineal inflammatory disease. Ann Plast Surg. 1997;38(6):653–7.
58. Dufresne RG, Ratz JL, Bergfeld WF, Roenigk RK. Squamous cell carcinoma arising from the follicular occlusion triad. J Am Acad Dermatol. 1996;35:475–7.
59. Malaguanera M, Pontillo T, Pistone G, Succi L. Squamous-cell cancer in Verneuil's disease (hidradenitis suppurativa). Lancet. 1996;348:1449.
60. Alikhan A, Lynch PJ, Eisen DB. Hidradenitis suppurativa: a comprehensive review. J Am Acad Dermatol. 2009;60:539–61.
61. Jemec GBE, Wendelboe P. Topical clindamycin versus systemic tetracycline in the treatment of hidradenitis suppurativa. J Am Acad Dermatol. 1998;39:971–4.
62. Shah N. Hidradenitis suppurativa: a treatment challenge. Am Fam Physician. 2005;72:1547–52.
63. Ritz JP, Runke N, Haier J, Buhr HJ. Extent of surgery and recurrence rate of hidradenitis suppurativa. Int J Colorectal Dis. 1998;13:164–8.
64. Greely PW. Plastic surgical treatment of chronic suppurative hidradenitis. Plast Reconstr Surg. 1951;7:143–6.

65. Paletta FX. Hidradenitis suppurativa: a pathologic study and the use of skin flaps. Plast Reconstr Surg. 1963;31:307–15.
66. Elwood ET, Bolitho DG. Negative-pressure dressings in the treatment of hidradenitis suppurativa. Ann Plast Surg. 2001;46:49–51.
67. Blackburn JH, Boemi L, Hall WW, Jeffords K, Hauck RM, Banducci DR, et al. Negative-pressure dressings as a bolster for skin grafts. Ann Plast Surg. 1998;40:453–7.
68. Ger R. Fecal diversion in management of large infected perianal lesions. Dis Colon Rectum. 1996;39:1327–29.
69. Beck DE. Miscellaneous disorders of the colon, rectum and anus: stricture, pruritus ani, proctalgia, colitis cystica profunda, solitary rectal ulcer, hidradenitis. In: Pemberton SH, editor. Shackleford's surgery of the alimentary tract, vol. 4. 5th ed. Philadelphia, PA: W.B. Saunders; 2002. p. 501–18.

16 Dermatology and Pruritus Ani

Charles O. Finne and John R. Fenyk

Introduction

Perianal skin is subject to virtually all of the diseases that affect skin and mucosa. The differential diagnosis of disease in perianal skin is broad (Table 16-1) and includes a variety of diagnoses. These diseases almost never present solely within the perianal area; however, there are common diseases such as psoriasis that may present in the perianal area without obvious ties to other areas of the body unless a careful search is made. Certain diseases have specific causes and well-recognized treatment protocols (e.g., psoriasis, candida, and Bowen's disease), other diseases have less well-defined causes and all too often where therapy is established it is poorly defined. Recognition of important treatable causes requires a disciplined, organized approach to diagnosis with careful and complete history, physical exam, and the frequent use of biopsy. This chapter's objective is to lay out a strategy to facilitate accurate diagnosis and successful treatment of perianal and anal skin conditions. Implicit in this strategy is (1) the ability to properly examine the anus with appropriate instruments and bright light and (2) to understand diseases peculiar to the anal area. Hence, the importance of the colorectal surgeon, who possesses the unique skills, experience and training needed to accomplish this task. The importance of complete, accurate evaluation is demonstrated by a St. Louis University series in which 209 patients with the presenting symptom of pruritus ani revealed 75% of those patients had coexisting anal or colorectal pathology. While the majority of patients had hemorrhoids or fissure diagnoses also included 11% with rectal cancer, 6% anal canal cancer, and 2% with colon cancer.[2]

Definitions

Accurate description of the morphology of skin lesions can aid in the diagnosis and follow-up of patients with pruritic complaints. Macules are flat spots. Papules are elevated circumscribed solid lesions. Vesicles are separations of the epidermis from the dermis filled with serum. Bullae are larger vesicles or blisters greater than or equal to 10 mm. Pustules contain pus. Ulcers are surface lesions with loss of continuity of the skin and may result from rupture of vesicular lesions, infection, or trauma. Intertrigo is inflammation seen between two opposing skin surfaces, often the result of mixed bacterial, fungal infection associated with moisture, obesity, and poor hygiene.

Pruritus ani is a term of Latin derivation, which means itchy anus. Pruritus ani is a symptom, a Medline MeSH searchable diagnosis, and is also used to designate a specific condition of multiple etiologies recognized since antiquity.[1,3] The term pruritus when used alone simply means itchy: there is no distinction between pruritus and itch (an unpleasant sensation that provokes the desire to scratch). To avoid confusion in this chapter, the syndrome will always be referred to as pruritus ani. Pruritus ani is classified as either primary or secondary. The primary form is the classic syndrome of idiopathic pruritus ani, whereas the secondary form implies an identifiable cause or a specific diagnosis.

Physiologic Considerations

There are different types of itch which may respond to different forms or modalities of therapy: (1) pruritoceptive (C-fiber mediated), (2) neuropathic (e.g., Post-zoster), and (3) central or neurogenic. Itch is a surface phenomenon mediated by unmyelinated C-fibers in the epidermis and subepidermis, these fibers may have a lower threshold for stimulation when reporting itch than when reporting pain. Itch receptors may be located more superficially than those dedicated to pain. Because receptors are superficial, innocuous, nondamaging stimuli such as wearing long fibered fabric (i.e., wool) or other minor mechanical stimuli may induce itching. In addition to histamine, kallikrein, bradykinin, papain, and trypsin experimentally produce itching, but these substances do not respond to blockade with classic histamine antagonists such as diphenhydramine; hence, topical antihistamines are not

D.E. Beck et al. (eds.), *The ASCRS Textbook of Colon and Rectal Surgery: Second Edition*,
DOI 10.1007/978-1-4419-1584-9_16, © Springer Science+Business Media, LLC 2011

TABLE 16-1. Differential diagnosis of anal dermatoses

Inflammatory diseases	*Nonsexual infectious disease*
Pruritus ani	Pilonidal disease
Psoriasis	Hidradenitis suppurativa
Lichen planus	Beta hemolytic streptococcus
Lichen sclerosus et atrophicus	Fistula-in-ano
Atrophoderma	Crohn's disease
Contact (allergic) dermatitis	Tuberculosis
Contact (irritant) dermatitis	Actinomycosis
Seborrheic dermatitis	Herpes zoster
Atopic dermatitis	Vaccinia
Radiation dermatitis	Fournier's gangrene
Behçet's syndrome	Tinea cruris
Lupus erythematosus	Candidiasis
Dermatomyositis	"deep" mycoses
Scleroderma	Amebiasis cutis
Erythema multiforme	Trichomoniasis
Darier's disease	Schistosomiasis cutis
Familial chronic pemphigus (Hailey-Hailey)	Bilhartziasis
	Oxyurasis (pinworm)
Pemphigus vulgaris	Creeping eruption (larva migrans)
Cicatricial pemphigoid	Larva currens
Bullous pemphigoid	Cimicosis (bed bugs)
Dermatitis herpetiformis	Pediculosis (lice)
	Scabies
Sexually transmitted disease	*Premalignant and malignant disease*
Gonorrhea	Acanthosis nigricans
Syphilis	Leukoplakia
Chancroid	Mycosis fungoides
Granuloma inguinale	Leukemia cutis
Lymphogranuloma venereum	Basal cell carcinoma
Molluscum contagiosum	Squamous cell carcinoma
Herpes simplex	Melanoma
Condyloma acuminata	Bowen's disease (AIN)
	Extramammary Paget's disease

(Modified from Corman ML, Colon and rectal surgery. 2nd ed. Philadelphia, PA: Lippincott, 1989. p. 287.[1])

always effective against itching.[4] Recent studies suggest that gastrin releasing peptide receptors may, at least in part, mediate itch. This finding could explain some of the impact of H2 blockers (nonclassic antihistamines) on itch. The phenomenon of hyperesthesia with chronic pain may have a parallel with itching; just as minimal stimulation of the skin may induce itching, scratching with subsequent injury may produce an expanding area of itchy skin. Scratching produces inadequate feedback to inhibit itching, more scratching occurs with cutaneous injury, which provides an additional stimulus to scratch in a self-defeating loop. Substituting heat, cold, painful, or stinging stimulus for the itch by applying alcohol or pepper extract (capsaicin) may provoke an inhibitory feedback not supplied by scratching alone and lead to inhibition of the urge to scratch. Cowhage induced itching does not produce an inflammatory reaction and is mediated by different neurons than histamine-induced itching and may be the type of itching blocked by use of capsaicin.[5,6] Antidepressant medications (such as paroxetine) and anticonvulsants (gabapentin) have antipruritic effects at the central nervous system level though mechanisms of action may not be clear.[7] Itching associated with healing probably results from the combination of histamine release, release of other kinins and prostaglandins involved in the inflammatory phase of healing, and regeneration of nerves which may be thinly myelinated in immature scars. Antihistamines, topical anti-inflammatory agents (steroids), topical anesthetics, moisturization, petrolatum, and aloe preparations (prostaglandin inhibitors) all have beneficial effects on the itching of healing wounds.[4]

Etiology of Pruritus

Because pruritus is a symptom that may have protean causes, it is useful to consider diagnoses which have been associated with pruritus ani. Table 16-2 is a list of diagnoses and conditions modified from Stamos and Hicks.[8] Specific causes are considered below.

Localized Itch Syndromes

Notalgia paresthetica is a defined syndrome with itching or pain of the upper mid-back to either side of the scapular region. This has been attributed to spinal nerve damage or entrapment, although an inherited form has been described. Skin biopsies have shown increases in sensory innervation in the area of notalgia paresthetica; other changes are seen in the biopsy which could be attributed to repeated rubbing and scratching. Treatment by application of pepper cream (capsaicin 0.025%) has been effective. Such treatment may exacerbate the symptoms during the first week of application, but thereafter both the symptoms and the side effects of the treatment subside. Topical application of eutectic mixture of local anesthetic (EMLA) (2.5% lignocaine + 2.5% prilocaine), a topical anesthetic cream, has also been effective.[4] Dermatographism has been reported as a cause of anogenital pruritus.[9,10] It is not unreasonable to propose that one etiology of the idiopathic forms of pruritus ani may be related to dermatographism or notalgia paresthetica, and that the skin changes are the sole result of skin trauma. The effectiveness of the anal tattooing procedures, discussed later, may lend some insight into the etiologies of idiopathic pruritus ani.

Fecal Contamination

Systematic, rigorous studies of anal pruritus are rare, but good evidence supports fecal contamination as one cause of symptoms. Caplan[11] performed a study in 27 Caucasian men on whom fresh autologous feces was applied as a patch test both perianally and on the inner arm, and perianal skin was also cultured for fungi. In ten control subjects fecal samples were collected and while the skin was spatulated, feces were not applied. The patch tested subjects ($n=27$) had several pH-adjusted samples applied to the skin in addition to the

TABLE 16-2. Proposed etiologies of idiopathic pruritus ani

Anatomic factors	Obesity, deep clefts, hirsutism, tight clothing
Anorectal disease	Fissure, fistula, tags, prolapsing papilla, hemorrhoids, mucosal prolapse, sphincter insufficiency, deforming scars
Antibiotics	
Contact dermatitis	Chemicals in topical preparations, toilet paper, wet wipes, alcohol, witch hazel, "caine" anesthetics, fecal soiling
Dermatoses	Psoriasis, seborrheic dermatitis, atopic dermatitis, lichen planus, lichen simplex, lichen sclerosis, dermographism
Diet	Coffee (caffeinated and decaffeinated), chocolate, spicy foods, citrus fruits, tomatoes, beer, dairy products, vitamin A and D deficiencies, fat substitutes, consumption of large volumes of liquids
Diarrhea	Infectious diarrhea, irritable bowel syndrome, Crohn's Disease, ulcerative colitis
Drugs	Quinidine, colchicine, IV steroids
Gynecologic conditions	Pruritus vulvae, vaginal discharge of infection
Idiopathic	
Infection	Viruses: herpes simplex, cytomegalovirus, papillomavirus; Bacteria: *Staphylococcus aureus*, beta hemolytic strep, mixed infections; Fungi: dermatophytes, Candida species; Parasites: pin worms, scabies, pediculosis; Spirochetes: syphilis
Neoplasms	Bowen's disease (AIN), extramammary Paget's disease, squamous cell carcinoma variants, secreting villous tumors
Personal hygiene	Poor cleansing habits, over meticulous cleansing producing mechanical trauma, use of soaps
Psychogenic/neurogenic	Anxiety, neurosis, psychosis, neurodermatitis, neuropathy, "itch syndromes"
Radiation	Radiation dermatitis, sphincter compromise or leakage due to radiation proctitis
Systemic disease	Jaundice, diabetes mellitus, chronic renal failure, iron deficiency, thyroid disorders, lymphoma, polycythemia vera

(Modified from Stamos MJ, Hicks TC, Pruritus ani: diagnosis and treatment. In: Perspectives in Colon and Rectal Surgery, 1998;11(1):1–20. Thieme Medical Publishers.[8])

unadulterated samples; 12 of the 27 had a history of pruritus ani prior to being enrolled in this study. pH of the perianal skin varied from 5.0 to 7.0 and was not different between the two groups. Five of twelve pruritus subjects (42%) grew yeast (non *Candida albicans*) but no dermatophytes, while 4 of 15 nonpruritus subjects (27%) grew *C. albicans* (3) or *Geotrichum*. Twelve of 27 (44%) with feces applied to the skin developed symptoms from the feces. Four of 12 (33%) of the pruritus group developed symptoms, 8 of 15 (53%) of the nonpruritus group developed symptoms, while none of the control group developed symptoms. Symptoms occurred within 1–6 h in all but one subject and were relieved by washing the skin. Only one of the 27 subjects reacted to feces on the arms patch test, suggesting that the skin in different locations reacts differently. The prompt appearance of symptoms and relief with cleansing was felt to indicate an irritant effect rather than an allergic effect.

Smith et al.,[12] in a rigorous study of 75 patients with pruritus, found that half of their patients had poorly formed stools and 41% of their patients complained of soiling from daily to several times a week. Seepage of liquid and mucous was felt to be an important factor in the etiology of the symptoms. Coffee consumption lowered anal resting pressure in 8 of 11 patients.

Allan et al.[13] showed that leakage during a saline infusion test occurred sooner in patients with pruritus ani than in nonpruritic controls (median leak point 600 ml vs. 1,300 ml in controls). This is consistent with findings by Farouk et al.[14] and Eyers and Thompson[15] who both found that the anal inhibitory reflex was more pronounced in patients with pruritus ani. Rectal distension makes these patients more prone to leak and soil, because the fall in anal pressure from baseline is greater in patients with pruritus ani.

Viral Infection

Condylomata accuminata is a common cause of itching, but the diagnosis is generally easy to recognize and should not be confused with idiopathic pruritus ani. Condylomata, human papilloma virus infection and anal intraepithelial neoplasia (AIN) will be discussed extensively elsewhere. Herpes syndromes are usually accompanied by pain or burning rather than itching and the clinical course is accompanied by a characteristic eruption consisting of red macules, which progress to vesicles that rupture, ulcerate, and may become secondarily infected. Culture or biopsy shows specific diagnostic findings. Likewise, molluscum contagiosum produces characteristic lesions, palpable papules, 2–5 mm diameter, with central umbilication, flesh colored to slightly pink and usually clustered. HIV-associated lesions are rarely associated with chronic itching except for secondary fungal infections.

Fungal Infection

Smith et al.[12] found no instances of fungal infection in their investigation of pruritus ani where each of 75 patients had scrapings and fungus cultures. In contrast, Dodi et al.[16] found *C. albicans* had no relationship to pruritus (culture positive in 23% of control subjects, 26% of those with pruritus, and 28% of those without pruritus), but ten patients who cultured dermatophytes all had itching. None of these patients had exposure to steroids or antibiotics. Their conclusion was that *C. albicans* was saprophytic in the absence of steroids, but that dermatophytes were always pathogenic. Prolonged courses of steroids are said to enhance pathogenicity of *C. albicans* and to mask Candida infection.[17]

Verbov[3] found 7 of 47 (15%) patients with pruritus ani had itching which was attributable to Candida. In a review of his dermatologic practice (3,000 patients surveyed on the basis of their primary complaint), Pirone et al.[18] reported that surgical treatment of anal disorders (hemorrhoids, fissure, spasm, mucosal prolapse) eliminated Candida and dermatophyte infections in all but 3 of 23 patients who were culture positive and symptomatic with itching before surgery. Two of these three failures responded to antifungal treatment, but the third patient continued to itch.

In another study of 200 patients evaluated by colorectal surgeons and dermatologists, thrush was found in 28 (14%), only one of whom was diabetic. Fourteen patients had Candida infection after local steroid therapy, and six occurred after a course of systemic antibiotics. Only one case of dermatophyte infection was found.[19]

Perianal dermatophyte infection, all *Trichophyton rubrum*, was reported to be infrequent by Alexander (four of nearly 300 cases).[17] Topical steroids may render direct scrapings negative for hyphae, though most frequently they facilitate dermatophyte growth.

Bacterial Infection

Several nonsexually transmitted bacterial infections are reported to cause longstanding pruritus. Weismann et al.[20] reported that 19 patients (16 males and 3 females) with pruritus of duration 1–20 years had beta hemolytic streptococci cultured (four also had *Staphylococcus aureus*) from the perianal area but not from nasal or throat swabs. Treatment with various regimen resulted in cure of 42% and amelioration of symptoms in the rest. Erythrasma was reported to cause pruritus in 15 of 81 (18%) patients who failed to respond to routine treatment.[21] Wood's light fluorescence (coral pink or red in the case of *Corynebacterium minutissimum*) was the most reliable diagnostic test, being positive in every case, whereas cultures for *C. minutissimum* were positive in only 4 of 15 cases. Groin, thighs, and toes were also involved in every case and cure was achieved in all patients with erythromycin. Smith et al.[12] found erythrasma in only one of their 75 patients, each of whom had Wood's light examination. *C. minutissimum* is probably present as normal skin flora, but moisture, diabetes, and obesity predispose to pathogenicity, which usually develops in the body folds (axillae, groin, intergluteal, inframammary) and toe webs.[22] The St. Mark's Hospital series found erythrasma in 16% of 200 cases, but in 27% of the patients who had been symptomatic for over 5 years *C. minutissimum* was identified.[19] These patients had disease in more than one site, in common with other quoted series.

S. aureus has been anecdotally implicated as a cause of treatable pruritus.[23] Intertrigo was reported in 27% of the St. Mark's Hospital series and was highly treatable with topical agents.[19]

Contact Dermatitis

Contact dermatitis may develop from a wide variety of preparations including topical anesthetics, topical antibiotics, topical antiseptics, topical antihistamines, nickel and topically applied steroids (discussed later).[19,24] Common sensitizing agents identified in the dermatologic literature are listed in Table 16-3. The role of feces and seepage as an irritant contact agent has been emphasized in almost every paper devoted to pruritus ani. Contact dermatitis may have an irritant or allergic basis but is recognized by being an eczematous inflammation characterized by erythema, scale, and vesicles.[25] Avoidance of contact with the inciting agent is the obvious treatment. Topical steroids may be useful unless secondary infection is present. It is preferable to avoid detergents and soaps. Bath oils and emollient creams may be useful for cleansing.

The cause of contact dermatitis is often obscure, requiring detailed history and examination to resolve. Dasan et al.[24] report one patient who had pruritus associated with bathing in a tub of water in which his wife shampooed her hair with paraphenylenediamine, a dye. When the patient's wife stopped shampooing her hair in the tub, his symptoms resolved.

A study of patch testing in 80 patients with pruritus ani in Sheffield, England emphasized the importance of allergic contact dermatitis as an aggravating factor in 55 patients who tested positive. Thirty-eight of the positives were to medicaments or their constituents including neomycin, fragrance mix, Balsam of Peru, and cinchocaine. After counseling, two-thirds of these 55 patients experienced improvement or resolution of their symptoms.[26] These authors disputed the recommendation to use "wet wipes" for cleansing due to possible sensitization. Bruynzeel[27] corroborates the potential sensitization from use of moist wipes containing methyldibromoglutaronitrile. Rohde[28] feels that excessive exposure

TABLE 16-3. Common sensitizing agents

Ethylenediaminetetraacetic acid
Formalin
Lanolin (wood wax alcohol)
Mercury ($Hg(NH_2)Cl$, thimerosal)
Neomycin
Nickel
Paraben mixtures
Paraphenylenediamine
Potassium dichromate
Rubber ingredients
Topical anesthetics (benzocaine, dibucaine)
Turpentine oil

to water and the act of excessive cleansing itself may incite symptoms, and recommends the use of oils for cleaning.

Alexander[17] found lanolin, neomycin, procaine, and parabens to be offending agents and emphasized the difficulty of identifying these types of products when incorporated with a local anesthetic or steroid because the anesthetic suppresses the itching and the steroid suppresses the inflammation giving paradoxical temporary relief. Temporary relief leads to increasing application of the offending agent over a wider area, escalating the process.

Psoriasis

Psoriasis has been an important underlying cause of itch in every published study on the subject of pruritus ani. In a combined colorectal dermatologic clinic established to prospectively evaluate patients with pruritus, 22 of 40 patients were found to have psoriasis.[24] Alexander[17] confirms that psoriasis may present as an isolated lesion in the perianal area, and emphasizes that lesions in this location may have an altered appearance secondary to maceration. Smith et al.[12] found six (8%) cases of psoriasis in his series of pruritus ani, five of which had not been previously diagnosed. The St. Marks Hospital series found 5.5% of their 200 patients had psoriasis.[19] They also emphasized the nontypical appearance of the perianal lesions. Lockridge[29] reported a series of 81 patients with pruritus ani who were ultimately diagnosed with psoriasis. All of his patients in this series responded to fluocinolone acetonide 0.025% (Synalar®) with normalization of the skin. He recommended a search for lesions elsewhere; including elbows, knees, ankles, extensor surfaces of the forearm, base of the scalp, ear canals, eyelids, nipples, penis, vulva, and navel. Biopsy was rarely diagnostic secondary to changes attributable to drugs or trauma and limited experience of pathologists with diagnosis of perianal skin. Psoriasis affects 1–3% of the general population.[30] Typical psoriasis involves the trunk and extensor surfaces such as knees, elbows, sacral area, and scalp, but psoriasis involving groin, genitals, axillae, umbilicus, and anus is referred to as inverse psoriasis because it involves the inverse of the usual distribution. The exact incidence is unknown, but a review of 709 patients with psoriasis in a Chinese dermatology clinic found 48 (6.8%) with this distribution and 54% of this group had involvement of the anus.[31] The National Psoriasis Foundation corroborates these figures and suggests that limited Type IB evidence supports short-term use of a low to mid-potency topical steroid (betamethasone valerate in one study) once daily for up to 4 weeks for induction of remission, with a switch to calcipotriene (Dovonex®; LEO Laboratories Ltd., Dublin, Ireland) or pimecrolimus, or tacrolimus for maintenance to avoid long-term side effects of steroids.[32] Calcipotriene may be used as a primary agent but may take 6–8 weeks for maximum effect to occur and may be accompanied by discomfort. A combination of these agents may be required.

Atopic Dermatitis

Atopic dermatitis or eczema may be the most common hereditary cause of pruritus ani. This disorder presents as nonspecific and diffuse erythema, often dramatically marked by evidence of excoriation. The probability of correctly diagnosing atopic dermatitis may be improved by documenting the associated findings of (1) keratosis pilaris (rough sandpaper-like texture over the posterior biceps and thighs), (2) Morgan's folds or Morgan–Dennie lines (redundant creases beneath the eyes), (3) "sniffers" or "snuffers" lines (a transverse often subtle crease across mid-nose), (4) urticaria, and (5) white dermatographism. Although generally informative and often helpful in making the diagnosis, biopsies are most frequently not diagnostic, showing a mixed inflammatory infiltrate with eosinophils.

This inherited disease has a frequency greater than psoriasis (15–20% of the population) and is caused by disruption of epidermal barrier function. The atopic diseases (hayfever, asthma, atopic dermatitis/eczema and the multiple sensitive/allergic patient) have direct genetic and epigenetic influences. Fillagrin appears integral to the development of the atopic diseases and the fillagrin gene (FLG) appears to have no expression rather than polymorphisms in atopic dermatitis.[33] Fillagrin (keratin filament aggregating protein) is the cement of the epidermis. Complete loss of FLG is seen in ichthyosis vulgaris,[34] a common keratinizing disorder frequently associated with atopic dermatitis and seen over the buttocks and on perianal skin. Polymorphisms of FLG are commonly seen in asthma and other "atopic" conditions. Absence of FLG results in a permeable epidermal barrier function which can be indirectly observed by following measurements of enhanced transepidermal water loss in affected patients.[35] With the loss of an adequate barrier bacterial growth and colonization increases, access to the dermis by irritants increases the inflammatory response.

Treatment of atopic dermatitis begins with providing a barrier such as Vaseline® (white petrolatum USP), use of aggressive moisturization techniques, and the use of anti-inflammatory agents (systemic and topical), antipruritic agents both topical and systemic (antihistaminics H1 and H2, leukotriene inhibitors, etc.). True allergies may be seen in association with atopic dermatitis, especially with longer duration of disease. Basically, the greater the risk of induction of allergy to topicals is seen with more frequent use of greater concentration of medicaments over a longer period of time (frequency, duration, and concentration). Suspicion of the development of truly allergic component in this process should be raised when in spite of the medications and therapy used, the condition continues to exacerbate.

Lichen Sclerosus

Lichen sclerosus (formerly lichen sclerosus et atrophicus) (LS) is a chronic disease of unknown cause, occurring more frequently in women (female/male: 10/1); when this process occurs on the penis it is termed balanitis xerotica obliterans. In females LS has a predilection for the vulva and perianal area. Characteristic appearance is a gradual progression from erythema with mild induration to white, atrophic, and wrinkled to the end stage of loss of normal perineal and perianal architecture clinically and histologically consistent with nothing more than a scar, lacking the lymphocytic interface dermatitis and other changes.[25,36–39] Involvement of the labia gives this condition a characteristic distribution that makes recognition easier once the diagnosis is considered. Biopsy is characteristic and may be especially indicated in a lesion not responding to treatment because of rare occurrence of squamous cell carcinoma.[40–42] Patients with LS in the vulva probably have a 4–6% incidence of squamous cell carcinoma arising in or adjacent to the LS.[43] Women with lichen sclerosus have a 300-fold increase in the likelihood of developing cancer compared with those who do not, and treatment of the disease does not appear to modify this risk.[41] Although in the paper by Funaro[44] topical testosterone was a popular treatment, it has now been shown to be without benefit. Treatment of LS with a potent topical steroid (clobetasol propionate 0.05%, Temovate®) for 6–8 weeks is highly successful, often resulting in normalization of the skin.[4,37,38] Other recent reports suggest that tacrolimus ointment may avoid skin atrophy which may accompany potent steroid use.[45,46] Secondary to the increased risk of squamous cell carcinoma, these patients should be followed periodically for raised lesions or ulcers that fail to heal. The exact role LS plays in the development of cancer is not certain but is thought to be independent of human papilloma virus.[42]

Food Factors

No controlled trials have been done to examine food stuffs or diet as a cause for itching, but strong opinions have garnered a revered place in the literature. Friend states that virtually all patients with idiopathic pruritus ani consume enormous quantities of liquids, are almost never constipated, and usually have loose stools.[47] Because it helps their symptoms, patients with severe pruritus usually maintain good anal hygiene. Friend states that there are six common foods that unequivocally cause idiopathic pruritus: coffee, tea, cola, beer, chocolate, and tomato (ketchup) and that total elimination will result in remission of itching in 2 weeks. After a 2 week elimination period the food may be reintroduced to determine the threshold for appearance of symptoms. Thresholds are typically between two and three cups of coffee, four cups of tea, less than two cans of beer.

As we reviewed briefly earlier in this chapter, Smith et al.[12] demonstrated that coffee lowered anal resting pressure in 8 of 11 patients tested. An elimination diet gave partial or complete relief in 27 of 56 (48%) of their patients. Specific dietary items identified by elimination as a cause were coffee (eight), alcohol (five), peanuts (three), chocolate (two), milk products (three), cola (one), citrus (one). Alcohol was an equivocal factor in this study because 41% did not consume alcohol and only a third of patients drank more than 1 ounce per day. Smith et al. confirm the importance of poorly formed stool and coffee which may contribute to seepage and recommend a bulk agent taken at the same time of day to promote regular, complete emptying of stool.[12]

Daniel et al.[2] reported that average coffee intake in patients with primary pruritus ani averaged six cups per day, compared to those with secondary pruritus who averaged about 3.5 cups per day. Akl[48] reported an 8-year-old boy with asthma, intolerant of milk with abdominal pain, whose pruritus ani disappeared after elimination of yogurt.

Coexisting Anal Disease

Coexisting surgical anal conditions (hemorrhoids, fissure, fistulas) may of themselves produce itching or aggravate any tendency to itch. Most authors agree that correcting these disorders in selected patients is indicated. Smith et al.[12] reported that 8 of his 75 patients required treatment of hemorrhoids (four operations, four Barron ligations) which by virtue of prolapse may induce soiling. These authors note, however, that correction of the hemorrhoids eliminated itching in only one patient. Another with scars from previous fissure surgery also had soiling not amenable to surgical correction. Murie et al.[49] in a study of 82 hemorrhoidal patients with and without pruritus felt that pruritus is more common in patients with hemorrhoids than in age- and sex-matched controls without hemorrhoids and that correction of the hemorrhoids usually eliminated itching along with the other symptoms of bleeding, pain, soiling, and protrusion. Bowyer and McColl[19] reported that hemorrhoids were the sole cause of itching in 16 of their 200 patients, contributory in 27 others, and that correction of fissure was required in five patients before symptoms were relieved. Five others had skin tags which when removed, eliminated symptoms. These patients could point to specific skin tag(s) as the source of their discomfort, raising the possibility of a causal relationship between skin tags and pruritus ani. Dasan et al.[24] in a study of 40 patients with pruritus found two that required surgery, one to remove complex skin tags and the other to correct a fistula. The St. Louis University group found that 52% of 109 patients with the sole presenting complaint of itching had anorectal disease as the cause.[2] The diagnoses included hemorrhoids, fissure, idiopathic proctitis, condyloma, ulcerative proctitis, abscess, and fistula.

Pirone et al.[18] as mentioned previously, believe that correction of hemorrhoids, fissure, mucosal prolapse and spasm can resolve fungal infection and the consequent pruritus.

Psychological Factors

Smith et al.[12] studied 25 of their patients who completed an Minnesota Multiphasic Personality Inventory (MMPI). They found no deviations on the clinical scales but a trend toward inhibition of aggression, and denial of feeling of social and emotional alienation. Anxiety, stress, and fatigue, as well as personality, coping skills, and obsessive compulsive disorders, probably play a role in the exacerbation of pruritus ani.[50] Because of this, psychotropic drugs may play a role in its management in isolated cases supporting the use of Doxepin HCl with its strong H1 and H2 effects, amitryptiline, nortryptiline, and gabapentin.

Steroid-Induced Itching

Anogenital itching has been reported following bolus administration of intravenous dexamethasone.[51] More commonly, itching occurs as a rebound phenomenon after withdrawal of steroids, leading to their reinstitution and chronic use. This syndrome has been characterized as steroid addiction[52] and can lead to permanent deformity and dependence.[53] Experimental application of potent steroids under occlusion for as little as 3 weeks has been shown to produce an acute dermatitis resembling that seen with a blister that has been unroofed and exposed to air.[52] Steroids should only be used to achieve specific effects. Potency and dosing should be tapered in a planned fashion with the goal of eliminating steroids altogether from a maintenance regimen. Allergic contact dermatitis to topically applied steroids has been well documented and is chemical class specific. Switching to desoximetasone (a less commonly used agent in steroid class) may be a solution. The ideal solution would be elimination of the steroid, if, however, elimination is not possible, alternate day therapy or intermittent therapy once or twice a week is to be preferred. The calcineurin inhibitors (macrolide anti-inflammatories) tacrolimus and pimecrolimus offer excellent anti-inflammatory effect without steroids or steroidal side effects.

Skin Trauma

Trauma can arise from physiological processes such as diarrhea or frequent stools which may be associated with frequent wiping and maceration. Scratching either consciously or nocturnally while asleep may result in the classic lesion of lichen simplex chronicus. Alexander-Williams puts it nicely, "Perianal dermatitis is a cross between a nappy rash, athlete's foot, and a self inflicted injury. In most patients the problem is due either to inadequate cleansing of the anus or to over vigorous attempts to polish it clean."[54] There is controversy about the best way to clean the anus. Rohde takes issue with the standard method using water or wet wipes (which can induce irritant or allergic contact dermatitis) and advocates a smooth dry article with olive oil if necessary, feeling that water breaks down the barrier function of the skin.[28] Most authors agree that contact dermatitis is a contributing cause of perianal irritation and that attempts to discontinue over-the-counter preparations (OTCs), perfumed or scented products including toilet paper, should be made because of potential sensitizing agents (Table 16-3). Bland emollients, Acid Mantle creams, and waterless cleansing agents are reasonable substitutes that may be used with tissue paper or cotton balls for cleansing and left on the skin. My own experience suggests that dilute white vinegar (one tablespoon in 8 ounces of water) and Burow's solution (Domeboro®, Bayer Corp.) are effective cleansing agents associated with little adverse reaction. Since Burow's solution and acetic acid have been found to be an effective antibacterial in chronic otitis externa with little toxicity, its use in perianal disease seems justified.[55–58]

Neoplasms

Perianal Paget's disease is rare and large series do not exist; however, more than half of patients with Paget's disease have itching, often lasting longer than 3 months.[59–61] Perianal Bowen's disease (intraepithelial squamous cell carcinoma in situ) is also rare, but in a series of 47 patients reviewed at the Cleveland Clinic, 28 (60%) had perianal itching as a presenting complaint.[62] AIN is the sequel to human papillomavirus infection (associated with itching) and refers to premalignant change in the area of the dentate line and anal transitional zone. Although pruritus has not been described in large series looking at AIN,[63,64] because of their study design it would seem prudent to be alert for neoplastic change in any patient with a history of warts who presents with pruritus. Itching was present either alone or with soreness in 77% of lichen sclerosus associated carcinoma and 73% of non-LS-associated vulvar carcinoma.[42] Higher grade tumors such as melanoma or squamous cell cancer usually present with bleeding or pain, not with pruritus.[65–67] Further discussion of neoplastic disease is provided in Chap. 20.

Diagnosis of Perianal Disease

Given the variety of possible diagnoses, it is important to identify the specific diagnoses that are treatable for cure, and to engage a strategy that will avoid mistakes. It is often helpful in the differential diagnosis of anal and perianal disease processes to divide them into the general classifications of mass (inflammatory or neoplastic), rash or fissure (primary or secondary). The morphology of a lesion is a starting point for diagnosis, but may not be specific, and the same disease may have several different appearances (Table 16-4). As an example, Candidiasis may be present as an erythematous lesion, a papular lesion, or as an ulcerative lesion. Specific techniques are necessary, therefore, to establish or eliminate a diagnosis. Bacterial culture is a time-honored technique for identification of organisms, but proper media and collection techniques must be used to avoid killing certain species.[68]

History and Physical Examination

History and physical examination are still the most basic maneuvers for diagnosis (see Table 16-5). Inquiry about other skin diseases, allergic conditions such as asthma or

Table 16-4. Morphology of perianal skin lesions

Ulcers	*Papules*
Herpes genitalis	Venereal warts
Syphilis	Scabies
Trauma	Molluscum contagiosum
Chancroid	Candidiasis
Fixed drug eruption	Syphilis
Lymphogranuloma venereum	
Tularemia	
Behcet's syndrome	
Malignancy	
Donovanosis (granuloma inguinale)	
Candidiasis	
Histoplasmosis	
Mycobacterioses	
Amebiasis	
Gonorrhea	
Trichomoniasis	
Diffuse erythema	*Crusts*
Candidiasis	Herpes genitalis
Trauma	Scabies
Contact dermatitis	
Fixed drug eruption	
Miscellaneous findings	
Linear tracks: scabies	
Reddish flecks: crab louse excreta	
Maculae ceruleae (sky-blue spots): crab lice	
Nits: crab lice	
Hypertrophic: donovanosis	

Table 16-5. Historical and physical factors aiding diagnosis of anal and perianal disease

Historical
- Other skin conditions, asthma, urticaria
- Prior treatments/OTC topicals
- Allergies
- Chemicals/clothes/laundry
- Antibiotic use
- Systemic disease
- Chronicity

Physical findings
- Multiple sites (elbows, groins, intertriginous areas, labia, toe webs)
- Mass or woody induration
- Hyperpigmentation
- Scale
- Lichenification
- Ulceration
- Groin adenopathy
- Defined edge or margin

urticaria, or sites of involvement may the first clue to diagnosis of unrecognized psoriasis or atopic dermatitis. Patients may not relate the itch on their elbow to the itch around their anus. Erythrasma usually involves the groin and toes, usually is chronic and often associated with hyperpigmentation. Patients frequently do not consider over-the-counter or nonprescription preparations as medicines, though these may modify the appearance of a condition or even cause it. Specific questions about the use of these products are necessary to uncover their use and patient exposure to unsuspected ingredients. Knowledge of a patient's allergies is important not only for avoidance but also may aid in uncovering an unsuspected exposure to an occult ingredient. Patients sometimes have had patch testing and allergy consultation, and may not volunteer that information unless specifically asked. Patch testing, dermatologic consultation, and withdrawal of medication may be in order. Specific questions about infections, colds, or diarrheal illnesses treated with pills may be necessary to uncover antibiotic use. Patients sometimes may not list prednisone in their list of medications until asked a question pertinent to an illness such as arthritis or asthma or myalgias. A condition that has come and gone for years or that has seasonal exacerbation may be a clue to anal fissure but could reflect dietary changes, type of clothes worn, or laundry practices.

Physical examination should specifically look for other sites of involvement. The groin is a classic intertriginous area that is easily accessible in the prone jack-knife or the lateral position and should be the first place one looks to confirm a suspected yeast or fungus diagnosis. Hyperpigmentation in the buttock cleft or other intertriginous area is a clue to a chronic inflammatory condition or the presence of chronically infected drainage or secretion. Effective treatment of a patient with changes in the groin as well as the cleft requires attention to each area of involvement. If a condition is infectious, steps to eliminate the infection will be more successful if the environment of the host is made inhospitable to the organism in each area of involvement. Broad areas of erythema with indistinct borders and findings suggestive of excoriation or chronic rubbing should generate thoughts of eczema or atopic dermatitis. A sharply defined border usually points to a definable diagnosis such as tinea, especially when accompanied by scale (Figure 16-1). Psoriasis usually has a sharply defined border but in the cleft may lack the classic scale seen in skin that is exposed to air and may, in fact, exhibit maceration. In the confined, occluded area of the cleft there usually is no scale (Figure 16-2). Neoplastic changes may appear sharply marginated, but margins may be microscopically involved, especially around the dentate line, even if grossly normal (Figure 16-3). Infiltrative processes may be less well defined as in Paget's disease of the anus with the same caveat about margins (Figure 16-4). Inflammatory changes of idiopathic nature often have borders that are indistinct and nondescript (Figures 16-5 and 16-6). Brilliant red erythema often is seen with perianal yeast (Figure 16-6), frequently "satellite" pustules will be present outside the main area of involvement. Erythema may be seen with chronic steroid use (Figure 16-7). Patient A had used hydrocortisone daily for 20 years or more and came in with recurrent warts and carcinoma in situ when the cortisone failed to control his symptoms. Treatment of his warts, carcinoma in situ, and withdrawal of his steroids resulted in resolution of his symptoms and normalization of his skin, with

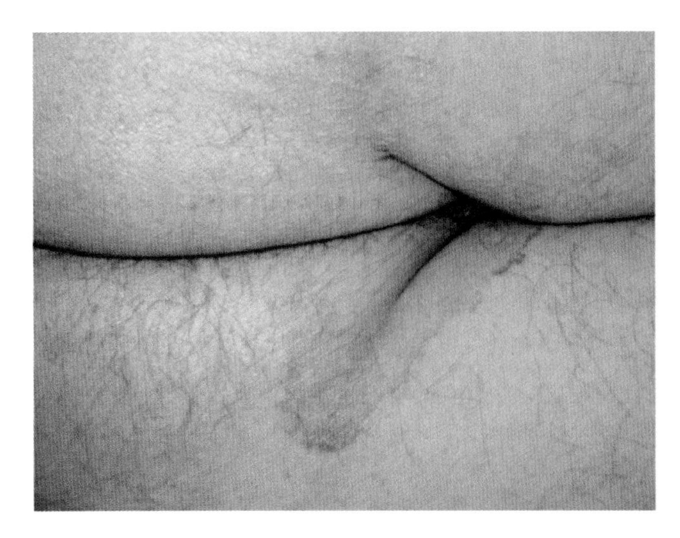

FIGURE 16-1. Dermatophyte infection. Note the sharp border, the scale at the edges and its involvement of the groin crease. As this type of infection moves into the anal cleft, the characteristic edge at the border of the cleft and involvement of the groin may be the only clues.

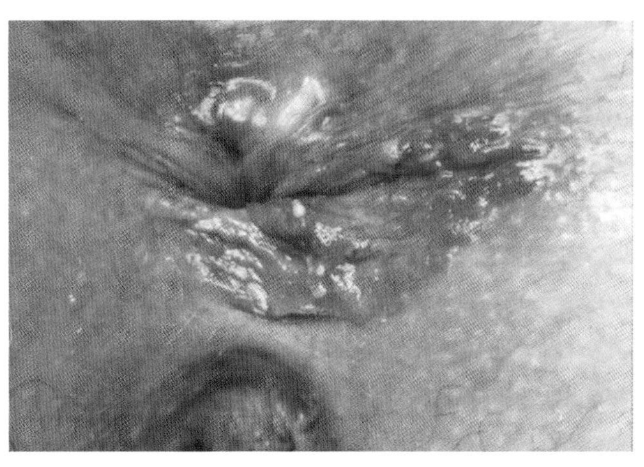

FIGURE 16-3. Anal Bowen's disease or squamous cell carcinoma in situ may have a varied appearance and be indistinguishable from Paget's disease (Figure 16-5) by clinical examination. The *white pearls* on the *red* background are often present and are a clue to the diagnosis. Despite sharp appearing edges, the process often involves normal-looking skin and requires frozen section to confirm negative margins.

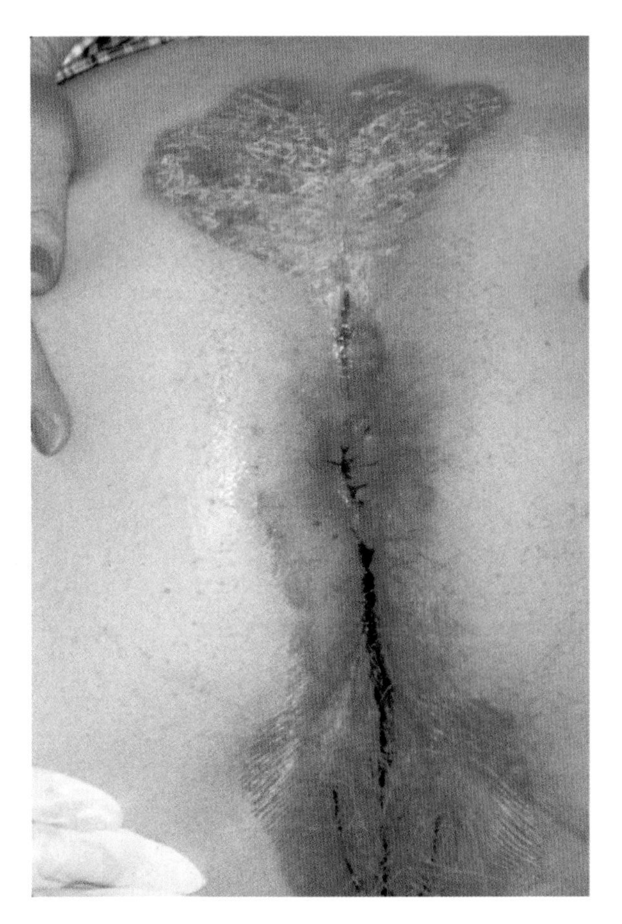

FIGURE 16-2. Psoriasis often appears atypical in the cleft and around the labia, lacking the silvery scale that is so characteristic. Isolated areas of involvement in the cleft occur and require biopsy confirmation by a competent skin pathologist.

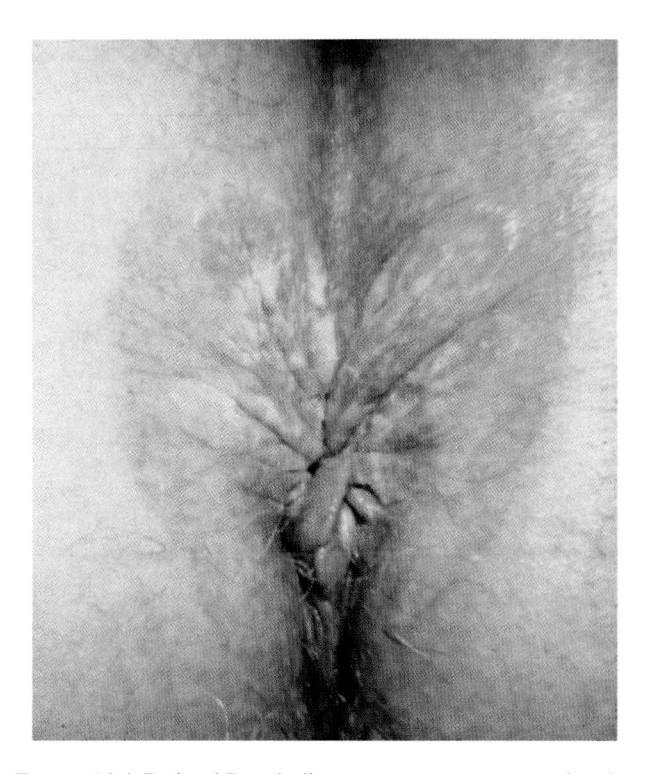

FIGURE 16-4. Perianal Paget's disease may present as a nondescript rash that itches. This clinical appearance is not specific and requires biopsy to confirm the diagnosis. Unlike Paget's of the breast, there is rarely an underlying invasive adenocarcinoma, and local excision with clear margins is the treatment of choice. Margins of excision require frozen section confirmation because clinically normal skin may be involved.

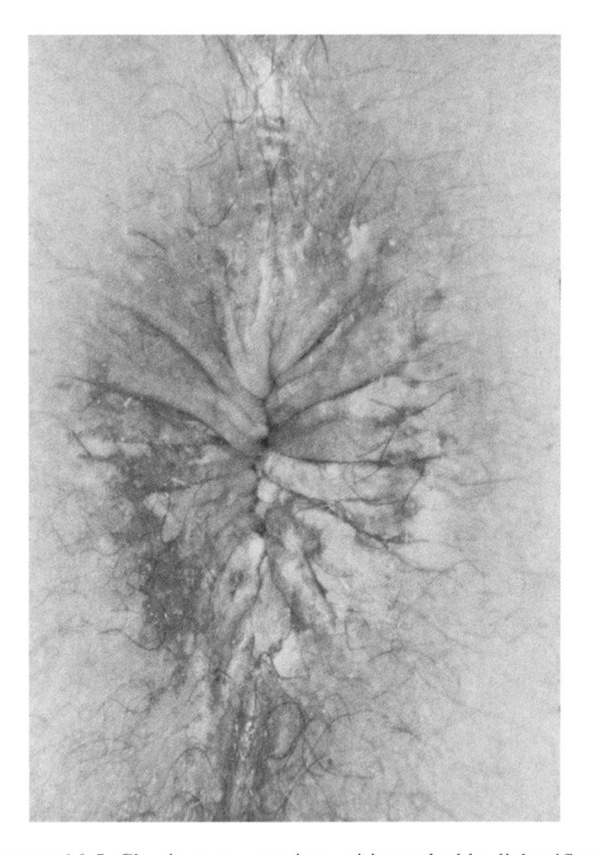

FIGURE 16-5. Classic severe pruritus ani is marked by lichenification (leathery thickening of the skin), accentuation of folds, fissuring of the skin, and erosions and an indistinct border. Changes this severe require short-term aggressive therapy with high potency steroids for 4–8 weeks which then are rapidly tapered to a maintenance program, if possible without steroids. It is important to rule out secondary infection, which requires specific treatment.

no reoccurrence of disease or symptoms to date, 7 years later. Patient B had used Mycolog® (a combination of nystatin and triamcinolone acetonide) cream daily for several years, after having radiation therapy for prostate cancer; both Mycolog® and topical steroids were withdrawn. Acute, severe injury from prolonged diarrhea with frequent wiping produced lichen simplex chronicus (Figure 16-8), which was treated by controlling the patient's diarrhea, cleansing with Burow's solution, and application of topical silver sulfadiazine to which cortisone was added. Chronic infected discharge may lead to hyperpigmentation of the cleft (Figure 16-9). In the example shown this hyperpigmentation is due to chronic pilonidal disease, but it may also occur with fistulas, chronic yeast or fungus infection, or hidradenitis. Complications of treatment can result in a rash, in this example a patient with contact dermatitis from clotrimazole (Figure 16-10) is shown. Severe symptoms, especially paresthesias, coupled with scattered lesions may be a clue to Herpes virus infection (Figure 16-11). Lichen sclerosus characteristically involves the perineum and labia in the female and has a distinctive appearance with wrinkling of the skin (Figure 16-12). Biopsy is characteristic.

Inguinal lymphadenopathy, and the presence or absence of pain, tenderness, or other symptoms, can have specific relevance to diagnosis of perianal and anal disease (Table 16-6), especially sexually transmitted diseases.

Laboratory Examination

Ideally, infected material should be aspirated with a syringe and expelled into a sterile container; next best is a swab of exudate collected from a deep portion of the

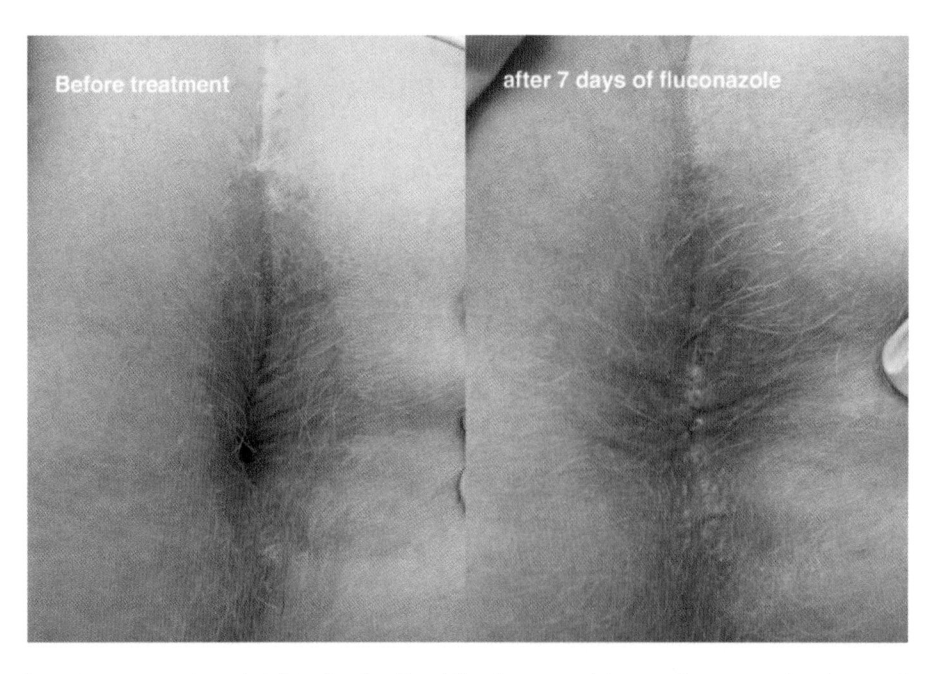

FIGURE 16-6. Perianal yeast may present as a *bright red rash* without the cheesy exudate sometimes seen elsewhere and may follow treatment with antibiotics for some other condition. This infection is easy to treat but has a tendency to recur. Rendering the cleft environment inhospitable by drying with a hair dryer after bathing and using athletes foot powder to coat the skin and absorb moisture can help maintain remission.

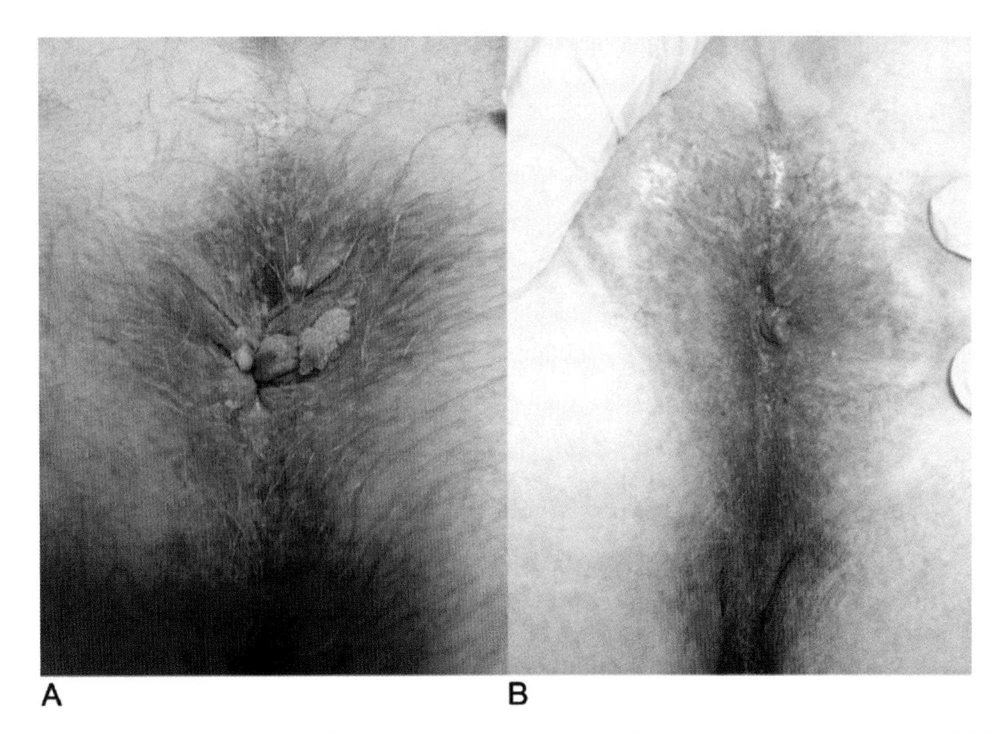

FIGURE 16-7. Chronic steroid use may cause itching or mask other processes. **A** shows an elderly man who had used 1% cortisone daily for over 20 years but had worsening of his symptoms despite increasing use. Treatment of his warts and carcinoma in situ along with withdrawal of steroids resolved his symptoms. The erythema has disappeared and he had remained free of symptoms for over a year. **B** shows a similar erythema superimposed on radiation dermatitis from treatment of prostate cancer. Withdrawal of Mycolog®, which had been used for years without interruption and substitution of a barrier cream with menthol relieved his symptoms.

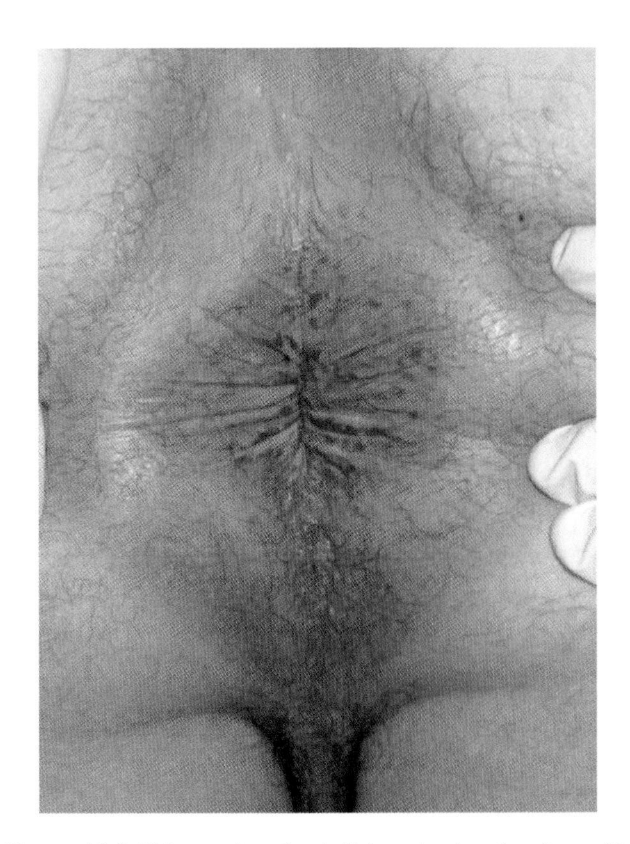

FIGURE 16-8. This man has classic lichen simplex chronicus with inflammation and erosion resulting from unremitting diarrhea of 3 weeks duration with wiping five times a day. Treatment of the patient's diarrhea and topical silver sulfadiazine with 2% cortisone achieved rapid healing and relief of symptoms.

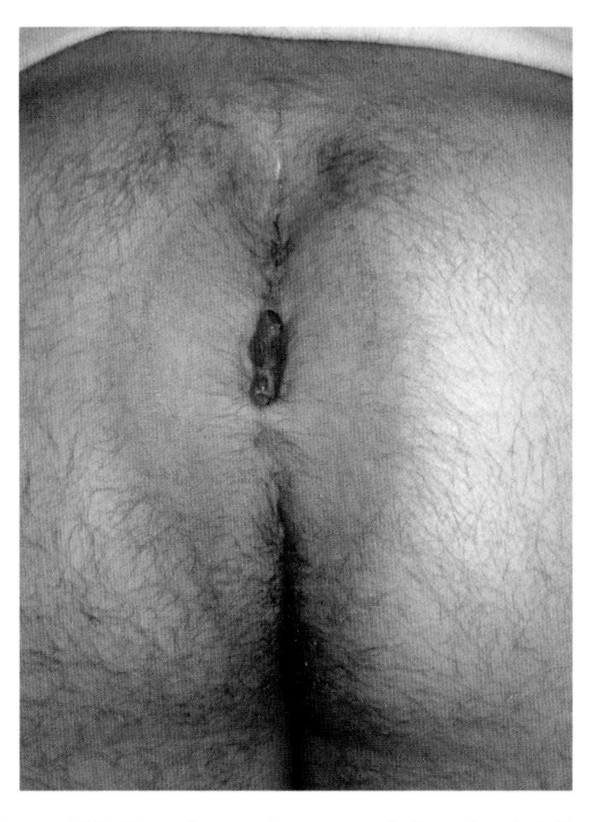

FIGURE 16-9. Hyperpigmentation may result from chronic inflammatory changes in the skin for whatever reason. In this particular case, infected drainage from a chronic pilonidal sinus was the cause, but fistula disease, chronic dermatophyte infection, erythrasma may produce the same picture. This finding should emphasize the need to modify environmental conditions within the cleft and surrounding area as an adjunct to healing.

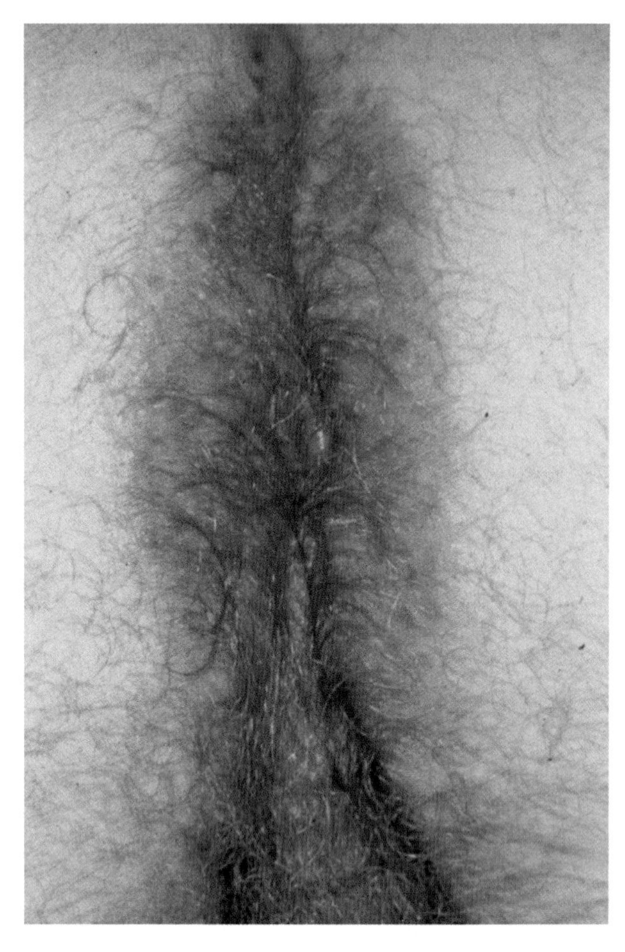

FIGURE 16-10. This patient had a reaction to topical clotrimazole in use for 1 week.

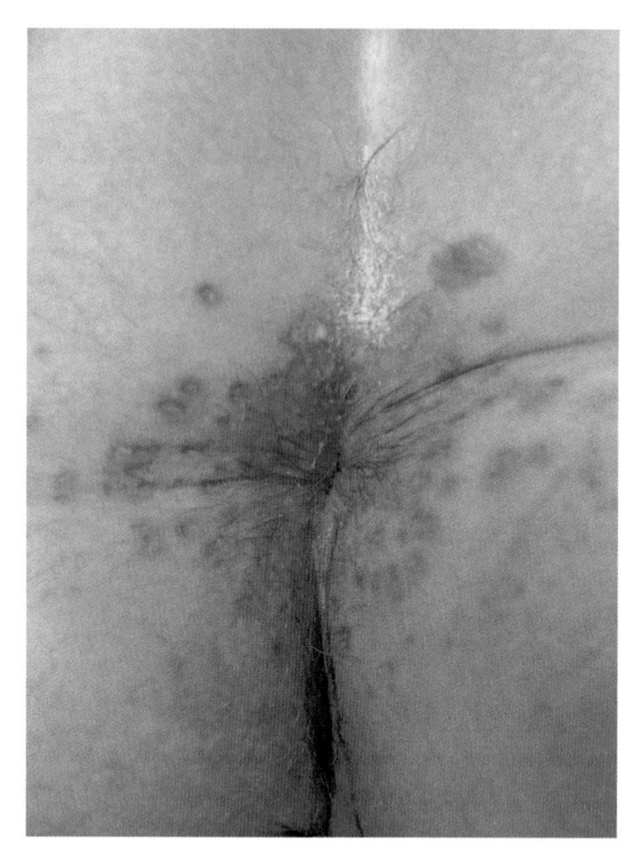

FIGURE 16-11. Scattered lesions, especially when accompanied by severe symptoms suggest Herpes virus infection. Herpes Simplex Type I was cultured from the base of these ulcerations that were 9 days old at the time of this picture. Treatment caused prompt resolution of symptoms.

lesion. Bacterial and fungal cultures should be placed into a bacterial transport medium and refrigerated if any delay in transport to the laboratory occurs. Anaerobic specimens require transport in a special anaerobic medium, and should not be refrigerated. Viral cultures require a viral transport medium and should be kept on ice. Vesicular lesions should be unroofed and cultures taken from the base of the vesicle. Microscope slides can be pressed against the base of the lesion for Tzanck smears, but inoculation of the fluid or exudate from the lesion base onto cell culture is more sensitive (viral culture).[68]

The office should have arrangements with a laboratory, which will supply culture swabs with transport media appropriate for aerobic, anaerobic, fungal, and viral culture. These become outdated and can result in rejection of specimens for processing. The practitioner should check the appropriateness of the media and its date before using it. Because staph and strep have been documented as causal agents, it is prudent to culture for pathogens in almost all cases whose treatment is not obvious. Conventional water soluble lubricant is bactericidal for some organisms (Neisseria gonorrhea). Swabs should be lubricated with saline, if lubricated at all. Ulcerated lesions should have the base vigorously swabbed. Biopsy should be accomplished early with a representative lesion and should include an area of adjacent normal skin. Specific query should be made to the pathologist about suspected diagnoses, and if possible a pathologist with skin expertise should be consulted. Highly reliable histologic criteria exist for viral lesions, pyoderma, syphilis, and neoplastic lesions. EMLA® cream, applied as a lubricant at the time of examination, may facilitate injection of local anesthetic, and biopsy may conveniently be done with either an 11 blade or skin punch blades (Keyes dermal punches) that come in numerous sizes in separate sterile packages (Figure 16-13). Bleeding from punch biopsy holes is readily controlled with sliver nitrate sticks or GELFOAM® (Pfizer Inc., New York, NY) packing.

Skin scrapings may be submitted for fungus culture, and if available examined by KOH prep for hyphae. Most colorectal offices are not set up for KOH prep; rarely are we trained in this technique and in the United States CLIA certification may be required; therefore, culture is preferable.

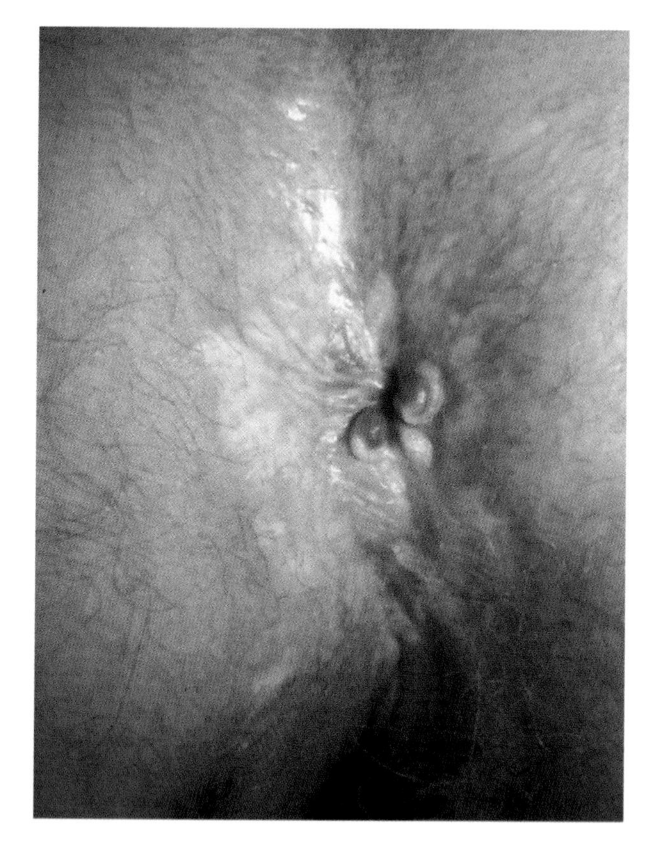

FIGURE 16-12. Lichen sclerosis has a distinctive appearance with cigarette paper thinning and wrinkling of the skin. It almost always involves the labial skin and perineum, making it easy to recognize. Biopsy is characteristic and is especially indicated for any areas which are raised, ulcerated, or unresponsive to treatment because of a 5% risk of squamous cell carcinoma developing within its distribution.

TABLE 16-6. Differential diagnosis of groin (inguinal) adenopathy

Benign reactive (shoeless walking)
Lymphoma
Carcinoma (penis, vulva, anal canal)
Sarcoidosis
Syphilis (nontender)
Leishmaniasis
Chancroid (tender)
Herpes genitalis (tender)
Lymphogranuloma venereum

Treatment of Pruritus Ani

A general strategy is presented in Table 16-7. Directed treatment for a specific, curable diagnosis is the ideal, and diagnostic efforts should be directed to avoid overlooking curable disease.

Many investigators have alluded to the importance of controlling seepage and fecal contamination of the skin. Diet may directly contribute to itching and it is prudent to give patients a list of potential foods implicated in itching for an elimination trial. Patients with loose stools may benefit from the addition of fiber to absorb moisture and add bulk and improve emptying with defecation. Many patients who have tried fiber without benefit may benefit from judicious use of Immodium® (McNEIL-PPC, Inc., Skillman, NJ) or Lomotil® (Pfizer Inc., New York, NY) to lessen frequency and firm up stools. Questran® (Bristol-Myers Squibb, Princeton, NJ), in varied doses, has been helpful in my practice to firm loose stools.

Environmental factors should be altered as much as possible with removal of irritants such as soaps, perfumes, dyes in clothes or wiping tissues, alcohol or witch hazel containing agents, moisture. Dove® (Unilever, London, UK) is free of conventional soap and is the preferred bathing agent. Bidets are not common in the USA, but detachable shower heads are

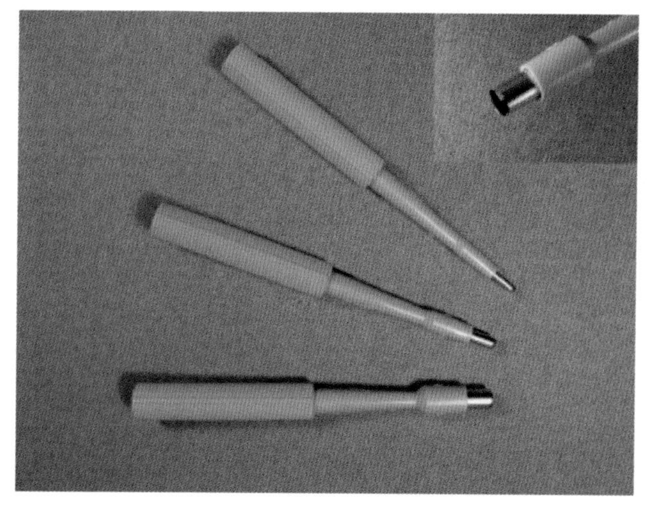

FIGURE 16-13. Skin punch biopsy tools come in various sizes up to 1 cm in diameter (2, 3, and 5 mm pictured). They may be purchased as autoclavable sets which may be sterilized and reused, or for the occasional user, disposable punches are supplied in individually wrapped sterile packages. One advantage of the disposable instruments is that they are always sharp.

TABLE 16-7. Treatment of pruritus ani

1.	Specific directed treatment for a diagnosis
2.	Eliminate offending agent (contact irritant (perfume, soap, toilet paper), organism)
3.	Eliminate scratching (especially noctural)
4.	Control symptoms
5.	Hygienic measures (Dove® soap, detachable showerhead, hair dryer to dry)
6.	Withdraw inappropriate steroids
7.	Treat infection (silver sulfadiazine cream, gentamicin or clindamycin topically, nystatin, clotrimazole)
8.	Protect skin (barrier creams, powders (esp. athlete's foot powder))
9.	Correct anal disease (fissure, hemorrhoids)
10.	Judicious use of appropriate steroids
11.	Emphasize control as a chronic condition
12.	Reassess diagnosis if response to treatment is not appropriate
13.	Anal tattooing in extreme cases

common and inexpensive and when equipped with long tubing and handle may be a useful item for cleansing the perianal skin and anal canal and eliminating soap residues by flushing with water in the squatting position. Subsequent drying with a hair dryer can eliminate moisture, and application of an athlete's foot powder or barrier cream will lubricate and prevent maceration of the skin in the cleft and anal canal. Zeasorb® (Stiefel Laboratories, Research Triangle Park, NC) is an alternate lubricating, drying agent in powder form. Cornstarch is to be avoided because it is culture medium for yeast. Cornmeal agar is used to identify different species of yeast in the laboratory.[57] Dilute white vinegar (one tablespoon in an 8 ounce glass of water) on a cotton ball is a cheap effective nonsoapy cleanser that can be kept at the toilet when bathing is not handy. Burow's solution, 1:40 (Domeboro® tablet one in 12 ounces water or one in six ounces for 1:20) is another nonirritating cleanser that can be kept refrigerated in a plastic squeeze bottle and used in lieu of soap or plain water. Burow's® may be used as an antibacterial soak for 5–15 min and then dried. Balneol® (Alaven Pharmaceutical, Marietta, GA) is a commercially available mineral oil-based preparation that can be kept in a pocket and squeezed onto toilet paper to make a soothing cleansing agent when using public facilities. Breaks in the skin caused by scratching or over vigorous cleansing efforts must be avoided, so an attempt to control symptoms with application of topical anesthetics, menthol, phenol, camphor, or a combination of ingredients may be appropriate. These agents may be used on combination with topical steroids, topical antifungal agents and topical antibacterials. Doxepin (Sinequan®, Pfizer, Inc., New York, NY – orally) is available topically as an effective antihistamine (Zonalon®, DPT Laboratories, Ltd. San Antonio, TX), but orally it is 1,000 times more potent that diphenhydramine (Benadryl®, McNEIL-PPC, Inc., Skillman, NJ) for elimination of itching and may a useful adjunct at bed time to avoid nocturnal scratching. Doxepin possesses both, anti-H1 and anti-H2 activity, a fact which may explain some of the enhanced effectiveness. Cimetidine, in 1 g/day dose, has been reported to eliminate itching induced by lymphoma and polycythemia vera, and oral gabapentin and paroxetine have been reported to have centrally acting antipruritic effects. Our combined experience with doxepin, cimetidine, gabapentin, and paroxetine has been quite rewarding.[7] Nocturnal scratching, of which the patient may be unaware, is probably a significant contributing factor in most cases of idiopathic pruritus ani. Patients who are awakened by the urge to scratch should be instructed to gently cleanse the area to eliminate any fecal seepage and reapply their steroid or barrier cream whichever is in effect at the time but not to scratch. Topical capsaicin may be useful in breaking the overwhelming urge to scratch by substituting a more powerful temporary burning stimulus.

No data exists on the influence of clothes or other formites on pruritus, but from a practical standpoint, loose underwear that allows air circulation and promotes dryness makes sense. Fresh clothes laundered without perfume or fabric softeners, perhaps with the addition of a small amount of chlorine bleach to secure lowered bacterial counts should be used daily.

Patients who come to the office with acute moderate to severe changes of the skin may be treated by application of Berwick's dye (combination of gentian violet and brilliant green) which has alcohol content and stings, often relieving the itch. The dye is dried with compressed air or a hair dryer. Benzoin tincture is applied over top of this as a barrier and dried similarly. This preparation will stay in place for several days if only water is used to cleanse and gives excellent temporary relief of symptoms and allows reepithelialization of broken skin. Berwick's is suitable as an office-applied remedy but is generally not for home application.

Patients who have mild to moderate symptoms with minimal skin changes will often respond to topical 1% hydrocortisone cream which can be combined with menthol, 0.5–1.0%, and topical antibiotics (gentamicin, clindamycin, or bacitracin) or antifungals (clotrimazole, nystatin). This preparation is applied at night and in the morning after bathing, being used daily until symptoms subside. Thereupon a tapering regimen is instituted, ending with substitution of a barrier cream such as Calmoseptine® (Calmoseptine, Inc., Huntington Beach, CA) to keep the skin covered. Elimination of the steroids and substitution of an innocuous agent to maintain attention to the hygiene is an important goal. Patients with thickened skin and chronic moderate or severe changes should be approached with higher intensity therapy, with a medium or high potency steroid for a limited, defined period of time (Table 16-8). When prescribing topical steroids, the use of brand name products allows control of both the delivery vehicle and specific active steroid salt (Table 16-8). The choice of solution, lotion, cream, or ointment is of major therapeutic importance. For instance, betamethasone as Diprolene® (Schering Laboratories, Kenilworth, NJ) is over 1,000 times more potent than Valisone® (Schering Laboratories, Kenilworth, NJ) cream, with Valisone® (Schering Laboratories, Kenilworth, NJ) ointment somewhere in between. These differences can lead to a great deal of confusion when prescribing by generic name without spelling out every tiny detail. It is important to emphasize to patients that a high potency steroid should be used for a limited period of time, generally 4–8 weeks. When normalization of the skin has been achieved, patients are switched to a mild steroid such as hydrocortisone 1% or Locoid® (Ferndale Laboratories, Inc., Ferndale, MI) 0.1% with tapering frequency of application down to once or twice a week or to total elimination. Patients who have frankly eroded or denuded skin may benefit from topical antibiotics. Silver sulfadiazine cream to which hydrocortisone or triamcinolone and menthol has been added may be soothing and promote regrowth of epidermis over ulcerated areas while suppressing the inflammation that can cause fissuring in the skin.

Skin atrophy is a serious problem with prolonged use of potent steroids, but each of the steroid preparations differs in

TABLE 16-8. Relative potency of topical steroids (descending order)

Group 1 (most potent)	Group 4
Betamethasone dipropionate 0.05% (Diprolene®)	Desoximetasone 0.05% (Topicort LP®)
Clobetasol propionate 0.05% (Temovate®)	Flurandrenolide 0.05% (Cordran®)
Group 2	Group 5
Desoximetasone 0.25% (Topicort®)	Betamethasone valerate cream 0.1% (Valisone®)
Fluocinonide 0.05% (Lidex®)	Hydrocortisone butyrate 0.1% (Locoid®)
	Triamcinolone acetonide 0.1% (Kenalog®)
Group 3	Group 6 (least potent)
Betamethasone valerate ointment 0.1% (Valisone®)	Alclometasone dipropionate 0.05% (Aclovate®)
Triamcinolone acetonide 0.5% (Aristocort®)	Hydrocortisone 1%

TABLE 16-9. Nonsteroidal topical therapy for Itching

Berwick's dye (crystal violet 1%+brilliant green 1%+95% ethanol 50%+distilled H_2O q.s.ad. 100%) with benzoin barrier
Burow's solution 1:40
Calmoseptine®
Camphor (0.1–3%)
Calcipotriene (Dovonex®)
Capsaicin (Zostrix® 0.025%, Dolorac 0.25%)
Cold compress (ice cube)
Doxepin 5% (Zonalon®)
EMLA (eutectic mixture of local anesthetics)
Hot compress (120°F)
Macrolide topical agents (tacrolimus and pimecrolimus)
Menthol (0.125–1%)
Phenol (0.125–2%)
Pramoxine
Shake lotions (Calamine+additives)
Topical "caines"

its tendency to cause trouble. Creams cause comparatively greater atrophy than ointment preparations containing identical ingredients.[69] Newer, double-ester, nonfluorinated steroids may prove to be less atrophogenic than the older preparations,[70,71] but the FDA required informational inserts for prednicarbate and mometasone furoate still quote 8 and 6% incidence of mild skin atrophy for these compounds. Macrolide topical immune modulators (tacrolimus and pimecrolimus) appear to be free of the problem of skin atrophy, a fact that enhances their appeal for use on the opposed skin of the cleft.[72] Use of topically applied picolimus and tacrolimus has not been approved for skin diseases other than atopic dermatitis. As such, its use is off-label. Burning sensation after application has been relatively common in my experience, but tends to subside (Table 16-9). The FDA issued a black box warning regarding risk of lymphoma and skin cancer in 2005, but recent long-term safety data in large cohorts of patients with up to 4 years duration of treatment have not revealed an increase in either skin or internal cancer associated with topical use.[73] European and US use of these agents

TABLE 16-10. Adverse reactions to topical steroids

Skin atrophy with telangiectasia, pseudoscars, purpura, striae, spontaneous bleeding
Ulceration
Tinea, impetigo, scabies incognito
Allergic contact dermatitis
Systemic absorption with adrenal suppression
Burning, itching, dryness from vehicle
Rebound worsening after withdrawal

topically now approaches 17 years and anecdotally, safety has not appeared as a problem. These compounds may have some intrinsic antifungal activity as well.[74] I (COF) have had limited but very good clinical experience with these compounds. There is currently no published data on topical macrolide use in pruritus ani. Table 16-10 lists the potential complications of topical steroids, which are not to be taken lightly, and are all the more important as they are preventable complications of treatment.

Anal Tattooing

Every practice has a small number of patients who respond poorly to any treatment and whose symptoms are severe enough to alter life and happiness. These refractory patients may benefit from a technique originally described by a Russian surgeon, but espoused in the USA by Wollock and Dintsman[75] who described nine patients, eight of whom had relief after one treatment, one requiring a second injection to obtain a good result. Eusebio et al.[76] reported 23 patients: 13 with complete relief, 8 with incomplete relief but much improved, and 2 who were not improved but who had initially presented with burning, not itching. Three cases of skin necrosis resulted in modification of their technique and treatment of an additional 11 patients was without complication and with good result.[77] The modified technique consists of the intradermal and subcutaneous injection of the following solution with the patient under intravenous sedation in the prone jack-knife position: 10 ml 1% methylene blue+5 ml normal saline+7.5 ml 0.25% bupivacaine with epinephrine (1/200,000)+7.5 ml 0.5% lidocaine. Farouk and Lee[78] reported six patients treated with a similar volume to Eusebio's modified technique. Five patients got substantial relief of symptoms with follow-up of 2–5 years. Three of the six required a repeat injection at 1, 3, and 5 years after the initial treatment.

The authors have personally used this technique on four patients, infiltrating the skin with the same solution as Eusebio et al. using a modified technique. I use a 30 or 27 gauge needle and infiltrate the skin as I would for cutaneous anesthesia with multiple injection sites sufficient to cover the perianal involved skin up to the dentate line (Figure 16-14). All four of my patients had positive results lasting at least 1 year, during which time all have had relative cutaneous hypoesthesia. They describe the sensation as similar to having the side of one's face numb after a dental block. Certain individuals have

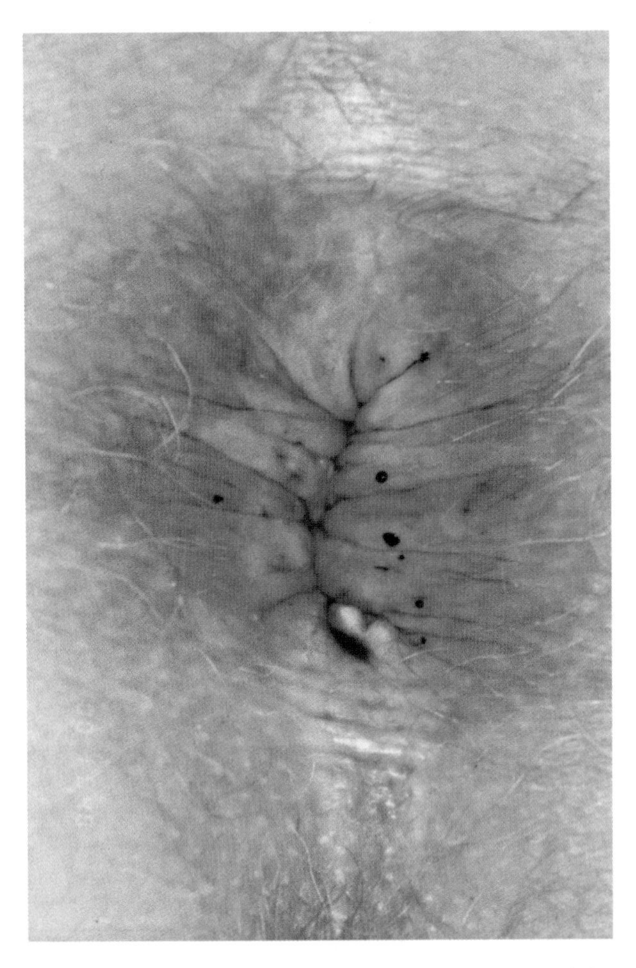

FIGURE 16-14. Tattooing with methylene blue is a simple technique to treat intractable itching that does not respond to traditional vigorous therapy. Patients experience hypalgesia and numbness of the perianal skin that can be bothersome, but rapid resolution of itching occurs and the chronic skin changes normalize quickly.

found this sensation very disagreeable, so I am careful to warn them in detail before treatment. The skin changes of severe pruritus in all cases rapidly and dramatically regressed and resolved. One patient who initially responded to injection, experienced recurrence of much milder symptoms which then responded to institution of topical therapy and did not require repeat injection. The response of these patients during the time of hypalgesia lends some credence to the idea that some forms of pruritus ani may be a neurodermatitis resulting from noctural scratching of which patients are not aware.

Conclusion

Diseases of the perineum, anus, and perianal areas are laden with social stigma and a real reticence on the part of the patient to seek medical assistance. These skin conditions are nonetheless quite common and often poorly diagnosed and treated. This anatomic region represents only about 1% of the total body surface area, yet the discomfort both physical and psychological is immensely disproportionate. The colorectal surgeon should welcome the opportunity to provide relief from disease that all too often does not come to the attention of any other specialty.

The appearance of a lesion is rarely pathognomonic, a systematic approach to evaluation of disease in this area will lead to a successful outcome. Extension of physical examination beyond the peri-area, and expanded and often extensive past medical history, family history, social history, and review of systems, as well as follow-up of treatment plans, reevaluation of patients, and reconsideration of ongoing prescriptions, should be standard practice and will help to avoid misdiagnosis (or at least give a second chance at the correct diagnosis). The most important rule in evaluation or reevaluation is never believe anyone's diagnosis, least of all your own.

References

1. Corman ML. Colon and rectal surgery. 2nd ed. Philadelphia, PA: Lippincott; 1989. p. 287.
2. Daniel GL, Longo WE, Vernava III AM. Pruritus ani causes and concerns. Dis Colon Rectum. 1994;37:670–4.
3. Verbov J. Pruritus ani and its management – a study and reappraisal. Clin Exp Dermatol. 1984;9:46–52.
4. Bernhard JD. Itch: mechanisms and management of pruritus. New York: McGraw-Hill; 1994.
5. Davidson S, Zhang X, Yoon CH, Khasabov SG, Simone DA, Giesler Jr GJ. The itch-producing agents histamine and cowhage activate separate populations of primate spinothalamic tract neurons. J Neurosci. 2007;27:10007–14.
6. Johanek LM, Meyer RA, Hartke T, Hobelmann JG, Maine DN, LaMotte RH, et al. Psychophysical and physiological evidence for parallel afferent pathways mediating the sensation of itch. J Neurosci. 2007;27:7490–7.
7. Stander S, Weisshaar E, Luger TA. Neurophysiological and neurochemical basis of modern pruritus treatment. Exp Dermatol. 2008;17:161–9.
8. Stamos MJ, Hicks TC, Pruritus ani: diagnosis and treatment. In: Perspectives in Colon and Rectal Surgery, 1998;11(1):1–20. Thieme Medical Publishers.
9. Bernhard JD, Kligman AM, Shelley WB. Dermographic pruritus: invisible dermographism. J Am Acad Dermatol. 1995;33:322.
10. Sherertz EF. Clinical pearl: symptomatic dermatographism as a cause of genital pruritus. J Am Acad Dermatol. 1994;31: 1040–1.
11. Caplan RM. The irritant role of feces in the genesis of perianal itch. Gastroenterology. 1966;50:19–23.
12. Smith LE, Henrichs D, McCullah RD. Prospective studies on the etiology and treatment of pruritus ani. Dis Colon Rectum. 1982;25:358–63.
13. Allan A, Ambrose NS, Silverman S, Keighley MR. Physiological study of pruritus ani. Br J Surg. 1987;74:576–9.
14. Farouk R, Duthie GS, Pryde A, Bartolo DC. Abnormal transient internal sphincter relaxation in idiopathic pruritus ani:

physiological evidence from ambulatory monitoring. Br J Surg. 1994;81:603–6.

15. Eyers AA, Thomson JP. Pruritus ani: is anal sphincter dysfunction important in aetiology? Br Med J. 1979;2:1549–51.
16. Dodi G, Pirone E, Bettin A, Veller C, Infantino A, Pianon P, et al. The mycotic flora in proctological patients with and without pruritus ani. Br J Surg. 1985;72:967–9.
17. Alexander S. Dermatological aspects of anorectal disease. Clin Gastroenterol. 1975;4:651–7.
18. Pirone E, Infantino A, Masin A, Melega F, Pianon P, Dodi G, et al. Can proctological procedures resolve perianal pruritus and mycosis? A prospective study of 23 cases. Int J Colorectal Dis. 1992;7:18–20.
19. Bowyer A, McColl I. A study of 200 patients with pruritus ani. Proc R Soc Med. 1970;63(Suppl):96–8.
20. Weismann K, Sand Petersen C, Roder B. Pruritus ani caused by beta-haemolytic streptococci. Acta Derm Venereol. 1996; 76:415.
21. Bowyer A, McColl I. Erythrasma and pruritus ani. Acta Derm Venereol. 1971;51:444–7.
22. Sindhuphak W, MacDonald E, Smith EB. Erythrasma. Overlooked or misdiagnosed? Int J Dermatol. 1985;24:95–6.
23. Baral J. Pruritus ani and *Staphylococcus aureus*. J Am Acad Dermatol. 1983;9:962.
24. Dasan S, Neill SM, Donaldson DR, Scott HJ. Treatment of persistent pruritus ani in a combined colorectal and dermatological clinic. Br J Surg. 1999;86:1337–40.
25. Habif TP. Clinical dermatology: a color guide to diagnosis and therapy. 3rd ed. St. Louis: Mosby; 1996.
26. Harrington CI, Lewis FM, McDonagh AJ, Gawkrodger DJ. Dermatological causes of pruritus ani. BMJ. 1992;305:955.
27. Bruynzeel DP. Dermatological causes of pruritus ani. BMJ. 1992;305:955.
28. Rohde H. Routine anal cleansing, so-called hemorrhoids, and perianal dermatitis: cause and effect? Dis Colon Rectum. 2000;43:561–3.
29. Lochridge Jr E. Pruritus ani – perianal psoriasis. South Med J. 1969;62:450–2.
30. Habif TP. Clinical dermatology: a color guide to diagnosis and therapy. 4th ed. Philadelphia, Pa: Mosby, 2004.
31. Wang G, Li C, Gao T, Liu Y. Clinical analysis of 48 cases of inverse psoriasis: a hospital-based study. Eur J Dermatol. 2005;15:176–8.
32. Kalb RE, Bagel J, Korman NJ, Lebwohl MG, Young M, Horn EJ, et al. Treatment of intertriginous psoriasis: from the Medical Board of the National Psoriasis Foundation. J Am Acad Dermatol. 2009;60:120–4.
33. Smith FJ, Irvine AD, Terron-Kwiatkowski A, Sandilands A, Campbell LE, Zhao Y, et al. Loss-of-function mutations in the gene encoding filaggrin cause ichthyosis vulgaris. Nat Genet. 2006;38:337–42.
34. Segre JA. Epidermal differentiation complex yields a secret: mutations in the cornification protein filaggrin underlie ichthyosis vulgaris. J Invest Dermatol. 2006;126:1202–4.
35. Segre JA. Epidermal barrier formation and recovery in skin disorders. J Clin Invest. 2006;116:1150–8.
36. Meffert JJ, Davis BM, Grimwood RE. Lichen sclerosus. J Am Acad Dermatol. 1995;32:393–416. quiz 417–398.
37. Neill SM, Tatnall FM, Cox NH. Guidelines for the management of lichen sclerosus. Br J Dermatol. 2002;147:640–9.
38. Powell JJ, Wojnarowska F. Lichen sclerosus. Lancet. 1999; 353:1777–83.
39. Wong YW, Powell J, Oxon MA. Lichen sclerosus: a review. Minerva Med. 2002;93:95–9.
40. Byren I, Venning V, Edwards A. Carcinoma of the vulva and asymptomatic lichen sclerosus. Genitourin Med. 1993;69:323–4.
41. Carli P, Cattaneo A, De Magnis A, Biggeri A, Taddei G, Giannotti B. Squamous cell carcinoma arising in vulval lichen sclerosus: a longitudinal cohort study. Eur J Cancer Prev. 1995;4:491–5.
42. Carli P, De Magnis A, Mannone F, Botti E, Taddei G, Cattaneo A. Vulvar carcinoma associated with lichen sclerosus. Experience at the Florence, Italy, Vulvar Clinic. J Reprod Med. 2003;48:313–8.
43. Val I, Almeida G. An overview of lichen sclerosus. Clin Obstet Gynecol. 2005;48:808–17.
44. Funaro D. Lichen sclerosus: a review and practical approach. Dermatol Ther. 2004;17:28–37.
45. Assmann T, Becker-Wegerich P, Grewe M, Megahed M, Ruzicka T. Tacrolimus ointment for the treatment of vulvar lichen sclerosus. J Am Acad Dermatol. 2003;48:935–7.
46. Bohm M, Frieling U, Luger TA, Bonsmann G. Successful treatment of anogenital lichen sclerosus with topical tacrolimus. Arch Dermatol. 2003;139:922–4.
47. Friend WG. The cause and treatment of idiopathic pruritus ani. Dis Colon Rectum. 1977;20:40–2.
48. Akl K. Yogurt-induced pruritus ani in a child. Eur J Pediatr. 1992;151:867.
49. Murie JA, Sim AJ, Mackenzie I. The importance of pain, pruritus and soiling as symptoms of haemorrhoids and their response to haemorrhoidectomy or rubber band ligation. Br J Surg. 1981;68:247–9.
50. Koblenzer CS. Psychologic and psychiatric aspects of itching. In: Bernhard JD, editor. Itch: mechanisms and management of pruritus. New York: McGraw-Hill; 1994. p. 347–65.
51. Andrews D, Grunau VJ. An uncommon adverse effect following bolus administration of intravenous dexamethasone. J Can Dent Assoc. 1986;52:309–11.
52. Kligman AM, Frosch PJ. Steroid addiction. Int J Dermatol. 1979;18:23–31.
53. Goldman L, Kitzmiller KW. Perianal atrophoderma from topical corticosteroids. Arch Dermatol. 1973;107:611–2.
54. Alexander-Williams J. Pruritus ani. Br Med J (Clin Res Ed). 1983;287:159–60.
55. Dibb WL. In vitro efficacy of Otic Domeboro against Pseudomonas aeruginosa. Undersea Biomed Res. 1985;12:307–13.
56. Thorp MA, Gardiner IB, Prescott CA. Burow's solution in the treatment of active mucosal chronic suppurative otitis media: determining an effective dilution. J Laryngol Otol. 2000;114:432–6.
57. Thorp MA, Kruger J, Oliver S, Nilssen EL, Prescott CA. The antibacterial activity of acetic acid and Burow's solution as topical otological preparations. J Laryngol Otol. 1998; 112:925–8.
58. Thorp MA, Oliver SP, Kruger J, Prescott CA. Determination of the lowest dilution of aluminium acetate solution able to inhibit in vitro growth of organisms commonly found in chronic suppurative otitis media. J Laryngol Otol. 2000;114:830–1.
59. Helwig EB, Graham JH. Anogenital (extramammary) Paget's disease: a clinicopathological study. Cancer. 1963;16:387–403.

60. Jensen SL, Sjolin KE, Shokouh-Amiri MH, Hagen K, Harling H. Paget's disease of the anal margin. Br J Surg. 1988;75:1089–92.
61. Sarmiento JM, Wolff BG, Burgart LJ, Frizelle FA, Ilstrup DM. Paget's disease of the perianal region – an aggressive disease? Dis Colon Rectum. 1997;40:1187–94.
62. Marchesa P, Fazio VW, Oliart S, Goldblum JR, Lavery IC. Perianal Bowen's disease: a clinicopathologic study of 47 patients. Dis Colon Rectum. 1997;40:1286–93.
63. Chang GJ, Berry JM, Jay N, Palefsky JM, Welton ML. Surgical treatment of high-grade anal squamous intraepithelial lesions: a prospective study. Dis Colon Rectum. 2002;45:453–8.
64. Goldstone SE, Winkler B, Ufford LJ, Alt E, Palefsky JM. High prevalence of anal squamous intraepithelial lesions and squamous-cell carcinoma in men who have sex with men as seen in a surgical practice. Dis Colon Rectum. 2001;44: 690–8.
65. Brady MS, Kavolius JP, Quan SH. Anorectal melanoma. A 64-year experience at Memorial Sloan-Kettering Cancer Center. Dis Colon Rectum. 1995;38:146–51.
66. Enker WE, Heilwell M, Janov AJ, Quan SH, Magill G, Stearns Jr MW, et al. Improved survival in epidermoid carcinoma of the anus in association with preoperative multidisciplinary therapy. Arch Surg. 1986;121:1386–90.
67. Goldman S, Glimelius B, Pahlman L. Anorectal malignant melanoma in Sweden. Report of 49 patients. Dis Colon Rectum. 1990;33:874–7.
68. McClatchey KD. Clinical laboratory medicine. 2nd ed. Philadelphia, PA: Lippincott Williams & Wilkins; 2002.
69. Kerscher MJ, Korting HC. Comparative atrophogenicity potential of medium and highly potent topical glucocorticoids in cream and ointment according to ultrasound analysis. Skin Pharmacol. 1992;5:77–80.
70. Hoffmann K, Auer T, Stucker M, Hoffmann A, Altmeyer P. Comparison of skin atrophy and vasoconstriction due to mometasone furoate, methylprednisolone and hydrocortisone. J Eur Acad Dermatol Venereol. 1998;10:137–42.
71. Kerscher MJ, Korting HC. Topical glucocorticoids of the non-fluorinated double-ester type. Lack of atrophogenicity in normal skin as assessed by high-frequency ultrasound. Acta Derm Venereol. 1992;72:214–6.
72. Robinson N, Singri P, Gordon KB. Safety of the new macrolide immunomodulators. Semin Cutan Med Surg. 2001;20:242–9.
73. Becker EM, Koo JY. Clinical focus: the spectrum of topical agents for the treatment of psoriasis. Medscape CME; 2009
74. Ling MR. Topical tacrolimus and pimecrolimus: future directions. Semin Cutan Med Surg. 2001;20:268–74.
75. Wolloch Y, Dintsman M. A simple and effective method of treatment for intractable pruritus ani. Am J Proctol Gastroenterol Colon Rectal Surg. 1979;30:34–6.
76. Eusebio EB, Graham J, Mody N. Treatment of intractable pruritus ani. Dis Colon Rectum. 1990;33:770–2.
77. Eusebio EB. New treatment of intractable pruritus ani. Dis Colon Rectum. 1991;34:289.
78. Farouk R, Lee PW. Intradermal methylene blue injection for the treatment of intractable idiopathic pruritus ani. Br J Surg. 1997;84:670.

17
Sexually Transmitted Diseases

Charles B. Whitlow, Lester Gottesman, and Mitchell A. Bernstein

Introduction

There are over 25 diseases primarily spread by sexual means with an annual incidence of approximately 15 million cases in the USA.[1] In 1994, the overall cost related to major sexually transmitted diseases (STDs) was estimated to be 17 billion dollars. In the UK, the incidence of STDs has substantially increased over the past 6 years and has led to a new government strategy to counteract these increases.[2,3]

Site and route of infection determine the symptoms caused by STDs. Infections of the distal anal canal, anoderm, and perianal skin are similar to lesions in other parts of the genitalia and perineum caused by the same organisms. These infections are typically the result of anal receptive intercourse but in some instances represent contiguous spread from genital infections. Proctitis from sexually transmitted organisms is almost always acquired from anal intercourse. Direct or indirect fecal–oral contact produces infection with organisms which cause proctocolitis or enteritis but which are generally thought of as food or waterborne diseases instead of STDs. Included in this group are *Entameba histolytica*, *Campylobacter*, *Shigella*, *Giardia lamblia*, and hepatitis A. While it appears that male homosexual activity and the use of the anorectum for sexual gratification is increasing, data regarding the frequency of these behaviors both past and present are limited. Current estimates are that less than 2% of adult males regularly practice anal receptive intercourse while between 2 and 10% participate in homosexual activity at any point in their life.[4] Between 5 and 10% of females engage in anal receptive intercourse "with some degree of regularity" and females appear to be more likely than men to have unprotected anal intercourse.[4]

Difficulty in correct diagnosis and appropriate treatment of STD of the anorectum is caused by several factors. (1) The signs and symptoms of infection are more organ related than organism related so that no symptom or symptom complex or physical finding is diagnostic for many STDs. (2) The presence of more than one organism is not uncommon, especially with anogenital ulcerations. (3) Determining true pathogen from colonizing organism may be difficult. (4) Lastly, there is a lack of rapid sensitive diagnostic tests for many STDs so that empiric treatment is frequently required.

This chapter discusses the STDs that are most commonly seen by colorectal surgeons. Entire texts are devoted to STDs; however, we confine most of our comments to the diagnosis, treatment, and prevention of the anorectal component of these infections. Infections, which manifest as one of the colitides, are covered in Chap. 34.

Overview of Anorectal Immunology

The optimal state of health of the anus requires the integrity of the skin, which acts as the primary protection against invasive pathogens. The mucosa shed from the rectum contains IgA, which traps foreign antigens and expels them with stool, preventing them from reaching the rectal crypt cells.[5] Cellular immunity is controlled by the Langerhan's, or denditric cells which communicate with the T cells through a complicated mechanism and essentially prime the T cells to identify foreign cells.[6] This process allows the entire complement of cell-mediated immunity to destroy alien substances. Although study of anal immunology is still in its infancy, it appears that certain pathogens may alter the balance of cellular elements. It is known that while Human papillomavirus (HPV) increases Langerhan's cells, human immunodeficiency virus (HIV) may damage their effectiveness. In addition, pathogens like HPV and herpes simplex virus (HSV) invade into the host cell, combining with cellular elements or the genome, evading surveillance mechanisms. In addition, in the case of HPV, the identifying foreign antigens are placed onto the frame of the new virus near the epidermis, where the virus normally sheds and where an attack by the host has little value.[7]

HIV is known to impair cell-mediated immunity by depletion of T cells and destruction of Langerhan's cells. This process allows propagation of oncogenic processes such as HPV to become dysplastic. Although both exact switches and the

D.E. Beck et al. (eds.), *The ASCRS Textbook of Colon and Rectal Surgery: Second Edition*,
DOI 10.1007/978-1-4419-1584-9_17, © Springer Science+Business Media, LLC 2011

mechanism(s) have not yet been elucidated, they appear to be related to the coexistence of perhaps HSV and the highly active antiretroviral therapy (HAART) drugs.

Failure of the mucous complex to protect the rectum is seen in various diseases contracted through anal intercourse. The act of intercourse abrades the mucous lining and delivers pathogens directly to the crypt and columnar cells allowing for easy entry. Depending on their mechanism of action, they may burrow into the cells (ameba) or proliferate on the cells without damaging them (*G. neisseria*). Invasive pathogens (*LGV*) unleash nefarious cytokines which destroy the cell. The immune response is usually too late to contain an acute attack. In the case of recurrent viral attacks, it appears that the level of functioning T cells may have an impact on recurrence of warts or herpes outbreaks. The mechanics of anoreceptive intercourse, as compared to vaginal intercourse, almost demands denuding of the protecting cellular and mucous protection of the anus and rectum.

Latex allergies may also cause severe invasive and erosive proctitis and should be in the differential of a caustic burn to the rectum after protected sexual anoreceptive intercourse.

Diagnosis and Management of Bacterial Pathogens

Gonorrhea

Neisseria gonorrhea, the gram-negative diplococcus (Figure 17-1) responsible for gonorrhea was first described by Albert Neisser in 1879 from exudates from urethritis and cervicitis.[8] It is probably the most common bacterial STD affecting the anorectum. While gonorrhea rates decreased over the last several decades, in the mid-1990s the incidence slowly increased to the current rate of about 650,000 cases per year. Similar recent increases have been noted in Canada and the UK.[9] Peak incidence for all forms of gonorrhea is in the late teens for females and early 20s for males. African Americans have a 30-fold higher rate of infection than do white Americans.

Infection from *N. gonorrhoeae* occurs in columnar, cuboidal, or noncornified epithelial lined cells of the urethra, endocervix, rectum, and pharynx and is frequently asymptomatic. The incubation period ranges from 3 days to 2 weeks. Untreated infection may lead to disseminated gonococcal infection with transient bacteremia, arthritis, and dermatitis. Rare but severe sequelae include endocarditis and meningitis.

Anorectal transmission in homosexual males and in some females is by anoreceptive intercourse with an infected partner. Thirty-five to fifty percent of women with gonococcal cervicitis have concomitant rectal infection which is believed to be from contiguous spread from the genital infection.[10] Oral–anal sex has been suggested as another mode of anorectal gonococcal infection.[11] A large percentage of patients who culture positive for rectal gonorrhea are asymptomatic – up to 50% of males and 95% of females. Asymptomatic rectal infection constitutes the main reservoir of gonococcal disease in homosexual men.

Symptomatic anorectal gonococcal infection results in pruritis, tenesmus, bloody discharge, mucopurulent discharge, or severe pain. External inspection of the anus is generally unremarkable; however, nonspecific erythema and superficial ulceration may occur (Figure 17-2). Anoscopy reveals a thick purulent discharge, which classically is expressed from the anal crypts as pressure is applied externally on the anus. Nonspecific proctitis may be present with erythema, edema, friability, and pus. Diagnosis is confirmed by culture on selective media (Thayer-Martin or Modified New York City) incubated in a CO_2-rich environment and Gram's stain of directly visualized discharge.[12] The use of lubricants other than water may introduce antibacterial agents during anoscopy and decrease diagnostic yield. Nonculture detection of gonorrhea is being used more frequently especially in

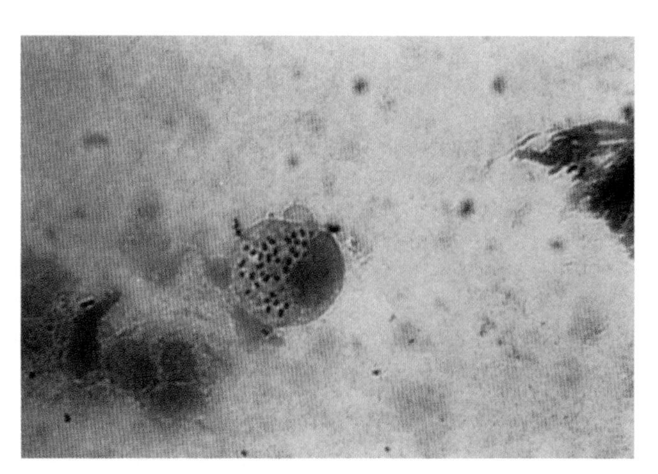

FIGURE 17-1. Gram-negative intracellular diplococcus.

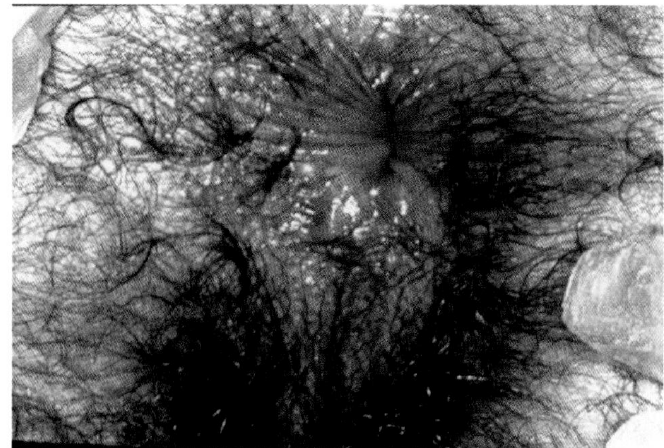

FIGURE 17-2. Anorectal gonorrhea.

TABLE 17-1. Treatment of anorectal gonococcal infection[14]

One of the following as a single dose:
Ceftriaxone – 125 mg IM
Ciprofloxacin – 500 mg orally
Ofloxacin – 400 mg orally
Levofloxacin – 250 mg orally
Cefixime – 400 mg orally

urethral and cervical infections. Nucleic acid amplification tests (NAATs), such as polymerase chain reaction (PCR), ligase chain reaction (LCR), and nonamplified DNA probes, provide sensitivities of greater than 95% but do not provide antibiotic susceptibility data. There are no NAATs currently licensed for the detection of rectal gonorrhea.[13]

Because of the prevalence of penicillinase-producing *N. gonorrhoeae* (PPNG) starting in the 1970s, penicillin G is no longer the drug of choice for gonorrhea. The most current recommended treatment regimen from the Centers for Disease Control (CDC) was published in 2002 and is listed in Table 17-1. Since publication of these guidelines cefixime has become unavailable in the US alternative regimens include spectinomycin (2 g as a single intramuscular injection), other cephalosporins (ceftizoxime, cefoxitin, and cefotaxime), and other quinolones. Only a few isolates reported by the Gonococcal Isolate Surveillance Report (GISP) in the past 10 years showed decreased susceptibility to the cephalosporins listed in Table 17-1.[15] Quinolone resistant *N. gonorrhea* (QRNG) have been detected in the past decade with increasing frequency in Asia and the Pacific. In the USA, this is particularly important in Hawaii (where QRNG may account for as much as 14% of gonorrhea isolates) and California. In the UK, the overall rate of QRNG was reported at 9.8% for 2002.[16] Concurrent HIV infection does not alter treatment for anorectal gonorrhea. Because of the high rate of concomitant infection with chlamydia, patients treated for gonococcal infections should be given appropriate treatment for chlamydia at the same visit or measures to exclude chlamydial infection should be taken.

Routine follow-up at 3 months is no longer necessary since current treatment provides near 100% efficacy. Patients with persistent symptoms after treatment should be followed and cultured as should those treated with nonstandard antibiotics. Sexual partners from the past 60 days should be treated and patient should abstain from intercourse until treatment is completed and symptoms resolved.

Chlamydia/Lymphogranuloma Venereum (LGV)

Chlamydia trachomatis is an obligate intracellular bacterium that is sexually transmitted and results in clinical infections that are similar to those caused by *N. gonorrhea*. Simultaneous infection with both organisms is common. Chlamydia is the most commonly reported STD in the USA with an annual incidence of about three million cases per year.[17] Aggressive screening programs have been credited with the decline of the Chlamydia infection rate from its peak of over four million per year in the early 1970s.

Anorectal transmission of chlamydia is through anoreceptive intercourse although secondary involvement can occur as a late manifestation of genital infection. Different serovars of *C. trachomatis* produce differing clinical illness. Serovars D through K (non-LGV) are responsible for proctitis and common genital infections. Lymphogranuloma venereum is caused by LGV serovars L1-L3. The incubation period for chlamydia is 5 days to 2 weeks. Non-LGV serovars are less invasive and cause mild proctitis (manifest by tenesmus, pain, and discharge) but asymptomatic infection is common. LGV serovars produce a much more aggressive infection with perianal, anal, and rectal ulceration. The proctitis produced can be difficult to distinguish from Crohn's disease (including microscopic findings of granulomas) with resulting rectal pain and discharge. Anoscopy and sigmoidoscopy demonstrate friable rectal mucosa, which is more severe in appearance (and extends above the rectum in some cases) in LGV strains.[18–20] Perianal abscesses, fistulas, and strictures may also occur. Lymphadenopathy develops in draining nodal basins, including the iliac, perirectal, inguinal, and femoral regions several weeks after initial infection. Large indurated matted nodes (Figure 17-3) and overlying erythema may produce a clinical picture similar to syphilis.

Diagnosis of chlamydia as the causative agent in proctitis can be difficult. Proper specimen collection increases diagnostic yield and consists of a cotton or Dacron swab with an inert shaft (plastic or metal). Specimen for tissue culture should be transported on specific medium and kept refrigerated or on ice until inoculated onto culture plates. Specimens that are to be tested by a nonculture technique are transported and stored in accordance with the test manufacturers guidelines. In patients with a clinical presentation consistent with chlamydia proctitis, rectal Gram's stain showing polymorphonuclear leukocytes without visible gonococci is presumptive for a diagnosis of chlamydia.[20]

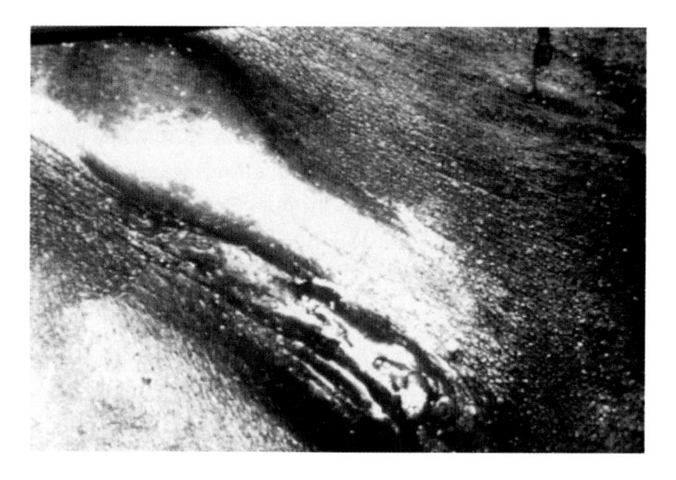

FIGURE 17-3. Inguinal adenopathy of LGV; *LGV* lymphogranuloma venereum.

Tissue culture for chlamydia is relatively insensitive and is not widely available because of cost and technical requirements.[21]

Antigen detection by direct fluorescent antibody (DFA) or enzyme immunoassay DFA is highly specific, widely available and does not require rapid transportation or refrigeration. A trained microscopist is needed for interpretation. As with gonorrhea, newer NAATs are available. Their use is increasing in genital infection but unproven for anorectal chlamydia. A pilot study using both PCR and LCR techniques showed that these techniques can be effective for making this diagnosis but there are little additional data on the use of NAATs in anorectal chlamydia.[22]

The two recommended treatment regimens for rectal chlamydia (non-LGV) are azithromycin, 1 g orally as a single dose or doxycycline, 100 mg orally, twice a day for 7 days.[14] Alternative regimens include erythromycin (less effective, more GI side effects), ofloxacin (7-day course, more expensive), or levofloxacin (7-day course, no data on efficacy). Treatment of lymphogranuloma venereum is with doxycycline or erythromycin for 21 days. In patients with HIV and LGV prolonged therapy may be required. Management of sexual contacts is the same as for gonorrhea. Abstinence from sexual intercourse should last until 7 days after treatment with azithromycin or completion of 7 days of doxycycline.

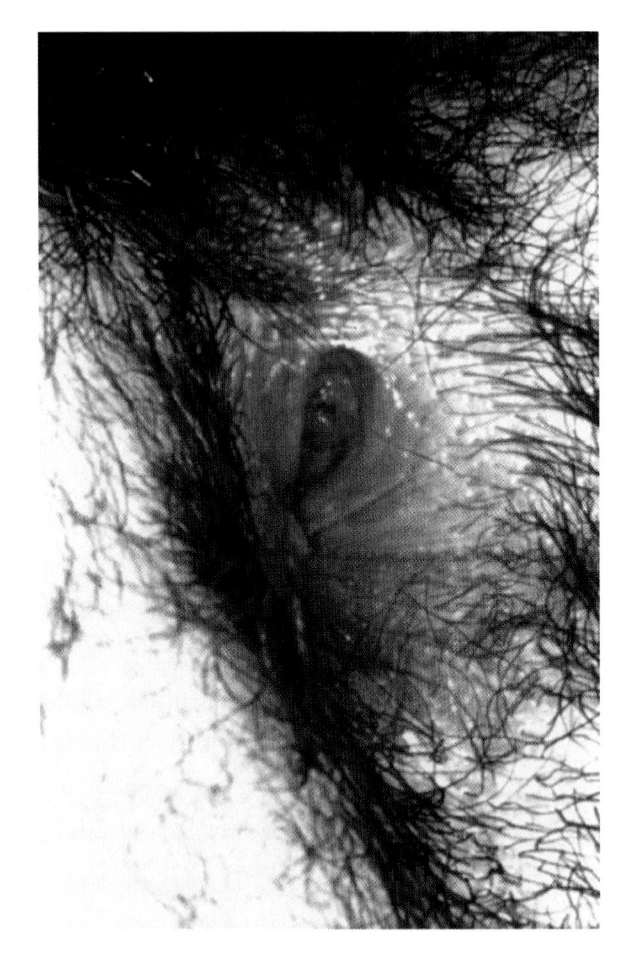

FIGURE 17-4. Solitary anal chancre.

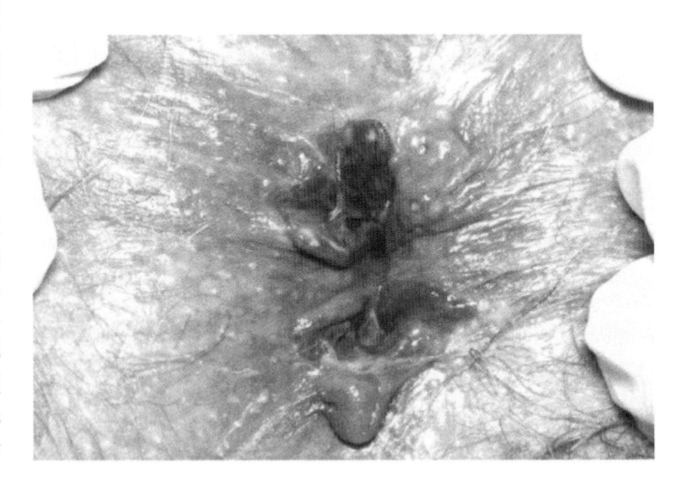

FIGURE 17-5. Multiple anal chancres.

Syphilis

Syphilis is an STD caused by the spirochete *Treponema pallidum* that can present in one of several progressive stages – primary (chancre or proctitis), secondary (condyloma lata), or tertiary. The incidence of syphilis had its recent peak of 107 cases per 100,000 people in the USA in 1991, but decreased to 2.2 per 100,000 in 2001, meaning that only 6,103 cases were reported. A slight increase in primary and secondary syphilis cases reported occurred in 2002.[23] These low rates have led to a national plan for eliminating syphilis.[24]

The primary stage of anorectal syphilis appears within 2–10 weeks of exposure via anal intercourse. The chancre begins as a small papule that eventually ulcerates. Anal ulcers are frequently painful (in contrast to genital ulcers) and without exudates. They may be single or multiple (Figures 17-4 and 17-5) and located on the perianal skin, in the anal canal or distal rectum. Differentiation from idiopathic anal fissures may be difficult. Painless but prominent lymphadenopathy is common. Proctitis from syphilis may occur with or without chancres.[18] Untreated lesions in this stage usually heal in several weeks.

Hematogenous dissemination of untreated syphilis leads to a secondary stage that occurs 4–10 weeks after primary lesions appear. Nonspecific systemic symptoms from this infection include fever, malaise, arthralgias, weight loss, sore throat, and headache. A maculopapular rash is seen on the trunk and extremities. Condyloma lata, another secondary manifestation, are gray or whitish, wart-like lesions that appear adjacent to the primary chancre and are laden with spirochetes. Untreated, the symptoms of syphilis usually resolve after 3–12 weeks – of these patients, approximately one-fourth have a relapse of symptoms in the first year, a stage known as early latent syphilis.

Diagnosis in the primary or secondary stage is made by visualization of spirochetes on dark-field microscopic exam

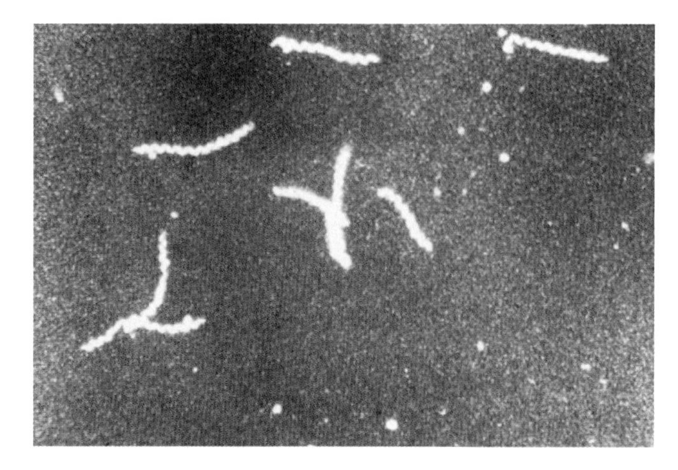

FIGURE 17-6. Spirochetes demonstrated on dark-field microscopy.

of scrapings from chancres (Figure 17-6). Alternatively, spirochetes may be demonstrated on Warthin-Starry silver stain of biopsy specimens. A DFA test for *T. pallidum* (DFA-TP) is performed by some labs.[18,25] Serologic tests, rapid plasma regain (RPR) and Venereal Disease Research Laboratory (VDRL), have a false negative rate of up to 25% in primary syphilis and are called nontreponemal tests because they are not specific for *T. pallidum* infection. Positive nontreponemal tests should be confirmed by a treponemal test, such as the fluorescent treponemal antibody absorption test (FTA-ABS), which remains positive for life.

A single intramuscular injection of 2.4 million units of benzathine penicillin G is the treatment for primary and secondary syphilis. Penicillin-allergic patients are treated with doxycyline (100 mg orally, twice daily for 14 days) or tetracycline (500 mg orally, four times a day for 14 days). Follow-up serology (VDRL or RPR) should be checked at 6 months after therapy for HIV negative patients and every 3 months for HIV positive patients.[14] Treatment failures are retreated with the same dose of penicillin but at weekly intervals for a total of 3 weeks. Partner notification, testing, and treatment depends on stage at diagnosis of the index case. At-risk partners include sexual contacts (a) within the prior 3 months plus duration of symptoms for patients with primary syphilis; (b) within the prior 6 months plus duration of symptoms for patients with secondary syphilis and; (c) within the prior year for those with early latent syphilis.[26]

Chancroid

Chancroid is an ulcerating STD caused by the gram-negative, facultative anaerobic bacillus *Hemophilus ducreyi*. While there were approximately 5,000 cases reported per year in the late 1980s and early 1990s in the USA, there were fewer than 200 cases reported in 1999.[1] It is much more common in developing countries with a global incidence estimated at six million.[27]

Transmission of *H. ducreyi* is strictly via sexual contacts through breaks in the skin during intercourse and results in genital ulcers. The initial manifestation (hour to days after exposure) is as infected tender papules with erythema that subsequently develop into pustules and then (days to weeks) become ulcerated and eroded. Multiple ulcers are common and are generally painful, especially in males. While chancroid ulcers are most commonly located on the genitalia, perianal abscesses and ulceration may occur. Anal ulcerations in females may be the result of drainage from adjacent genital infections. Differentiation of other ulcerating STDs cannot be made on gross appearance in most cases.[28] Painful inguinal adenopathy accompanies half of cases in males and is usually unilateral. Females are less likely to develop adenopathy from *H. ducreyi* infection.[29] Abscess formation may result, necessitating drainage. Besides causing genital ulcers, *H. ducreyi* facilitates transmission of HIV and vice versa.

Diagnosis of chancroid is made by Gram stain and culture of *H. ducreyi* (on selective medium agar) from the base of ulcers. Gram stain is only 40–60% sensitive relative to culture and demonstrates nonmotile Gram-negative rods in small groups. *H. ducreyi* is difficult to culture and many labs in the USA are not equipped to perform this test. PCR is more sensitive than culture for detecting *H. ducreyi* but is not commercially available at this time.[30] Treatment for *H. ducreyi* is single dose treatment with azithromycin (1 g, orally) or ceftriaxone (250 mg, intramuscularly). Alternatively, regimens include ciprofloxacin, 500 mg orally twice a day for 3 days or erythromycin 500 mg three times a day for 1 week.[14]

Granuloma Inguinale (Donovanosis)

Donovanosis is an ulcerating infection of the genitalia and anus caused by *Calymmatobacterium granulomatis* (also called *Donovania granulomatis*). Transmission is believed to occur from both sexual and nonsexual contact. It is rarely seen in the USA but is common in parts of Africa, South America, and Australia. Morphologic manifestations include and ulcerogranulomatous form (nontender, fleshy, beefy red ulcers), hypertrophic or verrucous lesions, necrotic ulcers, or cicatrical. Genital involvement is most common but contiguous involvement of the anorectum occurs. Development of sclerotic lesions causes anal stenosis.[31]

C. granulomatis cannot be cultured by routine techniques. Diagnosis can be made by tissue smear or biopsy that reveals Donovan bodies (small inclusions) within macrophages. Several antibiotic regimens have been recommended, although the most recent CDC guidelines are doxycycline (100 mg orally, twice daily for 1 week) or trimethoprim-sulfamethoxazole (one 800 mg/160 mg tablet orally, twice a day for at least 3 weeks).[14] Alternative treatments include at least 3 weeks of ciprofloxacin, azithromycin, or erythromycin. Some authors believe azithromycin to be the preferred treatment.[31]

Diagnosis and Management of Viral Pathogens

Herpes Simplex Virus

HSV is a DNA virus of the family Herpesviridae that includes Varicella-Zoster virus, Epstein–Barr virus, and Cytomegalovirus (CMV). Herpes is the most prevalent STD in the USA with current the seroprevalence rate for HSV-2 estimated to be 20% for the general population.[32] Black females are the subgroup with the highest seroprevalence at 55%. Two serotypes of HSV are described. HSV-2 has been most associated with anogenital herpes infections. HSV-1 infection most commonly presents as labial oral or ocular lesions but accounts for about 30% of genital infections. Several recent reports have shown an increasing percentage of genital infections due to HSV-1;[33,34] asymptomatic infection with HSV is common.

Transmission is via close contact with an individual who is shedding the virus and infection results from penetration of mucosal surfaces or breaks in the skin. Productive infection causes viral replication within cells and cell death. Clinical infection presents first with systemic symptoms, such as fever, headache, and myalgias, followed by local symptoms, including pain and pruritis. Vesicles appear over the anogenital area, increase in number and size, and eventually ulcerate and coalesce (Figures 17-7 and 17-8). These vesicles and ulcerations generally heal over a mean time of 3 weeks.

Anorectal involvement by HSV-2 is acquired by anorectal intercourse and is second only to gonorrhea as a cause of proctitis in homosexual men. Herpetic infection of the anorectum results in severe anal pain, tenesmus, hematochezia, dysuria, and rectal discharge. The proctitis seen is typically limited to the distal 10 cm of the rectum with diffuse friability. Simultaneous with infection, HSV moves through peripheral sensory nerves to sensory or autonomic nerve root ganglia. Sacral radiculopathy of the lower sacral roots from this infection causes sacral paresthesias and neuralgias, urinary retention, constipation, and impotence. Tender inguinal adenopathy occurs in half of patients with HSV proctitis.[35]

Herpes has the ability to persist in their host because of latency – the viral genome maintained in a stable condition in host cell nuclei. For HSV, the site of latent infection is the sensory ganglia of nerves innervating the site of infection. Reactivation of latent virus results in recurrent infection but the stimuli for this process are poorly understood.[36] Recurrent attacks are generally milder, shorter in duration, and without the constitutional symptoms that occur with initial infection.

Diagnosis is frequently made by clinical evidence although cultures taken from ulcerations, rectal swabs, or biopsies confirm the diagnosis. Multinucleated giant cells with intranuclear inclusion bodies (ground-glass appearance) on Pap smear or Tzank prep are less sensitive than viral culture. Direct immunofluorescence has also been used for diagnosing HSV.[18] For cases in which cultures are not available, paired type-specific serology demonstrating seroconversion is diagnostic. In the past 5 years, the Food and Drug Administration (FDA) have approved several commercially available HSV serology tests. These tests have specificities and sensitivities greater than 90% and are sure to become more commonly used in the diagnosis of HSV.[37,38] It should be noted that seroconversion may take several weeks after initial infection and repeat testing intervals are dependent on the particular serology kit used.[39]

Treatment of patients with anorectal herpes includes comfort measures, such as warm soaks and oral analgesics. The only prospective randomized trial of antiviral treatment for herpes proctitis demonstrated a shortened duration of symptoms and period of viral shedding with oral acyclovir 400 mg, five times a day for 10 days.[40] A three times per day dosing has been shown to be effective for genital herpes but has not been evaluated for herpes proctitis.[41] Other antiviral agents, such as valacyclovir and famciclovir used for genital herpes, are most likely effective for HSV proctitis at

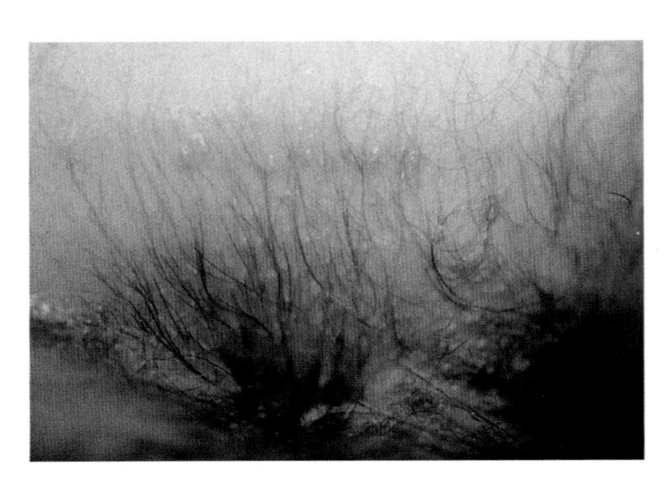

FIGURE 17-7. Perianal herpes.

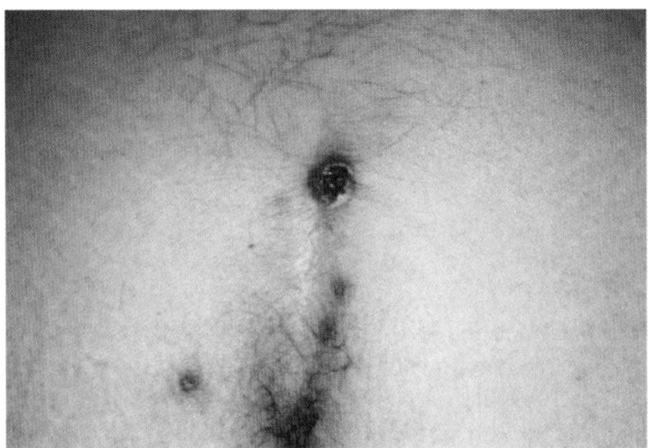

FIGURE 17-8. Perianal herpes.

the same doses used for genitourinary infection but clinical studies for this indication are lacking. Severe mucocutaneous HSV infection in which the patient cannot tolerate oral medication warrants intravenous acyclovir. Topical acyclovir has limited efficacy and is not recommended. Treatment of initial episodes of HSV do not prevent latency, asymptomatic viral shedding, or the course of subsequent episodes. Recurrent episodes may be treated with oral antiviral agents. Valacyclovir (500 mg twice a day) and acyclovir (200 mg five times a day) have demonstrated equal efficacy in treating genitourinary HSV recurrences.[42] Prompt initiation of treatment at the onset of symptoms of HSV recurrence reduces the duration of symptoms and healing times. Patients who experience more than five recurrences per year are considered for suppressive treatment. Valacyclovir, acyclovir, and famciclovir have all demonstrated 70% or greater reduction compared to placebo.

As with all STDs, counseling of patients with HSV is an important part of treatment and prevention.[41,42] Specific items that should be addressed are (1) infectivity is not isolated to symptomatic outbreaks; most sexual HSV transmission occurs during asymptomatic periods; (2) latent infection and the risk of recurrence; suppressive therapy does not eliminate latent infection or viral shedding; (3) abstinence is recommended while lesions are present. Condoms are advised for all other times although they most likely provide incomplete protection. Most recently, once-daily administration of valacyclovir has been shown to reduce the risk of HSV-2 transmission between HSV-2 seropositive patients and there seronegative sexual partners.[43]

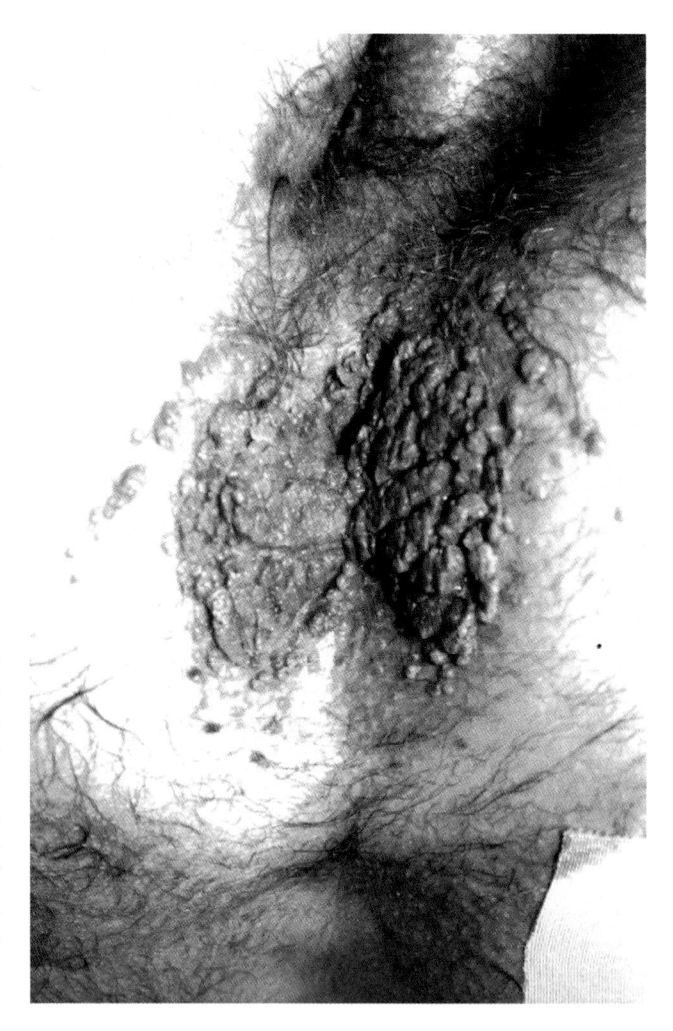

FIGURE 17-9. Perianal condyloma.

Human Papilloma Virus

HPV is a DNA papovirus. It is the most common STD in the USA with an estimated incidence of over five million cases per year.[1] There are over 80 subtypes of HPV, almost one-third of which cause anogenital warts. Subtypes 6 and 11 are the most common of the low-risk HPV subtypes while subtypes 16 and 18 have the greatest associated risk of anal dysplasia and anal cancer. Transmission is vial sexual contact with infected individuals with or without gross lesions and asymptomatic infection is common. Perianal involvement can occur in the absence of receptive anal intercourse.

Presenting complaints of perianal or anal condyloma accuminata include the presence of a growth, pruritis, bleeding, chronic drainage, pain, and difficulty with hygiene. Physical examination is generally all that is required for diagnosis and shows the characteristic gray or pink fleshy, cauliflower-like growths of variable size in the perianal region (Figure 17-9). Anoscopy is an integral part of the evaluation. In the anal canal, the lesions tend to be small papules and involvement above the dentate line is rare. Examination should focus on the genitalia, including vaginal speculum exam and Pap smear, as well as evaluation of the perineum and groin folds.

The goal of treatment of condyloma accuminata is destruction or removal of all obvious disease while minimizing morbidity, although this process does not ensure eradication of infection. Tangential excision, cryotherapy, or fulguration of small lesions can be performed as an office procedure with a local anesthetic, and causing little discomfort or inconvenience to the patient. Larger lesions are treated by electrodessication. The patient is placed in the lateral or prone jack-knife position. Depending on the size and number of lesions local, spinal, or general anesthesia is used. The superficial-most layer of the condyloma is fulgurated with the electrosurgery tip until the lesion takes on a gray–white appearance. This step is followed by curettage or simply abrading the fulgurated tissue with gauze. The process is repeated until the condylomas are completely removed without burning into the deep dermis or subcutaneous fat. Pedunculated warts are simply transected at their base. Tissue from HIV+ patients, recurrent lesions, flat lesions, or those suspicious lesions which may be ulcerated, friable, or hypervascular should be sent for histopathologic evaluation. Topical 5% lidocaine is helpful in decreasing postoperative pain. Oral analgesics and daily cleansing with mild soap and water are all that is required for postoperative care in most patients. Silver sulfadiazine or mupirocin are applied in cases in which postoperative bacterial infection is suspected. Overall condyloma clearance rates for surgical techniques range from 60 to 90% with recurrence rates of 20–30%.[44]

The patient can apply topical agents like podofilox and imiquimod although neither agent is approved for use in the anal canal. Podofilox is the purified active component of the antimitotic plant resin podophyllin and is available as a 0.5% gel or solution. A treatment cycle consists of twice daily application for 3 days followed by no treatment for 4 days utilized for up to 1 month. Toxicity concerns are less than those issues with podophyllin while clearance rates for condyloma of 35–80% have been reported. Recurrence rates in patients treated with podofilox are 10–20%.[44–48] Imiquimod is an immune response modifier that increases local production of interferon. A complete response can be expected in 50% of patients treated with imiquimod with 11% of patients experiencing a recurrence.[44,49–51] It is applied at bedtime three times a week, left in place for 6–8 h and then removed by washing; treatment may take up to 16 weeks. One study demonstrated no benefit to increased dosing frequency from one to two or even three times daily.[52] Side effects of imiquimod include pain burning, itching, and ulceration which may require cessation of therapy. Imiquimod is used (1) as initial treatment with electrodessication reserved for those who have incomplete response or (2) following destructive treatment and epithelial healing to treat remaining disease or decrease recurrence (no randomized data to support this use). Currently, imiquimod is not approved for anal canal use but this application is being investigated.[53] Trichloracetic acid is applied topically and is useful for treating small lesions in the anal canal. Topical and intralesional interferon have been used to treat condyloma accuminata with mixed results. Other agents that have been used to treat anogenital condyloma but are not in widespread use include 5-FU cream, cidofovir and autologous vaccine.

Bushke and Loewenstein first described giant condyloma accuminata (GCA) in 1925.[54] They are most associated with HPV types 6 and 11 but histologically demonstrate some differences from ordinary condyloma – marked papillomatosis, acanthosis, thickened rete ridges, and increased mitotic activity. The substantial percentage of cases with in situ or invasive squamous cell cancers has lead to speculation that GCA represents part of a continuum from condyloma to invasive squamous cell cancer.

Wide local excision with a 1 cm margin is the treatment of choice for these lesions. Local tissue flaps or grafted skin may be required to repair surgical defects. Abdominal–perineal resection has been used for GCA involving the anal sphincters. Chemoradiation is also an option in the treatment of GCA, especially in those patients who are poor surgical candidates or in whom clear surgical margin are not attainable.[55] Complete regression of GCA with chemoradiation has been reported.[56]

HPV, Anal Intraepithelial Dysplasia, and Anal Cancer

While it is clear that HPV plays a significant role in the development of cervical cancer, its significance in the development of anal cancer (Figure 17-10) and its presumed precursor, anal intraepithelial dysplasia, is not as well defined. Parallels can be drawn between the anal canal and the cervical canal as they share embryologic and histologic features. Furthermore, both canals derive from the embryonic cloacal membrane and both are areas where ectodermal and endodermal tissues fuse to form a transition zone from columnar epithelium to squamous epithelium.

Epidemiologic parallels can be drawn as well. Studies prior to the HIV infection epidemic showed the incidence of anal cancer in homosexual males to be 12.5–37 per 100,000 in the USA[57] This incidence is similar to the incidence of cervical cancer prior routine Pap testing. The risk of anal cancer developing in an HIV+ homosexual male is estimated to be 38 times that of the general population and twice the risk of an HIV– homosexual male.[57,58] HPV infection has been reported in 93% of HIV+ homosexual males compared to 60% of HIV– homosexual males.[55]

Anal cytology has been suggested as a screening tool for detecting patients with anal dysplasia. Applying the current cervical cytology terminology specimens are designated normal, atypical squamous cells of indeterminate significance (ASCUS), low-grade squamous intraepithelial lesions (LSIL), or high-grade squamous intraepithelial lesions (HSIL). The benefit and best timing of this screening is undetermined. Evaluation and treatment algorithms as well as recommended testing schedules have been reported.[59,60] One such evaluation and treatment algorithm recommends high-resolution (with acetowhitening and staining with Lugol's solutions) anoscopy with biopsy.[60] Subsequent treatment is based on histologic findings which are typically reported as normal or anal epithelial neoplasia (AIN) I, II, or III. Options for treatment include local destruction (with topical agents,

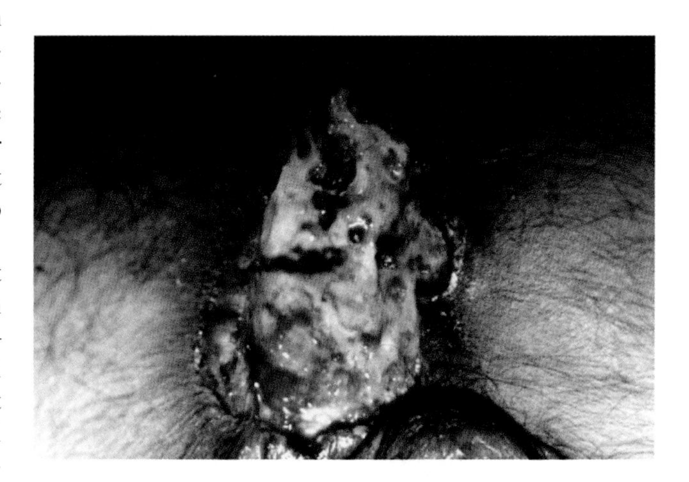

FIGURE 17-10. Anal cancer in HIV-positive patient; *HIV* human immunodeficiency virus.

cryotherapy, or fulguration), excision, or observation. However, there are limitations of our understanding of the relationship between HPV, AIN, and anal cancer that prevent the dogmatic recommendation and widespread acceptance of such an approach. First, the incidence and predictability of the progression of AIN to invasive cancer is unclear.[61,62] The lack of inter- and intraobserver agreement in the interpretation of AIN no doubt contributes to this lack of understanding.[63] Second, data demonstrating efficacy, which is defined as long-term removal of AIN and prevention of anal cancer of treatment is lacking. The absence of established benefit combined with the morbidity of treatment leads us and others to the recommendation that AIN, regardless of grade, be observed unless there are gross visual or palpable lesions or ulcerations present.

Two additional comments with regard to the association of HPV, HIV, and AIN should be made. First, the use of HAART (discussed further later in the section on HIV) does not reduce the incidence of AIN.[64] The clinical implications of this fact are: (a) anal cytology screening should not be stopped just because a patient is treated with HAART and (b) with HIV patients living longer secondary to HAART, the incidence of anal cancers may increase. Second, the prevalence of HPV and AIN is high in HIV positive males with CD4+ counts less than 500×10^6 cells/L even in the absence of a history of anal intercourse.[65] These patients should also be considered for cytologic screening.

Molluscum Contagiosum

The molluscum contagiosum virus is a member of the poxvirus family and causes a benign papular condition of the skin. Transmission is by sexual and nonsexual contact. The incubation period is 1–6 months, followed by the development of 2–6 mm flesh-colored, umbilicated papules.[66] Symptoms are uncommon though pruritis or tenderness may occur. Immunocompromised hosts, such as those with HIV, are more prone to infection with molluscum contagiosum (compared to HIV negative) and may have a more severe form of the disease with hundreds of lesions. Diagnosis is usually made on clinical grounds but excisional biopsy demonstrates enlarged epithelial cell with intracytoplasmic molluscum bodies. Treatment is generally through eradication with curettage, electrodessication or cryotherapy. Podophyllotoxin (0.5%) and imiquimod (5%) have both been used as self-applied topical preparations with success,[67,68] although neither compound is FDA approved for this use.

HIV and the Acquired Immunodeficiency Syndrome

Infection from the HIV (originally called human t-lymphotropic virus) related to acquired immunodeficiency syndrome (AIDS) was first described in 1983.[69] The most current data available show that in 2005 there were approximately 433,760 people in the USA with AIDS and another 215,653 with HIV infection not meeting the criteria for AIDS.[70] Cumulative totals showed a total of 984,155 cases of AIDS in the USA through 2005 and a death rate of 51% in this group. While the incidence of HIV infection has apparently stabilized, the numbers of new AIDS cases and deaths from AIDS have decreased. This fact is in large part due to HAART – combinations of potent anti-HIV drugs which are nucleoside analogs, nonnucleoside reverse transcriptase inhibitors, or protease inhibitors. Table 17-2 shows the current classification system for patients who are HIV positive.

TABLE 17-2. Revised classification system for HIV and AIDS[72]

CD4+ T-lymphocyte categories
Category 1: greater than or equal to 500 cells/μL
Category 2: 200–499 cells/μL
Category 3: less than 200 cells/μL
Clinical categories
Category A: HIV positive; asymptomatic; persistent generalized lymphadenopathy
Category B: Symptomatic conditions not listed in clinical category C; are conditions that are attributed to HIV infection; or conditions that have a clinical course or require management that is complicated by HIV infection. Examples include: bacillary angiomatosis, oropharyngeal or vulvovaginal candidiasis, cervical dysplasia, diarrhea (greater than 1 month in duration), more than one episode of herpes zoster, pelvic inflammatory disease, peripheral neuropathy
Category C: Diagnoses included in the AIDS surveillance case definition – candidiasis (pulmonary or esophageal), invasive cervical cancer, Coccydiomycosis, extrapulmonary cryptococcosis, chronic intestinal Cryptosporidiosis, Cytomegalovirus disease (other than liver, spleen, nodes) or retinitis, HIV-encephalopathy, HSV (chronic ulcers, pulmonary or esophageal), Histoplasmosis (disseminated or extrapulmonary), Isosporiasis (chronic intestinal), Kaposi's sarcoma, Burkitt's lymphoma, immunoblastic lymphoma, primary brain lymphoma, Mycobacterium avium complex or any mycobacterium species other than M. tuberculosis (extrapulmonary or disseminated), Mycobacterium tuberculosis, Pneumocystis carinii pneumonia, progressive focal leukoencephalopathy, recurrent Salmonella speticemia, Toxoplasmosis of the brain, HIV wasting syndrome

	Clinical categories		
CD4+ categories	A1	B1	***C1***
	A2	B2	***C2***
	A3	***B3***	***C3***

Bold italic groups are defined as AIDS.

Surgery for anorectal diseases is the most common indication for surgery in HIV infected patients and in 5% of patients, their anorectal complaint is the presenting symptom of their HIV infection.[71] Most of the indications for surgery are common to the population at large but some are unique to AIDS patients. Several studies demonstrate poor wound healing and increased morbidity in the surgical treatment of anorectal disease in AIDS patients.[72–74] Delayed or failed wound healing has been associated with the presence of AIDS, decreased absolute leukocyte count, and decreased CD4 count. Morandi et al. found that at 32 weeks after hemorrhoidectomy, 50% of AIDS patients had incompletely healed wounds. The overall complication rate was significantly higher in the AIDS group than in HIV+ patients without AIDS.[73] Conversely, Lord reported decreased wound healing in HIV+ patients with T-lymphocyte count of less than 50.[75] Others have shown longer interval and decreased complete wound healing in HIV+ patients with CD4+ T-lymphocyte counts of less than 200.[74] The studies reviewed above describe patients who were not treated with HAART. There is a lack of data describing wound healing in anorectal surgery since the widespread use of HAART; however, the observation of the authors is that compensated HIV+ patients are at no significant risk of increased complications from anorectal surgery. Other factors to be considered in selecting appropriate treatment include any untreatable diarrheal conditions, degree of existing fecal incontinence, and the effect of the proposed surgical procedure on incontinence.

Anal fissures that occur in HIV+ patients must be distinguished from idiopathic AIDS-related anal ulcers (Figure 17-11) and ulcerating STDs, such as HSV or syphilis. Anal fissures in this patient population are indistinguishable from those in the general population and their treatment is similar – initial conservative management with surgery for treatment failures.[76,77] Treatment of fissures in HIV+ patients is modified by the factors described previously and include controlling diarrhea when possible and encouraging abstinence from anoreceptive intercourse.

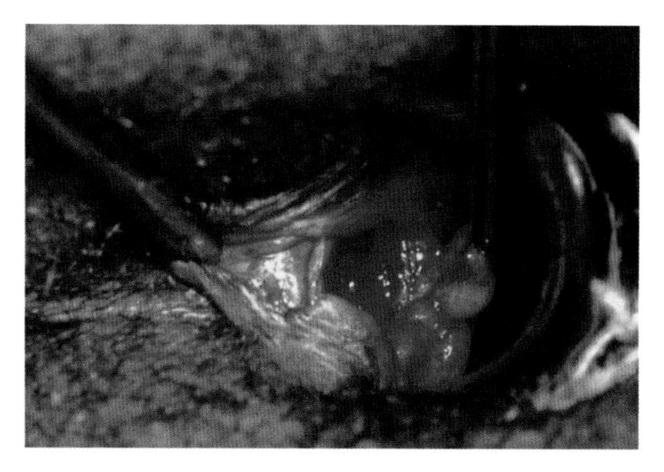

FIGURE 17-11. AIDS and ulcer.

While data on the incidence of AIDS-related anal ulcers is lacking, it appears that they are less common with HAART because the lesions are most frequently associated with clinical AIDS and lower CD4+ counts. These ulcers can be distinguished from typical anal fissures because they are more proximal in the anal canal (frequently above the dentate line or anorectal ring), broader based, deeply ulcerating with the destruction of sphincter planes, and may demonstrate mucosal bridging. Debilitating pain is a common presenting symptom of these ulcers. Surgical debridement allows for adequate drainage of feculent or purulent material trapped in the ulcer and removal of necrotic debris. Biopsy and culture identifies potentially treatable causes for ulceration – malignancy, acid-fast bacilli, HSV, *H. ducreyi*, *T. pallidum*. CMV has been cultured from these ulcers by some authors but is apparently not causal and therefore does not require treatment. Intralesional injection with steroids (methylprednisolone 80–160 mg, in 1 cc 0.25% bupivacaine) provides relief in the majority of patients but not healing.[78] Patients who have persistent pain are reinjected at their ulcer sites.

Perianal suppurative diseases are common conditions in AIDS patients. Abscesses should be drained using small incisions and the placement of a mushroom catheter lessens recurrent sepsis. Broad spectrum antibiotics should be given in immune compromised especially if cellulitis is present. Culture (to include mycobacterium) and histopathologic evaluation identifies infection from atypical organisms and malignancy.

Naldal et al. reported on fistulotomies performed in 31 HIV+ patients. Seven patients had failure of wound healing and all had clinical AIDS, CD4+ counts of less than 200, and absolute leukocyte counts of less than 3,000/mm^3.[74] Based on this, the authors treat anal fistulas in AIDS patients with high viral loads and low CD4+ counts similar to Crohn's patients. Draining setons are placed liberally with selective use of fistulotomy for low uncomplicated fistulas. Fistulotomy in HIV+ patients with AIDS and normal CD4+ counts is based on criteria similar to HIV− patients.

Thrombosed external hemorrhoids in patients with AIDS are treated the same as for HIV− patients. Acute thrombosis (24–48 h after onset of symptoms) is treated with excision. Subacute thrombosis (longer than 48 h from symptom onset) is treated conservatively with Sitz baths and oral analgesics.

Internal hemorrhoids present with symptoms of bleeding or prolapse. Initial treatment in patients with AIDS is with a high fiber diet and bulking agents. Proximal colonic sources of bleeding should be excluded via colonoscopy. Patients who fail initial conservative measures are treated with rubber band ligation or infrared coagulation. Other nonoperative techniques, such as bipolar coagulation, cryotherapy, or injection sclerotherapy, are acceptable. There are conflicting recommendations for operative treatment of hemorrhoids published within the last decade. In a retrospective study, Hewitt et al. found no difference in wound healing between HIV+ and HIV− patients.[79] The mean CD4+ count was 301 but they classified 81% of patients as having AIDS based on symptoms or CD4 count less than 200. In the discussion, the authors comment that the majority of their patients were well nourished and otherwise healthy. They conclude that HIV status should not alter the indications for surgery in patients with symptomatic hemorrhoids. In contrast, as mentioned, Morandi et al. prospectively evaluated healing time after hemorrhoidectomy.[73] Functional status and the presence of AIDS were the two factors that correlated with poor wound healing. AIDS patients with nonhealing had a mean CD4+ count of 79. Unfortunately, they do not comment relief of hemorrhoid symptoms. It appears that asymptomatic HIV+ patients and who do not meet the clinical or CD4+ count diagnostic criteria for AIDS (Table 17-2) can be treated with hemorrhoidectomy with the expectation that they have good symptomatic relief and normal wound healing. AIDS patients with more advanced disease (clinical category C) or low CD4+ counts (especially less than 100) are at increased risk for wound healing problems. The benefit of symptomatic relief may still warrant performing surgical treatment in this group.[76]

References

1. Centers for Disease Control and Prevention. Tracking the hidden epidemics. Trends in STDs in the USA. Atlanta: Centers for Disease Control and Prevention; 2001. p. 1–26.
2. British Medical Association. Sexually transmitted infections. February 2002;1–25.
3. Kinghorn G. A sexual health and HIV strategy for England. Br Med J. 2001;323:243–4.
4. Halperin DT. Heterosexual anal intercourse: prevalence, cultural factors, and HIV infection and other health risks, Part 1. AIDS Patient Care STDs. 1999;13:717–30.
5. Kozlowski PA, Neutra MR. The role of mucosal immunity in prevention of HIV transmissions. Curr Mol Med. 2003;3:217–28.
6. Sobhani I, Walker F, Aparicio T, et al. Effect of anal epidermoid cancer-related viruses on the dendritic (Langerhans') cells of the human anal mucosa. Clin Cancer Res. 2002;8:2862–9.
7. Middleton K, Peh W, Southern S, et al. Organization of human papillomavirus productive cycle during neoplastic progression provide a basis for selection of diagnostic markers. J Virol. 2003;77:10186–201.
8. Kampmeier RH. Identification of the gonococcus by Albert Neisser. Sex Transm Dis. 1978;5:71.
9. Hansen L, Wong T, Perrin M. Gonorrhoea resurgence in Canada. Int J STD AIDS. 2003;14:727–31.
10. Hook III EW, Handsfield HH. Gonococcal infection in the adult. In: Holmes KK, Sparling PR, Mardh PA, et al., editors. Sexually transmitted diseases. New York: McGraw-Hill; 1999. p. 451–66.
11. McMillan A, Young H, Moyes A. Rectal gonorrhoea in homosexual men: source of infection. Int J STD AIDS. 2000;11:284–7.
12. Ison C, Martin D. Gonorrhea. In: Morse SA, Ballard RC, Holmes KK, Moreland AA, editors. Atlas of sexually transmitted diseases and AIDS. Edinburgh: Mosby; 2003. p. 109–25.
13. Young H, Manavi K, McMillan A. Evaluation of ligase chain reaction for the non-cultural detection of rectal and pharyngeal gonrrhea in men who have sex with men. Sex Transm Infect. 2003;79:484–6.
14. Centers for Disease Control and Prevention. Sexually transmitted diseases treatment guidelines 2002. MMWR. 2002; 51(RR-6):1–77.
15. Centers for Disease Control and Prevention. Sexually transmitted disease surveillance 2002 supplement. Gonococcal isolate surveillance project annual report. Atlanta: US Department of Health and Human Services; 2003.
16. Fenton KA, Ison C, Johnson AP, et al. Ciprofloxacin resistance in *Neisseria gonorrhoeae* in England and Wales in 2002. Lancet. 2003;361:1867–8.
17. Cates W. Estimates of the incidence and prevalence of sexually transmitted diseases in the United States. Sex Transm Dis. 1999;26(Suppl):S2–7.
18. Rampalo AM. Diagnosis and treatment of sexually acquired proctitis and proctocolitis: an update. Clin Infect Dis. 1999;28 Suppl 1:S84–90.
19. Gregory A, Gottesman L. Sexually transmitted and infectious diseases. In: Beck DE, Wexner SD, editors. Fundamentals of anorectal surgery. London: WB Saunders; 1998. p. 414–31.
20. Stamm W. *Chlamydia trachomatis* infections of the adult. In: Holmes KK, Sparling PR, Mardh PA, et al., editors. Sexually transmitted diseases. New York: McGraw-Hill; 1999. p. 407–22.
21. Schacter J, Stephens R. Infections caused by *Chlamydia trachomatis*. In: Morse SA, Ballard RC, Holmes KK, Moreland AA, editors. Atlas of sexually transmitted diseases and AIDS. Edinburgh: Mosby; 2003. p. 73–96.
22. Golden MR, Astet SG, Galvan R, et al. Pilot study of COBAS PCR and ligase chain reaction for detection of rectal infections due to *Chlamydia trachomatis*. J Clin Microbiol. 2003;41:2174–5.
23. Centers for Disease Control and Prevention. Primary and secondary syphilis – United States 2002. MMWR. 2003; 52:1117–20.
24. Centers for Disease Control and Prevention. The national plan to eliminate syphilis from the United States. Atlanta: US Department of Health and Human Services; 1999. p. 1–84. http://www.cdc.gov/stopsyphilis/plan.pdf.
25. Cox D, Liu H, Moreland A, Levine W. Syphilis. In: Morse SA, Ballard RC, Holmes KK, Moreland AA, editors. Atlas of sexually transmitted diseases and AIDS. Edinburgh: Mosby; 2003. p. 23–51.
26. Kohl KS, Farley T, Ewell J, Scioneaux J. Usefulness of partner notification for syphilis control. Sex Transm Dis. 1999; 26:201–7.
27. Spinola SM, Bauer ME, Munson RS. Immunopathogenesis of *Haemophilus ducrei* infection (Chancroid). Infect Immun. 2002;70:1667–76.
28. DiCarlo RP, Martin DH. The clinical diagnosis of genital ulcer disease in men. Clin Infect Dis. 1997;25:292–8.
29. Ballard R, Morse S. Chancroid. In: Morse SA, Ballard RC, Holmes KK, Moreland AA, editors. Atlas of sexually transmitted diseases and AIDS. Edinburgh: Mosby; 2003. p. 53–71.
30. Orle KA, Gates CA, Martin DH, et al. Simultaneous PCR detection of *Haemophilus ducreyi*, *Treponema pallidum*, and herpes simplex virus types 1 and 2 from genital ulcers. J Clin Microbiol. 1996;34:49–54.
31. O'Farrell N. Donovanosis. Sex Transm Dis. 2002;78:452–7.
32. Fleming DT, McQuillan GM, Johnson RE, et al. Herpes simplex virus type 2 in the United States, 1976 to 1994. N Engl J Med. 1997;337:1105–11.

33. Roberts CM, Pfister JR, Spear SJ. Increasing proportion of herpes simplex virus type 1 as a cause of genital herpes infection in college students. Sex Transm Dis. 2003;30:797–800.
34. Lafferty WE. The changing epidemiology of HSV-1 and HSV-2 and implications for serological testing. Herpes. 2002;9:51–5.
35. Goodell SE, Quinn TC, Mkrtichian E, et al. Herpes simplex virus proctitis in homosexual men. Clinical, sigmoidoscopic, and histopathological features. N Engl J Med. 1983;308:868–71.
36. Pertel PR, Spear PG. Biology of herpesviruses. In: Holmes KK, Sparling PR, Mardh PA, et al., editors. Sexually transmitted diseases. New York: McGraw-Hill; 1999. p. 269–83.
37. Wald A, Ashley-Morrow R. Serological testing for herpes simplex virus (HSV)-1 and HSV-2 infection. Clin Infect Dis. 2002;35 Suppl 2:S173–82.
38. Slomka MJ. Current diagnostic techniques in genital herpes: their role in controlling the epidemic. Clin Lab. 2000;46: 591–607.
39. Ashley RL. Performance and use of HSV type-specific serology test kits. Herpes. 2002;9:38–45.
40. Rompalo AM, Mertz GJ, Davis LG, et al. A double-blind study of oral acyclovir for the treatment of first episode herpes simplex virus proctitis in homosexual men. JAMA. 1988;259:2879–81.
41. Wald A. New therapies and prevention strategies for genital herpes. Clin Infect Dis. 1999;28(Suppl):S4–13.
42. Patel R. Progress in meeting today's demands in genital herpes: an overview of current management. J Infect Dis. 2002;186 Suppl 1:S47–56.
43. Corey L, Wald A, Patel R, et al. Once-daily valacyclovir to reduce the risk of transmission of genital herpes. N Engl J Med. 2004;350:11–20.
44. Wiley DJ, Douglas J, Beutner K, et al. External genital warts: diagnosis, treatment, and prevention. Clin Infect Dis. 2002;35 Suppl 2:S210–24.
45. von Krogh G, Longstaff E. Podophyllin office therapy against condyloma should be abandoned. Sex Transm Infect. 2001;77:409–12.
46. von Krogh G, Lacey CJN, Gross G, et al. European course on HPV associated pathology: guidelines for primary care physicians for the diagnosis and management of anogenital warts. Sex Transm Infect. 2000;76:162–8.
47. Greenberg MD, Rutledge LH, Reid R, et al. A double-blind, randomized trial of 0.5% podofilox and placebo for the treatment of genital warts in women. Obstet Gynecol. 1991;77:735–9.
48. Edwards L, Ferenczy A, Eron L, et al. Self-administered topical 5% imiquimod cream for external anogenital warts. Arch Dermatol. 1998;134:25–30.
49. Tyring S, Edwards L, Cherry LK, et al. Safety and efficacy of 0.5% podofilox gel in the treatment of anogenital warts. Arch Dermatol. 1998;134:33–8.
50. Maitland JE, Maw R. An audit of patients who have received imiquimod cream 5% for the treatment of anogenital warts. Int J STD AIDS. 2000;11:268–70.
51. Beutner K, Tyring SK, Trofatter Jr KF, et al. Imiquimod, a patient-applied immune-response modifier for treatment of external genital warts. Antimicrob Agents Chemother. 1998;42:789–94.
52. Fife KH, Ferenczy A, Douglas JM, et al. Treatment of external warts in men using 5% imiquimod cream applied three times a week, once daily, twice daily, or three times a day. Sex Transm Dis. 2001;28:226–31.
53. Kaspari M, Gutzmer R, Kaspari T, et al. Application of imiquimod by suppositories (anal tampons) efficiently prevents recurrences after ablation of anal canal condyloma. Br J Dermatol. 2002;147:757–9.
54. Buschke A, Lowenstein L. Uber carcinomahnliche condylomata acuminata. Klin Wochenschr. 1925;4:1726.
55. Trombetta LJ, Place RJ. Giant condyloma acuminatum of the anorectum: trends in epidemiology and management. Report of a case and review of the literature. Dis Colon Rectum. 2001;44:1878–86.
56. Butler TW, Gefter J, Kleto D, et al. Squamous-cell carcinoma of the anus in condyloma acuminatum: successful treatment with pre-operative chemotherapy and radiation. Dis Colon Rectum. 1987;30:293–5.
57. Frisch M, Biggar RJ, Goedert JJ. Human papillomavirus-associated cancers in patients with immunodeficiency virus infection and acquired immunodeficiency syndrome. J Natl Cancer Inst. 2000;92:1500–10.
58. Goedert JJ, Cote TR, Virgo P, et al. Spectrum of AIDS-associated cancers in patients with human immunodeficiency virus infection and acquired immunodeficiency syndrome. Lancet. 1998;351:1833–9.
59. Chin-Hong PV, Palefsky JM. Natural history and clinical management of anal human papillomavirus disease in men and women infected with human immunodeficiency virus. Clin Infect Dis. 2002;35:1127–34.
60. Palefsky JM. Anal human papillomavirus infection and anal cancer in HIV-positive individuals: an emerging problem. AIDS. 1994;8:293–5.
61. Cleary RK, Shaldebrand JD, Fowler JJ, et al. Perianal Bowen's disease and anal intraepithelial neoplasia. Dis Colon Rectum. 1999;42:945–51.
62. Caruso ML, Valentini AM. Different human papillomavirus genotypes in anogenital lesions. Anticancer Res. 1999;19:3049–53.
63. Colquhoun P, Nogeras JJ, Dipasquale B, et al. Interobserver and intraobserver bias exists in the interpretation of anal dysplasia. Dis Colon Rectum. 2003;46:1338.
64. Piketty C, Darragh TM, Heard I, et al. High prevalence of anal squamous intraepithelial lesions in HIV-positive men despite the use of highly active antiretroviral therapy. Sex Transm Dis. 2004;31:96–9.
65. Piketty C, Darragh TM, Da Costa M, et al. High prevalence of anal human papillomavirus infection and anal cancer precursors among HIV-infected persons in the absence of anal intercourse. Ann Intern Med. 2003;183:453–9.
66. Douglas Jr JM. Molluscum contagiosum. In: Holmes KK, Sparling PR, Mardh PA, et al., editors. Sexually transmitted diseases. New York: McGraw-Hill; 1999. p. 385–9.
67. Skinner RB. Treatment of mollscum contagiosum with imiquimod 5% cream. J Am Acad Dermatol. 2002;47:S221–4.
68. Syed TA, Lundin S, Ahmad M. Topical 0.3% and 0.5% podophyllotoxin cream for self-treatment of molluscum contagiosum in males. A placebo-controlled, double-blind study. Dermatology. 1994;189:65–8.
69. Barre-Sinoussi F, Chermann JC, Rey F, et al. Isolation of a T-lymphotropic retrovirus from a patient at risk for acquired immune deficiency syndrome (AIDS). Science. 1983;220:868–71.

70. Centers for Disease Control and Prevention. HIV/AIDS surveillance report 2005 (modified June, 2007);17:12.
71. Centers for Disease Control and Prevention. MMWR 1992; 41(RR-17)
72. Barrett WL, Callahan TD, Orkin BA. Perianal manifestations of human immunodeficiency virus infection. Experience with 260 patients. Dis Colon Rectum. 1998;41:606–12.
73. Morandi E, Merlini D, Salvaggio A, et al. Prospective study of healing time after hemorroidectomy. Influence of HIV infection, acquired immunodeficiency syndrome, and anal wound infection. Dis Colon Rectum. 1999;42:1140–4.
74. Nadal SR, Manzione CR, Galvao VM, et al. Healing after fistulotomy. Comparative study between HIV+ and HIV− patients. Dis Colon Rectum. 1998;41:177–9.
75. Lord RVN. Anorectal surgery in patients infected with human immunodeficiency virus. Factors associated with delayed wound healing. Ann Surg. 1997;226:92–9.
76. Brar HS, Gottesman L, Surawicz C. Anorectal pathology in AIDS. Gastrointest Endosc Clin N Am. 1998;8:913–31.
77. Bernstein M. Anal fissure and the human immunodeficiency virus. Semin Colon Rectal Surg. 1997;8:40–5.
78. Modesto VL, Gottesman L. Surgical debridement and intralesional steroid injection in the treatment of idiopathic AIDS-related anal ulcerations. Am J Surg. 1997;174: 439–41.
79. Hewitt WR, Sokol TP, Fleshner RP. Should HIV status alter indications for hemorrhoidectomy? Dis Colon Rectum. 1996; 39:615–8.

18
Fecal Incontinence

Dana R. Sands and Mari A. Madsen

Introduction

Fecal incontinence is a socially devastating condition, affecting between 1.4 and 18% of the population and up to 50% of all nursing home residents.[1,2] It has been defined as "recurrent uncontrolled passage of fecal material for at least 1 month,"[3] while partial incontinence is typically described as inability to control the passage of flatus and fecal soiling.

Populations at risk for fecal incontinence include: parous females, patients with cognitive impairment, neurologic disorders, and nursing home residents.[4,5] In fact, fecal incontinence is the second leading reason for admission to nursing homes.[6] As a result of the social stigma and the fear for loss of autonomy, the true incidence of this problem is believed to be vastly under reported. It has been dubbed the "silent affliction."[7]

Etiology

It is important to realize that fecal incontinence is not a diagnosis, but a symptom of which there are multiple causes. Normal bowel continence requires a complex integration of function between the anal sphincters, pelvic floor, stool volume/consistency, rectal compliance, and neurologic function. It is first necessary to determine if the patient is having true fecal incontinence. Pseudo incontinence can be caused by a variety of anorectal conditions including hemorrhoidal prolapse, incomplete evacuation, poor hygiene, fistula-in-ano, dermatologic conditions, anorectal sexually transmitted diseases (STDs), and anorectal neoplasms. Fecal urgency from a noncompliant rectum can also cause incontinence. Consideration should be given to other disease states such as inflammatory bowel disease and radiation proctitis. The diagnosis of overflow incontinence from incomplete rectal evacuation should also be entertained in patients whose history indicates this condition.

A thorough history will allow the examiner to diagnose a diarrheal state as the etiology of the incontinence. Any change in bowel habits with diarrhea should be excluded. Various systemic disease states can affect continence. In the appropriate patient, central nervous system pathology including spinal cord injury and neoplasm should be part of the differential diagnosis. Autonomic neuropathies such as diabetes can also cause derangements in continence.

Perhaps the more common etiologies of incontinence treated by the colorectal surgeon are those that pertain to abnormal pelvic floor function. Anal sphincter injury can be the result of obstetric injury, direct trauma, neoplasm, or rectal prolapse. Obstetric injury is a common occurrence with occult tears of the anal sphincter reported in 25–35% of women after vaginal delivery.[8,9] The incidence of obstetric tears has been reported from 0.6 to 9% in the literature.[10,11] Factors that affect the risk for developing obstetric tears are use of forceps, mediolateral episiotomy, and primiparity.[12,13]

Denervation injuries to the pelvic floor are also common sequelae of childbirth; 60% of patients with an obstetric tear also have evidence of pudendal nerve damage.[14,15] The mechanism of pelvic floor denervation appears to be a result of compression or traction injury to the pudendal nerves during vaginal delivery, particularly when it is prolonged or requires forceps assistance. High birth weight is also a risk factor for compression injury. The end stage of denervation injury is pelvic floor failure and descending perineum syndrome.

Iatrogenic injury to the anal sphincter musculature is also a cause of fecal incontinence. Incontinence after surgery for fissure with lateral internal sphincterotomy is not uncommon.[16,17] Fistulotomy is also associated with seepage and soiling and incontinence rates reported as high as 35–45%.[18,19] Local sphincter lesions and intra-anal scarring (keyhole deformity) are not the sole explanation for the high incidence of incontinence since it also occurs after non-muscle-cutting anorectal surgery such as anal stretch,[20] hemorrhoidectomy,[21] and transanal advancement flaps.[22]

Patients who have suffered from congenital malformations including spina bifida, imperforate anus, and myelomeningocele often have severe alterations of continence and evacuatory function. The difficulty is related not only to the function of the pelvic floor musculature but also to the

D.E. Beck et al. (eds.), *The ASCRS Textbook of Colon and Rectal Surgery: Second Edition*,
DOI 10.1007/978-1-4419-1584-9_18, © Springer Science+Business Media, LLC 2011

proprioceptive response of the rectum. Radiation therapy can result in fecal incontinence from both a direct damage to the anal sphincter as well as through its effect on the compliance of the rectum.

Diagnosis

History

The first step in the evaluation of any medical condition is to attain a thorough patient history. Patients with fecal incontinence are often embarrassed and reluctant to provide details of the problem unless specifically asked. It is important to create a comfortable environment for the patient during the history and physical examination. The onset of the symptoms can provide useful insight into the etiology of the problem. A thorough obstetric and surgical history is imperative. Other neurologic conditions should be considered as well. Changes in bowel consistency are a common cause of fecal incontinence which can be overlooked by many physicians. Any cause of diarrhea should be explored as a potential etiology of the patients' symptoms especially if there is a temporal relationship.

After appropriate questioning, the physician will often be able to determine if the patient has active or passive incontinence. Active (urge) incontinence, or the loss of stool despite the patients' best efforts to control it, will lead the physician to consider etiologies which involve an intact sensory mechanism with a derangement in the external anal sphincter function.[23] Passive incontinence, or the loss of stool without the patient's awareness, will lead the examiner to consider internal anal sphincter pathology or neurologic etiologies.

It is helpful to quantify the degree of the fecal incontinence. Numerous scoring systems have been used to evaluate incontinence. When utilizing these tools, it is important to take into account the impact of the patient's perception of the severity of their symptoms and their response to treatment.[24] The Cleveland Clinic Florida Fecal Incontinence Score (CCF-FIS) is an independently validated tool which has the benefit of ease of use combined with incorporation of a quality of life component (Table 18-1).[25]

Table 18-1. Cleveland Clinic Florida Fecal Incontinence Score (CCF-FIS)

Type of incontinence	Frequency				
	Never	Rarely	Sometimes	Usually	Always
Solid	0	1	2	3	4
Liquid	0	1	2	3	4
Gas	0	1	2	3	4
Pad usage	0	1	2	3	4
Lifestyle impact	0	1	2	3	4

0 = perfect continence.
20 = complete incontinence.
Never = 0, rarely = <1/month, sometimes = >1/month, <1/week, usually = >1/week, <1/day, always = >1/day.

An often overlooked component of the history of the patient suffering from fecal incontinence is the presence of other pelvic floor complaints. Physicians should be sure to inquire about the presence of any form of rectal prolapse as well as the presence of urinary incontinence or genital organ prolapse. It has been noted that there is a significant overlap of symptoms in this complex patient population.

Physical Examination

A complete physical examination will include inspection of the perianal skin for scars from prior surgeries, trauma or birthing injuries, fistulae, excoriation from chronic soiling, or large prolapsing hemorrhoids. A specific evaluation of the perineal body in parous females should include palpation to determine if it is thinned. At rest, the anal canal should be well approximated, not patulous. A patulous anus suggests a possible rectal prolapse, which is best reproduced by asking the patient to Valsalva while sitting on a toilet or squatting. Checking the perianal sensation to pinprick as well as the anocutaneous "wink" reflex will serve as a simple assessment of neurologic function.

Digital rectal examination can reveal masses or a fecal impaction. It also provides a gross assessment of both resting tone and voluntary squeeze. With some attention, it is possible to discern contraction of the puborectalis in the upper canal versus constriction of the external anal sphincter. Lastly, anoscopy or potentially a rigid vs. flexible proctosigmoidoscopy may reveal inflammatory bowel disease, infectious proctitis, or neoplastic process if suspected.

Diagnostic Studies

Endoanal Ultrasound

Endosonography has become the diagnostic cornerstone of the anorectal physiologic evaluation of fecal incontinence. Endoluminal ultrasonography has been utilized extensively to delineate anal canal anatomy. Pulsed sound waves emitted from a luminally placed transducer create transverse images of the anal canal. The efficacy of this technique was demonstrated by Sultan et al.[26] who have used cadaveric and surgical specimens to correlate ultrasonographic findings with anatomic dissection. Their findings were further confirmed with histopathologic evaluation of the dissected specimens. This test is well tolerated and provides physicians with important information about the anatomy of patients suffering from incontinence, fistulous disease, and anal pain. The ultrasound provides excellent imaging of the internal anal sphincter which appears hypoechoic (Figure 18-1). The external sphincter is hyperechoic and scar tissue often has a mixed echogenecity appearance. Obviously, the most important parameter is to determine if the musculature is intact or if there are traumatic defects present. When present, defects

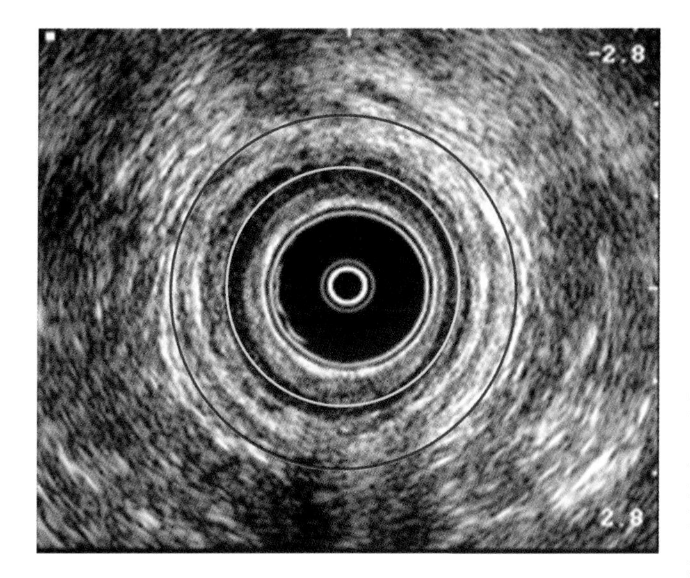

FIGURE 18-1. Normal endoanal ultrasound. The *red line* illustrates the lateral border of the external anal sphincter (hyperechoic) while the *yellow depicts* the lateral border of the internal anal sphincter (hypoechoic).

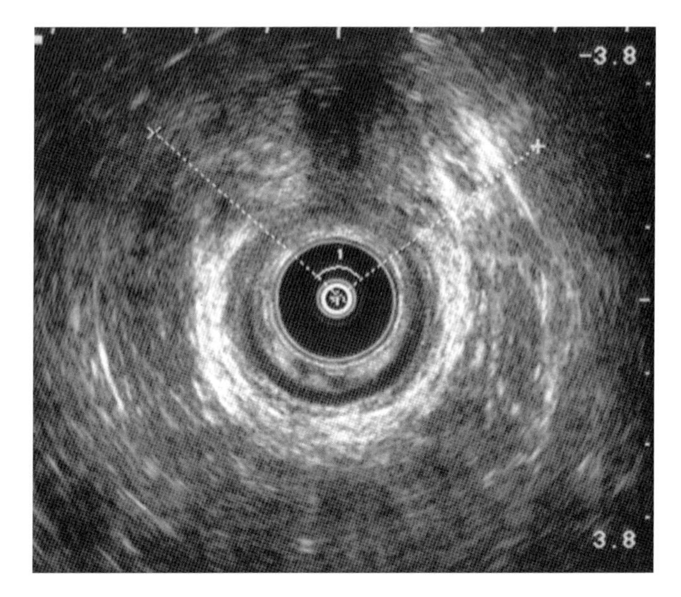

FIGURE 18-2. Endoanal ultrasound with anterior sphincter defect (internal and external).

in the musculature should be measured. Additionally, the perineal body thickness (PBT) should be measured. PBT less than 10 mm is considered abnormal, and those patients with PBT greater than 12 mm are considered unlikely to have a sphincter defect in the absence of prior reconstructive surgery (Figure 18-2).[27]

Anorectal Manometry

Anorectal manometry provides important information about the functional status of the anal sphincters and distal rectum. There is no standardized method of manometric evaluation. Several methods have been described.[28] Microtransducers can be used in the anal canal and are well tolerated by patients. Multichannel water-perfused catheters are perhaps the most common tool used to perform anal manometry. Flow rates of 0.3 mL per channel per minute are required to adequately measure outflow pressure.[29] Higher flow rates can result in accumulation of fluid and distortion of the measurements.

The resistance of flow of fluid from the catheter determines pressure measurements. Measurements can be taken in a continuous fashion (continuous pull through) or at set levels within the anal canal (station pull through). The continuous pull-through technique requires the catheter to be removed at a continuous speed from the anal canal. A computerized motor is used for this purpose. This technique can provide a detailed recording of both the radial and longitudinal pressure profiles. Computer analysis can then generate a three dimensional representation of the anal canal. The stationary pull-through technique measures anal canal pressures at 1 cm increments in the anal canal. It has been theorized that this method provides a more accurate assessment of anal pressures because there is a stabilization period before each reading, thereby reducing artifact.[30]

Measurements

Resting Pressure. The mean resting pressure in healthy volunteers ranges from 40 to 70 mmHg. The internal anal sphincter generates the majority of the resting pressure.[31] This smooth muscle is in a continuous state of maximal contraction accounting for 55–60% of resting tone. The external anal sphincter contributes less to the resting anal tone. The final determinant of resting anal tone is the contribution of the hemorrhoidal plexi. Patients with alterations in continence related to the internal anal sphincter often have low baseline resting pressure.

Squeeze Pressure. The maximal squeeze pressure in healthy individuals is two to three times the baseline resting value. The external anal sphincter is the main contributor to the generation of these pressures. Traumatic defects of the external anal sphincter, whether from obstetric or surgery, often result in decreased squeeze pressures.

High-Pressure Zone. The high-pressure zone is defined as the length of the internal anal sphincter, through which pressures are greater than half of the maximal resting pressure. The high-pressure zone is approximately 2–3 cm in women and 2.5–3.5 cm in men.[28]

Rectoanal Inhibitory Reflex. The rectoanal inhibitory reflex (RAIR) is thought to play a role in the fine adjustments of continence. Rectal distension, usually with small volumes (10–30 mL), causes a contraction of the external anal sphincter followed by a pronounced internal anal sphincter relaxation. This reflex enables the sensory mucosa of the anal canal to "sample" the contents of the distal rectum and the patient to distinguish between gas, liquid, and solid stool. This reflex is absent or abnormal in patients with Hirschsprung's disease, Chagas' disease, dermatomyositis, and scleroderma.

Rectal Sensation. Alterations in rectal sensation can lead to decreased fecal continence. Rectal sensation is measured with an intrarectal balloon and incremental instillation of known volumes of air. Sensation is generally achieved with 40 mL air. Overflow incontinence can result from a decrease in rectal sensation and subsequent fecal impaction.

Rectal Compliance. Compliance is determined by the change in pressure associated with a change in volume ($C=V/P$). This is calculated by subtracting the volume of first sensation from the maximum tolerable volume and dividing by the change in pressure at these two points. A noncompliant rectum can contribute to fecal incontinence as the patient is not able to accommodate the amount of stool presented to the rectum. This is common in conditions which cause proctitis.

Pudendal Nerve Terminal Motor Latency

Pudendal neuropathy has been implicated in the etiology of fecal and urinary incontinence. Assessment of the pudendal nerve terminal motor latency (PNTML) is an important component to the evaluation of the patient with fecal incontinence. A disposable electrode is attached to the examiner's finger which is then directed toward the ischial spine and electrical impulses are delivered to the pudendal nerve. The time for response at the level of the external anal sphincter is measured. Normal response is within 2.0 ± 0.2 ms. Pudendal neuropathy has been implicated in poor outcome after anterior overlapping sphincteroplasty.[32,33] The presence of pudendal neuropathy in the setting of an external anal sphincter defect does not preclude repair[34]; however, the patient can be appropriately counseled in the preoperative and the possible need for future intervention can be discussed.

Electromyography

Anal electromyography (EMG) relies on the use of a concentric needle electrode to record electrical activity generated by the anal sphincter muscle fibers. Sequential recordings of the motor unit potentials are taken circumferentially around the anal canal. This technique is used to "map" the external anal sphincter and document neuromuscular integrity.[35] While this test is more uncomfortable than anal ultrasound, it can provide useful data about the physiologic status of the specific portions of the anal sphincter. This is a useful adjunct when there is excessive scarring on the anal ultrasound.[36]

Defecography

Defecography is the radiological visualization of the act of defecation. It provides a picture of the successive phases of defecation and gives a dynamic impression of pelvic floor activity during these actions. Changes in the rectal configuration and the anorectal angle become visible and the degree of evacuation can be studied. It has become evident that it can demonstrate abnormalities that were unsuspected on clinical examination. While typically utilized in the evaluation of patients suffering from constipation, the value of defecography in the evaluation of fecal incontinence is to demonstrate the presence of incomplete evacuation thereby leading the physician to consider overflow incontinence as the cause of the patient's symptoms.

Colonoscopy

Endoscopic evaluation of the colon can rectum should be undertaken in the evaluation of patients suffering from fecal incontinence. This will allow for the exclusion of any lesions within the lumen of the bowel as well as to ensure that there is no evidence of any inflammatory conditions which could be causing a change in the stool consistency or rectal compliance.

Treatment

Nonoperative Management

Medical Therapies

There are a variety of pharmacotherapies available for the medical management of fecal incontinence, but ultimately the number of randomized, placebo-controlled trials is limited. In fact, the Cochrane Database systemic review on the subject stated "there is little evidence with which to assess the use of drug therapies for the management of fecal incontinence."[37] That said, medical management therapies are broadly broken down into the following categories: bulking agents, constipating agents, and laxative regimen with scheduled disimpactions.

As is suggested by the wide differential diagnosis leading to fecal incontinence, the first step for controlling the incontinence is determination of the underlying cause. Certain etiologies, such as chronic diarrhea, chronic constipation, certain neurologic conditions and systemic diseases, such as diabetes, are best targeted through medical management. At a minimum, use of medical therapies is an important adjunct to mitigate the impact of fecal incontinence.

Bulking Agents

Fiber, both natural and synthetic, has long been a staple in treatment of minor fecal incontinence. It has the benefit of adding bulk and has the ability to absorb additional fluid, providing a more solid stool in the face of mild chronic diarrhea. In laboratory studies calcium polycarbophil (Konsyl®, FiberCon®) a synthetic, insoluble fiber was able to absorb 70 times its weight in fluid, thereby reducing fecal water content.[38] Conversely, in constipation, calcium polycarbophil increases stool frequency and weight without leading to diarrhea.[39] Bliss et al.[40] were able to demonstrate a 50% reduction in incontinence episodes by adding daily fiber supplementation in 39 patients for 1 month.

Constipating Agents

In patients with chronic diarrhea, up to 50% also suffer from incontinence.[41] In patients with diarrhea-predominant irritable bowel syndrome, it is estimated that 20% have associated fecal incontinence.[42] It therefore stands to reason that use of constipation inducing drugs, such as loperamide, codeine, dephenoxylate plus atropine, difenoxin plus atropine, and amitriptyline, are of utility for this group of patients. Loperamide is a synthetic opioid which inhibits small and large intestinal peristalsis via the m (Mu) receptors in the gut. It has also been shown to increase anal resting sphincter pressure, improve rectal sensation, and retention of fluid load, as well as increase the RAIR.[43,44] Amitriptyline has also been suggested as therapy based on its anticholinergic properties leading to a reduction in the frequency and amplitude of rectal motor complexes.[45]

Laxative Regimen with Scheduled Disimpactions

In contrast to patients with diarrhea, patients with constipation and fecal impaction experience fecal incontinence secondary to overflow incontinence. Chassagne et al.[46] compared a regimen of 30 g lactulose daily to 30 g of lactulose daily with the addition of a daily glycerin suppository and a weekly tap-water enema in 206 institutionalized elderly patients with a history of prior fecal impaction and at least weekly episodes of fecal incontinence. The patients receiving the suppositories and weekly enemas in addition to the lactulose had a 35% reduction in fecal incontinence episodes and a 42% reduction in soiled laundry.

Biofeedback

The goal of biofeedback is to use visual, auditory, or other forms of sensory information to improve a patient's ability to sense rectal distention and reinforce appropriate sphincter contraction. In 1974, Engel et al.[47] pioneered the technique and published their results on six patients with fecal incontinence using a Miller–Abbott balloon as a sensor attached to a polygraph to improve the quality of Kegel exercises. Heymen et al.[48] designed a randomized controlled trial in three phases comparing manometric biofeedback to pelvic floor exercises for fecal incontinence, with the aim of reducing the impact of confounding factors by providing all patients with a 4-week pretreatment education and a similar schedule of training visits for both groups. At the completion of the study 44% of patients in the biofeedback group were able to achieve complete continence vs. 21% in the pelvic floor exercise group ($P = 0.008$). A greater increase in anal canal squeeze pressure was seen in the biofeedback group ($P = 0.014$) and at 3 months 76% of patients treated with biofeedback compared to 41% of patients treated with pelvic floor exercises reported adequate relief of their fecal incontinence ($P < 0.001$). It is interesting to note that both groups showed a significant improvement in episodes of fecal incontinence after the 4-week pretreatment phase ($P < 0.001$) and only a trend in favor of the biofeedback group at 3 month posttreatment follow-up ($P = 0.083$).

Published studies typically demonstrate improvement in continence for both adults and children[49,50] as a result of biofeedback in over 70% of the patients.[51–54] Current described methods are widely variable and include weekly or bi-weekly sessions of 30 or 60 min, use of home practice machines, EMG, manometry, and even ultrasound.[55] The Cochrane Database systemic review of the subject included 11 randomized controlled trials and concluded that there is no one method of biofeedback which has been demonstrated superior over the others, nor that biofeedback is conclusively better than conservative measures such as pelvic floor exercises, dietary measures, and pharmacologic agents.[55]

Long-term, the benefits of biofeedback are less clear, with many authorities suggesting an attenuation of results and the need for "refresher" training sessions. Regardless, a trial of biofeedback is considered an important noninvasive, first-line therapeutic option for highly motivated patients who have failed medical management.[56] Factors associated with short-term treatment success are completion of a full six training sessions, female gender, older age (<61), and more severe incontinence.[54]

Secca® Procedure

The Secca® procedure involves the use of radiofrequency delivered as an alternating current at high frequency leading to frictional movement of ions and generation of heat, or thermal energy. As a result of the delivered thermal energy, there is immediate contraction of collagen fibers which are then permanently shortened via remodeling resulting in a tightening of the muscle.[57] Radiofrequency has been used for treatment of gastroesophageal reflux disease (GERD),[58] joint capsule instability,[59] benign prostatic hypertrophy,[60] and even sleep apnea.[61]

The technique is a modification of the Stretta procedure, developed for the treatment of gastroesophageal reflux. In Secca®, the radiofrequency is delivered to the anal sphincter under constant monitoring of the temperature and tissue impedance while simultaneously cooling the probes at the surface to minimize mucosal damage. The current is automatically ceased if the tissue temperature rises above 85°C at the electrode tip or above 42°C at the anoderm surface.

The patients selected are generally those with mild to moderate complaints of fecal incontinence who have failed conservative measures including dietary modification, pharmacotherapy and biofeedback, and do not have a demonstrable

TABLE 18-2. Secca® procedure for treatment of fecal incontinence

Author (year)	No. of patients	CCF-FIS Preoperative	CCF-FIS Postoperative	*P* value	Duration of follow-up (months)
Takahashi (2002)[63]	10	13.5	5.0	<0.001	12
Takahashi (2003)[64]	10	13.5	7.3	0.002	24
Efron (2003)[65]	50	14.5	11.1	<0.0001	6
Takehashi-Monroy (2008)[62]	19	14.37	8.26	<0.00025	60

CCF-FIS = Cleveland Clinic Florida Fecal Incontinence Score.

sphincter defect. To date, the studies have been limited by either small sample size or length of follow-up. Complications have been minor, and include bleeding and ulceration at an application site which can be immediate or delayed requiring a return to the operating room for oversewing.[62]

The Secca® procedure is typically performed in an outpatient, ambulatory setting under intravenous sedation with local anesthetic. Prophylactic antibiotics are given. The patient is positioned in either prone jack-knife or lithotomy, following which, the handpiece is inserted into the anal canal and lined up so the four needle electrodes will be deployed at the level of the dentate line. Radiofrequency is then delivered for 90 s to one quadrant. The process is then repeated for each of the four quadrants and at 5 mm level increments proximal to the dentate line. Dependant on the length of the anal canal, there should be 16–20 application sites.

Takehashi et al.[62] recently published their results on 19 patients at 5 years of follow-up, showing a durable improvement in mean CCF-FIS from 14.37 to 8.26 ($P<0.00025$). In 16 of the patients there was a >50% improvement in their incontinence score. The results are encouraging, but additional studies are warranted. Table 18-2 summarizes the results of the Secca® procedure for fecal incontinence.[62–65]

Injectables

Injection of a biocompatible bulking agent has been adapted from its initial reported successful application in the treatment of urinary incontinence.[66] Its chief application is for the treatment of minor fecal incontinence due to internal anal sphincter dysfunction.[56] This option gains significance because surgical repair of the internal anal sphincter has not been shown to be effective,[67–69] whereas more aggressive operations and their attendant complications are typically out of proportion to the complaints of this specific patient population. Proponents of this therapy cite the fact that it is a safe, minimally invasive therapy, typically administered on an outpatient basis, in some instances in an office setting with minimal complications under local anesthetic alone or with intravenous sedation.[70–73]

The technique involves injection of a bulking agent either into the anal submucosal or intersphincteric space. Currently the two most studied materials are silicone biomaterial and carbon-coated microbeads. The mechanism of action is not fully understood, but Davis et al.[74] suggested an increase in anal resting pressure secondary to augmentation of the anal cushions and restoration of anal canal symmetry. Other proposed mechanisms include bulking of the anal canal providing increased resistance to the passage of stool, allowing for improved sensation and that fibrosis over time contributes to increased sphincter muscle volume. Typically, the maximal improvement in fecal continence is observed within the first 1–6 months and appears durable up to 1–2 years later.[74–76] Because of concerns of absorption and migration of the bulking agent, further long-term data are still needed. Additionally, the ideal number and location of injections, utility of ultrasound guidance for said localization as well as which materials and volume are most suitable for injection have yet to be definitively determined. Table 18-3 summarizes the results of the use of injectables for the treatment of fecal incontinence.[77–81]

Operative Procedures

Anterior Overlapping Sphincteroplasty

Anterior overlapping sphincteroplasty is the mainstay surgical treatment for patients suffering from severe fecal incontinence in conjunction with an external sphincter defect (Table 18-4).[82–87] The patient is given a full mechanical bowel preparation. After induction of anesthesia, the patient is placed in the prone jack-knife position. Tapping of the buttocks provides excellent exposure. A transverse incision is made on the thin or absent perineal body. Lateral dissection allows for identification of the normal ends of the external anal sphincter musculature. Care should be taken not to proceed too far posterior due to the potential for injury to the nerves entering in this location. Once the muscle is isolated on each side, the dissection should proceed medial to the anterior aspect of the anal canal. Preservation of the scar tissue in this location is important for the ensuing repair as it is helpful in holding the sutures. There has been suggestion that the presence of overlapped scar tissue correlates with improved short-term outcome as well.[82] Care should be taken to avoid injury to either the vaginal wall or anal canal. At the proximal extent of the dissection, the levators are identified and plicated anteriorly. Following this, the medial scar is divided and the external anal sphincter muscles are

TABLE 18-3. Injectable anal sphincter bulking agents for treatment of minor fecal incontinence

Author (year)	N	Bulking agent	Significant improvement of fecal incontinence	Mean follow-up (months)
Shafik (1995)[77]	14	Autologous fat	Yes[a]	18.6
Kumar et al. (1998)[70]	17	GAX collagen	P value not reported	8
Kenefick et al. (2002)[71]	6	Silicone	Yes $P=0.04$	18
Weiss et al. (2002)[78]	10	Carbon-coated microbeads	Yes ($P=0.012$) FIS 13 to 10	6
Davis (2003)[74]	18	Carbon-coated microbeads	Yes ($P=0.003$) FIS 11.89 to 8.07	28.5
Tjiandra et al. (2004)[72]	82	Silicone	Yes ($P<0.001$)	6
Van der Hagen (2007)[79]		Silicone	Yes ($P<0.001$)	12
Altomare (2008)[75]	33	Carbon-coated microbeads	Yes ($P<0.001$) FIS 12 to 8	20.8
Aigner (2009)[76]	11	Carbon-coated microbeads	Yes ($P=0.003$) FIS 12.27 ± 0.97 to 4.91 ± 0.87	26.1
Tjiandra (2009)[80]	20	Silicone	Yes $P<0.0001$ at 6 months	12
	20	Carbon-coated microbeads	Yes $P<0.0001$ at 6 months	
Danielson (2009)[81]	34	Hyaluronic acid	Yes ($P=0.004$)	12

[a] All patients had complete continence at 2–3 months – following which all but three had deterioration of their results.

TABLE 18-4. Long-term results of anterior overlapping sphincteroplasty

Year	Author	N	Months follow-up	Results
2000	Karoui et al.[84]	74	40	45% Continent to solid and liquid
2002	Halverson and Hull[85]	49	69	4 Stomas 46% Continent to solid and liquid
2006	Barisic et al.[86]	65	60	48% "Good or excellent"
2009	Oom et al.[87]	120	69	37% "Good or excellent"

overlapped in the anterior midline (Figure 18-3A–C). Outcome after end-to-end repair is somewhat inferior to overlapping repair, whereas overlapping repair might be associated with more evacuation difficulties.[83] The initial results of anterior sphincteroplasty are promising; however, numerous authors have noted diminishing efficacy over time with disappointing long-term continence.

Parks Posterior Anal Repair

The Parks posterior anal repair has been described for the treatment of neurogenic fecal incontinence in those patients without a sphincter defect. The initial premise was that it lengthened the anal canal and corrected the anorectal angle.[88] A curved incision is made behind the anus and an anterior skin flap is dissected. The intersphincteric space is identified and dissected free up to the upper part of the anal canal where Waldeyer's fascia, a dense fibrous structure, is encountered. Division gives access to the pelvis. The rectum can be dissected free from the levator ani by blunt dissection. A lattice is constructed by plicating the pubococcygeus and, in a second layer, the puborectalis. Additional sutures are placed in the deep and superficial part of the external sphincter (Figure 18-4). Part of the skin is left open to prevent sepsis. This operation has not gained widespread support in the USA, possibly because of the published poor long-term results with continence rates of only 33% at 5 years.[89]

Sacral Nerve Stimulation

Sacral nerve stimulation (SNS) or neuromodulation was initially developed for the management of urinary incontinence. It was subsequently noted that in patients with fecal incontinence treated with SNS for urinary incontinence the fecal incontinence also improved. This observation prompted Matzel et al.[90] to successfully attempt treatment of three patients with fecal incontinence using SNS.

Unlike other therapeutic modalities, SNS is a staged procedure. The first stage is the percutaneous nerve evaluation (PNE) which serves as feasibility trial period lasting 2 weeks. Patients who experience an improvement of 50% or greater decrease in the number of incontinence episodes progress to the final stage and are offered placement of a permanent stimulator.

The electrode placement is performed under sterile conditions with fluoroscopic guidance. Stimulation of the S2, S3, and S4 nerve roots via their sacral foramina is tested. The goal is to elicit contraction of the levator ani and external anal sphincter with plantar flexion of the first two toes, seen with stimulation of S3. The purpose of direct stimulation of the sacral nerves is to recruit additional inactive motor

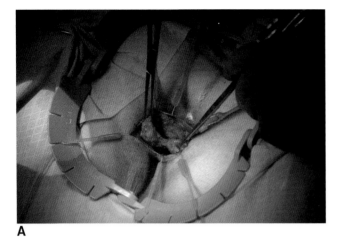

A

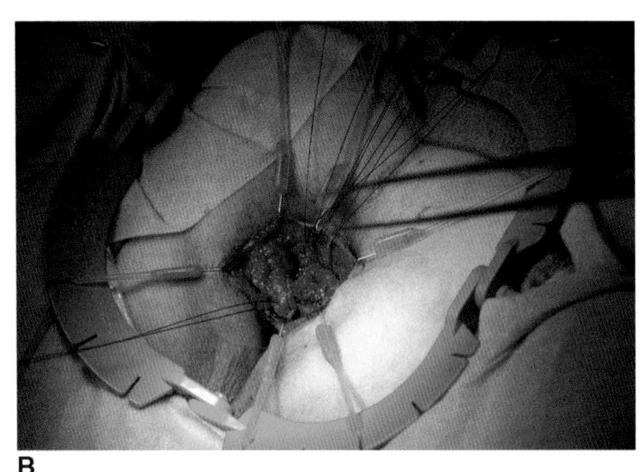

B

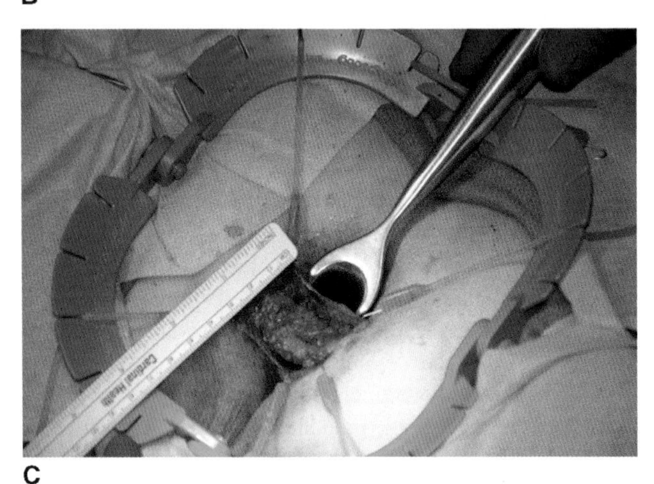

C

FIGURE 18-3. **A** Anterior overlapping sphincteroplasty. Overlapping and suturing of the external anal sphincter in the *midline*; **B** anterior overlapping sphincteroplasty. **C** Final repair with recreation of the perineal body.

units to improve muscle strength, resulting in an increase in resting anal pressure as demonstrated by Kenefick et al.[91] Additionally, SNS has been shown to improve the rectal sensory threshold and balloon expulsion time.[92]

Both the initial PNE and subsequent placement of the permanent stimulator are performed on an outpatient basis. Complications are rare and have all been minor with lead migration being most typical. Other complications include infection leading to explantation of the stimulator and pain attributed to either the leads of the stimulator.[93]

The obvious benefit of sacral nerve stimulation is that it avoids creation of an incision around or near the anal canal. This is important because it avoids further anal scarring as well as significantly decreases the risk of infection. When comparing sacral nerve stimulation to the artificial bowel sphincter, it has been proposed that SNS should be considered the first-line option due to the observed improved continence and decreased rate of outlet obstruction.[94]

Most recently, the results of the largest prospective randomized trial of the use of sacral nerve stimulation have been published. Sixteen centers in North America and Australia participated in the trial which included 129 patients who underwent the subchronic stimulation phase. Of the 129 patients, 120 qualified for permanent implantation by achieving a decrease in the incontinent episodes by at least 50% during the test phase. The mean follow-up period was 28 months. Persistent benefits of a 50% decrease in the weekly incontinence episodes, incontinent days and urgent incontinent episodes were noted in over 75% of the patients at all follow-up periods up to 36 months, with most of interval measurements over 80% success.[95] There was also a consistent improvement in quality of life throughout the study period.

While the device has still to obtain FDA approval in the USA, it has been used extensively in other countries. Promising short and long-term success has been reported with significant and sustained decreases in the CCF-FIS. The results of sacral nerve stimulation and summarized in Table 18-5.[96–104]

Artificial Bowel Sphincter

The artificial bowel sphincter was first reported in 1987.[105] A man with neurogenic incontinence had an artificial urinary sphincter inserted and he was able to have "complete control of defecation." The device was subsequently modified for the use around the anus. The procedure involves creating a subcutaneous tunnel around the anus, typically through a transverse perineal incision. The cuff is situated around the anus. The pump is tunneled through a pfannensteil incision down to either the labia or scrotum, while the reservoir is placed in the space of retzius (Figure 18-5A and B). All of the tubing is tunneled subcutaneously. The device provides continence by keeping the perianal cuff full in the resting state. When the patient needs to evacuate, he/she needs to actively pump fluid from the cuff to the reservoir. The cuff will then passively refill. When considering a patient for artificial bowel sphincter, it is important to ensure that there is not a significant soft tissue loss on the perineum which could preclude adequate coverage and guarantee erosion. It is also imperative to ensure that the patient will have the manual dexterity to activate the device.

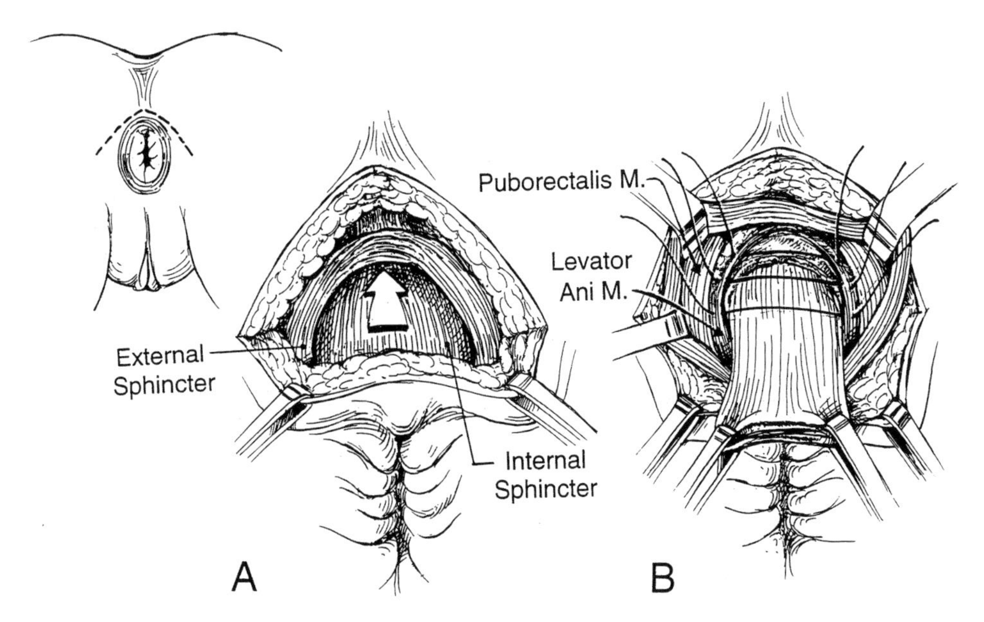

FIGURE 18-4. Postanal repair (with permission from Beck DE and Wexner SD, eds. Fundamentals of anorectal surgery, 2nd ed.).

TABLE 18-5. Results of sacral neuromodulation

			Fecal incontinence episodes/week		Cleveland Clinic Fecal Incontinence Score			
Author (year)	Patients (*N*)	Patients with permanent implant (*N*)	Baseline	Follow-up	Baseline	Follow-up	*P* value	Follow-up (months)
Leroi (2001)[96]	11	6	3.0	0.5				6
Rosen (2001)[97]	20	16	2.0	0.67				15
Uludag (2002)[98]	44	34	8.66	0.67				11
Matzel (2003)[99]	16	16	40% of movements	0% of movements	17	5	0.003	32.5
Jarrett (2003)[100]	59	46	7.5	1.0	14	6	<0.0001	12
Hetzer (2007)[101]	44	37			16	5	<0.001	13
Holzer (2007)[102]	36	29	2.33	0.67				
Tjandra (2008)[103]	60	53	9.5	3.1	16	1.2	<0.0001	12
Altomare (2009)[104]	94	60	3.5	0.7	15	5	<0.001	74
Wexner (2010)[95]	129	120	87% of patients decreased incontinent episodes per week by 50%					28

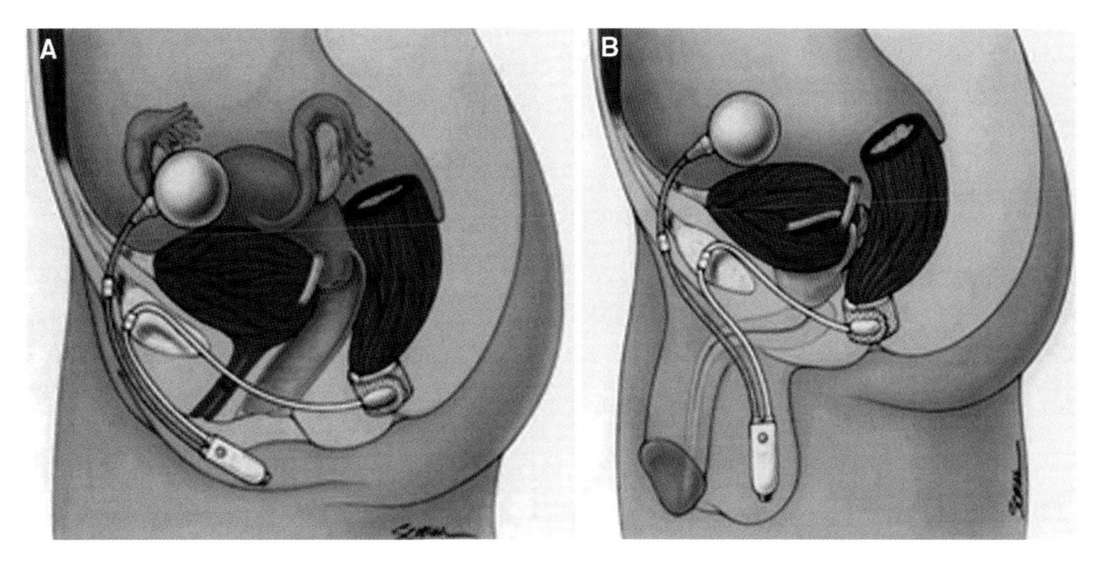

FIGURE 18-5. Artificial bowel sphincter. Artificial bowel sphincter implanted in the **A** female and **B** male patient (with permission from Acticon®, American Medical Systems®, Inc., Minnetonka, MN, http://www.AmericanMedicalSystems.com).

Infection has been the greatest challenge for patients and surgeons utilizing the artificial bowel sphincter. The results of a multicenter trial were published by Wong et al.[106] in 2002; 112 patients were implanted. There were 384 device-related adverse events in 99 patients. 246 required either no or noninvasive intervention. 73 revisional operations were performed in 51(46%) patients. Twenty-five percent of patients developed infection requiring surgical revision and 41(37%) patients had devices completely explanted. While the intention to treat success rate was low at 53%, 85% of patients with a functional device had a successful outcome. Recent reports of the long-term outcome for patients with the artificial bowel sphincter have been published.[107] Seventeen consecutive patients underwent sphincter implantation. The mean follow-up was 68 months (range: 3–133). All of the patients had some complication and 65% required at least one reoperation. As with other published series, 53% of the patients had an implanted device at follow-up. Those patients enjoyed the benefit of improved quality of life and significantly decreased fecal incontinence scores. Some factors associated with failure have been proposed. The experience from the Cleveland Clinic Florida suggested that early failures were more common with patients who had an early first postoperative bowel movement and who had a history of perineal sepsis. Early failure was more often related to infectious complications, while late failure was related to device associated mechanical complications.[108] There was a 41% infection rate noted in the series of 51 implantations, of these, 35% were early and 6% late. The major challenge of this treatment for fecal incontinence is infection followed by late device-related complications.

Muscle Transposition

The concept of substituting the anal sphincter was first reported by Chetwood in 1902[109] using the gluteus maximus. The ideal muscle for substitution of the sphincter complex should have a negligible role in movement and posture, yet it should be able to provide sufficient bulk. The muscle itself must have a reliable neurovascular bundle, so that it will not be damaged in the process of dissection.

The advantages of the gluteus maximus muscle are that it has a location in close proximity to the anal canal and provides excellent strength and bulk to the anal canal; however, its use poses significant functional impairment to the patient while standing or climbing stairs. The majority of data are case series, wherein a bilateral gluteus flap is performed; however, Devesa et al.[110] have suggested that a unilateral gluteus flap is simpler and yields superior results because of reduced tension on the muscular neosphincter. The major technical difficulty of this procedure is obtaining sufficient length to adequately encircle the anal canal.[111]

Gracilis Muscle Transposition

Gracilis muscle transposition was first reported by Pickrell in 1952[109] for the treatment of children with fecal incontinence due to neurologic and congenital anomalies. It is generally a treatment option best for those patients whose incontinence results from either trauma or congenital anomaly, where the additional muscle bulk can supplement deficient native tissue. A history of diarrhea, severe refractory constipation, obstetric injury, and advanced age generally predict a poor outcome and therefore are relative contraindications for this technique.

The essence of the operation is mobilization of the gracilis muscle followed by transposition of the muscle around the anus and fixation to the contralateral ischial tuberosity. In concept the gracilis acts as a barrier to the passage of stool by acting as a living Thiersch. The patient is placed in the lithotomy position and prepped beyond the knee. Because the blood supply for the gracilis is based proximally, the distal end of the gracilis can be freely mobilized. The gracilis is first identified by palpating and marking its course from the pubic arch to the upper medial tubercle of the tibia. Generally the muscle is mobilized via three separate incisions over the course of the muscle, with division of the gracilis tendon at its insertion on the tibia. Special care is taken at the cephalad dissection to identify and preserve the neurovascular bundle, which defines the proximal limit of dissection. A tunnel is then created between the proximal incision and two incisions placed approximately 1.5–2.0 cm from the anal verge located anteriorly and posteriorly. A circumferential tunnel is also created in the ischirectal fossae between the perianal incisions. The distal portion of the gracilis is then passed around the anus, under the anterior and posterior raphe and encompassing any existing native sphincter muscle. The muscle is then anchored to the contralateral ischial tuberosity with a nonabsorbable suture. The completed graciloplasty should admit one finger snuggly.

Functionally, most patients are only able to control the passage of solid stool. The additional limitation is that skeletal muscle is more easily fatigued, leading Salmons[112] to suggest use of a stimulator to convert fast-twitch (type II) muscle fibers in the gracilis into slow-twitch (type I) that comprise 80% of the external sphincters found in cadavers.[113] Complications associated with graciloplasty include evacuatory dysfunction, pain in the perineum or with contraction of gracilis, and infection. Additional complications specific to the stimulated graciloplasty include lead displacement and erosion, nerve fibrosis, and implant infection. A randomized, controlled trial comparing unstimulated to stimulated graciloplasty has not been done. In the USA, the stimulator is not available for implantation; however, it remains a viable option for a highly selected group patients in other countries.

Fecal Diversion

Creation of a colostomy or ileostomy is typically the therapeutic option of last resort, when all other reasonable options have been exhausted. The majority of patients will be best

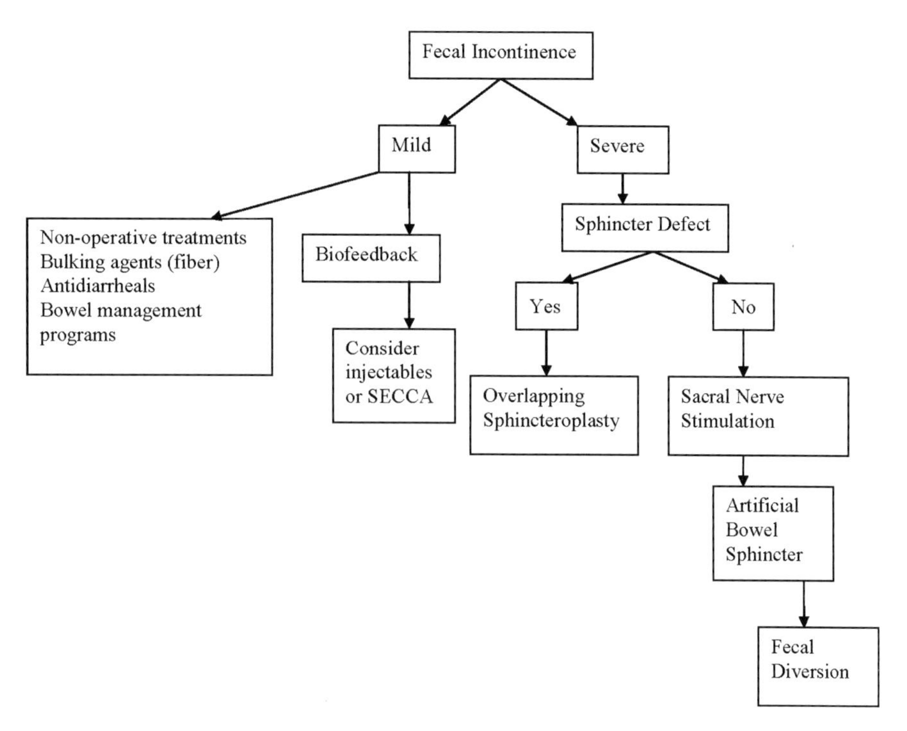

FIGURE 18-6. Algorithm for the management of fecal incontinence.

served with an end sigmoid colostomy, but some patients with chronic constipation and slow transit may be best served with an ileostomy. Predictably, strong resistance even in the face of severe and debilitating incontinence is common. Patient education in the form of a visit with an enterostomal therapist and perhaps a patient already living with an ostomy can greatly ease anxiety. It is important to emphasize there is no time-limit for the decision to convert an uncontrolled perineal stoma to a more easily managed abdominal one.

Conclusion

Fecal incontinence is a socially devastating condition which is extremely common and under reported. There are many options available for patients who can treat or significantly improve their symptoms. The first step for the physician is to diagnose the problem. This will often not take place until the examiner specifically asks the patient as they will often not offer the information. Through a detailed history, the physician can formulate a differential diagnosis. Anorectal physiologic testing can add specific information with regards to the functional status to the sphincter musculature. Many patients quality of life can be improved with noninvasive modalities focused on improving stool consistency and strengthening of the musculature with biofeedback.

If there is a significant impact on quality of life and the patient is a candidate for invasive therapy, surgical intervention should be considered. The overlapping sphincteroplasty remains the mainstay of surgical treatment when a sphincter defect is present. When a defect is absent or the sphincteroplasty has failed, sacral nerve stimulation and the artificial bowel sphincter are options. For less severe forms of incontinence, injectables and SECCA may be of benefit. Figure 18-6 provides a generalized algorithm for the management of fecal incontinence.

Acknowledgments. This chapter was written by Cornelius Baeten and Hans Kuijpers in the previous version of this textbook.

References

1. Kuehn BM. Silence masks prevalence of fecal incontinence. JAMA. 2006;295:1362–3.
2. Nelson RL. Epidemiology of fecal incontinence. Gastroenterology. 2004;126:s3–7.
3. Whitehead WE, Wald A, Norton NJ. Treatment options for fecal incontinence. Dis Colon Rectum. 2001;44:131–44.
4. Nelson R, Norton N, Cautley E, et al. Community-based prevalence of anal incontinence. JAMA. 1995;274:559–61.
5. Bharucha AE, Zinmeister AR, Locke GR, et al. Prevalence and burden of fecal incontinence: a population-based study in women. Gastroenterology. 2005;129:42–9.
6. Sangwan YP, Coller JA. Fecal incontinence. Surg Clin North Am. 1994;74:1377–98.
7. Johanson JF, Lafferty J. Epidemiololgy of fecal incontinence: the silent affliction. Am J Gastroenterol. 1996;91:33–6.
8. Zetterstrom J, Mellgren A, Jensen LL, et al. Effect of delivery on anal sphincter morphology and function. Dis Colon Rectum. 1999;42(10):1253–60.

9. Damon H, Henry L, Barth X, Mion F. Fecal incontinence in females with a past history of vaginal delivery: significance of anal sphincter defects detected by ultrasound. Dis Colon Rectum. 2002;45(11):1445–50. discussion 1450–1.
10. Suilleabhain CB, Horgan AF, McEnroe L, et al. The relationship of pudendal nerve terminal motor latency to squeeze pressure in patients with idiopathic fecal incontinence. Dis Colon Rectum. 2001;44(5):666–71.
11. Davis K, Kumar D, Stanton SL, et al. Symptoms and anal sphincter morphology following primary repair of third-degree tears. Br J Surg. 2003;90(12):1573–9.
12. Bollard RC, Gardiner A, Duthie GS, Lindow SW. Anal sphincter injury, fecal and urinary incontinence: a 34-year follow-up after forceps delivery. Dis Colon Rectum. 2003;46(8):1083–8.
13. Sultan AH, Kamm MA, Hudson CN, et al. Anal-sphincter disruption during vaginal delivery. N Engl J Med. 1993;329(26):1905–11.
14. Snooks SJ, Henry MM, Swash M. Faecal incontinence due to external anal sphincter division in childbirth is associated with damage to the innervation of the pelvic floor musculature: a double pathology. Br J Obstet Gynaecol. 1985;92(8):824–8.
15. Jacobs PP, Scheuer M, Kuijpers JH, Vingerhoets MH. Obstetric fecal incontinence. Role of pelvic floor denervation and results of delayed sphincter repair. Dis Colon Rectum. 1990;33(6):494–7.
16. Nyam DC, Pemberton JH. Long-term results of lateral internal sphincterotomy for chronic anal fissure with particular reference to incidence of fecal incontinence. Dis Colon Rectum. 1999;42(10):1306–10.
17. Garcia-Aguilar J, Belmonte C, Wong WD, et al. Open vs. closed sphincterotomy for chronic anal fissure: long-term results. Dis Colon Rectum. 1996;39(4):440–3.
18. van Tets WF, Kuijpers HC. Continence disorders after anal fistulotomy. Dis Colon Rectum. 1994;37(12):1194–7.
19. Garcia-Aguilar J, Belmonte C, Wong WD, et al. Anal fistula surgery. Factors associated with recurrence and incontinence. Dis Colon Rectum. 1996;39(7):723–9.
20. Konsten J, Baeten CG. Hemorrhoidectomy vs. Lord's method: 17-year follow-up of a prospective, randomized trial. Dis Colon Rectum. 2000;43(4):503–6.
21. Hetzer FH, Demartines N, Handschin AE, Clavien PA. Stapled vs excision hemorrhoidectomy: long-term results of a prospective randomized trial. Arch Surg. 2002;137(3):337–40.
22. Zimmerman DD, Briel JW, Gosselink MP, Schouten WR. Anocutaneous advancement flap repair of transsphincteric fistulas. Dis Colon Rectum. 2001;44(10):1474–80.
23. Gee ASS, Durdey P. Urge incontinence of faeces is a marker of severe external anal sphincter dysfunction. Br J Surg. 1995;82:1179–82.
24. Deutekom M, Terra MP, Dobben AC, et al. Selecting an outcome measure for evaluating treatment in fecal incontinence. Dis Colon Rectum. 2005;48(12):2294–301.
25. Jorge JM, Wexner SD. Etiology and management of fecal incontinence. Dis Colon Rectum. 1993;36:77–97.
26. Sultan AH, Nicholls RJ, Kamm MA, et al. Anal endosonography and correlation with in vitro and in vivo anatomy. Br J Surg. 1993;80:508–11.
27. Oberwalder M, Thaler K, Baig MK, et al. Anal ultrasound and endosonographic measurement of perineal body thickness: a new evaluation for fecal incontinence in females. Surg Endosc. 2004;18(4):650–4.
28. Roberts PL. Principles of manometry. Semin Colon Rectal Surg. 1992;3(2):64–7.
29. Jorge JM, Wexner SD. Anorectal manometry: techniques and clinical applications. South Med J. 1993;86(8):924–31.
30. Coller JA. Clinical application of anorectal manometry. Gastroenterol Clin North Am. 1987;16:17–33.
31. Lestar B, Pennicykxx F, Kerremans R. The composition of anal basal pressure. Int J Colorectal Dis. 1989;4:118–22.
32. Gilliland R, Altomare DF, Moriera H, et al. Pudendal neuropathy is predictive of failure following anterior overlapping sphincteroplasty. Dis Colon Rectum. 1998;41(12):1516–22.
33. Sangwan YP, Coller JA, Barrett RC, et al. Unilateral pudendal neuropathy. Impact on outcome after anal sphincter repair. Dis Colon Rectum. 1996;39(6):686–9.
34. Chen AS, Luchtefeld MA, Senagore AJ, et al. Pudendal nerve latency. Does it predict outcome after anal sphincter repair? Dis Colon Rectum. 1998;41(8):1005–9.
35. Rosato GO, Lumi C, Miguel MA. Anal sphincter electromyography and pudendal nerve terminal motor latency assessment. Semin Colon Rectal Surg. 1992;3(2):68–74.
36. Burnett SJD, Speakman CTM, Kamm MA, et al. Confirmation of endosonographic detection of external anal sphincter defects by simultaneous electromyographic mapping. Br J Surg. 1991;78:448–50.
37. Cheetham M, Brazzelli M, Norton C, et al. Drug treatment for fecal incontinence in adults. Cochrane Database Syst Rev. 2003;4:1–26.
38. Saito T, Mizutani F, Iwanaga Y, et al. Calcium polycarbophil, a water-absorbing polymer, increases bowel movement and prevents sennoside-induced diarrhea in dogs. Jpn J Pharmacol. 2000;83:206–14.
39. Saito T, Mizutani F, Iwanaga Y, et al. Laxative and antidiarrheal activity of polycarbophil in mice and rats. Jpn J Pharmacol. 2002;89:133–41.
40. Bliss DZ, Jung HJ, Savok K, et al. Supplementation with dietary fiber improves fecal incontinence. Nurs Res. 2001;50:203–13.
41. Goode PS, Burgio KL, Halli AD, et al. Prevalence and correlates of fecal incontinence in community-dwelling older adults. J Am Geriatr Soc. 2005;53:629–35.
42. Drossman DA. What can be done to control incontinence associated with irritable bowel syndrome. Am J Gastroenterol. 1989;84:365–6.
43. Hallgren T, Fasth S, Delbro DS, et al. Loperamide improves anal sphincter function and continence after restorative proctocolectomy. Dig Dis Sci. 1994;39:2612–8.
44. Read M, Read NW, Barber DC, et al. Effects of loperamide on anal sphincter function in patients complaining chronic diarrhea with fecal incontinence and urgency. Dig Dis Sci. 1982;27:807–14.
45. Santoro GA, Eitan BZ, Pryde A, et al. Open study of low-dose amitriptyline in the treatment of patients with idiopathic fecal incontinence. Dis Colon Rectum. 2000;43:1676–82.
46. Chassagen P, Jego A, Gloc P, et al. Does treatment of constipation improve fecal incontinence in institutionalized elderly patients? Age Ageing. 2000;29:159–64.
47. Engel BT, Nikoomanesh P, Schuster MM. Operant conditioning of rectosphincteric responses in the treatment of fecal incontinence. N Engl J Med. 1974;290:646–9.
48. Heymen S, Scarlett Y, Jones K, et al. Randomized controlled trial shows biofeedback to be superior to pelvic floor exercises for fecal incontinence. Dis Colon Rectum. 2009;52:1730–7.

49. Olness K, McParland FA, Piper J. Biofeedback: a new modality in the management of children with fecal soiling. J Pediatr. 1980;96:505–9.
50. Solomon MH, Pager CK, Rex J, et al. Randomized, controlled trial of biofeedback with anal manometry, transanal ultrasound, or pelvic floor retraining with digital guidance alone in the treatment of mild to moderate fecal incontinence. Dis Colon Rectum. 2003;46:703–10.
51. Heymen S, Jones KR, Ringel Y, et al. Biofeedback treatment of fecal incontinence: a critical review. Dis Colon Rectum. 2001;44:728–36.
52. Norton C, Kamm MA. Anal sphincter biofeedback and pelvic floor exercises for faecal incontinence in adults: a systematic review. Aliment Pharmacol Ther. 2001;15:1147–54.
53. Norton C, Chelvanayagam S, Wilson-Barnett J, et al. Randomized controlled trial of biofeedback for fecal incontinence. Gastroenterology. 2003;125:1320–9.
54. Byrne CM, Solomon MJ, Young JM, et al. Biofeedback for fecal incontinence: short-term outcomes of 513 consecutive patients and predictors of successful treatment. Dis Colon Rectum. 2007;50:417–27.
55. Norton C, Cody JD, Hosker G. Biofeedback and/or sphincter exercises for the treatment of faecal incontinence in adults. Cochrane Database Syst Rev. 2006; CD002111.
56. Tjandra JJ, Dykes SL, Kumar RR, et al. Practice parameters for the treatment of fecal incontinence. Dis Colon Rectum. 2007;50:1497–507.
57. Gustavson KH. On the chemistry of collagen. Fed Proc. 1964;23:613–7.
58. Triadafilopoulous G, Di Basie JK, Nostrant TT, et al. The Stretta procedure for the treatment of GERD: 6 and 12 month follow-up of the US open label trial. Gastrointest Endosc. 2002;55:149–56.
59. Hecht P, Hayashi K, Lu Y, et al. Monopolar radiofrequency energy effects on joint capsular tissue: potential treatment for join instability. An in vivo mechanical, morphological, and biochemical study using an ovine model. Am J Sports Med. 1999;27:761–71.
60. Dawkins GP, Harrison NW, Ansell W. Radiofrequency heat-treatment to the prostate for bladder outlet obstruction associated with benign prostatic hyperplasia: a 4-year outcome study. Br J Urol. 1997;79:910–4.
61. Powell NB, Riley RW, Troell RJ, et al. Radiofrequency volumetric tissue reduction of the palate in subjects with sleep-disordered breathing. Chest. 1998;113:1163–74.
62. Takahashi-Monroy T, Morales M, Garcia-Osogobio S, et al. Secca procedure for the treatment of fecal incontinence: results of five-year follow-up. Dis Colon Rectum. 2008;51:355–9.
63. Takahashi T, Garcia-Osogobio S, Valdovinos MA, et al. Radio-frequency energy delivery for the treatment of fecal incontinence. Dis Colon Rectum. 2002;45:915–9.
64. Takahashi T, Garcia-Osogobio S, Valdovinos MA, et al. Extended two-year results of radio-frequency energy delivery for the treatment of fecal incontinence. Dis Colon Rectum. 2003;46:711–5.
65. Efron JE, Corman ML, Fleshman J, et al. Safety and effectiveness of temperature-controlled radio-frequency energy delivery to the anal canal (Secca procedure) for the treatment of fecal incontinence. Dis Colon Rectum. 2003;46:1606–18.
66. Lightner D, Calvosa C, Andersen R, et al. A new injectable bulking agent for treatment of stress urinary incontinence: results of a multicenter, randomized, controlled, double-blind study of Durasphere. Urology. 2001;58:12–5.
67. Felt-Bersma RJ, Cuesta MA, Koorevaar M. Anal sphincter repair improves anorectal function and endosonographic image. A prospective clinical study. Dis Colon Rectum. 1996;39:878–85.
68. Leroi AM, Kamm MA, Weber J, et al. Internal anal sphincter repair. Int J Colorectal Dis. 1997;12:243–5.
69. Morgan R, Patel B, Beynon J, et al. Surgical management of anorectal incontinence due to internal anal sphincter deficiency. Br J Surg. 1997;84:226–30.
70. Kumar D, Benson MJ, Bland JE. Glutaraldehyde cross-linked collagen in the treatment of fecal incontinence. Br J Surg. 1998;85:987–9.
71. Kenefick NJ, Vaizey CJ, Malouf AJ, et al. Injectable silicone biomaterial for faecal incontinence due to internal anal sphincter dysfunction. Gut. 2002;51:225–8.
72. Tjiandra JJ, Lim JF, Hiscock R, et al. Injectable silicone biomaterial for fecal incontinence caused by internal anal sphincter dysfunction is effective. Dis Colon Rectum. 2004;47:2138–46.
73. Vaizey CJ, Kamm MA. Injectable bulking agents for treating faecal incontinence. Br J Surg. 2005;92:521–7.
74. Davis K. Preliminary evaluation of an injectable anal sphincter bulking agent (Durasphere) in the management of faecal incontinence. Aliment Pharmacol Ther. 2003;18:237–43.
75. Altomare DF, La Torre F, Rinaldi M, et al. Carbon-coated microbeads anal injection in outpatient treatment of minor fecal incontinence. Dis Colon Rectum. 2008;51:432–5.
76. Aigner F, Conrad F, Margreiter R, et al. Anal submucosal carbon bead injection for treatment of idiopathic fecal incontinence: a preliminary report. Dis Colon Rectum. 2009;52:293–8.
77. Shafik A. Perianal injection of autologous fat for treatment of sphincteric incontinence. Dis Colon Rectum. 1995;38:583–7.
78. Weiss EG, Efron JE, Nogueras JJ, et al. Submucosal injection of carbon-coated beads is a successful and safe office-based treatment for fecal incontinence. Dis Colon Rectum. 2002;45:A46.
79. Van der Hagen SJ, van Gemert WG, et al. PTQ implants in the treatment of faecal soiling. Br J Surg. 2007;94:222–3.
80. Tjiandra JJ. Injectable silicone biomaterial (PTQ) is more effective than carbon-coated beads (Durasphere) in treating passive faecal incontinence – a randomized trial. Colorectal Dis. 2009;11:382–9.
81. Danielson J, Karlbom U, Sonesson AC, et al. Submucosal injection of stabilized nonanimal hyaluronic acid with dextranomer: a new treatment option for fecal incontinence. Dis Colon Rectum. 2009;52:1101–6.
82. Moscovitz I, Rotholtz NA, Baig MK, et al. Overlapping sphincteroplasty does preservation of the scar influence immediate outcome? Colorectal Dis. 2002;4(4):275–9.
83. Tjandra JJ, Han WR, Goh J, et al. Direct repair vs. overlapping sphincter repair: a randomized, controlled trial. Dis Colon Rectum. 2003;46(7):937–42. discussion 942–3.
84. Karoui S, Leroi AM, Koning E, et al. Results of sphincteroplasty in 86 patients with anal incontinence. Dis Colon Rectum. 2000;43(6):813–20.
85. Halverson AL, Hull TL. Long-term outcome of overlapping anal sphincter repair. Dis Colon Rectum. 2002;45(3):345–8.
86. Barisic GI, Krivokapic ZV, Markovic VA, et al. Outcome of overlapping anal sphincter repair after 3 months and after a mean of 80 months. Int J Colorectal Dis. 2006;21(1):52–6.

87. Oom DM, Gosselink MP, Schouten WR. Anterior sphincteroplasty for fecal incontinence: a single center experience in the era of sacral neuromodulation. Dis Colon Rectum. 2009;52(10):1681–7.
88. Browning GG, Parks AG. Postanal repair for neuropathic faecal incontinence: correlation of clinical result and anal canal pressures. Br J Surg. 1983;70(2):101–4.
89. Carraro PS, Kamm MA, Nichols RJ. Longterm results of postanal repair for neurogenic fecal incontinence. Br J Surg. 1994;81:140–4.
90. Matzel KE, Stadelmaier U, Hohenfellner M, et al. Electrical stimulation of sacral spinal nerves for treatment of faecal incontinence. Lancet. 1995;346:1124–7.
91. Kenefick NJ, Emmanuel A, Nicholls RJ, et al. Effect of sacral nerve stimulation on autonomic nerve function. Br J Surg. 2003;90:1256–60.
92. Ganio E, Masin A, Ratto C, et al. Short-term sacral nerve stimulation for functional anorectal and urinary disturbances: results in 40 patients: evaluation of a new option for ano-rectal functional disorders. Dis Colon Rectum. 2001; 44:1261–7.
93. Jarrett ME, Mowatt G, Glazener CM, et al. Systematic review of sacral nerve stimulation for faecal incontinence and constipation. Br J Surg. 2004;91:1559–69.
94. Meurette G, La Torre M, Regenet N, et al. Value of sacral nerve stimulation in the treatment of severe faecal incontinence: a comparison to the artificial bowel sphincter. Colorectal Dis. 2009;11(6):631–5. Epub 2008 Jul 15.
95. Wexner SD, Coller JA, Devroede G, et al. Sacral nerve stimulation for fecal incontinence: results of a 120-patient prospective multicenter study. Ann Surg. 2010;251(3):441–9.
96. Leroi AM, Michot F, Grise P, et al. Effect of sacral nerve stimulation in patients with fecal and urinary incontinence. Dis Colon Rectum. 2001;44:779–89.
97. Rosen HR, Urbarz C, Holzer B, et al. Sacral nerve stimulation as a treatment for fecal incontinence. Gastroenterology. 2001;121:536–41.
98. Uludag O, Dejong HC. Sacral neuromodulation for faecal incontinence. Dis Colon Rectum. 2002;45:A34–6.
99. Matzel KE, Bittorf B, Stadelmaier U, et al. Sacral nerve stimulation in the treatment of faecal incontinence. Chirurg. 2003;74:26–32.
100. Jarrett ME, Varma JS, Duthie GS, et al. Sacral nerve stimulation for faecal incontinence in the UK. Br J Surg. 2003;91:755–61.
101. Hetzer FH, Hahnloser D, Clavien PA, et al. Quality of life and morbidity after permanent sacral nerve stimulation for fecal incontinence. Arch Surg. 2007;142:8–13.
102. Holzer B, Rosen HR, Novi G, et al. Sacral nerve stimulation for neurogenic faecal incontinence. Br J Surg. 2007;94:749–53.
103. Tjandra JJ, Chan MK, Yeh CH, et al. Sacral nerve stimulation is more effective than optimal medical therapy for severe fecal incontinence: a randomized, controlled study. Dis Colon Rectum. 2008;51:494–502.
104. Altomare DF, Ratto C, Ganio E, et al. Long-term outcome of sacral nerve stimulation for fecal incontinence. Dis Colon Rectum. 2009;52:11–7.
105. Christiansen J, Lorentzen M. Implantation of artificial sphincter for anal incontinence. Lancet. 1987;2(8553):244–5.
106. Wong WD, Congliosi SM, Spencer MP, et al. The safety and efficacy of the artificial bowel sphincter for fecal incontinence: results from a multicenter cohort study. Dis Colon Rectum. 2002;45(9):1139–53.
107. Ruiz Carmona MD, Alós Company R, Roig Vila JV, et al. Long-term results of artificial bowel sphincter for the treatment of severe faecal incontinence. Are they what we hoped for? Colorectal Dis. 2009;11(8):831–7. Epub 2008 Jul 25.
108. Wexner SD, Jin HY, Weiss EG, et al. Factors associated with failure of the artificial bowel sphincter: a study of over 50 cases from Cleveland Clinic Florida. Dis Colon Rectum. 2009;52(9):1550–7.
109. Chetwood CH. Plastic operation of the sphincter ani with report of a case. Med Rec. 1902;61:529.
110. Devesa JM, Vincente E, Enriquez JM, et al. Total fecal incontinence: a new method of gluteus maximum transposition. Preliminary results and report of previous experience with similar procedures. Dis Colon Rectum. 1992;35:339.
111. Prochiantz A, Gross P. Gluteal myoplasty for sphincter replacement: principles, results and prospects. J Pediatr Surg. 1982;17:25.
112. Salmons S. The adaptive response of skeletal muscle to increased use. Muscle Nerve. 1981;4:94–105.
113. Konsten J, Baeten CGMI, Haventih MG, et al. Morphology of dynamic graciloplasty compared with the anal sphincter. Dis Colon Rectum. 1993;36:559–63.

19 Pelvic Floor Disorders

Patrick Y.H. Lee and Guillaum Meurette

Pelvic floor disorders are mostly a continuum of a disease process resulting from the loss of pelvic floor support. Although these diseases are commonly believed to afflict primarily women, the ease in examination of the pelvic floor in women makes the identification of pelvic floor disorders easier in women than in men. Anatomical differences in the size of the genital hiatus between the sexes also make women more prone to pelvic floor prolapse. Epidemiologic studies on pelvic floor prolapse suggest that it is a disease that will become more prevalent as the population ages. Olsen et al.[1] reported the findings of pelvic organ prolapse on 149,554 women aged 20 years or older at Kaiser Permanente; their study showed that 11.1% of these women will have a lifetime risk of undergoing an operation related to pelvic prolapse or incontinence by the age of 80. Surgical repair related to the rectum or posterior compartment constituted 45% of the operations. Reoperation for prolapse was 29.9%, and the time interval between repeat procedures decreased with each successive repair.[1] According to the government census, the population in the USA is projected to reach 440 million by 2050, and the population of 75 years old or older is projected to increase from 6% to 11%.[2] These findings and trends help highlight the importance of pelvic floor disorders and the role of the colorectal specialist in the management of pelvic floor disorders.

Despite the incomplete knowledge on the etiology of pelvic floor laxity and prolapse, surgical management is one of the most important modalities in the repair of the pelvic floor in women. Hence, successful repair of the pelvic floor requires a good understanding not only of the pelvic floor anatomy, but also of the dynamic interaction between pelvic floor muscles and organs. The anatomy discussed here will primarily focus on how pelvic organs are supported and the pathologic changes of pelvic floor prolapse. The pelvic floor disorders that will be discussed are rectocele, defecatory dysfunction, and rectal and genital prolapse. The disease processes will be correlated with the anatomic changes seen on physical exams and radiologic studies. Restoration of function is the ultimate goal in any treatment, and how that is accomplished with the current surgical techniques will be discussed.

Grant's Atlas and Netter's anatomic drawings of the pelvis need no introduction,[3,4] but they provide very little in the understanding of the dynamic interaction between pelvic musculature and ligamentous connective tissue in the stabilization of pelvic organs. The levator ani complex and the supporting or endopelvic fascia are the two most important dynamic structures of the pelvis that are extensively discussed in the gynecologic, urologic, and colorectal literatures. In the resting state, the levator ani muscle group (puborectalis, pubococcygeus, and iliococcygeus) is in a constant state of contraction.[5] Magnetic resonance imaging (MRI) of the normal pelvic floor in a woman shows the levator ani complex to have a hyperbolic or biconcave shape posteriorly and a sling-like appearance around the rectum, vagina, and urethra anteriorly (Figure 19-1A and B).[6,7] Anatomically, the iliococcygeus forms the posterior biconvex shape on the MRI and functions to support the rectum. The puborectalis slings around the rectum, vagina, and urethra. Singh et al.[8] describe the puborectalis as a belt, which encases the pelvic organs and contracts in a dorsoventral direction to close the levator hiatus and thus maintain continence. Lawson[9] in his dissection of the pelvis of neonates and infants, describes the pubococcygeus as a vertical sling, which has very little fiber going to the coccyx and has muscle fibers which interdigitate with the anorectum, vagina, urethra, and perineal body.[10] The exact etiology of the loss of the levator ani muscle integrity resulting in pelvic floor prolapse is unclear. Animal models show that chronic stretching of the pelvic muscles leads to myopathic injury.[11]

The supporting or endopelvic fascia is a more complex and controversial structure than the levator ani. Located between the visceral peritoneum and parietal fascia of the levator ani is fibroareolar tissue containing neurovascular bundles, smooth muscles, collagen, and elastin, which is often called the endopelvic or endovisceral fascia.[12] In Figure 19-2, the endopelvic fascia is drawn as a layer which fans out to envelop the pelvic organs and anchors them to

D.E. Beck et al. (eds.), *The ASCRS Textbook of Colon and Rectal Surgery: Second Edition*,
DOI 10.1007/978-1-4419-1584-9_19, © Springer Science+Business Media, LLC 2011

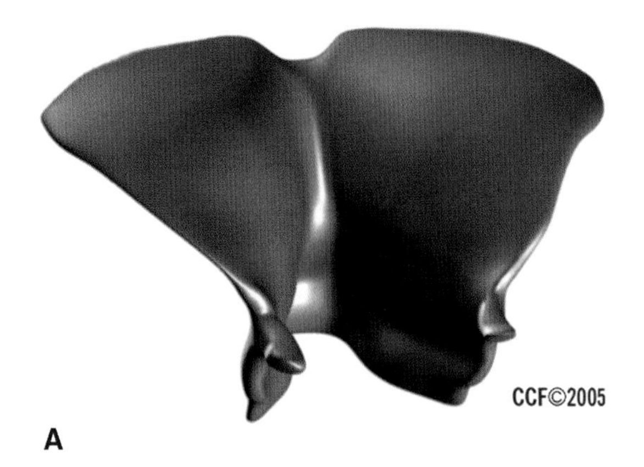

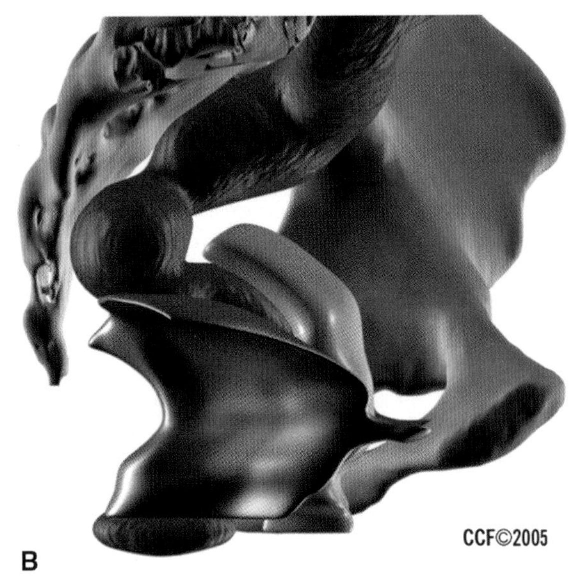

FIGURE 19-1. **A** and **B**. Digitally enhanced MRI reconstruction of the levator ani at rest in a 23-year-old nulliparous woman. The levator ani gives a biconcave shape posteriorly and the puborectalis show as a sling imbedded in the muscle of the pelvic floor. (Reprinted with permission from Cleveland Clinic Center for Medical Art and Photography© 2004–2009 and Matthew Barber, MD).

the surrounding pelvic side wall structures such as the uterosacral ligament, arcus tendineus fascia pelvis, and perineal body.[6] DeLancey calls the endopelvic fascia the viscero-fascial layer because it is a combination of the pelvic viscera and endopelvic fascia and plays a key role in the support of the vagina and uterus.[10,13,14] Norton[15] has described the interaction between levator ani and endopelvic fascia as the "boat in the dry dock." The levator ani is like the water in a dry dock that floats the boat, and the ligaments are like the mooring that holds the boat in place. When the water in the dock begins to recede, the moorings are strained to hold the boat in place. Similarly, as the levator ani begins to lose its integrity, the ligaments are stretched and at some point will lose their ability to hold the pelvic organs in place. Norton postulated that collagen composition changes with injury and results in a higher concentration of the weaker type III than stronger type I collagen. It is unknown if this transformation of collagen type is permanent. The replacement of collagen type and the loss of elasticity in the endopelvic fascia are believed to result in the loss of fascial ability to return the pelvic organs to their appropriate anatomic alignment.

Clinical studies of patients with collagen and elastin defects like those found in patients with Marfan and Ehlers–Danlos syndrome show a 42 and 50% incidence of urinary incontinence and a 33 and 75% incidence of pelvic organ prolapse, respectively.[16] Similarly, patients with hypermobile joints have a higher prevalence of cystocele, 89% versus 58% ($p=0.001$); rectocele, 84% versus 48% ($p=0.0002$); and uterine or vault prolapse, 66% versus 29% ($p=0.0002$).[17] Soderberg et al.[18] showed that women younger than 53 years of age with genital prolapse had a 30% lower collagen concentration than age-matched controls ($p=0.01$). In patients with complex multiorgan prolapse, Sullivan et al.[19] found a 44% incidence of arthritis in women with pelvic floor prolapse, suggesting an underlying collagen vascular disease. Their findings are supported by epidemiologic studies of women in Sweden which showed that genital prolapse, urinary and fecal incontinence were associated with obesity, chronic bronchitis, vaginal delivery, age, heredity, and diseases suggestive of collagen vascular disorders.[20]

Despite a well-established consensus in the gynecologic literature that the endopelvic fascia exists, there remains controversy over its existence or significance. Berglass and Rubin[21] in 1953 confirmed the works of earlier anatomists that there are no histologic findings to support a well-defined sheath around the rectum, vagina, and bladder to be termed "fascia." In 2004, Fritsch et al.[22] published their extensive anatomical and histologic study of the pelvis of 11 adults (6 female and 5 male), 7 newborns, and 79 fetuses and concluded that the endopelvic fascia does not exist. They concluded that pelvic floor support is dependent on intact pelvic floor muscles, undisturbed topography of the pelvic organs, and intact perineum. Regardless of the controversies on the existence and significance of the endopelvic fascia, all anatomists and surgeons agree that lying between the rectum and vagina or prostate is a fascial septum that is attached to the perineal body; in women that is known as the rectovaginal fascia and in men Denonvilliers' fascia. The importance of this fascia and the perineal body will become apparent in the findings and repair of pelvic organ prolapse.

Equally important to the understanding of pelvic anatomy is an understanding of the dynamic changes of the pelvic organs. Visualization of the dynamic changes between pelvic floor and pelvic organs was first described by Burhenne in 1963,[23] when he performed cinefluorography on the rectum during defecation. These studies have evolved to include evaluation of the bladder, vagina, and small bowel during evacuation. Kelvin and associates[24] popularized the use of four-contrast study to outline the small bowel, bladder, vagina, and rectum. The dynamic evaluation of the pelvic floor before, during, and after evacuation of the contrasts in the rectum and bladder not only yields a tremendous amount

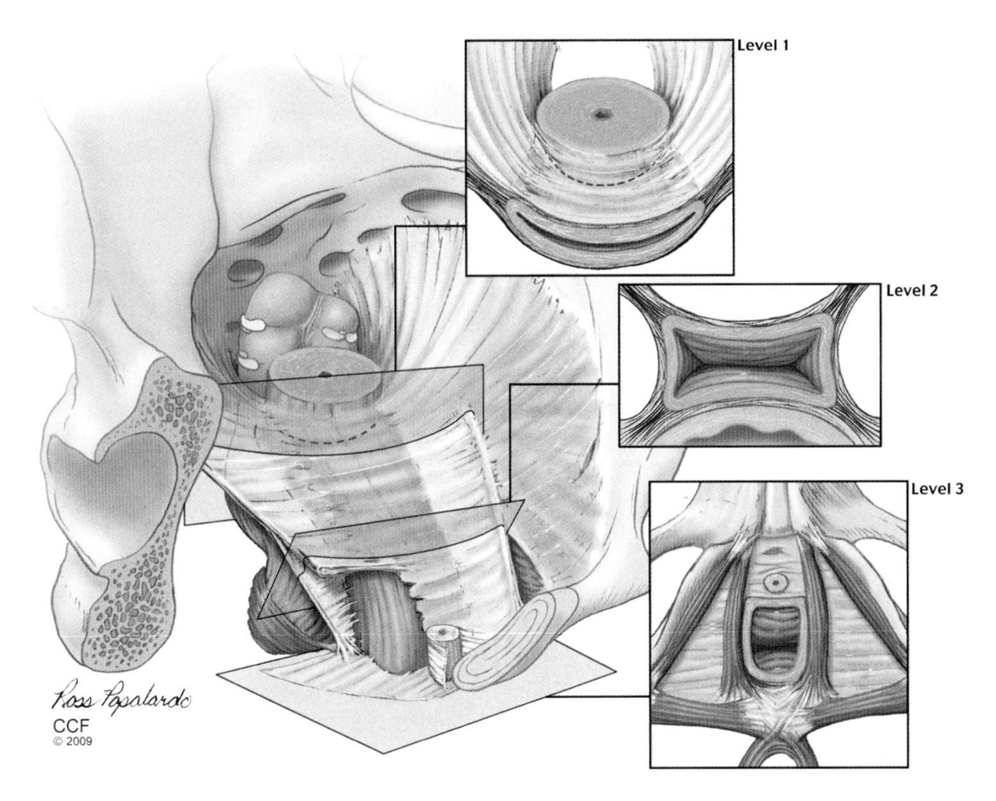

FIGURE 19-2. Illustration of the endopelvic fascia as it fans out to cover the pelvic floor and provide support to the surrounding organs. The levels 1, 2, and 3 depict the vaginal support (Reprinted with permission from Cleveland Clinic Center for Medical Art and Photography© 2004–2009 and Matthew Barber, MD).

of information about the function of the pelvic organs and the surrounding structures which support them, but it also complements physical examination for enterocele, one of the findings in advanced pelvic floor prolapse.[25,26] Kelvin et al.[24], using their four-contrast study to evaluate 74 women with pelvic floor prolapse, found 14 (19%) to have enteroceles, 50% of which were missed on physical exam. These dynamic studies also helped to identify other pelvic organ dysfunctions. In a study of 100 women referred for evaluation of pelvic floor prolapse, dynamic cystoproctography or cystodefecography found that of the 20 patients with anterior compartment systems (urinary), 45% had middle compartment findings of vaginal vault prolapse; of posterior compartment findings, 90% had rectocele, 40% had enterocele, and 35% had rectal intussusception. Similarly, of the 45 patients with symptoms of middle compartment defects (genital), 91% had anterior compartment findings of cystocele and 56% of hypermobile bladder neck; of posterior compartment findings, 82% had findings of rectocele and 58% of enterocele. Of the 17 patients with posterior compartment symptoms (anorectal), 71% had cystocele, 65% had hypermobile bladder neck, and 35% had vaginal prolapse. Their study concluded that 95% of the women with pelvic floor dysfunction had abnormalities of all three compartments.[27]

This study underscores the global nature of pelvic floor disorders and the need to understand the pelvic floor as a unit rather than as compartments.[27] The usefulness of cystodefecography was further validated by Mellgren et al.[28] who evaluated the defecation complaints of 2,816 patients and found 31% with rectal intussusceptions (13% rectal prolapse), 27% with rectocele, 19% with enterocele, and 21% with two or more of these combinations. Halligan and Bartram,[29] in a study to determine the usefulness of evacuation proctography in the management of patients with rectal dysfunction, found a change of diagnosis in 18%, a change of surgical to nonsurgical management in 14%, and a change from nonsurgical to surgical management in 4%. Hence, it is imperative that a patient who presents with symptoms of defecation dysfunction, anal or urinary incontinence, and/or prolapse of the rectum, bladder, or vagina and unexplained PELVIC pressure undergo a cystodefecography to evaluate their pelvic floor and organs.

The loss of pelvic organ alignment as seen on cystodefecography of the bladder, vagina, uterus, and rectum is obvious, but the significance of an enterocele remains controversial. Kinzel[30] described an enterocele as a "true" hernia because it contains a hernia sac (the pouch of Douglas), neck and contents. Delancey[31] postulates that enterocele sac develop as a result of the loss of suspension of the upper vagina and muscle integrity of the levator ani muscles that leads to the herniation of the cul-de-sac between the rectum and vagina. Enteroceles are often classified as congenital, pulsion, traction, and iatrogenic. A congenital enterocele is a result of the failure of the fusion of the anterior and posterior peritoneum during fetal development, resulting in a deep pouch of Douglas. Pulsion type is caused by chronic increase abdominal pressure. While traction type is caused by the loss of pelvic floor support and resulting in the pulling or traction of the pelvic organ on the surrounding structures out of the pelvis such as the vagina. Iatrogenic is caused by surgical injury.[32] Except for the congenital and iatrogenic types of enterocele, pulsion and traction enteroceles are probably a reflection of the degree of pelvic floor laxity rather than of a different etiology. The clinical presentations of an enterocele are dependent on the extent of the herniation and may present from no physical findings to bulging of the perineum or posterior vagina during strain. Clinical examination of the vagina, or bidigital exam of the rectum and vagina during maximum strain can help detect the spreading of the rectovaginal plane between the fingers as the enterocele enters into the rectovaginal plane, however, physical examination is unreliable in detecting enterocele. Kelvin et al.[33] reported their findings on 170 patients with symptoms of pelvic floor dysfunction who were evaluated by urogynecologist, and found 47 patients (28%) with an enterocele, only 24 (51%) of these patients were found by physical exam.

Others have advocated the use of peritoneal contrast, peritoneography, to increase the sensitivity of detecting significant pelvic floor prolapse. Peritoneocele, as defined by Bremmer et al.[34] is an extension of the pouch of Douglas below the upper third of the vagina, and are classified as rectal, septal, or vaginal depending on their location. Peritoneocele can be further classified into small (<100 cc), medium (100–300 cc), and large (>300 cc). Bremmer et al.[34] reported their findings on the formation and transformation of peritoneocele and enterocele on 46 patients with defecation disorder symptoms with known peritoneocele on defaeco-peritoneography. Thirty two patients (70%) had no peritoneocele at the start and developed them during maximum strain. None of the patients had an enterocele at the start, but during maximum strain, 21 patients (45%) developed an enterocele, and 15 of these patients (71%) had a persistent enterocele after evacuation at rest. Their study suggests that peritoneocele precedes the development of enterocele and that peritoneogram is more sensitive in detecting the early transformation of the herniation of the pouch of Douglas than the findings of enteroceles found on defecography. These findings are supported by Halligan et al.[35] who evaluated 47 patients with constipation symptoms using simultaneous proctography and peritoneography, and found peritoneal descent to be greater compared to controls during strain ($p<0.0001$), 42% had peritoneal sac without enteric content.[35] Interestingly, their study showed that patients with enterocele, evacuated better ($p<0.008$) than those with peritoneocele.[35] The degree of the peritoneocele and the presence of enterocele not only reflects on the herniation of the pouch of Douglas, but also on the association of pelvic organ prolapse. Baessler and Schuessler[36] found that when the percentage of the depth of the pouch of Douglas, as calculated as the percentage of the depth of the pouch to the total vaginal length, is greater than 50%, the odds of posterior vaginal wall prolapse is 14.2. Mellgren et al.[37] found a 93% association of rectal intussusception, or rectal prolapse in patients with enteroceles. Similarly, Takahashi et al.[38] found concomitant abnormalities such as perineal descent, rectocele, and rectal intussusception in 76% of the patients with enteroceles. It is not clear how the detection of a peritoneocele or enterocele changes the surgical management.

There are, however, controversies about the significance of enterocele containing small bowel versus sigmoid colon. Wexner[39] in his letter to the editor of Diseases Colon and Rectum about the study by Gosselink et al.[40] on the treatment of enterocele by mesh obliteration of the pelvic inlet, contends that enteroceles containing sigmoid colon results in defecatory dysfunction whereas enteroceles containing small bowel are more reflective of pelvic floor prolapse. Wexner's group[41] reported their findings on 24 patients with sigmoidoceles, representing 5.2% of the total cinedefecography studies, and found that patients who had enterocele containing sigmoid colon classed as second and third degree sigmoidoceles did better with sigmoid resection than medical management 100% versus 33%, with a mean follow-up of 23 months. It is not clear why the resection of the sigmoid colon without realignment of the rectum in the pelvis improved the defecatory symptoms. Was the obstructive effect of the sigmoid colon anatomical, or functional, and did the enterocele cause or a result of the sigmoid dysfunction? Their findings highlight some of the difficulties encountered in understanding the interrelationship between colorectal function and pelvic floor prolapse. Answering these complex questions may require the use of radiopaque marker and cystodefecography before and after surgical interventions.

MRI has been reported to be useful in the detection of enteroceles. Gousse et al.[42] reported that MRI had a sensitivity of 87%, specificity of 80%, and a positive predictive value of 91% compared to intraoperative findings. Typical findings of the pelvic floor on MRI of patients with pelvic organ prolapsed are shown in Figure 19-3. The MRI pictures illustrate the difference in the area of the levator hiatus between normal and prolapsed states. An angle can be measured when two lines drawn along each side of the puborectalis, bisects in the posterior midline, forming what we call the levator hiatus angle. This angle can also be measured by endorectal ultrasound (ERUS). The authors have found that when the levator hiatus angle measured by ERUS is greater than 75 degrees, we begin to see enterocele and other findings of pelvic floor prolapse on MRI and cystodefecography.[43]

MRI is helpful in evaluating not only the size of the levator hiatus in prolapse, but also changes in the anatomy of the levator ani muscle. Singh et al.[7] used a three-dimensional MRI reconstruction to assess the size of the levator hiatus and morphology of the levator ani muscle. They found that

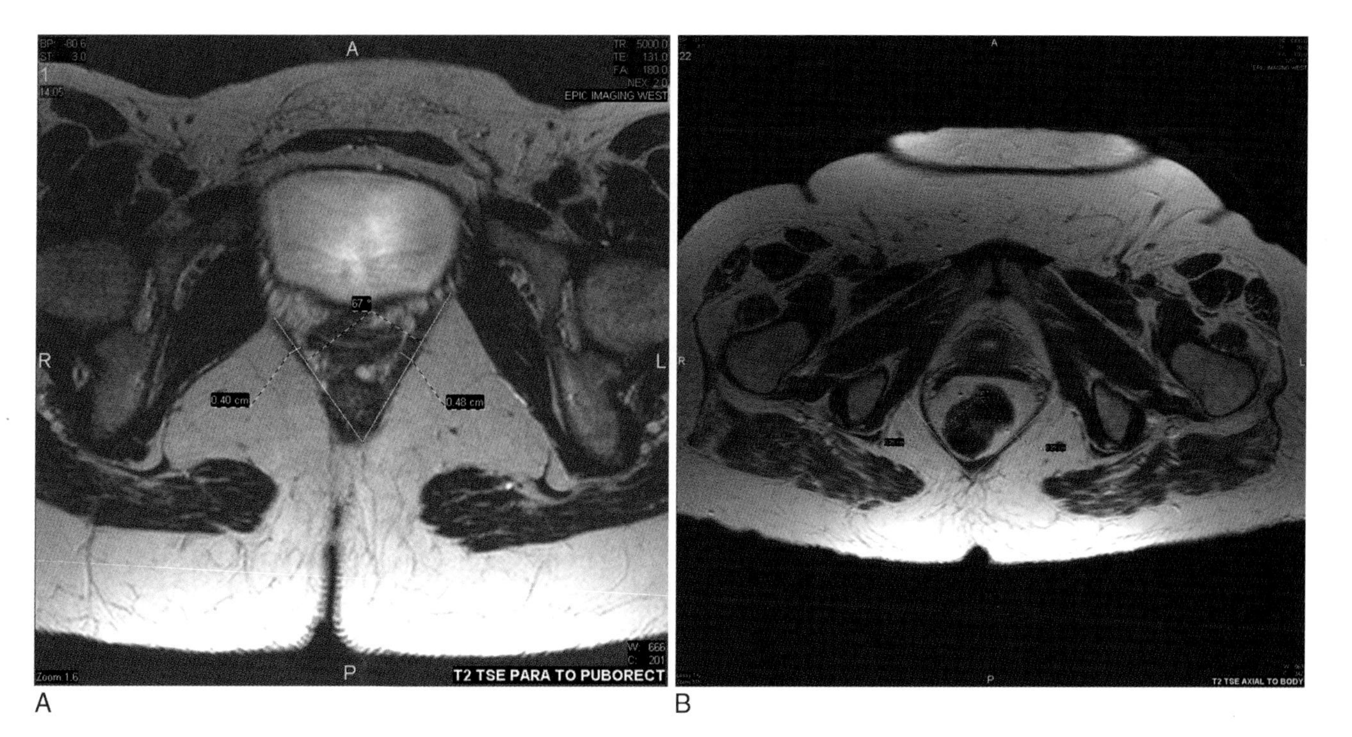

FIGURE 19-3. MRI of the levator hiatus, normal on the *left* **A** and enlarged on the *right* **B**. The angle between the two lines drawn along the puborectalis muscle and bisecting in the posterior midline of the levator ani defines the levator hiatus angle. This angle can also be measured by endorectal ultrasound and is found to correlate with findings of enterocele and pelvic floor prolapse findings on MRI and cystodefecography.

increasing stage of prolapse correlated with increasing size of the levator hiatus, but not with the morphology of the levator ani. They proposed that patients who have pelvic organ prolapse with normal levator ani morphology may only need fascial repair, compared to those who show morphologic changes of muscle injury.[7] Pannu et al.[44] showed that levator hiatus enlargement is best obtained during strain. Eguare et al.[45] using dynamic MRI in the evaluation of 85 patients with combined urinary and fecal incontinence, showed statistically significant findings of increase in the width of the levator hiatus compared to control (48.3 ± 8 mm versus 46.5 mm ± 8 mm, $p = 0.001$). Comparisons of MRI versus cystodefecography by Kelvin et al.[46] showed similar detection rates for pelvic floor prolapse, but MRI underestimated the extent of cystoceles and enteroceles though it was better at delineating the pelvic floor musculature. Kaufman et al.[47] showed that dynamic MRI, when combined with cystocolpoproctography (CCP) or cystodefecography, resulted in a change of the initial operative plan in 9 of 22 patients (41%); MRI accounted for 5 of the 9 patients (55%) and CCP for 4 of the 9 patients (44%). Currently, the MRI remains the best imaging technique in looking at the anatomy of the pelvic floor, while cystodefecography provides for dynamic images of the pelvic organs during defecation and urination. The increasing use of open-configuration MRI to allow the patient to assume a sitting position has shown this to be equivalent to the supine MRI in the evaluation of pelvic floor laxity.[48] In the future, the open-configuration MRI may offer superior imaging findings compared to cystodefecography.

The MRI and cystodefecography studies have helped confirm what is already clinically known about the enlargement of the levator hiatus in pelvic organ prolapse. What is not known is at what point in the levator hiatus enlargement does pelvic organ dysfunction or prolapse occur, and why. Such questions can only be answered in the future with longitudinal studies. The mechanism of enlargement of the levator hiatus was shown by Berglas and Rubin[49] in 1953 with the use of barium injected into the levator ani, called levator myography. Their studies showed that the degree of uterine prolapse was associated with the incline of the "levator plate": the greater the incline, the greater the longitudinal diameter and the total area of the levator hiatus. This enlargement of the levator opening was associated with descent or prolapse of the uterus (Figure 19-4). Moschowitz[50] had long recognized the importance of the levator hiatus in pelvic organ prolapse; in 1912, Moschowitz[50] published his theory on the pathophysiology of rectal prolapse as a pelvic floor hernia and described how the loss of fascial support of the rectum leads to a "hernia par glissement," meaning a sliding out of the rectum. He was able to prevent the rectum from prolapsing out by placing two fingers on the anterior rectal wall, while the same did not hold true when he placed his fingers on the posterior wall of the rectum. His findings

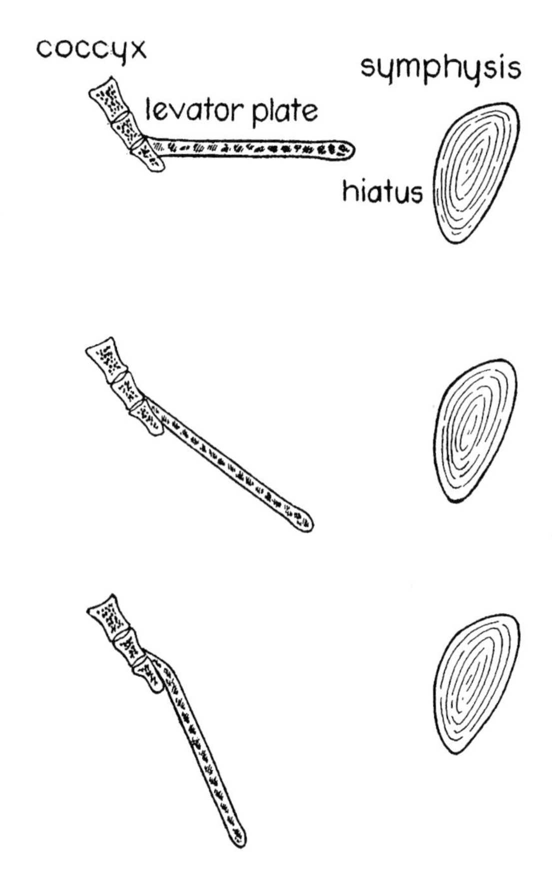

FIGURE 19-4. Illustration of the incline of the levator plate and enlargement of the levator hiatus resulting in pelvic organ prolapse. (With permission from Berglas B, Rubin IC. Study of the supportive structures of the uterus by levator myography. Surg Gynecol Obstet 1953;97:677–92).[38]

suggested that stabilization of the anterior rectal wall by his fingers restored a reanchoring of the rectum to some type of fascia, which he called "transversalis." He likely was referring to the rectovaginal septum, which is believed to play an important role in the anchoring of the rectum and vagina to the pelvic side wall and perineal body.[51–53] The importance of the ability of the anterior rectal wall was further confirmed in 1967 by Broden and Snellman,[54] who demonstrated with the use of cystodefecography that rectal prolapse begins with an anterior wall intussusception beginning about 6–8 cm up the rectum. DeLancey and Hurd[55] in 1998 reported that not only is the grade of prolapse associated with the increase in size of the levator hiatus, but that successful repair of prolapse correlated to a smaller levator hiatus.

The true incidence or prevalence of colorectal diseases associated with pelvic floor disorder is unknown. This is in part due to our failure to recognize the early signs of pelvic floor laxity and in part due to the poor correlation between the degree of pelvic organ prolapse and symptoms.[56–59] In an attempt to identify patients with pelvic organ prolapse by history, Barber et al. found that when patients with high probability of prolapse were asked, "Do you usually have a bulge or something falling out that you can see or feel in your vagina?" an affirmative answer had a 96% sensitivity (95% CI 92–100) and 79% specificity (95% CI 77–92) for stage III and IV vaginal prolapse defined by the Pelvic Organ Prolapse Quantification (POP-Q).[60,61] Interestingly, the degree of colorectal symptoms associated with vagina and bladder prolapse seems to be higher in early stages than in late. In a study of 322 women presenting for sacrocolpopexy who were assessed with the Colorectal-Anal Distress Inventory (CRADI), a questionnaire, which measured 17 symptom items divided into 4 subscales (obstructive, incontinence, pain/irritation, and rectal prolapse),[62] they found that although there were no correlations between stages of genital prolapse and bowel symptoms, there was a higher incidence of defecation complaints with early than with late stages of prolapse.[63] This may not be too surprising when one considers the role of the anal sphincter and anal canal resistance. As the resistance of the anal canal is overcome by the stretching of the anal sphincter by the prolapsed rectum, defecation may actually improve and the symptoms of rectal pressure, pain, tissue prolapse, and fecal incontinence become more dominant. Hence, the lack of correlation between the degree of prolapse and symptoms may be related to the spectrum of pelvic floor disorders and the failure of the questions to identify changes in symptoms.

The progression of enlargement of the levator hiatus appears to be in a ventral-caudal direction. This view is not only supported by cystodefecography and MRI studies, but by numerous clinical studies showing the higher incidence of urinary and vaginal prolapse over rectal prolapse in women with pelvic floor prolapse.[10,64,65] Furthermore, patients with rectal prolapse have on average 1.5–3.3 operations related to bladder and vaginal prolapse prior to their presentation with anorectal symptoms.[19,66] Peters et al.[66] studied 55 women with rectal prolapse; 95% had other pelvic floor defects. The five most common complaints were vaginal prolapse/pressure (92%), rectal prolapse/pressure (69%), constipation (71%), fecal incontinence (40%), and obstructive defecation (38%). Their study underscores the importance of colorectal evaluation in patients with vaginal prolapse/pressure. Although there are no longitudinal studies to validate the progression of pelvic floor prolapse resulting in rectal symptoms, the clinical studies along with the cystodefecography and MRI support the postulate that as the rectum descends and loses its anatomical alignment in the pelvis, a spectrum of colorectal symptoms will emerge. In the early phase, the symptoms of worsening "hemorrhoids" and mucous discharge may be related to rectal mucosal prolapse. As the rectum descends further from the pelvic floor, symptoms of incomplete evacuation of stool and needing to splint or use fingers to extract the stool are often associated with rectocele and internal rectal prolapse. In the advanced phase of rectal prolapse, symptoms of tissue protrusion out of the anus or vagina, along with pressure and pain in the local and regional areas of the pelvis, may represent the rectal and vaginal prolapse with enterocele.[37] In the extreme form of pelvic floor prolapse, the rectum, vagina, uterus, and bladder are prolapsed out, as shown in Figure 19-5. Sullivan et al.[67] described this condition as The Tetralogy of Fallout.

The continuum of pelvic floor laxity leading to anorectal symptoms makes it difficult to evaluate the effectiveness of medical versus surgical management, but medical management becomes less effective than surgery when the patient's complaints and physical findings of rectal and other pelvic organ prolapse become evident. The medical management of symptoms not specific to pelvic floor prolapse, such as constipation, pruritus ani, hemorrhoids, and fecal incontinence, has been addressed elsewhere in this book and will not be repeated here. The presence of rectocele and multi-pelvic-organ prolapse is specific to pelvic floor disorders and manifests as complaints of rectal pressure, defecation difficulty, incomplete emptying, fecal seepage, low back and pelvic pain, "hemorrhoids," and tissue "falling out" of the rectum and vagina.

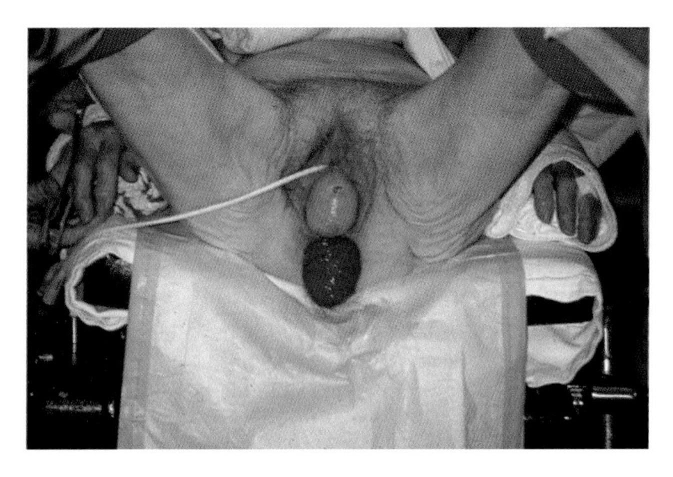

FIGURE 19-5. Extreme form of multiorgan prolapse with rectum, uterus, vagina, and bladder prolapsed out of the levator hiatus.

The evaluation and determination of when a rectocele becomes significant for surgical intervention are hampered by the lack of a unified agreement on the pathogenesis and diagnostic evaluation of rectoceles.[68] They are usually described as herniation or defect of the rectovaginal septum,[69,70] but clinical findings of perineal laxity and cystodefecography findings of increased length between the pubis and anus during strain, as shown in Figure 19-6A and B, suggest that rectoceles also have a component of rectal descent in addition to rectovaginal defect. The evidence of rectal descent is even more compelling in men with rectocele. Chen et al.[71] evaluated 234 men with defecation complaints and found 40 men (17%) with rectocele; 40% had prostatectomies. Rectoceles were anterior in 48% and posterior in 52%, nonrelaxing or partially relaxing puborectalis muscle 66%, perineal descent 65%, intussusception 23%, and sigmoidocele 15%. Their findings support the view that rectoceles rarely occur in isolation. Furthermore, rectoceles are not all equal in their effect on defecation dysfunction. Pucciani et al.[72] described two types of rectocele in women, type I (distension) and type II (displacement), and found that type II was associated with higher incidence of vaginal prolapse, more frequent manual evacuation, lower anal pressure, and greater mucosal intussusception than type I. The displacement type of rectocele is likely a result of the descent of the rectum. Brubaker[73] described the displacement of the rectum as the "rectal width," and correlated this to stool entrapment. The loss of rectal alignment in the pelvis means that intraabdominal pressure is ineffectively transferred during defecation, leading to obstructive defecation complaints. Halligan et al.[74] showed that patients who

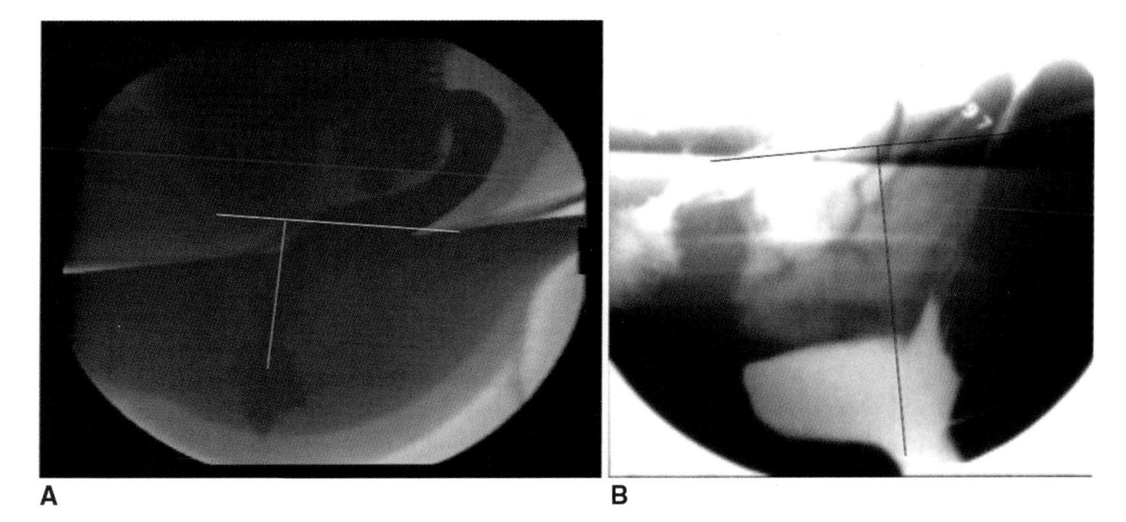

FIGURE 19-6. Cystodefecographies show the widening of the distance between the pubis and anal opening in patients on the *right* (**A**) compared to the normal on the *left* (**B**). Measurement of the distance can be made by drawing a perpendicular line from the pubococcygeal line to the anal opening during the defecation phase.

were able to expel a 10 cc pressure transduced balloon had higher intrarectal pressure than those who did not (median 208 versus 143 cm H_2O).[74] Evacuation ability of the rectal balloon correlated with defecography findings of prolonged and incomplete evacuation.[74] Interestingly, they found eight patients who had prolonged evacuation time, low intrarectal pressure, and very little change in pelvic floor descent, and concluded that these patients lacked the ability to generate intraabdominal pressure. It is unclear if these eight patients had extreme pelvic descent such that they could not have any further excursion of their pelvic floor during the evacuation phase of their defecography. Karlbom et al.[75] showed that successful improvement of rectal emptying after rectocele repair is associated with elevation of the pelvic floor.

Surgical repairs of rectoceles are generally divided into transanal and transvaginal approaches. Transabdominal approaches for rectocele are usually done in conjunction with other more severe pelvic organ prolapse findings. The most common transanal approach to rectocele repair is the modified Delorme procedure popularized by Sullivan et al.[76] in which the anterior rectal wall was plicated after the mucosa was lifted up from the muscularis propria. The recognition that up to 70% of rectal mucosal intussusceptions or internal rectal mucosal prolapses were associated with rectocele[77] led to the return of Delorme's original description of the repair, which involved the circumferential stripping of the rectal mucosa and plication of the rectal musculature.[78,79] Currently, the technique begins with the patient in a prone jackknife position with buttocks taped apart. The rectal mucosa about 1–2 cm proximal to the dentate line is infiltrated with a 1:1 mixture of 1% xylocaine with epinephrine and 0.5% bupivacaine, injected circumferentially. The rectal mucosa is then circumferentially divided with electrocautery and dissected free from the rectal musculature, resulting in a mucosal tube for a distance of about 10–15 cm, or corresponding to the proximal edge of the rectocele. A series of imbricating 2-0 polyglycolic acid sutures on a swagged needle is placed initially in four quadrants and is then further reinforced by additional sutures between the quadrants. This technique in essence corrects the rectal intussusceptions and rectocele and lifts up the rectum back into alignment in the pelvis. The effectiveness of transanal repair of rectocele in alleviating defecation dysfunction or outlet obstruction is usually 80–98%.[80–82] However, long-term outcomes of transanal rectocele repair are associated with 50% recurrence at 5.5 years.[83] It is unclear if recurrence means return of symptoms of obstructive defecation, or anatomical recurrence of rectocele, or both. Other techniques using a stapler to obliterate the rectocele and reduce intussusception, such as the single-stapled transanal prolapsectomy with perineal levatorplasty (STAPL) and double-stapled transanal rectal resection (STARR), had 76 and 88% improvement of obstructive defecation symptoms at 20 months, respectively.[84] Again, the lack of postsurgical defecography or MRI studies makes it difficult to explain why reduction of the rectocele results in improvement of symptoms. Van Laarhoven et al.[85] showed that there is no correlation between patients' symptoms and size of rectocele reduction, suggesting that other factors may be at play for patients' improved symptoms.

Transvaginal techniques of rectocele repair or posterior colporrhaphy are primarily performed by gynecologists using one of the four techniques: (1) levator ani (puborectalis) or rectovaginal muscularis reapproximation,[86] (2) site-specific repair of the rectovaginal septum,[107] (3) reapproximation of the rectovaginal septum to the levator ani fascia,[87] (4) posterior repair of the rectovaginal defect with grafts or mesh.[88] All these techniques involve an incision in the posterior wall of the vagina and separating the plane between the rectum and vaginal wall. Once the exposure is complete, then various techniques of reinforcement of the septum are performed. In general, the approximation of the levator ani results in up to 50% incidence of dyspareunia.[70] This technique has been mostly abandoned and replaced with rectovaginal septal repair by reapproximating it either longitudinally or transversally, with or without grafts or mesh. The concept of site-specific repair of the rectovaginal septum is best described by Richardson,[70] who described "breaks" in the rectovaginal septum resulting in rectocele formation. Depending on the location and extent of the breaks, various types of rectocele emerge, and with higher "breaks" enteroceles may enter into the rectovaginal plane. The use of biologic grafts and synthetic mesh in rectocele repair is reserved for large rectoceles (with >4 cm depth), presence of vaginal prolapse, poor native tissue, and associated vagina and bladder prolapse.[90–93] In general, the use of grafts or mesh in the repair of rectocele is safe, but its superiority and efficacy over established repair remains inconclusive.

The best study on the benefits of transvaginal repair of rectocele was done by Mellgren et al.[94] who reported on 25 patients prospectively for a mean period of 1 year. Constipation was present in 88% preoperatively and relieved in 84% postoperatively. Paraiso et al.[95] reported their randomized trial evaluating three surgical techniques of posterior colporrhaphy (rectovaginal muscularis reapproximation, site-specific repair, and site-specific repair with a xenograft) and found all three methods had similar improvement in symptoms, quality of life, and sexual function. Interestingly, they found a 46% anatomical failure rate with the xenograft, but without any difference in outcome compared to the other two techniques.[95] No cystodefecography studies were performed before or after the repairs to document the effects of the surgical intervention, which makes it difficult to explain the unexpected outcomes of any pelvic floor repair. An attempt to compare transanal versus transvaginal repair of rectocele for symptoms of obstructive defecation by Nieminen et al.[96] on 30 patients suggests that at 1 year postoperative follow-up, more transvaginal repair patients remain asymptomatic compared to the transanal repair group (93% versus 73%; $p=0.08$). Again, there were no postoperative studies to explain the discrepancy of their results.

Progression of pelvic floor laxity leads to complex, multi-pelvic-organ prolapse similar to what Sullivan et al.[67] described as the Tetralogy of Fallout. Central to the successful restoration of the pelvic organs to their anatomic position is stabilization of the perineal body and reinforcement of the rectovaginal septum or posterior vaginal fascia. In men this septum or fascia is known as Denonvilliers' fascia. Sears[53] in 1933 published anatomic findings of the rectovaginal septum and described it as a double-layer sheet of fascia arising from the levator ani and uterosacral ligament. One of the layers (lateral) forms the urogenital diaphragm, and the other (medial) fuses to the fibers of the posterior vagina and perineal body (Figure 19-7).[53] Milley and Nichols[97] provided further evidence of the relationship between the rectovaginal septum and perineal body in 143 specimens, whose ages ranged from 8 weeks fetus to 100 years. Lane in 1962[98] was the first to use mesh in the pelvis to reinforce the rectovaginal septum in the repair of vaginal vault prolapsed. Although there has been a plethora of mesh development, Lane's technique of the transabdominal sacrocolpopexy has undergone very little modification. Nygaard et al.[99] summarized the published data on abdominal sacrocolpopexy from 1966 to 2004

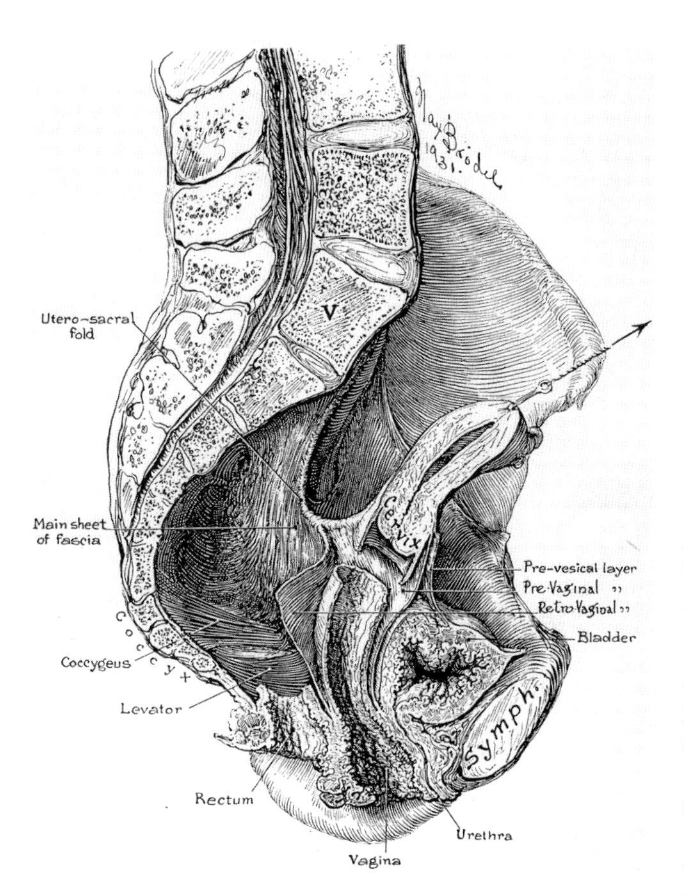

FIGURE 19-7. The endopelvic layer arising from the pelvic sidewall and fanning out between the rectum and vagina to form the rectovaginal septum and anchoring to the perineal body. (With permission from Sears NP. The fascia surrounding the vagina, its origin and arrangement. Am J Obstet Gynecol 1933;25:484–92).

and reported the range of success rates for apical prolapse was 78–100%, organ prolapse 58–100%, reoperation for prolapse median 4.4% (range 0–18.2%), and mesh erosion 3.4%. They concluded that sacrocolpopexy with mesh is an effective technique for vaginal apical prolapse, but reported an increase in constipation complaints from 29% to 52%. Pilsgaard and Mouritsen[100] reported their experience with 35 patients who underwent sacrocolpopexy with mesh with a mean follow-up period of 2 years (6 months to 4.5 years) and reported a 30% increase in the symptoms of defecation difficulty. The exact etiology of the increased defecation dysfunction or constipation is unclear. Addison et al.[101] reported on 3 cases of sacrocolpopexy with mesh failure and suggested mesh avulsion from the apex of the vagina or herniation below the mesh repair as a cause of recurrent symptoms of prolapse. They advocated placement of the mesh throughout the length of the vagina. Sullivan et al.[19] in 2001 published the largest long-term result on pelvic floor prolapse repair with their technique called total pelvic mesh repair (TPMR). Over a 10-year period, 236 women had TPMR, and 205 were available for a median follow-up of 5.3 years. They reported resolution of defecation difficulty in 76% and of fecal incontinence in 85%, and patient satisfaction of 74% at 6 years or greater. Their procedure incorporates the current understanding of perineal stabilization and reinforcement of the rectovaginal septum by placing a mesh for the full length of the vagina and anchoring it to the perineal body. The mesh is made of polypropylene, cut into the shape of a trapezoid, placed below the visceral peritoneum, to the left of the rectum, and anchored to the sacrum at the level of S1 and S2. Two additional strips of mesh are secured onto the lateral edges of the sacroperineal mesh, tunneled deep to the peritoneum lateral to the vagina and bladder, and secured to Cooper's ligament about two fingers' breadth from the pubic symphysis (Figure 19-8). Cundiff et al.[102] developed a similar technique of anchoring the perineal body to the sacrum with polyester mesh, called the abdominal sacral colpoperineopexy. The procedure combines a transvaginal and transabdominal approach of securing a polyester mesh to the perineal body and vagina, and tying it down to the sacrum. Nineteen patients had this procedure and were followed for a mean of 11 weeks. All the patients had improvement in their stage of prolapse by at least one level as determined by the POP-Q. Bowel symptoms of fecal incontinence and constipation improved in 8 of the 12 patients (66%).[102] These two studies highlight the importance of perineal body stabilization and rectovaginal septum reinforcement with mesh in the support of pelvic floor prolapse.

The use of mesh slings have proliferated beyond the initial use for urinary incontinence and have been advocated for the treatment of fecal incontinence and rectal prolapse. However, this is not a new concept, Nigro[103] borrowing urologic concepts of fascial sling in the urethral support of urinary incontinence, reported his technique of Teflon mesh via a transcoccygeal–suprapubic approach in five patients with

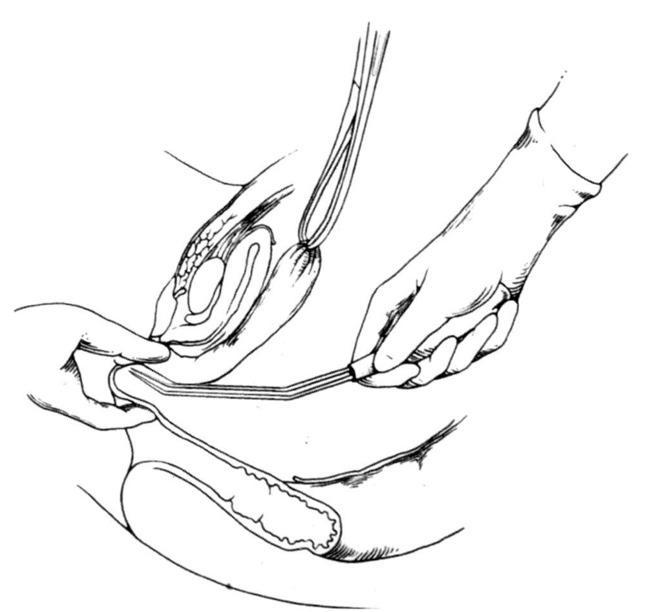

FIGURE 19-8. In the Total Pelvic Mesh Repair (TPMR), a Cobb-Ragde needle (V. Mueller, Deerfield, IL) is placed in back of the rectovaginal sulcus and pushed through into the introitus to secure the perineal body. A polypropylene suture is placed through the eye of the Cobb-Ragde needle and pulled into the pelvis to secure the mesh between the sacrum and the perineal body. Two additional strips of mesh are then placed on each side of the sacroperineal mesh, tunneled deep to the peritoneum, and secured lateral to the vagina and bladder to Cooper's ligament in the space of Retzius.

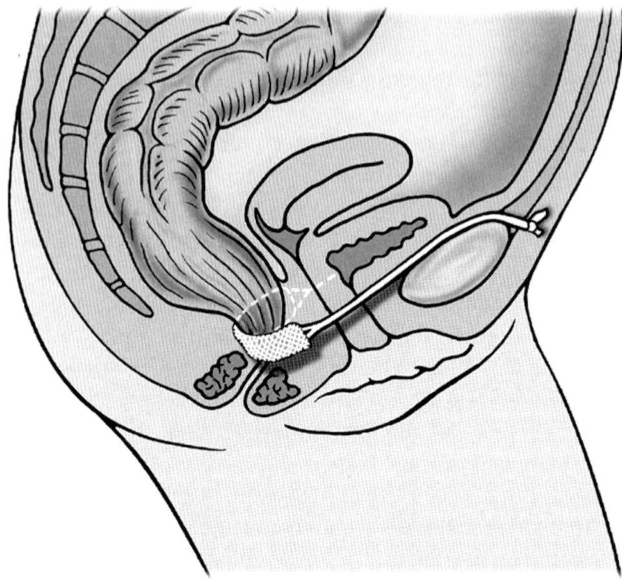

FIGURE 19-9. Transperineal trocar system to place a posterior rectal sling for fecal incontinence.

rectal prolapse. He reported no recurrence with follow-up of 2 months to 5 years. In 1970, Nigro[104] reported a transabdominal approach in 6 patients, and updated on 15 patients with the transcoccygeal–suprapubic approach and revealed 2 out of 15 failures. More recently, Yamana et al.[105] reported the use of a transperineal trocar system to place a posterior rectal sling for fecal incontinence (Figure 19-9) in 8 patients, 1 developed infection requiring the removal of the sling, and the remaining 7 had improvement of their Fecal Incontinence Severity Index from 27 to 9, Cleveland Clinic Florida Fecal Incontinence Score improved from 13 to 5, Fecal incontinence Quality of Life Scale was improved in all four categories.

Although mesh placement, regardless of whether it is a transabdominal, transvaginal, or transperineal approach, seems to offer a better outcome than non-mesh repairs, there are no conclusive evidence to suggest that patients with early symptoms and findings of pelvic floor laxity will require more advance repairs with mesh than those patients reported by Sullivan et al.[19] Cundiff et al.[102] and others.[40] The current techniques of local repair of the bladder, vagina, and rectum may be adequate, provided that clinical and radiologic findings show them to be truly isolated pelvic organ prolapse, but as discussed earlier such isolated prolapse is uncommon, and the failure to recognize and repair multiorgan prolapse is a primary source of patient dissatisfaction.[106]

Unlike diseases which are surgically addressed with one technique such as appendicitis, the pathogenesis of pelvic floor prolapse is chronic and result in progressive constellation of symptoms and findings. The global transformation of the pelvic floor may result in surgical treatments that are successful for a limited period of time and fail not because of the technique, but because of the progression of the pelvic floor prolapse. The exact etiology of pelvic floor prolapse remains unknown, and it is for this reason that dynamic imaging with cystodefecography, MRI, and other modalities are so important in documenting the disease process of pelvic floor disorders. Undoubtedly there will be new technologies and techniques that will evolve to replace the old, but as Moschowitz[50] most elegantly put it in his axiom, or generally accepted truth, about treatments of rectal prolapse, "the more remedies there are suggested for the cure of a malady, the less the likelihood of the efficacy of any particular one." A corollary to this axiom would be, "the more remedies there are for a disease, the more reflective of our lack of understanding of its pathogenesis."

Acknowledgment. This chapter was written by Frank Harford and Linda Brubaker in the first edition of this textbook.

References

1. Olsen AL, Smith VJ, Bergstrom JO, Colling JC, Clark AL. Epidemiology of surgically managed pelvic organ prolapse and urinary incontinence. Obstet Gynecol. 1997;89:501–6.
2. National Center for Health Statistics. Health, United States, 2009: With Special Feature on Medical Technology. Hyattsville, MD. Accessed on November 2010. http://www.cdc.gov/nchs/data/hus/hus09.pdf

3. Agur AMR, Dalley AF. Grant's atlas of anatomy, Pennsylvania. 12th ed. Lippincott Williams & Wilkins; 2008.
4. Netter FH. Atlas of Human Anatomy, New Jersey. Ciba Geigy; 1990.
5. Parks AG, Porter NH, Melzak J. Experimental study of the reflex mechanism controlling the muscles of the pelvic floor. Dis Colon Rectum. 1962;5:407–14.
6. Barber MD. Contemporary views on female pelvic anatomy. Cleve Clin J Med. 2005;72(4):S2–11.
7. Singh K, Jakab M, Reid WM, Berger LA, Hoyte L. Three-dimensional assessment of levator ani morphology features in different grades of prolapse. Am J Obstet Gynecol. 2003;188: 910–5.
8. Singh K, Reid WM, Berger LA. Magnetic resonance imaging of normal levator ani anatomy and function. Obstet Gynecol. 2002;99:433–8.
9. Lawson JON. Pelvic anatomy I. Pelvic floor muscles. Ann R Coll Surg Engl. 1974;54:244–52.
10. Ashton-Miller JA, DeLancey JO. Functional anatomy of the female pelvic floor. Ann NY Acad Sci. 2007;1101:266–96.
11. Yiou R, Delmas V, Carmeliet P, Gherardi RK, Meimon GB, Chopin DK, et al. The pathophysiology of pelvic floor disorders: evidence from a histomorphologic study of the perineum and a mouse model of rectal prolapse. J Anat. 2001;199:599–607.
12. Uhlenhuth E, Day E, Smith RD, Middleton EB. The visceral endopelvic fascia and the hypogastric sheath. Surg Gynecol Obstet. 1948;86:9–28.
13. DeLancey JOL. The anatomy of the pelvic floor. Curr Opin Obstet Gynecol. 1994;6:313–6.
14. DeLancey JOL. Anatomy and biomechanics of genital prolapse. Clin Obstet Gynecol. 1993;36:897–909.
15. Norton PA. Pelvic floor disorders: the role of fascia and ligaments. Clin Obstet Gynecol. 1993;36:926–38.
16. Carley ME, Schaffer J. Urinary incontinence and pelvic organ prolapse in women with Marfan or Ehlers- Danlos Syndrome. Am J Obstet Gynecol. 2000;182:1021–3.
17. Norton PA, Baker JE, Sharp HC, Warenski JC. Genitourinary prolapse and joint hypermobility in women. Obstet Gynecol. 1995;85:225–8.
18. Soderberg MW, Falconer C, Brystrom B, Malmstrom A, Ekman G. Young women with genital prolapse have a low collagen concentration. Acta Obstet Gynecol Scand. 2004;83:1193–8.
19. Sullivan ES, Longaker CJ, Lee PYH. Total pelvic mesh repair, a ten year experience. Dis Colon Rectum. 2001;44:857–63.
20. Fornell EU, Wingren G, Kjolhede P. Factors associated with pelvic floor dysfunction with emphasis on urinary and fecal incontinence and genital prolapse: an epidemiological study. Acta Obstet Gynecol Scand. 2004;83:383–9.
21. Berglas B, Rubin IC. Histologic study of the pelvic connective tissue. Surg Gynecol Obstet. 1953;97:277–89.
22. Fritsch H, Lienemann A, Brenner E, Ludwikowski B. Clinical anatomy of the pelvic floor. Adv Anat Embryol Cell Biol. 2004;175(III-IX):1–64.
23. Burhenne HJ. Intestinal evacuation study: a new roentgenologic technique. Radiol Clin. 1963;33:79–83.
24. Kelvin FM, Maglinte DD, Hornback JA, Benson JT. Pelvic prolapse: assessment with evacuation proctography (defecography). Radiology. 1992;184:547–51.
25. Kelvin FM, Maglinte DD, Benson TJ. Evacuation proctography (defecography): an aid to the investigation of pelvic floor disorders. Obstet Gynecol. 1994;83:307–14.
26. Maglinte DDT, Kelvin FM, Hale DS, Benson JT. Dynamic cystoproctography: a unifying diagnostic approach to pelvic floor and anorectal dysfunction. AJR. 1997;169:759–67.
27. Maglinte DD, Kelvin FM, Fitzgerald K, Hale DS, Benson JT. Association of compartment defects in pelvic floor dysfunction. AJR. 1999;172:439–44.
28. Mellgren A, Bremmer S, Johansson C, Dolk A, Uden R, Ahlback SO, et al. Defecography: results of investigation in 2,816 patients. Dis Colon Rectum. 1994;37:1133–41.
29. Harvey CJ, Halligan S, Bartram CI, Hollings N, Sahdev A, Kingston K. Evacuation proctography: a prospective study of diagnostic and therapeutic effects. Radiology. 1999;211: 223–7.
30. Kinzel GE. Enterocele: a study of 265 cases. Am J Obstet Gynecol. 1961;1:1166–74.
31. Delancey JOL. Pelvic organ prolapse. In: Scott J et al., editors. Danforth's obstetrics and gynecology. 9th ed. Philadelphia: Lippincott Williams Wilkins; 2003. p. 791–817.
32. Holley R. Enterocele: a review. Obstet Gynecol Surv. 1994; 49:284–93.
33. Kelvin FM, Hale DS, Maglinte DDT, Patten BJ, Benson JT. Female pelvic organ prolapse: diagnostic contribution of dynamic cystoproctography and comparison with physical examination. AJR. 1999;173:31–7.
34. Bremmer S, Mellgren A, Holmstrom B, Uden R. Peritoneocele and enterocele. Formation and transformation during rectal evacuation as studied by means of defaeco-peritoneography. Acta Radiol. 1998;39:167–75.
35. Halligan S, Bartram C, Hall C, Wingate J. Enterocele revealed by simultaneous evacuation proctography and peritoneography: does "defecation block" exist? AJR. 1996;167:461–6.
36. Baessler K, Schuessler B. The depth of the pouch of Douglas in nulliparous and parous women without genital prolapse and in patients with genital prolapse. Am J Obstet Gynecol. 2000;182:540–4.
37. Mellgren A, Johansson C, Dolk A, Anzen B, Bremmer S, Nilsson BY, et al. Enterocele demonstrated by defaecography is associated with other pelvic floor disorders. Int J Colorectal Dis. 1994;9:121–4.
38. Takahashi T, Yamana T, Sahara R, Iwadare J. Enterocele: what is the clinical implication. Dis Colon Rectum. 2006;49: S75–81.
39. Wexner SD. Letter to the editor: treatment of enterocele by obliteration of the pelvic intel. Dis Colon Rectum. 2000;43:115–6.
40. Gosselink MJ, van Dam JH, Huisman WM, Ginai AZ, Schouten WR. Treatment of enterocele by obliteration of the pelvic inlet. Dis Colon Rectum. 1999;42:940–4.
41. Jorge JMN, Yang YK, Wexner SD. Incidence and clinical significance of sigmoidoceles as determined by a new classification system. Dis Colon Rectum. 1994;37:1112–7.
42. Gousse AE, Barbaric ZL, Safir MH, Madjar S, Marumoto AK, Raz S. Dynamic half Fourier acquisition, single shot turbo spin-echo magnetic resonance imaging for evaluating the female pelvis. J Urol. 2000;164:1606–13.
43. Lee PYH et al. Levator hiatus angle: a new parameter measured by endorectal ultrasound in the evaluation of pelvic floor prolapse; manuscript pending.
44. Pannu HP, Kaufman HS, Cundiff GW, Genadry R, Bluemke DA, Fishman E. Dynamic MR imaging of pelvic organ prolapse: spectrum of abnormalities. Radiographics. 2000;20:1567–82.

45. Eguare EI, Neary P, Crosbie J, Johnston SM, Beddy P, McGovern B, et al. Dynamic magnetic resonance imaging of the pelvic floor in patients with idiopathic combined fecal and urinary incontinence. J Gastrointest Surg. 2004;8:73–82.
46. Kelvin FM, Maglinte DD, Hale DS, Benson JT. Female pelvic organ prolapse: a comparison of triphasic dynamic MR imaging and triphasic fluroroscopic cystocolpoproctography. AJR. 2000;174:81–8.
47. Kaufman HS, Buller JL, Thompson JR, Pannu HK, DeMeester SL, Genadry RR, et al. Dynamic pelvic magnetic resonance imaging and cystocolpoproctography alter surgical management of pelvic floor disorders. Dis Colon Rectum. 2001;44:1575–84.
48. Fieldings JR, Griffiths DJ, Versi E, Mulkern RV, Lee MLT, Jolesz FA. MR imaging of pelvic floor continence mechanisms in the supine and sitting positions. AJR. 1998;171:1607–10.
49. Berglas B, Rubin IC. Study of the supportive structures of the uterus by levator myography. Surg Gynecol Obstet. 1953;97:677–92.
50. Moschowitz AV. The pathogenesis, anatomy and cure of prolapse of the rectum. Surg Gynecol Obstet. 1912;15:7–12.
51. Uhlenhuth E, Wolfe WM, Smith EM, Middleton EB. The rectogenital septum. Surg Gynecol Obstet. 1948;86:148–63.
52. Smith GE. Studies in the anatomy of the pelvis with special reference to the fasciae and visceral supports. J Anat Physiol. 1908;42:198–218.
53. Sears NP. The fascia surrounding the vagina, its origin and arrangement. Am J Obstet Gynecol. 1933;25:484–92.
54. Broden B, Snellman B. Procidentia of the rectum studied with cineradiography: a contribution to the discussion of causative mechanism. Dis Colon Rectum. 1968;11:330–47.
55. DeLancey JO, Hurd WM. Size of the urogenital hiatus in the levator ani muscles in normal women and women with pelvic organ prolapse. Obstet Gynecol. 1998;91:364–8.
56. Ellerkmann RM, Cundiff GW, Melick CF, et al. Correlation of symptoms with location and severity of pelvic organ prolapsed. Am J Obstet Gynecol. 2001;185:1332–7.
57. Swift SE, Tate SB, Nicholas J. Correlation of symptoms with degree of pelvic organ support in a general population of women: what is pelvic organ prolapse? Am J Obstet Gynecol. 2003;189:372–9.
58. Ghetti C, Gregory T, Edwards R, Otto LN, Clark AL. Pelvic organ descent and symptoms of pelvic floor disorders. Am J Obstet Gynecol. 2005;193:53–7.
59. Barber MD. Symptoms and outcome measures of pelvic organ prolapse. Clin Obstet Gynecol. 2005;48:648–61.
60. Barber MD, Neubauer NL, Klein-Olarte V. Can we screen for pelvic organ prolapse without a physical examination in epidemiologic studies? Am J Obstet Gynecol. 2006;195:942–8.
61. Bump RC, Mattiasson A, Bo K, et al. The standardization of terminology of female pelvic organ prolapse and pelvic floor dysfunction. Am J Obstet Gynecol. 1996;175:10–7.
62. Barber MD, Walters MD, Cundiff GW, the PESSRI Trial Gp. Responsiveness of the pelvic floor distress inventory (PFDI) and pelvic floor impact questionnaire (PFIQ) in women undergoing vaginal surgery and pessary treatment for pelvic organ prolapse. Am J Obstet Gynecol. 2006;194:1492–8.
63. Bradley C, Brown M, Cundiff GW, Goode P, Kenton KS, Nygaard IE, et al. Bowel symptoms in women planning surgery for pelvic organ prolapse. Am J Obstet Gynecol. 2006;195:1814–9.
64. Bump RC, Norton PA. Epidemiology and natural history of pelvic dysfunction. Obstet Gynecol Clin North Am. 1998;4:723–46.
65. Gonzalez-Argente FX, Jain A, Norgueras JJ, Davila GW, Weiss EG, Wexner SD. Prevalence and severity of urinary incontinence and pelvic genital prolapse in females with anal incontinence or rectal prolapse. Dis Colon Rectum. 2001;44:920–6.
66. Peters WA, Smith MR, Drescher CW. Rectal prolapse in women with other defects of pelvic floor support. Am J Obstet Gynecol. 2001;184:1488–95.
67. Sullivan ES, Strandburg CO, Sandoz IL, Tarnasky JW, Longaker CJ. Repair of total pelvic prolapse: an overview. Perspect Colon Rectal Surg. 1990;3:119–31.
68. Halligan S, Bartram CI. Is barium trapping in rectoceles significant? Dis Colon Rectum. 1995;38:764–8.
69. Mollen RMHG, Van Laarhoven CJHM, Kuijpers JHC. Pathogenesis and management of rectoceles. Semin Colon Rectal Surg. 1996;7:192–6.
70. Richardson AC. The rectovaginal septum revisited: its relationship to rectocele and its importance in rectocele repair. Clin Obstet Gynecol. 1993;36:976–83.
71. Chen HH, Iroatulam A, Alabaz O, Weiss EG, Nogueras JJ, Wexner SD. Associations of defecography and physiologic findings in male patients with rectocele. Tech Coloproctol. 2001;5:157–61.
72. Pucciani F, Rottoli L, Bologna A, Buri M, Cianchi F, Paglial P, et al. Anterior rectocele and anorectal dysfunction. Int J Colorectal Dis. 1996;11:1–9.
73. Brubaker L. Rectocele. Curr Opin Obstet Gynecol. 1996;8:376–9.
74. Halligan S, Thomas J, Bartram C. Intrarectal pressures and balloon expulsion related to evacuation proctography. Gut. 1995;37:100–4.
75. Karlbom U, Graf W, Nilsson S, Pahlman L. Does surgical repair of a rectocele improve rectal emptying? Dis Colon Rectum. 1996;39:1296–302.
76. Sullivan ES, Leaverton GH, Hardwick CE. Transrectal perineal repair: an adjunct to improved function after anorectal surgery. Dis Colon Rectum. 1968;11:106–14.
77. Janssen LWM, Van Dijke CF. Selection criteria for anterior rectal wall repair in symptomatic rectocele and anterior rectal wall prolapse. Dis Colon Rectum. 1994;37:1100–7.
78. Uhlig BE, Sullivan ES. The modified Delorme operation: its place in surgical treatment for massive rectal prolapse. Dis Colon Rectum. 1979;22:513–21.
79. Corman ML. Classic articles in colonic and rectal surgery. Edmond Delorme 1847–1929. Dis Colon Rectum. 1985;28:544–53.
80. Murthy VK, Orkin BA, Smith LE, Glassman LM. Excellent outcome using selective criteria for rectocele repair. Dis Colon Rectum. 1996;39:374–8.
81. Khubchandani IT, Sheets JA, Stasik JJ, Hakki AR. Endorectal repair of rectocele. Dis Colon Rectum. 1983;26:792–6.
82. Sehapayak S. Transrectal repair of rectocele: an extended armamentarium of colorectal surgeons. A report of 355 cases. Dis Colon Rectum. 1985;28:422–33.

83. Roman H, Michot F. Long-term outcomes of transanal rectocele repair. Dis Colon Rectum. 2005;48:510–7.
84. Boccasanta P, Venturi M, Salamina G, Cesana BM, Bernasconi F, Roviato G. New trends in the surgical treatment of outlet obstruction. Clinical and functional results of the two novel trans-anal stapled techniques from a randomized controlled trial. Int J Colorectal Dis. 2004;19:359–69.
85. Van Laarhoven CJHM, Kamm MA, Bartram CL, Halligan S, Hawlet PR, Phillips RKS. Relationship between anatomic and symptomatic long-term results after rectocele repair for impaired defecation. Dis Colon Rectum. 1999;42:204–11.
86. Jeffcoate TNA. Posterior colpoperineorrhaphy. Am J Obstet Gynecol. 1959;77:490–502.
87. Maher CF, Qatawneh AM, Baessler K, Schluter PJ. Midline rectovaginal fascial plication for repair of rectocele and obstructed defecation. Obstet Gynecol. 2004;104:685–9.
88. Nichols DH. Sacrospinous fixation for massive eversion of the vagina. Am J Obstet Gynecol. 1982;142:901–4.
89. Francis WJ, Jeffcoate TN. Dyspareunia following vaginal operations. J Obstet Gynecol Br Emp. 1961;68:1–10.
90. Sung V, Rogers R, Schaffer J, Balk EM, Uligh K, Lau J, et al. Graft use in transvaginal pelvic organ prolapse repair. A systematic review. Obstet Gynecol. 2008;112:1131–42.
91. Birch C. The use of prosthetics in pelvic reconstructive surgery. Best Pract Res Clin Obstet Gynaecol. 2005;19: 979–91.
92. Le TH, Kon L, Bhatia NN, Ostergard DR. Update on the utilization of grafts in pelvic reconstruction surgeries. Curr Opin Obstet Gynecol. 2007;19:480–9.
93. Huebner M, Hsu Y, Fenner DE. The use of graft materials in vaginal pelvic floor surgery. Int J Gynecol Obstet. 2006;92:279–88.
94. Mellgren A, Anzen B, Nilsson BY, Johansson C, Dolk A, Gillgren P, et al. Results of rectocele repair. A prospective study. Dis Colon Rectum. 1995;38:7–13.
95. Paraiso MFR, Barber MD, Muir TW, Walters MD. Rectocele repair: a randomized trial of three surgical techniques including graft augmentation. Am J Obstet Gynecol. 1006;195: 1762–71.
96. Nieminen K, Hiltunen KM, Laitinen J, Oksal J, Heinonen PK. Transanal or vaginal approach to rectocele repair: a prospective randomized pilot study. Dis Colon Rectum. 2004;47: 1636–42.
97. Milley PS, Nichols DH. A correlative investigation of the human rectovaginal septum. Anat Rec. 1969;163:443–51.
98. Lane F. Repair of posthysterectomy vaginal-vault prolapse. Obstet Gynecol. 1962;20:72–7.
99. Nygaard IE, McCreery R, Brubaker L, Connolly A, Cundiff G, Weber AM, et al. Abdominal sacrocolpopexy: a comprehensive review. Obstet Gynecol. 2004;104:805–23.
100. Pilsgaard K, Mouritsen L. Follow-up after repair of vaginal vault prolapse with abdominal colposacropexy. Acta Obstet Gynecol Scand. 1999;78:66–70.
101. Addison WA, Timmons MC, Wall LL, Livengood CH. Failed abdominal sacral colpopexy: observation and recommendations. Obstet Gynecol. 1989;74:480–2.
102. Cundiff GW, Harris RL, Coates K, Low VHS, Bump RC, Addison WA. Abdominal sacral colpoperineopexy: a new approach for correction of posterior compartment defects and perineal descent associated with vaginal vault prolapse. Am J Obstet Gynecol. 1997;177:1345–55.
103. Nigro ND. Restoration of the levator sling in the treatment of rectal procidentia. Dis Colon Rectum. 1958;1:123–7.
104. Nigro ND. A sling operation for rectal prolapse. Proc R Soc Med. 1970;63:106–7.
105. Yamana T, Takahashi T, Iwadare J. Perineal puborectalis sling operation for fecal incontinence: preliminary report. Dis Colon Rectum. 2004;47:1982–9.
106. Blanchard KA, Vanlangendonck R, Winters CJ. Recurrent pelvic floor defects after abdominal sacral colpopexy. J Urol. 2006;175:1010–3.
107. Cundiff GW, Weidner AC, Visco AG, Addison WA, Bump RC. An anatomic and functional assessment of the discrete defect rectocele repair. Am J Obstet Gynecol. 1998;179:1451–7.

20 Anal Cancer

Mark Lane Welton and Nalini Raju

Introduction

This chapter reviews the anatomy that defines anal and perianal squamous cell carcinomas (SCC), discusses the cancers and precursor lesions that are most commonly found in these regions, and concludes with brief discussions of the less common malignancies of the anus and perineum.

New Anatomic Considerations

Approximately 5,290 new cases of anal cancer were diagnosed in the USA in 2009 according to the American Cancer Society.[1] This number may actually somewhat overestimate the true incidence, as it is our impression that perianal or anal margin cancers are often classified as anal canal cancers due to proximity to the anus without actual involvement of the anal canal. While colorectal surgeons are quite familiar with the landmarks that define the anal canal and anal margin, other health care providers involved in the diagnosis and treatment of this disease are less familiar with these landmarks in that their primary practices are internal medicine, gastroenterology, radiation oncology, medical oncology, dermatology, HIV medicine, etc. Given these limitations, new terminology based on landmarks that all healthcare providers can easily visualize and understand was developed and published in the previous version of this text and largely adopted in the latest version of the American Joint Committee on Cancer (AJCC) Staging Manual.[2] The new terminology is necessary because true anal canal lesions may have a more aggressive biology requiring chemoradiotherapy while lesions of the perianal skin may simply be treated with local excision. Thus, if the two classes of lesions are unwittingly grouped together, the response rates of anal cancer to chemoradiation therapy may be overstated.

The classification system divides the region into three easily identifiable regions, anal canal, perianal, and skin (Figure 20-1A, B).[3] *Anal canal* lesions are lesions that cannot be visualized at all, or are incompletely visualized, with gentle traction placed on the buttocks. In contrast, *perianal lesions* are completely visible and fall within a 5 cm radius of the anal opening when gentle traction is placed on the buttocks. Finally, *skin lesions* fall outside of the 5 cm radius of the anal opening. A key component of this classification system is that all clinicians, including gastroenterologists, surgeons, nurse practitioners, and medical and radiation oncologists can perform this simple exam in their offices without the aid of an anoscope or a clear understanding of the anatomic landmarks (dentate line and anal verge) of the region.

Identification of a new zone, the *transformation zone*, was also proposed to help clinicians and pathologists understand how anal squamous cell carcinomas (SCC) may be found 6, 8, or even 10 cm proximal to the dentate line in the anatomic rectum. The transition zone is a well-known region. It is an area, zero to 12 mm in length beginning at the dentate line, where a "transitional urothelium-like" epithelium may be found in the rectal mucosa instead of the standard columnar mucosa of the rectum. The *transformation zone* of the rectum is a region in which squamous metaplasia may be found overlying the normal columnar mucosa. This immature metaplastic tissue may extend up the rectum in a fluid and dynamic fashion involving at times 10 cm or more of distal rectal mucosa. The *transformation zone* is an important region, where metaplastic tissue susceptible to human papiloma virus (HPV) infection, in particular HPV 16, may be found.

Locations of all lesions within the above referenced zones should be clearly reported. Frequently, accurate reconstruction of the exact location of a lesion removed by a referring caregiver is not possible. This may lead to overtreatment of perianal and even skin lesions. In the distal rectum, it may still be necessary to refer to one established anatomic landmark, the dentate line (mucocutaneous junction), to accurately reflect how far proximally in the rectum a lesion was found. In contrast to the dentate line, the anal verge is poorly understood, poorly visualized and often confused with anal margin, which represents a region, not an anatomic boundary.

D.E. Beck et al. (eds.), *The ASCRS Textbook of Colon and Rectal Surgery: Second Edition*,
DOI 10.1007/978-1-4419-1584-9_20, © Springer Science+Business Media, LLC 2011

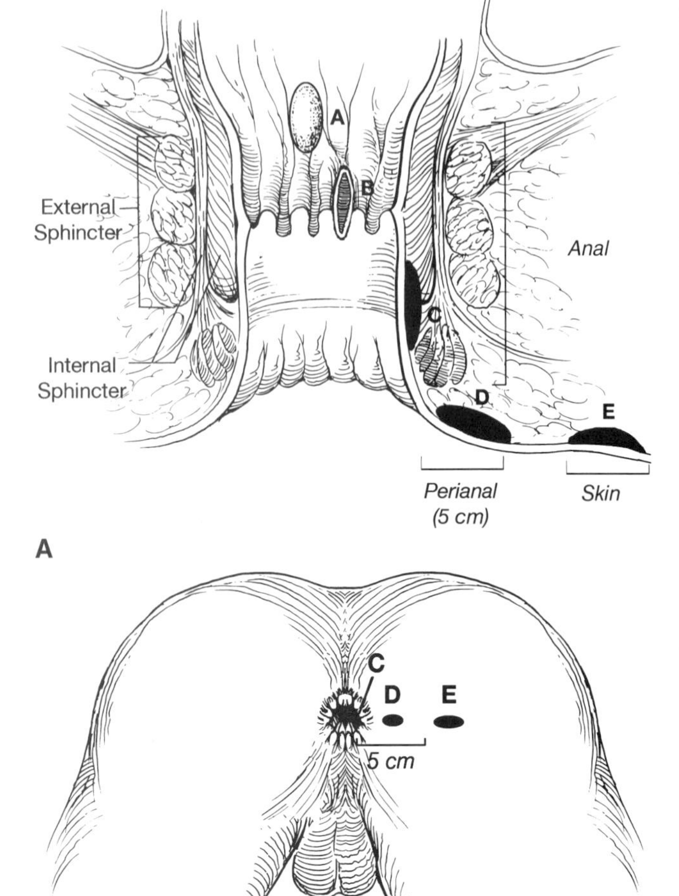

FIGURE 20-1. **A** and **B**. Terminology for location of anal and perianal lesions. Tumors **A**, **B** and **C** represent **ANAL** lesions that are not visible or are incompletely visible while gentle traction is placed on the buttocks. Tumor **D** is a perianal tumor because it is completely visible with gentle traction on the buttocks and lesion **E** is a skin cancer.

Terminology

The terminology used by pathologists when reporting premalignant lesions of the anus and perineum is often confusing to the treating clinicians. The terms squamous cell carcinoma in situ (CIS), anal intraepithelial neoplasia (AIN), anal dysplasia, squamous intraepithelial lesion (SIL), and Bowen's disease may all be used to refer to the same histopathology. The training of the pathologist often dictates the terms chosen. An additional point of confusion is that AIN terminology derives from histologic exams (microscopic evaluation of thin slices of tissue) while SILs are cytologic diagnoses (microscopic evaluation of cell scrapings or needle aspiration). AIN and dysplasia have both historically been broken into AIN I, II, and III and low-, moderate-, and high-grade dysplasia. However, as with other pathologic staging systems, the intra- and inter-observer variability is too high with this many categories. Therefore, when referring to anal canal, perianal, and skin lesions of the buttock the tissue should be classified as either normal, low-grade squamous intraepithelial lesions (LSIL), high-grade squamous intraepithelial lesions (HSIL), or invasive cancer as is done in the AJCC Staging Manual.[2]

Lymphatic Drainage

Lymphatic drainage above the dentate line occurs via the superior rectal lymphatics to the inferior mesenteric lymph nodes and laterally to the internal iliac nodes. Below the dentate line, drainage is not only primarily to the inguinal nodes, but may also involve the inferior or superior rectal lymph nodes.

Etiology and Pathogenesis of Anal Dysplasia and Anal Squamous Cell Carcinoma

The HPV is a necessary but not sufficient cause for the development of anal SCC and SIL.[4,5] HPV is a DNA papovavirus with an 8 kb genome and is the most common viral sexually transmitted infection.[6–8] Although most patients clear the virus with only 1% of the patients developing genital warts with low oncogenic potential (HPV serotypes 6 and 11),[9–11] an estimated 10–46% of patients develop subclinical infections that may harbor malignant potential (HPV serotypes 16, 18, 31, 33, 35).[12–15]

Transmission is not prevented by condoms as the virus pools at the base of the penis and scrotum. Thus, abstinence is the only effective means of prevention. In women, the virus may pool and extend from the vagina to the anus. Anoreceptive intercourse may be associated with the development of intra-anal disease but the presence of condylomata or dysplasia within the anus does not indicate that anoreceptive intercourse has occurred.[16]

In the rare patient who develops chronic infection, a variety of events must occur starting with the virus entering the basal and parabasal cells. This may occur through a disruption in the normal mucosal barrier that developed as a result of anoreceptive intercourse, other sexually transmitted diseases (ulcers from syphilis, gonorrhea), friable prolapsing hemorrhoidal tissues or a firm bowel movement. As noted above, the squamous metaplastic tissue above dentate line is a relatively "immature" incompletely developed squamous epithelium overlying the columnar epithelium and may not require trauma to disrupt an intact "barrier" making it particularly susceptible to HPV infection.[17] If high-risk viral DNA eludes immune surveillance and gains access to the nuclei of replicating cells (wound repair or metaplasia), the infection can become widespread and persistent lasting for decades resulting in an increased risk of cancer.

Cell-mediated immunity appears to be important to the cellular response prohibiting the virus from establishing a prolonged presence. This hypothesis is supported by the observation that cervical dysplasia patients with established high-risk lesions had a decreased ability to mount a T helper cell type 1 (Th1 IL-2) response in contrast to those patients with low-risk lesions.[18] Further support comes from the increased anal cancer rates observed in kidney transplant and HIV (+) patients, both populations with blunted cell-mediated responses.[19–25]

Oncogenic viruses lead to cellular proliferation in the latency phase by interfering with cell cycle control mechanisms.[17,26] Two "early region" viral genes, E6 and E7, inhibit cell cycle control resulting in increased proliferation. E7 binds directly to the retinoblastoma (Rb) tumor suppressor protein products p105, p107, and p130 related proteins leading to a complicated cascade of events involving E2F transcriptions factors, cyclin complexes and other regulatory proteins allowing the cell to progress through G1 into S phase.[27] Cell cycle release by E7 allows for immortalization of the cells but is not sufficient for the transformation of the infected cell. Accumulation of genetic errors appears necessary for transformation, which is consistent with the clinical scenario of a long-standing low-grade infection preceding the development of malignancy.[28] The genetic errors may accumulate as a result of the E6 protein which binds to p53 with E6-associated protein (E6AP) leading to degradation of the complex through the ubiquitin pathway.[27,29] The unblocked p53 protein is an important cell cycle regulating protein that leads to cell cycle arrest and apoptosis when genetic errors have accumulated thus allowing for DNA repair and avoidance of replication of errors.

The E2 protein allows the HPV DNA to avoid intracellular detection by facilitating the attachment of the HPV DNA to the host chromatin. This also assures replication in a steady state with each cell division.[17,30–32] In uninfected epithelium, division occurs in the basal layers and maturation results in pyknotic condensed cells that slough from the tissue surface. In infected tissues, the viral DNA replication process is reactivated leading to the presence of specific proteins and viral particles that can be detected in the upper cell layers. In summary, through the combined effect of E7, E6, and E2, cells with genetic errors may proliferate, accumulate and involve the entire thickness of the epithelium.[17] This may result in carcinogenesis.

As the infection with oncogenic viruses persists the anal tissues may progress through low-grade to high-grade dysplasia and cancer. With this disease progression is an associated increased proliferation and angiogenesis, and decreased apoptosis.[33] In contrast to the mechanisms responsible for the increased proliferation and decreased apoptosis outlined in the above discussion, the mechanisms involved in increased angiogenesis are less well defined. However, in the cervix, angiogenic changes have long been recognized as an important and visible step in the progression of dysplasia to cancer. Colposcopy, a magnified view of the cervix with the aid of acetic acid and Lugol's solution, allows for direct visualization of characteristic vascular patterns seen with LSIL and HSIL. Gynecologists are trained to recognize these vascular patterns and target their therapeutic destruction in the cervix accordingly. This therapeutic intervention, in combination with screening Pap smears, has led to the belief that cervical cancer is a largely preventable cancer.

Fortunately, the angiogenic changes associated with the development of anal HSIL are also visible with the aid of acetic acid and Lugol's solution in the perianal skin, anus and distal rectum through an operative microscope, colposcope, or loupes in the office or operating room (Figure 20-2A–D).[15] Targeted destruction is safe and may result in the same decrease in anal cancer incidence as was seen with cervical cancer when cervical Pap smears and targeted destruction were introduced for cervical disease.[34,35]

The cost-effectiveness of such an anal cytology screening system to prevent anal cancer has been demonstrated using an economic model in both HIV-positive[36] and HIV-negative men who have sex with men (MSM).[37] These studies demonstrated that screening to identify patients with HSIL to be referred for treatment would be cost-effective if performed annually for HIV-positive MSM and every 2–3 years for HIV-negative MSM.

Although the association of MSM and anal cancer is clear[16,38,39], the association of HIV with the development and progression of anal cancer has been hard to separate from other confounding factors. Initial studies accumulating anal cancer rates from the pre HAART (highly active antiretroviral therapy) era failed to show a correlation presumably because patients succumbed to complications of the HIV.[40,41] HPV is an indolent infection that leads to cancer in a minority of patients who generally suffer from a long-term infection. Thus, as might be expected, more recent studies reporting anal cancer rates in patients who are now surviving longer with effective HAART suggest an association with HIV and anal cancer.[19,20,42–45] Supporting this association is the observed rise in anal cancer and dysplasia rates seen in HIV positive MSM, and HIV positive heterosexual men and women who do not report anoreceptive intercourse.[19–21] Further, HIV positive patients are more likely to have HSIL, are more likely to progress from LSIL to HSIL over a two-year time period, and both of these findings are increased in the patients with a lower CD4 count (<200 cells/mm).[42–44] Low CD4 counts are a surrogate measure for immunosuppression from the HIV infection, and it is therefore suggested that HIV infection is associated with an increased risk of progression of anal disease.

Although the above articles suggest a permissive role for HIV in the development of anal cancer in HIV positive men and women, one cancer registry report comparing anal cancer rates before and after the individual's AIDS diagnosis found no correlation.[46] Nonetheless, data is accumulating that suggests that as men and women live longer in the HAART era, the indolent HPV infection results in an increased risk for the development of anal cancer, and this effect is the most significant in the most immunocompromised patients.[45]

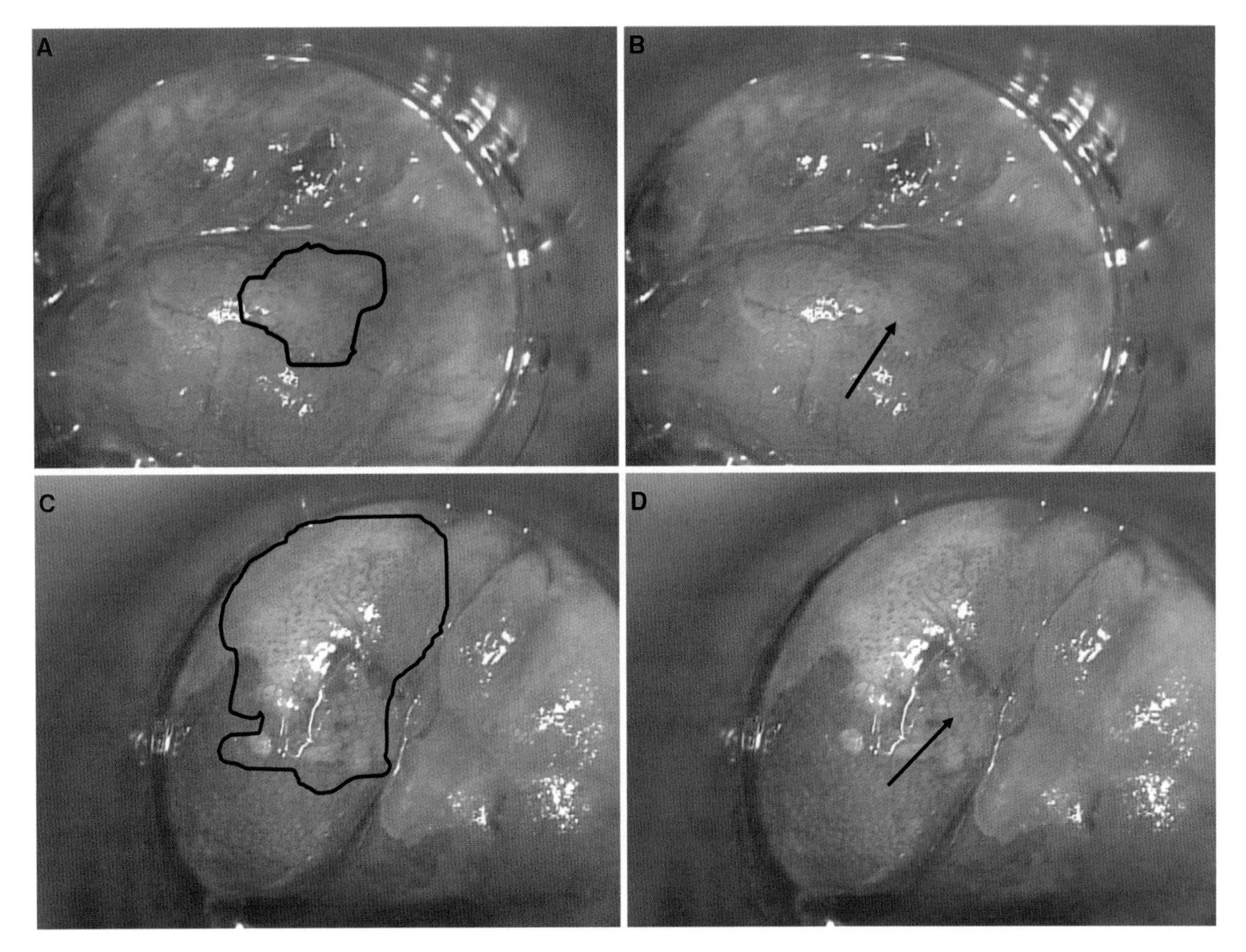

FIGURE 20-2. LSIL and HSIL visualized in the office with a colposcope after the application of acetic acid. The *arrows* in both images depict where the biopsy of the lesion was taken. **A** and **B** Anal LSIL in the distal rectal mucosa with subtle punctate vessel changes. The geography of the lesion in highlighted in the left frame. **C** and **D** Anal HSIL in the distal rectal mucosa with the left image highlighting serpiginous, cerebriform vessels and the outline of the entire lesion and the right image highlighting the mosaic pattern created by the vessels in the aceto-white background.

Epidemiology

The incidence of anal SCC has been increasing in frequency in over the last 30 years in the USA, Europe, and South America. This increase has been quite pronounced over the last 8 years, where there has been an increase from 3,900 new cases for 2002 to 5,290 new cases for 2009.[1,47] The California Cancer Registry found a statewide increase in anal cancers in non-Hispanic white men of approximately 2% per year between 1988 and 1999 with 1.0 case per 100,000 population in 1988 and 1.4 cases per 100,000 population in 1999.[22] There was not a comparable increase for women over the same time period. Most alarming was the increase in the age adjusted incidence for San Francisco white men age 40–64, where the rates rose from 3.7 per 100,000 for 1973–1978 to 8.6 per 100,000 in 1984–1990 and ultimately to 20.6 per 100,000 in 1996–1999. This is the first report ever of anal cancer rates higher among men under age 40 compared to women of the same age group.[22] Previous reports have consistently shown a higher rate in women in all age groups.[48]

In Denmark during the years 1943–1987, there was a 1.5-fold increase in men and a threefold increase in women.[49] A significant decrease in the mean age of men diagnosed with anal SCC from 68 to 63 years of age was also found. An even greater increase was found in city populations, where a threefold increase in the incidence of anal cancers in Copenhagen and its suburbs was observed. A significant rise in incidence for the entire male population was still seen with the incidence observed between the years 1983 and 1987 representing an increase of 30–40% of that seen in the 5-year span of 1943–1947. The rates in Copenhagen and surrounding areas were equal to the national level in 1943–1947, but in 1983–1987 the incidence in the city was 2.5-fold higher than that seen in the rest of the country. The average age of women patients with SCC did not change, but the incidence did increase threefold over the entire country with a significantly greater increase in Copenhagen when compared to the entire country. Men with anal cancer were significantly less likely to have been married when compared to men with colon cancer and stomach cancer. The same was not true of women with anal cancer. Similar findings were reported from Sweden, where a dramatic increase in incidence of anal cancer was observed around 1960, with a greater change in women than men (2:1), and the steepest increase in the heavily populated cities.[48] A study from Vermont shows that the trend seen in the cities is also present in more rural settings.[50]

In another Copenhagen study, women with anal cancer were noted to have a higher risk of having had cervical neoplasia or cancer.[51] Risk factors for developing HSIL and anal cancer also included HIV seropositivity, low CD4 count, persistent infection with high-risk HPV genotypes (16, 18, 31, 33, 35), infection with multiple genotypes, cigarette smoking, anal receptive intercourse, and immunosuppression for organ allograft. Multiple partners was not a significant independent risk factor.[28,42,43,52–58]

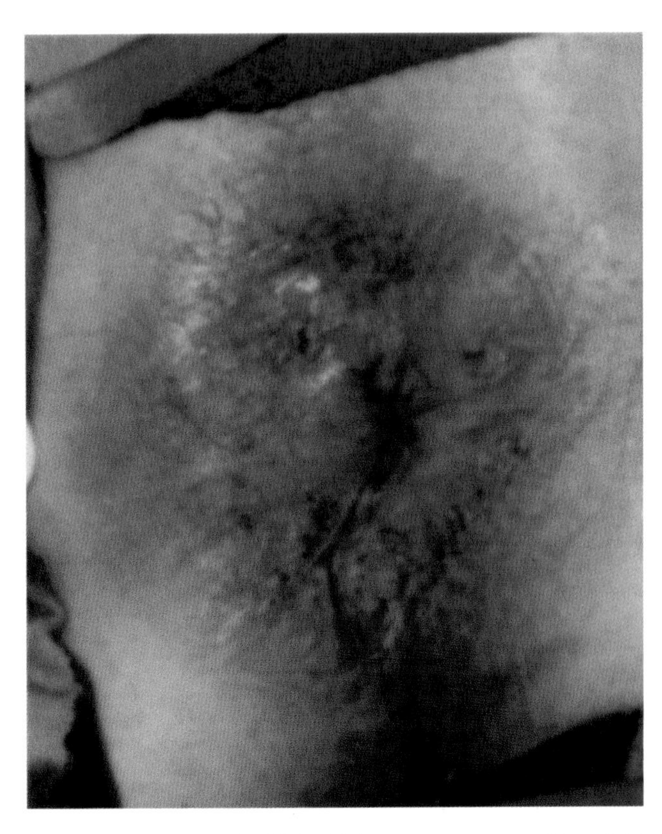

FIGURE 20-3. Perianal HSIL. With permission from Beck DE, Wexner SD. Anal neoplasms. In: Beck DE, Wexner SD, editors. Fundamentals of anorectal surgery. London: W. B. Saunders; 1998. p. 261–277.

Anal Canal and Perianal High-Grade Squamous Intraepithelial Lesions (Formerly Bowen's Disease)

As mentioned earlier in the chapter, the distinction between Bowen's disease and HSIL is unclear and appears to have more to do with the pathologist's training, histopathology versus cytopathology, than any biologic difference. Bowen's disease is anal SCC in situ, AIN II and III and HSIL. The term Bowen's disease is applied to SCC in situ in both keratinizing and nonkeratinizing tissues. Thus, we feel the term is archaic and confusing, and should be abandoned in favor of HSIL. Throughout this chapter, we use the term HSIL to refer to what has previously been termed Bowen's Disease.

HSIL is commonly found as an incidental histologic finding after surgery for an unrelated problem, often hemorrhoids. The lesion is clinically unapparent, but histologic assessment of the specimen reveals HSIL (Figure 20-3). Alternatively, patients may present with complaints of perianal burning, pruritis, or pain. Physical examination may reveal scaly, discrete, erythematous or pigmented lesions (Figure 20-4).

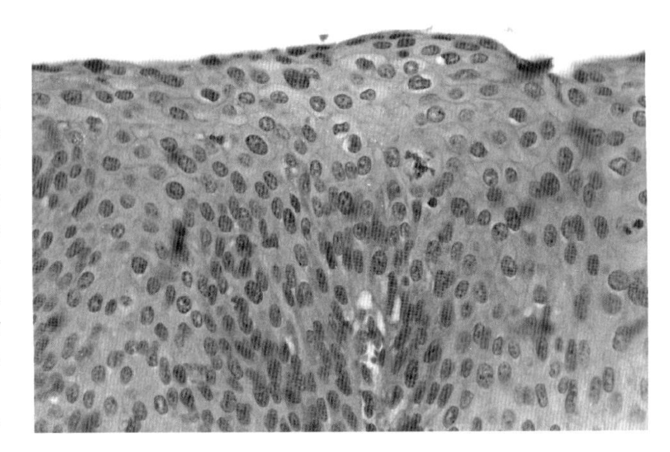

FIGURE 20-4. Perianal HSIL. (Photomicrograph hematoxylin and eosin ×400). With permission from Beck DE, Wexner SD. Anal neoplasms. In: Beck DE, Wexner SD, editors. Fundamentals of anorectal surgery. London: W. B. Saunders; 1998. p. 261–277.

The natural history of HSIL is poorly defined. In the immunocompetent, fewer than 10% progress to cancer.[59] However, in immunocompromised patients, the progression rate appears greater as evidenced by the higher rates of anal cancers observed in the HIV (+) and immunosuppressed transplant patients.[19–24] As we are as yet unable to identify those patients that progress, the authors favor treatment of HSIL. An exception to this recommendation would be patients with advanced AIDS with poor performance statuses despite maximal medical therapy. This was a common problem in the early 1990s but since the advent of HAART, the vast majority of our AIDS patients are candidates for surgical intervention. The other exception might be the elderly patient with an asymptomatic lesion and a short life expectancy. Unlike perianal Paget's disease, there is no association with other visceral malignancies.[60]

The preferred treatment is fairly controversial and should be tailored to the given patient. An older recommendation for the unsuspected lesion found after hemorrhoidectomy is to return the patient to the operating for random biopsies taken at 1 cm intervals starting at the dentate line and around the anus in a clock-like fashion. Frozen sections establish the presence of HSIL and these areas are widely locally excised with 1 cm margins. Large defects are covered with flaps of gluteal and perianal skin. Although this technique has been shown to provide excellent local control, it does not prevent recurrences.[61] Recurrence rates in one series were as high as 23% despite this radical approach.[62] Although no cancers developed in this group, HIV status was not noted and complications, including incontinence, stenosis, and sexual function were not reported. In another study of wide local excision, the authors noted a 63% persistence rate at 1 year and a 13% recurrence rate at 3 years. Eleven percent of the patients developed incontinence or stenosis.[63] The unknown risk of disease progression, high recurrence rate, and the significant morbidity associated with extensive wide excisions have led many authorities (including the authors and a few editors) to rarely use or recommend this option.

A less radical approach involves taking patients to the operating room to perform High Resolution Anoscopy (HRA) with the aid of an operating microscope, acetic acid, and Lugol's solution. The lesions are visualized and targeted for electrocautery destruction. Like cervical disease, the HSIL is visible because of its characteristic vascular pattern identifying the at-risk tissue for selective destruction (Figure 20-2).[15] This technique minimizes the morbidity of the procedure and saves the normal anal mucosa and perianal skin that would otherwise be sacrificed. Postoperative pain is significant as with any perianal procedure. One author (MLW) reviewed 247 patients with HSIL treated with HRA.[35] The majority of these patients had extensive circumferential or near circumferential disease and were immunocompromised (HIV or other.) Although recurrent HSIL lesions occurred in 57% of patients, most were retreated with high-resolution directed office-based therapies. Initial extent of disease was the only factor that correlated with recurrence. During the 10-year study period, only 3 (1.2%) patients progressed to SCC. Patients were followed for an average of 19 months (range 3–92) and 78% had no evidence of HSIL at their last office visit.[35] HSIL identified with HRA may also simply be locally excised taking care to stay close to the lesion margin directly visualized with the operative microscope. The deep margin is kept equally close as wide local excision seems of limited benefit and increases morbidity. The resulting minimal defects heal in secondarily. High-risk patients, the immunocompromised, and patients practicing anoreceptive intercourse should be followed with Pap smears at yearly and three yearly intervals for the immunocompromised and immunocompetent, respectively.[36,37]

Other therapeutic modalities include topical 5-Fluorouracil (5-FU) cream, Imiquimod, photodynamic therapy, radiation therapy, laser therapy, and combinations of the above. The reports are generally small series with limited follow-up, but there may be anecdotal success with each approach, and the options may be kept in mind for challenging cases. Initial reports of the use of 5-FU cream were generally disappointing.[64] However, two small subsequent studies have shown encouraging results.[65] One of these reports suggests that Erbium:YAG laser pretreatment may improve the response of HSIL.[66] Reports of the use of Vidarabine and cidofovir support their consideration but the series are small with limited follow-up.[67,68] Imiquimod has been reported to be of benefit alone[69] and in combination with 5% 5-FU therapy in the immunosuppressed transplant and HIV (+) patient population.[70,71] Radiotherapy with a special skin patch or conventional external beam has also been reported.[72,73] Photodynamic therapy has been tried with success[74,75] and compared favorably to topical 5-FU in a randomized comparison.[76]

Perianal Squamous Cell Carcinoma (Formerly Anal Margin)

SCC arises from both the perianal skin and the anal canal. The distinction between the two locations has become more important as they are increasingly considered different entities with separate treatments and prognosis. Immunohistochemical studies of squamous cell tumors from the anal margin and anal canal demonstrate differences in expression of cadherin, cytokeratins and p53 confirming that these tumors are of distinct histogenetic origin.[77] Perianal lesions are completely visible and fall within a 5 cm radius of the anal opening when gentle traction is placed on the buttocks.

Clinical Characteristics

Perianal tumors resemble SCC of other areas of skin and are therefore staged and often treated in a similar fashion.[78] They have rolled, everted edges with central ulceration, and may have a palpable component in the subcutaneous tissues although the sphincter complex is not usually involved. Patients present in the seventh decade of life with equal incidence in men and women.[79,80] Presenting symptoms include a painful lump, bleeding, pruritis, tenesmus, discharge or even fecal incontinence.[81] In general, perianal tumors are characterized by a delay in diagnosis due to their location and indistinct features, and SCC is no exception. Patients have been noted to have symptoms anywhere from 0 to 144 months prior to diagnosis (median of 3 months),[82] and almost a third are misdiagnosed at their first physician

TABLE 20-1. American Joint Committee on Cancer (AJCC) Staging of Squamous Cell Carcinoma (SCC)

Primary Tumor (T)				
Tx	Primary tumor cannot be assessed			
T0	No evidence of primary tumor			
T*is*	Carcinoma in situ (Bowen's disease, high-grade squamous intraepithelial lesion (HSIL), anal itraepithelial neoplasia II-III (AIN II-III)			
T1	Tumor less ≤2 cm in greatest dimension			
T2	Tumor 2–5 cm in greatest dimension			
T3	Tumor ≥5 cm in greatest dimension			
T4	Tumor of any size invades adjacent organ(s), e.g., vagina, urethra, bladder* *Direct invasion of the rectal wall, perirectal skin, subcutaneous tissue, or the sphincter muscle(s) is not classified as T4.			
Nodal Status (N)				
Nx	Regional lymph nodes cannot be assessed			
N0	No regional lymph node metastasis			
N1	Metastasis in perirectal lymph node(s)			
N2	Metastasis in unilateral internal iliac and/or inguinal lymph node(s)			
N3	Metastasis in perirectal and inguinal lymph nodes and/or bilateral internal iliac and/or inguinal lymph nodes			
Distant Metastasis (M)				
M0	No distant metastasis			
M1	Distant metastasis present			
Stage Grouping				
Stage 0	T*is*	N0	M0	
Stage I	T1	N0	M0	
Stage II	T2, 3	N0	M0	
Stage IIIA	T1, 2, 3	N1	M0	or T4 N0 M0
Stage IIIB	Any T	N2, 3	M0	or T4 N1 M0
Stage IV	Any T	Any N	M1	

visit.[81] Patients were given erroneous diagnoses of hemorrhoids, anal fissures, fistulas, eczema, abscesses, or benign tumors. For perianal tumors, however, there was no significant difference in survival between correctly diagnosed and misdiagnosed patients.[81]

Staging

The staging of perianal SCC is based on the size of the tumor and lymph node involvement, both of which correlate with prognosis. Lymphatic drainage of the perianal skin extends to the femoral and inguinal nodes and then to the external and common iliac nodes. Venous drainage occurs through the inferior rectal vein. Lymph node involvement is associated with the size and differentiation of the tumor.[82–84] In one study, the incidence of inguinal lymph node metastasis was noted to be 0% for tumors <2 cm, 23% for tumors 2–5 cm in size, and 67% for tumors >5 cm.[84] Distant visceral metastasis at presentation is rare but should be evaluated with a CT scan of the abdomen and pelvis, to assess for liver metastases, as well as the presence of nodal disease. A chest X-ray or CT may be performed to evaluate for lung metastases. These tumors are generally slow growing and histologically are well differentiated with well-developed patterns of keratinization.[79,85] The AJCC staging system is described in Table 20-1.[2]

TABLE 20-2. Results of local excision of perianal tumors

Author	Year	*N*	Local recurrence	Survival
Beahrs and Wilson[91]	1976	27	0	100
Al Jurf et al.[88]	1979	10	50	90
Schraut et al.[89]	1983	11	18	80
Greenall et al.[87]	1985	31	42	68
Jensen et al.[86]	1988	32	63	–
Pintor et al.[90]	1989	41	–	68

Treatment Options

Treatment of perianal SCC traditionally consisted of surgical resection with wide local excision for smaller-sized tumors and abdominoperineal resection (APR) for larger, invasive tumors. However, it is well documented that wide local excision alone results in high locoregional recurrence rates (18–63%) (Table 20-2)[79,86–91] and should be reserved for those lesions that can be excised with a 1 cm margin, are T*is* or T1, and do not involve enough sphincter to compromise function.[80] A series of 27 patients with T*is* and T1 lesions treated with wide local excision had a 100% 5-year survival[91] and in

TABLE 20-3. Radiation therapy for perianal tumors by T stage

Author	Year	N	Local control (%) T1	T2	T3	Cancer specific 5-year survival (%)
Cummings et al.[95]	1986	29	100	100	60	–
Cutuli et al.[96]	1988	21	50	71	37	72
Papillon and Chassard[84]	1992	54	100	84	50	80
Touboul et al.[93]	1995	17	100	60	100	86
Peiffert et al.[92]	1997	32	88	73	57	89

another study, all patients with small or superficial tumors locally excised had a survival of 100%, whereas those with deep invasion did not survive 5 years.[89] Since it was introduced in the early 1970s, radiation therapy has become the mainstay of therapy for SCC of the anal canal and its application to perianal tumors is increasing. In patients with T1 or early T2 lesions, local excision or radiation therapy provides similar local control rates (60–100%),[84,92,93] but for less favorable lesions, chemoradiation is now utilized as the first line therapy using perineal and inguinal fields, even without clinically detectable disease in the groin.[84,93] Pelvic lymph nodes are also treated for those patients with T3 and T4 tumors.[79,80,84,94] Local control rates for radiation therapy reported by T stage are as follows T1:50–100%, T2: 60–100%, T3:37–100% (Table 20-3).[84,92,93,95,96] In one study, the T3 lesions were separated into tumors 5–10 cm in size and those greater than 10 cm with local control rates of 70% versus 40%, respectively.[95] Patients with persistent tumor can be treated with local excision or APR with a 50% salvage rate.[86,97] Those with recurrence after successful radiation can also be salvaged for cure with surgery.[98–101] The absolute 5-year survival rate for patients treated with local excision or APR ranges from 60 to 100% but is lower in patients with larger tumors.[87,88,102] Similarly, absolute 5-year survival in patients treated with radiation ranges from 52 to 90% with sphincter preservation in about 80%.[80] The use of chemoradiation specifically pertaining to perianal SCC has not been well examined. However, one study did show an improvement in local control (64% vs. 88%) with the addition of 5-FU and mitomycin to radiation.[95] In extrapolation of data from a randomized, multicenter study, including early stage tumors, anal canal, and perianal cancers, it would be postulated that chemoradiation is superior.[101] More recently, Mendenhall et al.[80] report local control in 19 patients treated with radiotherapy alone or combined with adjuvant chemotherapy over a 21-year period. One patient with T1 disease died secondary to regional and distant disease. Four patients died of intercurrent disease and the remaining 14 patients were disease-free at 25, 29, 37, and 113 months following treatment. No patients required salvage APR or salvage surgical therapy.

In summary, the choice of treatment is dependent on the stage of tumor, the anticipated functional result as a result of therapy and the risk of complications. Although surgery may result in alteration of sphincter function, or a permanent colostomy, radiation therapy may also cause skin changes or proctitis that produces urgency, incontinence, or the need for diversion. For T1 and early T2 tumors, wide local excision may be less morbid and time consuming than radiation therapy and therefore a superior choice. However, if the excision will result in damage to the sphincters with impairment of sphincter function, radiation provides similar local control and survival. Larger T2 tumors should be treated with radiation therapy to the primary lesion and inguinal fields due to poor local control with excision and the significant risk of lymph node metastasis. This treatment modality is much less morbid than resection of the primary and bilateral lymph node dissection with similar control rates.[83] Those with T3, T4, or poorly differentiated tumors should receive radiation to the primary lesion and include inguinal and pelvic fields to treat regional nodes in these areas. APR should be reserved for those patients with persistent or recurrent disease after radiation therapy.[80,94]

Squamous Cell Carcinoma of the Anal Canal

SCC incorporates all large-cell keratinizing, large-cell nonkeratinizing (transitional) and basaloid histologies. The terms epidermoid, cloacogenic, and mucoepidermoid carcinoma are all encompassed in the squamous cell carcinoma group.[2,103] SCC of the anal canal is five times more common than perianal SCC, but its incidence is one-tenth that of rectal cancer. The incidence, epidemiology and etiology were described earlier in this chapter.

Clinical Characteristics

The most common presenting symptom is bleeding, which occurs in over 50% of patients with many complaining of anal pain. Other symptoms include palpable lump, pruritis, discharge, tenesmus, change in bowel habits, fecal incontinence, and rarely, inguinal lymphadenopathy.[81,104,105] A small number of patients are asymptomatic. Unfortunately, most patients are diagnosed late with up to 55% of patients being misdiagnosed at the time of presentation.[81] In another study of 172 patients with SCC, only 17 were diagnosed with tumors confined to the epithelium and subepithelial connective tissue.[106]

Evaluation

Physical examination should include a complete anorectal examination with external inspection of the anoderm, digital exam, anoscopy, proctoscopy, when necessary, and examination of inguinal nodes. Lesions are characteristically hard and ulcerated and, if large, may extend outside the anal canal (Figure 20-5). Careful notation should be made of the size, location, and mobility of the mass, associated perirectal lymphadenopathy, and in women, a pelvic examination should be performed to look for any associated lesions or invasion of tumor into the vagina. Complete examination and biopsy may require anesthesia for those patients with significant pain. Additional workup may include an endoanal/endorectal ultrasound to assess the depth of the tumor, presence of perirectal lymph nodes, and invasion of adjacent organs as an adjunct to the physical examination although this may be limited by pain.[107–110] Ultrasound has been found to be superior to physical exam in assessing the involvement of internal and external anal sphincter muscle and perirectal lymph nodes. This has an impact on staging as physical exam often under-stages tumors. One study demonstrated that endorectal ultrasound T and N stage were significant predictors of relapse, whereas the corresponding clinical staging was not.[109] A study of three-dimensional ultrasound has demonstrated improved accuracy in detecting perirectal lymph nodes and some suggestion of improved evaluation of tumor invasion.[111] Inguinal nodal involvement at the time of presentation can be difficult to determine. The sensitivity of radiologic imaging and clinical exam are poor.[112] Enlarged lymph nodes can be reactive to secondary inflammation in some cases and therefore should be biopsied with direct fine-needle aspiration (FNA) or ultrasound-guided FNA if detected by imaging. Excisional lymph node biopsy is rarely required but may be done if FNA is inconclusive. Studies of sentinel lymph node biopsy have demonstrated that the technique is safe and may result in more accurate staging[113], but the actual impact on initial and subsequent management remains unclear as long as inguinal fields are included during radiation therapy. CT scan or MRI of the abdomen and pelvis can add to locoregional staging as well as evaluating for liver metastasis. A chest CT or chest X-ray is used as a screening tool for lung lesions. PET scans are primarily useful for assessing persistent or residual disease after treatment. Sigmoidoscopy can exclude any associated lesions proximal to the anal canal. Lastly, a HIV test should be performed for those at higher risk. HIV positive patients with CD4 counts <200 need better monitoring of opportunistic infections, closer attention to toxic effects of chemoradiation with possible alterations in dosage, and management of antiretroviral therapy.[104,105,114,115]

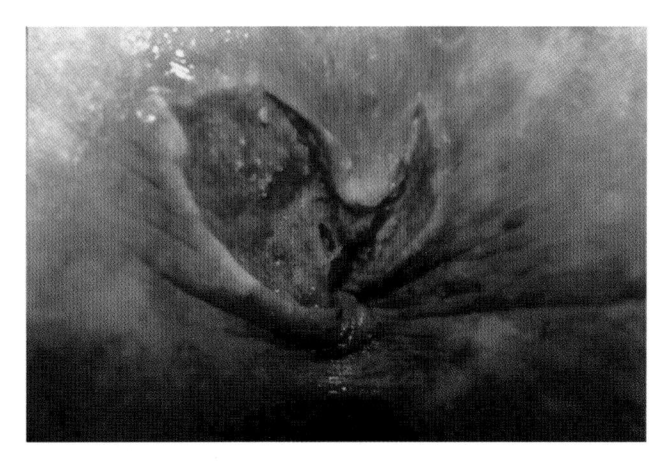

FIGURE 20-5. Anal canal carcinoma.

Staging

The staging of anal canal SCC is based on the size of the tumor and lymph node metastasis. The TNM staging is listed in Table 20-1. The risk of nodal metastasis correlates with the size, depth of invasion, and the histologic grade of the tumor. In a series of 305 patients with SCC, lymph node metastasis was present in 16%. Nodal metastasis by T stage was as follows: T1 (0%), T2 (8.5%), T3 (29%), T4 (35%). Lymph node metastasis occurred in 47% of patients with T4 tumors greater than 5 cm in size.[116] Inguinal metastases have been detected in 10–30% of patients at the time of diagnosis[90,106,117,118] with an additional 5–22% of patients developing clinically apparent lymph node metastases over time.[118] Nodal metastasis was almost double (58% vs. 30%) in those tumors invading beyond the external sphincter compared to invasion of the internal sphincter.[119] Lymphatic drainage of the anal canal above the dentate line proceeds along the superior rectal vessels. At the dentate line, the drainage basin includes the internal pudendal, internal iliac, and obturator nodes. Below the dentate line, the lymphatic drainage is through the inguinal, femoral, and external iliac lymph nodes.[120] Mesenteric lymph nodes are more common in tumors of the proximal anal canal (50%) than the distal anal canal (14%).[104] An anatomic study of lymph node metastasis demonstrated that they most often occur above the peritoneal reflection and not in the perianal area. Additionally, almost half of the positive lymph nodes were less that 5 mm in size.[120] Distant visceral metastasis occurs in 10–17% of patients at presentation and can be found in the liver, lung, bone, and subcutaneous tissues.[100,101] Subsequent metastasis is more common and was the cause of 40% of cancer-specific deaths in one series.[101]

Treatment

Surgery

The treatment of anal canal SCC was historically operative with APR being the standard of care. Unfortunately, local recurrence rates ranged from 27 to 47% and 5-year survival was 40–70%.[89,90,103,104,106,112,121] The presence of pelvic lymph nodes decreased the 5-year survival to below 20%.[105] Local excision was performed in those patients who could not tolerate an abdominal operation, refused a permanent colostomy, or had small, well-differentiated tumors. The recurrence rates and 5-year survival ranged from 20 to 80% and 45 to 85%, respectively.[85,86] However, in well-selected patients with early tumors, the 5-year survival was 100%.[89,90,106]

Radiation Therapy

Primary radiation therapy is quite effective in treating SCC as this tumor is extremely radiosensitive. It can be given as external beam radiation, brachytherapy or in combination. Response is dose-dependent with the best chance of tumor eradication occurring with at least 54 Gy of external beam radiation (Table 20-4).[122,123] However, this benefit is lost when radiation is administered in a split-course fashion.[124,125] Local control and cure can be achieved in 70–90 % of selected patients with 60–70% retaining sphincter function.[117,122] However, when tumors are larger than 5 cm or lymph nodes are involved the cure rate decreases to 50%.[78,100,117,122] Better results with higher doses of radiation must be exchanged with increased radiation-induced complications when more than 40 Gy is administered. Serious late complications include anal necrosis, stenosis, and ulcerations, diarrhea, urgency and fecal incontinence, cystitis, urethral stenosis, and small bowel obstruction. Significant impairment of bowel control due to anal complications can lead to the placement of a colostomy. Studies have found a dose-dependent effect on morbidity with the requirement of a colostomy in 6–12% of patients.[117,126,127] However, one study examining risk factors predictive of requiring a colostomy for management of anal cancers found that tumor size was the only risk factor. Although radiation toxicities did occur, patients were not at an increased risk for requiring a stoma.[128] Brachytherapy used alone or in conjunction with external beam radiation is also effective with local control rates of 75–79% and 5-year survival of 61–65%, but 3–6% of patients had serious complications that required surgery. The high rate of anal necrosis seen when both modalities are used has dampened the enthusiasm for this approach.[129,130] At this time, radiation therapy alone is not commonly utilized but may have a role in treating T1 tumors.[126,131]

Table 20-4. Response to radiation based on dosage

		Local control (%)	
Author	Year	<54 Gy	>54 Gy
Hughes et al.[122]	1989	50	90
Constantinou et al.[123]	1997	61	77

Chemoradiation Therapy

The introduction of chemoradiation therapy by Nigro in 1974 revolutionized the treatment of anal canal SCC by demonstrating equivalent local control and survival rates with the preservation of sphincter function and thus avoidance of a colostomy.[132–134] Since that time, multiple studies have confirmed these results and chemoradiation is the standard therapy for SCC of the anal canal. Nigro described using 30-Gy external beam radiation with 5-Fu and mitomycin C, and demonstrated a complete pathological response in 21 of 26 patients treated (81%). Since that time various radiation doses (30–60 Gy) and chemotherapeutic regimens have been used with similar complete pathologic responses (45–100%) and survival rates (70–90%) (Table 20-5). As a result, operative treatment for anal canal SCC was largely abandoned and reserved for those patients with persistent or recurrent disease

Table 20-5. SCC of the anal canal: results of combination of radiation and 5-FU plus mitomycin C

Author (s)	No. of patients	Dose (Gy)	Complete regression (%)	Follow-up (mo)	5-year survival (%)
Flam et al. (1987)[189]	30	41–50	87	9–76->	–
Nigro (1987)[190]	104	30	93	24–132->	83
Habr-Gama ét al. (1989)[191]	30	30–45	73	12–60->	–
Sischy et al. (1989)[192]	79	40.8	90	20–55->	–
Cho et al. (1991)[193]	20	30	85	Av. 34	70
Cummings et al. (1991)[126]	69	50	85–93	>36	76
Lopez et al. (1991)[194]	33	30–56	88	Med., 48	79
Doci et al. (1992)[195]	56	36+18	87	2–45	81
Johnson et al. (1993)[196]	24	40.5–45	100	Med., 41	87
Tanum et al. (1993)[197]	86	50	T1*97 T2*80	46%>36	72
Beck and Karulf (1994)[198]	35	30–45	97	4–155	87
Smith et al. (1994)[199]	42	30	T1*90 T2*87	31 31	90 87
Bartelink et al. (1997)[100]	51	30–45	80	Med. 42	Overall survival 58% $P=0.17$
UKCCCR (1996)[101]	292	45	Not specifically reported	Med. 42	3-year – 65%
Ajani et al. (2008)[200]	324	45–59	Not specifically reported	Med., 30	75

TABLE 20-6. Result of two randomized trials examining radiation therapy alone and radiation therapy with chemotherapy for anal canal SCC

	N	Follow-up	Local control (%)			Overall survival (%)		
			XRT	Chemo XRT	P value	XRT	Chemo XRT	P value
EORTC[100]	110	5 years	50	68	0.02	57	52	0.17
UKCCCR[101]	585	3 years	39	61	<0.001	58	65	0.25

after chemoradiation. Although much controversy existed as to the benefit of chemoradiation therapy compared to primary radiation therapy, two randomized controlled studies have demonstrated the superiority of chemoradiation therapy with 5-FU and mitomycin C to radiation alone.[100,101] Using 45 Gy with a boost for good response, both studies exhibited better local control rates with chemoradiation (Table 20-6) but no significant difference in survival. However, one study noted a higher complete response rate (80% vs. 54%) and an improvement in colostomy-free survival (72% vs. 47% at 3 years) which is significant.[100] Chemotherapy-related deaths occurred in 5.4% of patients in one series leading to changes in the protocol which included a reduction of the dose for patients older than 70, bed-bound, frail, or with evidence of tumor-related sepsis.[101] The role of mitomycin C was also examined in a randomized trial which demonstrated better complete pathologic response rate (92% vs. 85%), local control rate (84% vs. 66%), colostomy-free survival rate (71% vs. 59%), and disease-free survival (73% vs. 51%) when mitomycin C was used in conjunction with 5-FU and radiation compared to 5FU and radiation alone.[135] However, treatment toxicity was increased in the mitomycin C group (23% vs. 7%) with a 4% chemotherapy-related mortality and overall survival was equivalent.

Although the use of mitomycin C has provided excellent results, cisplatin has gained favor as it is a radiation sensitizer, is less myelosuppressive than mitomycin C and has been used for those patients who failed to respond to mitomycin C. In series of patients treated with 45–55 Gy of radiation, 5-FU, and cisplatin, the reported rates of local control (80–83%), disease-free survival (77–90%), and colostomy-free survival (71–82%) were comparable to the best results obtained from mitomycin C regimens. Additionally, there were fewer severe toxicities reported.[136,137] A pilot study of the CALGB using cisplatin demonstrated a complete response rate of 80%, colostomy-free survival of 56% and overall survival of 78%.[105,115] Although the initial studies were encouraging, more recent data suggests that mitomycin C remains the mainstay of chemotherapy. The US Gastrointestinal Intergroup trial RTOG 98-11 was a randomized controlled trial conducted between October 1998 and June 2005 that compared treatment with cisplatin, 5-FU, and radiotherapy to mitomycin C, 5-FU, and radiotherapy.[101] A total of 682 patients with anal canal carcinoma were enrolled in the trial. The primary end point was defined as 4-year disease-free survival. Secondary endpoints were overall survival and time to relapse. Cisplatin-based therapy did not improve disease-free survival compared with mitomycin-based therapy. Additionally, cisplatin-based therapy was associated with a higher rate of colostomy.

Although the presence of inguinal metastasis at presentation indicates a worse prognosis, the overall 5-year survival is 48% (range 30–66%). Those with lymph nodes greater than 2 cm in size, T3 or T4 tumors or anal margin involvement had a worse survival (29–32%).[118] For patients with obvious evidence of inguinal node metastasis, local control can be achieved in 90% of patients receiving chemoradiation compared to 65% receiving radiation alone. Surgical management with radical groin dissection can lead to significant complications and may be successful only 15% of the time.[112] The management of synchronous inguinal node metastasis is not standardized and different centers use primary radiation therapy (45–65 Gy), chemoradiation, and selective lymph node dissection followed by radiation which has been reported to maintain disease-free intervals in up to 60% of patients.[79] For those with subclinical lymph nodes in the groin, chemoradiation is advocated with doses as low as 30–34 Gy. This minimizes toxicity but is effective in treating small volume disease based on previous studies of small sized tumors.[105] Whether or not inguinal fields should always be included when treating patients for anal canal SCC remains controversial.

Follow-up

No consensus has been reached on appropriate follow-up after the treatment of SCC. It is generally agreed that early intervention for persistent disease and recurrent locoregional disease can lead to successful salvage therapy. Routine examination with digital rectal exam and anoscopy every 3 months in the first 2 years, and every 6 months until 5 years has been recommended. Ultrasound examination has also become popular in detecting recurrence although the literature is mixed on its benefit.[109,138] CT scan or MRI performed after the completion of chemoradiation may also be useful as a baseline for future comparison. MRI is useful for distinguishing surrounding tissues and detecting persistent or recurrent disease.

Treatment of Residual or Recurrent Disease

Persistent or recurrent disease localized to the pelvis after chemoradiation can be treated with salvage therapy. Patients need to be restaged with a CT of the chest, abdomen, and pelvis. MRI may be useful to assess resectability of pelvic recurrence and PET scan may help to differentiate tumor from radiation-induced tissue changes or other undetectable metastases. APR can be performed for tumor localized to the pelvis with a 5-year survival of 24–47%.[139–144] Those with positive margins, nodal disease at salvage and persistent disease after chemoradiation have poorer outcomes.[144,145] Morbidity for APR in this setting is significant with an increased risk of perineal wound complications. This has prompted the use of plastic surgery reconstruction using rotational or advancement flaps or alternatively, use of the vacuum assisted closure (VAC) to promote healing. The benefit of adjuvant chemotherapy after APR is currently unknown. Symptomatic inguinal disease after chemoradiation of the primary tumor can be treated with radical groin dissection if radiation has already been administered. Additional radiotherapy can be considered if maximal doses of radiation were not delivered. Radical groin dissection in selected patients can result in a 5-year survival of 55%.[146] Distant metastasis have been found in 10–17% of patients treated with chemoradiation,[100,101] and are usually treated with systemic chemotherapy, such as cisplatin or 5-FU for palliation. If the metastases are isolated in the liver or lung and the primary disease is controlled, resection can be considered.

Uncommon Anal Canal Neoplasms

Adenocarcinoma

Anal canal adenocarcinomas are classified into three types. The first group may arise from the mucosa of the transitional zone in the upper canal and are indistinguishable from rectal adenocarcinoma. The second derives from the base of the anal glands, which are lined with mucin-secreting columnar epithelium. The last can develop in the setting of a chronic anorectal fistula.[85] Adenocarcinomas account for 5–19% of all anal cancers[147–149] and have a more aggressive natural history than SCC.[150] The average age at presentation ranges from 59 to 71 years with equal gender distribution.[148,151] Patients may present with pain, induration, abscess/fistula, or a palpable mass. Other symptoms include bleeding, pruritis, seepage, prolapse, and weight loss.[85]

Due to the rarity and heterogeneity of this tumor, the role of surgery and chemoradiation has been difficult to assess, thus making definitive recommendations for treatment impossible. Many patients present with advanced local or metastatic disease making curative treatment challenging. The local disease may tend to be more advanced in those that arise in glands and fistulous tracts because these locations are outside the bowel wall, and therefore the disease originates in a locally advanced location. Wide local excision may be feasible for those patients with a "rectal-type" tumor that is small, well differentiated, and does not invade the sphincter complex. All other tumors require APR. Chemoradiation alone has not been shown to be as effective for adenocarcinoma compared to SCC due to high local recurrence rates (54% vs. 18%) and poor survival rates (64% vs. 85%).[150] However, in another study analyzing treatments for anal canal adenocarcinoma, including APR, surgery with radiation, and chemoradiation, similar locoregional recurrence rates (20%, 37%, 36%) and better overall survival was seen in the chemoradiation group (21%, 29%, 58%).[151] Other studies have suggested that a combined modality approach of surgery with chemoradiation does improve outcome with survival rates exceeding 60%.[147,148] Although no large series of patients has been treated in any uniform manner to substantiate the approach of chemoradiation therapy followed by surgery, the success of this approach for rectal adenocarcinoma would support its use.

Melanoma

Anorectal melanoma is characterized by lesions that are often difficult to differentiate from benign pathology. For this reason, and its rarity, many patients present with advanced stage disease. Although the anorectum is the most common site for primary melanoma of the gastrointestinal tract, it comprises only 0.5–5% of all malignancies there. Fewer than 500 cases have been reported in the literature.[152] Patients are frequently female, Caucasian and in their sixties. Isolated cases have been reported in African American and Asian populations.[78,153,154]

Anorectal bleeding is the most common symptom described. However, anal pain, change in bowel habits, or tenesmus may also be reported. Weight loss and malaise may be indicative of advanced disease. A mass in the anal canal is the most frequent sign with palpable inguinal lymph nodes common. These tumors arise from the transitional epithelium of the anal canal, the anoderm or the mucocutaneous junction. Although some lesions may seem to arise within the rectal mucosa, it is postulated that this is due to heterotopic epithelium within the rectum or mucosal spread from a primary foci within the anal canal.[153]

Most lesions are pigmented, with early lesions appearing polypoid and larger lesions having ulcerations, raised edges or significant growth into the rectal vault. An early lesion may be indistinguishable from a thrombosed hemorrhoid, and some cases have been incidentally diagnosed from a hemorrhoidectomy specimen. Approximately two-thirds of the lesions are grossly pigmented or show histological evidence of melanin.[155] Amelanotic lesions can be difficult to differentiate from undifferentiated squamous cell carcinoma.

Surgical management of anorectal melanoma provides the only chance for cure. However, the choice of operation continues to be controversial since the prognosis is so poor. Up to 35% of patients present with metastatic disease,[156,157] and those patients with tumors greater than 10 mm in thickness are not cured by any treatment.[157] Additionally, long-term survival rates, which range from 0 to 29%,[152,155–159] do not seem to differ when wide local excision or APR is performed. However, some studies have shown fewer locoregional recurrences with a more radical operation,[155,156,160] thereby supporting the use of APR for earlier stage tumors. In a study of anorectal melanomas stratified by tumor thickness, tumors greater than 4 mm had inadequate local tumor control with wide local excision alone and APR was advocated.[157] Despite this, anorectal melanoma is largely a fatal disease and so the choice of treatment has little influence on the eventual outcome. Therefore, many authors advocate local excision to spare patients the morbidity of an APR and a colostomy. If the tumor is bulky and negative margins (1–2 cm) cannot be achieved, it involves the sphincter complex, or local resection will result in incontinence, then an APR is the recommended treatment option. If the patient already has signs of regional or systemic metastasis, radical excision should not be performed. The use of endoanal ultrasound and sentinel lymph node biopsies may further guide treatment for this disease.[152,158]

Adjuvant therapy for cutaneous melanoma has been studied extensively; however, the applicability of this data to anorectal melanoma remains uncertain. Many immunotherapeutic and chemotherapeutic agents such as dacarbazine, bacillus Calmette-Guerin, levamisole, and interferon-α have demonstrated no benefit.[158] Cytotoxic chemotherapy, including cisplatin, vinblastine, and dacarbazine, combined with interleukin-2 or interferon-α2b has shown some improvement in survival, however, patients suffered significant treatment-related toxicity.[161] Radiation therapy has also been utilized to improve local and regional control yet due to the small numbers of patients with anorectal melanoma, its efficacy is unknown. Due to its predilection for developing systemic metastasis, it is unclear whether efforts to achieve better local control are useful.

Gastrointestinal Stromal Tumors

Gastrointestinal stomal tumors (GIST) of the anus are extremely uncommon with only 17 cases reported in the literature up to 2003.[162] GISTs are tumors of mesenchymal origin that are not derived from smooth muscle or Schwann cells. They are identified by immunohistochemical studies that stain positive for CD34 and CD117 antigens. It is important to differentiate them from true smooth muscle tumors, with which they were previously combined, as they have a different pathogenesis and biological outcome. However, most series that have reported on leiomyomas and leiomyosarcomas in the past did not make this distinction, but in fact, reflect a large proportion of GISTs.[162,163] Due to the rarity of anal GISTs, they have only been studied with lesions of the rectum as a single entity.

Patients present in the fifth to seventh decade of life are more commonly men. Most patients are asymptomatic but bleeding, anal pain, change in bowel habits, or urinary symptoms can occur. Pathologic factors implicated in aggressive tumors with metastatic potential are size greater than 5 cm in diameter and high mitotic counts, pleomorphism, infiltration of muscularis propria, and coagulative necrosis. The presence of symptoms is also associated with a worse prognosis.

Treatment involves local excision for tumors less than 2 cm and APR for those with larger tumors or worse pathologic features.[162] In a study of anorectal stromal tumors, recurrence rates for local excision and radical resection were 60% and 0%, respectively.[164] The natural history of GISTs is indolent with a long latency period (greater than 4 years) to recurrence or metastasis, which is usually by a hematogenous route.[163] The role of adjuvant therapy in anal GIST is uncertain given the small numbers of patients affected. However, the success of Gleevec® (imitanib mesylate) in treating other GISTs would suggest it as a first line therapy for c-Kit (+) (CD117) GIST of the anus and rectum where compromised bowel control or permanent stoma is an issue.

Small-Cell Carcinoma/Neuroendocrine Tumors

Small cell or neuroendocrine tumors comprise less than 1% of all colorectal malignancies and are extremely rare in the anal canal. In a series of neuroendocrine carcinomas of the lower gastrointestinal tract, 16% were found in the anal canal.[165] Diagnosis involves identification of the classic histopathologic pattern. Hyperchromatic nuclei, pale nucleoli, high mitotic count, in addition to tumor growth in loose, noncohesive sheets are seen, similar to small cell or oat cell carcinoma of the lung. Sixty-five to 80% of patients with extrapulmonary small cell tumors present with metastatic disease. Therefore, it is important to stage them accurately. Those with disease limited to the anal canal are treated in a similar fashion to those with adenocarcinoma, including chemoradiation and radical surgery. Those with disseminated disease may benefit from combination chemotherapy regimens used for small cell lung cancer, such as cisplatin and etopside.[153,165]

Uncommon Perianal Neoplasms

Basal Cell Carcinoma

The incidence of basal cell carcinomas (BCC) of the anus, in comparison to sun-exposed areas of the body, is extremely low. It comprises about 0.1% of all BCC diagnosed and fewer than 200 cases of BCC have been reported on the perianal and genital area.[166] BCCs of the anal margin account for only 0.2% of all anorectal cancers. The largest series of perianal BCC thus far reported includes only 34 cases.[167]

The etiology of perianal BCC is likely different from BCC arising in sun-exposed skin. Although preexisting skin conditions, such as basal cell nevus syndrome and xeroderma pigmentosum, immunodeficiency, and genetics, may contribute to both types, radiation, chronic irritation or infection, and history of trauma or burn have all been implicated in perianal lesions.[166,168] The majority of these carcinomas occur in men (60–80%) and the average age at presentation is 65–75 years. Approximately one-third have a previous or concomitant history of BCC at other skin sites.[166,167,169]

The average size at presentation is less than 2 cm, although they can be as large as 10 cm and extend into the anal canal.[167] The clinical appearance can range from erythematous papules to nodules, plaques, and ulcers.[166] They tend to be mobile and superficial with little invasive or metastatic potential. Histologically, they are similar to BCC of other areas of the body and do not contain HPV.[166] It is extremely important to differentiate BCC from basaloid carcinoma histologically as these entities behave in a different manner.

It was previously thought that anorectal BCC was more aggressive than other cutaneous BCC, but it is[169] likely that perianal BCC was not adequately differentiated from the more aggressive basaloid tumors thus suggesting a worse prognosis.

Treatment is wide local excision ensuring adequate margins, which is possible in lesions less than 2 cm. Larger lesions may require excision with skin grafting or use of Mohs micrographic surgery to preserve uninvolved tissue. Recurrence rates for local excision range from 0 to 29%.[167,169] Cancer specific survivals in both series were 100% at 5 years. Recurrences can be treated with re-excision. Large lesions extending into the anal canal may be better treated with radiation or APR.

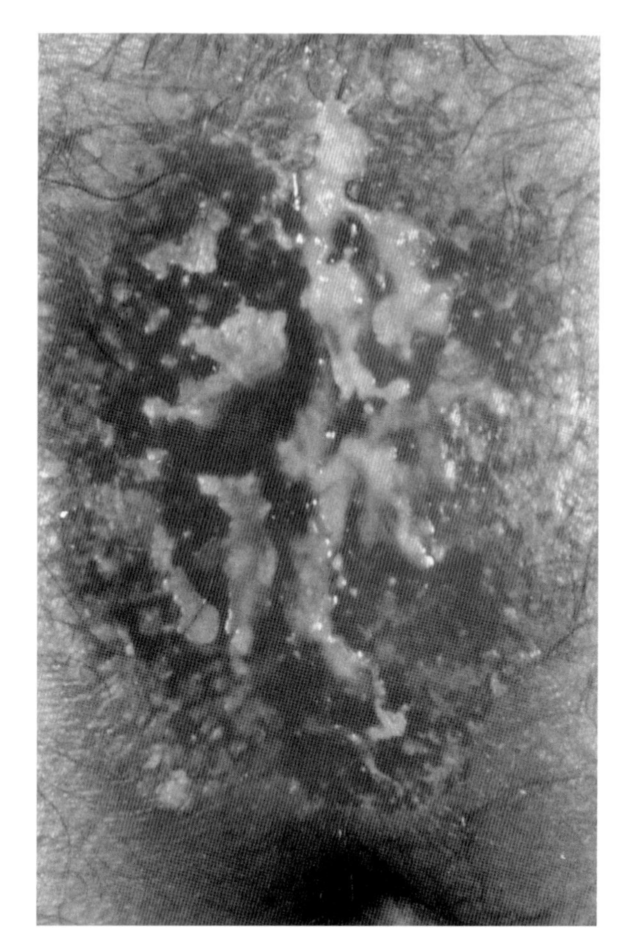

FIGURE 20-6. Perianal Paget's Disease. With permission from Beck DE, Wexner SD. Anal neoplasms. In: Beck DE, Wexner SD, editors. Fundamentals of anorectal surgery. London: W. B. Saunders; 1998. p. 261–277.

Paget's Disease

Paget's disease can be divided into two groups, mammary and extra mammary. The former was identified on the nipple of the female breast with an underlying carcinoma by Sir James Paget in 1847.[170] The latter was described specifically in the perianal area by Darier and Couillaud in 1893[171] and comprises about 20% of the extramammary type.[153] Other sites of Paget's disease include the axilla, scrotum, penis, vulva, groin, thigh, and buttock where apocrine glands are found.

It is currently believed that Paget's cells represent an intraepithelial adenocarcinoma with a prolonged preinvasive phase that eventually develops into an adenocarcinoma of the underlying apocrine gland given enough time. The origin of these cells is not completely understood. One theory suggests that a pluripotent basal cell is the progenitor of the Paget's cell with the adenocarcinoma arising in the epidermis and extending into the dermis. The other theory supports the origin of Paget's cells from the apocrine glands that spreads into the overlying epidermis. The latter hypothesis may be more likely given the fact that the lesions tend to occur in areas of high density apocrine glands.[79,153,172]

This is a rare condition with fewer than 200 cases reported in the literature to date.[173] Patients present in the seventh decade of life with equal distribution among men and women. The most common presenting symptom is intractable itching followed by bleeding, palpable mass, inguinal lymphadenopathy, weight loss, anal discharge and constipation. The median duration of symptoms is 3 years.[174,175] The lesions themselves often have an erythematous, eczematous appearance with well-demarcated borders mimicking a rash (Figure 20-6). They may look ulcerated or plaque-like with oozing or scaling. A third of cases involve the entire anus.[176] These lesions are often misdiagnosed because of their similarity to other conditions. The differential includes HSIL, Crohn's disease, condyloma acuminatum, hidradentits suppurativa, pruritis ani, and squamous cell carcinoma. Biopsy is essential to confirm the diagnosis.

Histologically, Paget's cells have large, round, eccentric, hyperchromic nuclei with pale-staining, vacuolated cytoplasm (Figure 20-7). The cytoplasm stains positive with periodic acid-Schiff stain due to the abundance of mucin

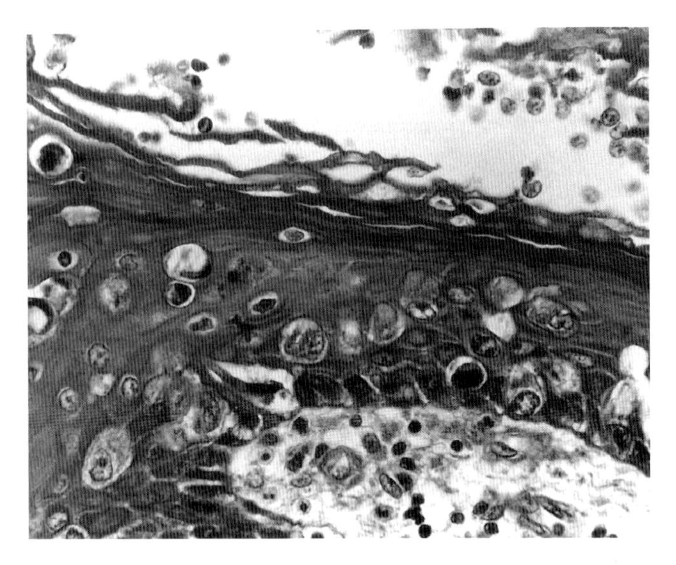

FIGURE 20-7. Perianal Paget's Disease (Photomicrograph hematoxylin and eosin ×400). With permission from Beck DE, Wexner SD. Anal neoplasms. In: Beck DE, Wexner SD, editors. Fundamentals of anorectal surgery. London: W. B. Saunders; 1998. p. 261–277.

and also stains positive for mucicarmine, cytokeratin 7, and alcian blue, which stain mucoproteins, and differentiates it from HSIL. Both mammary and extramammary Paget's disease have similar histologic features but mammary Paget's consistently presents with an associated invasive carcinoma, whereas in perianal Paget's disease, less than half (30–44%) present with invasive adenocarcinoma.[172,176,177] However, the incidence of associated visceral malignancies in perianal Paget's disease is elevated with various series reporting rates of 30–50%. The most common sites include the gastrointestinal tract, anus, skin, prostate, neck, and nasopharynx.[172,176–178] There may also be synchronous lesions in the axillary or anogenital area in patients diagnosed with perianal disease, and therefore a careful survey of other sites for malignancy and secondary disease is necessary.[153]

The treatment for perianal Paget's disease depends on the presence of invasion and other associated anorectal malignancies. For noninvasive lesions, wide local excision is the procedure of choice. In addition to resecting the lesion with grossly negative margins, it is important to map the extent of involvement of the lesion microscopically. This can be performed either by taking random biopsies 1 cm from the edge of the lesion in all four quadrants, including the dentate line, anal verge, and perineum[173,178] or by using toluidine blue and acetic acid to stain the Paget's cells, thereby directing the site for biopsy.[79] The use of intraoperative frozen sections ensures that any disease that extends beyond the gross lesion is excised to reduce the chance of recurrence. Positive margins requiring re-excision are not uncommon when this technique is not utilized. In a series of 27 patients, nine had positive margins and 12 required further surgery. Of the five patients who had mapping with 1 cm biopsies, none developed recurrence.[172] Another study reported positive margins in 53% of patients.[179] Preoperative mapping can also be performed using dermatologic punch biopsies. If the defect is small, the skin may be closed primarily. For larger lesions that require circumferential excision of the perianal skin, split-thickness skin grafts or sliding and rotational flaps may be required. Recurrence rates range from 37 to 100%.[172,177,180] Most recurrences were treated with wide re-excision with excellent results. For those who developed invasion, more radical surgery or adjuvant therapy was utilized.

Patients who have an invasive component or an associated anorectal malignancy should be considered for radical excision with APR. If positive inguinal lymph nodes are present, then an inguinal lymphadenectomy should be added. Unfortunately, patients with invasive disease present with metastasis 25% of the time and all patients who die of this disease have an invasive component.[79,172] Too few cases of perianal Paget's disease exist to allow for a comparison of invasive and noninvasive groups. Disease-specific survival for all perianal Paget's disease at 5 years ranges from 54 to 70%[172,176–178] and at 10 years decreases to 39–45%.[172,176]

The role of adjuvant chemoradiation therapy remains uncertain. It is currently used in some cases of invasive or aggressive recurrent disease. Concurrent anorectal malignancies may be another indication. Radiation has been associated with an increased rate of local complications when used for perianal Paget's disease[179] and is therefore reserved for patients who are not candidates for further surgical resection.[172]

Verrucous Carcinoma

The term verrucous carcinoma was initially coined in 1948 to describe a low-grade carcinoma of the oral mucosa that resembled viral warts. It has now been expanded to include those lesions described as giant condyloma acuminatum or Buschke-Lowenstein tumors. Abraham Buschke first described the latter in 1896 with respect to two invasive condylomata of the penis. Buschke and Lowenstein[181] then further delineated these lesions of the anus in 1925. Condylomatous features characterized these tumors with growth to a large size, local invasion and destruction of surrounding tissues, and the absence of metastases. Although it is a well-recognized entity, fewer than 60 cases have been reported in the literature to date.[182] HPV is frequently detected.

These tumors are more commonly found in men with a 2.7:1 male to female ratio. The average age of patients is 45 years and is slowly decreasing. Patients present most commonly with the complaint of an anal growth. Pain, perianal discharge/abscess, anorectal bleeding, pruritis, and a change in bowel habits may also occur.[182,183] The lesions themselves are generally slow growing with a soft, cauliflower like appearance that can become nodular as it penetrates the underlying tissues. One theory suggests that direct expansion of the tumor causes erosion and even necrosis of the surrounding tissues thereby predisposing to the development of fistulas that drain purulent fluid. Another suggests that condylomatous disease complicates existing abscess fistulous disease leading to the appearance of tissue erosion, necrosis, and invasion. The tumors arise most commonly from the perianal skin but can also present in the anal canal and distal rectum. At presentation, they tend to be quite large measuring anywhere from 1.5 to 30 cm.[182] Regional lymphadenopathy may also occur secondary to infection.

The tumor, which is clinically difficult to distinguish from a malignancy, is histologically benign. Papillomatosis, acanthosis with hyperplasia of the prickle cell layer, variable hyperkeratosis, parakeratosis, and underlying inflammation are often found.[181] However, of all the cases of giant condyloma acuminatum reported, only 42% were histologically diagnosed as condyloma without any invasion. A malignant transformation was identified in 58% of the tumors; 8% had carcinoma-in situ, and 50% had invasion that was termed verrucous carcinoma, SCC or basaloid carcinoma.

The standard treatment for verrucous carcinoma is radical local excision. For those patients with extensive deep tissue involvement, multiple fistulas, or involvement of the anal sphincter, APR is indicated. Cure can be achieved only by radical excision. Neoadjuvant radiation therapy may be useful for those tumors with invasive carcinoma and to render a tumor resectable due to its large size; however, some controversy exists as to whether radiation promotes malignant transformation of the tumors. The most current studies do not support this concept, as the incidence of invasive lesions after radiation is extremely low.[183] It has been hypothesized that the high recurrence rates after radical excision may be attributable to spillage of residual tumor, which could potentially be prevented by reducing the tumor size with preoperative chemoradiation. Certainly, size and local extent of tumor invasion, not malignant histology, has the greatest impact on morbidity, recurrence, and mortality. The authors favor the hypothesis that local recurrence is related to transection of the complicated infected fistulous tracts commonly associated with this process. Unfortunately, the rarity of this condition makes it difficult to study this issue prospectively.

HIV-Related Anal Cancer

Kaposi's Sarcoma

Although Kaposi's sarcoma is the most common cutaneous malignancy in patients with AIDS,[184] the incidence of perianal lesions is quite small and decreasing with the increasingly effective antiretroviral therapy available today.[185] A study of 180 consecutive HIV-seropositive patients seen for anorectal symptoms revealed two perianal Kaposi's sarcomas. They were both small, round, purplish lesions that could easily have been mistaken for hemorrhoids. Both were treated with chemotherapy although radiation has been used for localized cutaneous lesions.[186]

Lymphoma

The incidence of non-Hodgkin's lymphoma (NHL) has been increasing in AIDS patients as treatment improves and life expectancy increases. NHL is the second most common AIDS-related neoplasm after Kaposi's sarcoma. Compared to lymphomas found in the general population, these tumors are characterized by B-cells of a higher histologic grade that originate from extranodal tissue. They are also more aggressive, prone to dissemination, and resistant to treatment. Most lymphomas are found in the central nervous system and the gastrointestinal tract. However, anorectal lymphomas are extremely rare, comprising less than 1% of all anorectal neoplasms in the general population.[187] Although the anorectal area is devoid of lymphoid tissue, it is postulated that the exposure to chronic infections from anal receptive intercourse or an immunocompromised state may result in an "acquired" mucosa-associated lymphoid tissue (MALT).

The most common presenting symptoms are pain, pruritis, drainage, or a palpable mass. Some patients may have more constitutional symptoms, such as fever, night sweats, or weight loss.[187] After appropriate staging, patients are treated with a standard regimen for NHL of chemotherapy and radiation therapy of the affected area.

There is no role for surgical treatment. Usual chemotherapeutic agents include cyclophosphamide, actinomycin, vincristine, and corticosteroids (CHOP). There are too few cases of anorectal lymphoma reported to discuss overall prognosis. However, younger patients without constitutional symptoms may fare better. Additionally, low CD4 counts and performance status may affect a patient's ability to endure aggressive therapy.[153] Isolated reports of immunocompetent patients with anorectal lymphoma have been reported with excellent response to treatment.[188]

References

1. Jemal A et al. Cancer statistics, 2009. CA Cancer J Clin. 2009;59(4):225–49.
2. Edge SB, Byrd DR, Compton CC, Fritz AG, Greene FL, Trotti A. AJCC cancer staging manual. 7th ed. Springer: New York, NY; 2010.
3. Welton ML, Sharkey FE, Kahlenberg MS. The etiology and epidemiology of anal cancer. Surg Oncol Clin N Am. 2004;13(2):263–75.
4. Frisch M et al. Sexually transmitted infection as a cause of anal cancer. N Engl J Med. 1997;337(19):1350–8.
5. Munoz N et al. Epidemiologic classification of human papillomavirus types associated with cervical cancer. N Engl J Med. 2003;348(6):518–27.
6. Strickler HD, Schiffman MH. Is human papillomavirus an infectious cause of non-cervical anogenital tract cancers? BMJ. 1997;315(7109):620–1.
7. Koutsky L. Epidemiology of genital human papillomavirus infection. Am J Med. 1997;102(5A):3–8.

8. O'Mahony C et al. New patient-applied therapy for anogenital warts is rated favourably by patients. Int J STD AIDS. 2001;12(9):565–70.
9. Bauer HM et al. Genital human papillomavirus infection in female university students as determined by a PCR-based method. JAMA. 1991;265(4):472–7.
10. Pecoraro G, Morgan D, Defendi V. Differential effects of human papillomavirus type 6, 16, and 18 DNAs on immortalization and transformation of human cervical epithelial cells. Proc Natl Acad Sci USA. 1989;86(2):563–7.
11. Woodworth CD, Doniger J, DiPaolo JA. Immortalization of human foreskin keratinocytes by various human papillomavirus DNAs corresponds to their association with cervical carcinoma. J Virol. 1989;63(1):159–64.
12. van der Snoek EM et al. Human papillomavirus infection in men who have sex with men participating in a Dutch gay-cohort study. Sex Transm Dis. 2003;30(8):639–44.
13. Palefsky JM et al. Anal intraepithelial neoplasia and anal papillomavirus infection among homosexual males with group IV HIV disease. JAMA. 1990;263(21):2911–6.
14. Palefsky JM et al. Detection of human papillomavirus DNA in anal intraepithelial neoplasia and anal cancer. Cancer Res. 1991;51(3):1014–9.
15. Jay N et al. Colposcopic appearance of anal squamous intraepithelial lesions: relationship to histopathology. Dis Colon Rectum. 1997;40(8):919–28.
16. Holly EA et al. Anal cancer incidence: genital warts, anal fissure or fistula, hemorrhoids, and smoking. J Natl Cancer Inst. 1989;81(22):1726–31.
17. Bosch FX et al. The causal relation between human papillomavirus and cervical cancer. J Clin Pathol. 2002;55(4):244–65.
18. Hildesheim A et al. Immune activation in cervical neoplasia: cross-sectional association between plasma soluble interleukin 2 receptor levels and disease. Cancer Epidemiol Biomarkers Prev. 1997;6(10):807–13.
19. Palefsky JM et al. Prevalence and risk factors for anal human papillomavirus infection in human immunodeficiency virus (HIV)-positive and high-risk HIV-negative women. J Infect Dis. 2001;183(3):383–91.
20. Holly EA et al. Prevalence and risk factors for anal squamous intraepithelial lesions in women. J Natl Cancer Inst. 2001; 93(11):843–9.
21. Sobhani I et al. Prevalence of high-grade dysplasia and cancer in the anal canal in human papillomavirus-infected individuals. Gastroenterology. 2001;120(4):857–66.
22. Cress RD, Holly EA. Incidence of anal cancer in California: increased incidence among men in San Francisco, 1973–1999. Prev Med. 2003;36(5):555–60.
23. Penn I. Cancers of the anogenital region in renal transplant recipients. Analysis of 65 cases. Cancer. 1986;58(3):611–6.
24. Penn I. Cancer in the immunosuppressed organ recipient. Transplant Proc. 1991;23(2):1771–2.
25. Vajdic CM et al. Cancer incidence before and after kidney transplantation. JAMA. 2006;296(23):2823–31.
26. McGlennen RC. Human papillomavirus oncogenesis. Clin Lab Med. 2000;20(2):383–406.
27. zur Hausen H. Immortalization of human cells and their malignant conversion by high risk human papillomavirus genotypes. Semin Cancer Biol. 1999;9(6):405–11.
28. Martin F, Bower M. Anal intraepithelial neoplasia in HIV positive people. Sex Transm Infect. 2001;77(5):327–31.
29. Werness BA, Levine AJ, Howley PM. Association of human papillomavirus types 16 and 18 E6 proteins with p53. Science. 1990;248(4951):76–9.
30. Chow LT, Broker TR. Papillomavirus DNA replication. Intervirology. 1994;37(3–4):150–8.
31. Dollard SC et al. Production of human papillomavirus and modulation of the infectious program in epithelial raft cultures. OFF. Genes Dev. 1992;6(7):1131–42.
32. Flores ER, Lambert PF. Evidence for a switch in the mode of human papillomavirus type 16 DNA replication during the viral life cycle. J Virol. 1997;71(10):7167–79.
33. Litle VR et al. Angiogenesis, proliferation, and apoptosis in anal high-grade squamous intraepithelial lesions. Dis Colon Rectum. 2000;43(3):346–52.
34. Chang GJ et al. Surgical treatment of high-grade anal squamous intraepithelial lesions: a prospective study. Dis Colon Rectum. 2002;45(4):453–8.
35. Pineda CE et al. High-resolution anoscopy targeted surgical destruction of anal high-grade squamous intraepithelial lesions: a ten-year experience. Dis Colon Rectum. 2008;51(6):829–35. discussion 835–7.
36. Goldie SJ et al. The clinical effectiveness and cost-effectiveness of screening for anal squamous intraepithelial lesions in homosexual and bisexual HIV-positive men. JAMA. 1999;281(19):1822–9.
37. Goldie SJ et al. Cost-effectiveness of screening for anal squamous intraepithelial lesions and anal cancer in human immunodeficiency virus-negative homosexual and bisexual men. Am J Med. 2000;108(8):634–41.
38. Daling JR et al. Sexual practices, sexually transmitted diseases, and the incidence of anal cancer. N Engl J Med. 1987; 317(16):973–7.
39. Scholefield JH et al. Anal and cervical intraepithelial neoplasia: possible parallel. Lancet. 1989;2(8666):765–9.
40. Rabkin CS, Yellin F. Cancer incidence in a population with a high prevalence of infection with human immunodeficiency virus type 1. J Natl Cancer Inst. 1994;86(22):1711–6.
41. Koblin BA et al. Increased incidence of cancer among homosexual men, New York City and San Francisco, 1978–1990. Am J Epidemiol. 1996;144(10):916–23.
42. Critchlow CW et al. Prospective study of high grade anal squamous intraepithelial neoplasia in a cohort of homosexual men: influence of HIV infection, immunosuppression and human papillomavirus infection. AIDS. 1995;9(11):1255–62.
43. Palefsky JM et al. Anal squamous intraepithelial lesions in HIV-positive and HIV-negative homosexual and bisexual men: prevalence and risk factors. J Acquir Immune Defic Syndr Hum Retrovirol. 1998;17(4):320–6.
44. Palefsky JM et al. Virologic, immunologic, and clinical parameters in the incidence and progression of anal squamous intraepithelial lesions in HIV-positive and HIV-negative homosexual men. J Acquir Immune Defic Syndr Hum Retrovirol. 1998;17(4):314–9.
45. Chaturvedi AK et al. Risk of human papillomavirus-associated cancers among persons with AIDS. J Natl Cancer Inst. 2009;101(16):1120–30.
46. Frisch M, Biggar RJ, Goedert JJ. Human papillomavirus-associated cancers in patients with human immunodeficiency

virus infection and acquired immunodeficiency syndrome. J Natl Cancer Inst. 2000;92(18):1500–10.
47. Jemal A et al. Cancer statistics, 2003. CA Cancer J Clin. 2003;53(1):5–26.
48. Goldman S et al. Incidence of anal epidermoid carcinoma in Sweden 1970–1984. Acta Chir Scand. 1989;155(3):191–7.
49. Frisch M, Melbye M, Moller H. Trends in incidence of anal cancer in Denmark. BMJ. 1993;306(6875):419–22.
50. Ciobotaru B et al. Prevalence and risk factors for anal cytologic abnormalities and human papillomavirus infection in a rural population of HIV-infected males. Dis Colon Rectum. 2007;50(7):1011–6.
51. Melbye M, Sprogel P. Aetiological parallel between anal cancer and cervical cancer. Lancet. 1991;338(8768):657–9.
52. Holmes F et al. Anal cancer in women. Gastroenterology. 1988;95(1):107–11.
53. Palefsky JM, Shiboski S, Moss A. Risk factors for anal human papillomavirus infection and anal cytologic abnormalities in HIV-positive and HIV-negative homosexual men. J Acquir Immune Defic Syndr. 1994;7(6):599–606.
54. Caussy D et al. Interaction of human immunodeficiency and papilloma viruses: association with anal epithelial abnormality in homosexual men. Int J Cancer. 1990;46(2):214–9.
55. Friedman HB et al. Human papillomavirus, anal squamous intraepithelial lesions, and human immunodeficiency virus in a cohort of gay men. J Infect Dis. 1998;178(1):45–52.
56. Palefsky JM et al. High incidence of anal high-grade squamous intra-epithelial lesions among HIV-positive and HIV-negative homosexual and bisexual men. AIDS. 1998;12(5):495–503.
57. Ogunbiyi OA et al. Prevalence of anal human papillomavirus infection and intraepithelial neoplasia in renal allograft recipients. Br J Surg. 1994;81(3):365–7.
58. Daling JR et al. Cigarette smoking and the risk of anogenital cancer. Am J Epidemiol. 1992;135(2):180–9.
59. Marfing TE, Abel ME, Gallagher DM. Perianal Bowen's disease and associated malignancies. Results of a survey. Dis Colon Rectum. 1987;30(10):782–5.
60. Arbesman H, Ransohoff DF. Is Bowen's disease a predictor for the development of internal malignancy? A methodological critique of the literature. JAMA. 1987;257(4):516–8.
61. Margenthaler JA et al. Outcomes, risk of other malignancies, and need for formal mapping procedures in patients with perianal Bowen's disease. Dis Colon Rectum. 2004;47(10):1655–60. discussion 1660–1.
62. Marchesa P et al. Perianal Bowen's disease: a clinicopathologic study of 47 patients. Dis Colon Rectum. 1997;40(11):1286–93.
63. Brown SR et al. Outcome after surgical resection for high-grade anal intraepithelial neoplasia (Bowen's disease). Br J Surg. 1999;86(8):1063–6.
64. Bargman H, Hochman J. Topical treatment of Bowen's disease with 5-Fluorouracil. J Cutan Med Surg. 2003;7(2):101–5.
65. Graham BD et al. Topical 5-fluorouracil in the management of extensive anal Bowen's disease: a preferred approach. Dis Colon Rectum. 2005;48(3):444–50.
66. Wang KH et al. Erbium:YAG laser pretreatment accelerates the response of Bowen's disease treated by topical 5-fluorouracil. Dermatol Surg. 2004;30(3):441–5.
67. Snoeck R et al. Treatment of a bowenoid papulosis of the penis with local applications of cidofovir in a patient with acquired immunodeficiency syndrome. Arch Intern Med. 2001;161(19):2382–4.
68. Okamoto A et al. Combination therapy with podophyllin and vidarabine for human papillomavirus positive cervical intraepithelial neoplasia. Oncol Rep. 1999;6(2):269–76.
69. Micali G, Nasca MR, Tedeschi A. Topical treatment of intraepithelial penile carcinoma with imiquimod. Clin Exp Dermatol. 2003;28 Suppl 1:4–6.
70. Smith KJ, Germain M, Skelton H. Squamous cell carcinoma in situ (Bowen's disease) in renal transplant patients treated with 5% imiquimod and 5% 5-fluorouracil therapy. Dermatol Surg. 2001;27(6):561–4.
71. Pehoushek J, Smith KJ. Imiquimod and 5% fluorouracil therapy for anal and perianal squamous cell carcinoma in situ in an HIV-1-positive man. Arch Dermatol. 2001;137(1):14–6.
72. Panizzon RG. Radiotherapy of skin tumors. Recent Results Cancer Res. 2002;160:234–9.
73. Chung YL et al. Treatment of Bowen's disease with a specially designed radioactive skin patch. Eur J Nucl Med. 2000;27(7):842–6.
74. Webber J, Fromm D. Photodynamic therapy for carcinoma in situ of the anus. Arch Surg. 2004;139(3):259–61.
75. Varma S et al. Bowen's disease, solar keratoses and superficial basal cell carcinomas treated by photodynamic therapy using a large-field incoherent light source. Br J Dermatol. 2001;144(3):567–74.
76. Salim A et al. Randomized comparison of photodynamic therapy with topical 5-fluorouracil in Bowen's disease. Br J Dermatol. 2003;148(3):539–43.
77. Behrendt GC, Hansmann ML. Carcinomas of the anal canal and anal margin differ in their expression of cadherin, cytokeratins and p53. Virchows Arch. 2001;439(6):782–6.
78. Gervasoni Jr JE, Wanebo HJ. Cancers of the anal canal and anal margin. Cancer Invest. 2003;21(3):452–64.
79. Skibber J, Rodriguez-Bigas MA, Gordon PH. Surgical considerations in anal cancer. Surg Oncol Clin N Am. 2004;13(2):321–38.
80. Newlin HE et al. Squamous cell carcinoma of the anal margin. J Surg Oncol. 2004;86(2):55–62. discussion 63.
81. Jensen SL et al. Does an erroneous diagnosis of squamous-cell carcinoma of the anal canal and anal margin at first physician visit influence prognosis? Dis Colon Rectum. 1987;30(5):345–51.
82. Winburn GB. Anal carcinoma or "just hemorrhoids"? Am Surg. 2001;67(11):1048–58.
83. Mendenhall WM et al. Squamous cell carcinoma of the anal margin treated with radiotherapy. Surg Oncol. 1996;5(1):29–35.
84. Papillon J, Chassard JL. Respective roles of radiotherapy and surgery in the management of epidermoid carcinoma of the anal margin. Series of 57 patients. Dis Colon Rectum. 1992;35(5):422–9.
85. Nivatvongs S. Perianal and anal canal neoplasms. In: Gordon PH, Nivatvongs S, editors. Prinicples and practice of surgery for the colon, rectum, and anus. St. Louis: Quality Medical Publishing; 1999. p. 448–71.
86. Jensen SL et al. Long-term prognosis after radical treatment for squamous-cell carcinoma of the anal canal and anal margin. Dis Colon Rectum. 1988;31(4):273–8.
87. Greenall MJ et al. Epidermoid cancer of the anal margin. Pathologic features, treatment, and clinical results. Am J Surg. 1985;149(1):95–101.
88. Al-Jurf AS, Turnbull RP, Fazio VW. Local treatment of squamous cell carcinoma of the anus. Surg Gynecol Obstet. 1979;148(4):576–8.

89. Schraut WH et al. Depth of invasion, location, and size of cancer of the anus dictate operative treatment. Cancer. 1983;51(7):1291–6.
90. Pintor MP, Northover JM, Nicholls RJ. Squamous cell carcinoma of the anus at one hospital from 1948 to 1984. Br J Surg. 1989;76(8):806–10.
91. Beahrs OH, Wilson SM. Carcinoma of the anus. Ann Surg. 1976;184(4):422–8.
92. Peiffert D et al. Conservative treatment by irradiation of epidermoid carcinomas of the anal margin. Int J Radiat Oncol Biol Phys. 1997;39(1):57–66.
93. Touboul E et al. Epidermoid carcinoma of the anal margin: 17 cases treated with curative-intent radiation therapy. Radiother Oncol. 1995;34(3):195–202.
94. Mendenhall WM et al. Squamous cell carcinoma of the anal margin. Oncology (Huntingt). 1996;10(12):1843–8. discussion 1848, 1853–4.
95. Cummings BJ et al. Treatment of perianal carcinoma by radiation(RT) or radiation plus chemotherapy(RTCT). Int J Radiat Oncol Biol Phys. 1986;12:170.
96. Cutuli B et al. Anal margin carcinoma: 21 cases treated at the Institut Curie by exclusive conservative radiotherapy. Radiother Oncol. 1988;11(1):1–6.
97. John MJ et al. Feasibility of non-surgical definitive management of anal canal carcinoma. Int J Radiat Oncol Biol Phys. 1987;13(3):299–303.
98. Roelofsen F, Bartelink H. Combined modality treatment of anal carcinoma. Oncologist. 1998;3(6):413–8.
99. Allal AS et al. The impact of treatment factors on local control in T2-T3 anal carcinomas treated by radiotherapy with or without chemotherapy. Cancer. 1997;79(12):2329–35.
100. Bartelink H et al. Concomitant radiotherapy and chemotherapy is superior to radiotherapy alone in the treatment of locally advanced anal cancer: results of a phase III randomized trial of the European Organization for Research and Treatment of Cancer Radiotherapy and Gastrointestinal Cooperative Groups. J Clin Oncol. 1997;15(5):2040–9.
101. UKCCCR. Epidermoid anal cancer: results from the UKCCCR randomised trial of radiotherapy alone versus radiotherapy, 5-fluorouracil, and mitomycin. UKCCCR Anal Cancer Trial Working Party. UK Co-ordinating Committee on Cancer Research. Lancet. 1996;348(9034):1049–54.
102. Bieri S, Allal AS, Kurtz JM. Sphincter-conserving treatment of carcinomas of the anal margin. Acta Oncol. 2001;40(1):29–33.
103. Dougherty BG, Evans HL. Carcinoma of the anal canal: a study of 79 cases. Am J Clin Pathol. 1985;83(2):159–64.
104. Rousseau Jr DL, Petrelli NJ, Kahlenberg MS. Overview of anal cancer for the surgeon. Surg Oncol Clin N Am. 2004;13(2):249–62.
105. Clark MA, Hartley A, Geh JI. Cancer of the anal canal. Lancet Oncol. 2004;5(3):149–57.
106. Boman BM et al. Carcinoma of the anal canal. A clinical and pathologic study of 188 cases. Cancer. 1984;54(1):114–25.
107. Roseau G et al. Endoscopic ultrasonography in the staging and follow-up of epidermoid carcinoma of the anal canal. Gastrointest Endosc. 1994;40(4):447–50.
108. Drudi FM et al. TRUS staging and follow-up in patients with anal canal cancer. Radiol Med (Torino). 2003;106(4):329–37.
109. Giovannini M et al. Anal carcinoma: prognostic value of endorectal ultrasound (ERUS). Results of a prospective multicenter study. Endoscopy. 2001;33(3):231–6.
110. Goldman S et al. Transanorectal ultrasonography in anal carcinoma. A prospective study of 21 patients. Acta Radiol. 1988;29(3):337–41.
111. Christensen AF et al. Three-dimensional anal endosonography may improve staging of anal cancer compared with two-dimensional endosonography. Dis Colon Rectum. 2004;47(3):341–5.
112. Fuchshuber PR et al. Anal canal and perianal epidermoid cancers. J Am Coll Surg. 1997;185(5):494–505.
113. Perera D et al. Sentinel node biopsy for squamous-cell carcinoma of the anus and anal margin. Dis Colon Rectum. 2003;46(8):1027–9. discussion 1030–1.
114. Hoffman R et al. The significance of pretreatment CD4 count on the outcome and treatment tolerance of HIV-positive patients with anal cancer. Int J Radiat Oncol Biol Phys. 1999;44(1):127–31.
115. Eng C, Abbruzzese J, Minsky BD. Chemotherapy and radiation of anal canal cancer: the first approach. Surg Oncol Clin N Am. 2004;13(2):309–20. viii.
116. Deniaud-Alexandre E et al. Results of definitive irradiation in a series of 305 epidermoid carcinomas of the anal canal. Int J Radiat Oncol Biol Phys. 2003;56(5):1259–73.
117. Touboul E et al. Epidermoid carcinoma of the anal canal. Results of curative-intent radiation therapy in a series of 270 patients. Cancer. 1994;73(6):1569–79.
118. Gerard JP et al. Management of inguinal lymph node metastases in patients with carcinoma of the anal canal: experience in a series of 270 patients treated in Lyon and review of the literature. Cancer. 2001;92(1):77–84.
119. Cummings BJ. Treatment of primary epidermoid carcinoma of the anal canal. Int J Colorectal Dis. 1987;2(2):107–12.
120. Wade DS et al. Metastases to the lymph nodes in epidermoid carcinoma of the anal canal studied by a clearing technique. Surg Gynecol Obstet. 1989;169(3):238–42.
121. Ryan DP, Mayer RJ. Anal carcinoma: histology, staging, epidemiology, treatment. Curr Opin Oncol. 2000;12(4):345–52.
122. Hughes LL et al. Radiotherapy for anal cancer: experience from 1979–1987. Int J Radiat Oncol Biol Phys. 1989;17(6):1153–60.
123. Constantinou EC et al. Time-dose considerations in the treatment of anal cancer. Int J Radiat Oncol Biol Phys. 1997;39(3):651–7.
124. John M et al. Dose escalation in chemoradiation for anal cancer: preliminary results of RTOG 92-08. Cancer J Sci Am. 1996;2(4):205.
125. Myerson RJ et al. Radiation therapy for epidermoid carcinoma of the anal canal, clinical and treatment factors associated with outcome. Radiother Oncol. 2001;61(1):15–22.
126. Cummings BJ et al. Epidermoid anal cancer: treatment by radiation alone or by radiation and 5-fluorouracil with and without mitomycin C. Int J Radiat Oncol Biol Phys. 1991;21(5):1115–25.
127. Allal AS et al. Impact of clinical and therapeutic factors on major late complications after radiotherapy with or without concomitant chemotherapy for anal carcinoma. Int J Radiat Oncol Biol Phys. 1997;39(5):1099–105.
128. Nguyen WD, Mitchell KM, Beck DE. Risk factors associated with requiring a stoma for the management of anal cancer. Dis Colon Rectum. 2004;47(6):843–6.

129. Ng Ying Kin NY et al. Our experience of conservative treatment of anal canal carcinoma combining external irradiation and interstitial implant: 32 cases treated between 1973 and 1982. Int J Radiat Oncol Biol Phys. 1988;14(2):253–9.
130. Papillon J, Montbarbon JF. Epidermoid carcinoma of the anal canal. A series of 276 cases. Dis Colon Rectum. 1987;30(5):324–33.
131. Mitchell SE et al. Squamous cell carcinoma of the anal canal. Int J Radiat Oncol Biol Phys. 2001;49(4):1007–13.
132. Nigro ND, Vaitkevicius VK, Considine Jr B. Combined therapy for cancer of the anal canal: a preliminary report. Dis Colon Rectum. 1974;17(3):354–6.
133. Buroker TR et al. Combined therapy for cancer of the anal canal: a follow-up report. Dis Colon Rectum. 1977;20(8):677–8.
134. Nigro ND. An evaluation of combined therapy for squamous cell cancer of the anal canal. Dis Colon Rectum. 1984;27(12):763–6.
135. Flam M et al. Role of mitomycin in combination with fluorouracil and radiotherapy, and of salvage chemoradiation in the definitive nonsurgical treatment of epidermoid carcinoma of the anal canal: results of a phase III randomized intergroup study. J Clin Oncol. 1996;14(9):2527–39.
136. Hung A et al. Cisplatin-based combined modality therapy for anal carcinoma: a wider therapeutic index. Cancer. 2003;97(5):1195–202.
137. Gerard JP et al. Treatment of anal canal carcinoma with high dose radiation therapy and concomitant fluorouracil-cisplatinum. Long-term results in 95 patients. Radiother Oncol. 1998;46(3): 249–56.
138. Lund JA et al. Endoanal ultrasound is of little value in follow-up of anal carcinomas. Dis Colon Rectum. 2004;47(6):839–42.
139. van der Wal BC et al. Results of salvage abdominoperineal resection for recurrent anal carcinoma following combined chemoradiation therapy. J Gastrointest Surg. 2001;5(4):383–7.
140. Zelnick RS et al. Results of abdominoperineal resections for failures after combination chemotherapy and radiation therapy for anal canal cancers. Dis Colon Rectum. 1992;35(6):574–7. discussion 577–8.
141. Pocard M et al. Results of salvage abdominoperineal resection for anal cancer after radiotherapy. Dis Colon Rectum. 1998;41(12):1488–93.
142. Ellenhorn JD, Enker WE, Quan SH. Salvage abdominoperineal resection following combined chemotherapy and radiotherapy for epidermoid carcinoma of the anus. Ann Surg Oncol. 1994;1(2):105–10.
143. Allal AS et al. Effectiveness of surgical salvage therapy for patients with locally uncontrolled anal carcinoma after sphincter-conserving treatment. Cancer. 1999;86(3):405–9.
144. Akbari RP et al. Oncologic outcomes of salvage surgery for epidermoid carcinoma of the anus initially managed with combined modality therapy. Dis Colon Rectum. 2004;47(7):1136–44.
145. Nilsson PJ et al. Salvage abdominoperineal resection in anal epidermoid cancer. Br J Surg. 2002;89(11):1425–9.
146. Greenall MJ et al. Recurrent epidermoid cancer of the anus. Cancer. 1986;57(7):1437–41.
147. Klas JV et al. Malignant tumors of the anal canal: the spectrum of disease, treatment, and outcomes. Cancer. 1999;85(8):1686–93.
148. Beal KP et al. Primary adenocarcinoma of the anus treated with combined modality therapy. Dis Colon Rectum. 2003;46(10):1320–4.
149. Basik M et al. Prognosis and recurrence patterns of anal adenocarcinoma. Am J Surg. 1995;169(2):233–7.
150. Papagikos M et al. Chemoradiation for adenocarcinoma of the anus. Int J Radiat Oncol Biol Phys. 2003;55(3):669–78.
151. Belkacemi Y et al. Management of primary anal canal adenocarcinoma: a large retrospective study from the Rare Cancer Network. Int J Radiat Oncol Biol Phys. 2003;56(5):1274–83.
152. Malik A, Hull TL, Floruta C. What is the best surgical treatment for anorectal melanoma? Int J Colorectal Dis. 2004;19(2):121–3.
153. Billingsley KG et al. Uncommon anal neoplasms. Surg Oncol Clin N Am. 2004;13(2):375–88.
154. Chang AE, Karnell LH, Menck HR. The National Cancer Data Base report on cutaneous and noncutaneous melanoma: a summary of 84, 836 cases from the past decade. The American College of Surgeons Commission on Cancer and the American Cancer Society. Cancer. 1998;83(8):1664–78.
155. Brady MS, Kavolius JP, Quan SH. Anorectal melanoma. A 64-year experience at Memorial Sloan-Kettering Cancer Center. Dis Colon Rectum. 1995;38(2):146–51.
156. Thibault C et al. Anorectal melanoma – an incurable disease? Dis Colon Rectum. 1997;40(6):661–8.
157. Weyandt GH et al. Anorectal melanoma: surgical management guidelines according to tumour thickness. Br J Cancer. 2003;89(11):2019–22.
158. Bullard KM et al. Surgical therapy for anorectal melanoma. J Am Coll Surg. 2003;196(2):206–11.
159. Moozar KL, Wong CS, Couture J. Anorectal malignant melanoma: treatment with surgery or radiation therapy, or both. Can J Surg. 2003;46(5):345–9.
160. Roumen RM. Anorectal melanoma in The Netherlands: a report of 63 patients. Eur J Surg Oncol. 1996;22(6):598–601.
161. Eton O et al. Sequential biochemotherapy versus chemotherapy for metastatic melanoma: results from a phase III randomized trial. J Clin Oncol. 2002;20(8):2045–52.
162. Tan GY et al. Gastrointestinal stromal tumor of the anus. Tech Coloproctol. 2003;7(3):169–72.
163. Miettinen M et al. Gastrointestinal stromal tumors, intramural leiomyomas, and leiomyosarcomas in the rectum and anus: a clinicopathologic, immunohistochemical, and molecular genetic study of 144 cases. Am J Surg Pathol. 2001;25(9):1121–33.
164. Walsh TH, Mann CV. Smooth muscle neoplasms of the rectum and anal canal. Br J Surg. 1984;71(8):597–9.
165. Bernick PE et al. Neuroendocrine carcinomas of the colon and rectum. Dis Colon Rectum. 2004;47(2):163–9.
166. Gibson GE, Ahmed I. Perianal and genital basal cell carcinoma: a clinicopathologic review of 51 cases. J Am Acad Dermatol. 2001;45(1):68–71.
167. Nielsen OV, Jensen SL. Basal cell carcinoma of the anus – a clinical study of 34 cases. Br J Surg. 1981;68(12):856–7.
168. Espana A et al. Perianal basal cell carcinoma. Clin Exp Dermatol. 1992;17(5):360–2.
169. Paterson CA, Young-Fadok TM, Dozois RR. Basal cell carcinoma of the perianal region: 20-year experience. Dis Colon Rectum. 1999;42(9):1200–2.
170. Paget J. On disease of the mammary areola preceding cancer of the mammary gland. St Barth Hosp Rep. 1874;10:87–9.
171. Darier J, Couillaud P. Sur un cas de maladie de Pager de la region kerineo-anal er scrotale. Ann Dermatole dr Syph. 1893;4:25–31.

172. McCarter MD et al. Long-term outcome of perianal Paget's disease. Dis Colon Rectum. 2003;46(5):612–6.
173. Beck D. Paget's disease and Bowen's disease of the anus. Semin Colon Rectal Surg. 1995;6:143–9.
174. Berardi RS, Lee S, Chen HP. Perianal extramammary Paget's disease. Surg Gynecol Obstet. 1988;167(4):359–66.
175. Tulchinsky H et al. Extramammary Paget's disease of the perianal region. Colorectal Dis. 2004;6(3):206–9.
176. Jensen SL et al. Paget's disease of the anal margin. Br J Surg. 1988;75(11):1089–92.
177. Sarmiento JM et al. Paget's disease of the perianal region – an aggressive disease? Dis Colon Rectum. 1997;40(10):1187–94.
178. Beck DE, Fazio VW. Perianal Paget's disease. Dis Colon Rectum. 1987;30(4):263–6.
179. Besa P et al. Extramammary Paget's disease of the perineal skin: role of radiotherapy. Int J Radiat Oncol Biol Phys. 1992;24(1):73–8.
180. Marchesa P et al. Long-term outcome of patients with perianal Paget's disease. Ann Surg Oncol. 1997;4(6):475–80.
181. Grussendorf-Conen EI. Anogenital premalignant and malignant tumors (including Buschke-Lowenstein tumors). Clin Dermatol. 1997;15(3):377–88.
182. Trombetta LJ, Place RJ. Giant condyloma acuminatum of the anorectum: trends in epidemiology and management: report of a case and review of the literature. Dis Colon Rectum. 2001;44(12):1878–86.
183. Chu QD et al. Giant condyloma acuminatum (Buschke-Lowenstein tumor) of the anorectal and perianal regions. Analysis of 42 cases. Dis Colon Rectum. 1994;37(9):950–7.
184. Frisch M et al. Cancer in a population-based cohort of men and women in registered homosexual partnerships. Am J Epidemiol. 2003;157(11):966–72.
185. Gates AE, Kaplan LD. AIDS malignancies in the era of highly active antiretroviral therapy. Oncology (Huntingt). 2002;16(4):441–51. 456, 459.
186. Yuhan R et al. Anorectal disease in HIV-infected patients. Dis Colon Rectum. 1998;41(11):1367–70.
187. Place RJ, Huber PJ, Simmang CL. Anorectal lymphoma and AIDS: an outcome analysis. J Surg Oncol. 2000;73(1):1–4. discussion 4–5.
188. Smith 2nd DL, Cataldo PA. Perianal lymphoma in a heterosexual and nonimmunocompromised patient: report of a case and review of the literature. Dis Colon Rectum. 1999;42(7):952–4.
189. Flam MS et al. Definitive combined modality therapy of carcinoma of the anus. A report of 30 cases including results of salvage therapy in patients with residual disease. Dis Colon Rectum. 1987;30(7):495–502.
190. Nigro ND. Multidisciplinary management of cancer of the anus. World J Surg. 1987;11(4):446–51.
191. Habr-Gama A et al. Epidermoid carcinoma of the anal canal. Results of treatment by combined chemotherapy and radiation therapy. Dis Colon Rectum. 1989;32(9):773–7.
192. Sischy B et al. Definitive irradiation and chemotherapy for radiosensitization in management of anal carcinoma: interim report on Radiation Therapy Oncology Group study no. 8314. J Natl Cancer Inst. 1989;81(11):850–6.
193. Cho CC et al. Squamous-cell carcinoma of the anal canal: management with combined chemo-radiation therapy. Dis Colon Rectum. 1991;34(8):675–8.
194. Lopez MJ et al. Squamous cell carcinoma of the anal canal. Am J Surg. 1991;162(6):580–4.
195. Doci R et al. Combined chemoradiation therapy for anal cancer. A report of 56 cases. Ann Surg. 1992;215(2):150–6.
196. Johnson D et al. Carcinoma of the anus treated with primary radiation therapy and chemotherapy. Surg Gynecol Obstet. 1993;177(4):329–34.
197. Tanum G, Tveit KM, Karlsen KO. Chemoradiotherapy of anal carcinoma: tumour response and acute toxicity. Oncology. 1993;50(1):14–7.
198. Beck DE, Karulf RE. Combination therapy for epidermoid carcinoma of the anal canal. Dis Colon Rectum. 1994;37(11):1118–25.
199. Smith DE et al. Cancer of the anal canal: treatment with chemotherapy and low-dose radiation therapy. Radiology. 1994;191(2):569–72.
200. Ajani JA et al. Fluorouracil, mitomycin, and radiotherapy vs fluorouracil, cisplatin, and radiotherapy for carcinoma of the anal canal: a randomized controlled trial. JAMA. 2008;299(16):1914–21.

21 Presacral Tumors

Eric J. Dozois and Maria Dolores Herreros Marcos

Introduction

The presacral or retrorectal space may be the site of a group of heterogeneous and rare tumors that display indolent growth and produce ill-defined symptoms. As detection is often difficult and delayed, patients frequently present with tumors that have reached considerable size and involve multiple organ systems, complicating their treatment. The diagnosis and management of these tumors has evolved in recent years due to improved imaging modalities, a better understanding of tumor biology, adjuvant chemoradiation therapy and a more aggressive surgical approach. Few surgeons have the opportunity to treat these complex lesions, and the care of these patients can be greatly optimized by an experienced, multidisciplinary team.

Anatomy and Neurophysiology

A thorough understanding of pelvic anatomy, including soft tissue, neurologic, and osseous structures is essential in the evaluation and management of presacral tumors. The boundaries of the retrorectal region include the posterior wall of the rectum anteriorly and the sacrum posteriorly (Figure 21-1). This space extends superiorly to the peritoneal reflection and inferiorly to the rectosacral fascia and the supralevator space. Laterally, the area is bordered by the ureters, the iliac vessels, and the sacral nerve roots (Figure 21-2A). Several important vascular and neural structures are located in this area and injury to them may have important physiologic rectoanal sequelae, as well as neurologic and musculoskeletal consequences. If all sacral roots on one side of the sacrum are sacrificed, the patient will continue to have normal anorectal function. Likewise, if the upper three sacral nerve roots are left intact on either side of the sacrum, the patient's ability to spontaneously defecate and to control anorectal contents will remain essentially intact. If, however, both S-3 nerve roots are sacrificed, the external anal sphincter will no longer contract in response to gradual balloon dilation of the rectum and this will translate clinically into variable degrees of anorectal incontinence and difficult defecation.[1] If sacrectomy is to be performed, the surgeon must be familiar with the relationship among thecal sac, sacral nerve roots, sciatic nerve, piriformis muscle thecal sac, and sacrotuberous and sacrospinous ligaments (Figure 21-2B). Structurally, the majority of the sacrum can be resected, if more than half of the S-1 vertebral body remains intact, pelvic stability will be maintained. However, preoperative radiation to the sacrum may ultimately lead to stress fractures if only S-1 remains. As such, spinopelvic stability may be augmented with fusion in select patients. Knowledge of anatomy of the thigh and lower extremity is also required in complex cases requiring muscle or other soft tissue flaps. It is important to discuss with patients preoperatively the potential neuromuscular and visceral losses that may occur during the operation and how this will influence their function and quality of life.

Classification

General Considerations

Presacral lesions are rare. Reports from various large referral centers have indicated that their incidence may be as low as 1 in 40,000 hospital admissions (0.014%).[2] Spencer and Jackman found precoccygeal cysts in only 3 of 20,851 proctologic exams.[3] While Jao et al.[4] reported 120 patients over a 19-year period.

Lesions found in the presacral space can be broadly classified as congenital or acquired, benign or malignant. Two-thirds of lesions are congenital, two-thirds of which are benign and one-third neoplastic. Overall, 45–50% of the presacral masses are malignant or have areas of malignant change within them.[4–6] The presacral space has a complex embryologic development, and this potential space is primarily composed of connective tissue, nerves, fat, and blood vessels. As this area contains totipotential cells that differentiate into three germ cell layers, a multitude of tumor types may be encountered.

D.E. Beck et al. (eds.), *The ASCRS Textbook of Colon and Rectal Surgery: Second Edition*,
DOI 10.1007/978-1-4419-1584-9_21, © Springer Science+Business Media, LLC 2011

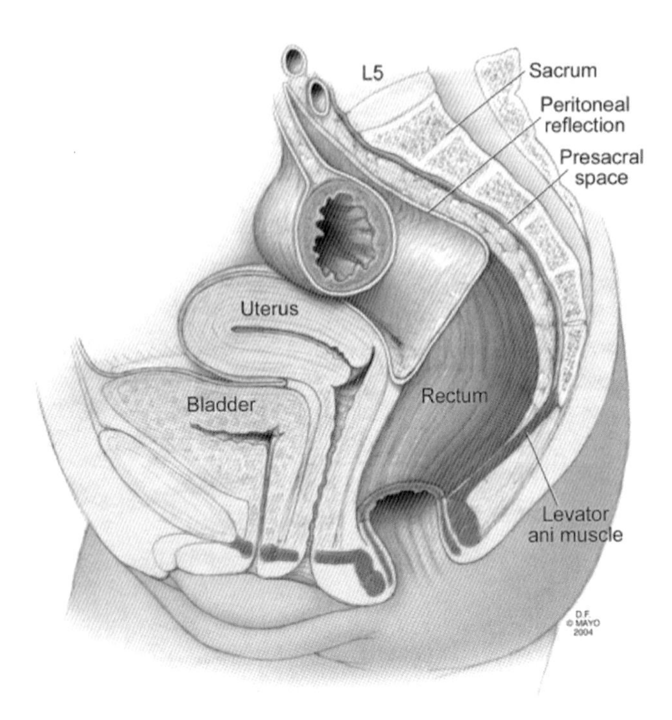

FIGURE 21-1. Relationship of pelvic structures to presacral space.

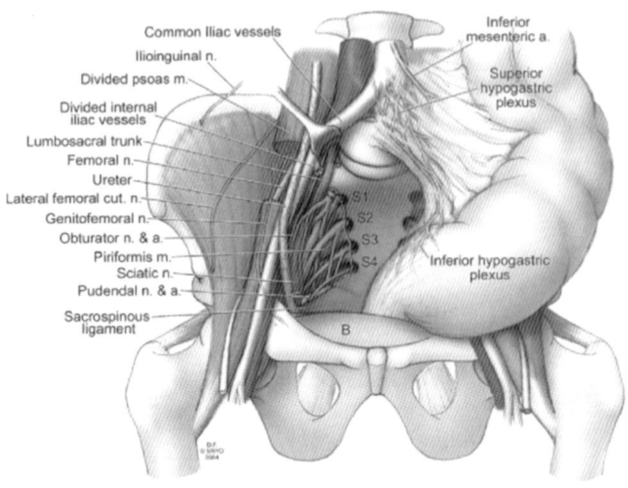

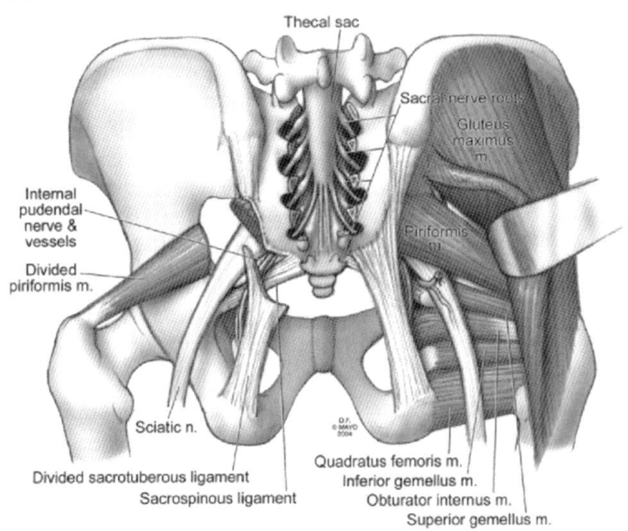

FIGURE 21-2. **A** Anterior view of pelvic anatomy. **B** Posterior view or pelvic anatomy with sacral elements removed.

The classification first described by Uhlig and Johnson[7] has been used for many years and divides tumors into broad categories; congenital, neurogenic, osseous, and miscellaneous. We have modified and updated this system to subcategorize tumors into malignant and benign entities, as this greatly impacts therapeutic approaches (Table 21-1).

Gross and Histologic Appearance

Epidermoid cysts result from defects during the closure of the ectodermal tube. They are histologically composed of stratified squamous cells, do not contain skin appendages, and are typically benign.

Dermoid cysts also arise from the ectoderm, but histologically they contain stratified squamous cells and skin appendages. These are also generally benign. Epidermoid and dermoid cysts tend to be well circumscribed, round and have a thin outer layer. Occasionally, they communicate with the skin surface producing a characteristic postanal dimple. They are most common in females and the infection rate may be high as they are often misdiagnosed as a perirectal abscess and operatively manipulated.

Enterogenous cysts are lesions thought to originate from sequestration of the developing hindgut, if related with the rectum they are called rectal duplication cysts. Because they originate from endodermal tissue, they can be lined with squamous, cuboidal, or columnar epithelium. Transitional epithelium may also be found. These lesions tend to be multilobular with one dominant lesion and smaller satellite cysts. Like dermoid and epidermoid cysts, they can become infected and are more common in women. These are generally benign, but case reports have described malignant transformation within rectal duplications.[8]

Tailgut cysts, which are sometimes referred to as cystic hamartomas, are congenital lesions arising from remnants of normally regressing postanal primitive gut. They are more common in females and can be seen as multiloculated or biloculated cysts on magnetic resonance imaging (MRI) (Figure 21-3).[9] These cysts are composed of squamous, columnar, or transitional epithelium that may have a morphologic appearance similar to that of the adult or fetal intestinal tract. The presence of glandular or transitional epithelium differentiates this lesion from an epidermoid or dermoid cyst. Malignant transformation has been reported in up to 13% in some series.[10,11]

Teratomas are true neoplasms derived from totipotential cells and include all three germ layers. They may undergo

TABLE 21-1. Classification of presacral tumors

- *Congenital*
  - Benign
    - Developmental cysts (teratoma, epidermoid, dermoid, mucus-secreting)
    - Duplication of rectum
    - Anterior sacral meningocele
    - Adrenal rest tumor
  - Malignant
    - Chordoma
    - Teratocarcinoma
- *Neurogenic*
  - Benign
    - Neurofibroma
    - Neurilemmoma (schwannoma)
    - Ganglioneuroma
  - Malignant
    - Neuroblastoma
    - Ganglioneuroblastoma
    - Ependymoma
    - Malignant peripheral nerve sheath tumors (malignant schwannoma, neurofibrosarcoma, neurogenic sarcoma)
- *Osseous*
  - Benign
    - Giant-cell tumor
    - Osteoblastoma
    - Aneurysmal bone cyst
  - Malignant
    - Osteogenic sarcoma
    - Ewing's sarcoma
    - Myeloma
    - Chondrosarcoma
- *Miscellaneous*
  - Benign
    - Lipoma
    - Fibroma
    - Leiomyoma
    - Hemangioma
    - Endothelioma
    - Desmoid (locally aggressive)
  - Malignant
    - Liposarcoma
    - Fibrosarcoma/malignant fibrous histiocytoma
    - Leiomyosarcoma
    - Hemangiopericytoma
    - Metastatic carcinoma
  - Other
    - Ectopic kidney
    - Hematoma
    - Abscess

Modified from Uhlig BE et al. Presacral tumors and cysts in adults. Dis Colon Rectum. 1975;18:581–96.[7]

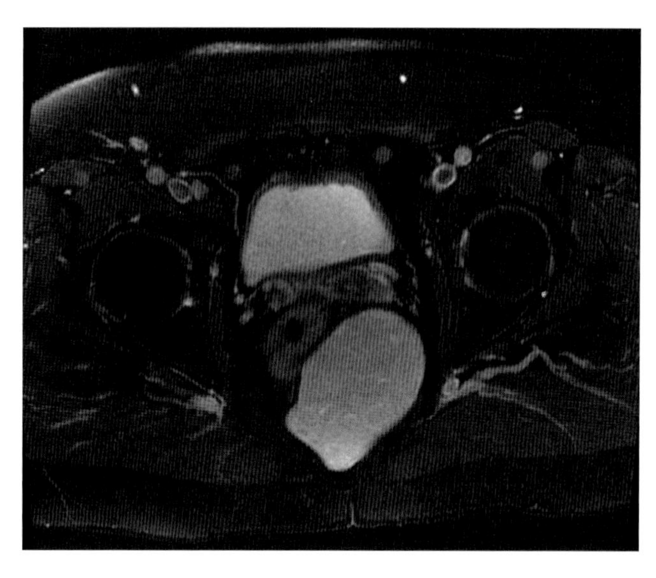

FIGURE 21-3. Tailgut cyst.

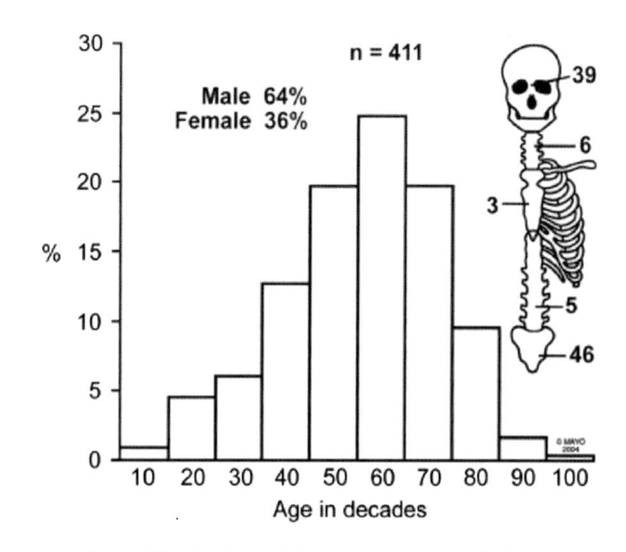

FIGURE 21-4. Distribution of chordomas (Mayo Clinic orthopedic database).

malignant transformation to squamous cell carcinoma arising from the ectodermal tissue, or rhabdomyosarcoma arising from the mesenchymal cells. Anaplastic tumors are also seen in which the tissue of origin may not be distinguishable. Histologically, these tumors are referred to as either "mature" or "immature" reflecting the degree of cellular differentiation. Teratomas are more common in females and in the pediatric age group, and are often associated with other anomalies of the vertebra, urinary tract, or anorectum.[12] In adults, malignant degeneration can occur in 40–50%.[13] Incomplete or intralesional resection increases the likelihood of malignant degeneration.[14] These lesions can also become infected and be misdiagnosed as a perirectal abscess or fistula. Diagnosis is often delayed and these tumors may reach considerable size.

Sacrococcygeal chordoma is the most common malignancy in the presacral space. These tumors are believed to originate from the primitive notochord which embryologically extends from the base of the occiput to the caudal limit in the embryo. They can occur anywhere along the spinal column, but have a predilection for the pheno-occipital region at the base of the skull and for the sacrococcygeal region in the pelvis. Over half occur in the sacrum (Figure 21-4). They predominate in men and are rarely encountered in patients younger than 30 years of age.[15] These tumors may be soft, gelatinous, or firm and may invade, distend, or destroy bone and soft tissue. The center of these tumors contains extracellular mucin. Hemorrhage and necrosis within tumors may lead to secondary calcification and pseudocapsule formation. Common symptoms include pelvic, buttock, and lower back pain aggravated by sitting and alleviated by standing or walking. Diagnosis is often delayed and these tumors may reach a considerable size. Although chordomas are low to intermediate-grade malignant lesions, a radical surgical approach that achieves negative margins greatly improves survival.[15]

Anterior sacral meningoceles are a result of a defect in the thecal sac and may be seen in combination with presacral cysts or lipomas. Typical symptoms include constipation, low back pain, and headache exacerbated by straining or coughing. Anterior sacral meningocele may be associated with other congenital anomalies, such as spina bifida, tethered spinal cord, uterine and vaginal duplication, or urinary tract or anal malformations. Surgical management consists of ligation of the dural defect.

Neurogenic tumors include neurilemmomas, ganglioneuromas, ganglioneuroblastomas, neurofibromas, neuroblastomas, ependymomas, and malignant peripheral nerve sheath tumors (neurofibrosarcoma, malignant schwannomas, and neurogenic sarcomas). In a Mayo Clinic series, schwannomas were the most common benign tumor and malignant peripheral nerve sheath tumors the most common malignant lesions.[16] Benign schwannomas are usually solitary, well circumscribed, encapsulated tumors.[17] Malignant transformation of benign schwannoma is very rare and only nine cases have been reported.[18] Although neurogenic tumors tend to slowly grow, they may eventually reach considerable size. Preoperative differentiation between benign and malignant pathology can be difficult without a tissue biopsy, but is of paramount importance to guide the operative approach.

Osseous tumors include chondrosarcoma, osteosarcoma, myeloma, and Ewing's sarcoma. These tumors arise from bone, cartilage, fibrous tissue, and marrow. Due to relatively rapid growth, these lesions often reach considerable size and pulmonary metastases are common. All osseous tumors of the presacral space are associated with sacral destruction. Although benign, giant cell tumors are locally destructive and can metastasize to the lungs ("benign metastasizing giant cell tumor").

Miscellaneous lesions in this region include metastatic deposits, inflammatory lesions related to Crohn's disease or diverticulitis, hematomas, and anomalous pelvic ectopic kidneys. Carcinoid tumors of the presacral space are unusual but have been reported.[19] Most represent direct extension or metastatic spread from rectal carcinoids. There is no gender predilection. Half of them are associated with development cyst, being malignant about 30% of the cases. Sigmoidoscopy and biopsy is required to differentiate a primary presacral carcinoid with a rectal lesion that has metastasized.

Overall, most presacral tumors occur in females and are cystic. Most solid tumors are chordomas and more commonly seen in males. Benign lesions are frequently asymptomatic and are incidentally discovered during routine gynecologic examination which may explain the greater incidence in females. By contrast, malignant tumors are more often symptomatic, but still commonly found late due to their vague symptomatology. Some presacral tumors present as part of a congenital syndrome, such as Currarino syndrome, which is a combination of presacral mass, anorectal malformations, and sacral anomalies.[20] In Currarino syndrome, the most frequent component of the presacral mass is meningocele, but teratomas have been identified in 20–40% of reported cases.[21]

Diagnosis and Management

History and Physical Examination

Due to their indolent course, presacral tumors are commonly found incidentally at the time of periodic pelvic or rectal examination. Symptomatic patients typically complain of vague, longstanding pain in the perineum or low back. Pain may be aggravated by sitting and improved by standing or walking. In a Mayo Clinic series, pain was more common when the tumor was malignant as compared to benign (88 vs. 39% repeatedly).[4] Occasionally, patients complain of longstanding perineal discharge and their symptoms may be confused with anal fistula or pilonidal disease.[22] Several clues may alert the clinician to the presence of a retrorectal cystic lesion, including repeated operations for anal fistula, the inability of the examiner to uncover the primary source of infection at the level of the dentate line, a postanal dimple, or fullness and fixation of the precoccygeal area. All patients in the Mayo series with osseous tumors complained of low back pain, perineal pain, or both.[4] Some patients may give a history of referral to a psychiatrist because of clinicians' inability to ascertain the origin of their chronic, ill-defined pain. Patients with larger tumors may complain of constipation and/or rectal and urinary incontinence, and sexual dysfunction due to the sacral nerve root involvement.

Patients should be carefully examined, focusing on the perineum, rectal examination and assessing for a postanal dimple. In a series from our institution, 97% of presacral tumors could be palpated on rectal exam.[4] Digital rectal exam (DRE) typically reveals the presence of an extrarectal mass displacing the rectum anteriorly with a smooth and intact overlying mucosa. Rectal examination is also critical in assessing the level of the uppermost portion of the lesion, degree and extent of fixation, and relationship to other pelvic organs, such as the prostate. Rigid or flexible sigmoidoscopy can be used to assess the overlying mucosa and rule out transmural penetration of the tumor. A careful neurologic exam focusing on the sacral nerves and musculoskeletal reflexes is mandatory, and may also aid in the diagnosis of extensive local tumor invasion.

Diagnostic Tests

The presence of a presacral tumor can be confirmed with imaging modalities such as computerized tomography (CT), MRI, and endorectal ultrasound (ERUS). Simple anterior–posterior and lateral radiographs (AP/LAT) of the sacrum can identify osseous expansion, destruction, and/or calcification of soft tissue masses, but are typically not helpful in rendering a specific diagnosis. A chordoma is the most common tumor causing these findings, but sarcomas or benign, locally aggressive tumors, such as giant cell tumor, neurilemmoma (schwannoma) and aneurysmal bone cysts, may also cause extensive bony destruction. The characteristic "scimitar sign" on plain radiographs denotes the presence of an anterior sacral meningocele, a diagnosis that can be confirmed with conventional myelography or MRI with gadolinium.

In recent years, state-of-the-art imaging, such as CT, MRI, and positron emission tomography (PET) scan, has dramatically changed the way in which these tumors are evaluated. Computerized tomography and MRI complement each other and are the most important radiographic studies in evaluating a patient with a presacral lesion. Computerized tomography can determine whether a lesion is solid or cystic and whether adjacent structures, such as the bladder, ureters, and rectum, are involved (Figure 21-5A–C). CT is also the best study to evaluate cortical bone destruction. MRI is highly recommended because of its multiplanar capacity and improved soft tissue resolution that is essential for planning specific lines of resection (Figure 21-6A and B). Sagittal views assist in decision making in regards to need for and level of sacrectomy (Figure 21-6C). MRI is also more sensitive than is CT in spinal imaging, showing associated cord anomalies, such as a meningocele, nerve root, and foraminal encroachment by tumor, or thecal sac compression.[23] Angiography and venogram can be added to the MRI (MR angiogram, venography) to delineate vascular involvement and anatomy grossly distorted by tumor mass effect. This information is helpful to the vascular, plastic, and orthopedic surgeons for operative planning. Gadolinium-enhanced MRI imaging before, during, and/or after neoadjuvant therapy may also show the effectiveness of this treatment in terms of volume of tumor that appears vascularized and viable.

In patients with presacral cystic lesions thought to be the source of a chronically draining sinus, fistulogram may occasionally help clarify the diagnosis. ERUS has been used by some to characterize retrorectal tumors and its relationship to the muscularis propria of the rectum.[24]

Preoperative Biopsy

Historically, the role of preoperative biopsy of presacral tumors has been a controversial topic. Methodology, and even its very necessity, varies among authors. In the past, some authors have considered any presacral tumor deemed resectable as a contraindication to preoperative biopsy,[4,25–27] with only a minority of authors stating that all solid tumors should be preoperatively sampled by biopsy.[28] This recommendation in part, may have to do with the fact that the literature on this topic is sparse and outdated, especially when one considers the availability of modern imaging, better knowledge of tumor biology, and new opportunities for neoadjuvant therapy. Indeed, some patients substantially benefit from preoperative chemotherapy and radiation, especially in osseous tumors, such as Ewing's sarcoma, osteogenic sarcoma, and neurofibrosarcoma. Likewise, very large tumors, such as pelvic desmoids, can be more easily removed after reducing their size with radiation. Preoperative tissue diagnosis *is* essential to the management of solid and heterogeneously cystic presacral tumors.[11,16] For example, the surgical approach and necessary margins is dramatically different when faced with a neurofibroma as compared to a neurofibrosarcoma. When performed correctly, preoperative biopsy can only improve the overall management, rather than harm it.

What is clear about preoperative biopsies of presacral tumors is that they should never be transrectally or transvaginally performed. In the presence of a cystic lesion, such an approach is likely to result in infection rendering its future complete excision more difficult and increasing the likelihood of postoperative complications and recurrence. More importantly, inadvertent transrectal needling of a meningocele may lead to disastrous sequelae, such as meningitis and even subsequent death. Moreover, as the biopsy tract needs to be removed en bloc with the specimen, transrectal biopsy would mandate proctectomy in a patient whose rectum may otherwise have been spared.

There is rarely an indication to biopsy a purely cystic presacral lesion. From a technical standpoint, a presacral tumor biopsy should be done by a radiologist with experience in the evaluation and management of pelvic tumors. In planning the approach for a biopsy, the surgeon should always consider the resection margins so that the needle tract can be removed en bloc with the specimen. The transperineal or parasacral approach is usually ideal and falls within the field of the pending surgical resection (Figure 21-7A and B). Transperitoneal, transretroperitoneal, transvaginal, and transrectal biopsy should be avoided. Biopsy tracts should never traverse neurovascular planes. Normal coagulation studies are required prior to biopsy, as hematoma formation and/or bleeding potentially contaminate(s) involved areas. PET-CT scan can be useful to guide biopsy needles into small focal areas of high tumor density.

Role of Preoperative Neoadjuvant Therapy

Modern protocols and the wide availability of neoadjuvant tumor irradiation and systemic chemotherapy have

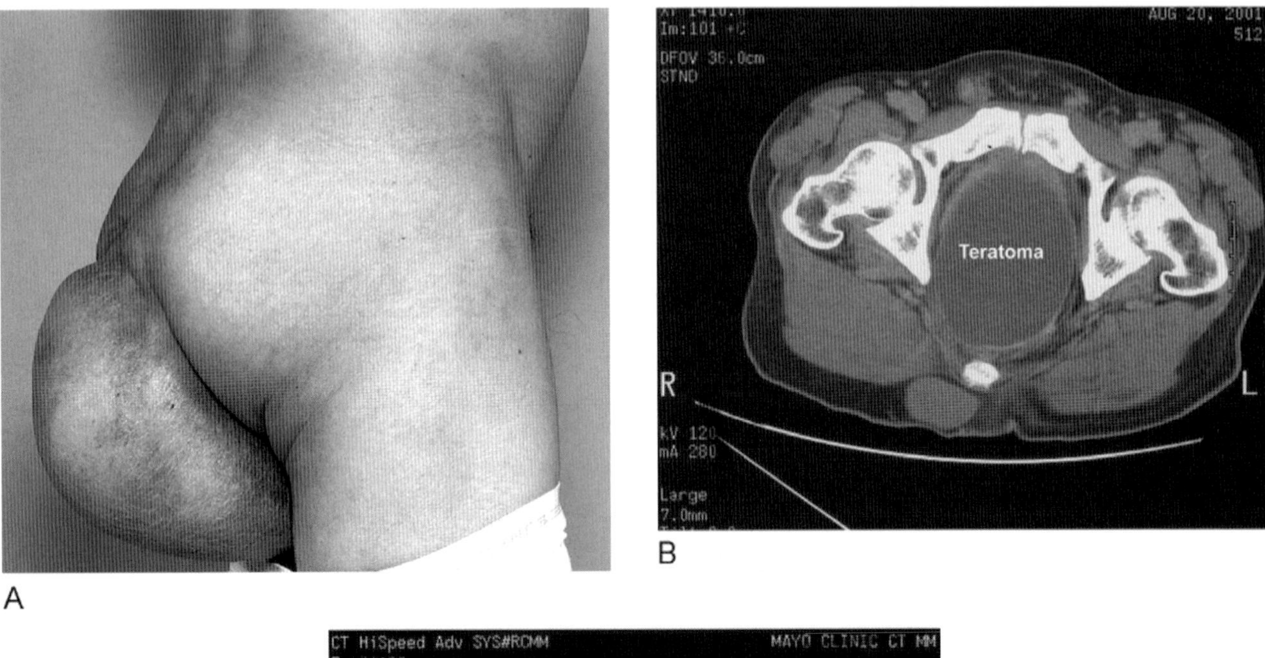

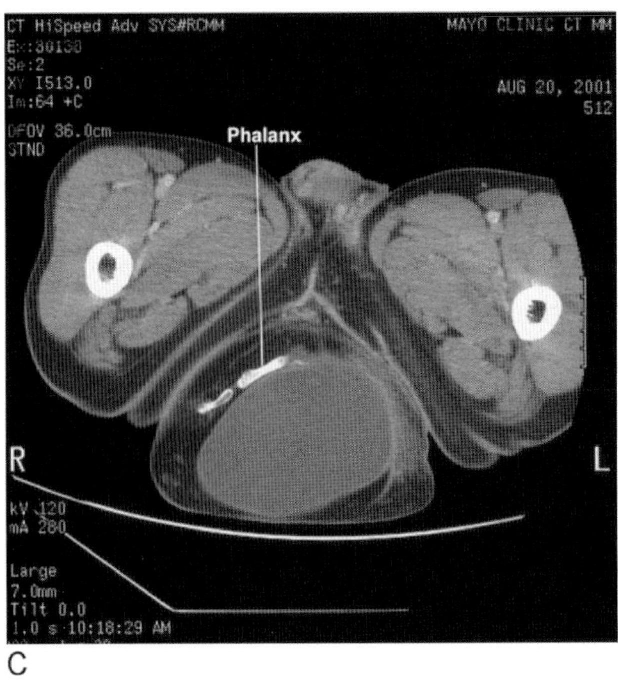

FIGURE 21-5. Massive cystic teratoma with sacral appendage. **A** CT image of teratoma, intrapelvic portion, **B** extrapelvic portion, **C** including fully developed phalanx.

revolutionized the management of patients with complex malignancies. It is in large part due to these new treatment modalities prior to surgery that a preoperative diagnosis is of paramount importance. Although some tumors, such as chondrosarcoma and chordoma, are poorly responsive to both chemotherapy and irradiation, there are a number of tumors seen in the presacral space whose rate of local recurrence can be markedly decreased with the addition of irradiation. Preoperative, as opposed to postoperative, irradiation can be extremely helpful in the face of large pelvic tumors. One of the significant advantages of preoperative irradiation is that it allows treatment to a smaller radiation field. Postoperative irradiation for a pelvic tumor would require irradiation of the entire surgical bed, previous tumor site, all contaminated surgical planes and the sites of all skin incisions. This increased radiation exposure is associated with increased morbidity. Furthermore, should "spillage" occur during resection of a radiosensitive tumor, this contamination may be with previously irradiated necrotic, nonviable cells. A third, and perhaps most important, advantage of

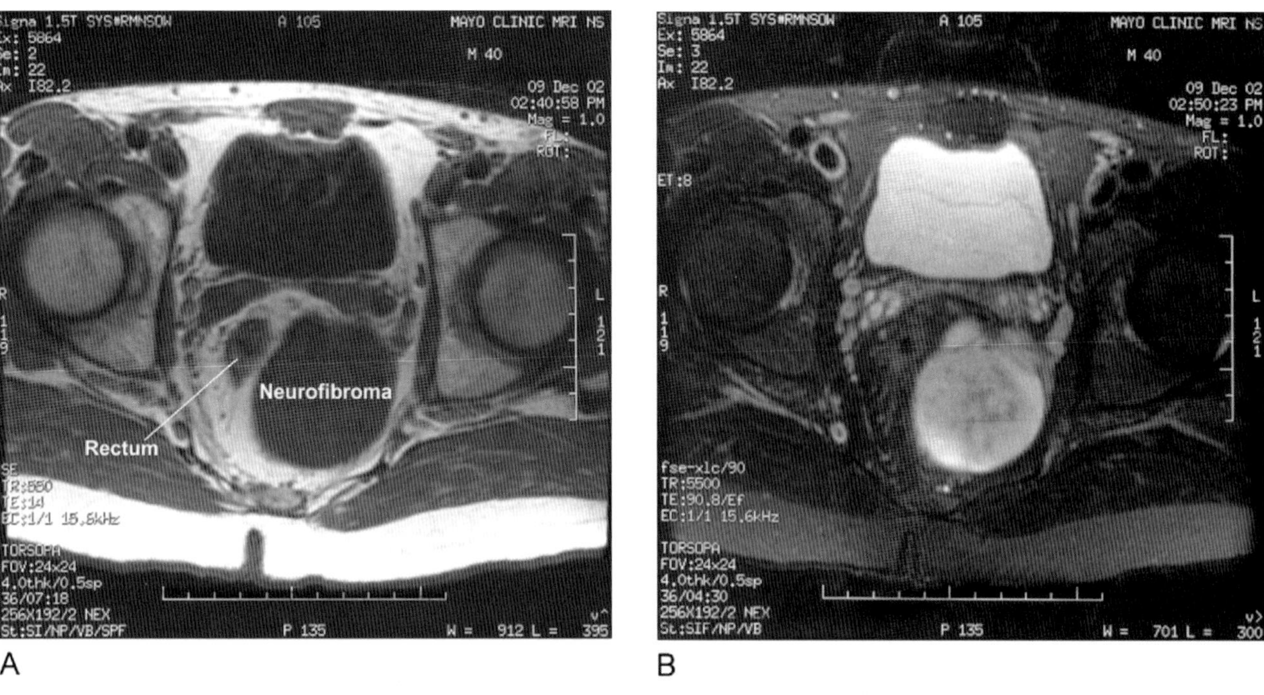

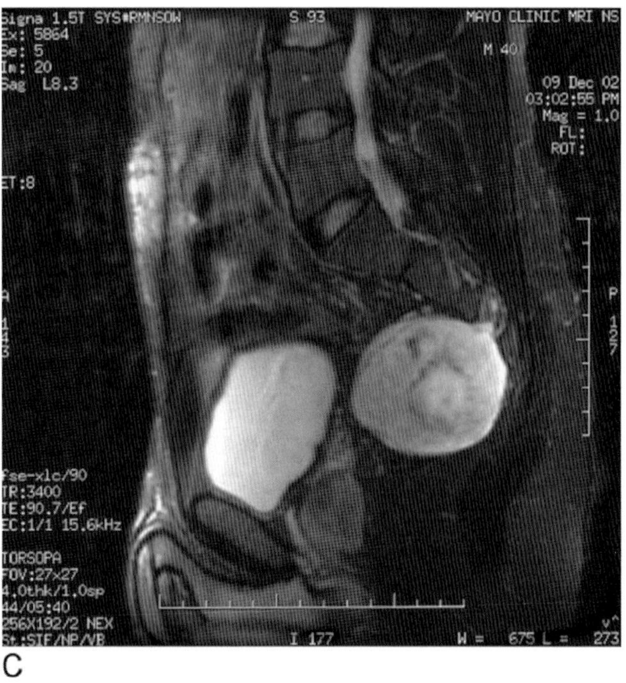

FIGURE 21-6. MRI of pelvic neurofibroma displacing the rectum anterior and lateral. **A** T1 weighted coronal image, **B** T2 weighted coronal image, **C** sagittal view with tumor exiting the 3rd sacral foramen.

preoperative irradiation in sensitive tumors, is the fact that decreased tumor size is often observed. A decrease in tumor size in a pelvic tumor may allow the surgeon to spare vital structures, which would have had to be sacrificed in order for wide margins to be achieved without prior radiation. Additionally, a smaller tumor often means a surgery of a lesser magnitude and therefore less risk for intraoperative complications.

Large tumors in the presacral space, especially sarcomas, are notorious for systemic metastasis. Neoadjuvant chemotherapy is the cornerstone of treatment for diagnoses such as Ewing's sarcoma and osteogenic sarcoma. A wide resection of a pelvic tumor of this type, which would cause a delay in systemic chemotherapy treatment, is not in the patient's best interest. Micrometastatic disease must be treated in patients with diagnoses such as these preoperatively, unless the

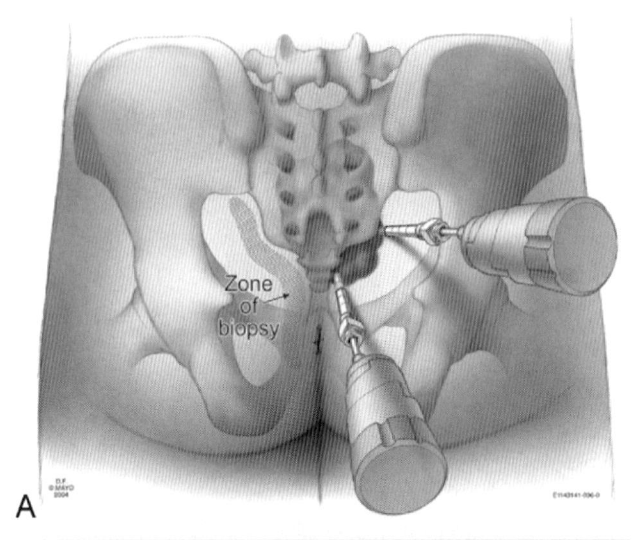

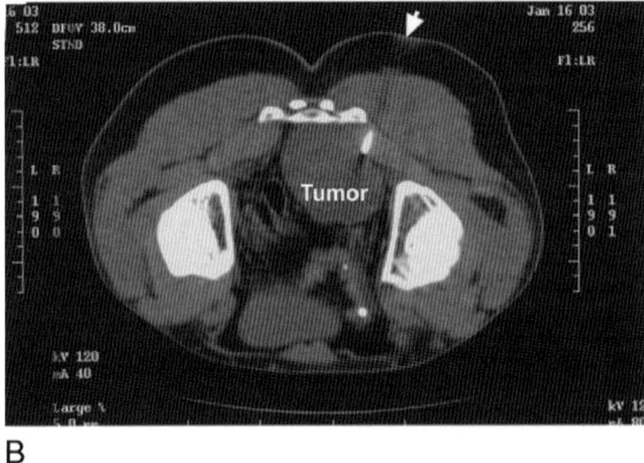

FIGURE 21-7. **A** Preoperative biopsy technique using CT guidance, **B** Parasacral approach to presacral neurogenic tumor.

tumor has caused an immediate complication that requires emergent surgery. Furthermore, one could argue, that lymphoma or Ewing's sarcoma, can be completely treated with chemoradiation, and that surgery may not be necessary at all.

Most non-chordoma malignant presacral tumors are sarcomas. The use of adjuvant therapy for presacral sarcomas in our recent review followed protocols typically for other types of soft-tissue sarcomas (unpublished data).[29] Use of adjuvant radiation and chemotherapy in patients with pelvic sarcomas remains controversial due to small samples sizes, mixed pathology, and lack of randomized data. Radiation therapy has been shown to significantly decrease local relapse following surgery for both extremity and retroperitoneal sarcomas, and by extrapolation, would be expected to decrease local relapse in patients with pelvic sarcomas if adequate dose can be safely delivered.[30,31] Similar findings using chemotherapy alone, or in combination with radiation, have been seen for extremity and retroperitoneal sarcomas, resulting in decreased local and distant relapse with trends toward improved survival.[16,29,32,33] Due to the small sample sizes in most series, meaningful conclusions as to the utility of adjuvant therapy in this surgical setting cannot be drawn. However, given that improved survival in patients with soft-tissue sarcomas, especially those with high-grade lesions, has been limited by high rates of local and distant relapse, an aggressive multimodality approach seems warranted.[16,29]

Regarding malignant neurogenic tumors, the use of adjuvant therapy has been recently reported by our institution.[16] Preoperative chemotherapy was given to 21% of patients, 33% of whom also had it in the postoperative period. The vast majority of patients had doxorubicin-, ifosfamide-, or doxorubicin/ifosfamide-based regimen. Radiation therapy, pre-, intra-, or postoperatively, was given to 72% of patients. The median preoperative radiation dose was 5,040 cGy (range 4,500–5,560 cGy) and the median postoperative dose was 3,000 cGy (range 1,402–6,400 cGy). For those patients who received intraoperative radiation with electrons, the median dose was 1,250 cGy (range 1,000–1,750 cGy).

Surgical Treatment

Rationale for Aggressive Approach

The rationale for an aggressive surgical approach for presacral tumors is based on several arguments. The lesion may already be malignant or transform into a malignant state if left in place. In patients with teratomas, especially those patients in the pediatric age group, the risk of malignant transformation is considerable and continues to dramatically increase if removal is delayed or incomplete.[13] Untreated anterior sacral meningoceles may become infected and lead to meningitis, which is associated with high mortality.[34] Cystic lesions may become infected making their excision difficult and increasing the possibility of postoperative infection and future recurrence. A presacral mass in a young woman may cause dystocia at the time of delivery. Lastly, benign and malignant tumors left untreated may grow to considerable size making surgical resection much more complicated.

In the past, many surgeons have adopted a rather defeatist attitude toward sacrococcygeal chordomas and other tumors in this area based on a number of erroneous misconceptions. Presacral tumors may produce vague symptoms, which leads to a delay in diagnosis for months or even years. Thus, patients may seek medical treatment late in the course of their disease and the presence of a large mass in this often unfamiliar and complex anatomic area makes some surgeons reluctant to consider aggressive surgical approach for fear of serious operative and postoperative complications.

Finally, and most importantly, tumors in this area have been inadequately treated in the past because of tumor violation, their large size and location, and fear of neurologic complication and/or musculoskeletal instability. Preoperative tumor violation can take place when such tumors are biopsied, or intraoperatively when margins of resection are inadequate or tumor cells are spilled in an effort to be too conservative. When a surgeon is attempting to avoid injury to the rectal wall or important neurological structures, they may inappropriately restrict excision and compromise oncologic outcome. For malignant lesions wide, en bloc removal of adjacent organs, soft tissue, and bone (if locally adherent) is the goal of resection.

Role of Multidisciplinary Team

It is of great importance that an experienced team consisting of a colorectal surgeon, orthopedic oncologic surgeon, spine surgeon, urologist, plastic surgeon, vascular surgeon, musculoskeletal radiologist, medical oncologist, radiation oncologist, and specialized anesthesiologist evaluate and surgically treat tumors that are large and extend to or destroy the hemipelvis or the upper half of the sacrum. The importance of a multispecialty approach for presacral tumors was first described in 1953 by a Mayo Clinic team of surgeons. They found an improvement in outcome in this difficult to manage group of patients with the combined effort of multiple specialists.[35] This quote from their publication describes their convictions:

> The surgical management of presacral and sacral tumors has been in general unsatisfactory. We feel that progress in treating these lesions may have been impeded rather than enhanced by the individual surgical specialists who came into contact with these lesions. Consequently, we have united our efforts in solving the problem and thereby utilizing the special assets of the three surgical specialties – neurologic, orthopedic and general Surgery – in meeting this problem.

Surgical Approach

Careful surgical planning is important in deciding how to approach these tumors whether it be an anterior approach (abdominal), posterior approach (perineal), or a combined abdominoperineal approach. Computerized tomography and MRI help define the margins of resection and the relationship of the tumor to the sacral level (Figure 21-8). Small and low-lying lesions can be removed transperineally through a parasacral incision, whereas tumors extending above the S-3 level, especially if large, often require a combined anterior and posterior approach.

For large malignant lesions requiring extended resection, a plastic surgeon plays a significant role, as adequate soft tissue coverage can often be difficult. Most often, the authors use the transabdominal rectus abdominus myocutaneous (TRAM) flap, which fills dead space and can cover large cutaneous defects left by the resection. Healthy, well-vascularized tissue flaps, placed in the surgical bed, markedly decrease the incidence of wound-related complications.

Preoperative Considerations

Optimizing patients for surgery is of extreme importance in a majority of these cases. Adequate nutritional repletion with total parenteral nutrition or with a feeding tube may be necessary in patients who present severely debilitated.

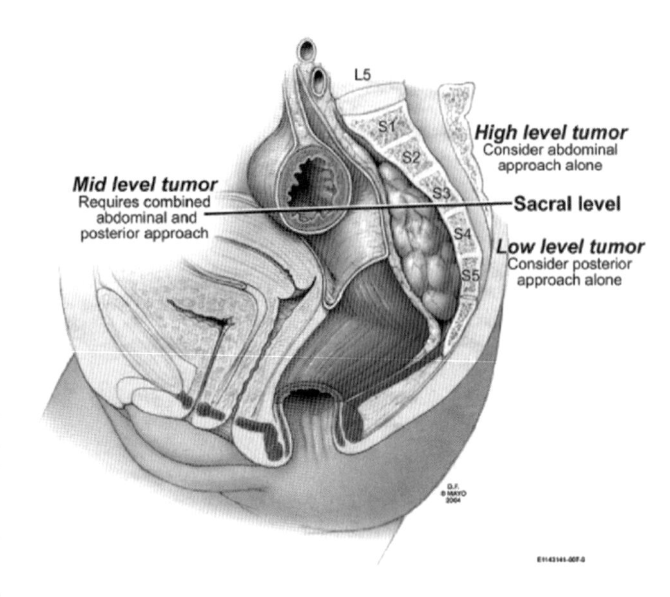

FIGURE 21-8. Relationship of tumor to sacral level and proposed approach.

In technically complex cases, when we expect a long operative time and significant debilitation postoperatively, we consider placement of a temporary intravena caval filter, since the risk of deep venous thrombosis and pulmonary embolus is high and postoperative anticoagulation may be contraindicated. Preoperative selective coil embolization done by an interventional radiologist may be useful in patients with large, vascular tumors to decrease intraoperative bleeding.[36] A multidisciplinary team should preoperatively review films and plan surgical strategy avoids confusion during the day of surgery. An operating theater capable of managing massive transfusion requirements is mandatory, as is an anesthesiologist comfortable with the physiologic management needed during the procedure.

Posterior Approach

For low-lying tumors, the patient is placed in the prone jackknife position with the buttocks spread with tape (Figure 21-9A). An incision is made over the lower portion of the sacrum and coccyx down to the anus taking care to avoid damage to the external sphincter. Resection of the tumor may be facilitated by transection of the anococcygeal ligament and coccyx (Figure 21-9B). The lesion can then be dissected from the surrounding tissues, including the rectal wall, in a plane between the retrorectal fat and the tumor mass itself. In the case of very small lesions, the surgeon may double-glove the left hand and with the index finger in the anal canal and lower rectum, push the lesion outward, away from the depths of the wound (Figure 21-9C) facilitating dissection of the lesion off the wall of the rectum without injury. If necessary, the lower sacrum or coccyx or both can be excised en bloc with the lesion to facilitate excision.

An intersphincteric approach has been described for very low-lying tumors.[37] It is performed in a lithotomy position.

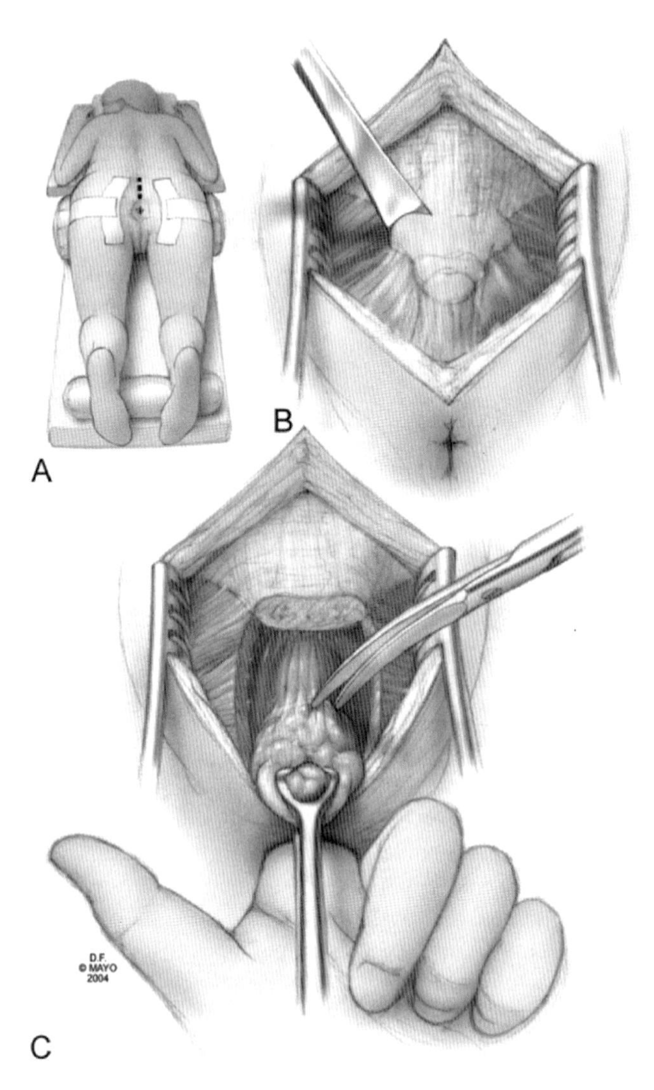

FIGURE 21-9. **A** Positioning for posterior approach. **B** Coccygectomy. **C** Index finger in anal canal to "push" tumor outward facilitating dissection.

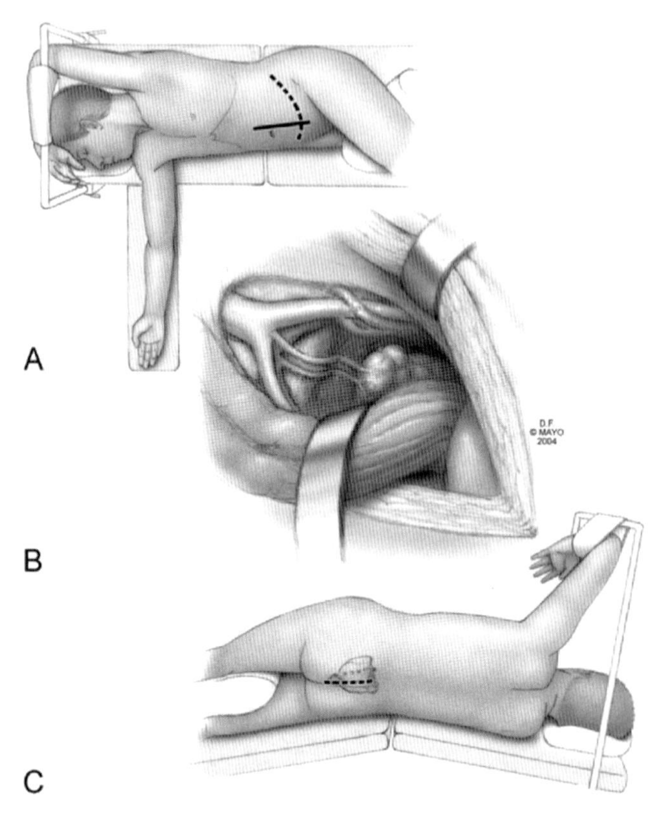

FIGURE 21-10. **A** Modified lateral position for anterior exposure via a midline (*large arrow*) or ileoinguinal (*smaller arrow*) incision. **B** Anterior exposure of vessels and tumor. **C** Posterior approach to sacrum.

Through a V-shaped, or radial incision posterior to the anus, the intersphincteric plane is opened and bluntly dissected. The anal canal and internal sphincter are separated from the external sphincter up to the level of the puborectalis sling. The dissection is continued upward in the retrorectal fatty space. The division of Waldeyer's fascia may be necessary to expose the upper surface of the levator ani muscles.

Combined Abdominal and Sacral–Perineal Approach

If the upper pole of the tumor extends clearly above the S-3 level, an anterior and posterior approach is usually indicated. Patients may be placed in the supine or lateral position, depending on the surgeon's preference and previous experience. A variety of techniques and positioning to the abdominal perineal approach have been described.[38] If an anterior–posterior approach is necessary, the patient can be placed in a "sloppy-lateral" position to facilitate a simultaneous two-team approach (Figure 21-10A–C). We always recommend cystoscopy and bilateral ureteral stent placement before laparotomy. Through a midline incision the abdomen should be carefully examined to rule out metastasis or other important pathology. After the lateral attachments to the sigmoid have been mobilized and the presacral space is entered just below the promontory, the posterior rectum can be dissected from the upper sacrum down to the upper extension of the tumor. The ureters and hypogastric nerves are identified and protected. The rectum can then be mobilized laterally, and if necessary, anteriorly.

If a malignant tumor can be safely separated from the posterior wall of the rectum without compromising a wide margin, the lesion can be dissected in a plane between its capsule and the mesorectal fat to preserve the rectum. If the tumor is extremely large, markedly compressing and displacing the rectum, making dissection between the rectal vault and the tumor hazardous, one should remove the rectum en bloc with the tumor and the involved segments of the sacrum. It is mandatory in malignant cases that no structures attached to the specimen should be separated with dissection, and that they are removed en bloc with the primary tumor mass. In this situation, the upper rectum is transected with a stapler at the level of the promontory. Under these circumstances, it is imperative that the anterior wall of the rectum be completely freed from the seminal vesicles and prostate in men and the upper two-thirds of the vagina in women. The pelvic floor can then be reconstructed over the anal remnant and the sigmoid colostomy established in the left lower abdominal wall.

In the presence of very large tumors, blood loss during the procedure can be substantial. This potentially adverse sequelae may be minimized by ligating the middle and lateral sacral vessels and both internal iliac arteries and veins (Figure 21-11). When ligating the internal iliac artery, in order to reduce the risk of perineal necrosis it is best to preserve the anterior division from which the inferior gluteal artery arises. This maneuver is often performed in conjunction with permissive hypotension. A vascular surgeon can be helpful during this portion of the procedure especially in patients that have had prior irradiation or have distorted vascular anatomy. In a situation in which a large tissue defect is expected, one may elect to mobilize one rectus muscle on its vascular pedicle and place it in the presacral area for later use in the closure of the perineal wound when the patient is prone. In the anterior–posterior approach, when a flap is used, a thick piece of silastic mesh is placed posterior to the vital structures and anterior to the bony structures to protect vital structures from injury during bony resection while in the prone or lateral position. After the abdominal incision is closed and the colostomy is matured, the anesthetized patient can then be moved from the supine to the prone position. The perineal approach is similar to that used for benign low-lying cystic or solid tumors, except that wider and more proximal dissection is necessary. After an incision has been made over the sacrum and coccyx down to the anus, the anococcygeal ligament is transected and the levator muscles are laterally retracted. If the rectum is to be preserved, the tumor can be separated from the rectum by careful dissection of the plane between the rectum and the tumor. The orthopedic surgeon can then proceed with the separation of gluteus maximus muscles on both sides, detachment of the sacrospinous and sacrotuberous ligaments, and division of the piriformis muscles bilaterally to protect the sciatic nerves (Figure 21-12A). A posterior laminectomy may be required to expose and ligate nerve roots (Figure 21-12B) to be sacrificed and/or the thecal sac (Figure 21-12C). In this manner, the lesion can be removed en bloc with the lower sacrum and coccyx and involved sacral roots. If the surgeon previously elected to excise the rectum en bloc, it is preferable to remove the anus and anal canal with the rectal specimen. The wound is then closed in layers over suction silastic drain, or a rectus abdominus myocutaneous flap is inserted and sewn

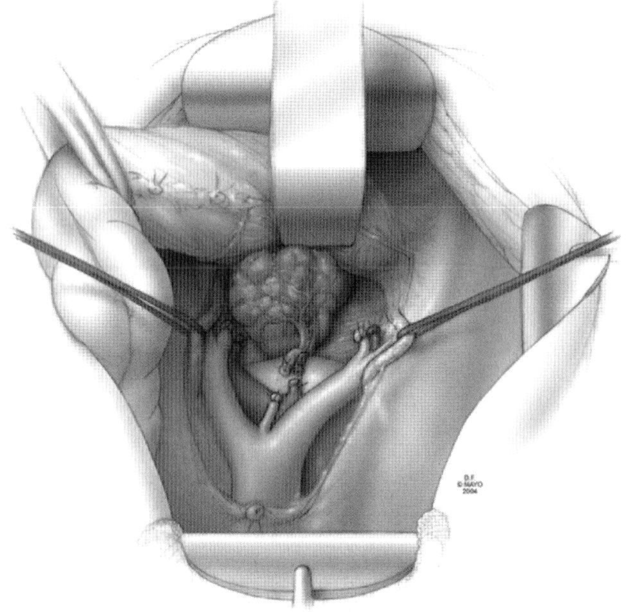

FIGURE 21-11. Ligation of middle sacral and internal iliac vessel.

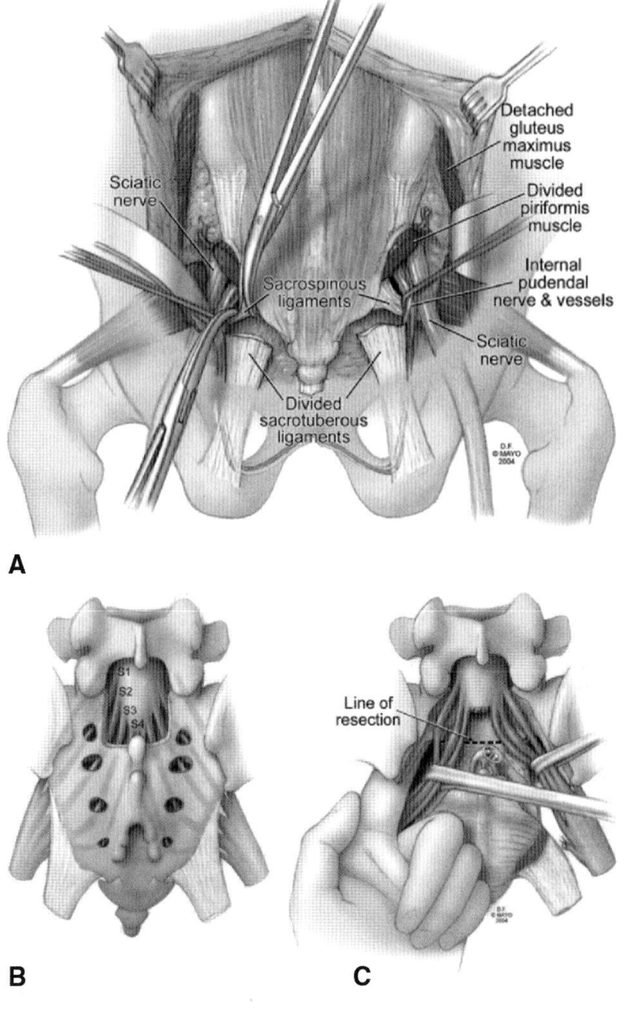

FIGURE 21-12. **A** Posterior approach and exposure of sciatic nerves, **B** sacral nerve roots, **C** and ligation of the thecal sac.

into place by the plastic surgeon. More complex soft tissue procedures may be required if the tumor involves the posterior soft tissue elements.

Recently, there have been reports using minimally invasive laparoscopic techniques as an approach for presacral tumor resection, both for anterior-only and for anterior–posterior approaches.[39–42] If the anterior portion of a combined anterior–posterior approach can be done laparoscopically (rectum divided, colostomy made, tumor partially mobilized, vasculature ligated), it should decrease the morbidity of the overall operation significantly. Leygyel et al.[42] described a laparoscopic approach to treat advanced rectal cancer with similar surgical steps to the malignant presacral tumor laparoscopic resection. The operation was performed in two phases: a laparoscopic abdominal phase with the patient in the modified Lloyd-Davies position, followed by a transsacral phase with the patient in the prone jackknife position. The key features of the abdominal (laparoscopic) component were lateral-to-medial mobilization of the rectum, ligation of the inferior mesenteric vessels, careful identification and preservation of the pelvic nerves and sacral nerve roots, and division of the colon with construction of the colostomy and completion of the proctectomy.

Follow-Up Considerations

The authors recommend an annual visit, including a digital rectal examination, to assess for recurrence of a benign lesion. If digital rectal examination reveals a mass, a CT scan is done. We recommend a baseline CT at 1 year following surgery and then repeated at every 5 years, even if examination is normal.[11]

In the case of malignant tumors, the patients are closely followed with particular attention to local recurrence and pulmonary metastasis. An annual pelvic MRI and chest CT-scan is performed for the first 5 years. If the patient rectum was left in place, annual DRE with possible anoscopy is performed by the colorectal surgeon. Patients are offered repeat resection for locally advanced tumors and for pulmonary metastasis if all disease can be removed operatively.

Results of Treatment

Malignant Lesions

Results of surgical treatment of presacral lesions depend on both the natural behavior of the tumor and the adequacy of resection. If wide margins were not achieved during resection of a malignant lesion or if the tumor is violated, one can expect a high local recurrence rate and a poor overall outcome. In general, most malignant tumors reported in the literature have had a rather poor prognosis, but many such tumors had been incompletely resected or excised piecemeal, breaking oncologic principles.[4,16] Kaiser et al.[43] found that local recurrence rate increased from 28 to 64% if chordomas are perioperatively violated in patients.

Fuchs et al.[15] reported one of the largest series of sacral chordoma. Fifty-two patients underwent surgical treatment for sacrococcygeal chordoma in a 21-year period. Posterior approach was performed in 22 patients while a combined anteroposterior approach was used in 30. A wide surgical margin was achieved in 21 patients, it was defined as a cuff or normal tissue at least 1–2 cm except anteriorly. At an average of 7.8 years of follow-up, 23 patients were alive with no evidence of disease. Twenty-three patients (44%) had local recurrence. The rate of recurrence-free survival was 59% at 5 years and 46% at 10 years. The overall survival rates were 74, 52, and 47% at 5, 10, and 15 years, respectively. The most important predictor of survival was a wide margin. All patients with a wide margin survived, and this survival rate was significantly different from that for patients who had either marginal or intralesional excision ($p=0.0001$). Of the 21 patients with a wide margin, 17 (81%) had undergone a combined anteroposterior approach and only four had been treated with a posterior approach. Overall, lung metastasis developed in 16 (31%) of the 52 patients, and all but three of those patients also had a local recurrence.

On the contrary, surgical management of non-chordoma malignant retrorectal tumors has only been reported in small series or single case reports, and therefore limited data exist on the long-term oncologic outcomes.[4,44] In a recent analysis of presacral sarcomas at the authors' institution (unpublished data), 37 patients underwent resection, with an R0 margin in 84% and R1 in 16%. Overall, 76% of the patients required en bloc resection of adjacent pelvic organs and bony structures. The most frequent sarcomas found were malignant peripheral nerve sheath tumors and chondrosarcomas. Postoperative chemotherapy was given to 70% of the patients, and IORT was administered to 22% of the patients. Thirty-day mortality occurred in one patient and overall survival at 2, 5, and 10 years was 75, 55, and 47%, respectively. Disease-free survival at 5 years was 51%.

Cody et al.[44] reported their experience with malignant presacral tumors, nine (38%) of which had chordomas. Excision of these tumors was described as "en bloc" or "in fragments." Forty-eight percent developed local recurrence; 60% of patients underwent open biopsy. For all treated patients, survival at 5, 10, 15, and 20 years was 69, 50, 37, and 20%, respectively.

Lev-Chelouche et al.[25] reported on 21 patients with malignant presacral tumors, nine of which were chordomas. No patients underwent preoperative biopsy; nearly all patients had a palpable lesion on rectal exam. Fifteen of 21 malignant lesions were completely excised. Most recurrences were seen in patients with incomplete resection and 50% of these patients died of disease.

Wang et al.[5] reported their series of 22 patients with malignant presacral tumors, five of which were chordomas, and seven of which were leiomyosarcomas, tumor size ranged from 1.5 to 40 cm. The average size of malignant tumors was 17 cm, 96% were palpable by rectal exam. Computerized tomography was felt to be the best test to identify the lesions and define extent and degree of tumor invasion, but the diagnosis remained nonspecific. No patients underwent preoperative biopsy. Five patients had complete resection and 17 had incomplete resection. The overall 5-year survival rate for malignant tumors was 41%. No patients underwent preoperative adjuvant therapy. Postoperative chemotherapy and radiotherapy was used in selected patients with malignant tumors.

Bohm et al.[27] reported their series of 24 patients with congenital presacral tumors. They had four patients with chordomas and 20 with developmental cysts. All patients with chordoma underwent excision. Three of four chordoma patients had recurrence at 25, 32, and 55 months. Patients with recurrence presented with pain and neurologic disturbance. Complete local re-excision was done in the three patients with recurrence. Only 3/20 patients with developmental cysts developed recurrence, all of which underwent successful re-excision.

Few data exist regarding the outcomes in patients undergoing surgery for presacral tumors of neurogenic origin. The largest surgical series reported to date of pelvic neurogenic tumors included several in the presacral space.[16] In that series, 89 patients were identified, of whom 44 were male. Median age was 38 years. Malignant lesions were found in 43 patients (48%). Schwannomas were the most common benign tumor (61%) and malignant peripheral nerve sheath tumors the most common malignant lesion (81%). Malignant tumors had histopathologic evidence of infiltration of surrounding structures in 49% of cases. Intralesional resection was the most common surgical technique for both benign and malignant tumors. Five-year local recurrence rates for benign and malignant lesions were 35.9 and 35.0%, respectively. Survival in those with malignant lesions at 1, 5, and 10 years was 79.5, 47.9, and 29.6%, respectively. For all patients, the overall probability of being disease free at 1, 5, and 10 years was 72.6, 40.0, and 30.0%, respectively. Five-year disease-free survival for malignant tumors was 25.9%.

Congenital Cystic Lesions

In general, cystic lesions can be treated adequately by complete excision via a posterior approach. Large cystic lesions such as teratomas extending high into the pelvis can be excised via a combined abdominal–perineal approach. There continues to be some debate as to whether or not a coccygectomy needs to be done for all resections of congenital cystic lesions.[22] Several authors advocate coccygectomy stating that this approach improves surgical exposure and decreases the risk of recurrence as the coccyx may harbor a nidus of totipotential cellular remnants that may later evolve into a recurrent cyst.[6,12,45] The concern of increased recurrence though is not supported by any published data. In fact, some authors state that if the cyst is not adherent to the coccyx, and can be removed entirely without coccygectomy, the coccyx should be left in place.[27] Likely the cyst itself, and not the coccyx per se, harbors the aberrant remnants of the postanal gut leading to the formation of the cyst, and if the cyst is not adherent to the coccyx, there would be no advantage to a coccygectomy. It is clear from our recent series that our approach followed this perspective, and most surgeons elected to preserve the coccyx unless en bloc resection was required for malignancy or if the cyst was densely adhered to the coccyx.[11]

In a Mayo Clinic series, 49 congenital cystic lesions were described, including 15 epidermoid cysts, 16 mucus-secreting cysts, 15 teratomas, and 2 meningoceles.[4] Three teratocarcinomas were seen. Most lesions were in females with only three in males. Average size of cysts was 4–7 cm. Almost all cystic lesions were treated with a posterior approach. Of 66 patients with benign tumors, ten had recurrence (four had giant cell tumors, six had congenital benign cysts), most of which were treated successfully with re-excision.

Presacral tailgut cyst surgical outcomes at Mayo Clinic have been recently reported.[11] Thirty-one patients were identified and complete cyst excision was achieved in all patients, using a posterior (20/31), anterior (9/31), or combined (2/31) approach. Coccygectomy or distal sacrectomy was performed in 26% of the patients. Malignant transformation was present in four patients (13%), adenocarcinoma in three and carcinoid in one. A fistula to the rectum was found in four patients (13%). One benign recurrence was detected during follow-up and there has no mortality. Long-term complications were noted in five patients and included: delayed wound healing ($n=2$), pelvic floor dysfunction ($n=2$) and sexual dysfunction ($n=1$) in a male reoperated for recurrence.

Lev-Chelouche et al.[25] reported 21 benign presacral lesions. Complete excision of benign lesions was possible in all cases with no recurrences during the 10 year follow-up. Singer et al.[22] reported on seven patients with presacral cysts (six females, one male). All patients had previously been misdiagnosed and treated for pilonidal cysts, perirectal abscesses, fistula in ano, psychogenic disorder, proctalgia fugax and posttraumatic or postpartum pain before the correct diagnosis was made. Patients underwent an average of 4.1 prior operative procedures. All patients were successfully treated with resection through a parasacrococcygeal approach after the correct diagnosis was made with CT fistulogram.

Based on the experience at our institution, we have established a decision-making algorithm to guide the management of presacral tumors (Figure 21-13).

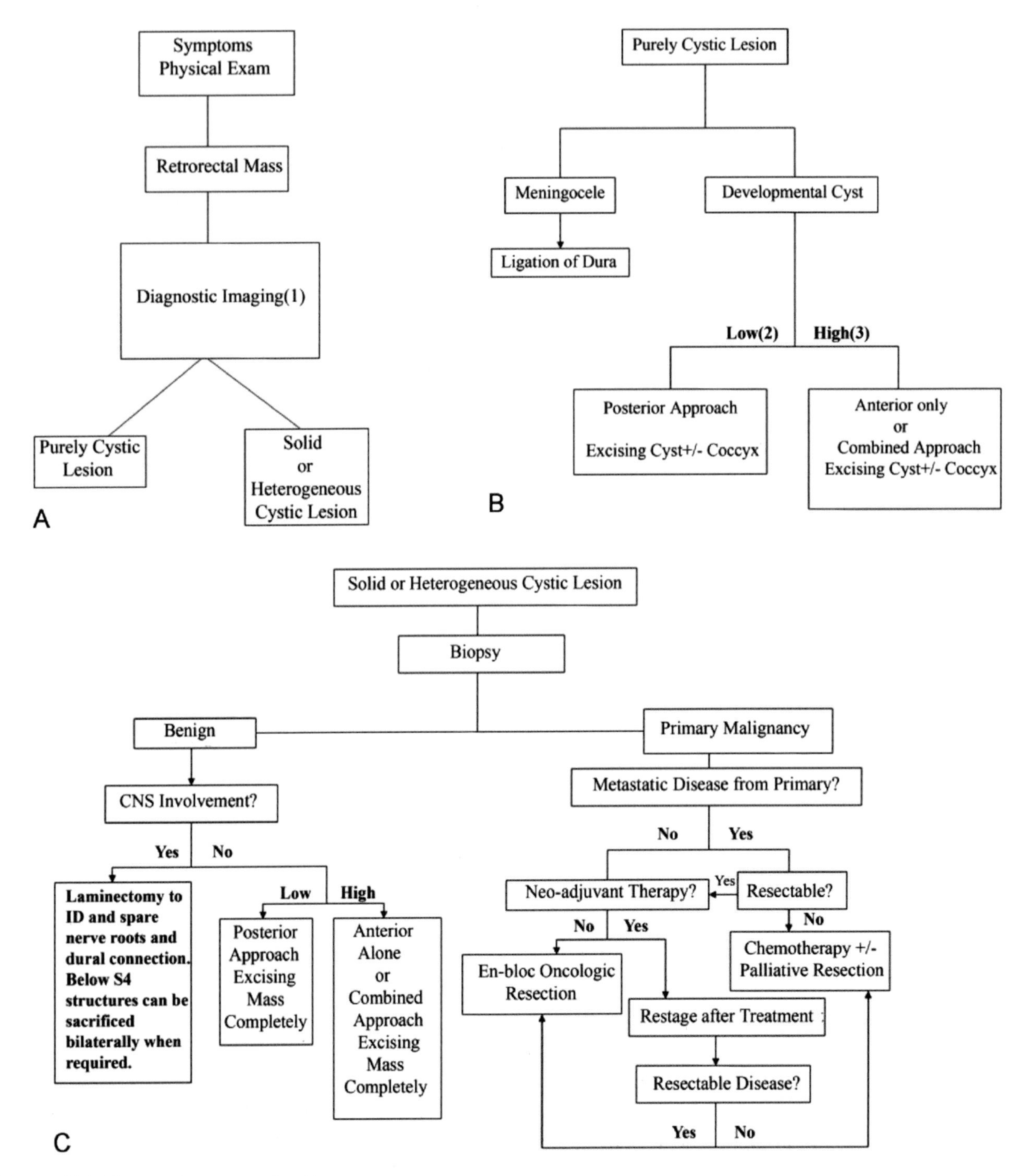

FIGURE 21-13. Proposed treatment algorithm.

Conclusion

Presacral tumors are rare, the differential diagnosis extensive, and their discovery is notoriously difficult and late. A high index of suspicion is needed to identify these patients. Once a benign or malignant presacral lesion is discovered and histologically diagnosed, it should be treated, even if the patient is asymptomatic. CT and MRI imaging can help differentiate between benign and malignant, cystic and solid and accurately define the extent of adjacent organ and bony involvement to guide operative planning. Completely cystic lesions, in general, do not require preoperative biopsy unless malignancy is suspected. All solid tumors and heterogeneous cysts should be considered for biopsy to rule out malignancy, guide neoadjuvant therapy, and plan the extent of resection.

An aggressive approach, by an experienced, multidisciplinary team, that can achieve a tumor-free, en bloc resection, avoid tumor violation, restore spinopelvic stability, and minimize intraoperative and postoperative complications, should decrease the risk of local recurrence and improve survival. Minimally invasive approaches may improve overall recovery and the quality of life in selected patients in the future.

References

1. Gunterberg B, Kewenter J, Petersen I, Stener B. Anorectal function after major resections of the sacrum with bilateral or unilateral sacrifice of sacral nerves. Br J Surg. 1976;63(7):546–54.
2. Whittaker LD, Pemberton JD. Tumors ventral to the sacrum. Ann Surg. 1938;107(1):96–106.
3. Spencer RJ, Jackman RJ. Surgical management of precoccygeal cysts. Surg Gynecol Obstet. 1962;115:449–52.
4. Jao SW, Beart Jr RW, Spencer RJ, Reiman HM, Ilstrup DM. Retrorectal tumors. Mayo Clinic experience, 1960-1979. Dis Colon Rectum. 1985;28(9):644–52.
5. Wang JY, Hsu CH, Changchien CR, et al. Presacral tumor: a review of forty-five cases. Am Surg. 1995;61(4):310–5.
6. Wolpert A, Beer-Gabel M, Lifschitz O, Zbar AP. The management of presacral masses in the adult. Tech Coloproctol. 2002;6(1):43–9.
7. Uhlig BE, Johnson RL. Presacral tumors and cysts in adults. Dis Colon Rectum. 1975;18(7):581–9.
8. Springall RG, Griffiths JD. Malignant change in rectal duplication. J R Soc Med. 1990;83(3):185–7.
9. Yang DM, Park CH, Jin W, et al. Tailgut cyst: MRI evaluation. AJR Am J Roentgenol. 2005;184(5):1519–23.
10. Caropreso PR, Wengert Jr PA, Milford HE. Tailgut cyst – a rare retrorectal tumor: report of a case and review. Dis Colon Rectum. 1975;18(7):597–600.
11. Mathis KL, Dozois EJ, Grewal MS, Metzger P, Larson DW, Devine RM. Local recurrence and risk of malignant transformation in presacral tailgut cyst: surgical outcomes in 31 patients. Br J Surg. 2010;97(4):575–9.
12. Izant Jr RJ, Filston HC. Sacrococcygeal teratomas. Analysis of forty-three cases. Am J Surg. 1975;130(5):617–21.
13. Waldhausen JA, Kolman JW, Vellios F, Battersby JS. Sacrococcygeal teratoma. Surgery. 1963;54:933–49.
14. Hickey RC, Martin RG. Sacrococcygeal teratomas. Ann NY Acad Sci. 1964;114:951–7.
15. Fuchs B, Dickey ID, Yaszemski MJ, Inwards CY, Sim FH. Operative management of sacral chordoma. J Bone Joint Surg Am. 2005;87(10):2211–6.
16. Dozois EJ, Wall JC, Spinner RJ, et al. Neurogenic tumors of the pelvis: clinicopathologic features and surgical outcomes using a multidisciplinary team. Ann Surg Oncol. 2009;16(4):1010–6.
17. Daneshmand S, Youssefzadeh D, Chamie K, et al. Benign retroperitoneal schwannoma: a case series and review of the literature. Urology. 2003;62(6):993–7.
18. Woodruff JM, Selig AM, Crowley K, Allen PW. Schwannoma (neurilemoma) with malignant transformation. A rare, distinctive peripheral nerve tumor. Am J Surg Pathol. 1994;18(9): 882–95.
19. Luong TV, Salvagni S, Bordi C. Presacral carcinoid tumour. Review of the literature and report of a clinically malignant case. Dig Liver Dis. 2005;37(4):278–81.
20. Currarino G, Coln D, Votteler T. Triad of anorectal, sacral, and presacral anomalies. AJR Am J Roentgenol. 1981; 137(2):395–8.
21. Kochling J, Pistor G, Marzhauser Brands S, Nasir R, Lanksch WR. The Currarino syndrome – hereditary transmitted syndrome of anorectal, sacral and presacral anomalies. Case report and review of the literature. Eur J Pediatr Surg. 1996; 6(2):114–9.
22. Singer MA, Cintron JR, Martz JE, Schoetz DJ, Abcarian H. Retrorectal cyst: a rare tumor frequently misdiagnosed. J Am Coll Surg. 2003;196(6):880–6.
23. Lee KS, Gower DJ, McWhorter JM, Albertson DA. The role of MR imaging in the diagnosis and treatment of anterior sacral meningocele. Report of two cases. J Neurosurg. 1988;69(4):628–31.
24. Scullion DA, Zwirewich CV, McGregor G. Retrorectal cystic hamartoma: diagnosis using endorectal ultrasound. Clin Radiol. 1999;54(5):338–9.
25. Lev-Chelouche D, Gutman M, Goldman G, et al. Presacral tumors: a practical classification and treatment of a unique and heterogeneous group of diseases. Surgery. 2003; 133(5):473–8.
26. Luken 3rd MG, Michelsen WJ, Whelan MA, Andrews DL. The diagnosis of sacral lesions. Surg Neurol. 1981;15(5):377–83.
27. Bohm B, Milsom JW, Fazio VW, Lavery IC, Church JM, Oakley JR. Our approach to the management of congenital presacral tumors in adults. Int J Colorectal Dis. 1993;8(3):134–8.
28. Eilbert F. Expert commentary on retrorectal tumors: spectrum of disease, diagnosis and surgical management. Perp Col Rec Surg. 1990;3:252–5.
29. Raut CP, Pisters PW. Retroperitoneal sarcomas: combined-modality treatment approaches. J Surg Oncol. 2006;94(1):81–7.
30. Yang JC, Chang AE, Baker AR, et al. Randomized prospective study of the benefit of adjuvant radiation therapy in the treatment of soft tissue sarcomas of the extremity. J Clin Oncol. 1998;16(1):197–203.
31. Feng M, Murphy J, Griffith KA, et al. Long-term outcomes after radiotherapy for retroperitoneal and deep truncal sarcoma. Int J Radiat Oncol Biol Phys. 2007;69(1):103–10.
32. Rosenberg SA, Tepper J, Glatstein E, et al. The treatment of soft-tissue sarcomas of the extremities: prospective randomized evaluations of (1) limb-sparing surgery plus radiation therapy compared with amputation and (2) the role of adjuvant chemotherapy. Ann Surg. 1982;196(3):305–15.
33. Adjuvant chemotherapy for localised resectable soft-tissue sarcoma of adults: meta-analysis of individual data. Sarcoma Meta-analysis Collaboration. Lancet. 1997;350(9092): 1647–54.
34. Amacher AL, Drake CG, McLachlin AD. Anterior sacral meningocele. Surg Gynecol Obstet. 1968;126(5):986–94.
35. MacCarty CS, Waugh JM, Coventry MB, Cope Jr WF. Surgical treatment of sacral and presacral tumors other than sacrococcygeal chordoma. J Neurosurg. 1965;22(5):458–64.
36. Dozois EJ, Malireddy KK, Bower TC, Stanson AW, Sim FH. Management of a retrorectal lipomatous hemangiopericytoma by preoperative vascular embolization and a multidisciplinary surgical team: report of a case. Dis Colon Rectum. 2009;52(5):1017–20.
37. Buchs N, Taylor S, Roche B. The posterior approach for low retrorectal tumors in adults. Int J Colorectal Dis. 2007; 22(4):381–5.

38. Localio SA, Eng K, Ranson JH. Abdominosacral approach for retrorectal tumors. Ann Surg. 1980;191(5):555–60.
39. Yang CC, Chen HC, Chen CM. Endoscopic resection of a presacral schwannoma. Case report. J Neurosurg Spine. 2007;7(1):86–9.
40. Gunkova P, Martinek L, Dostalik J, Gunka I, Vavra P, Mazur M. Laparoscopic approach to retrorectal cyst. World J Gastroenterol. 2008;14(42):6581–3.
41. Konstantinidis K, Theodoropoulos GE, Sambalis G, et al. Laparoscopic resection of presacral schwannomas. Surg Laparosc Endosc Percutan Tech. 2005;15(5):302–4.
42. Lengyel J, Sagar PM, Morrison C, Gonsalves S, Lee P, Phillips N. Multimedia article. Laparoscopic abdominosacral composite resection. Dis Colon Rectum. 2009; 52(9):1662–4.
43. Kaiser TE, Pritchard DJ, Unni KK. Clinicopathologic study of sacrococcygeal chordoma. Cancer. 1984;53(11):2574–8.
44. Cody 3rd HS, Marcove RC, Quan SH. Malignant retrorectal tumors: 28 years' experience at Memorial Sloan-Kettering Cancer Center. Dis Colon Rectum. 1981;24(7):501–6.
45. Miles RM, Stewart Jr GS. Sacrococcygeal teratomas in adult. Ann Surg. 1974;179(5):676–83.

22 Diverticular Disease

Alan G. Thorson and Jennifer S. Beaty

The term "diverticular disease" of the colon represents a continuum of anatomic and pathophysiologic changes within the colon related to the presence of diverticula. These changes most commonly occur in the sigmoid colon but may involve the entire colon. The continuum can range from the presence of a single diverticulum (a sac or pouch in the wall of an organ) to many diverticula (which may be too numerous to count). It can refer to an asymptomatic state (diverticulosis) or to any one of a number of combinations of inflammatory symptoms, changes, and complications (diverticulitis).

Symptoms may result from: simple physiologic changes in colonic motility related to altered neuromuscular activity in the sigmoid colon, varying degrees of localized inflammatory response, or complex inflammatory interactions leading to diffuse peritonitis and septic shock. These more complex symptoms and resulting complications arise from breaches in the integrity of the wall of one or more diverticula.

This chapter will deal with inflammatory diverticular disease and its associated complications. Bleeding diverticular disease is discussed in Chap. 24.

Incidence

Diverticulosis was first described in the mid nineteenth century as more of a curiosity than a significant disease entity. However, since the early twentieth century, an increasing prevalence of the disease has been recognized in industrialized countries. The incidence increases with age and with the adoption of a diet high in red meat, refined sugars, and milled flour but low in whole grains, fruits, and vegetables. Although the exact incidence is not well established, numerous autopsy, radiographic and endoscopic series have shown that the incidence has increased dramatically over the past 75 years,[1–4] from around 5% near the turn of the century to 50% or more by 1975.[2,3] It is now estimated that the risk of developing diverticular disease in the USA approximates 5% by age 40 and may rise to over 80% by age 80.[5]

This increase in observed incidence was originally attributed to new imaging techniques (the introduction of the barium enema in the early twentieth century) and bias inherent to estimates based on a population presenting with symptoms requiring an investigation.[6] It is now clear that not only is the incidence of diverticulosis increasing but also the incidence of related complications is increasing as well. This is exemplified by increasing costs in the treatment of diverticular disease which accounts for nearly 450,000 hospital admissions, two million office visits, 112,000 disability cases, and 3,000 fatalities each year in the USA.[7] It is estimated that costs will continue to increase as the population continues to age over the next several decades.

Proportionately, few people become symptomatic from the presence of diverticula. Roughly 10–20% of people with diverticula develop symptoms of diverticulitis. Only 10–20% of these will require hospitalization. Of those that require hospitalization, 20–50% will require operative intervention. The percentage of hospitalized patients requiring operation has been increasing as outpatient management becomes more common and those admitted as inpatients are more seriously ill.[8] Overall, less than 1% of patients with diverticula will ultimately require surgical management.[9]

National Census data estimates that as of July 2006, there would be 89,327,640 adults aged 50 or greater.[10] That would mean that approximately 15 million people would develop diverticulitis and of those, 2.5 million would be admitted. If the 1% average is correct and taking into account the percentage of patients with diverticulosis based on age, approximately 539,015 people will ultimately require an operation for diverticular disease.

There is some evidence that males are more frequently affected at a younger age compared to females; however, significant bias may influence this impression. Young females may frequently be under diagnosed due to confusion with gynecologic diseases in women who are of child-bearing age. Older females may be over diagnosed due to confusion with irritable bowel syndrome (IBS). There also appears to be a dichotomy in age and sex with regard to complications of

D.E. Beck et al. (eds.), *The ASCRS Textbook of Colon and Rectal Surgery: Second Edition*,
DOI 10.1007/978-1-4419-1584-9_22, © Springer Science+Business Media, LLC 2011

diverticular disease, particularly perforation. The incidence of perforation is higher in males under age 50. In contrast, the incidence of perforation is higher in females over age 50.[11]

Pathophysiology

Diverticulosis is associated with high intraluminal pressures. Pressures in patients with diverticular disease have been found to be as high as 90 mmHg during peak contraction. This represents a value nearly nine times higher than seen in patients with normal colons.[12] It has been theorized that abnormally high pressures lead to segmentation. Segmentation refers to a process whereby the colon effectively functions as a series of separate compartments rather than as one continuous tube.

The high pressures that each compartment is capable of producing are directed toward the colonic wall rather than as propulsive waves. These pressures predispose to herniation of mucosa through the muscular defects that occur where blood vessels penetrate to reach the submucosa and mucosa (vasa recta brevia). Most of these penetrations occur between the mesenteric and anti-mesenteric tinea where, coincidentally, most diverticula are found. As the mucosa herniates, it does so without dragging the muscular layer along, leaving the diverticula denuded of muscle, which is consistent with the definition of an acquired process. Diverticula may be true, containing all layers of the bowel wall (congenital), or false, lacking the muscular layer (acquired or pulsion diverticula). Thus, the most common diverticula are acquired or pulsion diverticula.

These high pressures are consistent with the sigmoid colon being the most common site of involvement. This can be explained by the Law of Laplace which states that the tension in the wall of a hollow cylinder is proportional to its radius multiplied by the pressure within the cylinder. As the narrowest segment of colon, the sigmoid has the highest pressures and, consequently, the highest risk of diverticulum formation. It is hypothesized that at least a part of the protective effect of dietary fiber is stool bulking, which maintains a larger lumen within the bowel. The stool bulking and larger lumen prevent segmenting contractions and, therefore, decrease high pressures.

Complementary to these theories of pathogenesis is the consistent muscle abnormality associated with sigmoid diverticular disease. Both the circular and longitudinal muscle walls are typically thickened resulting in a reduction in the size of the lumen and a shortening of the sigmoid colon. The reduced lumen size may be further enhanced by secondary pericolic fibrosis.

The source of this muscular thickening is not clear. It has been observed that in the normal process of left colon peristalsis, smooth muscle in the rectosigmoid will relax in response to a stimulus, causing contractions in the colon above and in the rectum below. A combination of poor diet, aging, and constipation could lead to malfunction of this relaxation response leading to a functional obstruction and the hypertrophy seen in the muscle.[13] Cellular hypertrophy, cellular hyperplasia, and elastosis have all been described. Elastosis appears to precede the development of diverticulosis. It is not found in any other inflammatory conditions of the colon.

Several alternative concepts have been advanced to explain the differences in presentation of diverticular disease. Although the most common finding in diverticular disease is the muscular changes already discussed, some patients fail to demonstrate this characteristic. These patients are more likely to have diffuse diverticula throughout the colon. There is a higher incidence of bleeding with diffuse involvement. There may be an underlying connective tissue abnormality, which could explain the development of diverticula in the absence of high intraluminal pressures. The high incidence of bleeding in these patients could be related to an associated inadequate vascular support in the diverticular wall.

Pain associated with diverticular disease may be related to muscle spasm as well as inflammation. Perforation can occur in the absence of inflammation and may be secondary to the extremely high intraluminal pressure.[14]

Etiology

The etiology of diverticular disease remains complex and relatively poorly understood. Pathophysiologic studies reveal that complications do not occur until there is microperforation through the wall of a diverticulum into the pericolic tissue. A single diverticulum experiences a change in the permeability of its isolated mucosa from physical, biochemical, or physiologic means. It is postulated that perforation then occurs leading to a characteristic response which results in varying degrees of inflammation. The perforation might cause microabscess, phlegmon, large abscess, fistulas, or even free perforation. Free perforations occur rarely, while fistulas are more likely, with the bladder being the most common site of fistula formation.[15]

The original communication between the diverticular perforation with the lumen of the bowel, is usually rapidly obliterated by the inflammatory process. Occasionally, failure of the diverticular neck to obliterate may lead to a free communication between the bowel and the peritoneal cavity with resultant fecal peritonitis. Rupture of a noncommunicating abscess may lead to purulent peritonitis.[16]

Low-grade inflammation of colonic mucosa, induced by changes in bacterial microflora, can affect the enteric nervous system and alter gut function, leading to symptom development. This explanation for symptoms in IBS can be easily extrapolated to diverticular disease since some patients with diverticular disease demonstrate bacterial overgrowth.[17]

Recent clinical investigations have shown that disturbances in cholinergic activity may contribute to diverticular disease. Cholinergic stimulation in patients with diverticular disease leads to unsynchronized slow waves of relatively low frequency as opposed to bursts of action potentials normally associated with peristalsis.[18,19] This suggests a possible role for cholinergic denervation hypersensitivity in colonic smooth muscle with upregulation of smooth muscle muscarinic receptors.[20]

A colon with diverticular disease has more cholinergic innervation than a normal colon. In addition, there is less noncholinergic, nonadrenergic inhibitory nerve activity. This increased cholinergic activity and the relative paucity of inhibitory activity may contribute to the high intraluminal pressures and segmentation seen in colonic diverticular disease.[21]

Epidemiology

Diet

Large cohort and case–control studies in the USA and Greece have shown that diets high in red meat and low in fruit and vegetable fiber increase diverticular symptoms by as much as threefold.[22,23] Vegetables and brown grains have been shown to be protective.[23] Fiber may be protective by increasing stool weight and water content which decreases colonic segmentation pressures and transit times.[24] Fiber, through the process of fermentation, also provides short chain fatty acids to the colonic epithelial cells, an important source of fuel and mucosal health.[25–27]

Patients with diverticulosis were often told to avoid seeds, nuts, and popcorn. A large cohort study of US health-care professionals evaluated 47,228 men between the ages of 40–75 who were free of diverticulosis at baseline, and they were followed for 18 years.[28] There were inverse correlations between nut and popcorn consumption and the risk of diverticulitis.[28] The consumption of nuts, corn, and popcorn did not increase the risk of diverticulosis or diverticular complications and therefore the recommendation to avoid these foods to prevent diverticular complications should be reconsidered.[28]

Red meat has been associated with heterocyclic amines, a factor in colon mucosal apoptosis.[29] Dietary heme has been shown to be highly cytotoxic to rat colons.[30]

Age and Gender

Female patients present with complications requiring surgery an average of 5 years later than male patients. Men have a higher incidence of bleeding than women; however, women have a higher incidence of fistula formation compared to men. Younger men present with fistula more frequently, while older men present more frequently with bleeding. Young females are more likely to present with perforation while older females are more likely to present with chronic disease and stricture. Overall, patients younger than 50 present more often with chronic or recurrent diverticulitis.[31,32]

Nonsteroidal Anti-inflammatory Drugs

Nonsteroidal anti-inflammatory drugs (NSAIDs) have been linked to increased rates of complications related to diverticular disease. The plausible mechanism of action is indirect through known inhibition of cyclo-oxygenase and resultant decreased prostaglandin synthesis in the gut. Prostaglandins are important in the maintenance of mucosal blood flow and in providing an effective colonic mucosal barrier. A direct mechanism also exists through mucosal damage caused by NSAIDs which leads to increased translocation of toxins and bacteria.[33,34]

Immune Status

The use of corticosteroids is associated with a higher risk of perforation and more severe inflammatory complications. The postulated mechanism is immunosuppressive and anti-inflammatory effects hinder confinement of perforation in its early stages, resulting in more serious sequelae. The use of other immunosuppressive drugs has also been associated with such increased risks. The main risk appears to be more virulent complications once complications occur.[35]

Opiates

The use of opiate pain medications has been shown to raise intracolonic pressure and slow intestinal transit, both of which increase the risk of complications from diverticular disease. Case series have shown a higher percentage of perforation in patients who were taking opiate analgesics.[32,36] Although, patients who require narcotic pain medication may be at higher risk of perforation based on severity of abdominal symptoms.

Smoking

A recent large case–control study demonstrated that smokers had three times the risk of developing complications from diverticular disease than did nonsmokers.[37] However, a large cohort study involving over 46,000 men in the USA did not find this same association.[38]

Alcohol

A Danish cohort study showed the risk of diverticulitis was three times higher in female alcoholics compared to the general population and two times higher in male alcoholics. However, the data may be biased due to dietary and smoking habits associated with alcoholics.[39]

Clinical Manifestations

Clinical Patterns

Diverticular disease may be classified into diverticulosis (asymptomatic) and diverticulitis (symptomatic) (Table 22-1). Diverticulosis refers to the presence of diverticula with no related symptoms. This applies to the vast majority (80–90%) of patients with diverticular disease. Diverticulitis can be subclassified into noninflammatory, acute (simple or complicated), chronic (atypical or recurring/persistent), or complex disease. The term "malignant diverticulitis" has been used to describe a particularly severe form of fibrosing disease with phlegmonous inflammation extending below the peritoneal reflection. This is associated with frequent fistula formation, obstruction, and high postoperative morbidity and mortality.[40] Many consider this form to be misdiagnosed Crohn's disease.

Noninflammatory Diverticular Disease

Noninflammatory diverticular disease describes those patients with symptoms of diverticulitis but without associated inflammation.[41] The diagnosis is made at the time of elective operation when no inflammatory changes are found in the specimen. This has been reported in 15–35% of resections.[41] Some would consider this a missed diagnosis (IBS). However, if that were always the case, then one would expect a very low resolution of symptoms following resection. In fact, although a lack of inflammatory changes in the resected specimen has been associated with lesser degrees of symptom relief, the success rate is not zero.[41–44] One could conclude that resections are being performed for the right indication but the wrong pathology.

The term "atypical" has been applied to patients with chronic symptoms who never develop the necessary clinical and laboratory criteria to be judged as having acute diverticulitis. Up to 24% of these patients are found to lack inflammatory changes in the resected specimen thus fulfilling the criteria for noninflammatory diverticular disease. The remaining members of this group could be considered as having had acute diverticulitis based on histologic findings of inflammation. A high percentage of atypical patients (88%) became pain free after resection on short term (12 months) follow-up.[44]

Table 22-1. The classification of diverticular disease

Diverticulosis	Asymptomatic
Diverticulitis	
Noninflammatory	Symptoms without inflammation
Acute	Symptoms with inflammation
Simple	Localized
Complicated	With perforation
Chronic	Persistent, low grade
Atypical	Symptoms without systemic signs
Recurring, persistent	Symptoms with systemic signs (may be intermittent)
Complex	With fistula, stricture, obstruction
Malignant	Severe, fibrosing

Acute Diverticulitis

Acute diverticulitis is represented by signs and symptoms of acute inflammation and may be simple (limited to the colonic wall and adjacent tissues) or complicated (with perforation or fistula). Simple acute disease is usually accompanied by systemic signs of fever and leukocytosis while complicated acute disease may have the added signs of tachycardia and hypotension.

Complicated acute diverticulitis can be classified according to the extent of spread of the inflammatory process. A common classification for diverticulitis with perforation was first described in 1963 by Hughes et al.[45] and slightly revised and popularized by Hinchey et al.[16] in 1978. Stage I diverticulitis is a localized pericolic or mesenteric abscess, Stage II is a confined pelvic abscess, Stage III is generalized purulent peritonitis, and Stage IV is generalized fecal peritonitis (Table 22-2).

Chronic Diverticulitis

Patients with chronic diverticulitis remain symptomatic (left lower quadrant pain) despite standard treatment. It is considered atypical if systemic signs never develop. With systemic signs, chronic disease may manifest as recurring, intermittent episodes of acute disease or as persistent, symptomatic low-grade disease. This is frequently associated with the presence of a phlegmon. If resection is performed, there will be evidence of inflammatory changes within the specimen.

Complex Diverticular Disease

Complex diverticulitis refers to disease in those patients who manifest sequelae of chronic inflammation including fistula, stricture, and obstruction. Each of these complications will be addressed later in this chapter.

Presenting Symptoms

Patients with acute diverticulitis typically complain of left lower quadrant abdominal pain. However, in a patient with a redundant sigmoid colon an inflamed segment might present with pain in the right lower quadrant, thus complicating the differential diagnosis with appendicitis. The pain is generally

Table 22-2. The Hinchey classification (proposed by Hinchey et al. in 1978)[16]

Hinchey I	Localized abscess (para-colonic)
Hinchey II	Pelvic abscess
Hinchey III	Purulent peritonitis (the presence of pus in the abdominal cavity)
Hinchey IV	Feculent peritonitis

constant in nature, not colicky. Radiation may occur to the back, ipsilateral flank, groin, and even the leg. The pain may be preceded or accompanied by episodes of constipation or diarrhea. It commonly is progressive in nature if appropriate treatment is not instituted.

Historically, age was used as a primary determinant in distinguishing the most likely etiology of such pain. However, as increasing numbers of young people are found to have diverticular disease, the overlap between age groups has broadened and the need for diagnostic acumen has significantly sharpened.

Nausea and vomiting are unusual in the absence of obstruction. Bleeding is not an associated finding. Symptoms of dysuria or urgency suggest possible bladder involvement due to an adjacent inflammatory mass or a colovesical fistula. Pneumaturia, fecaluria, or passage gas and stool through the vagina suggest a colovesical or colovaginal fistula, respectively. Fever is common and proportional to the amount of inflammatory response present. A high fever suggests a perforation with abscess or peritonitis.

Occasionally, diverticular disease will present in unusual ways. These include lower extremity joint infections of a chronic nature that culture positive for enteric bacteria. Other unusual presentations include female adnexal masses on the left, inflammation/necrosis of the perineum and genitalia including Fournier's gangrene, subcutaneous emphysema of the lower extremities, neck and abdominal wall, isolated hepatic abscess due to enteric organisms, brain abscess due to enteric organisms, and cutaneous lesions mimicking pyoderma gangrenosum.[46,47]

Physical Findings

Patients presenting with acute diverticulitis will be tender to palpation in the left lower quadrant and left iliac region. There may be limited rigidity or localized guarding to deeper palpation. With resolution of the acute phase, palpation may reveal a mass in the left lower quadrant. Classically, there is no prodromal epigastric pain with diverticulitis as one might expect to see with appendicitis.

In the event of a perforation with development of fecal or purulent peritonitis, the area of pain will spread throughout the abdomen. Guarding will become prominent and the abdominal wall will become rigid.

Diagnostic Evaluation

Abdominal X-Rays

The primary value of abdominal X-rays is to rule out pneumoperitoneum or to assess for a possible obstruction, therefore plain films of the abdomen should include supine and upright or left lateral decubitus views. Computed tomography (CT) scan is often the evaluation of choice in the face of acute abdominal pain, so in many centers, the plain abdominal film is rarely used.

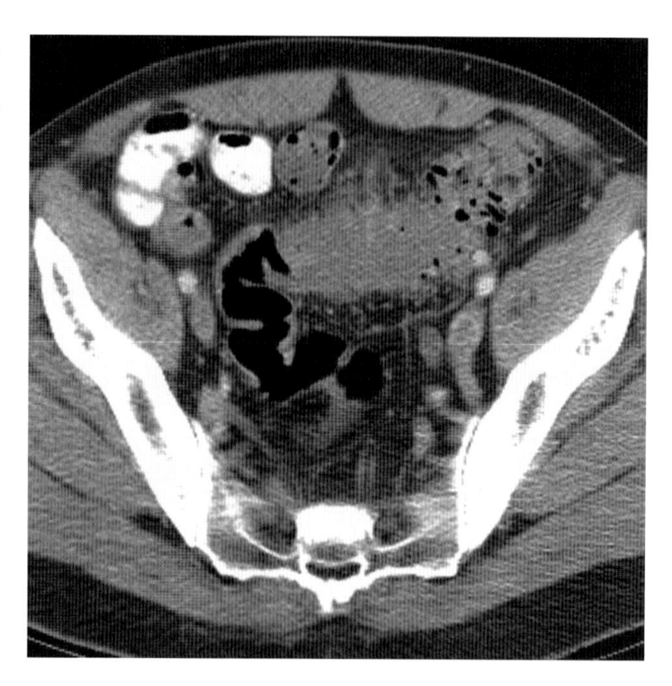

FIGURE 22-1. CT scan reveals uncomplicated diverticulitis with bowel wall thickening and streaky fat in the mesentery.

Contrast Studies

Barium or water soluble contrast studies have their proponents for utilization; however, CT scans provide a significantly more thorough evaluation, making it the preferred imaging study in many centers (Figure 22-1). Nonetheless, due to costs, some clinicians will utilize CT scan only if there is clinical suspicion of an abscess or other complicating feature for which an alternative to standard bowel rest and antibiotics might be applied. A water soluble contrast study can evaluate the lumen of the bowel if there is concern about distal bowel obstruction. It may be an important part of the assessment for the possible use of a colonic stent if malignant disease is suspected.

Contrast studies have been shown to identify fistulas, most commonly colovaginal or coloenteric. Some clinicians prefer the anatomic view of the entire colon provided by barium enema since it distinguishes the extent of diverticulosis throughout the colon and can assess for stricture and colonic length. In most centers, contrast studies, if used at all, are used in a limited fashion to evaluate the anatomy of the colon prior to an operation.

CT Scan

An important advantage of a CT scan is the ability to document diverticulitis, even if uncomplicated, when the diagnosis is in doubt. Studies utilizing CT scan as the initial diagnostic test have shown that up to 5% of patients admitted for acute diverticulitis have been hospitalized for the incorrect clinical diagnosis.[48]

It has been demonstrated that CT can recognize and stratify patients according to the severity of their disease. It can distinguish uncomplicated disease with a predictably short length of hospital stay from complicated disease as defined by abscess, fistula, peritonitis or obstruction and a predictably long length of stay. It also provides information about extracolonic pathology and anatomic variation which is useful for surgical planning. Early CT guided drainage of abscesses allows down-staging of complicated diverticulitis, converting an otherwise urgent or emergent operation with its attendant increases in morbidity and mortality to the safety of an elective operation.[48] In some selected cases there may be no need for elective resection.

Colonography

Preliminary studies utilizing magnetic resonance imaging (MRI) colonography have shown a high correlation with CT findings in patients with diverticular disease without exposure to ionizing radiation. Three-dimensional rendered models and virtual colonoscopy can be performed only in the nonacute setting. These comprehensive 3-D models, rather than barium enema, may have a role in presurgical planning with concurrent assessment of the residual colon.[49]

Ultrasonography

Transrectal ultrasound (TRUS) has been utilized in the evaluation of diverticular disease in conjunction with transabdominal ultrasound (TAUS). Combining TRUS with TAUS reveals complications not visualized on TAUS alone including inflamed diverticula. TRUS may be an accurate adjunct for confirming clinically suspected acute colonic diverticulitis when the rectosigmoid or perirectal tissues are affected as one might see in the case of malignant diverticulitis. It helps avoid false-negative results and defines the severity of disease in the lower sigmoid colon better than TAUS alone. TRUS may prove to be a useful adjunct in selected cases of rectosigmoid diverticulitis and perirectal involvement by diverticular disease in centers where CT scanning is not readily available.[50]

Endoscopy

Endoscopy in the face of acute diverticulitis must be undertaken with extreme caution due to risk of perforation and decreased chance of successful cecal intubation. It can provide important information prior to operation but will change acute management in less than 1% of cases.[51] Generally, in the absence of an urgent indication, colonoscopy should be delayed until resolution of the acute episode is complete.

In the case of elective colonoscopy, the unexpected finding of acute diverticulitis (manifested as erythema, edema, pus, or granulation tissue at a diverticula opening) is distinctly unusual, occurring in just 0.8% of patients. Treatment with antibiotic therapy for such findings is generally unnecessary as follow-up has shown that symptoms of diverticulitis do not develop following the colonoscopy.[52]

Differential Diagnosis

The differential diagnosis for diverticular disease includes IBS, carcinoma, inflammatory bowel disease (IBD), appendicitis, bowel obstruction, ischemic colitis, gynecologic disease, and urologic disease. Of these, IBS is perhaps the most difficult to differentiate in many patients.

Irritable Bowel Syndrome

In many ways, the distinction between chronic diverticulitis and noninflammatory diverticular disease relies upon the pathologist while the distinction between noninflammatory diverticular disease and IBS relies on the diagnostic acumen of the clinician and the long-term outcomes of resection. Due to the prevalence of diverticular disease many patients with IBS will have concomitant diverticular disease. However, due to the fact that diverticular disease is most commonly asymptomatic, the presence of diverticulosis in these patients will often not be the source of their symptoms but rather just a source of confusion in the differential. It is helpful to be familiar with the Rome II criteria (Table 22-3) for the diagnosis of IBS in order to sort through this differential.

Colonic Neoplasia

Distinguishing diverticular disease from cancer can be difficult. Imaging techniques can provide significant diagnostic

TABLE 22-3. The Rome II criteria for irritable bowel syndrome

Irritable Bowel Syndrome can be diagnosed based on at least 12 weeks (which need not be consecutive), in the preceding 12 months, of *abdominal discomfort or pain that has two of three of these features*:
1. Relieved with defecation, and/or
2. Onset associated with a change in frequency of stool, and/or
3. Onset associated with a change in form (appearance) of stool

Symptoms that cumulatively support the diagnosis of IBS:
1. Abnormal stool frequency (>3 stools per day or <3 stools per week)
2. Abnormal stool form (lumpy/hard or loose/watery stool)
3. Abnormal stool passage (straining, urgency, or feeling of incomplete evacuation)
4. Passage of mucus
5. Bloating or feeling of abdominal distension.

Red Flag symptoms which are NOT typical of IBS:
Pain that often awakens/interferes with sleep
Diarrhea that often awakens/interferes with sleep
Blood in stool (visible or occult)
Weight loss
Fever
Abnormal physical examination

assistance but occasionally a resection is necessary. Several features of barium enema (BE) support a diagnosis of diverticular disease including preservation of the mucosa, long strictures, and the presence of diverticula. A BE is preferred by some clinicians to assess the extent of the diverticulosis and evaluate the length of the colon prior to resection. Although colonoscopy can frequently resolve this issue, it is not always possible due to acute angulations or narrowing of the lumen. CT evaluates the entire abdomen, which can identify concurrent disease and may give clues to underlying colonic pathology.

The increasing incidence of colonic neoplasia with increasing age parallels that of diverticular disease. Polyps and cancer must be considered whenever a diagnostic workup for diverticular disease is begun. Although unusual, cases of adenocarcinoma arising within a diverticulum have been reported.[53] Since colonic diverticula are thin walled, containing only mucosa and serosa, early penetration by cancer is likely, leading to advanced stages with small primary lesions.

Although historically diverticular disease was not felt to have an etiologic link to colon cancer, a causal association has been identified between left-sided colon cancer and diverticulitis. In a review of 7,159 patients from the Swedish Cancer Registry, patients with diverticulitis had a long-term increased risk of left-sided colon cancer compared to patients with asymptomatic diverticulosis (odd's ratio = 4.2).[54–56]

Inflammatory Bowel Disease

Crohn's disease can be a particularly difficult diagnosis to make. Both Crohn's and diverticular disease may present with similar complications including fistulas, phlegmons, and abscesses. Rectal involvement, anal disease, extracolonic signs, and bleeding suggest Crohn's disease. Recurrent "diverticulitis" requiring a repeat resection should always raise the question of possible Crohn's disease.[57] Ulcerative colitis is rarely a significant differential diagnostic dilemma since bleeding is not a prominent symptom of diverticulitis and a simple endoscopic exam showing inflammation within the rectum should suffice to rule out diverticular disease. In the unusual circumstance where diverticulitis and ulcerative colitis both exist, treatment should be targeted toward both entities simultaneously.

Other Colitides, Appendicitis, Gynecologic, and Urologic Disease

Endoscopy can be an important adjunct in differentiating IBD, ischemic colitis, and other forms of colitis although caution must be used in the acute setting. A major advantage of the CT scan is the ability to evaluate for many of the other potential differentials including appendicitis, gynecologic, and urologic disease.

Special Considerations

Diverticulitis in Young Patients

There continues to be some debate as to the issue of recurrence in patients younger than 50 years old. It does appear that there is an increased incidence in younger patients presenting with diverticulitis. In a recent study by Etzioni et al.[58] evaluating the nationwide inpatient sample data for changing patterns of diverticular disease and treatment, a 73% increase in the rate of admission for patients aged 18–44 years with diverticulitis was found between 1998 and 2005. While an increase was also found in patients aged 45–74 year, the increase was only 29%.

Historically, diverticular disease in patients less than age 50 has been described as more virulent and with more serious complications.[59–63] Despite the increased number of younger patients with the disease, its virulence does not appear to be any different compared to older counterparts.[64] It is now doubtful that age itself should be a primary consideration in the decision to operate. The literature is mixed with proponents of a more aggressive approach to the disease in young patients[59–66] and those that feel age alone does not significantly increase risk.[67–74] Other factors apply, most of which are not age related.

Young patients with diverticular disease are more commonly male,[59,66] obese[60,74] and have a higher incidence of right-sided diverticulitis.[69,70] Young patients undergoing operation are frequently misdiagnosed preoperatively[60,68,70] with appendicitis being the most common misdiagnosis.[70] Many recommend that patients less than age 50 have an elective resection after a single episode of acute disease. Recent evidence is mixed.

In some series, young people present with more severe disease at first presentation[61–63,65] but less frequently have a resection at that time. Reasons for this include missed diagnoses and rapid response to therapy. With fewer resections for more complex disease, a higher percentage of young patients return with delayed complications and the appearance of more aggressive disease. Elective resection following the first episode of diverticulitis is thus advised.[61–63]

Others have recommended elective resections at a younger age to avoid the increased morbidity and mortality associated with urgent or emergent surgery in the elderly (0% vs. 34.9%).[71] Some recommendations for elective resection in the young patient are based on cost savings related to definitive surgical management vs. the higher costs of ongoing medical treatment for recurring disease.[66] These types of recommendations assume a high risk of recurrent disease.

There is evidence that diverticular disease in young patients is changing. It is not as rare as in the past[62,72,73] and continues to become more prevalent.[73] And recent evidence suggests there is no increased risk of complications from diverticular disease in the young.[68–73] Based on these findings, resection following a single episode of diverticulitis is not recommended.

Data is difficult to interpret because the presentations of diverticular disease are so varied and most studies are small and retrospective with risks of unrecognized selection bias. However, it does appear that diverticular disease is more common in young patients than generally recognized. Obesity may be a risk factor related to diet. Diets high in fiber are less likely to result in obesity compared to diets associated with diverticular disease.

The issue of male predominance could be a result of missed diagnoses in females. Young females frequently have a gynecologic focus of attention placed on causes of abdominal pain other than diverticular disease. This is further compounded by the general poor recognition of the prevalence of diverticular disease in younger patients.

Current recommendations for resection are based on the predicted risk of developing a serious complication that would lead to emergency surgery with increased morbidity and mortality. To improve management we must become better at predicting who is at risk for recurrent disease. Age alone does not appear to be a reliable factor. The use of CT to identify "severe" or "complex" diverticular disease seems most promising.

In a recent study, the incidence of remote complications was the highest (54% at 5 years) for young patients with severe diverticulitis on CT and the lowest (19% at 5 years) for older patients with mild disease. Young age and severe diverticulitis taken separately were both statistically significant factors for poor outcome ($P=0.007$ and 0.003, respectively), although age was no longer significant after stratification for disease severity on CT ($P=0.07$).[75] Other studies have shown similar risks associated with complex disease on CT.[76,77]

Giant Colonic Diverticulum

Giant diverticula of the colon are rare entities associated with sigmoid diverticular disease. They are generally pseudodiverticula with inflammatory rather than colonic mucosal walls. They usually arise off of the antimesenteric border of the sigmoid colon. The mechanism of formation is unknown but they have been reported to be as large as 30–40 cm[78,79]; 12% occur in patients under the age of 50.

Diagnosis is by plain film of the abdomen which demonstrates a large, solitary, gas-filled cavity. Communication with the colon can be demonstrated with contrast enema. The differential diagnosis includes congenital duplication of the colon, cholecystenteric fistula, colonic volvulus, emphysematous cholecystitis, infected pancreatic pseudocyst, pneumatosis cystoides intestinalis, Meckel's diverticulum, intra-abdominal abscess, giant duodenal diverticulum, dilated intestinal loop, gastric dilatation, tubo-ovarian abscess, and mesenteric cyst.[80]

Most patients will present with vague symptoms of abdominal discomfort or pain and a soft, mobile abdominal mass. A few patients will present with one of the known complications which include perforation, sepsis, intestinal obstruction, or volvulus. The natural history is slow enlargement over time. The treatment of choice is resection of the diverticulum and adjacent colon at time of diagnosis if the patient is symptomatic.

Rectal Diverticula

Rectal diverticula are rare. They are typically true diverticula since they include the muscular layer of the rectum in their wall. They are frequently solitary. Inflammation can generally be managed with antibiotics, rarely surgical resection is required.

Cecal and Right-Sided Diverticulitis

Right-sided diverticular disease is much more common in the Far East than in the west, representing 35–84% of diverticula in that region. Patients present an average of 20 years younger than with sigmoid diverticulitis. Classically, cecal diverticula are described as true diverticula containing all layers of the bowel wall. However, most cecal diverticula actually are false and frequently not solitary.

It is estimated that 13% of patients with cecal diverticulosis develop diverticular inflammation. Cecal diverticulitis can be graded according to the extent of the inflammation. Grade I disease refers to an easily recognizable projecting inflamed cecal diverticulum. Grade II is an inflamed cecal mass. Grade III encompasses a localized abscess or fistula. Grade IV is a free perforation or ruptured abscess with diffuse peritonitis. Cecal diverticulitis is correctly diagnosed preoperatively only 5% of the time. Appendicitis is the preoperative diagnosis in more than two-thirds of cases.[81]

Intraoperative diagnosis is relatively easy with Grade I and to a lesser extent with Grade II disease. Most episodes of cecal diverticulitis presenting with Grade III or Grade IV disease are misdiagnosed intraoperatively as perforated carcinoma.

If a correct diagnosis of uncomplicated cecal diverticulitis can be made preoperatively, then antibiotics and treatment similar to left-sided disease are appropriate. However, this is rare. Intraoperatively, the options for treatment include (1) appendectomy, nonresection of the diverticulum and postoperative antibiotic therapy; (2) appendectomy with diverticulectomy for Grade I and identifiable Grade II disease; or (3) right hemicolectomy is the procedure of choice for not readily identifiable Grade II, Grade III, and Grade IV disease, failed treatment or possible cancer. Appendectomy should always accompany nonresection or diverticulectomy whenever the base of the appendix is not inflamed to avoid confusion at a later date.[81–83]

Diverticular Disease of the Transverse Colon

This is an exceedingly rare condition. Clinical presentation most often mimics appendicitis, cholecystitis or, less frequently, ischemic or Crohn's colitis. It is reported to occur in a younger age group than sigmoid disease and is more common in females. Treatment parallels that of sigmoid diverticulitis; however, resection is more commonly performed since a pre-operative diagnosis is more difficult to make and a carcinoma frequently cannot be ruled out.

Saint's Triad

Saint's triad is a described association of diverticulosis, cholelithiasis and hiatal hernia. Although it has been suggested that the triad occurs in 3–6% of the general population,[82] it is of unknown clinical significance and likely represents the normal concomitant distribution of these common maladies.

Polycystic Kidney Disease

There is a such a high incidence of diverticulosis among patients with autosomal dominant polycystic kidney disease that some consider it an extra-renal manifestation.[84] These patients undergoing renal transplantation are at particularly high risk for devastating infectious complications due to their immunocompromised state. Many transplant centers recommend prophylactic sigmoid resection in those polycystic kidney patients scheduled for transplantation with a documented history of diverticulitis.[84–86]

Treatment of Acute Diverticulitis

Dietary Management

The primary management of asymptomatic diverticular disease is diet. The goal of dietary manipulation is to increase the bulkiness of stool thus increasing lumen size, decreasing transit time, and decreasing intraluminal pressures. This decreases segmentation which has been described as a significant factor in the development of diverticular disease. The ideal amount of fiber is not known; however, the recommended daily amount is 20–30 gm. In general, fiber can be obtained by consuming foods high in fiber or through supplementation with one or more of a large variety of bulk laxatives. Epidemiologic evidence strongly suggests a diet high in fiber can reduce the risk of developing diverticulosis. What is less clear is whether a high fiber diet can prevent diverticulitis and its complications in patients who already have diverticulosis. Recent evidence is building in support of this concept.[87–90]

Medical Management

In the absence of systemic signs and symptoms (high fever, marked leukocytosis, tachycardia, and hypotension), most patients experiencing symptoms of diverticulitis will respond to a regimen of bowel rest and antibiotics as outpatients. Diet is usually restricted to low residue or clear liquids during the acute illness but with resolution of the acute symptoms, a high fiber diet should be instituted. There is no need to restrict the ingestion of seeds or hulls since there is no data to substantiate this practice.

Appropriate antibiotics should be instituted. The most predominant organisms cultured from acute diverticular abscess and peritonitis include the aerobic and facultative bacteria *Escherichia coli* and *Streptococcus* spp. The most frequently isolated anaerobes include *Bacteroides* spp. (*B. fragilis* group), *Peptostreptococcus*, *Clostridium*, and *Fusobacterium* spp.[91]

The use of anticholinergics as adjunctive therapy is based on theoretically reducing pain related to spasm and hypermotility in the sigmoid colon. Efficacy has not been proven.

Signs of more advanced disease including marked leukocytosis, high fever, tachycardia, or hypotension as well as a physical examination demonstrating more advanced intra-abdominal pathology, dictate a need for inpatient management. Patients admitted for inpatient care will usually undergo a baseline CT scan which can confirm the diagnosis, rule out potential alternative diagnoses, and evaluate for complicated disease that would require a change in initial management.[48]

Antibiotics should be administered via an intravenous route. Generally the patient will be placed nil per os (NPO) until there is evidence of clinical improvement making surgical intervention less likely. The diet is then gradually advanced from clear liquids to a low residue diet for a variable period of time before reinstituting a high fiber diet. Symptoms should improve within 24–48 h. Failure to improve requires further diagnostic workup including repeat CT and re-evaluation of the need for surgery.

Surgical Management

The surgical management of acute diverticular disease is replete with varied options that allow for customizing an operation to meet the needs of the individual patient. A thorough knowledge of these options and the indications for each is necessary for the surgeon managing these cases. The goal should always be to manage a complex patient in a way which will maximize the opportunity to avoid an emergency operation in favor of an elective resection.

Surgical options include primary resection with anastomosis with or without proximal diversion, resection with proximal colostomy and oversewing of the rectal remnant (Hartmann's procedure) or mucous fistula (Mikulicz operation), simple diversion with drainage of the affected segment, diversion with oversewing of the perforation site and, rarely, subtotal colectomy. Adjunctive measures include on-table lavage and the option of a laparoscopic approach.

The historical discussion of these options would include the use of a three-stage approach with diversion and drainage followed by a second operation for resection and a third operation for reestablishment of intestinal continuity.

A modification of this approach includes oversewing of a visible site of perforation with an omental patch as a part of the initial operation.[92] Alternatives include a two-stage approach consisting of a Hartmann's or Mikulicz procedure followed by a second operation for re-establishment of intestinal continuity and resection with primary anastomosis, with or without proximal diversion, as a single operation. For the most part, current discussions revolve around the relative merits of a single stage vs. a two-stage approach in acute cases requiring urgent or emergent surgery.[93–95] The three-stage approach is unlikely to be used except in the most extreme cases of medical instability.[96,97]

The following sections will discuss the applications of these approaches to the various presentations of diverticular disease including both chronic and acute forms. Special consideration will be given to the management of intra-abdominal abscesses.

Intra-abdominal Abscess

For a patient found to have an abscess, there is a large volume of clinical evidence supporting the advantages of percutaneous drainage and the conversion of an emergent operation with its attendant increased morbidity and mortality to the relative safety of an elective operation.[48,98] An abscess not responding to medical management should be drained percutaneously or transrectally as appropriate to its location (Figure 22-2).

If drainage cannot be accomplished nonoperatively, or if drainage is performed but fails to resolve systemic signs and symptoms, operation is indicated. Generally, the clinical scenario in this situation would be that of an advanced Hinchey Class II. Although it is possible that intraoperative findings would support a resection with primary anastomosis with or without proximal diversion, it is more likely that a Hartmann's resection will be required.

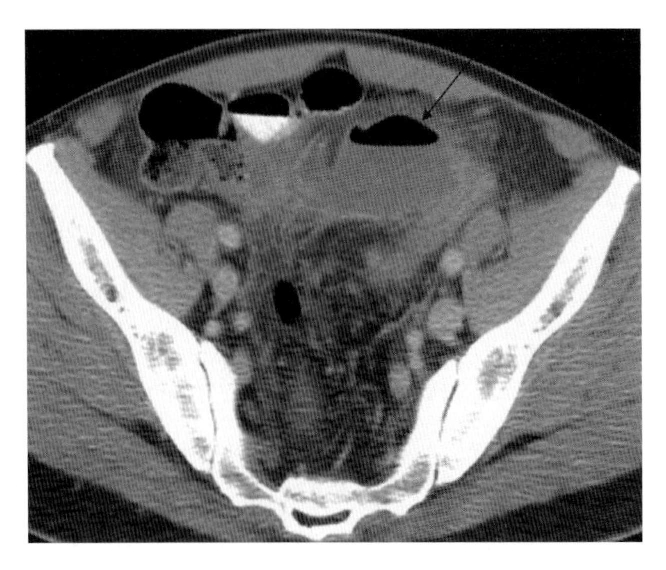

FIGURE 22-2. CT reveals pericolic abscess (Hinchey Stage I).

In a recent study of 511 patients diagnosed with complicated diverticulitis, 99 were diagnosed by CT scan with abscess, and 16 of these underwent percutaneous drainage.[99] Of these patients with continued nonoperative treatment, even after percutaneous drainage a recurrence rate of 42% was noted with an associated increased probability of emergent procedure. Based on these findings it is recommended that all patients with complicated findings undergo at best an elective operation.[99]

This therapy of treating patients with percutaneous drainage and medical management until it was feasible to perform an elective operation has also been evaluated. Salem reviewed all hospitalized patients for the state of Washington and found after evaluating over 25,000 patients that percutaneous drainage was associated with a decrease in emergency operative interventions.

Ricciardi et al.[100] evaluated the nationwide inpatient sample data from 1991 to 2005 analyzing the incidence of complicated diverticulitis admissions. Despite a significant decline in surgical treatment for diverticulitis during this time period, there was no change in the proportion of patients discharged with complicated diverticulitis.

Indications for Surgery for Acute Disease

The indications for surgery of acute disease include (1) failure of phlegmon or abscess to respond to nonoperative management with clinical deterioration (increasing fever, leukocytosis, tachycardia, hypotension, signs of sepsis, or a worsening physical examination), (2) free perforation with peritonitis, and (3) obstruction. Perforation without peritonitis may not require operation (Figure 22-3).

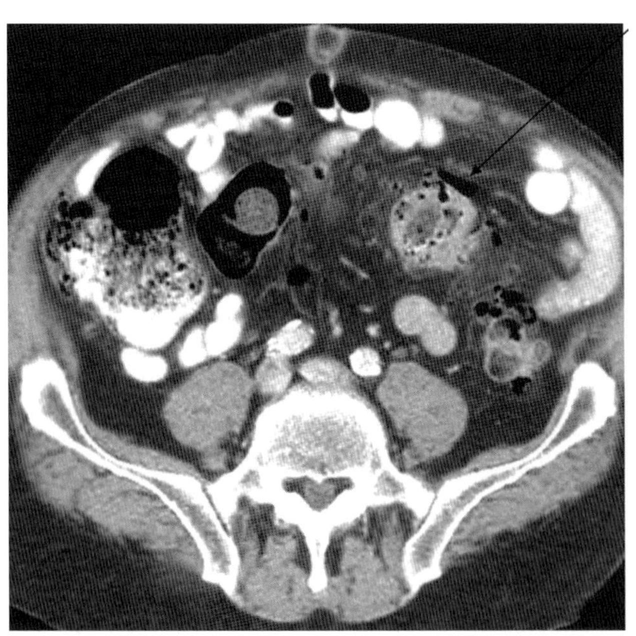

FIGURE 22-3. 3-Diverticulitis with localized perforation. The patient was treated with antibiotics and improved without the need for emergency surgery.

Surgical Procedures

For acute disease, the choice of operation is highly dependent upon the degree of inflammatory response encountered at the time of operation. Since most acute diseases can be managed nonoperatively (including the percutaneous drainage of most abscesses), the fact that an operation has become necessary suggests rather advanced pathology and the need to be conservative. In general, most Hinchey Class I and some Class II disease can be managed with a one-stage procedure (resection and anastomosis) if the patient is stable, the extent of contamination is limited and adequate bowel preparation is possible[93,101] recognizing, however, the necessity of mechanical bowel preparation in colon resections has been questioned.[102] Proximal diversion may be necessary. Most cases of Hinchey Class III and IV disease will require a two-stage approach. Some recent evidence suggests a possible role for resection with primary anastomosis and proximal diversion in highly selected cases without gross fecal contamination.[100–106]

In a recent review by Salem and Flum,[106] who reviewed 98 articles on the outcome of complicated diverticulitis based on the type of operation performed, 1,051 patients were identified who had a Hartmann procedure from 54 studies, and 569 patients who had a primary anastamosis from 50 studies. Of the 569 cases, 16% had covering stomas and 10% underwent on-table lavage. The mortality rates were higher in the Hartmann group, 19.6% vs. 9.9% for primary anastamosis. Anastomotic leak rate ranged from 6.3 to 19.3% in patients undergoing a primary anastamosis. When primary anastomosis was performed with a covering stoma, the lowest rate of leak rate (6.3%) and the lowest wound infection rate (4%) was demonstrated. Wound infections were also more frequently seen in the Hartman group 24.2% vs. 9.6%. Hartmann patients also required a larger second operation than those who had a primary anastamosis with or without a covering stoma. The conclusion was the primary anastomosis is no worse than a Hartmann and has several advantages including higher restoration of continuity rate, less hospitalization, and fewer infectious complications (Table 22-4).

A major disadvantage of a two-stage procedure is that 35–45% of patients never have their colostomy closed.[103] However, in patients with preexisting incontinence, a Hartman's pouch should be the procedure of choice. Women are more likely than men to not have closure.[103,104] For patients who do not undergo closure of their stoma, it is critical that their rectal stump undergo scheduled surveillance for neoplasia as the remaining rectum maintains at the same risk for neoplasia as other patients of equal age.[105]

Hartmann Reversal

Reversal of a Hartmann's colostomy carries significant risks that must be entertained when considering this operation for patients who will desire continuity in the future. Failure to reverse the colostomy has been reported in 20–50% [106] of patients and leak rates on reversal range from 2 to 30%.[106,107] Mortality has been reported anywhere from 0 to 10% and wound infection rates range from 12 to 50%.

TABLE 22-4. Outcomes of primary anastomosis and Hartmann's procedure

	Patients	Mortality (%)	Wound infection (%)	Leaks (%)
Hartmann procedure	1,051	18.8	24.2	NA
Primary anastomosis	295	8.1	16.4	19.3
Primary anastamosis with stoma	<109	9.2	4	9.6

Modified from: Salem L, Flum DR. Primary anastomosis or Hartmann's procedure for patients with diverticular peritonitis. A systemic review. Dis Colon Rectum. 2004;47:1953–64.[106]

Maggard et al.[108] reviewed 1,176 patients who had a Hartmann's procedure for diverticular disease, only 65% had a reversal at a mean of 143 days. Younger men were more likely to have their ostomy reversed as opposed to older patients and women. Patients with more comorbidities also had fewer reversals. When evaluating all patients, 35% never had their ostomy reversed during the 4-year study. The complication rate following Hartmann reversal was 57.4%, including infection (9.1%), aspiration pneumonia (8.7%), pulmonary edema (6%), and acute renal failure (4.9%).[108]

Complications from Surgical Resection

Predictors of complications after resection for diverticular disease include advanced age (greater than 70–75 years), two or more co-morbid conditions, obstipation at initial examination, the use of steroids, sepsis, and obesity.[96,109,110] Complications of resection include anastomotic leak and hemorrhage.[111] The prevalence of leak from a low intraperitoneal anastomosis is generally considered to be between 2 and 5%.[112] Anastomotic leaks may lead to localized abscess, stricture, peritonitis and sepsis. The diagnosis is dependent upon a high index of suspicion on the part of the surgeon and quick response to any unusual signs of sepsis. Fever, vague abdominal pain, diarrhea, obstruction and sepsis all should raise the question of a leak. The diagnosis is most commonly confirmed by water soluble contrast enema or by CT scan with intravenous, oral and rectal contrast.

An anastomotic leak without an abscess can usually be managed with intravenous antibiotics and response assessed. Failure to respond to treatment within 24–48 h or initial severe sepsis or peritonitis requires exploration with resection of the anastomosis and proximal diversion. Repair of the anastomosis with proximal diversion is usually unsatisfactory because of the high risk for recurrent leak in this inflammatory setting. An exception would be a "pin-hole" leak with limited inflammatory response which may be managed with repair, colonic lavage, and proximal diversion.

An anastomotic leak resulting in an abscess can generally be managed with percutaneous or transrectal drainage. Again, failure to respond will require laparotomy, take down of the anastomosis and proximal diversion.

A colocutaneous fistula related to a diverticular resection will usually respond to nonoperative measures. Provided there is no distal obstruction, no foreign body, and no underlying Crohn's disease, spontaneous closure should be anticipated. Important steps to facilitate closure of colocutaneous fistulas include draining any undrained abscess; maximizing nutrition; and delivering appropriate wound care, which may require the help of enterostomal therapy nurses.

Strictures are an unusual complication related to diverticular resection, unless the underlying process is Crohn's disease. In the rare instance when stricture does occur, the most likely etiologies include ischemia or localized sepsis due to confined leak. Such strictures can most commonly be managed by dilatation with a balloon or rigid proctoscopy but occasionally will require a formal resection with recreation of anastomosis.

Ureteral injuries are reported to occur in 1–10% of abdominal surgeries.[112] Early identification of any injury is the key to preventing significant morbidity. Although ureteral stents have not been shown to decrease the rate of injury, they do improve intraoperative identification of the ureters and the early identification of any ureteral injury.[113] The decision to place ureteral stents prior to operation should be a function of clinical suspicion and the extent of inflammation on CT scan.

General postoperative complications related to colon and rectal surgery and specifics related to the recognition and management of the specific complications mentioned above are discussed more thoroughly in Chap. 10.

Recurrence After Resection

Recurrence of diverticulitis or its symptoms following resection has been reported in 3–13% of elective cases.[114] Factors contributing to recurrence of diverticulitis include shorter resection length and anastomosis to sigmoid colon rather than to rectum.[114,115] Thaler et al.[116] demonstrated that the level of the anastomosis is the only significant determinant of recurrence after laparoscopic resection for diverticular disease.

Treatment of Chronic and Recurrent Diverticulitis

Most patients who develop a first episode of symptomatic diverticulitis have been asymptomatic until 1 month prior to presentation. Most will respond to bowel rest and antibiotics as an outpatient. It is difficult to reliably estimate how many outpatients will have recurrence because outpatient data is generally not reflective of a primary care population. However, it has been reported that up to 10% of patients with a first episode who have responded to outpatient management will develop recurrent or persistent symptoms which will require hospitalization.[59]

Data is more readily available on recurrence for patients who were initially treated as inpatients. But our understanding of the natural history continues to evolve as antibiotics become more effective and inpatient status reflects increasingly severe disease. This makes historical data regarding these issues of less value. Presently, inpatients might be expected to be at a greater risk for recurrence. In fact, 20% or more of these patients will develop a recurrence.[59] Some, but not all, will require a second hospitalization. The interval between acute events may be prolonged (median 5 years).[117] Following a second hospital admission, up to 70% will continue with symptoms and over half of those that require another admission will do so within 1 year. The more complicated the attack, the higher the risk of recurrence.[4,15,118–121]

It has been estimated that up to 1% of all patients with diverticulosis will eventually require operative intervention.[9] However, with an increasing denominator in the number of individuals affected with diverticulosis and better antibiotics for managing infections, this estimate may now be too high.

The risk of recurrence following an attack of uncomplicated diverticulitis has been shown to be quite low. The range of recurrence following an attack is 1.4–18%.[122–124] It has been estimated that only 1 in 2,000 patient/years of follow-up will require an urgent Hartmann's procedure after resolution of diverticulitis.[125] In the 1950s, it was reported that morbidity and mortality were higher with recurrent attacks of acute inflammation, and early interval resection was a means of avoiding those problems.[75,126–128] Recent studies have shown repeatedly that prophylactic operation to prevent the need of a colostomy is unfounded. In patients with uncomplicated diverticulitis, Chautems et al.[75] followed 118 patients after a first uncomplicated attack of diverticulitis for 9.5 years. Of these patients, 71% had no recurrent episodes and of those who did, none required emergent surgery. More recently, Anaya and Flum[129] with a large population-based study of over 20,000 patients admitted with nonoperatively managed diverticulitis, found that only 5.5% progressed to require an emergent colectomy or colostomy. Younger patients in this study were found to be at higher risk than their older counterparts.[129]

Anaya and Flum[129] published a review of 25,058 patients hospitalized for an initial episode of diverticulitis. Of the 20,136 patients treated nonoperatively, 19% developed a recurrence, with those less than 50 years of age having a slightly higher incidence (27% vs. 17% $P<0.001$). These numbers are significantly lower than previous estimations of recurrence rates greater than 30%.

Very few patients presenting and requiring an emergent operation had been previously diagnosed with diverticulitis. An estimated 75–96% of patients presenting with peritonitis requiring an emergent operation had never been diagnosed with diverticulitis. This supports the notion that operating to prevent complications of diverticulitis is ineffective at achieving the goal.[8,130–132] Patients with multiple, recurrent episodes of acute diverticulitis documented by CT scan should be considered for resection. Traditional teaching with respect to diverticulitis dictated elective sigmoid resection for patients suffering more than one episode of uncomplicated diverticulitis. In fact, most of the consensus data on elective resection after two documented episodes comes from literature that was published prior to the use of CT scanning and modern day antibiotic therapy. Because of these and other studies, the American Society of Colon and Rectal Surgeons (ASCRS) revised its previous recommendations for resection of diverticular disease. The 2006 revised practice parameters now reads as follows: "The decision to recommend surgery should be influenced by the age and medical condition of the patient, the frequency and severity of the attacks, and whether there are persistent symptoms after the acute episode."[133]

Recent data has suggested that the recommendation for resection following two episodes of diverticulitis treated as an inpatient may result in too many patients undergoing resection, thereby increasing the total cost of health care. Performing resection after the third episode of diverticulitis results in significant cost savings.[134] Performing resection following four documented episodes rather than after two results in fewer deaths, fewer colostomies, and an additional cost savings of over $5,000 per patient in those less than 50 years of age.[135] Others question the role of elective resection at all due to the high success rate of nonoperative management and the large percentage of patients presenting with urgent surgical disease that have no previous history of diverticulitis.[130,136]

The ultimate goal is to perform an operation electively rather than as an emergency. This requires correctly predicting those patients who are most likely to have serious complications as a result of their disease. CT evidence of complicated or "severe" disease has shown some promise in predicting risk. The risk of complications within 5 years of a first attack of diverticulitis exceeds 50% if CT shows severe diverticulitis at the initial episode.[75] Mild findings on CT can be defined as localized thickening of colonic wall and inflammation of pericolic fat. Severe findings are defined as abscess and/or extraluminal air and/or extraluminal gastrograffin. Abscess, extraluminal air, and extraluminal gastrograffin have been associated with an increased risk of poor outcome from medical management regardless of age.[76,77]

Another approach is to identify specific groups of patients (other than age) who are at increased risk. Immunocompromised patients are at particular risk for a poor outcome.[35] The risk is due to a higher incidence of perforation and more severe inflammatory complications when perforation does occur.

Surgical Procedures

Patients undergoing resection for chronic disease will almost always be candidates for single stage resection with primary anastomosis. This includes patients returning for closure of a colostomy following initial diversion and drainage, diversion with oversewing of perforation or diversion with resection via either Hartmann's or a Mikulicz procedure.

Techniques for Appropriate Resection

The practice parameters of the ASCRS set out several general recommendations regarding resection of diverticular disease. For elective resections, all thickened, diseased colon but not necessarily the entire proximal diverticula-bearing colon should be removed. It may be acceptable to retain proximal diverticular colon as long as the remaining bowel is not hypertrophied. All of the sigmoid colon should be removed. When anastomosis is elected it should be made to normal rectum and must be free of tension and well vascularized.[133] The single most important predictor of recurrence following sigmoid resection for uncomplicated diverticulitis is an anastomosis to the sigmoid colon rather than to the rectum.[137] In urgent or emergent cases, resection and diversion are generally required. In selected cases where sepsis can be removed, definitive resection with anastomosis (with or without proximal stoma) may be appropriate. On-table colonic lavage may be a useful adjunct to resection and anastomosis.[116]

Laparoscopic Surgery

The role of laparoscopy in the management of diverticular disease is evolving. Recent data suggest decreased overall costs associated with laparoscopic resections when compared to open resections.[137,138] Patients who are converted from laparoscopic to open procedures are a concern with regard to added costs but conversion rates are below 20%,[137–142] predictable[141,143], and thus probably avoidable in many instances.[140] Higher conversion rates are associated with more complex disease.[144] Recurrence rates match those for open procedures.[140,143,144] Laparoscopic resection results in a shorter length of stay[137,138] and fewer complications.[138] Hand-assisted laparoscopic colectomy has also been compared against straight laparoscopic colectomy and has been found to be equivalent in patient outcomes.[145,146] Marcello et al.[147] in a multicenter prospective randomized trial found the benefit of hand-assisted laparoscopic sigmoid resection compared to laparoscopic resection includes shorter operating time with similar length of hospital stay (Table 22-5).[147]

TABLE 22-5. Results of a multicenter prospective randomized trial of hand-assisted laparoscopic sigmoid resection compared to laparoscopic resection in diverticular disease

	HA (n=33)	LAP (n=33)	P value
Operative time (min)	175±58	208±55	0.021
Estimated blood loss (mL)	211±160	198±175	0.074
Ureteral stents	3	4	0.99
Incision size (cm)	8.2±1.5	6.1±2.1	<0.01
Passage flatus (days)	2.7±1.6	2.9±1	0.64
Length of stay (days)	5.7±3.4	5.2±2.6	0.55

HA hand-assisted colectomy, *LAP* straight laparoscopic colectomy. Data are means±standard deviations.

Adapted from Marcello PW, Fleshman JW, Milsom JW. Hand-assisted laparoscopic vs. laparoscopic colorectal surgery: a multicenter, prospective, randomized trial. Dis Colon Rectum. 2008;51:818–28.[147]

Despite the recent eruption of literature and discussion of laparoscopic colectomies, only 5–10% of all colectomies are currently performed using a laparoscopic technique.[145] As data continues to accumulate, it appears that laparoscopic surgery is set to play a significant role in the management of diverticular disease.

A therapy unique to laparoscopic surgery is the use of laparoscopic lavage. A new approach has been described by Myers et al.[148] from Ireland as an alternative to resection and Hartman's pouch in perforated diverticular disease. They describe using laparoscopic peritoneal lavage for generalized peritonitis for perforated diverticulitis in 100 patients prospectively. They converted 8 patients to a Hartmann's procedure who had feculent peritonitis, the remaining 92 were followed with only a 4% morbidity and 3% mortality. Only two patients required additional procedures for pelvic abscesses and two patients had recurrent diverticulitis, one at 12 months and the other at 84 months postprocedure. Additional studies are needed to determine what role this management option may play in acute diverticular disease.

Complications of Diverticular Disease

Bleeding

Bleeding is not recognized as a feature of diverticulitis. Bleeding related to diverticulosis is discussed in Chap. 24.

Perforation

Perforation can occur at two levels. If an abscess forms and then ruptures, purulent peritonitis is the result. If a large perforation occurs through the diverticulum directly into the peritoneum, fecal peritonitis is the result. Mixed fecal and purulent peritonitis may result from the rupture of an abscess which has an ongoing communication with the bowel lumen and then perforates. Clinically, the presentation is that of either abrupt onset of abdominal pain for a free perforation or an abrupt exacerbation of progressive localized pain in the case of a ruptured abscess. A pneumoperitoneum is seen on abdominal films or CT scan. Rapid progression to diffuse abdominal pain and rigidity can be expected.

Abscess

An abscess most commonly results from the mechanism described above. Small abscesses less than 1 cm in diameter will frequently resolve with antibiotic therapy. Larger abscesses may require drainage. CT-guided percutaneous drainage is the preferred approach when possible as it can convert the high risks of an urgent operation to a much safer elective operation.

Fistula

The incidence of fistulization reported in the literature ranges from 5 to 33% depending largely upon the type of referral center making the report.[47] Colovesical fistula is the most common fistula associated with diverticular disease and diverticular disease is the most common cause of colovesical fistula (Figure 22-4A and B). Other relatively common fistulas associated with diverticular disease include colocutaneous, colovaginal, and coloenteric. Most patients who develop a colovaginal fistula have had a previous

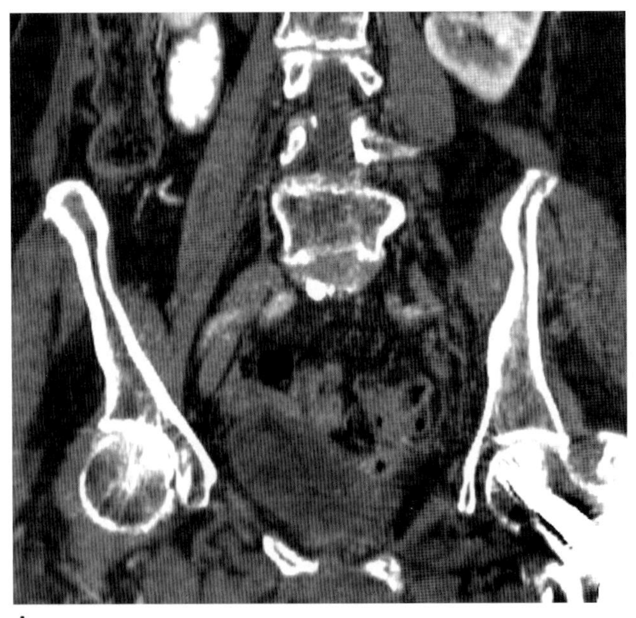
A

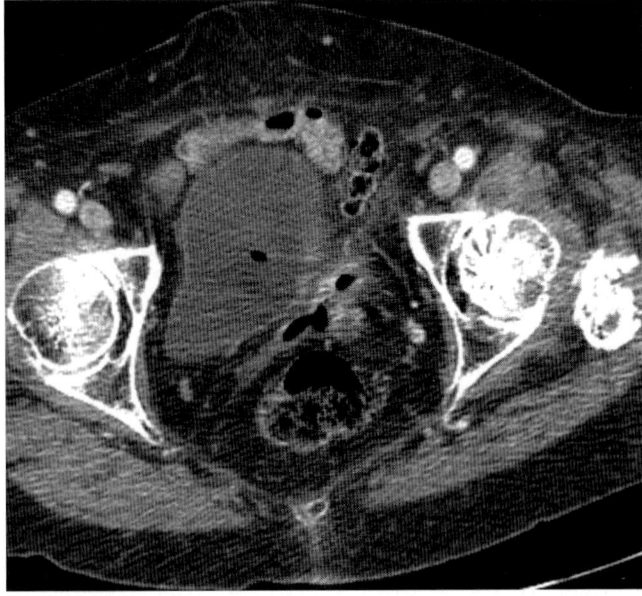
B

FIGURE 22-4. **A/B** CT scan reveals air in the bladder consistent with a colovesical fistula.

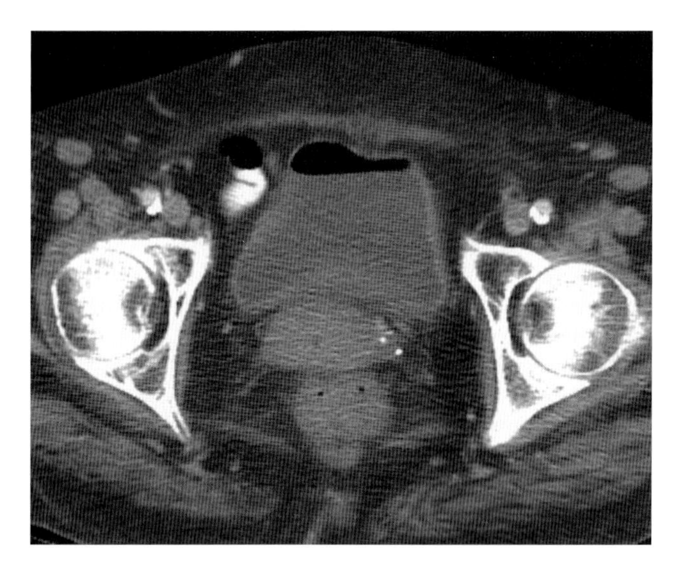

FIGURE 22-5. Colovaginal fistula occur almost exclusively in patient who have undergone prior hysterectomy.

hysterectomy (Figure 22-5). Other fistulas have rarely been described and include colocolic, ureterocolic, colouterine, colosaphingeal, coloperineal, sigmoido-appendiceal, colovenous, and even fistulas to the thigh (a variant of a colocutaneous fistula).

The diagnosis of diverticular fistula is generally clinical. Many fistulas will not be identifiable by imaging studies. Thus, excess efforts should not be undertaken to try to radiographically demonstrate a fistula. The primary aim of a diagnostic workup is not to see the fistula but to determine the etiology (diverticulitis, cancer, IBD, etc.) so that appropriate therapy can be initiated. The general principle of management is resection of the colon, usually with primary anastomosis, with varying treatment for the organ involved. For the bladder, simple drainage of the bladder for 7 days is advised. No treatment of the vagina is required in most circumstances. Cutaneous fistulas will usually require cutaneous closure by delay or secondary intention. Enteric fistulas require closure or resection of the involved small bowel or colon. Ureteral drainage for fistulas to the ureter, observation or hysterectomy for uterine fistulas, salpingo-oophorectomy for fistulas to the fallopian tubes, and appendectomy for appendiceal fistulas are the most common treatments for uncomplicated fistulas of the other named varieties. If there is any question of cancer, an en-bloc resection of a portion of the involved organ must accompany the resection.

Occasionally, nonoperative management is appropriate when symptoms are minor or when the patient is at otherwise too great a risk for other health reasons. The use of long-term suppressive antibiotic therapy in selected patients with colovesical fistula has been shown to eliminate symptoms and prevent complications related to the fistula until death from other causes.[149]

Stricture

The development of a phlegmon with repeated attacks of acute disease or long-term persistent disease may result in a stricture. Although a relatively uncommon complication, patients will present with constipation, abdominal pain, and bloating. It is necessary to rule out carcinoma as the true cause of the stricture. Colonoscopy is the first choice to help make this distinction; however, it is not uncommon for associated bowel angulation and fixation to prevent endoscopic visualization. Contrast studies may assist in the evaluation in such instances, but resection may be necessary to make a diagnosis.

Obstruction

On rare occasions complete obstruction may occur. If this is due to diverticular disease, most patients will respond to initial medical management allowing for an elective resection at a later date. Persistence of an obstruction may require a Hartmann's procedure or primary anastomosis with proximal diversion for management. The successful use of colonic stents to relieve obstruction secondary to diverticulitis has been described. [150,151] In this setting, the colonic stent is used as a bridge to surgery with later elective resection. However, the use of stents in benign disease is not an indicated use. There is a high incidence of complications leading to emergency surgery for removal of the stent and management of complications.[152]

Ureteral Obstruction

The ureter is infrequently involved with diverticular disease. When involved, it is most frequently the left ureter. Rarely, diverticular disease has been reported as fistulizing to the ureter. A stricture may occur but compression is more common. This can result from retroperitoneal fibrosis secondary to diverticular inflammation. Most commonly this resolves as the underlying diverticular disease process resolves, although occasionally ureterolysis has been advised.[153]

Phlegmon

A phlegmon represents an inflammatory mass without a surrounding central abscess. A phlegmon can significantly complicate the technical aspects of surgical resection. Many phlegmons will resolve with antibiotic therapy. If resection is planned due to recurrent episodes of disease, it is best to treat the acute phlegmon to resolution if possible, prior to resection. Occasionally, operation may become necessary in the face of an acute phlegmon. This situation may be the source of some descriptions of "malignant" diverticulitis as earlier described.

References

1. Almy TP, Howell DA. Diverticula of the colon. N Engl J Med. 1980;302:324–31.
2. Rankin FW, Brown PW. Diverticulitis of the colon. Surg Gynecol Obstet. 1930;50:836–47.
3. Heller SN, Hackler LR. Changes in the crude fiber content of the American diet. Am J Clin Nutr. 1978;31:1510–4.
4. Parks TG. Natural history of diverticular disease of the colon. Clin Gastroenterol. 1975;4:53–69.
5. Colcock BF. Diverticular disease of the colon. Philadelphia: WB Saunders; 1971.
6. Schoetz Jr DJ. Diverticular disease of the colon: a century-old problem. Dis Colon Rectum. 1999;42:703–9.
7. Corman ML. Colon and rectal surgery. 5th ed. Philadelphia: Lippincott Williams & Wilkins; 2005.
8. Somasekar K, Foster ME, Haray PN. The natural history of diverticular disease: is there a role for elective colectomy? J R Coll Surg Edinb. 2002;47:481–4.
9. Roberts PL, Veidenheimer MC. Current management of diverticulitis. Adv Surg. 1994;27:189–208.
10. U.S. Census Bureau. 2010. http://www.census.gov. Accessed 21 July 2010.
11. Morris CR, Harvey IM, Stebbings WS, et al. Epidemiology of perforated colonic diverticular disease. Postgrad Med J. 2002;78:654–8.
12. Painter NS, Truelove SC, Ardran GM, et al. Segmentation and the localization of intraluminal pressures in the human colon, with special reference to the pathogenesis of colonic diverticula. Gastroenterology. 1965;49:169–77.
13. Mann CV. Problems in diverticular disease. Proctology. 1979;1:20–5.
14. Ryan P. Two kinds of diverticular disease. Ann R Coll Surg Engl. 1991;73:73–9.
15. Floch MH, Bina I. The natural history of diverticulitis: fact and theory. J Clin Gastroenterol. 2004;38(Suppl):S2–7.
16. Hinchey EJ, Schaal PG, Richards GK. Treatment of perforated diverticular disease of the colon. Adv Surg. 1978;12: 85–109.
17. Colecchia A, Sandri L, Capodicasa S, et al. Diverticular disease of the colon: new perspectives in symptom development and treatment. World J Gastroenterol. 2003;9:1385–9.
18. Huizinga JD, Waterfall WE, Stern HS. Abnormal response to cholinergic stimulation in the circular muscle layer of the human colon in diverticular disease. Scand J Gastroenterol. 1999;34:683–8.
19. Maselli MA, Piepoli AL, Guerra V, et al. Colonic smooth muscle responses in patients with diverticular disease of the colon: effect of the NK2 receptor antagonist SR48968. Dig Liver Dis. 2004;36:348–54.
20. Golder M, Burleigh DE, Belai A, et al. Smooth muscle cholinergic denervation hypersensitivity in diverticular disease. Lancet. 2003;361:1945–51.
21. Tomita R, Fujisaki S, Tanjoh K, et al. Role of nitric oxide in the left-sided colon of patients with diverticular disease. Hepatogastroenterology. 2000;47:692–6.
22. Aldoori WH, Giovannucci EL, Rimm EB, et al. A prospective study of diet and the risk of symptomatic diverticular disease in men. Am J Clin Nutr. 1994;60:757–64.
23. Manousos O, Day NE, Tzonou A, et al. Diet and other factors in the aetiology of diverticulosis: an epidemiological study in Greece. Gut. 1985;26:544–9.
24. Cummings JH, Stephen AM. The role of dietary fibre in the human colon. Can Med Assoc J. 1980;123:1109–14.
25. Edwards C. Physiology of the colorectal barrier. Adv Drug Deliv Rev. 1996;28:173–90.
26. Anonymous. Dietary fibre: importance of function as well as amount [editorial]. Lancet. 1992;340:1133–4.
27. Mariadason JM, Catto-Smith A, Gibson PR. Modulation of distal colonic epithelial barrier function by dietary fibre in normal rats. Gut. 1999;44:394–9.
28. Strate LL, Liu YL, Syngal S, et al. Nut, corn and popcorn consumption and incidence of diverticular disease. JAMA. 2008;300(8):407–14.
29. Hirose Y, Sugie S, Yoshimi N, et al. Induction of apoptosis in colonic epithelium treated with 2-amino-1-methyl-6-phenylimidazo[4, 5-b]pyridine (PhIP) and its modulation by a P4501A2 inducer, beta-naphthoflavone, in male F344 rats. Cancer Lett. 1998;123:167–72.
30. Sesink AL, Termont DS, Kleibeuker JH, et al. Red meat and colon cancer: the cytotoxic and hyperproliferative effects of dietary heme. Cancer Res. 1999;59:5704–9.
31. McConnell EJ, Tessier DJ, Wolff BG. Population-based incidence of complicated diverticular disease of the sigmoid colon based on gender and age. Dis Colon Rectum. 2003;46: 1110–4.
32. Hart AR, Kennedy HJ, Stebbings WS, et al. How frequently do large bowel diverticula perforate? An incidence and cross-sectional study. Eur J Gastroenterol Hepatol. 2000;12:661–5.
33. Schwartz HA. Lower gastrointestinal side effects of nonsteroidal anti-inflammatory drugs. J Rheumatol. 1981;8:952–4.
34. Day TK. Intestinal perforation associated with osmotic slow release indomethacin capsules. BMJ. 1983;287:1671–2.
35. Tyau ES, Prystowsky JB, Joehl RJ, et al. Acute diverticulitis. A complicated problem in the immunocompromised patient. Arch Surg. 1991;126:855–8.
36. Painter NS, Truelove SC. The intraluminal pressure patterns in diverticulosis of the colon. Part II: the effect of morphine. Gut. 1964;5:207–13.
37. Papagrigoriadis S, Macey L, Bourantas N, et al. Smoking may be associated with complications in diverticular disease. Br J Surg. 1999;86:923–6.
38. Aldoori WH, Giovannucci EL, Rimm EB, et al. A prospective study of alcohol, smoking, caffeine, and the risk of symptomatic diverticular disease in men. Ann Epidemiol. 1995;5:221–8.
39. Tonnesen H, Engholm G, Moller H. Association between alcoholism and diverticulitis. Br J Surg. 1999;86:1067–8.
40. Morganstern L, Weiner R, Michel SL. "Malignant" diverticulitis. A clinical entity. Arch Surg. 1979;114:1112–26.
41. Killingback M. Surgical treatment of diverticulitis. In: Fazio VW, Church JM, Delaney CP, editors. Current therapy in colon and rectal surgery. 2nd ed. Philadelphia: Elsevier/Mosby; 2005. p. 284–95.
42. Breen RE, Corman ML, Robertson WG, et al. Are we really operating on diverticulitis? Dis Colon Rectum. 1986;29:174.
43. Thorn M, Graf W, Stefansson T, Pahlman L. Clinical and functional results after elective colonic resection in 75 consecutive patients with diverticular disease. Am J Surg. 2002;183:7–11.

44. Horgan AF, McConnell EJ, Wolff BG, et al. Atypical diverticular disease: surgical results. Dis Colon Rectum. 2001;44:1315–8.
45. Hughes ESR, Cuthbertson AM, Carden ABG. The surgical management of acute diverticulitis. Med J Aust. 1963; 1:780–2.
46. Polk HC, Tuckson WB, Miller FB. The atypical presentations of diverticulitis. In: Welch JP, Cohen JL, Sardella WV, Vignati PV, editors. Diverticular disease, management of the difficult surgical case. Baltimore: Williams and Wilkins; 1998. p. 384–93.
47. Gordon PH. Diverticular disease of the colon. In: Gordon PH, Nivatvongs S, editors. Principles and practice of surgery for the colon, rectum and anus. 2nd ed. St. Louis: Quality Medical Publishing; 1999. p. 975–1043.
48. Hachigian MP, Honickman S, Eisenstat TE, et al. Computed tomography in the initial management of acute left-sided diverticulitis. Dis Colon Rectum. 1992;35:1123–9.
49. Schreyer AG, Furst A, Agha A, et al. Magnetic resonance imaging based colonography for diagnosis and assessment of diverticulosis and diverticulitis. Int J Colorectal Dis. 2004;19:474–80.
50. Hollerweger A, Rettenbacher T, Macheiner P, et al. Sigmoid diverticulitis: value of transrectal sonography in addition to transabdominal sonography. AJR Am J Roentgenol. 2000;175:1155–60.
51. Sakhnini E, Lahat A, Melzer E, et al. Early colonoscopy in patients with acute diverticulitis: results of a prospective pilot study. Endoscopy. 2004;36:504–7.
52. Ghorai S, Ulbright TM, Rex DK. Endoscopic findings of diverticular inflammation in colonoscopy patients without clinical acute diverticulitis: prevalence and endoscopic spectrum. Am J Gastroenterol. 2003;98:802–6.
53. Cohn KH, Weimar JA, Fani K, et al. Adenocarcinoma arising within a colonic diverticulum: report of two cases and review of the literature. Surgery. 1993;113:223–6.
54. Stefansson T, Ekbom A, Sparen P, et al. Association between sigmoid diverticulitis and left-sided colon cancer: a nested, population-based, case control study. Scand J Gastroenterol. 2004;39:743–7.
55. Stefansson T, Ekbom A, Sparen P, et al. Increased risk of left sided colon cancer in patients with diverticular disease. Gut. 1993;34:499–502.
56. Stefansson T, Ekbom A, Sparen P, et al. Cancers among patients diagnosed as having diverticular disease of the colon. Eur J Surg. 1995;161:755–60.
57. Berman IR, Corman ML, Coller JA, et al. Late-onset Crohn's disease in patients with colonic diverticulitis. Dis Colon Rectum. 1979;22:524.
58. Etzioni DA, Mack TM, Beart Jr RW, Kaiser AM. Diverticulitis in the United States: 1998–2005: changing patterns of disease and treatment. Ann Surg. 2009;249(2):210–7.
59. Makela J, Vuolio S, Kiviniemi H, et al. Natural history of diverticular disease: when to operate? Dis Colon Rectum. 1998;41:1523–8.
60. Schauer PR, Ramos R, Ghiatas AA, et al. Virulent diverticular disease in young obese men. Am J Surg. 1992;164:443–6.
61. Ambrosetti P, Robert JH, Witzig JA, et al. Acute left colonic diverticulitis: a prospective analysis of 226 consecutive cases. Surgery. 1994;115:546–50.
62. Ambrosetti P, Robert JH, Witzig JA, et al. Acute left colonic diverticulitis in young patients. J Am Coll Surg. 1994;179: 156–60.
63. Anderson DN, Driver CP, Davidson AI, et al. Diverticular disease in patients under 50 years of age. J R Coll Surg Edinb. 1997;42:102–4.
64. Nelson RS, Velasco AF. Management of diverticulitis in younger patients. Dis Colon Rectum. 2006;49:1341–5.
65. Minardi Jr AJ, Johnson LW, Sehon JK, et al. Diverticulitis in the young patient. Am Surg. 2001;67:458–61.
66. Cunningham MA, Davis JW, Kaups KL. Medical versus surgical management of diverticulitis in patients under age 40. Am J Surg. 1997;174:733–5.
67. Acosta JA, Grebenc ML, Doberneck RC, et al. Colonic diverticular disease in patients 40 years old or younger. Am Surg. 1992;58:605–7.
68. Schweitzer J, Casillas RA, Collins JC. Acute diverticulitis in the young adult is not "virulent". Am Surg. 2002;68:1044–7.
69. Reisman Y, Ziv Y, Kravrovitc D, et al. Diverticulitis: the effect of age and location on the course of disease. Int J Colorectal Dis. 1999;14:250–4.
70. Spivak H, Weinrauch S, Harvey JC, et al. Acute colonic diverticulitis in the young. Dis Colon Rectum. 1997;40:570–4.
71. Biondo S, Pares D, Marti Rague J, et al. Acute colonic diverticulitis in patients under 50 years of age. Br J Surg. 2002;89: 1137–41.
72. Guzzo J, Hyman N. Diverticulitis in young patients: is resection after a single attack always warranted? Dis Colon Rectum. 2004;47:1187–90.
73. West SD, Robinson EK, Delu AN, et al. Diverticulitis in the younger patient. Am J Surg. 2003;186:743–6.
74. Vignati PV, Welch JP, Cohen JL. Long-term management of diverticulitis in young patients. Dis Colon Rectum. 1995;38:627–9.
75. Chautems RC, Ambrosetti P, Ludwig A, et al. Long-term follow-up after first acute episode of sigmoid diverticulitis: is surgery mandatory?: a prospective study of 118 patients. Dis Colon Rectum. 2002;45:962–6.
76. Poletti PA, Platon A, Rutschmann O, et al. Acute left colonic diverticulitis: can CT findings be used to predict recurrence? AJR Am J Roentgenol. 2004;182:1159–65.
77. Ambrosetti P, Robert J, Witzig JA, et al. Prognostic factors from computed tomography in acute left colonic diverticulitis. Br J Surg. 1992;79:117–9.
78. Scerpella PR, Bodensteiner JA. Giant sigmoid diverticula. Report of two cases. Arch Surg. 1989;134:1244–6.
79. Mainzer F, Minagi H. Giant sigmoid diverticulum. Am J Roentgenol. 1971;113:352–3.
80. de Oliveira NC, Welch JP. Giant diverticula of the colon. In: Welch JP, Cohen JL, Sardella WV, Vignati PV, editors. Diverticular disease, management of the difficult surgical case. Baltimore: Williams and Wilkins; 1998. p. 410–8.
81. Lo CY, Chu KW. Acute diverticulitis of the right colon. Am J Surg. 1996;171:244–6.
82. Komuta K, Yamanaka S, Okada K, et al. Toward therapeutic guidelines for patients with acute right colonic diverticulitis. Am J Surg. 2004;187:233–7.
83. Thorson AG, Ternent CA. Cecal diverticulitis. In: Welch JP, Cohen JL, Sardella WV, Vignati PV, editors. Diverticular

disease, management of the difficult surgical case. Baltimore: Williams and Wilkins; 1998. p. 428–41.

84. Lederman ED, McCoy G, Conti DJ, et al. Diverticulitis and polycystic kidney disease. Am Surg. 2000;66:200–3.

85. Dominguez FE, Albrecht KH, Heemann U, et al. Prevalence of diverticulosis and incidence of bowel perforation after kidney transplantation in patients with polycystic kidney disease. Transpl Int. 1998;11:28–31.

86. Pirenne J, Lledo-Garcia E, Benedetti E, et al. Colon perforation after renal transplantation: a single-institution review. Clin Transplant. 1997;11:88–93.

87. Aldoori W, Ryan-Harshman M. Preventing diverticular disease. Review of recent evidence on high-fibre diets. Can Fam Physician. 2002;48:1632–7.

88. Aldoori WH, Giovannucci EL, Rockett HR, et al. A prospective study of dietary fiber types and symptomatic diverticular disease in men. J Nutr. 1998;128:714–9.

89. Aldoori WH, Giovannucci EL, Rimm EB, et al. Prospective study of physical activity and the risk of symptomatic diverticular disease in men. Gut. 1995;36:276–82.

90. Marlett JA, McBurney MI, Slavin JL. Position of the American Dietetic Association: health implications of dietary fiber. J Am Diet Assoc. 2002;102:993–1000.

91. Brook I, Frazier EH. Aerobic and anaerobic microbiology in intra-abdominal infections associated with diverticulitis. J Med Microbiol. 2000;49:827–30.

92. Kronborg O. Treatment of perforated sigmoid diverticulitis: a prospective randomized trial. Br J Surg. 1993;80:505–7.

93. Bahadursingh AM, Virgo KS, Kaminski DL, et al. Spectrum of disease and outcome of complicated diverticular disease. Am J Surg. 2003;186:696–701.

94. Schilling MK, Maurer CA, Kollmar O, et al. Primary vs. secondary anastomosis after sigmoid colon resection for perforated diverticulitis (Hinchey Stage III and IV): a prospective outcome and cost analysis. Dis Colon Rectum. 2001;44:699–703.

95. Farthmann EH, Ruckauer KD, Haring RU. Evidence-based surgery diverticulitis – a surgical disease? Langenbecks Arch Surg. 2000;385:143–51.

96. Chandra V, Nelson H, Larson DR, et al. Impact of primary resection on the outcome of patients with perforated diverticulitis. Arch Surg. 2004;139:1221–4.

97. Zeitoun G, Laurent A, Rouffet F, et al. Multicentre, randomized clinical trial of primary versus secondary sigmoid resection in generalized peritonitis complicating sigmoid diverticulitis. Br J Surg. 2000;87:1366–74.

98. Rothenberger DA, Wiltz O. Surgery for complicated diverticulitis. Surg Clin North Am. 1993;73:975–92.

99. Kaiser AM, Jiang JK, Lake JP, et al. The management of complicated diverticulitis and the role of computed tomography. Am J Gastroenterol. 2005;100:910–7.

100. Ricciardi R, Baxter NN, Read TE, et al. Is the decline in surgical treatment for diverticulitis associated with an increase in complicated diverticulitis? Dis Colon Rectum. 2009;52(9):1558–63.

101. Maggard MA, Chandler CF, Schmit PJ, et al. Surgical diverticulitis: treatment options. Am Surg. 2001;67:1185–9.

102. Guenaga KF, Matos D, Castro AA, et al. Mechanical bowel preparation for elective colorectal surgery. Cochrane Database Syst Rev. 2003;2:CD001544.

103. Maggard MA, Zingmond D, O'Connell JB, et al. What proportion of patients with an ostomy (for diverticulitis) get reversed? Am Surg. 2004;70:928–31.

104. Desai DC, Brennan Jr EJ, Reilly JF, et al. The utility of the Hartmann procedure. Am J Surg. 1998;175:152–4.

105. Haas PA, Fox Jr TA. The fate of the forgotten rectal pouch after Hartmann's procedure without reconstruction. Am J Surg. 1990;159:106–10.

106. Salem L, Flum DR. Primary anastomosis or Hartmann's procedure for patients with diverticular peritonitis? A systemic review? Dis Colon Rectum. 2004;47:1953–64.

107. Wigmore SJ, Duthie GS, et al. Restoration of intestinal continuity following Hartmann's procedure: the Lothian experience 1987–1992. Br J Surg. 1995;82:27–30.

108. Maggard MA, Zingmond D, et al. What proportion of patients with an ostomy for diverticulitis get reversed? Am Surg. 2004;70:928–31.

109. Pessaux P, Muscari F, Ouellet JF, et al. Risk factors for mortality and morbidity after elective sigmoid resection for diverticulitis: prospective multicenter multivariate analysis of 582 patients. World J Surg. 2004;28:92–6.

110. Elliott TB, Yego S, Irvin TT. Five-year audit of the acute complications of diverticular disease. Br J Surg. 1997;84:535–9.

111. Vernava III AM, Longo WE. Postoperative anastomotic complications. In: Hicks TC, Beck DE, Opelka FG, Timmcke AE, editors. Complications in colon and rectal surgery. Baltimore: Williams and Wilkins; 1996. p. 82–98.

112. Roach MB, Donaldson DS. Urologic complications of colorectal surgery. In: Hicks TC, Beck DE, Opelka FG, Timmcke AE, editors. Complications in colon and rectal surgery. Baltimore: Williams and Wilkins; 1996. p. 99–117.

113. Leff EI, Groff W, Rubin RJ, et al. Use of ureteral catheters in colonic and rectal surgery. Dis Colon Rectum. 1982;25:457–60.

114. Munson KD, Hensien MA, Jacob LN, et al. Diverticulitis: a comprehensive follow-up. Dis Colon Rectum. 1996;39:318–22.

115. Benn PL, Wolff BG, Ilstrup DM. Level of anastomosis and recurrent colonic diverticulitis. Am J Surg. 1986;151:269–71.

116. Thaler K, Baig MK, Berho M, et al. Determinants of recurrence after sigmoid resection for uncomplicated diverticulitis. Dis Colon Rectum. 2003;46:385–8.

117. Chautems R, Ambrosetti P, Ludwig A, et al. Long-term follow-up after first acute episode of sigmoid diverticulitis: is surgery mandatory? Dis Colon Rectum. 2001;44:A12.

118. Boles RS, Jordan SM. The clinical significance of diverticulosis. Gastroenterology. 1958;35:579–81.

119. Fearnhead NS, Mortensen NJ. Clinical features and differential diagnosis of diverticular disease. Best Pract Res Clin Gastroenterol. 2002;16:577–93.

120. Farmakis N, Tudor RG, Keighley MR. The 5-year natural history of complicated diverticular disease. Br J Surg. 1994;81:733–5.

121. Horner JL. Natural history of diverticulosis of the colon. Am J Dig Dis. 1958;3:343–50.

122. Salem TA, Molloy RG, O'Dwyer PJ. Prospective, five year follow-up study of patients with symptomatic uncomplicated diverticular disease. Dis Colon Rectum. 2007;50:1460–4.

123. Broderick-Villa G, Burchette RJ, et al. Hospitalization for acute diverticulitis does not mandate routine elective colectomy. Arch Surg. 2005;140:576–83.

124. Shaikh S, Krukowski AH. Outcome of a conservative policy for managing acute sigmoid diverticulitis. Br J Surg. 2007;94: 876–9.
125. Janes S, Meagher A, Frizelle FA. Elective surgery after acute diverticulitis. Br J Surg. 2005;92:133–42.
126. Bartlett MK, McDermott WV. Surgical treatment of diverticulitis of the colon. N Engl J Med. 1953;248:497–9.
127. Colcock BP. Surgical management of complicated diverticulitis. N Engl J Med. 1958;259:570–3.
128. Welch CE, Allen AW, Donaldson GA. An appraisal of resection of the colon for diverticulitis of the sigmoid. Ann Surg. 1953;138:332–43.
129. Anaya DA, Flum DR. Risk of emergency colectomy and colostomy in patients with diverticular disease. Arch Surg. 2005;140:681–5.
130. Lorimer JW. Is prophylactic resection valid as an indication for elective surgery in diverticular disease? Can J Surg. 1997;40(6):445–8.
131. Alexander J, Karl RC, Skinner DB. Results of changing trends in the surgical management of complications of diverticular disease. Surgery. 1983;94:683–90.
132. Nylamo E. Diverticulitis of the colon: role of surgery in preventing complications. Ann Chir Gynaecol. 1990;79:139–42.
133. Wong WD, Wexner SD, Lowry A, et al. Practice parameters for the treatment of sigmoid diverticulitis – supporting documentation. The Standards Task Force. The American Society of Colon and Rectal Surgeons. Dis Colon Rectum. 2000;43:290–7.
134. Richards RJ, Hammitt JK. Timing of prophylactic surgery in prevention of diverticulitis recurrence: a cost-effectiveness analysis. Dig Dis Sci. 2002;47:1903–8.
135. Salem L, Veenstra DL, Sullivan SD, et al. The timing of elective colectomy in diverticulitis: a decision analysis. J Am Coll Surg. 2004;199:904–12.
136. Sarin S, Boulos PB. Long-term outcome of patients presenting with acute complications of diverticular disease. Ann R Coll Surg Engl. 1994;76:117–20.
137. Dwivedi A, Chahin F, Agrawal S, et al. Laparoscopic colectomy vs open colectomy sigmoid diverticular disease. Dis Colon Rectum. 2002;45:1309–14.
138. Senagore AJ, Duepree HJ, Delaney CP, et al. Cost structure of laparoscopic and open sigmoid colectomy for diverticular disease: similarities and differences. Dis Colon Rectum. 2002;45:485–90.
139. Gervaz P, Pikarsky A, Utech M, et al. Converted laparoscopic colorectal surgery. Surg Endosc. 2001;15:827–32.
140. Schlachta CM, Mamazza J, Seshadri PA, et al. Predicting conversion to open surgery in laparoscopic colorectal resections. A simple clinical model. Surg Endosc. 2000;14:1114–7.
141. Schwandner O, Farke S, Fischer F, et al. Laparoscopic colectomy for recurrent and complicated diverticulitis: a prospective study of 396 patients. Langenbecks Arch Surg. 2004;389:97–103.
142. Schwandner O, Farke S, Bruch HP. Laparoscopic colectomy for diverticulitis is not associated with increased morbidity when compared with non-diverticular disease. Int J Colorectal Dis. 2004;20(2):165–72. Epub 2004 Sep 30.
143. Vargas HD, Ramirez RT, Hoffman GC, et al. Defining the role of laparoscopic – assisted sigmoid colectomy for diverticulitis. Dis Colon Rectum. 2000;43:1726–31.
144. Thaler K, Weiss EG, Nogueras JJ, et al. Recurrence rates at minimum 5-year follow-up: laparoscopic versus open sigmoid resection for uncomplicated diverticulitis. Surg Laparosc Endosc Percutan Tech. 2003;13:325–7.
145. Lee SW, Yoo J, Dujovny N, et al. Laparoscopic vs hand assisted laparoscopic sigmoidectomy diverticulitis. Dis Colon Rectum. 2006;49:464–9.
146. Chang YJ, Marcello PW, Rusin LC, et al. Hand assisted laparoscopic sigmoid colectomy. Surg Endosc. 2005;19:656.
147. Marcello PW, Fleshman JW, Milsom JW. Hand-assisted laparoscopic vs. laparoscopic colorectal surgery: a multicenter, prospective, randomized trial. Dis Colon Rectum. 2008;51(6):818–28.
148. Myers E, Hurley M, O'Sullivan GC, et al. Laparoscopic peritoneal lavage for generalized peritonitis due to perforated diverticulits. Br J Surg. 2008;95(1):97–101.
149. Moss RL, Ryan Jr JA. Management of enterovesical fistulas. Am J Surg. 1990;159:514–7.
150. Davidson R, Sweeney WB. Endoluminal stenting for benign colonic obstruction. Surg Endosc. 1998;12:353–4.
151. Tamim WL, Ghellai A, Counihan TC, et al. Experience with endoluminal colonic wall stents for the management of large bowel obstruction for benign and malignant disease. Arch Surg. 2000;135:434–8.
152. Paúl L, Pinto I, Gómez H, et al. Metallic stents in the treatment of benign diseases of the colon: preliminary experience in 10 cases. Radiology. 2002;223:715–22.
153. Siminovitch JMP, Fazio VW. Obstructive uropathy secondary to sigmoid diverticulitis. Dis Colon Rectum. 1980;23:504–7.

23 Colonic Volvulus

Jan Rakinic

Introduction

Volvulus, from the Latin *volvere*, means "to twist." Volvulus may occur in any part of the gastrointestinal tract where there is sufficient length of gut to twist about a fixed point. Colonic volvulus is the cause of 10–15% of colon obstruction in USA.[1,2] Colonic volvulus occurs when a mobile portion of the colon has a mesentery with a narrow, fixed base. The colonic segment twists around this fixed point, producing a closed loop obstruction. The mesenteric narrowing may be congenital or acquired, often by surgical scarring near the mesenteric root. As may be anticipated, the most common sites of colonic volvulus are the sigmoid colon and cecum, which are the most mobile parts of the colon. In a series of 546 cases of colonic volvulus in USA, the site-specific incidence was found to be cecum, 34.5%; transverse colon, 3.6%; splenic flexure, 1%; and sigmoid colon, 60.9%.[3] A more recent Australian study had incidence as follows: cecum, 39%; transverse colon, 2%; and sigmoid colon, 59%.[4] Factors that place patients at elevated risk for colonic volvulus include chronic constipation, previous abdominal surgery, and megacolon.

More than half of the patients with colonic volvulus present acutely with crampy abdominal pain, marked tympanitic abdominal distention, and absence of flatus or stool. Some institutionalized patients may not complain of pain; rather, a caregiver may notice an unusually long interval between bowel movements associated with significant abdominal distention. There may not be a preceding history of worsening constipation or thinner stools, as can be seen with progressive mechanical obstruction, since volvulus is a more acute process. Vomiting is an uncommon early symptom. Pain becomes more constant when ischemia worsens due to compression of the vessels within the twisted mesentery. There is a group of patients who have recurring subacute episodes of volvulus, with often painless abdominal distention and tympany. These episodes resolve spontaneously with passage of copious amounts of liquid stool and gas, described as "explosive." These patients should be evaluated for colonic dysmotility and megacolon, as these findings alter the surgical therapy. Total abdominal colectomy is the procedure of choice if megacolon is found, due to the high risk of recurrent volvulus if abnormal colon is retained.[5–8]

In children, colonic volvulus is rare, with a male predominance. Recurrent subacute episodes are most common. Mortality varies, but is higher when gangrenous bowel is present. Many of the children who develop colonic volvulus have medical comorbidities or developmental abnormalities. A report from Turkey described 19 pediatric patients treated for sigmoid volvulus over a 36-year period. The mean age was 10 years; 90% were male; two (10.5%) had volvulized previously. Gangrenous bowel was found in 15 patients (79%). Mortality was 21% (4/19).[9] A retrospective study from Texas over a 60-year span found 63 cases of colonic volvulus in children, with a median age of 7 years and a male:female ratio of 3.5:1. Of the 63 patients, 11 (17.5%) had Hirschsprung's disease. A number of the children had recurrent preoperative symptoms consistent with repeated episodes of volvulus. Overall mortality was 6%; operative mortality was 8.1%.[10] A series from England reported seven cases of pediatric colonic volvulus over a 6-year period; five of the children had cerebral palsy, and one had moyamoya disease with spastic paraplegia. Mean age was 8.3 years; six were female. Segmental resection was done in all cases; there was no mortality.[11]

Volvulus in the pregnant patient merits special consideration. While intestinal obstruction is rare in pregnancy, nearly 45% is caused by sigmoid volvulus, and it is estimated that 10% of patients with reports of cecal volvulus are pregnant at presentation. It has been postulated that the enlarging uterus lifts the sigmoid colon and cecum out of the pelvis, and that these segments become more prone to torsion about the pelvic sidewall attachments.[12,13] Volvulus in pregnancy carries a high mortality rate, often because diagnosis is delayed due to avoidance of radiography and because of similarity of symptoms to other clinical entities. A high index of suspicion for volvulus must be maintained when a pregnant patient presents with symptoms of "constipation" and abdominal pain.

D.E. Beck et al. (eds.), *The ASCRS Textbook of Colon and Rectal Surgery: Second Edition*,
DOI 10.1007/978-1-4419-1584-9_23,

Urgent intervention is often required in the setting of volvulus due to the risk to both mother and fetus.

Sigmoid Volvulus

Epidemiology/Pathogenesis

The sigmoid colon is the most common site for colonic volvulus in USA. American patients with sigmoid volvulus are generally elderly, institutionalized patients on psychoactive medications with chronic constipation, and approximately 80% are male.[14] In regions where a high fiber diet is the norm, including Africa, India, Pakistan, and the Middle East, the incidence of sigmoid volvulus is much higher than in the West, and patients are several decades younger, with persistence of male preponderance.[15–18] An anatomic study of the sigmoid mesocolon showed the female mesosigmoid to be wider than long, or brachymesocolic, whereas the male mesosigmoid was more likely to be dolichomesocolic, or longer than wide. This finding may explain the male predominance seen in sigmoid volvulus.[19]

The geographic variation in the incidence of sigmoid volvulus is believed to be linked to the ingestion of a high fiber diet, which lengthens the sigmoid colon and its mesentery, fostering an anatomic predisposition to volvulize.[20] Perry observed that while the bowel elongates as it distends, the antimesenteric border of the bowel elongates by 30%, whereas the mesenteric border elongates only by 10%.[21] In the setting of a long, narrow mesentery, distention of the bowel induces it to twist about the mesenteric axis. Several authors have described patients with other colonic disorders such as constipation and pseudo-obstruction developing sigmoid volvulus.[6,8] One researcher has suggested that sigmoid volvulus may itself be a variant of Hirschsprung's disease, which is marked by the absence of parasympathetic ganglion cells in the intramural and submucosal plexuses.[22] A VA study from 1996 investigated the density of ganglion cells in the Auerbach's plexus in dilated and nondilated segments of colons resected for volvulus. Fewer ganglion cells per high-powered field were found in the dilated portions. However, no correction was made for the acutely enlarged diameter of the affected colon segments.[23] Furuya et al. studied ganglion cell density comparing volvulized and non-volvulized sigmoid colons, and found no difference after correcting for the acute dilation. There was also no difference in ganglion cell density comparing sigmoid colons resected at the first instance of volvulus, and those re-resected ($N=2$) for recurrent volvulus after what was thought to be an adequate initial volvulus resection.[24] This would seem to imply that there is no absolute loss of ganglion cells in sigmoid volvulus unaccompanied by megacolon.

The twist of the sigmoid volvulus is most commonly counterclockwise around the mesocolic axis. Torsion must be at least 180° to produce clinically significant obstruction. The sigmoid colon can tolerate more intraluminal pressure than other parts of the colon, and so the bowel wall can remain viable for a few days; however, strangulation will eventually occur, first with venous occlusion and then, followed by arterial occlusion, thrombosis, and necrosis. Gangrene may occur much more quickly due to a sudden, tight compression of the mesenteric vessels caused by rapid distention of the colon lumen.

Diagnosis

Exploratory laparotomy is mandatory if peritonitis is present. However, in the more usual presentation, the diagnosis is strongly suspected by history and physical examination. A plain abdominal film often confirms the clinical diagnosis, displaying the "bent inner-tube" or "omega loop" appearance of a massively distended bowel loop, with both ends closely adjacent in the pelvis (Figure 23-1). In up to 40% of cases, the plain film can be equivocal: there may be superimposition of distended transverse colon or small bowel; the sigmoid loop may be transversely oriented; or a massively dilated small bowel may mimic a sigmoid loop.

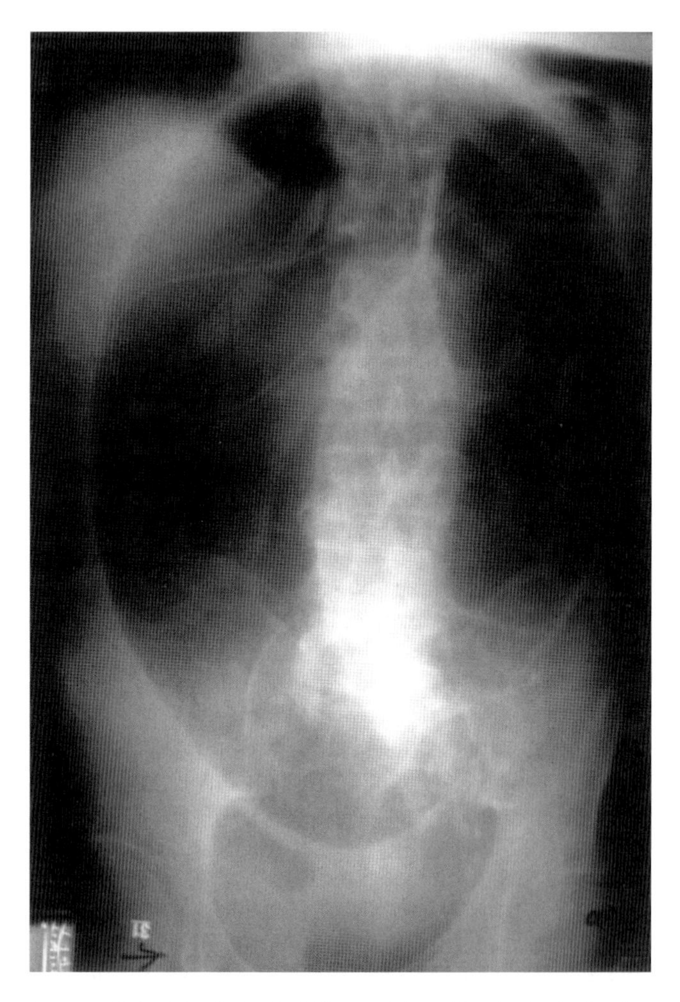

FIGURE 23-1. Plain abdominal X-ray of sigmoid volvulus indicating the "bent inner tube" sign.

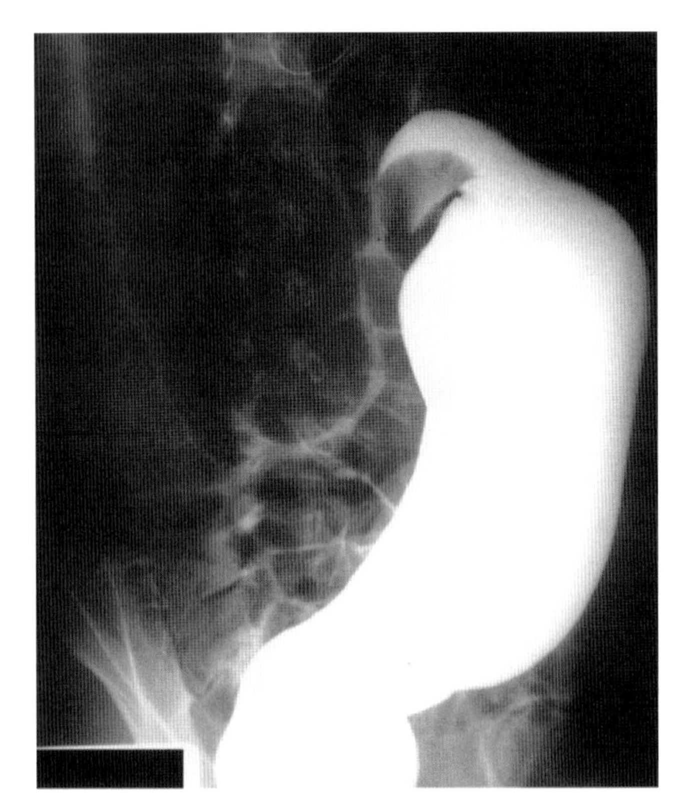

FIGURE 23-2. Barium enema study of a sigmoid volvulus indicating the bird's beak deformity and complete obstruction to retrograde flow of contrast.

In these situations, a contrast enema or CT scan may clarify the diagnosis.

If a contrast enema is desired, it should be done with water-soluble contrast material, as the mortality with barium is very high if a perforation is encountered. A water-soluble contrast enema classically shows the contrast column ending sharply in a "bird's beak" shape at the site of torsion (Figure 23-2). The major differential diagnoses that must be considered are obstruction due to colonic neoplasm and colonic ileus, or Ogilvie's syndrome, both of which can present in a similar way. The contrast study is helpful in diagnosis clarification. In the case of neoplasm, there may be a wisp of contrast through the lesion; if the obstruction is complete, the appearance is distinctly different from the classic "bird's beak" appearance. In Ogilvie's syndrome, the water-soluble contrast enema will show that there is no obstruction, and may also be therapeutic.

Abdominal CT scan can be quite helpful in the identification of colonic volvulus. Much information has been written on the "whirl sign" indicating twisted mesentery and intestinal volvulus,[25,26] although most reports refer to small bowel volvulus. More recent reports have noted that the "whirl sign" can be observed in settings other than intestinal volvulus[27,28] and so may not be pathognomonic for intestinal volvulus.

In the pregnant patient, the diagnosis of sigmoid volvulus is usually made clinically, with subsequent endoscopic confirmation, or intraoperatively due to patient deterioration. The size of the uterus presents a challenge for operating in the pelvis; this makes simple detorsion or sigmoidopexy appear more attractive when the sigmoid colon is viable, but exposes the patient to a high risk of recurrence and need for another, definitive operative procedure.

Treatment and Outcome

The first volvulus-specific maneuver in the stable patient with a sigmoid volvulus is attempted endoscopic detorsion. Successful detorsion converts a surgical emergency into an elective situation. If the patient is febrile or has localized tenderness over the distended loop, nonviable colon should be strongly suspected, and attempted detorsion should be abandoned. Attempted detorsion of nonviable bowel risks perforation and peritonitis, with the attendant complications thereof. While detorsion was historically done with the rigid proctoscope, the flexible sigmoidoscope or colonoscope has replaced it as the instrument of choice. Detorsion has also been described using a column of barium or a blindly passed rectal tube. Due to concern that the sigmoid could be gangrenous, only detorsion techniques that visualize the mucosa should be used. When decompression is successful, as it is in 60–80% of attempts,[4,15,20,29,30] there is evacuation of significant flatus and stool with visible lessening of abdominal distention. A decompressing tube should be placed into the detorsed loop to allow continued decompression and to prevent retorsion. A plain abdominal film should then be obtained to confirm relief of volvulus and absence of intraperitoneal free air.

Decompression alone as a management choice bears the risks of recurrent volvulus and death, which are not always mutually exclusive. A large study from the VA reported that of 50 patients managed with endoscopic decompression alone, six (12%) died during the index admission, and ten of the remaining 44 (23%) developed recurrent volvulus requiring treatment; two of those ten (20%) subsequently died.[20] Lau et al. reported 49 patients from Brisbane, Queensland, of whom 12 were treated initially with endoscopic decompression alone. Six of these patients suffered seven recurrences within 32 days (one patient recurred twice), and 4 (33.3%) required emergency operation.[4] A study from Finland reported results of endoscopic decompression as the initial therapy for 17 of 58 patients with sigmoid volvulus: mortality was 12% and recurrence rate was 29%.[29] A Taiwanese study showed recurrence of sigmoid volvulus in 12 of 14 patients (86%) who refused operation after successful endoscopic decompression.[5] A study from Greece reported on 15 of 33 patients with sigmoid volvulus who were treated with endoscopic decompression and discharged. Five of these patients (33.3%) suffered recurrent volvulus requiring emergency operation; of these patients, three (60%) died.[30]

A study from Riyadh, Saudi Arabia, reported that of seven patients with sigmoid volvulus who were initially decompressed endoscopically and then refused elective surgery, three recurred (43%); these underwent repeat decompression followed by elective resection.[15] A recent study from Ireland reported a recurrent volvulus rate of 86.6% (13 of 15) in sigmoid volvulus patients initially managed with endoscopic decompression alone who survived the initial hospitalization.[31]

The high rate of revolvulus after detorsion alone, coupled with a mortality rate over 20% for emergent surgery compared to 6% or less with elective resection[4,17,20,30], has prompted most surgeons to proceed with elective sigmoid resection during the same hospitalization for most patients. Complete colonoscopy should be performed prior to operation to rule out synchronous lesions that would alter management. The standard elective surgical procedure is sigmoid resection with primary anastomosis, which may be accomplished with open technique, or laparoscopic technique if the colon is sufficiently decompressed.[32,33] Patients successfully endoscopically decompressed prior to definitive resection have an incidence of recurrent volvulus close to zero.[4,17,20,30] However, in the setting of megacolon, total abdominal colectomy is the recommended procedure; otherwise, the patient is at very high risk of recurrent volvulus. Ryan reported 66 consecutive patients with sigmoid volvulus from Melbourne, six of whom had megacolon. He noted that in the non-megacolon group, flatus tube decompression was usually successful, and sigmoid resection was curative of the volvulus. In the megacolon group, patients had recurrent episodes of volvulus, tube decompression was less successful, and symptoms including revolvulus occurred after sigmoidectomy.[7] Morrissey reported on the postoperative course of 29 patients after surgery for sigmoid volvulus. There was an overall recurrence rate of 36%. In patients who had an otherwise normal colon, the recurrence rate was 6%, but in those with megacolon who had undergone resection of only the sigmoid colon, recurrence was 82%. Morrissey noted that no recurrence occurred in those with megacolon who had undergone subtotal colectomy.[6] Chung et al. reported on 35 patients from Singapore with sigmoid volvulus. Of patients who underwent sigmoid resection, six had recurrent volvulus. Chung found that concomitant megacolon and megarectum were significant predictors of recurrence.[5] Strom et al. reported a 30-year experience with 129 patients suffering 163 episodes of sigmoid volvulus, noting that sigmoidectomy resolved volvulus "only if bowel atony was limited to the segment removed." Megacolon required subtotal colectomy to avoid volvulus recurrence.[8]

A number of non-resectional techniques have also been described for the treatment of sigmoid volvulus. These include surgical detorsion without resection or fixation, or detorsion with methods of either sigmoid or mesenteric fixation. The described techniques of sigmoid fixation include extraperitoneal sigmoidopexy[16]; nonsurgical endoscopic sigmoidopexy with or without tube fixation[34,35]; parallel colopexy to the transverse colon (Figure 23-3);[36] laparoscopic fixation;[37] fixation of the sigmoid colon to the abdominal wall with bands of prosthetic with or without percutaneous colon deflation;[38] and percutaneous endoscopic colostomy.[39] Mesenteric fixation techniques include mesosigmoplasty and mesenteric fixation (Figure 23-4A and B).[40,41]

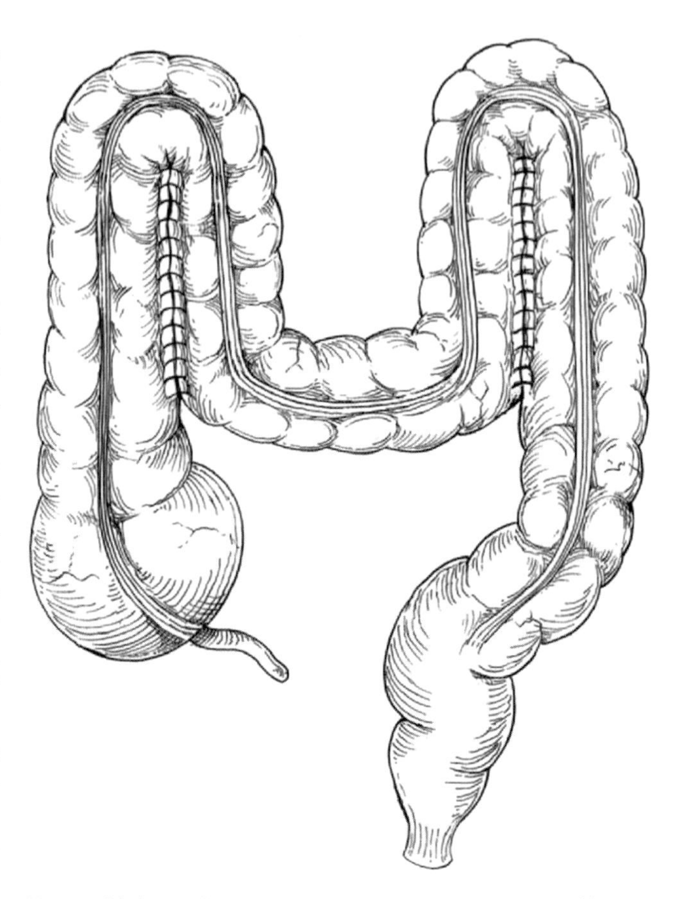

FIGURE 23-3. Parallel colopexy as described by Mortensen.[36]

All nonresectional techniques are associated with high morbidity and/or high recurrence rate. Hiltunen reported on 58 patients from Finland with sigmoid volvulus, of which 21 were treated with detorsion with or without fixation.[29] This group had 24% recurrence, compared to 5% recurrence after sigmoidectomy. A 2007 report from Turkey cited 36% of recurrent volvulus after surgical detorsion as the only treatment.[18] Remes-Troche et al. reported 25 cases of sigmoid volvulus, of which 12 were treated with surgical fixation only. Recurrence after fixation was 38% at 12 months and 69% at 24 months, with associated 50% mortality.[42] In a large series from Turkey, 31 patients treated with mesosigmoidopexy had a recurrence rate of 16.1%.[18] A retrospective review from Varanasi, India, showed a recurrence rate of 38.5% (5/13) after colopexy alone.[43] In a recent report of 27 patients who underwent percutaneous endoscopic colostomy (PEC) for a number of indications, no recurrence of sigmoid colon volvulus occurred in eight cases with a PEC tube in place. However, mortality was 26% in the overall group; two deaths were from fecal peritonitis. Morbidity was also

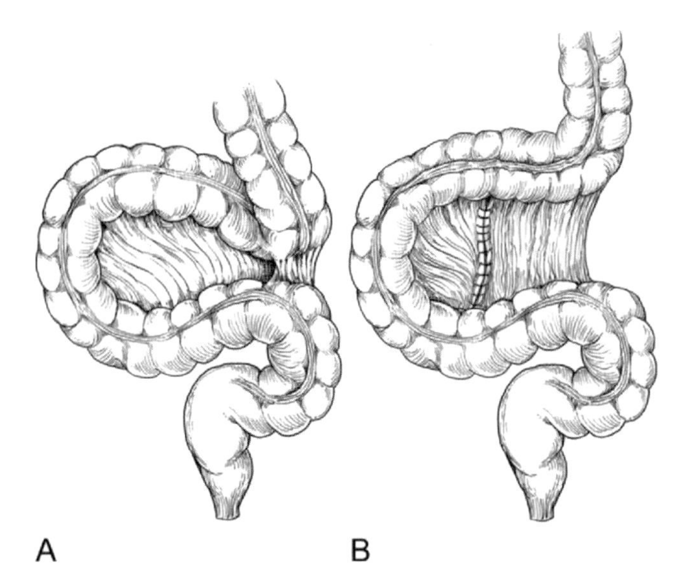

FIGURE 23-4. Mesosigmoidoplasty. **A** A longitudinal peritoneal incision made in the elongated, narrow mesentery. **B** The incision is then closed transversely, broadening the mesenteric base and shortening the height of the sigmoid loop.

significant; 77% had episodes of infection which led to tube removal in 44%.[39] The only prospective randomized trial in the literature comparing mesosigmoidopexy with resection and primary anastomosis in sigmoid volvulus without gangrene indicates that sigmoid resection bears the lowest risk of recurrence of sigmoid volvulus.[44]

It is important to understand that the search for alternatives to resection for sigmoid volvulus was based on *historical* rates of morbidity and mortality. Considering that modern surgical and anesthetic techniques have significantly reduced surgical complication rates, it seems clear that resection after decompression provides near-zero risk of recurrence with acceptable morbidity and mortality rates.[17,20,30]

If endoscopic decompression is unsuccessful or visualizes gangrenous mucosa, the situation is a surgical emergency and efforts at detorsion should be halted and preparation of the patient for surgery should be expeditiously done. Exploration should be done via a midline laparotomy incision, or potentially by laparoscopy if the patient is hemodynamically stable. If the bowel appears viable or possibly viable, the twist should be reduced. While some surgeons advocate sigmoidopexy for a viable sigmoid, the recurrence rate is high and so most surgeons favor sigmoid resection. The decision for anastomosis versus Hartmann's procedure should be based on standard surgical criteria: the presence of good blood supply, absence of (or minimal) peritoneal soilage, reasonable nutritional status, and absence of shock would suggest that anastomosis is reasonable. When considering stoma formation, it should be remembered that many of the stomas formed in this setting will be permanent, as infirm patients with other medical comorbidities will rarely become candidates for stoma closure. The usual maneuvers used for selecting stoma location are often difficult to employ preoperatively, given the abdominal contour and urgency of the patient's situation. The bowel is often quite dilated, and a large opening in the abdominal wall may be required for a colostomy. This leads to a higher incidence of parastomal hernia.

Both morbidity and mortality are higher for emergent operations for sigmoid volvulus, compared to those for the elective or semi-elective setting. Deaths and complications increase further if gangrenous colon is encountered. A study of volvulus in urban Australia showed a mortality of 36% in patients operated emergently for sigmoid volvulus.[4] Grossman's study of sigmoid volvulus in VA medical centers showed 24% mortality for emergency operations, compared to 6% for elective operations after decompression. Mortality was positively correlated with emergency surgery ($p<0.01$) and necrotic colon ($p<0.05$).[20] In a report on 33 sigmoid volvulus patients from Greece, mortality after emergency operations was 40% and that after elective operations was 5.9%. However, if the sigmoid colon is found to be viable, sigmoidectomy and primary anastomosis have a good outcome and avoid the morbidity of a second surgery for stoma closure.[30] A study from Guinea showed that emergency sigmoid resection with primary anastomosis was well tolerated in the absence of gangrenous sigmoid, with mortality of 12.5%; however, in the presence of gangrene, the mortality rose to 33.3%.[44] In a 2009 study from Ireland, six of ten patients undergoing emergency surgery for sigmoid volvulus without decompression had sigmoidectomy with primary anastomosis. There were no deaths, wound infections, or anastomotic leaks in this group.[31] Oren's study of sigmoid volvulus includes patients treated over a 38-year span. In this large group, 36 patients with gangrenous sigmoid colon had sigmoidectomy with primary anastomosis. While mortality in this group was 21.6%, Oren notes that all deaths occurred in the earliest years of the series.[18] Kuzu et al. reported 106 patients from Ankara, Turkey, who underwent emergency sigmoidectomy for volvulus without preoperative decompression; 57 patients had a primary anastomosis performed. Mortality was 6.6%, but rose to 11% if the bowel was gangrenous. A higher rate of wound infection and intra-abdominal abscess was also seen in the group with gangrenous bowel.[45] These studies support that good outcomes can be achieved with primary anastomosis at the time of emergent sigmoidectomy for sigmoid volvulus with careful patient selection.

Caring for the pregnant patient with sigmoid volvulus presents the challenge of managing two patients at once. An argument can be made for endoscopic detorsion in the first trimester if mucosa is viable, with an attempt to delay definitive management until the second trimester, when the risk to the fetus is less. In the case of sigmoid volvulus in the third trimester, nonoperative therapy should be pursued when possible until fetal maturity; then delivery and definitive volvulus management can be undertaken.[12] Ischemic sigmoid colon is managed with Hartmann's procedure.

Ileosigmoid Knotting

Epidemiology/Pathogenesis

Ileosigmoid knotting, also called "compound volvulus" or "double volvulus," although these are now considered misnomers, is unusual in the West. It is more common in certain areas of Africa, Asia, and the Middle East, although still quite rare. Patients with ileosigmoid knotting are younger than those with sigmoid volvulus, and the condition is more common in males.[46–48] In this condition, loops of ileum and sigmoid colon wrap about one another, causing a double obstruction of both the ileum and the sigmoid. Four patterns of ileosigmoid knot formation have been described, which differentiate between an active or passive segment of bowel and the direction of rotation (Figure 23-5A–D).[49,50] The ileum is most commonly the active component and wraps around the sigmoid.[49,51] Less commonly, the sigmoid wraps around the ileum. In either instance, the direction of the wrap may be clockwise or counterclockwise. Endoscopic reduction attempts are always unsuccessful, and the diagnosis of ileosigmoid knot should be considered when endoscopic reduction has failed. Theories of pathogenesis center on the typical diet of the regions where ileosigmoid knotting is most common: a large volume diet high in bulk and carbohydrates, associated with large volumes of concomitant liquid ingestion. It is postulated that as the stomach contents empty into the jejunum, the weight pulls the bowel into the left paracolic gutter. Empty distal loops of small bowel are then displaced around a narrow based sigmoid. Continued peristalsis leads to further rotation of the loop, internal herniation, and knot formation. Another theory suggests that relatively rapid ingestion of large amounts of food and liquid, as in regions where a single daily meal is the norm, allows the sigmoid colon to volvulize due to the abruptly increased weight of luminal contents.[49,52]

Diagnosis

Presentation is acute, with distention, nausea and vomiting, and severe abdominal pain which may be colicky in nature. In contrast to other forms of volvulus, there is an absence of previous similar episodes. Patients often present in shock with signs of an intra-abdominal catastrophe, including acidosis, hypotension, and tachycardia. Preoperative diagnosis is difficult due to the rarity and complexity of the problem. Characteristic radiographic features have been described, consisting of a double obstruction with a distended obstructed sigmoid loop pulled toward the right and a proximal small bowel obstruction on the left.[53] In practice, X-rays are often atypical and difficult to interpret. Only one of 15 patients in an Ethiopian review had radiologic findings

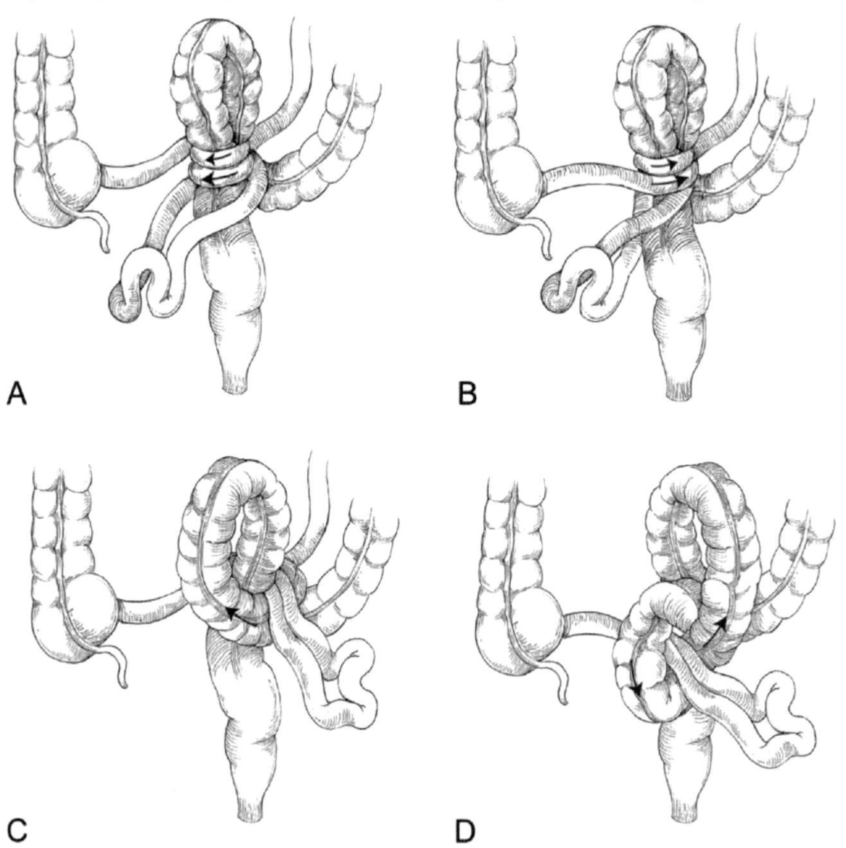

FIGURE 23-5. Ileosigmoid knotting: these schematic illustrations indicate the four terms of knotting. The active ileum may rotate around the sigmoid colon in either a clockwise **A** or a counterclockwise **B** direction. Much more frequently, the sigmoid colon may act as the active loop and rotate in either a clockwise **C** or a counterclockwise **D** direction around the ileum.

of combined small and large bowel obstruction,[47] and only three of seven in an Indian series.[54] A diagnostic triad has been proposed, consisting of a clinical small bowel obstruction, a radiographic colon obstruction, and the inability to pass a sigmoidoscope to decompress a suspected sigmoid volvulus.[48] In practice, the diagnosis is made correctly in fewer than 20% of patients, and over 70% have gangrenous bowel at surgery.[46–51]

Treatment and Outcome

Patients who present in this manner should be urgently resuscitated and taken for exploration. Treatment recommendations range from simple double detorsion to double resection. Advocates of enbloc resection without detorsion reason that attempts to untie the knot are time consuming and difficult, may contribute to systemic release of endotoxin with worsening of shock, and increase the risk of bowel perforation and peritoneal contamination. However, others have recommended detorsion if one or both segments are felt to be viable. Deflation of the involved segments has been shown to assist in detorsion and diminish the risk of perforation.[47,48,55] The data on recurrence after detorsion alone are conflicting. Some authors advocate sigmoid resection in all cases, even if the sigmoid is viable, to eliminate the risk of recurrent knot or simple sigmoid volvulus in future.[46,48,56]

Primary small bowel or ileocolic anastomosis is performed in nearly all patients with gangrenous ileum. Historically, Hartmann's procedure has been the most commonly performed operation when nonviable sigmoid colon is found,[47,51,55] although more surgeons are now performing primary colonic anastomoses in this setting.[48,50] There appears to be a risk of thrombosis of the superior rectal artery or inferior mesenteric artery, prompting some authors to recommend resection of the sigmoid well beyond the areas of twisting or gangrene to ensure adequate vascular supply.[46,48,49,54]

Overall surgical mortality ranges from 30 to 50%.[49,50,55] However, when the colon is not gangrenous, the mortality is lower, approximately10–30%. Several older studies have showed an inverse relationship between duration of symptoms and mortality,[49,52] although a smaller, more recent study from India did not bear that out.[48] In general, outcome is poorer when gangrenous colon is present. Finally, if extensive gangrenous small bowel is found, leaving less than 60 cm of viable small bowel, the mortality rate was 100%.[49]

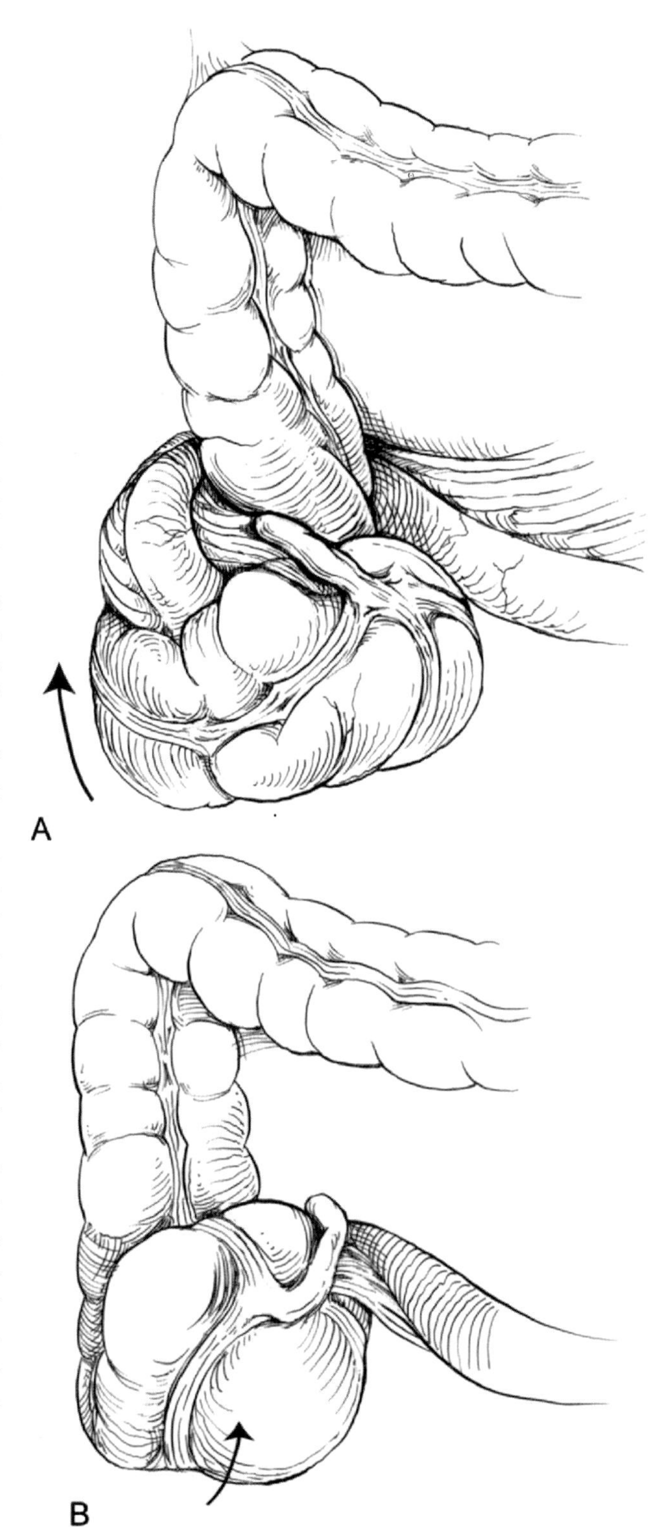

FIGURE 23-6. **A** Schematic illustration of a cecal volvulus; **B** Schematic illustration of a cecal bascule.

Cecal Volvulus

Epidemiology/Pathogenesis

Cecal volvulus is the second most common site of colonic volvulus, and technically consists of volvulus of the terminal ileum, cecum, and proximal right colon. Two variants exist: a true axial rotation of the terminal ileum, cecum, and proximal right colon around its mesentery (Figure 23-6A), and cecal bascule, which is an anteriosuperior folding of a mobile cecum over the proximal right colon without axial rotation (Figure 23-6B). The rotation of a cecal volvulus is most commonly clockwise around the mesenteric axis.

Cecal bascule accounts for approximately 10% of cases of cecal volvulus[2] and is less likely to present with vascular compromise. Individuals with cecal volvulus are several decades younger than patients with sigmoid volvulus, with a female:male ratio of 1.4:1.[57] While the gender ratio seems unchanged, more recent series have described a patient population that is increasing in age. The mean age in a 1984 series was 46.7 years,[58] whereas a 1990 series from Israel included patients of a mean age of 53 years.[57] While the seven patients in a 2000 Taiwanese report had a mean age of 63.4 + 17.3 years,[59] more recently a series from France reported a mean age of 64 years in their 45 patients[60] and a Spanish series of 18 cases reported a mean age of 63.3 years.[61]

Mobility of the cecum is required, but that feature alone is not sufficient to cause a clinically apparent volvulus: a cadaver study revealed an 11% incidence of freely mobile right colons and a 26% incidence of cecal mobility sufficient to allow anterior folding.[2] Previous abdominal surgery is felt to be a major risk factor for cecal volvulus: in published reports of cecal volvulus, 30–70% of patients had a history of abdominal surgery. Other risk factors include chronic constipation, obstructing colon lesions, and malrotation. Upward displacement of the cecum by an enlarged uterus or other pelvic mass may also promote cecal volvulus. Several series have reported that 10% of patients with cecal volvulus are pregnant at presentation.

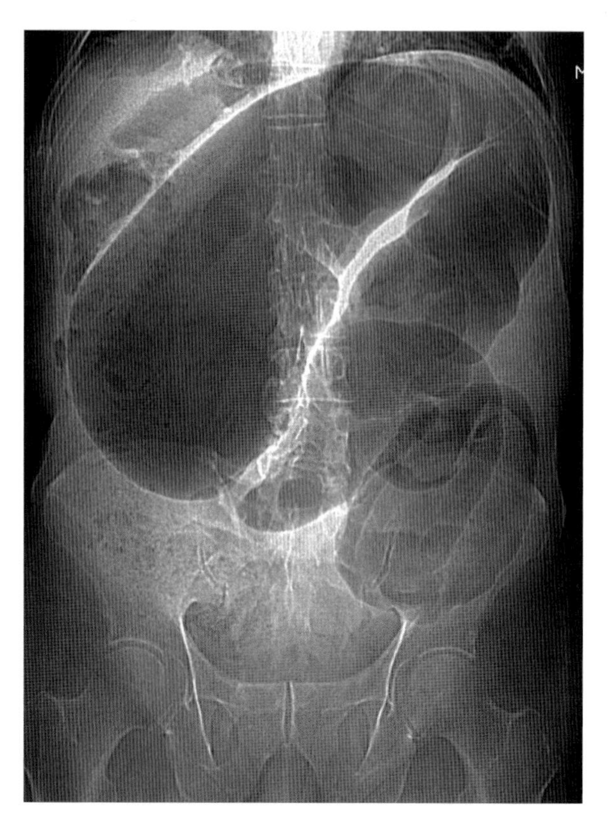

FIGURE 23-7. Plain abdominal X-ray of a cecal volvulus with "coffee bean" deformity evident in the *left upper quadrant*.

Diagnosis

As with sigmoid volvulus, presentation may be that of an acute obstruction or one of an intermittent, recurrent pattern. Abdominal distention is generally less marked than that with volvulus of more distal colonic segments. The acute presentation is of a closed loop obstruction with vascular compromise. Abdominal pain, distention, obstipation, nausea, and vomiting are common signs. If intervention is not timely, ischemia may progress to gangrene. With the intermittent pattern, duration of symptoms may be relatively brief, and diagnosis may, therefore, be difficult to gain.

Diagnosis is most often made on the basis of clinical presentation and plain films. Plain abdominal radiographs may identify the classic "coffee bean" deformity directed toward the left upper quadrant (Figure 23-7). While nearly half of the plain films suggest the diagnosis,[58,62] fewer than 20% are clearly diagnostic.[57,60] Contrast enema increases the preoperative diagnostic rate, showing a "bird's beak" type cutoff in the right colon (Figure 23-8), and may be employed in stable patients when the diagnosis is in question. CT scan has become much more common in the setting of nonspecific abdominal pain and distention (Figure 23-9). CT scan findings in cecal volvulus include the location of the cecum within the abdomen, the "bird's beak" cutoff, and the "whirl sign" of mesenteric torsion.[63] However, about half of the patients with cecal volvulus have the diagnosis made in the operating room.

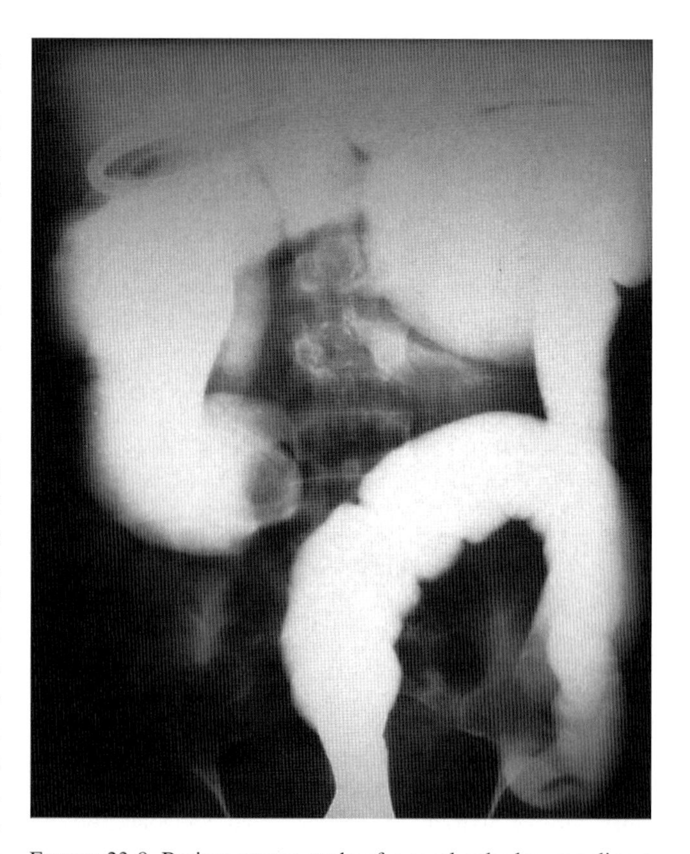

FIGURE 23-8. Barium enema study of a cecal volvulus revealing a bird's beak deformity.

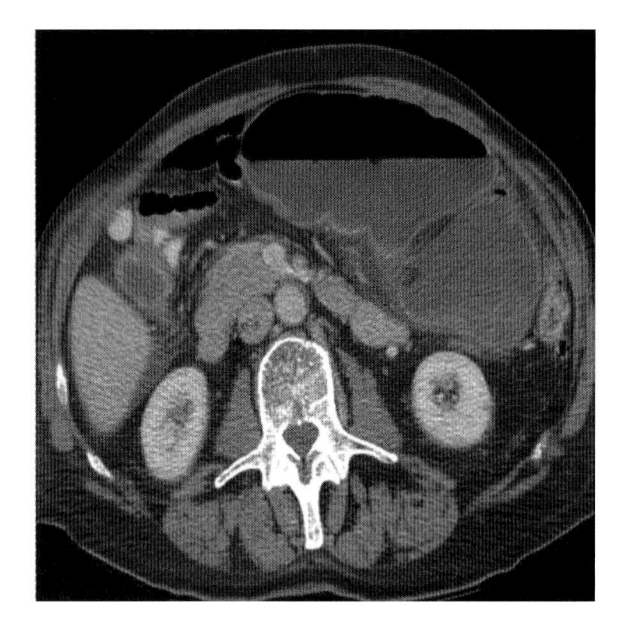

FIGURE 23-9. Typical CT findings in cecal volvulus include bird's beak cutoff and location of the cecum on the left side.

Diagnosis of cecal volvulus in the pregnant patient is most often made in the operating room after clinical deterioration. Radiologic studies normally performed in the evaluation of most patients with abdominal pain are often deferred. A case can be made for judicious use of radiologic evaluation of the pregnant abdomen when trying to diagnose the cause of abdominal pain and vomiting in the pregnant patient.[64,65] Diagnostic laparoscopy is also a viable alternative when the pregnant patient has an acute abdomen.[64]

Treatment and Outcome

While less efficacious than endoscopic detorsion of more distal colonic volvulus, colonoscopic reduction of cecal volvulus has been reported with some success. Reasons cited for limited use of this approach include difficulty in traversing the unprepared bowel to reach the right colon, difficulty in performing the detorsion, lack of clear diagnosis, and a higher rate of ischemia in cecal volvulus.[2,42,66] Some authors feel that this approach simply delays definitive surgical management and places the patient at higher risk for perforation. Proponents feel that when successfully employed, there may be a relatively low rate of recurrence, and the subsequent need for surgery may be debatable.[67]

Cecal gangrene mandates resection, and in most cases primary anastomosis can be safely done. In the circumstance of a malnourished and/or anemic patient or in the presence of other factors that may adversely affect healing, ileostomy with or without mucus fistula may be appropriate. Resection carries no risk of recurrence, and postoperative morbidity is similar to the morbidity following fixation techniques.[60] In a series of 45 patients from France, 51% had gangrenous colon. All 45 patients underwent right colectomy and 43 of these had a primary anastomosis. Mortality was 6.6% and morbidity was 20%, including two anastomotic leaks.[60]

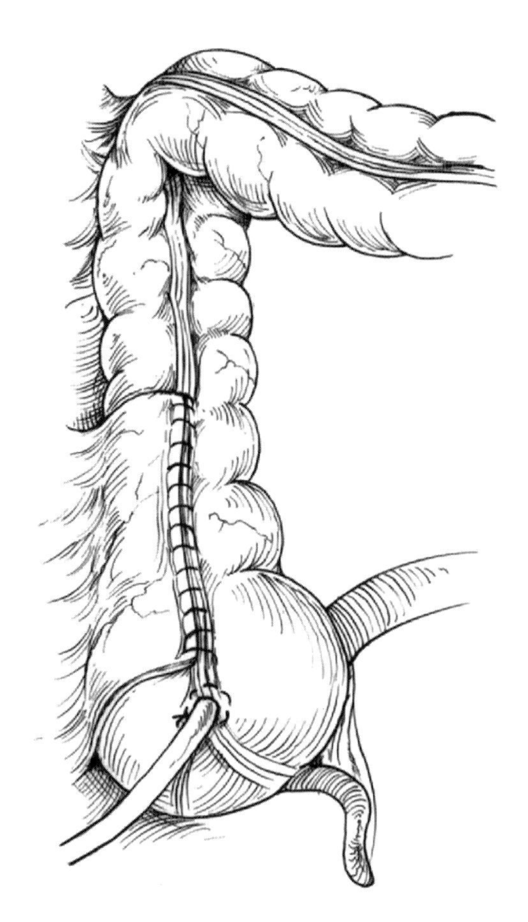

FIGURE 23-10. Cecopexy and cecostomy for cecal volvulus.

If the cecum is viable, detorsion with or without fixation may be considered. Detorsion alone carries a recurrence rate as high as 25%.[58] Fixation is generally performed by cecopexy and/or cecostomy tube placement (Figure 23-10). Cecopexy is done by raising a flap of peritoneum along the length of the right colon and suturing it to the serosa of the anterior right colon, effectively placing the right colon in a partially retroperitoneal position, eliminating the abnormal mobility. Tube cecostomy both anchors the cecum and provides a vent for the distended colon. Proponents of cecostomy find it easy to perform, and note that spontaneous closure of the cecocutaneous fistula is common after tube removal. However, the rate of recurrent cecal volvulus after cecostomy is significant, and management of the tube and its complications can be troublesome. Rabinovici's review of cecal volvulus cited a 12–14% rate of volvulus recurrence after operative detorsion, cecopexy, or cecostomy.[57] He also noted that patients undergoing cecostomy had a mortality rate of 32% – triple the rate of mortality after cecopexy (10%) or detorsion alone (13%). Ostergaard found a higher mortality after detorsion alone (14.2%), and also after cecostomy alone (66.6%) compared to that after cecal resection (7.2%). There were no deaths after cecopexy alone. He concluded that resection gave the best long-term results.[68]

Transverse Colon and Splenic Flexure Volvulus

Epidemiology/Pathogenesis

Volvulus of these colonic segments is exceptionally rare. Transverse colon volvulus is estimated to account for 1–4% of all colonic volvulus, and splenic flexure volvulus for approximately 1–2%. Patients with these disorders are younger than patients with cecal or sigmoid volvulus, with a two- to threefold female predominance.[2,66,69] Common historical points in patients with transverse colon volvulus include chronic constipation, previous abdominal surgery, institutionalization, high fiber diet, and recurrent distal obstruction. In patients with splenic flexure volvulus, previous abdominal surgery is common, and chronic constipation is also felt to increase risk, possibly by leading to redundancy and elongation of the colon. Reports in the literature speculate on associations with malrotation, Hirschsprung's disease, and Chilaiditi syndrome. Demetrius Chilaiditi first described hepato-diaphragmatic interposition of bowel in 1910 as an incidental radiographic finding. This radiographic entity is known as Chilaiditi's sign. When this interposed bowel is symptomatic, it is termed Chilaiditi syndrome. Chilaiditi syndrome is more prevalent in men, the elderly,[70] and perhaps the obese.[71] A retrospective study of 850 abdominal CT scans found hepato-diaphragmatic interposition of bowel in ten patients (0.12%). Eight of the ten patients were men; five had a BMI greater than 28.5, and three had had a BMI between 25 and 27.5 sometime in their lives. There are a number of case reports of Chilaiditi syndrome with transverse colon and splenic flexure volvulus in the surgical literature, cautioning a high index of suspicion for volvulus when this radiographic finding is noted in symptomatic patients.[72]

Clinical presentation of volvulus of the transverse colon or splenic flexure is that of a large bowel obstruction. As with sigmoid and cecal volvulus, presentation may be acute and fulminating, or may be a subacute recurring process, as is seen in up to 50% of patients. In the acute form, there is less distention than is seen in the subacute form, pain is more marked, and vomiting is usually present. Clinical deterioration is rapid in this setting. The subacute form usually has a gradual onset with milder pain, but significantly more abdominal distention, perhaps due to colon elongation from repeated episodes; vomiting is usually absent.

Diagnosis

Plain films are rarely diagnostic and may reveal a distended proximal colon with decompressed distal colon, and two air-fluid levels, representing the right colon or right transverse colon, and the left transverse colon.[73] More often, the films may be misinterpreted as a sigmoid volvulus due to the variable position of the transverse colon. Patients may then undergo colonoscopy with no clear transition point seen in the sigmoid colon. In this situation, further attempts to identify a transition point should be terminated, and a contrast study should be obtained. Contrast enema will show a bird's beak deformity at the site of the twist. However, definitive management of an acutely ill patient should not be unduly delayed to obtain these studies.

Treatment and Outcome

Successful endoscopic decompression has been reported with both transverse colon and splenic flexure volvulus. However, as with cecal volvulus, there are the same concerns of difficulty in traversing unprepared bowel, difficulty in performing detorsion, and the possibility that the diagnosis may not be clarified. There is a risk of excessive insufflation causing cecal distention and vascular compromise. Also, based on the outcomes of endoscopic detorsion elsewhere in the colon, it may be assumed that a high risk of post-decompression recurrence remains.

Operative procedures include resection, and detorsion with or without colopexy. Resection is mandatory if gangrenous bowel is found. Most authors recommend either transverse colectomy or extended right colectomy as definitive treatment for transverse colon volvulus, as this resection eliminates virtually all risk of recurrence. Mortality has been reported as high as 33% in the presence of gangrenous colon, but in most reports, it is much lower.[74,75] If the colon is viable, mortality is approximately 6%,[66] similar to that seen following resection of other volvulus of other colonic segments. The affected colon in splenic flexure volvulus is more likely to be redundant and dilated than in transverse colon volvulus. For this reason, patients with splenic flexure volvulus may be best served with an extended resection and ileosigmoid or ileorectal anastomosis.[76] Stomas should be reserved for cases in which perforation and peritoneal contamination are encountered, or for other high-risk cases.

Acknowledgments. This chapter was written by Michael D. Hellinger and Randolph M. Steinhagen in the first edition of this textbook.

References

1. Kerry RL, Ransom HK. Volvulus of the colon. Arch Surg. 1969;99:215–22.
2. Ballantyne GH, Brandner MD, Beart Jr RW, Ilstrup DM. Volvulus of the colon. Incidence and mortality. Ann Surg. 1985;202:83–92.
3. Ballantyne GH. Review of sigmoid volvulus. Clinical patterns and pathogenesis. Dis Colon Rectum. 1982;25:823–30.
4. Lau KC, Miller BJ, Schache DJ, Cohen JR. A study of large-bowel volvulus in urban Australia. Can J Surg. 2006;49:203–7.

5. Chung YF, Eu KW, Nyam DC, Leong AF, Ho YH, Seow-Choen F. Minimizing recurrence after sigmoid volvulus. Br J Surg. 1999;86:231–3.
6. Morrissey TB, Deitch EA. Recurrence of sigmoid volvulus after surgical intervention. Am Surg. 1994;60:329–31.
7. Ryan P. Sigmoid volvulus with and without megacolon. Dis Colon Rectum. 1982;25:673–9.
8. Strom PR, Stone HH, Fabian TC. Colonic atony in association with sigmoid volvulus: its role in recurrence of obstructive symptoms. South Med J. 1982;75:933–6.
9. Atamanalp SS, Yildirgan MI, Basoglu M, Kantarci M, Yilmaz I. Sigmoid colon volvulus in children: review of 19 cases. Pediatr Surg Int. 2004;20:492–5.
10. Salas S, Angel CA, Salas N, Murillo C, Swischuk L. Sigmoid volvulus in children and adolescents. J Am Coll Surg. 2000; 190:717–23.
11. Samuel M, Boddy SA, Nicholls E, Capps S. Large bowel volvulus in childhood. Aust N Z J Surg. 2000;70:258–62.
12. Alshawi JS. Recurrent sigmoid volvulus in pregnancy: report of a case and review of the literature. Dis Colon Rectum. 2005;48:1811–3.
13. Lord SA, Boswell WC, Hungerpiller JC. Sigmoid volvulus in pregnancy. Am Surg. 1996;62:380–2.
14. Ballantyne GH. Sigmoid volvulus: high mortality in county hospital patients. Dis Colon Rectum. 1981;24:515–20.
15. Alam MK, Fahim F, Al-Akeely MH, Qazi SA, Al-Dossary NF. Surgical management of colonic volvulus during same hospital admission. Saudi Med J. 2008;29:1438–42.
16. Bhatnagar BN, Sharma CL. Nonresective alternative for the cure of nongangrenous sigmoid volvulus. Dis Colon Rectum. 1998;41:381–8.
17. Heis HA, Bani-Hani KE, Rabadi DK, Elheis MA, Bani-Hani BK, Mazahreh TS, et al. Sigmoid volvulus in the Middle East. World J Surg. 2008;32:459–64.
18. Oren D, Atamanalp SS, Aydinli B, Yildirgan MI, Basoglu M, Polat KY, et al. An algorithm for the management of sigmoid colon volvulus and the safety of primary resection: experience with 827 cases. Dis Colon Rectum. 2007;50:489–97.
19. Bhatnagar BN, Sharma CL, Gupta SN, Mathur MM, Reddy DC. Study on the anatomical dimensions of the human sigmoid colon. Clin Anat. 2004;17:236–43
20. Grossmann EM, Longo WE, Stratton MD, Virgo KS, Johnson FE. Sigmoid volvulus in Department of Veterans Affairs Medical Centers. Dis Colon Rectum. 2000;43:414–8.
21. Perry EG. Intestinal volvulus: a new concept. Aust N Z J Surg. 1983;53:483–6.
22. Tomita R, Ikeda T, Fujisaki S, Tanjoh K, Munakata K. Hirschsprung's disease and its allied disorders in adults' histological and clinical studies. Hepatogastroenterology. 2003;50:1050–53.
23. Collure DW, Hameer HR. Loss of ganglion cells and marked attenuation of bowel wall in cecal dilatation. J Surg Res. 1996;60:385–8.
24. Furuya Y, Yasuhara H, Yanagie H, Naka S, Takenoue T, Shinkawa H, et al. Role of ganglion cells in sigmoid volvulus. World J Surg. 2005;29:88–91.
25. Frank AJ, Goffner LB, Fruaff AA, Losada RA. Cecal volvulus: the CT whirl sign. Abdom Imaging. 1993;18:288–9.
26. Shaff MI, Himmelfarb E, Sacks GA, Burks DD, Kulkarni MV. The whirl sign: a CT finding in volvulus of the large bowel. J Comput Assist Tomogr. 1985;9:410.
27. Blake MP, Mendelson RM. The whirl sign: a non-specific finding of mesenteric rotation. Australas Radiol. 1996;40:136–9.
28. Gollub MJ, Yoon S, Smith LM, Moskowitz CS. Does the CT whirl sign really predict small bowel volvulus? J Comput Assist Tomogr. 2006;30:25–32.
29. Hiltunen KM, Syrja H, Matikainen M. Colonic volvulus. Diagnosis and results of treatment in 82 patients. Eur J Surg. 1992;158:607–11.
30. Safioleas M, Chatziconstantinou C, Felekouras E, Stamatakos M, Papaconstantinou I, Smirnis A, et al. Clinical considerations and therapeutic strategy for sigmoid volvulus in the elderly: a study of 33 cases. World J Gastroenterol. 2007;13:921–4.
31. Larkin JO, Thekiso TB, Waldron R, Barry K, Eustace PW. Recurrent sigmoid volvulus – early resection may obviate later emergency surgery and reduce morbidity and mortality. Ann R Coll Surg Engl. 2009;91:205–9.
32. Cartwright-Terry T, Phillips S, Greenslade GL, Dixon AR. Laparoscopy in the management of closed loop sigmoid volvulus. Colorectal Disease. 2007;10:370–2.
33. Liang JT, Lai HS, Lee PH. Elective laparoscopically assisted sigmoidectomy for the sigmoid volvulus. Surg Endosc. 2006;20:1772–3.
34. Chiulli RA, Swantkowski TM. Sigmoid volvulus treated with endoscopic sigmoidopexy. Gastrointest Endosc. 1993;39:194–6.
35. Pinedo G, Kirberg A. Percutaneous endoscopic sigmoidopexy in sigmoid volvulus with T-fasteners: report of two cases. Dis Colon Rectum. 2001;44:1867–70.
36. Mortensen NJ, Hoffman G. Volvulus of the transverse colon. Postgrad Med J. 1979;55:54–7.
37. Miller R, Roe AM, Eltringham WK, Espiner HJ. Laparoscopic fixation of sigmoid volvulus. Br J SUrg. 1992;79:435.
38. Salim AS. Management of acute volvulus of the sigmoid colon: a new approach by percutaneous deflation and colopexy. World J Surg. 1991;15:68–72.
39. Cowlam S, Watson C, Eltringham M, Bain I, Barrett P, Green S, et al. Percutaneous endoscopic colostomy of the left side of the colon. Gastrointest Endosc. 2007;65:1007–14.
40. Akgun Y. Mesosigmoplasty as a definitive operation in treatment of acute sigmoid volvulus. Dis Colon Rectum. 1996;39:579–81.
41. Subrahmanyam M. Mesosigmoplasty as a definitive operation for sigmoid volvulus. Br J Surg. 1992;79:683–4.
42. Remes-Troche JM, Perez-Martinez C, Rembis V, Arch Ferrer J, Ayala Gonzalez M, Takahashi T. Surgical treatment of colonic volvulus. Ten year experience at the Instituto Nacional de la Nutricion Salvador Zubiran. Rev Gastroenterol Mex. 1997;62:276–80.
43. Khanna AK, Kumar P, Khanna R. Sigmoid volvulus: study from a north Indian hospital. Dis Colon Rectum. 1999;42:1081–4.
44. Bagarani M, Conde AS, Longo R, Italiano A, terenzi A, Venuto G. Sigmoid volvulus in west Africa: a prospective study on surgical treatments. Dis Colon Rectum. 1993;36:186–90.
45. Kuzu MA, Aslar AK, Soran A, Polat A, Topcu O, Hengirmen S. Emergent resection for acute sigmoid volvulus: results of 106 consecutive cases. Dis Colon Rectum. 2002;45:1085–90.
46. Akgun Y. Management of ileosigmoid knotting. Br J Surg. 1997;84:672–3.
47. Kotisso B, Bekele A. Ilio-sigmoid knotting in Addis Ababa: a three-year comprehensive retrospective analysis. Ethiop Med J. 2006;44:377–83.
48. Raveenthiran V. The ileosigmoid knot: new observations and changing trends. Dis Colon Rectum. 2001;44:1196–200.

49. Alver O, Oren D, Tireli M, Kayabasi B, Akdemir D. Ileosigmoid knotting in Turkey. Review of 68 cases. Dis Colon Rectum. 1993;36:1139-47.
50. Alver O, Oren D, Apaydin B, Yigitbasi R, Ersan Y. Internal herniation concurrent with ileosigmoid knotting or sigmoid volvulus: Presentation of 12 patients. Surgery. 2005;137:372–7.
51. Atamanalp SS, Oren D, Basoglu M, Yildirgan MI, Balik AA, Polat KY, et al. Ileosigmoid knotting: outcome in 63 patients. Dis Colon Rectum. 2004;47:906–10.
52. Shepherd JJ. The epidemiology and clinical presentation of sigmoid volvulus. Br J Surg. 1969;56:353–9.
53. Young WS, White A, Grave GF. The radiology of ileosigmoid knot. Clin Radiol. 1978;29:211–6.
54. Puthu D, Rajan N, Shenoy GM, Pai SU. The ileosigmoid knot. Dis Colon Rectum. 1991;34:161–6.
55. Kedir M, Kotiso B, Messele G. Ileosigmoid knotting in Gondar teaching hospital north-west Ethiopia. Ethiop Med J. 1998;36:255–60.
56. Gibney EJ, Mock CN. Ileosigmoid knotting. Dis Colon Rectum. 1993;36:855–7.
57. Rabinovici R, Simansky DA, Kaplan O, Mavor E, Manny J. Cecal volvulus. Dis Colon Rectum. 1990;33:765–9.
58. Burke JB, Ballantyne GH. Cecal volvulus. Low mortality at a city hospital. Dis Colon Rectum. 1984;27:737–40.
59. Yang SH, Lin JK, Lee RC, Li AF. Cecal volvulus: report of seven cases and literature review. Zhonghua Yi Xue Za Zhi (Taipei). 2000;63:482–6.
60. Tuech JJ, Pessaux P, Regenet N, Derouet N, Bergamaschi R, Arnaud JP. Results of resection for volvulus of the right colon. Tech Coloproctol. 2002;6:97–9.
61. Ruiz-Tovar J, Calero Garcia P, Morales Castineiras V, Martinez Molina E. Caecal volvulus: presentation of 18 cases and review of literature. Cir Esp. 2009;85:110–3.
62. Wright TP, Max MH. Cecal volvulus: review of 12 cases. South Med J. 1988;81:1233–5.
63. Delabrousse E, Sarlieve P, Sailley N, Aubry S, Kastler BA. Cecal volvulus: CT findings and correlation with pathophysiology. Emerg Radiol. 2007;14:411–5.
64. Chase DM, Sparks DA, Dawood MY, Perry E. Cecal volvulus in a multiple-gestation pregnancy. Obstet Gynecol. 2009;114:475–7.
65. Hogan BA, Brown CJ, Brown JA. Cecal volvulus in pregnancy: report of a case and review of the safety and utility of medical diagnostic imaging in the assessment of the acute abdomen during pregnancy. Emerg Radiol. 2008;15:127–31.
66. Friedman JD, Odland MD, Bubrick MP. Experience with colonic volvulus. Dis Colon Rectum. 1989;32:409–16.
67. Frizelle FA, Wolff BG. Colonic volvulus. Adv Surg. 1996;29:131–9.
68. Ostergaard E, Halvorsen JF. Volvulus of the caecum. An evaluation of various surgical procedures. Acta Chir Scand. 1990;156:629–31.
69. Loke KL, Chan CS. Case report: transverse colon volvulus: unusual appearance on barium enema and review of the literature. Clin Radiol. 1995;50:342–4.
70. Saber AA, Boros MJ. Chilaiditi's syndrome: what should every surgeon know? Am Surg. 2005;71:261–3.
71. Murphy JM, Maibaum A, Alexander G, Dixon AK. Chilaiditi's syndrome and obesity. Clin Anat. 2000;13:181–4.
72. Orangio GR, Fazio VW, Winkelman E, McGonagle BA. The Chilaiditi syndrome and associated volvulus of the transverse colon. Dis Colon Rectum. 1986;29:653–56.
73. Mindelzun RE, Stone JM. Volvulus of the splenic flexure: radiographic diagnosis. Radiology. 1991;181:221–3.
74. Anderson JR, Lee D, Taylor TV, Ross AH. Volvulus of the transverse colon. Br J Surg. 1981;68:179–81.
75. Gumbs MA, Kashan F, Shumofsky E, Yerubandi SR. Volvulus of the transverse colon. Reports of cases and review of the literature. Dis Colon Rectum. 1983;26:825–8.
76. Sanderson AJ, Elford J, Hayward SJ. Case report: volvulus of the splenic flexure in a patient with systemic sclerosis. Br J Radiol. 1995;68:537–9.

24 Lower Gastrointestinal Hemorrhage

Craig A. Reickert and Melissa Times

Lower gastrointestinal bleeding (LGIB) is defined as measurable bleeding from a source distal to the ligament of Treitz. LGIB is a broad term used to encompass the spectrum of symptoms ranging from minimal bleeding noticed on bathroom tissues associated with hemorrhoids to massive bleeding encountered with diverticular hemorrhage. Etiologies range from the rare small-bowel tumors to the frequently identified diverticular sources. To complicate matters further, the bleeding may be intermittent, leading to a challenging diagnostic and management dilemma.

Epidemiology

A population-based study examining the inpatient hospital records of 2,115 patients from 1990–1993 in a California health maintenance organization found the annual incidence rate of LGIB was 22.5 per 100,000 (0.02% of hospitalizations).[1] The three most common etiologies were diverticulosis (41.6%), colorectal malignancy (9.1%), and ischemic colitis (8.7%). The largest study and only nationwide analysis of LGIB is an examination of the Department of Veteran Affairs discharge data from 1988 to 1991 that found 17,941 patients or 0.7% of all discharges were for LGIB. The three most common etiologies were diverticulosis (60%), inflammatory bowel disease (13%), and anorectal sources (11%).[2]

Increasing age is cited frequently as a risk factor for LGIB with many studies reporting mean age greater than 60.[3–7] The common etiologies of LGIB such as diverticular disease are seen more frequently with advancing age.[8] Male gender is an inconsistent demographic factor with studies showing both a predominance of males with LGIB[1,9,10] and no statistical difference between males and females with LGIB.[7,11,12] Race has not been noted to be a predisposing factor for LGIB.[9,11,13] However, in the population-based study by Longstreth, The Acute Lower Gastrointestinal Bleeding Retrospective Analysis (ALGEBRA), and the American College of Gastroenterology Bleeding Registry, demographic information on race was not reported.[1,5,14]

Etiology

Diverticular Disease

The prevalence of diverticulosis at age 40 is less than 10% and increases to 50–66% at age 80.[15] LGIB from diverticulosis is noted in up to 17% of patients based on a review of over 6,000 patients with diverticular hemorrhage.[16] Diverticular bleeding as a source of LGIB occurs in 20–60% of cases.[2,8] In 75% of patients, bleeding will cease spontaneously.[17] Rebleeding rates after the first episode are 25%[18] and increase to 50% after two episodes.[19]

Diverticular bleeding relates to the development of pseudodiverticula in areas of weakness in the colonic wall where the vasa recta, the intramural branches of the marginal artery, course through the muscular layers to the mucosa and submucosa. At the site of the diverticulum, the vasa recta travel in the serosa with no significant tissue between the mucosa, the vasa recta, and the lumen of the bowel. Asymmetric and eccentric rupture of the vasa recta leads to intraluminal, and not peritoneal, hemorrhage.[20] Anecdotally, bleeding diverticula are attributed to mostly right-sided disease despite the greater propensity to have left-sided diverticula. However, it is difficult to find overwhelming support for this assumption. McGuire's[17] article from 1994 found nine patients with bleeding diverticula proximal and nine patients with bleeding distal to the splenic flexure. Longstreth's population-based study noted four patients with proximal bleeding and eight patients with left-sided colonic bleeding.[1] Information regarding location of diverticular bleeding is frequently not included in studies examining diverticular and lower gastrointestinal bleeding.[9,12,21,22]

Anorectal

Anorectal sources commonly include hemorrhoids, anal fissures, and rectal ulcers. They are the etiology of LGIB in 11–17% of patients.[2,6,7] Hemorrhoids were noted in 21% of patients with LGIB in an urban emergency medical center.[9]

D.E. Beck et al. (eds.), *The ASCRS Textbook of Colon and Rectal Surgery: Second Edition*,
DOI 10.1007/978-1-4419-1584-9_24, © Springer Science+Business Media, LLC 2011

Bleeding from hemorrhoids or fissures is uncommonly associated with hemodynamic instability or large volumes of blood loss. Rectal ulcers can cause severe hemorrhage associated with hemodynamic instability, with almost half of them being identified by stigmata of recent hemorrhage,[23] although the etiology of the ulcers is multiple and not frequently defined in the literature in bleeding patients. Careful historical elucidation of radiation treatment, sexually transmitted diseases (STDs), anorectal trauma, nonsteroidal anti-inflammatory drugs (NSAIDs) exposure, liver disease associated with rectal varices, and other uncommon etiologies must be included in evaluations.

Hemorrhoids are sinusoids and do not have muscular walls.[24] They are present at birth, and over time, the anal support weakens, causing internal hemorrhoids to move distally in the anal canal. The skin and mucosa are stretched causing growth of new fibrous and sinusoidal tissue. Eventually, the internal hemorrhoids slip past the anal verge and are subjected to trauma, which can lead to disruption of the sinusoids and arterial bleeding.[25,26] Hemorrhoidal bleeding is generally limited to bleeding with bowel movements, although patients may describe spraying or splattering of blood in the bowel (see Chap. 11).

Angiodysplasia

Studies from the late 1980s demonstrated rates of documented angiodysplasia varying from 15 to 27% of patients with LGIB.[27–30] However, more recent and larger studies have reported lower rates of angiodysplasia as an etiology of LGIB. A study of 1,112 patients in an urban setting reviewed the etiology of LGIB during two periods: 1988–1997 and 1998–2006. The rate of angiodysplasia decreased from 4.76% in the earlier period to 2.3% in the most recent period.[9] In the Veteran Affairs study, angiodysplasia was the source of LGIB in only 3% of patients.[2]

Angiodysplasias are vascular ectasias that can occur in the small- and large-bowel mucosa and submucosa. Small-bowel angiodysplasia is a common source of obscure gastrointestinal bleeding with up to a third of patients having this diagnosis.[31–33] Colonic angiodysplasia has a prevalence of 1% in the general population[34] with a tendency for right-sided lesions.[35–37] Angiodysplasia had been thought to be associated with aortic valvular disease and renal failure, but these associations have not been found in more statistically rigorous studies.[38,39]

Malignancy

Colorectal cancers are a source of LGIB in 9.1–13.6% of patients[1,2,9] and are associated with ulcerated tumors. As a symptom, rectal bleeding is seen in 6.5–17% of patients diagnosed with rectal cancer.[40,41] Colorectal cancer and adenomas greater than 1.0 cm were found in 13.3 and 20.5% of 405 patients who underwent a colonoscopy for bleeding,[42] although benign polyps are not commonly associated with bleeding and are simply identified during workup.

Ischemic Colitis

Ischemic colitis as an etiology of LGIB occurs in 9–18% of patients.[1,43,44] The annual incidence of acute large-bowel ischemia in a California-based HMO was 15.6/100,000 patient years with increasing incidence associated with age. Patients presented with abdominal pain (87%) and bloody bowel movements (84%) without diffuse peritonitis. There are multiple etiologies of ischemic colitis that affect both young and old patients: shock, autoimmune diseases, coagulopathies, long-distance running (with associated dehydration), mesenteric venous thrombosis, acute arterial thrombosis, emboli, small vessel disease, and cocaine use.[45,46] Despite the multitude of etiologies, the typical patient with colonic ischemia is either an elderly patient or a patient with multiple comorbidities such as cardiovascular disease, hypertension, and renal failure.[45,47,48] Further support for the typical patient description was noted in Longstreth's population-based study of gastrointestinal ischemia where the average age was 69 and patients who were admitted for another disease process had an odds ratio of 7.48 (95% CI 2.19–25.54) for developing severe lower gastrointestinal ischemia after admission.[1] Other hospitalized patients with increased risk for ischemic colitis are patients undergoing open and endovascular abdominal aortic aneurysm repair for nonruptured aneurysms. These patients have an incidence of ischemic colitis of 2–3% in open procedures and 1.3–2.9% in endovascular interventions.[49–54]

In the literature, the described location of ischemic colitis is variable: right-sided, 8–14%, splenic flexure 23–28%, and left-sided, 50–87%.[55–57] Knowledge of the arterial blood supply and areas of collateral circulation is necessary to understand the potential areas for insult and the high likelihood of anatomic variations. In a cadaver study by Nelson et al.[58] only 22, 24, and 16% of dissected specimens had the typical branching of the celiac, superior mesenteric, and inferior mesenteric arteries respectively. In addition, colonic blood supply is dependent on interconnection of the perfusing vessels by the marginal artery of Drummond, which connects the superior and inferior mesenteric arteries through a series of arcades. At the splenic flexure, there is an area without vasa recta in 11% of individuals, which makes the area more susceptible to ischemic insult. The arc of Riolan is an artery connecting the left branch of the middle colic artery to the inferior mesenteric artery. It is present in only 7% of individuals but can allow acceptable perfusion in the absence of other collaterals. The highly variable arterial anatomy of the colon makes it susceptible to ischemia as a complication of surgical and angiographic procedures used to treat LGIB, which can compound the management considerations.

Acute mesenteric ischemia (small-bowel ischemia) can be either occlusive or nonocclusive. Occlusive mesenteric ischemia due to either embolization or thrombosis constitutes 50 and 25% of the cases of acute ischemia, whereas nonocclusive mesenteric ischemia and venous thrombosis account for 20 and 5% of the cases. Differentiating between occlusive and nonocclusive disease is imperative, since occlusive disease is managed emergently with surgery.[59] Massive bleeding from small-bowel ischemia is not likely to resolve spontaneously and may be a manifestation of transmural ischemia of the small bowel.

Other Colonic Etiologies

Postpolypectomy bleeding after colonoscopy ranges from 0.08 to 0.87% with mortality in a large Canadian study of over 97,000 colonoscopies estimated at 1/14,000.[60,61] Postpolypectomy bleeding accounted for 4.1% of cases in Longstreth's population-based study.[1] In the large VA and urban emergency medical center studies, postpolypectomy bleeding was not reported as a source of LGIB.[2,9]

Bleeding from a colorectal anastomosis requiring endoscopic therapy or surgery is rare with a rate of 0.5–1.8%.[62–64] If bleeding persists after resuscitation, transfusion, and correction of any coagulopathy, endoscopy should be used to identify and stop the bleeding. Therapeutic interventions include cautery, endoclips, and epinephrine injection. If these measures fail, surgical management should be undertaken.

Gastrointestinal bleeding is a common presenting symptom in ulcerative colitis and Crohn's disease. However, acute hemorrhage with hemodynamic compromise is atypical. The studies evaluating gastrointestinal hemorrhage in inflammatory bowel disease have small numbers of patients with the largest study including 38 patients reflecting this unusual event. Acute hemorrhage occurs in 0.9–6% of patients with Crohn's disease[65–67] and 1.4–4.2% for patients with ulcerative colitis.[68–70] As a percentage of patients presenting with LGIB, Crohn's disease accounts for 2.3–13% of cases with increasing percentages associated with higher volume studies.[1,2,9,69] Bleeding occurred in both young and older patients and was not related to the duration of disease.[70,71] Acute hemorrhage was the initial presentation of Crohn's disease in 16–23.5% of patients and is generally associated with areas of active inflammation.[72,73] Malignant lesions must also be considered in patients with long-standing history of inflammatory bowel disease (IBD) and LGIB.

Patients with human immunodeficiency virus (HIV)/acquired immune deficiency syndrome (AIDS) have additional etiologies for LGIB. Two studies with 1,003 HIV+ patients found the most common etiologies to be HIV-associated diseases: cytomegalovirus (CMV) colitis, idiopathic colonic ulcers, lymphoma, and idiopathic colitis.[74,75] Recurrent bleeding occurred in 17.6–22% of patients with mortality rates as high as 54.5%. Overall, the 30-day mortality rate was three times higher (14.4 versus 5%) for patients with HIV and LGIB than for the routine population.

NSAIDs commonly cause complications in the upper gastrointestinal tract. Documented adverse effects of NSAIDs on the lower gastrointestinal tract include increased gut permeability (44–70%), gut inflammation (60–70%), malabsorption (40–70%), and blood loss and anemia (30%).[76] A systematic review demonstrated the blood loss from NSAIDs and aspirin 325 mg was 1–2 ml/day, which was increased from the baseline level of 0.5 ml/day;[77] 5% of patients taking NSAIDs lost at least 5 ml/day. The MEDAL study was a randomized comparison of a cyclooxygenase (COX)-2 selective NSAID and a traditional NSAID with the primary gastrointestinal endpoint being lower gastrointestinal clinical events.[78] Over 34,000 patients with osteoarthritis and rheumatoid arthritis were followed for 18 months. Lower gastrointestinal bleeding was noted in 0.27% of patients. A quarter of these patients had lesions presumed to be caused by NSAIDs such as ulcers, colitis, and enteritis. Diverticula were the most common source of bleeding. There was no placebo group in this large study, so the ability to estimate the increase in adverse events with NSAID use versus placebo was not available. A systematic review of 47 studies examining the use of NSAIDs and lower gastrointestinal (LGI) events found an increase in LGI events with NSAID use.[79] However, the studies included in the review were varied; some were not originally designed to address the proposed hypothesis of the systematic review, and the studies of LGIB and NSAID use were either case-controlled or were unable to demonstrate a relationship due to the small sample size.[79] NSAID use is common, and physicians should be cognizant of the potential harmful effects of their use on the lower gastrointestinal tract.

Rectal injury due to pelvic radiation usually presents as bleeding and occurs in 95% of patients within 1 year from treatment. In most patients, bleeding will resolve, but in the minority of patients who go on to develop chronic radiation proctitis (5%), management is problematic and repetitive. Thermal coagulation with argon or Nd:Yag laser have been used with positive results.[80,81] Topical formalin in 3, 4, and 10% also has been successful for cessation of bleeding.[82,83] Three or four percent formalin is instilled in 50-ml aliquots for a total of 500 ml. Due to the associated rectal discomfort, this method is usually employed with some type of analgesia. After each application, the rectum is irrigated with normal saline. Another option ("Dab" method) is to use 16 Fr cotton-tipped applicator that is soaked in 10% formalin. This is applied to the rectal mucosa through an anoscope or a proctoscope. The Dab method can be performed in the office without analgesia.

Success rates in both procedures range between 75 and 90%. Surgical management is used as a last resort with high morbidity (65–80%) and mortality rates (6.7–13%).[84–86] Surgical options include diverting stoma and limited resections.[87]

Obscure Gastrointestinal Bleeding

Obscure gastrointestinal bleeding (OGIB) is the bleeding not identified during colonoscopy or esophagogastroduodenoscopy (EGD). OGIB accounts for 1.19–9% of LGIB with lower rates noted in larger studies.[1,9,31,88] Angiodysplasia, small-bowel tumors, and ulcers/erosions are the three most common etiologies of OGIB.[31,88,89] When diagnosing the source, patients with OGIB undergo more procedures than patients with upper gastrointestinal and colonic bleeding, 5.3 versus 1.5 and 2.1, respectively (Table 24-1).[89]

The diagnosis of OGIB was limited to upper and lower endoscopy and conventional radiography until 2001, when capsule endoscopy and double balloon enteroscopy (DBE) were introduced. Prior to these two technical advances, intraoperative enteroscopy was used to identify bleeding in the small bowel. Indications for capsule endoscopy include OGIB, unexplained iron-deficiency anemia, and suspected Crohn's disease, small-bowel tumors, or refractory malabsorptive syndromes.[90] Contraindications are related to the structure and transmission signal of the capsule as well as the need for normal peristalsis for capsule efficacy. Therefore, patients with swallowing disorders, pacemakers or implanted devices, obstruction, fistula, or stricture are not candidates for capsule endoscopy. Entrapment of the capsule occurs in 3.3% of procedures and is associated with Crohn's disease, radiation, and NSAID-induced strictures.[91,92] Indications for DBE include a positive capsule endoscopy and a high suspicion of a small-bowel source in the setting of a normal capsule study.[93–96] DBE has the ability to perform therapies such as sclerotherapy, polypectomy, dilations, and clippings. DBE can be performed from anterograde (oral) or retrograde (rectal) approach. Patients undergoing the anterograde approach require a 6–8 h fast prior to the procedure, while those having a retrograde exam need a bowel preparation.

The diagnostic yield of capsule endoscopy and DBE is 38–83% and 58%, respectively.[97–99] Two meta-analyses comparing capsule endoscopy and DBE found similar diagnostic yields.[100,101] Recent articles have supported the position that the techniques are complementary and should be used together to identify small-bowel sources of bleeding.[102,103]

TABLE 24-1. Diagnosis by etiology for patients admitted to an urban emergency medical center, 1998–2006[8]

Etiology	N (%)
Diverticulosis	227 (37.34)
Hemorrhoids	128 (21.05)
Neoplasia	72 (11.84)
Colitis	65 (10.69)
Inflammatory bowel disease	33 (5.43)
Vascular ectasias	14 (2.30)
Other colonic disease	40 (6.58)
Small-intestine disease	8 (1.32)
Unknown	21 (3.45)
Total	608 (100)

Positive capsule endoscopy can direct the DBE approach (oral or rectal) depending if the lesion is in the proximal or distal small bowel based on capsule transit time.[104] Currently, capsule endoscopy should be the first study ordered for OGIB. DBE is relatively new, not widely available, and associated with higher complication rates than diagnostic colonoscopy.[105–107]

Clinical Presentation, Physical Exam, and Management

LGIB has many presentations reflecting the diverse pathology found in the upper and lower gastrointestinal tract. The variety of presentations creates a diagnostic and management quandary. Adding to the quandary is the variability noted in studies regarding the presentation, workup, and management. The lack of randomized trials regarding diagnosis and management compounds the variability encountered with the presentation of LGIB.

Evaluation of a patient's hemodynamic stability upon presentation is imperative. Patients presenting with syncope, chest pain, pallor, shortness of breath, tachycardia, and changes in blood pressure with positioning are hemodynamically unstable. Tachycardia and hypotension represent acute hemorrhagic shock associated with a blood loss of more than 500 ml, or 15% of the total blood volume.[108] These patients require two large bore IVs or central venous access for resuscitation if peripheral access cannot be obtained. Continuous monitoring of vitals and urine output with a urinary bladder catheter are standard. Nasogastric tube (NG) placement has been recommended routinely to rule out an upper gastrointestinal source of bleeding. In a retrospective cohort study, 220 patients without hematemesis had a NG placed.[109] Only 2% of patients had bright red blood, greater than 450 ml of blood, or difficulty clearing the gastric lavage. Eight patients had an aspirate of bile, which was considered negative. However, 5 of these eight patients were found to have an upper gastrointestinal source of bleeding. The largest study (n = 1,190) evaluating NG tube aspirate found that 60% of patients with a negative aspirate had a lower gastrointestinal source.[110] However, 39% of patients with a negative aspirate were classified as having an unknown source of bleeding. Despite the results of these two studies, NG placement is a fast and inexpensive diagnostic test that if positive (clots, coffee ground emesis, blood), can quickly direct the workup toward identification of an upper gastrointestinal source. Upper gastrointestinal sources are seen in 11% of patients who present with a LGIB.[111] The NG tube can be left in and used for the bowel preparation if an urgent colonoscopy is needed.

After intravenous access has been obtained, resuscitation should start immediately. However, there are no systematic reviews, and only one randomized controlled trial evaluating the role of transfusions in gastrointestinal bleeding is available.[112] A Cochrane systematic review evaluating the resuscitation of trauma, burn, and surgical patients with either crystalloid or colloids found no survival benefit using colloids instead of crystalloids.[113] Despite the lack of large, randomized trials evaluating transfusion requirements in patients with LGIB, there is mounting evidence that limiting or eliminating transfusions lead to improved outcomes such as decreased mortality and morbidity.[114–118] The trauma literature has demonstrated that blood transfusions are an independent predictor of infection, multisystem organ failure, increased intensive-care length of stay, and death.[119–121] Patients who managed nonoperatively for blunt splenic and hepatic injuries have increased mortality rates if they are transfused.[122] A recent, risk-adjusted prospective study demonstrated a dose-dependent relationship between blood products transfused (blood, fresh frozen plasma, platelets) and increased mortality and infection.[123] Based on studies in the medical and surgical literature, transfusion practices in LGIB should be evaluated, and the decision to transfuse a patient should occur after the risks and benefits are analyzed.

The patient's history should be taken simultaneously with the placement of intravenous access and monitors if the patient is hemodynamically unstable. Important aspects of the history that should be elucidated are given as follows: frequency, volume, color and duration of bloody stools, comorbid conditions such as liver and cardiovascular disease, medication use such as clopidogrel, warfarin, and NSAIDs, and date of last colonoscopy/EGD.

Visual inspection of the perineum for prolapsed or thrombosed hemorrhoids, anal fissures, or masses are the first part of the anorectal exam. After visual inspection, digital rectal exam and anoscopy are performed. It is imperative to assess the anus, anal canal, and distal rectum prior to further diagnostic tests. Anoscopy can be performed efficiently at the bedside, and if a source is found, such as internal hemorrhoids, therapy can be provided.

Laboratory studies should include a chemistry panel, complete blood count, coagulation profile, and a type and cross. Any identified coagulopathies must be corrected with appropriate factors or products. Patients with cardiovascular disease should undergo an electrocardiogram, and if it turns out to be abnormal, cardiac enzymes are obtained.

After the initial clinical evaluation and review of laboratory values, the volume of hemorrhage can be classified into one of the following three groups: (1) minor and self-limited, (2) major and self-limited, and (3) major and ongoing.[124] Patients with minor and self-limited lower gastrointestinal bleeding with no or minimal change in hematocrit are unlikely to be hemodynamically unstable. These patients can undergo a colonoscopy during their admission or as an outpatient. Patients with massive, ongoing bleeding who remain hemodynamically unstable after initial resuscitation need urgent diagnosis and treatment either with angiography or with surgery. Patients in the middle of the spectrum with major bleeding who are stable or their bleeding has ceased are the patients at the core of the diagnostic dilemma surrounding LGIB. The three common diagnostic tests that can be employed for identifying the etiology of a LGIB are colonoscopy, angiography, and nuclear scintigraphy.

Colonoscopy

Colonoscopy can be both diagnostic and therapeutic. The likelihood of identifying the source of bleeding with colonoscopy ranges from 45 to 95% with the majority of studies with greater than 100 patients showing diagnostic yield rates of 89–97%.[8] The timing of colonoscopy is debatable. Urgent colonoscopy has been performed within 24 h, within 12 h, and after a fast oral purge, making comparison between studies challenging.[13,21,43,88,111,125,126] In some studies, early colonoscopy has been associated with decreased length of stay.[12,44] All studies evaluating urgent colonoscopy except one had patients undergo a bowel preparation, which would improve visualization and decrease the difficulty of the procedure and any endoscopic therapy. Endoscopic interventions were performed in 10–15% of patients who underwent an urgent colonoscopy.[127] Interventions include heater probes, argon plasma coagulation, bipolar coagulation, topical and intramucosal epinephrine, and endoclips (Figure 24-1). Overall complication rate of colonoscopy in LGIB is 1.3%.[128]

Patients with major, self-limited hemorrhage who have been resuscitated should undergo a bowel preparation with a polyethylene glycol solution and colonoscopy within 24 h. The goal of colonoscopy is to identify a source of bleeding and if possible, treat it endoscopically. If a bleeding source

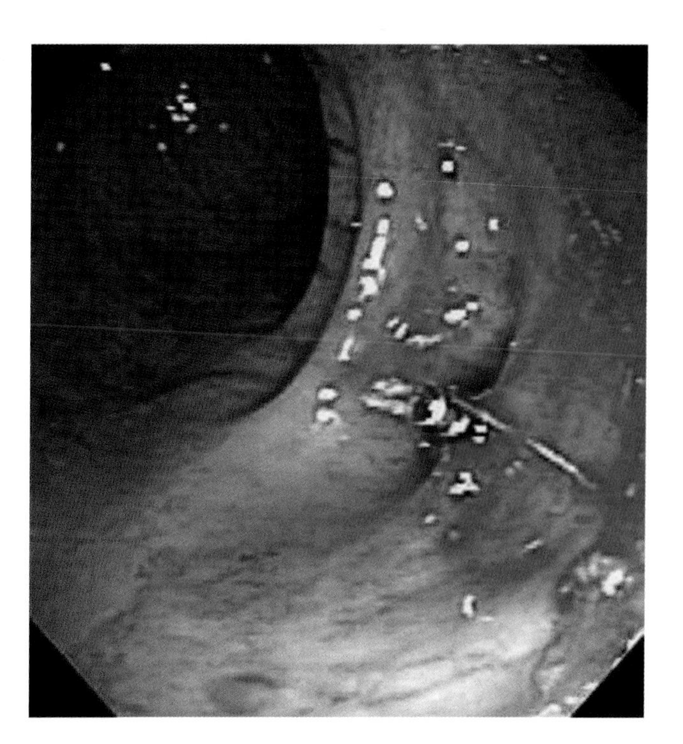

FIGURE 24-1. Clip applied to bleeding diverticular vessel.

is noted, the area should be marked, and the patients who rebleed require emergent surgery. Anatomic localization during endoscopy has known limitations and errors, and without a definitive mark (clip or tattoo) resection can be prone to error.

Angiography

Angiography can be both diagnostic and therapeutic (Figure 24-2). Angiography has both broad positivity (27–77%) and sensitivity (40–86%), with specificity being 100%.[18,128,129] For angiography to be positive, bleeding must occur at 0.5 ml/min or faster. Small, single-institution retrospective studies have shown blood pressure less than 90, transfusion requirement greater than 5 units, and a blush within 2 min on nuclear scintigraphy to be associated with positive angiograms.[130,131] Superselective embolization is the preferred treatment for positive angiograms. Recent studies have demonstrated success rates from 60 to 90%, rebleeding rates of 0–33%, and significant ischemia of less than 7%.[132,133] In addition, a meta-analysis found embolization of diverticular disease was three to four times more effective than embolization of nondiverticular sources.[132] Superselective embolization occurs at the level of the vasa recta or marginal artery.[134] Materials used for embolization include microcoils, polyvinyl alcohol particles, and gelfoam. They may be used individually or in combination. Microcoils are permanent materials with multiple sizes that are easily visible during fluoroscopy.[133,135] Polyvinyl alcohol particles are also permanent and will be carried by the circulation to the bleeding site which has the least resistance to flow.[136] These particles have decreased selectivity and are poorly visualized. Gelfoam is not a permanent agent with vessel recannulization in days to weeks.[137,138] but it is not routinely used. Material choice is decided by location, angiographer expertise, and microcatheter position in relation to the bleeding vessel.[139–142] Technical aspects that can lead to failure or inability to embolize are atherosclerosis, vascular tortuosity, and vasospasm.[134,139,143]

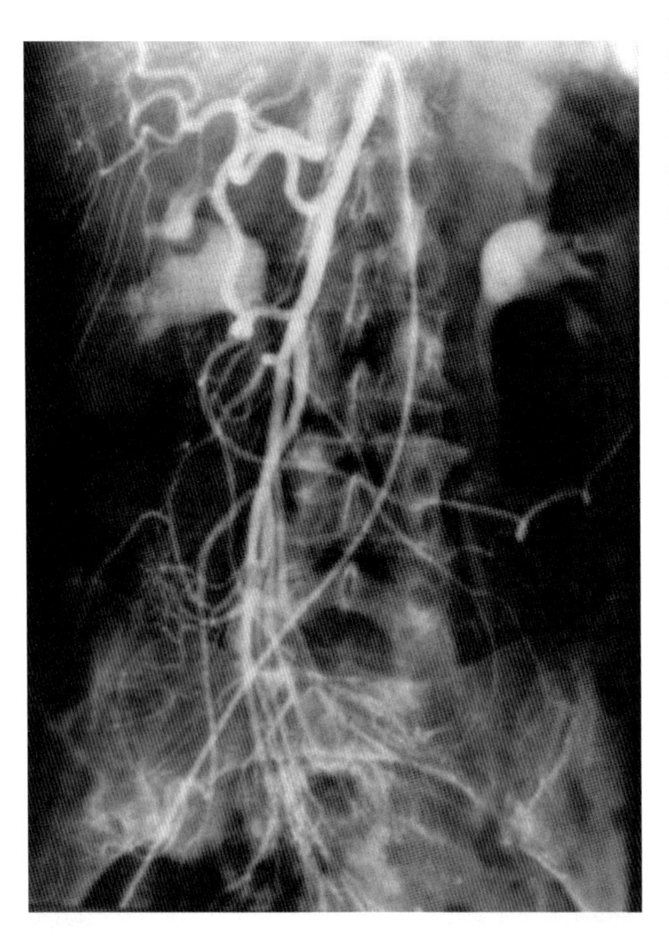

FIGURE 24-2. Angiogram demonstrating extravasation (hemorrhage) in cecum.

Patients with major, ongoing hemorrhage or patients who rebleed need angiography. Similar to colonoscopy, the goal of angiography is to localize the source of bleeding and provide directed therapy. If superselective embolization is unable to be performed, but a bleeding site is localized, angiographers can inject methylene blue into the artery providing a temporary marker for the surgeon.[144,145] Another option is highly selective, intra-arterial vasopressin infusion. The potent arterial contraction may reduce or halt the hemorrhage. Infusion rates of vasopressin being at concentrations of 0.2 U/min may progress to 0.4 U/min. The systemic effects and cardiac impact of vasopressin may limit maximizing the dosage. Vasopressin controls bleeding in as many as 91% of patients. However, bleeding may recur in as many as 50% of patients once the vasopressin is tapered.

In patients who have negative upper and lower endoscopy with continued evidence of bleeding, angiography can be used to localize the source. However, superselective embolization for sources other than diverticuli has higher failure rates.[132]

Since most LGIB is sporadic, it is not uncommon to be unable to localize the source, even after an EDG, a colonoscopy, and an angiography. Provocative angiography, which uses anticoagulants, vasodilators, or fibrinolytics to induce bleeding, can be used in these cases. Agents used in these procedures include urokinase, streptokinase, and tissue plasminogen activator. Studies evaluating provocative angiography are small and from single institutions with identification of the bleeding source varying from 20 to 80%.[146–148] If a bleeding site is identified, superselective embolization can be used for treatment.

Radionuclide Scintigraphy

Nuclear scintigraphy or the radioactive labeling of red blood cells is used to evaluate patients with LGIB (Figure 24-3A and B). In comparison to colonoscopy or angiography, it does not have any therapeutic capabilities. However, it is not invasive, does not require a bowel preparation, or require

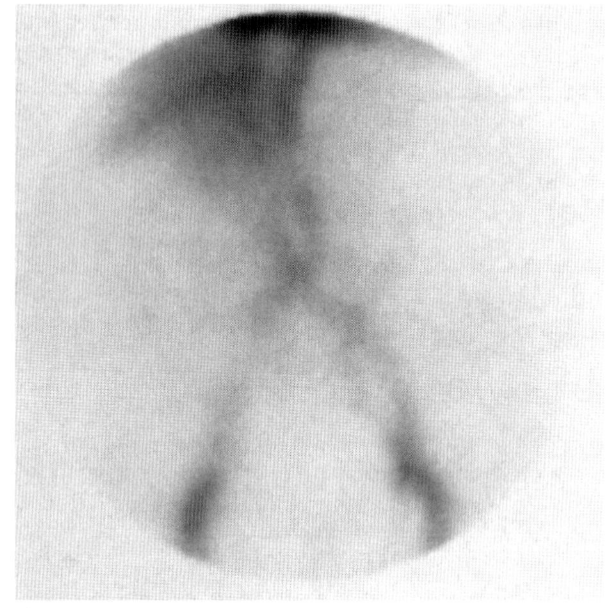

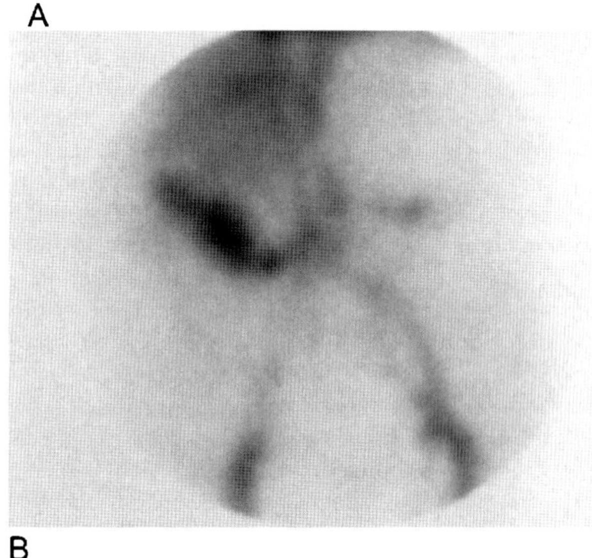

FIGURE 24-3. Selected images from a 99mTc-labeled RBC gastrointestinal bleeding study in a patient with known diverticulosis. Images acquired at 1 min **A** and 14 min **B**. Abnormal increased isotopic activity developed in the proximal transverse colon, which progressed antegrade to the descending colon.

specialists to be called in to perform the study. Bleeding at rates as low as 0.1 ml/min can be detected. Red blood cells are labeled with technetium or sulfur colloid. Technetium-labeled red blood cell (TRBC) scanning is positive in 16–91% of patients.[8,128] A number of studies have attempted to define characteristics of positive TRBC scans.[130,149,150] Scans that are positive early have shown increased positivity on angiography and accuracy rates in some studies, but not in others.[130,150–154] The largest study examining the predictive value of scintigraphy retrospectively reviewed 249 scans and 271 arteriograms. Using a positive scintigraphy as a requirement for angiography led to an increase in positive angiograms from 22 to 53%.[154] Common clinical parameters such as hemodynamic instability and the number of blood transfusions are not associated with a positive TRBC scan.[149,151,155] A more reliable indicator than the overall number of blood transfusions may be the number of units transfused within the 24 h preceding scintigraphy.[156] Multivariate analysis confirmed that patients who received more than 2 units of packed red blood cells within 24 h prior to the scan were twice as likely to have a positive study.

The role of radionuclide scintigraphy in the management of LGIB continues to be poorly defined. In patients who have major, self-limited hemorrhage and are stable to go to radiology, this test, if positive early, can direct further workup and management. However, if radionuclide scintigraphy is negative, rebleeding rates are not negligible. One advantage of TRBC is that rebleeding within 24 h can be restudied promptly without a second labeling procedure. This can allow a repeat study if the clinical condition changes during the evaluation period. A study from the Oschner Clinic where scintigraphy is the first diagnostic modality used after anoscopy/proctoscopy noted a rebleeding rate of 25% after a negative TRBC scan.[157] Colonoscopy performed after a negative scan found potential bleeding etiologies in 89% of patients.[130] More important than the rate of recurrent bleeding is the inability of scintigraphy to adequately localize the bleeding source to enable surgeons to reliably operate.[158–160] Surgical resection based on radionuclide scintigraphy is not recommended.

Multidetector Row CT

Multidetector row computed tomography (MDCT) may have an increasing role in the diagnostic workup of LGIB. In porcine models, blood flow can be detected at 0.3 ml/min, which is still less than those in angiography.[161] MDCT is considered positive when vascular contrast material is extravasated into the bowel lumen.[162] A meta-analysis of 94 patients demonstrated that 85% of MDCT abnormalities correlated with lesions identified during surgery and that 72% of patients who underwent angiography had confirmed bleeding sources.[163] Similar to angiography, scintigraphy, and colonoscopy, MDCT positivity and confirmation vary by study due to different inclusion criteria (upper and lower gastrointestinal bleeding versus only lower), number of CT slices (16 or 64), and sample size (all less than 60).[162–167] There are no randomized controlled or multicenter studies. Despite these limitations, MDCT offers the following advantages over radionuclide scintigraphy: (1) it is easy to perform and readily available in emergency rooms with CT scanners, (2) accurate localization of the bleeding site, which allows for a directed angiogram and less contrast use, (3) identification of other pathologies.[162,166]

Surgery

Emergent surgery is necessary in hemodynamically unstable patients who have massive ongoing bleeding and are unresponsive to the initial resuscitation, patients who have had the source of bleeding localized but no therapeutic measures were performed or they failed, and patients who have required at least 6 units of packed red cells within 24 h.[124] The need for emergent, exploratory surgery without a localized source of bleeding is uncommon, occurring in 4.8% of patients with LGIB at an urban medical center.[9] In Longstreth's study, 16% of patients underwent surgery.[1] Taking into account the patient's clinical status, comorbidities, and localization studies, the surgeon can devise an operative strategy to fit the patient.[124] Prior to surgery, ileostomy and colostomy sites should be marked when possible.

An open laparotomy through a midline incision that allows access to both the upper and lower gastrointestinal tract should be performed. Examination of the entire intra-abdominal gastrointestinal tract is required with focus on identifying blood within the bowel lumen. The stomach, duodenum, small bowel, and colon are visually examined and palpated.[124]

If there is no identifiable bleeding source and localization was not successful, push intraoperative enteroscopy (IOE) can be considered. Transillumination of the bowel may identify a source such as angiodysplasia or small tumors. IOE is technically challenging and time-consuming. The identification of bleeding pathology occurs in 70–87% of patients. However, rebleeding rates are 19–30%.[168–171] If a source of bleeding is identified, then resection is warranted.

If no bleeding site is identified in the upper gastrointestinal tract or small bowel and the source is presumed to be colonic, then a total abdominal colectomy should be performed. If the patient was on vasoactive medication or is hemodynamically unstable, then an end ileostomy should be created. Postoperatively, these patients will require further resuscitation and possibly continued or intermittent pressor use, which can jeopardize a bowel anastomosis. In addition, the majority of patients with LGIB are elderly with multiple comorbidities augmenting the complexity of their management.

The aim of the preoperative diagnostic workup is to localize the source of bleeding. If a colonic source is localized, then a segmental rather than subtotal colectomy can be performed. Nonlocalized segmental colectomy based on a clinical "best guess" is not a safe or reliable option. Mortality can be as high as 50% and rebleeding rates as high as 75%.[19,172,173] Mortality rates associated with segmental and subtotal colectomy for LGIB are 4–14% and 0–40%, respectively.[18]

Outcomes in Lower Gastrointestinal Bleeding

The heterogeneity of patients with LGIB and the lack of randomized data concerning the diagnostic workup have led to studies attempting to characterize prognostic indicators (Table 24-2). The following clinical data are independent predictors of severity in LGIB: initial heart rate greater than or equal to 100, initial systolic blood pressure less than or equal to 115 mmHg, initial hematocrit less than or equal to 35%, gross blood on rectal exam or rectal bleeding within the first 4 h of evaluation, aspirin use, and more than two active comorbid conditions.[4,9] Severe LGIB was defined by one or more of the following clinical characteristics: transfusion of greater than or equal to 2 units of blood, decrease of hematocrit by greater than or equal to 20% in the first 24 h, and recurrent rectal bleeding after 24 h of stability coinciding with a further decrease in hematocrit of greater than or equal to 20%, more transfusions, and readmission within 1 week of discharge.[174] Patients were considered high risk if they had greater than 3 risk factors and low risk if they had no risk factors. High-risk patients had increased rates of surgery and death, increased number of transfusions, and longer hospital stays.[174] Prognostic factors for urgent surgery are hypotension on arrival (systolic blood pressure 70–80 mmHg) and the etiology of the bleeding.[7] Urgent surgery and associated comorbidities (neuropathies, diabetes, hepatic, cardiovascular and pulmonary disease) were risk factors for morbidity and mortality.[7] Postoperatively, only transfusion needs greater than ten units predicted mortality and morbidity after multivariate analysis.[3] The average number of units transfused prior to surgery in this study was 9.3. These findings support an earlier study from 1991 where patients who received less than ten units had a 7% mortality

Table 24-2. Mortality of lower gastrointestinal bleeding by etiology[124]

Investigator [ref]	Diverticulosis (%)	Angiodysplasia (%)	Cancer/polyp (%)	Colitis/ulcer (%)	Anorectal (%)	Other (%)	Mortality (%)
Jensen and Machicado 1997[111]	23	40	15	12	5	4	NA
Longstreth 1997[1]	41	3	9	16	5	14	3.6
Bramley et al. 1996[6]	24	7	10	21	9	4	5.1
Richter et al. 1995[7]	48	12	11	6	3	6	2
Rossini et al. 1989[30]	15	4	30	22	0	11	NA
Jensen and Machicado 1988[28]	20	37	14	11	5	5	NA

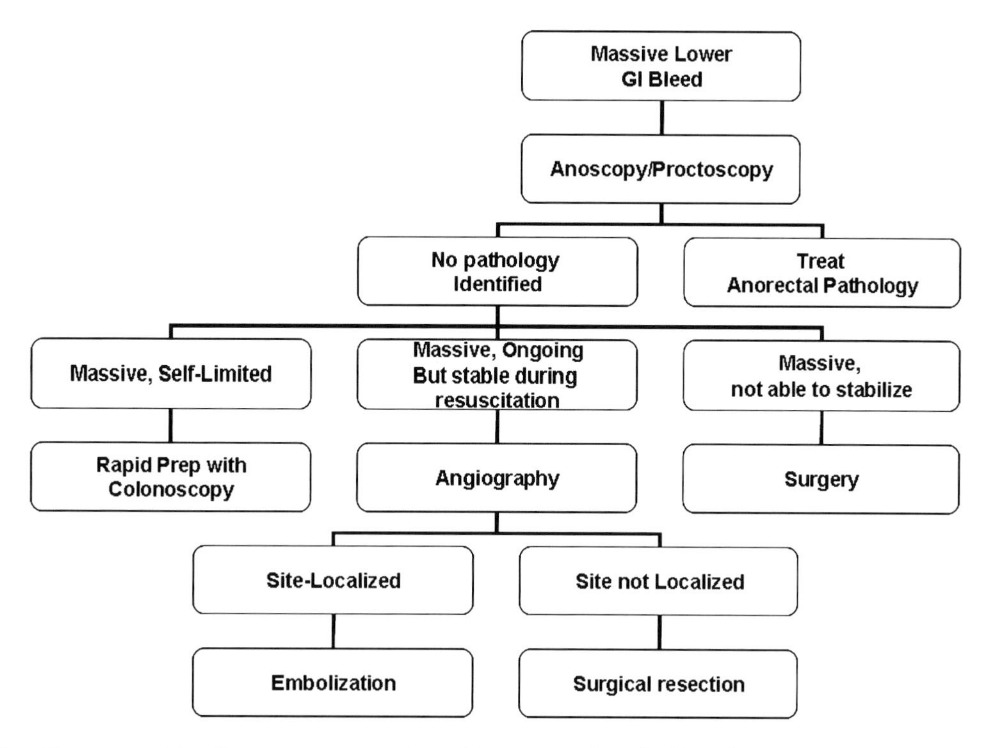

FIGURE 24-4. Algorithm summarizing the management options of lower gastrointestinal bleeding.

rate and patients who received greater than ten units had a mortality rate of 27%.[173]

The literature has shown that there are multiple options in the workup of LGIB that can be used interchangeably with adequate results. Urgent endoscopy can be performed as the first diagnostic step, followed by other localizing studies if not successful, but evaluation with TRBC followed by selective angiography if TRBC is positive can also be successful for localization. Studies have shown clearly that segmental colon resection after radionuclide scintigraphy alone is ill-advised and that blind resections have high rebleeding rates and lead to worse patient outcomes. The steps in the workup remain variable but should be tailored to a physician's expertise and hospital resources.

Billingham's[175] description, in 1997, of LGIB as a conundrum with five main problems continues to reflect the current management issues. First, bleeding can be from any location in the gastrointestinal tract. The second problem faced by surgeons is the sporadic nature of lower gastrointestinal bleeding. The third problem is the necessity of surgical intervention prior to localization. Fourth, rebleeding after extensive resections remains a concern. Finally, there are few consensus statements regarding diagnosis and management. Certainly, the conundrum has not been solved. However, a variety of new technologies and evolving methods of treatment are allowing clinicians to make progress with less dramatic interventions for patients. New imaging techniques such as MDCT may be able to efficiently identify sources of bleeding and guide management with less delay and better anatomic definition. Superselective angiography can provide safe and accurate diagnostic and therapeutic options. Capsule endoscopy can assist in locating obscure bleeding sources and has become the standard of care for workup in a nonacute setting. DBE will become more available and may provide multiple therapeutic options for lesions not reached by traditional endoscopic techniques, but is not advocated in the urgent or emergent setting at this time. Acceptance and practice of urgent colonoscopy and superselective angiography provide opportunities to identify the source prior to surgery and even avoid surgery entirely. In addition, the diagnostic and therapeutic options available with colonoscopy, capsule endoscopy, DBE, and superselective angiography offer a variety of options to localize and treat the source with minimal risk compared to emergent surgery. Nevertheless, LGIB can be a challenging event for the patient and physician. Successful treatment of LGIB requires the ability to perform massive resuscitation, expeditious workup, and skilled surgical assessment with prompt operative intervention when required. An algorithm summarizing the management is provided in Figure 24-4.

Acknowledgment. This chapter was written by Frank G. Opelka, J. Byron Bathright, and David E. Beck in the first edition of this textbook.

References

1. Longstreth GF. Epidemiology and outcome of patients hospitalized with acute lower gastrointestinal hemorrhage: a population-based study. Am J Gastroenterol. 1997;92:419–24.
2. Vernava AM, Longo WE, Virgo KS, Johnson FE. A nationwide study of the incidence and etiology of lower gastrointestinal bleeding. Surg Res Comm. 1996;18:113–20.
3. Czymek R, Kempf A, Roblick U, et al. Factors predicting the postoperative outcome of lower gastrointestinal hemorrhage. Int J Colorectal Dis. 2009;24:983–8.
4. Velayos FS, Williamson A, Sousa KH, et al. Early predictors of severe lower gastrointestinal bleeding and adverse outcomes: a prospective study. Clin Gastroenterol Hepatol. 2004;2:485–90.
5. Brackman MR, Gushchin VV, Smith L, et al. Acute lower gastroenteric bleeding retrospective analysis (The ALGEBRA Study): An analysis of the triage, management and outcomes of patients with acute lower gastrointestinal bleeding. Am Surg. 2003;69:145–9.
6. Strate LL, Orav EJ, Syngal S. Early predictors of severity in acute lower intestinal tract bleeding. Arch Intern Med. 2003;163:838–43.
7. Rios A, Montoya MJ, Rodriguez JM, et al. Severe acute lower gastrointestinal bleeding: risk factors for morbidity and mortality. Langenbecks Arch Surg. 2007;392:165–71.
8. Strate LL. Lower GI bleeding: epidemiology and diagnosis. Gastroenterol Clin N Am. 2005;34:643–64.
9. Gayer C, Chino A, Lucas C, et al. Acute lower gastrointestinal bleeding in 1, 112 patients admitted to an urban emergency medical center. Surgery. 2009;146:600–7.
10. Lanas A, Garcia-Rodriguez LA, Polo-Tomas M, et al. Time trends and impact of upper and lower gastrointestinal bleeding and perforation in clinical practice. Am J Gastroenterol. 2009;104:1633–41.
11. Strate LL, Syngal S. Predictors of utilization of early colonoscopy vs. radiography for severe lower intestinal bleeding. Gastrointest Endosc. 2005;61:46–52.
12. Schmulewitz N, Fisher DA, Rockey DC. Early colonoscopy for acute lower GI bleeding predicts shorter hospital stay: a retrospective study of experience in a single center. Gastrointest Endosc. 2003;58:841–6.
13. Green BT, Rockey DC, Portwood G, et al. Urgent colonoscopy for evaluation and management of acute lower gastrointestinal hemorrhage: a randomized controlled trial. Am J Gastroenterol. 2005;100:2395–402.
14. Peura DA, Lanza FL, Gostout CJ, et al. The American College of Gastroenterology bleeding registry: preliminary findings. Am J Gastroenterol. 1997;92:924–8.
15. Martel J, Raskin J. History, incidence and epidemiology of diverticulosis. J Clin Gastroenterol. 2008;42(10):1125–7.
16. Rushford AJ. The significance of bleeding as a symptom of diverticulitis. J R Soc Med. 1956;49:577–9.
17. McGuire Jr HH. Bleeding colonic diverticula. A reappraisal of natural history and management. Ann Surg. 1994;220:653–6.
18. Vernava AM, Moore BA, Longo WE, Johnson FE. Lower gastrointestinal bleeding. Dis Colon Rectum. 1997;40:846–58.
19. McGuire Jr JJ, Haynes Jr BW. Massive hemorrhage from diverticulosis of the colon: guidelines for therapy based on bleeding patterns observed in 50 cases. Ann Surg. 1972;175:847–53.
20. Meyers MA, Alonso DR, Baer JW. Pathogenesis of massively bleeding colonic diverticulosis: new observations. Am J Roentgenol. 1976;127:901–8.
21. Jensen DM, Machicado GA, Jutabha R, et al. Urgent colonoscopy for the diagnosis and treatment of severe diverticular hemorrhage. N Engl J Med. 2000;342:78–82.
22. Smoot RL, Gostout CJ, Rajan E, et al. Is early colonoscopy after admissión for acute diverticular bleeding needed? Am J Gastroenterol. 2003;98:1996–9.
23. Kanwal F, Dulai G, Jensen DM, et al. Major stigmata of recent hemorrhage on rectal ulcers in patients with severe hematochezia: endoscopic diagnosis, treatment, and outcomes. Gastrointest Endsoc. 2003;57:462–8.
24. Thompson WHF. The nature of hemorrhoids. Br J Surg. 1975;62:542–52.
25. Beck DE. Hemorrhoidal disease. In: Beck DE, Wexner SD, editors. Fundamentals of anorectal surgery. 2nd ed. London, UK: W.B. Saunders Company Ltd; 1998. p. 237–53.
26. Thulesius O, Gjores JE. Arterio-venous anastomosis in the anal region with reference to the pathogénesis and treatment of hemorrhoids. Acta Chir Scand. 1973;139:476–8.
27. Caos A, Benner KD, Manier J, et al. Colonoscopy after Golytely preparation in acute rectal bleeding. J Clin Gastroenterol. 1986;8:46–9.
28. Jenson DM, Machicado GA. Diagnosis and treatment of severe hematochezia: the role of urgent colonoscopy after purge. Gastroenterology. 1988;95:1569–74.
29. Leitman IM, Paull DE, Shires GT. Evaluation and management of massive lower gastrointestinal hemorrhage. Ann Surg. 1989;209:175–80.
30. Rossini FP, Ferrari A, Spandre M, et al. Emergency colonoscopy. World J Surg. 1989;13:190–2.
31. Okazaki H, Fujiwara Y, Sugimori S, et al. Prevalence of mid-gastrointestinal bleeding in patients with acute overt gastrointestinal bleeding: multi-center experience with 1, 044 consecutive patients. J Gastroenterol. 2009;44:550–5.
32. Sun B, Rajan E, Cheng S, et al. Diagnostic yield and therapeutic impact of double-balloon enteroscopy in a large cohort of patients with obscure gastrointestinal bleeding. Am J Gastroenterol. 2006;101:2011–5.
33. Pennazio M, Santucci R, Rondonotti E, et al. Outcome of patients with obscure gastrointestinal bleeding after capsule endoscopy: report of 100 consecutive cases. Gastroenterology. 2004;126:643–53.
34. Foutch PG, Rex DK, Lieberman DA. Prevalence and natural history of colonic angiodysplasia among healthy asymptomatic people. Am J Gastroenterol. 1995;90:564–7.
35. Boley SJ, DiBase A, Brandt LJ. Lower intestinal bleeding in the elderly. Am J Surg. 1979;137:57–64.
36. Nath RL, Sequeira JC, Weitzman AF, et al. Lower gastrointestinal bleeding: diagnostic approach and management conclusions. Am J Surg. 1981;141:478–81.
37. Santos JCM, Aprilli F, Guimaraes AS, et al. Angiodysplasia of the colon: endoscopic diagnosis and treatment. Br J Surg. 1988;75:256–8.
38. Bhutami MS, Gupta SC, Markert RJ, et al. A prospective controlled evaluation of endoscopic detection of angiodysplasia and its association with aortic valve disease. Gastrointest Endosc. 1995;42:389–402.

39. Imperiale TF, Ransohoff DF. Aortic stenosis, idiopathic gastrointestinal bleeding, and angiodysplasia: Is there an association? A methodologic critique of the literature. Gastroenterology. 1988;95:1670–6.
40. Ferraris R, Senore C, Fracchia M, et al. Predictive value of rectal bleeding for distal colonic neoplastic lesions in a screened population. Eur J Cancer. 2004;40:245–52.
41. Helfand M, Marton KI, Zimmer-Gembeck MJ, et al. History of visible rectal bleeding in a primary care population: initial assessment and 10-year follow-up. JAMA. 1997;277:44–8.
42. Lasson A, Kilander A, Stotzer P. Diagnostic yield of colonoscopy based on symptoms. Scan J Gastroenterol. 2008;43:356–62.
43. Ohyama T, Sakurai Y, Ito M, et al. Analysis of urgent colonoscopy for lower gastrointestinal tract bleeding. Digestion. 2000;61:189–92.
44. Strate LL, Syngal S. Timing of colonoscopy: impact on length of hospital stay in patients with acute lower intestinal bleeding. Am J Gastroenterol. 2003;98:317–22.
45. Longo WE, Oliver GC. Less common benign disorders of the colon and rectum. In: Wolff BG, Fleshman JW, Beck DE, Pemberton JH, Wexner SD, editors. The ASCRS textbook of colon and rectal surgery. NY: Springer Science + Business Media, LLC; 2007. p. 601–2.
46. Preventza OA, Lazarides K, Sawyer MD. Ischemic colitis in young adults: a single institution experience. J Gastrointest Surg. 2001;5:328–32.
47. Guttmorson NL, Burbrick MP. Mortality from ischemic colitis. Dis Colon Rectum. 1989;32:469–72.
48. Newman LA, Mittman N, Hunt Z, Alfonso AE. Survival among chronic renal failure patients requiring major abdominal surgery. J Am Coll Surg. 1999;188:310–4.
49. Miller A, Marotta M, Scordi-Bello I, et al. Ischemic colitis after endovascular aortoiliac aneurysm repair. A 10 year retrospective study. Arch Surg. 2009;144:900–3.
50. Mehta M, Roddy S, Darling III C, et al. Infrarenal abdominal aortic aneurysm repair via endovascular versus open retroperitoneal approach. Ann Vasc Surg. 2005;19:374–8.
51. Moore WS, Kashyap VS, Vescera CL, et al. Abdominal aortic aneurysm: a 6-year comparison of endovascular versus transabdominal repair. Ann Surg. 1999;230:298–306.
52. Dadian N, Ohki T, Veith FJ, et al. Overt colon ischemia after endovascular aneurysm repair: the importance of microembolization as an etiology. J Vasc Surg. 2001;34:986–96.
53. Zhang WW, Kulaylat MN, Anain PM, et al. Embolization as a cause of bowel ischemia after endovascular abdominal aortic aneurysm repair. J Vasc Surg. 2004;40:867–72.
54. Maldonado TS, Rockman CB, Riles E, et al. Ischemic complications alter endovascular abdominal aortic aneurysm repair. J Vasc Surg. 2004;40:703–9. discussion 709-710.
55. Longo WE, Ballantyne GH, Gusberg RJ. Ischemic colitis patterns and prognosis. Dis Colon Rectum. 1992;35:726–30.
56. Longstreth GF, Yao JF. Epidemiology, clinical features, high-risk factors, and outcomes of acute large bowel ischemia. Clin Gastroenterol Hepatol. 2009;7:1075–80.
57. Scharff JR, Longo WE, Vartanian SM, et al. Ischemic colitis: spectrum of disease and outcome. Surgery. 2003;134:624–30.
58. Nelson TM, Pollack R, Jonasson O, Abcarian H. Anatomic variants of the celiac, superior mesenteric and inferior mesenteric arteries and their clinical significance. Clin Anat. 1988;1:75–91.
59. Paterno F, Longo WE. The etiology and pathogenesis of vascular disorders of the intestine. Radiol Clin N Am. 2008;46:877–85.
60. Rabeneck L, Paszat LF, Hilsden RJ, et al. Bleeding and perforation after outpatient colonoscopy and their risk factors in usual clinical practice. Gastroenterology. 2008;135:1899–906.
61. Warren JL, Klabunde CN, Mariotto AB, et al. Adverse events after outpatient colonoscopy in the Medicare population. Ann Intern Med. 2009;150:849–57.
62. Martínez-Serrano MA, Parés D, Pera M, et al. Management of lower gastrointestinal bleeding after colorectal resection and stapled anastomosis. Tech Coloproctol. 2009;13(1):49–53.
63. Cirocco WC, Golub RW. Endoscopic treatment of postoperative hemorrhage from a stapled colorectal anastomosis. Am Surg. 1995;61(5):460–3.
64. Malik AH, East JE, Buchanan GN, Kennedy RH. Endoscopic haemostasis of staple-line haemorrhage following colorectal resection. Colorectal Dis. 2008;10(6):616–8.
65. Robert JH, Sachar DB, Greenstein AJ. Severe gastrointestinal hemorrhage in Crohn's disease. Ann Surg. 1991;213:207–11.
66. Cirocco WC, Reilly JC, Rusin LC. Life-threatening hemorrhage and exsanguination from Crohn's disease. Report of four cases. Dis Colon Rectum. 1995;38:85–95.
67. Driver CP, Anderson DN, Keenan RA. Massive intestinal bleeding in association with Crohn's disease. J R Coll Surg Edinb. 1996;41:152–4.
68. Robert JH, Sachar DB, Aufses AH, et al. Management of severe hemorrhage in ulcerative colitis. Am J Surg. 1990;159:550–5.
69. Edwards FC, Truelove SC. The course and prognosis of ulcerative colitis. III Complications. Gut. 1964;5:1–26.
70. Bruce D, Cole WH. Complications of ulcerative colitis. Ann Surg. 1962;155:768–81.
71. Barnacle AM, Aylwin AC, Jackson JE. Angiographic diagnosis of inflammatory bowel disease in patients presenting with gastrointestinal bleeding. Am J Roentgenol. 2006;187:976–85.
72. Pardi DS, Loftus EV, Tremaine WJ, et al. Acute major gastrointestinal hemorrhage in inflammatory bowel disease. Gastrointest Endosc. 1999;49:153–7.
73. Belaiche J, Louis E, D'Haens G, et al. Acute lower gastrointestinal bleeding in Crohn's disease: characteristics of a unique series of 34 patients. Am J Gastroenterol. 1999;94:2177–81.
74. Chalasani N, Wilcox CM. Etiology and outcome of lower gastrointestinal bleeding in patients with AIDS. Am J Gastroenterol. 1998;93:175–8.
75. Bini EJ, Weinshel EH, Falkenstein DB. Risk factors for recurrent bleeding and mortality in human immunodeficiency virus-infected with acute lower GI hemorrhage. Gastrointest Endosc. 1999;49:748–53.
76. Lanas A, Sopena F. Nonsteroidal anti-inflammatory drugs and lower gastrointestinal complications. Gastroenterol Clin N Am. 2009;38:333–52.
77. Moore RA, Derry S, Henry J, et al. Faecal blood loss with aspirin, nonsteroidal anti-inflammatory drugs & cyclo-oxygenase-2 selective inhibitors: systematic review of randomized trials using autologous chromium labelled erythrocytes. Arthritis Res Ther. 2008;10:R7.
78. Laine L, Curtis SP, Langman M, et al. Lower gastrointestinal events in a double-blind trial of the cyclo-oxygenase-2 selective inhibitor etoricoxib and the traditional nonsteroidal anti-inflammatory drug diclofenac. Gastroenterology. 2008;135:1517–25.

79. Laine L, Smith R, Min K, Dubois RW. Systematic review: the lower gastrointestinal adverse effects of non-steroidal anti-inflammatory drugs. Aliment Pharmacol Ther. 2006;24:751–67.
80. Postgate A, Saunders B, Tjandra J, Vargo J. Argon plasma coagulation in chronic radiation proctitis. Endoscopy. 2007;39: 361–5.
81. Tjandra JJ, Sengupta S. Argon plasma coagulation is an effective treatment for refractory hemorrhagic radiation proctitis. Dis Colon Rectum. 2001;44(12):1759–65.
82. DeParades V, Etienney I, Bauer P, et al. Formalin application in the treatment of chronic radiation-induced hemorrhagic proctitis-an effective but not risk-free procedure: a prospective study of 33 patients. Dis Colon Rectum. 2005;48:1535–41.
83. Counter SF, Froese DP, Hart MJ. Prospective evaluation of formalin therapy for radiation proctitis. Am J Surg. 1999;177:396–8.
84. Jao SW, Beart Jr RW, Gunderson LL. Surgical treatment of radiation injuries of the colon and rectum. Am J Surg. 1986;151:272–7.
85. Pricolo VE, Shellito PC. Surgery for radiation injury to the large intestine variables influencing outcome. Dis Colon Rectum. 1994;37:675–84.
86. Kimose HH, Fischer L, Spjeldnaes N, Wara P. Late radiation injury of the colon and rectum Surgical management and outcome. Dis Colon Rectum. 1989;32:684–9.
87. Denton AS, Andreyev JJ, Forbes A, Maher J. Non surgical interventions for late radiation proctitis in patients who have received radical radiotherapy to the pelvis. Cochrane Database of Systematic Reviews 2002, Issue 1. Art. No.: CD003455. DOI: 10.1002/14651858.CD003455.
88. Jensen DM, Machicado GA. Diagnosis and treatment of severe hematochezia. The role of urgent colonoscopy after purge. Gastroenterology. 1988;95:1569–74.
89. Prakash C, Zuckerman GR. Acute small bowel bleeding: a distinct entity with significantly different economic implications compared with GI bleeding from other locations. Gastrointest Endosc. 2003;58:330–5.
90. ASGE Technology status evaluation report: wireless capsule endoscopy. Gastrointest Endosc 2006;63 (4):539–545.
91. Cheifetz AS, Lewis BS. Capsule retention: is it a complication? J Clin Gastroenterol. 2006;40:688–91.
92. Sachdev MS, Leighton JA, Fleischer DE, et al. A prospective study of the utility of abdominal radiographs after capsule endoscopy for the diagnosis of capsule retention. Gastrointest Endosc. 2007;66:894–900.
93. Yamamoto H, Kita H. Double-balloon endoscopy: from concept to reality. Gastrointest Endosc Clin N Am. 2006;16(2): 347–61.
94. May A, Ell C. European experiences with push-and-pull enteroscopy in double-balloon technique (double-balloon endoscopy). Gastrointest Endosc Clin N Am. 2006;16(2):377–82.
95. Martins NB, Wassef W. Upper gastrointestinal bleeding. Curr Opin Gastroenterol. 2006;22(6):612–9.
96. Lo SK. Small bowel endoscopy: have we conquered the final frontier? Am J Gastroenterol. 2007;102(3):536–8.
97. Rondonotti E, Villa F, Mulder CJJ, et al. Small bowel capsule endoscopy in 2007: indications, risks and limitations. World J Gastroenterol. 2007;14:6140–9.
98. Pennazio M, Santucci R, Rondonotti E, et al. Outcome of patients with obscure gastrointestinal bleeding after capsule endoscopy: report of 100 consecutive patients. Gastroenterology. 2004;126:643–53.
99. Ohmiya N, Yano T, Yamamoto H, et al. Diagnosis and treatment of obscure GI bleeding at double balloon endoscopy. Gastrointest Endosc. 2007;66(3 Suppl):S72–7.
100. Pasha SF, Leighton JA, Das A, et al. Double-balloon enteroscopy and capsule endoscopy have comparable diagnostic yield in small-bowel disease: a metaanalysis. Clin Gastroenterol Hepatol. 2008;6:671–6.
101. Chen X, Ran ZH, Tong JL, et al. A meta-analysis of the yield of capsule endoscopy compared to double-balloon enteroscopy in patients with small bowel diseases. World J Gastroenterol. 2007;13:4372–8.
102. Alexander JA, Leighton JA. Capsule endoscopy and balloon-assisted endoscopy: competing or complementary technologies in the evaluation of small bowel disease? Curr Opin Gastroenterol. 2009;25:433–7.
103. Kamalaporum P, Cho S, Basset N, et al. Double-balloon enteroscopy following capsule endoscopy in the management of obscure gastrointestinal bleeding: outcome of combined approach. Can J Gastroenterol. 2008;22(5):491–5.
104. Gay G, Delvaux M, Fassler I. Outcome of capsule endoscopy in determining indication and route for push-and-pull enteroscopy. Endoscopy. 2006;38:49–58.
105. Gerson L, Kamal A. Cost effectiveness analysis of management strategies for obscure GI bleeding. Gastrointest Endosc. 2008;65:920–36.
106. Mensink PB, Haringsma J, Kucharzik T, et al. Complications of double balloon enteroscopy: a multicenter survey. Endoscopy. 2007;39:613–5.
107. Gerson L, Tokar J, Decker A, et al. Complications associated with double balloon enteroscopy: the U.S. experience. Am J Gastroenterol. 2008;103:AB S109.
108. Thompson ABR, Shaffer EA. First principles of gastroenterology: the basis of disease and an approach to management. 3rd ed. Toronto, Ontario, Canada: University of Toronto Press; 1992. 392.
109. Witting MD, Magder L, Heins AE, et al. Usefulness and validity of diagnostic nasogastric aspiration in patients without hematemesis. Ann Emerg Med. 2004;43:525–32.
110. Luk GD, Bynum TE, Hendrix TR. Gastric aspiration in localization of gastrointestinal hemorrhage. JAMA. 1979;241:576–8.
111. Jensen DM, Machicado GA. Colonoscopy for diagnosis and treatment of severe lower gastrointestinal bleeding. Routine outcomes and cost analysis. Gastrointest Endosc Clin N Am. 1997;7:477–98.
112. Blair SD, Janvrin SB, McCollum CN, et al. Effect of early blood transfusion on gastrointestinal haemorrhage. Br J Surg. 1986;73:783–5.
113. Perel P, Roberts I, Pearson M. Colloids versus crystalloids for fluid resuscitation in critically ill patients. Cochrane Database of Systematic Reviews 2008, Issue 3. Art. No.: CD000567.
114. Rahbari NN, Zimmermann JB, Schmidt T, et al. Meta-analysis of standard, restrictive, and supplemental fluid administration in colorectal surgery. Br J Surg. 2009;96:331–41.
115. Herbert PC, Wells G, Blajchman MA, et al. A multicenter, randomized, controlled clinical trial of transfusion requirements in critical care. N Engl J Med. 1999;340:409–17.
116. Vincent JL, Baron JF, Reinhart K, et al. Anemia and blood transfusion in critically ill patients. JAMA. 2002;288:1499–507.

117. Garcia-Tsao G, Sanyal AJ, Grace ND, et al. Prevention and management of gastroesophageal varices and variceal hemorrhage in cirrhosis. Am J Gastroenterol. 2007;102:2086–102.
118. Marik PE, Corwin HL. Efficacy of red blood cell transfusion in the critically ill: a systematic review of the literature. Crit Care Med. 2008;36:2667–74.
119. Malone DL, Dunne J, Tracy JK, et al. Blood transfusion, independent of shock severity, is associated with worse outcome in trauma. J Trauma. 2003;54:898–905.
120. Dunne JR, Malone DL, Tracy JK, Napolitano LM. Allogenic blood transfusion in the first 24 hours after trauma is associated with increased systemic inflammatory response syndrome (SIRS) and death. Surg Infect (Larchmont) 2004;Winter:395–404.
121. Moore FA, Moore EE, Sauaia A. Blood transfusion. An independent risk factor for post-injury multiple organ failure. Arch Surg. 1997;132:620–4. discussion 624-625.
122. Robinson 3rd WP, Ahn J, Stiffler A, et al. Blood transfusion is an independent predictor of increased mortality in nonoperatively managed blunt hepatic and splenic injuries. J Trauma. 2005;58:437–44. discussion 444-445.
123. Bochicchio GV, Napolitano L, Joshi M. Outcome analysis of blood product transfusion in trauma patients: a prospective, risk-adjusted study. World J Surg. 2008;32:2185–9.
124. Opelka FG, Gathright JB, Beck DE. Lower gastrointestinal hemorrhage. In: Wolff BG, Fleshman JW, Beck DE, Pemberton JH, Wexner SD, editors. The ASCRS textbook of colon and rectal surgery. NY: Springer Science + Business Media, LLC; 2007. p. 299–307.
125. Chaudhry V, Hyser MJ, Gracias VH, Gau FC. Colonoscopy: the initial test for acute lower gastrointestinal bleeding. Am Surg. 1998;64:723–8.
126. Angtuaco TL, Reddy SK, Drapkin S, et al. The utility of urgent colonoscopy in the evaluation of acute lower gastrointestinal tract bleeding: a 2-year experience from a single center. Am J Gastroenterol. 2001;96:1782–5.
127. Green BT, Rockey DC. Lower gastrointestinal bleeding-management. Gastroenterol Clin N Am. 2005;34:665–78.
128. Zuckerman GR, Prakash C. Acute lower intestinal bleeding. Part I: clinical presentation and diagnosis. Gastrointest Endosc. 1998;48:606–16.
129. Fiorito JJ, Brandt LJ, Kozicky O, et al. The diagnostic yield of superior mesenteric angiography: correlation with the pattern of gastrointestinal bleeding. Am J Gastroenterol. 1988;84:878–81.
130. Ng DA, Opelka FG, Beck DE, et al. Predictive value of technetium Tc 99m-labeled red blood cell scintigraphy for positive angiogram in massive lower gastrointestinal hemorrhage. Dis Colon Rectum. 1997;40:471–7.
131. Abbas SM, Bissett IP, Holden A, et al. Clinical variables associated with positive angiographic localization of lower gastrointestinal bleeding. ANZ J Surg. 2005;75:953–7.
132. Khanna A, Ognibene SJ, Koniaris LG. Embolization as first-line therapy for diverticulosis-related massive lower gastrointestinal bleeding: evidence from a meta-analysis. J Gastrointest Surg. 2005;9:343–52.
133. Weldon DT, Burke SJ, Sun S, et al. Interventional management of lower gastrointestinal bleeding. Eur Radiol. 2008;18:857–67.
134. Kuo WT, Lee DE, Saad WEA, et al. Superselective microcoil embolization for the treatment of lower gastrointestinal hemorrhage. J Vasc Interv Radiol. 2003;14:1503–9.
135. Kickuth R, Rattunde H, Gschossmann J, et al. Acute lower gastrointestinal hemorrhage: minimally invasive management with microcatheter embolization. J Vasc Interv Radiol. 2008;19:1289–96.
136. DeFreyne L, Vanlangenhove P, De Vos M, et al. Embolization as a first approach with unmanageable acute nonvariceal gastrointestinal hemorrhage. Radiology. 2001;218:739–48.
137. Darcy M. Embolization for lower GI bleeding. In: Golzarian J, Sun S, Sharafuddin MJ, editors. Vascular embolotherapy: a comprehensive approach. Berlin, Heidelberg, New York: Springer; 2006. p. 73–84.
138. Funaki B. Superselective embolization of lower gastrointestinal hemorrhage: a new paradigm. Abdom Imaging. 2004; 29:434–8.
139. Bandi R, Shetty PC, Sharma RP, et al. Superselective arterial embolization for treatment of lower gastrointestinal hemorrhage. J Vasc Interv Radiol. 2001;12:1399–405.
140. Funaki B. Microcatheter embolization of lower gastrointestinal hemorrhage: an old idea whose time has come. Cardiovasc Intervent Radiol. 2004;27:591–9.
141. Evangelista PT, Hallisey MJ. Transcatheter embolization for acute lower gastrointestinal hemorrhage. J Vasc Interv Radiol. 2000;11:601–6.
142. Coldwell DM, Stokes KR, Yakes WF. Embolotherapy: agents, clinical applications, and techniques. Radiographics. 1994;14:623–43.
143. Funaki B, Kostelic JK, Lorenz J, et al. Superselective microcoil embolization of colonic hemorrhage. Am J Roentgenol. 2001;177:829–36.
144. Remzi FH, Dietz DW, Unal E, et al. Combined use of preoperataive provocative angiography and highly selective methylene blue injection to localize an occult small-bowel bleeding site in a patient with Crohn's disease. Dis Colon Rectum. 2003;46(2):260–3.
145. McDonald ML, Farnell MP, Stanson AW, Ress AM. Preoperative highly selective catheter localization of occult small-intestinal hemorrhage with methylene blue dye. Arch Surg. 1995;130(1):106–8.
146. Bloomfeld RS, Smith TP, Schneider AM, Rockey DC. Provocative angiography in patients with gastrointestinal hemorrhage of obscure origin. Am J Gastroenterol. 2000;95:2807–12.
147. Koval G, Benner KG, Rosch J, Kozak BE. Aggressive angiographic diagnosis in acute lower gastrointestinal hemorrhage. Dig Dis Sci. 1987;32:248–53.
148. Malden ES, Hicks ME, Royal HD, Aliperti C, Allen BT, Picus D. Recurrent gastrointestinal bleeding: use of thrombolysis with anticoagulation in diagnosis. Radiology. 1998;207:147–51.
149. McKusick KA, Froelich J, Callahan RJ, et al. 99m TC red blood cells for detection of gastrointestinal bleeding: experience with 80 patients. Am J Roentgenol. 1981;137:1113–8.
150. Gupta S, Luna E, Kingsley S, et al. Detection of gastrointestinal bleeding by radionuclide scintigraphy. Am J Gastroenterol. 1984;79:26–31.
151. Dusold R, Burke K, Carptentier W, et al. The accuracy of technetium 99m labeled red cell scintigraphy in localizing gastrointestinal bleeding. Am J Gastroenterol. 1994;89:345–8.
152. Pennoyer WP, Vignati PV, Cohen JL. Mesenteric angiography for lower gastrointestinal hemorrhage. Are there predictors for a positive study? Dis Colon Rectum. 1997;40:1014–8.

153. Bentley DE, Richardson JD. The role of tagged red blood cell imaging in the localization of gastrointestinal bleeding. Arch Surg. 1991;126:821–4.
154. Gunderman R, Leef J, Ong K, et al. Scintigraphic screening prior to visceral arteriography in acute lower gastrointestinal bleeding. J Nucl Med. 1998;39:1081–3.
155. Prakash C, Zuckerman GR, Aliperti G, et al. Prospective analysis of work-up of acute lower gastrointestinal bleeding: can an optimal algorithm be designed [abstract]? Gastrointest Endosc. 1998;47:AB102.
156. Olds GD, Cooper GS, Chak A, et al. The yield of bleeding scans in acute lower gastrointestinal hemorrhage. J Clin Gastroenterol. 2005;39:273–7.
157. Hammond KL, Beck DE, Hicks TC, et al. Implications of negative technetium 99m-labeled red blood cell scintigraphy in patients presenting with lower gastrointestinal bleeding. Am J Surg. 2007;193:404–7.
158. Hunter JM, Pezim ME. Limited value of technetium 99m-labelled red cell scintigraphy in localization of lower gastrointestinal bleeding. Am J Surg. 1990;159:504–6.
159. Winzelberg GG, McKusick KA, Froelich JW, et al. Detection of gastrointestinal bleeding with 99m TC labeled red blood cells. Semin Nucl Med. 1982;12:139–46.
160. Voeller GR, Bunch G, Britt L. Use of technetium labeled red blood cell scintigraphy in the detection and management of gastrointestinal hemorrhage. Surgery. 1991;110:799–804.
161. Kuhle W, Sheiman G. Detection of active colonic hemorrhage with use of helical CT: findings in a swine model. Radiology. 2003;228:743–52.
162. Laing CJ, Tobias T, Rosenblum DI, et al. Acute gastrointestinal bleeding: emerging role of multidetector CT angiography and review of current imaging techniques. Radiographics. 2007;27:1055–70.
163. Anthony S, Milburn S, Uberoi R. Multi-detector CT: review of its use in acute GI haemorrhage. Clin Radiol. 2007;62:938–49.
164. Yoon W, Jeong YY, Shin SS, et al. Acute massive gastrointestinal bleeding: detection and localization with arterial phase multi-detector row helical CT. Radiology. 2006;239:160–7.
165. Jaeckle T, Stuber G, Hoffman MHK, et al. Detection and localization of acute upper and lower gastrointestinal (GI) bleeding with arterial phase multi-detector row helical CT. Eur Radiol. 2008;18:1406–13.
166. Zink SI, Ohki SK, Stein B, et al. Noninvasive evaluation of active lower gastrointestinal bleeding: comparison between contrast-enhanced MDCT and 99mTc-labeled RBC scintigraphy. Abdom Imaging. 2008;191:1107–14.
167. Lee S, Welman CJ, Ramsay D. Investigation of acute lower gastrointestinal bleeding with 16- and 64-slice multidetector CT. J Med Imaging Radiat Oncol. 2009;53:56–63.
168. Ress AM, Benacci JC, Sarr MG. Efficacy of intraoperative enteroscopy in diagnosis and prevention of recurrent, occult gastrointestinal bleeding. Am J Surg. 1992;163:94–8.
169. Desa LA, Ohri SK, Hutton KA, et al. Role of intraoperative enteroscopy in obscure gastrointestinal bleeding of small bowel origin. Br J Surg. 1991;78:192–5.
170. Hartmann D, Schmidt H, Schilling D, et al. Follow-up of patients with obscure gastrointestinal bleeding after capsule endoscopy and intraoperative enteroscopy. Hepatogastroenterology. 2007;54:780–3.
171. Douard R, Wind P, Berger A, et al. Role of intraoperative enteroscopy in the management of obscure gastrointestinal bleeding at the time of video-capsule endoscopy. Am J Surg. 2009;198:6–11.
172. Casarella WJ, Galloway SJ, Taxin RN, et al. Lower gastrointestinal tract hemorrhage: new concepts based on arteriography. Am J Roentgenol. 1974;131:357–68.
173. Eaton AC. Emergency surgery for acute colonic hemorrhage-a retrospective study. Br J Surg. 1981;68:109–12.
174. Strate LL, Saltzman JR, Ookubo R, et al. Validation of a clinical prediction rule for severe acute lower intestinal bleeding. Am J Gastroenterol. 2005;100:1821–7.
175. Billingham RP. The conundrum of lower gastrointestinal bleeding. Surg Clin N Am. 1997;77:241–52.

25 Endometriosis

Michael J. Snyder

Introduction

Endometriosis is a disease characterized by the presence of endometrial glands and stroma outside the uterine cavity. It is one of the most common conditions requiring surgery for women during their reproductive years. Endometriosis, while not fatal, may be associated with disabling pain and intractable infertility. The degree of symptoms varies widely and does not always correspond to the extent of pathology encountered at surgery. Small lesions may cause severe pain and infertility, while larger lesions may be asymptomatic and be found only incidentally during surgery for other diagnoses. Diagnosis is typically made or confirmed at laparoscopy or during laparotomy. Colon and rectal surgeons often become involved in the management of patients with intestinal endometriosis. This involvement may occur as a result of a combined procedure with a gynecologist or in the management of an endometrioma masquerading as a neoplastic or inflammatory lesion. Treatment for endometriosis is usually multimodal and may require surgery in those patients with infertility, pelvic pain, obstruction, or a poor response to hormonal suppression. While advances in diagnostic tests and therapy have been made, endometriosis remains a frustrating and incompletely understood disease for both the patient and her physicians.

Epidemiology

The true prevalence of endometriosis is unknown. There is no noninvasive screening test for endometriosis, and its diagnosis depends on the visual or pathologic identification of implants during laparoscopy or laparotomy. Various authors have estimated that up to 15% of all women of reproductive age and one-third of infertile women have endometriosis.[1,2] A study by Houston et al. is the only population-based study of endometriosis.[3] After reviewing the medical records for Caucasian women in Rochester, Minnesota during the 1970s, they estimated that 6.2% of premenopausal women have endometriosis.

While endometriosis is primarily a disease of the reproductive years, the widespread use of exogenous estrogens and increasing obesity in our society have made it more prevalent in postmenopausal women. Conversely, there is a decrease in the incidence of the disease when women use oral contraceptives or experience multiple pregnancies.[4] These observations coupled with the fact that the incidence of endometriosis increases over time after a woman's last childbirth suggest that uninterrupted menstrual cycles predispose susceptible individuals to the development of endometrial implants.[5] There is no racial predilection for endometriosis other than in Japanese women who have double the incidence of the disease than do Caucasian women.[6]

Etiology

The precise etiology that completely explains the cause and pathogenesis of endometriosis is unknown. The two most popular theories as to its etiology are coelomic metaplasia and the implantation of viable endometrial cells from retrograde menstruation through the fallopian tubes. Coelomic metaplasia, postulated by Meyers, suggests that under the correct hormonal milieu, the coelomic epithelium will undergo metaplastic changes and transform into endometrial tissue.[7] He based his theory on studies demonstrating that the peritoneum and uterine endometrium both originate from embryonic coelomic epithelium. While this theory offers a good explanation for endometriosis in men and nonmenstruating women, it does not adequately address the anatomical distribution and clinical pattern of endometriosis. The vast majority of endometriosis occurs in the pelvis, but the peritoneum at risk with this theory is evenly distributed throughout the abdominal cavity. In addition, metaplasia should worsen with age and endometriosis clearly does not.

Retrograde menstruation, first proposed by Sampson,[8] remains the most plausible explanation for the distribution of endometrial implants. This theory postulates that endometriosis

D.E. Beck et al. (eds.), *The ASCRS Textbook of Colon and Rectal Surgery: Second Edition*,
DOI 10.1007/978-1-4419-1584-9_25,

arises from retrograde menstruation through the fallopian tubes and into the peritoneal cavity. Viable endometrial tissue has been demonstrated in menstrual effluent, and endometriosis has been induced both in primates, with artificially produced retrograde menstruation,[9] and in women volunteers who permitted injection of menstrual tissue into their peritoneum.[10] This theory, however, is probably only part of the answer.

While retrograde menstruation is very common, occurring in virtually all women, endometriosis affects only a small minority. Clearly other factors must be involved to permit the implantation and growth of endometrial tissue. Several studies indicate a possible genetic aspect to endometriosis. Simpson et al.[11] demonstrated that the disease appears to occur more commonly within families. He found a 7% relative risk for blood relatives of affected individuals as opposed to a 1% relative risk for non-blood controls. Additionally, the clinical manifestations of the disease were more severe among the related group. It appears that the inheritance pattern is polygenic or a combination of genetic and environmental factors. This conclusion is consistent with the clinical associations with delayed childbearing and uninterrupted cyclic menstruation.

Dmowski et al.[12] have theorized that the genetic factor may involve the immune system. They demonstrated depressed cellular immunity in monkeys with spontaneous endometriosis. Other investigators have confirmed alterations in both cellular and humoral immunity in humans.[13,14] The most striking change observed in cellular immunity is the high concentration of activated macrophages and decreased functional capacity of natural killer cells. The most significant abnormality in humoral immunity is the presence of autoantibodies against different cellular components. These changes have been observed in both the peritoneal cavity and the systemic circulation, suggesting that endometriosis may be a systemic disease. It is still unclear whether these changes represent manifestations of the disease or a subsequent reaction to it. This research, however, suggests that mild subclinical immunosuppression may subsequently lead to endometriosis many years later.

Clinical Manifestations

The most common sites where endometriosis occurs are summarized in Table 25-1. The most frequent of these are in the pelvis. Potential sites of implantation in the abdomen include the appendix, small bowel, and diaphragm. Rarely, implantation may occur in the inguinal canal (in patients with hernias), surgical incisions, the vulva, vagina, cervix, or systemically in the lungs, bronchi, or kidneys.

As the majority of women have disease confined to the pelvis, the most common presenting complaints relate to menstrual irregularities, pelvic pain, and infertility. Many women with endometriosis may be completely asymptomatic and the natural history of the disease in these patients has never been well defined. In studies with placebo arms, a few interesting observations have been made. A trial involving infertile women with otherwise asymptomatic endometriosis revealed that laparoscopic scoring of the severity of the disease increased over the length of the study in almost 50% of the placebo group.[15] Another study compared pain scores in women receiving placebo versus gonadotropin-releasing hormone (GnRH) analogs.[16] The cumulative dysmenorrhea rate and severity of pain were significantly lower in the treatment group suggesting a progressive course of the disease. Other studies on infertile women revealed that mild endometriosis can spontaneously resolve and that medical therapy may only suppress the disease until hormonal stimulation resumes.[17]

TABLE 25-1. Sites and incidence of endometriosis[42]

Common	
Ovaries	60–75%
Uterosacral ligaments	30–65%
Cul-de-sac	20–30%
Uterus	4–20%
Rectosigmoid colon	3–10%
Less common	
Appendix	2%
Ureter	1–2%
Terminal ileum	1%
Bladder	<1%
Abdominal scars	<1%
Rare	
Diaphragm	
Inguinal canal	
Liver	
Spleen	
Kidney	

Pelvic Pain and Dysmenorrhea

Pain is the most common symptom of endometriosis, affecting up to 80% of patients subsequently diagnosed with the disease. Endometriosis has been discovered in 30–50% of women undergoing laparoscopy for pelvic pain.[18] Pelvic pain associated with endometriosis presents as dysmenorrhea, dyspareunia, or chronic noncyclic pelvic pain. There are women, however, with extensive endometriosis who experience little or no pain. Moreover, total lesion volume does appear to correlate directly to the degree of pain.[19] Instead, symptoms seem related to the depth of penetration of the lesion, the type of lesion, and its location. Implants involving the uterosacral ligaments and rectovaginal septum are most often implicated. The pain is typically most intense just prior to menstruation and lasts for the duration of menstruation. The pain is often associated with back pain, dyschezia, and levator muscle spasm and is more severe with advanced stages of endometriosis.

Dysmenorrhea occurs in most women with endometriosis. The association is not well understood, and some have hypothesized that high uterine pressures cause dysmenorrhea with retrograde menstruation a consequence of these elevated pressures.[20] Other investigators, however, have failed to show an increase in the prevalence of dysmenorrhea with early stage endometriosis.[21]

Dyspareunia, deep pelvic pain with vaginal penetration, is usually a symptom of advanced endometriosis. Dyspareunia is most pronounced just prior to menstruation and is associated with specific coital positions. The presence of dyspareunia is often indicative of the degree of fixation of the pelvic organs, especially in the cul-de-sac of Douglas, the uterosacral ligaments, and the rectovaginal septum.

Chronic noncyclic pelvic pain is pain present for longer than 6 months and may be intermittent or continuous. The pain is often associated with both perineural inflammation and uterosacral ligament involvement with endometriosis.[22] Gastrointestinal and urinary complaints may accompany the pain.

Pain in the shoulder during or just preceding menstruation may be due to endometrial implants involving the diaphragm. The diaphragm should always be viewed during laparoscopy, so these diaphragmatic deposits can possibly be treated with laser vaporization. Differentiation from adhesions associated with pelvic inflammatory disease (Fitz Hugh Curtis syndrome) is usually not difficult unless the two pathologies coexist.

The pathophysiology of pain arising from endometriosis is not completely clear. Pain may occur from the cyclic growth and subsequent increase in pressure within the capsule surrounding the implant. Alternatively, extravasation of menstrual debris into the surrounding tissue may occur with subsequent edema and release of inflammatory mediators. As the implant matures with surrounding unyielding scar tissue, the stretching of this scar by the products of the endometrial glands may produce pain. This scenario is probably particularly true for deeper implants. A study by Cornillie et al.[22] discovered that all women with implants deeper than 1 cm experienced severe pelvic pain.

Adhesions, very common in endometriosis, may also be associated with pain. Adherence of the colon and small bowel along with retroflexion of the uterus from extensive posterior adhesions may occur. Such retroflexion and fixation of the rectosigmoid can result in pressure on the sacrum with consequent back and rectal pain.

Since the 1960s, multiple investigators have attempted to define the role of prostaglandins in the pathogenesis of pelvic pain.[23,24] Macrophages are responsible for the removal of foreign material such as the endometrial implants. They are present around the endometrial implants and are potent producers of inflammatory mediators such as the prostaglandins. Both prostacyclin (PGI-2) and prostaglandin E-2 are able to sensitize pain receptors to chemical mediators. Leukotriene B-4, another macrophage product, is a potent chemotactic agent and leukocyte activator. These factors are thought to explain some of the pelvic pain, but not all the studies agree.[24] The relative transient nature of prostaglandin action and the inherent difficulty in measuring pain complicates attempts to quantify the impact of chemical mediators.

Infertility

The relationship between endometriosis and infertility is also unclear. Some studies have demonstrated a high percentage of infertile patients with endometriosis.[25] Certainly, those reports comparing rates of endometriosis for women undergoing elective laparoscopic sterilization versus laparoscopy for infertility have demonstrated a fourfold or greater increase in the infertile group. In women with known endometriosis, the infertility rate is 30–50%. Whether endometriosis causes infertility or is the product of uninterrupted menstruation is still hotly debated.

There is little disagreement that moderate-to-severe disease with mechanical distortion of the fallopian tubes, ovaries, and peritoneum can potentiate infertility. Pelvic endometriosis and the resulting inflammatory response can produce dense, fibrotic adhesions that may significantly interfere with both the oocyte release from the ovary and the ability of the fallopian tube to pickup and transmit the oocyte to the uterus. Blockage of the tube may produce a hydrosalpinx, and in one recent study, endometriosis was the etiology in 14% of patients undergoing tubal reconstruction for occlusion.[26] In moderate or severe endometriosis, the pregnancy rates following surgery are 50 and 40%, respectively, compared with only 7% when expectant management is practiced.[27,28] Surgical treatment of these patients is clearly beneficial.

Treatment of infertile patients with mild endometriosis is more problematic. A study by Inoue et al.[29] on 2,000 infertile women with mild endometriosis did not reveal any improvement in fertility with either medical or surgical therapy when compared with expectant management. Other studies have demonstrated a lower pregnancy per cycle rate in patients with endometriosis compared with those free of the disease.[30]

Intestinal Symptoms

Although some women with intestinal endometriosis may be asymptomatic, some degree of intestinal complaints are found in most women with moderate-to-severe disease. Bowel involvement occurs in 12–37% of cases of endometriosis. Depending on the site of involvement, the symptoms of endometriosis may vary somewhat. In patients with intestinal endometriosis, the rectosigmoid is involved in over 70%, followed by the small bowel and appendix. Rectosigmoid disease often results in alterations in bowel habits such as constipation, diarrhea, a decreased caliber of the stool, tenesmus, or, rarely, rectal bleeding. Such symptoms appear more often around the time of menses.

Colonic endometriosis can present with obstruction and may be difficult to differentiate from other causes of large bowel obstruction, such as Crohn's disease or neoplasm. This difficulty is of particular concern in the postmenopausal woman on hormone replacement therapy.

Intestinal perforation may occur with endometriosis. Colonic perforation has been reported during pregnancy from endometriosis.[31] Perforation also occurs with transmural appendiceal endometriosis.

For those patients with asymptomatic intestinal endometriosis, the natural history appears to be benign. Prystowsky et al.,[32] who followed 44 patients with known intestinal endometriosis for a period of 1–12 years, found that only one patient developed clinically significant gastrointestinal symptoms. Consequently, intestinal resection in these asymptomatic patients is probably unwarranted.

Confusion between small bowel endometriosis and Crohn's disease is common, as both can produce similar endoscopic and even histologic findings (Figure 25-1). Small bowel implants involving the terminal ileum are often noted incidentally at the time of laparoscopy and may often be asymptomatic. When symptoms occur they are usually nonspecific such as recurrent abdominal pain and bloating. Occasionally, acute or chronic small bowel obstruction develops from extensive fibrotic adhesions which are due to endometriosis.

The next most frequent site of intestinal endometriosis is the appendix. Endometrial implants are not infrequently found when the appendix is removed incidentally. The clinical significance of appendiceal endometriosis is less than that involving the small bowel and colon. Although endometrial implants may produce acute appendicitis with right lower quadrant abdominal pain, nausea, fever, and leukocytosis, historically most abdominal explorations for presumed acute appendicitis with a subsequent diagnosis of endometriosis have been due to ruptured endometrial cystic implants involving the ovary. Endometriosis of the appendix may also produce a chronic obstruction of the intestinal lumen with formation of a mucocele or periappendiceal inflammatory mass that is difficult to distinguish from a neoplasm. Finally, endometrial implants of the appendix and cecum may serve as lead points for an intussusception.

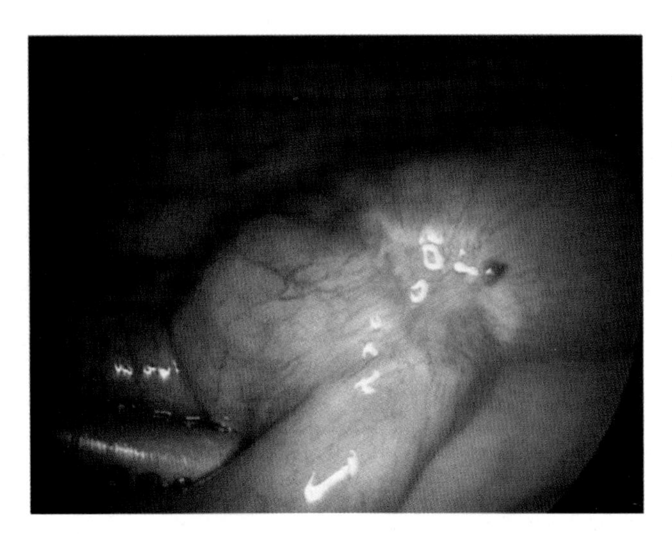

FIGURE 25-1. Endometriosis involving the small intestine.

Malignant Transformation

Malignant transformation of endometriosis is an uncommon complication of the disease. Almost 80% of the tumors are ovarian and two-thirds are endometriod carcinomas. Patients with ovarian neoplasms arising from endometriosis are younger than the typical ovarian cancer patient with most tumors occurring in the fourth decade of life.[33] Symptoms of pelvic pain and an enlarging pelvic mass are the most common symptoms. In women with known endometriosis, a cyst larger than 10 cm, cyst rupture, or a change in the nature of the chronic pelvic pain is potential signs of malignancy.

The rectosigmoid colon is the most common site for extragonadal tumors arising from endometriosis. Prolonged unopposed estrogen exposure is a significant risk factor, and rectal bleeding is the most common symptom. Recurrent symptoms of pelvic endometriosis following hysterectomy and bilateral salpingo-oophorectomy can be possible signs of malignant degeneration. Endometrial carcinoma is the most common tumor type. Histologically, the tumor must be shown to arise from the colon rather than invading it from another source. The diagnosis also requires that endometriosis or premalignant changes in endometrial glands be found contiguous with the invasive neoplasm.[34]

Treatment of both ovarian and extragonadal tumors is based on the particular stage of the tumor. The prognosis is generally good with tumors confined to the ovary or an extragonadal site having 5-year survivals greater than 60%. Even if a locally extensive tumor is encountered, there may be a benefit from aggressive local resection.

Diagnosis

Physical Examination

Patients with mild cases of endometriosis may have a normal physical examination and the diagnosis may not even be suspected unless the patient undergoes laparoscopy. For patients with pelvic pain, careful bimanual and rectal examination may reveal nodularity or induration especially in the uterosacral ligaments or cul-de-sac of Douglas. Fixed tender retroversion of the uterus in a patient without previous pelvic surgery may raise suspicion for endometriosis. Palpation of the ovaries may reveal an ovarian mass. As these ovarian masses are generally soft and cystic, those less than 5 cm in diameter may be difficult to palpate. Cyclical pain or bleeding from any location, especially coinciding with menses, should be adequately investigated for endometriosis. The inguinal canal, previous incisions, umbilicus, and lungs can all be potentially involved with endometrial implants.

Laboratory Evaluation

CA-125, an antigen expressed on tissues derived from human coelomic epithelium, is elevated in women with moderate-to-severe endometriosis. However, the sensitivity and specificity of this test is poor as the antigen may be mildly elevated in other diseases and within the normal range in women with mild endometriosis. The concentration of CA-125 does correlate with the severity of the disease and is probably most useful in gauging response to medical therapy. It may also be of value in following women post-resection who had elevated levels preoperatively and are again exhibiting symptoms of endometriosis. No other serum markers are commercially available, but assays of antiendometrial antibodies and endometrial secretory protein PP14 are currently being evaluated for clinical relevance.[35]

Endoscopy

As the lesions begin on the outside of the intestine, endoscopic evaluation of the large bowel is often normal except in severe disease or infiltrating nodular endometrial implants. Occasionally, serosal involvement with adhesions can lead to obstruction. Endoscopically, the mucosa is generally intact, occasionally associated with significant luminal narrowing. Infiltration of the submucosa, while uncommon, may produce nodularity and distortion of the overlying mucosa (Figure 25-2). These findings may be difficult to visually differentiate from Crohn's disease, ischemia, or malignancy. Pressure against these areas of distorted bowel may produce pain that suggests the diagnosis of endometriosis. In addition, biopsies of the mucosa, taken in areas of endometriosis, can resemble solitary rectal ulcer or prolapse syndromes. Rarely is the diagnosis of endometriosis definitively confirmed by endoscopy or from endoscopic biopsies. Colonoscopy is, however, useful in excluding colon cancer from the differential diagnosis, especially in older patients presenting with a rectosigmoid mass while on hormone replacement.

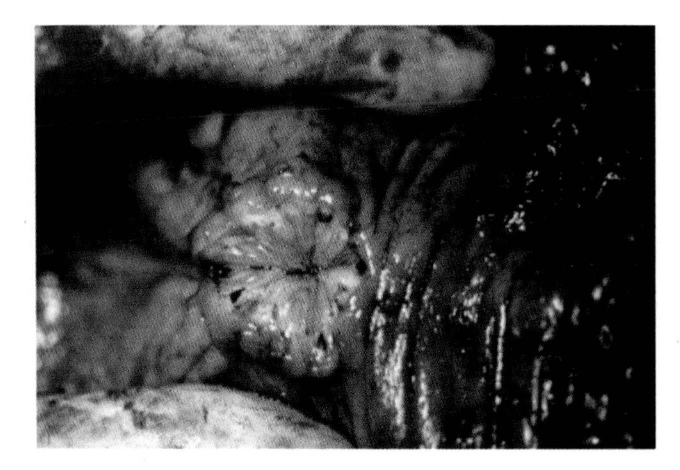

FIGURE 25-2. Polypoid endometrial implant of the colon.

Rigid proctoscopy is very helpful in predicting the depth of rectosigmoid involvement in patients with severe endometriosis of the cul-de-sac of Douglas. After two enemas are given to remove any fecal debris, the rigid proctoscope is deployed above the rectosigmoid and slowly withdrawn with care to maintain adequate insufflation. The mucosa is often fixed over area of submucosal or deep muscular involvement with tethering or puckering and loss of the normal mucosal mobility. In our experience, these mucosal findings have correlated with significant intestinal wall invasion by the endometrial implant and often a need for intestinal resection.

Imaging Techniques

Imaging techniques used to facilitate the diagnosis of endometriosis include ultrasonography, barium enema, computerized tomography (CT), magnetic resonance imaging (MRI), and immunoscintigraphy. Many of these tests are obtained for the evaluation of chronic pelvic pain and/or bleeding from the reproductive tract or colon. They are primarily utilized to rule out more common conditions, but there are some findings that may strongly suggest the diagnosis of endometriosis before visual or pathologic confirmation by laparoscopy or laparotomy.

Transvaginal ultrasound has been used for several years to evaluate ovarian endometriomas. It is a sensitive test and in experienced hands provides specificity greater than 90% for ovarian endometriosis. Ultrasound of the pelvis, however, is not very sensitive in detecting focal nonovarian endometrial implants. Endometriosis has been termed "the great mimicker" because the appearance on ultrasound is highly variable with some lesions being nearly sonolucent and others quite echogenic.

Endorectal ultrasound is a potentially valuable tool to determine rectal wall invasion by endometrial implants in the cul-de-sac. Chapron and colleagues[36] studied the reliability of endorectal ultrasound in assessing the depth of bowel invasion with rectovaginal endometriosis. In 17 patients with proven deep pelvic endometriosis, the ultrasound revealed infiltration of the bowel wall and suggested the need for intestinal resection. The ultrasound findings were subsequently confirmed at laparoscopy and evaluation of the pathologic specimen in 16 patients. Twenty-one other patients with endometriosis of the cul-de-sac of Douglas whose ultrasounds did not show infiltration of the rectal wall did not require intestinal resection and were able to have complete removal of the endometriosis with laparoscopic techniques without complications. The accuracy of ultrasound was recently confirmed by Doniec and colleagues who determined both the sensitivity and specificity of preoperative staging of rectal wall involvement by endometriosis to be

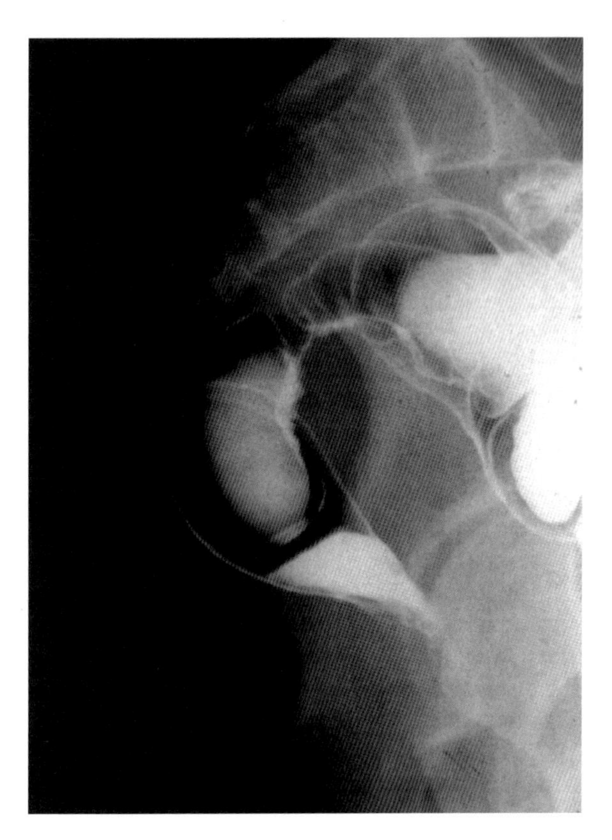

FIGURE 25-3. Barium enema demonstrating a rectosigmoid stricture.

97%.[37] The only real concern in evaluating patients having cul-de-sac endometriosis by endorectal ultrasound is the significant discomfort experienced by the patient when rectal distention from the balloon probe compresses the implant.

Barium enema examination is another imaging technique often obtained by gynecologists for the intestinal complaints associated with deep pelvic endometriosis. The lateral and prone cross-table views of the rectum offer excellent evaluation of the cul-de-sac of Douglas as long as care is taken in ensuring that the balloon is kept in the distal rectum (Figure 25-3). Studies in patients without bowel wall involvement are either normal or reveal smooth extrinsic compression with normal mucosa. Deep invasion of the bowel wall by endometriosis produces a variety of appearances on barium enema. Irregularities of the rectal wall such as tethering or even polypoid lesions may be difficult to distinguish from inflammatory bowel disease or neoplasm. Strictures of the rectosigmoid may also be identified on barium enema.

Computerized tomography is the imaging technique probably used most frequently for the evaluation of abdominal and pelvic pain. Unfortunately, there is no standard CT appearance for a mass caused by endometriosis to clearly differentiate it from pelvic masses due to other causes. Cystic lesions are more commonly seen on the ovaries while deeper pelvic disease usually consists of either solid lesions or mixed cystic/solid lesions. CT evaluation of the pelvic sidewall for endometrial implants is better than ultrasound, but there is still significant overlap between infectious and malignant pathology. CT scanning is probably most useful for patients with pelvic pain and a negative ultrasound to assess the musculoskeletal boundaries of the pelvis and the rectosigmoid colon.

When pelvic endometriosis is strongly suspected, MRI is more useful than CT scanning because of the benefit of imaging in multiple planes and the lack of ionizing radiation. MRI may be the best noninvasive modality for imaging suspected endometriosis. Colorectal involvement on MRI is strongly suspected when there is disappearance of the fat plane between the rectum and the vagina, loss of the hypointense signal of the anterior bowel wall on T2-weighted images, and a contrast enhanced mass on T1-weighted images involving the bowel wall.[38] Sagittal images are particularly valuable in imaging the cul-de-sac of Douglas. MRI is superior to CT scanning for extraperitoneal lesions and the evaluation of pelvic masses.[39] Identification of endometrial implants is dependent on the hemorrhage that occurs in these lesions. The time between imaging and the most recent hemorrhage may determine in which weighted images the masses are most intensely seen. The sensitivity and specificity of MRI for detecting and adequately evaluating colorectal endometriosis is approximately 78 and 98%, respectively.[38]

Immunoscintigraphy with radioactive iodine-labeled CA-125 monoclonal antibodies has been studied to clarify the extent of pelvic endometriosis, particularly in the face of severe pelvic adhesive disease.[40] In such a study of 28 women, 22 had a positive test with 16 confirmed to have endometriosis. Two of five women had a negative test despite having histologically confirmed endometriosis. As such, immunoscintigraphy is not currently recommended for screening and remains primarily a research tool.

Laparoscopy

The diagnosis of endometriosis usually requires direct visual and/or tactile assessment of the abdomen and pelvis. Laparoscopy is currently the initial approach to many patients suspected of having endometriosis and has revolutionized both its diagnosis and treatment. Most patients with severe pelvic pain and many patients with refractory infertility undergo laparoscopy. The timing of laparoscopy in relation to the menstrual cycle is unimportant except in patients being evaluated for infertility. In these patients, the procedure is performed in the luteal phase to provide additional valuable information concerning ovarian function.

The technique of diagnostic laparoscopy has become widespread in both the surgical and gynecologic literature. A camera, often attached to a video monitoring system with photographic and recording capabilities, is introduced at the level of the umbilicus or upper abdomen, while a second instrument is placed in a suprapubic location to allow manipulation of the pelvic and abdominal viscera. A thorough examination of the entire abdomen and especially the pelvis is critical to enable complete assessment of the disease. Both ovaries should be mobilized to evaluate the pelvic peritoneum, and the uterus should be manipulated to allow complete visualization of the cul-de-sac of Douglas, uterosacral ligaments, sigmoid colon, and ureters. It is important to view the base of the appendix as well as the distal small bowel.

Obtaining a complete assessment of the abdominal and pelvic viscera can be technically demanding. The accuracy of laparoscopy is completely dependent on the surgeon's visual evaluation of the abdomen and pelvis. The findings of endometriosis can be very subtle, and several studies have demonstrated that visually normal peritoneum may have microscopic evidence of endometriosis.[41] The extent of endometriosis should be carefully documented and staged. The current staging system has been formulated primarily for infertility and was revised by the American Society for Reproductive Medicine in 1998 (Figure 25-4).[42] This revision is certainly an improvement over previous staging systems

Patient's Name ______________________ Date ______________________

Stage I (Minimal) - 1–5
Stage II (Mild) - 6–15
Stage III (Moderate) - 16–40
Stage IV (Severe) - > 40
Total ______________

Laparoscopy ________ Laparotomy ________ Photography ____________
Recommended Treatment ______________________
____
Prognosis ______________________

	ENDOMETRIOSIS	< 1cm	1–3cm	> 3cm
PERITONEUM	Superficial	1	2	4
	Deep	2	4	6
OVARY	R Superficial	1	2	4
	Deep	6	16	20
	L Superficial	1	2	4
	Deep	4	16	20

	POSTERIOR CUL-DE-SAC OBLITERATION	Partial	Complete
		4	40

	ADHESIONS	< 1/3 Enclosure	1/3–2/3 Enclosure	<2/3 Enclosure
OVARY	R Filmy	1	2	4
	Dense	4	8	16
	L Filmy	1	2	4
	Dense	4	8	16
TUBE	R Filmy	1	2	4
	Dense	4•	8•	16
	L Filmy	1	2	4
	Dense	4•	8•	16

•If the fimbriated end of the fallopian tube is completely enclosed, change the point assignment to 16.
Denote appearance of superficial implant types as red [(R), red, red-pink, flamelike, vesicular blobs, clear vesicles], white [(W), opacifications, peritoneal defects, yellow-brown], or black [(B) black, hemosiderin deposits, blue]. Denote percent of total described as R___%,W___ % and B___%. Total should equal 100%.

Additional Endometriosis: ______________________

Associated Pathology: ______________________

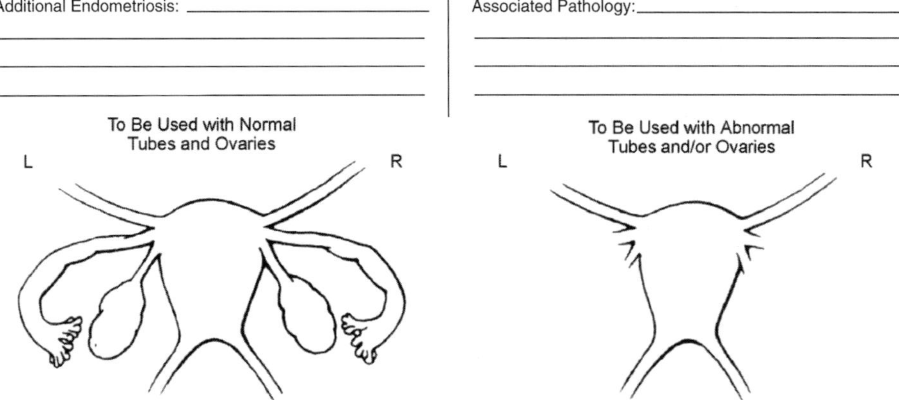

FIGURE 25-4. Revised American Society for Reproductive Medicine 1996 classification of endometriosis.

that were more concerned with adhesions than with implants. Virtually all patients with intestinal lesions requiring resection are Stage IV, especially if they have cul-de-sac involvement.

The current classification system, however, is often not useful for the gastrointestinal surgeon. The more critical information for the surgeon is the identification and location of intestinal lesions. There is no uniform type of endometrial lesion. The classic implant is nodular with a variable degree of fibrosis and pigmentation. The color may be black, white, brown, blue, or even red. The appearance of the lesion may be vesicular, popular, or hemorrhagic (Figure 25-5). Glandular tissue is found in the great majority of these lesions. Lesions may change color or consistency over time, with red lesions noted early in the course of the disease and blue/black ones typical of older implants. Healed implants appear as fibrotic nodules. There are also a wide variety of atypical lesions occasionally associated with positive biopsies. The inability to definitively identify endometriosis through purely visual means necessitates pathologic confirmation of the disease before a definitive diagnosis can be made, especially in mild disease.

Implants in the cul-de-sac of Douglas, which occur in nearly 20% of women with endometriosis, were initially described by Cullen in 1920. Ninety percent of these represent an important variant that is especially relevant for the intestinal surgeon. Histologically, these lesions are characterized by desmoplastic tissue composed of fibrous and smooth muscle cells with strands of endometrial glands and stroma. The major component of the lesion is the fibromuscular tissue and not the endometrial tissue typical of other locations. These implants are both proliferative and infiltrating and more than 25% extend at least 5 mm in depth.[43] The depth of invasion may be difficult to assess laparoscopically, and the full extent of the implant may not be appreciated until laparotomy. The progressive fibrosis leads to narrowing of the intestinal lumen and occasionally to bowel obstruction.

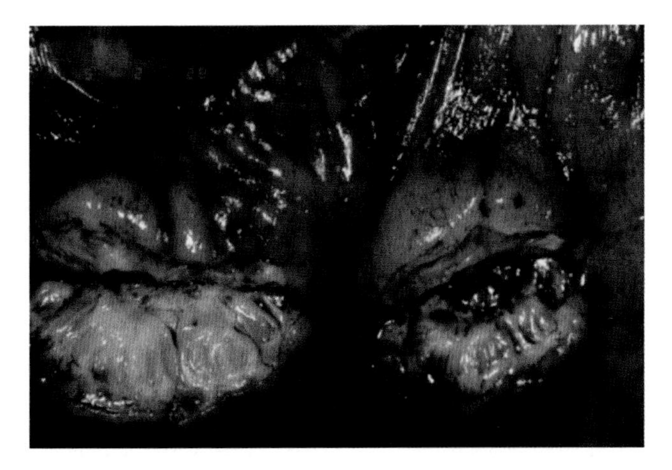

FIGURE 25-5. Endometrial implants with hemorrhagic centers and fibrosis.

These rectovaginal implants also behave differently during the menstrual cycle. There is poor to absent secretory changes during the luteal phase. Vasodilatation and not necrosis and bleeding occur at menstruation. Resistance to medical therapy is common with several studies demonstrating no significant decrease in mitotic activity in rectovaginal endometriosis after GnRH agonist treatment.[44] This resistance is thought to be due to estrogen receptor inactivity, inadequate drug access, or genetic programming that is only secondarily affected by estrogen.

Treatment

Treatment options for women with endometriosis are currently based upon the severity and type of symptoms. Currently, the prevention of endometriosis is not yet possible, and therefore treatment is primarily begun to ameliorate symptoms. Some women with endometriosis are completely asymptomatic and the implants are found incidentally at the time of surgery for other reasons. A study by Martin et al.[45] revealed that 25% of women undergoing elective tubal ligation had asymptomatic endometrial implants. This finding strongly suggests that not all women with endometriosis require treatment. Other authors have analyzed the prevalence of endometriosis in these asymptomatic women with regard to the time from their last pregnancy. They discovered that the odds of having endometrial implants increased significantly at 10 years following the last pregnancy.[5,46] Consequently, as the natural history appears unclear, long-term follow-up of these patient cohorts may demonstrate late development of symptoms and the need for more aggressive medical or surgical management.

Before the introduction of diagnostic laparoscopy in the 1960s, exploratory laparotomy was the only modality available for the diagnosis and treatment of endometriosis. Laparoscopy revolutionized the diagnostic evaluation of these women and allowed patients with limited disease to undergo medical therapy. With improvements in laparoscopic techniques and equipment in the past decade, notably the development of laparoscopic laser techniques, many if not most early endometrial lesions can now be ablated at the time of diagnosis. Even complex excisional surgery involving the bowel and ureter can be occasionally performed safely via a laparoscopic approach in many patients. As advanced laparoscopic techniques have become more widespread, the indications and use of medical therapy is also evolving.

Medical Management

Medical therapy is designed to treat the symptoms of endometriosis, notably pelvic pain. As pelvic pain may have causes other than the endometriosis seen during laparoscopy, a trial of ovarian suppression is often used to help determine the contribution of the pain from the endometrial implants. In those patients with infertility, with or without pelvic pain, the primary goal is an intrauterine pregnancy. After other causes of infertility have been excluded, ovarian suppression may allow for laparoscopic removal of smaller endometrial lesions with optimal preservation of ovarian tissue.

Despite the many advances in the surgical treatment of endometriosis, there are still some significant advantages to medical therapy. Surgery can remove only lesions that are both visible and accessible. Microscopic disease or disease on vital structures is often left behind. Subsequent recurrence is not surprising. Additionally, there are complications associated with ablative surgery in the pelvis, especially if the woman requires multiple attempts at control of her disease. For infertile women, the adhesions that can form after any pelvic surgery may further impair the ability to conceive. In addition, laser destruction of ovarian implants may destroy germinal tissue and conceivably limit the reproductive potential from the involved ovary. In limited disease, medical therapy is comparable with surgery in terms of relief of symptoms, recurrence of disease, and subsequent pregnancy rates. Finally, medical therapy does not require specialized training or equipment and is much less costly than surgery.

Medical therapy alone also has significant potential disadvantages. All the hormonal therapies subsequently discussed have side effects and often require prolonged treatment. For example, medical therapies manipulate the hormonal environment to suppress the cyclic secretion of ovarian estrogen and progesterone, and this suppression induces atrophy of the ectopic endometrium so that over several months the implants regress. Advanced lesions, especially those with a nodular, proliferative histology will often only partially regress. No current hormonal regimen can completely eradicate these lesions, and upon cessation of therapy, the lesions may again become symptomatic.

Oral Contraceptives

The first effective medical therapy for endometriosis was introduced by Kistner. He proposed the administration of high dose, continuous estrogen/progestogens in 1958. These agents result in the induction of pseudo-pregnancy with hyperhormonal amenorrhea. Pituitary and ovarian function is thereby suppressed, and in the later stages of the treatment regimen, endometrial implants resorb and resolve. The usual treatment regimen consists of daily administration of a tablet for 6–9 months. When Vercellini and colleagues[47] compared oral contraceptives with GnRH agonists, they found that deep dyspareunia and pelvic pain were reduced in both groups, with fewer side effects experienced by the oral contraceptive women. Pain relief appeared similar in the two groups at 1 year. Side effects rarely cause cessation of treatment, but exacerbation of endometriotic symptoms may occur early in the course of treatment.

Another drug regimen used for the treatment of endometriosis involves the administration of synthetic progestogens alone. This may induce a pseudo-pregnancy by acting in concert with endogenous estrogens. Ovarian suppression is often inconsistent. Both oral and depot preparations are available. In patients who do not desire pregnancy and in whom surgery is contraindicated, depot progestogens have been effective in ameliorating pelvic pain with equivalent efficacy to danazol.[48] Side effects include breakthrough vaginal bleeding, weight gain, and fluid retention.

Danazol

Danazol was first used extensively for endometriosis in the mid-1970s, and until the introduction of GnRH agonists (GnRH-a), was the most widely used drug for suppression of the ectopic endometrium. Danazol lowers peripheral estrogen and progesterone levels by a direct effect on ovarian steroidogenesis and pituitary production of FSH and LH. Danazol also binds directly to endometrial cellular receptors leading to atrophy and suppression of proliferation. In addition, danazol is a potent immunomodulator with beneficial effects on both humoral and cellular immunity.[49]

The side effects of danazol necessitate discontinuation in less than 5% of patients for short courses, but are poorly tolerated for long-term suppression.[50] Predictable manifestations of menopause are most common. Danazol also raises free testosterone levels and produces a hyperandrogenic state, especially at lower doses. Hirsutism, acne, weight gain, and deepening voice changes may occur. In addition, since danazol alters lipid metabolism and liver function, it should not be used in women with elevated liver enzymes, liver disease, or complications of atherosclerosis.

Gonadotropin-Releasing Hormone Agonists

The introduction of GnRH-a as a new treatment modality for endometriosis has improved results primarily by a reduction in side effects. GnRH-a is synthetic molecules derived from the ten peptide long GnRH. Continuous administration of GnRH-a completely suppresses pituitary release of FSH and LH. Administered either by injection or intranasally beginning in the mid-luteal phase of the menstrual cycle, the current recommended length of therapy is 6 months. Pain relief is complete in over 50% of women and significantly decreased in over 90%. Laparoscopic evaluation after 6 months of treatment indicates resolution or a significant decrease in size of the lesions in the majority of patients. Studies comparing danazol and GnRH-a indicate similar clinical efficacy.[51]

Side effects of GnRH-a are predictably, due to the sometimes, profound hypoestrogenic state many of these women experience. Cessation of therapy for side effects is uncommon. The degree of bone loss that can occur with the typical 6-month treatment regimen is unclear, but GnRH-a is not recommended for women with osteoporosis. Interestingly, a potentially serious complication can result when GnRH-a is inadvertently administered at the wrong point in the menstrual cycle, and a brief period of hypersecretion of FSH and LH occurs. Rarely, this upsurge in gonadotropin activity may precipitate an acute exacerbation in endometriotic symptoms, occasionally necessitating emergency surgical intervention.[52]

Surgical Management

Surgical treatment of endometriosis has evolved significantly over time. Before the advent of laparoscopy and suppressive medical therapy, most operations were performed for advanced disease and consisted of radical removal of the uterus and ovaries. While the most effective treatment of pelvic pain still consists of surgical castration along with resection of the endometrial implants, many of these young patients strongly desire to maintain their options for pregnancy. Currently, surgery is considered conservative only when reproductive potential is preserved. Therefore, the major goal of surgical therapy for endometriosis is to completely excise or ablate the endometrial implants. Secondary goals include the preservation of ovarian function and minimizing postoperative adhesion formation. Currently, we approach these patients in concert with gynecologists experienced with treating ovarian endometriosis to completely remove all gross disease, restore normal anatomy, and optimize fertility.

General Principles

Endometriosis is an invasive disease that can extend deeply into the retroperitoneum and is often surrounded by a rim of fibrosis that may make it difficult to completely assess the true extent of the implant. Removal of the lesions requires sharp excision or vaporization with electrocautery and/or the CO_2 laser. Both techniques have the potential for iatrogenic injury to the intestinal or urinary tracts. Recognizing when a lesion is completely ablated is highly dependent on surgical technique and the expertise of the surgeon. Utilizing techniques that minimize injury to the surrounding tissue, such as a cutting current to outline lesions to be removed by electrocautery and high-power density settings with the CO_2 laser are desirable. Laparoscopic hydrodissection is also very useful in identifying normal surrounding tissue.

Meticulous hemostasis and frequent irrigation are critical to maintaining good visualization of the operative field in both open and laparoscopic surgery. Tissue planes are often distorted, especially in the cul-de-sac of Douglas, and intraoperative instrumentation of the vagina or proctoscopic evaluation of the rectum may help to avoid iatrogenic injury to these structures. Finally, minimizing tissue trauma with gentle handling will decrease adhesions and maximize potential fertility.

All patients undergoing surgery for advanced endometriosis, either by an open or laparoscopic approach, should have a full mechanical and antibiotic bowel preparation. Prophylactic antibiotics and other appropriate practices for patients undergoing major abdominal or pelvic surgery are standard. Patients are positioned in the low-lithotomy position with access to both the vagina and rectum for instrumentation. Ureteral stents are liberally used and are especially useful in women with severe obliterative disease in the cul-de-sac and in reoperative pelvic surgical procedures.

Provided that complete removal of the endometriosis is performed, no specific technique or approach has been proven to be superior. With endometriosis, the surgeon's experience and skill are paramount. In experienced hands, laparoscopic removal of extensive endometriosis can be accomplished. However, removal of deep lesions in the rectovaginal septum necessitating bowel resection still often requires open laparotomy to safely and completely excise the endometrial implant with restoration of intestinal continuity.

The management and techniques concerning the surgical treatment of ovarian and ureteral endometriosis are extensively discussed in the appropriate gynecologic and urologic literature. This discussion on surgical therapy will concentrate on management of intestinal lesions.

Rectovaginal Endometriosis

Endometriosis of the cul-de-sac of Douglas that extends into the rectovaginal septum is the most common site of intestinal involvement and may require intestinal resection. These lesions are often deep fibrotic nodules that extend from the posterior vagina and anterior rectum to the uterosacral ligaments (Figure 25-6). Small superficial lesions involving the

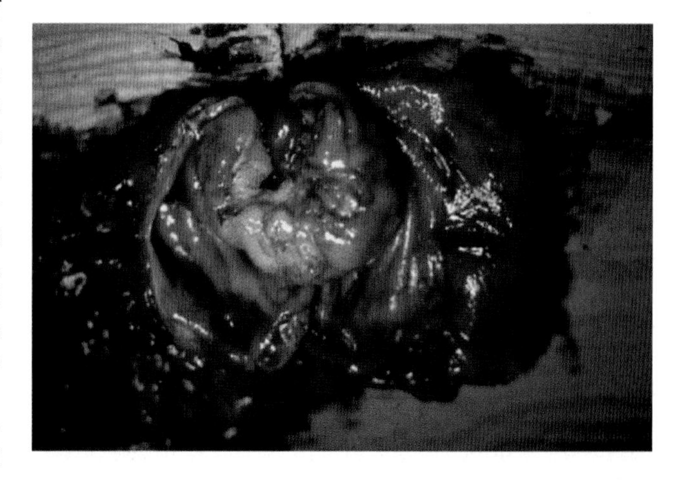

FIGURE 25-6. Deep infiltrating endometrial implant of the rectosigmoid.

intraperitoneal rectum may be vaporized with the CO_2 laser or electrocautery. When using either technique, it is critical to initially outline the lesion to be removed to ensure complete extirpation, because distortion of the planes and tissue can otherwise make it difficult to assess the completeness of excision. Cutting current as opposed to coagulating current is preferred. The former technique minimizes carbonization that can make it challenging to recognize when an adequate depth has been achieved by the appearance of normal tissue. After the lesion is removed, the bowel wall is carefully assessed. Since most of these superficial lesions can be removed without entering the mucosa, the defects can be closed with interrupted transversely placed Lembert stitches.

Surgical treatment of the deeper lesions is more controversial. Removal of the rectosigmoid with reanastomosis is technically demanding and should be performed by skilled intestinal surgeons to minimize complications in these young patients. As experience has grown, there has been a shift to more aggressive therapy, usually in conjunction with gynecologists who remove endometrial deposits on the ovaries, fallopian tubes, and uterosacral ligaments. Medical treatment has not proven adequate for infiltrating intestinal or urologic lesions, so it is no surprise that castration alone has also proven ineffective.[53] Many of these women suffer from chronic pain or partial colonic obstructive symptoms following bilateral salpingo-oophorectomy when the endometrial implant is not resected. As a result, excision of the implant either with a disk of rectal wall or a formal anterior resection is recommended for women with symptoms related to the endometriosis. Both procedures can occasionally be performed laparoscopically, if the endometriosis is completely removed. Unfortunately, laparoscopy may miss lesions that are not visually apparent and discernible only by palpation. It should be noted, however, that for severe disease laparoscopic ablation, when possible, had similar crude pregnancy rates in comparison to laparotomy, and both techniques were clearly superior to medical management alone.[54]

The infiltrating nodular endometrial implants involving the rectovaginal portion of the cul-de-sac often invade both the vagina and rectum. Since the removal of the implant will require resection of a portion of the rectal wall, dissection of the lesion from the vagina allows for en bloc removal of the lesion with the rectal wall. There is often no discernible plane between these lesions and the walls of the rectum or vagina. Care must be taken to avoid the penetration of the vaginal wall with possible injury to the cervix, especially in women desiring eventual pregnancy. Often it is advantageous to mobilize the rectum in the posterior and lateral tissue planes to adequately define the lesion before attempting the anterior dissection. Blunt dissection of the rectovaginal plane below the area of involvement may help clarify the distorted anatomy and avoid inadvertent entry into the bowel lumen. After careful dissection of the lesion from the vagina, the normal rectovaginal plane is reached,

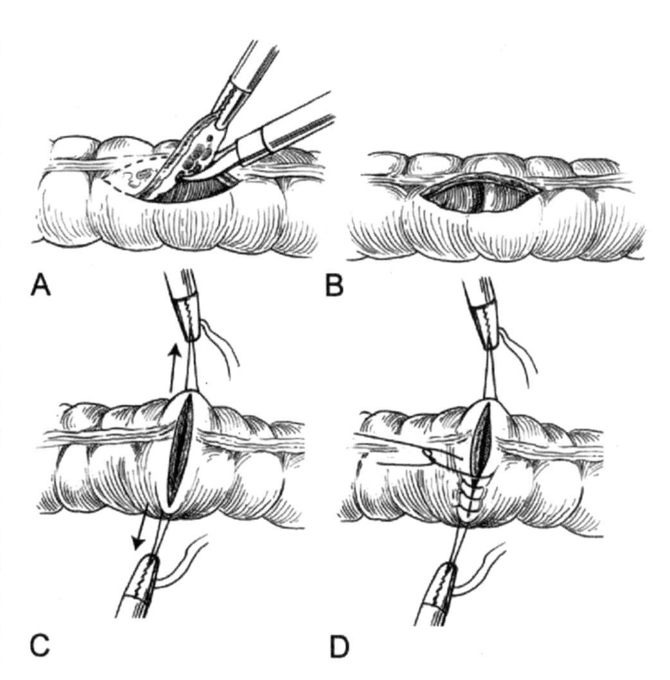

FIGURE 25-7. Disk excision of an endometrial implant.

and the fixed, hard mass may suddenly become mobile and amenable to resection.

Disk excision of the anterior rectal wall, by either laparoscopic or open technique, is performed for single lesions usually less than 3 cm in diameter (Figure 25-7A–D). After marking the lesions circumferentially with electrocautery, stay sutures are placed on either side of the endometrial implant. Full-thickness bowel wall excision is then performed with the cutting current electrocautery. Interrupted transverse absorbable sutures are subsequently placed to close the resulting defect. It is critical that a rim of normal bowel wall be removed with the lesion to ensure complete removal of the lesion. Remorgida et al.[55] in 2005 evaluated full-thickness disk excision of bowel implants and discovered that 40% were incomplete. They postulated that not all endometriotic lesions are surrounded by fibrosis and consequently not included in the specimen.

Segmental resection of the rectosigmoid is performed for larger lesions or when neoplasia is a concern. Margins are to grossly normal colon, and unless there are multiple lesions, a large colonic resection is not required. High ligation of the sigmoid vessels is also unnecessary, and the anastomosis may be either hand-sewn or stapled. When resection is performed laparoscopically, the involved segment may be removed by extending one of the port sites. Nezhat and colleagues[56] have described a technique of prolapsing the lesion outside the anus for resection. Redwine et al.[57] described a transvaginal approach for specimen removal. Open or laparoscopic excision of these deeply infiltrating rectovaginal lesions is very technically demanding. The lack of discernable tissue planes, the intimate association of the rectum and vagina, and the frequent occurrence of distal infiltration of endometriosis down to the mid-to-lower rectum makes laparoscopic resection possible only by surgeons very experienced in complex intestinal laparoscopy. Even in the hands of experienced laparoscopists, rectovaginal fistula requiring ileostomy has been reported to occur following these resections.[56] In fact, Darai et al.[58] in 2007 recommended that a protecting ileostomy be performed when combined resection of the vaginal and rectal walls is performed laparoscopically to minimize the high risk of anastomotic complications. Our current approach is to place omentum between the rectum and the vagina, if the suture lines are in contact. Proctoscopic insufflation to assess for leak is practiced routinely by the authors with all rectal anastomoses, whether performed open or laparoscopically.

Small Bowel and Appendiceal Endometriosis

While endometriosis involving the small bowel or appendix is much less common than rectosigmoid disease, careful inspection of these organs is critical in patients with advanced endometriosis to ensure complete removal of all gross disease and to minimize recurrence. Superficial small bowel implants may be treated with sharp excision, electrocautery, or the laser, as described above. Deeper implants may require small bowel resection, and, if within 5 cm of the ileocecal valve, may need an ileocecectomy. Appendiceal endometriosis is treated with appendectomy. Occasionally, a surgeon will encounter a patient with an endometrial implant while operating for another condition. While the lesion may exhibit a classic visual appearance consistent with endometriosis, a biopsy to confirm the diagnosis and exclude malignancy is important. Several studies have suggested that few patients with small asymptomatic endometrial implants of the appendix will become symptomatic, but no study has yet defined the natural history of these lesions. As a result, for those patients with asymptomatic endometriosis observation is probably sufficient, but hormone replacement therapy should be avoided.

Results After Surgical Therapy

Recurrence of endometriosis after surgical excision is difficult to assess because of a wide variability in the operative approach to endometriosis by various authors and the obvious need for postoperative laparoscopy to document asymptomatic recurrence. While there are no long-term prospective studies to date, the larger studies suggest a histologically confirmed rate of recurrent endometriosis of approximately 19%.[59] Gauging the response to surgery by the resolution of preoperative pelvic pain or infertility is easier to measure. The largest series of intestinal resections for advanced intestinal endometriosis by Bailey et al.[60] found that 86% of patients had complete or near complete relief of their preoperative pelvic pain. In addition, a 50% crude pregnancy rate was achieved which was comparable with rates found when treating much lower stages of disease. These results in over 130 cases with a median follow-up of 5 years were achieved with minimal morbidity, no anastomotic leaks, and no documented instance of recurrent colorectal endometriosis. Laparoscopic series of intestinal resections performed for extensive endometriosis have reported similar pregnancy rates albeit with smaller number of cases, higher complication rates, and shorter long-term follow-up.

Combined Medical and Surgical Therapy

Both medical and surgical therapies for endometriosis have potential reasons why each treatment alone may not be successful in eradicating the disease and minimizing recurrence. Medical therapy affects endometrial implants variably, and there is a high instance of recurrence following cessation of therapy. Surgery may not remove microscopic disease, and postsurgical adhesions may contribute to postoperative pelvic pain and infertility. For these reasons, combination therapy either pre- or postoperatively has been used for several years, although with a paucity of prospective randomized data to conclusively prove long-term improvement in recurrence and symptoms.

The rationale for preoperative medical therapy conducted over a period of 3–6 months is principally to decrease the inflammation and possibly the size of the endometrial implants. Presumably, this therapy will allow easier excision with diminished adhesion formation. Medical therapy may also reduce the vascularity of endometrial implants. A prospective study by Buttram et al.[61] in 1985 revealed an improvement in pregnancy rates with 6 months of danazol given preoperatively with all stages of endometriosis. The optimal length of therapy and long-term (and not just delayed) recurrence rates must still be elucidated. Postoperative treatment with danazol and oral contraceptive pills has not been shown to have durability, and the initial excitement over improved recurrence rates at 12 months has not been duplicated after longer follow-ups. Our current use of combined therapy is a 3–6 month course of a GnRH-a prior to definitive surgery.

Conclusion

The diagnosis and management of intestinal endometriosis has evolved tremendously over the last 20 years with the widespread availability of laparoscopy and a clear understanding of the necessity to remove all endometrial implants in symptomatic patients. With the advent of stapling devices that facilitate low pelvic anastomoses, the intestinal surgeon should be able to resect the endometrial implants and restore bowel continuity in virtually all patients with minimal morbidity and preserved fertility, when desired. Further improvements in outcomes will probably not occur until a better understanding of the precise etiology and growth of the endometrial implant is discovered.

References

1. Hasson HM. Incidence of endometriosis in diagnostic laparoscopy. J Reprod Med. 1976;16:135–8.
2. Drake TS, Grunert GM. The unsuspected pelvic factor in the infertility evaluation. Fertil Steril. 1980;34:27–31.
3. Houston DE, Noller KL, Melton III J, Selwyn BJ. The epidemiology of pelvic endometriosis. Clin Obstet Gynecol. 1988;31(4):787–800.
4. Halme J, Stovall D. Endometriosis and its medical management. In: Walch EE, Zacur HA, editors. Reproductive medicine and surgery. St. Louis: Mosby; 1995. p. 695–710.
5. Moen MH. Is a long period without childbirth a risk factor for endometriosis? Hum Reprod. 1991;6:1404–7.
6. Miyazawa K. Incidence of endometriosis among Japanese women. Obstet Gynecol. 1976;48:407–9.
7. Ridley JH. The histogenesis of endometriosis. A review of facts and fancies. Obstet Gynecol Surv. 1968;20:1–35.
8. Sampson JA. Perforating hemorrhagic (chocolate) cysts of the ovary, their importance and especially their relation to pelvic adenomas of endometrial type. Arch Surg. 1921;3:245–323.
9. Telinde RW, Scott RB. Experimental endometriosis. Am J Obstet Gynecol. 1950;60:1147–73.
10. Ridley JH, Edwards KI. Experimental endometriosis in the human. Am J Obstet Gynecol. 1958;76:783–90.
11. Simpson JL, Elias S, Malinak LR, Buttram VC. Heritable aspects of endometriosis. 1. Genetic studies. Am J Obstet Gynecol. 1980;137:327–31.
12. Dmowski WP, Steele RW, Baker GF. Deficient cellular immunity in endometriosis. Am J Obstet Gynecol. 1981;141: 377–83.
13. Vigano P, Vercellini P, DiBlasio AM, et al. Deficient anti-endometrium lymphocyte mediated cytotoxicity in patients with endometriosis. Fertil Steril. 1991;56:894–9.
14. Oosterlynck DJ, Cornillie FJ, Waer M, et al. Women with endometriosis show a defect in natural killer activity resulting in a decreased cytotoxicity to autologous endometrium. Fertil Steril. 1991;56:45–51.
15. Thomas EJ, Cooke ID. Impact of gestrinone on the course of asymptomatic endometriosis. Br Med J. 1987;294:272–4.
16. Bergqvist A, Thorbjorn B, Hogstrom L, et al. Effects of triptorelin versus placebo on the symptoms of endometriosis. Fertil Steril. 1998;69:702–8.
17. Evers JLH. The second-look laparoscopy for evaluation of the result of medical treatment of endometriosis should not be performed during ovarian suppression. Fertil Steril. 1987;47: 502–4.
18. Vercillini P, Fedele L, Molteni P, et al. Laparoscopy in the diagnosis of gynecologic chronic pelvic pain. Int J Gynaecol Obstet. 1990;32:261–5.
19. Koninckx PR, Meuleman C, Demeyere S, et al. Suggestive evidence that pelvic endometriosis is a progressive disease, whereas deeply infiltrating endometriosis is associated with pelvic pain. Fertil Steril. 1991;55:759–65.
20. Schulman H, Duvivier R, Blattner P. The uterine contractility index: a research and diagnostic tool in dysmenorrhea. Am J Obstet Gynecol. 1983;145:1049–58.
21. Liu DTY, Hitchcock A. Endometriosis: its association with retrograde menstruation, dysmenorrhea and tubal pathology. Br J Obstet Gynecol. 1986;93:859–62.
22. Cornillie FJ, Oosterlynck DJ, Lauweryns J, et al. Deeply infiltrating pelvic endometriosis: histology and clinical significance. Fertil Steril. 1990;53:978–93.
23. Badaway S, Marshall L, Gabal A, et al. The concentration of 13,14-dihydro-15-keto-prostaglandin F2alpha and prostaglandin E2 in peritoneal fluid of infertile patients with and without endometriosis. Fertil Steril. 1982;38:166–70.
24. Dawood M, Khan-Dawood F, Wilson L. Peritoneal fluid prostaglandins and prostanoids in women with endometriosis, chronic pelvic inflammatory disease, and pelvic pain. Am J Obstet Gynecol. 1984;148:391–5.
25. Hull MGR, Glazener CMA, Kelly NJ, et al. Population study of causes, treatment, and outcome of infertility. Br Med J. 1985;291:1693–7.
26. Fortier KJ, Haney AF. The pathologic spectrum of uterotubal junction obstruction. Obstet Gynecol. 1985;65:93–8.
27. Buttram Jr VC, Reiter RC. Endometriosis. In: Buttram Jr VC, Reiter RC, editors. Surgical treatment of the infertile female. Baltimore: Williams & Wilkins; 1985. p. 89–148.
28. Garcia CR, David SS. Pelvic endometriosis: infertility and pelvic pain. Am J Obstet Gynecol. 1977;129:740–7.
29. Inoue M, Kobayshi Y, Honda I, et al. The impact of endometriosis on the reproductive outcome of infertile patients. Am J Obstet Gynecol. 1992;167:278–82.
30. Jansen RPS. Minimal endometriosis and reduced fecundability: prospective evidence from an artificial insemination by donor program. Fertil Steril. 1986;46:141–3.
31. Floberg J, Backdahl M, Silfersward C, et al. Postpartum perforation of the colon due to endometriosis. Acta Obstet Gynecol Scand. 1984;63:183–4.
32. Prystowsky JB, Stryker SJ, Ujiki GT, Poticha SM. Gastrointestinal endometriosis. Arch Surg. 1988;123:855–8.
33. Aure JC, Hoeg K, Kolstad P. Carcinoma of the ovary and endometriosis. Acta Obstet Gynecol Scand. 1971;50:63–7.
34. Yantiss RK, Clement PB, Young RH. Neoplastic and preneoplastic changes in gastrointestinal endometriosis. Am J Surg Pathol. 2000;24:513–24.
35. Kennedy SH, Starkey PM, Sargent I, et al. Anti-endometrial antibodies in endometriosis measured by an enzyme-linked immunosorbent assay before and after treatment with danazol and nafarelin. Obstet Gynecol. 1990;75:914–7.
36. Chapron C, Dumontier I, Dousset B, et al. Results and role of rectal endoscopic ultrasonography for patients with deep pelvic endometriosis. Hum Reprod. 1998;13:2266–70.
37. Doniec JM, Kahlke V, Peetz F, et al. Rectal endometriosis: high sensitivity and specificity of endorectal ultrasound with an impact for the operative management. Dis Colon Rectum. 2003;46:1667–73.
38. Bazot M, Darai E, Hourani R, et al. Deep pelvic endometriosis: MR imaging for diagnosis and prediction of extension of disease. Radiology. 2004;232:379–89.
39. Kinkel K, Chapron C, Balleyguier C, et al. Magnetic resonance imaging characteristics of deep endometriosis. Hum Reprod. 1999;14:1080–6.
40. Kennedy SH, Soper ND, Mojiminiyi OA. Immunoscintigraphy of endomentriosis. A preliminary study. Br J Obstet Gynecol. 1988;95:693–7.
41. Vasquez G, Cornillie FJ, Brosens IO. Peritoneal endometriosis: scanning electron microscopy in visually normal peritoneum. Fertil Steril. 1986;42:696–703.

42. American Society for Reproductive Medicine. Revised American Society for Reproductive Medicine classification of endometriosis: 1996. Fertil Steril. 1997;67:817–21.
43. Donnez J, Nisolle M, Casanas-Roux F, et al. Stereometric evaluation of peritoneal endometriosis and endometriotic nodules of the rectovaginal septum. Hum Reprod. 1995;11:224–8.
44. Koninckx PR. Deeply infiltrating endometriosis. In: Brosens I, Donnez J, editors. Endometriosis: research and management. Carnforth: Parthenon Publishing; 1993. p. 437–46.
45. Martin DC, Hubert GD, Vander Zwaag R, et al. Laparoscopic appearances of peritoneal endometriosis. Fertil Steril. 1989;51:63–7.
46. Koninckx PR, Martin DC. Deep endometriosis: a consequence of infiltration or retraction or possibly adenomyosis externa? Fertil Steril. 1992;58:924–8.
47. Vercellini P, Aimi G, Panazza S, et al. A gonadotropin-releasing hormone agonist versus a low-dose oral contraceptive for pelvic pain associated with endometriosis. Fertil Steril. 1992;60:75–9.
48. Dmowski WP, Radwanska E, Rana N. Recurrent endometriosis following hysterectomy and oophorectomy: the role of residual ovarian fragments. Int J Gynaecol Obstet. 1988;26:93–103.
49. Dmowski WP, Gebel H, Braun DP. The role of cell mediated immunity in pathogenesis of endometriosis. Acta Obstet Gynecol Scand. 1994;159:7–14.
50. Noble AD, Letchworth AT. Medical treatment of endometriosis: a comparative trial. Postgrad Med J. 1979;55:37–9.
51. Wheeler JM, Knitte JD, Miller JD. Depot Leuprolide versus danazol in treatment of women with symptomatic endometriosis. Am J Obstet Gynecol. 1992;167:1367–71.
52. Hall LH, Malone JM, Ginsburg KA. Flare-up of endometriosis induced by gonadotropin-releasing hormone agonist leading to bowel obstruction. Fertil Steril. 1995;64:1204–6.
53. Redwine DB. Endometriosis persisting after castration: clinical characteristics and results of surgical management. Obstet Gynecol. 1994;83:405–13.
54. Olive DL, Lee KL. Analysis of sequential treatment protocols for endometriosis-associated infertility. Am J Obstet Gynecol. 1986;154:613.
55. Remorgida V, Ragni N, Ferrero S, et al. How complete is full thickness disc resection of bowel endometriotic lesions? A prospective surgical and histologic study. Hum Reprod. 2005;20:2317–20.
56. Nezhat C, Pennington E, Nezhat F, Silfen SL. Laparoscopically assisted anterior rectal wall resection and reanastomosis for deeply infiltrating endometriosis. Surg Laparosc Endosc. 1991;1:106–8.
57. Redwine DB, Koning M, Sharpe DR. Laparoscopically assisted transvaginal segmental resection of the rectosigmoid colon for endometriosis. Fertil Steril. 1996;65:193–7.
58. Darai E, Ackerman G, Bazot M, et al. Laparoscopic segmental colon resection for endometriosis: limits and complications. Surg Endosc. 2007;21:2039–43.
59. Wheeler JM, Malinak LR. Recurrent endometriosis. Contrib Gynecol Obstet. 1987;16:13–21.
60. Bailey HR, Ott MT, Hartendorp P. Aggressive surgical management for advanced colorectal endometriosis. Dis Colon Rectum. 1994;37:747–53.
61. Buttram VC, Reiter RC, Ward SM. Treatment of endometriosis with Danazol: report of a six year prospective study. Fertil Steril. 1985;43:353.

26
Trauma of the Colon and Rectum

David B. Hoyt and Michael E. Lekawa

Colon Injuries

Optimal management of colon injuries continues to be an evolving and controversial topic. Despite the dramatic reduction of colon-related mortality from about 60% during World War I to about 40% during World War II to about 10% during the Vietnam War and to lower than 3% in the last few decades, the colon-related morbidity remains high. The abdominal sepsis rate has remained significant at about 20% in a large prospective study in 2001 (Table 26-1).[1–6] No other organ injury is associated with a higher septic complication rate than colon injury. In the subgroups of patients with colon injuries with a Penetrating Abdominal Trauma Index (PATI) ≥25 or with multiple blood transfusions, the incidence of intraabdominal sepsis has been reported to be as high as 27%.[7] In patients with destructive colon injuries requiring resection, the reported incidence of abdominal complications is about 24%.[6] Many studies have attempted to identify risk factors for complications and create an optimal management strategy.

Epidemiology

The vast majority of colon injuries are due to penetrating trauma. In American urban centers, firearms are by far the most common cause of injury. In anterior or posterior abdominal gunshot wounds, the colon is the second most commonly injured organ after the small bowel, and it is involved in about 27% of cases undergoing laparotomy.[8,9] In anterior abdominal stab wounds, the colon is the third most commonly injured organ after the liver and small bowel, and an injury is found in about 18% of patients undergoing laparotomy. In posterior stab wounds, the colon is the most commonly injured organ and is injured in about 25% of patients undergoing laparotomy.[10] In abdominal gunshot wounds, the transverse colon is the most commonly affected segment. In stab wounds, the left colon is the most commonly injured segment, probably due to the predominance of right-handed assailants.

Blunt trauma to the colon is uncommon and is diagnosed in about 0.5% of all major blunt trauma or in 10.6% of patients undergoing laparotomy.[11,12] Most of these injuries are of partial thickness, and only 3% of patients undergoing laparotomy have full-thickness colon perforations.[11,13] Motor-vehicle trauma is the most common cause of blunt colon injury. Deceleration injuries may cause avulsion of the colon from the mesentery, resulting in ischemia but blowout perforations due to transient closed loop formation may occur as well. Seat belts increase the risk of hollow viscous perforations, and the presence of a seat-belt mark sign is a predictor of hollow viscous injury. In rare cases, colonic wall hematoma or contusion may result in delayed perforation, several days after the injury. The left colon is the most commonly injured segment followed by the right colon and the transverse colon.[11]

Diagnosis

The diagnosis of colon injury is almost always made intraoperatively. However, with the introduction of selective nonoperative management of penetrating abdominal trauma, there has been a concern of missing colon injuries. This is particularly important in penetrating injuries of the back because small retroperitoneal colon injuries may not give early clinical signs. A rectal examination may show blood in the stool, especially in cases with distal colon or rectal injuries. A preoperative upright chest film may show free air under the diaphragm. The colon can reliably be evaluated by water-soluble contrast enema studies or abdominal CT scan with soluble rectal contrast. Retroperitoneal gas or contrast extravasation is diagnostic and an exploratory laparotomy should be performed. Otherwise, one trial from Grady Memorial Hospital found that all significant injuries were clinically evident within 18 h.[14] Other investigations such as ultrasound or diagnostic peritoneal lavage are unreliable in the evaluation of suspected colon injuries due to its retroperitoneal location. The preoperative diagnosis of colon injury following blunt trauma can be a major challenge, especially

D.E. Beck et al. (eds.), *The ASCRS Textbook of Colon and Rectal Surgery: Second Edition*,
DOI 10.1007/978-1-4419-1584-9_26, © Springer Science+Business Media, LLC 2011

TABLE 26-1. Incidence of abdominal septic complications in colon injuries (prospective studies)

Author, year	Number of patients	Abdominal sepsis (%)
George, 1989[1]	102	33
Chappuis, 1991[2]	56	20
Demetriades, 1992[3]	100	16
Iratury, 1993[4]	252	17
Gonzalez, 1996[5]	114	24
Demetriades, 2001[6]	297	24
Overall	921	22

TABLE 26-2. American Association for the Surgery of Trauma (AAST) colon injury scale

Grade	Injury description
I	(a) Contusion of hematoma without devascularization (b) Partial thickness laceration
II	Laceration ≤50% of circumference
III	Laceration >50% of circumference
IV	Transection of the colon
V	(a) Transection of the colon with segmental tissue loss (b) Devascularized segment

if the patient is unevaluable due to associated head injuries. The diagnosis may be suspected by the presence of free air or thickened colonic wall on the routine abdominal CT scan. In some cases, the diagnosis may be delayed by many days with catastrophic consequences. Intraoperatively, every paracolic hematoma due to penetrating trauma should be explored and the underlying colon should be evaluated carefully. Failure to adhere to this important surgical principle may lead to serious complications. Paracolic hematomas due to blunt trauma should not undergo routine exploration unless there is evidence of colon perforation.

Colon Injury Scale

The American Association for the Surgery of Trauma (AAST) developed a grading system for organ injuries to have objective criteria for the classification of the severity of the injury and enable reliable comparisons of results. On the basis of the injury grade, an abbreviated injury score (AIS) is assigned and may be used for the calculation of the injury severity score (ISS). The AAST colon injury scale is shown in Table 26-2.

Operative Management

Historical Perspective

The first guidelines regarding the management of colon injuries were published by the United States Surgeon General in 1943 and mandated proximal diversion or exteriorization of all colon wounds.[15] This unusual directive was initiated because of the very high mortality of colorectal injuries during the early years of World War II. The mortality in both civilian and military reports exceeded 50%.[16,17] Although these guidelines were not based on any scientific evidence, they were credited for the significant reduction of mortality in the last years of the war. However, during this period, many other major changes in trauma care took place. Faster evacuation from the battlefield and early definitive care, improved resuscitation protocols, and the introduction of penicillin and sulfadiazine could all have contributed to the reduction of mortality. The policy of mandatory colostomy for all colon injuries remained the unchallenged standard of care until the late 1970s. Stone reported the first major scientific challenge of this policy in 1979.[18] In a prospective randomized study, which excluded patients with hypotension, multiple associated injuries, destructive colon injuries, and delayed operations, the authors concluded that primary repair was associated with fewer complications than colostomy. The exclusion criteria were perceived as risk factors for anastomotic leak and were absolute indications for diversion.

With mortality rates due to colon-related complications improving over the next few years, surgeons challenged the validity of the "standard" contraindications for primary repair or resection and anastomosis. A few prospective randomized studies with no exclusion criteria (class I evidence) confirmed the safety of primary repair, at least in nondestructive colon injuries. Another alternative to primary repair or colostomy was exteriorized repair, which was introduced in the 1970s. With this technique, the sutured colon was exteriorized and observed for 4–5 days. If the repair remained intact during this period of observation, the colon was returned to the abdominal cavity. If the repair leaked, it was converted to a loop colostomy.[19,20] The enthusiasm for this approach waned in the 1980s due to the overwhelming evidence of the superiority of primary repair.

In the 1990s and 2000s, primary repair became the standard of care in most cases, although there is still some skepticism by many surgeons, especially in the presence of certain risk factors such as destructive colon injuries, severe contamination, multiple injuries, and delays in treatment.

Nondestructive Colon Injuries

There is now enough class I evidence (prospective randomized studies) supporting primary repair in all nondestructive colon injuries (injuries involving <50% of the bowel wall and without devascularization, i.e., AAST Grade I or II, irrespective of risk factors.) In a randomized study of 56 patients with no exclusion criteria, Chappuis et al. concluded that primary repair should be considered in all colon injuries irrespective of risk factors.[2] In another landmark study, Sasaki et al.

randomized 71 patients with colon injuries to either primary repair or diversion, without any exclusion criteria.[21] The overall complication rate was 19% in the primary repair group and 36% in the diversion group. In addition, the complication rate for colostomy closure was 7%. The authors concluded that primary repair is the method of choice of treatment of all penetrating colon injuries in the civilian population despite any associated risk factors for adverse outcome.

In 1996, Gonzalez et al.[5] published another important prospective study in which 109 patients were randomized to primary repair or diversion, independent of any risk factors. The sepsis-related complication rate was 20% in the primary repair group and 25% in the diversion group. In the presence of certain risk factors, such as severe fecal contamination, shock on admission, blood loss of 1,000 ml, or more than two associated organ injuries, the diversion group still had a higher complication rate, although this difference did not reach statistical significance. The authors continued their study until the series increased to 176 patients with penetrating colon injury and concluded again that in civilian trauma, all penetrating colon injuries should be primarily repaired.[22]

Overall, collective review of all available prospective randomized studies (class I evidence) identified 160 patients with primary repair and a 13.1% incidence of abdominal sepsis complications. In the group of 143 patients treated with diversion, the abdominal sepsis complication rate was 21.7% (Table 26-3). In addition to the available class I evidence, numerous prospective observational studies (class II evidence) demonstrated the superiority of primary repair over diversion in nondestructive injuries.[1,3,4,23] In conclusion, there is sufficient class I and II data to support routine primary repair of all nondestructive colon injuries, irrespective of risk factors for abdominal complications. No study has ever shown that colostomy is associated with better results than primary repair.

Despite the available scientific evidence, there is still some skepticism about liberal primary repair, and many surgeons still consider colostomy as the procedure of choice in many colon injuries. In a survey of 317 Canadian surgeons in 1996, 75% of them chose colostomy in low-velocity gunshot wounds to the colon.[24] In a 1998 survey of 342 American trauma surgeons, members of the AAST, a colostomy was the procedure of choice in 3% of colon perforations with minimal spillage, in 43% of perforations with gross spillage, in 18% of colon injuries involving >50% of the wall, and in 33% of cases with colon transection.[25] More recently, in a review of 99 colon injuries treated at one center from 1996 to 2006, 31% of patients have been treated with diversion.[26] It is obvious that dogma still plays a significant role in modern trauma surgery.

TABLE 26-3. Primary repair versus diversion: prospective randomized studies with no exclusion criteria

	Primary repair		Diversion	
Study	No. of patients	Abdominal septic complications (%)	No. of patients	Abdominal complications (%)
Chappuis[2]	28	4 (14.3)	28	5 (17.9)
Sasaki[21]	43	1 (2.3)	28	8 (28.6)
Gonzalez[22]	89	16 (18)	87	18 (21)
Total	160	21 (1,301)	143	31 (21.7)

Destructive Colon Injuries

Until recently, there was no sufficient class I or II data regarding the management of destructive colon injuries requiring resection (loss of >50% of bowel wall or devascularization). Until the last decade, the available prospective randomized studies included only 36 patients with colon resection and anastomosis. The overall incidence of anastomotic leak was 2.5% and no deaths occurred. All these studies recommended primary anastomosis irrespective of the presence of any risk factors for abdominal complications.[2,21,22] In a 1998 prospective, but not randomized, study on colon injuries by Cornwell et al.,[7] there were 25 patients with destructive colon injuries treated by resection and anastomosis and two patients treated by resection and colostomy. All patients had a PATI ≥ 25 or were transfused with ≥6 units of blood, or the operation was delayed by ≥6 h from the time of injury. There were two anastomotic leaks (8%) and both were fatal. The study concluded that some high-risk patients with destructive colon injuries might benefit from diversion. Unfortunately, the study did not include enough patients with diversion for comparison with the primary anastomosis group. There are two retrospective studies, which included only destructive colon injuries requiring resection: Stewart et al.[27] analyzed 60 patients, 43 of which were managed by resection and anastomosis and 17 by diversion. The overall anastomotic leak rate was 14%, and in the subgroup of patients with blood transfusion >6 units the leak rate was 33%. The authors suggested that primary anastomosis should not be performed in patients receiving massive blood transfusions or in the presence of underlying medical illness. Another retrospective study from Los Angeles analyzed the complications in a series of 140 patients with destructive colon injuries requiring resection.[28] The incidence of intraabdominal sepsis was similar in the groups with primary anastomosis or diversion. Univariate analysis identified PATI ≥ 25 or hypotension in the emergency room to be associated with increased risk of anastomotic leak. The study suggested that a diversion procedure might be appropriate in these high-risk subgroups of patients.

In summary, until 2000, the available prospective randomized studies, which include only a small number of cases, recommend resection with anastomosis irrespective of risk factors. Two large retrospective studies advocate diversion in the subgroups of patients with certain risk factors such as PATI ≥ 25, multiple blood transfusions, or associated medical illness.[27,28] Subsequently, the guidelines of the Eastern Association for the Surgery of Trauma (EAST) published in 1998 supported resection and primary anastomosis in the subgroups of patients with destructive colon injuries if they (a) are hemodynamically stable intraoperatively, (b) have minimal associated injuries (PATI<25, ISS<25), (c) have no peritonitis, and (d) have no underlying medical illness. The guidelines suggest that patients with shock, significant associated injuries, peritonitis, or underlying disease should be managed with resection and colostomy.[29] However, these guidelines were based on class III evidence. In their review of the literature, there were only 40 patients in class I studies with resection and anastomosis, and the anastomotic leak rate was 2.5% without mortality. In class II studies, there were only 12 patients who underwent resection and anastomosis, and the leak rate was 8.3% without mortality. In class III retrospective studies, there were 303 patients with a leak rate of 5.2% and three deaths (1%) due to the leak.

In view of the lack of large prospective studies in the literature, the AAST sponsored a prospective multicenter study to evaluate the safety of primary anastomosis or diversion and identify independent risk factors for colon-related complications in patients with destructive colon injuries requiring resection.[6] This study, published in 2001, included 297 patients with penetrating injuries requiring colon resection (rectal injuries were excluded) that survived at least 72 h. The overall colon-related mortality was 1.3% (4 deaths) and all deaths occurred in the diversion groups ($P=0.01$). The overall incidence of abdominal complications was 24%, and the most common complication was an intraabdominal abscess (19% of patients) followed by fascia dehiscence (9%). The incidence of anastomotic leaks was 6.6%. Multivariate analysis identified three independent risk factors for abdominal complications: severe fecal contamination, ≥4 units of blood transfusions within the first 24 h, and single-agent antibiotic prophylaxis. If all the three risk factors were present, the incidence of abdominal complications was about 60%; if any two factors were present, the complications rate was 34%; if only one factor was present, this figure was about 20%, and with no risk factors it was 13%. The method of colon management, delay of operation >6 h, shock at admission, site of colon injury, PATI>25, ISS>20, or associated intraabdominal injuries were not found to be independent risk factors.

In a second analysis, the group of patients with primary anastomosis was compared with the group with diversion, using multivariate analysis that controlled for PATI>25, transfusion >6 units of blood, >6 h delay of operation, shock at admission, and severe fecal contamination. These factors have been described in previous studies as significant risks for abdominal complications. With colon diversion serving as reference (RR 1.00) for comparison, the adjusted relative risk of primary anastomosis was exactly the same (1.00).

In a similar analysis according to subgroups with ileocolostomy, colocolostomy, ileostomy, and colostomy, the adjusted relative risk of abdominal complications was similar. In another analysis, all patients were classified into either a high-risk group (if any of the following factors was present: hypotension at admission, blood transfusions >6 units, delay of operation >6 h, severe peritoneal contamination, or PATI>25) or a low-risk group if none of the above risk factors was present. These risk factors are considered by many surgeons as strong indications for diversion. The colon-related mortality in the high-risk patients was 4.5% (4 of 88 patients) in the diversion group and no deaths in the 121 patients who underwent primary anastomosis ($P=0.03$). Multivariate analysis showed that the adjusted relative risk of abdominal complication in patients with primary anastomosis or diversion was similar, in both the low-risk and high-risk patients (Table 26-4). There was a trend toward shorter ICU and hospital stay in the primary anastomosis group. The study concluded that "in view of these findings and the fact that colon diversion is associated with worse quality of life and requires an additional operation for closure, colon injuries requiring resection should be managed by primary repair, irrespective of risk factors".[6]

Damage control procedures with abdominal packing and temporary closure of the abdominal wall with a prosthetic material pose a special dilemma regarding the management of destructive colon injuries. No studies have ever addressed this issue, and the existing practices are based on personal beliefs and experience. The authors advocate primary anastomosis because of the theoretical disadvantages of having a colostomy, which is an open source of fecal material, near an open abdomen. The only conditions for which there is agreement for colostomy are the presence of severe colon edema or a questionable blood supply of the colon. In these situations, theoretically, a diversion procedure should be

TABLE 26-4. American Association for the Surgery of Trauma (AAST) colon resection study: comparison of abdominal complications between primary anastomosis and diversion in high- and low-risk patients

Patient population	Primary anastomosis: abdominal complications (%)	Diversion: abdominal complications (%)	Adjusted relative risk (95% CI)	*P* value
All patients	22	27	0.81 (0.55–1.41)	0.69
Low-risk* patients	13	8	1.26 (0.21–8.39)	0.82
High-risk* patients	28	30	0.90 (0.53–1.40)	0.67

*High-risk patients were those with PATI>25, severe fecal contamination, 6 h from injury to operation, transfusion of >6 units of blood preintraoperatively, or systolic blood pressure ≤90 mmHg.

*Low-risk patients were those without any of the above risk factors.

a safe option. Despite this evidence, the move away from colostomy formation is slow and ongoing.[26]

Risk Factors for Abdominal Complications

The abdominal complication rate in colon injuries is very high, with a sepsis rate of about 20% (Table 26-1). In destructive colon injuries requiring resection, the prospective AAST colon resection study of 298 patients recorded an overall incidence of 24% of abdominal complications. Many studies attempted to identify risk factors for complications and, on the basis of these risks, to modify the treatment.

Left- Versus Right-Colon Injuries

For many years and until recently, there was an anecdotal perception that left-colon injuries are associated with a higher risk of anastomotic leaks and septic complications than right colon injuries. This perception was based on theoretical reasons (different anatomy and blood supply, higher concentration of bacteria, and poorer healing properties in the left colon) rather than clinical evidence. This perception led surgeons to advocate liberal primary repair of right colon wounds and colostomy in left-colon wounds. However, no clinical or experimental study has ever demonstrated any healing differences between the two sides of the colon or any evidence that the two anatomical sides should be treated differently. Experimental work in baboons, which have very similar anatomy and bacteriology to humans, showed no difference of the healing properties between the right and left colon.[30] The study involved resection of a 10-cm segment of right colon and a 10-cm segment of left colon and primary anastomosis, without any mechanical or chemical preparation of the colon. The healing of the anastomosis was assessed at autopsy 7 days postoperatively for complications (leak, local abscess), mechanically by measuring the breaking strength of the anastomosis and biochemically by measuring the hydroxyproline concentrations at the anastomotic site. The study showed identical healing properties of the two sides of the colon.

In another study using the same model, one of the authors evaluated the effect of hypovolemia (blood loss of 20 ml/kg) on healing of the left and right sides of the colon, and again no differences were found (Figures 26-1 and 26-2).[31]

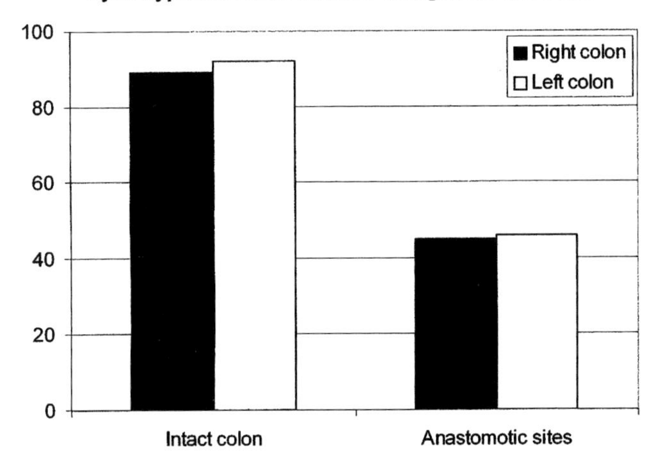

FIGURE 26-1. Hydroxyproline concentration (biochemical marker of wound healing) are similar in both sides of the colon *R* right colon, *L* left colon (values in µg/mg). (Adapted from Sofianos C, Demetriades D, Oosthuizen MM, et al. The effect of hypovolemia on healing of the right and left colon. An experimental study. S Afr J Surg. 1992;30:42–3.[31]).

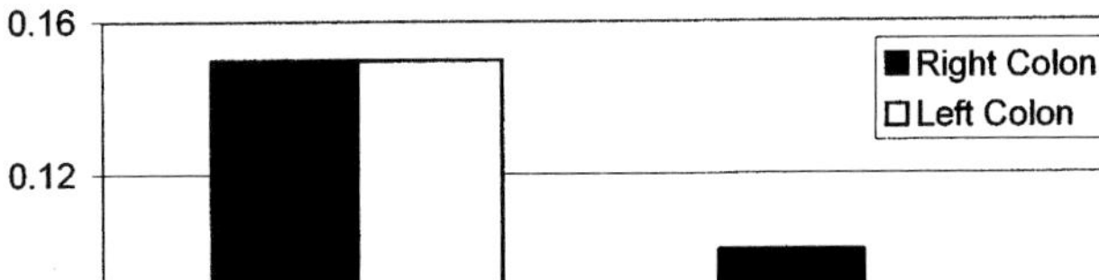

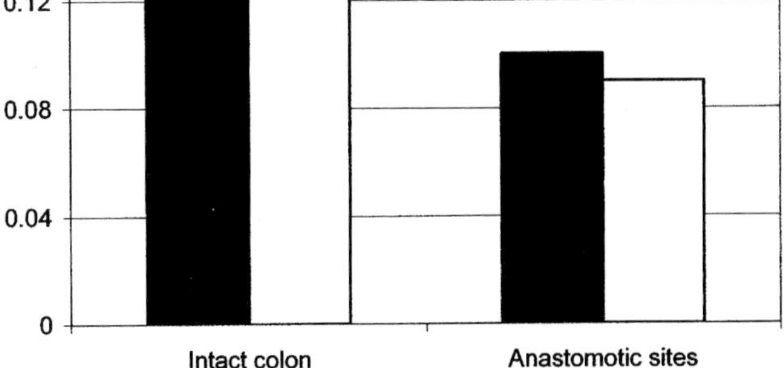

FIGURE 26-2. Breaking strength of the right and left colon are similar: *R* right colon *L* left colon (values in N/mm^2). (Adapted from Sofianos C, Demetriades D, Oosthuizen MM, et al. The effect of hypovolemia on healing of the right and left colon. An experimental study. S Afr J Surg. 1992;30:42–3.[31]).

Associated Abdominal Injuries

Early studies suggested that because multiple or severe associated intraabdominal injuries (PATI>25) are associated with a high incidence of septic complications, they were considered to be contraindications for primary repair of the colon.[4,7] This factor was considered even more critical in destructive colon injuries and was suggested as an indication for diversion.[29] However, class I and II studies have shown that although multiple associated intraabdominal injuries are significant risk factors for intraabdominal sepsis, the method of colon management does not affect the incidence of abdominal sepsis.[3,5–7,32] Some studies have suggested that the creation of an ostomy in these high-risk patients may independently contribute to abdominal sepsis.[32] The current class I and II literature supports primary repair or resection and anastomosis in patients with severe or multiple associated abdominal injuries.

Military Wounds

Recent results from colon injuries incurred during the conflict in South Asia reflect a continued reliance on temporary stoma creation. This is due to a number of issues, including the destructive nature of the injuries, and time to transport to tertiary care centers in Europe and the USA. This illustrates the continued difficulty with translation of clinical practice to military practice, and vice versa.[33–35]

Shock

There is now sufficient class I and II evidence that preoperative or intraoperative shock is neither an independent risk factor for abdominal sepsis nor a contradiction for primary colon repair or anastomosis.[3,5,6,30]

Blood Transfusions

Multiple blood transfusion (≥4 units of blood within the first 24 h) has been shown to be a major independent risk factor for abdominal septic complications.[6,32] In a large prospective AAST study of 297 patients with penetrating destructive colon injuries requiring resection, blood transfusion was the most critical independent factor for abdominal sepsis (adjusted RR 2.0; 95% CI, 1.31–2.83; $P=0.001$). However, the method of colon management did not influence the complication rate in this group of patients, and primary anastomosis was recommended.[6]

Injury Severity Score

The injury severity score (ISS) is not an independent risk factor for abdominal sepsis, and high ISS (>15) is not a contraindication for primary repair or anastomosis.[3,6]

Fecal Contamination

Severe fecal contamination of the peritoneal cavity is a major independent risk factor for abdominal sepsis.[1,6,11,28,32,36,37] This finding led some studies to suggest that the presence of severe contamination should be a contraindication for primary repair or anastomosis.[1,11,36,37] However, all prospective randomized studies and recent large prospective observational studies have shown that the method of colon management in this group of patients does not influence the septic complication rate and have recommended primary repair or anastomosis.[2,5,6]

Specific Associated Abdominal Injuries

There is class III evidence that the combination of colon injuries with pancreatic or ureteric injuries is associated with an increased incidence of septic complications.[38,39] However, there is no evidence that the presence of any of these injuries is a contraindication for primary repair or anastomosis.[6] Common sense may dictate that the colon anastomosis should be physically separated from the intraabdominal injury, if possible.

Time from Injury to Operation

The length of delay of surgical repair over which the septic complication rate increases is not well defined. Some studies suggest ≥6 h while others have suggested ≥12 h as the critical delays associated with an increased risk of infections.[7,23,28,40] It seems that the degree of contamination is much more important than the delay in surgical management, and the time delay in itself should not be used as a criterion for primary repair or diversion. In a prospective study of 297 destructive colon injuries, the incidence of abdominal complication was 11.4% (4/35) in the group of patients with preoperative time >6 h and 26.1% in patients with preoperative times ≤6 h. Multivariate analysis failed to identify time delay as an independent risk factor.[6]

Retained Missiles

Missiles that passed through the colon and remained lodged in the tissues are not associated with increased risk of local sepsis, and they should be removed only if the removal is technically easy and does not prolong the operation. In a study of 84 patients with gunshot wounds of the colon, the bullet remained in the body in 40 and was removed in 44. The incidence of local septic complications was 5% in patients with retained bullets and 7% in those without.[41]

Temporary Abdominal Wall Closure

Damage control laparotomy and temporary abdominal wall closure with prosthetic material seem to be associated with increased incidence of abdominal septic complications. The crude relative risk of abdominal sepsis in patients with temporary abdominal wall closure has been reported to be 2.12 (1.32–3.40; $P=0.005$) in a study of 297 of destructive colon injuries requiring resection. However, multivariate analysis failed to identify this method as an independent risk factor.[6] A recent evaluation of delayed primary anastomosis during damage control laparotomy by Miller et al. illustrated that 11 colon resections treated after damage control laparotomy with primary anastomosis had no suture line breakdown. They concluded that scheduled primary anastomosis is safe.[42] The Denver group also illustrated the safety of delayed primary anastomosis after damage control laparotomy.[26] Another recent retrospective review by Weinberg et al.[43] found that patients who underwent damage control laparotomy have a trend toward higher complications and anastomotic dehiscence than in single laparotomy patients. While this should give pause in making an absolute recommendation for anastomosis after damage control laparotomy, the trend away from colostomy continues in most centers. The anastomosis is usually done on the first return to the operating room.

Anastomotic Leaks

Colon leaks remain the most serious complication in repaired or anastomosed colons. The overall incidence of suture line failures is fairly low. In a collective review of 35 prospective or retrospective studies with 2,964 primary repairs, Curran reported 66 (2.2%) leaks.[44] In prospective studies including 534 patients with colon repair or resection and anastomosis, there were 17 (3.2%) leaks.[44] The leak rate after resection and anastomosis is significantly higher than in simple repairs. In a 1999 collective review of 362 patients with resection and anastomosis, the overall incidence of anastomotic leak was 5.5%.[44] The same year, in another large retrospective study of 112 patients with penetrating or blunt colonic injuries treated by resection and primary anastomosis, Murray et al.[28] reported a leak rate of 9%. In a more recent multicenter prospective study of 197 patients with penetrating colon injuries who underwent resection and primary anastomosis, the leak rate was 6.6%.[6]

The risk factors for anastomotic leak are not well defined. It seems that colocolostomies are associated with a higher incidence of anastomotic leaks than ileocolostomies. Murray et al.[28] reported a leak rate of 4% in 56 patients with ileocolostomies and 13% in 56 colocolostomies. Univariate analysis identified PATI $\geq$25, $\geq$6 units of blood transfusion and hypotension in the emergency room as risk factors for anastomotic leak. A multicenter prospective AAST study reported a leak rate of 4.2% for ileocolostomies and 8.9% for colocolostomies.[6] The leaks occurred in patients with or without multiple blood transfusions, severe contamination, and multiple associated injuries. No significant independent risk factors could be identified.

Many cases of anastomotic leak that do not result in diffuse peritonitis can be managed safely nonoperatively with a low-residue diet. In most cases, the leak results in a fecal fistula, which heals spontaneously within a few days. In other cases, the leak results in a local abscess which can be drained percutaneously. However, in some patients, the colonic leak causes severe intraabdominal sepsis, and a proximal diversion procedure may be required. Curran reported no deaths in a collective series of 66 patients who underwent repair for leaks.[44] However, Murray et al.[28] reported 2 colon-related deaths in a group of ten patients with anastomotic leak. The AAST multicenter study reported no deaths in the 13 patients with anastomotic leaks. The overall mortality due to colon leak-related complications in a collective review of 3,161 trauma patients treated with primary repair or resection and anastomosis was only 0.1%.[6,44]

In summary, colonic leaks occur more commonly in patients with colocolostomies than in patients with ileocolostomies. External fecal fistulas can safely be managed nonoperatively with low-residue diet. Localized abscesses are best drained percutaneously by interventional radiology, and the ensuing fecal fistula almost always closes spontaneously. Reexploration of the abdomen and creation of fecal diversion with or without resection of the leaking colon should be reserved only for patients with generalized peritonitis or failed percutaneous drainage.

Technique of Colon Repair

In nondestructive injuries, repair of the injured colon should be performed after debridement of the perforation. This step is critical in gunshot wounds when failure to debride may result in breakdown of the suture line. In destructive injuries, resection to normal and well-perfused edges should be performed, and the anastomosis should be tension-free. The method of anastomosis, hand-sewn or stapled, does not influence the incidence of abdominal complications or leak rate and it should be the surgeon's preference. In a prospective AAST study of 207 patients with penetrating destructive injuries who underwent resection and anastomosis, 128 cases were managed by hand-sewn anastomosis and 79 cases by stapled anastomosis. The incidence of anastomotic leak was 7.8% and 6.3%, respectively. Multivariate analysis adjusting for blood transfusions, degree of fecal contamination, and antibiotic coverage showed identical complication rates (stapled anastomosis adjusted RR = 0.99).[45] Further protection of the anastomosis with adjacent omentum is recommended whenever possible.

Rectal Injuries

The management of rectal trauma has undergone many changes in the same manner as colon injuries, with many of the principles of management evolving from wartime experiences. The mortality related to rectal trauma has decreased dramatically from 67% during World War I down to today's civilian reports of 0–10%.[46–51] Likewise, the morbidity, which was as high as 72% during the Vietnam War, is now as low as 10%.[51,52] The components of management, developed from lessons learned from combat experiences, have remained controversial and include (1) diversion of fecal stream, (2) distal rectal washout, (3) presacral drainage, and (4) debridement and closure of wounds when possible. Because of the paucity of class I and class II data, no consensus has been achieved with respect to the optimal management of rectal trauma.

Anatomy

The anatomy of the rectum makes it difficult to apply the principles of colon trauma management. The majority of the rectum is completely surrounded by the bony pelvis, making injuries infrequent and exposure difficult. The rectum varies in length from 12 to 15 cm, with only the upper two-thirds anteriorly and the upper one-third laterally covered by peritoneum (intraperitoneal rectum). The lower third of the rectum completely lacks peritoneal covering (extraperitoneal rectum), which makes exposure and repair of injuries difficult. Finally, the rectum is easily accessible from the anus, with the anterior peritoneal reflection only approximately 6 cm from the anal verge. This results in a not uncommon finding of intraperitoneal injury from rectal foreign bodies.

Epidemiology

For various anatomical reasons, injuries to the rectum occur infrequently and are usually the result of penetrating trauma. In most series, gunshot and shotgun wounds account for 80–85% of injuries, and stab wounds for 3–5%.[46,53,54] In a series of 59 patients with gunshot wounds to the buttocks, only 3.4% had rectal injuries.[55] In another series of 192 patients with gunshot wounds to the back, 2.6% had a rectal injury.[9] Interestingly, in a series of 309 anterior abdominal gunshot wounds and a series of 37 transpelvic gunshot wounds, no rectal injuries were identified, reiterating the infrequency of this injury.[8,56]

Other causes include iatrogenic injuries from urologic and endoscopic procedures, sex-related trauma, and anorectal foreign bodies. Blunt trauma accounts for 5–10% of cases, and it is usually the result of pelvic fractures or impalement.[46,49,53,54,57] Rectal injuries have been reported in nearly 2% of all pelvic fractures.[58]

Diagnosis

The diagnosis of intraperitoneal rectal injury, similar to colonic injuries, is usually made intraoperatively. Extraperitoneal rectal injuries may not always be obvious. A high index of suspicion is necessary with both blunt and penetrating mechanisms to avoid missing an injury. The cornerstone for diagnosing an extraperitoneal injury is the combination of a digital rectal exam and rigid proctoscopy. In most series, the diagnostic accuracy of the digital rectal exam and rigid proctoscopy ranges from 80 to 95%.[46,51,54,59–61] However, the false-negative rate of the two has been reported to be as high as 31%.[47] For this reason, any suggestion of a rectal injury, even with a normal rectal and proctoscopic exam, should prompt further evaluation. In hemodynamically stable patients with a mechanism suspicious for a rectal injury (gluteal, perineal, and transpelvic gunshot wounds, pelvic fractures, and foreign body insertion), a digital rectal exam and a rigid proctoscopy must be performed, and in the appropriate cases, further evaluation by means of a water-soluble contrast study should be considered. In mechanisms of injury other than foreign body insertion, intraluminal blood on proctoscopy should generally be considered positive for rectal injury, as the actual injury may be obscured in an unprepped rectum. The first pass of the proctoscope is the critical view, as blood seen on subsequent scans may be iatrogenic in nature.

Rectal Organ Injury Scale

The grading system developed by the AAST for rectal injuries is similar to that of colonic injuries (Table 26-2).

Operative Management

Historical Perspective

The history of rectal trauma parallels that of colon trauma with much of the early management principles evolving from lessons learned from wartime experiences. Mortality from rectal gunshot wounds was as high as 67% in World War I and the early part of World War II, until the Army Surgeon General mandated colostomy for fecal diversion for all colon and rectal injuries.[15,17,46] Subsequently, the mortality dropped down to 35%.[17] Retrorectal drainage was added in 1943, which appeared to bring the mortality down further to approximately 5%.[46,62] Shortly after World War II, several civilian series demonstrated satisfactory results with colostomy and presacral drainage.[63,64] During the Vietnam War, where more destructive injuries were encountered, colostomy and presacral drainage alone were found to be inadequate. Rectal repair and distal rectal washout were added to the management and were associated with improved results.[52] Early postwar civilian studies demonstrated acceptable results when colostomy, rectal repair, presacral drainage, and distal irrigation were all employed.[47,65] Interestingly, there were other studies that also demonstrated acceptable results when only colostomy and presacral drainage were utilized.[49,62,66] Presently, there is no acceptable gold standard for the treatment of rectal injuries, as most studies have been unable to demonstrate any advantage of the various treatment options.

Intraperitoneal Injuries

With no class I or class II data present regarding the management of intraperitoneal rectal injuries and limited class III data that combines both extraperitoneal and intraperitoneal injuries, it is difficult to draw a conclusion regarding management. However, several studies do indicate that injuries to the intraperitoneal rectum can be managed like left-colon injuries with primary repair, and without the need for colostomy.[50,54,59,61,67] No increase in abdominal complications was found in these series when primary repair without colostomy was performed, making primary repair in this group of patients a reasonable option.

Extraperitoneal Injuries

As previously mentioned, there is no agreement in terms of the optimal management of extraperitoneal rectal injuries, but the mainstay of treatment has included four main components: (1) fecal diversion with colostomy, (2) presacral drainage, (3) distal rectal washout, and (4) repair of the injury, when possible. Each component is addressed separately below.

Fecal Diversion with Colostomy

Ever since World War II, the mainstay of management of extraperitoneal injuries has been proximal colostomy.[46,49,50,57,59–61]

The only controversial aspect has been whether to perform a loop colostomy versus an end colostomy. Some argue that a loop colostomy does not offer complete fecal diversion, whereas proponents of loop colostomy argue that a properly constructed loop colostomy will function as a true diverting colostomy, with the added benefit of simple construction and rapid closure.[46,59] In fact, Rombeau et al.[68] demonstrated that a properly constructed loop colostomy, supported by a solid rod above the level of the skin, achieves complete fecal diversion. The authors believe that the type of colostomy performed should be dictated by the operative findings. Extensive destruction of the rectum that requires a resection may best be served with a Hartmann's procedure, whereas injuries that are not repaired or require limited dissection may be addressed by a loop colostomy.

Recently, there have been reports of primary repair without fecal diversion in selected extraperitoneal rectal injuries.[53,54,59,61,69] In a series of 30 patients with extraperitoneal rectal injuries, five were transanally repaired without fecal diversion and with no subsequent morbidity.[54] Similarly, injuries right at the peritoneal reflection, or injuries encountered with minimal dissection, may also be primarily repaired without the need for colostomy.[61]

Presacral Drainage

Presacral drainage was added to the armamentarium in World War II because it was thought to decrease the pelvic sepsis rate.[59,70] It has remained controversial, with many studies showing a benefit with its use,[46,47,49,59,71] whereas other studies have failed to show any benefit.[50,53,60,61,72] In a series published by Velmahos of 30 consecutive patients with extraperitoneal injuries, no benefit was found with the use of presacral drains.[60] Despite the conflicting data, many authors continue to recommend the use of presacral drains for most injuries.[61] This was challenged by a 1998 randomized prospective trial evaluating the importance of presacral drainage.[73] In this series of 48 patients, in which 23 randomized to presacral drainage and 25 randomized to no drainage, no difference in pelvic sepsis was encountered. This represents the first and only class I study involving rectal injuries. Although it was a study with relatively few patients, it convincingly demonstrated that the addition of presacral drainage is unnecessary. Over the last 15 years, the use of presacral drainage has diminished considerably. It involves an additional procedure and dissection into an uninvolved space. The drains that are placed may malfunction or become malpositioned, and most importantly, there is no evidence that their use improves outcome.

Distal Rectal Washout

Distal rectal irrigation was added to the management of rectal injuries during the Vietnam War, when Lavenson and Cohen reported a decrease in morbidity from 72% to 10% with its use.[52] Since then, there have been supporters of rectal washout[47,48,50,65] as well as nonsupporters.[46,49,53,59,72] The overall value of distal washout is questionable. It has been suggested that there may be a benefit in patients with high-velocity wounds,[46,51] and in patients with rectal injuries from pelvic fractures.[74,75] However, this remains controversial. In summary, there is no proven benefit, and it may be associated with a high risk of infection due to spillage of intraluminal contents out of unrepaired rectal injuries.[62]

Rectal Repair

The addition of rectal repair to colostomy was also introduced during the Vietnam War.[52] However, rectal repair with or without a diverting colostomy is infrequently performed for extraperitoneal injuries.[60] In the majority of cases, repair is not technically feasible, with some series reporting successful repair in only 20–37% of cases.[46,50,59] Even when repair is performed, no outcome advantage has been proven.[46,49,50] Attempts at repair are associated with extensive dissection and unnecessary contamination of the peritoneal cavity. Attempts at repair should only be made when the rectal injury is encountered during the exposure of an associated injury such as bladder or iliac vessel, or if the injury is easily accessible at the peritoneal reflection. As previously mentioned, injuries that are easily accessible from the transanal route may also be repaired with excellent results.[54]

Miscellaneous Options

Though extremely rare, abdominoperineal resection has been described for patients with severe bleeding, massive tissue loss, or devascularizing injuries.[47,69,76] Recent reports have introduced laparoscopy in the management of rectal injuries.[77,78] In a prospective study of 20 patients with extraperitoneal rectal injuries, laparoscopy (to rule out an intraperitoneal injury), followed by a diverting loop sigmoid colostomy without laparotomy yielded excellent results.[78]

Associated Injuries

Associated injuries are commonly seen with rectal injuries and have been reported to occur in as many as 77% of cases.[46,60] Genitourinary, and in particular bladder injuries, are usually the most commonly seen associated injuries, occurring in 30–64% of cases.[46,49,53] Every effort should be made to close both injuries and separate both sites with well-vascularized tissues such as omentum. This should reduce the high incidence of rectovesical fistula, which can occur in up to 24% of patients with combined bladder and rectal injuries (Figure 26-3).[59,79]

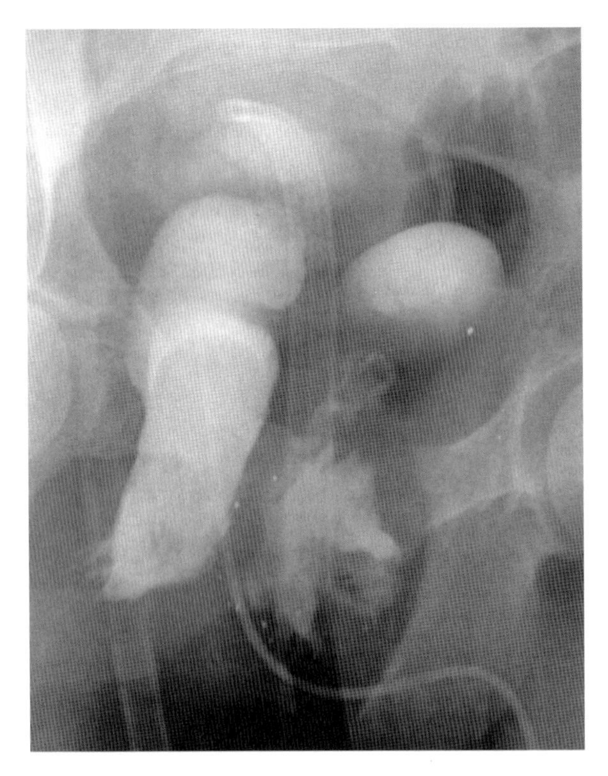

FIGURE 26-3. Rectovesical fistula following repair of a gunshot wound involving the rectum and the bladder. Every effort should be made to separate the two organs with vascularized tissues such as omentum, to reduce the risk of this complication.

Wound Management

The incidence of wound sepsis in patients with colon or rectal injury is high. In a prospective study of 100 patients with gunshot wounds and routine skin closure, the wound infection rate was 11%.[3] Primary wound closure in the presence of severe fecal spillage is a significant risk factor for wound sepsis and fascia dehiscence. This high-risk group of patients is best managed by delayed primary closure of the skin 3–5 days postoperatively, or closure by secondary intention.

Antibiotic Prophylaxis

In view of the high incidence of septic complications in patients with colon injuries, appropriate antibiotic prophylaxis is critical. It is a standard practice to cover against both aerobes and anaerobes. In early studies, the combination of penicillin/aminoglycoside/metranidazole was a popular antibiotic choice. Subsequent studies showed that in penetrating abdominal trauma, single agents were as good as combination antibiotics.[80,81] However, practically, all available studies included a large number of fairly minor or moderately severe abdominal injuries and only a small number of severe colon injuries with extensive fecal spillage. The reported overall incidence of intraabdominal abscess in abdominal trauma series is about 3%,[81] while in severe colon injuries it is about 19%.[6] The AAST destructive colon injury study identified single-antibiotic-agent prophylaxis as an independent risk factor for abdominal sepsis. The overall incidence of abdominal septic complications was 31% in patients who received single-agent prophylaxis and 16% in patients who received combination antibiotics (adjusted RR 1.78; 95% CI 1.12–2.67; $P=0.02$). Further comparison of the two agents used for single-antibiotic prophylaxis (cephalosporin versus ampicillin/sulbactam) showed an abdominal infection rate of 37% in the cephalosporin group and 22% in the ampicillin/sulbactam group. (crude RR 1.67; 95% C1, 0.93–2.99; $P=0.07$). It is possible that although single agents may be effective in minor or moderate trauma, they might be suboptimal in severe colon injuries. It is also possible that it might be necessary to cover against *Enterococcus*. Weigelt et al.[82] in a prospective randomized study of 595 abdominal trauma patients compared ampicillin/sulbactam with cefoxitin. The wound infection rate was significantly lower with ampicillin/sulbactam. The study suggested that the lower infection rate with ampicillin/sulbactam was due to better *Enterococcus* coverage.[82] The issue of antibiotic coverage in colon injuries merits further investigation. However, ampicillin/sulbactam (or similar antibiotics with *Enterococcus* coverage) prophylaxis in all suspected abdominal hollow viscous injuries is a reasonable choice.

The duration of antibiotic prophylaxis has been a controversial issue. There is now class I evidence that 24-h prophylaxis is at least as effective as prolonged prophylaxis for 3–5 days, even in the presence of major risk factors for abdominal sepsis, such as colon injury, multiple blood transfusions, and high abdominal trauma index. In a prospective randomized study of 63 patients with penetrating colon injuries and associate Abdominal Trauma Index ≥ 25 or ≥ 6 units of blood transfusions or delay of operation ≥ 6 h, Cornwell et al. reported an abdominal infection complication rate of 19% in patients who received 24 h antibiotic prophylaxis and 38% in patients who received 5 days prophylaxis.[7] With respect to rectal injuries, no study has addressed the type or length of antibiotic therapy. In the available studies that have even mentioned antibiotics, the length of therapy has been at least 2 days using single or double agents covering both aerobes and anaerobes.[46,73,78]

Stoma Related Complications

When deciding about the method of management of a colon or rectal injury, the surgeon should take into account the problems related to the creation of a stoma, and later on, the

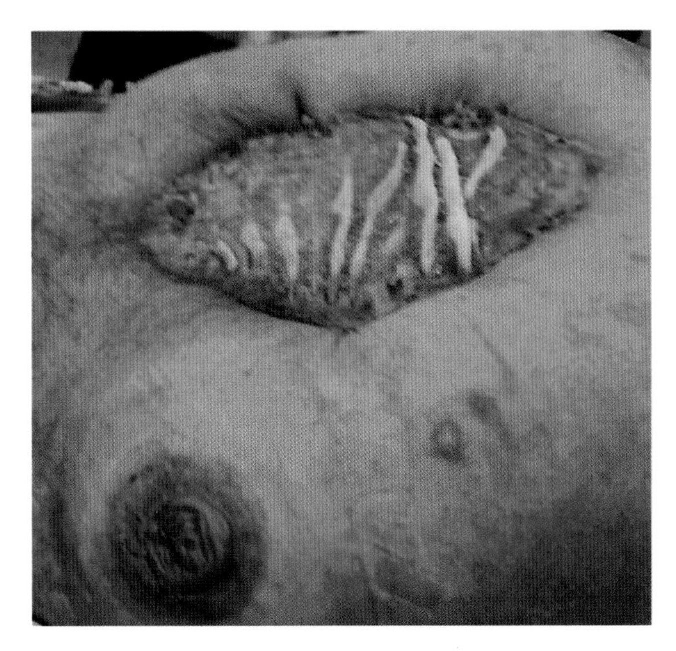

FIGURE 26-4. End Colostomy in the presence of a complicated abdominal wound with protruding mesh. Closure of this colostomy is a high-risk procedure.

complications associated with the subsequent operation for colostomy closure. The presence of an ostomy is, in itself, a significant emotional trauma, especially in an image-conscious young person. In addition, the incidence of complications directly related to the ostomy construction is a significant one. The most common serious complications include necrosis, retraction, prolapse, parastomal abscess, and parastomal hernia. Less serious complications include troublesome skin irritation and poor location with difficulties in the application of the collection bag. Park et al., in a series of 528 stomas created for trauma, reported an incidence 22% of severe or minor early complications and 3% of late complications directly related to the stoma.[83]

The morbidity of colostomy closure is significant (Figure 26-4). In a collective review of 809 colostomy closures in trauma patients during the period of 1970–1990, the overall incidence of colon-related complications was 13.1% (major complications 5.3%, minor complications 7.8%).[44] Another study of 110 colostomy closures reported an overall local complication rate of 14.5%, including 2.7% colon leaks.[84] In a more recent collective review of 1,085 colostomy closures, the overall complication rate was 14.8%.[85]

The timing of colostomy closure does not seem to play an important role in the incidence of complications. Early studies had suggested colostomy closure should be performed after 3 months from the original operation to allow time for the colostomy to "mature".[86,87] Subsequent studies showed that closure of the stoma earlier than 3 months is safe and not associated with increased complication rates.[84,88] Some studies even recommended closure during the same admission of the injury, which is usually within 2 weeks of the colostomy construction.[89] The optimal time for colostomy closure should be individualized, and time should be allowed for wound healing and nutritional recovery. This might require only a few weeks for some patients or many months in severely injured patients.

Rectal Foreign Bodies

Rectal foreign bodies represent an uncommon cause of rectal injury, accounting for less than 5% of cases.[46,49,59] More commonly, patients present to the hospital with a retained foreign body. These patients present a surprisingly common management dilemma.[90] Most objects can be safely removed in the emergency department. However, a small percentage of patients will require general anesthesia and operative management with or without laparotomy. In one review of 87 patients presenting with a retained foreign body, 75% were successfully retrieved at the bedside while 8% required laparotomy with colotomy for foreign body extraction.[91] The only independent risk factor for operative intervention was if the foreign body was located in the sigmoid colon (OR 2.25; 95% CI, 1.1–4.4; $P=0.04$). Abdominal films with AP and lateral views are helpful to define the foreign body and the orientation in the colon, in addition to excluding free intraperitoneal air.

Patients with a history of retained foreign body who present with peritonitis should be taken directly to the operating room. Without peritonitis, patients should have an attempt at retrieval at the bedside. If unsuccessful, patients should be taken to the operating room with an attempt at transanal extraction under intravenous sedation. As mentioned previously, patients most likely to require operative intervention are those with the foreign body located in the sigmoid colon.[91] The use of grasping forceps should be avoided, as it may lead to rectal mucosal injury. If transanal extraction is unsuccessful, then a laparotomy should be performed to maneuver the foreign body into the rectum for transanal removal.[91] If this is unsuccessful, then a colotomy may be necessary for foreign body retrieval.

One recently described method of distal foreign body removal is both effective and minimally invasive. Under general anesthesia, one or more lubricated Foley catheters or similar tubes may be passed transanally past the foreign body (Figure 26-5). The balloons are safely inflated to provide traction. Air is injected into the distal port, proximal to the foreign body to prevent "suction," while the foreign body is advanced. Once the foreign body reaches the anus, it is grasped with a clamp and removed.[92] This approach has proven successful in multiple patients at the author's institution. Following removal, sigmoidoscopy should be performed to exlude a mucosal injury or perforation.

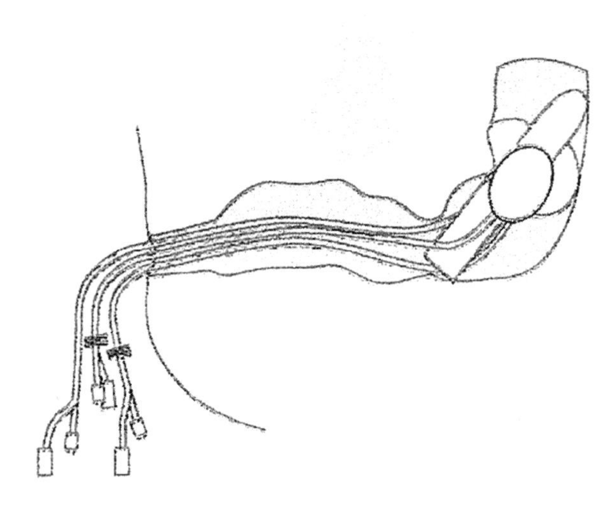

FIGURE 26-5. The "Blow as well as pull" technique for removal of rectal foreign body.

Acknowledgment. This chapter was written by Demetrios Demetriades and Ali Salim in the previous version of this textbook.

References

1. George SM, Fabian TC, Voeller GR, et al. Primary repair of colon injuries: a prospective trial in nonselected patients. Ann Surg. 1989;209:728–34.
2. Chappuis CW, Frey DJ, Dietzen CD, et al. Management of penetrating colon injuries. A prospective randomized trial. Ann Surg. 1991;213:492–7.
3. Demetriades D, Charalambides D, Pantanowitz D. Gunshot wounds of the colon: role of primary repair. Ann R Coll Surg Engl. 1992;74:381–4.
4. Ivatury RR, Gaudino J, Nallathambi MN, et al. Definitive treatment of colon injuries: a prospective study. Am Surg. 1993;59:43–9.
5. Gonzalez RP, Merlotti GJ, Holevar MR. Colostomy in penetrating colon injury: is it necessary. J Trauma. 1996;41: 271–5.
6. Demetriades D, Murray JA, Chan L, et al. Penetrating colon injuries requiring resection: diversion or primary anastomosis? An AAST prospective multicenter study. J Trauma. 2001;50:765–73.
7. Cornwell EE, Velmahos GC, Berne TV, et al. The fate of colonic suture lines in high-risk trauma patients: a prospective analysis. J Am Coll Surg. 1998;187:58–63.
8. Demetriades D, Velmahos G, Cornwell E, et al. Selective non-operative management of gunshot wounds of the anterior abdomen. Arch Surg. 1997;132:178–83.
9. Velhamos G, Demetriades D, Foianini E, et al. A selective approach to the management of gunshot wounds of the back. Am Surg. 1997;174:342–6.
10. Demetriades D, Rabinowitz B, Sofianos C, et al. The management of penetrating injuries of the back. A prospective study of 230 patients. Ann Surg. 1988;207:72–4.
11. Ross SE, Cobean RA, Hoyt DB, et al. Blunt colonic injury – a multicenter review. J Trauma. 1992;33:379–84.
12. Ciftci AO, Tanyel FC, Salman AB, et al. Gastrointestinal tract perforation due to blunt abdominal trauma. Pediatr Surg Int. 1998;13:259–64.
13. Munns J, Richardson M, Hewett P. A review of intestinal injury from blunt abdominal trauma. Aust NZ Surg. 1995;65:857–60.
14. Macleod J, Freiberger D, Lewis F, et al. What is the optimal observation time for a penetrating wound to the flank? Am Surg. 2007;73:25–31.
15. Office of the surgeon general. Circular Letter No 178. October 23, 1943.
16. Elkin DC, Ward WC. Gunshot wounds of the abdomen: Survey of 238 cases. Ann Surg. 1943;118:780–7.
17. Ogilvie WH. Abdominal wounds in the western desert. Surg Gynecol Obstet. 1944;78:225–38.
18. Stone HH, Fabian TC. Management of perforating colon trauma: randomization between primary closure and exteriorization. Ann Surg. 1979;190:430–6.
19. Schrock TR, Christensen N. Management of perforating injuries of the colon. Surg Gynecol Obstet. 1972;135:65–8.
20. Kirkpatrick JR. Management of colonic injuries. Dis Colon Rectum. 1974;17:319–21.
21. Sasaki LS, Allaben RD, Golwala R, et al. Primary repair of colon injuries: a prospective randomized study. J Trauma. 1995;39:895–901.
22. Gonzalez RP, Falimirsky ME, Holevar MR. Further evaluation of colostomy in penetrating colon injury. Am Surg. 2000;66:342–7.
23. Baker LW, Thomson SR, Chadwick SJ. Colon wound management and prograde colonic lavage in large bowel trauma. Br J Surg. 1990;77:872–6.
24. Pezim ME, Vestrup JA. Canadian attitudes toward use of primary repair in management of colon trauma: a survey of 317 members of the Canadian Association of General Surgeons. Dis Colon Rectum. 1996;39:40–4.
25. Eshraghi N, Mallins R, Mayberry JC, et al. Surveyed opinion of American Trauma Surgeons in management of colon injuries. J Trauma. 1998;44:93–7.
26. Woo K, Wilson MT, Killeen K, et al. Adapting to the changing paradigm of management of colon injuries. Am J Surg. 2007;194:746–50.
27. Stewart RM, Fabian TC, Groce MA, et al. Is resection with primary anastomosis following destructive colon wound always safe? Am J Surg. 1994;168:316–9.
28. Murray JA, Demetriades D, Colson M, et al. Colon resection in trauma: colostomy versus anastomosis. J Trauma. 1999; 46:250–4.
29. Pasquale M, Fabian TC, EAST Ad Hoc Committee. Practice management guidelines for trauma from the Eastern Association for the Surgery of Trauma. J Trauma. 1998;44:941–7.
30. Demetriades D, Lawson HH, Sofianos C, et al. Healing of the right and left colon. An experimental study. S Afr Med J. 1988;73:657–8.
31. Sofianos C, Demetriades D, Oosthuizen MM, et al. The effect of hypovolemia on healing of the right and left colon. An experimental study. S Afr J Surg. 1992;30:42–3.
32. Deute CJ, Tyburski J, Wilson RF, et al. Ostomy as a risk factor for posttraumatic infection in penetrating colonic injuries: univariate and multivariate analyses. J Trauma. 2000;49:628–37.
33. Vertrees AM, Wakefield M, Pickett C, et al. Outcomes of primary repair and primary anastomosis in war-related colon injuries. J Trauma. 2009;66:1286–93.

34. Welling DR, Hutton JE, Minken SL, et al. Diversion Defended – Military Colon Trauma. J Trauma. 2008;64:1119–22.
35. Duncan JE, Corwin CH, Sweeney WB, et al. Management of colorectal injuries during operation Iraqi freedom: patterns of stoma usage. J Trauma. 2008;64:1043–7.
36. Flint LM, Vitale GC, Richardson JD, et al. The injured colon: relationships of management to complications. Ann Surg. 1981;193:619–23.
37. Burch JM, Martin RR, Richardson RJ, et al. Evolution of the treatment of the injured colon in the 1980's. Arch Surg. 1991;126:979–84.
38. Ivatury RR, Nallathambi M, Rao P, et al. Penetrating pancreatic injuries. Analysis of 103 consecutive cases. Am Surg. 1990;56:90–5.
39. Velmahos GC, Degiannis E, Wells M, et al. Penetrating ureteral injuries: the impact of associated injuries on management. Am Surg. 1996;62:461–8.
40. Morgado PJ, Alfaro R, Morgado Jr PJ, et al. Colon trauma – clinical staging for surgical decision making. Analysis of 119 cases. Dis Colon Rectum. 1992;35:986–90.
41. Demetriades D, Charalambides D. Gunshot wounds of the colon: role of retained bullets in sepsis. Br J Surg. 1993;80:772–3.
42. Miller PR, Chang MC, Hoth JJ, et al. Colonic resection in the setting of damage control laparotomy: is delayed anastomosis safe? Am Surg. 2007;76:606–10.
43. Weinberg JA, Griffin RL, Vandromme MJ, et al. Management of colon wounds in the setting of damage control: a cautionary tale. J Trauma. 2009;67:929–35.
44. Curran TJ, Borzotta AP. Complications of primary repair of colon injury: literature review of 2,964 cases. Am J Surg. 1999;177:42–7.
45. Demetriades D, Murray JA, Chan LS, et al. Handsewn versus stapled anastomosis in penetrating colon injuries requiring resection: a multicenter study. J Trauma. 2002;52:117–21.
46. Burch JM, Feliciano DV, Mattox KL. Colostomy and drainage for civilian rectal injuries: is that all? Ann Surg. 1989;209:600–11.
47. Grasberger RC, Hirsch EF. Rectal trauma: a retrospective analysis and guidelines for therapy. Am J Surg. 1983;145:795–9.
48. Shannon FL, Moore EE, Moore FA, et al. Value of distal colon washout in civilian rectal trauma: reducing gut bacterial translocation. J Trauma. 1988;28:989–94.
49. Tuggle D, Huber PJ. Management of rectal trauma. Am J Surg. 1984;148:806–8.
50. Mangiante EC, Graham AD, Fabian TC. Rectal gunshot wounds: management options in penetrating rectal injuries. Am Surg. 1986;52:37–40.
51. Morken JJ, Kraatz JJ, Balcos EG, et al. Civilian rectal trauma: a changing perspective. Surgery. 1999;126:693–700.
52. Lavenson GS, Cohen A. Management of rectal injuries. Am J Surg. 1971;122:226–31.
53. Thomas DD, Levison MA, Dykstra BJ, Bender JS. Management of rectal injuries: dogma versus practice. Am Surg. 1990;56:507–10.
54. Levine JH, Longo WE, Pruitt C, et al. Management of selected rectal injuries by primary repair. Am J Surg. 1996;172: 575–9.
55. Velmahos GC, Demetriades D, Cornwell EE, et al. Gunshot wounds to the buttocks: predicting the need for operation. Dis Colon Rectum. 1997;40:307–11.
56. Velmahos GC, Demetriades D, Cornwell EE. Transpelvic gunshot wounds: routine laparotomy or selective management? World J Surg. 1998;22:1034–8.
57. Brunner RG, Shatney CH. Diagnostic and therapeutic aspects of rectal trauma: blunt versus penetrating. Am Surg. 1987;53:215–9.
58. Aihara R, Blansfield JS, Millham FH, et al. Fracture locations influence the likelihood of rectal and lower urinary tract injuries in patients sustaining pelvic fractures. J Trauma. 2002;52:205–9.
59. Ivatury RR, Licata J, Gunduz Y, et al. Management options in penetrating rectal injuries. Am Surg. 1991;57:50–7.
60. Velmahos GC, Gomez H, Falabella A, et al. Operative management of civilian rectal gunshot wounds: simpler is better. World J Surg. 2000;24:114–8.
61. McGrath V, Fabian TC, Croce MA, et al. Rectal trauma: management based on anatomic distinctions. Am Surg. 1998;64:1136–41.
62. Trunkey D, Hays RJ, Shires GT. Management of rectal trauma. J Trauma. 1973;13:411–5.
63. Taylor ER, Thompson JE. The early treatment, and results thereof, of injuries of the colon and rectum. Int Abstr Surg. 1948;87:209–28.
64. Woodhall JP, Ochsner A. The management of perforating injuries of the colon and rectum in civilian practice. Recent Adv Surg. 1949;20:305–21.
65. Vitale GC, Richardson JD, Flint LM. Successful management of injuries to the extraperitoneal rectum. Am Surg. 1983;49: 159–62.
66. Bartizal JF, Boyd DR, Folk FA, et al. A critical review of management of 392 colonic and rectal injuries. Dis Colon Rectum. 1974;17:313–8.
67. Maxwell RA, Fabian TC. Current management of colon trauma. World J Surg. 2003;27:632–9.
68. Rombeau JL, Wilk PJ, Turnbull RB, et al. Total fecal diversion by the temporary skin-level loop transverse colostomy. Dis Colon Rectum. 1978;21:223–6.
69. Haas PA, Fox TAJ. Civilian injuries of the rectum and anus. Dis Colon Rectum. 1979;22:17–23.
70. Armstrong RG, Schmitt HJ, Patterson LT. Combat wounds of the extraperitoneal rectum. Surgery. 1983;74:570–83.
71. Weil PH. Injuries of the retroperitoneum portions of the colon and rectum. Dis Colon Rectum. 1983;26:19–21.
72. Levy RD, Strauss P, Aladgem D, et al. Extraperitoneal rectal gunshot injuries. J Trauma. 1995;38:274–7.
73. Gonzalez RP, Falimirski ME, Holevar MR. The role of presacral drainage in the management of penetrating rectal injuries. J Trauma. 1998;45:656–61.
74. Maull KI, Sachatello CR, Ernst CB. The deep perineal laceration – an injury frequently associated with open pelvic fractures: a need for aggressive surgical management. J Trauma. 1977;17:685–96.
75. Richardson JD, Harty J, Amin M, et al. Open Pelvic fractures. J Trauma. 1982;22:533–8.
76. Getzen LC, Pollack EG, Wolfman EF. Abdominoperineal resection in the treatment of devascularizing rectal injuries. Surgery. 1977;82:310–3.
77. Navsaria PH, Graham R, Nicol A. A new approach to extraperitoneal rectal injuries: laparoscopy and diverting loop sigmoid colostomy. J Trauma. 2001;51:532–5.

78. Navsaria PH, Shaw JM, Zellweger R, et al. Diagnostic laparoscopy and diverting sigmoid loop colostomy in the management of civilian extraperitoneal rectal gunshot injuries. Br J Surg. 2004;91:460–4.
79. Franko ER, Ivatury RR, Schwalb DM. Combined penetrating rectal and genitourinary injuries: a challenge in management. J Trauma. 1993;34:347–53.
80. Hooker KD, Dipiro JT, Wynn JJ. Aminoglycoside combinations versus beta-lactams alone for penetrating abdominal trauma: a meta-analysis. J Trauma. 1991;31:1155–60.
81. Sims EH, Thadepalli H, Ganesan K, et al. How many antibiotics are necessary to treat abdominal trauma victims? Am Surg. 1997;63:525–35.
82. Weigelt JA, Easley SM, Thal ER, et al. Abdominal surgical wound infection is lowered with improved perioperative enterococcus and bacteroides therapy. J Trauma. 1993;34:579–85.
83. Park JJ, Pino AD, Orsay CP, et al. Stoma complications: the Cook County Hospital experience. Dis Colon Rectum. 1999;42:1575–80.
84. Demetriades D, Pezikis A, Melissas J, et al. Factors influencing the morbidity of colostomy closure. Am J Surg. 1988;155:594–6.
85. Berne JD, Velmahos GC, Chan LS, et al. The high morbidity of colostomy closure after trauma: further support for the primary repair of colon injuries. Surgery. 1998;123:157–64.
86. Frend H, Raniel J, Maggia-Sulaw W. Factors affecting the morbidity of colostomy closure. Dis Colon Rectum. 1982;25:712–5.
87. Parks S, Hastings P. Complications of colostomy closure. Am Surg. 1985;149:672–5.
88. Renz BM, Feliciano DV, Sherman R. Same admission colostomy closure (SACC) – a new approach to rectal wounds: a prospective study. Ann Surg. 1993;3:279–83.
89. Velmahos GC, Degiannis E, Weels M, et al. Early closure of colostomies in trauma patients: a prospective randomized trial. Surgery. 1995;118:815–20.
90. Barone JE, Yee J, Nealon TF. Management of foreign bodies and trauma of the rectum. Surg Gynecol Obstet. 1983;156:453–7.
91. Lake JP, Essani R, Petrone P, et al. Management of retained colorectal foreign bodies: predictors of operative intervention. Dis Colon Rectum. 2004;47:1694–8.
92. Manimaran N, Shorafa M, Eccersley J. Blow as well as pull: an innovative technique for dealing with a rectal foreign body. Colorectal Dis. 2009;11:325–6.

27
IBD: Diagnosis and Evaluation

Walter A. Koltun

History

In 1932, Crohn, Ginzburg, and Oppenheimer described 13 patients with "regional ileitis" included in a total of 52 cases of nonspecific granulomatous inflammation of the intestine.[1] Prior to their publication, numerous others had reported various cases of what were in retrospect, probably Crohn's disease (CD), as early as 1813,[2] but it was their published description that established the formal classification of the disease syndrome and association with noncaseating granulomas. The surgeon involved in the care of the majority of the patients, Dr. AA Berg, did not want his name included in the article. Because of the variable clinical and anatomic manifestations of the illness, "CD" has subsequently become as common a descriptor of this disease entity as the term "regional enteritis."

The difficulty in distinguishing the colonic form of CD and ulcerative colitis (UC) confused the diagnosis and treatment of these illnesses until their differences were clarified by classic publications by Brooke in 1959 and Lockart-Mummery in 1960.[3,4] These authors pointed out both the segmental and granulomatous nature of the colitis in CD. In addition, Brooke contributed significantly to the treatment of these inflammatory bowel diseases (IBD) by introducing pioneering surgical techniques in the 1950s that created a more functional ileostomy, which until that time was a miserable and disabling consequence of colectomy.[5] Truelove and Witts in 1959 reported on a double-blind, controlled study demonstrating the value of high-dose cortisone as treatment for severe colitis.[6] Other turning points in the management and treatment of CD include the demonstration of the therapeutic value of metronidazole[7], 6-mercaptopurine[8], and more recently, the tumor necrosis factor-alpha (TNF-α) antagonist, infliximab.[9]

Surgical management of UC has been a continuous evolution, starting with colectomy/ileostomy,[10,11] supplanted by the continent Koch ileostomy[12], and finally the definitive reconstruction procedure known as the ileal-pouch anal anastomosis (IPAA), first described by Parks and Nicholls in 1978 and subsequently refined by Utsunomiya.[13,14] The IPAA is now the standard of care for the surgical correction of UC.

Epidemiology

The causes of UC and CD remain unknown, and thus epidemiological data have been collected over many years in the hope of providing some clue to the etiologies of these illnesses. Much of this data must be viewed with caution, however. Variations in diagnostic criteria, definitions of disease, and biases resulting from surveys done in tertiary care specialty centers make universal conclusions difficult. However, some general statements can be made using such data that relate to disease prevalence and associated risk factors (Table 27-1).

The prevalence of IBD greatly varies throughout the world. Prevalence is the product of incidence and disease duration. Since IBD symptoms tend to wax and wane in severity, prevalence may be underestimated in some studies. IBD is found in the more temperate climates of North America and Europe. Studies from these regions show prevalence rates much higher than those in Asia, South America, or Africa. Prevalence rates as high as 300–400 per 100,000 population are found in Minnesota (USA), Manitoba (Canada), and UK. Conversely, prevalence rates of approximately 23/100,000 are found in Japan, 10/100,000 in Singapore, and 75–120/100,000 in Israel. The relative incidence of CD versus UC is, again, variable, with either being found greater than the other depending upon the geographic region studied.[15–19]

It is generally recognized that both CD and UC have been increasing in incidence to a remarkable degree over the past 20–30 years with two- to tenfold increases depending on the population and region studied.[18,20] These dramatic increases suggest an environmental effect, since a genetic factor would probably not influence disease rates so rapidly.

CD most commonly occurs in the third decade of life, while UC is more common in the fourth decade. There may

D.E. Beck et al. (eds.), *The ASCRS Textbook of Colon and Rectal Surgery: Second Edition*,
DOI 10.1007/978-1-4419-1584-9_27, © Springer Science+Business Media, LLC 2011

TABLE 27-1. Epidemiologic and associated risk factors for inflammatory bowel disease

Epidemiology
- Race/ethnicity:
  - Whites and Blacks > Hispanic, Native American, Asian
    - Jews > Non-Jews
- Geography:
  - Northern climates > Southern
  - Scandinavia, North America, Europe > Asia, Africa, South America, Japan, Spain
- Gender:
  - CD: Female > Male
  - UC: Male > Female
- Age:
  - CD: Third decade
  - UC: Fourth decade
- Residence:
  - Urban > Rural
  - Indoor > Outdoor

RISK factors
- Diet:
  - Sugar Consumption – ↑ CD
  - ETOH – ↓ UC
  - Margarine – no association
  - Coffee – no association
  - Fiber – no association
  - Food Additives – no association
- Childhood diarheal illness ↑ IBD
- Higher socioeconomical status ↑ IBD
- Oral contraceptive use ↑ IBD
- Cigarettes – ↑ CD
  - ↓ UC
- Appendectomy ↓ ulcerative colitis
- NSAIDS – ↑ symptoms of IBD

ETOH alcohol; UC ulcerative colitis; CD Crohn's disease; NSAIDS nonsteroidal anti-inflammatory drugs.

be a bimodal distribution of disease incidence with a second peak in the sixth or seventh decade, but this pattern remains unclear and may simply be due to difficulty in differentiating it from other colitides such as diverticulitis or ischemic colitis.

Though originally thought to be relatively rare in blacks, more recent case–control studies in USA suggest a similar incidence to whites, although Africa itself has a very low incidence of IBD.[17] There is great variability in the incidence of IBD in Jews around the world, but nonetheless seems to be consistently higher than that found in the non-Jewish population in most countries studied.[21] IBD is more common in urban, "indoor" populations of individuals of middle to upper socioeconomic status, suggesting the "hygiene" hypothesis that relates the lack of early exposure to environmental antigens to the later development of disease.[15,19,22]

There is very little evidence that a specific dietary factor causes disease, although increased sugar consumption is associated with CD and alcohol intake is inversely related to UC.[23,24] Childhood diarrheal illness, and oral contraceptive and nonsteroidal anti-inflammatory drugs (NSAIDs) use are measurable risk factors for IBD, with NSAIDs reported as precipitating relapse in patients with inactive disease.[25] Smoking has been clearly shown to worsen CD, with increased risk of developing the disease de novo and increased risk of recurrence after surgical resection. Conversely, smoking is protective for UC, as is prior appendectomy.[26,27]

Genetic Disease Determinants in IBD

Approximately 20% of patients with IBD will have a family member also afflicted, implying a genetic basis for the disease. The recent development of sophisticated genetic mapping techniques combined with the recruitment of large groups of clinically characterized IBD patients has led to genome-wide association studies (GWAS) identifying areas (loci) in the human genome that are associated with the various forms of IBD. Fine mapping of these loci has led to the identification of specific mutations [or so-called single nucleotide polymorphisms (SNPs)] affecting specific genes that predispose to the development of IBD. As of mid-2009, an excess of 32 loci (most containing several potential disease-causing genes) was found for CD alone. UC appears to have less of a genetic component to its pathobiology, but similarly has at least 15 loci associated with it (Figure 27-1).[28–32]

Such genetic work has allowed the identification of relevant genes and thus physiologic pathways that are altered in IBD. Patterns are emerging with some genes playing a role in both illnesses, while others are confined to playing a role in only CD or UC. Many of these genes, however, can be integrated into a mechanistic paradigm which suggests that IBD is the consequence of an altered host immune response to various environmental factors, most probably enteric or commensal bacteria within the gut. Other factors may also play a role, such as smoking or NSAID use that further alters the host immune system or affects its function (Figure 27-2).[33]

The bowel and its epithelium are in fact an interface between the host and a relatively hostile environment. This barrier is made up of the mucous layer, the epithelium itself (enterocytes, goblet cells, and mucin-secreting paneth cells), and the underlying immunologic apparatus that includes lamina propria dendritic cells, regulatory and effector lymphocytes, and an extracellular matrix that contains cytokines and surface receptors that help guide and regulate the host inflammatory process. Thus mutations in any of these components of either host immunity (innate or acquired) or the epithelial barrier can potentially result in an abnormal inflammatory response to enteric bacteria with resulting destruction of the relatively fragile intestinal mucosa.

The first CD-associated genetic mutation was found in the NOD2/CARD 15 gene on chromosome 16.[34] This gene's protein product recognizes muramyl dipeptide, a component of bacterial cell walls, and activates NF-kappa B, a potent second messenger involved in immune regulatory mechanisms. Though a homozygous (double) mutation in this gene increases the risk of CD approximately 30-fold, any one patient with a mutation will still only have

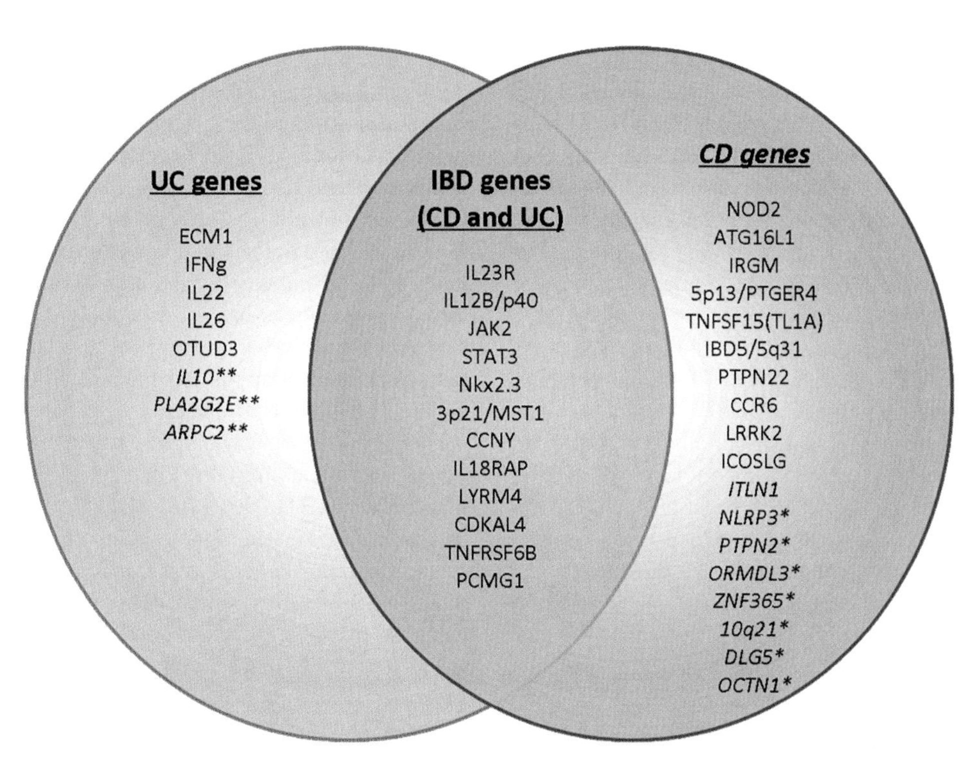

FIGURE 27-1. Genes implicated in the pathogenesis of Crohn's disease and ulcerative colitis (as of late 2009). Some genes seem to play a role in both diseases. Not all genes have been confirmed by second investigators.

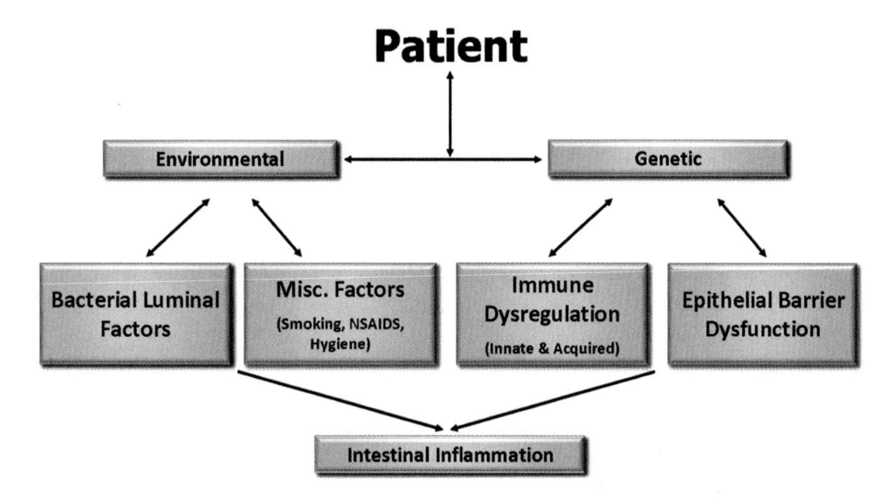

FIGURE 27-2. Pathogenesis of inflammatory bowel disease incorporating a genetic (predisposition) component and an environmental aspect, each of which may play a varying role in the individual patient.

a approximately 2.5% risk of developing CD, reflecting the role for other genetic determinants in the development of CD. Clinically, patients with this mutation tend to have earlier onset of disease in the ileocolic area.

The NOD2/CARD15 molecule is part of the innate immune system protecting the organism from invading enteric bacteria, but through the previously mentioned GWAS, several other genes affecting the innate immune system have been subsequently identified. Autophagy, i.e., the cell's ability to destroy and recycle defective cytoplasmic molecules including invading bacteria, is compromised by of mutations in the ATG16L1 and IRGM genes which have been associated with CD.[35] Similarly, mutations in the acquired immune system, especially those involving the IL-23 and IL-12 signaling pathways, have been found. A mutation in the IL23R (receptor) gene has been shown to be *protective* against CD and UC.[29] Various alleles in other molecules found in the IL-23 pathway including JAK2, STAT3, and IL12B have also been linked with CD and UC. Experimentally, blockade of the IL-23 pathway has been shown to compromise bacterial clearance in some models, again reinforcing the concept that IBD is the consequence of an abnormal immune response to commensal gut bacteria.[36]

IBD-associated mutations have been found in many other genes, including DLG5 (coding for an epithelial cytoplasmic scaffolding protein), NKX2-3 (a developmental protein found in the lymphoid tissue of gut and involved in the expression of lymphocyte trafficking molecules), PTPN2 (involved in T-cell-dependant B-cell function), and IL-10R (receptor). Exactly how these mutations then lead to disease is often complex and not obvious. However, the relevancy of such genetic effects on the etiology of IBD is periodically validated by direct clinical discoveries. Such was the case for IL-10R where a clinical report described a severe early onset form of CD in two family pedigrees and several other children that were shown to be caused by homozygous mutations in IL10 receptor genes. This resulted in a hyperinflammatory immune response (increased secreted levels of TNF) associated with the clinical findings of proctitis with perianal fistulization, which was cured in one child by a bone marrow transplant from an IL-10R wild-type donor.[37]

The future of IBD management will likely depend on the reclassification of individual patients based on the genetic determinants of disease etiology. Both medical and surgical care will then be dictated not only by phenotype, but also by genotype. Improved responses to care interventions will be achieved by identifying which genetic determinants predict better results with specific therapies.

Signs and Symptoms

Gastrointestinal Symptoms

Crohn's Disease

CD can affect any portion of the gastrointestinal (GI) tract from the mouth to the anus. It is usually discontinuous, commonly involving several areas of the bowel at once, with sections of normal intestine interposed. The inflammation of CD involves the entire bowel wall, from mucosa to serosa and even into adjacent structures. These features are responsible for its presenting symptomatology.

The most common complaints of any patient with CD are abdominal pain and diarrhea, being found in over 75% of patients. Weight loss, fever, and bleeding are present in approximately 40–60% of patients, while anal symptoms of abscess and/or fistula occur in 10–20% of patients. Many classification systems for CD have been suggested, but the anatomic one has direct practical relevance in explaining symptoms. CD is most frequently found in the ileo-cecal region, making up approximately 40% of patients. Abdominal pain most commonly correlates with disease in this region.[20] Colonic disease is found in approximately 30% of patients and most directly correlates with symptoms of diarrhea and bleeding. The remaining 30% of patients have disease confined to the small bowel proximal to the terminal ileum and correlates with abdominal pain, bloating, and a sense of postprandial nausea, especially if partial obstruction due to inflammation or stricture occurs. Anal disease is typically associated with patients having the terminal ileal and colonic distributions of disease.

The more recently developed Vienna classification of CD segregates patients into three categories based on behavior: inflammatory (B1), stricturing (B2), and fistulizing (B3).[38] This classification attempts to characterize disease biology but is imperfect. Patients will frequently change categories as disease progresses, since IBD commonly becomes stricturing or fistulizing disease. Louis et al.[39] over a 10-year period found that in 125 patients with CD, the B2 and B3 categories (stricturing and fistulizing) each increased from approximately 10% to approximately 30–40% with a compensatory decrease in the inflammatory, B1 category. Thus duration of disease plays a critical role in defining the category in this classification system.

Clinical severity of symptoms is widely variable, since CD typically has a waxing and waning course characterized by periods of disease activity interspersed with periods of remission. At any one time, approximately 50% of CD patients will be in clinical remission. The majority of patients (60–75%) will have alternating years of quiescence and disease activity. About 10–20% will have either a chronic, unremitting course or repetitive annual flaring of disease. Prolonged quiescence is found in about 10–15% of patients. The only useful predictor of future disease activity is past clinical behavior.

Ulcerative Colitis

The inflammation of UC characteristically starts in the rectum and extends proximally. The so-called backwash ileitis is the only possible area of the small bowel that can be affected in UC. If additional small bowel is involved, CD should be suspected. Clinical symptoms relate to the extent and location of disease. Thus rectal disease results in increased stool frequency, hematochezia, and tenesmus. Diarrhea is a frequent symptom and with tenesmus, it can result in incontinence, especially at night. In spite of severe rectal inflammation, constipation with a sense of incomplete evacuation can be a complaint in 20–25% of patients, but blood and mucous are nearly always present. With more proximal involvement, abdominal complaints increase including left lower quadrant pain and pain associated with peristalsis or stool evacuation. With increasing severity and extent of disease, nausea, vomiting, and weight loss ensue. Weight loss is due to both the loss of serum proteins through the diseased mucosa and the reluctance of the patient to eat in order to avoid exacerbation of symptoms. The development of systemic signs of illness such as tachycardia, fever, and increasing fluid requirement bespeaks severe disease. High-dose steroids may disguise worsening abdominal complaints, including peritonitis, in such circumstances and should not divert the clinician from recognizing the gravity of the development of such symptoms and signs. The so-called toxic megacolon is a moniker that should be discarded, since severe life-threatening colitis may occur without colonic dilatation, and urgent surgical intervention should be based upon the triad of toxicity defined by tachycardia, fever, and elevated white blood cell count.

Extraintestinal Manifestations

Musculoskeletal

The most common non-GI complaints in IBD patients relate to the musculoskeletal system. Osteopenia and osteoporosis are very common, in part due to therapeutic steroid use, occurring in as many as 50 and 15% of IBD patients, respectively. Such bone density loss is now recognized as leading to significant comorbidity and complications in IBD patients. One study found a 40% increased risk of bone fractures in IBD patients.[40] The arthropathies associated with IBD are found in up to 30% of patients and are divided into two broad categories. Peripheral arthritis usually affects multiple small joints and has little relation to gastrointestinal disease activity. Axial arthritis (ankylosing spondylitis) is associated with certain HLA subtypes (B27) and is found in approximately 5% of both CD and UC patients. Its severity commonly parallels disease activity. Recently, anti-tumor necrosis factor (TNF) therapies have been shown to be effective in both CD and the arthropathy of IBD.[41,42]

Cutaneous

Pyoderma gangrenosum and erythema nodosum occur in approximately 0.5–5% of patients with IBD. These, as well as oral lesions such as aphthous stomatitis and pyostomatitis vegetans, are more commonly associated with CD than UC and commonly parallel underlying gastrointestinal disease activity. The new appearance of pyoderma gangrenosum around the ileostomy of an IBD patient after colectomy is unexplained but is a clear clinical phenomenon.[43] There is a reported increased rate of psoriasis and eczema in IBD patients that does not parallel disease activity. One-third to one-half of patients with pyoderma gangrenosum have IBD.[44]

Hepatobiliary

Primary sclerosing cholangitis (PSC) has a reported incidence of approximately 3% in both CD and UC patients. It may present independent of intestinal disease activity, and colectomy in UC patients does not affect the progression of liver disease. The presence of PSC in the UC patient increases the risk for malignant disease in both the colon and the hepatobiliary system.[45]

Several studies have suggested an increased incidence of gallstones in IBD, especially CD, although this is disputed. The mechanism is presumed to be due to an altered enterohepatic biliary circulation due to ileal disease.[46]

Ophthalmologic

Iritis, uveitis, and episcleritis can affect 2–8% of patients with UC and CD, respectively, and are generally unrelated to disease activity. Iritis and uveitis present as blurred vision, eye pain, and photophobia and requires prompt treatment to avoid scarring and even blindness. Episcleritis is typically less threatening and is characterized by scleral injection, burning, and tearing.

Coagulopathy

There is an identified increased risk of deep venous thrombosis (DVT), mesenteric thrombosis, and pulmonary embolism (PE) in IBD patients that are not explained simply by increased hospitalization and surgery. Decreased protein S and antithrombin III levels due to mucosal loss and increased levels of acute-phase reactants including factors V and VIII have been implicated. Mortality due to postoperative mesenteric thrombosis in the IBD patient has been reported to be as high as 50%, but probably occurs more frequently than previously recognized with an overall lower mortality and milder forms of morbidity.[47–49] Anticoagulation and work-up for coagulation disorders are usually recommended.

Disease Severity Assessment

Crohn's Disease

The CD activity index (CDAI) is the most commonly used method for quantification of disease severity in CD. It was developed by Best et al. using multiple regression analysis and includes a total of eight items that are measured, multiplied by respective weighting factors, and then summated to yield a score (Table 27-2). It is generally accepted that a total score less than 150 points indicates quiescent disease, whereas over 450 indicates severe, active disease. Relapses are defined as a score rising to over 150 or an increase of 100 points over baseline. The CDAI is most commonly used in longitudinal clinical studies to evaluate the results of experimental interventions. It suffers from many deficiencies including its reliance on subjective complaints and that it is time consuming, requiring the patient to keep a diary for 7-day periods defining symptomatology. Some measured symptoms, such as diarrhea and belly pain, may reflect short gut due to prior surgery or strictures that do not represent active IBD.[50] Other indices have been developed

TABLE 27-2. The Crohn's disease activity index (CDAI)

Item calculation	Data collected weighing factor	
No. of liquid stools	7-Day diary 2	Sum of 7 days
Abdominal pain	0–3 Scale, 7-day diary 5	Sum of score for each day
General well-being	0–4 Scale, 7-day diary 7	Sum of score for each day
Symptoms[a]	At clinic visit 20	Sum (6 total) possible
Lomotil use	7-Day diary 30	Yes = 1, No = 2
Abdominal mass	At clinic visit 10	None = 0, questionable = 2, definite = 5
HCT	At clinic visit 6	M: (47 subtract patient's HCT) F: (42 subtract patient's HCT)
Weight	At clinic visit 1	% below ideal weight

HCT hematocrit.
[a]Symptoms include presence or absence of each of arthritis/arthralgia, iritis/uveitis, erythema nodosum/pyoderma gangrenosum/aphthous stomatitis, anal fissure/fistula/abscess, other fistula, or temperature >100°F.

TABLE 27-3. Truelove and Witts ulcerative colitis activity index

	Mild	Severe
Bowel frequency	<4	>6
Blood in stool	+	+++
Fever	Absent	>37.5
Pulse	<90	>90
Hgb	>75% nl	<75% nl
ESR	<30	>30

HgB hemoglogin; ESR erythrocyte sedimentation rate.

in an attempt to address these criticisms. The Harvey Bradshaw index (or modified CDAI) and the Van Hees Index, which relies entirely on nine objective factors such as ESR, albumin, temperature, and stool consistency, are two such measurement tools, but they are infrequently used, even in protocol settings.[51] The Vienna classification, discussed above, is an attempt to classify or categorize subsets of CD patients and is not used as a severity assessment tool.[38] A perianal CD activity index has also been described.[52]

Ulcerative Colitis

The benchmark study by Truelove and Witts in 1955 evaluating the effect of cortisone on UC also described the still most often used clinical assessment tool for severity assessment in UC (Table 27-3).[6] The simplicity and clinical relevancy of the factors in this index allow for its daily use as a clinical tool and also for clinical response in study protocols. Variations in its initial format have included the creation of a "moderate" category for patients displaying features intermediate in value between the mild and severe categories. This index also does not take into account variability in the anatomic extent or observed severity of disease within the colon. Modern clinical studies requiring disease assessment will thus often use a variation in the Truelove and Witts classification, which will include additional criteria based on colonoscopic appearance and possibly pathologic severity as well.[53,54]

Evaluation

Radiology

The diagnosis of IBD depends on the triad of clinical presentation, radiologic work-up, and histopathology of tissue biopsy. Thus radiologic studies are critical in the evaluation of the patient with suspected or confirmed IBD.

Plain X-Rays

Conventional radiologic studies play a significant role in the work-up and management of IBD. Plain abdominal radiographs can show signs of obstruction, perforation (free air), and at times thickening of the bowel or loss of haustral markings. The initial presentation of any patient with abdominal pain and a known or suspected diagnosis of IBD will incorporate a plain and upright film to look for these features. On the plain film, air can act as a contrast medium and can allow the identification of the more subtle findings of nodularity of the mucosa, suggesting ulceration or pseudopolyp formation. Chronic colitis may result in an ahaustral, tube-like colon that can be seen with air contrast (Figure 27-3). Fulminant colitis may result in toxic dilatation (toxic megacolon) that mandates surgical intervention and the specific avoidance of colonoscopy or contrast enema studies that may result in perforation. Incidental discoveries of gallstones or renal calculi that occur with increased incidence in patients with IBD may also be made.

Contrast Radiologic Studies

Contrast studies will more frequently be used in patients with CD than in those with UC due to its predisposition for small bowel involvement. For the colitic patient, whether due to CD or UC, colonoscopy is usually the preferred study, frequently obviating the need for barium enema. However, a double-contrast barium enema may still be used to discover or delineate the extent of disease in patients with gastrointestinal symptoms, especially when due to CD. Colonic contrast studies in the patient with CD can reveal segmental disease, strictures, and fistuli. Reflux into the terminal ileum occurs in approximately 85% of patients and can more effectively reveal ileal disease than small-bowel follow-through due to

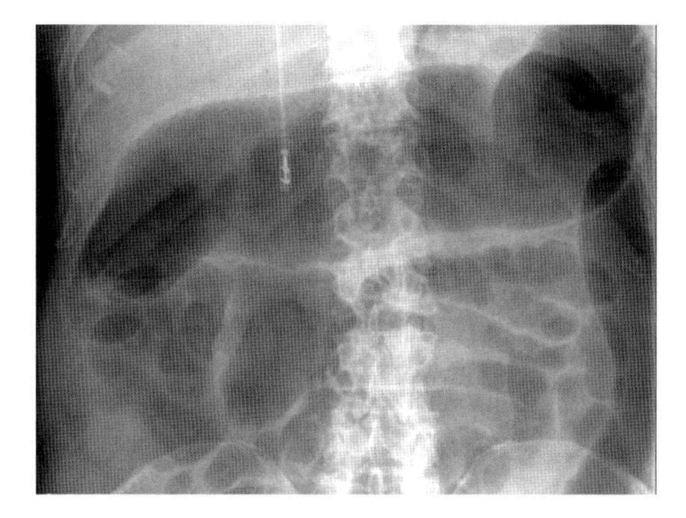

FIGURE 27-3. Plain radiographs of a patient with worsening symptoms of ulcerative colitis. Note the ahaustral left and transverse colon, signs of small bowel ileus and enlarged ("mega") transverse colon.

less interference by other intestinal loops. When fistuli or near obstructing strictures are suspected, a water-soluble dye such as Gastrografin is preferred. This contrast medium minimizes the complications associated with possible extravasation of the agent if a fistula or intestinal perforation is present or with subsequent impaction of barium proximal to a stricture. Frequently, in patients with CD, an unsuspected rectal fistula tracking to a diseased terminal ileum is found on rectal contrast study (Figure 27-4). Such a fistula can be easily overlooked during colonoscopy because it almost always originates with the diseased terminal ileum, while the rectum and sigmoid are normal.

The difficulty of reaching the small bowel using fiberoptic instruments necessitates the common use of small bowel contrast studies to assess the degree of CD involvement of the small bowel. A small bowel series can effectively show areas of stricturing and upstream dilatation but may be difficult to perform or interpret due to slow intestinal transit from strictures, overlying loops of bowel, and pain associated with compression spot views (Figure 27-5). Enteroclysis is preferred over simple small-bowel follow-through, although the need for the placement of a naso-intestinal tube makes patient cooperation and satisfaction with this study much less. High-density barium must be used as the contrast agent, since water-soluble dyes rapidly dilute in the small bowel, making detailed assessment of the intestinal mucosa difficult. After placement of the nasal tube beyond the pylorus, relatively small boluses of barium are injected that coat the walls of the intestine and then air is insufflated to distend the bowel, allowing detailed examination of the mucosa. Repetitive infusions of dye and air, with subsequent spot compression films, can result in remarkable detail being revealed but results are clearly dependent on operator expertise and patient cooperation.

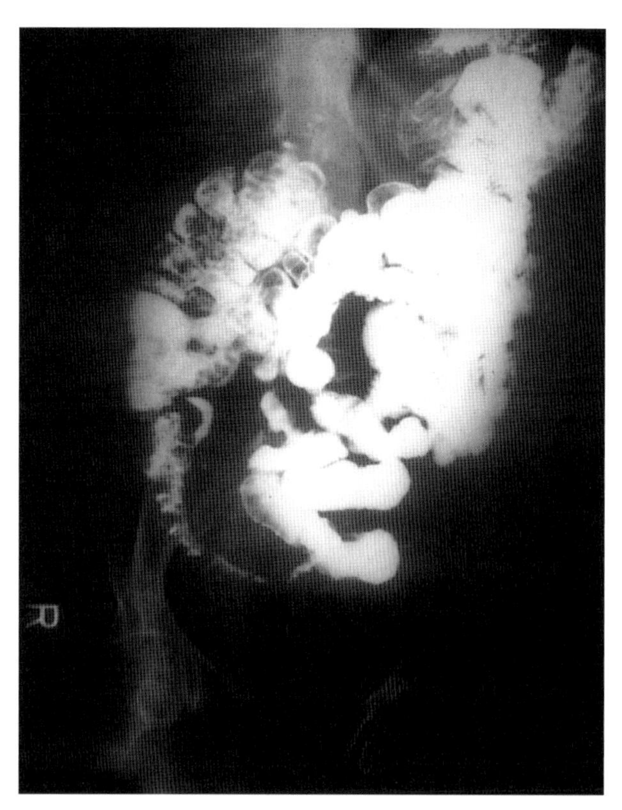

FIGURE 27-4. Small-bowel follow-through contrast study showing terminal ileal stricturing disease, with displacement of adjacent bowel loops due to ileal thickening.

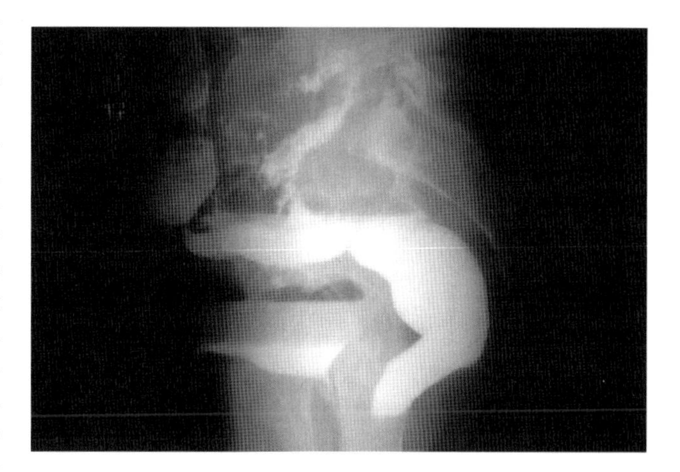

FIGURE 27-5. Colonic contrast study in Crohn's disease patient showing complex fistulizing disease. Contrast is present in the proximal, diseased ileum and air and contrast in the bladder due to fistulizing disease.

Gastrointestinal contrast studies surpass computed tomography (CT) for detecting enteroenteric and enterocolic fistuli.[55] The discovery of an enteric fistula can be made when orally consumed contrast material is seen in a distal portion of bowel without illuminating intervening intestine, such as can occur with ileal disease fistulizing into the rectum.

Sometimes the dye will directly illuminate the fistula or the involved organ, such as the bladder, as it tracks from the bowel irrespective of whether the contrast is given orally or rectally (Figure 27-4).

Sinography or fistulography can be used to delineate the path or origin of fistulous disease in patients with CD, whether involving the abdominal wall or the perineum. Such studies can also be done via the drainage catheter after percutaneous drainage of an abscess to document intestinal communication and should be done again with a water-soluble contrast agent. Such anatomic localization assists in directing subsequent surgical care (especially when fistulous disease involving the urinary tree is found) and assessing response to therapy.

Retrograde studies through a stoma, especially an ileostomy, can provide very good evaluation for disease. The effectively foreshortened intestine allows better delineation of disease with less overlapping bowel loops and better double-contrast definition.

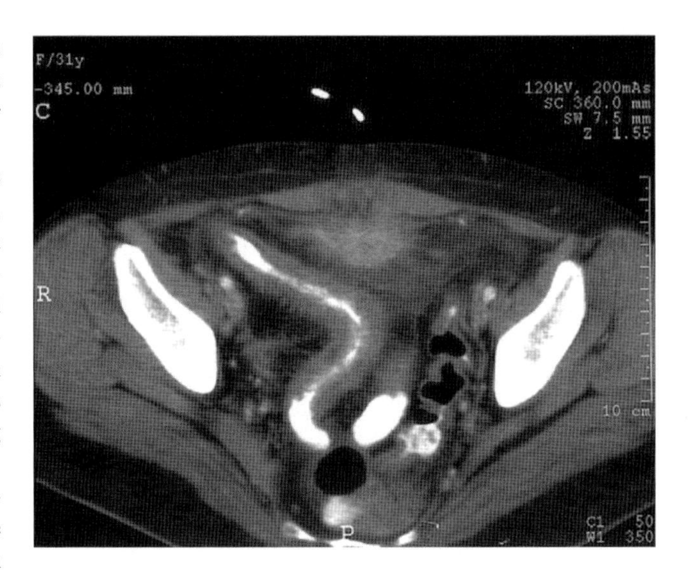

FIGURE 27-6. Computed tomography scan of Crohn's disease patient with severe terminal ileal thickening and early abscess formation under anterior abdominal wall.

Computed Tomography

Abdominal and pelvic CT is probably the most commonly obtained study in the acute evaluation of patients with IBD, especially CD. Such studies should be undertaken with orally ingested low-density barium or iodinated contrast material that has been allowed to traverse the entire GI tract. Due to strictures or slow transit time, rectal administration of contrast material will sometimes be necessary. CT scanning is especially useful for delineating enterovesical or colovesical fistuli, and scans should be obtained before administering intravenous contrast, as contrast originating from the bowel will be seen in the bladder defining the fistula. Air within the bladder without prior instrumentation is also a very sensitive sign defining the presence of a fistula.

The great advantage of CT is its ability to evaluate the entire thickness of the intestine and its adjacent structures. Thus, thickened intestine, phlegmon, abscess, air in extraintestinal structures, and fistula formation are signs of CD that can be found on CT scan (Figure 27-6). Percutaneous drainage of abscess collections done under CT guidance can also be performed. Though less commonly performed for UC, CT findings that can be seen include increased perirectal and presacral fat, inhomogenous areas of colonic thickening, target or "double halo" sign of the colon, and changes consistent with cancer development such as strictures or mass lesions.[55]

Magnetic Resonance Imaging

Magnetic resonance imaging (MRI) is playing an increasing role in the evaluation of IBD patients. Intestinal CD can be identified simply by thickened bowel loops on conventional MRI. However, MRI differs from CT, in that the intensity of T2-weighted signals from areas of disease correlates with the severity of inflammation, especially after gadolinium administration. Such signal intensity in both the mesentery and bowel decreases with resolution of acute inflammation and may hold promise for monitoring the response of patients to medical therapy.[56,57]

The value of MRI in defining perineal disease in the CD patient approaches – and may exceed – that achieved with examination under anesthesia.[57,58] Endorectal coil placement may improve sensitivity but is infrequently necessary and sometimes impossible in the diseased anus. Intravenous injection of gadolinium highlights the fistula tract and combined with MRI's ability to define soft tissue anatomy accurately, it can result in remarkable delineation of disease.[59,60] MRI testing is expensive, however, and is probably unnecessary in the conventional perineal CD patient since examination under anesthesia performed by a competent surgeon is usually as accurate and can also aid in providing simultaneous treatment.[58] However, MRI is finding a role in re-assessing the failed patient for unrecognized pathology and, more recently, in defining whether medical treatment with infliximab has truly healed a patient's fistulous disease. Several studies using gadolinium-enhanced MRI have shown that many fistuli that respond to exclusive medical management are, in fact, still present but quiescent.[61,62]

Ultrasound

The role of ultrasound in IBD is presently very limited. European centers are more familiar with its use for assessing the GI tract in patients with IBD where it is sometimes used to assess a patient's response to therapy longitudinally. In the hands of an experienced operator, so-called transabdominal bowel sonography (TABS) can look for bowel wall thickening and fistula formation, and can even assess functional effects of strictures by observing bowel peristalsis and distention in the vicinity of such pathology[63]. This method of noninvasive intestinal evaluation has not gained wide popularity in USA.

Intrarectal ultrasound can be used to document and map perianal fistula formation by injecting a solution of hydrogen peroxide into the external opening. The resulting bubbles are easily seen on ultrasound as they outline the path of the fistula tract. However, such uncomfortable and operator-dependent techniques of fistula assessment have been largely replaced by MRI scanning (see above).

Nuclear Medicine

The injection of radionuclide-labeled white cells allows subsequent scintigraphic imaging of the abdominal organs and is increasingly being used as a technique to visualize actively inflamed bowel. Most techniques use Indium[111] labeling of autologous leukocytes that are harvested from the patient, labeled, and then reinjected. Indium[111] has the advantage of a long half-life that allows scanning at 6, 12, and 24 h with any visualized bowel activity as being abnormal. A fixed area of activity suggests an abscess. Newer techniques using Technetium –99m-haxamethyl-propylamine-oxime (HMPAO) provide for better image quality due to its relatively selective labeling of granulocytes and also result in a lower radiation dose to the patient. Some studies using this tracer have shown very high sensitivity rates, but specificity is less due to its inability to differentiate between IBD and infectious causes of disease.[64] The advantage of such radionuclide scanning techniques relates mostly to their ability to differentiate between inflamed versus quiescent disease, and their use will probably increase as newer labeling agents are devised.

TABLE 27-4. Indications for colonoscopy in inflammatory bowel disease

• Diagnosis:	– Gross appearance – Tissue biopsy
• Disease extent	
• Disease complications:	– Fistuli – Stricture – Bleeding
• Preoperative "Staging"	
• Monitor response to therapy	
• Stricture management:	– Biopsy – Dilatation
• Cancer surveillance	

TABLE 27-5. Gross (Colonoscopic) features of colitis

	Ulcerative colitis	Crohn's disease
Early		
	Edema	Aphthous ulcers
	Confluent erythema	Patchy, asymmetric erythema
	Loss of vascular markings	Anal disease: waxy skin tags linear fissures
Intermediate		
	Granularity	Linear serpiginous ulcers
	Bleeding	Pseudopolyps
	Micropurulence	Anal disease: Fistulia abscesses
Advanced/late		
	Ulcerations, transmural disease	Confluent ulcers
	Pseudopolyp formation	Deep "bear claw" ulcerations
	Purulence	Strictures
	Variable thinning/thickening	Mucosal bridging of colon
	Mucosal bridging	

Endoscopy

Colonoscopy has strongly influenced the diagnosis and evaluation of the patient with IBD. It is the study of choice for the patient with suspected UC since it can directly visualize the entire extent of the disease process. It is similarly relevant for CD when involving the colon, and can also be used to intubate and evaluate the terminal ileum. Most significantly, colonoscopy provides biopsies, which allows a tissue diagnosis to be made by the pathologist. There are numerous indications for colonoscopy in the patient with IBD (Table 27-4) and as such, colonoscopy plays a significant role in the evaluation and management of these patients. The gross appearance of the colon as seen on colonoscopy can frequently differentiate between CD and UC (Table 27-5). Its use in the patient with severe disease is controversial. Although studies exist suggesting that it can be safely undertaken in the severely colitic patient, the risk of perforation due to insufflation, biopsy, or mechanical bending of the scope is generally acknowledged as being high and thus colonoscopy is generally avoided in the acute setting. However, such severely ill patients still need endoscopic evaluation to exclude concurrent diseases such as pseudomembranous or cytomegalovirus-induced colitis. Rigid or flexible proctoscopic evaluation is thus recommended, with biopsies done in the lower rectum below the peritoneal reflection in order to minimize the risk of free perforation.

The flexible sigmoidoscope is conveniently used for the evaluation of the unsedated, office patient, but is limited by its 65-cm length to visualize the colon up to approximately the splenic flexure. However, this evaluation can often be adequate and, in the case of UC, definitive. In the patient with typical presenting symptoms of bloody diarrhea and tenesmus, a flexible sigmoidoscopy with biopsies and stool culture for pathogens and ova/parasites may complete the work-up and make the diagnosis.

There is an increasing experience with through-the-scope (TTS) pneumatic dilatation of colonic or ileocolonic strictures in CD. The technique incorporates repetitive insufflation of the TTS balloon for 15–60-s periods, with the larger balloons (25 mm) being associated with more patient pain and complications than the smaller ones (12 mm). In a prospective study of 55 patients, long-term success (mean follow-up of 34 months) with complete relief of obstructive symptoms was achieved in 62% of patients, while 19 (38%) patients required operation and six (11%) suffered a perforation.[65]

Upper endoscopy or esophagogastroduodenoscopy (EGD) will infrequently be used in the management of CD since gastroduodenal CD occurs in less than 5% of patients. However, when CD does affect the stomach or duodenum, strictures are common, and therapeutic dilatation and biopsies to evaluate for malignancy via EGD are necessary. More commonly, EGD is useful in the evaluation of the differential diagnosis of upper abdominal pain or dysphagia in the IBD patient. Esophageal candidiasis brought on by immunosuppression, duodenal or gastric ulcerative disease due to steroids, or reflux disease from downstream partial obstruction occurs with increased frequency in the IBD patient and is well evaluated by EGD. The so-called push enteroscopy using specially designed flexible scopes has been developed to improve access of the endoscopist to the jejunum, but its use is very limited. The preferred study for the evaluation of small bowel CD is still small-bowel contrast follow-through, enteroclysis, or CT enterography.

Wireless Capsule Endoscopy

Wireless capsule endoscopy (WCE) is a recent unique development for the visualization of the small bowel. An 11×26 mm capsule is swallowed that transmits two video images per second to a receiver worn on the belt. Over the 8-h battery life of the device, more than 50,000 images are transmitted and stored that are subsequently evaluated at 25 frames per second by dedicated software and the human eye. Subtle small bowel lesions, usually out of the reach of the colonoscope or upper endoscope, can be appreciated. Its role in CD is still being clarified, but criteria for its use include the recommendation for prior colonoscopy and intubation of the terminal ileum. Many studies using WCE have found CD in the most common regions that can be easily reached by a colonoscope, obviating the need for the more expensive WCE. In addition, a small-bowel contrast series is also necessary since the size of the capsule may cause it to impact at a stricture, precipitating acute bowel obstruction requiring surgery. Other problems include its limited battery life in patients with slow transit, the inability to biopsy, and its imperfect localization of identified lesions. Nonetheless, this technology provides an added and potentially more sensitive tool in the diagnosis and management of patients with CD.[57,66,67]

Pathology

Ulcerative Colitis

UC begins in the rectum and extends proximally to a variable distance, with the worst disease being distal and the least disease being proximal. The disease may be limited to the rectum (ulcerative proctitis), or extend to only the left colon or completely to the cecum (pancolitis). The terminal ileum may be inflamed in continuity with the cecum (backwash ileitis). The disease is in continuity, and segmental or "skip" disease does not occur, although the so-called rectal sparing or some degree of patchiness can be seen in the actively treated patient, especially when enema therapy has been given. The gross appearance of the inflammatory process depends on the severity and duration of the disease (Table 27-5). In early disease, inflammation is restricted to the mucosa but in its severest, toxic form, it can become transmural and indistinguishable grossly and histopathologically from CD, with deep ulcerations, pseudopolyp formation, and variable areas of thickened and thinned colonic wall.

The histopathologic features of UC are listed in Table 27-6. There are no pathognomonic features of UC and in its extreme form, it can resemble CD. However, typical UC is associated with inflammation limited to the mucosa or lamina propria, including relatively uniform crypt distortion and crypt abscesses. Goblet cell mucin depletion is common and the inflammatory infiltrate is usually neutrophilic, two features that distinguish UC from CD where mucin depletion is uncommon and the inflammation is usually mononuclear. More severe UC leads to the entire loss of the crypt, with deeper submucosal and transmural inflammation and ulceration. In the chronic, more quiescent phase, UC will have mucosal reconstitution but will still have crypt distortion, foreshortening, and branching. Inflammation will be variably reduced, or even absent, but when present, it will be relatively uniform in distribution. Dysplasia in long-standing UC is common but can be interpreted only in the setting of

TABLE 27-6. Histology of inflammatory bowel disease

	Ulcerative colitis	Crohn's disease
Early		
	Crypt distortion, branching	Patchy crypt distortion
	Goblet cell mucin depletion	Minimal goblet cell mucin depletion
	Vascular congestion (without inflammation)	Aphthoid ulcers
	Mucosal inflammation	
Intermediate		
	Uniform crypt abscesses	Focal crypt abscesses
	Loss of mucosa with retention of crypts	Vasculitis (20%)
	Noncaseating granulomas	
	Lamina propria neutrophils	(20–60%) Mononuclear cell infiltrate
Advanced/late		
	Crypt destruction	Transmural inflammation
	Neuronal hyperplasia uncommon	Neuronal hyperplasia common
	Deeper submucosa inflammation	Mucosal and submucosal
	Pseudopolyp, mucosal thickening bridging	Fibrosis and strictures
	Dysplasia common	Dysplasia uncommon

non-inflamed bowel, since many of its features are common with inflammation, namely, crypt distortion, increased mitotic index, and nuclear atypia.

Crohn's Disease

The gross features of CD include its ability to affect any portion of the GI tract, its transmural inflammation, and its propensity to create fistulas and strictures, including in the perianal area. Skip lesions are common, resulting in multiple areas of bowel affected simultaneously with intervening segments of normal intestine. Diseased bowel may fistulize into adjacent bowel that is otherwise unaffected, a type of bystander injury that only requires surgical removal of the offending segment of intestine with primary repair of the fistula in the remaining, healthy bowel. Serositis is common in CD, as is fat wrapping or creeping fat, all nonspecific responses to the observed transmural inflammation. On the mucosal surface, the earliest changes are aphthous ulcers, which are tiny white pinpoint lesions representing mucosal ulcerations in the vicinity of enlarged lymphoid follicles. These lesions are thought to then enlarge and coalesce into the larger, deeper longitudinal serpiginous ulcers commonly found in CD. These areas will have a deep, fissuring appearance and will extend ever deeper into the bowel wall, infrequently perforating freely, but instead recruiting an inflammatory response from adjacent organs that tend to wall off the inflamed bowel and that can then lead to fistulization. Healing is associated with granulation tissue and stricture formation, features not commonly found in UC.

Microscopically, the inflammatory infiltrate is commonly mononuclear and there is minimal goblet cell dropout in the mucosa. When crypt abscesses occur, they are nonuniform, affecting some crypts and not others. Vasculitis is sometimes seen (20%) and neuronal hyperplasia is common, both features that are rarely seen in UC. The classic noncaseating granuloma is found in 20–60% of patient biopsies and is composed of epithelioid and giant cells of the Langhans type. Granulomas probably wax and wane in their presence and can also be found in adjacent tissues affected in continuity, such as bladder, lymph nodes, ovaries, and perianal squamous epithelial skin tags. Their significance remains unclear, with some suggesting that they indicate a less aggressive form of CD.

Indeterminate Colitis

Approximately 10–15% of patients with colitis will have either clinical or pathologic features that do not allow a clear diagnosis of either CD or UC to be definitively made. This dilemma is often attributable to rapidly deteriorating, fulminant colitis, where even UC can have transmural or irregular mucosal involvement. Sometimes the gross anatomic appearance is complicated by incomplete response to various medications, especially when delivered transanally as enemas, which can lead to relative "rectal sparing" and, therefore, suggest CD over UC. Frequently, the correct diagnosis involves the judgment of an experienced clinician who considers not only the histopathology, but also the clinical characteristics of the patient, the history of disease progression, and even more subtle data such as serum antineutrophil cytoplasmic antibody (ANCA) and ASCA testings (see Serum Tests for IBD). More than half of such indeterminate cases can usually be resolved with such consideration of the entire clinical picture. This is especially important in the patient who is a candidate for pelvic pouch reconstruction, where the results of such surgery are significantly worse in the misdiagnosed patient with CD.[68]

Serum Tests for IBD

Serum tests for IBD can be divided into several categories: acute phase reactants, nutritional parameters, and inflammatory markers. The prototypic acute phase reactant is the erythrocyte sedimentation rate (ESR), which is commonly used, especially in CD in spite of its imperfect correlation with disease activity. It is a necessary component to determine the CDAI (see section above). Some have suggested that ESR correlates better with colitis, either CD or UC, than with small bowel CD. This may be due to the fact that ESR may be normal in CD patients with noninflammatory disease who nonetheless may be very symptomatic due to the presence of "burned-out" fibrotic strictures.[69] Conversely, an acute abscess from a long-standing fistula in ano may elevate the ESR without any evidence for flaring of intestinal disease. Similar difficulties have been encountered in correlating disease status with other acute phase reactants, such as C-reactive protein (CRP), orosomucoid (alpha-1-acid glycoprotein), alpha-1-antitrypsin, and alpha-2-globulin.[70] The fecal excretion of alpha-1-antitrypsin when measured as a clearance ratio has some correlation to active intestinal disease, but difficulty with collection methodology makes this test rarely used. Presently, ESR and possibly CRP are the only two tests commonly used in the clinical arena.

Nutritional parameters are commonly used to assess the consequence of acute and subacute disease in IBD. Albumin, prealbumin, and iron (transferrin and serum iron) studies are reflective of the combined effects of decreased food intake (to minimize symptoms), compromised absorption (from inflammation or surgical shortening of the bowel), and increased losses (from loss of proteins and blood from mucosal ulceration). B12 is commonly decreased in CD patients with ileal disease or after surgical resection. Such nutritional tests are nonspecific, but extremely valuable in clinical decision making from either a surgical or a medical perspective. Other relevant serum studies include liver function testing that may reveal subclinical primary sclerosing cholangitis.

Research into the immune regulatory pathways that play a role in the inflammation seen in IBD has resulted in the identification of numerous chemokines that are altered in IBD.[45] Many of these, including IL-1, IL-2, IL-6, IL-8, TNF, CD45, soluble IL-2, and interferon-gamma, have not been used beyond investigative protocols for a number of reasons. Frequently, serum levels of these cytokines do not correlate with the abnormal levels found in the affected tissues, thus obviating their use as serum tests. A possible exception may be the soluble IL-2 receptor (sIL-2r). Increased serum levels of sIL-2r seem to correlate with mucosal inflammatory activity. Levels drop with response to therapy in parallel with the CDAI, and high levels have been predictive of clinical relapse.[71]

Perinuclear antineutrophil cytoplasmic antibody (pANCA) is an autoantibody found in the serum of approximately 50–70% of UC patients, but only in 20–30% of CD patients.[72] It does not correlate with disease activity, but is thought to indicate a more aggressive disease type, due to its association with patients who are relatively resistant to medical management and also with patients who commonly suffer pouchitis after IPAA.[73,74] Another serum antibody, to a common yeast, *Saccharomyces cerevisiae* (ASCA), has been shown to be present in 50–70% of CD patients but only in 10–15% of UC patients. Thus, the measurement of both ANCA and ASCA is increasingly being used to try to differentiate between CD and UC when the disease is limited to the colon and confusing features, such as rectal sparing, exist.

Recently, a number of genetic mutations have been discovered which are associated with Crohn's disease. The presence of these mutations can be assayed using the DNA of leukocytes harvested by peripheral blood draw. Three mutations affecting the CARD15/NOD 2 gene on the short arm of chromosome 16 have been identified as being associated with CD.[34,75] The NOD2/CARD15 gene codes for an intracellular protein that has high binding affinity for bacterial peptidoglycan and may play a role in innate immunoresponsiveness to enteric bacteria. Mutations in this gene are found in approximately 10–30% of CD patients versus 8–15% of healthy controls. The relative risk of developing CD if mutations are carried in both copies of this gene is 10–40 times that in the general population. The presence of this mutation in a patient with CD is associated with ileal disease, earlier age of onset, and possibly fibrostenosing characteristics.[76,77] Mutations can be easily assayed by polymerase chain reaction (PCR) techniques, and hold promise for possibly predicting responsiveness to medical or surgical therapies.

Evaluation of the Acute Patient with Acute Exacerbation of IBD

The clinical and laboratory evaluation of the patient presenting with IBD will depend on many factors. Obviously, a good history and physical examination will focus the clinical caregiver in one or another area that will then direct subsequent testing and care. Many of the testing regimens described previously in this chapter apply to a greater or lesser degree based on clinical circumstances. There is no one good test for IBD, so the clinical judgment, experience, and acumen of the physician are key in patient management. Nonetheless, there are some basic and fundamental testing regimens that should at least be considered, if not repetitively performed, whenever IBD is considered the possible diagnosis. A basic outline of evaluation of the acutely presenting IBD patient is found in Table 27-7. It is important to remember that the patient with a known diagnosis of IBD will frequently still require such a basic evaluation whenever the disease flares. This need is in part due to the recognition that these patients are at significant risk for the development of a superimposed secondary diagnosis not infrequently related to iatrogenic causes. These associated problems might include pseudomembranous or cytomegalovirus colitis, stress or steroid-induced gastric ulceration, fungal sepsis, or neutropenia. In addition, a patient known to have IBD who presents with worsening symptoms may have progression of the disease or the development of a directly related complication, such as an intraabdominal abscess, bowel obstruction, toxic colitis, or colovesical fistula. Thus the studies outlined in Table 27-7 should be regularly considered for the patient presenting with an acute exacerbation of IBD, tempered by the good clinical judgment of the caring physician.

Table 27-7. Evaluation of the patient with inflammatory bowel disease

	Test	Purpose
Serum labs	CBC	r/o anemia, leukocytosis
	Electrolytes, renal function	r/o electrolyte disturbance 2° diarrhea, dehydration
	ESR, +/– CRP	↑ in systemic disease
	LFT's, albumin	r/o PSC, nutritional compromise
Stool studies	C. difficile	r/o infectious causes
	O&P	r/o infectious causes
	Pathogens	r/o infectious causes
X-rays	Plain abdominal X-rays	r/o free air, toxic colitis, stones, obstruction
	SBFT/enteroclysis	For small bowel disease
	Barium/Gastrografin enema	For fistuli, strictures, and distribution of disease
	CT scan	For abscess, obstruction, fistuli, and adjacent organ involvement
Endoscopy	Flexible/rigid scope	For biopsy to r/o CMV, granulomas, pseudomembranes
	Colonoscopy	For biopsy, visualize extent and severity of disease

SBFT small-bowel follow-through; *r/o* rule out; *CMV* cytomegalovirus; *LFTs* liver function tests; *CT* computed tomography; *O&P* ova and parasites; *ESR* erythrocyte sedimentation rate; *CRP* C-reactive protein; *CBC* complete blood cell count; *PSC* primary sclerosing cholangitis.

References

1. Crohn BB, Ginzburg L, Oppenheimer GD. Regional Ileitis. AMA Am J Dis Child. 1932;99:1323–9.
2. Combe C, Saunders W. A singular case of stricture and thickening of the ileum. Med Trans Royal Soc Med 1806;16–18.
3. Brooke BN. Granulomatous disease of the intestine. Lancet 1959;2(7106):745–9.
4. Lockhart-Mummery HE, Morson BC. Crohn's disease (regional enteritis) of the large intestine and its distinction from ulcerative colitis. Gut. 1960;1:87–105.
5. Brooke BN. The management of an ileostomy including its complications. Dis Colon Rectum. 1993;36:512–6.
6. Truelove SC, Witts LJ, Bourne WA, et al. Cortisone and corticotropin in ulcerative colitis. Br Med J. 1959;1(5119):387–94.
7. Gitnick G. Inflammatory bowel disease: diagnosis and treatment. New York: Igaku-Shoin; 1991.
8. Korelitz BI. Immunosuppressive therapy of inflammatory bowel disease: a historical perspective. Gastroenterologist. 1995;3(2):141–52.
9. Targan SR, Hanauer SB, van Deventer SJ, et al. A short-term study of chimeric monoclonal antibody cA2 to tumor necros factor alpha for Crohn's disease. Crohn's disease cA2 study group. N Engl J Med. 1997;337(15):1029–35.
10. Dennis C. Ileostomy and colectomy in chronic ulcerative colitis. Surgery. 1945;18:435–52.
11. Strauss AA, Strauss SF. Surgical treatment of ulcerative colitis. Surg Clin North Am. 1944;24:211–24.
12. Koch NG. Intra-abdominal reservoir in patients with permanent ileostomy. Arch Surg. 1969;99:223–31.
13. Parks AG, Nicholls RJ. Proctocolectomy without ileostomy for ulcerative colitis. Br Med J. 1978;2:85–8.
14. Utsunomiya J. Restorative proctocolectomy for ileal reservoir. Int J Colorectal Dis. 1986;1:2–19.
15. Ekbom A, Helmick C, Zack M, et al. The epidemiology of inflammatory bowel disease: a large, population-based study in Sweden. Gastroenterology. 1991;100:350–8.
16. Yang SK, Hong WS, Min YI, et al. Incidence and prevalence of ulcerative colitis in the Songpa-Kangdong district, Seoul, Korea. J Gastroenterol Hepatol. 2000;15:1037–42.
17. Sonnenberg A, McCarty DJ, Jacobsen SJ. Geographic variation of inflammatory bowel disease within the United States. Gastroenterology. 1991;100:143–9.
18. Loftus Jr EV, Schoenfeld P, Sandborn WJ. The epidemiology and natural history of Crohn's disease in population-based patient cohorts from North America: a systemic review. Aliment Pharmacol Ther. 2002;16:51–60.
19. Blanchard JF, Bernstein CN, Wajda A, et al. Small-area variations and sociodemographic correlates for the incidence of Crohn's disease and ulcerative colitis. Am J Epidemiol. 2001;154:328–35.
20. Munkholm P, Langholz E, Nielsen OH, et al. Incidence and prevalence of Crohn's disease in the country of Copenhagen 1962-87: a sixfold increase in incidence. Scand J Gastroenterol. 1992;27:609–14.
21. Gilat T, Grossman A, Fireman Z, et al. Inflammatory bowel disease in Jews. Front Gastrointest Res. 1986;11:135–40.
22. Sonnenberg A. Occupational distribution of inflammatory bowel disease among German employees. Gut. 1990;31:1037–40.
23. Reif S, Klein I, Lubin F, et al. Pre-illness dietary factors in inflammatory bowel disease. Gut. 1997;40:754–60.
24. Boyko EJ, Perera DR, Koepsell TD, et al. Coffee and alcohol use and the risk of ulcerative colitis. Am J Gastroenterol. 1989;84:530–4.
25. Tanner AR, Raghunath AS. Colonic inflammation and nonsteroidal anti-inflammatory drug administration. An assessment of the frequency of the problem. Digestion. 1988;41:116–20.
26. Vessey M, Jewell D, Smith A, et al. Chronic inflammatory bowel disease, cigarette smoking, and use of oral contraceptives: findings in a large cohort study of women of childbearing age. Br Med J (Clin Res Ed). 1986;292:1101–3.
27. Calkins BM. A meta-analysis of the role of smoking in inflammatory bowel disease. Dig Dis Sci. 1989;34:1841–54.
28. Barrett JC, Hansoul S, Nicolae DL, et al. Genome-wide association defines more than 30 distinct susceptibility loci for Crohn's disease. Nat Genet. 2008;40(8):955–62.
29. Duerr RH, Taylor KD, Brant SR, et al. A genome-wide association study identifies IL23R as an inflammatory bowel disease gene. Science. 2006;314(5804):1461–3.
30. Silverberg MS, Cho JH, Rioux JD, et al. Ulcerative colitis-risk loci on chromosomes 1p36 and 12q15 found by genome-wide association study. Nat Genet. 2009;41(2):216–20.
31. Rioux JD, Xavier RJ, Taylor KD, et al. Genome-wide association study identifies new susceptibility loci for Crohn's disease and implicates autophagy in disease pathogenesis. Nat Genet. 2007;39(5):596–604.
32. The Wellcome Trust Case Control Consortium. Genome-wide association study of 14,000 cases of seven common diseases and 3,000 shared controls. Nature. 2007;447:661–78.
33. Lees CW, Satsangi J. Genetics of inflammatory bowel disease: implications for disease pathogenesis and natural history. Expert Rev Gastroenterol Hepatol. 2009;3(5):513–34.
34. Ogura Y, Bonen DK, Inohara N, et al. A frameshift mutation in NOD2 associated with susceptibility to Crohn's disease. Nature. 2001;411(6837):603–6.
35. Hampe J, Franke A, Rosenstiel P, et al. A genome-wide association scan of nonsynonymous SNP's identifies a susceptibility variant for Crohn's disease in ATG16L1. Nat Genet. 2007;39(2):207–11.
36. Cho JH. The genetics and immunopathogenesis of inflammatory bowel disease. Nat Rev Immunol. 2008;8(6):458–66.
37. Glocker EO, Kotlarz D, Boztug K, et al. Inflammatory bowel disease and mutations affecting the interleukin-10 receptor. N Engl J Med. 2009;361(21):2033–45.
38. Gasche C, Scholmerich J, Brynskov J, et al. A simple classification of Crohn's disease: report of the working party for the world congresses of gastroenterology Vienna 1998. Inflamm Bowel Dis. 2000;6:8–15.
39. Louis E, Collard A, Oger AF, et al. Behaviour of Crohn's disease according to the Vienna classification: changing pattern over the course of the disease. Gut. 2001;49:777–82.
40. Bernstein CN, Blanchard JF, Rawsthorne P, et al. The prevalence of extraintestinal diseases in inflammatory bowel disease: a population-based study. Am J Gastroenterol. 2001;96:1116–22.
41. Generini S, Giacomelli R, Fedi R, et al. Infliximab in spondyloarthropathy associated with Crohn's disease: an open study on the efficacy of inducing and maintaining remission

of musculoskeletal and gut manifestations. Ann Rheum Dis. 2004;63(12):1664–9.
42. Nahar IK, Shojania K, Marra CA, et al. Infliximab treatment of rheumatoid arthritis and Crohn's disease. Ann Pharmacother. 2003;37(9):1256–65.
43. Sheldon DG, Sawchuk LL, Kozarek RA, et al. Twenty cases of peristomal pyoderma gangrenosum: diagnostic implications and management. Arch Surg. 2000;135(5):564–8.
44. Powell FC, Schroeter AL, Su WPD, et al. Pyoderma gangrenosum: a review of 86 patients. Q J Med. 1985;217:173–86.
45. Poritz LS, Koltun WA. Surgical management of ulcerative colitis in the presence of primary sclerosing cholangitis. Dis Colon Rectum. 2003;46(2):173–8.
46. Cohen S. Liver disease and gallstones in regional enteritis. Gastroenterology. 1971;60:237–45.
47. Talbot RW, Heppel J, Dozois RR, et al. Vascular complications of inflammatory bowel disease. Mayo Clin Proc. 1986;61:140–5.
48. Fichera A, Cicchiello LA, Mendelson DS, et al. Superior mesenteric vein thrombosis after colectomy for inflammatory bowel disease: a not uncommon cause of postoperative acute abdominal pain. Dis Colon Rectum. 2003;46(5):643–8.
49. Remzi RH, Fazio VW, Oncel M, et al. Portal vein thrombi after restorative proctocolectomy. Surgery. 2002;132(4):655–61.
50. Best WR, Becktel JM, Singleton JW, et al. Development of a Crohn's disease activity index, national cooperative Crohn's disease study. Gastroenterology. 1976;70:439–44.
51. Poritz LS, Koltun WA. Techniques of disease activity assessment in Crohn's disease. Semin Colon Rectal Surg. 2001;12(1):16–21.
52. Pikarsky AJ, Gervaz P, Wexner SD. Perianal Crohn's disease: a new scoring system to evaluate and predict outcome of surgical intervention. Arch Surg. 2002;137:774–7.
53. Powell-Tuck J, Day DW, Buckell NA, et al. Correlations between defined sigmoidoscopic appearances and other measures of disease activity in ulcerative colitis. Dig Dis Sci. 1982;27:533–7.
54. Rutegard I, Ahsgren L, Stenling R, et al. A simple index for assessment of disease activity in patients with ulcerative colitis. Hepatogastroenterology. 1990;37:110–2.
55. Carucci LR, Levine MS. Radiographic imaging of inflammatory bowel disease. Gastroenterol Clin North Am. 2002;31(1):93–117.
56. Maccioni F, Viscido A, Broglia L, et al. Evaluation of Crohn's disease activity with magnetic resonance imaging. Abdom Imaging. 2000;25:219–28.
57. Schreyer AG, Golder S, Seitz J, et al. New diagnostic avenues in inflammatory bowel diseases. Capsule endoscopy, magnetic resonance imaging and virtual enteroscopy. Dig Dis. 2003;21(2):129–37.
58. Borley NR, Mortensen NJ, Jewell DP. MRI scanning in perianal Crohn's disease: an important diagnostic adjunct. Inflamm Bowel Dis. 1999;5(3):231–3.
59. Koelbel G, Schmiedl U, Majer MC, et al. Diagnosis of fistulae and sinus tracts in patients with Crohn disease: value of MR imaging. AJR Am J Roentgenol. 1989;152:999–1003.
60. O'Donovan AN, Somers S, Farrow R, et al. MR imaging of anorectal Crohn disease: a pictorial essay. Radiographics. 1997;17(1):101–7.
61. Bell SJ, Halligan S, Windsor AC, et al. Response of fistulating Crohn's disease to infliximab treatment assessed by magnetic resonance imaging. Aliment Pharmacol Ther. 2003;17 (3):387–93.
62. Van Assche G, Vanbeckevoort D, Bielen D, et al. Magnetic resonance imaging of the effects of infliximab on perianal fistulizing Crohn's disease. Am J Gastroenterol. 2003;98(2):332–9.
63. Gasche C, Moser G, Turetschek K, et al. Transabdominal bowel sonography for detection of intestinal complication in Crohn's disease. Gut. 1999;44:112–7.
64. Arndt JW, Grootscholten MI, van Hogezand RA, et al. Inflammatory bowel disease activity assessment using technetium-99m-HMPAO leukocytes. Dig Dis Sci. 1997;42:387–93.
65. Gevers AM, Couckuyt H, Coremans G, et al. Efficacy and safety of hydrostatic balloon dilation of ileocolonic Crohn's strictures: a prospective long-term analysis. Acta Gastroenterol Belg. 1994;57:320–2.
66. Iddan G, Meron G, Glukhovsky A, et al. Wireless capsule endoscopy. Nature. 2000;405:417.
67. Fireman Z, Mahajna E, Broide E, et al. Diagnosing small bowel Crohn's disease with wireless capsule endoscopy. Gut. 2003;52:390–2.
68. Guindi M, Riddell RH. Indeterminate colitis. J Clin Pathol. 2004;57:1233–44.
69. Camilleri M, Proano M. Advances in the assessment of diseases activity in inflammatory bowel disease. Mayo Clin Proc. 1989;64:800–7.
70. Brignola D, Lanfarnchi GA, Campieri M, et al. Importance of laboratory parameters in the evaluation of Crohn's disease activity. J Clin Gastroenterol. 1986;8:245–8.
71. Louis E, Belaich J, Kemseke CV, et al. Soluble interleukin-2 receptor in Crohn's disease: assessment of disease activity and prediction of relapse. Dig Dis Sci. 1995;40:1750–6.
72. Cambridge G, Rampton DS, Stevens TR, et al. Anti-neutrophil antibodies in inflammatory bowel disease: prevalence and diagnostic role. Gut. 1992;33:668–74.
73. Sandborn WJ, Landers CJ, Tremain WJ, et al. Association of antineutrophil cytoplasmic antibodies with resistance to treatment of left-sided ulcerative colitis: results of a pilot study. Clin Proc. 1996;71:431–6.
74. Sanborn WJ, Landers CJ, Tremain WJ, et al. Antineutrophil cytoplasmic antibody correlates with chronic pouchitis after ileal pouch anal anastomosis. Am J Gastroenterol. 1995;90:740–7.
75. Hugot JP, Chamaillard M, Zouali H, et al. Association of NOD2 leucine-rich repeat variants with susceptibility to Crohn's disease. Nature. 2001;411:559–603.
76. Ahmad T, Armuzzi A, Bunce M, et al. The molecular classification of the clinical manifestations of Crohn's disease. Gastroenterology. 2002;122:854–66.
77. Lesage S, Zouali H, Cezard JP, et al. CARD 15/NOD2 mutational analysis and genotype-phenotype correlation in 612 patients with inflammatory bowel disease. Am J Hum Genet. 2002;70:845–57.

28 IBD: Medical Management

Bruce E. Sands

Introduction

Crohn's disease (CD) and ulcerative colitis (UC) are inflammatory conditions characterized by periods of symptomatic relapse and remission. The cause of inflammatory bowel disease (IBD) is unknown but it is believed to be caused by a combination of environmental, genetic, and immunological factors in which an uncontrolled immune response within the intestinal mucosa leads to inflammation in genetically predisposed individuals. Multifactorial evidence suggests that a defect of innate immune response to microbial agents, as well as abnormalities in adaptive immunity and epithelial barrier function are involved in IBD.[1]

The goals of therapy for IBD include controlling symptoms, improving quality of life and minimizing short-term and long-term complications of disease and treatment. Therapy is guided by the anatomic extent of inflammation, the severity of clinical symptoms, patient response to treatment, adverse outcomes related to treatment and the occurrence of disease complications. There are two phases of treatment: (1) inducing remission in active disease and (2) maintaining remission. Surgery is usually reserved for treating medically refractory disease or for specific complications; however, appropriate timing for surgery requires considerable judgment about the anticipated risks, benefits, and outcomes of surgery.

Crohn's Disease: Medical Management

CD is a chronic inflammatory condition that can affect any area of the gastrointestinal tract from the mouth to the anus. The disease most commonly affects the ileum and colon. Inflammation in CD disease tends to be focal, asymmetric, transmural, and occasionally granulomatous. In addition, CD may be complicated further by penetrating (fistula, abscess) or cicatrizing (stricture) complications. Such complications are variable in their rate of occurrence, with some individuals presenting early with complicated disease behavior, and others never developing such complications over long periods of observation. Recurrent disease tends to manifest with the same complications. Therefore, a patient who requires a resection for ileal stricture is at increased risk for a second surgery for the same complication, and patients who demonstrate fistulizing disease behavior are likely to have recurrent fistulas. It is also possible to find both sorts of complications in the same individual. In particular, enteroenteric or enterocolonic fistulas may arise behind high grade strictures.

Given the variability of disease location and complications, symptoms and their severity are highly variable among individuals. Characteristic symptoms of CD include diarrhea, sometimes including nocturnal diarrhea, abdominal pain, and fatigue. Rectal bleeding may occur in CD but is less common than in UC. Clinical signs include fever, weight loss, pallor, an abdominal mass or tenderness, and perianal conditions, including fissure, fistula, or abscess. Extraintestinal manifestations are also common. These include arthralgias or frank arthritis; inflammatory conditions of the eye, including scleritis, iritis, or uveitis; skin conditions such as erythema nodosum or pyoderma gangrenosum; and mouth sores.

Mild-to-Moderate Crohn's Disease

Individuals with mild to moderate disease have fewer than four stools daily, are ambulatory, and able to tolerate solid foods and liquids. Often these individuals do not experience abdominal tenderness and do not have an abdominal mass. Severe complications such as intestinal obstruction are lacking, as are signs of systemic toxicity (fever, tachycardia, anemia, elevated erythrocyte sedimentation rate). Aminosalicylates and antibiotics are often used to treat mild-to-moderate Crohn's disease, although the topically acting steroid, budesonide, is increasingly used as a drug of choice for mild to moderate disease of the terminal ileum or proximal colon, with minimal steroid side effects.

D.E. Beck et al. (eds.), *The ASCRS Textbook of Colon and Rectal Surgery: Second Edition*,
DOI 10.1007/978-1-4419-1584-9_28, © Springer Science+Business Media, LLC 2011

Sulfasalazine and 5-Aminosalicylates

Sulfasalazine (SSZ) and 5-aminosalicylates (5-ASA) are often used as first-line therapy for the treatment of mild to moderate CD, despite thin evidence in support of their efficacy. The National Cooperative Crohn's Disease Study (NCCDS) and the European Cooperative Crohn's Disease Study (ECCDS) were large controlled clinical trials evaluating the efficacy of SSZ for the induction and maintenance of remission in patients with active CD.[2,3] The results of NCCDS demonstrated the benefits of SSZ 6 g/day over placebo for up to 16 weeks in patients with active ileocolonic and colonic CD.[2] In contrast, SSZ did not induce remission at 3 g/day as monotherapy but was shown to be beneficial in combination with methylprednisolone in the ECCDS.[3] Most studies have shown that SSZ is not consistently effective for patients with active disease limited to the small intestine.[3–5]

Mesalamine (5-ASA), an aminosalicylate without the sulfa component found in SSZ, was developed to increase tolerance and decrease the occurrence of side effects. Depending on the delivery system, 5-ASA is formulated to release at certain pH values or in a time-dependent manner in specific areas of the small and/or large intestine. Delayed-release formulations of mesalamine include Eudragit-S coated mesalamine (Asacol®) that releases 5-ASA in the terminal ileum and cecum at pH 7, and Eudragit-L coated mesalamine formulations (Salofalk®, Mesasal®, and Claversal®) that release in the mid-ileum at pH 6. Pentasa®, (a sustained-release formulation of mesalamine microgranules enclosed within a semipermeable membrane of ethylcellulose), is designed for controlled release throughout the small and large intestine, beginning in the duodenum. Newer azo-bonded formulations designed for release in the colon include the 5-ASA dimer, olsalazine (Dipentum®), and balsalazide (Colazal®), which are composed of 5-ASA molecules azo-bonded to the inert carrier molecule 4-aminobenzoyl-β alanine. Lialda® is a delayed-release tablet containing mesalamine that allows for once-daily dosing and releases at a pH 7 or above, normally in the terminal ileum. Apriso®, also a mesalamine compound, is an extended release capsule that is taken once daily and dissolves at a pH 6 starting in the small intestine and continuing throughout the colon.

Although commonly prescribed for the treatment of CD in clinical practice, 5-ASA has not consistently demonstrated efficacy in controlled clinical trials.[6] Table 28-1 describes dosing guidelines for SSZ and 5-ASA. Response to therapy should be evaluated after 6–12 weeks. Though occasionally used for disease limited to the rectum and left colon, topically delivered preparations of 5-ASA (suppositories, enemas) have not been evaluated in controlled trials in patients with distal colonic CD. SSZ and 5-ASA are not recommended for maintenance of remission.

Treatment-limiting adverse events occur frequently with SSZ. Headache and gastrointestinal upset are common dose-dependent side effects of SSZ. Patients who are slow-acetylators are at an increased risk of developing these side effects.[7] Rare side effects include hypersensitivity reactions, fever, rash, pneumonitis, hepatitis, pancreatitis, hemolytic anemia, and bone marrow suppression. SSZ depletes folate and should therefore be given with a folate supplement. Young men wishing to conceive should be alerted to the fact that SSZ may cause reversible sperm abnormalities, leading to relative infertility that reverses within 3 months of stopping the drug.

5-ASA preparations are well tolerated, and hypersensitivity reactions are rare. The majority of patients who cannot tolerate SSZ can tolerate a 5-ASA. Common side effects include headache, diarrhea, flatulence, nausea, and abdominal pain. Patients taking olsalazine may experience worsening of diarrhea resulting from increased ileal fluid secretion. This dose-dependent phenomenon usually improves with time.

Antibiotics

Antibiotics are used as alternative agents to SSZ or 5-ASA in CD. In addition to treating mild-to-moderate CD, antibiotics are valuable in treating perianal or perforating complications of CD. The two most commonly prescribed antibiotics are metronidazole and ciprofloxacin. The majority of studies demonstrate improvement with antibiotics when disease is limited to the colon.[8–11]

Clinical response is seen in patients taking up to 20 mg/kg of body weight daily of metronidazole.[8,9] Side effects occur in up to 50% of patients who take metronidazole short-term and include gastrointestinal intolerance, metallic taste, and

TABLE 28-1. Sulfasalazine and 5-aminosalicylates

Generic	Brand	Daily dose	Site of action
Sulfasalazine	Azulfidine	4–6 g daily in divided doses	Colon
	Azulfidine EN-Tabs	4–6 g daily in divided doses	Colon
Mesalamine	Canasa (suppositories)	500–1,000 mg daily QHS	Rectum
	Rowasa (enemas)	1–4 g daily QHS	Rectum/distal colon
	Asacol	2.4–4.8 g daily in divided doses	Terminal ileum/colon
	Pentasa	2–4 g daily in divided doses	Distal small bowel/colon
	Lialda	2.4–4.8 g daily in a single dose	Colon
	Apriso	1.5 g daily in a single dose QAM	Colon
Olsalazine	Dipentum	1.5–3 g daily	Colon
Balsalazide	Colazal	6.75 g daily	Colon

reaction to alcohol. Peripheral neuropathy, possibly irreversible, may occur with long-term use and patients should be counseled about this potential complication.

Ciprofloxacin, a quinolone antibiotic, has a suppressive effect on a variety of intestinal bacteria. Ciprofloxacin was shown in one study to be as effective as 5-ASA for achieving remission in mild-to-moderate active disease.[12] Combination treatment with metronidazole and ciprofloxacin may be an alternative to steroid treatment in mild-to-moderate active CD.[13] Ciprofloxacin is generally prescribed at a dose of 500 mg twice daily. Side effects include gastrointestinal upset, skin reactions, and an increase in transaminase levels. In addition, ciprofloxacin has been associated with rare cases of tendonitis and Achilles tendon rupture.

Rifaximin, a broad spectrum antibiotic with negligible intestinal absorption, was shown to be efficacious in an open-label study in patients with active CD.[14] A dose of 200–400 mg three times daily is usually prescribed. Described side effects include flatulence, headache, abdominal pain, tenesmus, and fecal urgency.

Budesonide

Enteric coated preparations of budesonide deliver corticosteroid topically with minimal systemic exposure. Multiple randomized controlled trials have demonstrated the efficacy of budesonide over placebo for the induction of remission in patients with mild to moderately active ileal or ileo-right colonic disease.[15–17] Budesonide has also been shown to be a more effective treatment than 5-ASA for patients with the correct disease locations.[18] Several studies have compared budesonide with prednisone and found that rates of clinical remission were similar in each group and the occurrence of corticosteroid-related side effects was considerably less.[19–22]

Approximately 90% of budesonide undergoes first-pass metabolism, which accounts for lower systemic exposure than traditional corticosteroids and minimizes adverse events. A course of therapy is initiated at 9 mg/day. After clinical response is achieved, usually in 4–8 weeks, the dose is tapered by 3 mg every 2 weeks. Budesonide, 6 mg/day, can delay clinical relapse rates for 3–6 months[23–26] but not at 1 year;[27] therefore, it is not recommended as a long-term maintenance agent.

Moderate-to-Severe Crohn's Disease

Patients with moderate-to-severe CD are considered to have failed treatment for mild-to-moderate disease, or have prominent symptoms of fever, significant weight loss of >10%, abdominal pain or tenderness, intermittent nausea or vomiting (without obstructive findings), or significant anemia. The treatment options for these patients include corticosteroids, biologic agents, and the early addition of immunomodulator therapy with azathioprine (AZA), 6-mercaptopurine (6-MP), or methotrexate (MTX) as an adjunct or a bridge to maintenance therapy.

Oral Corticosteroids

Oral corticosteroids are effective for the induction of remission in patients with moderate to severe CD. Approximately 60% of patients treated with prednisone in the NCCDS were in clinical remission at 17 weeks compared to 30% on placebo.[2] During the ECCDS, 80% of patients treated with methylprednisolone achieved clinical remission at 18 weeks compared to <40% of placebo patients.[3]

Prednisone doses of 40–60 mg daily are often prescribed for 2–6 weeks to induce remission, although no appropriate dose-ranging studies have been performed to date. Approximately 50–70% of patients will achieve remission at these doses.[2] Higher doses of prednisone (1 mg/kg) or methylprednisolone (1 mg/kg) have had somewhat higher response rates of 80–90%; however, there is an increased incidence of side effects.[3] Generally, prednisone doses are tapered by 5–10 mg/week until 20 mg and then by 2.5–5 mg weekly from 15 or 20 mg until discontinuation of therapy; however, taper schedules vary by clinician and according to patient response. The majority of patients treated with corticosteroids are unlikely to remain well over 1 year without specific effective maintenance therapy with other agents.[28,29] Corticosteroids are not recommended as maintenance agents.

Dependency and resistance are major concerns when treating patients with corticosteroids. On average, 50% of patients treated for active symptoms with a corticosteroid will become "steroid dependent" or "steroid resistant."[28,29] Studies suggest that younger patients, smokers, and/or those with colonic disease have the highest risk of becoming corticosteroid dependent.[30]

The occurrence and severity of most side effects associated with corticosteroids are related to the dose and duration of treatment. Common findings include insomnia, fluid retention, acne, moon face, abdominal striae, weight gain, hypertension, hyperglycemia, glaucoma, cataracts, and mood disturbances. Musculoskeletal complications, such as osteoporosis, osteonecrosis, and myopathy, are important side effects. In addition, adrenal suppression can arise in the course of treatment and contribute to physiologic dependence.

Immunomodulators

AZA and 6-MP are effective for maintaining a corticosteroid-induced remission and are beneficial as steroid sparing agents in steroid-dependent and steroid-refractory CD.[31,32] In clinical practice, AZA 2.0–2.5 mg/kg and 6-MP 1.0–1.5 mg/kg are used for maintenance therapy. Clinical benefit may not be evident for 3–4 months after initiation[31,32] but may be durable.

Adverse events include leukopenia, liver function abnormalities, pancreatitis (3–7%) and lymphoma.[33] Pancreatitis typically presents during the first 8 weeks of therapy. Reintroduction of either agent should be avoided if pancreatitis occurs as it will invariably reoccur. Routine monitoring of complete blood counts, initially every 1–2 weeks, then, at least every 3 months is recommended to avoid the risk of acute or delayed bone marrow suppression. Rare hypersensitivity reactions, including high fever, rash, liver function test abnormalities, may occur. Non-melanoma skin cancers and cervical cancer may also occur more frequently. There is a slightly increased risk of lymphoma estimated at nine cases in 10,000 patient-years of exposure.[34] Genetic polymorphisms of thiopurine methyltransferase (TPMT), the primary enzyme metabolizing 6-MP, have been identified and drug metabolite levels may be measured. Such clinical assays allow practitioners to more accurately monitor and dose these medications according to measurements of the metabolites 6-thioguanine and 6-methylmercaptopurine.[35] The value of therapeutic monitoring has not been adequately assessed in a prospective fashion. Prior to starting AZA or 6-MP, TPMT enzyme activity or genotype should be determined for each patient whenever possible. AZA and 6-MP should be avoided in patients deficient in TPMT. Patients with heterozygous genotype of intermediate activity should initiate therapy at reduced doses, generally, AZA 1.0–1.25 mg/kg or 6-MP 0.5–0.75 mg/kg daily. If TPMT activity or genotype cannot be assayed in advance of starting therapy, these drugs should be dosed with caution initially, with careful monitoring for leukopenia.

Methotrexate

MTX may be used to induce remission and as a steroid sparing agent in patients with corticosteroid-refractory or dependent CD.[36–40] MTX 25 mg administered once weekly subcutaneously (SC) or intramuscularly (IM) is the preferred dose. Folic acid 1 mg daily is routinely given as well. After remission has been achieved, a dose of 15 mg weekly may be effective. Oral doses ≤ 15 mg/week are sometimes used to prevent development of antibodies to anti-TNF agents, a regimen adapted from rheumatology practice but never validated in IBD. MTX is an alternative agent to AZA and 6-MP for maintenance of remission.[39,41,42]

The most frequent side effects reported with MTX are nausea, vomiting, stomatitis, and, less often than with AZA or 6-MP, leukopenia. Ondansetron (Zofran®) and other antiemetic agents may improve tolerance. Rare complications of therapy include hepatic fibrosis and hypersensitivity pneumonitis. MTX is contraindicated in pregnancy as it is teratogenic and abortifacient.

Biologic Therapy

Historically, biologic therapies (primarily anti-tumor necrosis factor antibodies) have been considered when CD is moderately to severely active despite therapy with aminosalicylates, corticosteroids, and/or immunomodulators, or if corticosteroids or immunomodulators are contraindicated, not tolerated, or ineffective. Biologic therapy may also be indicated if patients are corticosteroid dependent or refractory, or treatment with previous biologics was ineffective. Patients with complications such as draining fistulas or extraintestinal manifestations may derive particular benefit from biologic therapy.

Infliximab (chimeric monoclonal antibody) has been shown to effectively induce remission in patients with moderate to severe CD and to maintain remission in those patients.[43,44] Initial response to infliximab was seen in 58% of patients enrolled in the ACCENT I trial.[44] During long-term follow-up, 51% of patients receiving infliximab experienced a clinical response compared to 27% of patients taking placebo. In this same study, remission was achieved in 39% of patients receiving infliximab compared to 27% in the placebo group.[44]

Infliximab is also useful for treating patients with corticosteroid-dependent and fistulizing disease.[44,45] Patients treated with infliximab experience fewer hospitalizations and surgeries related to CD.[46] The occurrence of extraintestinal manifestations, such as spondyloarthropathy, arthralgias, and pyoderma gangrenosum may be reduced with infliximab.[47–49]

Approximately 30% of patients have no response to infliximab and not all responders have a complete response.[44,50,51] Elevated C-reactive protein (CRP), nonstricturing and pure colonic disease subtypes, and concomitant use of immunomodulators have been described as positive predictors for response to infliximab.[52] AZA and 6-MP are most commonly used as concomitant suppression. Methotrexate (MTX) may also be used.[53]

Adalimumab (human anti-TNF antibody) and certolizumab pegol (pegylated humanized anti-TNF Fab) are effective for inducing and maintaining remission in patients with moderate to severe CD who are naïve to anti-TNF agents or who have been exposed to infliximab, and for healing intestinal mucosa.[51,54–64] Adalimumab is also effective as a steroid sparing agent and in treating fistulas.[51,65,66]

Initial response rates to adalimumab and certolizumab pegol were 58% (CHARM) and 64% (PRECiSE 2), respectively.[51,67] During long-term follow up of over 1 year, adalimumab achieved a clinical response in 52% of patients compared to 27% patients taking placebo among patients who initially responded. Remission was achieved in 40% of those taking adalimumab compared with only 17% in the placebo group.[51]

During the PRECiSE 2 study 62.8% of patients receiving certolizumab pegol experienced a clinical response compared to only 36.2% of those assigned to placebo among patients who initially responded to induction therapy with certolizumab pegol. Remission was achieved in 47.9% of patients assigned to certolizumab pegol compared to only 28.6% of those receiving placebo.[67]

Newer treatment paradigms, referred to as "top-down therapy," have been investigated, with the suggestion that anti-TNF therapy may be more effective when given earlier in the course of disease, and when given in combination with an immunomodulator such as AZA. A landmark study from

Belgium and the Netherlands randomized patients with active CD, no history of complicated disease behavior, and no prior exposure to corticosteroids, immunomodulators or anti-TNF antibodies to receive either "step-up" therapy or early aggressive therapy. In the step-up arm, patients were given a steroid taper. If this proved unsuccessful in controlling symptoms, or if symptoms reoccurred upon taper, a second steroid taper was given. Failing this, patients received an immunomodulator (AZA, or MTX if AZA was not tolerated). Finally, patients refractory to each of these steps were given an infusion of infliximab. This arm of randomization represents the prevailing paradigm of treatment, where therapy is dictated by control of symptoms as trial and error escalation through therapies of increasing immune suppression. The second arm of randomization incorporated induction dosing with infliximab 5 mg/kg at weeks 0, 2, and 6, and simultaneous initiation of an immunomodulator. If the patient flared despite this regimen, an additional dose of infliximab could be given, and failing this, a tapering course of oral corticosteroids. The primary outcome measures were remission without corticosteroids and without bowel resection at weeks 26 and 52. At week 26, 60% of patients in the combined immunosuppression group were in remission without corticosteroids and without surgical resection compared to only 35.9% in the "step-up" group (absolute difference 24.1%, CI 7.3–40.8, $p=0.0062$). Similar benefits were seen at week 52, 61.5% receiving early immunosuppression achieved the clinical endpoints of corticosteroid-free remission and prevention of surgical resection compared to 42.2% taking corticosteroids (absolute difference 19.3%, 95% CI 2.4–36.3, $p=0.028$). The occurrence of serious adverse events was comparable in each group. The authors concluded that combined immunosuppression was more effective than conventional management for induction of remission and reduction of corticosteroid use in patients who had been recently diagnosed with CD. Initiation of more intensive treatment early in the course of disease may result in better outcomes.[68]

In a second randomized controlled trial, the benefits of monotherapy with an immunomodulator or anti-TNF antibody was compared to the combination of both in patients with relatively early and uncomplicated disease. The SONIC study was conducted to compare azathioprine monotherapy, infliximab monotherapy, and the combination of both agents in patients with CD naïve to immunomodulators and biologic therapy.[69] The primary endpoint of the study was corticosteroid-free clinical remission at 26 weeks. In the study, significantly more patients treated with infliximab alone or the combination of infliximab and azathioprine had relief of symptoms than patients treated with azathioprine alone. Approximately 31% of patients taking azathioprine alone significantly achieved corticosteroid-free clinical remission compared with 44.4% of patients on infliximab monotherapy and 56.8% of patients on combination therapy.[69] Patients with the highest levels of C-reactive protein and/or with endoscopic evidence of ulcers did better with infliximab alone or with combination therapy. Mucosal healing was seen in 44% of patients receiving infliximab combination therapy and 30% receiving infliximab monotherapy compared with 17% of patients receiving azathioprine alone.[69] Patients with CD who are naïve to immunomodulators and biologic agents are more likely to have enhanced mucosal healing when they are treated with infliximab and AZA, and attain a corticosteroid-free clinical remission. Adverse events were similar in all three arms of the study. There was no trend toward an increased risk of serious infections with infliximab alone or in combination with azathioprine.[69]

Additional data to support the "top-down" approach has shown that response to anti-TNF agents decreases with longer duration of disease. In the CHARM study 59% of patients diagnosed with CD for <2 years responded significantly to treatment with adalimumab compared to only 41% of patients having CD for ≥5 years.[70] Similar results were seen in the PRECiSE trial. Sixty-eight percent of patients with CD for <1 year responded to treatment with certolizumab pegol compared to only 44% of patients with a disease duration >5 years.[67]

Natalizumab is a humanized monoclonal antibody that targets human α_4 integrin, thereby interfering with trafficking of leukocytes into the mucosa. Natalizumab is indicated for the induction and maintenance of response or remission in patients with moderate to severely active CD with documented inflammation, such as an elevated serum CRP concentration. Natalizumab should only be used in patients who are refractory or intolerant to immunomodulators and anti-TNF therapy and for whom surgery is not an acceptable option. In addition, because of the risk of progressive multifocal leukoencephalopathy (PML), natalizumab should not be used concomitantly with immunomodulators or anti-TNF agents, and corticosteroids should be tapered off by 12 weeks from initiation of therapy with this agent.[71–74] See Table 28-2 for specific indications and Table 28-3 for dosing guidelines for biologic therapies.

Anti-TNF agents and natalizumab have been shown in randomized placebo-controlled trials to be effective for maintenance of remission in patients with moderate to severe CD.[44,51,67,73]

Loss of Response to Anti-TNF Agents

One-third of patients who initially respond to an anti-TNF agent will subsequently lose response over the course of 6–12 months.[44,51,67] Loss of response is attributed to the development of antibodies to therapy or loss of response to the mechanism of action of the TNF agent. The development of antibodies against biologic therapies can decrease the degree and duration of therapeutic response, and increase the likelihood of infusion reactions in the case of infliximab. Forty-eight percent of patients receiving infliximab in ACCENT I, 46% of patients taking adalimumab in CHARM and 37% of patients receiving certolizumab pegol in PRECiSE 2 no longer responded to treatment at 6 months.[44,51,67]

TABLE 28-2. Indications for biologic therapies

Indication	Crohn's disease				Ulcerative colitis
	Infliximab	Adalimumab	Certolizumab	Natalizumab	Infliximab
Induction of response and remission	X	X	X	X[1]	X
Maintenance of response and remission	X	X	X	X	X
Mucosal healing	X	X	X		X
Induction of response in adults with draining perianal fistulas	X	X			
Induction of response in adults with draining abdominal or rectovaginal fistulas	X				
Steroid sparing agent	X	X		X	X
Treatment of spondyloarthropathy, arthritis/arthralgia, pyoderma gangrenosum and erythema nodosum, uveitis and other ocular manifestations of Crohn's disease	X	X			X
Loss of response or intolerance to infliximab		X	X	X	

X[1] Must have also failed anti-TNF therapy and have evidence of inflammation.

TABLE 28-3. Dosing guidelines for biologic therapy

Biologic agent	Induction regimen	Maintenance dose	Attenuated response	Discontinue therapy
Infliximab	5 mg/kg IV at weeks 0, 2, and 6	5 mg/kg IV every 8 weeks beginning at week 14	10 mg/kg at 8-week intervals, or 5 mg/kg every 4 weeks	No response after 2 doses or infusions are required more frequently than every 4 weeks
Adalimumab	160 mg SC on day 1 of week 0, then 80 mg SC on day 1 of week 2	40 mg SC every other week	40 mg SC weekly or 80 mg every other week	No response to induction therapy or duration of response decreases to less than 1 week
Certolizumab	400 mg SC at weeks 0, 2, and 4	400 mg SC every 4 weeks	Extra dose of 400 mg SC 2 weeks after last dose	No response to induction therapy or when the duration of response decreases to 2 weeks
Natalizumab	300 mg IV at weeks 0, 4, and 8	300 mg IV every 4 weeks	Other dosing regimens have not been adequately evaluated	Lack of response or inability to discontinue steroids by week 12

Human anti-chimeric antibody (HACA) is produced in response to treatment with infliximab. It is associated with a shorter duration of response and increases risk of infusion reactions.[75] Patients who develop HACA will often be switched to an alternate anti-TNF agent. In a recent study, 92% of patients with loss of response to infliximab with detectable HACA had a clinical response to an alternative anti-TNF agent compared with only 17% of patients who underwent an alternative strategy of increasing the dose of infliximab. In contrast, those patients with detectable HACA and subtherapeutic serum concentrations of infliximab responded significantly better to increased doses of Infliximab (86%) rather than an alternative anti-TNF agent (40%).[76] Therefore, a reasonable approach to loss of response to infliximab is to test for HACA and levels of infliximab. Patients with detectable HACA (normal <1.69 mcg/ml, levels ≥ 8 mcg/ml associated with loss of response) should be changed to an alternative anti-TNF agent or, less desirably, the dose could be increased. Those patients with subtherapeutic levels of infliximab (levels ≥ 12.0 mcg/ml at 4 weeks postinfusion correlate with a longer duration of response) may benefit from an increase in dose or frequency of dosing. An alternative option for these patients is changing to a different anti-TNF agent.[75,76]

A recent study evaluated the use of adalimumab in patients with CD who had responded to infliximab initially then either lost that response or became intolerant to therapy. Patients were randomly assigned to receive induction doses of adalimumab, 160 and 80 mg, at weeks 0 and 2, respectively, or placebo at the same time points. The primary endpoint was induction of remission at week 4. Twenty-one percent of patients in the adalimumab group versus 7% of those in the placebo group significantly achieved remission at week 4. The absolute difference in clinical remission rates was 14.2%. Adalimumab induced remission more frequently than placebo in adult patients with CD who could not tolerate infliximab or had symptoms despite receiving infliximab therapy.[77]

Concomitant immune suppression with AZA, 6-MP, or MTX reduces the development of antibodies. Antibodies to infliximab (ATI) were found in 38% of patients receiving episodic doses of infliximab without an immunomodulator compared to only 16% receiving both episodic doses of infliximab and an immunomodulator during the ACCENT I study.[78] Maintenance doses of anti-TNF agents in combination with an immunomodulator have been shown to limit the development of ATIs.

Adverse Events Associated with Biologics

Anti-TNF agents share similar adverse events including infusion or injection site reactions, autoimmunity (positive ANA, anti-double-stranded DNA antibodies; rare lupus-like reactions), activation of latent tuberculosis and development of opportunistic infections. Fungal infections caused by *Histoplasma capsulatum* have been reported in 240 patients taking an anti-TNF agent, of which 12 deaths have occurred.[79] Given the risk of reactivation of latent tuberculosis, all patients should be screened for tuberculosis with tuberculin skin testing (and chest X-ray if skin testing is positive) prior to initiating therapy with infliximab. Hematologic complications may also occur, including such as leukopenia, neutropenia, thrombocytopenia, or pancytopenia. Rarely, liver toxicity may occur and present as acute liver failure, jaundice, hepatitis, and cholestasis. Neurologic disorders including optic neuritis, seizures, and new onset or exacerbation of central nervous system demyelinating disorders, including multiple sclerosis, have been reported with the use of anti-TNF agents.

Rare cases of hepatosplenic T-cell lymphoma, a lethal form of non-Hodgkin's lymphoma, have been reported in patients receiving infliximab and AZA/6-MP.[80] Cases of hepatosplenic T-cell lymphoma have been described almost exclusively in young males, and non-Hodgkin's lymphoma is more common among men in general. There is a slightly increased risk of non-Hodgkin's lymphoma estimated at 6.1 cases in 10,000 patient-years of exposure to anti-TNF agents in combination with immunomodulators, as compared to the general population risk of 1.9 per 10,000 patient-years.[81] An age-and gender-adjusted standardized incidence ratio is 3.23 per 10,000 patient years (95% CI 1.5–6.9).[81]

Natalizumab may cause headache or rare infusion reactions. Among patients receiving natalizumab for multiple sclerosis or CD, the risk of developing PML is approximately 1 in 1,000 patients for patients treated for at least 1 year.[82] Immunomodulators are contraindicated with natalizumab due to increased risk of PML. There are also rare reports of liver toxicity with natalizumab.[83]

Contraindications to Biologic Therapies

Contraindications to anti-TNF agents are consistent across the class and include the following:

1. Known hypersensitivity to agent, if severe
2. Active infection
3. Untreated latent tuberculosis
4. Preexisting demyelinating disorder
5. Moderate to severe congestive heart failure
6. Current or recent malignancy, without advice from an oncologist
7. Further treatment with infliximab is contraindicated when the patient presents with uncontrolled infusion reactions

Contraindications to natalizumab include

1. Known hypersensitivity to agent, if severe
2. Active infection
3. Current or past PML
4. Liver disease
5. Continued treatment with an immune modulator or anti-TNF antibody

Tacrolimus

Data on the use of tacrolimus in CD are limited and the drug is infrequently used to treat patients with significant disease and no other options. Various small studies have shown a trend toward clinical benefit especially in fistulizing disease.[84–90] Oral therapy is usually started with 0.1–0.2 mg/kg/day as a twice daily divided dose. Adverse effects of tacrolimus include renal insufficiency, liver function abnormalities, infection, hyperglycemia, hypertension, and myelosuppression. Drug levels, blood counts, liver enzymes, renal function, glucose level, and blood pressure need to be monitored on a regular basis in patients taking tacrolimus. Laboratory tests should be performed weekly initially and then less often after stable dosing is achieved. Trough drug levels should be maintained between 5 and 15 ng/mL.

Severe Crohn's Disease

Patients with severe to fulminant CD have ongoing symptoms despite treatment with oral corticosteroids or an anti-TNF agent. Symptoms include high fever, frequent vomiting, evidence of intestinal obstruction, rebound tenderness, cachexia, or evidence of an abscess. These patients often require hospitalization and resuscitative therapy with fluid and electrolytes for dehydration. Surgical evaluation is warranted for patients with intestinal obstruction or who have a tender abdominal mass suggestive of an abscess.

Severe disease may be treated with high-dose intravenous corticosteroids. Doses of hydrocortisone 100 mg IV three times daily or methylprednisolone up to 60 mg IV daily may be used to induce remission. AZA or 6-MP should be initiated in patients who respond to IV corticosteroids.[86] A patient who does not respond after 5–7 days of therapy may benefit from infliximab or intravenous (IV) cyclosporine (CSA). Failure to respond to medical therapy or worsening symptoms are indications for surgery.

Indications for Surgery in Crohn's Disease

Unlike UC, CD is not surgically curable. Approximately two-thirds of patients with CD will require surgery at some point during their disease course. Surgery is often performed to avoid medication side effects or to treat complications of disease such as hemorrhage, perforation, obstruction, or abscess. While surgical resection is most commonly done, the disease predictably recurs at the anastomotic site, and stricturoplasty is a reasonable surgical alternative if previous small bowel resections place the patient at risk of short bowel syndrome. Any patient who fails to respond to 7–10 days of intensive inpatient management should be strongly considered for surgery.

The indications for emergency surgery include primary free perforation or secondary rupture of an abscess into the peritoneal cavity and massive, uncontrollable hemorrhage. Urgent surgical procedures (performed within a few days after the diagnosis of a complication) are required for fulminant Crohn's colitis with or without toxic megacolon and severe perianal sepsis. Elective procedures (performed within weeks after the decision for surgery) are an option for definitive treatment of intra-abdominal abscesses, complete or incomplete obstruction of the bowel, or an intractable course of disease (including steroid-dependent or steroid-resistance) and neoplastic or pre-neoplastic lesions.[91]

Crohn's Disease: Maintenance Therapy After Medical Induction of Remission

The goal of maintenance therapy is to reduce hospitalizations, prevent surgery, and improve patients' quality of life. Although often given in clinical practice, randomized controlled trials investigating the use of SSZ[2,3] or 5-ASA[92] have not demonstrated significant maintenance benefits in CD. In particular, 5-ASA (at a dose of 4 g daily) has not been efficacious in preventing relapse after corticosteroid-induced remissions.[93] Immunomodulators, including AZA, 6-MP, and MTX, as well as anti-TNF agents and natalizumab may be effective maintenance agents, particularly among those patients who have initially responded to these agents.

Postoperative Reoccurrence of Crohn's Disease and Prophylaxis

Factors associated with an increased risk of early postoperative recurrence include smoking, absence of prophylactic postoperative therapy and extent of disease greater than 100 cm.[94] Many patients with long-standing strictures have a relatively good postoperative prognosis, whereas patients with rapid progression of perforating complications and smokers have a worse prognosis.

Despite multiple studies, the best postoperative prophylactic therapy remains uncertain. 5-ASA and, to a lesser extent, SSZ are often used in clinical practice to prevent postoperative reoccurrence of CD because of their well-known safety profile. SSZ has not been statistically superior to placebo in preventing postoperative relapse.[95] A meta-analysis of 15 randomized controlled studies of 5-ASA as a maintenance medication in CD found a modest pooled risk reduction of 13% for those patients with surgically induced remissions.[96] Some authors believe that 5-ASA may be more effective in preventing postoperative recurrence in patients with isolated small bowel disease.[97]

Data supporting the use of AZA and 6-MP for prevention of postoperative recurrence are limited; however, the data suggest possible efficacy.[98–100] Preliminary reports propose that infliximab may be used as a postoperative prophylactic agent.[101] It has been shown to prevent postoperative clinical and endoscopic recurrence after ileocecal resection.[102]

Imidazole antibiotics, including metronidazole, decrease short-term, but not long-term endoscopic recurrence and are limited by side effects.[103] Corticosteroids do not prevent postoperative relapse. At the moment, there is insufficient evidence to support the use of probiotics in preventing postoperative recurrence of CD. Overall, there are no consistent recommendations regarding medical therapy after surgical resection for Crohn's disease.

Perianal Crohn's Disease

Perianal disease may precede the onset of bowel symptoms in CD. Perianal complications include skin tags, anal fissures, fistulas, abscesses, and anal stenosis. The most common acute complication is a fistula-related abscess. An abscess requires surgical drainage with or without the placement of setons.

Perianal fistulae occur in up to 43% of patients.[104] Treatment often combines medication and surgery. Medications commonly used for the treatment of perianal fistulae include antibiotics, immunomodulators, and anti-TNF agents. There is no role for the use of 5-ASA or corticosteroids in the treatment of perianal fistulas.

Perianal fistulae typically respond to metronidazole alone[105–107] or in combination with ciprofloxacin; however, continuous therapy may be necessary to prevent recurrent drainage. Simple, superficial fistulae may respond completely to fistulotomy and antibiotics. However, patients with complex fistulae may respond best to combined medical/surgical approaches. Some patients may require chronic maintenance therapy with AZA or 6-MP. MTX has not been prospectively evaluated in perianal fistulizing CD, but several uncontrolled studies suggest a possible benefit.[108] Two pivotal studies have demonstrated that infliximab is effective at acutely closing fistula[45] and maintaining closure with maintenance dosing.[50]

Ulcerative Colitis: Medical Management

Ulcerative colitis is a chronic inflammatory condition that results in ulceration of the mucosal lining of the large intestine. Inflammation is diffuse and continuous, and uniformly affects the rectum but may extend proximally to involve part or all of the large intestine. Common symptoms of UC include frequent bloody bowel movements, diarrhea, urgency, and tenesmus.

Proctitis

Proctitis refers to inflammation of the rectum. This area can be effectively treated with topical therapies such as enemas or suppositories. Oral agents can also be effective if patients fail, cannot tolerate, or refuse topical therapies. Topical formulations of 5-ASA are considered first-line therapy for the treatment of proctitis. These agents are considered more effective than rectal steroids and have been shown to be more effective than oral 5-ASA.[109] Suppositories are preferred over enemas because they are more easily administered and are more viscous than enemas so leakage is less. Canasa (1.0–1.5 g daily) in the evening or in divided doses is highly effective for proctitis up to 20 cm.[109] The proportion of patients achieving remission increases with the duration of treatment and is not dose dependent. Response is usually seen within 2–3 weeks with increased response rates (63–79%) at 4–6 weeks.[110] For patients not responding to rectal 5-ASA alone, combination treatment with topical corticosteroids (foam or enema) is better than either therapy alone.[111] As an alternative, oral 5-ASA can be used with topical therapy for active proctitis.[109,112]

Distal Ulcerative Colitis

Patients with distal colitis can be treated with topical 5-ASA (suppositories, enemas) topical corticosteroids (suppositories, enemas), oral 5-ASA, or a combination of these agents. Rectal therapies may have a more rapid effect than oral therapies.[110] Rectal 5-ASA is considered superior to rectal corticosteroids for inducing remission,[113] however, combination therapy with a topical corticosteroid may be more effective than monotherapy.[3,111] Therapy with a combination of oral and rectal 5-ASA achieves higher remission rates than either therapy alone.[112] Remission rates for topical therapy increase with duration of treatment (63–72% after 4 weeks) and are independent of dose. There are no advantages to prescribing doses greater than 1 g daily of a topical 5-ASA.[110]

A small proportion of patients have a hypersensitivity to 5-ASA either given orally or rectally. It may present as worsening of rectal bleeding and urgency usually within 3–5 days of administration. 5-ASA should be discontinued and improvement should be seen within 72 h. Treatment with a topical corticosteroid is usually effective in achieving remission in this group.

Extensive Ulcerative Colitis

Extensive UC refers to inflammation which extends proximal to the splenic flexure and requires systemic medications. Supplementary topical medications are often beneficial to treat prominent rectal symptoms of urgency or tenesmus. Activity is defined as mild to moderate, moderate to severe, or severe to fulminant. Treatment is based on clinical activity.

Mild-to-Moderate Extensive Ulcerative Colitis

Signs and symptoms of mild disease include <4 stools daily with or without blood, no systemic signs of toxicity and normal erythrocyte sedimentation rate (ESR). Patients with moderate disease will experience somewhat more serious symptoms but are not yet considered to have severe UC by virtue of toxic features. Inflammation extends proximal to the splenic flexure and beyond the reach of topical therapy. Oral therapy is required for extensive disease.

Sulfasalazine and 5-Aminosalicylates

SSZ and oral 5-ASA are considered first-line agents for induction of remission in mild to moderate UC. The efficacy of SSZ has been well-established.[2] SSZ achieves remission in 64–80% of patients at doses of 2–6 g daily.[2] There is a dose–response for SSZ; the higher the doses the higher the rate of remission. However, 30–40% of patients are unable to tolerate increased doses due to systemic absorption of the sulfapyridine component.[114]

Clinical response can be achieved in up to 84% of patients taking a 5-ASA.[115] All formulations of 5-ASA work topically and have similar pharmacokinetic profiles. The dose of 5-ASA should be increased in patients who do not begin to improve within 2 weeks of starting therapy. Combining oral 5-ASA with topical 5-ASA preparations has been shown to be well tolerated and more efficacious in patients with extensive UC.[116]

Corticosteroids

Patients who do not respond to optimal doses of oral 5-ASA can be given an oral corticosteroid. Oral corticosteroids successfully induce remission in the majority of patients. Doses of prednisone 20–60 mg/day are often used, but doses greater than 60 mg/day have no additional benefit. There is no difference between once-daily and divided dosing. Once remission is achieved prednisone is tapered by 5–10 mg weekly until 15–20 mg then taper by 2.5–5 mg weekly while attempting to maintain remission with a 5-ASA. Budesonide is released in the distal ileum and proximal colon limiting its effectiveness in UC. Topical corticosteroids in addition to oral and/or rectal 5-ASA may be beneficial for relieving rectal symptoms associated with extensive UC.

Severe and Fulminant Extensive Ulcerative Colitis

Severe disease is defined as ≥6 bloody stools daily, abdominal tenderness with signs of systemic toxicity including fever (>37.5°C), tachycardia (>90 bpm), anemia (<75% of normal value), and increased ESR (>30 mm/h).[117] Fulminant disease is defined as >10 bloody stools per day, anemia requiring a transfusion, signs of systemic toxicity, abdominal distention and tenderness, fever and leukocytosis.

Intravenous Corticosteroids

Approximately 60% of patients with severe/fulminant colitis treated with IV corticosteroids respond fully.[117] Doses of hydrocortisone 100 mg IV three times daily or methylprednisolone 60 mg IV daily are used to induce remission. Continuous infusion of corticosteroids is not more efficacious than bolus dosing. Patients who fail to improve within 3–7 days (depending on severity of illness) should be considered for colectomy or rescue therapy with CSA or infliximab.

Azathioprine/6-Mercaptopurine

In patients with persistently active, steroid-dependent, or steroid-refractory UC, immunomodulators (AZA or 6-MP) should be considered.[118–120] AZA or 6-MP can induce a clinical remission or response in 30–50% of patients, improve overall symptoms, and allow the dose of steroids to be reduced or discontinued.[119,120] Induction of remission may take as long as 3–4 months to achieve. Doses of 2.5 mg/kg for AZA and 1.5 mg/kg for 6-MP are often used. Infliximab is an alternative agent for refractory disease.

Cyclosporine

Intravenous CSA is used as rescue therapy for severe corticosteroid-refractory UC. Patients failing to respond to 7 days of IV corticosteroids may benefit from IV CSA. Several studies report response rates between 70 and 80% in patients with this type of UC.[121–123]

CSA is initiated as a continuous infusion while continuing IV corticosteroids. Doses of 2–4 mg/kg daily are used clinically. General improvement is seen within 4–5 days of initiating treatment. If a response is noted the patient is transitioned to oral CSA 5 mg/kg/day divided BID and AZA is usually started as maintenance therapy. If no improvement is noted within 7 days or the condition deteriorates during treatment with CSA surgery should be considered. CSA is discontinued generally after 3–4 months if treatment proves effective.

Symptoms of CSA toxicity include infection, paresthesia, nausea, tremors, headache hypertension, and permanent or temporary renal toxicity. Patients who are noncompliant, have a history of uncontrolled seizures or active infection should not receive CSA. Patients with low cholesterol (serum cholesterol < 120 mg/dl) and low serum magnesium levels (serum magnesium < 1.5 mg/dl) are at increased risk of seizures. CSA is contraindicated in patients with multiple organ dysfunction.

Tacrolimus

One randomized controlled trial and multiple open-label trials of tacrolimus for the treatment of refractory UC have reported favorable results.[85,124,125] In the randomized controlled trial, patients with refractory active UC were assigned to one of three groups: (1) high trough concentration (10–15 ng/ml), (2) low trough concentration (5–10 ng/ml), or (3) placebo group ($n = 20$). Initially, each patient was prescribed a dose of 0.05 mg/kg tacrolimus or placebo twice daily. Improvement was seen in 68.4% of cases in the high trough group compared with 10.0% in the placebo group ($p < 0.001$). In the high trough group, 20.0% of patients had clinical remission and 78.9% had mucosal healing. Tacrolimus was shown to be a steroid sparring agent during the open-label portion of the study. The mean dose of prednisolone was reduced from 19.7 to 7.8 mg/day at week 10. The incidence of side effects was significantly increased in the high trough group compared to the placebo group. The most common event was mild finger tremor. The optimal target range appears to be 10–15 ng/ml in terms of efficacy with 2-week therapy.[125]

Infliximab

Infliximab is the only anti-TNF agent approved for use in UC. It has been shown to successfully induce and maintain remission in patients with moderate to severe and corticosteroid-dependent UC.[126] In ACT 1 and ACT 2, a clinical response was seen in ≥60% of patients receiving infliximab compared to ~30% of patients in the placebo group. In those same studies clinical remission was achieved in ≥30% of patients assigned to infliximab as compared to only 14.9% receiving placebo.[126] Infliximab is also used as a steroid sparing agent in patients with corticosteroid dependent or refractory UC. Infliximab appears to decrease the rate of colectomy at 3 months and 1 year.[117,127]

Ulcerative Colitis: Maintenance Therapy After Medical Induction of Remission

Remission is achieved when diarrhea, tenesmus, bleeding, urgency, and passage of mucopus have resolved. Rectal and oral 5-ASA are effective for maintaining remission of distal UC and proctitis[128] even when used on an intermittent basis.[129] Up to 90% of patients with extensive colitis can be maintained in remission using oral once-daily 5-ASA therapy.[130,131] AZA and 6-MP are useful as corticosteroid sparing agents,[132] for maintaining remission[133] in patients not adequately controlled by 5-ASA alone, and for maintaining CSA-induced remission.[134] Maintenance benefits have been shown for up to 2 years[135] but endure much longer for most patients. Infliximab was able to maintain remission in patients with UC for up to 54 weeks in a large randomized controlled trial.[126] The role of MTX in the treatment of UC is still controversial.

Indications for Surgery in Ulcerative Colitis

The goal of medical therapy has been to reduce the need for colectomy while avoiding fatal complications. Between 20 and 30% of UC patients will eventually require surgery. Indications for emergency surgery include massive hemorrhage, toxic megacolon, perforation and severe colitis unresponsive to medical therapy. Elective surgery may be performed for cancer/dysplasia, failure of therapy, adverse events resulting from medial therapy, malnutrition, growth retardation in children and control of certain extraintestinal manifestations.[117]

Preoperative Treatment Effect on Postsurgical Complications

Many patients with inflammatory bowel disease will require surgery during the course of their disease. For most patients requiring surgery, medical options have been exhausted. Preoperative treatment with corticosteroids, immunomodulators and biologic agents raises concerns about potential postoperative complications.

Studies have shown that corticosteroid use prior to surgery increases the risk of postoperative infectious complications.[136–138] Patients taking corticosteroids preoperatively may have double the risk of infectious complications compared to those not taking corticosteroids.[139] A meta-analysis was performed to estimate the risk of postoperative complications (infectious and noninfectious) in patients receiving corticosteroids prior to abdominal surgery. Patient taking corticosteroids preoperatively were more likely to experience postoperative complications including infections (all postoperative complications OR 1.41, 95% CI 1.07–1.87, infectious complications OR 1.68, 95% CI 1.24–2.28). Patients taking >40 mg had a considerably higher risk of developing postoperative complications (OR 2.04, 95% CI 0.28–3.26).[140] The risk of postoperative infections may be related to corticosteroid doses >10 mg/day and duration of treatment >1 month.[138,141]

Although the data are limited, most studies have shown that treatment with AZA or 6-MP prior to surgery is not a risk factor for postoperative complications.[136,137,142] The effect of preoperative infliximab on postsurgical complications is controversial. Two retrospective studies in patients with CD suggest that infliximab infused within 8–12 weeks before abdominal surgery is not associated with an increased rate of postoperative complications.[142,143] In contrast, analysis of a third retrospective series found that infliximab use within 3 months prior to surgery is associated with increased rates of postoperative sepsis, abscess, and hospital readmission in patients with CD.[144]

The data regarding postsurgical complications in UC patients receiving infliximab prior to surgery are limited. A retrospective review was conducted in patients with chronic UC treated with and without infliximab before IPAA to compare postoperative complications. Infliximab use prior to surgery was shown to be associated with an increased risk of pouch failure and infectious complications related to the pouch. The authors suggest that the pouch should be constructed as a three-stage procedure in this population.[145]

Pouchitis

Pouchitis is the most common long-term complication of ileal-pouch anal anastomosis (IPAA) for UC. Most often patients respond to 2 weeks of ciprofloxacin at 500 mg twice daily or metronidazole 750–1,200 mg/day.[146] Over 60% of those patients, however, will go on to develop a second episode and approximately 20% of patients will have refractory or relapsing symptoms.[147,148] These patients require a prolonged course of the same antibiotic or with a combined antibiotic regimen. If patients relapse at least three times within 1 year, chronic maintenance therapy with lower doses of antibiotics is recommended.[147,148]

Approximately 20% of patients develop chronic refractory pouchitis.[147] Longer courses of antibiotics are required for these patients and each new antibiotic should be tried for at least 1 month prior to making any changes. Combination antibiotic therapy may be the most effective.[149] Rifaximin alone or in combination with ciprofloxacin is an effective treatment for patients with active chronic, refractory pouchitis.[149–151]

Budesonide and infliximab may be used as alternative treatments.[152,153] Maintenance with VSL #3, a probiotic, is an option.[154] Patients who are refractory to all forms of medical treatment should be referred to a surgeon for a pouch revision or excision.

Irritable Pouch Syndrome

Irritable pouch syndrome (IPS) is often misdiagnosed as pouchitis because of its similar presentation. The major differentiating factor between IPS and pouchitis is that with pouchitis, mucosal inflammation is evident.[147] Treatment with anti-diarrheals such as diphenoxylate and loperamide, or anti-spasmodics, such as dicyclomine and hyoscyamine, may help to control symptoms.

Crohn's Disease of the Pouch

CD of the pouch is one of the most common long-term inflammatory complications of IPAA and one of the leading causes of pouch failure. It can occur weeks to years after an IPAA for UC. CD of the pouch may be treated with topical and oral 5-ASA, oral or topical corticosteroids, antibiotics, and immunomodulators. In patients whose disease is refractory to these agents, particularly when they have concurrent extraintestinal symptoms, biological agents such as infliximab and adalimumab can be used.[155,156]

Conclusion

Treating patients with IBD poses a significant challenge. Often it is a balancing act between controlling symptoms, improving quality of life, and minimizing complications of disease and treatment. Aminosalicylates are first-line agents for the treatment of mild to moderate disease and for maintaining remission; however, in the case of CD, evidence of efficacy is sparse. Antibiotics are somewhat effective in colonic CD but are not considered useful as treatment for UC, although efficacious for the treatment of pouchitis. Corticosteroids are effective for inducing remission in more severe disease but are associated with multiple side effects. Corticosteroids are not recommended as maintenance therapy. The immunomodulators, AZA, 6-MP, and MTX, are best employed as maintenance agents and, in the case of AZA and 6-MP, require approximately 3–4 months to be effective.

Recently, biologic agents have become the focus for treatment of moderate to severe CD. These agents are effective for inducing and maintaining remission and healing fistulas, as steroid sparing agents, and for the treatment of certain extraintestinal manifestations. Infliximab is the only anti-TNF agent approved for use in UC, thus far.

Acknowledgments. This chapter was written by Stephen B. Hanauer, Wee-Chian Lim, and Miles Sparrow in the previous version of this textbook. The author wishes to thank Stacey Grabert, Pharm.D., MS, for editorial assistance in preparing this manuscript.

References

1. Torres MI, Rios A. Current view of the immunopathogenesis in inflammatory bowel disease and its implications for therapy. World J Gastroenterol. 2008;14(13):1972–80.
2. Summers RW, Switz DM, Sessions Jr JT, et al. National Cooperative Crohn's Disease Study: results of drug treatment. Gastroenterology. 1979;77(4 Pt 2):847–69.
3. Malchow H, Ewe K, Brandes JW, et al. European Cooperative Crohn's Disease Study (ECCDS): results of drug treatment. Gastroenterology. 1984;86(2):249–66.
4. Van Hees PA, Van Lier HJ, Van Elteren PH, et al. Effect of sulphasalazine in patients with active Crohn's disease: a controlled double-blind study. Gut. 1981;22(5):404–9.
5. Anthonisen P, Barany F, Folkenborg O, et al. The clinical effect of salazosulphapyridine (Salazopyrin r) in Crohn's disease. A controlled double-blind study. Scand J Gastroenterol. 1974;9(6):549–54.
6. Feagan BG. Aminosalicylates for active disease and in the maintenance of remission in Crohn's disease. Eur J Surg. 1998;164(12):903–9.
7. Das KM, Eastwood MA, McManus JP, Sircus W. Adverse reactions during salicylazosulfapyridine therapy and the relation with drug metabolism and acetylator phenotype. N Engl J Med. 1973;289(10):491–5.
8. Sutherland L, Singleton J, Sessions J, et al. Double blind, placebo controlled trial of metronidazole in Crohn's disease. Gut. 1991;32(9):1071–5.
9. Ursing B, Alm T, Barany F, et al. A comparative study of metronidazole and sulfasalazine for active Crohn's disease: the cooperative Crohn's disease study in Sweden. II. Result. Gastroenterology. 1982;83(3):550–62.
10. Greenbloom SL, Steinhart AH, Greenberg GR. Combination ciprofloxacin and metronidazole for active Crohn's disease. Can J Gastroenterol. 1998;12(1):53–6.
11. Steinhart AH, Feagan BG, Wong CJ, et al. Combined budesonide and antibiotic therapy for active Crohn's disease: a randomized controlled trial. Gastroenterology. 2002;123(1):33–40.
12. Colombel JF, Lemann M, Cassagnou M, et al. A controlled trial comparing ciprofloxacin with mesalazine for the treatment of active Crohn's disease. Groupe d'Etudes Therapeutiques des Affections Inflammatoires Digestives (GETAID). Am J Gastroenterol. 1999;94(3):674–8.
13. Prantera C, Zannoni F, Scribano ML, et al. An antibiotic regimen for the treatment of active Crohn's disease: a randomized, controlled clinical trial of metronidazole plus ciprofloxacin. Am J Gastroenterol. 1996;91(2):328–32.
14. Shafran I, Johnson LK. An open-label evaluation of rifaximin in the treatment of active Crohn's disease. Curr Med Res Opin. 2005;21(8):1165–9.
15. Otley A, Steinhart AH. Budesonide for induction of remission in Crohn's disease. Cochrane Database Syst Rev. 2005;4:CD000296.
16. Greenberg GR, Feagan BG, Martin F, et al. Oral budesonide for active Crohn's disease. Canadian Inflammatory Bowel Disease Study Group. N Engl J Med. 1994;331(13):836–41.
17. Tremaine WJ, Hanauer SB, Katz S, et al. Budesonide CIR capsules (once or twice daily divided-dose) in active Crohn's disease: a randomized placebo-controlled study in the United States. Am J Gastroenterol. 2002;97(7):1748–54.
18. Thomsen OO, Cortot A, Jewell D, et al. A comparison of budesonide and mesalamine for active Crohn's disease. International Budesonide-Mesalamine Study Group. N Engl J Med. 1998;339(6):370–4.
19. Gross V, Andus T, Caesar I, et al. Oral pH-modified release budesonide versus 6-methylprednisolone in active Crohn's disease. German/Austrian Budesonide Study Group. Eur J Gastroenterol Hepatol. 1996;8(9):905–9.
20. Rutgeerts P, Lofberg R, Malchow H, et al. A comparison of budesonide with prednisolone for active Crohn's disease. N Engl J Med. 1994;331(13):842–5.
21. Bar-Meir S, Chowers Y, Lavy A, et al. Budesonide versus prednisone in the treatment of active Crohn's disease. The Israeli Budesonide Study Group. Gastroenterology. 1998;115(4):835–40.
22. Campieri M, Ferguson A, Doe W, Persson T, Nilsson LG. Oral budesonide is as effective as oral prednisolone in active Crohn's disease. The Global Budesonide Study Group. Gut. 1997;41(2):209–14.
23. Greenberg GR, Feagan BG, Martin F, et al. Oral budesonide as maintenance treatment for Crohn's disease: a placebo-controlled, dose-ranging study. Canadian Inflammatory Bowel Disease Study Group. Gastroenterology. 1996;110(1):45–51.
24. Ferguson A, Campieri M, Doe W, Persson T, Nygard G. Oral budesonide as maintenance therapy in Crohn's disease – results of a 12-month study. Global Budesonide Study Group. Aliment Pharmacol Ther. 1998;12(2):175–83.
25. Lofberg R, Rutgeerts P, Malchow H, et al. Budesonide prolongs time to relapse in ileal and ileocaecal Crohn's disease. A placebo controlled one year study. Gut. 1996;39(1):82–6.

26. Hanauer S, Sandborn WJ, Persson A, Persson T. Budesonide as maintenance treatment in Crohn's disease: a placebo-controlled trial. Aliment Pharmacol Ther. 2005;21(4):363–71.
27. Simms L, Steinhart AH. Budesonide for maintenance of remission in Crohn's disease. Cochrane Database Syst Rev. 2001;1:CD002913.
28. Faubion Jr WA, Loftus Jr EV, Harmsen WS, Zinsmeister AR, Sandborn WJ. The natural history of corticosteroid therapy for inflammatory bowel disease: a population-based study. Gastroenterology. 2001;121(2):255–60.
29. Munkholm P, Langholz E, Davidsen M, Binder V. Frequency of glucocorticoid resistance and dependency in Crohn's disease. Gut. 1994;35(3):360–2.
30. Franchimont DP, Louis E, Croes F, Belaiche J. Clinical pattern of corticosteroid dependent Crohn's disease. Eur J Gastroenterol Hepatol. 1998;10(10):821–5.
31. Pearson DC, May GR, Fick GH, Sutherland LR. Azathioprine and 6-mercaptopurine in Crohn disease. A meta-analysis. Ann Intern Med. 1995;123(2):132–42.
32. Candy S, Wright J, Gerber M, Adams G, Gerig M, Goodman R. A controlled double blind study of azathioprine in the management of Crohn's disease. Gut. 1995;37(5):674–8.
33. Kandiel A, Fraser AG, Korelitz BI, Brensinger C, Lewis JD. Increased risk of lymphoma among inflammatory bowel disease patients treated with azathioprine and 6-mercaptopurine. Gut. 2005;54(8):1121–5.
34. Beaugerie L, Brousse N, Bouvier AM, et al. Lymphoproliferative disorders in patients receiving thiopurines for inflammatory bowel disease: a prospective observational cohort study. Lancet. 2009;374(9701):1617–25.
35. Aberra FN, Lichtenstein GR. Review article: monitoring of immunomodulators in inflammatory bowel disease. Aliment Pharmacol Ther. 2005;21(4):307–19.
36. Hayee BH, Harris AW. Methotrexate for Crohn's disease: experience in a district general hospital. Eur J Gastroenterol Hepatol. 2005;17(9):893–8.
37. Alfadhli AA, McDonald JW, Feagan BG. Methotrexate for induction of remission in refractory Crohn's disease. Cochrane Database Syst Rev. 2005;1:CD003459.
38. Feagan BG, Rochon J, Fedorak RN, et al. Methotrexate for the treatment of Crohn's disease. The North American Crohn's Study Group Investigators. N Engl J Med. 1995;332(5):292–7.
39. Chong RY, Hanauer SB, Cohen RD. Efficacy of parenteral methotrexate in refractory Crohn's disease. Aliment Pharmacol Ther. 2001;15(1):35–44.
40. Lemann M, Chamiot-Prieur C, Mesnard B, et al. Methotrexate for the treatment of refractory Crohn's disease. Aliment Pharmacol Ther. 1996;10(3):309–14.
41. Lemann M, Zenjari T, Bouhnik Y, et al. Methotrexate in Crohn's disease: long-term efficacy and toxicity. Am J Gastroenterol. 2000;95(7):1730–4.
42. Feagan BG, Fedorak RN, Irvine EJ, et al. A comparison of methotrexate with placebo for the maintenance of remission in Crohn's disease. North American Crohn's Study Group Investigators. N Engl J Med. 2000;342(22):1627–32.
43. Targan SR, Hanauer SB, van Deventer SJ, et al. A short-term study of chimeric monoclonal antibody cA2 to tumor necrosis factor alpha for Crohn's disease. Crohn's Disease cA2 Study Group. N Engl J Med. 1997;337(15):1029–35.
44. Hanauer SB, Feagan BG, Lichtenstein GR, et al. Maintenance infliximab for Crohn's disease: the ACCENT I randomised trial. Lancet. 2002;359(9317):1541–9.
45. Present DH, Rutgeerts P, Targan S, et al. Infliximab for the treatment of fistulas in patients with Crohn's disease. N Engl J Med. 1999;340(18):1398–405.
46. Lichtenstein GR, Yan S, Bala M, Blank M, Sands BE. Infliximab maintenance treatment reduces hospitalizations, surgeries, and procedures in fistulizing Crohn's disease. Gastroenterology. 2005;128(4):862–9.
47. Generini S, Giacomelli R, Fedi R, et al. Infliximab in spondyloarthropathy associated with Crohn's disease: an open study on the efficacy of inducing and maintaining remission of musculoskeletal and gut manifestations. Ann Rheum Dis. 2004;63(12):1664–9.
48. Brooklyn TN, Dunnill MG, Shetty A, et al. Infliximab for the treatment of pyoderma gangrenosum: a randomised, double blind, placebo controlled trial. Gut. 2006;55(4):505–9.
49. Herfarth H, Obermeier F, Andus T, et al. Improvement of arthritis and arthralgia after treatment with infliximab (Remicade) in a German prospective, open-label, multicenter trial in refractory Crohn's disease. Am J Gastroenterol. 2002;97(10):2688–90.
50. Sands BE, Anderson FH, Bernstein CN, et al. Infliximab maintenance therapy for fistulizing Crohn's disease. N Engl J Med. 2004;350(9):876–85.
51. Colombel JF, Sandborn WJ, Rutgeerts P, et al. Adalimumab for maintenance of clinical response and remission in patients with Crohn's disease: the CHARM trial. Gastroenterology. 2007;132(1):52–65.
52. Rutgeerts P, Van Assche G, Vermeire S. Review article: Infliximab therapy for inflammatory bowel disease – seven years on. Aliment Pharmacol Ther. 2006;23(4):451–63.
53. Schroder O, Blumenstein I, Stein J. Combining infliximab with methotrexate for the induction and maintenance of remission in refractory Crohn's disease: a controlled pilot study. Eur J Gastroenterol Hepatol. 2006;18(1):11–6.
54. Sandborn WJ, Feagan BG, Stoinov S, et al. Certolizumab pegol for the treatment of Crohn's disease. N Engl J Med. 2007;357(3):228–38.
55. Rutgeerts PJ, Mellili LE, Li J, Pollack PF. Adalimumab maintains improvement in IBDQ scores over 1 year following the initial attainment of remission in patients with moderately severely active Crohn's disease: results of the Classic II study. Gastroenterology. 2006;130:A479.
56. Sandborn WJ, Hanauer S, Loftus Jr EV, et al. An open-label study of the human anti-TNF monoclonal antibody adalimumab in subjects with prior loss of response or intolerance to infliximab for Crohn's disease. Am J Gastroenterol. 2004;99(10):1984–9.
57. Papadakis KA, Shaye OA, Vasiliauskas EA, et al. Safety and efficacy of adalimumab (D2E7) in Crohn's disease patients with an attenuated response to infliximab. Am J Gastroenterol. 2005;100(1):75–9.
58. Hanauer SB, Sandborn WJ, Rutgeerts P, et al. Human antitumor necrosis factor monoclonal antibody (adalimumab) in Crohn's disease: the CLASSIC-I trial. Gastroenterology. 2006;130(2):323–33. quiz 591.

59. Sandborn W, Rutgeerts P, Enns RA, Hanauer SB, Colombel JF, Panaccione R, et al. Adalimumab rapidly induces clinical remission and response in patients with moderate to severe Crohn's disease who had secondary failure to infliximab therapy: results of the GAIN study. Am J Gastroenterol. 2006;101(Abstract):S448.
60. Schreiber S, Rutgeerts P, Fedorak RN, et al. A randomized, placebo-controlled trial of certolizumab pegol (CDP870) for treatment of Crohn's disease. Gastroenterology. 2005;129(3):807–18.
61. Schreiber S, Khaliq-Kareemi M, Lawrence I, Hanauer SB, McColm J, Bloomfield R, et al. Certolizumab pegol, a humanized anti-TNF pegylated FAb fragment is safe and effective in the maintenance of response and remission following induction in active Crohn's disease: a phase III study (PRECiSE II). Gut. 2005;54(Abstract):A82.
62. Winter TA, Wright J, Ghosh S, Jahnsen J, Innes A, Round P. Intravenous CDP870, a PEGylated Fab′ fragment of a humanized antitumour necrosis factor antibody, in patients with moderate-to-severe Crohn's disease: an exploratory study. Aliment Pharmacol Ther. 2004;20(11–12):1337–46.
63. Sandborn W, Feagan BG, Stoinov S, Honiball PJ, Rutgeerts P, McColm JA, et al. Certolizumab pegol administered subcutaneously is effective and well tolerated in patients with active Crohn's disease: results from a 26 week, placebo controlled phase II study (PRECiSE 1). Gastroenterology. 2006;130(Abstract):A107.
64. Rutgeerts P, D'Haens GR, Van Assche GA, et al. Adalimumab induces and maintains mucosal healing in patients with moderate to severe ileocolonic Crohn's disease – first results of the EXTEND trial. Program and abstracts from Digestive Disease Week, 30 May–4 June 2009, Chicago, IL. Abstract 751e.
65. Colombel JF, Schwartz DA, Sandborn WJ, et al. Adalimumab for the treatment of fistulas in patients with Crohn's disease. Gut. 2009;58(7):940–8.
66. Lofberg R, Louis E, Reinisch W, et al. Adalimumab induces sustained fistula healing in both anti-TNF-Naïve and anti-TNF-experienced patients with Crohn's disease: The Care Trial. Program and abstracts from Digestive Disease Week, 30 May–4 June 2009, Chicago, IL. Abstract S1144.
67. Schreiber S, Khaliq-Kareemi M, Lawrance IC, et al. Maintenance therapy with certolizumab pegol for Crohn's disease. N Engl J Med. 2007;357(3):239–50.
68. D'Haens G, Baert F, van Assche G, et al. Early combined immunosuppression or conventional management in patients with newly diagnosed Crohn's disease: an open randomised trial. Lancet. 2008;371(9613):660–7.
69. Sandborn W, Rutgeerts P, Reinisch W, et al. SONIC: A randomized double-blind, controlled trial comparing infliximab and infliximab and azathioprine to azathioprine in patients with Crohn's disease naive to immunomodulators and biologic therapy. Am J Gastroenterol. 2008;103:1117. Abstract 29.
70. Schreiber S, Reinisch W, Colombel JF, Sandborn WJ, Hommes DW, Li J, et al. Early Crohn's disease shows high levels of remission to therapy with adalimumab: sub-analysis of Charm. Gastroenterology. 2007;132(4 Suppl 2):A-147.
71. Panaccione RCJ, Enns R, Feagan B, Hanauer S, Lawrence I, Rutgeerts P, et al. Natalizumab maintains remission in patients with moderately to severely active Crohn's disease for up to 2 years: results from an open-label extension study. Gastroenterology. 2006;130(Abstract):A111.
72. Ghosh S, Goldin E, Gordon FH, et al. Natalizumab for active Crohn's disease. N Engl J Med. 2003;348(1):24–32.
73. Sandborn WJ, Colombel JF, Enns R, et al. Natalizumab induction and maintenance therapy for Crohn's disease. N Engl J Med. 2005;353(18):1912–25.
74. Targan S, Feagan B, Fedorak R, Lashner B, Panacionne R, Present D, et al. Natalizumab induces sustained response and remission in patients with active Crohn's disease: results from the ENCORE trial. Gastroenterology. 2006;130(Abstract):A108.
75. Baert F, Noman M, Vermeire S, et al. Influence of immunogenicity on the long-term efficacy of infliximab in Crohn's disease. N Engl J Med. 2003;348(7):601–8.
76. Afif W, Loftus EV Jr, Faubion W et al. Clinical utility of measuring infliximab and human anti-chimeric antibody concentrations in patients with inflammatory bowel disease. Am J Gastroenterol. 2010;105(5):1133–9.
77. Sandborn WJ, Rutgeerts P, Enns R, et al. Adalimumab induction therapy for Crohn disease previously treated with infliximab: a randomized trial. Ann Intern Med. 2007;146(12):829–38.
78. Hanauer SB, Wagner CL, Bala M, et al. Incidence and importance of antibody responses to infliximab after maintenance or episodic treatment in Crohn's disease. Clin Gastroenterol Hepatol. 2004;2(7):542–53.
79. FDA Consumer Resources Page. Food and Drug Administration Web site. http://www.fda.gov/Forconsumers/ConsumersUpdates/ucm107878.htm (2008). Accessed 12 Nov 2009.
80. Clark M, Colombel JF, Feagan BC, et al. American gastroenterological association consensus development conference on the use of biologics in the treatment of inflammatory bowel disease, June 21–23, 2006. Gastroenterology. 2007;133(1):312–39.
81. Siegel CA, Marden SM, Persing SM, Larson RJ, Sands BE. Risk of lymphoma associated with combination anti-tumor necrosis factor and immunomodulator therapy for the treatment of Crohn's disease: a meta-analysis. Clin Gastroenterol Hepatol. 2009;7(8):874–81.
82. Yousry TA, Major EO, Ryschkewitsch C, et al. Evaluation of patients treated with natalizumab for progressive multifocal leukoencephalopathy. N Engl J Med. 2006;354(9):924–33.
83. FDA Drug Safety Page. Food and Drug Administration Web site. http://www.fda.gov/Drugs/DrugSafety/DrugSafetyNewsletter/ucm120064.htm (2008). Accessed 15 Nov 2009.
84. van Dieren JM, Kuipers EJ, Samsom JN, Nieuwenhuis EE, van der Woude CJ. Revisiting the immunomodulators tacrolimus, methotrexate, and mycophenolate mofetil: their mechanisms of action and role in the treatment of IBD. Inflamm Bowel Dis. 2006;12(4):311–27.
85. Baumgart DC, Wiedenmann B, Dignass AU. Rescue therapy with tacrolimus is effective in patients with severe and refractory inflammatory bowel disease. Aliment Pharmacol Ther. 2003;17(10):1273–81.
86. Ierardi E, Principi M, Francavilla R, et al. Oral tacrolimus long-term therapy in patients with Crohn's disease and steroid resistance. Aliment Pharmacol Ther. 2001;15(3):371–7.
87. Lowry PW, Weaver AL, Tremaine WJ, Sandborn WJ. Combination therapy with oral tacrolimus (FK506) and azathioprine or 6-mercaptopurine for treatment-refractory Crohn's disease perianal fistulae. Inflamm Bowel Dis. 1999;5(4):239–45.
88. Sandborn WJ, Present DH, Isaacs KL, et al. Tacrolimus for the treatment of fistulas in patients with Crohn's disease: a randomized, placebo-controlled trial. Gastroenterology. 2003;125(2):380–8.

89. de Oca J, Vilar L, Castellote J, et al. Immunodulation with tacrolimus (FK506): results of a prospective, open-label, non-controlled trial in patients with inflammatory bowel disease. Rev Esp Enferm Dig. 2003;95(7):465–70. 459–64.
90. Casson DH, Eltumi M, Tomlin S, Walker-Smith JA, Murch SH. Topical tacrolimus may be effective in the treatment of oral and perineal Crohn's disease. Gut. 2000;47(3):436–40.
91. Lukas M. What is the time for surgery in severe Crohn's disease? Inflamm Bowel Dis. 2008;14:S271–2.
92. Akobeng AK, Gardener E. Oral 5-aminosalicylic acid for maintenance of medically-induced remission in Crohn's disease. Cochrane Database Syst Rev. 2005;(1):CD003715.
93. Modigliani R, Colombel JF, Dupas JL, et al. Mesalamine in Crohn's disease with steroid-induced remission: effect on steroid withdrawal and remission maintenance, Groupe d'Etudes Therapeutiques des Affections Inflammatoires Digestives. Gastroenterology. 1996;110(3):688–93.
94. Blum E, Katz JA. Postoperative therapy for Crohn's disease. Inflamm Bowel Dis. 2009;15(3):463–72.
95. Achkar JP, Hanauer SB. Medical therapy to reduce postoperative Crohn's disease recurrence. Am J Gastroenterol. 2000;95(5):1139–46.
96. Camma C, Giunta M, Rosselli M, Cottone M. Mesalamine in the maintenance treatment of Crohn's disease: a meta-analysis adjusted for confounding variables. Gastroenterology. 1997;113(5):1465–73.
97. Lochs H, Mayer M, Fleig WE, et al. Prophylaxis of postoperative relapse in Crohn's disease with mesalamine: European Cooperative Crohn's Disease Study VI. Gastroenterology. 2000;118(2):264–73.
98. Hanauer SB, Korelitz BI, Rutgeerts P, et al. Postoperative maintenance of Crohn's disease remission with 6-mercaptopurine, mesalamine, or placebo: a 2-year trial. Gastroenterology. 2004;127(3):723–9.
99. Ardizzone S, Maconi G, Russo A, Imbesi V, Colombo E, Bianchi Porro G. Randomised controlled trial of azathioprine and 5-aminosalicylic acid for treatment of steroid dependent ulcerative colitis. Gut. 2006;55(1):47–53.
100. Ardizzone S, Maconi G, Sampietro GM, et al. Azathioprine and mesalamine for prevention of relapse after conservative surgery for Crohn's disease. Gastroenterology. 2004;127(3):730–40.
101. Sorrentino D, Terrosu G, Avellini C, Beltrami CA, Bresadola V, Toso F. Prevention of postoperative recurrence of Crohn's disease by infliximab. Eur J Gastroenterol Hepatol. 2006;18(4):457–9.
102. Regueiro M, Schraut W, Baidoo L, et al. Infliximab prevents Crohn's disease recurrence after ileal resection. Gastroenterology. 2009;136(2):441–50.e1. quiz 716.
103. Rutgeerts P, Hiele M, Geboes K, et al. Controlled trial of metronidazole treatment for prevention of Crohn's recurrence after ileal resection. Gastroenterology. 1995;108(6):1617–21.
104. Schwartz DA, Pemberton JH, Sandborn WJ. Diagnosis and treatment of perianal fistulas in Crohn disease. Ann Intern Med. 2001;135(10):906–18.
105. Bernstein LH, Frank MS, Brandt LJ, Boley SJ. Healing of perineal Crohn's disease with metronidazole. Gastroenterology. 1980;79(2):357–65.
106. Brandt LJ, Bernstein LH, Boley SJ, Frank MS. Metronidazole therapy for perineal Crohn's disease: a follow-up study. Gastroenterology. 1982;83(2):383–7.
107. Jakobovits J, Schuster MM. Metronidazole therapy for Crohn's disease and associated fistulae. Am J Gastroenterol. 1984;79(7):533–40.
108. Mahadevan U, Marion JF, Present DH. Fistula response to methotrexate in Crohn's disease: a case series. Aliment Pharmacol Ther. 2003;18(10):1003–8.
109. Gionchetti P, Rizzello F, Venturi A, et al. Comparison of oral with rectal mesalazine in the treatment of ulcerative proctitis. Dis Colon Rectum. 1998;41(1):93–7.
110. Cohen RD, Woseth DM, Thisted RA, Hanauer SB. A meta-analysis and overview of the literature on treatment options for left-sided ulcerative colitis and ulcerative proctitis. Am J Gastroenterol. 2000;95(5):1263–76.
111. Mulder CJ, Fockens P, Meijer JW, van der Heide H, Wiltink EH, Tytgat GN. Beclomethasone dipropionate (3 mg) versus 5-aminosalicylic acid (2 g) versus the combination of both (3 mg/2 g) as retention enemas in active ulcerative proctitis. Eur J Gastroenterol Hepatol. 1996;8(6):549–53.
112. Safdi M, DeMicco M, Sninsky C, et al. A double-blind comparison of oral versus rectal mesalamine versus combination therapy in the treatment of distal ulcerative colitis. Am J Gastroenterol. 1997;92(10):1867–71.
113. Lee FI, Jewell DP, Mani V, et al. A randomised trial comparing mesalazine and prednisolone foam enemas in patients with acute distal ulcerative colitis. Gut. 1996;38(2):229–33.
114. Nielsen OH. Sulfasalazine intolerance. A retrospective survey of the reasons for discontinuing treatment with sulfasalazine in patients with chronic inflammatory bowel disease. Scand J Gastroenterol. 1982;17(3):389–93.
115. Sutherland L, Macdonald JK. Oral 5-aminosalicylic acid for induction of remission in ulcerative colitis. Cochrane Database Syst Rev. 2006;(2):CD000543.
116. Marteau P, Probert CS, Lindgren S, et al. Combined oral and enema treatment with Pentasa (mesalazine) is superior to oral therapy alone in patients with extensive mild/moderate active ulcerative colitis: a randomised, double blind, placebo controlled study. Gut. 2005;54(7):960–5.
117. Sands BE. Fulminant colitis. J Gastrointest Surg. 2008;12(12):2157–9.
118. George J, Present DH, Pou R, Bodian C, Rubin PH. The long-term outcome of ulcerative colitis treated with 6-mercaptopurine. Am J Gastroenterol. 1996;91(9):1711–4.
119. Adler DJ, Korelitz BI. The therapeutic efficacy of 6-mercaptopurine in refractory ulcerative colitis. Am J Gastroenterol. 1990;85(6):717–22.
120. Fraser AG, Orchard TR, Jewell DP. The efficacy of azathioprine for the treatment of inflammatory bowel disease: a 30 year review. Gut. 2002;50(4):485–9.
121. Naftali T, Novis B, Pomeranz I, et al. Cyclosporine for severe ulcerative colitis. Isr Med Assoc J. 2000;2(8):588–91.
122. Lichtiger S, Present DH, Kornbluth A, et al. Cyclosporine in severe ulcerative colitis refractory to steroid therapy. N Engl J Med. 1994;330(26):1841–5.
123. Svavoni F, Bonassi U, Bonassi F. Effectiveness of cyclosporine in the treatment of refractory ulcerative colitis. Gastroenterology. 1998;114:A1096.
124. Hogenauer C, Wenzl HH, Hinterleitner TA, Petritsch W. Effect of oral tacrolimus (FK 506) on steroid-refractory moderate/severe ulcerative colitis. Aliment Pharmacol Ther. 2003;18(4):415–23.

125. Ogata H, Matsui T, Nakamura M, et al. A randomised dose finding study of oral tacrolimus (FK506) therapy in refractory ulcerative colitis. Gut. 2006;55(9):1255–62.
126. Rutgeerts P, Sandborn WJ, Feagan BG, et al. Infliximab for induction and maintenance therapy for ulcerative colitis. N Engl J Med. 2005;353(23):2462–76.
127. Sandborn WJ, Rutgeerts P, Feagan BG, et al. Colectomy rate comparison after treatment of ulcerative colitis with placebo or infliximab. Gastroenterology. 2009;137(4):1250–60. quiz 1520.
128. Hanauer S, Good LI, Goodman MW, et al. Long-term use of mesalamine (Rowasa) suppositories in remission maintenance of ulcerative proctitis. Am J Gastroenterol. 2000;95(7): 1749–54.
129. Mantzaris GJ, Hatzis A, Petraki K, Spiliadi C, Triantaphyllou G. Intermittent therapy with high-dose 5-aminosalicylic acid enemas maintains remission in ulcerative proctitis and proctosigmoiditis. Dis Colon Rectum. 1994;37(1):58–62.
130. Dignass A, Veerman H. Once versus twice daily mesalazine (Pentasa) for the maintenance of remission in ulcerative colitis: the result from a multinational study. Gut. 2008;57 Suppl 1:A1.
131. Kruis W, Gorelov A, Kiudelis G. Once daily dosing of 3g mesalamine is therapeutic equivalent to a three times daily dosing of 1g mesalamine for the treatment of active ulcerative colitis. Gastroenterology. 2007;132:A130.
132. Ardizzone S, Molteni P, Imbesi V, Bollani S, Bianchi Porro G. Azathioprine in steroid-resistant and steroid-dependent ulcerative colitis. J Clin Gastroenterol. 1997;25(1):330–3.
133. Timmer A, McDonald JW, Macdonald JK. Azathioprine and 6-mercaptopurine for maintenance of remission in ulcerative colitis. Cochrane Database Syst Rev. 2007;(1):CD000478.
134. Sutherland L, MacDonald JK. Oral 5-aminosalicylic acid for induction of remission in ulcerative colitis. Cochrane Database Syst Rev. 2003;(3):CD000543.
135. Hawthorne AB, Logan RF, Hawkey CJ, et al. Randomised controlled trial of azathioprine withdrawal in ulcerative colitis. BMJ. 1992;305(6844):20–2.
136. Aberra FN, Lewis JD, Hass D, Rombeau JL, Osborne B, Lichtenstein GR. Corticosteroids and immunomodulators: postoperative infectious complication risk in inflammatory bowel disease patients. Gastroenterology. 2003;125(2):320–7.
137. Mahadevan U, Loftus Jr EV, Tremaine WJ, et al. Azathioprine or 6-mercaptopurine before colectomy for ulcerative colitis is not associated with increased postoperative complications. Inflamm Bowel Dis. 2002;8(5):311–6.
138. Reding R, Michel LA, Donckier J, de Canniere L, Jamart J. Surgery in patients on long-term steroid therapy: a tentative model for risk assessment. Br J Surg. 1990;77(10):1175–8.
139. Stein RB, Hanauer SB. Comparative tolerability of treatments for inflammatory bowel disease. Drug Saf. 2000;23(5): 429–48.
140. Subramanian V, Saxena S, Kang JY, Pollok RC. Preoperative steroid use and risk of postoperative complications in patients with inflammatory bowel disease undergoing abdominal surgery. Am J Gastroenterol. 2008;103(9):2373–81.
141. Stuck AE, Minder CE, Frey FJ. Risk of infectious complications in patients taking glucocorticosteroids. Rev Infect Dis. 1989;11(6):954–63.
142. Colombel JF, Loftus Jr EV, Tremaine WJ, et al. Early postoperative complications are not increased in patients with Crohn's disease treated perioperatively with infliximab or immunosuppressive therapy. Am J Gastroenterol. 2004;99(5): 878–83.
143. Kunitake H, Hodin R, Shellito PC, Sands BE, Korzenik J, Bordeianou L. Perioperative treatment with infliximab in patients with Crohn's disease and ulcerative colitis is not associated with an increased rate of postoperative complications. J Gastrointest Surg. 2008;12(10):1730–6. discussion 1736–7.
144. Appau KA, Fazio VW, Shen B, et al. Use of infliximab within 3 months of ileocolonic resection is associated with adverse postoperative outcomes in Crohn's patients. J Gastrointest Surg. 2008;12(10):1738–44.
145. Selvasekar CR, Cima RR, Larson DW, et al. Effect of infliximab on short-term complications in patients undergoing operation for chronic ulcerative colitis. J Am Coll Surg. 2007;204(5):956–62. discussion 962–3.
146. Madden MV, McIntyre AS, Nicholls RJ. Double-blind crossover trial of metronidazole versus placebo in chronic unremitting pouchitis. Dig Dis Sci. 1994;39(6):1193–6.
147. Maser EA, Present DH. Pouch-ouch. Curr Opin Gastroenterol. 2008;24(1):70–4.
148. Gionchetti P, Rizzello F, Venturi A, et al. Oral bacteriotherapy as maintenance treatment in patients with chronic pouchitis: a double-blind, placebo-controlled trial. Gastroenterology. 2000;119(2):305–9.
149. Gionchetti P, Rizzello F, Venturi A, et al. Antibiotic combination therapy in patients with chronic, treatment-resistant pouchitis. Aliment Pharmacol Ther. 1999;13(6):713–8.
150. Isaacs KL, Sandler RS, Abreu M, et al. Rifaximin for the treatment of active pouchitis: a randomized, double-blind, placebo-controlled pilot study. Inflamm Bowel Dis. 2007;13(10):1250–5.
151. Baidoo L, Kundu R, Su C. Rifaximin is an effective antibiotic for the treatment of pouchitis. Gastroenterology. 2005;128:A797.
152. Gionchetti P, Rizzello F, Poggioli G, et al. Oral budesonide in the treatment of chronic refractory pouchitis. Aliment Pharmacol Ther. 2007;25(10):1231–6.
153. Gionchetti P, Morselli C, Rizzello F, et al. Infliximab in the treatment of refractory pouchitis. Gastroenterology. 2005; 128:A578.
154. Gionchetti P, Rizzello F, Helwig U, et al. Prophylaxis of pouchitis onset with probiotic therapy: a double-blind, placebo-controlled trial. Gastroenterology. 2003;124(5):1202–9.
155. Colombel JF, Ricart E, Loftus Jr EV, et al. Management of Crohn's disease of the ileoanal pouch with infliximab. Am J Gastroenterol. 2003;98(10):2239–44.
156. Shen B, Remzi FH, Shen L. Efficacy and safety of adalimumab in the treatment of Crohn's disease of the ileal pouch. The annual meeting of the American College of Gastroenterology, Orlando, FL; 2008. Abstract:620.

29
Ulcerative Colitis: Surgical Management

Zuri Murrell and Phillip Fleshner

Ulcerative colitis (UC) is a diffuse inflammatory disease of the mucosal lining of the colon and rectum that manifests clinically as diarrhea, abdominal pain, fever, weight loss, and rectal bleeding. Since removal of the affected organ is curative, surgery has assumed a pivotal position in the management of these patients. Although removal of the entire colon and rectum with a permanent ileostomy had been the standard operation for decades, increased experience with anal sphincter preservation has demonstrated the feasibility of performing surgical procedures which spare sphincter function while still removing all disease. This chapter considers the surgical alternatives, decision making, and techniques surrounding these procedures.

Indications for Surgery

Approximately 10% of UC patients will undergo surgery for very specific reasons, including: an acute flare unresponsive to medical measures, development of a life-threatening complication such as toxic colitis, perforation, or hemorrhage, medical intractability, risk of malignancy, disabling extracolonic disease, and growth retardation in children. During an acute exacerbation of colitis, the patient should be aggressively treated with intravenous steroids and bowel rest. The role of parenteral hyperalimentation in this situation is controversial. Encouraging results have been reported with the use of either cyclosporine[1] or infliximab[2] in the acute setting, yet long-term effectiveness of these treatment modalities remains undefined. While there is no reported increase in the incidence of perioperative complications after subtotal colectomy in patients treated before surgery with cyclosporine,[3,4] there is some controversy as to whether infliximab increases the perioperative complication rate after restorative proctocolectomy as these patients usually have more advanced active disease than do the patients who are not receiving active infliximab treatment.[5,6] The *combined* use of cyclosporine and infliximab is not advised as there may be a higher incidence of infectious complications in patients who ultimately require colectomy.[5]

Patients with life-threatening complications are generally easy to recognize and define. Nevertheless, these patients are frequently taking large doses of steroids and may appear deceptively well; consequently, appreciation of the severity of the disease and the timing of operation are of paramount importance. Medical intractability is the most common indication for operation and may seem difficult to define. In fact, there is probably no strict definition that a physician can uniformly apply. It is important to recognize that medical intractability is a problem that the patient identifies in conjunction with the physician. Although a physician may feel that 12 months of steroids or other immunosuppressive management without complete resolution of symptoms is an adequate medical trial, the patient must be convinced that surgery is indicated. Only the patient can decide that he or she feels fatigued, has missed too much work or school, or is unable to do things he or she would like to do because of the systemic effects of active colitis and/or its medical treatment. If the surgeon waits until the patient has arrived at the conclusion that the disease is not satisfactorily controlled medically, the patient will graciously accept alternatives the surgeon has to offer. We feel this is a particularly important strategy for the surgeon to employ if the patient is to be satisfied.

Patients with UC are also prone to the development of colorectal cancer. The risk of cancer is relatively low for the first 10 years after disease onset, but then begins to increase so that by the time the patients has had the disease for 20 years, the cumulative risk of colorectal cancer may be as high as 10%. The overall prevalence of colorectal cancer in any UC patient is approximately 4%.[7] The question of timing of surgery for cancer prophylaxis remains undefined. Certainly, surgical treatment of carcinoma is mandatory. More controversial, however, is the management of patients with dysplasia. Most surgeons contend that during a surveillance biopsy program identification of dysplasia of any grade by an experienced pathologist, especially in the absence of severe inflammation,

D.E. Beck et al. (eds.), *The ASCRS Textbook of Colon and Rectal Surgery: Second Edition*,
DOI 10.1007/978-1-4419-1584-9_29,

is an indication for colectomy. The management of patients with UC who are found to have a sporadic adenoma (by definition a dysplastic lesion) is also contentious, as the simultaneous discovery of both lesions is not uncommon. If the lesion is detected in an area of colonic mucosa unaffected by UC, such a lesion may be reliably diagnosed as a sporadic adenoma. Alternatively, dysplastic mass lesions detected within should be viewed with a high degree of suspicion for malignant potential.[8]

Elective colectomy may be indicated for some categories of severe extraintestinal manifestations of the disease. Persistent or recurrent monoarticular arthritis, uveitis, or iritis all respond favorably to colectomy. However, primary sclerosing cholangitis, ankylosing spondylitis, and sacroilitis are not improved by colectomy. The response of pyoderma gangrenosum to colectomy is unpredictable.

Growth retardation is a common feature in children with UC. Contrary to popular belief, steroid therapy cannot be entirely blamed for delayed growth. Inadequate protein intake and excess loss in the colon are also contributory.[9] A rapid growth spurt is often observed after definitive surgery.

Emergency Versus Elective Procedures

Operative management of UC largely depends on whether the surgery is elective or emergent. Under elective conditions, the four available surgical options are: (1) total proctocolectomy and Brooke ileostomy, (2) total proctocolectomy and continent ileostomy, (3) abdominal colectomy with ileorectal anastomosis (IRA), and (4) ileal pouch–anal anastomosis (IPAA). Total proctocolectomy and Brooke ileostomy has been traditionally regarded as the optimal surgical approach and remains the operation with which alternative procedures should be compared. The technique has been well described, and the immediate and late results are very satisfactory. Furthermore, patients avoid any risk for cancer, steroid medications are eliminated, and physician visits and reoperations are kept to a minimum. Although quality-of-life studies[10] have demonstrated excellent results, the loss of fecal continence and its attendant physical and psychological sequelae continue to be significant drawbacks of the procedure. In addition, problems with nonhealing of the perineal wound, and the high incidence of small bowel obstruction (SBO) and ileostomy revision, are not to be minimized,

Total proctocolectomy and continent ileostomy couples the benefit of complete large bowel excision with a reduction in some of the untoward aspects of an ileostomy, since no external appliance is needed and the stoma can be placed in a less conspicuous position on the abdominal wall. Continent ileostomy can be performed at anytime in UC patients having previously undergone total proctocolectomy and Brooke ileostomy if they find a standard ileostomy unsatisfactory. Due to increased surgical experience and improved surgical techniques, the morbidity associated with the continent pouch has decreased since its initial clinical description. Most patients are ultimately happy with the results of the operation.[11] Nonetheless, troublesome complications leading to incontinence continue to plague the postoperative course of a substantial number of patients.[11,12] The continent ileostomy may also be a viable treatment option in selected patients who have failed an IPAA.[13]

There are many attractive features of total colectomy and IRA. The procedure avoids the perineal complications of total proctocolectomy, the risk of sexual dysfunction is minimal, is technically easy to perform, may provide perfect control of feces and flatus, and is well accepted by most patients. However, unlike the three other surgical options, ileorectostomy does not achieve total excision of colorectal mucosa. Many surgeons have not used this operation for patients with UC, arguing that in excess of 25% patients will require subsequent rectal excision for persistent proctitis, a small percentage of patients will develop cancer in the rectal remnant, and only one-half of the patients have satisfactory long-term functional results. While we concur that this operation should not be advised in most patients with UC, IRA does have a role in certain clinical situations. For example, an elderly patient with a long history of UC who develops a transverse colon cancer may be well served with an IRA in lieu of total proctocolectomy. An IRA may also be offered to females of childbearing age to preserve fertility.[14] Decisions must be made on an individualized basis, taking into account the compliance of the rectum and the integrity of the sphincter mechanism.

Ileal pouch–anal anastomosis has the attractive features of complete excision of the colorectal mucosa, avoidance of a permanent intestinal stoma, continence via a normal route of defecation, and no prospect for a troublesome nonhealing perineal wound. Continence is usually preserved and the frequency of defecation is diminished with incorporation of a pelvic pouch into the operative procedure. Although the operation is associated with minimal mortality, the morbidity of this complex procedure is relatively high, and problems such as small bowel obstruction and pouchitis continue to be a cause for concern.

Under emergent conditions, surgical alternatives are limited. If the patient is septic, the diseased or perforated bowel should be removed. If the colon is bleeding, the colon should be removed. Traditionally, it has been taught that the rectum should also be removed. However, with currently available sphincter-saving alternatives, careful preoperative proctoscopic evaluation to exclude a rectal etiology for the bleeding and a subsequent abdominal colectomy with end ileostomy can be safely performed. A subsequent procedure can then restore intestinal continuity. Similarly, with toxic colitis, it is seldom necessary to perform a proctectomy at the time of colectomy. In general, concerns over healing of the perineal wound in these frequently malnourished patients receiving high-dose steroids should deter surgeons from undertaking proctectomy in the emergent setting. Many surgeons have not found it necessary to use the blow-hole technique of Turnbull, but this alternative is a philosophically acceptable approach in that it does not preclude subsequent continence-preserving alternatives.

A few technical issues regarding subtotal colectomy in these patients must be stressed. Mesenteric dissection in the vicinity of the ileocecal valve should be flush with the colon in order to preserve ileal branches of the ileocolic artery and vein. These branches are necessary to facilitate subsequent construction of an ileal pouch. Distally, it is unnecessary to mobilize the rectum within the pelvis. In fact, dissection of the sigmoid to the sacral promontory, without violation of presacral planes, and a Hartmann procedure are recommended. This precaution has shown to decrease the incidence of pelvic sepsis and facilitate subsequent pelvic surgery. A transanal rectal drain may prevent leakage from the diseased Hartmann pouch closure site. Laparoscopic-assisted or hand-assisted subtotal colectomy is both feasible and safe in these patients.[15]

There is a trend to avoid subjecting patients to multiple surgical procedures and to perform a definitive procedure at the time of emergent surgery. Although an IPAA can be successfully performed in patients undergoing surgery for emergent complications, this approach is generally not safe. These patients are usually on high doses of steroids and are nutritionally depleted. Patients with UC receiving high-dose steroids (more than 40 mg/day) have a significantly greater risk of developing pouch-related complications after colectomy than patients with UC receiving 1–40 mg/day and patients with UC who are not receiving corticosteroids.[16] From a practical standpoint, surgical options are limited in emergent situations. Salvage of the patient should be the primary concern. Abdominal colectomy is safe in these very ill, nutritionally depleted patients[17] and the procedure does not preclude the future of any of the other surgical alternatives. Additionally, the patient is able to live with an ileostomy and assess its impact on his or her life, thus allowing for an informed decision regarding subsequent continence-restoring surgery.

Brooke Ileostomy

The preoperative period should include effective patient education. A patient must be fully informed of the effects of an ileostomy on his or her quality of life. An ileostomy visitor, preferably age and sex matched and who has completely recovered from surgery, is invaluable during this period. Resistance to a permanent ileostomy can be tempered by stressing the beneficial aspects of this operation such as curing the disease. It is also essential, when possible, to select the stoma site preoperatively with the help of an enterostomal therapist. As discussed in Chap. 31 the stoma should be placed in a flat area away from bony prominences, scars, and significant skin creases. Attention to these details will ensure a well-functioning ileostomy.

Operative Technique

A colectomy is performed in the standard fashion with the patient in a modified lithotomy-Trendelenburg position. A minimally invasive approach is often preferred.[18] The proctectomy phase of the procedure is remarkable for keeping the dissection close to the rectal wall, especially anteriorly in the area of Denonvilliers' fascia. Meticulous dissection to minimize the risk of injury to pelvic autonomic nerves is essential. Perineal dissection should be performed in the intersphincteric plane. After the colorectum is removed, a 2-cm circular piece of skin is excised at the marked stoma site and a two finger-wide aperture is made through the lateral one-third of the rectus muscle. It is most important that this opening be of correct size to avoid chronic stomal obstruction or parastomal hernia. The mesentery of the ileum should be well mobilized to allow at least 5–6 cm of the ileum to protrude through the abdominal wall defect. The ileum may be anchored to the abdominal wall fascia with nonabsorbable sutures to prevent retraction of the stoma in the postoperative period. These sutures may also help prevent parastomal herniation, but there is no controlled study demonstrating that they are effective in preventing this complication. After the bowel is brought through the abdominal wall, a defect remains lateral to the small bowel mesentery. It is unclear whether this defect needs to be routinely closed. This area can be closed either by eliminating the defect laterally or by suturing the mesentery to the anterior abdominal wall. If the stoma is thought to be temporary, closing this mesenteric defect could possibly complicate subsequent small bowel mobilization.

The technical contribution of Brooke[19] was primary maturation of the ileostomy. Previously, the immature protruding ileostomy was left to protrude from the abdominal wall. Exposure of the serosa resulted in ileitis characterized by symptoms of small bowel obstruction. By folding the ileum back on itself, one covers the serosa and minimizes these symptoms. The stoma is routinely matured by removing 3–5 cm of mesentery from the end of the ileum and folding the edge of the bowel upon itself (see Chap. 31). To anchor the edge of the bowel, we use the "three-bite" suture that includes the full thickness of the bowel, seromuscular layer of the bowel, and the dermis of the skin. It is important to avoid placing a suture through the epidermis, in which mucosal cells can be implanted and cause difficulty with appliance security. An appliance is then placed over the stoma. Bowel function is expected in 1–3 days.

In some situations, the end of the ileum does not reach far enough through the abdominal wall to allow primary maturation. In these situations, the mesentery is usually a limiting factor and selection of a more proximal site in the bowel may allow better mobilization. Alternatively, a loop ileostomy rather than an end ileostomy may reach more easily. In these unusual situations, a segment of intact bowel is brought through the abdominal wall defect. Some surgeons prefer to suture the bowel to the fascia with nonabsorbable sutures rather than to use a rod to support the bowel in place.

Regardless of how the bowel is secured, the stoma should be primarily matured. This step is done by dividing the bowel distally through 85% of its circumference. The bowel is then folded back upon the proximal bowel and primarily sutured with the three-bite technique already described.

Postoperative Complications

Brooke ileostomy is a safe procedure with a predictable long-term outcome. It is, however, not entirely free of complications. Delayed healing of the perineal wound is not uncommon and can be quite problematic.[20] Failure of the wound to close should prompt investigation to exclude the presence of retained mucosa, foreign material, or Crohn's disease (CD). Sexual complications of proctocolectomy in men are much less common than in patients having a radical resection for cancer, yet permanent impotence or retrograde ejaculation can occur. Almost 30% of women complain of dyspareunia after this operation, presumably due to perineal scarring.[21] Intestinal obstruction is a troublesome complication that can be managed conservatively in most patients. Gentle irrigation of the stoma is an important therapeutic maneuver. Prolonged nonoperative treatment should not be pursued for fear of infarction. Although problems from the ileostomy have diminished markedly with the use of modern appliances and the Brooke modification, skin irritation, stomal stenosis, prolapse, and herniation remain significant causes of postoperative morbidity. Treatment of these problems can be as simple as reeducating a patient about the proper maintenance of the ileostomy. However, up to one-third of these patients ultimately require operative revision.[22] Despite the fact that these patients have undergone major abdominal surgery and have a permanent stoma, their quality of life as measured by validated questionnaires is very good and similar to that of the general population.[10] Over 90% of patients are happy with their current lifestyle. However, significant problems do remain. Almost 25% of patients are restricted in their social and recreation activities, and nearly 15% of patients who are knowledgeable of alternative procedures would consider conversion. In short, the Brooke ileostomy is generally well accepted, although a number of patients experience significant psychosocial and mechanical difficulties. This procedure is commonly performed using minimally invasive techniques. Current indications for the procedure include elderly patients, individuals with distal rectal cancer, patients with severely compromised anal function, and patients who choose this operation after appropriate education.

Continent Ileostomy

Physicians involved with patients requiring an ileostomy should be aware of the continent ileostomy. Although this procedure is less commonly performed today, it remains a viable alternative in patients who have discrete problems with an appliance. The surgeon should not primarily advise this procedure after a proctocolectomy. The continent ileostomy should be reserved for patients who have failed Brooke ileostomy or those individuals who are candidates for an IPAA, but cannot have a pouch because of rectal cancer, perianal fistulas, poor anal sphincter function, or occupations that may preclude frequent visits to the toilet.

Preoperatively, exclusion of CD using barium examination of the stomach and small intestine and/or CT-enterography and/or capsule endoscopy is important. Suspicion of CD contraindicates construction of a continent ileostomy, since the risk of recurrent disease in the pouch is increased; this could necessitate resection of 45 cm of valuable small bowel and render the patient unable to maintain nutrition. Obesity and age over 40 years are associated with an increased risk of pouch dysfunction and represent relative contraindications to the continent ileostomy.[23]

The period before surgery must also include an open discussion with the patient, stressing that although continence is likely, major complications often occur. These setbacks generally must be corrected surgically, sometimes leading to pouch excision and creation of a standard Brooke ileostomy. The patient must comprehend that by learning to care for and intubate the reservoir; he or she plays an important role in its functional outcome. Only highly motivated, emotionally stable individuals should consider this procedure.

Operative Technique

Patients undergoing combined total proctocolectomy/continent ileostomy have a proctocolectomy performed in the usual fashion. Excision of a very short segment of terminal ileum and a diligent search for CD during the procedure are essential. In patients with a standard ileostomy undergoing conversion to continent ileostomy, the stoma is mobilized from the abdominal wall. Construction of the reservoir in these two patient groups is then performed in an identical fashion.

The technique of constructing a continent ileostomy is conceptually difficult (Figure 29-1). Using the terminal 45 cm of the ileum, an aperistaltic reservoir is created by making an S pouch or a pouch originally described by Kock.[23] In the classic technique, two 15-cm limbs ileum are sutured together with continuous absorbable sutures to form a pouch. The antimesenteric border is incised and then folded over to form a reservoir. The ileum immediately distal to the reservoir is then scarified with electrocautery and 5 cm of adjacent mesentery is removed and intussusception of this terminal 15 cm of ileum into the pouch is performed. The intussusception is secured with multiple nonabsorbable sutures and staples. The end of the ileum is then brought

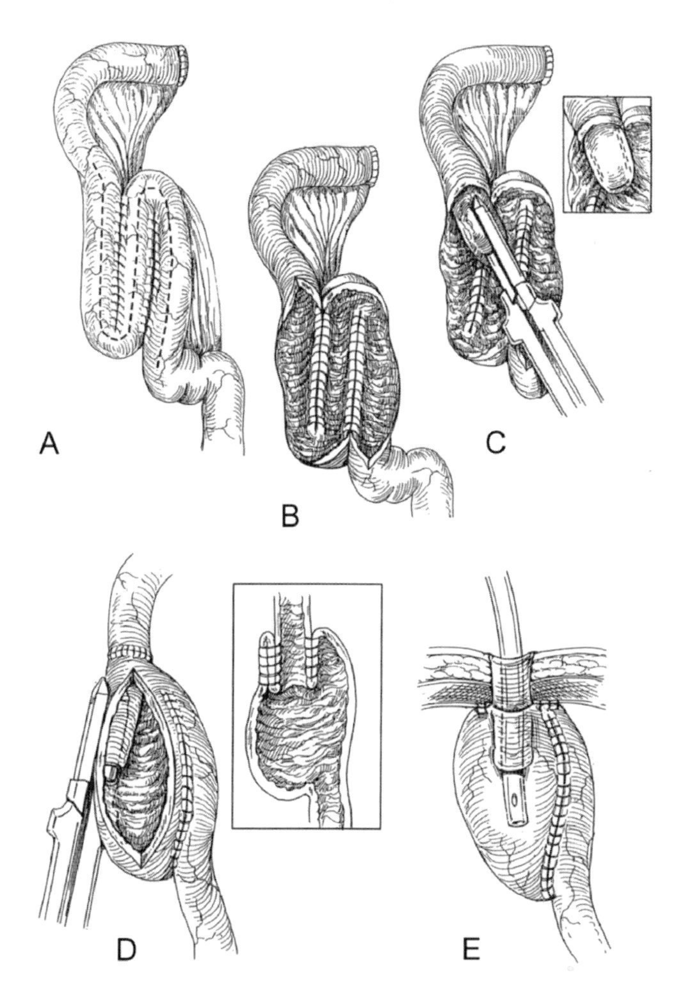

FIGURE 29-1. Continent ileostomy. **A** Three limbs of small bowel are measured and the bowel wall is sutured together. **B** After opening the bowel (see the *dotted lines* in **A**), the edges are sewn together to form a two-layered closure. **C** A Valve is created by intussuscepting the efferent limb into the pouch and fixing it in place with a linear noncutting stapler. (*Inset*: staples in place on valve.) **D** The valve is attached to the pouch sidewall with the linear noncutting stapler (a cross section of the finished pouch is shown). **E** After closure of the last suture line, the pouch is attached to the abdominal wall and a catheter is inserted to keep the pouch decompressed during healing.

through the abdominal wall at the preoperatively identified site just above the escutcheon. The stoma is sutured flush with the skin and the pouch firmly anchored to the posterior rectus sheath. A wide plastic tube with large openings is placed into the pouch to allow gravity drainage of the pouch in the early postoperative period. This tube is occluded for progressively longer periods beginning 10 days after surgery until it can be removed for 8 h without distress. At this point, the pouch is significantly expanded, the tube is removed, and drainage is achieved by intubating the pouch three times a day. A 6-week period of the indwelling catheter is not uncommon.

Postoperative Complications

Postoperative complications that frequently occur are nipple valve slippage, pouchitis, intestinal obstruction, and fistula. Nipple valve slippage[24,25] occurs because of the tendency of the intussuscepted segment to slide and extrude on its mesenteric aspect. Difficult pouch catheterization, chronic outflow tract obstruction, and incontinence ensue. Because of the frequency of this problem, many techniques other than simple surgical stapling have been described to stabilize the valve. Wrapping the valve with prosthetic materials does prevent valve slippage, but also is accompanied by a potentially unacceptably high incidence of parastomal abscess and fistula formation.[12] Despite these technical modifications, nipple valve slippage remains the most common complication after continent ileostomy, occurring in almost 30% of patients.[12,24,25] Although nonoperative approaches have been attempted to correct this problem, surgical correction is virtually inevitable. Repair of the existing malfunctioning valve or creation of a new valve from the afferent ileal limb is performed.

Pouchitis is recognized in 25% of patients, making this the second most common postoperative complication after continent ileostomy.[12,24,25] Pouchitis refers to nonspecific inflammation that develops in the reservoir, and is thought to result from stasis and overgrowth of anaerobic bacteria. Patients present with a combination of increased ileostomy output, fever, weight loss, and stomal bleeding. The diagnosis is made by history and confirmed by pouch endoscopy. Pouchitis usually responds to a course of antibiotics and continuous pouch drainage.

Other complications include an incidence of intestinal obstruction after continent ileostomy of about 5%. Surgical intervention is mandatory when nonoperative therapy has been unsuccessful. The incidence of fistulas after creation of a continent ileostomy is approximately 10%. Fistulas most commonly originate in the pouch itself or at the base of the nipple valve. Pouch fistulas results from dehiscence of suture lines or, rarely ileostomy tube erosion. These tracts may close with bowel rest, parenteral nutrition, and continuous pouch drainage. Fistulas from the base of the valve lead to incontinence, since ileal contents bypass the high-pressure zone of the nipple valve. These fistulas commonly arise with tearing of the sutures anchoring the pouch to the anterior abdominal wall. Valve fistulas rarely heal without operation. At laparotomy, the valve is excised, the pouch rotated, and a new continent valve constructed from the afferent tract.

Patient satisfaction with a continent ileostomy has been reported by some authors as being very high.[11,26] Most patients note a marked improvement in their lifestyle, and almost all patients work and participate in social and recreational activities without restriction.[11,24] These observations are understandable in that 90% of patients eventually have total continence after one or more procedures. Conversely, their enthusiasm is surprising considering that complications

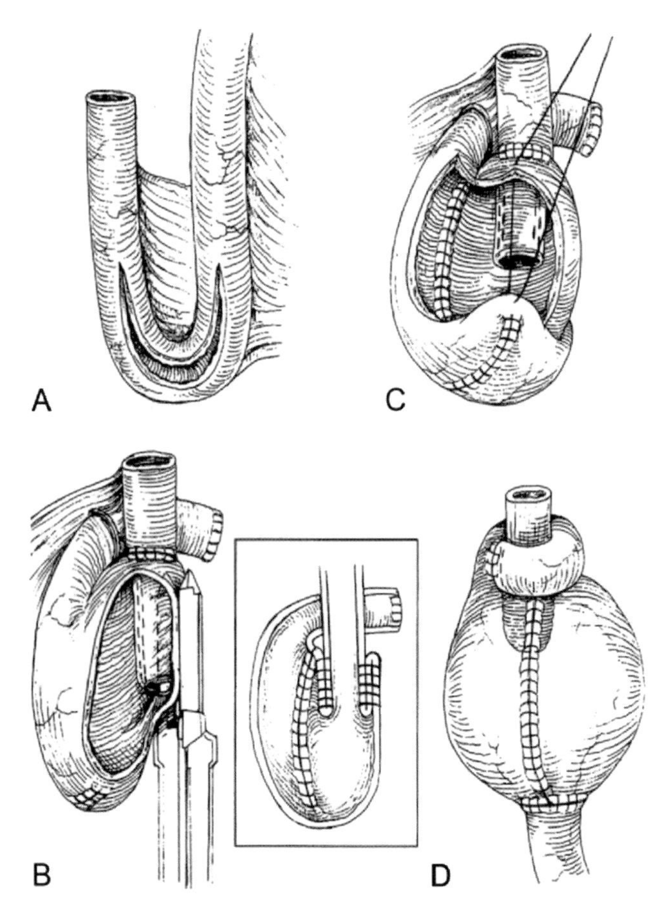

FIGURE 29-2. Barnet continent ileostomy reservoir (BCIR). **A** Two limbs of small intestine are sewn together and opened. **B** The afferent limb in intussuscepted to form a valve and the valve is stapled and stapled to the side of the reservoir. **C** The pouch is folded back and sutured closed. *Inset* shows cross section of pouch. **D** Completed BCIR. The afferent limb of bowel has been divided and reattached to the apex of the pouch and the efferent limb is wrapped around the valve to form a collar.

are quite frequent and often require major surgical intervention.[11,26] The often advertised Barnett modification of the Kock pouch (Figure 29-2) uses the afferent limb of small bowel to construct the nipple valve and wraps a portion of the residual efferent limb around the nipple valve.[27] Although designed to reduce the incidence of valve slippage and fistula formation, there are no controlled data to suggest that this modification is any better than the standard procedure most centers are using.

Ileorectal Anastomosis

Before the advent of IPAA, abdominal colectomy with IRA was performed in UC patients who might otherwise have been offered a permanent ileostomy. Currently, IRA is mainly considered in patients with indeterminate colitis (IC), in high-risk or older patients who are not good candidates for IPAA, or if there is mild rectal disease where rectal compliance remains adequate. The use of the operation may also be indicated in the teenager or young adult in order to rapidly regain good health, avoid a stoma and return to school or work quickly. In addition, it can also be considered in young females in an attempt to preserve fertility.[14] Functional results depend on the level of the anastomosis as well as the state of the rectum. Contraindications to IRA include a very diseased and noncompliant rectum, dysplasia or nonmetastatic cancer, perianal disease, and a severely compromised anal sphincter.

Postoperative Complications

Ileorectal anastomosis is a safe operation; mortality is low, particularly when it is performed as an elective procedure. The early morbidity of IRA is low, with the incidence of anastomotic leak being less than 10%, and major sepsis is very uncommon. Sexual function is well preserved. The overall complication rate is much lower than that of an IPAA.[28] Although the frequency of defecation after IRA is variable, most patients pass between two and four semi-liquid stools a day. Nocturnal defecation is quite common, but true incontinence is rare.[29]

The main concerns surrounding IRA for UC are the long-term issues regarding cancer risk in the retained rectum and the incidence of persistent rectal inflammation. The overall risk of cancer developing in the rectum after IRA approximates 6%, but this depends on the duration of follow up.[30] Few of these cancers develop less than 10 years after operation, with most cancers appearing 15–20 years after operation. Rectal cancer following IRA produces few symptoms and early lesions are not always easily identified at sigmoidoscopy. Patients being offered IRA must realize the need for semi-annual sigmoidoscopy with multiple biopsies to detect dysplasia, polyps, or invasive cancer. This recommendation is particularly important in young adults or children since these patients have the highest risk of developing cancer and are much more likely to be lost to follow up.

The rectal stump may be the site of recurrent or persistent inflammation in 20–45% of patients. Clinical features include severe diarrhea, tenesmus, bleeding and urgency. Rectal excision is needed in those cases that do not respond to topical or systemic therapies. About one-quarter of patients require proctectomy after IRA for severe proctitis.[28,30] The only clinical factor which predicts a successful outcome is the degree of inflammation in the rectum preoperatively, minimal proctitis being associated with an excellent prognosis.[28] A great advantage of the IRA is that should a failure occur, other options remain. Conversion from an IRA to an IPAA may be required when there is a poor functional outcome because of poor rectal compliance, persistent and disabling proctitis, and with development of an upper rectal cancer. If conversion to IPAA is required, it can be performed safely, although poorer bowel function may be expected. However, quality of life is similar before and after conversion in these patients.[31]

Ileal-Pouch Anal Anastomosis

The most attractive of the continence-preserving alternatives is the IPAA, which consists of near total proctocolectomy, creation of an ileal reservoir, and preservation of the anal sphincter complex. The original operation as described by Sir Alan Parks included a complete stripping of the anal mucosa of the anal canal.[32] In an attempt to improve functional outcome, some surgeons[33,34] preserve the anal transition zone and perform a stapled anastomosis between the ileal pouch and the anal canal immediately cephalad to the dentate line (double-staple technique). Both of these techniques remove the colorectum without creating a perianal wound, preserve innervation to the anus, bladder, and genitals, and retain the usual pathway for defecation. Preoperatively, the rectum should be evaluated sigmoidoscopically. Active rectal disease requires topical 5-aminosalicylic acid or steroid enemas to minimize rectal inflammation and facilitate mucosectomy. The anorectal sphincter mechanism must be intact to prevent leakage of watery ileal contents. Use of this procedure in patients with poor sphincter function or fecal incontinence must be carefully individualized. Preoperative evaluation also allows the surgeon to be certain that patients undergoing this operation are highly motivated and willing to cope with potential postoperative complications.

Recent surgical advances have allowed both laparoscopic and hand-assisted proctocolectomy and IPAA. Laparoscopic ileal pouch surgery is associated with longer operating time and less blood loss, but may have short term benefits such as diminished postoperative pain, reduced narcotic requirements, and shorter hospital stay compared to open surgery.[35,36] A prospective randomized controlled trial of hand-assisted laparoscopic colonic mobilization and open rectal dissection (via an 8-cm Pfannenstiel incision) versus open surgery through the midline showed no difference in postoperative quality-of-life measurements.[36]

Operative Technique

The patient is brought to the operating room and placed in the modified lithotomy position. A midline incision is made and the abdomen explored to rule out evidence of CD. The colon is mobilized in the usual fashion. A few technical points should be stressed. Omentectomy may be inappropriate, since there is a lower incidence of postoperative sepsis when the omentum is preserved.[37] Stapling of the distal ileum flush with the cecum is very important, as is preservation of the ileal branches of the ileocolic artery and vein. These vessels provide perfusion of the pouch after mesenteric division. The pelvic peritoneum is incised and rectal mobilization begun. Dissection is carried ventrally to the level of the prostate in men and the mid-portion of the vagina in women. Posteriorly, the dissection is carried past the end of the coccyx. Mobilization of the rectum should be flush with the fascia propria to minimize damage to nearby autonomic nerves traveling to urinary bladder and sexual organs.

Laparoscopic-assisted IPAA is performed using four to five trocars and a 4-cm to 5-cm periumbilical, Pfannenstiel, or lower midline incision with the patient in low modified lithotomy position. The lateral attachments are divided, and most commonly the mesenteric vessels are divided with a bipolar vessel sealing and cutting device. If a temporary diverting ileostomy is planned, a disc of skin and subcutaneous fat can be excised from the chosen stoma site for the placement of the trocar in the right lower quadrant. Exteriorization of the mobilized colon and rectum can be achieved through a 4-cm to 5-cm incision placed at the umbilicus, or in the suprapubic region as either a Pfannenstiel or a short vertical suprapubic incision. Resection and pouch construction is performed extracorporeally similar to the open procedure or in a laparoscopic intracorporeal manner. The pouch is then returned to the abdomen and under laparoscopic control anastomosed to the anal canal. A diverting loop ileostomy is constructed in the right lower quadrant.

Hand-assisted laparoscopic (HAL) colectomy begins with an 8-cm Pfannenstiel or lower midline incision after which the hand device is positioned into the incision (Figure 29-3).

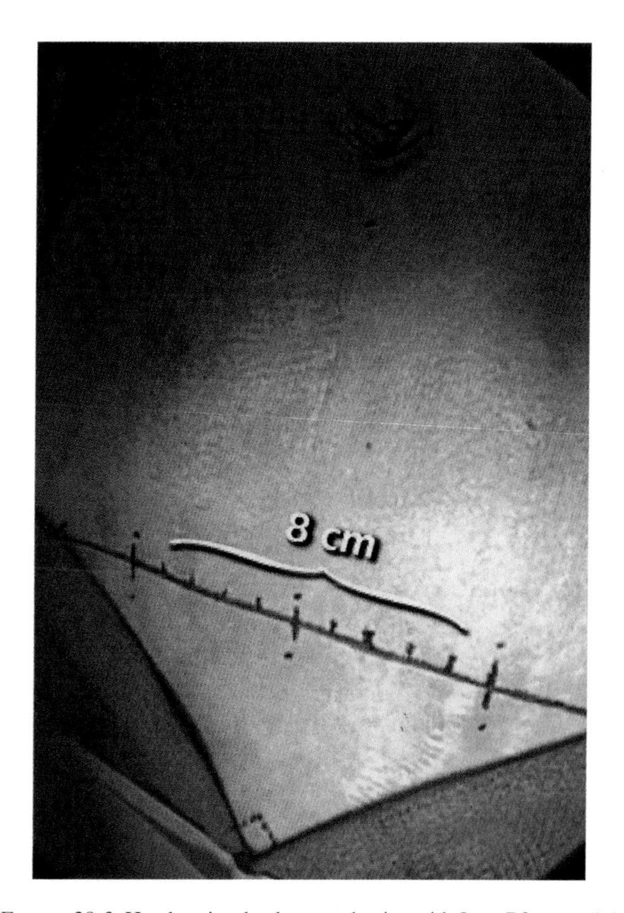

FIGURE 29-3. Hand-assisted colectomy begins with 8 cm Pfannenstiel or lower midline incision. Note how positioning of towels from the root of penis or top of the introitus to the anterior superior iliac spine creates a right angled triangle, assuring a straight transverse incision.

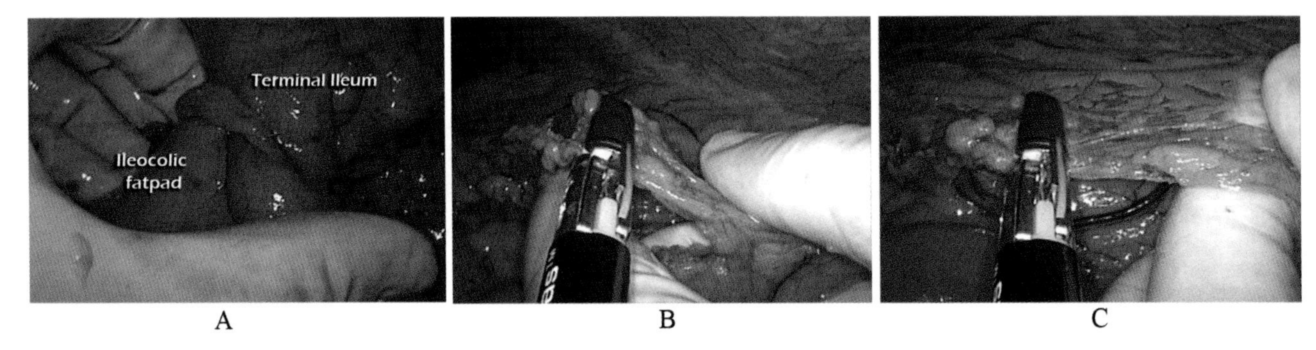

FIGURE 29-4. Technical maneuvers during hand-assisted laparoscopic total colectomy. **A** Traction of the ileocolic fat pad with traction towards the right lower quadrant will facilitate identification and preservation of the ileocolic artery. The omentum and transverse colon mesentery are divided either together **B** or separately after entry into the lesser sac **C**.

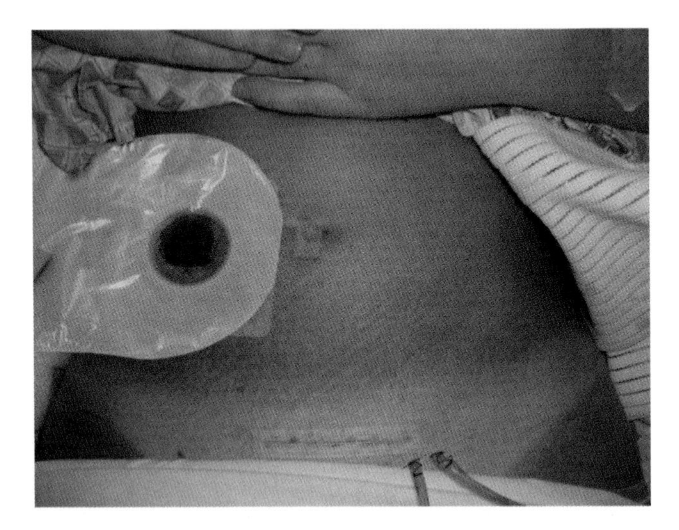

FIGURE 29-5. Typical wound appearance at completion of surgery.

A 12-mm trocar is inserted just below the umbilicus for the laparoscope and pneumoperitoneum. Additional 5-mm or 10-mm trocars are inserted as needed to facilitate the dissection. The surgeon's left hand is placed into the peritoneal cavity and the following procedures assisted. The greater omentum is dissected, the hepatocolic and splenocolic ligaments are taken down to mobilize the transverse colon, and the mesocolon is divided using a vessel sealing device (Figure 29-4). Although some authors advocate HAL rectal mobilization, the chapter authors advocate continuing the surgery open directly through the hand-device. The remainder of the procedure is continued akin to the open approach. This procedure provides the patient with a cosmetically acceptable outcome (Figure 29-5).

If desired, mucosal stripping is performed from a perineal approach. The use of a Lone Star™ (Lone Star Medical Products, Stafford, TX) retractor facilitates exposure and minimizes damage to the sphincter mechanism (Figure 29-6). A solution of dilute epinephrine is injected into the submucosal plane to facilitate mucosectomy and minimize bleeding

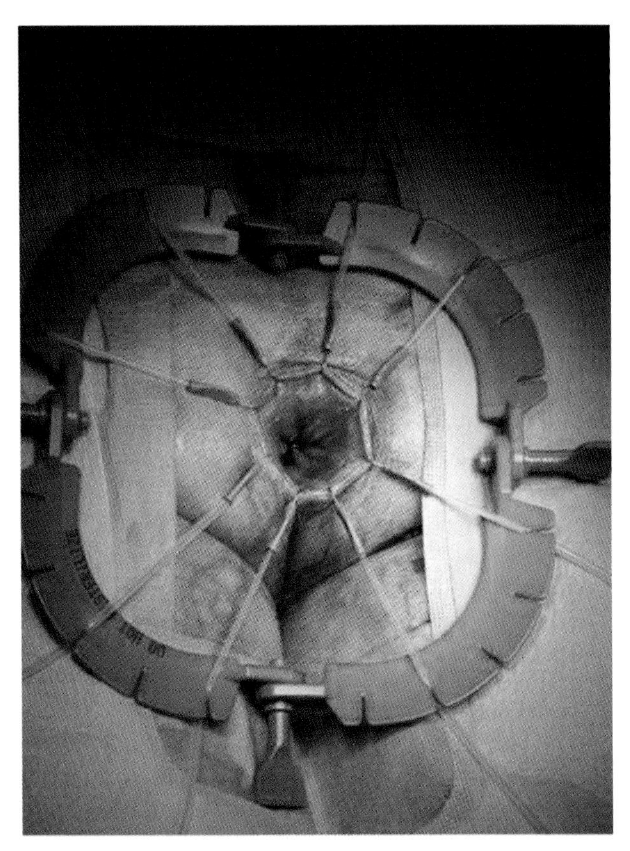

FIGURE 29-6. Lone Star™ retractor.

(Figure 29-7). The excised mucosa and remaining proximal rectum are removed, leaving a short cuff of denuded rectal muscle distally for about 4 cm above the dentate line. Attention is then directed towards creation of the ileal reservoir. The terminal ileum is aligned in a J configuration and the pouch constructed with either a continuous absorbable suture or stapling device (Figures 29-8 to 29-11). Both limbs of the J are approximately 15–25 cm in length, the exact length guided by where the pouch reaches deepest into the pelvis. The prospective apex of the pouch must reach beyond

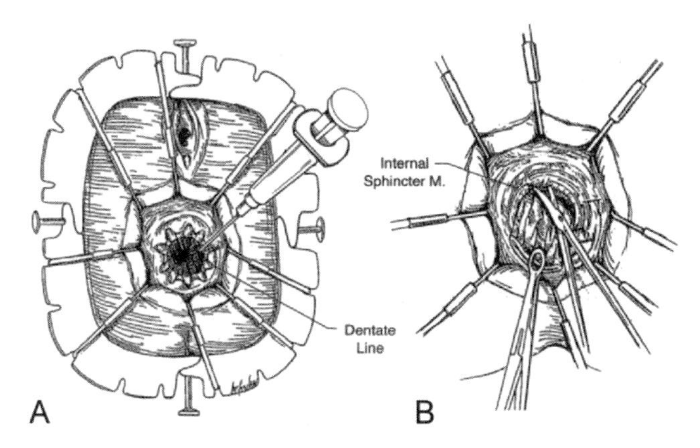

FIGURE 29-7. Mucosectomy. In **A**, a spinal needle is used to inject saline solution with epinephrine (1:200,000) into the submucosa from the dentate line to the levators. A circumferential incision through the mucosa is made at the dentate line. A sleeve of mucosa is dissected free from the internal sphincter using sharp dissection **B**.

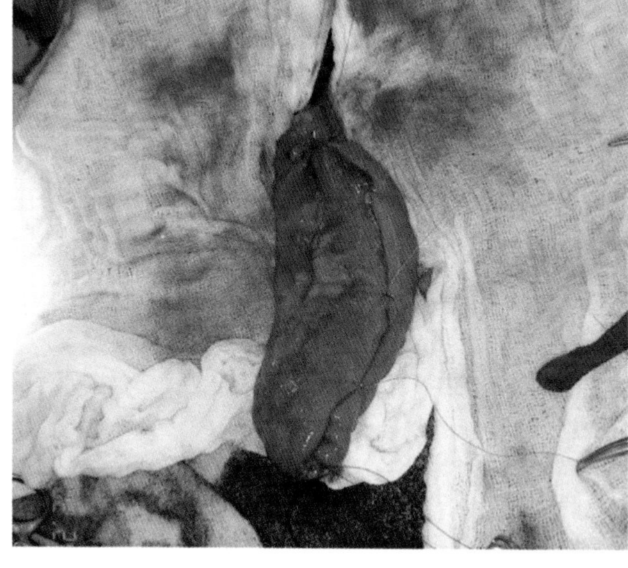

FIGURE 29-9. Ileal J-Pouch. Intraoperative photograph showing the two limbs of the ileum properly oriented using stay sutures.

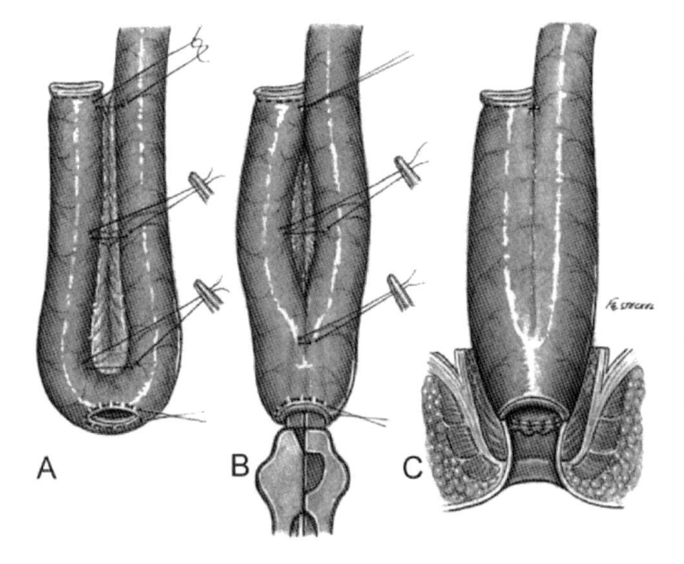

FIGURE 29-8. Ileal J-pouch creation. **A** The limbs of the ileum are oriented using stay sutures. **B** The common wall of the two limbs is then divided using a linear cutting stapler placed through an apical antimesenteric enterotomy. **C** The J-reservoir is then placed within the rectal muscular sleeve and sutured to the dentate line. (From Veidenheimer MC. Mucosal proctectomy, ileal J-reservoir, and ileoanal anastomosis. In: Braasch JW, Sedgwick CE, Veidenheimer MC, Ellis FH Jr., editors. Atlas of abdominal surgery. Philadelphia: WB Saunders; 1991).

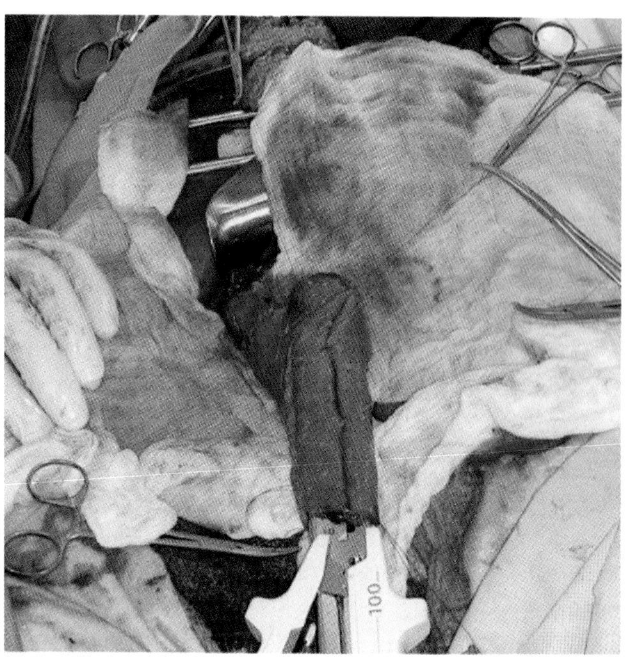

FIGURE 29-10. Ileal J-Pouch. Intraoperative photograph showing application of the linear stapler through the apical enterotomy. Note how the stay sutures are helpful in advancing the bowel over the stapler.

the symphysis pubis in order to accomplish a tension-free ileoanal anastomosis. Selective division of mesenteric vessels to the apex of a proposed J-pouch will allow for more length (Figure 29-12). Superficial incision on the anterior and posterior aspects of the small bowel mesentery along the course of the superior mesenteric artery, and mobilization of the small bowel mesentery up to and anterior to the duodenum, are two additional important lengthening maneuvers. The pouch is then pulled into the pelvis and the anastomosis carried out between the apex of the pouch and the dentate line, approximating full-thickness of the pouch wall to the internal sphincter and anal mucosa (Figure 29-13). A proximal defunctioning loop ileostomy is created. One or two suction drains can be placed in the presacral space and brought

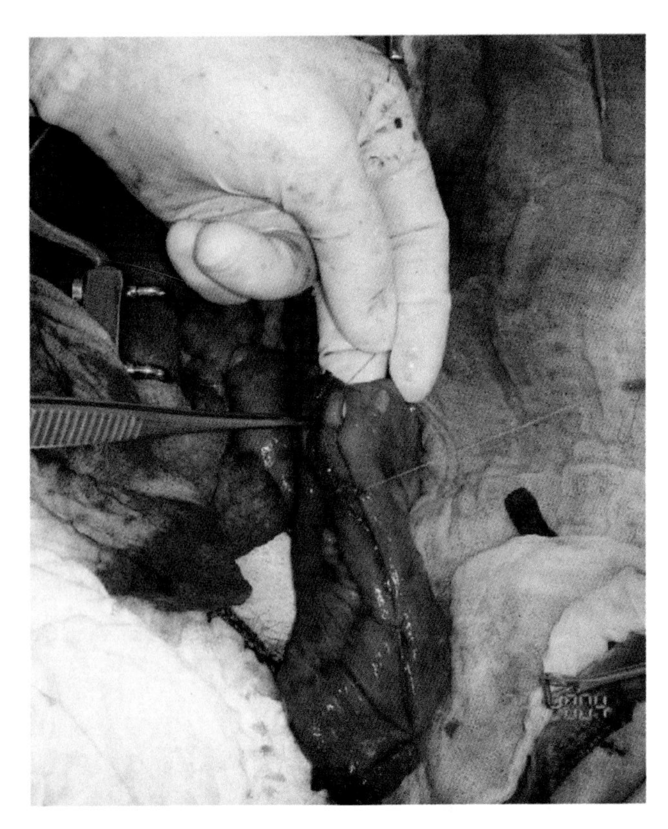

FIGURE 29-11. Ileal J-Pouch. Intraoperative photograph showing the completed J-Pouch.

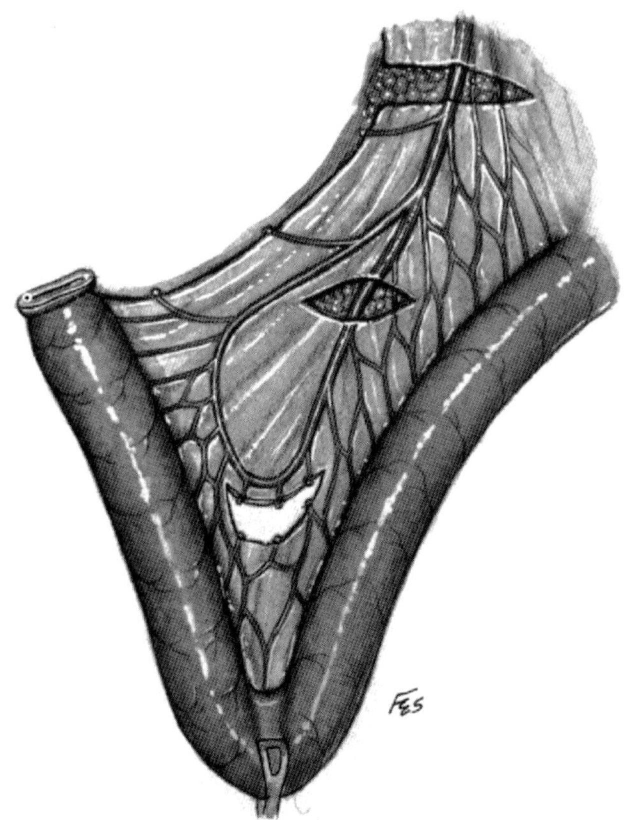

FIGURE 29-12. Ileal J-pouch. The peritoneum is scored to lengthen the mesentery. Selective division of mesenteric arcades is used to produce additional length (From Veidenheimer MC. Mucosal proctectomy, ileal J-reservoir, and ileoanal anastomosis. In: Braasch JW, Sedgwick CE, Veidenheimer MC, Ellis FH Jr., editors. Atlas of abdominal surgery. Philadelphia: WB Saunders; 1991).

out through the lower abdominal quadrant. Placement of an anti-adhesion barrier around the stoma and underneath the incision should be considered to reduce the incidence and severity of postoperative abdominal adhesions.[38]

In the double-stapled technique, the anorectum is divided by the abdominal operator approximately 2 cm above the dentate line using a right-angle linear stapler (Figure 29-14). After the pouch is created, the anvil of the mid-sized circular stapler device is tied in to the apex of the ileal pouch. Before proceeding with the anastomosis, integrity of the rectal staple line is tested using air insufflation. The stapler is placed transanally and the trocar advanced through the transverse staple line. The stapler is then closed as the abdominal surgeon ensures that no extraneous tissues are trapped within the stapling device.

Postoperative management is similar to that in patients who have had a low anterior resection. Ileostomy output can be quite high, since the stoma is more proximal than a traditional Brooke ileostomy. Patients should be encouraged to keep themselves well hydrated. In some instances, antidiarrheal medication is prescribed.

Patients are usually discharged after 7–10 days in the hospital and return 6–8 weeks later to have the temporary ileostomy closed. Before closure, however, the pouch is thoroughly investigated. Digital rectal examination is used to assess anal sphincter tone and detect anastomotic strictures or defects. The pouch is examined endoscopically

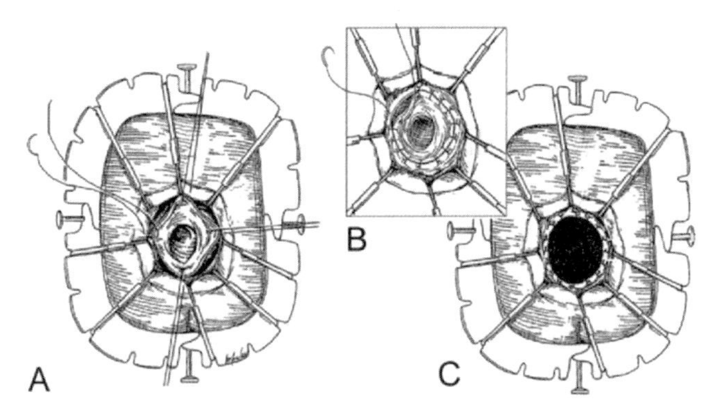

FIGURE 29-13. Handsewn ileoanal anastomosis. After the pouch is gently pulled through the anal canal by the perineal surgeon, four sutures incorporating full thickness of the pouch and a generous bite of the internal sphincter are placed at right angles to anchor the efferent limb within the anal canal **A**. The anastomosis is completed by placing sutures between each anchoring suture **B**. Completed anastomosis **C**.

to ensure that the suture lines are healed, and a contrast study is performed to detect pouch leaks, fistulas and sinus tracts. Only after confirmation that pouch abnormalities are

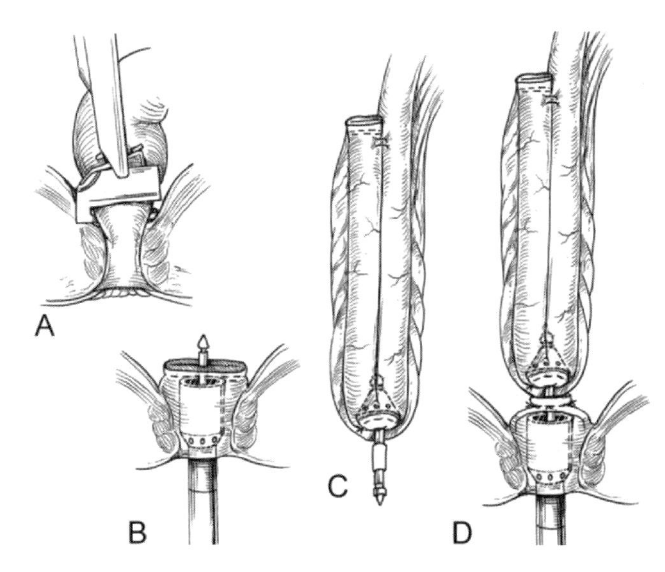

Figure 29-14. Double-stapled J pouch anastomosis. The anvil of a mid-sized circular stapler is tied into the apex of the J pouch **A**. The anorectum is divided with a stapler within the levator muscles about 1–2 cm above the dentate line. Adjacent tissue such as the bladder or vagina must be excluded from incorporation in the staple line. The integrity of the staple line should be tested with air insufflation through an anoscope **B**. The perineal operator advances the mid-sized circular stapler against the anorectal transaction site and advances the trocar through the transverse staple line **C**. The anvil mechanism is positioned onto the rod of the circular stapler. Before completing the anastomosis, the abdominal operator must prevent extraneous tissue from being trapped into the stapling device **D**.

not present is the ileostomy closed. Sphincter strengthening exercises should be encouraged in the period leading up to ileostomy closure, since they appear to improve functional results. In over 90% of patients, the ileostomy can be closed through a peristomal incision. However, in the remainder the midline abdominal incision must be reopened.

Postoperative Complications

Performing an IPAA is safe, with reported mortality rates ranging 0–1%.[39] In distinct contrast to mortality, however, morbidity after IPAA remains considerable. Small bowel obstruction occurs in 20% of patients and results from adhesion formation to the large number of raw surfaces after colectomy and from kinking at the ileostomy site. Most of the obstructive episodes occur in the immediate period after either procedure. Although an initial trial of nonoperative therapy is appropriate, surgical intervention may ultimately be required.[40] Several strategies have been devised to prevent adhesion formation. Intraoperative application of a bioresorbable adhesion barrier may reduce the incidence of clinical adhesive SBO.[41]. It is also anticipated that the incidence of adhesive SBO will be reduced with the increasing use of laparoscopic IPAA.

Although the incidence has steadily decreased with increasing surgical experience, pelvic sepsis still occurs in 5% of patients after IPAA. Septic complications result from anastomotic dehiscence or an infected pelvic hematoma. Pelvic sepsis may present in the immediate postoperative period or it may be delayed, manifesting as abscess formation (usually presacral) or a perineal fustula. The symptoms suggestive of early pelvic sepsis are fever, anal pain, tenesmus, and discharge of pus or secondary hemorrhage through the anus. Diagnosis is confirmed using computed tomography (CT) or magnetic resonance imaging (MRI), which demonstrates the presence of an abscess or of edematous tissues. As patients who develop sepsis in the early postoperative period have a higher likelihood of subsequent pouch failure,[42] an aggressive therapeutic approach should be adopted in these patients. Although most patients respond to intravenous antibiotics within 24–36 h, patients with ongoing sepsis and an organized abscess should undergo early operative endoanal or imaging-guided percutaneous drainage. If drainage of the cavity is unsatisfactory, an attempt should be made to deroof the abscess and curette the cavity through the anus, creating a large communication between the abscess and the reservoir. A catheter should be placed into the cavity to promote drainage and irrigation. Sometimes several local procedures are needed to eradicate sepsis. Although relaparotomy is reserved for cases in which CT-guided drainage or minor surgery has failed to control sepsis and also for patients who deteriorate quickly with signs of generalized peritonitis, this approach is rarely needed.

The reported incidence of ileoanal anastomotic stricture has varied between 5 and 38%,[43–46] and depends in part on the definition of stricture used by different authors. For some, a stricture is a narrowing of the anastomosis that requires at least two dilations[44,45] whereas for others, a stricture is narrowing associated with pouch-outlet obstruction and poor evacuation that requires repeated dilations. The etiology is usually anastomotic tension that also predisposes to infection from leakage. Full mobilization of the mesentery and avoidance of traction on the reservoir are key technical maneuvers to avoid stricture formation. Anchoring the pouch to surrounding tissues may prevent direct tension on the anastomosis itself. Avoidance of sepsis is paramount to a successful outcome. An apparent stricture may be noted when digital examination is carried out for the first time after the operation. These asymptomatic web-like strictures can be easily disrupted by gentle passage of the finger. More fibrotic strictures can usually be fractured digitally, but occasionally the insertion of graded dilators under anesthesia is necessary. Operative management usually requires repeated dilatations yet reasonable function can be expected in over 50% of patients.[44,45,47] Rarely, a transanal approach involving excision of the stricture and pouch advancement distally is necessary.[48]

Anastomotic separation is seen in approximately 10% of patients. If this complication is recognized during preileostomy closure contrast studies or as a defect on digital examination, ileostomy closure should be delayed until complete clinical and radiographic evidence of healing. Local drainage procedures for an associated abscess or a direct repair of the separation are sometimes necessary.[49] This aggressive approach will almost always be successful, allowing ileostomy closure.

The reported incidence of pouch-vaginal fistula ranges from 3 to 16%.[50–53] The patient complains of a vaginal discharge and clinical examination usually demonstrates the fistula. Occasionally, it is only detected by radiological contrast enema (pouchogram). It is important to exclude a pouch-vaginal fistula by careful operative examination of the vagina as well as the anal canal before closing the defunctioning ileostomy. The fistula may present before ileostomy closure or after stoma closure.[50] The internal opening is usually located at the ileoanal anastomosis, but less often it may arise at the dentate line, perhaps as a form of cryptoglandular sepsis. Causative factors may include injury to the vagina or rectovaginal septum during the rectal dissection or anastomotic dehiscence with pelvic sepsis. The latter is probably the major predisposing factor as pelvic sepsis rates are significantly higher in patients with pouch–vaginal fistula than in those without.[54] CD has been reported to be more common in patients with pouch–vaginal fistula, yet is difficult to prove in the majority of cases. Management depends on the severity of symptoms. When these are minimal and acceptable to the patient, no action or the placement of a seton may be all that is necessary.[52] In those with a clinically significant degree of incontinence, a diverting ileostomy should be established if not already present. The defunctioning, sepsis is drained with or without placement of a seton suture and, once it has settled, repair is indicated. Simple defunctioning alone does not often lead to fistula closure.[55] Medical therapy is not indicated in managing these fistulas, although one recent series showed efficacy of infliximab.[56] Surgical options are divided into abdominal and local procedures. The former includes abdominal revision with advancement of the ileoanal anastomosis, and the latter fistulectomy with or without sphincter repair, endoanal advancement flap repair, and endovaginal or transvaginal repair. The height of the ileoanal anastomosis is the essential feature that influences the choice of operative approach. Pouch–vaginal fistula from an anastomosis at or above the anorectal junction should be approached abdominally with pouch dissection, repair of the vaginal defect, and creation of a new ileoanal anstomosis. Several reports have reported an approximately 80% success rate using this approach.[55,57,58] A fistula arising from an anastomosis within the anal canal should not be treated with an abdominal procedure as there is not sufficient distal anal canal length to be clear of the fistula. A local procedure is necessary in such circumstances and most surgeons have used either an endoanal ileal advancement flap procedure[50,51,53,54] or a transvaginal technique.[59] Although both approaches result in fistula closure in 50–60% of cases, the transvaginal repair may have an advantage over the endoanal technique as it allows a direct approach to the fistula without the possibility of sphincter damage. Another alternative is the use of a gracilis muscle interposition.[60]

The most frequent long-term complication after IPAA for UC is a nonspecific inflammation of the ileal pouch commonly known as pouchitis.[61–63] There are two clinical forms of pouchitis. Acute pouchitis responds rapidly to oral antibiotic treatment. In a smaller number of patients, chronic pouchitis can develop, a condition requiring long-term therapy with antibiotics or other agents.[64] Clinical factors associated with acute pouchitis include the use of steroids before colectomy and smoking. Factors directly related to chronic pouchitis are the presence of extraintestinal disease such as primary sclerosing cholangitis, elevated platelet count, and length of follow-up after IPAA. Smoking appears to protect against the development of chronic pouchitis.[65,66] Expression of the serologic factors, perinuclear antineutrophil cytoplasmic antibody (pANCA) and CBir1, before colectomy predict the development of acute and chronic pouchitis after IPAA.[67,68] The etiology of this nonspecific inflammation is unclear, but as with the continent ileostomy may be due to an overgrowth of anaerobic bacteria. Presenting symptoms include abdominal cramps, fever, pelvic pain, and sudden increase in stool frequency. Treatment of pelvic reservoir pouchitis relies primarily on the use of antibiotics such as metronidazole and ciprofloxacin.[69,70] A mixture of probiotics is useful in most IPAA patients after resolution of the acute symptoms to prevent recurrence of pouchitis.[71] Although these regimens are almost always successful, occasionally steroid enemas or 5-aminosalicylates will be necessary. Uncommonly, an ileostomy with or without pouch excision is required for severe refractory pouchitis.

The number of bowel movements after successful ileoanal pouch procedures averages six per 24 h. Most patients are not particularly concerned with how often they defecate since most can postpone defecation to accommodate social and recreational activities. Major incontinence is very unusual, although minor incontinence to mucus or stool, particularly at night, is observed in approximately 30% of patients. These patients are managed effectively with good perianal hygiene and the occasional use of a perineal pad. Although continence is clearly altered after pelvic pouch surgery, quality of life is extremely well preserved.[72] Quality-of-life studies have disclosed that more than 95% of patients are satisfied with their pouch[73] and would not go back to an ileostomy. In order to obtain these results, however, approximately one half of patients regularly take a bulking agent or antidiarrheal medication to help regulate their bowels. Many patients also tend to eat less in the evening than at midday in order to minimize bowel movements when they are going out or while sleeping. Total failure, defined as removal of the pouch, occurs in only 5–8% of cases and is usually caused by pelvic sepsis, undiagnosed CD, or an unacceptable functional outcome.

Issues related to fertility, pregnancy, and the preferred method of delivery are of great importance in the female IPAA patient, many of whom are young and within their reproductive years. Two large studies showed a significant decrease in postoperative fertility.[74,75] Results of a recent systematic review were more promising, revealing an infertility rate of 12% before restorative proctocolectomy and only 26% after surgery based on 7 studies and 945 evaluable patients.[76] The decrease in postoperative fertility was attributed to probable tubal occlusion from adhesions, a phenomenon observed in another study.[77] However, physician recommendations against conception and patient concerns about having children affected with UC could not be discounted.[74] There are a number of strategies to improve fertility in these patients. Application of an anti-adhesion membrane around the fallopian tubes and ovaries during surgery is recommended. Surgeons may also consider delaying proctectomy until a family has been established. Finally, since laparoscopy appears to reduce the number of peritubal adhesions after IPAA,[78] minimally invasive surgery should be strongly considered in all young females.

The optimal method of delivery remains controversial. Cesarean section decreases the risk of incontinence resulting from damage to the anal sphincters and yet is associated with complications inherent to abdominal surgery, including injury to the pelvic pouch and adhesion formation. Vaginal delivery may damage the pudendal nerve and the anal sphincter mechanism, but it reduces the problems associated with abdominal surgery and recovery is more rapid. Recent reports show a higher incidence of an anterior sphincter defects and lower mean squeeze anal pressures following vaginal delivery compared with cesarean delivery in women with an IPAA.[79] In the short-term, vaginal delivery does not seem substantially to influence pouch function or quality of life.[76,80] However, vaginal delivery has been shown to cause occult sphincter damage[81] and injury to the innervation of the pelvic floor in normal females.[82] These factors could lead to an increased risk of fecal incontinence with age, which would be particularly devastating in a patient with a pelvic pouch.

Controversies

In approximately 10% of colitis patients, there are inadequate diagnostic criteria to make a definite distinction between UC and CD, especially in the setting of fulminant colitis.[83,84] Although some studies have found higher rates of perineal complications, development of CD, and eventual pouch loss in IC patients,[85] other papers have suggested that IC patients have outcomes comparable to UC patients.[86,87] These conflicting results in part arise from the retrospective design, small patient number, suboptimal patient follow-up and referral center bias typical of these studies. The disparate results also arise from widespread confusion over the precise diagnosis of IC. Even though the term IC was initially applied to resection specimens,[83] it has in recent years been also used in patients having atypical preoperative radiographic or endoscopic features, including biopsy specimens. This had resulted in many studies including patients with indeterminate features preoperatively, postoperatively, or both. Recently published World Congress of Gastroenterology recommendations recommend that the diagnosis of IC should be made only after colectomy, and that the term inflammatory bowel disease-unclassified (IBDU) be used in all other cases where definitive features of CD and UC are absent.[88] A large, prospective study recently reported the incidence of acute pouchitis, chronic pouchitis, and de novo CD after ileal pouch–anal anastomosis do not differ significantly between patients with UC, IBDU, or IC.[86] Patients with IBDU and IC can undergo ileal pouch–anal anastomosis and expect a long-term outcome equivalent to patients with UC.

Another debated issue is whether IPAA should be offered to elderly patients. Two reasons to avoid these procedures in older patients relate to the higher incidence of anal sphincter dysfunction with increasing age and the morbidity of reoperations in these potentially medically compromised patients. However operations for rectal cancer with anastomosis to the anal sphincter are regularly undertaken in patients in their seventh and eighth decades, and thus many surgeons contend that an IPAA should also be made available. Many groups have demonstrated that IPAA in the elderly patient is safe and feasible.[89,90] It appears that chronologic age should not itself be used as an exclusion criterion. Pouch procedures are feasible in suitably motivated elderly individuals who understand the risks and problems of this procedure. Although bowel frequency remains constant in the first decade after the surgical procedure,[91,92] it is unclear what will occur as the patient continues to age. Perhaps the use of a double-stapled technique with preservation of the anal transition zone might improve function over time, but this remains unproven.

Another controversy relates to the use of the IPAA in UC patients who have an established colorectal cancer. The presence of distant metastatic disease is generally a contraindication to IPAA. These unfortunate patients should be managed with segmental colectomy or abdominal colectomy with IRA to facilitate early discharge and allow them to spend the rest of their lives relatively free of complications. Patients with middle and low rectal tumors, in accordance with basic principles of cancer surgery, may not be eligible for this procedure. Radiation therapy, if indicated, should be performed preoperatively; a pelvic pouch should not be subjected to radiation because of a high incidence of pouch loss. UC patients with cecal cancers represent another unique subgroup of patients. The sacrifice of a long segment of adjacent distal ileum with its mesenteric vessels may limit positioning of the reservoir into the pelvis. If a tension-free anastomosis cannot be ensured, a Brooke ileostomy may be necessary.

Studies examining the use of the ileoanal pouch in patients with locally invasive cancers of the colon and upper rectum have been conflicting. In one series,[93] UC patients with a carcinoma had postoperative complications and functional results identical to UC patients without cancer. Metastatic disease developed in a small number of patients. In contrast, another study revealed that almost 20% of UC patients with cancer who had an IPAA died of metastatic disease.[94] Since both of these patients had T3 cancers at surgery, it is unclear that their course was adversely influenced by performing IPAA. This conservative management approach is also encouraged by surgeons at the Lahey Clinic,[95] where UC patients with a T3 cancer initially undergo an abdominal colectomy with ileostomy. An observation period of at least 12 months is recommended to ensure that no recurrent disease develops. Another reason to postpone IPAA in these patients is to allow adjuvant chemoradiation therapy to proceed unhindered without any added morbidity from a pouch–anal anastomosis and a relatively proximal ileostomy.

A number of innovations of the IPAA operation spurred by a desire to decrease complications and improve function have led to a series of technical controversies. Some authors feel that the entire rectal mucosa does not need to be removed. They favor leaving 1–2 cm of distal mucosa behind, transecting the rectum just above the puborectalis muscle and stapling the pouch to the rectal remnant. The potential advantages of the double-stapled approach include technical ease as it avoids a mucosectomy and the perineal phase of the operation, less tension on the anastomotic line, and improved functional results because sphincter injury is minimized and the anal transition zone with its abundant supply of sensory nerve endings is preserved.[96] On the other hand, surgeons who oppose this operative approach not only contend that residual diseased mucosa is at risk of malignancy, but are also concerned about the potential for continuing proctitis in the residual mucosa (i.e., cuffitis). A recent review of cases of adenocarcinoma occurring after IPAA suggested that cancer can occur when either a mucosectomy or a double-staple technique was used, whether there was dysplasia preoperatively, or whether the rectum was initially involved.[97] Although inflammation in the rectal cuff after double-stapled IPAA is commonly seen, only about 10% of these patients are symptomatic.[98] One small, uncontrolled study with significant patient dropout suggested that mesalamine suppositories might be an effective treatment for symptomatic cuffitis.[99] In an effort to resolve the handsewn versus stapled controversy, three small prospective randomized trials and one meta-analysis of those three trials failed to demonstrate any significant differences in perioperative complications or functional results in those patients where a mucosectomy was done versus those patients where the distal rectal mucosa was preserved.[100–103] It is important that the surgeon performing an IPAA be familiar with both techniques in the event of failure or inability to use the stapler or when a handsewn anastomosis is contemplated but where

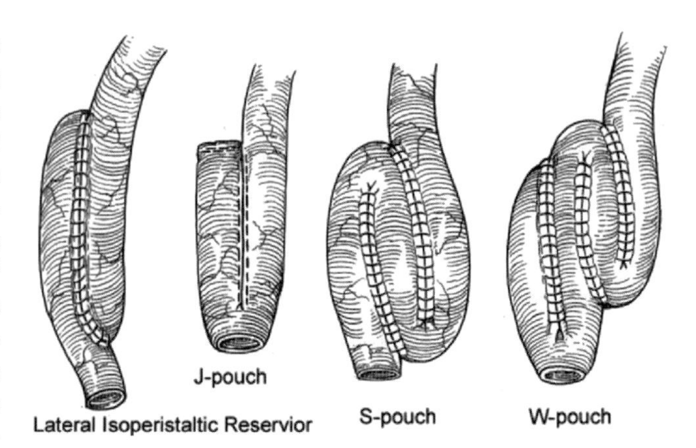

FIGURE 29-15. Different ileal pouch configurations.

anastomotic tension is excessive. It must be stressed that if a stapled technique is used, care should be taken to create an ileal pouch to anal anastomosis and not an ileal-to-rectum anastomosis. In addition, the patient must also be made aware of the need for long-term surveillance of the cuff, particularly if surgery was performed for carcinoma or dysplasia.[104] Alternatively, if mucosectomy is selected, the patients must understand that a cancer or colitis can occur in the isolated viable mucosal islands inside of the muscular cuff, but outside of the pouch serosa. Therefore these areas cannot be visualized or biopsied.

Another technical controversial issue is the shape and size of the reservoir. Although the initial ileal reservoir created by Parks in the late 1970s was a triple-loop S pouch,[32] other pouch configurations have been described in an attempt to reduce pouch complications and improve functional outcome (Figure 29-15). Three other configurations that have been described are the double-loop J pouch, the quadruple-loop W pouch, and the lateral isoperistaltic H pouch.[105–107] S pouches were initially plagued with evacuation problems associated with a long (5-cm or more) exit conduit, frequently requiring pouch catheterization.[32] With shortening of the exit conduit to 2 cm or less, mandatory catheterization has been substantially reduced.[108] The long outlet tract formed in the H pouch was also associated with pouch distention, stasis and pouchitis.[109] The W pouch has been favored by some surgeons[107] because its theoretically greater capacity may lead to fewer daily bowel movements. However, two randomized trials comparing the W and J pouch did not confirm this hypothesis.[110,111] In one study,[110], the median number of stools per day was the same in patients with a J or W pouch, and there was no difference in functional outcome between the two reservoirs in rates of incontinence, urgency, soiling, and the use of antidiarrheal agents. Johnston and coworkers[111] also demonstrated similar functional results between J and W pouches 1-year after surgery. At present, most centers perform a J pouch since it is easier and faster to construct.[110,112] An S pouch can provide additional length (2–4 cm) compared with the J pouch and can be useful in minimizing anastomotic tension. However, the 2-cm exit conduit of the S pouch may lengthen over time and obstructive defecation may develop.

A controversy that merits discussion relates to the routine use of a diverting loop ileostomy. Proponents of routine fecal diversion[113,114] contend that postoperative septic complications are minimized. Loop ileostomy also obviates the problem of immediate severe diarrhea through an edematous ileal pouch and a sphincter that has been damaged surgically by mucosectomy or double-stapling. On the other hand, many surgeons believe that the loop ileostomy is counterproductive.[115,116] Notwithstanding the additional operation and increased hospitalization associated with its closure, the morbidity of ileostomy closure is not insignificant, as small bowel obstruction and anastomosis leaks can occur. In addition, these ileostomies may be proximal in the small bowel and thus represent high-output stomas that can cause clinical dehydration. Some surgeons contend that omission of the ileostomy is safe when the anastomosis appears intact and under no tension, the procedure is not complicated by excessive bleeding or other technical difficulties, the terminal ileum is not affected by backwash ileitis, and the patients are not on high steroid doses prior to surgery. These criteria, however, have not been clearly studied in a prospective randomized fashion. It should be stressed that problems associated with the ileostomy or its closure such as dehydration, anastomotic leak, or bowel obstruction are easily managed with medical or surgical means. The development of a pouch specific complication in those patients without an ileostomy is a particularly morbid event requiring repeat laparotomy and fecal diversion in a septic patient. Clearly, more work is needed to further resolve the issue of whether an ileostomy should be routinely used in this procedure. It is clear that although associated with more skin irritation and stomal nursing care, a loop ileostomy is preferred over an end ileostomy for temporary fecal diversion after IPAA because of the ease of loop stoma closure.[117]

Many of the pelvic complications of the ileal pouch can be effectively managed by a perineal procedure. In some cases, however, these local procedures are not successful. The role of abdominal salvage surgery aimed at avoiding pouch excision or indefinite fecal diversion in patients with refractory pelvic sepsis, poor pouch function or inflammation of retained rectal mucosa remains to be defined. Successful outcomes after salvage surgery have been reported in up to 90% of UC patients.[118–121] Others, however, have reported poorer results.[42,47,122] This great variability in success rates may be explained by variation in the severity of sepsis and its location in relation to the anastomosis.[42] The duration of follow-up is also an important factor, as failure after salvage continues steadily with time.[42,47] Various factors need to be considered when advising an abdominal salvage procedure, including feasibility of success, magnitude of operation, overall duration of treatment, and the patient's wishes. Counselling is essential and the patient must be given a realistic appraisal of the prospect of a successful outcome. The potential morbidity of removal of the reservoir resulting in a permanent ileostomy should also be discussed, including the possibility of a high-output ileostomy, pelvic nerve damage, and an unhealed perineal wound.

Conclusion

The approach to the patient with UC who requires surgical intervention must begin with an honest and thorough discussion concerning the pros and cons of each procedure. Surgeons should individualize treatment based on the patients' desires, fears, and expectations. In general, those patients desiring a minimum of complications without regard for continence should undergo total proctocolectomy with Brooke ileostomy. Those patients wanting to preserve fecal incontinence, but also willing to accept a number of potential postoperative complications that in some cases may necessitate a stoma should consider an IPAA. The risk of complications and the unknown long-term effects of continence-preserving surgery require that patients be willing to undergo careful and regular follow-up. Patients not expected to comply with or take care of a continent ileostomy or IPAA should not be offered these procedures. The Standards Practice Task Force of the American Society of Colon and Rectal Surgeons has published practice parameters for the surgical treatment of UC.[123]

References

1. Lichtiger S, Present DH, Kornbluth A, et al. Cyclosporine in severe ulcerative colitis refractory to steroid therapy. N Engl J Med. 1994;330:1841–5.
2. Rutgeerts P, Sandborn WJ, Feagan BG, et al. Infliximab for induction and maintenance therapy for ulcerative colitis. N Engl J Med. 2005;353:2462–76.
3. Fleshner PR, Michelassi F, Rubin M, et al. Morbidity of subtotal colectomy in patients with severe ulcerative colitis unresponsive to cyclosporin. Dis Colon Rectum. 1995;38:1241–5.
4. Hyde GM, Jewell DP, Kettlewell MGW, et al. Cyclosporin for severe ulcerative colitis does not increase the rate of perioperative complications. Dis Colon Rectum. 2001;44:1436–40.
5. Schluender SJ, Ippoliti A, Dubinsky M, et al. Does infliximab influence surgical morbidity of ileal pouch-anal anastomosis in patients with ulcerative colitis? Dis Colon Rectum. 2007;50:1747–53.
6. Selvasekar CR, Cima RR, Larson DW, et al. Effect of infliximab on short-term complications in patients undergoing operation for chronic ulcerative colitis. J Am Coll Surg. 2007;204:956–63.
7. Eaden JA, Abrams KR, Mayberry JF. The risk of colorectal cancer in ulcerative colitis: a meta-analysis. Gut. 2001;48:526–35.
8. Goldblum JR. The histologic diagnosis of dysplasia, dysplasia-associated lesion or mass, and adenoma: a pathologist's perspective. J Clin Gastroenterol. 2003;36(Suppl):S6–69.

9. Motil KJ, Grand RJ, Davis-Kraft L, et al. Growth failure in children with inflammatory bowel disease: a prospective study. Gastroenterology. 1993;105:681–91.
10. Camilleri-Brennan J, Steele RJ. Objective assessment of quality of life following panproctocolectomy and ileostomy for ulcerative colitis. Ann R Coll Surg Engl. 2001;83(5):321–4.
11. Nessar G, Fazio VW, Tekkis P, et al. Long-term outcome and quality of life after continent ileostomy. Dis Colon Rectum. 2006;49:336–44.
12. Fazio VW, Church JM. Complications and function of the continent ileostomy at the Cleveland Clinic. World J Surg. 1988;12:148–54.
13. Lian L, Fazio VW, Remzi FH, Shen B, Dietz D, Kiran RP. Outcomes for patients undergoing continent ileostomy after a failed ileal pouch-anal anastomosis. Dis Colon Rectum. 2009;52:1409–16.
14. Mortier PE, Gambiez L, Karoui M, et al. Colectomy with ileorectal anastomosis preserves female fertility in ulcerative colitis. Gastroentérol Clin Biol. 2006;30:594–7.
15. Holubar SD, Larson DW, Dozois EJ, Pattana-arun J, Pemberton JH, Cima RR. Minimally invasive subtotal colectomy and ileal pouch-anal anastomosis for fulminant ulcerative colitis: a reasonable approach? Dis Colon Rectum. 2009;52:187–92.
16. Heuschen UA, Hinz U, Allemeyer EH, et al. Risk factors for ileoanal J pouch-related septic complications in ulcerative colitis and familial adenomatous polyposis. Ann Surg. 2002;235(2):207–16.
17. Alves A, Panis Y, Bouhnik Y, et al. Subtotal colectomy for severe acute colitis: a 20-year experience of a tertiary care center with an aggressive and early surgical policy. J Am Coll Surg. 2003;197:379–85.
18. Holubar SD, Privitera A, Cima RR, Dozois EJ, Pemberton JH, Larson DW. Minimally invasive total proctocolectomy with Brooke ileostomy for ulcerative colitis. Inflamm Bowel Dis. 2009;15:1337–42.
19. Brooke BN. The management of an ileostomy, including its complications. Lancet. 1952;2:102–4.
20. Frizelle A, Pemberton JH. Removal of the anus during proctectomy. Br J Surg. 1997;84:68–72.
21. Wickland M, Jansson I, Asztely M, et al. Gynaecological problems related to anatomical changes after conventional proctocolectomy and ileostomy. Int J Colorectal Dis. 1990;5:49–52.
22. Carlsen E, Bergan A. Technical aspects and complications of end ileostomies. World J Surg. 1995;19:632–6.
23. Kock NG, Darle N, Kewenter J, et al. Ileostomy. Curr Probl Surg. 1977;14:1–52.
24. Litle VR, Barbour S, Schrock TR, Welton ML. The continent ileostomy: long-term durability and patient satisfaction. J Gastrointest Surg. 1999;3:625–32.
25. Lepisto AH, Jarvinen HJ. Durability of Kock continent ileostomy. Dis Colon Rectum. 2003;46(7):925–8.
26. Beck DE. Clinical aspects of continent ileostomies. Clin Colon Rectal Surg. 2004;17:57–63.
27. Mullen P, Behrens D, Chalmers T, et al. Barnett continent intestinal reservoir. Multicenter experience with an alternative to the Brooke ileostomy. Dis Colon Rectum. 1995;38(6): 573–82.
28. Leijonmarck CE, Lofberg R, Hellers G. Long-term results of ileorectal anastomosis in ulcerative colitis in Stockholm County. Dis Colon Rectum. 1990;33:195–200.
29. Newton CR, Baker WNW. Comparison of bowel function after ileorectal anastomosis for ulcerative colitis and colonic polyposis. Gut. 1975;16:785–91.
30. Baker WNW, Glass RE, Richie JK, et al. Cancer of the rectum following colectomy and ileorectal anastomosis for ulcerative colitis. Br J Surg. 1978;65:862–8.
31. Soravia C, O'Connor BI, Berk T, et al. Functional outcome of conversion of ileorectal anastomosis to ileal pouch-anal anastomosis in patients with familial adenomatous polyposis and ulcerative colitis. Dis Colon Rectum. 1999;42:903–8.
32. Parks AG, Nicholls RJ. Proctocolectomy without ileostomy for ulcerative colitis. BMJ. 1978;2:85–8.
33. Johnston D, Holdsworth PJ, Nasmyth DG, et al. Preservation of the entire anal canal in conservative proctocolectomy for ulcerative colitis: a pilot study comparing end-to-end ileo-anal anastomosis without mucosal resection with mucosal proctectomy and endo-anal anastomosis. Br J Surg. 1987;74:940–4.
34. Wexner SD, James K, Jagelman DG. The double-stapled ileal reservoir and ileoanal anastomosis: a prospective review of sphincter function and clinical outcome. Dis Colon Rectum. 1991;34:487–94.
35. Rivadeneira DE, Marcello PW, Roberts PL, Rusin LC, Murray JJ, Coller JA, et al. Benefits of hand-assisted laparoscopic restorative proctocolectomy: a comparative study. Dis Colon Rectum. 2004;47:1371–6.
36. Maartense S, Dunker MS, Slors JF, et al. Hand-assisted laparoscopic versus open restorative proctocolectomy with ileal pouch anal anastomosis: a randomized trial. Ann Surg. 2004;240:984–91.
37. Ambroze Jr WL, Wolff BG, Kelly KA, et al. Let sleeping dogs lie: role of the omentum in the ileal pouch-anal anastomosis procedure. Dis Colon Rectum. 1991;34:563–5.
38. Salum MR, Wexner S, Nogueras JJ, et al. Does sodium hyaluronate and carboxymethylcellulose based bioresorbable membrane (Seprafilm) decrease operative time for loop ileostomy closure? Tech Coloproctol. 2006;10:187–91.
39. Michelassi F, Lee J, Rubin M, et al. Long-term functional results after ileal pouch anal restorative proctocolectomy for ulcerative colitis: a prospective observational study. Ann Surg. 2003;238:433–41.
40. MacLean AR, Cohen Z, MacRae HM, et al. Risk of small bowel obstruction after the ileal pouch-anal anastomosis. Ann Surg. 2002;235:200–6.
41. Fazio VW, Cohen Z, Fleshman JW, et al. Reduction in adhesive small-bowel obstruction by Seprafilm adhesion barrier after intestinal resection. Dis Colon Rectum. 2006;49:1–11.
42. Heuschen UA, Allemeyer EH, Hinz U, et al. Outcome after septic complications in J pouch procedures. Br J Surg. 2002;89:194–200.
43. Marcello PW, Roberts PL, Schoëtz Jr DJ, et al. Long-term results of the ileoanal pouch procedure. Arch Surg. 1993;128:500–3.
44. Lewis WG, Kuzu A, Sagar PM, et al. Stricture at the pouch-anal anastomosis after restorative proctocolectomy. Dis Colon Rectum. 1994;35:120–5.
45. Senapati A, Tibbs CJ, Ritchie JK, et al. Stenosis of the pouch anal anastomosis following restorative proctocolectomy. Int J Colorectal Dis. 1996;11:57–9.
46. Prudhomme M, Dozois RR, Godlewski G, et al. Anal canal strictures after ileal pouch-anal anastomosis. Dis Colon Rectum. 2003;46:20–3.

47. Galandiuk S, Scott NA, Dozois RR, et al. Ileal pouch-anal anastomosis. Reoperation for pouch-related complications. Ann Surg. 1990;212:446–52.
48. Fazio VW, Tjandra JJ. Pouch advancement and neoileoanal anastomosis for anastomotic stricture and anovaginal fistula complicating restorative proctocolectomy. Br J Surg. 1992;79:694–6.
49. Fleshman J, McLeod RS, Cohen Z, Stern H. Improved results following use of an advancement technique in the treatment of ileoanal anastomotic complications. Int J Colorectal Dis. 1988;3:161–5.
50. Wexner SD, Rothenberger DA, Jensen L, et al. Ileal pouch vaginal fistulas: incidence, etiology, and management. Dis Colon Rectum. 1989;32:460–5.
51. Groom JS, Nicholls RJ, Hawley PR, et al. Pouch-vaginal fistula. Br J Surg. 1993;80:936–40.
52. Keighley MR, Grobler SP. Fistula complicating restorative proctocolectomy. Br J Surg. 1993;80:1065–7.
53. Ozuner G, Hull T, Lee P, et al. What happens to a pelvic pouch when a fistula develops? Dis Colon Rectum. 1997;40:543–7.
54. Lee PY, Fazio VW, Church JM, et al. Vaginal fistula following restorative proctocolectomy. Dis Colon Rectum. 1997;40:752–9.
55. Paye F, Penna C, Chiche L, et al. Pouch-related fistula following restorative proctocolectomy. Br J Surg. 1996;83:1574–7.
56. Colombel JF, Ricart E, Loftus Jr EV, et al. Management of Crohn's disease of the ileoanal pouch with infliximab. Am J Gastroenterol. 2003;98:2239–44.
57. Cohen Z, Smith D, McLeod R. Reconstructive surgery for pelvic pouches. World J Surg. 1998;22:342–6.
58. Wilkinson ZR, Nicholls RJ KH. Ileal pouch-vaginal fistula treated by abdominoanal advancement of the ileal pouch. Br J Surg. 2003;90:1434–5.
59. Burke D, van Laarhoven CJ, Herbst F, et al. Transvaginal repair of pouch-vaginal fistula. Br J Surg. 2001;88:241–5.
60. Wexner SD, Ruiz DE, Genua J, Nogueras JJ, Weiss EG, Zmora O. Gracilis muscle interposition for the treatment of rectourethral, rectovaginal, and pouch-vaginal fistulas: results in 53 patients. Ann Surg. 2008;248:39–43.
61. Lohmuller JL, Pemberton JH, Dozois RR, et al. Pouchitis and extraintestinal manifestations of inflammatory bowel disease after ileal pouch-anal anastomosis. Ann Surg. 1990;211:622–7.
62. Fazio VW, Ziv Y, Church JM, et al. Ileal pouch-anal anastomoses complications and function in 1005 patients. Ann Surg. 1995;222:120–7.
63. Meagher AP, Farouk R, Dozois RR, et al. J ileal pouch-anal anastomosis for chronic ulcerative colitis: complications and long-term outcome in 1310 patients. Br J Surg. 1998;85: 800–3.
64. Mahadevan U, Sandborn WJ. Diagnosis and management of pouchitis. Gastroenterology. 2003;124:1636–50.
65. Fleshner PR, Ippoliti A, Dubinsky MC, et al. A prospective multivariate analysis of perioperative clinical factors associated with acute or chronic pouchitis after ileal pouch-anal anastomosis. Clin Gastroenterol Hepatol. 2007;5:952–8.
66. Sandborn W, LaRusso N, Schleck C, et al. Pouchitis after ileal pouch-anal anastomosis for ulcerative colitis occurs with increased frequency in patients with associated primary sclerosing cholangitis. Gut. 1996;38:234–9.
67. Fleshner PR, Vasiliauskas EA, Kam LY, et al. High level perinuclear antineutrophil cytoplasmic antibody (pANCA) in ulcerative colitis patients before colectomy predicts the development of chronic pouchitis after ileal pouch-anal anastomosis. Gut. 2001;49:671–7.
68. Fleshner PR, Vasiliauskas EA, Dubinsky M, et al. Both preoperative pANCA and anti-CBir1 expression in ulcerative colitis patients influence pouchitis development after ileal pouch-anal anastomosis. Clin Gastroenterol Hepatol. 2008;6:561–8.
69. Madden MV, McIntyre AS, Nicholls RJ. Double-blind crossover trial of metronidazole versus placebo in chronic unremitting pouchitis. Dig Dis Sci. 1994;39:1193–6.
70. Shen B, Achkar JP, Lashner BA, et al. A randomized trial of ciprofloxacin and metronidazole in treating acute pouchitis. Inflamm Bowel Dis. 2001;7:301–5.
71. Gionchetti P, Rizzello F, Venturi A, et al. Oral bacteriotherapy as maintenance treatment in patients with chronic pouchitis: a doubleblind, placebo-controlled trial. Gastroenterology. 2000;119:305–9.
72. Holubar S, Hyman N. Continence alterations after ileal pouch-anal anastomosis do not diminish quality of life. Dis Colon Rectum. 2003;46:1489–91.
73. Köhler LW, Pemberton JH, Zinsmeister AR, et al. Quality of life after proctocolectomy. A comparison of Brooke ileostomy, Kock pouch, and ileal pouch-anal anastomosis. Gastroenterology. 1991;101:679–84.
74. Olsen KO, Joelsson M, Laurberg S, et al. Fertility after ileal pouch-anal anastamosis in women with ulcerative colitis. Br J Surg. 1999;86:493–5.
75. Olsen KO, Juul S, Berndtsson I, et al. Ulcerative colitis: female fecundity before diagnosis, during disease, and after surgery compared with a population sample. Gastroenterology. 2002;122:15–9.
76. Cornish JA, Tan E, Teare J, et al. The effect of restorative proctocolectomy on sexual function, urinary function, fertility, pregnancy and delivery: a systematic review. Dis Colon Rectum. 2007;50:1128–38.
77. Oresland T, Palmblad S, Ellstrom M, et al. Gynaecological and sexual function related to anatomical changes in the female pelvis after restorative proctocolectomy. Int J Colorectal Dis. 1994;9:77–81.
78. Indar AA, Efron JE, Young-Fadok TM. Laparoscopic ileal pouch-anal anastomosis reduces abdominal and pelvic adhesions. Surg Endosc. 2009;23:174–7.
79. Remzi FH, Gorgun E, Bast J, et al. Vaginal delivery after ileal pouch-anal anastomosis: a word of caution. Dis Colon Rectum. 2005;48:1691–9.
80. Ravid A, Richard CS, Spencer LM, et al. Pregnancy, delivery, and pouch function after ileal pouch-anal anastomosis for ulcerative colitis. Dis Colon Rectum. 2003;45:1283–8.
81. Sultan AH, Kamm MA, Hudson CN, et al. Anal-sphincter disruption during vaginal delivery. N Engl J Med. 1993;329: 1905–11.
82. Snooks SJ, Setchell M, Swash M, et al. Injury to innervation of pelvic floor sphincter musculature in childbirth. Lancet. 1984;2:546–50.
83. Price AB. Overlap in the spectrum of non-specific inflammatory bowel disease – "colitis indeterminate". J Clin Pathol. 1978;31:567–77.
84. Marcello PW, Schoetz Jr DJ, Roberts PL, et al. Evolutionary changes in the pathologic diagnosis after the ileoanal pouch procedure. Dis Colon Rectum. 1997;40:263–9.

85. Yu CS, Pemberton JH, Larson D. Ileal pouch-anal anastomosis in patients with indeterminate colitis. Long-term results. Dis Colon Rectum. 2000;43:1487–96.
86. Dayton MT, Larsen KR, Christiansen DD. Similar functional results and complications after ileal pouch-anal anastomosis in patients with indeterminate colitis vs ulcerative colitis. Arch Surg. 2002;137:690–5.
87. Murrell ZA, Melmed GY, Ippoliti A, et al. A prospective evaluation of the long-term outcome of ileal pouch-anal anastomosis in patients with inflammatory bowel disease-unclassified and indeterminate colitis. Dis Colon Rectum. 2009;52:872–8.
88. Silverberg MS, Satsangi J, Ahmad T, et al. Toward an integrated clinical, molecular and serological classification of inflammatory bowel disease. Report of a Working Party of the 2005 Montreal World Congress of Gastroenterology. Can J Gastroenterol. 2005;19(Suppl A):5–36.
89. Takao Y, Gilliland R, Nogueras JJ, et al. Is age relevant to functional outcome after restorative proctocolectomy for ulcerative colitis? Prospective assessment of 122 cases. Ann Surg. 1998;227:187–94.
90. Chapman JR, Larson DW, DW WBG, et al. Ileal pouch-anal anastomosis: does age at the time of surgery affect outcome? Arch Surg. 2005;140:534–40.
91. McIntyre PB, Pemberton JH, Wolff BG, et al. Comparing functional results one year and ten years after ileal pouch-anal anastomosis for chronic ulcerative colitis. Dis Colon Rectum. 1994;37:303–7.
92. Bullard KM, Madoff RD, Gemlo BT. Is ileoanal pouch function stable with time? Dis Colon Rectum. 2002;45:299–304.
93. Taylor BA, Wolff BG, Dozois RR. Ileal pouch-anal anastomosis for chronic ulcerative colitis and familial polyposis coli complicated by adenocarcinoma. Dis Colon Rectum. 1988;31:358–62.
94. Stelzner M, Fonkalsrud EW. The endorectal ileal pullthrough procedure in patients with ulcerative colitis and familial polyposis with carcinoma. Surg Gynecol Obstet. 1989;169:187–94.
95. Wiltz O, Hashmi HF, Schoetz Jr DJ, et al. Carcinoma and the ileal pouch-anal anastomosis. Dis Colon Rectum. 1991;34:805–9.
96. Becker JM, Lamonte WS, Marie G, et al. Extent of smooth muscle resection during mucosectomy and ileal pouch anal anastomosis affects anorectal physiology and functional outcome. Dis Colon Rectum. 1997;40:653–60.
97. Branco BC, Sachar DB, Heimann TM, Sarpel U, Harpaz N, Greenstein AJ. Adenocarcinoma following ileal pouch-anal anastomosis for ulcerative colitis: review of 26 cases. Inflamm Bowel Dis. 2009;15:295–9.
98. Thompson-Fawcett MW, Warren BF. "Cuffitis" and inflammatory changes in the columnar cuff, anal transitional zone, and ileal reservoir after stapled pouch-anal anastomosis. Dis Colon Rectum. 1999;42:348–55.
99. Shen B, Lashner BA, Bennett AE. Treatment of rectal cuff inflammation (cuffitis) in patients with ulcerative colitis following restorative proctocolectomy and ileal pouch-anal anastomosis. Am J Gastroenterol. 2004;99:1527–31.
100. Seow-Choen A, Tsunoda A, Nicholls RJ. Prospective randomized trial comparing anal function after handsewn ileoanal anastomosis versus stapled ileoanal anastomosis without mucosectomy in restorative proctocolectomy. Br J Surg. 1991;78:430–4.
101. Luukkonen P, Jarvinen H. Stapled versus hand sutured ileoanal anastomosis in restorative proctocolectomy: a prospective randomized trial. Arch Surg. 1993;128:437–40.
102. Reilly WT, Pemberton JH, Wolff BG, et al. Randomized prospective trial comparing ileal pouch-anal anastomosis performed by excising the anal mucosa to ileal pouch-anal anastomosis. Ann Surg. 1997;225:666–76.
103. Schluender S, Mei L, Yang H, Fleshner P. Can a meta-analysis answer the question: is mucosectomy with handsewn or double-stapled anastomosis better in ileal pouch-anal anastomosis? Am Surg. 2006;72:912–6.
104. Remzi FH, Fazio VW, Delaney CP, et al. Dysplasia of the anal transitional zone after ileal pouch-anal anastomosis: results of prospective evaluation after a minimum of ten years. Dis Colon Rectum. 2003;46:6–13.
105. Fonkalsrud EW. Total colectomy and endorectal ileal pullthrough with internal ileal reservoir for ulcerative colitis. Surg Gynecol Obstet. 1980;150:1–8.
106. Utsunomiya J, Iwama T, Imago M, et al. Total colectomy, mucosal proctectomy and ileoanal anastomosis. Dis Colon Rectum. 1980;23:459–66.
107. Nicholls RJ, Lubowski DZ. Restorative proctocolectomy: the four loop (W) reservoir. Br J Surg. 1987;74:546–66.
108. Rothenberger DA, Buls JG, Nivatvongs S, et al. The Parks S ileal pouch and anal anastomosis after colectomy and mucosal proctectomy. Am J Surg. 1985;149:390–4.
109. Stone MM, Lewin K, Fonkalsrud EW. Late obstruction of the lateral ileal reservoir after colectomy and endorectal ileal pullthrough procedures. Surg Gynecol Obstet. 1986;162:411–7.
110. Keighley MRB, Yoshioka K, Kmiot W. Prospective randomized trial to compare the stapled double lumen pouch and the sutured quadruple pouch for restorative proctocolectomy. Br J Surg. 1998;75:1008–11.
111. Johnston D, Williamson MER, Lewis WG, et al. Prospective controlled trial of duplicated (J) versus quadrupled (W) pelvic ileal reservoirs in restorative proctocolectomy for ulcerative colitis. Gut. 1996;39:242–7.
112. Fazio VW, Tjandra JJ, Lavery IC. Techniques of pouch construction. In: Nicholls RJ, editor. Restorative proctocolectomy. Cambridge, MA: Blackwell Scientific; 1993.
113. Galandiuk S, Wolff BG, Dozois RR, et al. Ileal pouch-anal anastomosis without ileostomy. Dis Colon Rectum. 1991;34:870–3.
114. Tjandra JJ, Fazio VW, Milsom JW, et al. Omission of temporary diversion in restorative proctocolectomy – is it safe? Dis Colon Rectum. 1993;36:1007–14.
115. Gorfine SR, Gelernt IM, Bauer JJ, Harris MT, Kreel I. Restorative proctocolectomy without diverting ileostomy. Dis Colon Rectum. 1995;38:188–94.
116. Mowschenson PM, Critchlow JF, Peppercorn MA. Ileoanal pouch operation: long-term outcome with or without diverting ileostomy. Arch Surg. 2000;135:463–5.
117. Fonkalsrud EW, Thakur A, Roof L. Comparison of loop versus end ileostomy for fecal diversion after restorative proctocolectomy for ulcerative colitis. J Am Coll Surg. 2000;190:418–22.
118. Ogunbiyi OA, Korsgen S, Keighley MR. Pouch salvage. Long-term outcome. Dis Colon Rectum. 1997;40:548–52.
119. Fazio VW, Wu JS, Lavery IC. Repeat ileal pouch-anal anastomosis to salvage septic complications of pelvic pouches: clinical outcome and quality of life assessment. Ann Surg. 1998;228:588–97.

120. MacLean AR, O'Connor B, Parkes R, Cohen Z, McLeod RS. Reconstructive surgery for failed ileal pouch-anal anastomosis: a viable surgical option with acceptable results. Dis Colon Rectum. 2002;45:880–6.
121. Tekkis PP, Heriot AG, Smith JJ, Das P, Canero A, Nicholls RJ. Long-term results of abdominal salvage surgery following restorative proctocolectomy. Br J Surg. 2006;93:231–7.
122. Shawki S, Belizon A, Person B, Weiss E, Sands D, Wexner SD. What are the outcomes of reoperative restorative proctocolectomy and ileal pouch-anal anastomosis surgery? Dis Colon Rectum. 2009;52:884–90.
123. Cohen JL, Strong SA, Hyman NH, et al. Practice parameters for the surgical treatment of ulcerative colitis. Dis Colon Rectum. 2005;48:1997–2009.

30
Crohn's Disease: Surgical Management

Scott A. Strong

Introduction

Crohn's disease is a chronic, unremitting inflammatory condition of uncertain etiology that can affect the entirety of the alimentary tract. Appropriate diagnosis and management of the disease requires collaboration among physicians, radiologists, pathologists, and surgeons who work to safely maintain a satisfactory quality of life in patients who suffer from this incurable disorder. Depending upon the patient age, disease location, disease behavior, and other clinical parameters, the surgeon uses intestinal bypass, strictureplasty, and/or bowel resection to manage disease that is confounded by complications or refractory to conventional medical therapy. Particular care must be taken during surgery to address all areas of symptomatic disease while minimizing the risk for future complications arising from recurrent disease.

Prevalence

Increasing trends in the worldwide prevalence of Crohn's disease have been observed with a broad north–south gradient still prevailing in Europe.[1] The highest incidence areas are still seen in distinct regions of Canada, France, New Zealand, Netherlands, Scandinavia, and Scotland. While affluence and an industrialized status are common associations between endemic areas, an etiological role cannot be clearly supported based upon the current evidence.

Crohn's disease is recognized to demonstrate a bimodal age distribution with the first peak occurring between the ages of 15 and 30 years and the second between 60 and 80 years. However, most patients experience the onset of disease symptoms before 30 years of age. The disorder is more common in whites than in blacks, Hispanics, or Asians, and a two to fourfold increase in the prevalence has been found among the Jewish population in the USA, Europe, and South Africa compared to other ethnic groups.[2,3]

In a sample of nine million Americans, Kappelman and colleagues[4] recently reported the prevalence of Crohn's disease in patients aged younger and older than 20 years to be 43 and 201 per 100,000, respectively. A slight male predominance was seen in the pediatric population and a converse female predominance was noted in adulthood. Overall, only subtle regional differences in the prevalence were seen with the lowest prevalence observed in the South. However, the amount of geographic variation was less than that seen reported in Canada and Europe.

Etiopathology

The development of Crohn's disease likely involves host genetics, an environmental trigger, and altered immune responses. A recent review[5] of eight genome-wide association studies performed in Crohn's disease have identified several loci influencing disease susceptibility and a meta-analysis[6] implicated another 20–30 loci. Many of the new findings in Crohn's disease segregate into particular biological pathways and functions. Two particular pathways have generated significant interest.[7] The first of these involves autophagy, which is responsible for the recycling of cellular organelles and long-lived proteins, and plays an important role in tissue homeostasis as well as intracellular bacteria processing. The second is the IL-23/Th17 pathway. IL-23 stimulates the Th17 cell population to produce IL-17 and other pro-inflammatory cytokines involved in intestinal inflammation.

Environmental triggers of Crohn's disease have been long sought and research is based upon epidemiological, clinical, and experimental studies. To date, three hypotheses associate environmental factors with the etiopathology of Crohn's disease and they include the hygiene, infection, and cold chain hypotheses. Although the role of smoking as a risk factor has been reasonably well established,[8] many other environmental factors have been investigated, including diet, drugs, infectious agents, social status, and stress. Among these other factors, antibiotics, oral contraceptives, and selected microbes could potentially play a role in the triggering of Crohn's disease.[9–11]

D.E. Beck et al. (eds.), *The ASCRS Textbook of Colon and Rectal Surgery: Second Edition*,
DOI 10.1007/978-1-4419-1584-9_30, © Springer Science+Business Media, LLC 2011

In normal intestine, the immunologic character is typified by suppression or tolerance of immune responses against nonpathogens present within the gut lumen. These nonpathogens include both commensal flora and dietary antigens. Conversely, this tolerant state, at least to specific components of the flora, is lost in patients with Crohn's disease. Tolerance is mediated by regulatory cells that control immune responses, and these cells may be ineffectively activated or maintained in Crohn's disease. Although the cellular constituents are responsible for the inflammation, the cellular products and their effect on other local cell populations lead to the actual disease manifestations and the particular disease behavior is likely dictated by the distinct pathway involved in the abnormally regulated inflammatory response. Mounting evidence also suggests that the inflammatory mediators may transition over time because of the natural disease course or in response to medical therapy.[7]

Therefore, Crohn's disease likely arises in a genetically susceptible individual exposed to an ordinarily harmless trigger that initiates a dysregulated inflammatory response causing an aggressive and persistent inflammatory response that becomes progressively resistant to medical therapy during the patient's lifetime.

Classification

The original classification of Crohn's disease was described nearly four decades ago,[12] but inaccuracies associated with this and subsequent systems led to the development of the Vienna classification[13] and its modification, the Montreal classification.[14] The Vienna schema was generated by a World Congress of Gastroenterology Working Party that prospectively designed a simple phenotypic classification system based on objective and reproducible clinical variables that include age at disease diagnosis (A), anatomic location of disease (L), and disease behavior (B).

The ability of experts to independently agree on disease phenotype using the Vienna classification in controlled trials ranged from poor to fair.[15] Accordingly, the Montreal classification was introduced. The new schema did not alter the three principal categories, but modifications within each of the variables were introduced (Table 30-1).[14]

With respect to age of onset, the Montreal classification introduced a subgroup for patients with early onset of disease because several studies have demonstrated that specific serotypes or genotypes are more frequently found in early onset Crohn's disease.

Regarding disease location, the major limitation of the Vienna classification was that the four locations were mutually exclusive, and experience suggests that upper gastrointestinal disease can commonly coexist with more distal disease. Therefore, the upper gastrointestinal disease description is now used alone or as a modifier of the ileal, colonic, or ileocolonic subgroups. Ileal disease is defined as disease limited to the lower third of the small bowel (terminal ileum) with or without cecal involvement. Colonic disease is any colon involvement between the cecum and rectum without terminal ileal disease. Ileocolonic disease is disease of the terminal ileum with colon involvement noted between the cecum and rectum. Lastly, upper gastrointestinal disease is defined as any disease location proximal to the terminal ileum.

TABLE 30-1. Montreal classification system of Crohn's disease[14]

Age of diagnosis	A1 <16 years
	A2 17–40 years
	A3 >40 years
Location	L1 Ileal
	L2 Colonic
	L3 Ileo-colic
	L4 Isolated upper
Behavior	B1 nonstricturing nonpenetrating
	B2 Stricturing
	B3 Penetrating
	P Perianal disease

The behavior variable was edited because several reports indicate that perianal fistulizing disease is not inevitably associated with penetrating intestinal disease, and it was convincingly argued that perianal disease alone required a separate subclassification.

Initial application of the Vienna classification to clinical practice demonstrated that the Crohn's disease phenotype markedly changes for a given patient over time.[16] While only 15% of patients experience an alteration in anatomic location, nearly 80% of individuals with inflammatory disease ultimately demonstrate stricturing or penetrating behavior. It is unclear whether the various classification systems fail because of the heterogeneity of the disease or the inherent shortcomings of the schema itself. Although these failings may limit the utility of the Montreal classification in clinical trials and disease management, advances in determining the genetic linkages associated with Crohn's disease will eventually lead to a classification system that combines genotype and phenotype characteristics. In order to improve clinical utility, a classification system specific for perianal Crohn's disease has been described and is shown in Table 30-2.[17]

Symptoms and Signs

The symptoms and signs of patients suffering from Crohn's disease can vary depending upon multiple factors that include the anatomic location and behavior of the disease. Chronic diarrhea is the most common presenting symptom and is defined as a decrease in fecal consistency for more than 6 weeks to adequately differentiate this from self-limited infectious diarrhea. Abdominal pain and weight loss are seen in about 70% and 60% of patients before diagnosis, respectively. Blood or mucus in the stool can be seen in 40–50% of patients with Crohn's disease of the colon, but is unusual in patients with ileal or isolated upper gastrointestinal disease.

TABLE 30-2. Perianal Crohn's disease activity index[17]

Feature	Score
Abscess	
None *or*	0
First occurrence, single abscess *or*	1
First occurrence, multiple abscesses *or*	3
First recurrence, single or multiple abscesses *or*	4
Multiple recurrence, single or multiple abscesses	5
Maximum abscess score	8
Fistula	
None	0
Short-term (<30 days) fistula *or*	1
Long-term (>30 days) fistula *or*	2
Persistent postsurgery fistula *or*	3
Recurrent fistula	3
Multiple fistulas	3
Rectovaginal/rectourethral fistula *or*	4
Recurrent rectovaginal/rectourethral fistula	6
Maximum fistula score	14
Ulcer and fissure	
None	0
Short-term (<30 days) ulcer/fissure *or*	1
Long-term (>30 days) ulcer/fissure *or*	2
Single ulcer/fissure *or*	1
Multiple ulcers/fissures	2
Maximum ulcer/fissure score	4
Stenosis	
None	0
Short-term (<30 days) stenosis *or*	1
Long-term (>30 days) stenosis	2
Recurrent stenosis	4
Maximum stenosis score	6
Incontinence score	
No incontinence *or*	0
Incontinence score of 1–6 *or*	1
Incontinence score of 7–14 *or*	3
Incontinence score >14	5
Maximum incontinence score	5
Concomitant disease[a]	
None *or*	0, 0, 0
Moderate *or*	3, 2, 1
Severe	4, 3, 2
Active fistula	4, 3, 2
Maximum concomitant disease score	18

[a]Scores are for rectal, colonic, and small-bowel disease, respectively.

The most common of the recognized extra-intestinal manifestations, are abnormalities involving the axial and peripheral joints of the musculoskeletal system, which are most frequently seen when Crohn's disease affects the colon.[18]

Diagnosis

The initial diagnosis of Crohn's disease is based on an amalgamation of clinical, laboratory, imaging, endoscopic, and histologic findings. Although no single diagnostic test provides an unequivocal verdict, differing studies used in varying combinations can usually provide the information required to diagnose Crohn's disease. Accordingly, the current view is that the diagnosis is established by a defined combination of findings from clinical presentation, radiology, endoscopy, surgery, histology, and perhaps serology. Lennard-Jones and colleagues[19] were among the first to define macroscopic and microscopic criteria required to establish the diagnosis.

With evolving therapies that now allow physicians and surgeons to effectively treat nearly all forms of Crohn's disease, the success of these treatments depends upon the clinician's ability to recognize the extent and nature of disease. Therefore, the investigative studies must not only correctly identify the diagnosis of Crohn's disease, but also accurately assess its location, behavior, and severity. This knowledge is especially important in many scenarios such as distinguishing colonic Crohn's disease from ulcerative colitis and other colitides, inflammatory sites of narrowing from fibrotic strictures, intra-abdominal abscesses from phlegmons, and complex fistulas from simple fistulas.

A thorough history and physical examination might suggest the form of disease as earlier suggested, but laboratory testing can help identify patients with complicating disorders, such as anemia, inflammation, or malnutrition, or monitor response to therapy. Anemia and thrombocytosis represent the most common changes in the complete blood count in patients with Crohn's disease.[18] The C-reactive protein (CRP) and erythrocyte sedimentation rate (ESR) are standard laboratory surrogates of the acute phase response to inflammation. CRP broadly correlates with disease severity as assessed by standard indices, and the CRP level can be monitored to measure serial changes in inflammatory activity because of its relatively short half-life of 19 hours.[20,21] The ESR less accurately measures intestinal inflammation because it reflects changes in both plasma protein concentration and packed cell volume. Although the ESR level parallels disease activity, it better correlates with colonic than with ileal disease.[22]

The usage of imaging studies has greatly expanded in recent years with the advent of computed tomographic (CT) enterography and enteroclysis. These modalities differ from standard CT imaging of the abdomen and pelvis by using intraluminal bowel distention with neutral enteric contrast, mutidetector CT with narrow slice thickness and reconstruction interval, and intravenous contrast administration followed by delayed scans that optimize bowel wall enhancement (Figure 30-1). CT enterography has largely supplanted barium examinations because the CT study is more sensitive and allows improved visualization of small bowel loops within the pelvis.[23] Contrast-enhanced magnetic resonance imaging (MRI) enterography and enteroclysis also accurately display bowel wall changes in early Crohn's disease and appear to provide results comparable to those seen with CT studies without the risk of exposure to ionizing radiation.[23] Similar to the advances seen with imaging studies, endoscopic evaluation techniques have evolved from traditional ileocolonoscopy and esophagogastroduodenoscopy to now include capsule endoscopy and double-balloon

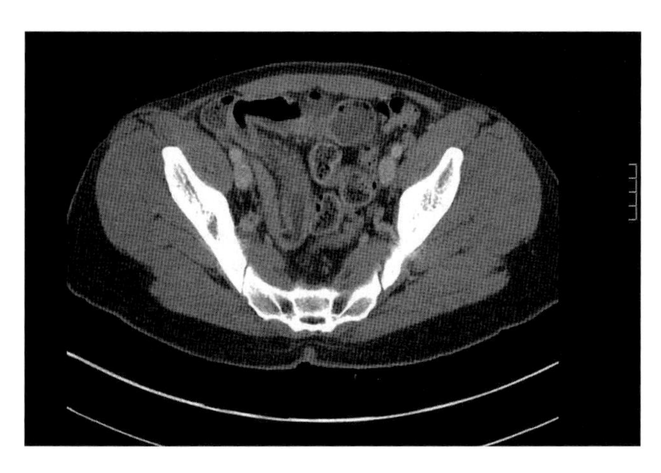

FIGURE 30-1. CT enterography.

enteroscopy, which allow visualization of small bowel that was previously impossible to view.

Microscopic features can be only partly judged on mucosal biopsy, but completely assessed on an operative specimen. The diagnosis of Crohn's disease typically depends on the finding of discontinuous and often granulomatous intestinal inflammation. The European Crohn's and Colitis Organization recently offered a consensus statement detailing the microscopic features required for the histologic diagnosis of Crohn's disease based upon findings associated with endoscopic biopsies and surgical specimens.[18]

Natural History

A recent comprehensive review of the natural history of Crohn's disease revealed that patients' initial presentations are equally distributed among ileitis, colitis, and ileocolitis, and the disease location remained relatively stable over time as earlier discussed.[24] Conversely, the majority of patients have nonstricturing, nonpenetrating disease at the time of diagnosis, but tend to evolve into a stricturing or penetrating phenotype over their lifetime.

Prior to the wide-spread usage of immunomodulators and introduction of biologic agents, approximately 1% of patients suffered continually active disease, 10% enjoyed prolonged remission, and one-half experienced a full year of remission within 3 years of diagnosis, but surgery was commonly required to achieve remission.[24] It is too early to accurately understand how advancements in medical therapy have impacted long-term disease activity and relapse rates.

Before the current medication era, steroids were prescribed to nearly one-half of patients at some time during the course of their disease. Nonresponders, sustained responders, and steroid-dependent responders comprised approximately one-fifth, one-third, and one-third of the patients receiving steroids, respectively, and one-third of patients required surgery despite treatment with steroids.[24] However, it is important to recognize that, the cumulative risk for surgery within 10 years of diagnosis is 40–55% and the risk of a second operation has been estimated to be 16%, 28%, and 35% at 5, 10, and 15 years following the initial procedure, respectively.[25]

Among unselected patients with Crohn's disease in a systematic review and meta-analysis of population-based studies focused on overall and cause-specific standardized mortality rates, overall mortality was slightly but significantly higher than that seen in the general population.[26] Regarding the cause-specific mortality, a significantly increased risk of cancer death, especially pulmonary cancer, was observed. Moreover, chronic obstructive pulmonary disease, gastrointestinal diseases, and genitourinary diseases were more commonly implicated as a cause of death in this cohort of patients.

Operative Indications

The indications for operative management of Crohn's disease include acute disease complications, chronic disease complications, and failed medical therapy. The acute complications are hemorrhage, perforation, and severe colitis with or without associated megacolon, whereas the chronic disease complications include extra-intestinal manifestations, growth retardation, and neoplasia. Failed medical therapy can take several forms, including unresponsive disease, incomplete response, medication-related complications, and noncompliance with medication.

Hemorrhage

Crohn's disease may be responsible for life-threatening lower gastrointestinal hemorrhage and even exsanguination, but fortunately this complication infrequent.[28] More commonly, entities unrelated to disease involvement, including peptic ulcer disease and gastritis, may precipitate intestinal bleeding. Accordingly, gastric aspiration and possibly esophagogastroduodenoscopy are required to exclude sources of hemorrhage indirectly associated with Crohn's disease. The principal management of disease-related hemorrhage is determined by the severity and persistence of bleeding as well as the risk for recurrence. Localization of the bleeding site is essential regardless the planned therapy.[27] In a stable patient with colonic disease, endoscopic evaluation is preferred because this approach allows for disease assessment and therapeutic attempts at control of the identified bleeding site. However, indiscriminate usage of colonoscopy for bleeding colitis should be discouraged because this form of hemorrhage typically accompanies severe colitis, and colectomy with ileostomy is advised in this instance, regardless of the endoscopic findings.

A patient who requires ongoing resuscitation to maintain hemodynamic stability or in whom a small bowel source of active bleeding is suspected should undergo emergent mesenteric angiography to localize the source of hemorrhage and arrest ongoing bleeding through superselective angiographic embolization.[28] If the hemorrhage is localized but cannot be controlled by this interventional modality, the catheter is left in position and intra-operative angiography is performed to accurately identify the bleeding site and guide a limited bowel resection.[29] Otherwise, wide resection might be unnecessarily performed to manage hemorrhage from a small ulcerated area within an extensive segment of diseased bowel.

An operation is warranted if the patient's hemodynamic state cannot be sustained, bleeding persists despite 6 units of transfused blood, hemorrhage recurs, or another indication for surgery exists. Resection with or without anastomosis is usually required for ongoing hemorrhage, whereas intraoperative enteroscopy with endoscopic therapy might be employed in less emergent settings.

Perforation

Free perforation of the small bowel is unusual and typically occurs at or immediately proximal to a stricture site.[30] The most appropriate treatment is resection of the involved bowel with or without anastomosis. A primary anastomosis without proximal diversion should be typically avoided, especially in the setting of delayed treatment, malnutrition, significant comorbidity, or severe sepsis. Instead, resection and proximal ileostomy with or without anastomosis is often recommended because it has an associated mortality rate of 4% compared to 41% with simple suture closure alone.[31] Perforation of the colon is also rare and typically requires subtotal colectomy for optimal management as these cases often occur in the setting of severe colitis or steroid usage.[32]

Severe Colitis

Severe colitis occurs in 4–6% of patients with colonic Crohn's disease and is a potentially fatal complication particularly if accompanied by megacolon. While several methods exist to accurately identify severe colitis, one reasonably simple schema employs a definition that includes a disease flare accompanied by at least six or more bloody stools per day with evidence of systemic toxicity as demonstrated by anemia (<10.5 g/dL), elevated ESR (>30 mm/h), fever (>37.8°C), or tachycardia (>90 beats/min). Use of this relatively objective definition may aid in the diagnosis and care of these patients whose severe condition can be underappreciated because of high dosages of corticosteroids, immunomodulators, or biologic agents.

Initial management in this setting is directed at reversing physiologic deficits with intravenous hydration, correction of electrolyte imbalances, and blood product transfusions. Free perforation, increasing colonic dilatation, massive hemorrhage, peritonitis, and septic shock are indications for emergent operation after the patient has been adequately resuscitated. In the absence of these features, stool studies are performed to exclude routine pathogens and *Clostridium difficile* as the cause of the acute flare. Gentle endoscopy can be used to judge the severity of disease, which potentially predicts the likelihood of treatment response. Furthermore, cautious endoscopic biopsies and serum studies are used to exclude cytomegalovirus as a cause of the fulminant symptoms.

For a presumed diagnosis of severe colonic Crohn's disease, medical therapy is initiated with high dosages of intravenous corticosteroids, immunomodulators, and/or biologic agents.[33] Broad spectrum antibiotics directed against intestinal flora are prescribed to minimize the risk of sepsis secondary to transmural inflammation or micro-perforation. Anticholinergics, antidiarrheals, and narcotics are avoided as they may worsen already impaired colonic motility or conceal ominous symptoms. The patient is closely observed with serial examinations and abdominal roentgenograms. Any worsening of the clinical course over the ensuing 24–72 h mandates urgent operation. Early surgical intervention before the occurrence of perforation typically avoids the onset of multiple organ dysfunction syndrome. Moreover, this approach reduces operative mortality rates to 2–8% compared to rates that approach 40% if perforation has occurred.[34]

If the patient minimally improves after approximately 5 days of conventional therapy, the medical therapy should be altered and hyperalimentation started if the patient is otherwise unable to maintain adequate nutritional requirements or surgery should be advised. No controlled data exists related to treatment with ciclosporin, tacrolimus, infliximab, or adalimumab in this setting.[35] Therefore, the clinician should be candid when counseling the patient about the potential risks and benefits associated with medication versus surgery. The medication's associated risk of treatment failure and serious opportunistic infections should be carefully weighed against the likelihood of operative complications or requiring a permanent ileostomy.[36] If medical therapy is pursued, patients not responding within 5–7 days should be referred for surgery, patients who do respond should be closely monitored for infections.

The principal operative options in patients with severe or fulminant colitis complicating Crohn's disease include subtotal colectomy with end ileostomy, total proctocolectomy with end ileostomy, and loop ileostomy with decompressive blowhole colostomy. Subtotal colectomy with end ileostomy is the most widely practiced of these options. The most difficult aspect of the surgery is managing the distal bowel stump. The distal limb may be closed with sutures or staples and left in the pelvis. Alternatively, if left sufficiently long, it can be delivered to the anterior abdominal wall where it can lie without tension in the subcutaneous fat of the lower midline wound. With this approach, dehiscence of the closure during the postoperative period results in a mucous fistula instead of a pelvic abscess as encountered when the closed stump is left within the peritoneal cavity. If the bowel wall is too friable to hold sutures or staples, a mucous fistula is primarily created. Rarely, instead of creating the fistula, the rectosigmoid stump must be exteriorized and wrapped in gauze to prevent retraction with a mucous fistula safely fashioned in 7–10 days.

Postoperatively, the patient typically improves over the ensuing few days and can be typically discharged within a week of the operation. An ileoproctostomy can be recommended 6 months later in selected persons who demonstrate minimal mucosal inflammation, adequate rectal compliance, absence of significant perianal disease, and sufficient sphincter strength. Otherwise, the diseased rectum is left in place and the patient is counseled about the risk of neoplasia and the need for appropriate surveillance endoscopy.[37] In these individuals, proctectomy is usually recommended if disease-related symptoms prove to be too bothersome, neoplasia is identified, surveillance is limited because of stricturing, or abdominal surgery is warranted for other reasons. Disease-related symptoms are likely to occur in patients with prior perianal disease and proctectomy is often required within the first few postoperative years.[36,38]

Proctocolectomy with end ileostomy is rarely performed in the severely ill patient with severe colitis because of the excessive rates of morbidity and mortality.[39,40] Proctectomy increases the difficulty of the procedure and risks pelvic bleeding as well as autonomic nerve damage. In rare instances of profuse colorectal hemorrhage or rectal perforation, or in the less severely ill patient who would not be a candidate for future ileoproctostomy, proctocolectomy may be a viable option. The surgeon must be cautioned, however, that primary proctocolectomy would nullify the option of a future restorative procedure.

The need for loop ileostomy combined with decompression blowhole colostomy has virtually disappeared with improved medical recognition and more sophisticated management of severe colitis. The operation is still useful in extremely ill patients or those in whom colectomy would be especially hazardous such as patients with a contained perforation, high-lying splenic flexure or pregnancy. Contraindications to the procedure include colorectal hemorrhage, intra-abdominal abscess, and free perforation. The operation is considered only a temporizing procedure, and a definitive operation is commonly performed approximately 6 months later.

Extra-intestinal Manifestations

Extra-intestinal manifestations of Crohn's disease occur in nearly 30% of patients with Crohn's disease and the occurrence of one manifestation seems to predispose to others.[41,42] Some extra-intestinal manifestations are temporally related to intestinal Crohn's disease activity, while others follow a course independent of disease activity. Some forms of peripheral arthritis, episcleritis erythema nodosum, and oral aphthous ulcers typically belong in the former group, while primary sclerosing cholangitis, pyoderma gangrenosum, spondylarthropathy, and uveitis are characteristic of the latter. Other disorders such as cholelithiasis, metabolic bone disease, and nephrolithiasis are disease complications that likely arise from altered intestinal function or medication usage.

Growth Retardation

Abnormal linear growth secondary to delayed skeletal maturation is frequently encountered in children and adolescents with Crohn's disease, especially children with upper gastrointestinal disease.[43] Specifically, nearly one-half of children may have a subnormal height velocity and approximately one-quarter have short stature.[43,44] Fortunately, surgical resection is often accompanied by growth response and pubertal progression.

Neoplasia

Overall, persons with Crohn's disease are at increased risk for developing cancer compared to the general population. In a recent meta-analysis[45] that identified 34 studies of 60,122 patients with Crohn's disease, the incidence and relative risk of cancer were calculated for patients with Crohn's disease and compared with the baseline population of patients without Crohn's disease. The relative risk of small bowel, colorectal, extra-intestinal cancer, and lymphoma compared with the baseline population was 28.4 (95% CI: 14.46–55.66), 2.4 (95% CI: 1.56–4.36), 1.27 (95% CI: 1.1–1.47), and 1.42 (95% CI: 1.16–1.73), respectively. On subgroup analysis, patients had an increased risk of colon cancer, but not of rectal cancer. Furthermore, a significant association was noted between the anatomic location of the diseased bowel and the risk of cancer in that segment.

The first endoscopic surveillance case series in patients with colonic Crohn's disease included patients with one-third or more of the colon involved by disease.[46] In this study, 259 patients were entered into a surveillance colonoscopy program. Dysplasia or cancer was identified in 16% of patients, including 10 with indefinite dysplasia, 23 with low-grade dysplasia, 4 with high-grade dysplasia, and 5 with cancer. Subsequent follow-up to this study, reported the cumulative risk of detecting any positive dysplasia or cancer after a negative screening colonoscopy to be 25% by the tenth surveillance examination.[47] Accordingly, it is recommended that patients with Crohn's disease with one-third or more of the colon involved and 8 years or more of chronic colitis should be enrolled in an endoscopic surveillance program.[46–49] The finding of multifocal low-grade dysplasia, high-grade dysplasia, or invasive cancer would likely warrant review by a second experienced pathologist and confirmation would prompt a colectomy.

Patients with primary sclerosing cholangitis are a notable exception to the practice of limiting surveillance to patients with 8 or more years of disease because of the heightened risk of colorectal cancer in these patients. Accordingly, yearly surveillance is recommended after a diagnosis of primary sclerosing cholangitis is made in the background of colonic Crohn's disease.

Failed Medical Therapy

Probiotics, antibiotics, 5-aminosalicylate compounds, corticosteroids, immunomodulators, and biologic agents all play a potential role in the management of Crohn's disease depending upon the clinical presentation. Each medication within these therapeutic groups possesses appropriate dosing parameters, associated side effects, and an optimal time interval during which beneficial effects should appear. Prior to initiating treatment with any medication, the patient should be counseled about these features and objective criteria for disease response should be discussed and then sought after an established time interval. If the desired response is not achieved, prohibitive side effects arise, or noncompliance is problematic, the medication has failed and another medication should be trialed. When all appropriate medical therapy has failed, operative intervention is warranted. The continuation of ineffective medical management risks the development of further disease complications that may detrimentally impact surgical outcome. Alternatively, some patients request an operation before exhausting all available medical therapies. A recent survey of outpatients with Crohn's disease, gastroenterologists, and colorectal surgeons underscores this attitude.[50] All participants were interviewed to quantify their preferences for six scenarios by using a prospective preference measure, and significant differences were seen between patients and gastroenterologists for three of six scenarios. Overall, 76% of gastroenterologists were willing to gamble to avoid an ileocolic resection compared with only 37% of colorectal surgeons and 39% of patients.

Operative Considerations

Some fundamental observations that must be considered when operating for Crohn's disease are as follows:

- Crohn's disease is incurable;
- Surgery is most often indicated for intestinal complications;
- Operative options are influenced by myriad factors;
- Asymptomatic disease should be ignored;
- Nondiseased bowel can be affected;
- Resection margins should be conservative (2 cm) as only a grossly normal and not microscopically normal margin is necessary;
- Mesenteric division can be difficult.

Crohn's disease is a chronic inflammatory disorder that cannot be cured by medical therapy or operative intervention. Accordingly, therapy focuses on safely alleviating disease symptoms and restoring life quality while attempting to maintain continuity of the intestinal tract. Of the various operative indications, intestinal complications, including stricturing or penetrating disease that is unresponsive to medical therapy, constitute the bulk of the indications, and the operative options depend upon multiple variables, including patient age, anatomic location, disease behavior, symptoms, prior therapies, nutritional status, comorbid conditions, and associated sepsis. The patient's symptoms are especially important because the disease encountered at the time of surgery is often unanticipated despite preoperative evaluation.[51] In these instances, the findings must be compared to the presenting symptoms and signs, and any extensive disease that does not appear to be contributing to symptoms should be typically ignored. Exceptions to this axiom include the management of out-of-circuit bowel and short, uncomplicated small bowel strictures, which should be addressed in most patients.

Nondiseased bowel can be affected by the disease process through inflammatory adhesions or internal fistulas. Every attempt should be made to conserve the nondiseased bowel, although this goal can be especially difficult when managing enteroparietal or interloop abscesses. Most internal fistulas are best managed by wedge excision and primary closure of the fistula site in the secondarily affected small bowel. However, a short segmental resection with primary anastomosis may be required for fistulas targeting the rectosigmoid region as these often enter the bowel at the mesenteric margin and simple wedge excision may be vulnerable to dehiscence of the suture line.[52,53]

Small bowel disease is best identified by digital palpation because the earliest feature of luminal disease is mesenteric ulceration, which corresponds to areas of paraintestinal neovasculature that obscure the normally distinct mesenteric edge of the bowel wall. In other words, the small bowel lumen will be macroscopically free of disease if the mesenteric margin can be palpated (Figure 30-2). Conversely, the extent of large bowel involvement is best determined by endoscopic inspection of the mucosa. Regardless the site of involvement, the bowel can be divided with a limited (2 cm) margin of grossly normal bowel without significantly jeopardizing risk for recurrent disease.[54] Frozen section analysis has no role and microscopic finding of disease at the margin need not necessitate any additional surgical intervention.

The disease process also typically causes the mesentery to be quite friable and abnormally thickened secondary to tissue

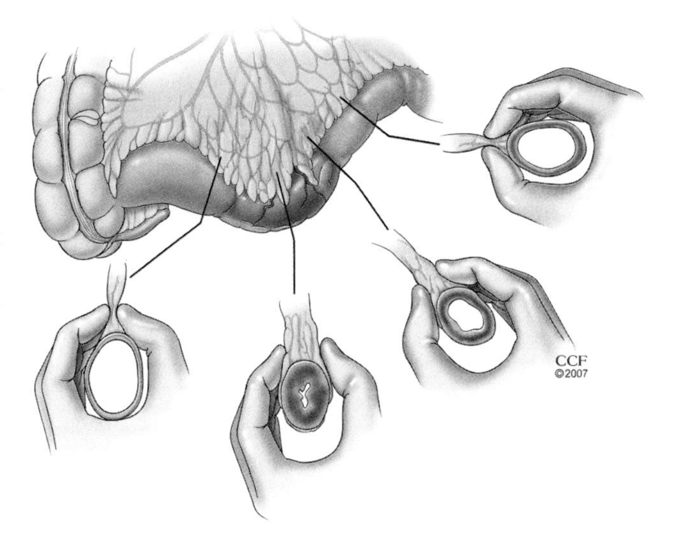

FIGURE 30-2. Mesenteric thickness associated with intestinal disease.

edema, fat deposition, and nodal enlargement. Mesenteric thickening near the vessel origin can make identification, isolation, and division of the ileocolic, middle colic, or inferior mesenteric vessels quite challenging and associated with dire consequences. Furthermore, the vasculature of diseased jejunum or proximal ileum cannot be ligated near its origin because of concerns of devascularizing nondiseased bowel that would mandate a more extensive intestinal resection.

Operative Options

The surgical procedures performed for intestinal Crohn's disease can be divided into groups depending upon whether resection of an intestinal segment is performed. The nonresectional procedures include internal bypass, external bypass, and strictureplasty, whereas the resectional procedures include resection of bowel. Patients often undergo multiple procedures at the time of their single operation and these can be a combination of nonresectional as well as resectional procedures.

Internal Bypass

Internal bypass was the procedure of choice in the early days of surgery for Crohn's disease when mortality rates associated with resection were high because of the lack of transfusion technology, antimicrobial medications, adequate anesthetic agents, and nutritional support services. However, with the advent of these modalities and recognition of complications, such as recrudescent disease, mucoceles, and malignancy arising in diverted segments, this procedure was largely abandoned. However, bypass operations may still be reasonable or even desirable in specific highly unique circumstances. A complicated ileocecal phlegmon with dense attachment to the iliac vessels or retroperitoneum can be aptly managed by an exclusion bypass if the proximal end of the excluded ileal segment is exteriorized as a small mucus fistula and definitive resection is planned to subsequently occur. Continuity bypass is sometimes the preferred method of managing symptomatic gastroduodenal Crohn's disease that is refractory to medical treatment, where resection would entail extensive reconstruction of the upper intestinal tract or pancreaticobiliary system.

External Bypass

External bypass can be permanent or temporary. Many of the stomas created to permanently bypass unresected disease fail to control symptoms secondary to the out-of-circuit bowel, and resection is ultimately warranted. High complex fistulas and deep ulcerations are among the disease characteristics likely to mandate proctectomy with permanent ostomy for persistent disease symptoms despite fecal diversion.[55] Similarly, temporary diversion intended to heal distal disease or its sequelae is usually unsuccessful unless combined with a secondary procedure, such as a rectal mucosal advancement flap that directly addresses the problem.[56] Even for free perforation of the small bowel, exteriorization of the proximal bowel alone is rarely the procedure of choice.

Strictureplasty

The incurable and pan-intestinal nature of Crohn's disease has led to a more conservative operative approach. Intestinal conservation may be maximally achieved for patients with multiple strictures of the small bowel by surgically widening the narrowed segment by performing a strictureplasty. This technique was initially described by Katariya[57] for the successful treatment of tubercular small bowel strictures, and later utilized in strictures secondary to Crohn's disease.[58] The procedure safely relieves obstructive symptoms[59–62] with the operated patients demonstrating weight gain accompanied by improved food tolerance as well as discontinuation or reduction of steroid usage.[63] Although patients undergoing strictureplasty alone experience significantly shorter recurrence-free survival than those undergoing resection and tend to be more likely to develop surgical recurrence, the procedure still plays a prominent role in the management of patients with small bowel Crohn's disease.[61]

The situations for which strictureplasty may be considered are:

- Diffuse involvement of the small bowel with multiple strictures;
- Stricture(s) in a patient who has undergone previous major resection(s) of small bowel (>100 cm);
- Rapid recurrence of Crohn's disease presenting as an obstruction;
- Stricture in a patient with short bowel syndrome;
- Nonphlegmonous fibrotic stricture.

The contraindications to strictureplasty are:

- Free or contained perforation of the small bowel;
- Phlegmonous inflammation, internal fistula, or external fistula involving the affected site;
- Multiple strictures within a short segment;
- Stricture in close proximity to a site chosen for resection;
- Hypoalbuminemia (<2.0 g/dL).

Multiple strictures in a patient with an albumin value <2.5 g/dL, preoperative weight loss, or advanced age may be regarded by some as a situation where strictureplasty should be avoided because of concerns of sepsis, but a proximal diverting stoma with multiple strictureplasties should be considered in this instance.[60] Factors that do not appear to be associated with increased operative risk include perforative or phlegmonous disease remote from the strictureplasty site, steroid dosage, synchronous resection, number of strictureplasties, and length of stricture.

The length of the strictured segment dictates the type of strictureplasty technique utilized (Figure 30-3). Short (<10 cm) strictures are best managed by a Heineke-Mickulicz-type of

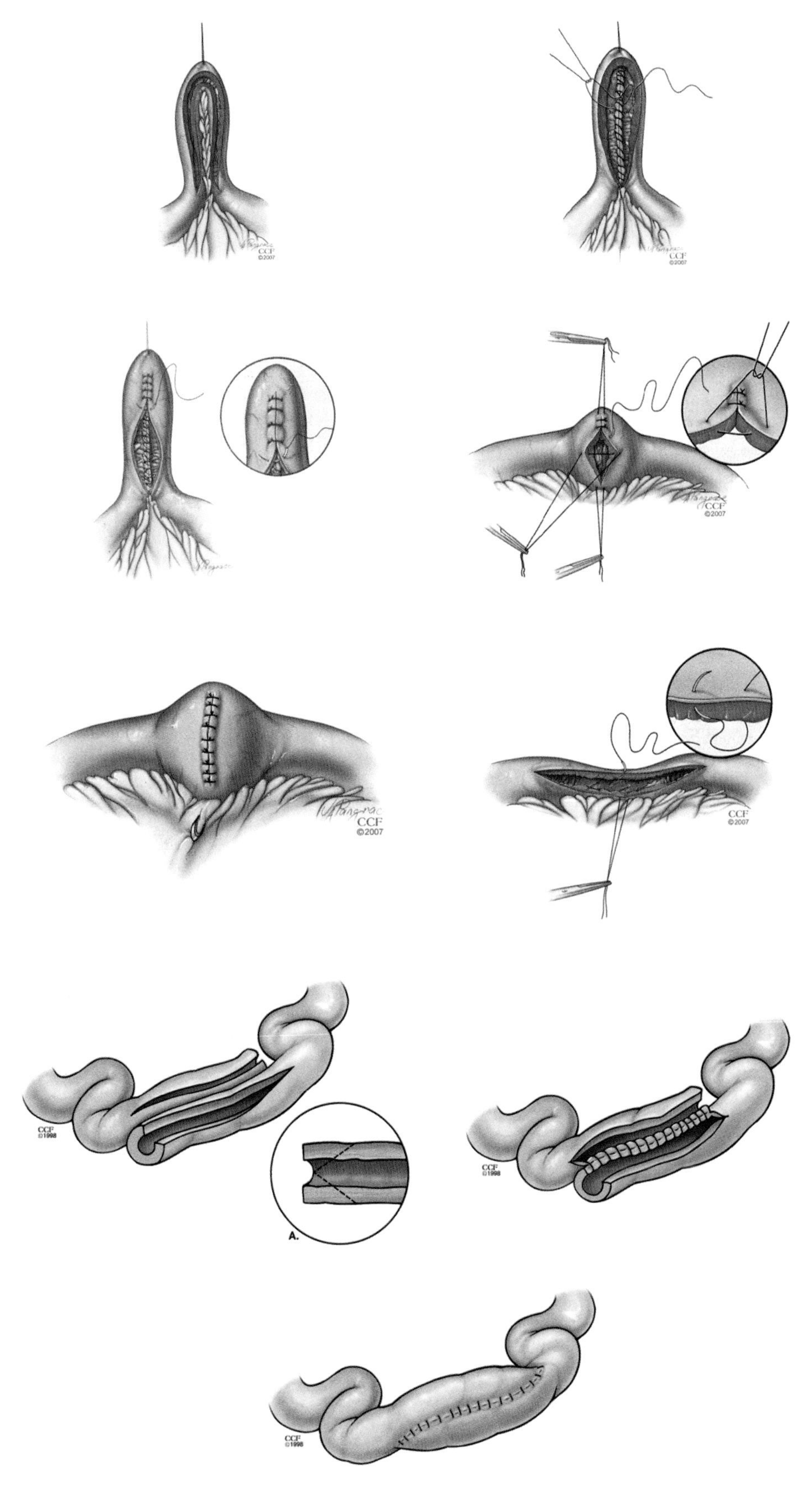

FIGURE 30-3 Strictureplasty techniques.

strictureplasty, while medium length (10–20 cm) strictures can be corrected by a Finney-type strictureplasty.[62] Long (>20 cm) strictures are best managed by a side-to-side isoperistaltic strictureplasty.[64] Regardless the technique, the bowel is incised along its antimesenteric margin extending 1–2 cm beyond the diseased segment, which is identified by the presence of mesenteric ulceration. Biopsy of any suspicious mucosa is performed to exclude carcinoma[65] and closure is achieved using an absorbable suture in a one- or two-layer fashion. The mesentery at each of the strictureplasty sites is then labeled with metallic clips to allow discrimination among the multiple sites in the unlikely event that postoperative hemorrhage occurs. Selective mesenteric angiography with intra-arterial vasopressin infusion controls most bleeding episodes, but the radio-opaque metal clips help avoid the need to open each of the strictureplasty sites to localize the bleeding site if reoperation is required.[66]

Many centers have safely and successfully employed a Finney-type strictureplasty for the the treatment of recurrent terminal ileal disease with the anastomosis created between the terminal ileum and proximal colon.[67–69]

Resection

The basic principles of resection should be followed whether an open or laparoscopic approach is utilized, and include mobilization of both diseased intestine as well as sufficient nondiseased bowel to facilitate the subsequent creation of a tension-free anastomosis or construction of an ostomy. Extensive mobilization may facilitate operations for terminal ileal disease complicated by fused ileal loops or a phlegmonous mass adherent to matted loops of small bowel, omentum, or retroperitoneal structures. Delivery of the ascending colon and terminal ileum into the wound or to the anterior abdominal wall enables separation of the involved intestinal loops and permits closer inspection to determine which segments require resection. Enteric fistulas commonly originate from diseased bowel that communicates with nondiseased intestine. While the primary site usually requires resection, the secondarily affected bowel segments are typically treated by conservative wedge excision and simple closure of the resultant defect or sometimes closure without wedge resection. The diseased bowel should be resected with conservative margins and the mesentery divided using the methods later described. The specimen should be opened after it has been delivered from the operative field to assure macroscopic disease-free resection margins.

After the diseased bowel has been resected, the surgeon must decide whether to create an end stoma, an anastomosis, or a diverted anastomosis. In general, an end stoma is desirable in patients who are critically ill, have fecal peritonitis, or suffer from coagulopathy. An anastomosis can be safely created in most other instances assuming a few general principles are respected specifically:

- Adequate blood supply must be assured;
- Tension or torsion are unacceptable;
- Luminal size needs to be equivalent;

A temporary diverting stoma should be considered to protect the anastomosis in instances of incompletely drained sepsis, excessive blood loss following a long operation, severe hypoalbuminemia (<2.5 g/dL), or significant immunosuppression.

Disease Locations

The operative approach to Crohn's disease is predicated upon many variables, including disease location and the particular nuances introduced by features unique to that location. The various disease locations include ileal, colonic, ileocolonic, upper gastrointestinal, and perianal disease.

Ileal Disease

Terminal ileal disease is defined as disease limited to the lower third of the small bowel with or without cecal involvement. Approximately one-third of patients with Crohn's disease express this phenotype, and usually present with symptoms suggestive of inflammation or obstruction. In the majority of cases, resection with construction of an ileal-ascending colon anastomosis is feasible and desirable. All nondiseased ascending colon should be preserved to provide the largest possible surface area for water absorption and to avoid a complex fistula involving retroperitoneal structures and a perianastomotic recurrence that overlies the second portion of the duodenum.

With mesenteric division, managing the small bowel vessels with simple ties can be catastrophic because the transected vessels might retract into the thickened mesentery and the resultant hematoma can rapidly dissect to the root of the superior mesenteric vessels; control of this bleeding potentially results in excision of extended lengths of nondiseased small intestine. Instead, clamps and suture ligatures should be applied in an overlapping fashion to best assure adequate hemostasis (Figure 30-4). Enlarged lymph nodes should be included in the excised specimen, unless extirpation of these nodes risks damage to the vessels associated with nondiseased intestine. On occasion and contingent upon the thickness and rigidity of the mesentry and the surgeons expertise, one of the newer energy sources may be an acceptable means of achieving vascular control.

Following operations for terminal ileal disease, the neo-terminal ileum tends to be the usual site of disease recurrence. Accordingly, many surgeons have hypothesized the anastomotic configuration and materials can influence recurrence. A recent meta-analysis reviewed outcomes associated with an end-to-end anastomosis and other anastomotic configurations after intestinal resection for patients with Crohn's disease.[70] The anastomotic leak rate was significantly reduced with a side-to-side anastomosis compared

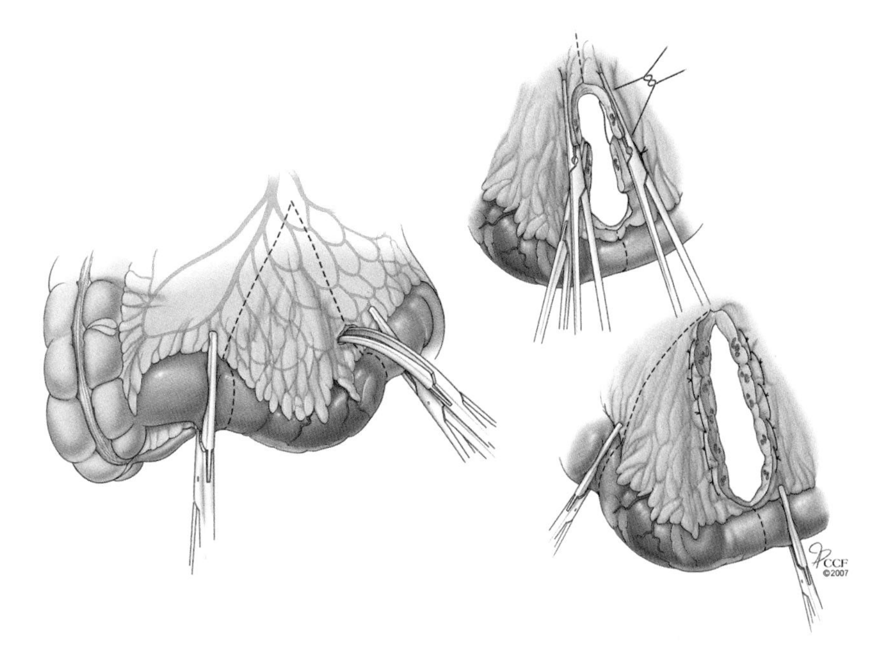

FIGURE 30-4. Ligation of thickened mesentery.

to an end-to-end anastomosis and persisted when studies included only ileocolostomies. Overall postoperative complications, complications other than anastomotic leak, and postoperative hospital stay were significantly reduced in the side-to-side anastomosis group versus the end-to-end anastomosis cohort. Furthermore, no significant difference was noted between the groups in perianastomotic recurrence and reoperation needed because of perianastomotic recurrence.

A separate review of the literature comparing stapled side-to-side ileocolostomy versus hand-sewn anastomosis concluded the stapled anastomosis is associated with fewer leaks than the hand-sewn anastomosis, but too few patients with Crohn's disease were included to allow subgroup analysis.[71] A more recent randomized trial found no difference in the leak or complication rates associated with a stapled side-to-side versus hand-sewn end-to-end anastomosis in patients with Crohn's disease undergoing ileocolostomy.[72] Regardless, it is important to utilize a hand-sewn technique when the bowel wall is abnormally thickened because the stapling instruments are not designed to safely construct an anastomosis under these conditions.

Some centers have adopted an approach to terminal ileal disease whereby they avoid bowel resection by creating a large Finney-type ileocolostomy encompassing the entirety of the diseased bowel.[68,73] Interestingly, subsequent endoscopic and imaging studies have revealed complete morphologic disease regression.

Terminal ileal disease with sparing of the ileocecal valve and cecum is ideally treated with resection and enteroenterostomy provided there is sufficient length (5–7 cm) of normal-appearing distal ileum after definitive ileal resection. Preservation of the ileocecal valve helps to minimize the risk of postoperative diarrhea. In many instances, a hand-sewn anastomosis is preferred because the distal segment may be too short to accommodate a stapled anastomosis.

Laparoscopic resection can be employed with usually comparable or improved results compared to open surgery. A recent meta-analysis[74] reviewed laparoscopic versus open ileocolic resection for Crohn's disease involving 783 patients, 338 of whom underwent laparoscopic resection. The overall conversion rate was relatively low at 6.8%, but many studies excluded patients with recurrent disease, multiple disease sites, fixed masses, or complex fistulas. Although the operative time was significantly longer in the laparoscopic group, total costs of hospitalization were comparable. Analysis of early postoperative complications found no significant difference between the groups in terms of bowel obstruction, chest infection, intra-abdominal abscess, postoperative anastomotic leak, or wound infection. Times to the first liquid and solid diets, times to the first flatus and bowel movement, and hospital stay were all significantly shorter in the laparoscopic group compared to the open group. Many centers have also described good results with laparoscopic resection of complex disease, including recurrent disease, multifactorial disease, fistulas, and abscesses, showing that such an approach is both feasible and safe.[75–77]

Long-term monitoring suggests that patients undergoing laparoscopic resection are not at any greater risk for disease recurrence than those undergoing an open resection.[78–80] In one series, however, only one-half of the recurrences occurring after laparoscopic ileocolic resection and one-third of recurrences following open ileocolic resection were amenable to successful treatment using laparoscopic techniques.[78]

Colonic Disease

Colonic disease is any colon involvement between the cecum and rectum without terminal ileal disease. Nearly one-third of patients suffer from this disease distribution, and often complains of inflammatory disease symptoms, including abdominal cramping, bloody diarrhea, and urgency.

Persons presenting with segmental disease are best treated with segmental resection to protect against dehydration and electrolyte imbalances associated with loss of the large intestine's physiologic role. A meta-analysis[81] comparing segmental colectomy to subtotal/total colectomy revealed no significant difference between the groups regarding the incidence of postoperative complications, disease recurrence, or need for a permanent stoma. However, the time to recurrence was shorter in the segmental resection group by 4.4 years and patients with two or more affected colonic segments tended to be best treated by subtotal or total colectomy.

In patients with disease limited to the ascending colon, the transverse colon is divided at the level of the middle colic vessels so that the mesenteric root naturally separates the anastomosis from the retroperitoneum, minimizing the risk for recurrent disease complicated by complex fistulas. Alternatively, a more proximal anastomosis may be wrapped with a pedicle of omentum, thereby preventing the anastomosis from lying in direct contact with the retroperitoneum. Disease involving the ascending and transverse colon is treated in a similar manner except an extended right colectomy is recommended as the mesentery of the ileum is more easily approximated to the mesentery of the sigmoid colon than the descending colon. Resection of the additional colonic segment avoids an internal hernia and does not adversely affect the functional outcome. Crohn's disease of the transverse, descending, or sigmoid colon presents a situation where segmental resection and colocolonic or colorectal anastomosis is most commonly employed. Resection with coloproctostomy is used for patients with left-sided disease, and a cecorectal anastomosis is constructed if the transverse colon is also involved. In younger patients and those without prior small bowel resection, the diseased segment and uninvolved proximal colon are resected and an ileosigmoid or ileorectal anastomosis is constructed.

Laparoscopic colectomy can also be safely employed in patients with colonic Crohn's disease. The options for division of the larger vascular pedicles of the large bowel include laparoscopic staplers, laparoscopic clip appliers, suture ligatures, and electrothermal bipolar vessel sealers; ultrasonic shears are not commonly recommended for dividing larger pedicles. The laparoscopic clip appliers and bipolar thermal energy devices can safely manage arteries and veins ≤7 mm in diameter, such as the ileocolic and inferior mesenteric vessels, but the thickness of the surrounding tissue that must be additionally incorporated may limit the utility of these approaches in selected settings. The laparoscopic staplers, on the other hand, can manage arteries <17 mm and veins <22 mm in diameter, which may be more useful because of the surrounding mesenteric tissue.[82] However, great care must be exercised because if the vessels retract unsealed within the thick mesentry, a significant rapidly expanding hematoma may occur. Comparing laparoscopic versus open colectomy, da Luz Moreira and associates[83] reported a conversion rate of 26% in cohorts well matched for age, gender American Society of Anesthesiologists score, type, and year of surgery. The incidence of postoperative complications was similar between the two groups, but patients treated by laparoscopic colectomy trended toward experiencing shorter time to first bowel movement and lesser lengths of hospital stay.

Colonic strictureplasty has been described for short strictures and appears to be associated with a morbidity rate, risk for surgical recurrence, and postoperative quality of life comparable to that seen with resection.[84] However, given the 7% incidence of malignancy arising in a colonic stricture,[85] some surgeons argue that resection should be exclusively encouraged if all of the outcome measures are comparable.

Patients with extensive colonic involvement, relative rectal sparing, and adequate fecal continence without active perianal sepsis or compromised rectal compliance are candidates for colectomy with ileoproctostomy. Rectal compliance can be subjectively judged by distending the rectum during proctoscopy or objectively quantified with anorectal physiology testing; patients whose maximum tolerated rectal volume measures <150 ml do poorly with an ileoproctostomy.[86] A rare patient presents with pan-colonic disease, significant upper rectal involvement, and sparing of the mid- and distal-rectum. Resection of all disease in this setting leaves an anastomosis only 6–8 cm above the anal verge, and is often associated with impaired function secondary to compromised compliance. Instead, in very carefully selected situations an ileal J-pouch can be configured with 10 cm limbs and joined to the spared mid-rectum after subtotal proctocolectomy.[87] Despite an increased disease recurrence compared to that seen with total proctocolectomy and ileostomy, the patient may enjoy several years without a stoma.

Patients with proctocolitis who warrant operative treatment usually require a total proctocolectomy with the creation of an end ileostomy, especially those persons with colitis whose proctitis, sphincter dysfunction, or perianal sepsis is too severe for rectal preservation and ileoproctostomy. If proctectomy is required, the entirety of the rectum should be excised in a single or staged procedure because of the significant risk of cancer developing in the defunct rectal stump despite surveillance proctoscopy.[88] An unhealed perineal wound that persists 6–12 months following endoanal proctectomy should be evaluated to exclude concomitant pyoderma gangrenosum, perineal sinus, enteroperineal fistula, and malignancy. A simple shallow wound usually responds to repeated wound debridement and diligent wound care with vacuum dressings and split-thickness skin grafts providing additional benefit. Wounds complicated by a perineal sinus or enteroperineal fistula require more extensive procedures that often include omental, muscle, or myocutaneous flaps.[89–91]

At least two centers have chosen to offer selected patients with Crohn's disease isolated to the colon and rectum a total proctocolectomy with ileal pouch–anal anastomosis.[53,92] They have reported that the rate of Crohn's disease-related pouch excision is 10–15% after 10 years of follow-up. Other reports that suggest 45–52% of patients with Crohn's disease subsequently require pouch excision 10 years following restorative proctocolectomy are looking at a cohort that includes patients who develop post-IPAA symptoms associated with an increased risk for pouch loss.[93–95]

Ileocolonic Disease

Ileocolonic disease affects the terminal ileum with colonic involvement noted distal to the cecum. This disease phenotype occurs as commonly as terminal ileal disease, and the operative approach to these patients is similar to that already outlined for individuals with terminal ileal or colon disease. Specifically, the surgeon must conserve as much of the nondiseased colon as possible and avoid large mesenteric defects. This result might require the construction of two anastomoses, which does not seem to significantly increase operative morbidity.

Upper Gastrointestinal Disease

Upper gastrointestinal disease is defined as any disease location proximal to the terminal ileum occurring in isolation or with concomitant disease located elsewhere. This phenotype is often the most difficult to manage because of its predilection for extensive disease and predominantly stricturing or penetrating behavior.

Small bowel disease proximal to the terminal ileum is often typified by several stenotic segments separated from one another by noninvolved bowel. These diseased segments range in length and can measure >50 cm. The prognosis for Crohn's disease diffusely involving the small bowel is significantly worse than that of localized disease.[96] The operative options in a symptomatic patient with diffuse jejunoileitis include internal intestinal bypass, strictureplasty, and resection. Intestinal bypass is rejected by most clinicians because of concerns about bacterial overgrowth and malignant degeneration. Resection risks immediate or future short bowel syndrome and is not generally recommended. An operation that consists of multiple strictureplasties is the procedure of choice using the previously discussed techniques to safely conserve small bowel and relieve symptoms secondary to luminal stenosis. The involved segments can be ignored only in the rare instance, where the diseased intestine appears to be inflamed without evidence of stricture or penetration.

Gastroduodenal Crohn's disease is relatively rare, and its most common presenting complaints are upper abdominal pain and symptoms of duodenal obstruction. Endoscopy demonstrates macroscopic abnormalities in the majority of patients with the antrum most frequently involved.[97] Isolated gastric disease is exceedingly rare and any reports of successful treatment are purely anecdotal.[98] For duodenal disease, medical therapy is the mainstay of treatment for inflammatory and penetrating disease, while strictures present a different challenge.[99] Ulcer-like lesions are nonspecific, rarely cause stenosis, spontaneously regress, and are usually associated with other diseased sites. Contrarily, stenotic duodenal segments are typically unifocal and often respond poorly to medical management. Endoscopic balloon dilatation has been safely used to treat short duodenal strictures, and the procedure appears to be well tolerated while providing marked symptom relief.[100] In the past, the operative management of duodenal strictures was restricted to gastrojejunostomy, but success with duodenal strictureplasty has been reported by several centers, and the technique appears to be the procedure of choice if the affected bowel is sufficiently supple and devoid of associated sepsis.[101–103] As seen with small bowel strictures, occult malignancies can complicate stricture sites involving the stomach and duodenum.[104]

Perianal Disease

A variety of perianal manifestations can complicate Crohn's disease, including perineal skin lesions such as skin tags and hemorrhoids, anal canal lesions including fissures, ulcers, strictures/stenoses, anoperineal abscesses or fistulas, anovaginal fistulas, and neoplasia. The fissures and ulcers are considered primary disorders, whereas the others are secondary abnormalities.[105]

Perianal disease involvement in patients with known intestinal Crohn's disease is generally obvious, but individuals without a history of Crohn's disease can present a diagnostic challenge as many of the findings are seen in normal individuals or patients with other gastrointestinal maladies. Crohn's disease is the more likely diagnosis if multiple abnormalities, such as laterally located fissures, cavitating anal canal ulcers, and anorectal ring stenosis, are noted. Endoanal ultrasound can be a useful tool for the diagnosis of anorectal sepsis, and may guide combined medical and operative therapy to significantly improve outcome.[106] Pelvic MRI is a similarly valuable means of identifying abscesses and classifying fistulas.[107] Direct comparison of endoanal ultrasound, MRI, and examination under anesthesia has suggested that ultrasound might be most accurate, but ultrasound and MRI used together or separately in combination with examination under anesthesia are 100% accurate.[108]

For many perianal conditions, local measures can provide some symptomatic relief and medical therapy, including antibiotics, immunomodulators, and biologic agents, is often beneficial. Uncontrolled studies have shown a reduction in fistula-associated pain and drainage in adults treated with metronidazole or ciprofloxacin after 6–8 weeks of therapy, but symptoms typically recur immediately after antibiotic discontinuation.[109] Immunomodulation with optimized azathioprine or 6-mercaptopurine is as effective as de novo therapy in nearly one-half of patients, but response is often slow or incomplete. Immunomodulators have also been found to successfully delay fistula recurrence following antibiotic discontinuation in patients initially responding to treatment.[110] Continuous therapy with biologic agents, such as infliximab which is an antitumor necrosis factor antibodies, is associated with complete arrest of fistula drainage in nearly one-half of adults.[111]

The appropriate operative treatment of perianal Crohn's disease must be individualized to the specific patient with adherence to certain management tenets. In general, a conservative surgical approach is adopted because a more aggressive attitude often results in outcomes that are worse than the disease itself. Surgical treatment of skin tags, whether conservative or aggressive, is often associated with morbidity due to chronic, nonhealing anal or perianal ulcers. Fissures should be relatively asymptomatic and nearly one-half heal with medical treatment, especially those that are painless or acute in nature. Refractory symptoms from an uncomplicated fissure may respond to lateral internal sphincterotomy, especially if anal hypertonicity is present and rectal inflammation is absent. Symptoms secondary to large, cavity forming ulcers can often be controlled with debridement of overhanging edges and intra-lesion corticosteroid injection.

An anorectal abscess, regardless of its etiology, is best treated with simple incision and drainage unless perineal sepsis complicates the presentation. The management of anal fistulas is a challenging dilemma, and is based upon the patient's presentation considering the fistula's location and complexity, the presence or absence of concomitant proctitis, and the severity of accompanying anal canal disease. In addition, the surgeon should be cognizant of the known potential for malignant degeneration of the chronic fistula tract and the patient should be counseled regarding this risk.[112] Medical therapy to optimize control of disease-related inflammation is typically recommended to increase the likelihood of healing without adversely impacting surgical outcomes.[113] Most low-lying, simple fistulas without concomitant proctitis can be appropriately managed by fistulotomy. If partial sphincter division would compromise fecal continence, a noncutting seton or rectal mucosal advancement flap is indicated for low-lying, simple fistulas without significant proctitis. Noncutting setons establish drainage of the fistula, minimize the risk for future abscesses arising from the fistula tract, rarely cause discomfort, and do not interfere with personal hygiene. Alternatively, the rectal mucosal advancement flap is a versatile procedure that can be used when rectal inflammation is limited and no cavitating ulceration or anal stenosis is present because the flap procedure does not significantly jeopardize continence or risk proctectomy (Figure 30-5). In the event that the above scenario is complicated by anal canal ulceration or stricturing, a rectal sleeve advancement with temporary fecal diversion can be performed in selected patients. If moderate or severe proctitis complicates a low-lying, simple fistula, concomitant sepsis is excluded and medical therapy is then employed with or without a noncutting seton.[114] In a patient with a high, complex fistula and no evidence of Crohn's proctitis, a rectal advancement flap can be performed with the expectation that one-third of complex fistulas treated in this fashion completely heal. If the anal canal is diseased, rectal sleeve advancement may be attempted. The presence of proctitis with a high, complex fistula relegates the patient to medical therapy in combination with seton drainage, temporary fecal diversion, or proctectomy.

More recently described procedures for the management of fistulas in adults with Crohn's disease entail occlusion of the fistula tract with fibrin sealant[115] or collagen plug.[116] Results with fibrin sealant for fistulas related to Crohn's disease have been inconsistent partially because complex fistulas tend to be less responsive to treatment, but the largest series to date revealed more than one-half of treated fistulas remained drainage-free after nearly two years of follow-up.[115] Similar to the fibrin sealant experience, some centers[117] have reported high success rates (>80%) in patients with fistula tracts treated by collagen plug occlusion while others[116] have encountered somewhat discouraging outcomes.

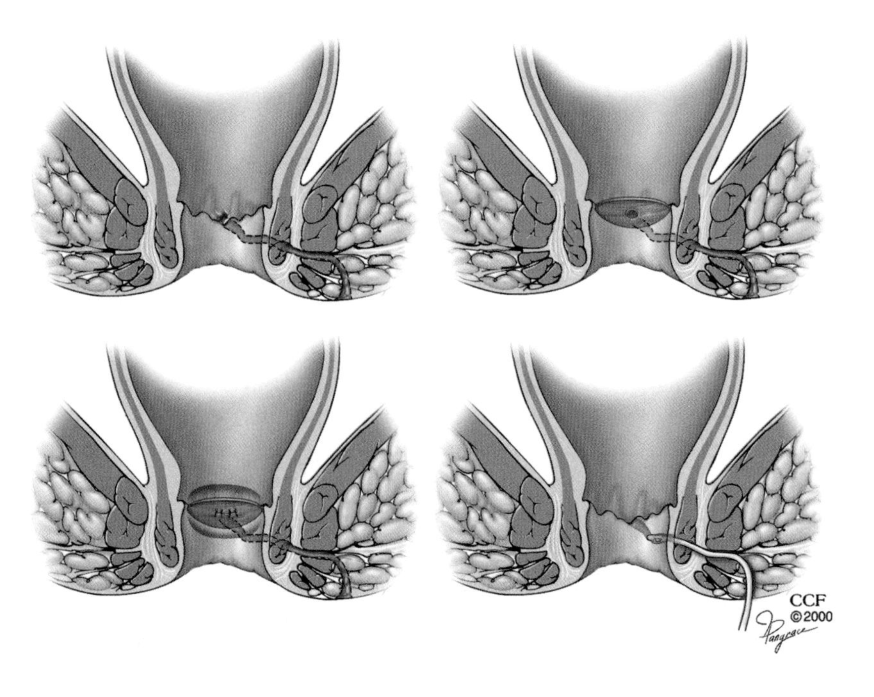

FIGURE 30-5. Rectal mucosal advancement flap.

In selected patients with severe perianal disease, fecal diversion is required. While patients undergoing temporary diversion enjoy an improved quality of life,[118] a temporary ileostomy does not generally influence the long-term outcome of perianal Crohn's disease because less than one-quarter of individuals have intestinal continuity restored.[55] The majority of patients who undergo successful closure of their stoma require a secondary procedure (e.g., rectal mucosal advancement flap) to achieve stoma closure. However, the creation of a loop ileostomy as a planned definitive procedure is rarely indicated. Instead, an endoanal proctectomy is necessary in approximately 5% of Crohn's disease patients solely to control perianal disease, especially if high, complex fistulas, deep ulcerations, colonic disease, or anal canal stenosis is present.

Prophylaxis Against Recurrent Disease

Recurrent disease following surgical management of Crohn's disease is commonplace and leads to the need for reinstatement of medical therapy in most instances and eventual surgery in some cases. Accordingly, multiple trials have been conducted using medications intended to decrease the recurrence rate with varying degrees of success. A recent review of the literature[119] revealed 23 studies that appropriately investigated this issue and the pooled results were presented. Probiotics were not superior to placebo for any outcome measured. The use of nitroimidazole antibiotics appeared to reduce the risk of clinical and endoscopic recurrence when compared to placebo; however, these agents were associated with higher risk of serious adverse events. Mesalamine therapy was associated with a significantly reduced risk of clinical and severe endoscopic recurrence relative to placebo. Azathioprine and 6-mercaptopurine were also associated with a significantly reduced risk of clinical and severe endoscopic recurrence when compared to placebo, and neither agent had a higher risk than placebo of serious adverse events. Lastly, mesalamine relative to azathioprine and 6-mercaptopurine was associated with a higher risk of endoscopic recurrence, but a lower risk of serious adverse events. A study not included in this review looked at the impact of postoperative infliximab compared to placebo, and found infliximab therapy after intestinal resection was significantly effective at preventing endoscopic and histologic recurrence without increasing the occurrence of adverse events.[120]

Summary

The operative management of Crohn's disease is predicated upon a thorough understanding of the patient and the nature of their disease. The surgeon must be knowledgeable about the potential disease complications and medical treatment options to appropriately judge which patients are legitimate candidates for surgical intervention. Furthermore, despite recent advances in radiographic and endoscopic diagnostics, the findings at the time of surgery are commonly different than those suggested by the preoperative studies. The surgeon must be accordingly cognizant of the various operative options and confident with their usage when it is necessary to deviate from the planned procedure. Lastly, the surgeon must address not only the immediate issue, but also employ measures that minimize the risk of future complications caused by the recurrent behavior of the disease. The Standards Practice Task Force of the American Society of Colon and Rectal Surgeons has published practice parameters for the surgical treatment of Crohn's disease.[121]

References

1. Economou M, Pappas G. New global map of Crohn's disease: genetic, environmental, and socioeconomic correlations. Inflamm Bowel Dis. 2008;14:709–20.
2. Binder V. Epidemiology of IBD during the twentieth century: an integrated view. Best Pract Res Clin Gastroenterol. 2004;18:463–79.
3. Loftus Jr EV. Clinical epidemiology of inflammatory bowel disease: incidence, prevalence, and environmental influences. Gastroenterology. 2004;126:1504–17.
4. Kappelman MD, Rifas-Shiman SL, Kleinman K, Ollendorf D, Bousvaros A, Grand RJ, et al. The prevalence and geographic distribution of Crohn's disease and ulcerative colitis in the United States. Clin Gastroenterol Hepatol. 2007;5:1424–9.
5. Melum E, Franke A, Karlsen TH. Genome-wide association studies – a summary for the clinical gastroenterologist. World J Gastroenterol. 2009;15:5377–96.
6. Barrett JC, Hansoul S, Nicolae DL, et al. Genome-wide association defines more than 30 distinct susceptibility loci for Crohn's disease. Nat Genet. 2008;40:955–62.
7. Mayer L. Evolving paradigms in the pathogenesis of IBD. J Gastroenterol. 2010;45:9–16.
8. Mahid SS, Minor KS, Soto RE, Hornung CA, Galandiuk S. Smoking and inflammatory bowel disease: a meta-analysis. Mayo Clin Proc. 2006;81:1462–71.
9. Rutgeerts P, Goboes K, Peeters M, Hiele M, Penninckx F, Aerts R, et al. Effect of fecal diversion on recurrence of Crohn's disease in the neoterminal ileum. Lancet. 1991;338:771–4.
10. Ekbom A, Montgomery SM. Environmental risk factors (excluding tobacco and microorganisms): critical analysis of old and new hypotheses. Best Pract Res Clin Gastroenterol. 2004;18:497–508.
11. Jantchou P, Monnet E, Carbonnel F. Environmental risk factors in Crohn's disease and ulcerative colitis (excluding tobacco and appendicectomy). Gastroentérol Clin Biol. 2006;30:859–67.
12. Farmer RG, Hawk WA, Turnbull RB. Clinical patterns in Crohn's disease: a statistical study of 615 cases. Gastroenterology. 1975;68:627–35.
13. Gasche C, Scholmerich J, Brynskov J, D'Haens G, Hanauer SB, Irvine EJ, et al. A simple classification of Crohn's disease: report of the Working Party for the World Congresses of Gastroenterology, Vienna 1998. Inflamm Bowel Dis. 2000;6:8–15.
14. Silverberg MS, Satsangi J, Ahmad T, et al. Toward an integrated clinical, molecular and serological classification of

inflammatory bowel disease: report of a Working Party of the 2005 Montreal World Congress of Gastroenterology. Can J Gastroenterol. 2005;19(Suppl A):5–36.
15. Fedorak RN. Is it time to re-classify Crohn's disease? Best Pract Res Clin Gastroenterol. 2004;18 Suppl:99–106.
16. Papi C, Festa V, Fagnani C, Stazi A, Antonelli G, Moretti A, et al. Evolution of clinical behaviour in Crohn's disease: predictive factors of penetrating complications. Dig Liver Dis. 2005;37:247–53.
17. Pikarsky AJ, Gervaz P, Wexner SD. Perianal Crohn disease: a new scoring system to evaluate and predict outcome of surgical intervention. Arch Surg. 2002;137:774–7.
18. Stange EF, Travis SP, Vermeire S, European Crohn's and Colitis Organisation, et al. European evidence based consensus on the diagnosis and management of Crohn's disease: definitions and diagnosis. Gut. 2006;55 Suppl 1:1–15.
19. Lennard-Jones JE, Shivananda S. Clinical uniformity of inflammatory bowel disease a presentation and during the first year of disease in the north and south of Europe. EC-IBD Study Group. Eur J Gastroenterol Hepatol. 1997;9:353–9.
20. Nielsen OH, Vainer B, Madsen SM, Seidelin JB, Heegaard NH. Established and emerging biological activity markers of inflammatory bowel disease. Am J Gastroenterol. 2000;95:359–67.
21. Vermeire S, Van Assche G, Rutgeerts P. C-reactive protein as a marker for inflammatory bowel disease. Inflamm Bowel Dis. 2004;10:661–5.
22. Sachar DB, Luppescu NE, Bodian C, Shlien RD, Fabry TL, Gumaste VV. Erythrocyte sedimentation as a measure of Crohn's disease activity: opposite trends in ileitis versus colitis. J Clin Gastroenterol. 1990;12:643–6.
23. Huprich JE, Rosen MP, Fidler JL, Gay SB, Grant TH, Greene FL, et al. ACR Appropriateness Criteria on Crohn's disease. J Am Coll Radiol. 2010;7:94–102.
24. Peyrin-Biroulet L, Loftus Jr EV, Colombel JF, Sandborn WJ. The natural history of adult Crohn's disease in population-based cohorts. Am J Gastroenterol. 2010;105:289–97.
25. Dhillon SL, Loftus Jr EV, Tremaine WJ, et al. The natural history of surgery for Crohn's disease in a population-based cohort from Olmsted County, Minnesota. Am J Gastroenterol. 2005;100:S305.
26. Duricova D, Pedersen N, Elkjaer M, Gamborg M, Munkholm P, Jess T. Overall and cause-specific mortality in Crohn's disease: a meta-analysis of population-based studies. Inflamm Bowel Dis. 2010;16:347–53.
27. Korzenik JR. Massive lower gastrointestinal hemorrhage in Crohn's disease. Curr Treat Options Gastroenterol. 2000;3:211–6.
28. Kazama Y, Watanabe T, Akahane M, Yoshioka N, Ohtomo K, Nagawa H. Crohn's disease with life-threatening hemorrhage from terminal ileum: successful control by superselective arterial embolization. J Gastroenterol. 2005;40:1155–7.
29. Fazio VW, Zelas P, Weakley FL. Intraoperative angiography and the localization of bleeding from the small intestine. Surg Gynecol Obstet. 1980;151:637–40.
30. Werbin N, Haddad R, Greenberg R, Karin E, Skornick Y. Free perforation in Crohn's disease. Isr Med Assoc J. 2003;5:175–7.
31. Greenstein AJ, Sachar DB, Mann D, Lachman P, Heimann T, Aufses Jr AH. Spontaneous free perforation and perforated abscess in 30 patients with Crohn's disease. Ann Surg. 1987;205:72–6.
32. Bundred NJ, Dixon JM, Lumsden AB, Gilmour HM, Davies GC. Free perforation in Crohn's colitis. A ten-year review. Dis Colon Rectum. 1985;28:35–7.
33. Santos JV, Baudet JA, Casellas FJ, Guarner LA, Vilaseca JM, Malagelada JR. Intravenous cyclosprine for steroid-refractory attacks of Crohn's disease. Short- and long-term results. J Clin Gastroenterol. 1995;20:207–10.
34. Sheth SG, LaMont JT. Toxic megacolon. Lancet. 1998; 351:509–13.
35. Lichtenstein GR, Hanauer SB, Practice Parameters Committee of American College of Gastroenterology. Management of Crohn's disease in adults. Am J Gastroenterol. 2009;104:465–83.
36. Yamamoto T, Keighley MR. Long-term outcome of total colectomy and ileostomy for Crohn disease. Scand J Gastroenterol. 1999;34:280–6.
37. Lavery IC, Jagelman DG. Cancer in the excluded rectum following surgery for inflammatory bowel disease. Dis Colon Rectum. 1982;25:522–4.
38. Guillem JG, Roberts PL, Murray JJ, Coller JA, Veidenheimer MC, Schoetz Jr DJ. Factors predictive of persistent or recurrent Crohn's disease in excluded rectal segments. Dis Colon Rectum. 1992;35:768–72.
39. Scott HW, Sawyers JL, Gobbel Jr WG, Graves HA, Shull HW. Surgical management of toxic dilatation of the colon in ulcerative colitis. Ann Surg. 1974;179:647–56.
40. Koudahl G, Kristensen M. Toxic megacolon in ulcerative colitis. Scand J Gastroenterol. 1975;10:417–21.
41. Bernstein CN, Blanchard JF, Rawsthorne P, Yu N. The prevalence of extraintestinal diseases in inflammatory bowel disease: a population-based study. Am J Gastroenterol. 2001;96: 1116–22.
42. Caprilli R, Gassull MA, Escher JC, et al. European evidence based consensus on the diagnosis and management of Crohn's disease: special situations. Gut. 2006;55 Suppl 1:i36–58.
43. Shamir R, Phillip M, Levine A. Growth retardation in pediatric Crohn's disease: pathogenesis and interventions. Inflamm Bowel Dis. 2007;13:620–8.
44. Savage MO, Beattie RM, Camacho-Hubner C, Walker-Smith JA, Sanderson IR. Growth in Crohn's disease. Acta Paediatr Suppl. 1999;88:89–92.
45. von Roon AC, Reese G, Teare J, Constantinides V, Darzi AW, Tekkis PP. The risk of cancer in patients with Crohn's disease. Dis Colon Rectum. 2007;50:839–55.
46. Friedman S, Rubin PH, Bodian C, et al. Screening and surveillance colonoscopy in chronic Crohn's colitis. Gastroenterology. 2001;120:820–6.
47. Friedman S, Rubin PH, Bodian C, Harpaz N, Present DH. Screening and surveillance colonoscopy in chronic Crohn's colitis: results of a surveillance program spanning 25 years. Clin Gastroenterol Hepatol. 2008;6:993–8.
48. Winawer S, Fletcher R, Rex D, Bond J, Burt R, Ferrucci J, et al. Colorectal cancer screening and surveillance: clinical guidelines and rationale – update based on new evidence. Gastroenterology. 2003;124:544–60.
49. Itzkowitz SH, Present DH. Consensus conference: colorectal cancer screening and surveillance in inflammatory bowel disease. Inflamm Bowel Dis. 2005;11:314–21.
50. Byrne CM, Solomon MJ, Young JM, Selby W, Harrison JD. Patient preferences between surgical and medical treatment in Crohn's disease. Dis Colon Rectum. 2007;50:586–97.
51. Otterson MF, Lundeen SJ, Spinelli KS, Sudakoff GS, Telford GL, Hatoum OA, et al. Radiographic underestimation of small bowel stricturing Crohn's disease: a comparison with surgical findings. Surgery. 2004;136:854–60.

52. Young-Fadok TM, Wolff BG, Meagher A, Benn PL, Dozois RR. Surgical management of ileosigmoid fistulas in Crohn's disease. Dis Colon Rectum. 1997;40:558–61.
53. Melton GB, Fazio VW, Kiran RP, He J, Lavery IC, Shen B, et al. Long-term outcomes with ileal pouch-anal anastomosis and Crohn's disease: pouch retention and implications of delayed diagnosis. Ann Surg. 2008;248:608–16.
54. Fazio VW, Marchetti F, Church J, Goldblum J, Lavery I, Hull T, et al. Effect of resection margins on the recurrence of Crohn's disease in the small bowel. A randomized controlled trial. Ann Surg. 1996;224:563–73.
55. Yamamoto T, Allan RN, Keighley MR. Effect of fecal diversion alone on perianal Crohn's disease. World J Surg. 2000;24:1258–62.
56. van Dongen LM, Lubbers EJC. Perianal fistulas in patients with Crohn's disease. Arch Surg. 1986;121:1187–90.
57. Katariya RN, Sood S, Rao PG, Rao PL. Stricture-plasty for tubercular strictures of the gastro-intestinal tract. Br J Surg. 1977;64:496–8.
58. Lee ECG, Papaioannou N. Minimal surgery for chronic obstruction in patients with extensive or universal Crohn's disease. Ann R Coll Surg Engl. 1982;64:229–33.
59. Tichansky D, Cagir B, Yoo E, Marcus SM, Fry RD. Strictureplasty for Crohn's disease: meta-analysis. Dis Colon Rectum. 2000;43:911–9.
60. Dietz DW, Laureti S, Strong SA, Hull TL, Church J, Remzi FH, et al. Safety and longterm efficacy of strictureplasty in 314 patients with obstructing small bowel Crohn's disease. J Am Coll Surg. 2001;192:330–7.
61. Reese GE, Purkayastha S, Tilney HS, von Roon A, Yamamoto T, Tekkis PP. Strictureplasty vs. resection in small bowel Crohn's disease: an evaluation of short-term outcomes and recurrence. Colorectal Dis. 2007;9:686–94.
62. Yamamoto T, Fazio VW, Tekkis PP. Safety and efficacy of strictureplasty for Crohn's disease: a systematic review and meta-analysis. Dis Colon Rectum. 2007;50:1968–86.
63. Yamamoto T, Allan RN, Keighley MR. Long-term outcome of surgical management for diffuse jejunoileal Crohn's disease. Surgery. 2001;129:96–102.
64. Michelassi F, Taschieri A, Tonelli F, Sasaki I, Poggioli G, Fazio V, et al. An international, multicenter, prospective, observational study of the side-to-side isoperistaltic strictureplasty in Crohn's disease. Dis Colon Rectum. 2007;50:277–84.
65. Menon AM, Mirza AH, Moolla S, Morton DG. Adenocarcinoma of the small bowel arising from a previous strictureplasty for Crohn's disease: report of a case. Dis Colon Rectum. 2007;50:257–9.
66. Ozuner G, Fazio VW. Management of gastrointestinal hemorrhage after strictureplasty for Crohn's disease. Dis Colon Rectum. 1995;38:297–300.
67. Tjandra JJ, Fazio VW. Strictureplasty for ileocolic anastomotic strictures in Crohn's disease. Dis Colon Rectum. 1993;36:1099–103.
68. Sampietro GM, Cristaldi M, Maconi G, Parente F, Sartani A, Ardizzone S, et al. A prospective, longitudinal study of nonconventional strictureplasty in Crohn's disease. J Am Coll Surg. 2004;199:8–20.
69. Futami K, Arima S. Role of strictureplasty in surgical treatment of Crohn's disease. J Gastroenterol. 2005;40 Suppl 16:35–9.
70. Simillis C, Purkayastha S, Yamamoto T, Strong SA, Darzi AW, Tekkis PP. A meta-analysis comparing conventional end-to-end anastomosis vs. other anastomotic configurations after resection in Crohn's disease. Dis Colon Rectum. 2007;50:1674–87.
71. Choy PY, Bissett IP, Docherty JG, Parry BR, Merrie AE. Stapled versus handsewn methods for ileocolic anastomoses. Cochrane Database Syst Rev. 2007:CD004320.
72. McLeod RS, Wolff BG, Ross S, Parkes R, Investigators of the CAST Trial. Recurrence of Crohn's disease after ileocolic resection is not affected by anastomotic type: results of a multicenter, randomized, controlled trial. Dis Colon Rectum. 2009;52:919–27.
73. Poggioli G, Stocchi L, Laureti S, Selleri S, Marra C, Magalotti C, et al. Conservative surgical management of terminal ileitis: side-to-side enterocolic anastomosis. Dis Colon Rectum. 1997;40:234–7.
74. Tilney HS, Constantinides VA, Heriot AG, Nicolaou M, Athanasiou T, Ziprin P, et al. Comparison of laparoscopic and open ileocecal resection for Crohn's disease: a metaanalysis. Surg Endosc. 2006;20:1036–44.
75. Wu JS, Birnbaum EH, Kodner IJ, Fry RD, Read TE, Fleshman JW. Laparoscopic-assisted ileocolic resections in patients with Crohn's disease: are abscesses, phlegmons, or recurrent disease contraindications? Surgery. 1997;122:682–8.
76. Evans J, Poritz L, MacRae H. Influence of experience on laparoscopic ileocolic resection for Crohn's disease. Dis Colon Rectum. 2002;45:1595–600.
77. Goyer P, Alves A, Bretagnol F, Bouhnik Y, Valleur P, Panis Y. Impact of complex Crohn's disease on the outcome of laparoscopic ileocecal resection: a comparative clinical study in 124 patients. Dis Colon Rectum. 2009;52:205–10.
78. Lowney JK, Dietz DW, Birnbaum EH, Kodner IJ, Mutch MG, Fleshman JW. Is there any difference in recurrence rates in laparoscopic ileocolic resection for Crohn's disease compared with conventional surgery? A long-term, follow-up study. Dis Colon Rectum. 2006;49:58–63.
79. Eshuis EJ, Polle SW, Slors JF, Hommes DW, Sprangers MA, Gouma DJ, et al. Long-term surgical recurrence, morbidity, quality of life, and body image of laparoscopic-assisted vs. open ileocolic resection for Crohn's disease: a comparative study. Dis Colon Rectum. 2008;51:858–67.
80. Stocchi L, Milsom JW, Fazio VW. Long-term outcomes of laparoscopic versus open ileocolic resection for Crohn's disease: follow-up of a prospective randomized trial. Surgery. 2008;144:622–7.
81. Tekkis PP, Purkayastha S, Lanitis S, Athanasiou T, Heriot AG, Orchard TR, et al. A comparison of segmental vs. subtotal/total colectomy for colonic Crohn's disease: a meta-analysis. Colorectal Dis. 2006;8:82–90.
82. Harold KL, Pollinger H, Matthews BD, Kercher KW, Sing RF, Heniford BT. Comparison of ultrasonic energy, bipolar thermal energy, and vascular clips for the hemostasis of small-, medium-, and large-sized arteries. Surg Endosc. 2003;17:1228–30.
83. da Luz Moreira A, Stocchi L, Remzi FH, Geisler D, Hammel J, Fazio VW. Laparoscopic surgery for patients with Crohn's colitis: a case-matched study. J Gastrointest Surg. 2007;11:1529–33.
84. Broering DC, Eisenberger CF, Koch A, Bloechle C, Knoefel WT, Durig M, et al. Strictureplasty for large bowel stenosis in Crohn's disease: quality of life after surgical therapy. Int J Colorectal Dis. 2001;16:81–7.
85. Yamazaki Y, Ribeiro MB, Sachar DB, Aufses AH, Greenstein AJ. Malignant strictures in Crohn's disease. Am J Gastroenterol. 1991;86:882–5.

86. Keighley MRB, Buchmann P, Lee JR. Assessment of anorectal function in selection of patients for ileo-rectal anastomosis in Crohn's colitis. Gut. 1982;23:102–7.
87. Kariv Y, Remzi FH, Strong SA, Hammel JP, Preen M, Fazio VW. Ileal pouch rectal anastomosis: a viable alternative to permanent ileostomy in Crohn's proctocolitis patients. J Am Coll Surg. 2009;208:390–9.
88. Cirincione E, Gorfine SR, Bauer JJ. Is Hartmann's procedure safe in Crohn's disease? Report of three cases. Dis Colon Rectum. 2000;43:544–7.
89. Rius J, Nessim A, Nogueras JJ, Wexner SD. Gracilis transposition in complicated perianal fistula and unhealed perineal wounds in Crohn's disease. Eur J Surg. 2000;166:218–22.
90. Hurst RD, Gottlieb LJ, Crucitti P, Melis M, Rubin M, Michelassi F. Primary closure of complicated perineal wounds with myocutaneous and fasciocutaneous flaps after proctectomy for Crohn's disease. Surgery. 2001;130:767–72.
91. Yamamoto T, Mylonakis E, Keighley MR. Omentoplasty for persistent perineal sinus after proctectomy for Crohn's disease. Am J Surg. 2001;181:265–7.
92. Regimbeau JM, Panis Y, Pocard M, Bouhnik Y, Lavergne-Slove A, Rufat P, et al. Long-term results of ileal pouch-anal anastomosis for colorectal Crohn's disease. Dis Colon Rectum. 2001;44:769–78.
93. Sagar PM, Dozois RR, Wolff BG. Long-term results of ileal pouch-anal anastomosis in patients with Crohn's disease. Dis Colon Rectum. 1996;39:893–8.
94. Mylonakis E, Allan RN, Keighley MR. How does pouch construction for a final diagnosis of Crohn's disease compare with ileoproctostomy for established Crohn's proctocolitis? Dis Colon Rectum. 2001;44:1137–42.
95. Braveman JM, Schoetz Jr DJ, Marcello PW, Roberts PL, Coller JA, Murray JJ, et al. The fate of the ileal pouch in patients developing Crohn's disease. Dis Colon Rectum. 2004;47:1613–9.
96. Cooke WT, Swan CH. Diffuse jejunoileitis of Crohn's disease. Quart J Med. 1974;72:583–601.
97. Nugent FW, Roy MA. Duodenal Crohn's disease: an analysis of 89 cases. Am J Gastroenterol. 1989;84:249–54.
98. Cary ER, Tremaine WJ, Banks PM, Nagorney DM. Case report: isolated Crohn's disease of the stomach. Mayo Clin Proc. 1989;64:776–9.
99. Poggioli G, Stocchi L, Laureti S, Selleri S, Marra C, Salone MC, et al. Duodenal involvement of Crohn's disease: three different clinicopathologic patterns. Dis Colon Rectum. 1997;40:179–83.
100. Kimura H, Sugita A, Nishiyama K, Shimada H. Treatment of duodenal Crohn's disease with stenosis: case report of 6 cases. Nippon Shokakibyo Gakkai Zasshi. 2000;9:697–702.
101. Eisenberger CF, Izbicki JR, Broering DC, Bloechle C, Steffen M, Hosch SB, et al. Strictureplasty with a pedunculated jejunal patch in Crohn's disease of the duodenum. Am J Gastroenterol. 1998;93:267–9.
102. Worsey MJ, Hull T, Ryland L, Fazio V. Strictureplasty is an effective option in the operative management of duodenal Crohn's disease. Dis Colon Rectum. 1999;42:596–600.
103. Yamamoto T, Bain IM, Connolly AB, Allan RN, Keighley MR. Outcome of strictureplasty for duodenal Crohn's disease. Br J Surg. 1999;86:259–62.
104. Tonelli F, Bargellini T, Leo F, Nesi G. Duodenal adenocarcinoma arising at the strictureplasty site in a patient with Crohn's disease: report of a case. Int J Colorectal Dis. 2009;24:475–7.
105. Hughes LE. Clinical classification of perianal Crohn's disease. Dis Colon Rectum. 1992;35:928–32.
106. Spradlin NM, Wise PE, Herline AJ, Muldoon RL, Rosen M, Schwartz DA. A randomized prospective trial of endoscopic ultrasound to guide combination medical and surgical treatment for Crohn's perianal fistulas. Am J Gastroenterol. 2008;103:2527–35.
107. Schaefer O, Lohrmann C, Langer M. Assessment of anal fistulas with high-resolution subtraction MR-fistulography: comparison with surgical findings. J Magn Reson Imaging. 2004;19:91–8.
108. Schwartz DA, Wiersema MJ, Dudiak KM, Fletcher JG, Clain JE, Tremaine WJ, et al. A comparison of endoscopic ultrasound, magnetic resonance imaging, and exam under anesthesia for evaluation of Crohn's perianal fistulas. Gastroenterology. 2001;121:1064–72.
109. Wise PE, Schwartz DA. Related management of perianal Crohn's disease. Clin Gastroenterol Hepatol. 2006;4:426–30.
110. Dejaco C, Harrer M, Waldhoer T, Miehsler W, Vogelsang H, Reinisch W. Antibiotics and azathioprine for the treatment of perianal fistulas in Crohn's disease. Aliment Pharmacol Ther. 2003;18:1113–20.
111. Present DH, Rutgeerts P, Targan S, Hanauer SB, Mayer L, van Hogezand RA, et al. Infliximab for the treatment of fistulas in patients with Crohn's disease. N Engl J Med. 1999; 340:1398–405.
112. Thomas M, Bienkowski R, Vandermeer TJ, Trostle D, Cagir B. Malignant transformation in perianal fistulas of Crohn's disease: a systematic review of literature. J Gastrointest Surg. 2010;14:66–73.
113. Kamm MA, Ng SC. Perianal fistulizing Crohn's disease: a call to action. Clin Gastroenterol Hepatol. 2008;6(1):7–10.
114. Regueiro M, Mardini H. Treatment of perianal fistulizing Crohn's disease with infliximab alone or as an adjunct to exam under anesthesia with seton placement. Inflamm Bowel Dis. 2003;9:98–103.
115. Vitton V, Gasmi M, Barthet M, Desjeux A, Orsoni P, Grimaud JC. Long-term healing of Crohn's anal fistulas with fibrin glue injection. Aliment Pharmacol Ther. 2005;21:1453–7.
116. Safar B, Jobanputra S, Sands D, Weiss EG, Nogueras JJ, Wexner SD. Anal fistula plug: initial experience and outcomes. Dis Colon Rectum. 2009;52:248–52.
117. O'Connor L, Champagne BJ, Ferguson MA, Orangio GR, Schertzer ME, Armstrong DN. Efficacy of anal fistula plug in closure of Crohn's anorectal fistulas. Dis Colon Rectum. 2006;49:1569–73.
118. Kasparek MS, Glatzle J, Temeltcheva T, Mueller MH, Koenigsrainer A, Kreis ME. Long-term quality of life in patients with Crohn's disease and perianal fistulas: influence of fecal diversion. Dis Colon Rectum. 2007;50:2067–74.
119. Doherty G, Bennett G, Patil S, Cheifetz A, Moss AC. Interventions for prevention of post-operative recurrence of Crohn's disease. Cochrane Database Syst Rev. 2009:CD006873.
120. Regueiro M, Schraut W, Baidoo L, Kip KE, Sepulveda AR, Pesci M, et al. Infliximab prevents Crohn's disease recurrence after ileal resection. Gastroenterology. 2009;136:441–50.
121. Strong SA, Koltun WA, Hyman NH, Buie WD, Standards Practice Task Force of the American Society of Colon and Rectal Surgeons. Practice parameters for the surgical management of Crohn's disease. Dis Colon Rectum. 2007;50:1735–46.

31
Intestinal Stomas

Laurence R. Sands and Floriano Marchetti

Introduction

Intestinal stomas have long been used by surgeons for fecal diversion and remain an important tool for both the general and colon and rectal surgeon. They are considered a vital element as either a permanent means for stool evacuation or as a temporary bridge in order to treat complicated abdominal problems or to heal more distal anastomoses. The surgeon must always regard fecal diversion as a means to salvage patients from abdominal catastrophy and should never consider stoma creation as a defeat even though many patients may regard it as such.

The History of the Stoma

The colostomy was initially described by Littre in 1710, whereby he fashioned a diverting stoma for a patient with an obstructing colon cancer.[1] The next report of a colostomy actually appeared many years later when it occurred spontaneously due to a strangulated umbilical hernia, whereby the skin sloughed leaving the bowel exposed and draining.[2] Later on, bowel exteriorization became much more popularized with battlefield injuries and was associated with long-term survival.

The ileostomy history is much more short-lived, however. They did not become popular until devices became available that allowed better seals of the devices to the skin because of the more liquid nature of the effluent. Ulcerative colitis made it necessary to use the ileostomy. Initial reports of ablative surgery for fulminating colitis seemed to be unsuccessful and it soon became recognized that patients would either die of their disease or need to function with an ileorectal anastomosis, a rather unsatisfying operation for ulcerative colitis in the face of severe proctitis. As such, Dr. John Young Brown of St. Louis introduced the ileostomy as part of the therapy for ulcerative colitis in 1913.[3] This stoma was used in order to obtain colonic rest in the course of this disease. Once total proctocolectomy was popularized as a cure for ulcerative colitis by Gavin Miller, surgeons were then forced to deal with the long-lasting effects of the ileostomy.[4] At that time, ileostomies were constructed by creating a flush connection of the bowel to the skin. They were fraught with complications of irritated skin, inflammation, subsequent parastomal scarring, and ultimately stomal narrowing secondary to the severe skin reaction and fibrosis. A chemistry student by the name of Koernig who had an ileostomy for ulcerative colitis developed a bag and seal of rubber with a latex preparation in order to help protect his skin from the caustic effects of the ileostomy effluent. It wasn't until 1952 when Brooke designed the everted stoma, whereby the appliances were now able to easily catch the stoma effluent and stop leakage, thereby preventing surrounding skin irritation and its complications.[5] This rather simple but ingenious design truly revolutionized the ability of surgeons to use an ileostomy as a means of stool diversion on a permanent or temporary basis.

Stoma Incidence

Stomas are used as often as is necessary. The true incidence of stomas is generally unknown. An estimate in the late 1970s within the United Kingdom suggested that there were 10,000 patients with an ileostomy at that time and that 400–500 ileostomies per year were being created.[6] It has also been estimated that about 4,000 ileostomies were created in 1968 alone within the USA.[7] There is no reason to suspect that these numbers have declined over the years since the indications for stoma creation have essentially not changed since then.

What Is an Ostomy?

An ostomy is a surgically created opening between a hollow organ and the body surface or between any two hollow organs. The word, *ostomy*, comes from the Latin word,

D.E. Beck et al. (eds.), *The ASCRS Textbook of Colon and Rectal Surgery: Second Edition*,
DOI 10.1007/978-1-4419-1584-9_31, © Springer Science+Business Media, LLC 2011

ostium, meaning mouth or opening. The suffix *-tomy* implies an intervention, either by surgery or injury. The word, stoma, comes from the Greek word for mouth and is used interchangeably with ostomy. An ostomy is further named by the organ involved. An ileostomy is an opening from the ileum to the skin, a colostomy is from the colon, a gastrostomy is from the stomach, and so forth. When two organs are joined the descriptive term incorporates both. For instance, an anastomosis between the small bowel and colon might be called an ileocolostomy, between colon and the rectum, a colorectostomy or coloproctostomy. A loop ostomy is formed by bringing an intact loop of bowel through the skin and then dividing the antimesenteric side and maturing it so that there are two open lumens, the proximal and the distal.

Indications and Types of Stomas

There are many indications for a stoma (Table 31-1). Permanent stomas are fashioned when there is a need for removal of the anus along with its associated musculature. This procedure may be necessary in patients with distal rectal cancers who require an abdominoperineal resection or those individuals with severe inflammatory bowel disease with involvement of the sphincter mechanisms. In addition, patients of any age with weak sphincter muscles and/or fecal incontinence may be better served with permanent fecal diversion in order to prevent perineal skin breakdown, improve perineal hygiene, and prevent decubitus ulcer formation.

Stomas may also be used on a temporary basis. Temporary stomas are indicated in cases of intra-abdominal catastrophes and may act as a lifesaving bridge in critically ill patients. Patients with diffuse peritonitis from a perforated colon due to an inflammatory condition such as diverticulitis or Crohn's disease are often at risk of anastomotic leak should the surgeon be tempted to perform such an anastomosis.

TABLE 31-1. Indications for a stoma

- Protection of distal anastomosis
- Treatment of anastomotic leak
- Large bowel obstruction
- Bowel perforation
- Abdominal or perineal trauma
- Rectal injury
- Diverticular disease
- Complex anorectal disease
- Complications from radiation
- Fecal incontinence
- Inflammatory bowel disease
- Motility and functional disorders including idiopathic megarectum and megacolon
- Infections – necrotizing fasciitis, Fournier's gangrene
- Congenital disorders – imperforate anus, Hirschsprung's disease, necrotizing enterocolitis, intestinal atresias

These patients are often best served with a temporary stoma in order to allow intra-abdominal healing and resolution of the inflammatory state.

Perhaps one of the most common indications for the creation of a temporizing stoma is for patients undergoing deep pelvic dissections, total mesorectal excisions, a low-lying ileo-anal or colo-anal bowel anastomosis, or in patients who undergo a high-risk distal bowel anastomosis. These stomas serve as a protection for anastomotic dehiscence. Temporary stomas are also often used in patients who undergo a restorative proctectomy after they have completed preoperative chemotherapy and radiation for advanced rectal cancer. The benefits of this type of fecal diversion will be discussed later in the context of this chapter.

Some surgeons may consider performing a diverting stoma at the time of diagnosis of advanced rectal cancer. While preoperative therapy often will shrink a large rectal cancer and improve patient's symptoms, there are many patients who may be so symptomatic that fecal diversion should be considered as the initial management for these patients. A recent British study evaluated whether stoma creation was indicated in patients with rectal cancer prior to undergoing neoadjuvant therapy. In this study, they performed a diverting stoma in nine patients, eight of whom had an inability to have their tumors cannulated at the time of colonoscopy and one who had fecal incontinence. Three of these patients never underwent definitive surgery for their rectal cancer after they completed neoadjuavant therapy because they had progression of their disease or had poor overall fitness to undergo the more definitive surgical procedure. They concluded that the only two indications for initial diversion were the inability to perform a colonoscopy past the lesion and fecal incontinence while worsening diarrhea or bowel function during the neoadjuvant therapy were not good indications for diverting stoma.[8]

Temporary stomas may be created as either an ileostomy or a colostomy, with the type of stoma used, dictated by the circumstances found at the time of the initial surgery as well as the preference of the surgeon. Many surgeons prefer a protective loop ileostomy for low-lying anastomoses because of the relative ease of reversal, easier stoma management by the patient, lower incidence of parastomal hernia formation, and a lower incidence of peristomal sepsis.[9,10]

A study comparing loop transverse colostomy to loop ileostomy for fecal diversion for low colo-rectal or colo-anal anastomoses demonstrated that the patients undergoing loop colostomy had more complications than those patients undergoing loop ileostomy such as parastomal and incisional hernias, stomal prolapse, and fecal fistulas. They suggested that loop ileostomy provided a better means of diversion.[11]

Stomas may be created as either a loop stoma or an end stoma. Loop stomas are often used when they are intended to be temporary since such a creation will often facilitate reversal. They may also be used in cases of distal intestinal obstruction, whereby the primary cause of the obstruction is left undisturbed. A loop stoma is required in these cases in order to decompress both sides of the bowel and to prevent a closed loop obstruction distally if an end stoma were created instead. Alternatively, an end stoma with a distal mucous fistula may be created in order to provide distal bowel decompression. Loop stomas are often larger than end stomas since both limbs of bowel must be exteriorized through the same fascial defect. This large size may make it more difficult for the patients to care for the stoma with an appropriate appliance. In addition, loop stomas may be more prone to develop parastomal hernias because of the larger abdominal wall defect and may ultimately result in stomal prolapse. These arguments against a loop stoma may make a proximal end stoma and a distal mucous fistula a more desirable option.

End stomas are often smaller and easier to manage. They are rarely associated with stomal prolapse and may have a lower incidence of parastomal hernia formation. However, if the end stoma is done on a temporary basis, they often require more extensive surgery for reversal since the other end of the bowel is often buried within the abdominal cavity. Many surgeons opt to tack the distal limb of bowel near the site of the end stoma if possible in order to facilitate reversal.

Another alternative in stoma creation is the loop end stoma. This may be performed in the obese patient where it is difficult to bring up an end stoma because of the large thick abdominal wall and the greater stretch applied to the bowel mesentery in these patients. The stretched mesentery may result in ischemia of the end of the bowel if it is brought up as a simple end stoma. In such cases, many surgeons prefer to bring the bowel up to the skin as a loop with the distal end being closed off in order to improve vascularity of the stoma itself since this will no longer be the end of the bowel.

Stoma Physiology

The physiological changes that occur in patients with ostomies are primarily related to the loss of continence and reduced colonic absorptive surface area. These affect fluid and electrolyte balance and lifestyle but generally have little effect on nutrition. However, once more than 50 cm of terminal ileum has been removed or taken out of continuity, nutritional consequences are likely.

Output

Ostomy output is directly related to the location of the opening in the bowel. Distal left or sigmoid colostomies normally produce formed stools that are of similar consistent to that of the anorectum. The more proximal the colostomy, the less surface area is available for water and electrolyte absorption and so the more liquid the stools. Right sided colostomies not only produce a high volume but also have the additional disadvantage of a malodorous output because of the effects of colonic bacteria.

Initially after creation the output from an ileostomy tends to be fairly watery and green or bilious in color. Within a few days to a week of resumption of a regular diet, the material becomes thicker and more yellow-brown, although a greenish tinge often remains. The typical consistency is of watery porridge or applesauce. It is affected by diet, fluid intake, medications, and on-going problems such as Crohn's disease or adhesions. If a substantial amount of small bowel has been removed the output is looser and the patient is more prone to dehydration. It is not uncommon for some food to pass out in a recognizable state. Notable foods for this occurrence include corn, other vegetables, and nuts. Some pills may also not be broken down in the small bowel, decreasing the bioavailability of these medications. Most patients with an ileostomy notice little odor from the output; however, certain foods, such as eggs and fish, may produce an offensive smell.[12]

Volume

In the healthy control subject, about 1,000–2,000 ml of fluid passes through the ileocecal valve daily. This quantity is reduced by 80–90% to 100–200 ml of fluid volume in normal stool as it passes through the colon. Unless the patient has diarrhea, left-sided colostomy output is similar to the feces that would be passed trans-anally, and there is little loss of total body fluid or sodium.[13]

Although postoperative ileostomy output may be high, it quite rapidly settles down to a more acceptable volume. "Ileostomy dysfunction," although a general sounding term, refers to increased ileostomy output due to partial obstruction caused by inflammation and stenosis. This term was coined in the era of secondary maturation. Historically, high outputs were anticipated for weeks after creation of an ileostomy, but this was found to be due to inflammation of the exposed small bowel serosa (serositis). Once primary maturation was adopted, this problem essentially disappeared.[5,14]

Postoperative colostomy output is also often liquid, but it rapidly becomes formed with the resumption of a normal diet and the return of ordered motility. The average colostomy produces about 200–700 ml with a median of about 500 ml per day. Total bowel rest results in a decrease in output by at least one-half and may be as low as 50–100 ml per day.[13]

The volume of ileostomy output fairly widely varies among patients but only mildly varies from day to day in an individual patient. Although the average output is about 500 ml per day, a healthy, functioning ileostomy may produce up to 1,000–1,500 ml in a day. Output above this level are usually associated with dehydration.[15–19] Large amounts of fluid intake usually do not alter the output volume very much as most of it is absorbed and excreted through the kidneys.[17]

Ileostomates may generally eat a regular diet without restrictions. Decreased fluid intake slows the output and thickens it, while fatty food and large amounts of liquid increase transit and the fluidity of the effluent.[12] Prunes and cabbage may also increase the output.[17] Ileostomy effluent is generally weakly acidic at a pH of about 6.3.[13] When the terminal ileum has been resected but colon remains in situ, more of the bile salts will enter the colon, which may result in a secretory diarrhea. This problem may be ameliorated by the use of oral bile binding agents such as cholestyramine (Questran).

Transit

An ileostomy continuously functions and its output is not eliminated by the timing of meals or rest. Yet, in most patients the output increases with meals and certain foods. Surgical resection of the anorectum and/or colon has effects on the function of the proximal gastrointestinal tract and the integration of hormonal and neuroenteric activity. These interactions are complex and not well understood in health, much less in postoperative patients. Although the data are limited, it appears that small bowel transit times decrease after ileostomy, possibly related to mucosal hypertrophy and adaptation. The specific mechanisms are not known. Gastric emptying has been a subject of several studies but the results are conflicting. Soper and his colleagues[20] found that gastric emptying is not altered in ileostomy patients. Yet, small bowel transit is longer than in control subjects (348 vs. 243 min). In a more recent study, Robertson and his colleagues[21] found that gastric emptying of liquids is not altered but emptying of solids is slowed.

Ileostomy output and dehydration may be decreased by prolonging the transit time to allow for more absorption. Codeine, loperamide, and Lomotil® have all been shown to have this effect.[22,23]

Fluid and Electrolyte Balance

The average ileostomy puts out about 500 ml of water and 60 mmol of sodium per day, amounts approximately two to three times higher volumes than found in normal fecal output.[13] Consequently, the ileostomate must compensate by increasing intake or conserving other losses. Urinary volume is relatively decreased in patients with ileostomies by as much as 40%, while renal sodium losses may be decreased by 55%.[24,25] Yet, in spite of the efforts of the kidneys to maintain balance, total body water and sodium reductions may be a chronic condition in ileostomy patients.[26–28]

The chronic dehydration and loss of fluid and electrolytes make ileostomy patients prone to dehydration. Rehydration is best accomplished with fairly large amounts of normal saline.[13] There is a direct relationship between absorption of nutrients and electrolytes and transit time.[29]

Flora

The normal terminal ileum harbors few organisms in the healthy individual. After creation of an ileostomy, the distal ileum is rapidly colonized with a variety of bacteria. The microflora of an individual is fairly stable over time, whereas there is great variability between individuals.[30] Staphylococci, streptococci, and fungi are increased while Bacteriodes fragilis is rarely found in ileostomy effluent. The major variations in the flora of effluent from ileostomies, transverse colostomies, and feces per anum are in the relative numbers of anaerobes with log differences increasing from proximal to distal.[31,32]

Nutrition

The colon plays little role in the maintenance of normal nutrition, working primarily to absorb fluid and to store feces so that the frequency of bowel evacuation may be limited. Thus, removal of the colon alone has little effect on nutrition. Patients who require a total proctocolectomy for diseases such as ulcerative colitis or Crohn's disease are often malnourished due to their underlying problem. Postoperatively, they are able to gain weight and return to a much better level of nitrogen balance and general nutrition.

Loss of more than a few feet of the terminal ileum, may result in loss of bile acids and poor absorption of fat and fat-soluble vitamins[17,33] Specifically, Vitamin B12, necessary for normal hemoglobin synthesis, may not be adequately absorbed in patients with terminal ileal loss or significant Crohn's disease. This loss results in pernicious or macrocytic anemia, and these patients may require monthly administration of Vitamin B12 (intramuscular or nasal). Absorption may also be impeded by distal ileal bacterial overgrowth.[34–36] Kidney stones may be a consequence of chronic dehydration and acidic urine. Adding sodium bicarbonate to the diet as well as increasing fluid intake may help to prevent uric acidic stone formation.[37–39]

Preoperative Considerations

Stomas need to be constructed in both the elective and emergency situations. If stomas are to be electively created during scheduled surgical cases then proper preoperative planning needs to be initiated. This planning includes both preoperative counseling and stoma marking. The counseling must encompass several critical aspects for the patient. First, the patient must understand the need for the stoma and whether the surgeon plans for the stoma to be placed on a permanent or temporary basis. Second, the patient should be provided with ample opportunity to ask questions related to the stoma and the overall surgery. Most patients will experience a great deal of anxiety related to the creation of a stoma. Third, the patients should be offered reading material, videos, and online Web sites that may help relieve this anxiety and answer their many questions. The patients should be shown the appliances and stoma-related products in advance of the surgery as well. Often times it is beneficial for the patient to speak to other willing patients in a similar situation who have a stoma so that many of their questions may be appropriately addressed by those dealing with a stoma. Support group participation may be very valuable. Lastly, the patients should be properly marked by the enterostomal therapist for the ideal site(s) of the stoma on the abdominal wall since stoma sites may greatly vary in individuals based upon body habitus. Stoma sites should be modified to avoid scars, skin creases, and other skin disorders. Stoma markings should be done with the patient in both the sitting and standing positions and attention must be given to the beltline and pant height. The site must be checked to ensure skin folds or crevices do not interfere with appliance fitting. In obese individuals, the stoma must not be hidden below a large abdominal pannus or stoma care will be very difficult (Figure 31-1). In this circumstance a supraumbilical stoma is often more functional. Stomas should be placed through the rectus sheath and not lateral to it in order to have the rectus muscle provide support and reduce the incidence of parastomal hernias.

Once proper placement is ascertained, the spot is marked with indelible ink. This may be done with a water-resistant marker if the marking is done close to the surgery date, or it may be done by using ink and then puncturing the skin under the ink thereby forming a permanent tattoo. In complex cases, a stoma appliance can be fixed to the proposed site and worn for 24 h to test placement. Hernias can also be used for temporary marking.

Siting a stoma through the umbilicus is a reasonable alternative when there is no other good location. Raza and colleagues[40] felt that this was a good option based on their series of 101 patients; only four needed revision and there were no parastomal hernias or prolapse. Fitzgerald et al.[41] noted that after closure in infants and children, the scar resembles a normal umbilicus and is cosmetically superior to that of an ostomy placed elsewhere.

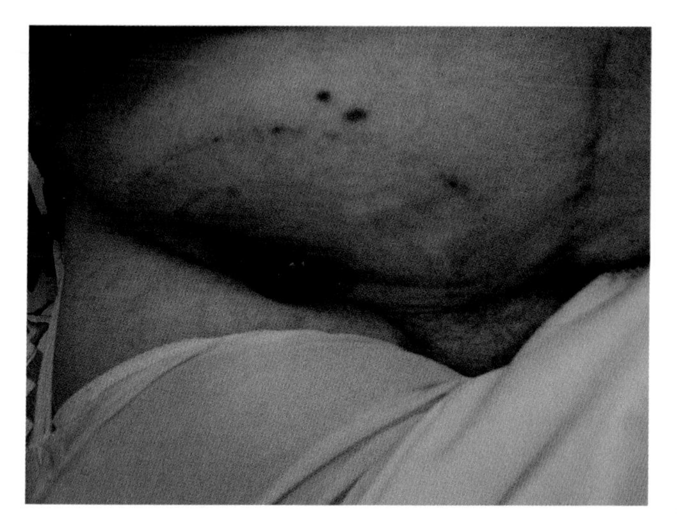

FIGURE 31-1. Example of poorly placed stoma.

Stoma counseling is an important part of stoma acceptance. This finding has been confirmed in a study that used multiple regression analysis to show that stoma adjustment was related to learning how to care for the stoma by the patient, interpersonal relationships that the patient has developed, and better stoma placement. The authors concluded that addressing the psychosocial concerns of the patient should become a part of the care routinely given to stoma patients and preoperative counseling plays a major role in this care.[42] Another randomized controlled trial comparing preoperative stoma teaching with postoperative stoma teaching after elective colorectal surgery showed far greater proficiency with the stoma, shorter hospital stays, and lower overall hospital costs if patients were educated about the stoma in advance of the surgery.[43]

Quality of Life with a Stoma

While many surgeons may feel that patients were "let down" after stoma creation a recent study evaluating the quality of life of patients who underwent surgery for rectal cancer showed that those patients undergoing stoma creation reported a higher global health status and fewer GI problems after surgery.[44] This result may be due to the fact that the patients were so debilitated with their initial disease that having a stoma significantly improved their overall status.

However, a Danish study evaluated the quality of life of colorectal cancer patients with and without a stoma. As one might expect, they found that those patients with a stoma experienced far great signs of depression, worse social functioning, greater issues with body image, greater problems voiding, and more sexual problems particularly in male patients. They also found that if the stoma was created at a later time rather than at the initial surgery, the patients also experienced a poorer quality of life.[45]

A study comparing the quality of life of patients with temporary ileostomy vs. temporary colostomy revealed that both groups of patients had a significant impairment in quality of life assessments. These authors found that the ileostomy effluent was more tolerable and that these patients had fewer issues with personal hygiene and better appetites than those with a colostomy. There were no differences in the two groups in terms of travel, daily activities, or sexual activity.[46]

While we may believe that patients are pleased to have their stomas reversed a study from Germany may suggest otherwise. They evaluated the quality of life of patients who underwent temporary stoma reversal. While they found that the patient's body image and leisure activities improved, there was no change in overall quality of life since many of the patients experienced an increase in gastrointestinal problems after stoma reversal. Many patients actually felt overall worse than before the stoma was reversed. The authors concluded that the surgeon should engage in preoperative counseling of patients prior to stoma reversal.[47]

In summary, there is no doubt that patients would prefer to live their lives without a stoma. However, with proper education and counseling by the surgeon, enterostomal therapists, and support groups both before and after the surgery, patients can learn to adapt and maintain a healthy and happy existence with a stoma.

Techniques of Stoma Creation

The basic surgical principles that apply to stoma creation include the following:

1. The bowel to be exteriorized must be well vascularized and the mesentery must not be stretched to the point of inducing stomal ischemia or necrosis.
2. The bowel must reach the skin without tension in order to prevent stomal retraction.
3. The intestine must be brought through the rectus sheath and the facial opening should be just two fingers breadth in width in order to reduce the incidence of parastomal hernia and prevent obstruction of the bowel as it exits through the opening.
4. A disc of skin should be excised where the stoma is to be placed rather than simply creating a slit in the skin. This will prevent stomal stenosis and obstruction.

A disc of skin is removed in the site where the stoma will be placed. The anterior and posterior fascia is then opened in an up and down manner in order to accommodate the portion of bowel. Some surgeons prefer a cruciate fascial incision instead. Care should be taken to avoid the inferior epigastric vessels as one approaches the posterior rectus sheath. The bowel is then grasped with a babcock clamp and then exteriorized. In loop stomas some surgeons prefer making a mesenteric window just underneath the bowel edge and placing an umbilical tape around the bowel and then pulling this through the abdominal wall with the bowel (Figures 31-2–31-4).

After exteriorization of the bowel the abdomen is closed and then the stoma is matured. A stoma rod is typically

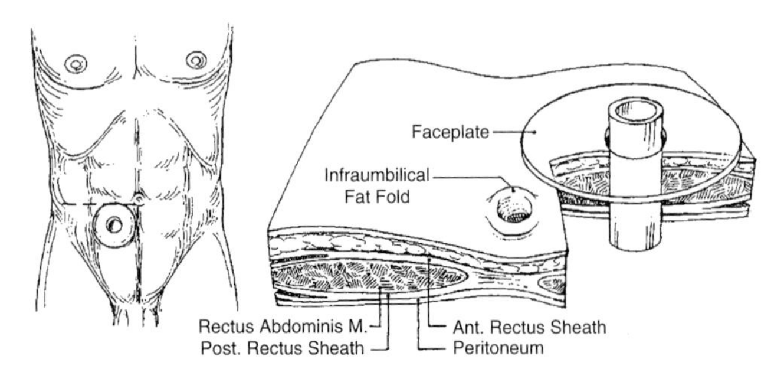

FIGURE 31-2. Stomal placement. The site is selected to bring the stoma through the rectus abdominus muscle (with permission from Beck DE. Intestinal stomas. In: Beck DE, editor. Handbook of colorectal surgery. 2nd ed. Taylor and Francis; 2003).

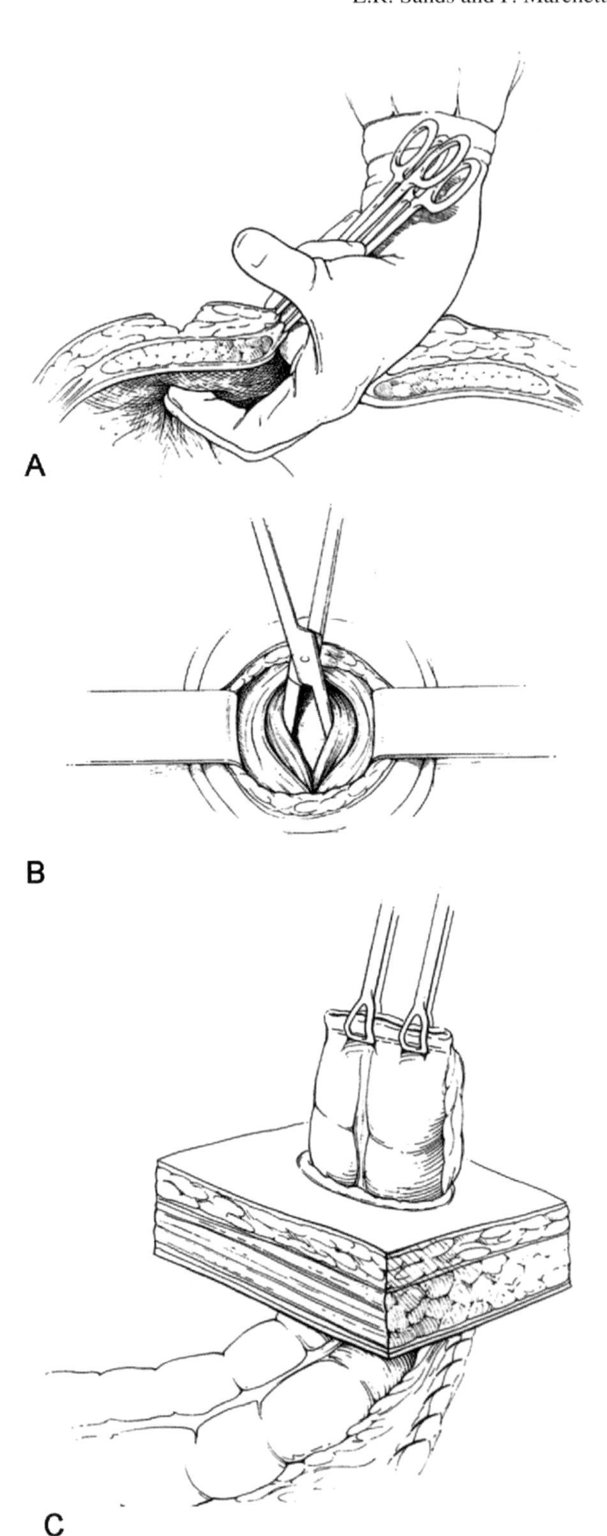

FIGURE 31-3. Colostomy creation: **A** Circular skin disk is removed. **B** Fascia is divided. **C** End of colon is brought through the fascia and skin opening (with permission from Beck DE. End sigmoid colostomy. In: MacKeigan JM, Cataldo PA, editors. Intestinal stomas. Principles, techniques, and management. Taylor and Francis; 1993).

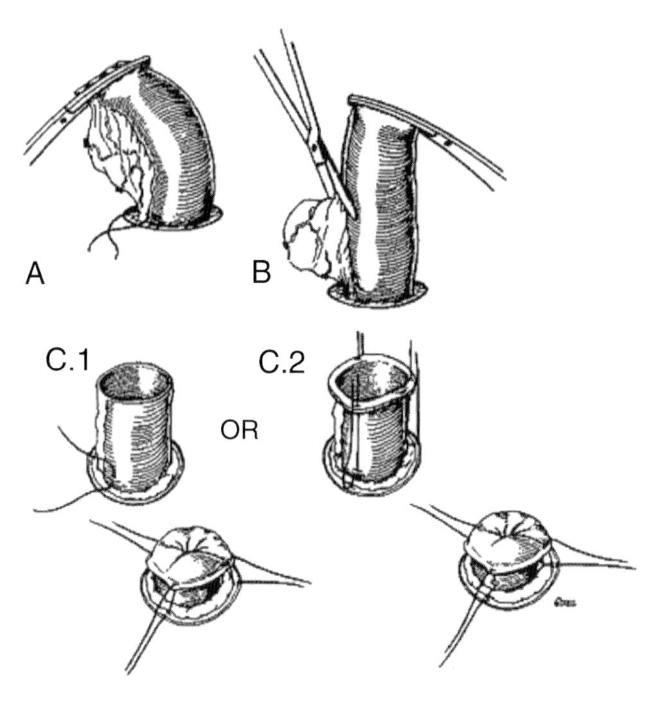

FIGURE 31-4. Ileostomy maturation. **A** Ligation. **B** Trimming of the ileal mesentery. **C.1** Serosa is attached to Scarpa's fascia and the mucosal edge sutured to the dermis. **C.2** Triangular stitch from ileal end to serosa to dermis; tying sutures inverts the ileum to the skin (with permission from Beck DE. Intestinal stomas. In: Beck DE, editor. Handbook of colorectal surgery. 2nd ed. Taylor and Francis; 2003).

placed under a loop stoma while end stomas are matured with a simple eversion technique using an absorbable suture material such as 3-0 chromic suture. While eversion is essential in ileostomies because of the greater liquid and voluminous effluent, not all colostomies need to be everted.

Some surgeons may choose to tack the mesentery to the lateral sidewall to prevent internal hernia formation around the stoma site while others may suture the stoma to the undersurface of the fascia in an attempt to prevent parastomal hernia formation or prolapse. While there is no data to suggest that these techniques may in fact be effective, Goligher in the 1950s advocated delivering the bowel via an extraperitoneal approach in order to reduce the incidence of these complications.[48] More recent innovations have included a variety of biologic and synthetic meshes employed in a prophylactic setting at the time of stoma construction. A range of sublayer underlay and overlay techniques have been described.

Laparoscopic Stoma Creation

Today many stomas are created laparoscopically. Laparoscopy has emerged as a frontrunner in terms of stoma creation because of the minimally invasive technique and the rather quick recovery. The advantages of laparoscopy include smaller incisions, less postoperative pain, reduced use of pain medication thereby reducing postoperative ileus and the time to first stool. The laparoscopic technique is ideally suited to stoma creation since it often does not require much dissection or specimen extraction, thereby making this one of the easiest laparoscopic procedures to perform. In addition, there are no incisions except for the port sites thereby facilitating the placement of the appliance over the stoma site.

If the patient is undergoing a colonic resection with a planned stoma, then the surgeon will often place a port at the site of the stoma marking and exteriorize the bowel through this area at the completion of the surgery. However, some care must be taken upon using this laparoscopic technique with regard to bowel orientation. Since many surgeons prefer placing the proximal portion of a loop stoma at the upper aspect of the skin and abdominal wall defect, one must ensure that the bowel is properly oriented upon delivery through the abdominal wall and that the bowel is not twisted or kinked. Twisting of the bowel at this level may result in a mechanical obstruction at the level of the stoma site.

More importantly one must assure that the proximal portion of the bowel is exteriorized in those patients undergoing an end stoma. Division of the bowel and maturation of the incorrect limb will result in a complete bowel obstruction and will ultimately require a return to the operating room to correct this problem. While this problem would rarely occur in open stoma creation, it is a possibility in the laparoscopic technique if one fails to identify the proper orientation of the bowel especially in cases of colonic redundancy. This problem may be avoided by ensuring complete visualization of the bowel and, in the case of an end colostomy, by identifying the upper aspect of the rectum noted by the convergence of the teniae coli and following the bowel proximally from that point. Another technique that may be used is to insufflate the rectum with air at the time of stoma creation in order to identify which end is most distal. If one is still having trouble identifying the proximal and distal portions of the bowel, then a loop stoma should be performed in order to prevent maturation of the incorrect side. Alternatively, one can always convert to an open procedure if there is still uncertainty about the correct anatomy. Conversion to an open procedure often shows good judgment rather than defeat.

There have been a variety of techniques described for laparoscopic stoma creation using zero, one, or more ports. Hellinger and his colleagues at the University of Miami have described a laparoscopic technique through a trephine incision and without a port and without gas insufflation for stoma creation in those patients who may not be able to tolerate a pneumoperitoneum. This technique simply uses abdominal wall retraction and placement of the laparoscope within the trephine opening in order to identify and orient the bowel. In addition, this technique allows for visualization and possible mobilization of the colon along the white line of Toldt should that be necessary.[49]

Most laparoscopic stomas are created using two or more ports. One port is typically placed at the site of the stoma

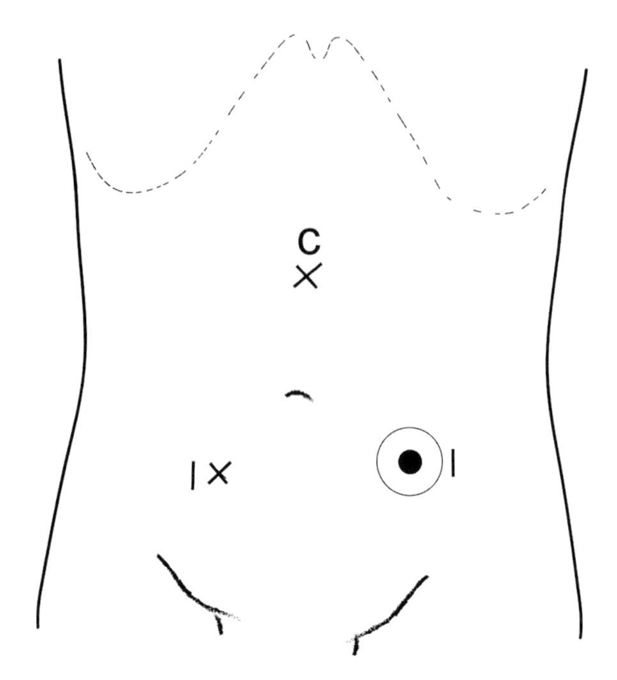

FIGURE 31-5. Port placement for stoma creation.

while the other ports are placed either peri-umbilical or on the opposite side of the abdomen in a triangular manner (Figure 31-5). This port configuration facilitates working within the abdominal cavity and allows the surgeon to identify and raise the limb of bowel for the stoma. The white line of Toldt is identified and dissected if bowel redundancy does not exist in order to allow the bowel greater mobility to be brought up for a stoma. As in any laparoscopic case, care must be taken to avoid inadvertent injury to other loops of bowel as well as the ureters in the retroperitoneum. Another laparoscopic technique for colostomy creation has been described by placing the camera in the right side of the abdomen, thereby facilitating dissection of the colon on the left side and detaching it from the white line of Toldt and thereby allowing it to easily reach a preselected stoma site in the left side of the abdomen.[50]

Laparoscopic stoma creation has been compared to open stoma creation in several studies. A study from Germany showed fewer operative complications from open stoma creation compared to laparoscopic stoma creation. However, the mortality associated with the laparoscopic group was considerably lower. They concluded that for palliative stoma creation there were significant advantages using the laparoscopic technique for stoma creation.[51]

The Cleveland Clinic Florida colorectal surgery team reported their experience with laparoscopic stoma creation in 1997. In their early study of 32 patients who mostly underwent loop ileostomy, they converted to open surgery in five patients. Two of these conversions were related to a noted enterotomy at the time of surgery that was repaired. In addition, two other patients required reoperation for stoma outlet obstruction, one of which was twisted at the level of the fascia. The mean operative time was 76 min and the mean length of stay was 6.2 days.[52]

Many surgeons now believe that laparoscopy should be the primary means of stoma creation and a recent study of a 10-year period confirmed this conclusion. In this review of 80 patients who mostly suffered from advanced unresectable colorectal cancer, all but one patient underwent successful laparoscopic stoma creation. While the majority of patients underwent loop stoma formation of either the ileum or colon, only five patients suffered complications requiring re-operation including parastomal abscess, stomal retraction, small bowel obstruction, postoperative bleeding, and port site hernia. The average length of stay was 10.3 days. While this length of stay may seem long it is most often related to proper patient teaching in stoma use and care.[53]

Morbidly obese patients present a significant challenge in stoma creation. Some have advocated a loop end stoma in this patient group.[54] Another technique has been described to assist in the stoma creation in the morbidly obese patient. This method involves the use of an Alexis wound protector placed in the abdominal wall, facilitating the bowel to pass through the abdominal wall with less friction and resistance because of the extensive subcutaneous tissues in these patients.[55]

Controversies of Intestinal Stomas

When Should Stomas Be Used to Provide Distal Anastomotic Protection

One of the most controversial topics regarding stomas relates to their use in protecting distal bowel anastomoses. While there are many advocates of diverting proximal stomas, there are also many others who believe that the complications of the stoma itself as well as the potential difficulties encountered in stoma reversal make the stoma extremely undesirable. This topic of fecal diversion to prevent distal leak is so controversial in that some surgeons believe that all distal anastomoses should be diverted while others feel that it should almost never be done. Still, there are others that believe there may be subsets of patients who should be diverted while others may avoid diversion altogether.

A recent meta-analysis of both retrospective and prospective series reviewed the results of a defunctioning stoma in patients undergoing surgery for distal rectal cancer. While the retrospective studies did not show any difference in the anastomotic failure rate with a defunctioning stoma in place, they did prove that there were far fewer major problems once these leaks occurred. The prospective series revealed a lower leak rate with a diverting stoma in place. The study concluded that there were true benefits from proximal anastomotic diversion in patients undergoing surgery for low rectal cancer.[56]

A surgical group from Italy tried to determine whether patients should receive a protective stoma after undergoing neoadjuvant therapy for rectal cancer and then definitive surgery. They studied 55 patients who underwent surgery without diversion; they experienced 15 anastomotic leaks, five of which were considered requiring major immediate surgery for diversion. One of these patients ultimately died of sepsis. They concluded that a diverting stoma was only necessary in 10% of their patients and therefore most patients may avoid the additional surgery, morbidity, or high complication rate of a temporizing stoma.[57]

Another study assessing diverting stoma compared two groups of patients who either underwent or did not undergo fecal diversion. Two patients in the undiverted group died of complications from anastomotic leakage. In addition, four patients in whom initial fecal diversion was not undertaken ultimately required permanent stomas. Conversely, no patients in whom initial diversion was undertaken required a permanent stoma. The authors concluded that there were clear and significant advantages to a proximal stoma in patients undergoing low resection for distal rectal cancer.[58]

The group from UC Irvine compared their patients who underwent surgery for rectal cancer, most of whom underwent neoadjuvant chemotherapy and radiation therapy for their disease. Most of their patients underwent a single-stage procedure with a lower overall and a lower anastomotic-associated complication rate than those who underwent fecal diversion at the initial procedure both of which reached statistical significance. However, most of their single-stage procedures involved a higher level anastomosis (3.8 cm above the anal verge vs. 2.6 cm) compared to the anastomoses constructed in patients who underwent fecal diversion. They felt that many patients may be safely operated on with a single-stage procedure and that fecal diversion may be reserved in selected patients.[59]

A publication from Germany evaluating 881 patients undergoing a low anterior resection with a protective stoma revealed virtually identical leak rates compared to the 1,848 patients who did not have fecal diversion. While both groups of patients had a leak rate of roughly 14%, the number of patients requiring operative intervention for a leak were significantly lower in the diverted group. In addition, the mortality was lower in the diverted patients. They also found that the morbidity associated with colostomy reversal was lower than it was for ileostomy reversal suggesting that patients may be better served with a colostomy rather than an ileostomy.[60]

Some surgeons have advocated anterior resection of rectal cancer without bowel preparation and without fecal diversion. In a study from the Netherlands of 144 patients who underwent anterior resection of the rectum without mechanical bowel preparation or fecal diversion, the authors reported a leak rate of only 4.9%. They found a trend toward higher leak rates amongst men with lower anastomoses and more advanced cancers. They concluded that performing anterior resection without bowel preparation or diversion is safe.[61]

One must clearly take into account the morbidity of a stoma as well. In a recent study from Norway where a protective stoma was used in 72 patients who underwent surgery for rectal cancer over a 12-year period, the authors found that five patients developed stomal complications immediately after the primary surgery, and another 20% developed problems after hospital discharge. Only 62 patients underwent stoma reversal, five of whom had problems with the reversal while in the hospital. In addition, two patients died of complications from the reversal surgery. In total 19 patients (26%) suffered complications of the stoma in general and eight of these patients required re-operation. They concluded that there was considerable morbidity to the stoma creation, many patients may never undergo reversal of the stoma, and the stoma does not prevent anastomotic leak.[62]

The need for a defunctioning stoma after low anterior resection was recently evaluated in a large meta-analysis of over 11,000 patients. Four randomized control trials and 21 nonrandomized studies were reviewed in this analysis. Both sets of studies showed a lower clinical anastomotic leak rate and a lower re-operation rate while the nonrandomized trials also showed a lower mortality rate in the stoma group. They concluded that stomas should routinely be used in patients undergoing low anterior resection.[63]

This study was reinforced by yet another randomized controlled trial that intraoperatively assigned to either receive a diverting stoma or be left in continuity while undergoing a low anterior resection; 34 patients were enrolled in the study and the symptomatic anastomotic leak rate was significantly higher in the undiverted group (37.5%) compared to the diverted group (5.5%). Six patients in the undiverted group required reoperation. The authors concluded that protective stomas are a necessary part of the healing process after proctectomy with total mesorectal excision.[64]

Stomal Complications

The difficulties of a stoma should not be underestimated. The true incidence of stoma-related complications is unknown since there is great debate as to what actually defines a stoma-related problem. As most patients will experience some sort of skin irritation from the stoma or the stoma appliance, this represents the largest subset of stoma-related issues.

The prevalence of intestinal stoma complications was assessed from a colorectal group in Chicago. They reported the incidence of stoma complications in 1,616 patients. A total of 34.2% of these individuals suffered a complication related to their stoma, 27.7% of those individuals having an early complication, and only 6.5% suffering a late complication. The authors noted that the highest complication rate was in patients with a loop ileostomy.[65]

In a study from the United Kingdom, patients who underwent laparoscopic colectomy had a significantly prolonged hospital stay (6 days vs. 10 days) from the mere presence of a stoma due to the teaching and comfort level that patients needed to attain with the stoma. Interestingly, conversion to open surgery did not pose a significant increase in length of stay compared to the presence of a stoma.[66]

A surgical group from Italy compared the complications of loop ileostomy, loop colostomy, and end colostomy. In this retrospective review, there was no correlation in complication rates associated with stomas created either on an elective or emergent basis, the indications for surgery, the patient's gender, or the stoma site. There was an overall stoma complication rate of 60% mostly related to dermatitis, parastomal hernia, leakage from the appliance, and stomal stenosis. The fewest complications were noted in end colostomies and in patients less than 68 years of age.[67]

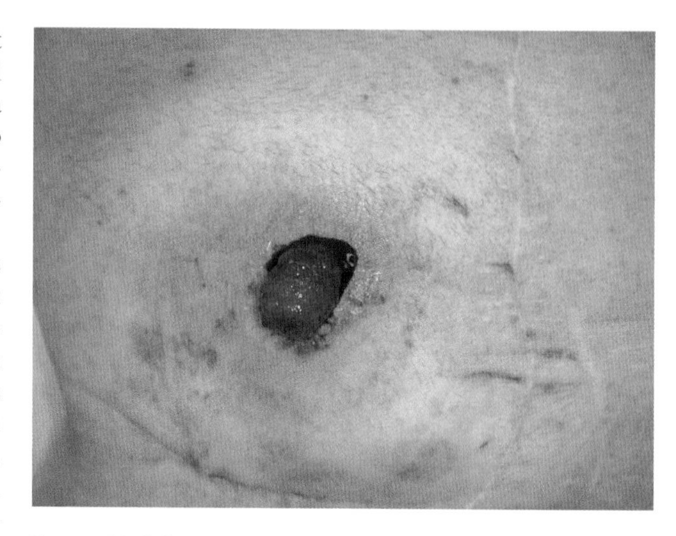

FIGURE 31-6. Stoma with severe skin problems.

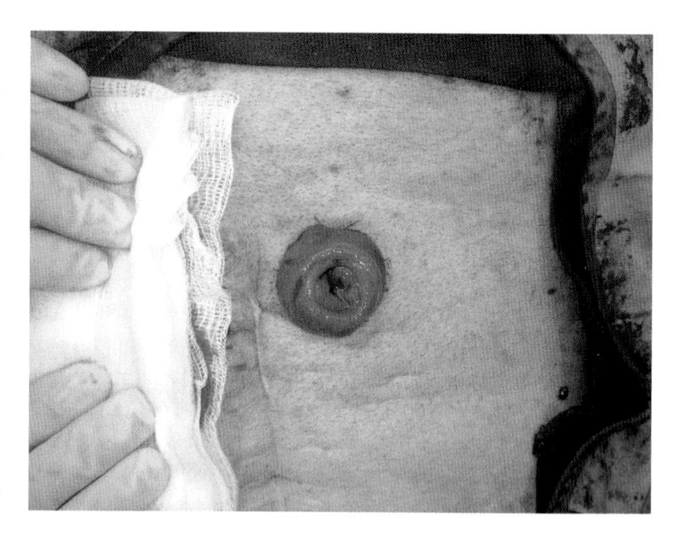

FIGURE 31-7. Stoma revision.

Skin Irritation and Leakage

While many surgeons would consider skin irritation and leakage commonplace issues relating to stomas, most surgeons consider this a complication only if the problem is so severe that it warrants surgical correction. Most of the skin issues related to the stoma do not require surgery. Many surgeons will refer their patients to an enterostomal therapist in order to help with this problem. However, many institutions may not employ an enterostomal therapist. Therefore, many colorectal training programs today provide their trainees an opportunity to work one on one with an enterostomal therapist in order to learn how to care for stomal-related problems. Often times the surgeon may be required to mark the patients in advance of surgery for proper stomal placement. It is imperative that surgeons have a good understanding of stomal care. Many of the skin problems from a stoma may be traced back to poor site selection in the first place whereby the stoma was placed under a skin crease. In these cases, it is important to try various other appliances of a convex nature in order to raise the lip of the stoma to get a better fit. In addition, a good seal may be achieved by using a variety of adhesives, powders, or sealants. Eakin cohesive seal rings form a waterproof barrier around the skin and the applied pouch and are designed to prevent pouch leakage in addition to extending the wear time of the pouch. They may also be useful to fill in uneven skin surfaces around the stoma site.

One study showed that 51% of patients questioned, reported problems with a rash and 36% had experienced leakage. Both problems were seen more often in patients with ileostomies rather than colostomies. In addition, nearly one-third to one-half of the patients also experienced a reaction to the stoma adhesive. However, only 8% of ostomates reported significant difficulty associated with skin irritation.[68]

Surgical correction for severe skin problems from the stoma may need to be done if enterostomal care has failed. If the stoma was used on a temporary basis then the stoma should be reversed as soon as it is feasible to do so. If, however, the stoma was created on a permanent basis, then stoma revision may need to be performed. Oftentimes the stoma will need to be resited to a more desirable area on the abdominal wall (Figures 31-6 and 31-7).

Parastomal Hernia

Parastomal hernia remains a major problem following stoma creation. While the true incidence of parastomal hernia is unknown, this complication is so frequent that most surgeons do not classify this as a complication until it becomes necessary to surgically repair the hernia. In fact, the creation of a defect in the abdominal wall for a stoma by definition places a weakness in the abdominal wall where there once was complete continuity. The truth is that many patients with parastomal hernia often have some disability related to this problem. The problems may be as minor as skin breakdown near the stoma site or an inability to fit an appliance around the stoma, or it can be as devastating as incarcerating a loop of bowel within the hernia and requiring emergency surgery for resection and repair.

A recent prospective audit of parastomal hernias found that the overall rate of parastomal hernia was 33% and that aperture size and patient age were independent predictors of this problem. They found that for every additional millimeter increase in aperture size there was a 10% increase in risk of developing a hernia and for every additional year of patient age the risk increased by 4%. In addition, colostomies were at higher risk for hernia formation than ileostomies.[69]

As a result, many surgeons have advocated prophylactic mesh placement at the time of the stoma creation in order to prevent parastomal hernias. These meshes have been placed at varying levels in the abdominal wall and the use of the newer biologic and synthetic meshes may be more promising. A recent prospective study using polypropylene mesh simply placed in the pre-peritoneal space without sutures was performed in a total of 42 patients. While the majority of the created stomas were end colostomies, five patients in this study underwent surgery for stoma resiting. In the postoperative follow-up there were four parastomal hernias noted (9.52%), three of which were asymptomatic while the fourth required re-repair due to a poorly fitting appliance. There were no complications related to the mesh itself. The authors concluded that these results justify the placement of a parastomal mesh on a prophylactic basis.[70]

One randomized trial of 54 patients undergoing permanent intestinal stoma revealed that none of the patients who underwent prophylactic mesh placement developed a parastomal hernia while 8 of 27 without mesh did develop a hernia.[71]

Guzman-Valdivia retrospectively reviewed incisional hernias occurring at the previous stoma site in 70 patients after stoma reversal. While all of these patients underwent identical, relatively simple procedures for stoma reversal, the authors found an incisional hernia rate of 31% at the previous stoma site leading the author to conclude that the mere presence of a stoma had some degree of morbidity in its own right. The rate of incisional hernia formation was higher in the first year of follow-up and in patients with comorbidities particularly diabetes.[72]

Another study evaluating risk factors for parastomal hernia after APR evaluated 41 patients who underwent either laparoscopic (22) or open (19) procedures. Parastomal hernias developed in nearly half the patients and in nearly equal numbers in both groups of patients. The authors concluded that the only risk factor for parastomal hernia formation after controlling for surgical approach, age, sex, or adjuvant therapy was obesity and waist circumference. They found that waist circumference over 100 cm was associated with a 75% probability of developing a parastomal hernia.[73]

Parastomal hernia prevention is perhaps the best method of treatment. As a general rule, stomas should be placed through the rectus sheath for additional muscular support, fascial openings should be of the appropriate size for the portion of exteriorized bowel, prophylactic use of mesh may be considered for those patients requiring a permanent stoma, and extraperitoneal tunneling of the bowel may also be considered.

Once parastomal hernias are present and repair is necessary, there are several surgical options available. The stoma may be resited to an area on the opposite side of the abdomen that has never been used. This operation may be performed by mobilizing the stoma via a parastomal incision and simply pushing the bowel over to the opposite side of the abdomen. This may be easily done if there are no adhesions to the anterior abdominal wall and if the bowel has sufficient length.

Other options for parastomal hernia repair include a laparoscopic approach with mesh implantation around the stoma and covering the fascial defect or an open technique around the stoma itself with either suture closure of the fascial defect or with the placement of mesh. Biologic meshes may be more suitable for this approach since the operation is considered a clean contaminated field.

A recent review from Hershey Medical Center regarding parastomal hernia repair evaluated their results in 25 patients over a 7-year period. Twelve patients underwent laparoscopic repair successfully completed in 11 patients while the remaining patients underwent open repairs. While the operative times were longer for the laparoscopic repairs (172 min vs. 137 min), the length of stay was shorter (3.1 days vs. 5.1 days). However, the recurrence rates were high in both groups occurring in four laparoscopic cases (33.3%) and seven open cases (53.8%).[74]

High Output Stomas

The long debate as to which stoma is best for the patient, colostomy or ileostomy will likely continue for years to come. The advantages of the colostomy include more formed stool with the ultimate possibility of stomal irrigation and not using an appliance. Many claim that the more solid effluent is easier to manage and there are far fewer cases of dehydration associated with the colostomy. However, others feel that the ileostomy with its smaller size and ease of reversal may be better. But the more voluminous and more liquid effluent typical of the ileostomy may make these patients more prone to electrolyte disturbances and dehydration with marked diarrhea and dehydration occurring in 5–20% of ileostomy patients particularly in the early postoperative period. An ileostomy typically begins to function by the third or fourth postoperative day with peaks of over 3 l of output by the fourth postoperative day.[75] Hyponatremia may ensue since the ostomy effluent is rich in sodium. In fact, even healthy patients with an ileostomy have been shown to in a chronic state of sodium and water depletion.[15] The normal ileostomy may lose in the range of 600 ml per day and 75 mmol of sodium per day. Therefore, serum electrolytes must be checked postoperatively and replenished with appropriate intravenous fluid selection. The small bowel often adapts quickly and the stoma output will thicken up especially when a diet is resumed. Patients should be told to drink plenty of fluids should they have a stoma with many of the popular sport drinks being suitable for fluid and electrolyte replenishment.

Once patients become dehydrated they also become uremic, often resulting in nausea secondary to the uremia. As such they have less desire to drink more fluids causing them to become more uremic and then more nauseated. This vicious cycle will continue until the patient is hospitalized and the intravascular volume is replenished with intravenous fluids. The stoma output will need to be controlled with anti-diarrheal agents or bile salt binders. Opiates may also be used to slow down small bowel transit. In extreme cases, injections of somatostatin may be used to reduce salt and water excretion and slow gastrointestinal tract motility.[76] Elements of the diet that increase stoma output such as foods high in sugar, salt, or fat should also be avoided.

Stone Formation

Another problem in patients with an ileostomy is the development of urinary stones. It has been estimated that up to 12% of patients with an ileostomy may develop urinary stones and the numbers seem to be higher in those patients who have had small bowel resected in addition to having an ileostomy.[77] While serum calcium, Vitamin D, and urinary calcium are often normal in these patients, it appears that a high level of uric acid is the main cause of the stone formation. As such, serum uric acid levels should be monitored in these patients and they should be started on allopurinol prophylactically if the levels remain high.[78,79]

The mechanism of urinary stone formation seems to be multifactorial. However, it is likely related to the fact that the uric acid crystals act as a nucleus for the precipitation of calcium salts. In addition, the hyperuricemia may allow the calcium oxalate crystals to form more readily by lowering the saturation index.[80] This may also be facilitated by the excess loss of fecal water, sodium, and bicarbonate, all of which reduces urinary pH and volume.[81] The acidic urine also favors the precipitation of uric acid. Patients should be advised to increase their fluid intake and possibly eliminate foods rich in oxalate such as spinach and some leafy vegetables.[82]

Whether there is a higher incidence of gallstone formation in patients with an ileostomy remains controversial. There does seem to be, however, a higher incidence of gallstones if there has been a resection of more than 10 cm of terminal ileum because of the increased loss of bile salts. This loss leads to a reduction in the bile salt pool causing instability in the solubility of cholesterol, thereby causing gallstone formation.[83]

Intestinal Obstruction

Intestinal obstruction may occur after any abdominal surgical procedure. Therefore, the true incidence of intestinal obstruction after stoma formation is not really known. In addition, how many obstructions are directly related to the stoma itself is not clear. However, there have been papers reporting bowel obstruction occurring in up to 20% of patients with an ileostomy. As in most cases, adhesions are probably the most common cause, but small bowel volvulus, internal hernia, or even incarcerated parastomal hernias may also be contributing factors. Some surgeons have suggested closing off the lateral peritoneal reflection around the stoma site or even bringing the bowel up to the skin in an extraperitoneal fashion in order to prevent internal hernia formation and torsion. However, there has never been proven true benefit to any of these methods.

Intestinal obstruction in patients with a stoma is handled as in any other case of bowel obstruction. The patients should be supported with intravenous fluids and nasogastric tube decompression of the bowel with serial abdominal exams and X-rays. Unresolving obstructions will need operative exploration and lysis of adhesions. If patients present with peritonitis with a bowel obstruction or signs of bowel ischemia then patients should be quickly resuscitated and taken to the operating room emergently for exploration. In this setting, many surgeons prefer a laparotomy to a laparoscopic approach since bowel distension may make laparoscopy difficult. If one suspects torsion of the bowel around the stoma site then it is unlikely that this will resolve without operative intervention.

Mention must be made of food bolus obstruction. Many patients with an ileostomy will develop signs and symptoms of bowel obstruction owing to the accumulation of poorly masticated or digested food (e.g., popcorn, peanuts, fresh fruits, meat, and vegetables). A careful history may reveal dietary indiscretions. Further, the possibility of a food bolus obstruction should be considered in any patient with an ileostomy who has radiologic evidence of a distal obstruction. A well-lubricated finger can be gently inserted into the stoma to feel for impacted material. A red rubber catheter is inserted gently into the ostomy and saline irrigation initiated. If suspicious concretions begin to pass into the stoma, the irrigations may be carefully repeated until the obstruction is relieved. A water soluble contrast enema through the obstructed stoma may also be both diagnostic and therapeutic by dislodging the bolus. Most of these food bolus obstructions resolve on their own and do not require surgery.

Ischemic Stomas

Many stomas may initially appear edematous and congested after stomal creation due to mechanical trauma and the compression of the small mesenteric vessels as they traverse the abdominal wall. This often resolves within a few days to weeks after surgery. However, true stomal ischemia is a much more serious problem and often occurs due to tension of the mesentery as the bowel exits the abdominal wall. It may also be related to the exteriorized portion of bowel being excessively stripped of its mesentery. Stoma creation becomes challenging in the morbidly obese patient and these patients in particular will require extensive mobilization of the bowel prior to exteriorization in order to avoid tension. In addition, the fascial opening will need to be of sufficient size in order not to compromise the mesenteric blood supply. If there is concern about bowel viability after surgery, one can simply insert a glass test tube or sigmoidoscope into the stoma in order to determine if the bowel is viable beneath the tip of the stoma. If the stoma is viable at the fascial level, then the patient may be carefully observed. However, if there is question about the viability of the stoma at the fascial level, the patient should be returned to the operating room in order to undergo stoma revision.

Proper stoma creation remains one of the most vital parts of the surgical procedure even though it is often the last part of a possibly long operation. Patient lifestyle and comfort depends on a well formed and viable stoma. The few extra efforts made during the stoma construction is often worth the days, weeks, or months of misery for the patient from a poorly done and ischemic stoma. While early stomal ischemia has been reported in 1–10% of colostomies and 1–5% of ileostomies,[84] stoma viability does not often get better once the patient is awake.

Stoma Prolapse

Stomal prolapse is a more common complication of loop than end stomas. This problem often occurs in patients with redundant segments of bowel and in those with a large enough fascial opening to permit such prolapse and intussusception. These patients commonly have parastomal hernias associated with the prolapse. Once again, the most conservative manner in which to manage this problem may be found with good enterostomal care. Often the appliances are cut to fit appropriately around the enlarged stoma with particular attention to providing good skin care around the stoma. A study investigating the cause of loop transverse colostomy prolapse revealed that the prolapse is the result of a redundant colon that invades the stoma with increased abdominal pressure. A suggestion of fixating the colon to the fascia may prevent this complication.[85]

The best way to treat a stomal prolapse is to reverse the stoma. If the stoma was initially planned as a temporizing stoma then the enterostomal therapist should assist the patient with managing the prolapse until the patient is ready to have the stoma reversed. Stoma reversal in these patients is usually straightforward and is often easily accomplished through a parastomal incision. Since these stomas are often loop stomas, both sides of the bowel are easily accessible and the bowel may be reanastomosed with sutures or stapling devices. However, if the stoma is a permanent one, then a technique to correct this problem under local anesthesia by amputating the excess bowel and reconstructing the stoma at the desired level with a linear stapler has been described.[86]

Stomal Irrigation and Continence

For those patients not desiring to wear an appliance, colostomy irrigation may provide an alternative. Colostomy irrigation may be learned by patients and may improve their quality of life and reduce overall costs. A study from Singapore in 26 patients who underwent abdominoperineal resection and ultimately learned stomal irrigation reported an improvement in stomal continence, sleep, sex, and skin complications compared to patients who did not learn or practice this technique and were clearly more satisfied. In addition, this study showed a cost reduction with this technique since the patients no longer needed appliances.[87]

However, colostomy irrigation requires a level of motivation, intelligence, and dexterity on the part of the patient. The device to irrigate consists of a reservoir with tubing that is placed via a stoma cone into the colostomy. About 500 ml to 1 l of room temperature water is infused into the bowel depending on patient tolerance. Then a drainage sleeve is placed over the stoma to allow for stool drainage. An earlier study reported that 71% of patients were continent with stomal irrigation while only 20% complained of leakage of gas.[88]

Many patients with a permanent stoma would prefer continence rather than wearing an appliance. Continent colostomy reservoirs have been tried but have largely been abandoned due to high rates of failure, sepsis, and generalized poor results. Attempts at using the cecum for such a reservoir with its less solid stool have also proven to be relatively unsuccessful as well.

The Kock pouch, or continent ileostomy, today remains the best option for patients seeking to maintain some degree of continence of liquid stool and gas. Dr. Nils Kock designed this pouch in 1969. He then described a continent internal reservoir from the patient's small intestine by involuting a segment of small bowel to make a "nipple valve." Patients are required to empty these pouches with a catheter several times a day via a flat slit created in the abdominal wall.[89] While there have been reports of improved lifestyle particularly in younger patients, problems remain with nipple valve slippage and nearly 50% of these patients will require another operation rate as a result of this. A relatively recent study evaluating the benefits of continent stomas constructed with various segments of bowel showed that while there are good outcomes there is an overall complication rate of 23.5%.[90]

Stoma Reversal

Stoma reversal may be either one of the easiest or most challenging procedures to perform depending on the type of stoma and the length of time the stoma has been in place. The procedure may be associated with significant morbidity as well. While most patients recover well from such surgery, severe complications can result in death. A recent systematic review of 48 studies of ileostomy reversal included over 600 patients from 18 countries. The overall morbidity after loop ileostomy reversal was 17.3% with a mortality rate of 0.4%. Less than 4% of patients required a laparotomy in order to facilitate the reversal. The most common postoperative complications were small bowel obstruction (7.2%) and wound infection (5.0%). The authors of this review concluded that while stoma creation may be considered necessary for anastomotic protection, the reversal is certainly far from a risk-free procedure.[91] Another study confirmed these same results reporting complications in as many as one-third of the patients who underwent ileostomy reversal with 3% of the patients dying after the surgery.[92]

Prior to stoma reversal the patients must be appropriately studied to ensure that it is safe to reverse the stoma. If the stoma was an end stoma, the surgeon must ensure that there is adequate length of bowel distally in which to perform the anastomosis. The patient may require a sigmoidoscopic evaluation of this portion of the bowel or a contrast enema. In addition, the proximal colon should always be evaluated prior to end colostomy reversal to ensure that there are no lesions present. This assessment may be done endoscopically or radiographically.

If the patient has a loop stoma that was performed to protect a distal anastomosis, one must ensure that this anastomosis is healed prior to the stoma reversal. If the anastomosis is low enough, it may be examined by digital rectal examination. Nevertheless, many surgeons prefer to visualize it with a sigmoidoscopic examination as well as a contrast enema to ensure anastomotic integrity. However, a prospective study reviewing contrast radiology of colonic j-pouches in 48 patients revealed that 46 of these patients had no clinical or radiographic evidence of leak. The authors concluded that the radiologic tests did not add much to the clinical assessment of these patients and was not necessary.[93]

The easiest stomas to reverse are traditionally the loop stomas. As discussed previously, both limbs of bowel are present and as such they simply need to be reanastomosed and returned to the abdominal cavity. This is often accomplished through a parastomal incision. However, if the bowel is stuck to the underlying tissues, the fascia or other loops of bowel within the abdominal cavity, then a formal laparotomy may need to be performed. Since the visibility around the stoma site is often limited, it is important to ensure that there are no inadvertent injuries made to any other loops of bowel. Once fully mobilized, loop stomas may be closed with the use of linear staplers by converting the bowel into a side to side or functional end to end bowel anastomosis. Alternatively, they may be closed by leaving the back wall intact and sewing the anterior wall of the bowel together. Many surgeons prefer using the side to side technique since this often leaves a wider anastomosis. After returning the bowel to the abdominal cavity the fascia is simply closed leaving the skin open for drainage and packing.

Hartman's stoma reversal is often more challenging. The abdominal cavity must be explored in order to locate the distal portion of the bowel. The distal bowel is often atrophied and may be friable from long standing diversion. This may make it difficult to use staplers especially circular stapling devices. Care must be taken in order not to tear or injure the serosa of the distal limb of bowel. In some select difficult cases, the surgeon may opt to redivert the patient with a proximal loop stoma after performing end stoma reversal if there is concern about the anastomosis. Salem and his colleagues found that the length of time from stoma creation to reversal made a difference in terms of whether or not another stoma was used in the reversal procedure suggesting that increased time made the reversal a more difficult operation.[94] Other surgeons have shared this feeling anecdotally as well.

Laparoscopic end stoma reversal may be a very difficult procedure to perform particularly if the initial stoma was created for a severe inflammatory process. The abdomen may be filled with adhesions making it harder to identify the distal segment of bowel and requiring an extensive laparoscopic adhesiolysis. A recent study from Israel comparing their results of laparoscopic to open Hartman's reversal revealed a conversion rate of 19.5% mainly due to dense adhesions and difficulty in identifying the rectal remnant. There were no mortalities, no anastomotic leaks, slightly shorter operative times (193 min vs. 209 min), less blood loss, shorter time to return of bowel function (4.1 days vs. 5.2 days), and shorter hospital stay (6.4 days vs. 8.0 days) in the laparoscopic group. They concluded that there were significant advantages in the laparoscopic approach for Hartman's reversal.[95] Another study comparing laparoscopic to open Hartman's reversal reported a high morbidity for both procedures while it was significantly lower for the laparoscopic group. While the operative times were longer in the laparoscopic group, the hospital length of stay was shorter in the laparoscopic group (4.8 days vs. 6.8 days). They too concluded that laparoscopic Hartman's reversal was a reasonable procedure with some obvious advantages over the open reversal.[96]

Not all patients are candidates for Hartman's reversal. In fact, many studies have suggested that many patients may never undergo stoma reversal because of their comorbidities. A recent review from the Cleveland Clinic showed that 30% of their patients studied did not undergo Hartman's reversal. They reviewed several variables including American Association of Anesthesiologist's score, patient age, pulmonary comorbidities, patient's use of anticoagulants, preoperative blood transfusion, and initial surgery due to bowel perforation in order to derive at a predictive score to determine if patient's should be considered for stoma reversal. This may help surgeons use objective criteria to select the best patient's for stoma reversal in order to improve surgical outcomes.[97]

Summary

Intestinal stomas remain a surgical option used for many different reasons but most importantly as a measure to treat or attempt to prevent complications. However, ironically, intestinal stomas are also associated with significant complications and as with any procedure the surgeon must weigh the risks and benefits of stoma creation in order to decide if it is truly necessary for the disease process being treated.

Acknowledgment. This chapter was written by Bruce Orkin, Peter Cataldo, Neil Hyman, and Richard Nelson, in two separate chapters in the previous version of this textbook.

References

1. Bryant TA. Case excision of a stricture of the descending colon through an incision made for a left lumbar colostomy: with remarks. Proc R Med Chir Soc. 1882;9:149–53.
2. Cheselden W. Colostomy for strangulated umbilical hernia. In Anatomy of the Human Body. 5th ed. London: William Bowyer; 1740.
3. Brown JY. The value of complete physiologic rest of the large bowel in the treatment of certain ulcerative and obstructive lesions of this organ. Surg Gynecol Obstet. 1913;16:610–3.
4. Miller GG, Gardner CMcG, Ripstein CB. Primary resection of the colon in UC. Can Med Assoc J. 1949;60:584–5.
5. Brooke BN. The management of an ileostomy including its complications. Lancet. 1952;2:102–4.
6. Hawley PR, Ritchie JK. Complications of ileostomy and colostomy following excisional surgery. Clin Gastroenterol. 1979;8:403–14.
7. Grogan JE, Smith MC. The economic cost of UC: a national estimate for 1968. Inquiry. 1973;10:61–8.
8. Paranby CN, Jenkins JT, Weston V, et al. Defunctioning stomas in patients with locally advanced rectal cancer prior to preoperative chemoradiotherapy. Colorectal Dis. 2009;11(1):26–31.
9. Rowbatham J. Stomal care. New Eng J Med. 1981;279:90–2.
10. Fazio VW. Invited commentary: loop ileostomy. World J Surg. 1984;8:405–7.
11. Edwards DP, Leppington-Clarke A, Sexton R, et al. Stoma-related complications are more frequent after transverse colostomy than loop ilesotomy: a prospective randomized clinical trial. Br J Surg. 2001;88(3):360–3.
12. Gazzard BG, Saunders B, Dawson AM. Diets and stoma function. Br J Surg. 1978;65(9):642–4.
13. Hill GL. Physiology of conventional ileostomy. In: Dozois RR, editor. Alternatives to conventional ileostomy. Chicago: Yearbook Medical Publishers; 1985. p. 31–5.
14. Turnbull Jr RB. Intestinal stomas. Surg Clin North Am. 1958;38:1361.
15. Crawford N, Broooke BN. Ileostomy chemistry. Lancet. 1957; 1:864–7.
16. Smiddy FG, Gregory SD, Smith IB, et al. Faecal loss of fluid, electrolytes and nitrogen in colitis before and after ileostomy. Lancet. 1960;1:14–9.
17. Kramer P, Kearney MM, Ingelfinger FJ. The effect of specific foods and water loading on the ileal excreta of ileostomized human subjects. Gastroenterology. 1962;42:535–46.
18. Kanaghinis T, Lubran M, Coghill NF. The composition of ileostomy fluid. Gut. 1963;4:322.
19. Hill GL, Millward SF, King RFGJ. Normal ileostomy output: close relation to body size. Br Med J. 1979;2:831–2.
20. Soper NJ, Orkin BA, Kelly KA, et al. Gastrointestinal transit after proctocolectomy with ileal pouch-anal anastomosis or ileostomy. J Surg Res. 1989;46:300.
21. Robertson MD, Mathers JC. Gastric emptying rate of solids is reduced in a group of ileostomy patients. Dig Dis Sci. 2000;45(7):1285–92.
22. Newton CR. Effect of codeine phosphate, Lomotil and Isogel on ileostomy function. Gut. 1978;19:377–83.
23. King RFGJ, Norton T, Hill GL. A double-blind cross-over study or the effect of loperimide hydrochloride and codeine phosphate on ileostomy output. Aust NZ J Surg. 1982;52(2):121–4.
24. Gallagher ND, Harrison DD, Skyring AP. Fluid and electrolyte disturbances in patients with long established ileostomies. Gut. 1962;3:219–23.
25. Bambach CP, Robertson WG, Peacock M, et al. Effect of intestinal surgery on the risk of urinary stone formation. Gut. 1981;22:257–63.
26. Clarke AM, Chirnside A, Hill GL, et al. Chronic dehydration and salt depletion in patients with established ileostomies. Lancet. 1967;2:740–3.
27. Hill GL, Goligher JC, Smith AH, et al. Long term changes in total body water, total exchangeable sodium and total body potassium before and after ileostomy. Br J Surg. 1975;62:524–7.
28. Cooper JC, Laughland A, Gunning EJ, Burkinshaw L, Williams NS. Body composition in ileostomy patients with and without ileal resection. Gut. 1986;27(6):680–5.
29. Holgate AM, Read NW. Relationship between small bowel transit time and absorption of a solid meal: influence of metachlopromide, magnesium sulfate, and lactulose. Dig Dis Sci. 1983;28:812.
30. Vince A, O'Grady F, Dawson AM. The development of ileostomy flora. J Infect Dis. 1971;128:638–41.
31. Finegold SM, Sutter VL, Boyle JD, Shimada K. The normal flora of ileostomy and transverse colostomy effluents. J Infect Dis. 1970;122(5):376–81.
32. Gorbach SL, Nahas L, Wenstein L. Studies of intestinal microflora: IV. The microflora of ileostomy effluent: a unique microbial ecology. Gastroent. 1967;53:874–80.
33. Percy-Robb IW, Jalan KN, McManus JP, et al. Effect of ileal resection on the bile salt metabolism in patients with ileostomy following proctocolectomy. Clin Sci. 1971;41:371–82.
34. Gorbach SL, Tabaqchali S. Bacteria, bile and the small bowel. Gut. 1969;10:963–72.
35. Hulten L, Kewenter J, Persson E, et al. Vitamin B12 absorption in ileostomy patients after operation for ulcerative colitis. Scan J Gastroent. 1970;5:113–5.
36. Dotevall G, Kock NG. Absorption studies in regional enteritis. Scan J Gastroent. 1968;3:293–8.
37. Modlin M. Urinary calculi and ulcerative colitis. Br Med J. 1972;3(821):292.
38. Fukushima T, Sugita A, Masuzawa S, Yamazaki Y, Takemura H, Tsuchiya S. Prevention of uric acid stone formation by sodium-bicarbonate in an ileostomy patient: a case report. Jap J Surg. 1988;18:465–8.

39. Christl SU, Scheppach W. Metabolic consequences of total colectomy. Scand J Gastroenterol Suppl. 1997;222:20–4.
40. Raza SD, Portin BA, Bernhoft WH. Umbilical colostomy: a better intestinal stoma. Dis Colon Rectum. 1977;20(3):223–30.
41. Fitzgerald PG, Lau GY, Cameron GS. Use of the umbilical site for temporary ostomy: review of 47 cases. J Pediatr Surg. 1989;24(10):973.
42. Simmons KL, Smith JA, Bobb KA, et al. Adjustment to colostomy; stoma acceptance, stoma care self efficacy and interpersonal relationships. J Adv Nurs. 2007;60(6):627–35.
43. Chaudhri S, Brown L, Hassan I, et al. Preoperative intensive, community-based vs. traditional stoma education: a randomized, controlled trial. Dis Colon Rectum. 2005;48(3):504–9.
44. Bloemen JG, Visschers RG, Truin RGJ, et al. Long-term quality of life in patients with rectal cancer: association with severe postoperative complications and presence of a stoma. Dis Colon Rectum. 2009;52(7):1251–8.
45. Ross L, Abild-Nielsen AG, Thomsen BL, et al. Quality of life of Danish colorectal cancer patients with and without a stoma. Support Care Cancer. 2007;15(5):505–13.
46. Silva MA, Ratnayake G, Deen KI. Quality of life of stoma patients: temporary ileostomy versus colostomy. World J Surg. 2003;27(4):421–4.
47. Siassi M, Hohenberger W, Losel F, et al. Quality of life and patient's expectations after closure of a temporary stoma. Int J Colorectal Dis. 2008;23(12):1207–12.
48. Goligher JC. Extraperitoneal colostomy or ileostomy. Br J Surg. 1958;46:97–103.
49. Hellinger M, Martinez S, Parra-Davilla E, et al. Gasless laparoscopic assisted intestinal stoma creation through a single incision. Dis Colon Rectum. 1999;42(7):1228–31.
50. Sakai T, Yamshita Y, Maekawa T, et al. Techniques for determining the ideal stoma site in laparoscopic colostomy. Int Surg. 1999;84(3):239–40.
51. Scheidbach H, Ptok H, Schubert D, et al. Palliatve stoma creation: comparison of laparoscopic vs. conventional procedures. Lagenbecks Arch Surg. 2009;394(2):371–4.
52. Oliveira L, Reissman P, Nogueras JJ, et al. Laparoscopic creation of stomas. Surg Endosc. 1997;11:19–23.
53. Liu J, Bruch HP, Farke S, et al. Stoma formation for fecal diversion: a plea for the laparoscopic approach. Tech Coloproctol. 2005;9(1):9–14.
54. Fazio VW. Loop ileostoym and loop-end ileostomy. In: Dudley H, Pories W, Carter D, editors. Rob and Smiths operative surgery. 4th ed. London: Butterworth; 1983. p. 54–64.
55. Meagher AP, Owen G, Gett R. Multimedia article. An improved technique for end stoma creation in obese patients. Dis Colon Rectum. 2009;52(3):531–3.
56. Huser N, Michalski CW, Erkan M, et al. Systemic review and meta-analysis of the role of defunctioning stoma in low rectal cancer surgery. Ann Surg. 2008;248(1):52–60.
57. Pappalardo G, Spoletini D, Proposito D, et al. Protective stoma in anterior resection of the rectum: when, how, and why? Surg Oncol. 2007;16 Suppl 1:S105–8.
58. Lefebure B, Tuech JJ, Bridoux V, et al. Evaluation of selective defunctioning stoma after low anterior resection for rectal cancer. Int J Colorectal Dis. 2008;23(3):283–8.
59. Kong AP, Kim J, Holt A, et al. Selective treatment of rectal cancer with single- stage coloanal or ultralow colorectal anastomosis does not adversely affect morbidity and mortality. Int J Colorectal Dis. 2007;22(8):897–901.
60. Gastinger I, Marusch F, Steinart R, et al. Protective defunctioning stoma in low anterior resection for rectal carcinoma. Br J Surg. 2005;92(9):1137–42.
61. Vlot EA, Zeebregts CJ, Gerritsen JJ, et al. Anterior resection of rectal cancer without bowel preparation and diverting stoma. Surg Today. 2005;35(8):629–33.
62. Mala T, Nesbakken A. Morbidity related to the use of a protective stoma in anterior resection for rectal cancer. Colorectal Dis. 2008;10(8):785–8.
63. Tan WS, Tang CL, Shi L, Eu KW. Meta-analysis of defunctioning stomas in low anterior resection for rectal cancer. Br J Surg. 2009;96(5):462–72.
64. Ulrich AB, Seiler C, Rahbari N, et al. Diverting stoma after low anterior resection: more arguments in favor. Dis Colon Rectum. 2009;52(3):412–8.
65. Park JJ, del Pino A, Orsay CP, Nelson RL, et al. Stoma complications. Dis Colon Rectum. 1999;42:1575–80.
66. Cartmell MT, Jones OM, Moran BJ, et al. A defunctioning stoma significantly prolongs the length of stay in laparoscopic colon resections. Surg Endosc. 2008;22(12):2643–7.
67. Caricato M, Ausania F, Ripetti V, et al. Retrospective analysis of long term defunctioning stoma complications after colorectal surgery. Colorectal Dis. 2007;9(6):559–61.
68. Nugent KP, Daniels P, Stewart B, et al. Quality of life in stoma patients. Dis Colon Rectum. 1999;42:1569–74.
69. Pilgrim CH, McIntyre R, Bailey M. Prospective audit of parastomal hernia: prevalence and associated comorbidities. Dis Colon Rectum. 2010;53(1):71–6.
70. Vijayasekar C, Marimuthu K, Jadhav V, et al. Parastomal hernia: is prevention better than cure? Use of a polypropylene mesh at the time of stoma formation. Tech Coloproctol. 2008;12(4):309–13.
71. Janes A, Cengiz Y, Israelsson LA. Randomized clinical trial of the use of a prosthetic mesh to prevent parastomal hernia. Br J Surg. 2004;91:280–2.
72. Guzman-Valdivia G. Incisional hernia at the site of a stoma. Hernia. 2008;12(5):471–4.
73. De Raet J, Delvaux G, Haentjens P, et al. Waist circumference is an independent risk factor for the development of parastomal hernia after permanent colostomy. Dis Colon Rectum. 2008;51(12):106–9.
74. Pastor DM, Pauli EM, Koltun WA, et al. Parastomal hernia repair: a single center experience. JSLS. 2009;13(2):170–5.
75. Tang CL, Yunos A, Leong AP, et al. Ileostomy output in the early postoperative period. Br J Surg. 1995;82:607.
76. Cooper JC, Williams NS, King RFGJ, et al. Effects of a long-acting somatostatin analogue in patients with severe ileostomy diarrhea. Br J Surg. 1986;73:128–31.
77. Maratka Z, Nedbal J. Urolithiasis as a complication of the surgical treatment of UC. Gut. 1964;5:214–7.
78. Kennedy HJ, Lee EGS, Claridge G, et al. Urinary stones in subjects with a permanent ileostomy. Q J Med. 1982;203:341–57.
79. Darren JJ, Parish JG, Lewitt MF, et al. Nephrolithiasis as a complication of UC and regional enteritis. Ann Intern Med. 1962;56:843–53.
80. Prien EL, Prien Jr EL. Composition and structure of urinary stones. Am J Med. 1968;45:654–72.
81. Christie PM, Knight GS, Hill GL. Comparison of relative risks of urinary stone formation after surgery for ulcerative colitis: conventional ileostomy vs. J-pouch. A comparative study. Dis Colon Rectum. 1996;39:50–4.

82. Christie PM, Knight GS, Hill GL. Metabolism of body water and electrolytes after surgery for ulcerative colitis conventional ileostomy versus J-pouch. Br J Surg. 1990;77:149–51.
83. Cohen S, Kaplan M, Gottlieb C, et al. Liver disease and gallstones in regional enteritis. Gastroenterology. 1971;60:237–45.
84. Shellito PC. Complications of abdominal stoma surgery. Dis Colon Rectum. 1998;41:1562–72.
85. Maeda K, Maruta M, Utsumi T, et al. Pathophysiology and prevention of loop stomal prolapse in the transverse colon. Tech Coloproctol. 2003;7(2):108–11.
86. Tepetes K, Spyridakis M, Hatzitheofilou C. Local treatment of a loop colostomy prolapse with a linear stapler. Tech Coloproctol. 2005;9(2):156–8.
87. Leong AF, Yunos AB. Stoma management in a tropical country: colostomy irrigation versus natural evacuation. Ostomy wound manage. 1999;45(11):52–6.
88. Terranova O, Sandei F, Rebuffat C, et al. Irrigation versus natural evacuation of left colostomy. Dis Colon Rectum. 1979;22:32–4.
89. Kock NG. Intra-abdominal "reservoir" in patients with permanent ileostomy. Preliminary observations on a procedure resulting in fecal "continence" in five ileostomy patients. Arch Surg. 1969;99(2):223–31.
90. Castellan MA, Gosalbez R, Labbie A, et al. Outcomes of continent catheterizable stomas for urinary and fecal incontinence: comparison among different tissue options. BJU Int. 2005;95(7):1053–7.
91. Chow A, Tilney HS, Paraskeva P, et al. The morbidity surrounding reversal of defunctioning ileostomies: a systematic review of 48 studies including 6, 107 cases. Int J Colorectal Dis. 2009;24(6):711–23.
92. Mansfield SD, Jensen C, Phair AS, et al. Complications of loop ileostomy closure: a retrospective cohort analysis of 123 patients. World J Surg. 2008;32(9):2101–6.
93. MacLeod I, Watson AJ, Hampton J, et al. Colonic pouchography is not routinely required prior to stoma closure. Colorectal Dis. 2004;6(3):162–4.
94. Salem L, Anaya DA, Roberts KE, et al. Hartmann's colectomy and reversal in diverticulitis: a population-level assessment. Dis Colon Rectum. 2005;48(5):988–95.
95. Mazeh H, Greenstein AJ, Swedish K, et al. Laparoscopic and open reversal of Hartmann's procedure – a comparative retrospective analysis. Surg Endosc. 2009;23(3):496–502.
96. Chouillard E, Pierard T, Campbell R, et al. Laparoscopically assisted Hartman's reversal is an efficacious and efficient procedure: a case control study. Minerva Chir. 2009;64(1):1–8.
97. Riansuwan W, Hull TL, Millan MM, et al. Nonreversal of Hartmann's procedure for diverticulitis: derivation of a scoring system to predict nonreversal. Dis Colon Rectum. 2009;52(8):1400–8.

32 Constipation and Functional Bowel Disorders

Madhulika G. Varma and Brooke H. Gurland

Definition and Prevalence

Constipation is one of the most common complaints voiced to primary care physicians, internists, gastroenterologists, and colorectal surgeons alike, with prevalence in North America estimated between 2 and 27%.[1,2] This broad range reflects a lack of agreement between how patients and physicians perceive constipation because definitions are variable and may refer to infrequent or hard bowel movements, or to difficulty with evacuation. In addition, complaints of constipation are two to three times more common in women than men. Knowles et al. reported that of 2,004 patients evaluated by transit study at three European tertiary referral centers for intractable constipation, 92% were women.[3] In a cohort of 2,000 women aged 40–69 years, 60% self-reported symptoms of difficult rectal evacuation over the last 12 months while 12% reported these symptoms weekly.[4] This difference can be explained by the vast diversity of how women define normal female bowel habits. Zutshi et al.[5] identified that women were more inclined to view their own habits as normal and perceive other habits unlike theirs as abnormal through self-reported questionnaires.

The incidence of constipation increases with age, and it is higher in nonwhites than whites, in people from a lower socioeconomic and educational status, and in the southern USA. A study done by Talley et al.[6] looking at elderly residents of Olmstead County in Minnesota further underscored the enormity of the problem by finding that nearly one in two women and one in three men over the age of 65 either had complaints of constipation or took laxatives.

The ROME Criteria were established to develop definitions, to augment research, and to evaluate treatment outcomes for functional gastrointestinal disorders.[7] Criteria for constipation are as follows:

- Less than three bowel movements per week.
- Straining more than 25% of the time.
- Hard stools more than 25% of the time.
- Incomplete evacuation more than 25% of the time.

When utilizing the standardized definitions of the Rome Criteria,[7] the prevalence of constipation in North America is estimated at 15%.

Validated symptom severity scores for constipation have also been developed, which are useful to assess the response to treatment, but their role in routine clinical practice has not been defined yet.[8–11] The Bristol stool scale is a visual representation of stool form and helps to subtype functional bowel disorders (Figure 32-1).[8]

Etiologies of Constipation

Constipation can be secondary to a myriad of conditions and medications. Physiologically, a number of complex interactions are necessary for the development of formed stool, the passage of stool through the colon, and the elimination of the stool bolus. The normal process of defecation requires the coordinated effort of colonic motility, rectal sensation, and pelvic floor relaxation.

Diet affects the size, consistency, and frequency of bowel movements; dietary fiber intake is highly correlated with stool bulk. For instance, inhabitants of countries with higher fiber intake pass more voluminous stool than those in countries with a lower intake of dietary fiber. Inhabitants of Western countries typically ingest inadequate amounts of fiber, secondary to reliance on processed grains. Since colonic distension triggers peristalsis, bulkier stools are a stronger and more efficient stimulus for colonic propulsion than smaller stools.

Many medical conditions are also recognized to affect bowel function. Metabolic and endocrine disorders such as hypothyroidism and diabetes, connective tissue disorders such as lupus and scleroderma, neurologic illness, immobilization, and psychiatric disease are a few of a long list of medical maladies associated with elevated rates of constipation. More colorectal-specific conditions, such as intrinsic colonic disease, can lead to decreased motility. Hirschsprung's disease and Chagas' disease alter the function of the colon through damage to the enteric nervous system. Colonic stricture,

D.E. Beck et al. (eds.), *The ASCRS Textbook of Colon and Rectal Surgery: Second Edition*,
DOI 10.1007/978-1-4419-1584-9_32, © Springer Science+Business Media, LLC 2011

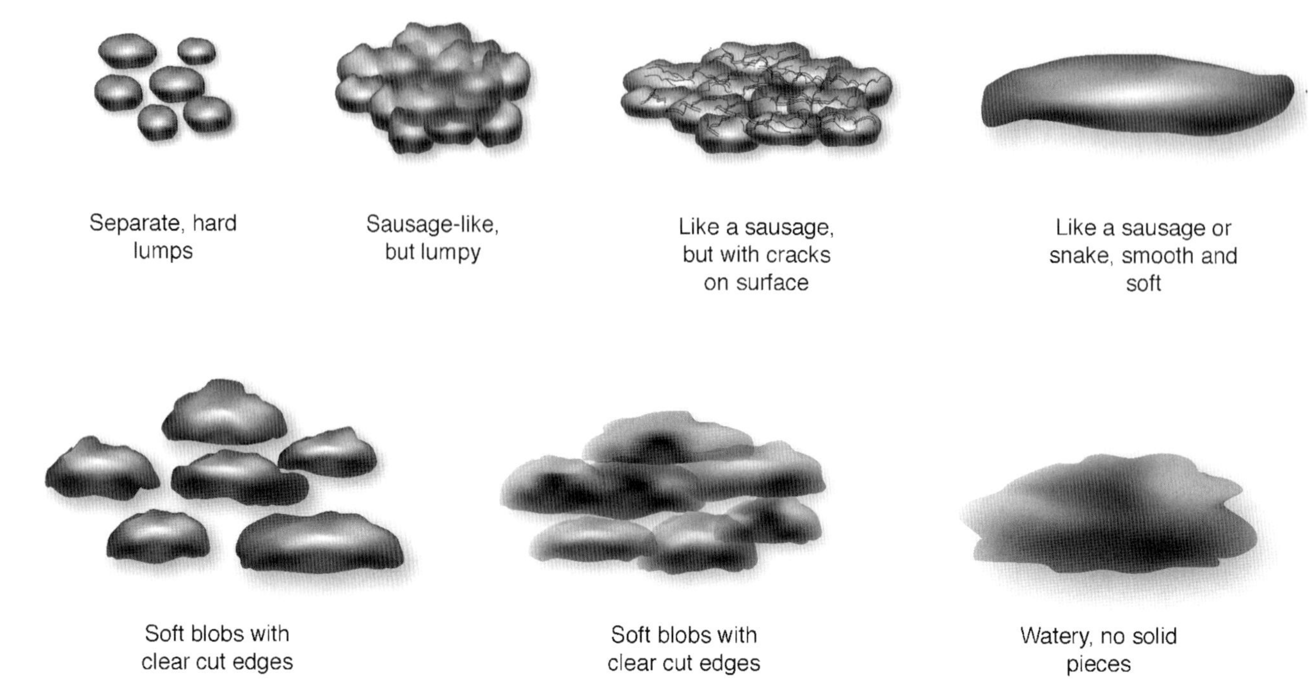

FIGURE 32-1. Bristol Stool Scale. (Adapted with permission from Lewis and Heaton, © 1997 Informa Healthcare. Reproduced with permission).

secondary to carcinoma, inflammatory bowel disease, radiation, or endometriosis, can cause colonic obstruction and altered function. Additionally, there is an ever-increasing list of medications for certain medical disorders like hypertension that can actually promote the development of constipation. Opiate and anticholinergic use, as well as laxative abuse, may also be associated with constipation. Factors associated with constipation are summarized in Table 32-1.

Subtypes of Constipation

Patients can be further classified by associated findings such as slow transit (motility disorders), irritable bowel syndrome (IBS), and pelvic floor dysfunction, also described as obstructed defecation syndrome (ODS) or mixed disorders. Motility disorders can be isolated to the colon (colonic inertia aka slow-transit constipation) or can affect the stomach and small bowel. Colonic inertia (CI) is frequently associated with constipation since childhood, fewer than 3 BMs per week, and laxative dependence. IBS-C (constipation subtype) is associated with abdominal pain, irregular bowel habits, and pain relieved by defecation. ODS refers to a constellation of symptoms such as prolonged repeated straining at bowel movements, sensation of incomplete evacuation, and the need for digital manipulation. Overlap between the various subtypes of constipation can coexist. Although clinical history can be suggestive as to which type of constipation motility disorders and ODS can coexist in the same patient, diagnostic testing is confirmatory.

History and Physical Examination

The evaluation of constipation begins with a thorough history. Specific details of the patients' complaints, stool size, frequency, consistency, and ease and efficacy of evacuation should be noted. The age at onset of symptoms, diet and exercise details, medical history, surgical history, and medications should be recorded. A patient diary of dietary intake, evacuation frequency, stool consistency, and any associated symptoms can be very helpful to both the patient and the medical provider. Query into psychiatric illness and sexual and physical abuse must be performed as they are often associated with defecation difficulties.[9] Multicompartment pelvic floor symptoms such as urinary dysfunction, pelvic organ and prolapse, and sexual dysfunction needs to be elicited, and appropriate referrals to other pelvic floor specialists in urology and urogynecology should be made for combined treatment.

Physical examination in patients with motility disorders and IBS-C will be frequently unremarkable, but abdominal distension may be noted. Evaluation for pelvic floor dysfunction includes vaginal, perineal, and rectal examination. Bulging of the posterior vaginal wall beyond the hiatus is consistent with advanced prolapse and may represent a rectocele, enterocele, or sigmoidocele. Examination in the standing position with a finger in the rectum and vagina may be performed to elicit the maximal prolapse of the pelvic organs as they descend through the pouch of Douglas and genital hiatus. A gaping patulous anus may indicate neurological injury, intraanal intussusception, or full-thickness

TABLE 32-1. Factors associated with constipation

Lifestyle
Inadequate fluid intake
Inadequate fiber intake
Inactivity
Laxative abuse
Medications
Opiates
Anticholinergics
Iron
Medical illness
Neurologic
Spinal cord dysfunction/damage
Parkinson's disease
Multiple sclerosis
Endocrine/metabolic dysfunction
Diabetes mellitus
Hypothyroidism
Electrolyte abnormalities
Uremia
Hypercalcemia
Porphyria
Psychological
Depression
Anorexia
Psychiatric illness
Sexual abuse
Colonic structure/function
Cancer
Crohn's disease
Irradiation
Endometriosis
Hirschsprung's disease
Chagas' disease
Pelvic floor abnormality
Nonrelaxing puborectalis
Anal stenosis
Rectocoele/enterocoele

rectal prolapse. Flattening of the perineum during Valsalva beyond the ischial tuberosities is suggestive of excessive perineal descent. Sphincter coordination is noted on anorectal examination when patients are asked to squeeze, relax, and push. Digital examination evaluates resting anal tone and squeeze strength, and can identify a large rectocele, sphincter defect, or no movement of the pelvic floor muscles. Valsalva maneuver or simulated defecation on a commode is useful to elicit full-thickness rectal prolapse. Anoscopy is performed to evaluate patients for mucosal abnormalities and rectoanal intussusception.

Diagnostic Testing

The subtypes of constipation are not mutually exclusive, and careful evaluation is important to guide treatment. Laboratory testing with thyroid studies and calcium levels are useful to exclude metabolic etiologies of constipation. Obstructing colon lesions and inflammatory conditions such as IBD or diverticulitis must be excluded by colonoscopy or GI contrast studies before considering functional etiologies.

Additional testing is reserved for patients who fail medical therapy. Radiological and anorectal studies are very useful to determine different pathologic mechanisms and to distinguish between normal versus slow transit and outlet dysfunction constipation.

Diagnostic Studies to Evaluate Intestinal Transit

Intestinal transit time can be estimated through various modalities. The most widely available technique for determining colonic transit uses radiopaque markers and radiographs of the abdomen. The concept of assessing transit using markers was first developed by Hinton et al.[10] modified by Martelli et al.,[11] and further changed by Metcalf et al.[12]

The patient should refrain from all enemas, laxatives, and most medications for 2 days prior to the ingestion of 24 radiopaque markers. The patient is required to ingest 30 g of fiber daily during the test and must continue to refrain from taking medication and laxatives. An abdominal radiograph is obtained on the fifth day, and the distribution and number of markers present in the colon is noted. Eighty percent of normal patients will have passed all the markers by 5 days. If the markers remain scattered throughout the colon and more than 20% of the markers remain in the colon, colonic inertia can be diagnosed. If the markers are found to have accumulated in the rectum, traditional teaching suggests that this is a diagnostic of outlet obstruction constipation (Figure 32-2). However, Cowlam et al.[13] refuted this hypothesis after evaluating the distribution of markers in 108 patients with functional constipation. They found no correlation between the pattern of marker distribution and any of the parameters denoting outlet obstruction.

There are many variations described for marker distribution. A more precise assessment of transit delay can be obtained by having the patient ingest radiopaque markers for three sequential days while following the same instructions and obtaining a radiograph on the fourth and seventh day. The number and distribution of the markers are tabulated and totaled. The resultant numeric values can then be compared to the established value for normal controls. The mean colon transit time through the entire colon in humans has been shown to be 31 h in males and 39 h in women. In the general population, 95% of patients will have a transit time of less than 65 h in men and 75 h in women. Patients with normal transit constipation will have a colon transit time that is in the normal range.

Another variation is to have the patient ingest a marker capsule (with 24 markers) on Sunday night and obtain abdominal films on Monday, Wednesday, and Friday morning. All markers in the colon on the Monday morning film provides a gross assurance that gastric and small intestinal transit are normal. The other two films provide additional documentation of colonic transit. The transit study can also be performed

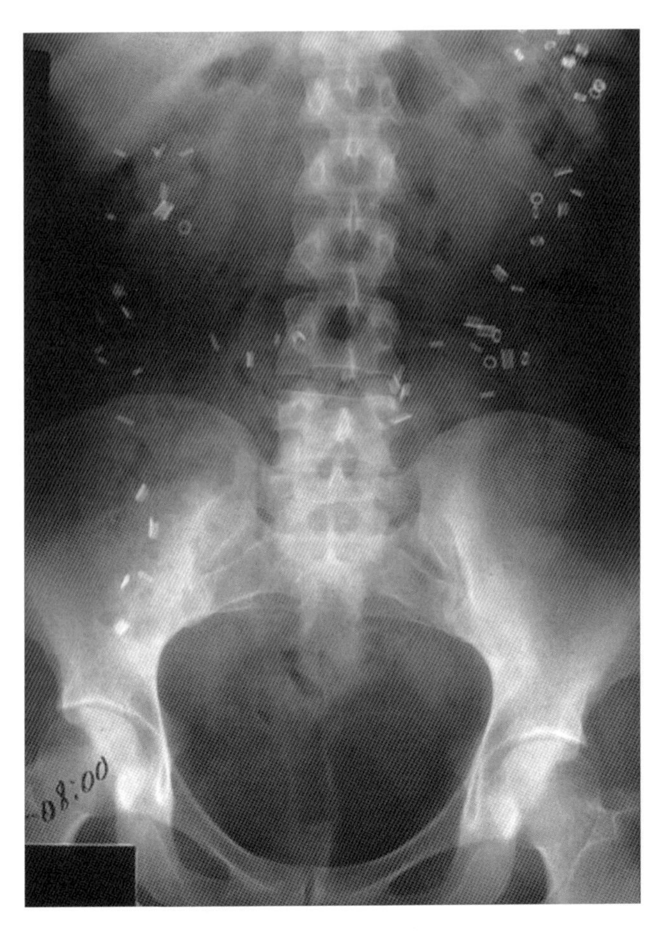

FIGURE 32-2. Marker study revealing colonic inertia.

with ingestion of one capsule and a single X-ray image on either day 5, 6, or 7. More than 20% of the markers remaining in the colon may suggest colonic dysmotility.

Scintigraphic evaluation of intestinal transit, though not as widely available as other evaluative tools, is useful in the assessment of transit in the colon and proximal gut.[14] Transit times obtained through scintigraphy are generated by following the passage of a radiolabeled meal. Small-bowel and gastric emptying rates can also be estimated with this examination.

Small-bowel transit time may also be measured with a lactulose hydrogen breath test. The principle of this examination is that hydrogen produced through lactulose fermentation only occurs in the colon. If one records the time from ingestion of lactulose to hydrogen production, small-bowel transit time can be inferred.

A wireless capsule, Smartpill® (Smartpill Corp., Buffalo, NY), is now available in the USA to measure intestinal motility. The SmartPill® Capsule collects pH, pressure, and temperature data throughout the entire gastrointestinal tract estimating total gut transit.[15] However, the availability, reimbursement, and expertise in interpretation of the SmartPill® Capsule make it difficult to determine its ultimate use in clinical practice.

Diagnostic Studies to Evaluate Pelvic Floor Dysfunction

Anal manometry evaluates resting and squeeze pressure of the sphincter over the length of the anal canal and any rectal sensory deficits. Often with constipation, patients exhibit internal sphincter hypertonia with poor incremental squeeze pressures. The volume noted at first sensation can be blunted, i.e., requiring larger volumes to obtain a sensory response, and the maximum tolerated volume can also be blunted. The presence of the rectal anal inhibitory reflex (RAIR) is useful to exclude Hirschsprung's disease. Electromyography aids in the diagnosis of puborectalis syndrome by indicating a paradoxical or nonrelaxing muscle. Balloon expulsion is an inexpensive method to assess ability to evacuate. Normal studies indicate the ability to evacuate a 50–100 cc balloon in less than 1 min.[16]

Defecography is the gold standard to confirm evacuatory dysfunction due to intussusception, rectal prolapse, enterocele, sigmoidocele, rectocele, and perineal descent. Defecography is done with contrast in the small bowel to demonstrate an enterocele, or in the vagina, rectum, and sigmoid to demonstrate a sigmoidocele and to evaluate the anorectal angle, rectocele, and the residual content after evacuation.[17] Some centers use a dynamic MRI, but the technique varies. For the best images, complete evacuation of the contrast during the MRI after valsalva will most likely simulate defecation. Defecating MRI has advantages over traditional defecography because it involves less radiation and provides multicompartment images. However, defecating in the supine position is not physiologic, and the sitting MRI is not universally available. [18]

Pelvic floor findings may be asymptomatic or may be secondary to chronic straining as a result of underlying motility disorders, and clinical correlation is highly recommended prior to considering surgery based on radiologic diagnoses. For patients with pelvic floor dysfunction who demonstrate dysnergic defecation, randomized controlled trials show that biofeedback is superior to laxatives, sham treatments, and alternative therapies.[19] In the setting of rectal intussusception, rectocele and mucosal prolapse, stapled transanal rectal resection (STARR) can be offered. STARR employs a double stapled circumferential full-thickness resection of the lower rectum using specialized stapling guns (Ethicon Endosurgery, Cincinnati, OH, USA). Modifications to the design of the staples and the device since its initial reports involve a reloadable curved cutter stapler, the Countour® Transtar™ (Ethicon Endosurgery, Cincinnati, OH, USA), for perineal proctectomy.[20] The first staple line placed anteriorly reduces the intussusception and the bulging rectocele, correcting the anterior wall defect, and the second staple line placed posteriorly is aimed at correcting the intussusception. Prospective multicenter trials reveal initial and long-term symptom improvement of obstructed defecation after STARR.[21–24] A randomized controlled trial of STARR versus biofeedback revealed that STARR is more effective for treatment of evacuatory dysfunction.[25] For patients with a clinical or radiologic rectocele and retained rectal contrast, rectocele repair can be suggested. A rectocele occurs due to a defect in the rectal vaginal septum and protrusion of the anterior rectum into the posterior vagina wall. Rectocele repair can be performed via transvaginal, transperineal, or transperineal approach with 75–80% reported bowel symptoms improvements.[26] Enterocele involves descent of small bowel into the lower pelvic cavity, leading to mechanical obstruction of the rectum. An enterocele results from a defect in the integrity of the endopelvic fascia at the vaginal apex, and repair can be performed via a transabdominal, laparoscopic, or vaginal route and is usually performed in conjunction with other pelvic floor procedures. A sigmoidocele refers to descent of the sigmoid colon into the lower pelvic cavity leading to compression and mechanical obstruction of the rectum. Sigmoid resection or sigmoidopexy in conjunction with posterior compartment repair has been shown to be effective in relieving symptoms of obstructed defecation in a limited number of patients.[27,28]

Medical Treatment of Constipation

Treatment of constipation is initiated with careful listening and validation of the patient's disability. Unfortunately, the community and health-care providers often fail to recognize or acknowledge the severe debilitation associated with this condition, and thus many patients do not get the attention or credibility associated with other diseases. Medical providers should strive to decrease patient anxiety over the act of defecation, to dispel the fear of malignancy, and to reassure the patient that a daily bowel movement is not requisite to good health.

Initial treatment of constipation focuses on review and modification of medications, lifestyle changes, and the intake of agents that affect the formation and composition of stool. Simple measures that can influence the passage of colonic content are increasing physical activity and fluid intake. Exercise, as limited as even gentle walking, can facilitate the elimination of stool. Fluid intake can cause the stool to be softer and easier to pass, along with other agents that can act to stimulate the colon to propel stool. Osmotic laxatives, stimulants, and enemas should be reserved for treatment of acute bouts of discomfort.

Lack of dietary fiber intake is a major factor in the development of constipation symptoms. Bulk forming agents are a first line therapy in the prevention and treatment of constipation. These agents facilitate an increase in the size of the stool bolus as well as make the stool softer. Bulking agents promote these changes by delivering a mass of nondigestible substrate to the colon and due to their hydrophilic nature, facilitate the absorption and retention of fluid in the stool. These substrates are derived from the nondigestible components of plants or are synthetic methylcellulose derivatives. Common bulk agents are psyllium (Metamucil®, Konsyl®), methylcellulose (Citrucel®), and calcium polycarbophil (Fibercon®). Side effects of fiber therapy include bloating and flatulence.

Osmotic laxatives are a class of medications that promote the accumulation of large volumes of fluid in the colon lumen through the delivery of osmotically active molecules into the small and large bowel. The osmotically active particles can be derived from sugars or salts such as sucrose-based sorbitol and lactulose. Lactulose is degraded in the colon yielding the production of fatty acids, hydrogen, and carbon dioxide. MiraLAX® (polyethylene glycol 3350) is an over-the-counter osmotic laxative that increases the frequency of bowel moments and softens the stool, so it is easy to pass. It is one of the most commonly recommended laxatives found to be safe and effective for everyday use.

Osmotic laxatives can also be based on nonabsorbable ions, commonly derived from magnesium or phosphate. Examples are magnesium hydroxide (Milk of Magnesia®) or sodium phosphate (Fleets® Phosphosoda). Caution must be exercised in patients with renal insufficiency as hypermagnesemia and renal failure can result. Other polyethylene glycol-based products such as NuLYTELY® or GoLYTELY® are used in many bowel cleansing regimes. Chronic use can lead to electrolyte disturbances and dehydration.

Colonic irritants are a class of agents that diminish constipation through stimulation of colonic motility. Examples are anthracene derivatives, which include senna and cascara and are found in Senekot® and Pericolace®. Long-term anthracene intake can generate a characteristic brown discoloration of the mucosa called pseudomelanosis coli. Bisacodyl is another irritant and can be found in the agent Dulcolax®. Long-term utilization of anthracene irritants may lead to poor colon function; therefore, such use is discouraged.

Mineral oil and docusate sodium (Colace®) are laxatives that act through the manipulation of stool composition. Mineral oil coats the stool bolus, preventing fluid loss. Docusate sodium lowers the surface tension at the stool–water interface, allowing greater penetration of the stool with fluid.

Enemas and suppositories are used to stimulate bowel movements. Strategies include promotion of defecation through distension (saline enema), rectal irritation (soapsuds, bisacodyl), or physical softening of the stool (glycerine). Enema therapy can be habituating and therefore should be used with caution to avoid dependency.

There have been a number of promotility agents that were initially available but were later recalled based on their toxicity profile. Lubiprostone (Amitizia®) is still commercially available for use in patients with functional constipation and IBS-C.[29,30] Lubiprostone (a bicyclic fatty acid) is a chloride channel activator that induces intestinal secretion without elevating serum electrolyte levels. It activates ClC-2 chloride channels in the apical membrane of the intestinal epithelium. It is Food and Drug Administration (FDA) approved for the treatment of chronic idiopathic constipation in the adult population (including patients > 65 years old) at the dose of 25 μg bid and for IBS constipation subtype patients at 8 μg bid. The most commonly reported adverse reactions include nausea, diarrhea, and headaches, causing patients to discontinue treatment. The cost of the medications can also be prohibitive for some patients.

Colonic Inertia

Colonic inertia (CI) represents a severe functional disturbance of colonic motility, which results in significant disability to the patient. In CI, there is ineffective colonic propulsion and a failure of a meal or stimulant to enhance colonic phasic contractile activity.[31] Patients with CI have heterogeneous clinical presentations and, like patients with normal transit and obstructed defecation syndrome, exhibit infrequent defecation and may suffer from abdominal pain, bloating, nausea, difficulty with and incomplete evacuation of stool. In the majority of patients, symptoms have been present since childhood, while others present with symptoms later in life without a sentinel event. However, some women report a change in bowel habits following hysterectomy or childbirth.[32]

Surgical management of constipation has changed little since its initial reports in 1908 when Lane described improvement in two thirds of patients after the removal of the abdominal colon.[33] Surgical intervention can be a good tool, but precise evaluation of colonic motility and pelvic floor function using the testing paradigm (described earlier in this chapter) is critical to identify which patients are most likely to benefit from surgical intervention. Issues like slow-transit constipation may be part of a more widespread disease affecting the whole gut, and patients with gastric and small-bowel dysmotility have less favorable results after surgical intervention than patients with colonic inertia alone.[34] Glia et al.[35] demonstrated a trend toward worse outcomes in patients with abnormal antroduodenal manometry.

Patients with slow-transit constipation and concomitant pelvic floor dysfunction represent a challenging subgroup to treat. Bernini et al.[36] evaluated 16 patients who had a combination of colonic inertia and nonrelaxing pelvic floor. All patients completed preoperative biofeedback training and could demonstrate relaxation of the pelvic floor musculature. Postoperative symptoms of difficult evacuation persisted, and nearly one-half were dissatisfied with their surgery. Hassan et al.[37] reports contradictory results. Patients with CI and pelvic floor dysfunction treated with preoperative biofeedback had equivalent long-term functional results and quality of life compared to patient with isolated CI. Psychological evaluation and management is important, especially in patients in whom surgery is being contemplated. Significant abnormalities have been documented with simple psychologic testing with instruments such as the Minnesota multiphasic personality inventory.[38]

Colectomy

The following surgical options for CI have been reported in the literature: total abdominal colectomy with ileorectal anastomosis, subtotal colectomy with ileosigmoid anastomosis, and subtotal colectomy with cecorectal anastomosis. All three of these procedures are effective at increasing the number of bowel movements, but may vary with regard to functional results such as diarrhea and fecal incontinence. All three of them are also generally amenable to being laparoscopically performed. It is thought that sparing of the cecum, the ileocecal valve, and the distal ileal loop will leave a physiologic reservoir with colonic flora that promotes normal stool consistency and normal absorption of fluid and electrolytes.[39] However, the possibility of recurrent constipation still exists. Feng et al.[40] compared ileosigmoid anastomosis to cecal rectal anastomosis in 79 patients with a 2-year follow-up and found that ileosigmoid anastomosis resulted in higher defecation frequency, less use of laxatives and enemas, and higher patient satisfaction.

Knowles et al.[41] reviewed 32 series published in the English language whose publications included ten or more patients treated with colectomy for colonic inertia through the year 1999. None of the studies were controlled with respect to the outcome from other surgical or medical interventions. Inconsistent functional results were reported, and it was difficult to compare outcomes because patient selection was not well defined. A median success rate was reported at 86% (range 39–100%), and results of subtotal colectomy proved to be inferior to those with total abdominal colectomy with ileorectal anastomosis. Postoperative fecal incontinence was reported in 16 series with a median incidence of 14% (range 0–52%). Persistent abdominal pain was reported in 14 series. Recurrent constipation following surgery was still present in 15 series with a median incidence of 9% (range 0–33%). The median incidence for small-bowel obstruction was 18% (2–71%) with a median reoperation rate of 14% (0–50%) (Table 32-2). In addition, permanent ileostomies were created in 5% of patients due to poor functional outcome (0–28%).

Preoperative functional evaluation is very important but does not guarantee successful outcome following colectomy for constipation.[45] Routine evaluation of the entire GI tract is recommended by some authors due to data that suggests that gastric and small-bowel dysmotility have less favorable results after surgical intervention than patients with colonic inertia alone.[34,35,46] However, Zmora et al.[49] identified good results after colectomy in patients with delayed small-bowel transit compared to those patients with normal small-bowel transit. Thus, the presence of delayed gastric or small-bowel motility on preoperative testing is not an absolute contraindication but may be a poor prognostic indicator resulting in persistent symptoms and continuous use of promotility and antinausea medications.

Furthermore, patients with prior sexual trauma have been shown to have more functional diagnosis, more precolectomy operations, and require more postcolectomy medical care for abdominal complaints.[50] Patients should be extensively counseled prior to surgery about the postoperative persistence of preoperative symptoms and the occurrence of new symptoms.

TABLE 32-2. Surgical therapy for constipation

Authors	*N*	Surgery/anastomosis type	Study design	Study subjects F	Study subjects M	Study subjects age Mean/median	Follow-up time Mean/median	#BM Mean/median	Patient reported outcomes	30-Day complications
Nyam et al.[42]	74	TAC w/ileorectostomy CI Group: 52 patients CI + PFD group: 22 patients	R	68	6	M: 43 (23–71)	M: 56 (2–101) month	Md: CI: 4 (0–20)/day CI+PFD: 2 (1–6)/day	72 (97%) patients satisfied	*23 (31%) patients* 9 (12%): ileus 7 (9.45%): SBO 4 (5%): wound infection 3 (4%): UTI
Pikarsky et al.[43]	30	TAC w/IRA	R	21	9	M: 60 (28–85)	M: 106 month	M: 2.5 (1–6) day	Good/excellent: 100%	6 (20%): SBO
Webster et al.[44]	55	50 (91%) patients: TAC w/ileoproctostomy 5 (9%) patients: TAC w/Brooke ileostomy	R	47	8	M: 40 (13–78)	FU: 12 month	M: 3/day	Good/excellent: 89% Poor: 11%	*23 (42%) patients* 24% Ileus 8% SBO 4% Anastomotic leak 6% Other
Mollen et al.[45]	21	TAC w/IRA	R*	19	2	M: 42.8 (16–75)	FU: 12 month	2.8/day	52%	*7 (33%) patients* 3 (14%) patients: SBO
Verne et al.[46]	13	ST: 7 patients: ISA 6 patients: IRA	R	13	0	M: 46.2 (26–67)	Not reported	M: 15 (±4.5) week	85% patients satisfied	Not reported
FitzHarris et al.[47]	75	ST w/primary anastomosis	R	75	0	Not reported	M: 3.9 (0.5–9.6) year	69 (92%) patients: 2–3/week	70 (93%) patients: willing to have SC again	*40 (53%) patients* 29 (37%): SBO 11 (15%): wound infection
Thaler et al.[48]	17	TAC w/IRA	R*	17	0	M: 47.8 (±14.3)	M: 58.3 (±27.3) month	M: 3.7 (±2.8) day	Good/exc: 100%	*6 (35.2%) patients* 2 (12%): hernias]4 (23.5%): SBO
Hassan et al.[37]	110	TAC w/IRA	P	104	6	Md: 40 years	Md: 11 (1.5–16.5) year	Md: 4/day	Good/improved: 90%	Not reported
Zutshi et al.[5]	69	TAC w/IRA	R	67	2	M: 38.6 (20–79)	Md: 10.8 year	M: 21/week	77% patients the surgery was beneficial	*20 (29%) patients* 11 (16%): ileus 4 (6%): prolonged fever 3 (4%): diarrhea 1 (1.5%): bleeding 1 (1.5%): anastomotic leak

TAC total abdominal colectomy, ST subtotal colectomy, ISA ileosigmoid anastomosis, IRA ileorectal anastomosis, CI colonic inertia, PFD pelvic floor dysfunction, R retrospective study, P prospective study, R* data prospectively collected, M mean, Md Median, SBO small-bowel obstruction.

Segmental Colon Resection

Segmental colon resection has also been suggested to avoid the diarrhea associated with abdominal colectomy. In a consecutive series of 28 patients with slow-transit constipation, as determined by scintigraphic transit study, who were subsequently treated with segmental colectomy, 23 patients were pleased with the outcome.[51] The median stool frequency increased from 1 to 7 per week with a median follow-up of 50 months. Since the ability to define segmental colonic transit is inexact and not universally available, total abdominal colectomy remains the most widely accepted surgical treatment option in the treatment of CI.

Proctocolectomy and Ileal Pouch Anal Anastomosis

Proctocolectomy with ileoanal pouch reconstruction has been described as a salvage operation for patients with recurrent constipation after abdominal colectomy with ileorectal anastomosis for slow-transit constipation. Keighly et al.[52] reported the results of eight patients, 50% required pouch excision for recurrent constipation. Furthermore, two of fifteen patients required pouch excision within eighteen months because of intractable pelvic pain.[53] Proctocolectomy has also been used as initial treatment for slow-transit constipation and rectal inertia. Overall, significant improvements in lifestyle scores were recorded in the categories of physical function, social function, pain, and general health for the group during the follow-up period following proctocolectomy.

Stoma

Fecal diversion with a permanent stoma is a last resort for the patients who fail other modalities. There is little data published to guide choice of ileostomy or colostomy, and symptoms such as distention and abdominal pain may persist.[54] Although very drastic, this is sometimes the only option for patients who fail all other management.

Sacral Nerve Stimulation

Sacral nerve stimulation (SNS) involves low-level chronic electrical stimulation to the sacral plexus, producing a physiologic effect on the end organs. As a coincidental finding in patients undergoing SNS for lower urinary tract dysfunction, many patients experienced improved fecal continence, an increase in bowel frequency, and improved defecation. Small series have investigated its efficacy in patients with slow-transit constipation and evacuation dysfunction refractory to medical therapy.[55–58] In general, the number of weekly BMs increased, and difficulty with evacuation (here defined as unsuccessful visits to the toilet) and time necessary to evacuate decreased. The exact mode of action is not known; however, it is postulated that sacral neuromodulation may involve afferent cortical stimulation, leading to increased motility and rectal sensitivity. The mechanism of SNS is poorly understood, making it difficult to give precise indications for eligible patients. However, there is a potential to alter colonic motility, pelvic floor and anal sphincter function, and afferent sensation. SNS is presently not approved for use in the USA for patients with bowel dysfunction as their primary indication.

Antegrade Colonic Enema

Patients with severe bowel dysfunction who are contemplating a permanent colostomy may find the antegrade colonic enema (ACE) procedure as an affirmative viable option. This procedure allows easy access to the colon through the abdominal wall with intermittent catheterization, irrigation of the colon, and rapid, controlled bowel purging (Figure 32-3).

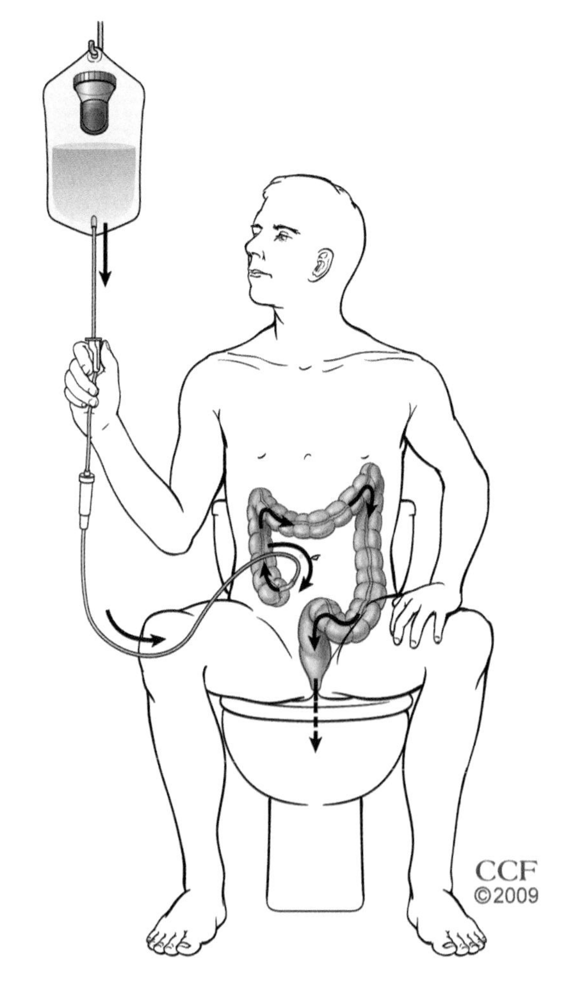

FIGURE 32-3. Antegrade colonic enema (ACE) procedure for colonic inertia. This procedure allows easy access to the colon through the abdominal wall with intermittent catheterization, irrigation of the colon, and rapid, controlled bowel purging (Reprinted with permission, Cleveland Clinic Center for Medical Art and Photography © 2009. All Rights Reserved).

The patient can avoid a stoma bag while independently managing their own bowel activities. The ACE technique was first described by Malone in 1990, using the appendix as the conduit, but since then the cecum, ileum, and left colon have been utilized as the continence mechanism.[59–61] These procedures have become an increasingly popular treatment option for children with spinal dysraphism and anorectal malformations and are well reported in pediatric literature.[62] The ACE procedure is also gaining recognition in the adult population for patients who would like to avoid a colostomy bag. Success has been reported in adults with neurologic dysfunction, obstructed defecation, and fecal incontinence.[63–68] Complications are related to the cutaneous stoma, which may sometimes need multiple revisions.

Irritable Bowel Syndrome

Irritable bowel syndrome (IBS) is a functional bowel disorder in which abdominal pain or discomfort is associated with defecation or a change in bowel habits with features of disordered defecation. Organic pathology is absent, and diagnosis is made on clinical symptoms and exclusion of other disease states. Although there is overlap between patients in this category and those individuals described in the previous section, the key features include chronic symptoms such as abdominal pain relieved by defecation and/or associated with a change in the consistency or frequency of stools. These symptoms are variably associated with mucorrhea and/or abdominal bloating. IBS can be categorized into the following: constipation predominant (IBS-C), diarrhea (IBS-D), or mixed (IBS_M). The Rome criteria for a clinical diagnosis of IBS are listed in Table 32-3.

Epidemiology

Population-based studies in Western countries report an overall prevalence of IBS of 10–20%.[69] The prevalence is similar in Western minority populations, with the exception of Hispanics in Texas and Asians in California, who may have a lower rate.[70,71] Overall, the incidence in Western countries is 1–2% per year. In non-Western countries in Asia and Africa, some studies suggest that IBS incidence may be lower. In Western countries, women are two to three times more likely to develop IBS than men; in India, this phenomenon is reversed.[72] Retrospectively, many patients report childhood symptoms, and 50% of patients have symptoms before age 35.[73]

Table 32-3. Rome criteria for irritable bowel syndrome[7]

Abdominal pain or discomfort characterized by the following
Relieved by defecation
Associated with a change in stool frequency
Associated with a change in stool consistency
Two or more of the following characteristics at least 25% of the time
Altered stool frequency
Altered stool form
Altered stool passage
Mucorrhea
Abdominal bloating or subjective distension

It has been recognized for many years that there are a variety of disorders associated with a clinical diagnosis of IBS. These include nonulcer dyspepsia, fibromyalgia, chronic fatigue syndrome, dysmenorrhea, urinary tract symptoms, and psychiatric disorders. Patients with IBS who present for evaluation are also at least twice as likely to meet criteria for psychiatric disorders as patients with organic disease with elevated scores of depression, anxiety, somatization, and neuroticism on standardized tests. However, no specific pattern of personality traits in patients has been identified. The most frequent of these disorders are depression and generalized anxiety. Interestingly, individuals with clinical symptoms of IBS who do not seek medical care have a similar prevalence of psychiatric disorders as the general population.[74] This suggests that the psychiatric disorder may be more important in health-care-seeking behavior than as an etiologic agent of the syndrome.

It has been estimated that only 10% of patients with IBS symptoms consult a physician for evaluation or treatment of their symptoms. With the exception of countries like India, women are more likely than men to present for physician evaluation. The socioeconomic impact of this disorder is also significant. There are 3.5 million physician visits estimated in the USA, and IBS is the most common diagnosis in gastroenterologist practice. Patients with IBS have more work absenteeism, more physician visits, and report a lower quality of life.[75]

Pathophysiology

The pathophysiology of IBS remains uncertain and several theories are listed below. Despite extensive investigations, no specific physiologic abnormality has been identified, and IBS remains a diagnosis of exclusion.

Gastrointestinal Motility

The current theories regarding the pathophysiology of IBS are of a complex interaction between altered gut motility and or visceral hyperalgesia and neuropsychopathology. Many studies measuring myoelectric activity in the colon have demonstrated abnormalities in patients with IBS. Normal colonic myoelectric activity consists of background slow waves with superimposed spike potentials. Bueno et al. demonstrated increased long spike bursts in patients with constipation and irregular short spike burst in patients with diarrhea.[76] Myoelectric studies in the small bowel have demonstrated shorter intervals between the migrating motor complex, which is of course, the predominant interdigestive small-bowel motor pattern.[77] Patients with IBS have variations in the colonic slow wave frequency and a blunted late peaking postprandial response of spike potentials in the colon. Transit studies in the small bowel have demonstrated delayed meal transit in patients with constipation-predominant IBS and accelerated meal transit in patients with diarrhea predominant IBS.[78,79] Overall, these studies and others suggest an underlying generalized hyper-responsiveness of smooth muscle in patients with IBS.

Visceral Hypersensitivity

Visceral hyperalgesia appears to be another component of this disorder. Studies measuring the perception of gut distension using various techniques have demonstrated abnormally high sensitivity in both the small and large bowel.[80,81] It appears that patients with a diagnosis of IBS have both an increased awareness of gut distension and experience such distension as painful at lower volumes and pressures as normal subjects – this is especially in response to rapid distension.[82] While there has been some argument regarding a reporting bias in patients with IBS (i.e., routinely reporting pain at lower subjective intensities than normal controls), such differences do not account for all of the sensory abnormalities seen.[83] Furthermore, patients with IBS have widened dermatomal referral pain patterns than normal controls from gut distension,[84] though this visceral hypersensitivity is not associated with a somatic hypersensitivity.[85] It is thought that patients with IBS may have sensitization of the intestinal afferent nocioreceptive pathways in the spinal cord.

The central nervous system modulates gut function for optimal digestive function. The limbic system, medial prefrontal cortex, amygdala, and hypothalamus communicate emotional changes to the gut via the autonomic nervous system. In turn, signals from the gut to the brain can affect reflex regulation and mood states.[86] Recent studies have suggested that patients with IBS may process visceral afferent input in the central nervous system in an abnormal way, and this response may be modified by attentional factors acknowledging that stress, anxiety, and prior unpleasant life events increase the perception of painful events.[80,87] On a biochemical level, patients with IBS have been demonstrated to have increased hypothalamic corticotropin-releasing factor in response to stress, as well as an exaggerated colonic motility response.[88]

Small Intestinal Overgrowth Syndrome

Small intestinal bacterial overgrowth syndrome (SIBO) ($>10^5$ bacteria/ml) has been implicated as possible etiology for IBS. There is a striking similarity between the symptoms of bloating and abdominal pain associated with IBS and SIBO. Pimental et al.[89,90] showed that 78% of patients with IBS had abnormal hydrogen breath test, and a 7-day course of neomycin was associated with improvement of their symptoms. Using jejunal aspirates to detect SIBO, Posserud et al.[91] found higher bacterial counts in IBS patients compared to placebo (43% vs. 12%). Treatment with oral antibotics has become an accepted course of therapy for some patients with suspected SIBO and IBS.

Mucosal Inflammation

The presence of low-grade inflammation and immune activation suggests that alterations in the indigenous intestinal flora may play a role.[92] A correlation between abdominal pain in IBS and the presence of activated mast cells in proximity to colonic nerves has been reported.[93] Probiotics may be helpful to restore the depleted bifidobacteria species found in the human intestine.

Psychological Abnormalities

The relationship between psychopathology and IBS is unclear. As previously noted, patients with IBS have a higher incidence of panic disorder, major depression, anxiety disorder, and hypocondriasis than do normal populations.[94] In addition, they report a higher prevalence of physical or sexual abuse.[95] Two thirds of patients with IBS report the onset of GI complaints with an Axis 1 disorder.[96]

Genetics

The relationship between learned behavior and genetics in IBS is under investigation. Twin studies found that concordance rates for IBS were as high in monozygotic twins compared to dizygotic twins.[97] It has also been hypothesized that genetic differences in serotonic reuptake may play a role in the pathophysiology of IBS.

Symptoms

The altered stool habits reported by patients with IBS can be constipation, diarrhea, or alternating constipation and diarrhea. Constipation can be described as hard and/or infrequent stools, or painful defecation requiring laxative use. Diarrhea is usually described as small-volume, frequent, urgent, and watery stool and when present is often postprandial in nature. Usually patients have either constipation or diarrhea alone; however, alternation between each can be present. What differentiates these patients from those with functional constipation is the presence of significant abdominal pain and bloating. Abdominal pain is usually perceived as diffuse and is most common in the lower abdomen, especially on the left. Sharp pain may be superimposed on a more chronic duller component. Pain may be precipitated by meals and is often relieved by defecation. Patients often report increasing bloating and gas through the daytime hours, which may or may not be associated with objective evidence such as mucorrhea, either white or clear. Patients with IBS are more likely to report upper gastrointestinal symptoms of nausea, vomiting, and heartburn. Overall symptoms may be worse in times of stress. Symptoms not typical of IBS that should alert the clinician to organic disease include the following: onset in middle age or older, progressive or nocturnal symptoms, anorexia, weight loss, fever, hematochezia, and painless diarrhea or steatorrhea.

Treatment of IBS-C

Although there are emerging novel medications for IBS that may prove useful, much of the current medical therapy depends on diet modification and reassurance. Explanation and patient education play an important role in the management of this chronic disorder. Treatment strategies depend not only on the type of symptoms present but also on their severity and chronicity.

Medical Therapy

Fiber supplementation may improve symptoms of either constipation or diarrhea, although studies are inconclusive due to a strong placebo effect. Many physicians feel that polycarbophil based bulking agents may be tolerated better than psyllium-based compounds due to an exacerbation of bloating symptoms in some patients with the latter. Similarly, ingesting more water, avoiding caffeine and legumes are all reasonable patient advice. For patients with constipation-predominant IBS who do not respond to fiber supplementation (20 g/day) or do not tolerate it, osmotic laxatives such as MiraLAX®, Milk of Magnesia®, or sorbitol may be tried.

Tegaserod (Zelnorm®), a partial 5HT-4 agonist, accelerates transit in the small bowel and colon. It was shown to improve constipation and global IBS symptoms in women with constipation-predominant IBS.[98] However, Tegaserod is no longer available because its use can induce cardiac conduction abnormalities.[98]

Lubiprostone (Amitizia®) chloride channel activator has been approved for patients with IBS-C at a lower dose 8 mcg bid to decrease constipation, abdominal discomfort, and bloating.[30]

Antibiotics have been recommended to treat patients with SIBO and IBS. The following oral antibiotics have been suggested: neomycin orally for 10 days; levofloxacin or ciprofloxacin for 7 days; metronidazole for 7 days; rifaximin (Xifaxan®) for 10 days at higher than normal doses of (1,200 mg/day) compared to standard lower doses (800 or 400 mg/day).[99] Retrospective studies suggest that rifaximin is superior to other oral antibiotics, but the cost and the unwillingness of insurance companies to cover the higher dose make it a challenge for the patients and prescribing physician.[100]

Probiotics

Probiotic bacteria may inhibit other symptom-causing bacteria in the intestine, or the probiotic bacteria may act on the host's intestinal immune system to suppress inflammation. The most common probiotic bacteria are lactobacilli (also used in the production of yogurt) and bifidobacteria. Both of these bacteria are found in the intestine of normal individuals. Probiotics are thought to have both qualitative and quantitative effects restoring the type of bacteria and the amount of normal bacteria (i.e., small intestinal bacterial overgrowth). Commercially available probiotics are available and have been shown to be effective; there is no evidence on the superiority of any particular strain.[101]

Other agents undergoing evaluation primarily focusing on symptoms of pain include clonidine (an alpha adrenergic agonist), fedotozine (a kappa opioid agonist) and ammonium derivatives (an antimuscarinic and neurokinin-receptor antagonist). Of these, fedotozine is clinically available for this indication and has shown to be helpful in reducing symptoms of pain in patients with IBS.[102]

An adjunctive therapy to medication is psychological treatment. Psychologic treatment is appropriate when there is evidence that stress or psychological factors are contributing to an exacerbation of symptoms, or patients have failed to respond to medical treatment. A clear explanation of the rationale for such treatment is important in patient acceptance of such therapy.

Conclusion

Constipation is an extremely prevalent problem that can often be treated with minimal changes to diet and lifestyle, but there is a subset of patients who will have severe symptoms that are difficult to treat or are associated with irritable bowel syndrome. The magnitude of the problem requires the colon and rectal surgeon to understand the etiology of constipation, be facile with the tests utilized in the evaluation of the constipated patient, and be able to recommend both medical and surgical therapies when appropriate. The Standards Practice Task Force of the American Society of Colon and Rectal Surgeons has published practice parameters for the evaluation and management of constipation.[103]

Acknowledgment. This chapter was authored by Amanda Metcalf and Howard Michael Ross in the previous edition of this textbook.

References

1. Higgins PD, Johanson JF. Epidemiology of constipation in North America: a systematic review. Am J Gastroenterol. 2004;99(4):750–9.
2. Sonnenberg A, Koch TR. Epidemiology of constipation in the United States. Dis Colon Rectum. 1989;32(1):1–8.
3. Knowles CH, Scott SM, Rayner C, Glia A, Lindberg G, Kamm MA, et al. Idiopathic slow-transit constipation: an almost exclusively female disorder. Dis Colon Rectum. 2003;46(12):1716–7.
4. Varma MG, Hart SL, Brown JS, Creasman JM, Van Den Eeden SK, Thom DH. Obstructive defecation in middle-aged women. Dig Dis Sci. 2008;53(10):2702–9.
5. Zutshi M, Hull TL, Bast J, Hammel J. Female bowel function: the real story. Dis Colon Rectum. 2007;50(3):351–8.
6. Talley NJ, Fleming KC, Evans JM, O'Keefe EA, Weaver AL, Zinsmeister AR, et al. Constipation in an elderly community:

a study of prevalence and potential risk factors. Am J Gastroenterol. 1996;91(1):19–25.
7. Drossman DA, Corazziari E, Talley NJ, Thompson WG, Whitehead WE, editors. ROME III. The functional gastrointestinal disorders diagnosis, pathophysiology, and treatment. A multinational consensus. 2nd ed. McLean, VA: Degnon Associates; 2000.
8. Lewis SJ, Heaton KW. Stool form scale as a useful guide to intestinal transit time. Scand J Gastroenterol. 1997;32(9):920–4.
9. Devroede G. Psychophysiological considerations in subjects with chronic idiopathic constipation. In: Wexner SD, Bartolo DC, editors. Constipation: etiology, evaluation and management. 1st ed. Oxford, UK: Butterworth-Heinemann; 1995. p. 103.
10. Hinton JM, Lennard-Jones JE, Young AC. A new method for studying gut transit times using radioopaque markers. Gut. 1969;10(10):842–7.
11. Martelli H, Devroede G, Arhan P, Duguay C, Dornic C, Faverdin C. Some parameters of large bowel motility in normal man. Gastroenterology. 1978;75(4):612–8.
12. Metcalf AM, Phillips SF, Zinsmeister AR, MacCarty RL, Beart RW, Wolff BG. Simplified assessment of segmental colonic transit. Gastroenterology. 1987;92(1):40–7.
13. Cowlam S, Khan U, Mackie A, Varma JS, Yiannankou Y. Validity of segmental transit studies used in routine clinical practice, to characterize defaecatory disorder in patients with functional constipation. Colorectal Dis. 2008;10(8):818–22.
14. Bonapace ES, Maurer AH, Davidoff S, Krevsky B, Fisher RS, Parkman HP. Whole gut transit scintigraphy in the clinical evaluation of patients with upper and lower gastrointestinal symptoms. Am J Gastroenterol. 2000;95(10):2838–47.
15. Maqbool S, Parkman HP, Friedenberg FK. Wireless capsule motility: comparison of the SmartPill GI monitoring system with scintigraphy for measuring whole gut transit. Dig Dis Sci. 2009;54(10):2167–74.
16. Fleshman JW, Dreznik Z, Cohen E, Fry RD, Kodner IJ. Balloon expulsion test facilitates diagnosis of pelvic floor outlet obstruction due to nonrelaxing puborectalis muscle. Dis Colon Rectum. 1992;35(11):1019–25.
17. Jorge JM, Wexner SD, Ger GC, Salanga VD, Nogueras JJ, Jagelman DG. Cinedefecography and electromyography in the diagnosis of nonrelaxing puborectalis syndrome. Dis Colon Rectum. 1993;36(7):668–76.
18. Bertschinger KM, Hetzer FH, Roos JE, Treiber K, Marincek B, Hilfiker PR. Dynamic MR imaging of the pelvic floor performed with patient sitting in an open-magnet unit versus with patient supine in a closed-magnet unit. Radiology. 2002;223(2):501–8.
19. Rao SS, Seaton K, Miller M, Brown K, Nygaard I, Stumbo P, et al. Randomized controlled trial of biofeedback, sham feedback, and standard therapy for dyssynergic defecation. Clin Gastroenterol Hepatol. 2007;5(3):331–8.
20. Romano G, Bianco F, Caggiano L. Modified perineal stapled rectal resection with contour transtar for full-thickness rectal prolapse. Colorectal Dis. 2009;11(8):878–81.
21. Boccasanta P, Venturi M, Stuto A, Bottini C, Caviglia A, Carriero A, et al. Stapled transanal rectal resection for outlet obstruction: a prospective, multicenter trial. Dis Colon Rectum. 2004;47(8):1285–96. discussion 1296–7.
22. Ommer A, Albrecht K, Wenger F, Walz MK. Stapled transanal rectal resection (STARR): a new option in the treatment of obstructive defecation syndrome. Langenbecks Arch Surg. 2006;391(1):32–7.
23. Frascio M, Stabilini C, Ricci B, Marino P, Fornaro R, De Salvo L, et al. Stapled transanal rectal resection for outlet obstruction syndrome: results and follow-up. World J Surg. 2008;32(6):1110–5.
24. Arroyo A, Gonzalez-Argente FX, Garcia-Domingo M, Espin-Basany E, De-la-Portilla F, Perez-Vicente F, et al. Prospective multicentre clinical trial of stapled transanal rectal resection for obstructive defaecation syndrome. Br J Surg. 2008;95(12):1521–7.
25. Lehur PA, Stuto A, Fantoli M, Villani RD, Queralto M, Lazorthes F, et al. Outcomes of stapled transanal rectal resection vs. biofeedback for the treatment of outlet obstruction associated with rectal intussusception and rectocele: a multicenter, randomized, controlled trial. Dis Colon Rectum. 2008;51(11):1611–8.
26. Nieminen K, Hiltunen KM, Laitinen J, Oksala J, Heinonen PK. Transanal or vaginal approach to rectocele repair: a prospective, randomized pilot study. Dis Colon Rectum. 2004;47(10): 1636–42.
27. Jorge JM, Yang YK, Wexner SD. Incidence and clinical significance of sigmoidoceles as determined by a new classification system. Dis Colon Rectum. 1994;37(11):1112–7.
28. Fenner DE. Diagnosis and assessment of sigmoidoceles. Am J Obstet Gynecol. 1996;175(6):1438–41. discussion 1441–2.
29. Lubiprostone (amitiza) for chronic constipation. Med Lett Drugs Ther. 2006;48(1236):47–8.
30. Lubiprostone (Amitiza) for irritable bowel syndrome with constipation. Med Lett Drugs Ther. 2008;50(1290):53–4.
31. Bassotti G, Gaburri M, Imbimbo BP, Rossi L, Farroni F, Pelli MA, et al. Colonic mass movements in idiopathic chronic constipation. Gut. 1988;29(9):1173–9.
32. MacDonald A, Baxter JN, Finlay IG. Idiopathic slow-transit constipation. Br J Surg. 1993;80(9):1107–11.
33. Classic articles in colonic and rectal surgery. Sir William Arbuthnot Lane 1856–1943. The results of the operative treatment of chronic constipation. Dis Colon Rectum. 1985;28(10):750–7.
34. Redmond JM, Smith GW, Barofsky I, Ratych RE, Goldsborough DC, Schuster MM. Physiological tests to predict long-term outcome of total abdominal colectomy for intractable constipation. Am J Gastroenterol. 1995;90(5):748–53.
35. Glia A, Akerlund JE, Lindberg G. Outcome of colectomy for slow-transit constipation in relation to presence of small-bowel dysmotility. Dis Colon Rectum. 2004;47(1):96–102.
36. Bernini A, Madoff RD, Lowry AC, Spencer MP, Gemlo BT, Jensen LL, et al. Should patients with combined colonic inertia and nonrelaxing pelvic floor undergo subtotal colectomy? Dis Colon Rectum. 1998;41(11):1363–6.
37. Hassan I, Pemberton JH, Young-Fadok TM, You YN, Drelichman ER, Rath-Harvey D, et al. Ileorectal anastomosis for slow transit constipation: long-term functional and quality of life results. J Gastrointest Surg. 2006;10(10):1330–6. discussion 1336–7.
38. Heymen S, Wexner SD, Gulledge AD. MMPI assessment of patients with functional bowel disorders. Dis Colon Rectum. 1993;36(6):593–6.
39. Sarli L, Iusco D, Donadei E, Costi R, Sgobba G, Violi V, et al. The rationale for cecorectal anastomosis for slow transit constipation. Acta Biomed. 2003;74 Suppl 2:74–9.

40. Feng Y, Jianjiang L. Functional outcomes of two types of subtotal colectomy for slow-transit constipation: ileosigmoidal anastomosis and cecorectal anastomosis. Am J Surg. 2008;195(1):73–7.
41. Knowles CH, Scott M, Lunniss PJ. Outcome of colectomy for slow transit constipation. Ann Surg. 1999;230(5):627–38.
42. Nyam DC, Pemberton JH, Ilstrup DM, Rath DM. Long-term results of surgery for chronic constipation. Dis Colon Rectum. 1997;40(3):273–9.
43. Pikarsky AJ, Efron J, Hamel CT, Weiss EG, Nogueras JJ, Wexner SD. Effect of age on the functional outcome of total abdominal colectomy for colonic inertia. Colorectal Dis. 2001;3(5):318–22.
44. Webster C, Dayton M. Results after colectomy for colonic inertia: a sixteen-year experience. Am J Surg. 2001;182(6):639–44.
45. Mollen RM, Kuijpers HC, Claassen AT. Colectomy for slow-transit constipation: preoperative functional evaluation is important but not a guarantee for a successful outcome. Dis Colon Rectum. 2001;44(4):577–80.
46. Verne GN, Hocking MP, Davis RH, Howard RJ, Sabetai MM, Mathias JR, et al. Long-term response to subtotal colectomy in colonic inertia. J Gastrointest Surg. 2002;6(5):738–44.
47. FitzHarris GP, Garcia-Aguilar J, Parker SC, Bullard KM, Madoff RD, Goldberg SM, et al. Quality of life after subtotal colectomy for slow-transit constipation: both quality and quantity count. Dis Colon Rectum. 2003;46(4):433–40.
48. Thaler K, Dinnewitzer A, Oberwalder M, Weiss EG, Nogueras JJ, Efron J, et al. Quality of life after colectomy for colonic inertia. Tech Coloproctol. 2005;9(2):133–7.
49. Zmora O, Colquhoun P, Katz J, Efron J, Weiss EG, Nogueras JJ, et al. Small bowel transit does not correlate with outcome of surgery in patients with colonic inertia. Surg Innov. 2005; 12(3):215–8.
50. O'Brien S, Hyman N, Osler T, Rabinowitz T. Sexual abuse: a strong predictor of outcomes after colectomy for slow-transit constipation. Dis Colon Rectum. 2009;52(11):1844–7.
51. Lundin E, Karlbom U, Pahlman L, Graf W. Outcome of segmental colonic resection for slow-transit constipation. Br J Surg. 2002;89(10):1270–4.
52. Keighley MR, Grobler S, Bain I. An audit of restorative proctocolectomy. Gut. 1993;34(5):680–4.
53. Kalbassi MR, Winter DC, Deasy JM. Quality-of-life assessment of patients after ileal pouch-anal anastomosis for slow-transit constipation with rectal inertia. Dis Colon Rectum. 2003;46(11):1508–12.
54. Scarpa M, Barollo M, Keighley MR. Ileostomy for constipation: long-term postoperative outcome. Colorectal Dis. 2005;7(3):224–7.
55. Kenefick NJ, Vaizey CJ, Cohen CR, Nicholls RJ, Kamm MA. Double-blind placebo-controlled crossover study of sacral nerve stimulation for idiopathic constipation. Br J Surg. 2002;89(12):1570–1.
56. Kenefick NJ. Sacral nerve neuromodulation for the treatment of lower bowel motility disorders. Ann R Coll Surg Engl. 2006;88(7):617–23.
57. Malouf AJ, Wiesel PH, Nicholls T, Nicholls RJ, Kamm MA. Short-term effects of sacral nerve stimulation for idiopathic slow transit constipation. World J Surg. 2002;26(2):166–70.
58. Ganio E, Masin A, Ratto C, Altomare DF, Ripetti V, Clerico G, et al. Short-term sacral nerve stimulation for functional anorectal and urinary disturbances: results in 40 patients: evaluation of a new option for anorectal functional disorders. Dis Colon Rectum. 2001;44(9):1261–7.
59. Malone PS, Ransley PG, Kiely EM. Preliminary report: the antegrade continence enema. Lancet. 1990;336(8725):1217–8.
60. Williams NS, Hughes SF, Stuchfield B. Continent colonic conduit for rectal evacuation in severe constipation. Lancet. 1994;343(8909):1321–4.
61. Kiely EM, Ade-Ajayi N, Wheeler RA. Caecal flap conduit for antegrade continence enemas. Br J Surg. 1994;81(8):1215.
62. Sinha CK, Grewal A, Ward HC. Antegrade continence enema (ACE): current practice. Pediatr Surg Int. 2008;24(6):685–8.
63. Gerharz EW, Vik V, Webb G, Leaver R, Shah PJ, Woodhouse CR. The value of the MACE (Malone antegrade colonic enema) procedure in adult patients. J Am Coll Surg. 1997;185(6): 544–7.
64. Lees NP, Hodson P, Hill J, Pearson RC, MacLennan I. Long-term results of the antegrade continent enema procedure for constipation in adults. Colorectal Dis. 2004;6(5):362–8.
65. Worsoe J, Christensen P, Krogh K, Buntzen S, Laurberg S. Long-term results of antegrade colonic enema in adult patients: assessment of functional results. Dis Colon Rectum. 2008;51(10): 1523–8.
66. Teichman JM, Harris JM, Currie DM, Barber DB. Antegrade continence enema for adult neurogenic patients. Can J Urol. 1998;5(3):603–6.
67. Poirier M, Abcarian H, Nelson R. Malone antegrade continent enema: an alternative to resection in severe defecation disorders. Dis Colon Rectum. 2007;50(1):22–8.
68. Hirst GR, Arumugam PJ, Watkins AJ, Mackey P, Morgan AR, Carr ND, et al. Antegrade continence enema in the treatment of obstructed defaecation with or without faecal incontinence. Tech Coloproctol. 2005;9(3):217–21.
69. Longstreth GF, Wolde-Tsadik G. Irritable bowel-type symptoms in HMO examinees. Prevalence, demographics, and clinical correlates. Dig Dis Sci. 1993;38(9):1581–9.
70. Zuckerman MJ, Guerra LG, Drossman DA, Foland JA, Gregory GG. Comparison of bowel patterns in Hispanics and non-Hispanic whites. Dig Dis Sci. 1995;40(8):1763–9.
71. Taub E, Cuevas JL, Cook 3rd EW, Crowell M, Whitehead WE. Irritable bowel syndrome defined by factor analysis. Gender and race comparisons. Dig Dis Sci. 1995;40(12):2647–55.
72. Jain AP, Gupta OP, Jajoo UN, Sidhwa HK. Clinical profile of irritable bowel syndrome at a rural based teaching hospital in central India. J Assoc Physicians India. 1991;39(5):385–6.
73. Kay L, Jorgensen T, Jensen KH. The epidemiology of irritable bowel syndrome in a random population: prevalence, incidence, natural history and risk factors. J Intern Med. 1994;236(1):23–30.
74. Whitehead WE, Bosmajian L, Zonderman AB, Costa Jr PT, Schuster MM. Symptoms of psychologic distress associated with irritable bowel syndrome. Comparison of community and medical clinic samples. Gastroenterology. 1988;95(3):709–14.
75. Drossman DA, Camilleri M, Mayer EA, Whitehead WE. AGA technical review on irritable bowel syndrome. Gastroenterology. 2002;123(6):2108–31.
76. Bueno L, Fioramonti J, Ruckebusch Y, Frexinos J, Coulom P. Evaluation of colonic myoelectrical activity in health and functional disorders. Gut. 1980;21(6):480–5.

77. Kellow JE, Phillips SF, Miller LJ, Zinsmeister AR. Dysmotility of the small intestine in irritable bowel syndrome. Gut. 1988;29(9):1236–43.
78. Cann PA, Read NW, Brown C, Hobson N, Holdsworth CD. Irritable bowel syndrome: relationship of disorders in the transit of a single solid meal to symptom patterns. Gut. 1983;24(5):405–11.
79. Lu CL, Chen CY, Chang FY, Lee SD. Characteristics of small bowel motility in patients with irritable bowel syndrome and normal humans: an Oriental study. Clin Sci. 1998;95(2):165–9.
80. Accarino AM, Azpiroz F, Malagelada JR. Attention and distraction: effects on gut perception. Gastroenterology. 1997;113(2):415–22.
81. Zighelboim J, Talley NJ, Phillips SF, Harmsen WS, Zinsmeister AR. Visceral perception in irritable bowel syndrome. Rectal and gastric responses to distension and serotonin type 3 antagonism. Dig Dis Sci. 1995;40(4):819–27.
82. Sun WM, Read NW, Prior A, Daly JA, Cheah SK, Grundy D. Sensory and motor responses to rectal distention vary according to rate and pattern of balloon inflation. Gastroenterology. 1990;99(4):1008–15.
83. Whitehead WE, Palsson OS. Is rectal pain sensitivity a biological marker for irritable bowel syndrome: psychological influences on pain perception. Gastroenterology. 1998;115(5):1263–71.
84. Munakata J, Naliboff B, Harraf F, Kodner A, Lembo T, Chang L, et al. Repetitive sigmoid stimulation induces rectal hyperalgesia in patients with irritable bowel syndrome. Gastroenterology. 1997;112(1):55–63.
85. Cook IJ, van Eeden A, Collins SM. Patients with irritable bowel syndrome have greater pain tolerance than normal subjects. Gastroenterology. 1987;93(4):727–33.
86. Silverman DH, Munakata JA, Ennes H, Mandelkern MA, Hoh CK, Mayer EA. Regional cerebral activity in normal and pathological perception of visceral pain. Gastroenterology. 1997;112(1):64–72.
87. Keogh E, Ellery D, Hunt C, Hannent I. Selective attentional bias for pain-related stimuli amongst pain fearful individuals. Pain. 2001;91(1–2):91–100.
88. Fukudo S, Nomura T, Hongo M. Impact of corticotropin-releasing hormone on gastrointestinal motility and adrenocorticotropic hormone in normal controls and patients with irritable bowel syndrome. Gut. 1998;42(6):845–9.
89. Pimentel M, Chow EJ, Lin HC. Eradication of small intestinal bacterial overgrowth reduces symptoms of irritable bowel syndrome. Am J Gastroenterol. 2000;95(12):3503–6.
90. Pimentel M, Chow EJ, Lin HC. Normalization of lactulose breath testing correlates with symptom improvement in irritable bowel syndrome. A double-blind, randomized, placebo-controlled study. Am J Gastroenterol. 2003;98(2):412–9.
91. Posserud I, Stotzer PO, Bjornsson ES, Abrahamsson H, Simren M. Small intestinal bacterial overgrowth in patients with irritable bowel syndrome. Gut. 2007;56(6):802–8.
92. Chadwick VS, Chen W, Shu D, Paulus B, Bethwaite P, Tie A, et al. Activation of the mucosal immune system in irritable bowel syndrome. Gastroenterology. 2002;122(7):1778–83.
93. Barbara G, Stanghellini V, De Giorgio R, Cremon C, Cottrell GS, Santini D, et al. Activated mast cells in proximity to colonic nerves correlate with abdominal pain in irritable bowel syndrome. Gastroenterology. 2004;126(3):693–702.
94. Drossman DA, McKee DC, Sandler RS, Mitchell CM, Cramer EM, Lowman BC, et al. Psychosocial factors in the irritable bowel syndrome. A multivariate study of patients and nonpatients with irritable bowel syndrome. Gastroenterology. 1988;95(3):701–8.
95. Drossman DA, Leserman J, Nachman G, Li ZM, Gluck H, Toomey TC, et al. Sexual and physical abuse in women with functional or organic gastrointestinal disorders. Ann Intern Med. 1990;113(11):828–33.
96. Creed F, Craig T, Farmer R. Functional abdominal pain, psychiatric illness, and life events. Gut. 1988;29(2):235–42.
97. Levy RL, Jones KR, Whitehead WE, Feld SI, Talley NJ, Corey LA. Irritable bowel syndrome in twins: heredity and social learning both contribute to etiology. Gastroenterology. 2001;121(4):799–804.
98. Layer P, Keller J, Mueller-Lissner S, Ruegg P, Loeffler H. Tegaserod: long-term treatment for irritable bowel syndrome patients with constipation in primary care. Digestion. 2005;71(4):238–44.
99. Pimentel M. Review of rifaximin as treatment for SIBO and IBS. Expert Opin Investig Drugs. 2009;18(3):349–58.
100. Yang J, Lee HR, Low K, Chatterjee S, Pimentel M. Rifaximin versus other antibiotics in the primary treatment and retreatment of bacterial overgrowth in IBS. Dig Dis Sci. 2008;53(1):169–74.
101. Wilhelm SM, Brubaker CM, Varcak EA, Kale-Pradhan PB. Effectiveness of probiotics in the treatment of irritable bowel syndrome. Pharmacotherapy. 2008;28(4):496–505.
102. Corazziari E. Role of opioid ligands in the irritable bowel syndrome. Can J Gastroenterol. 1999;13(Suppl A):71A–5.
103. Ternent CA, Bastawrous AL, Morin NA, Standards Practice Task Force of the American Society of Colon and Rectal Surgeons, et al. Practice parameters for the evaluation and management of constipation. Dis Colon Rectum. 2007;50:2013–22.

33 Rectal Prolapse

Steven Mills

Rectal prolapse is a telescoping of the rectum out of the anus; an intussusception is when the telescoping does not protrude through the anal canal. Either condition can be uncomfortable or less commonly painful, and are often associated with varying degrees of embarrassment for the patient. They rarely present with ischemia or necrosis of the rectum; these advanced states represent an emergent situation.

Many patients have other associated pathologies of the pelvic floor and often there is a long history of straining and constipation. Fecal incontinence is also a common associated symptom. Further, there is a frequent association with anterior compartment pathologies such as urinary incontinence, voiding disorders, cystocele, or rectocele. Careful history and physical examination can lead to their diagnosis, which is essential as repair of the rectal prolapse without concurrent treatment of the associated anterior pathology can worsen symptoms.

Many theories have been proposed in an effort to explain the etiology of rectal prolapse. Nearly 100 years ago, Moschcowitz[1] suggested that rectal prolapse occurs as a sliding hernia through a defect within the pelvic fascia. Later, Broden and Snellman[2] demonstrated, with the aid of cinedefecography, that rectal prolapse is an intussusception of the rectum.

Rectal prolapse is more common in women than in men, likely due to childbirth, prolonged straining at stool, and/or anatomical considerations such as a wider pelvis. In women, the disorder increase in frequency with age whereas men with prolapse tend to be younger, around 20–40 years old, and often have a predisposing condition (such as anal atresia or prior surgery). In women, the pudendal nerves can be damaged during childbirth and/or chronic straining at stool, resulting in pelvic floor disturbances such as incontinence or prolapse. Whereas rectal prolapse is almost always treated surgically, every effort should be made to avoid surgery for rectoanal intussusception.

A wide variety of different procedures have been described to treat rectal prolapse (Table 33-1). The surgeon must determine which procedure is the best for an individual patient. Multiple patient and procedural factors need to be considered in determining which of the over 100 operations to perform. Important patient factors include gender and age of the patient, the patient's overall medical condition, bowel function, and whether or not fecal incontinence is also present. Procedural factors to consider include extent of prolapse, impact of procedure on bowel function and incontinence, morbidity of procedure, recurrence rates, and the individual surgeon's experience.

Unfortunately, a dearth of high quality data exists regarding the optimum method by which to treat rectal prolapse. An attempt in 2008 to perform a comprehensive review of randomized trials found that there were insufficient data to analyze, though a few patterns did emerge.[3] The method of fixation during rectopexy did not change outcome. Division of the lateral stalks was associated with a higher incidence of constipation whereas resection and rectopexy was associated with less constipation. Finally, laparoscopy was associated with a shorter hospitalization and less morbidity.

Patient Evaluation

Most patients with rectal prolapse present to the surgeon with complaints associated with the prolapse itself. They often describe a sensation of "something falling out," especially at the time of bowel movements. Many will complain of the feeling that they are "sitting on a ball" until spontaneous or manual reduction occurs. There is a common association with soiling of their undergarments or a feeling of mucous discharge. As constipation and straining, fecal incontinence, and erratic bowel habits are commonly associated with prolapse as well as other functional bowel diseases and mucosal abnormalities, evaluation prior to surgical management is necessary.

Physical examination can be variable for patients with rectal prolapse. While a spontaneous prolapse is obvious (Figure 33-1),[4] other patients may require straining to demonstrate the prolapse. In these cases, the prolapse usually is best examined in the squatting or sitting position. The patient

D.E. Beck et al. (eds.), *The ASCRS Textbook of Colon and Rectal Surgery: Second Edition*,
DOI 10.1007/978-1-4419-1584-9_33, © Springer Science+Business Media, LLC 2011

Table 33-1. Operations described for rectal prolapse

Transabdominal procedures
1. Repair of the pelvic floor
Abdominal repair of levator diastasis
Abdominoperineal levator repair
2. Suspension-fixation
Sigmoidopexy (Pemberton–Stalker)
Presacral rectopexy
Lateral strip rectopexy (Orr–Loygue)
Anterior sling rectopexy (Ripstein)
Posterior sling rectopexy (Wells)
Puborectal sling (Nigro)
3. Resection procedures
Proctopexy with sigmoid resection
Anterior resection
Perineal procedures
Perineal rectosigmoidectomy (Altemeier)
Rectal mucosal sleeve resection (Delorme)
Perineal suspension-fixation (Wyatt)
Anal encirclement (Thiersch + modification)

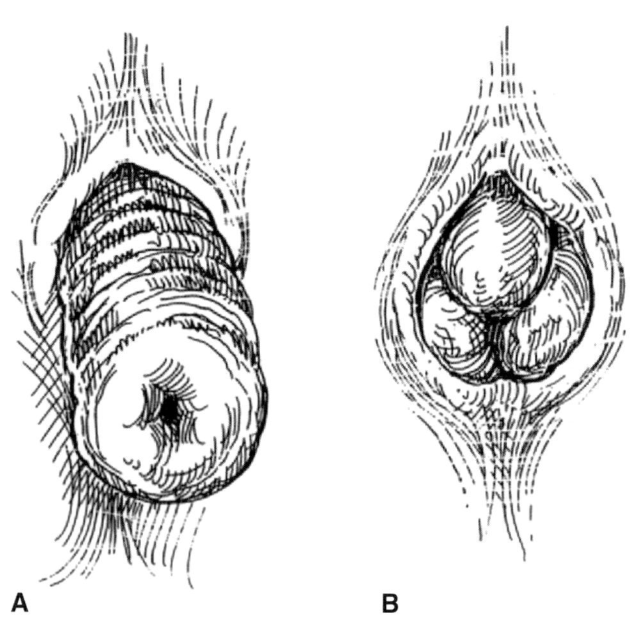

Figure 33-1. Mucosal versus full-thickness prolapse. **A** Circumferential full-thickness prolapse with concentric mucosal folds. **B** Radial folds seen with hemorrhoidal prolapse. [From Beck and Whitlow.[4] Copyright 2003 by Taylor & Francis Group LLC (B). Reproduced with permission of Taylor & Francis Group (B) in the format Textbook via Copyright Clearance Center].

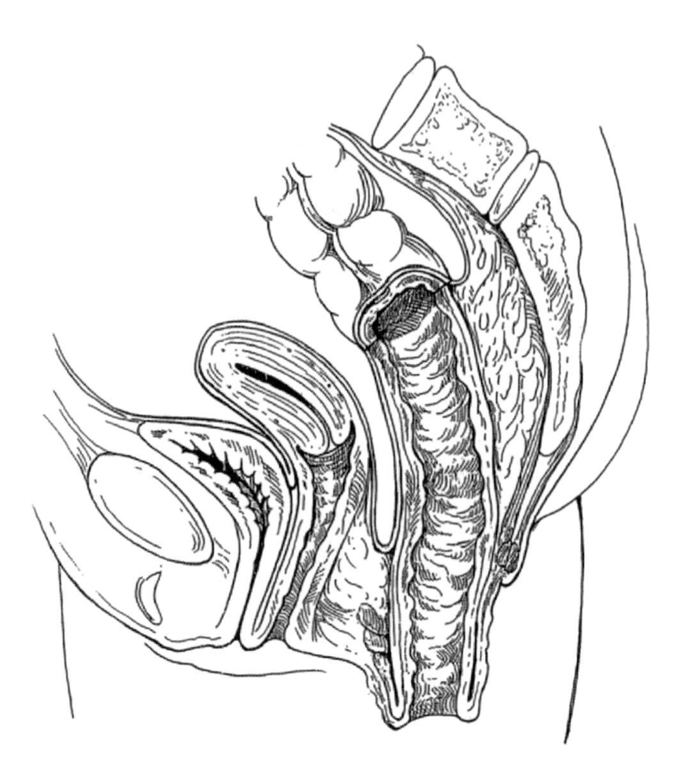

Figure 33-2. Sagittal view of full-thickness rectal prolapse. [From Beck and Whitlow.[4] Copyright 2003 by Taylor & Francis Group LLC (B). Reproduced with permission of Taylor & Francis Group (B) in the format Textbook via Copyright Clearance Center].

can be examined while he or she is on the toilet by having the patient lean forward. Alternatively, one can place a long rod to which a mirror is attached between the patient's legs to view the prolapse. A third option is to place a flexible endoscope into the toilet with the viewing end pointed toward the perineum. A more modern alternative might be a digital video or a digital photograph demonstrating the prolapse. Interestingly numerous patients present to the office with this rather unusual imagery already captured and eager to share with the surgeon.

Prior to choosing the appropriate procedure for prolapse, differentiation between full-thickness and mucosal prolapse is necessary. Full-thickness prolapse is identified by its concentric rings and grooves as opposed to the radially oriented grooves associated with mucosal prolapse (Figure 33-2). During the examination, one should also evaluate for any maceration or excoriation of the perianal skin. A thorough digital rectal examination is important to detect concomitant anal pathology and to evaluate adequacy of resting tone and squeeze pressure of the anal sphincters and function of the puborectalis muscle.

Further evaluation is indicated for patients with rectal prolapse. Either colonoscopy or flexible sigmoidoscopy with air contrast barium enema should be performed to exclude or otherwise address any associated mucosal abnormalities. Defecography is often unnecessary in the evaluation of full-thickness prolapse because it is diagnostically obvious; however, it can be an essential part of the evaluation of internal or occult procidentia (rectorectal intussusception) or as part of pelvic floor musculature evaluation. Anal manometry can help assess sphincter function, as chronic prolapse typically damages the internal anal sphincter, resulting in poor resting pressures.[5] In such patients, synchronous levatorplasty should be considered at the time of prolapse repair and may further improve continence.[6] In a manometric study evaluating patients with rectal prolapse, Spencer[5] reported that the anorectal inhibitory reflex was frequently absent or abnormal, that resting anal pressures were abnormally low, and that squeeze pressures were normal. Anal electromyography and pudendal nerve terminal motor latency are generally not clinically useful for this disorder unless there is a history of severe straining. In such a case, anal electromyography can be used to evaluate for the presence of inappropriate or paradoxical puborectalis contraction (anismus, nonrelaxing puborectalis or spastic pelvic floor). When discovered, biofeedback or botulinum toxin can be employed for therapy. Colonic transit times should be performed in patients with a history of severe constipation so that an appropriate operation can be chosen. Individuals with slow transit constipation typically benefit from a synchronous sigmoid colectomy with rectopexy versus rectopexy alone or even perineal rectosigmoidectomy. However, certain well-selected patients with concomitant slow transit constipation may be better served by a subtotal colectomy and ileorectal anastomosis at the time of rectopexy.

Surgical Procedures

There are two general approaches for surgery for rectal prolapse – abdominal operations and perineal operations. Men are at risk for neurologic injury resulting in sexual dysfunction from an abdominal operation; therefore, this option should be cautiously chosen. The risk of impotence for abdominal rectopexy should approach 1–2% in skilled hands and thus young males should be counseled to consider banking sperm prior to surgery.

The most common abdominal operations for prolapse are rectopexy with or without concomitant sigmoid resection. The typical perineal procedures are perineal rectosigmoidectomy (Altemeier) or a mucosal sleeve resection (Delorme). The specific operation must be tailored to the condition and pathology of each patient but some generalizations can be made. Elderly, high-risk patients are best treated with perineal procedures which can be performed under a regional anesthetic or even under a local anesthetic with IV sedation. Healthy adults with normal bowel habits can undergo either rectopexy with or without sigmoid resection or perineal rectosigmoidectomy with or without levatorplasty. Bowel function plays a role in determining the surgical plan. Constipated patients should usually undergo sigmoid resection and rectopexy, whereas incontinent patients should undergo either abdominal rectopexy or perineal rectosigmoidectomy with levatorplasty. Recurrent prolapse mandates knowledge of the prior repair as that information will dictate future options; the prior dissection may limit the available alternatives because of the remaining blood supply.

Perineal Procedures

Perineal Rectosigmoidectomy (Altemeier Procedure)

Perineal rectosigmoidectomy was popularized by Altemeier and his name is the eponym attached to the procedure.[7] The operation can be performed under a general or spinal anesthetic. Generally, the patient receives a full bowel preparation. The prone position is preferred; however, the left lateral (Simm's) or lithotomy position can also be effectively used. After prolapsing the rectum, the rectal wall is injected with an epinephrine-containing compound for hemostasis. A circumferential incision is made in the rectal wall approximately 1–2 cm above the dentate line (Figure 33-3). The incision is deepened until the full-thickness of the rectal wall

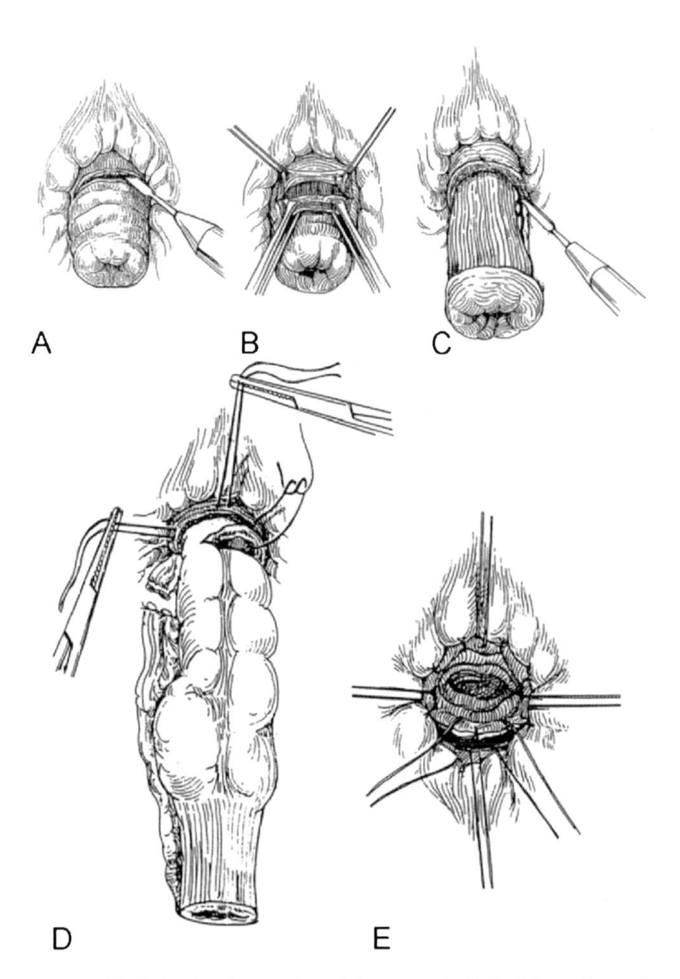

FIGURE 33-3. Perineal rectosigmoidectomy. **A**, **B** Incision of rectal wall. **C** Division of vessel adjacent to bowel wall. **D** The prolapsed segment is amputated. Stay sutures previously placed in distal edge of outer cylinder are placed in cut edge of inner cylinder. **E** Anastomosis of distal aspect of remaining colon to the short rectal stump. [From Beck and Whitlow.[4] Copyright 2003 by Taylor & Francis Group LLC (B). Reproduced with permission of Taylor & Francis Group (B) in the format Textbook via Copyright Clearance Center].

TABLE 33-2. Results of perineal rectosigmoidectomy

Authors	Number of patients	Recurrence (%)	Mortality (%)	Morbidity (%)
Altemeier et al.[7]	106	3	0	24
Friedman et al.[10]	27	50	0	12
Gopal et al.[11]	18	6	6	17
Finlay and Aitchison[12]	17	6	6	18
Williams et al.[13]	114	11	0	12
Johansen et al.[14]	20	0	5	5
Kim et al.[15]	183	16	0	14
Azimuddin et al.[16]	36	16	–	–
Zbar et al.[17]	80	4	–	–
Habr-Gama et al.[18]	44	7	0	9
Altomare et al.[19]	93	18	0	8

has been divided. Once a full-thickness incision has been made, the rectum is withdrawn out of the body while progressively dividing and ligating the mesorectum, advancing more cephalad. An energy source device can expedite this phase of the operation. Anteriorly, the peritoneal reflection (hernia sac) is opened. The dissection continues until there is no further redundancy remaining in the rectum/sigmoid colon, a judgment requiring some experience. After the redundant rectum has been adequately mobilized, it is divided and a hand-sutured coloanal anastomosis is performed. A colonic J pouch has also been described which may potentially improve function during the immediate postoperative period.[8] Alternatively, a circular stapler can be used to perform the anastomosis. In cases of severe fecal incontinence, a levator plication can be performed prior to the coloanal anastomosis which has been reported to improve continence in two-thirds of patients.[6,9] Following the procedure, patients are allowed to ambulate and eat regularly on postoperative day 1.

Several studies have been reported on perineal rectosigmoidectomy as summarized in Table 33-2. Mortality has been low with morbidity ranging from 5 to 24%.[7,10–19] Most of the reported morbidity stems from preexisting medical problems; however, a small number of patients do suffer anastomotic complications. Recurrence rates ranging from 0 to 10% are reported with a follow-up ranging from 6 months to 5 years; recurrence rates are higher for series with longer follow-up. An improvement in incontinence is reported in the majority of patients in whom levatorplasty was performed.[20] Indeed, levatorplasty may even be more beneficial as Chun et al.[21] reported a lower recurrence rate when perineal rectosigmoidectomy was combined with levatorplasty compared to perineal rectosigmoidectomy alone.

Mucosal Sleeve Resection (Delorme Procedure)

Another perineal option is the mucosal proctectomy first described by Delorme in 1900.[22] It is ideally suited to those patients with a less extensive prolapse (e.g., about 5 cm in length) or with full-thickness prolapse limited to partial circumference (e.g., anterior wall).

The Delorme procedure differs from the perineal rectosigmoidectomy (Altemeier) in that only the mucosa and submucosa are excised from the prolapsed segment (Figure 33-4). Delorme's procedure can be performed under general, spinal, or local anesthesia. Prone position is preferred; however, lithotomy position can also be successfully utilized. The bowel is prolapsed and the submucosa infiltrated with epinephrine solution; 1 cm cranial (proximal) to the dentate line the outer cylinder is incised through the mucosa only. The mucosa and submucosa are dissected off the underlying muscle (muscularis propria of the rectal wall). The mucosectomy may be more difficult in patients with prior anal surgery or a history of diverticulitis. The plane of dissection may be facilitated by continued submucosal injection of epinephrine solution as the dissection continues toward the apex of the prolapse. Four absorbable sutures (2-0) are placed sequentially in the rectal muscle at the anterior, posterior, and lateral positions as the dissection continues. These sutures plicate the muscle and provide traction. The dissection is carried inside the apex and the mucosa, which has been dissected free, is transected. After the mucosa is transected, the previously placed absorbable sutures (2-0) are used to reconnect the edges of the bowel. Four additional sutures are used to approximate the bowel between the placating sutures. Additional 3-0 sutures are placed in an interrupted fashion to complete the circumferential approximation of the mucosal edges.

Results of Delorme's procedure are summarized in Table 33-3. Reported operative mortality rates from a series of patients treated by Delorme's procedure range from 0 to 2.5%.[23–30] Morbidity rates were wide ranging (0–76%), with most morbidity associated with preexisting medical conditions. Surgery-specific morbidity includes hemorrhage, anastomotic dehiscence, and stricture. Recurrence rates (6–26% at 1–13 years postoperatively) are generally higher than with a perineal rectosigmoidectomy. Incontinence is improved in 40–50% of patients.[20] Constipation was not a problem in most series.

An alternative to the mucosal resection with muscular plication is the mucosal plication procedure (Gant–Miwa Procedure). Though not frequently performed in the USA, it has been associated with good results in Japan.[31] The best results seem to be when the mucosal plication is combined with an anal encircling procedure (see section "Thiersch Procedure" below).

Thiersch Procedure

Anal encirclement was first described by Thiersch in 1891.[32] He placed a silver wire subcutaneously around the anus under local anesthesia. The goal of this procedure was to mechanically supplement or replace the anal sphincter and stimulate a foreign body reaction in the perianal area, thereby increasing resistance at the anus. There were several reports of the use of this procedure in the early part of this century, especially in Europe.[33]

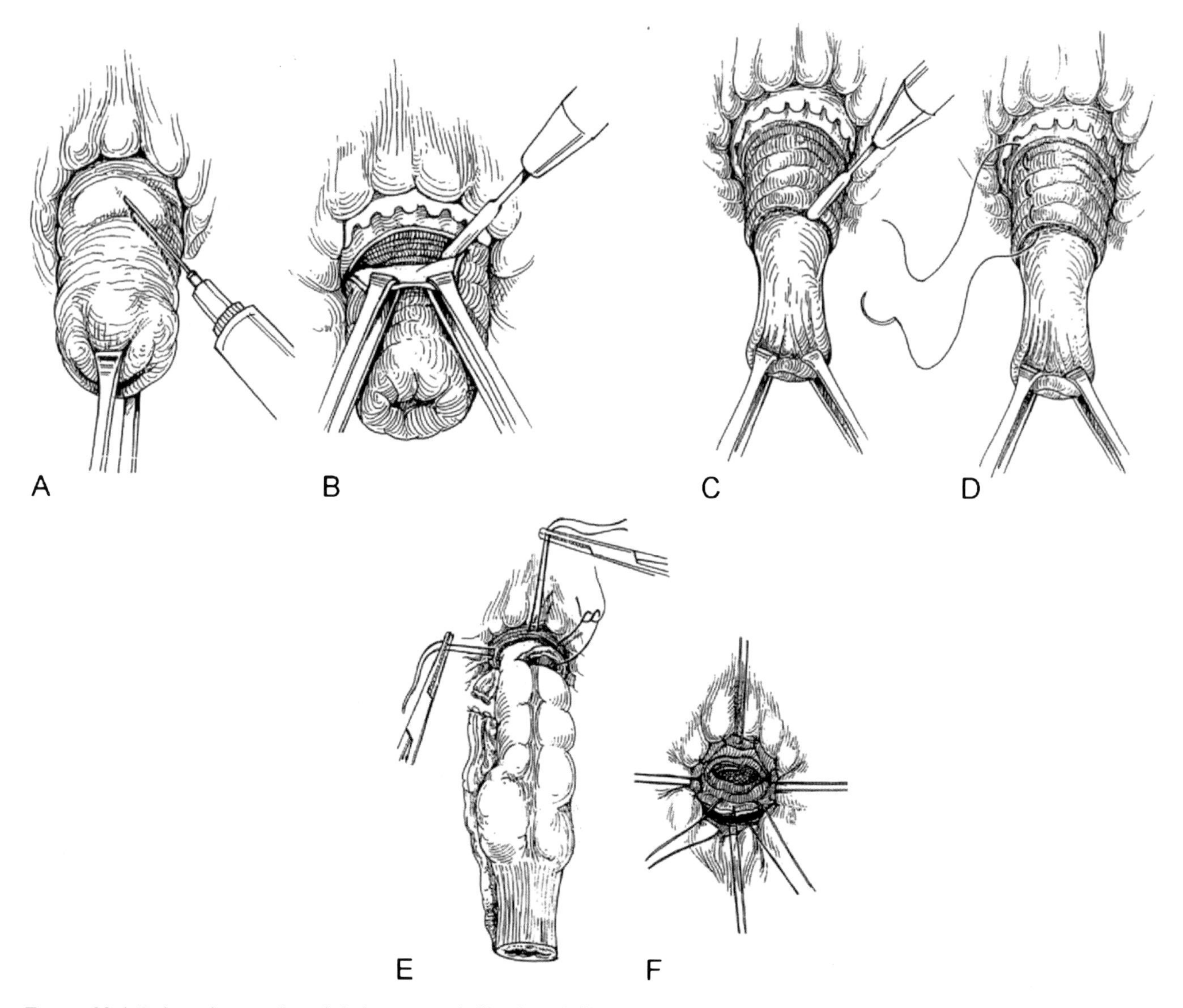

FIGURE 33-4. Delorme's procedure. **A** Subcutaneous infiltration of dilute epinephrine solution. **B** Circumferential mucosal incision. **C** Dissection of mucosa off muscular layer. **D** Plicating stitch approximating cut edge of mucosa, muscular wall, and mucosa just proximal to dentate line. **E** Plicating stitch tied. **F** Completed anastomosis. [From Beck and Whitlow.[4] Copyright 2003 by Taylor & Francis Group LLC (B). Reproduced with permission of Taylor & Francis Group (B) in the format Textbook via Copyright Clearance Center].

TABLE 33-3. Results of Delorme's procedure

Authors	Number of patients	Recurrence (%)	Mortality (%)	Morbidity (%)
Ulig and Sullivan[23]	44	7	0	34
Monson et al.[24]	27	7	0	0
Senapati et al.[25]	32	13	0	6
Oliver et al.[26]	41	22	2	62
Tobin and Scott[27]	43	26	0	12
Graf et al.[28]	14	21	0	–
Watkins et al.[29]	52	6	0	77
Lieberth et al.[30]	76	14	0	25

William Gabriel is credited with reviving interest in Thiersch's operation in the 1950s.[33] He reported on 25 cases of incontinence or minor rectal prolapse. He did not recommend this operation for major degrees of prolapse.

Anal encirclement is performed with the patient placed in the prone jackknife, lithotomy, or left lateral position (Figure 33-5). A local anesthetic is administered and a radial incision made on both sides of the anus about 2 cm from the anal verge. A curved hemostat is used to tunnel from one incision to the other, keeping "outside" of the external anal sphincter. The encircling material is brought through the tunnel so that the two ends meets. It is then secured by tying snuggly over an index finger in the anus. A variety of materials used for encirclement include nylon, silk, Silastic rods, silicone, Marlex mesh, Mersilene mesh, fascia, tendon, and Dacron.[34]

Complications of this procedure include breakage of the suture or wire, fecal impaction, sepsis, and erosion of the encircling material into the skin or anal canal. The Thiersch operation is not intended to correct the prolapse,

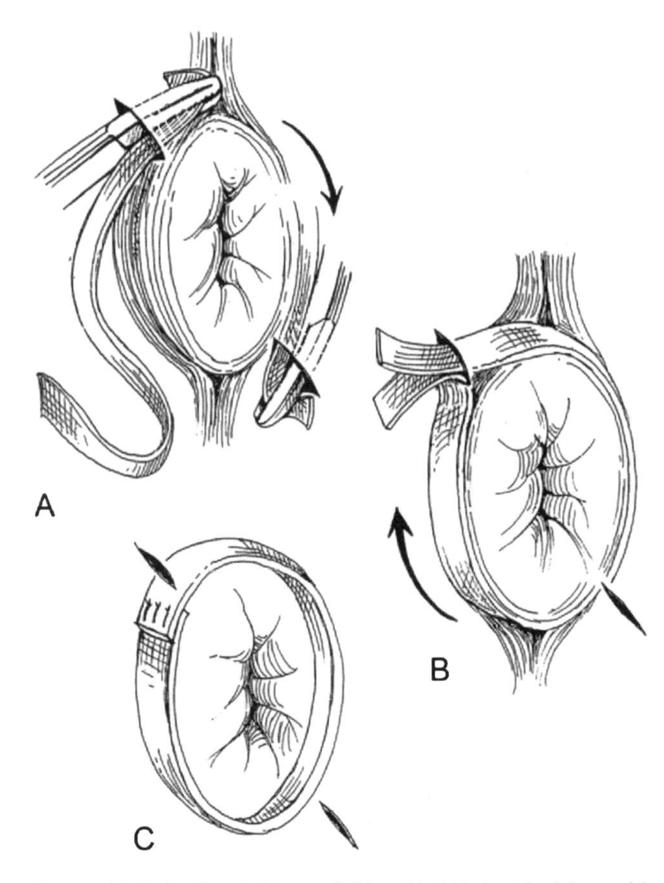

FIGURE 33-5. Anal encirclement (Thiersch). **A** Lateral incisions with prosthetic mesh tunneled around the anus. **B** Mesh completely encircling the anal opening. **C** Completed anal encirclement procedure. [From Beck and Whitlow.[4] Copyright 2003 by Taylor & Francis Group LLC (B). Reproduced with permission of Taylor & Francis Group (B) in the format Textbook via Copyright Clearance Center].

TABLE 33-4. Results of thiersch procedure

Authors	Number of patients	Recurrence (%)	Mortality (%)	Morbidity (%)
Jackaman et al.[36]	52	33	–	–
Labow et al.[34]	9	0	–	0
Hunt et al.[37]	41	44	–	37
Poole et al.[38]	15	33	–	33
Vongsangnak et al.[39]	25	39		59
Earnshaw and Hopkinson[40]	21	33	–	–
Khanduja et al.[41]	16	0	–	25
Sainio et al.[42]	14	15	–	–

but rather to narrow the anus enough to confine the prolapsing rectum above the anus. This goal is accomplished in 54–100% of cases.[35] Because of its failure to correct prolapse and the potential morbidity of this procedure, it is reserved for the most seriously ill patients who are unable to undergo one of the previously described perineal procedures. Results of the Thiersch procedure are summarized in Table 33-4.[36–42]

Abdominal Procedures

Abdominal Rectopexy and Sigmoid Colectomy

Abdominal rectopexy and sigmoidectomy was initially described in 1955 by Frykman[43] for management of full-thickness rectal prolapse, and it remains one of the main treatment options. The operation consists of four essential components (1) Complete mobilization of the rectum down to the levator musculature, leaving the lateral stalks intact, (2) elevation of the rectum cephalad with suture fixation to the presacral fascia just below the sacral promontory, (3) obliteration of the cul-de-sac, and (4) sigmoid colectomy with anastomosis. The current operation is essentially the same with the exception that some surgeons no longer obliterate the cul-de-sac (Figure 33-6). This procedure has become one of the most commonly performed operations for rectal prolapse. Results of sigmoid resection and rectopexy are summarized in Table 33-5. Morbidity is low (0–23%) with recurrence ranging from 0 to 3% (one study had recurrence as high as 9%).[44–51]

Abdominal Rectopexy

Simple suture rectopexy without sigmoid colectomy has been reported as an effective surgical treatment for rectal prolapse.[52,53] As rectopexy without resection can lead to worsening of constipation, this operation is typically utilized in patients who do not have associated constipation. The rectal mobilization and fixation is similar to that described above (complete to the pelvic floor musculature, preserving the lateral stalks) and is illustrated in Figure 33-7. Results are summarized in Table 33-6. Recurrence rates are under 5%.[52–54]

Ripstein Procedure

Described in 1963 by Ripstein and Lanter,[55] the Ripstein operation had been one of the most popular procedures for management of rectal prolapse. It is less frequently used today, likely due to the success of alternate therapies, the incidence of postoperative constipation, and because this particular operation requires the use of prosthetic material.

The rectum is mobilized posteriorly down to the coccyx, again preserving the lateral stalks. A 5-cm piece of prosthetic mesh (Marlex or Prolene) is sutured to the presacral fascia within the sacral hollow, about 5 cm below the sacral promontory in the midline. The rectum is retracted cephalad and the sling is wrapped around the rectum and sutured to it. Finally, the sling is sutured posteriorly from the opposite side (Figure 33-8). Care must be taken to avoid making the wrap too tight thus causing an obstruction. The results are summarized in Table 33-7. Recurrence rates are low, but morbidity is 13–33%.[55–60]

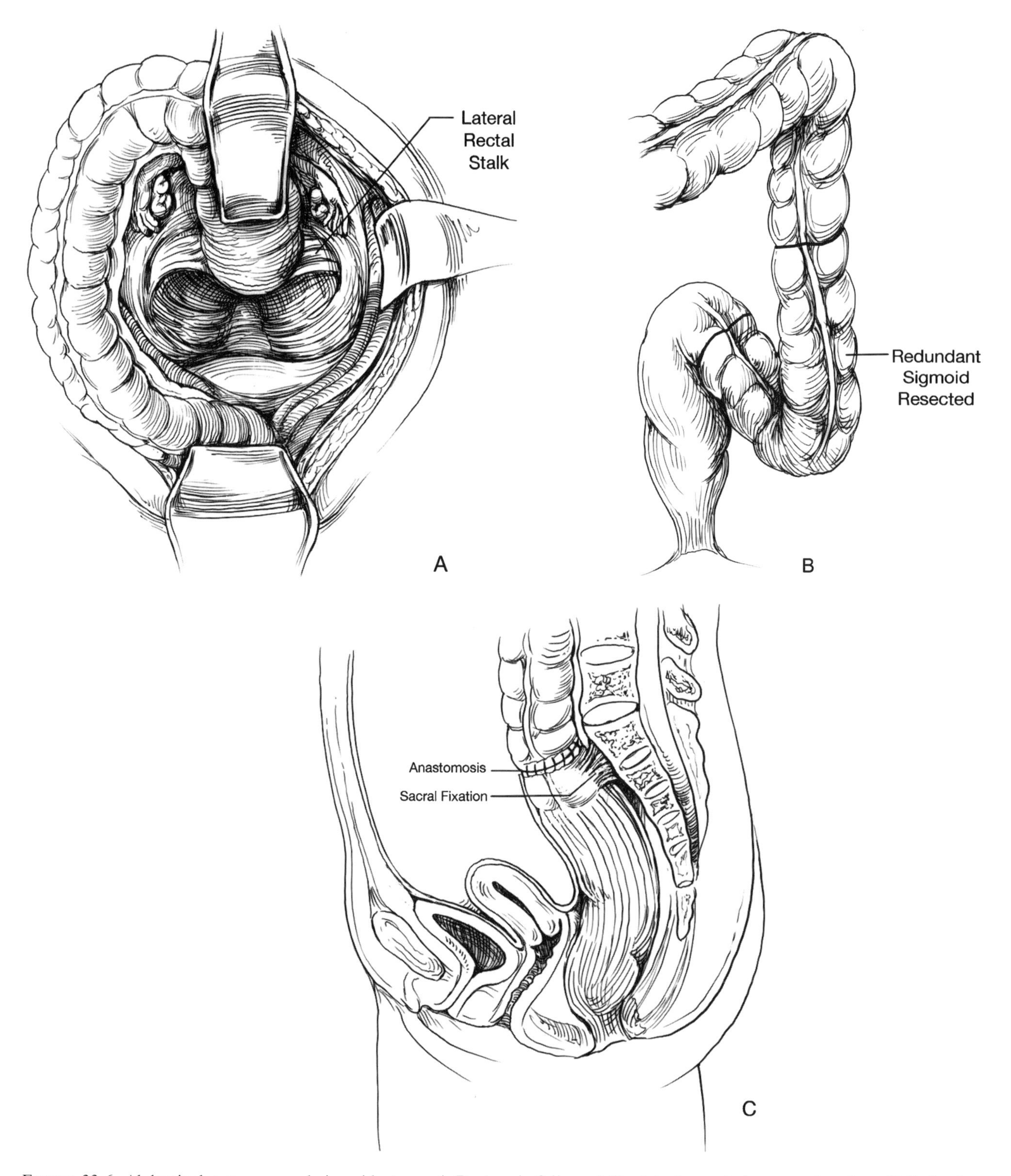

FIGURE 33-6. Abdominal rectopexy and sigmoidectomy. **A** Rectum is fully mobilized in the posterior avascular plane. **B** Redundant sigmoid colon is resected. **C** Anastomosis is completed and rectopexy sutures are placed. [From Beck and Whitlow.[4] Copyright 2003 by Taylor & Francis Group LLC (B). Reproduced with permission of Taylor & Francis Group (B) in the format Textbook via Copyright Clearance Center].

TABLE 33-5. Results of abdominal rectopexy and sigmoid colectomy

Authors	Number of patients	Recurrence (%)	Mortality (%)	Morbidity (%)
Watts et al.[44]	102	2	0	4
Husa et al.[45]	48	9	2	0
Sayfan et al.[46]	13	0	0	23
McKee et al.[47]	9	0	0	0
Luukkonen et al.[48]	15	0	7	20
Canfrere et al.[49]	17	0	0	–
Huber et al.[50]	39	0	0	7
Ashari et al.[51a]	117	2.5	0.8	9

[a] Laparoscopic approach.

Ivalon Sponge/Posterior Mesh Rectopexy

The Ivalon sponge wrap operation was first described in 1959 by Wells.[61] Traditionally, Ivalon (polyvinyl alcohol) sponge was used for the wrap, but other prosthetic meshes such as Prolene and Marlex (polypropylene) have also been successfully used. The operation begins with mobilization of the rectum posteriorly down to the levator ani. The rectum is also mobilized anteriorly, but the lateral stalks are again preserved. A piece of Ivalon sponge or mesh is then placed in the sacral hollow and sutured to the presacral fascia with nonabsorbable sutures. The lateral edges of the Ivalon or mesh are then wrapped around the rectum which has been retracted cephalad. The sponge/mesh is then sutured to the rectum such that only three-fourth of the rectum is wrapped (the anterior rectum is left free of the wrap material). The peritoneum is then closed over the sponge excluding it from the peritoneal cavity. Results of posterior wraps are summarized in Table 33-8. Recurrence rates are less than 3% with morbidity under 20%.[46,48,54,62]

Anterior Mesh Procedures

Multiple other mesh procedures have been described, some of which employ an anterior suspension technique. Among the most popular of these has been the Orr–Loygue procedure.[63] In this procedure, two ribbons of synthetic mesh is sutured to the anterior-lateral rectum (one on each side) after mobilization of the rectum as described earlier. The opposite ends of these mesh ribbons are then sutured to the sacral promontory under enough tension to hold the rectum from prolapsing. Loygue[63] reported on more than 250 patients treated for rectal prolapse using this procedure. Their recurrence rate was 5.6% (follow-up period up to 23 years) and 84% of patients with preoperative anal incontinence had continence restored.

Laparoscopic Approaches

Laparoscopic approaches to colorectal surgery have gained in popularity in recent years and have been shown to be appropriate for many indications. A laparoscopic approach to treat full-thickness rectal prolapse has been employed for multiple abdominal prolapse repairs, namely rectopexy, resection with rectopexy, and mesh repairs.[51,62,64–68] In general, success and morbidity are comparable to traditional approaches, with the benefit of shorter hospitalizations and a rapid recovery.

Ashari et al.[51] reported a 10-year, single-institution experience with laparoscopically assisted resection rectopexy in 117 patients with rectal prolapse. Mortality occurred in 1 (0.8%) patient and morbidity in 10 (9%) patients; 77 of the 117 patients (66%) were followed a median period of 62 months. Recurrent full-thickness rectal prolapse occurred in 2.5% while mucosal prolapse occurred in 18%.

Dulucq et al.[62] evaluated 77 patients who underwent laparoscopic posterior mesh rectopexy (modified Wells procedure). They only encountered one conversion to open for severe adhesions and two minor intraoperative complications which were managed laparoscopically with success. Only one patient had recurrence and 90% of patients were satisfied at long-term follow-up (34 months).

Solomon et al.[67] reported a trial involving 40 patients with full-thickness rectal prolapse. They were randomized to laparoscopic versus open posterior mesh rectopexy. They demonstrated a decrease in morbidity and shorter hospitalization in the laparoscopic group, though operative times were longer in that group. At 24 months follow-up, they reported one recurrence in the open group and none in the laparoscopic group.

A meta-analysis of six studies and 195 patients (98 open and 97 laparoscopic) comparing laparoscopic versus open suture rectopexy was reported by Purkayastha et al.[68] in 2005. They found no significant difference in terms of morbidity or recurrence of prolapse between the two approaches. Though operative time was longer in the laparoscopic group, there was a decrease in the length of hospitalization by 3.5 days as compared to the open group.

The use of robotics has recently increased in colon and rectal surgery. Although robotics have been considered by many surgeons to be an extension of laparoscopic surgery, some technical aspects of the robot (e.g., the need for "re-docking" when changing fields of operation and a steep learning curve), have lead to slow widespread acceptance of the robot. However, surgery for rectal prolapse has been considered by some surgeons to be ideal for utilizing the robot as the operation is only performed in the pelvis (obviating the need to move the robot). Multiple small series have been reported.[69–73] To this point, there is not adequate length of follow-up to show long-term success, but results seem to be as good as those with laparoscopy. de Hoog et al.[73] reported on 82 patients treated with open, laparoscopic, or robotic repair and found higher recurrence with both laparoscopic and robotic approaches compared to the open procedure. They suggested that randomized trials were needed.

All in all, laparoscopic approaches to performing abdominal surgeries for rectal prolapse are acceptable for surgeons

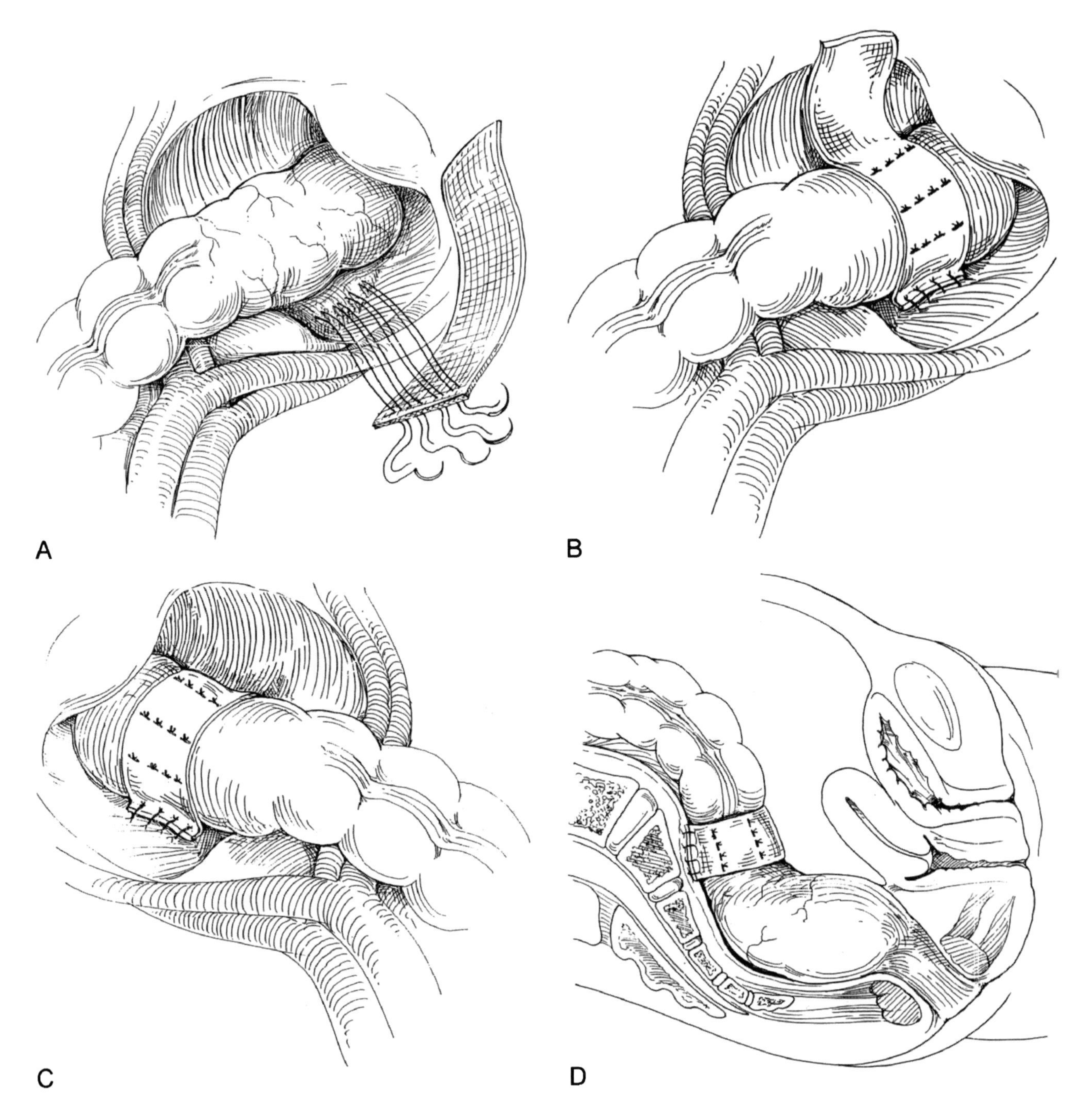

FIGURE 33-7. Mesh rectopexy (Ripstein). **A** Posterior fixation of sling on one side. **B** Sling brought anteriorly around mobilized rectum. **C** Sling fixed posteriorly on the opposite side. **D** Sagittal view of the completed rectopexy. [From Beck and Whitlow.[4] Copyright 2003 by Taylor & Francis Group LLC (B). Reproduced with permission of Taylor & Francis Group (B) in the format Textbook via Copyright Clearance Center].

TABLE 33-6. Results of abdominal rectopexy

Authors	Number of patients	Recurrence (%)	Mortality (%)	Morbidity (%)
Loygue et al.[52]	140	4	1	
Blatchford et al.[53]	42	2	0	20
Novell et al.[54]	32	3	0	9

with skill and experience performing complex laparoscopic surgery. In the near future, robotics will likely play a more significant role in prolapse surgery as adoption of robotic techniques increases. Further down the line, natural orifice transluminal endoscopic surgery (NOTES) procedures may become feasible for treating prolapse.

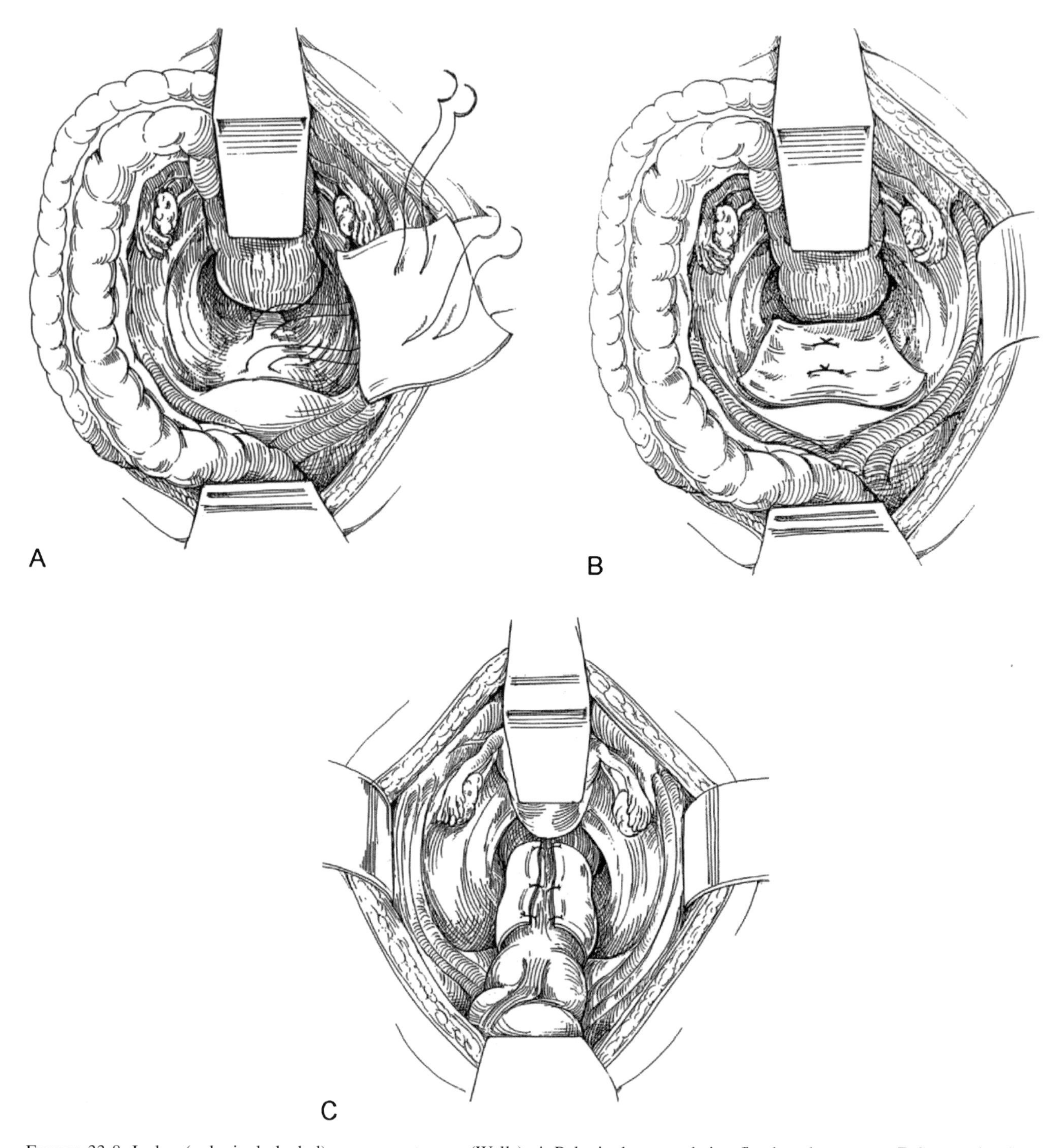

FIGURE 33-8. Ivalon (polyvinyl alcohol) sponge rectopexy (Wells). **A** Polyvinyl sponge being fixed to the sacrum. **B** Sponge in place before fixation to the rectum. **C** Incomplete encirclement of the rectum anteriorly with the sponge sutured in place. [From Beck and Whitlow.[4] Copyright 2003 by Taylor & Francis Group LLC (B). Reproduced with permission of Taylor & Francis Group (B) in the format Textbook via Copyright Clearance Center].

TABLE 33-7. Results of Ripstein procedure

Authors	Number of patients	Recurrence (%)	Mortality (%)	Morbidity (%)
Ripstein and Lanter[55]	289	0	0.3	–
Gordon and Hoexter[56]	1111	2	–	17
Eisenstadt et al.[57]	30	0	0	13
Tjandra et al.[58]	134	8	0.6	21
Winde et al.[59]	35	0	0	28
Schultz et al.[60]	69	1.6	1.6	33

TABLE 33-8. Results of Ivalon sponge/posterior mesh rectopexy operation

Authors	Number of patients	Recurrence (%)	Mortality (%)	Morbidity (%)
Sayfan et al.[46]	16	0	0	13
Luukkonen et al.[48]	15	0	0	13
Novell et al.[54]	31	3	0	19
Dulucq et al.[62a]	77	1	0	4

[a] Laparoscopic posterior mesh rectopexy.

Recurrent Prolapse

Though rectal prolapse has historically had a high recurrence rate (up to 50% or more), recent reports note recurrent prolapse following resection with rectopexy to be less than 10%. In general, perineal operations for prolapse have a higher risk of recurrence compared to abdominal approaches. Over a 30-year period, Hool et al.[74] reported recurrent rectal prolapse in 24/234 (10%) patients. In their retrospective report, the recurrent prolapse was repaired more often with an abdominal operation (86% of cases).

When full-thickness rectal prolapse recurs it is important to re-evaluate the patient for both constipation and other pelvic floor abnormalities in order to tailor the management best to address those issues. Therefore, patients with recurrent prolapse may require evaluation with manometry and/or defecography. It is important to inform the patient that although the recurrent rectal prolapse is repaired, the associated bowel dysfunction, including constipation and diarrhea, is largely unimproved following correction of the recurrence.[74–76]

One of the most important considerations in determining the best surgical option to treat recurrent prolapse is the residual blood supply of the remaining large bowel. The initial operative procedure performed for prolapse plays a dominant role in determining the selection of the next operation, as a prior resection will leave an interrupted colonic blood supply. Any patient who has undergone a prior rectal or sigmoid resection with anastomosis requires very careful evaluation prior to undergoing a secondary procedure, including a thorough review of the first operative report. The obvious risk to a secondary resection is ischemia to the segment of large intestine between two anastomoses. For example, if the patient has undergone an initial perineal rectosigmoidectomy, then a repeat perineal rectosigmoidectomy or abdominal rectopexy (without resection) can be safely performed. However, in such cases, abdominal rectopexy with sigmoid colectomy should be avoided because of the risk of ischemia to the retained rectal segment. For those patients who have undergone prior abdominal rectopexy but who now have recurrent prolapse, a redo abdominal rectopexy is an acceptable approach.

Recurrent full-thickness rectal prolapse can be successfully managed using the same operative options applied to initial disease. Reports in the literature place successful treatment of recurrence at between 85 and 100%.[75,76] Unfortunately, while most authors indicate the initial operative technique, the recurrence, and the secondary operative technique, they fail to describe adequately their rationale for selection of the secondary procedure. For that reason, there are a paucity of data upon which to base an intelligent treatment decision for management of recurrent rectal prolapse. There is no specific algorithm available which can be applied to select the best operation for treating recurrence, except that many reports suggest treating young patients using an abdominal approach and elderly patients employing a perineal approach. With that (lack of) information in mind and with consideration of remaining blood flow, a treating surgeon can make an individualized recommendation based upon the options summarized in Table 33-9.

Fengler et al.[75] reported the results of management of recurrent full-thickness rectal prolapse in 14 patients (13 repaired with perineal approach). The average length of time to recurrence was 14 months. Salvage operations performed to manage the recurrence included nine perineal operations and five abdominal operations. Patients were followed for 50 months after treatment for their recurrence. One patient died from an unrelated problem. None of the 13 remaining patients suffered a re-recurrence of the prolapse. Pikarsky et al.[76] reported on 27 patients with recurrent full-thickness rectal prolapse in a case-match study. Re-recurrence of prolapse occurred in 4/27 (15%) after a median follow-up period of 24 months, with similar results for abdominal and perineal approaches.

Steele et al.[77] performed a large retrospective study of 78 patients with recurrent rectal prolapse selected from a cohort of 685 patients who had undergone primary repairs. By evaluating re-recurrence after second and even third repairs, they demonstrated that approach (abdominal versus perineal) was associated with recurrence rate. Abdominal operations

TABLE 33-9. Management options for recurrent rectal prolapse

Initial operation	Options for management of recurrence
Perineal rectosigmoidectomy	Redo perineal rectosigmoidectomy Abdominal rectopexy (avoid resection)
Abdominal rectopexy	Redo abdominal rectopexy (+/– sigmoidectomy) Perineal rectosigmoidectomy
Abdominal rectopexy + resection	Redo abdominal rectopexy (+/– re-resection) Avoid perineal rectosigmoidectomy

to treat a recurrent rectal prolapse were associated with a lower re-recurrence rate. They concluded that when possible, abdominal approaches should be used for recurrent rectal prolapse repairs.

Solitary Rectal Ulcer Syndrome and Colitis Cystica Profunda

Solitary rectal ulcer syndrome (SRUS) and colitis cystica profunda (CCP) are uncommon and controversial conditions associated with rectal prolapse.[78] SRUS is a clinical condition characterized by rectal bleeding, copious mucous discharge, anorectal pain, and difficult evacuation. Despite its name, patients with this condition can have single, multiple, or no rectal ulcers. When present, the ulcers usually occur on the anterior rectal wall just above the anorectal ring. They generally are shallow with a "punched out" gray-white base surrounded by hyperemia.

CCP is a benign condition characterized by mucin-filled cysts located within the submucosa.[79] These lesions generally appear as nodules or masses, most commonly on the anterior rectal wall. Patients can be asymptomatic (with the lesions identified on screening endoscopy) or complain of rectal bleeding, mucous discharge or anorectal discomfort. Most patients complain of some difficulty with bowel movements. CCP is a pathologic diagnosis whose most important aspect is to differentiate it from adenocarcinoma, especially a well-differentiated mucinous adenocarcinoma. Obtaining the correct diagnosis can prevent unnecessary radical operations to treat a benign process.

CCP and SRUS are closely related diagnoses and some authors consider them interchangeable. The etiology of these conditions remains unclear, but a common feature is chronic inflammation and/or trauma. The inflammation may result from inflammatory bowel disease, resolving ischemia, trauma associated with internal intussusception or prolapse of the rectum, direct digital trauma, or the forces associated with evacuating a hard stool. Some suggest that CCP is the result of trapping of mucosal cells at the time of healing of an ulceration.

An endoscopic evaluation of the distal colon and rectum in symptomatic patients will reveal the above-described lesions. Defecography is generally abnormal in most patients.[80,81] The differential diagnosis of both CCP and SRUS includes polyps, endometriosis, inflammatory granulomas, infectious disorders, drug-induced colitides, and mucus-producing adenocarcinoma. Differentiation based upon histopathologic evaluation is possible, though snare excision or large biopsies via rigid scopes may be needed to obtain adequate tissue. SRUS is associated with characteristic obliteration of the lamina propria by fibrosis and a thickened muscularis mucosa with muscle fibers extending to the lumen.[80] Mucous cysts lined by normal columnar epithelium located deep to the muscularis mucosa characterize CCP pathologically.[79] The overlying mucosa may be normal or ulcerated and the submucosa surrounding the cysts is fibrotic and contains a mixed inflammatory infiltrate. By comparison, the epithelium in adenocarcinoma, is dysplastic and the surrounding stroma is reactive.

Treatment is directed at reducing symptoms or preventing some of the proposed etiologic mechanisms. Conservative therapy (high fiber diet and modifying bowel movements to avoid straining) will reduce symptoms in most patients and should be tried first. Patients without rectal intussusception should be offered biofeedback to retrain their bowel function.[82] If symptoms persist, a localized resection may be considered in selected patients.[83] Those few patients potentially suitable for localized resection should be highly symptomatic, be good surgical risks, have failed all conservative nonoperative management and have localized, accessible areas of disease. Patients with prolapse are considered for surgical treatment via an appropriate procedure as outlined previously. Those without prolapse may be offered excision which varies from a transanal excision to a major resection with coloanal pull through.

Conclusion

Optimal management of patients with rectal prolapse requires careful patient evaluation for synchronous functional bowel disorders. Although, the precise etiology of rectal prolapse remains unclear, the condition is frequently associated with constipation and straining; intuitively, these coexisting symptoms seem to play a role in the development of prolapse in many patients. Management of any associated constipation seems important to the ultimate outcome of treatment, although it remains unclear as to whether successful management of constipation results in a lower risk of recurrent prolapse. The preoperative evaluation of any associated anterior compartment problems such as urinary incontinence, voiding disorders, cystocele, and rectocele is essential. If those preexisting conditions are unrecognized and remain untreated correction of the rectal prolapse may exacerbate them. Fecal incontinence is a frequent complication of full-thickness rectal prolapse; unfortunately successful treatment of the prolapse results in only a 50% chance of improvement in preexisting fecal incontinence.

Operative management can be divided into abdominal approaches and perineal approaches. Generally, abdominal procedures have a higher morbidity but a lower rate of recurrence compared to the perineal approaches. Selection of the best specific procedure for a given patient is at the surgeon's discretion and remains highly dependant upon such variables as the patient's general medical condition, comorbid disorders, the presence of incontinence or constipation, and any prior history of colon resection. Typically, the surgeon balances the risk of recurrent prolapse against the operative morbidity in deciding between abdominal and perineal approaches. The use of mesh is acceptable, whereas anal encirclement is rarely used. Laparoscopic approaches to treat rectal prolapse have been shown to be safe and effective. The use of robotic-assisted surgery for rectal prolapse will likely increase.

SRUS and CCP are uncommon colorectal conditions often associated with prolapse. As they are benign conditions, efforts are directed to establishing the diagnosis, excluding malignancy, and treating symptoms. Initial conservative therapy is to modify bowel movements and habits and is associated the most success. If these measures fail, surgical therapy to correct any coexisting rectal prolapse or to excise locally the lesions may be considered.

Acknowledgments. This chapter was authored by Anthony M. Vernava, III and David E. Beck in the previous edition of this textbook.

References

1. Moschcowitz AV. The pathogenesis, anatomy and cure of prolapse of the rectum. Surg Gynecol Obstet. 1912;15:7–21.
2. Broden B, Snellman B. Procidentia of the rectum studied with cineradiography: a contribution to the discussion of causative mechanism. Dis Colon Rectum. 1968;11:330–47.
3. Tou S, Brown SR, Malik AI, Nelson RL. Surgery for complete rectal prolapse in adults. Cochrane Database Syst Rev. 2008;8:CD001758.
4. Beck DE, Whitlow CB. Rectal prolapse and intussusception. In: Beck DE, editor. Handbook of colorectal surgery. 2nd ed. New York: Marcel Dekker; 2003. p. 301–24.
5. Spencer RJ. Manometric studies in rectal prolapse. Dis Colon Rectum. 1984;27:523–5.
6. Prasad ML, Pearl RK, Abcarian H, Orsay CP, Nelson RL. Perineal proctectomy, posterior rectopexy, and postanal levator repair for the treatment of rectal prolapse. Dis Colon Rectum. 1986;29:547–52.
7. Altemeier WA, Culbertson WR, Schowengerdt CJ, Hunt J. Nineteen years' experience with the one stage perineal repair of rectal prolapse. Ann Surg. 1971;173:993–1006.
8. Baig MK, Galliano D, Larach JA, Weiss EG, Wexner SD, Nogueras JJ. Pouch perineal rectosigmoidectomy: a case report. Surg Innov. 2005;12:373–5.
9. Ramanujam PS, Venkateh KS. Perineal excision of rectal prolapse with posterior levator ani repair in elderly high risk patients. Dis Colon Rectum. 1988;31:704–6.
10. Friedman R, Mugga-Sullam M, Freund HR. Experience with the one stage perineal repair of rectal prolapse. Dis Colon Rectum. 1983;26:789–91.
11. Gopal FA, Amshel AL, Shonberg IL, Eftaiha M. Rectal procidentia in elderly and debilitated patients. Experience with the Altemeier procedure. Dis Colon Rectum. 1984;27:376–81.
12. Finlay IG, Aitchison M. Perineal excision of the rectum for prolapse in the elderly. Br J Surg. 1991;78:687–9.
13. Williams JG, Rothenberger DA, Madoff RD, Goldberg SM. Treatment of rectal prolapse in the elderly by perineal rectosigmoidectomy. Dis Colon Rectum. 1992;34:209–16.
14. Johansen OB, Wexner SD, Daniel N, Nogueras JJ, Jagelman DG. Perineal rectosigmoidectomy in the elderly. Dis Colon Rectum. 1993;36:767–72.
15. Kim D, Tsang C, Wong W, Lowry A, Goldberg S, Madoff R. Complete rectal prolapse: evolution of management and results. Dis Colon Rectum. 1999;42:460–9.
16. Azimuddin K, Khubchandani I, Rosen L, Stasik J, Riether R, Reed J. Rectal prolapse: a search for the "best" operation. Am Surg. 2001;67:622–7.
17. Zbar A, Takashim S, Hasegawa T, Kitabayashi K. Perineal rectosigmoidectomy (Altemeier's procedure): a review of physiology, technique and outcome. Tech Coloproctol. 2002;6:109–16.
18. Habr-Gama A, Jacob CE, Jorge JM, et al. Rectal procidentia treatment by perineal rectosigmoidectomy combined with levator ani repair. Hepatogastroenterology. 2006;53:213–7.
19. Altomare DF, Binda G, Ganio E, et al. Long-term outcome of Altemeier's procedure for rectal prolapse. Dis Colon Rectum. 2009;52:698–703.
20. Whitlow CB, Beck DE, Opelka FG, Gathright JB, Timmcke AE, Hicks TC. Perineal procedures for prolapse. La State Med J. 1997;149:22–6.
21. Chun SW, Pikarsky AJ, You SY, et al. Perineal rectosigmoidectomy for rectal prolapse: role of levatorplasty. Tech Coloproctol. 2004;8:3–8.
22. Delorme E. Sur le traitement des prolapsus du rectum totaux pour l'excision de la muqueuse rectale ou rectocolique. Bull Mém Soc Chir Paris. 1900;26:499–578.
23. Uhlig BE, Sullivan ES. The modified Delorme operation: its place in surgical treatment for massive rectal prolapse. Dis Colon Rectum. 1979;22:513–21.
24. Monson JR, Jones AN, Vowden P, Brennan TG. Delorme's operation: the first choice in complete rectal prolapse? Ann R Coll Surg Engl. 1986;68:143–6.
25. Senapati A, Nicholls RJ, Chir M, et al. Results of Delorme's procedure for rectal prolapse. Dis Colon Rectum. 1994;37:456–60.
26. Oliver GC, Vachon D, Eisenstar TE, et al. Delorme's procedure for complete rectal prolapse in severely debilitated patients. Dis Colon Rectum. 1994;37:461–7.
27. Tobin SA, Scott IHK. Delorme operation for rectal prolapse. Br J Surg. 1994;81:1681–4.
28. Graf W, Ejerblad S, Krog M, et al. Delorme's operation for rectal prolapse in elderly or unfit patients. Eur J Surg. 1992;158:555–7.
29. Watkins BP, Landercasper J, Belzer GE, et al. Long-term follow-up of the modified Delorme procedure for rectal prolapse. Arch Surg. 2003;138:498–502.
30. Lieberth M, Kondylis LA, Reilly JC, Kondylis PD. The Delorme repair for full-thickness rectal prolapse: a retrospective review. Am J Surg. 2009;197:418–23.
31. Yamana T, Iwadare J. Mucosal plication (Gant–Miwa procedure) with anal encircling for rectal prolapse – a review of the Japanese experience. Dis Colon Rectum. 2003;46:S94–9.
32. Goldman J. Concerning prolapse of the rectum with special emphasis on the operation by Thiersch. Dis Colon Rectum. 1988;31:154–5.
33. Gabriel WB. Thiersch's operation for anal incontinence and minor degrees of rectal prolapse. Am J Surg. 1953;86:583–90.
34. Labow S, Rubin R, Hoexter B, Salvati E. Perineal repair of procidentia with an elastic fabric sling. Dis Colon Rectum. 1980;23:467–9.

35. Williams JG. Perineal approaches to repair of rectal prolapse. Semin Colon Rectal Surg. 1991;2:198–204.
36. Jackaman FR, Francis JN, Hopkinson BR. Silicone rubber band treatment of rectal prolapse. Ann R Coll Surg Engl. 1980;62:386–7.
37. Hunt TM, Fraser IA, Maybury NK. Treatment of rectal prolapse by sphincteric support and using silastic rods. Br J Surg. 1985;72:491–2.
38. Poole Jr GV, Pennell TC, Myers RT, Hightower F. Modified Thiersch operation for rectal prolapse. Techniques and results. Am Surg. 1985;51:226–9.
39. Vongsangnak V, Varma JS, Smith AN. Reappraisal of Thiersch's operation for complete rectal prolapse. J R Coll Surg Edinb. 1985;30:185–7.
40. Earnshaw JJ, Hopkinson BR. Late results of silicone rubber perianal suture for rectal prolapse. Dis Colon Rectum. 1987;30:86–8.
41. Khanduja KS, Hardy TG, Aguilar PS, et al. A new silicone prosthesis in the modified Theirsch operation. Dis Colon Rectum. 1988;31:380–3.
42. Sainio AP, Halme LE, Husa AI. Anal encirclement with polypropylene mesh for rectal prolapse and incontinence. Dis Colon Rectum. 1991;34:905–8.
43. Frykman HM. Abdominal proctopexy and primary sigmoid resection for rectal procidentia. Am J Surg. 1955;90:780–9.
44. Watts JD, Rothenberger DA, Buls JG, Goldberg SM, Nivatvongs S. The management of procidentia: 30 years experience. Dis Colon Rectum. 1985;28:96–102.
45. Husa A, Sainio P, Smitten K. Abdominal rectopexy and sigmoid resection (Frykman-Goldberg) operation for rectal prolapse. Acta Chir Scand. 1988;154:221–4.
46. Sayfan J, Pinho M, Alexander-Williams J, Keighley MRB. Sutured posterior abdominal rectopexy with sigmoidectomy compared with Marlex rectopexy for rectal prolapse. Br J Surg. 1990;77:143–5.
47. McKee RF, Lauder JC, Poon FW, Aichison MA, Finlay IG. A prospective randomized study of abdominal rectopexy with and without sigmoidectomy in rectal prolapse. Surg Gynecol Obstet. 1992;174:145–8.
48. Luukkonen P, Mikkonen U, Jarvinen H. Abdominal rectopexy with sigmoidectomy vs rectopexy alone for rectal prolapse: a prospective randomized study. Int J Colorectal Dis. 1992;7:219–22.
49. Canfrere VG, des Barannos SB, Mayon J, Lehar PA. Adding sigmoidectomy to rectopexy to treat rectal prolapse: a valid option? Br J Surg. 1994;581:2–4.
50. Huber FT, Stein H, Siewert JR. Functional results after treatment of rectal prolapse with rectopexy and sigmoid resection. World J Surg. 1995;19:138–43.
51. Ashari LH, Lumley JW, Stevenson AR, Stitz RW. Laparoscopically-assisted resection rectopexy for rectal prolapse: ten years' experience. Dis Colon Rectum. 2005;48:982–7.
52. Loygue J, Hugier M, Malafosse M, Biotois H. Complete prolapse of the rectum: a report on 140 cases treated by rectopexy. Br J Surg. 1971;58:847–8.
53. Blatchford GJ, Perry RE, Thorson AG, Christensen MA. Rectopexy without resection for rectal prolapse. Am J Surg. 1989;158:574–6.
54. Novell JR, Osborne MJ, Winslet MC, Lewis AAM. Prospective randomized trial of Ivalon sponge versus sutured rectopexy for full thickness rectal prolapse. Br J Surg. 1994;81:904–6.
55. Ripstein CB, Lanter B. Etiology and surgical therapy of massive prolapse of the rectum. Ann Surg. 1963;157:259–64.
56. Gordon PH, Hoexter B. Complications of Ripstein procedure. Dis Colon Rectum. 1978;21:277–80.
57. Eisenstadt TE, Rubin RJ, Salvati EP. Surgical treatment of complete rectal prolapse. Dis Colon Rectum. 1979;22:522–3.
58. Tjandra JJ, Fazio VW, Church JM, Milsom JW, Oakley JR, Lavery IC. Ripstein procedure is an effective treatment for rectal prolapse without constipation. Dis Colon Rectum. 1993;36:501–7.
59. Winde G, Reers B, Nottberg H, Berns T, Meyer J, Bunt H. Clinical and functional results of abdominal rectopexy with absorbable mesh graft for treatment of complete rectal prolapse. Eur J Surg. 1993;159:301–5.
60. Schultz I, Mellgren A, Dolk A, Johansson C, Holmstrom B. Long-term results and functional outcome after Ripstein rectopexy. Dis Colon Rectum. 2000;43:35–43.
61. Wells C. New operation for rectal prolapse. Proc R Soc Med. 1959;52:602–3.
62. Dulucq JL, Wintringer P, Mahajna A. Clinical and functional outcome of laparoscopic posterior rectopexy (Wells) for full-thickness rectal prolapse. A prospective study. Surg Endosc. 2007;21:2226–30.
63. Loygue J, Nordlinger B, Cunci O, Malafosse M, Huguet C, Parc R. Rectopexy to the promontory for the treatment of rectal prolapse. Report of 257 cases. Dis Colon Rectum. 1984;27:356–9.
64. Baker R, Senagore AJ, Luchtefeld MA. Laparoscopic-assisted vs. open resection. Rectopexy offers excellent results. Dis Colon Rectum. 1995;38:199–201.
65. Heah SM, Hartley JE, Hurleey J, Duthie GS, Monson JR. Laparoscopic suture rectopexy without resection is effective treatment for full-thickness rectal prolapse. Dis Colon Rectum. 2000;43:638–43.
66. Kairaluoma MV, Viljakka MT, Kellokumpu IH. Open vs. laparoscopic surgery for rectal prolapse: a case-controlled study assessing short-term outcome. Dis Colon Rectum. 2003;46:353–60.
67. Solomon MJ, Young CJ, Eyers AA, Roberts RA. Randomized clinical trial of laparoscopic versus open abdominal rectopexy for rectal prolapse. Br J Surg. 2002;89:35–9.
68. Purkayastha S, Tekkis P, Athanasiou T, et al. A comparison of open vs. laparoscopic abdominal rectopexy for full-thickness rectal prolapse: a meta-analysis. Dis Colon Rectum. 2005;48:1930–40.
69. Munz Y, Moorthy K, Kudchadkar R, et al. Robotic assisted rectopexy. Am J Surg. 2004;187:88–92.
70. Ayav A, Bresler L, Brunaud L, Boissel P. Early results of on-year robotic surgery using the Da Vinci system to perform advanced laparoscopic procedures. J Gastrointest Surg. 2004;8:720–6.
71. Ayav A, Bresler L, Hubert J, Brunaud L, Boissel P. Robotic-asisted pelvic organ prolapse surgery. Surg Endosc. 2005;19:1200–3.
72. Heemskerk J, de Hoog DE, van Gemert WG, Baeten CG, Greve JW, Bouvy ND. Robot-assisted vs conventional laparoscopic rectopexy for rectal prolapse: a comparative study on costs and time. Dis Colon Rectum. 2007;50:1825–30.
73. de Hoog DE, Heemskerk J, Nieman FH, van Gemert WG, Baeten CG, Bouvy ND. Recurrence and functional results after open versus conventional laparoscopic versus robot-assisted laparoscopic rectopexy for rectal prolapse: a case-control study. Int J Colorectal Dis. 2009;24:1201–6.

74. Hool GR, Hull TL, Fazio VW. Surgical treatment of recurrent complete rectal prolapse. Dis Colon Rectum. 1997;40:270–2.
75. Fengler SA, Pearl RK, Prasad ML, et al. Management of recurrent rectal prolapse. Dis Colon Rectum. 1997;40:832–4.
76. Pikarsky AJ, Joo JS, Wexner SD, et al. Recurrent rectal prolapse: what is the next good option? Dis Colon Rectum. 2000;43:1273–6.
77. Steele SR, Goetz LH, Minami S, Madoff RD, Mellgren AF, Parker SC. Management of recurrent rectal prolapse: surgical approach influences outcome. Dis Colon Rectum. 2006;49:440–5.
78. Beck DE. Colitis cystica profunda. In: Johnson LR, editor. Encyclopedia of gastroenterology. San Diego: Elsevier Science; 2003. p. 374–5.
79. Guest CB, Reznick RK. Colitis cystica profunda. Review of the literature. Dis Colon Rectum. 1989;32:983–8.
80. Torres C, Khaikin M, Bracho J, et al. Solitary rectal ulcer syndrome: clinical findings, surgical treatment, and outcomes. Int J Colorectal Dis. 2007;22:1389–93.
81. Ortega AE, Klipfel N, Kelso R, et al. Changing concepts in the pathogenesis, evaluation, and management of solitary rectal ulcer syndrome. Am Surg. 2008;74:967–72.
82. Vaizey CJ, van den Bogaerde JB, Emmanuel AV, Talbot IC, Nicholls RJ, Kamm MA. Solitary rectal ulcer syndrome. Br J Surg. 1998;85:1617–23.
83. Beck DE. Surgical therapy for colitis cystica profunda and solitary rectal ulcer syndrome. Curr Treat Options Gastroenterol. 2002;5:231–7.

34 Other Benign Colorectal Disorders

Justin A. Maykel and Scott R. Steele

Introduction

Multiple different disease processes may affect the colon and rectum, each challenging in varying aspects for both patient and physician alike. Though considered benign, they encompass a wide spectrum of pathology ranging from infectious, radiation-induced, and vascular etiologies to more obscure and difficult to diagnose conditions such as collagen vascular and microscopic colitides. Confounding the situation, patients may present with a variety of clinical symptoms spanning from chronic, nonspecific diarrhea, vague abdominal pain, and low-grade fevers, to florid sepsis. As such, clinicians caring for these patients must be aware of not only the many subtleties associated with each condition, but also possess a sound, and often stepwise, approach for evaluation and treatment. In this chapter, we review the extensive gamut encompassing these less common conditions, highlighting the critical diagnostic and therapeutic strategies to maximize patient outcomes.

Bacterial Enteritis/Colitis

Escherichia coli

Escherichia coli normally resides in the human gastrointestinal (GI) tract. Five pathologic variants exist including enterotoxigenic *E. coli* (ETEC), enteropathogenic *E. coli* (EPEC), enterohemorrhagic *E. coli* (EHEC, also called Shiga toxin-producing *E. coli* or STEC), enteroinvasive *E. coli* (EIEC), and enteroaggregative *E. coli* (EAEC or EAggEc). These strains are not commonly distinguishable with standard laboratory testing, although EHEC H7-O157 is the only strain readily identified in the clinical laboratory. Typically, infection from all strains leads to variable degrees of diarrhea, from mild to severe, resulting in large volume GI tract losses and electrolyte abnormalities. Subtle differences can help distinguish between the strains clinically. Enteropathic *E. coli* (EPEC) primarily causes outbreaks of severe diarrhea in nurseries. The bacteria adhere to the mucosa of the small bowel and secrete a toxin that results in watery diarrhea, vomiting, and fever. ETEC is a major cause of traveler's diarrhea, with 30–50% of travelers from industrialized nations spending 3 weeks or more in developing nations experiencing this infection.[1] EHEC has occurred in the United States (US) during outbreaks associated with undercooked hamburger meat. Cases caused by EHEC can result in severe dysentery more commonly with bloody diarrhea than the other strains. Treatment in all cases is typically supportive, although antibiotics (fluoroquinolone or trimethoprim-sulfamethoxazole) are added for complicated and persisting cases, and in those with underlying immunosuppression. Additionally, there is some evidence that the duration of diarrhea from EAEC is decreased with antibiotics (i.e., ciprofloxacin) administration.[2]

Shigella

Named after the Japanese scientist Shiga who discovered them over 100 years ago, *Shigella* is the classic cause of dysentery in developing and industrialized countries. From the several variety of species of *Shigella* bacteria, *Shigella flexneri* (~1/3) and *Shigella sonnei* (~2/3) are far and away the most common causes of Shigellosis around the world that may be transmitted via person-to-person or through contaminated food, milk, or water. These bacteria are resistant to the low gastric pH, multiply in the small bowel, and eventually infiltrate colonocytes, resulting in clinical infection. *Shigella* is capable of colonizing the intestinal epithelium by exploiting epithelial-cell functions and circumventing the host innate immune response.[3] Patients commonly present with high fevers, abdominal cramps, tenesmus, and initially watery (though later bloody/mucoid) diarrhea. Malnourished and immunocompromised patients are most at risk for developing the debilitating and septic complications of infection.[4,5] In addition to the clinical presentation, diagnosis is confirmed by elevated fecal leukocytes and stool cultures. Endoscopic exam reveals a nonspecific friable, edematous, erythematous mucosa with focal ulcerations and bleeding. The most

D.E. Beck et al. (eds.), *The ASCRS Textbook of Colon and Rectal Surgery: Second Edition*,
DOI 10.1007/978-1-4419-1584-9_34,

often affected area is the rectum and sigmoid, although more severe infections often result in more proximal progression. Symptoms typically last 4–7 days, but vary depending on the infecting bacterial subtype and underlying immune status of the patient. Intestinal complications including rectal prolapse (particularly in infants and young children), toxic megacolon (3%),[6] intestinal obstruction (2.5%),[7] and perforation may also develop. Systemic complications may include bacteremia (in children and immunosuppressed), metabolic disturbances (i.e., SIADH hyponatremia, protein-losing enteropathy), leukemoid reaction, seizures (fever-related), reactive arthritis, and hemolytic uremic syndrome. Treatment is generally supportive, while in the immunocompromised host or when dysentery develops, trimethoprim-sulfamethoxazole, ciprofloxacin, and ampicillin have demonstrated effectiveness at shortening the duration and severity of illness.[8] Paradoxically, antidiarrheal agents such as loperamide (Imodium™) or diphenoxylate with atropine (Lomotil™) can make the illness worse, and should be avoided.

Salmonella

Salmonella, named for the pathologist Salmon who first isolated *Salmonella choleraesuis* from porcine intestine,[9] are gram-negative bacilli that grow under both aerobic and anaerobic conditions. They are the most commonly isolated pathogens from the stool of patients with gastroenteritis.[10] *Salmonella enteritidis* (which most frequently causes gastroenteritis) and *Salmonella typhi* (which more often causes enteric fever in underdeveloped countries) are also quite different in their epidemiology. In the US, the incidence rate of nontyphoidal *Salmonella* infection has doubled in the last two decades, with an estimated 1.4 million cases occurring annually.[11] *Salmonella* live in the intestinal tracts of humans and animals, and are usually transmitted to humans by eating foods contaminated with animal feces, including beef, poultry, milk, or eggs. Unlike *Shigella*, the organism is ingested and is susceptible to destruction by normal gastric acidity, pancreatic enzymes, and enteric secretions.[1] Gastroenteritis due to *Salmonella* is clinically indistinguishable from gastroenteritis caused by many other pathogens, commonly presenting with nausea, vomiting, fever, diarrhea, and cramping. *Salmonella* gastroenteritis is usually self-limited. Fever generally resolves within 48–72 h, though diarrhea takes longer at 4–10 days. Hemorrhage, obstruction, and perforation may occur, albeit infrequently, requiring emergent surgical intervention with resection and proximal diversion.[12] Up to 8% of patients with nontyphoidal *Salmonella* gastroenteritis develop bacteremia.[13] Of these, 5–10% also develop severe localized infections, including endocarditis, mycotic aneurysm, and osteomyelitis.[14] Similar to other bacterial infections, the clinical diagnosis is confirmed via stool culture. Treatment remains controversial and depends in part on the host immune status. In general, fluid and electrolyte replacement are administered. Based on available data, antibiotic therapy is not recommended in healthy immunocompetent individuals.[15] However, for those with severe disease (typically requiring hospitalization) or for those who are immunocompromised, antibiotics are recommended. Fluoroquinolones are the most frequent first line therapy, followed by trimethoprim-sulfamethoxazole, and are given for a 3- to 7-day course, with a longer minimum 14-day period in the immunosuppressed. Unfortunately, some *Salmonella* spp. bacteria have become resistant to antibiotics, largely as a result of the use of commercially used antibiotics to promote the growth of food-source animals. This should be kept in mind for patients not responding in the expected fashion.

Campylobacter

This spiral or "twisted" gram-negative rod is the most frequently identified cause of acute diarrheal illness in the US and industrialized nations. Of the various species, *Campylobacter jejuni* is the most common. Outbreaks generally occur during warm weather and are most frequently traced back to poor handling or preparation of beef or chicken products at barbecues. The organism can produce a spectrum of disease from watery diarrhea to dysentery, depending upon the strains' ability to produce enterotoxin, cytotoxin, or directly invade the mucosa.[5] Most cases present with fever, abdominal pain, diarrhea, nausea, and malaise within 2–5 days after exposure. Symptoms are generally self-limited, resolving within 1 week, though may linger up to 3 weeks or longer. The terminal ileum and cecum are most commonly involved sites. Rarely, when the organism elaborates mucosal invasive properties, mesenteric lymphadenopathy may simulate appendicitis or produce an enteric fever-like syndrome. Immunocompromised patients are at even greater risk for severe complications including perforation, obstruction, and sepsis. Long-term consequences of infection include arthritis, Reiter's syndrome, and Guillain–Barre syndrome.[16,17] Endoscopic findings range from segmental colonic ulcerations to a diffuse colitis. Further complicating this diagnosis, disease limited to the ileocecal region may also mimic Crohn's disease. Stool studies may reveal leukocytes or the characteristic organisms that are identifiable only by dark-field or phase-contrast microscopy.[18] Definitive diagnosis requires stool cultures as the disease clinically resembles both *Salmonella* and *Shigella*. As in other bacterial colitis, treatment with ciprofloxacin or erythromycin should be reserved for severely ill or immunocompromised patients. Otherwise, treatment is simply supportive with bowel rest, intravenous fluid, and correction of metabolic abnormalities. Surgical intervention may rarely necessary to treat complications such as megacolon, hemorrhage, or perforation; though more commonly occurs as a result of suspected appendicitis.

Yersinia

Three species of *Yersinia* produce human illness: *Yersinia pestis* (the causative agent of human plague), *Yersinia pseudotuberculosis* (rare in the US), and *Yersinia enterocolitica* (i.e., yersiniosis). Contaminated food (typically pork) and water serve as the major routes of transmission of infection, and typically affect children and young adults. After invading the intestinal epithelium, these gram-negative coccobacilli localize to lymphoid tissues of the intestinal mucosa (i.e., Peyer's patches) and regional mesenteric lymph nodes. Symptoms associated with yersiniosis include diarrhea, abdominal pain (especially right lower quadrant), fever, and less frequently nausea and vomiting. Symptoms typically develop 4–7 days after exposure and may last 1–3 weeks or longer. Similar to *Campylobacter* infection, this clinical presentation may be confused with other conditions such as appendicitis and Crohn's disease, often called pseudoappendicitis or mesenteric adenitis. As the bacteria tend to infect lymphoid tissue throughout the body, concomitant tonsillar symptoms of pharyngitis symptoms can help distinguish *Yersinia* from other causes of colitis. Gastrointestinal complications of acute yersiniosis include suppurative appendicitis, diffuse ulcerative ileitis and colitis, intestinal perforation, peritonitis, intussusception, toxic megacolon, small bowel necrosis, cholangitis, and mesenteric vein thrombosis.[19] Stool cultures remain the gold standard for diagnosis, although specific culture for *Campylobacter* is normally not standard, and typically requires a special request. Serologic tests are commercially available to help in diagnosis as well. While antimicrobial treatment has been shown to decrease fecal shedding,[20] there are no studies that have demonstrated a benefit in uncomplicated enterocolitis, and are generally not given. If clinically indicated for the treatment of complicated illness (i.e., septicemia),[19] therapy with a fluoroquinolone (adult) or trimethoprim-sulfamethoxazole (children) are first line choices, with a third-generation cephalosporin combined with gentamicin intravenously used in more severe disease. Following treatment, chronic sequelae are frequent, including erythema nodosum and reactive arthritis.[19] These usually develop approximately 1 month following the initial episode of diarrhea, and generally resolve spontaneously after 1–6 months.

Tuberculosis

Tuberculosis affecting the gastrointestinal tract in the US is almost always due to either *Mycobacterium tuberculosis* or *Mycobacterium bovis*. In general, infection is unusual in Western countries, outside of immigrants and people infected with HIV.[21] Tuberculous enterocolitis is generally contracted via consumption of unpasteurized milk or from swallowing sputum infected from pulmonary tuberculosis. From the time of exposure to the organism, clinical manifestations can be delayed for up to a year, further confounding the diagnosis. Gastrointestinal tuberculosis manifestations can be divided into three categories: the ulcerative form (60%), hypertrophic form (10%), and mass-like lesions (30%) that mimic malignancies. Which type the patient exhibits depends in part on the host's immune system.[22] Distal small bowel and cecal infections are most common and present with abdominal pain, weight loss, and fever, often mimicking Crohn's disease or malignancy.[23] Ulcers of varying depth, fistulas, and stenosis may also result from the infectious process, thus causing further difficultly in distinguishing this entity from inflammatory bowel disease. Clinically, tuberculosis can present in a wide variety of ways. Physical findings include generalized wasting, with up to 50% of patients having a palpable mass in the right lower quadrant. Barium enema, ultrasound, and CT may suggest the diagnosis, but findings are too often nonspecific.[24] Significant lymph node reaction may be seen, so-called tuberculous peri-colonic adenitis, producing extrinsic compression leading to symptoms of partial or complete intestinal obstruction. Tuberculous peritonitis can present as a surgical emergency mimicking acute appendicitis or a perforated hollow viscous. Colonoscopic biopsy or fine needle aspiration have permitted detection of acid-fast bacilli or caseating granulomas while awaiting culture reports. Diagnostic laparoscopy demonstrated tuberculous peritonitis with 95% accuracy in one series in select patients.[25] Anorectal involvement results in ulceration and stricture formation, often mimicking malignancy. Stool cultures for viable *Mycobacterium* organisms rarely demonstrate growth, but may be more likely positive in active cases of pulmonary tuberculosis. Serology tests have been developed and demonstrate sensitivity for intestinal tubercular disease of over 80%, though still are difficult in differentiating from Crohn's disease.[26] A positive tuberculin skin test may be useful, but not necessarily diagnostic, as this may result from remote disease or a prior exposure without any current clinical activity.

Treatment is usually medical with multidrug regimens. Isoniazid and rifampin are first line treatment, with pyrazinamide and streptomycin or ethambutol often required until sensitivity analysis can be determined in the immunocompromised host.[27] In more established cases, obstruction of the bowel secondary to sclerosing lesions or fistulous disease may require surgical intervention. It is still recommended that a medical trial be attempted as many patients will improve and resolve without surgery.[28] Rectal tuberculosis, while rare, can result in stricturing. Most cases will improve with antituberculous drugs, though dilation may be required, and operative treatment only for severe or recalcitrant symptoms.

Neisseria gonorrhea

First identified in 1879 by the German physician Albert Neisser, *Neisseria gonorrhea*, a gram-negative diplococcus, remains the second most common sexually transmitted infection in the United States and Europe.[28] Gonococcus can lead to genital or extragenital infections, particularly the pharynx and the rectum, occurring more commonly in men having sex with men (MSM). Gonococcal urethritis presents with purulent penile discharge and dysuria. Cervical gonococcus also results in pruritis and/or discharge, but may be asymptomatic in 50% of cases. Anorectal gonorrheal infections typically occur among men who engage in anoreceptive

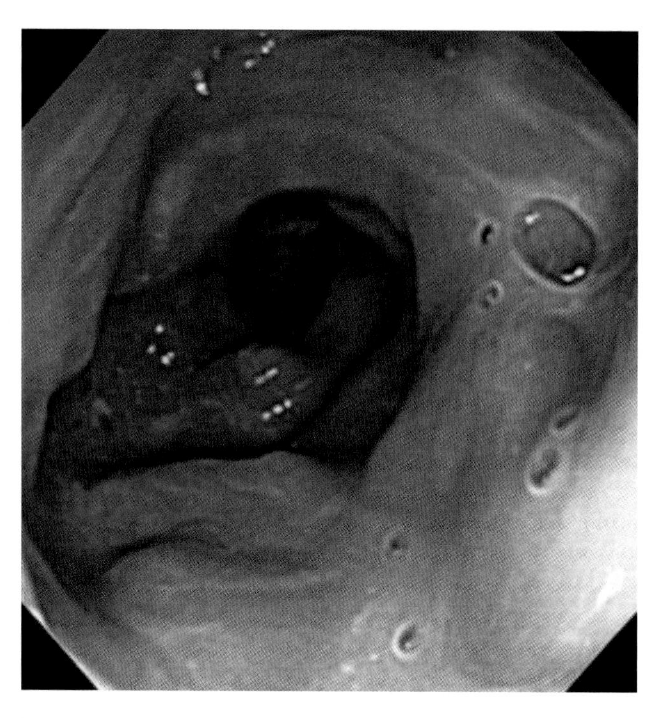

FIGURE 34-1. Endoscopic appearance of Gonoccocal proctitis. Notice the mucopurulent discharge.

intercourse. Symptoms of proctitis start 5–7 days after exposure and include a mucopurulent rectal discharge, tenesmus, constipation, and classically co-existent moderate to severe pain; although infection may infrequently be asymptomatic.[29] Physical examination may reveal edema, erythema, or fissuring of the anorectal mucosa (Figure 34-1). A mucopurulent discharge is the most common finding.[30] Culture for *N. gonorrhoeae* requires a Thayer–Martin chocolate agar and remains the "gold standard" for diagnosis. Cultures are taken with a cotton swab from the urethra, anal canal/rectum, or pharynx. Other options include gram stain (urethra), DNA probe, DNA amplification, and real-time PCR. Antimicrobial treatment must consider not only drug resistance, but co-pathogens such as *Chlamydia trachomatis* as well. Third generation cephalosporins (single dose 125 mg ceftriaxone, intramuscularly) are considered first-line therapy. Based on susceptibility, sulfonamides, penicillin, tetracycline, and fluoroquinolones are no longer recommended for the treatment of gonorrhoeae in the United States due to resistance patterns. Co-infection with *C. trachomatis* should be treated empirically with either doxycycline (100 mg BID for 7 days) or azithromycin (1 g in a single dose).[31] Patients should also alert their sexual partners for evaluation and treatment, to prevent disease spread or continued reinfection.

Lymphogranuloma Venereum

Although endemic to Africa, Southeast Asia, the Caribbean, and Central and South America, lymphogranuloma venereum (LGV) has become an increasingly common cause of proctitis in Western Europe and the United States, particularly among MSM (mainly in HIV-infected patients undertaking high-risk sexual activities).[32,33] LGV is caused by *C. trachomatis* serovars L1, L2, and L3. As LGV is primarily a disease of the lymphatics, infection extends from the primary inoculation site to the draining lymph nodes, producing a lymphangitis, with subsequent nodal necrosis and abscess formation.[33] The primary lesion of LGV occurs at the site of inoculation 3–30 days after sexual contact in the form of a painless pustule, shallow ulcer, or erosion. A secondary stage can occur 3–6 months after exposure and manifests as acute proctitis and inguinal lymphadenopathy that can suppurate and ulcerate. Excruciating pain helps to distinguish it from many other forms of proctitis. Left untreated, a chronic inflammatory response along with tissue destruction occurs, resulting in late sequelae including pelvic abscess, fibrosis, rectal stricture, fistula, and ulceration. Lymphedema and genital elephantiasis, with persistent suppuration and pyoderma, can also be seen.[33] The anal findings include ulcers, fistulas, and strictures, which, along with endoscopic findings, closely resemble Crohn's disease. Accordingly, treating physicians should consider this diagnosis in the proper clinical scenario. Specific LGV-associated serovars of *chlamydia* can be detected in those with positive PCR by genotyping. However, the diagnosis is usually initially based on clinical findings in association with a positive rectal *chlamydia* culture as genotyping results are not readily or immediately available.[34] The preferred treatment is doxycycline 100 mg twice daily for 3 weeks, with erythromycin used as an alternative. Administration of antibiotics both cures the infection and helps prevent further damage to tissues, although long-term scarring can ensue in areas of tissue reaction, particularly if diagnosis and treatment are delayed.

Syphilis

Treponema pallidum is a spirochete that invades subcutaneous tissues through abrasions caused during sexual intercourse. The spirochete establishes a painless ulcer (chancre), replicates, and infects draining lymph nodes (Figures 34-2 and 34-3). The painless nature of the chancre distinguishes it from the other major causes of a genital ulceration, herpes simplex virus (genital herpes), *C. trachomatis* (lymphogranuloma venereum), and *Hemophilus ducreyi* (chancroid). While the host immune system targets and heals the initial chancre within weeks, widespread dissemination of spirochetes occurs at the same time, leading to subsequent clinical manifestations of secondary or tertiary syphilis in untreated patients. Weeks to a few months later, approximately 25% of individuals with untreated infection develop a systemic illness that represents secondary syphilis, with symptoms including a rash on the palms, soles, and mucosal surfaces, fever, headache, malaise, anorexia, and diffuse lymphadenopathy. Similar to primary disease, these manifestations of secondary syphilis typically resolve spontaneously, even

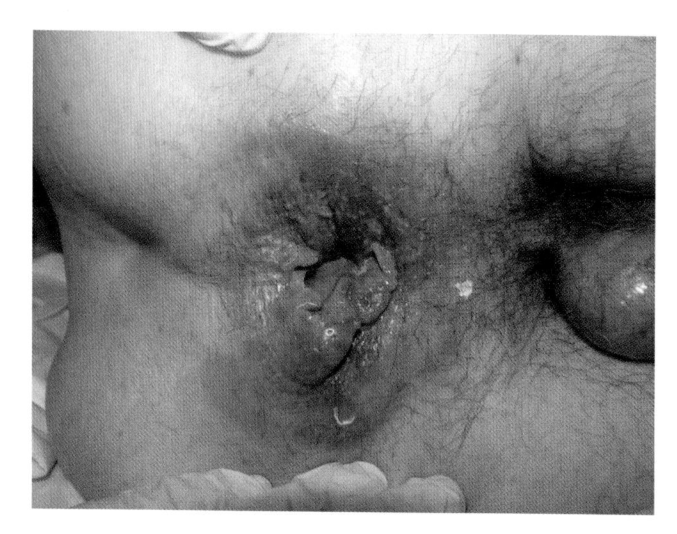

FIGURE 34-2. Painless posterior-lateral ulceration (chancre) of anal syphilis.

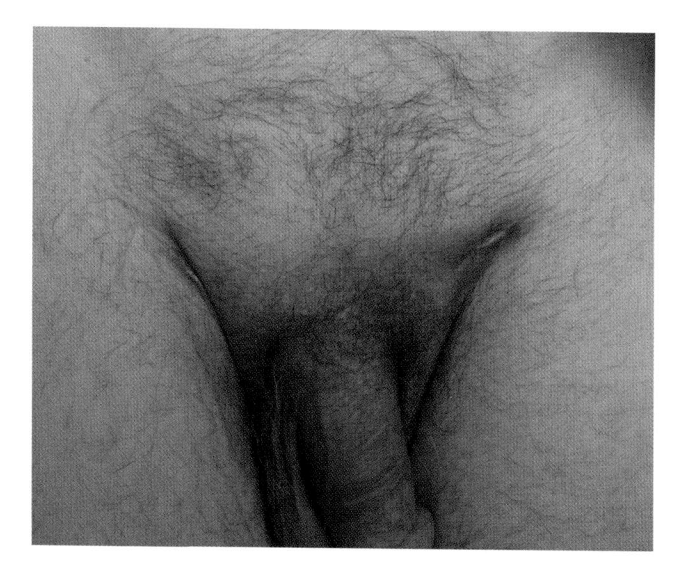

FIGURE 34-3. Suppurative inguinal lymphadenopathy of syphilis.

without therapy. When patients are untreated during the earlier stages of syphilis, they are at risk for the manifestations of late or tertiary syphilis, including central nervous system, cardiovascular, and gummatous syphilis. Condylomata lata occurring in the perianal region appear as moist wart-like lesions that may be confused for human papilloma virus infection. While the chancre of primary syphilis is best diagnosed by darkfield microscopy, serologic testing is the mainstay of diagnosis, traditionally involving a nonspecific nontreponemal antibody test followed by a more specific treponemal test for diagnostic confirmation.[35] Since *T. pallidum* divides slowly, long-acting penicillin preparations are the preferred drugs for the treatment of all stages of syphilis. A single dose of benzathine penicillin G (2.4 million units intramuscularly) remains the standard therapy for primary, secondary, or early latent syphilis. Late latent syphilis or latent syphilis of unknown duration requires three doses of 2.4 million units intramuscularly each at 1-week intervals.[36] Fortunately, there have been no cases of penicillin resistance reported. Options for the treatment of syphilis in penicillin allergic patients include tetracyclines, macrolides, or ceftriaxone.

Brucellosis

Brucellosis is a bacterium that is transmitted through unpasteurized goats' milk or cheese, contact with infected animals, or inhalation of aerosols. The constellation of symptoms is similar to the flu and may include fever, sweats, headaches, back pains, and weakness. It is encountered predominantly in underdeveloped nations, and is rarely seen in the US, with only 100–200 cases reported each year. Symptoms are that of a nonspecific colitis. Cultures of the exudate will reveal the organism and are required for confirmation. Endoscopic examination reveals inflammatory changes that are incapable of discriminating from other causes. Serologic tests are available to aid in early diagnosis and installation of treatment. Single agent therapy has an unacceptably high relapse rate so that currently, doxycycline 100 mg orally twice daily for 3–6 weeks and streptomycin 1 g IM q 12–24 h for 14 days are preferred. A more recent metaanalysis suggests that triple therapy by adding an aminoglycoside may result in lower failure rates.[37] Overall mortality is low (<2%), and is usually associated with the development of endocarditis.[38]

Actinomycosis

Actinomycosis is an uncommon, chronic granulomatous disease caused by *Actinomyces israelii*, an anaerobic gram-positive bacteria. The bacteria exists in the gastrointestinal tract, but can invade necrotic tissue and cause infections leading to granulomatous tissue, extensive reactive fibrosis and necrosis, abscesses, draining sinuses, and fistulas.[39] While infection in the cervicofacial area is most common (~50%), abdominal actinomycosis typically involves the appendix and ileocecal region. Similar to many of these infections, actinomycosis is a difficult disease to diagnose as its presentation mimics more common conditions such as malignancy, Crohn's disease, and tuberculosis. Therefore, the diagnosis is often made postoperatively. Colonoscopic findings can include thickened appearing mucosa, colitis, ulceration, nodularity, and a button-like elevation of an inverted appendiceal orifice.[40] Diagnosis is confirmed upon histological identification of characteristic yellow sulfur granules and/or culture of *A. israelii*. Medical treatment consists of a prolonged course of penicillin, intravenously for 4–6 weeks, followed by oral therapy for 6–12 months to prevent relapse. Surgical options are most often for disease complications such as resection of an obstructive segment or abscess drainage, which occur most often prior to a confirmative diagnosis. When necessary, surgery is coupled with systemic antibiotic therapy.[41]

Viral Enteritis/Colitis

Cytomegalovirus

Cytomegalovirus (CMV) is a member of the *herpes* virus family, and is considered an opportunistic infection in immunocompromised hosts. Yet it can also manifest as a spectrum of diseases in the immunocompetent host. In both of these patient populations, infections are not rare, as seroprevalence for CMV worldwide ranges from approximately 60 to 100%,[42] thus making the differentiation between endogenous reactivation and exogenous reinfection difficult. Infection typically occurs late in the course of HIV infection when CD4 cell counts plummet or in immunosuppressed transplant patients.[43] Involvement is most common in the colon, although concomitant disease may occur in the proximal gastrointestinal tract. The clinical manifestations of CMV colitis vary greatly, from asymptomatic carriers to fulminate life-threatening infections. Symptoms include fever, weight loss, abdominal pain, and diarrhea, which may be bloody. As the disease progresses, frank ulceration, toxic megacolon, and perforation may occur. The diagnosis of CMV colitis may be challenging, although fairly reliable findings on endoscopic examination include patchy erythema with or without ulcerations of variable size and depth. Biopsies should be obtained for histopathologic examination to evaluate for the characteristic inclusion bodies (Figure 34-4). Currently, there are several agents available for the systemic therapy of CMV infection, including ganciclovir, val-ganciclovir, foscarnet, and cidofovir. Surgical therapy is generally relegated to complications such as bleeding and perforation, where a subtotal colectomy with ileostomy is often required.

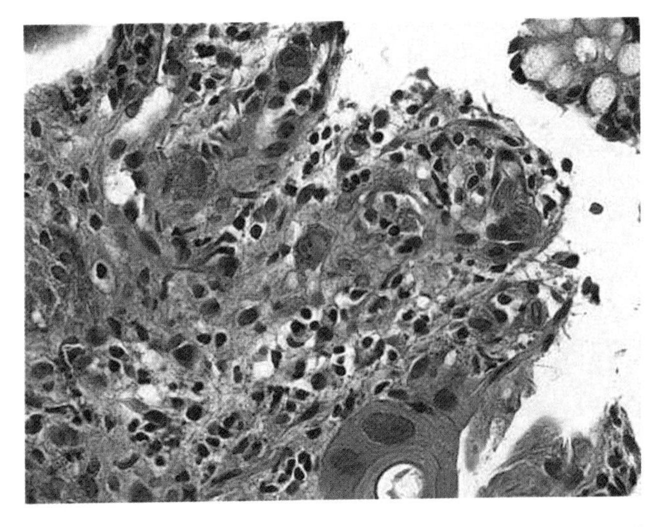

FIGURE 34-4. Cytomegalovirus colitis. Infected cells are enlarged with eosinophilic intranuclear and intracytoplasmic inclusions. (Courtesy of Jeanette R. Burgess, MD).

Herpes Simplex Virus Proctitis

Most colorectal infections are as a result of *herpes simplex virus* (HSV) type 2. HSV 1 is not common, accounting for 13% of rectal HSV infections, though most likely represents oro-anal transmission.[44] Gastrointestinal tract involvement usually manifests as proctitis following anal intercourse in MSM who are more commonly HIV positive. Presenting symptoms include anorectal pain, discharge, tenesmus, and rectal bleeding as well as difficulty in urinating, temporary impotence, fecal incontinence, and sacral parasthesias. The diagnosis is established by a suggestive history in combination with physical examination findings including herpetic vesicles, pustules, and ulcerations that affect the perianal skin and anal canal, though rarely extend into the rectum. Sigmoidoscopic exam demonstrates an acute proctitis. Laboratory evaluation of rectal samples allows the virus to be isolated by culture. A variety of immunoassays currently exist to aid in diagnosis. Oral acyclovir has been demonstrated to be effective in alleviating symptoms although other formulations may allow for twice or once daily dosing regimens. Immunocompromised patients should be treated with intravenous acyclovir followed by chronic suppressive therapy.[45]

Parasitic Enteritis/Colitis

Amebiasis

Entamoeba histolytica, while uncommon in the United States, is highly prevalent worldwide with approximately 40–50 million cases annually, accounting for 40,000 deaths.[46] This protozoan exists in either the cyst or trophozoite stages. Cysts are ingested in contaminated food or water, or via fecal–oral sexual transmission, and become trophozoites in the small intestine. Upon reaching the colon, they adhere to a specific lectin on the epithelial cell and penetrate the mucosa causing colitis and bloody diarrhea. The rates are much higher in developing countries and in homosexual males. Approximately 90% of *E. histolytica* infections are asymptomatic, with invasive disease depending on host genetic susceptibility, age, and immunocompetence.[47] In most patients, symptoms range from mild diarrhea to severe dysentery. Cases of fulminant colitis with bowel necrosis, perforation, and peritonitis occur in ~0.5%, but are associated with a mortality rate of more than 40%.[48] Localized colonic infection may also occur that results in a mass of granulation tissue, or an ameboma, which can mimic colon cancer. Perianal cutaneous amebiasis and rectovaginal fistulae are other reported rare complications. The diagnosis can be aided via antigen testing or serology tests. Colonoscopy classically demonstrates characteristic flask-shaped amebic ulcers where scrapings or biopsy specimens, best taken from the edge of ulcers, may be positive for cysts or trophozoites on microscopy. Treatment consists of oral metronidazole administered to eliminate the invading trophozoites and to eradicate intestinal carriage of the organism, with success reported in approximately 90% of cases.[46] Surgical intervention is reserved for complications including toxic megacolon, uncontrolled abscesses, and intestinal perforation.[49]

Balantidiasis

Balantidium coli is the largest and least common protozoal pathogen affecting humans and is the only ciliate that produces important human disease.[50] While rare in the US, it is most commonly found in tropical and subtropical regions, thus travel history is an important aspect in diagnosis. Communities that live in close association with pigs have an increased prevalence of disease due to the high rate of carriage of this organism by these animals. *B. coli* infection is spread to humans by ingestion of cysts spread by contaminated water and food. Similar to other protozoa, the trophozoite invades the distal ileal and colonic mucosa to produce intense mucosal inflammation and ulceration. In the symptomatic patient, diarrhea with blood and mucus is accompanied by nausea, abdominal discomfort, and weight loss. If allowed to progress, it can develop into fatal fulminant colitis with peritonitis and colonic perforation. The diagnosis is made by the identification of trophozoites excreted in the stool or from the margin of rectal ulcers associated with infection. The most commonly used treatment is tetracycline 500 mg four times daily for 10 days.[51,52]

Cryptosporidiosis

Cryptosporidium is an intracellular protozoan parasite that infects and the epithelial cells of the digestive or respiratory tracts, causing a secretory diarrhea that can be associated with malabsorption, and biliary tract disease (i.e., stricturing and cholangitis).[53] Cryptosporidiosis presents in one of three main settings: (1) sporadic: often water-related outbreaks of self-limited diarrhea in immunocompetent hosts; (2) chronic: life-threatening illness in immunocompromised patients (i.e., HIV infection); and (3) diarrhea with malnutrition in young children in developing countries. Transmission of *cryptosporidium* occurs via spread from an infected person or animal or from a fecal-contaminated food or water source.[54] The pathogenesis of *cryptosporidium* infection involves ingestion of oocysts, excyst to sporozoites in the small bowel lumen, and invasion of the epithelial cells. Clinically, this may result in an asymptomatic carrier state, mild diarrhea, or severe enteritis. The illness usually resolves without therapy in 10–14 days in immunologically healthy people, yet excretion of oocysts can continue for prolonged periods.[55] In immunocompromised AIDS patients, a number of other clinical manifestations have been described, including cholecystitis, cholangitis, hepatitis, pancreatitis, and respiratory tract involvement. Biliary tract involvement most commonly with acalculous cholecystitis or sclerosing cholangitis affects 10–30% of these patients with underlying AIDS.[56] The diagnosis of cryptosporidiosis is made by microscopic identification of the oocysts in stool or tissue, via microscopy, histopathology, ELISA, and PCR. Immunocompetent hosts generally recover within 2 weeks without antimicrobial therapy, only requiring simple supportive treatment. Treatment with nitazoxanide has been shown to speed clinical improvement and clear posttreatment *cryptosporidium* oocysts from stool samples.[57,58] This is recommended for persisting symptoms and in the pediatric age group. For HIV-infected patients, it is essential to initiate appropriate HAART treatment. In addition, nitazoxanide is recommended when CD4 counts are less than 100 cells/μL. Prognosis in this latter group is poor, particularly if the immune system cannot recover with HAART therapy. Ultimately, the majority of patients develop chronic disease with 10% acquiring a fulminant form with a corresponding high mortality rate.[59]

Giardiasis

Giardia lamblia is a flagellated protozoan gastrointestinal parasite that is commonly encountered in the United States. This is a common cause of water-borne and food-borne diarrhea encountered in day-care center outbreaks, internationally adopted children, and diarrhea in international travelers. Similar to *cryptosporidium*, after ingestion, the *Giardia* cysts excyst in the upper small bowel and release trophozoites which absorb to the mucosal surface of the jejunum, but do not invade the epithelium (Figure 34-5). Infection persists as the trophozoites revert to cysts in the large intestine. The mechanism how this leads to diarrhea and malabsorption is poorly understood; however, alterations in epithelial structure occur which may play a factor. Interesting to the surgeon,

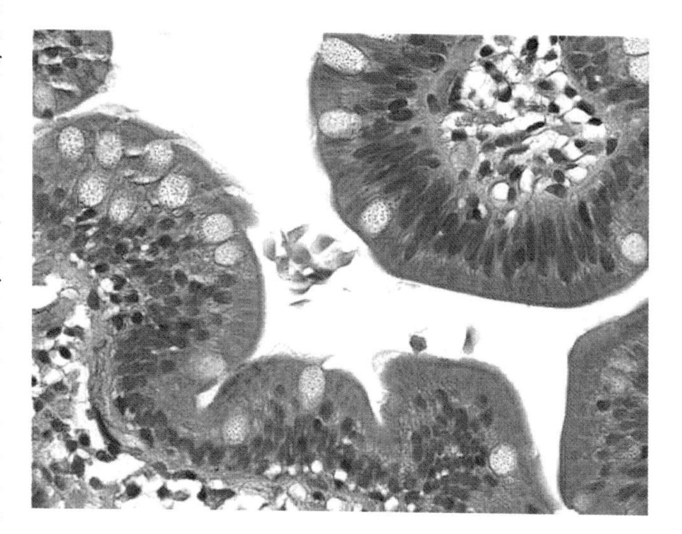

FIGURE 34-5. Duodenal giardiasis. Pale pink organisms are identified in the lumen. No architectural distortion or inflammation is seen. (Courtesy of Jeanette R. Burgess, MD).

hypochlorhydria is a risk factor for infection, particularly after gastrectomy or in patients on acid suppressive medications. Transmission occurs via person-to-person (infectious cysts in stool), in uncooked foods, and contaminated water supplies (common in hikers and bikers who drink from mountain lakes).[60] The clinical presentation of infection varies greatly, ranging from asymptomatic infection in up to 60% to a self-limited acute or long-lasting chronic infection.[61] Classic symptoms of an acute infection include a prolonged 2- to 4-week course of diarrhea along with weight loss.[62] Chronic infection can occur in up to 30–50% of symptomatic patients, resulting in loose stools, significant malabsorption, weight loss, and fatigue. In addition, malabsorption may lead to approximately 40% of patients developing lactose intolerance. As this may take many weeks to normalize, confusion may occur in differentiating lactose intolerance symptoms with recurrence after treatment. Proper identification involves stool samples for ova and parasite (O and P), which reveals trophozoites and cysts in 50–70% of cases with a single specimen, and approximately 90% after three specimens.[63] Immunoassays with antibodies directed against either cyst or trophozoite antigens can confirm the diagnosis. Most asymptomatic patients do not require treatment, while all symptomatic patients are given antimicrobial therapy. Metronidazole is the first-line therapy in the United States, resulting in resolution of infection in 80–95% of cases. While not commonly use, other options include tinidazole, quinacrine, albendazole, and nitazoxanide.

Trypanosomiasis

Trypanasoma cruzi is the organism responsible for Chagas' disease or trypanosomiasis. Chagas' disease is transmitted via the bite of the reduvid bug, also known as the "kissing bug." Chagas' disease occurs primarily in central Brazil, but also is found in nonendemic areas where it may be acquired by blood transfusion, congenital transmission, or organ transplantation.[64] Clinical syndromes present in two stages – acute and chronic. Most patients infected with *T. cruzi* are asymptomatic during the acute stage of infection, while others develop a wide range of symptoms including fever, swollen face or eyelids (Romana's sign), peripheral edema, conjunctivitis, hepatosplenomegaly, lymphadenopathy, and less commonly, myocarditis and meningoencephalitis.[65] Organ damage during the acute phase is due to both high-grade parasitemia and direct tissue parasitism, mainly in the gastrointestinal tract, central nervous system, and heart. Approximately 50% of infected individuals develop chronic disease, typically following a long period of clinical latency called the "indeterminate form," which lasts for years to decades. This may ultimately lead to cardiomyopathy, megaesophagus, and megacolon. Involvement of the colon results in abnormal basal colonic motility and an impaired relaxation response in the anal sphincter.[66] The colonic wall becomes thickened and dilated, most commonly at the sigmoid colon. Patients develop constipation, which can be severe, resulting in impaction of desiccated feces. The atonic colon occurs as result of denervation in both the submucosal (Meissner) and myenteric (Auerbach) plexuses. In the chronic form, parasites often cannot be detected circulating in the blood or visualized in biopsies of involved organs; as such, the diagnosis is made on linking clinical symptoms with a presence of an endemic area along with supportive radiological findings. Treatment of colonic complications includes fiber supplementation, enemas, and often, frequent disimpaction. Severe complications such as toxic megacolon and volvulus usually require either endoscopic treatment or surgical intervention. All patients with acute infection and all immunosuppressed individuals should be treated medically as well. The two main agents that are used are nifurtimox and benznidazole, although both have extensive side effect profiles that impact compliance. Finally, it is controversial whether patients in the indeterminate phase or late stage benefit of antiparasitic therapy and thus should be determined on a case-by-case basis.[67]

Ascariasis

Ascaris lumbricoides is one of the most common helminthic human infections worldwide, infecting an estimated 25% of the world population. Infection is more prevalent in children, tropical climates, and areas with poor sanitation. This is impacted by the fact that ova can survive in the environment for years and asymptomatic infected patients can shed ova for years.[68] Transmission typically occurs via ingestion of contaminated water or food. The life cycle entails the ova hatching in the small intestine and releasing larvae, which penetrate the intestinal wall and migrate hematogenously or via lymphatics. These larvae mature in the lungs, migrate up the bronchial tree, and are swallowed back into the GI tract. The mature worms are generally found in the jejunum, although they can live anywhere from esophagus to rectum. Adult worms live 1–2 years, and while not replicating in the host, one person can carry anywhere from 100 to 1,000 worms, depending on egg exposure. Although most patients are asymptomatic, large worm loads are responsible for the development of symptoms. Additionally, symptoms have been attributed to the immunologic response to the foreign body, luminal obstruction, or nutritional deficiencies. For the colorectal surgeon, a mechanical intestinal obstruction can occur from a mass conglomeration of worms, particularly at the ileocecal valve and in the pediatric population.[69] Worm migration into the biliary tree can cause biliary tract infections and strictures. Diagnosis is typically made by stool microscopy. One should note that the worms' eggs are not seen in the stool early in infection cycle or if the infecting worms are all male. Peripheral eosinophilia can be seen, particularly during the pulmonary infection stage.[70] Imaging including plain films, contrast studies, and CT scans often detect worm, either in the GI or biliary tracts. The mainstays for treatment are mebendazole and albendazole, typically administered as a single dose.[71] However, because they are teratogens, pyrantel pamoate is given during pregnancy. As these therapies are directed against the adult worm, as opposed to the larvae, patients should be rechecked in 2–3 months to rule out reinfection, which is unfortunately seen in up to 80% of individuals.[68]

Schistosomiasis

Schistosomiasis is caused by infection with parasitic blood flukes/trematode known as *schistosomes*. Infection is very common, manifests in an array of clinical presentations, and can result in significant illness. Several species exist and occur in geographic patterns. Their lifecycle is complex, beginning with infection via contaminated fresh water and subsequent hematogenous spread, where they survive for many years.[72] Most of the adult worms feed off circulating blood products, but do not cause disease. Rather, the eggs invade tissues, release toxins, and provoke an immune response.[73] In the bowel, granulomatous inflammation around the invading eggs can result in intestinal schistosomiasis characterized by ulceration and scarring.[74] A similar granulomatous fibrosing reaction causes injury in the biliary tract and urinary tract. Acute infection includes dermatitis and Katayama fever, which resembles serum sickness. Severity of chronic infection is related to the number of eggs trapped in tissues, their anatomic distribution, and the duration and intensity of infection.[75] This includes intestinal, hepatic, urinary, spinal cord, cerebral or cerebellar, and pulmonary schistosomiasis. Regarding intestinal schistosomiasis, most patients present with intermittent abdominal pain, poor appetite, and diarrhea. Intestinal polyps, ulcers, and strictures can also arise due to granulomatous inflammation surrounding eggs that are deposited in the bowel wall. The diagnosis is made by microscopy with egg identification, serology, or radiological findings in the appropriate clinical scenario. Rectal biopsy may also reveal the presence of eggs in the mucosa or submucosa. All infected patients should be treated, regardless of symptomatology, as the adult worms can live for years.[76] Praziquantel paralyzes worms by altering permeability of calcium channels, causing the worms dislodge from the intestines, and are ultimately passed by peristalsis. Cure rates exceed 85%, with even treatment failures still decreasing the intensity of infection in those not cured.[77]

Strongyloidiasis

Strongyloides stercoralis infection results in a wide range of clinical presentations, from a peripheral eosinophilia to septic shock, depending on host immune status. Cases are seen in the southeastern Appalachian region of the United States and in tropical endemic regions. Contact with contaminated soil allows the filariform larvae to penetrate the skin and spread hematogenously to the lungs, where they penetrate the alveolae, travel up the tracheobronchial tree, and are swallowed, similar to *Ascaris*. These larvae mature into adult worms and penetrate the mucosa of the duodenum and jejunum. Uniquely, the adult Strongyloides worms can produce rhabditiform larvae, which mature into filariform larvae within the gastrointestinal tract. These filariform larvae can then penetrate the perianal skin or colonic mucosa to complete the cycle. This maturation results in autoinfection and maintenance of parasitism.[78] As a result of this autoinfection, disease can persist for many years. Clinical manifestations include peripheral eosinophilia, cutaneous rashes (entry site most commonly sole of foot), gastrointestinal disturbances including duodenitis, enterocolitis, malabsorption, pulmonary, and hyperinfection syndrome that involve massive hematogenous dissemination (particularly in the immunosuppressed host) to the lungs, liver, heart, central nervous system, and endocrine glands.[79] The diagnosis of strongyloidiasis is made either by detecting rhabditiform larvae in the stool or via serologic testing. Ivermectin is the treatment of choice for strongyloidiasis, while albendazole is a less reliable option.[80]

Trichuriasis

Trichuriasis is a common intestinal helminthic infection, seen particularly in warm, moist climates.[81] *Trichuris trichiura* is also called "whipworm" because the adult worm is shaped like a whip. Eggs are ingested orally and release larvae that mature into adult worms in the intestinal tract where they attach to the bowel mucosa (Figure 34-6). Most infections are asymptomatic, although heavy worm loads can result in diarrhea with blood, mucous, and rectal prolapse, in which case the adult worms are visible on the prolapsed rectal mucosa. The diagnosis is made by seeing the characteristic barrel-shaped eggs harvested from stool samples, or visualizing the

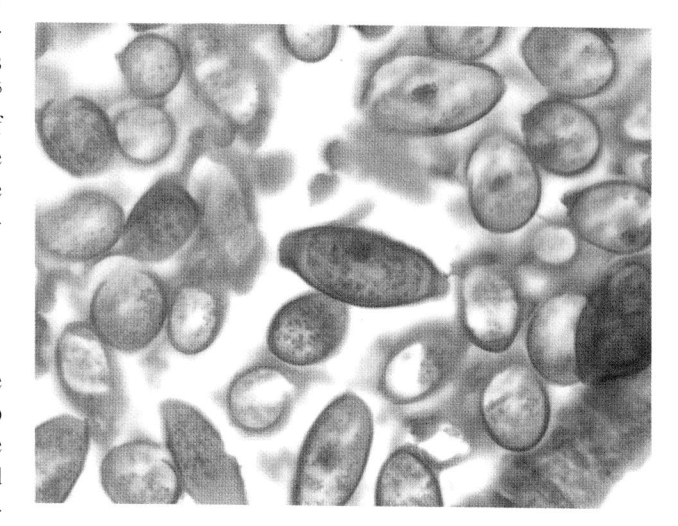

FIGURE 34-6. Characteristic microscopic appearance of *T. trichiura* (whipworm) egg.

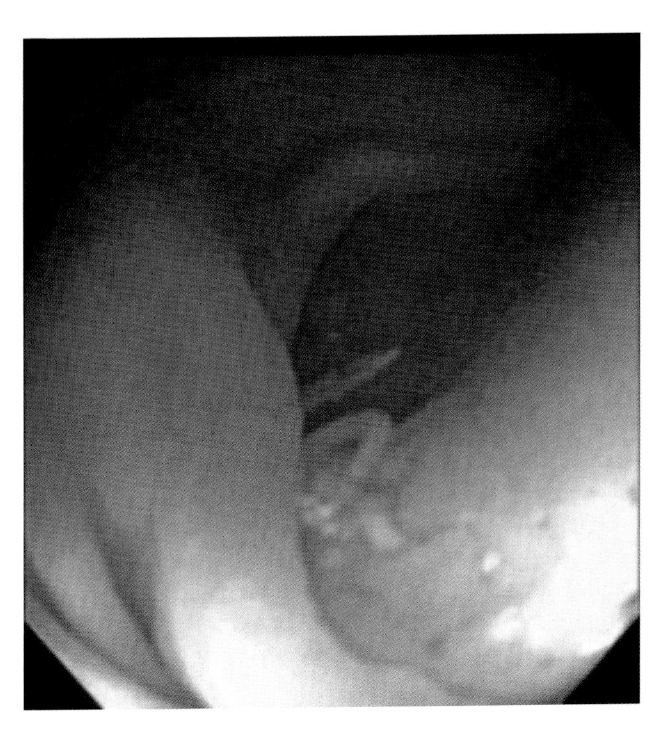

FIGURE 34-7. Endoscopic photograph of *T. trichiura* (whipworm) at appendiceal orifice. (Courtesy of Jean M. Houghton MD, PhD and Arumugam Velayudham, MD).

adult worms endoscopically (Figure 34-7). Mebendazole is the treatment of choice, administered in a dose of 100 mg twice daily for 3 days.[82]

Enterobiasis

Enterobius is a common nematode that is found worldwide. Otherwise known as "pinworm," infection occurs most frequently in school children aged 5–10 years. The adults live in the human gastrointestinal tract mainly in the cecum and appendix, and migrate out through the rectum onto the perianal skin at night to deposit eggs. As these larvae mature over the next 6 h, they cause local symptoms of pruritis ani secondary to an inflammatory reaction to the adult worms and eggs on the perianal skin. Scratching actually aids the worms by promoting reinfection and spread via oral ingestion. Rarely, with high worm burden, eosinophilic enterocolitis can develop.[83] Rarely, the adult worm can migrate locally and cause vulvovaginitis, salpingitis, oophoritis, or cervical granulomas.[84] The diagnosis of enterobiasis is best made using a "scotch tape" test, as adhesive tape will capture the eggs. These can be visualized under a microscope with their characteristic "bean-shaped" appearance. Adult pinworms may also be visualized endoscopically. Both mebendazole and albendazole are equally efficacious in curing 95% of patients, either with a single dose or repeated dose 1 week later aimed at treating reinfection.[85] Pyrantel pamoate is recommended for symptomatic pinworm infections in pregnant women again to the teratogenic effects of the former two medications. Due to the likelihood of reinfection, all family members should be treated along with washing of all sheets and clothes.

Anisakiasis

Anisakis is a roundworm that uses marine mammals as their natural hosts. Infection is most commonly encountered in Japan and areas where raw fish is ingested. The larvae enter the intestinal mucosa where they die, resulting in an inflammatory reaction and abscess formation. Patients usually present with relatively acute onset of epigastric or abdominal pain, nausea, and vomiting and subsequent bloody diarrhea. Intestinal complications include obstruction and perforation, along with eosinophilic enterocolitis. When the ileocecal region is involved, patients may be misdiagnosed with appendicitis.[86] Allergic reactions ranging from mild urticaria to anaphylactic shock can also occur. Diagnosis is made by visualizing the worm at the base of intestinal ulcerations, contrast studies with worm-like filling defects, or via serologic testing. Worms can be spontaneously regurgitated or removed endoscopically. Surgical treatment is typically reserved for complications such as perforation or obstruction.

Tapeworm

A number of adult tapeworms parasitize the intestinal tract of humans. They are classified as hermaphroditic flatworm parasites, and consist of a head, neck, and segmented body. Infection is acquired through the ingestion of raw or inadequately cooked infected flesh of the intermediate host. The clinical symptoms of all tapeworm species are variable, and include abdominal discomfort, nausea, vomiting, cutaneous sensitivity, headache, and malaise. Yet, most humans who carry an adult tapeworm are asymptomatic. *Diphyllobothrium latum* is the fish tapeworm that results from the ingestion of raw fish. The worm produces megaloblastic anemia due to vitamin B12 deficiency and fatigue. *Taenia solium* is the pork tapeworm acquired by eating inadequately cooked pork. Cysticercosis occurs when humans ingest the egg of *T. solium* and may present with a variety of neurological symptoms. *Taenia saginata* is the organisms responsible for beef tapeworm, which is found throughout the world and can achieve many meters in length. Patients may intermittently pass proglottids either with their stool (*T. solium*) or spontaneously (*T. saginata*). Often these are noted in the toilet bowel or patients may feel the spontaneous movement of proglottids through the anus. Segments occasionally enter the appendix, common bile duct, or pancreatic duct and cause obstruction. Finding the ova in fecal samples makes the diagnosis of tapeworm infection. Treatment for all tapeworms is with either niclosamide or praziquantel. Until all eggs and scolex portions of the tapeworm are eliminated, infection can reoccur; therefore, stools should be re-evaluated at 1–3 months following therapy.

Fungal Enteritis/Colitis

Fungal colidites may occur, but are highly unusual in an immunologically normal patient. This is separate from *Candida* colonization in healthy adults, found in 30–50% of oropharyngeal cultures and in 40–65% of normal fecal flora.[87] Clinical settings in which true fungal infection must be considered include human immunodeficiency virus (HIV) infections, immunocompromised states such as postsplenectomy, transplant patients, chronic liver disease, chronic steroid therapy, as well as in debilitated patients being treated with broad spectrum antibiotics. The major pathogens in this category include *Candida* species, *Histoplasma capsulatum*, and *Cryptococcus neoformans*. Outside the United States, other fungi may predominate such as is seen with *Penicilium marneffei* in Southeast Asia.

Candida

Certain conditions can promote the involvement of the lower GI tract by *Candida* species, including age (i.e., extremes of infancy and elderly), HIV infection, neoplasms, diabetes, endocrinopathies, and localized lesions of the GI tract.[88] Despite the high physiologic concentration of *Candida* species, infection does not occur under normal circumstances due to the innate defense mechanisms. *Candida* colitis is found predominantly in patients in the intensive care unit. Most commonly, the infection is systemic involving septicemia, the pulmonary tract, the urinary tract as well as the gastrointestinal tract. Colonic involvement may be diffused with resulting diarrhea, fever, and abdominal pain. Endoscopic findings include small creamy-white, curd-like patches on the surface of edematous, and inflamed mucosa. Perforation may occur with resultant peritonitis or fistulization – portending a poor prognosis. Stool cultures coupled with endoscopic biopsies are diagnostic when typical spores, yeast, or pseudomycelia are demonstrated. Medical treatment is first-line therapy in the absence of peritonitis. Mild candidiasis may only require oral nystatin 500,000–1,000,000 units four times daily. Yet, typically sicker patients need diflucan or ketoconazole 200–400 mg daily. For extremely ill patients or those with multiresistant disease, amphotericin B (0.3–0.6 mg/kg) or caspofungin (50 mg daily) can be administered intravenously. Surgical intervention may be required in the face of free perforation or clinical findings of peritonitis. Despite aggressive surgical intervention, mortality is very high due to the severity of the associated conditions.

Histoplasmosis

H. capsulatum is found endemically throughout the Midwestern United States. While principally being a pathogen of the reticuloendothelial system, like other fungal infections, it can cause systemic infection in the immunocompromised host. Pulmonary disease is most common, yet ileocolitis does occur as a granulomatous process causing bleeding, ulceration, stricture formation, and perforation.[89] Endoscopic examination can be confusing as the lesions may appear to resemble adenocarcinoma or inflammatory bowel disease. Skip areas, pseudopolyps, ulcerations, and plaque-like lesions may be seen, although biopsies will reveal intracellular budding yeasts within the mucosa when this organism is present.[89] Serologic tests and fungal cultures may also confirm the diagnosis. While perforation is rare, emergent surgery with resection of the grossly affected tissue and proximal diversion may be necessary. As these patients are often critically ill, intravenous amphotericin B may be indicated in severe cases, while ketoconazole has been used effectively in more mild disease and long-term to prevent relapse.

Cryptococcus

Cryptococcosis most commonly affects the central nervous system when *C. neoformans* is acquired via inhalation of soil contaminated with this encapsulated yeast. Isolated gastrointestinal infection is rare outside of immunocompromised patients. Colitis with perforation can occur spontaneously or following endoscopic biopsy, therefore, surgical intervention is generally reserved to manage life-threatening complications. A high index of suspicion must be maintained when patients present with symptoms of colitis and a concomitant history of immune suppressive therapy or infection with HIV. Early medical therapy provides the best means of avoiding surgery in these very ill patients. Diagnosis is confirmed by biopsy of infected mucosa demonstrating encapsulated budding yeasts or via stool culture. Similar to other fungal infections, ketoconazole is effective in mild disease forms, while amphotericin B is standard therapy in severely ill or immunocompromised patients.

AIDS Diarrhea

Diarrhea in the AIDS or HIV-positive patient can be the result of many causes, but is often a source of significant morbidity. Chronic diarrhea is defined as that persisting for more than 4 weeks. This was a much more prevalent symptom prior to the use of highly active antiretroviral therapy (HAART). It should be noted that diarrheal disease in HIV-infected individuals is frequently caused by infectious agents, but may also be due to medications or infiltrative diseases such as lymphoma, Kaposi's sarcoma, or GI tract infection of the HIV itself.[90] The specific infectious pathogen varies with the degree of immunocompromise in the host; therefore, it is important to ascertain the most recent CD4 cell count.[91] HIV-infected patients are often prescribed antibiotics, therefore *Clostridium difficile* or small bowel overgrowth syndrome is also potential diagnostic considerations. Diarrhea may also be a result of small or large bowel involvement. Symptoms may provide insight into location, with large volume, watery stools and associated bloating, cramping, and weight loss seen most typically with small bowel involvement. On the other hand, hematochezia, tenesmus, and lower abdominal cramps are more likely seen with colon involvement. Diagnostic work-up is broad-based, with the goal of finding a treatable source of infection. Stool studies including ova and parasites, *C. difficile* toxin assay, and bacterial culture, and with blood cultures, and endoscopy may all be required. In addition, upper endoscopy with small bowel biopsy is helpful in diagnosing opportunistic organisms such as *Cryptosporidium*, *Microsporidium*, *Histoplasmosis*, *Mycobacterium avium* complex, or lymphoma. Colonoscopy with biopsy can reveal *CMV* or *Kaposi* sarcoma. Malabsorption of nutrients can lead to even further significant malnutrition, which remains a strong predictor of morbidity and mortality in the setting of HIV. Treatment should be tailored to the specific organism, while empiric treatment with a quinolone and metronidazole after a negative diagnostic workup remains controversial. This antibiotic regimen is able to cover the most common causes of AIDS diarrhea including small bowel overgrowth, culture-negative *Campylobacter*, or *Giardia*; yet, may lead to development of resistant organisms. Surgery is reserved for acute abdominal emergencies and in of itself carries a substantial mortality.[92]

Clostridium difficile

C. difficile (CD) is a gram-positive rod bacterium that resides naturally within the human colon. Following antibiotic treatment, alterations of the normal colonic flora occur that allow preexisting colonization of CD to overgrow, become pathologic, and result in *C. difficile* or pseudomembranous colitis.[93] Symptoms of the disease may vary on a spectrum ranging from abdominal pain, distention and diarrhea, to outright sepsis with toxic megacolon requiring colectomy. In extreme cases, the process is nonreversible, resulting in hemodynamic instability and death. Although the bacteria are present in stool cultures of approximately 3% of normal healthy adults and up to 16–35% of hospitalized patients, increasing rates are now reported following exposure to antibiotics in asymptomatic carriers as well as those with severe underlying disease.[94,95] Overall, reported cases of CD colitis in the USA rose 200% between 2000 and 2005.[96] Similar alarming trends in CD colitis occurrence following pre-operative prophylactic antibiotics was illustrated in a large cohort study from a tertiary care hospital in Quebec showing an increase from 0.7 cases per 1,000 from 1999 to 2002 to 14.9 cases per 1,000 from 2003 to 2005.[97] This recent rise in the rate of CD colitis in hospitalized patients is even more concerning in light of reports of the increased virulence of particular strains, and has led to a greater concern about this disease worldwide. One such strain, known as B1/NAP/027, has shown capacity for hypersporulation, increased resistance to fluoroquinolones, a 16- to 23-fold increase in toxin production, and a severe disease pattern leading more frequently to fulminant CD colitis.[98–100]

Certain conditions are required to allow proliferation of bacteria such as *C. difficile*. In the most frequent mechanism, normal intraluminal homeostasis of gastrointestinal flora is altered via antibiotic-mediated destruction. While any single antibiotic can cause the change in this bacterial milieu leading to the pathologic state, certain drugs such as penicillin, clindamycin, fluoroquinolones, and third-generation cephalosporins are traditionally more commonly associated with development of CD colitis.[101] However, all antibiotics have been associated with *C. difficile* infection and recurrence, even those most often used for treatment of the infection.[102–104] In addition, pre-operative bowel preparations may alter this normal balance of colonic flora, leading to conditions amenable for secondary CD infection. Other risk factors reported to be associated with the development of *C. difficile* infection include concomitant multiple antibiotic use, advanced age, high gastrointestinal output, and prior GI surgery.[105]

Despite the underlying cause, this transformation in the typical bacterial environment allows the normally inhibited bacteria to flourish. The pathogenesis of CD infection relates to two major toxins that are released by the bacteria. The first, toxin A, acts as a chemoattractant for neutrophils and causes inflammation and fluid secretion of the colonic mucosa. Toxin A also causes the release of PGE2, which activates the Fas–Fas ligand system causing enterocyte and colonocyte apoptosis.[106] Additionally, both toxins A and B activate inflammatory cytokine release from monocytes, further inciting this inflammatory cascade.[107] Continued toxin production leads to connective tissue degradation causing colitis, watery diarrhea, and a pseudomembrane formation that can clinically result in a wide spectrum of enteric disease ranging from asymptomatic bacterial growth or bowel thickening and dilation, to sepsis and death.

Clinically, *C. difficile* colitis results in copious gastrointestinal output reflective of the natural history of the underlying disease process, and is present in 90–95% of cases. In fact, *C. difficile* is presently the leading cause of hospital-acquired diarrhea. This profuse diarrhea is often accompanied by low-grade fevers, abdominal pain, and often-significant leukocytosis. Varying degrees of abdominal tenderness may also be present, though in many patients the abdominal examination is unremarkable. A small percentage of patients go on to develop fulminant colitis with high fever, severe abdominal pain, and have diffuse peritonitis on abdominal examination. While hypotension, oliguria, sepsis, and toxic megacolon may be seen in this critically ill stage, the diarrhea may be paradoxically absent when the disease reaches its peak.[108]

While many clinicians prefer to initiate treatment empirically, the clinical diagnosis is often confirmed in the laboratory by sending stool for *C. difficile* cytotoxin and antigen assays. Several combinations currently in practice are based upon both the antigen and toxin assays, with antigenic positivity representing a marker for presence of the bacterium, while presence of the toxin is thought to signify clinically relevant intestinal disease. Similarly, stool cultures of the bacterium do not distinguish between carriers and those with acute infection. Diagnosis may also be made clinically by endoscopic examination and/or biopsy with the characteristic presence of pseudomembranes, inflammatory mucosal changes, and erythema (Figure 34-8).[109] Yet, the mucosal findings vary with the severity of the disease. In those with mild or moderate disease, endoscopy most often reveals normal mucosa or nonspecific inflammatory changes. On the other hand, severe disease often demonstrates the classic pseudomembranes appearing as round, punctate yellow or whitish lesions (Figure 34-9). Although the finding of pseudomembranes suggests the diagnosis of pseudomembranous colitis, biopsy of these lesions is recommended to definitively establish the diagnosis.[110]

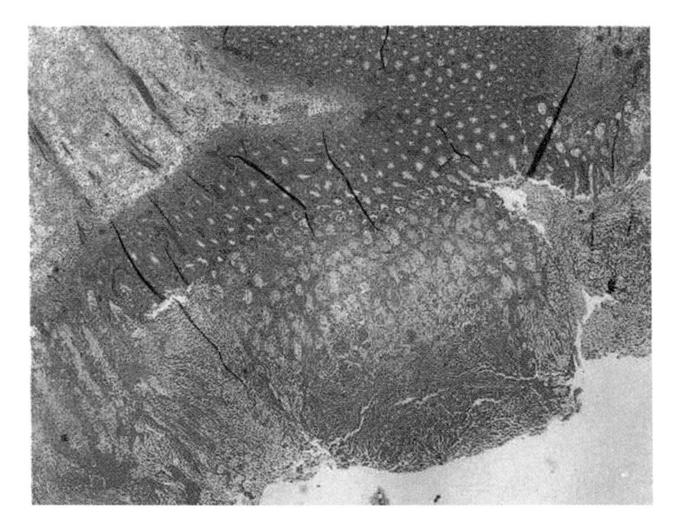

FIGURE 34-8. Low power view of pseudomembranous colitis. A thick pseudomembrane adheres to the colonic mucosa. (Courtesy of Jeanette R. Burgess, MD).

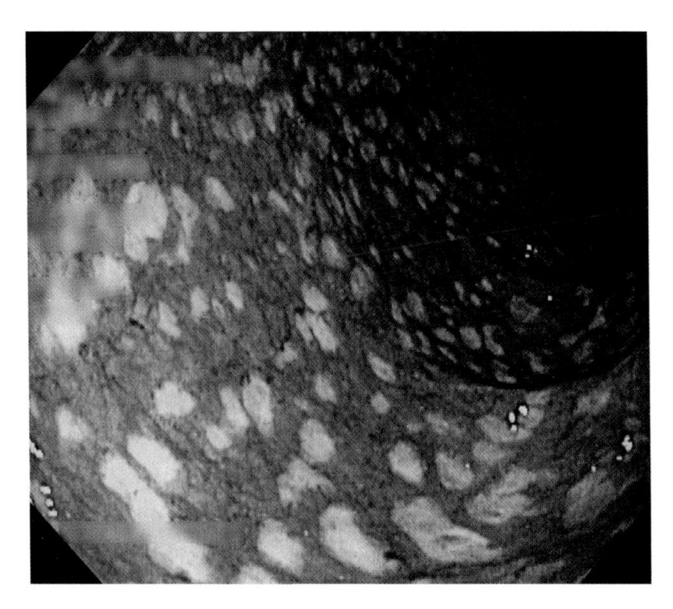

FIGURE 34-9. Classic pseudomembranous appearance of *C. difficile* on endoscopy.

Proper timing of therapy has been examined extensively in recent publications, due to failure of traditional medical management as a result of more virulent disease. Thus early identification and initiation of therapy along with recognition of a worsening course are paramount. Furthermore, small studies have demonstrated a cost savings approach through the implementation of empiric treatment alone when given a classical history.[111–113] However, a full evaluation for confirmatory diagnosis when encountering this clinical constellation is still recommended, especially those with recalcitrant symptoms. Attempts to verify the diagnosis of *C. difficile* colitis through laboratory evaluation may be performed while therapy is being instituted.

Once diagnosed, the most important initial intervention is to stop the inciting antibiotic or switch to alternative antibiotics with similar spectrum of antimicrobial properties. In cases of *Clostridial* infection of the colon, this will cause remission of the disease in 20–25% of patients without additional treatment. Vigorous fluid resuscitation and electrolyte replacement are often necessary in patients with high-volume watery diarrhea, as this may precipitate systemic cardiovascular, renal, and metabolic morbidity. Additionally, patients should be placed on contact precautions to prevent spread to other patients. The most effective and commonly used antibiotics against *C. difficile* are metronidazole and vancomycin, with cure rates of 76 and 97%, and recurrence in 14 and 15%, respectively.[114] The initial antibiotic chosen is often metronidazole, in part due its cost-effectiveness and that of contact isolation, but also as an attempt to prevent vancomycin-resistant *Enterococci* with extended use of the latter. This is despite higher cure rates with vancomycin. Additionally, metronidazole may be used intravenously in patients who are unable to have oral intake, as it is excreted through the hepatobiliary system. In patients with *C. difficile* infection of the distal colon and rectum, ileostomies, or even those with prior restorative proctocolectomies, metronidazole and vancomycin enemas may also be effective for treatment as primary therapy or as an adjunct – especially in cases that are refractory to or cannot take oral metronidazole.[115] Other agents that may be useful are teicoplanin and fusidic acid with clinical cure rates of 96 and 93%, respectively.[116,117] Bacitracin, when rarely used, has been shown to be as effective treatment as vancomycin when 20,000–25,000 units are used four times daily for 7 days.[118] Anion exchange resins have also been used successfully to treat *C. difficile* infection. Cholestyramine and colestipol act via binding to the *C. difficile* toxin in the lumen, thereby limiting the damage caused by the toxins. It is important to note that these agents have not proved to be as reliable as antimicrobials, and are therefore not recommended for use as sole treatment except in cases of mild infection. Furthermore, there are reports that these resins may bind to antimicrobials in the intestinal lumen when given concomitantly with the antibiotics, and additional consideration should be given to proper timing of medications.[119]

The medical treatment of *C. difficile* is recommended for a minimum of 10 days.[112] In most patients, significant improvement will often be witnessed within 2–5 days of initiation of therapy. Repeat stool assays are unnecessary if there is clinical response, as the assay may be positive for weeks in up to 50% of patients.[120] When possible, patients with a history of *C. difficile* should attempt to avoid the previously associated antibiotic as the use may precipitate recurrent disease. Furthermore, all patients with a history of *C. difficile* infection should have an annotation in their chart of the associated antibiotic to help avoid the peri-operative use and potential recurrence.

Indications for surgical management of CD colitis have been well documented, including severe disease refractory to medical management and the development of life-threatening complications such as perforation or toxic megacolon. Clinical signs that should trigger progression toward operative intervention include peritonitis and persistent hemodynamic instability.[121] Some authors advocate early colectomy for those who fail initial treatment with antibiotics. While mortality rates remain high among patients who undergo surgical treatment for complications of CD colitis, data suggests total abdominal colectomy with end ileostomy before onset of multisystem organ failure resulting from CD colitis is associated with improved morbidity and mortality.[122] Rarely, colectomy with primary ileorectal anastomosis with proximal diversion may be considered; however, bowel wall thickening, tenuous anastomosis, and hemodynamic instability often preclude this technique and are generally discouraged. Despite improvements in early recognition, implementation of therapy, and postoperative care, mortality rates following emergent colectomy for fulminant colitis has been reported to be 35–57%.[123,124]

Recurrence of *C. difficile* infection is not uncommon, occurring in 13–28% of patients, and is associated with multiple patient and therapeutic factors.[125] Reported factors include an inadequate immune response to the *C. difficile* toxin and a persistent disruption in the normal colonic flora. Other variables include advanced age, continuation of other antibiotics, and prolonged inpatient length of hospital stay.[126] When recurrence takes place, most authors suggest a second and longer course of antimicrobials for patients who have a symptomatic relapse. Current recommendations involve the first recurrence to be treated with the same agent as used for the initial occurrence; though with severe clinical disease vancomycin has been associated with better outcomes. Some authors recommend an additional course of cholestyramine or colestipol after the antimicrobials. There is also additional data suggesting probiotics may lessen the rate of subsequent recurrence, although the bulk of the current literature does not currently support their use.[127] Recurrent infection is often as responsive to antimicrobial treatment as are primary infections. Unfortunately, up to one-third of patients who relapse once will have further subsequent recurrences. Therefore, any patient with an unexplained abdominal illness who in the recent past has either been in the hospital or has received antibiotics should be suspected to have a *C. difficile* infection, even in the absence of diarrhea.[128]

A large body of literature also exists documenting poor outcomes associated with CD infections in hospitalized patients, even in the absence of surgery. Unfortunately, as depicted, surgery for fulminant colitis also portends a poor prognosis, thus leaving the clinician with a difficult conundrum. This is likely to only get worse, as population-based series have reported rising prevalence, mortality, and need for colectomy following development of CD colitis.[129] Even more concerning, the evolution of CD resistance to first-line therapy such as metronidazole, and higher recurrence rates suggest development of this disease may carry even greater morbid outcomes than previously reported. Finally, although many patient-related and peri-operative factors may play a role in eventual outcome, postoperative mortality following the development of severe CD colitis is highest when respiratory failure, renal failure, or vasopressor requirements occur.[111–113,130]

Ischemic Colitis

Gangrenous alterations to the colon have been recognized for over 100 years, yet it was not until the 1950s that the full spectrum of colonic changes from lack of blood flow was reported. These phenomena were initially described following high ligation of the inferior mesenteric artery during abdominal aortic aneurysm repair as well as with colectomy for carcinoma.[131,132] After performing a series of clinical and experimental animal studies, Boley first reported in 1963 that colonic ischemia was a reversible process secondary to vascular occlusion.[133] The actual term "ischemic colitis" was coined by Marston and colleagues after depicting its three stages of evolution (transient ischemia, late ischemic stricture, and gangrene) along with the natural history of the disease in 1966.[134] The original reports of ischemic colitis detailed the high mortality rate associated with this condition; which unfortunately, have not shown much improvement through the years. Currently, ischemic colitis is the most common form of gastrointestinal ischemia, accounting for 50–60% of all cases, approximately 1 in 2,000 hospital admissions, and as such, necessitates physician familiarity.[135]

The causes of ischemic colitis are numerous, though the exact etiology of the initial insult is rarely elucidated – particularly as this disease is most often witnessed in elderly, debilitated patients with multiple contributing co-morbidities. The differential diagnosis remains vast, with inflammatory and infectious colitis manifesting similarly, and making the true incidence of ischemic colitis unknown. Regardless of its etiology, patient outcome rests on the severity, extent, and rapidity of the ischemic insult, and is strongly influenced by prompt diagnosis and appropriate clinical management. Although the colon and rectum derive their blood supply from branches of three major vessels [superior mesenteric artery (SMA), the inferior mesenteric artery (IMA), and the paired internal iliac arteries], it is the extensive collateral circulation that allows this ischemic process to be avoided in many cases. The two main collateral routes are via the marginal artery of Drummond that parallels the colon and gives rise to the vasa recta, and the meandering mesenteric artery (or Arc of Riolan) which, while not always present, can represent another potential connection between the SMA and IMA systems. In addition, the IMA and internal iliac arteries communicate via the superior and middle hemorrhoidal arteries and the left colic branch off the IMA contributes to overlap the transverse colon that is supplied mostly by branches of the SMA.

In its most basic terms, ischemic colitis occurs when blood flow is interrupted or diminished, and supply does not equal colonic demand. Ischemic colitis may also be divided into two groups based on etiology: occlusive or non-occlusive. Occlusive ischemia can result from either arterial inflow or venous outflow obstruction, although the latter is very rare.[136] Most commonly, ischemia is not associated with occlusion of any of the major abdominal vessels, as the aforementioned collateral circulation of the colon is able to compensate. Nonocclusive ischemia occurs following a precipitating event such as hypotension, medication-induced vasoconstriction, shock, cardiac failure, hemorrhage, or sepsis that results in a low-flow state. Patients with nonocclusive ischemia may have preexisting vascular abnormalities that contribute to a worsening phenotypical manifestation.[137] Yet, with any source of inadequate flow, the earliest manifestation is witnessed at the mucosal level, furthest away from the vasa recta, and creates a secondary disruption of the mucosal barrier that can potentially lead to bacterial translocation and sepsis.[141,142] When occurring in the context of major vascular repair, the pathogenesis may be unique in that an isolated interruption of inferior mesenteric artery blood flow may be the sole underlying cause in many cases.[138] Other factors that have been shown to have a higher association with the development of colonic ischemia are increased intraoperative blood loss, hypotension, and prior pelvic radiation.[139,140] As radiation damage is both cumulative over time and progressive, this may be a precipitating factor not only in early disease, but also with chronic changes such as colonic stricture.

Although any area of the colon may be affected by inadequate flow, the watershed areas of the rectosigmoid (Sudeck's point) and splenic flexure (Griffith's point) are commonly involved due to frequent incomplete anastomoses of the marginal artery in those locations. The next most common area afflicted is the cecum, secondary to low blood flow in the terminal branches of the ileocolic artery combined with varying competency of the right colic artery.[141–143] Longo and colleagues[144] found a much higher rate of right colonic involvement than most other studies, with 46% of their 47 patients having this portion affected.

The diagnosis of ischemic colitis remains somewhat of a challenge, especially in its mild form, as the majority of symptoms are often self-limited and nonspecific. As such, the diagnosis is aided by the combination of early and repeated clinical evaluations, radiological studies, and colonoscopic visualization. Complete history and physical examination, focusing on the abdomen and evaluation for peritoneal signs is of utmost importance. Most commonly, patients present with abdominal pain, fever, distension, and diarrhea.[142] Sudden onset of crampy abdominal pain is present in two-thirds of all patients.[137] While generally poorly localized, ischemia arising in the left colon and rectum tends to be referred to the left lower quadrant and flank areas, while ischemia arising in the transverse and right colon refers symptoms to the central abdomen.[136] This pain is soon followed by an urge to defecate and subsequent passage of either bright red blood or maroon blood mixed with stool, typically within 24 h of onset. Occasionally the patient may also have nonbloody stools, depending on the location, degree, and extent of the colon affected. Abdominal examination may show widely variable findings ranging from mild localized tenderness to diffuse peritonitis. Rectal examination may be completely normal or demonstrate blood ranging from bright red to melena.

Laboratory examination is often noteworthy for a leukocytosis and metabolic acidosis. Occasionally, electrolyte and renal abnormalities may be present secondary to lack of oral intake combined with volume loss from diarrhea. Serum lactate levels may be elevated, though generalized systemic hypoperfusion or tissue hypoxia may also cause this, and is therefore not a specific marker. Unfortunately, no biochemical marker exists to date that is reliable in identifying colonic ischemia. Reports of measuring serum levels of D-lactate (a stereoisomer of lactate) have shown some promise. In healthy individuals, the serum levels are negligible,[145] whereas with colonic ischemic injury, mucosal permeability will increase, allowing D-lactate to enter the portal and systemic circulation. Elevated D-lactate was found to have a sensitivity of 82–90% and a specificity of 77–87% in predicting early colonic ischemia in small series.[145–147] What remains clear is that identifying patients at the onset of their clinical course entails a high index of suspicion.

Colonoscopy remains the most sensitive and specific study available for diagnosis of ischemic colitis. Ischemia has a wide extent of changes and characteristics when viewed endoscopically (Table 34-1). In early ischemia, the mucosa appears pale and edematous with interspersed areas of hyperemia.[148] As the ischemic process progresses, evidence of submucosal edema and hemorrhage can be seen as bluish-black

TABLE 34-1. Endoscopic findings of ischemic colitis

Stage	Endoscopic findings
Acute	Hyperemia, edema, friable mucosa, superficial ulcerations, petechial hemorrhage, gangrene[a]
Subacute	Edema, exudate, ulceration
Chronic	Stricture, mass, segmental involvement

[a]Irreversible damage characterized by gray, green, or black appearance.

blebs or nodules protruding into the lumen of the bowel.[136] These lesions create the characteristic thumbprinting sign on radiographic studies, which often disappear within days as the submucosal hemorrhages are either resorbed or evacuated into the colon when the overlying mucosa ulcerates and sloughs.[135] Occasionally, extensive areas of gray-green or black mucosa and submucosa are identified that can signify transmural infarction.[142] Endoscopy also allows the examiner to sample the colonic mucosa for pathologic assessment to help differentiate inflammatory, infectious, and ischemic etiologies. However, biopsy is hardly ever useful and is more likely to demonstrate either nonspecific ischemic or inflammatory changes, and rarely shows the ghost cells that are classic for ischemia.[142] The decision to pursue colonoscopy should be undertaken with caution, as air insufflation may result in distention of the bowel to pressures greater than 30 mmHg, diminishing colonic blood flow and may actually worsen the colonic ischemia.[144] In addition, the ischemic wall of the colon is fragile and at risk of perforating with the application of even minimal force, so any examination should proceed with great vigilance. The classic pattern of rectal and distal sigmoid sparing along with varying degrees of mucosally based changes more proximal is quite helpful in this select patient population.[149] In this light, endoscopy is used more to corroborate the clinical examination.

Other radiological tests may provide additional insight as to the diagnosis or the degree of insult to the bowel. Plain radiographs have limited use in the diagnosis of colonic ischemia. In approximately 20% of patients, specific signs of colonic ischemia may be present, including thumbprinting and rarely pneumatosis coli, a sign of advanced disease.[150] However, the majority of plain films are nonspecific, showing only dilation and/or air-fluid levels. The main utility in obtaining plain radiographs is to rule out visceral perforation and the presence of pneumoperitoneum. On the other hand, computed tomographic (CT) imaging has been used much more frequently to diagnose ischemic colitis, with associated changes in the bowel wall more often offering clues to the diagnosis (Figure 34-10).[151] By providing the ability to evaluate the bowel as well as the surrounding tissue, a diagnosis is aided by findings such as wall thickening, mesenteric fat stranding, mucosal enhancement, intramural air, dilatation, or even more ominous signs such as portal venous gas. It can also be a very useful test in ruling out other diagnoses.[152] In general, angiography does not help in patients with acute ischemic changes, although it may be occasionally useful in the patient who has previously undergone reimplantation of the inferior mesenteric artery to evaluate for patency or collateral circulation. Findings on air contrast or barium/air contrast enemas can be predictive of ischemic colitis, but often they do not exclude other forms of colitis such as inflammatory bowel disease or pseudomembranous colitis.[136] In the acute setting their use is extremely limited, and normally should be avoided. The risk of worsening the ischemic process with over-distention of the colon leading to perforation clearly outweighs the potential benefitis.[137] Finally, color Doppler and duplex ultrasound have been used to determine whether an arterial signal or color Doppler flow can be detected. When absent, ischemia should be a strong consideration and inflammatory sources virtually excluded. However, only 50% of patients with ischemia demonstrated this finding, and in general the sensitivity does not allow it to be a reliable primary diagnostic tool as patients may have preexisting thrombus independent of the acute event.[153]

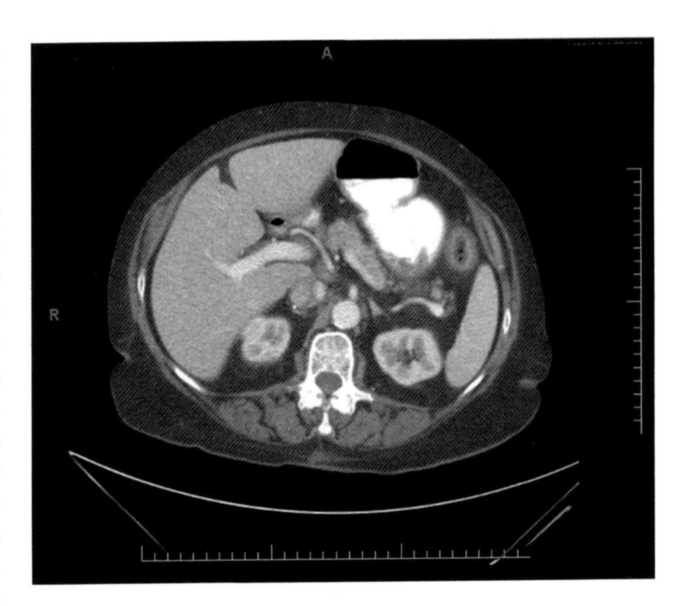

FIGURE 34-10. CT image of splenic flexure ischemic colitis demonstrating bowel wall thickening and peri-colonic fat stranding.

The mainstay of therapy for ischemic colitis remains supportive therapy with adequate fluid hydration and blood pressure support. As most patients present with only mucosal ischemia, their clinical course is often relatively benign. Intravenous fluids should be started and the patient placed at bowel rest. Cardiac function and oxygen delivery should be optimized and, if possible, any medications that are known to cause mesenteric vasoconstriction should be discontinued. If an ileus is present or the colon is markedly dilated, a nasogastric and/or rectal tube should be placed, although rectal tubes are generally discouraged in this setting and only be used with great caution.[154] Vasopressor support is controversial as it is also a contributing factor. Although low flow states and sepsis may require improvement in blood pressure, due to the vasoconstriction of the splanchnic vessels, vasopressors may amplify the ischemic process, worsening the already low-flow situation. Should pressor support be necessary, beta-adrenergic agonists that also improve cardiac output are preferred, while making every attempt to avoid alpha-agonists when possible. Additionally, broad spectrum antibiotics have been shown to decrease bacterial translocation and morbidity, and should be empirically added.[155–157]

With rare exceptions, all patients with evidence of bowel infarction or perforation require surgical therapy and exploration should rapidly follow. Surgical options generally fall into two categories: bowel resection and vascular reconstruction. Typically when patients require operative intervention, the surgeon must first determine bowel viability. Caution however must ensue, as often times the serosal appearance of the bowel does not accurately reflect the degree of ischemic changes to the entire bowel wall in cases with less than full thickness injury and frank necrosis. Intraoperatively, several different methods have been described to provide surgeons with additional useful information regarding blood flow. The surgeon must balance the need to avoid leaving behind necrotic bowel with the potential morbidity of overzealous resection leading to short bowel syndrome, although the intraoperative judgment of the well-trained surgeon remains one of the most important factors. Palpation of mesenteric pulses, detecting Doppler signals on the antimesenteric portion of the bowel wall, and Wood's lamp evaluation of the bowel wall following administration of fluorescein dye intravenously are all described techniques to help separate perfused from nonperfused bowel. Yet, in most cases, surgical resection involves a total abdominal colectomy with end ileostomy. Although primary anastomosis after a subtotal or partial colectomy with a proximal diversion may be considered in isolated hemodynamically stable patients with healthy bowel margins, this is almost uniformly a poor choice. Regardless of the approach, patients treated operatively in the acute setting have mortality rates as high as 40%, particularly when they carry other diagnoses such as atherosclerosis or chronic renal failure.[158] Surgeons have classically mandated a second look operation in 12–48 h regardless of the patient's clinical condition to evaluate the need for further resection and aid in being less aggressive at resecting potentially viable bowel at the initial surgery.[159] Yet, all clearly nonviable bowel needs to be resected at the initial operation, as mortality rates of 50–89% have been reported for patients requiring surgical resection of infarcted bowel at the second operation.[141]

Vascular repair involves first determining the patency of the vessel supplying the at risk portion of the colon. In addition, determining whether there is antegrade flow to the iliac vessels that may provide potential pelvic collaterals is crucial. Although the technical aspects of vascular reconstruction are beyond the scope of this chapter, options for dealing with the inferior mesenteric artery or other major visceral vessel include resection of the base of the vessel along with a small cuff of aortic wall (Carrell patch) and reimplanting it in the aorta or graft, patch angioplasty of the stenotic opening, bypass grafting, or endarterectomy of the atherosclerotic plaque.[160–162]

In most cases of ischemic colitis, the signs and symptoms of disease disappear within 24–48 h. More severe initial ischemic insults may result in necrosis of the overlying mucosa resulting in a future stenosis or stricture of the colon. A follow-up colonoscopy is advisable to either confirm complete resolution or to document the development of a stricture and/or persistent colitis. Another 20–30% of patients will go on to develop chronic colitis from irreversible ischemic injury, manifested by persistent diarrhea, rectal bleeding, and/or weight loss.[163] If suspected, this too will likely require surgical intervention. Recurrent episodes of attacks in otherwise asymptomatic patients are felt to be a result of unhealed areas of segmental colitis and should also be considered for elective resection. Other patients may develop chronic visceral ischemia. This is manifested by abdominal pain, especially with eating as a result of supply not equaling demand, and leads to relative bowel ischemia. Ultimately this may result in food fear and weight loss. Complete visceral artery revascularization of celiac, superior mesenteric, and inferior mesenteric arteries is often required to alleviate symptoms.[160] For this to be a success, requires a well-developed pattern of collateral circulation for the IMA system and should be evaluated prior to considering this option.

Finally, ischemic proctosigmoiditis is a rare condition affecting approximately 3% of patients with colorectal ischemia.[164] Excellent collateral blood supply almost always precludes this as an isolated entity, and it usually occurs in conjunction with more proximal colonic involvement. It is important to differentiate isolated ischemic proctosigmoiditis from inflammatory bowel disease, as the use of steroids may adversely affect those patients with ischemic proctosigmoiditis. Theories to its etiology include hemodynamic disturbance superimposed on atherosclerotic narrowing of the aorto-iliac vessels.[164] Most cases can be managed conservatively, as with ischemic colitis, and only rarely is proctectomy required.

Radiation Colitis

Radiation therapy is a frequent and successful modality used in the primary and adjuvant treatment of many malignancies including gynecological, anal, rectal, and prostate cancer. Despite this, radiation therapy is not without its hazards, due in part to a known dose-dependent relationship with cell death. Toxicity is focused on surrounding organs – especially the distal colon and rectum.[165,166] Other gastrointestinal sites may also be affected, particularly the terminal ileum in patients with prior adhesions that fixate the bowel in the pelvis.

Radiation therapy causes changes via two major mechanisms: (1) direct damage to DNA and (2) production of oxygen-free radicals.[167] Although the maximal radiation dose tolerance levels for the colon and rectum average 6,000–8,000 cGY, varying doses given over shorter intervals are associated with complication rates of 25–50%.[168] In the acute phase, changes within the bowel occur during the course of radiotherapy, though may become apparent over the course of several weeks and up to 6 months. In this setting, rapidly dividing crypt cells are most sensitive to radiation damage, and patients will experience atrophy of the villi, degeneration of the mucosal lining, diarrhea, mucous discharge, tenesmus, bleeding, and even incontinence.[169]

Chronic radiation injury appears most often at 6–12 months following radiation, and is secondary to a progressive fibrosis of the microvasculature (i.e., obliterative arteritis). This endothelial thickening in the small blood vessels eventually leads to thrombosis or reduced flow leading to ischemia. Clinically, this may manifest in a wide spectrum of findings including nonhealing ulcerations and telangiectasias of the bowel wall (Figure 34-11), fistulas and sepsis, as well as more common findings of thickening, stricture, and obstruction.[168,170–172] Additionally, there are reported higher rates of secondary colorectal cancer.

The method of delivery also impacts the types of symptoms. With external beam radiation therapy (EBRT), common complaints include pain, bleeding, tenesmus, incontinence, and an increase in stool frequency.[165] These may be further divided by the Radiation Therapy Oncology Group (RTOG) classification system (Table 34-2).[165] While the majority of symptoms are self-limiting, overall rates remain high, ranging from 41 to 57% for acute grade 2 symptoms, and 1–5% for acute grade 3 symptoms. Late grade 2 symptoms have also shown wide variability from 95 to 33%, while late grade 3 symptoms are reported in 0–6%.[173,174] Radiation may also be given via brachytherapy (BT) for certain malignancies such as prostate cancer, in which radioactive seeds are directly implanted. Radiation toxicity differs slightly with BT, as the majority of colorectal side effects are from local effects on the anterior rectal wall, as opposed to the field effects of EBRT.[175] As such, more concentrated effects have resulted in rates of 4–24% for rectal bleeding following this modality.[176,177] An additional potential complication of BT is the development of a rectal–urethral fistula, with reported incidences of 0.2–1%.[175,178] Patients classically present with recurrent urinary tract infections, pneumaturia, or fecaluria – symptoms which should prompt physicians to embark on a thorough work-up to exclude its presence in those patients with prior radiation therapy. Finally, anal stenosis with bleeding and obstructive symptoms has been described.[179]

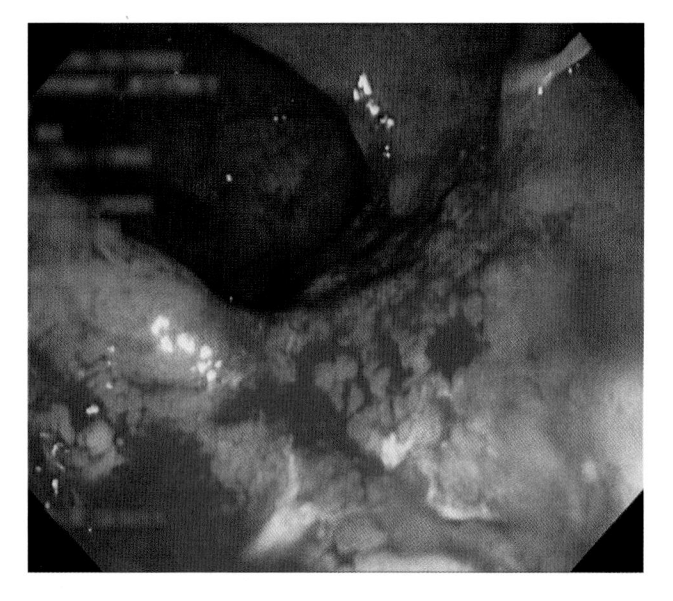

FIGURE 34-11. Endoscopic view of radiation colitis.

Although the vast majority of patients may be adequately treated with oral or topical medicines alone, some will require endoscopic or surgical therapy for complications. In patients with hemorrhagic proctitis, multiple different techniques have been described to include electrocautery, mesalamine, steroid, and carafate enemas.[180] Sucralfate has been associated with improved clinical response rate over anti-inflammatory agents, and may show further improved rates when used concomitantly with metronidazole.[181] Second-line therapy includes the use of Nd YAG and Argon lasers through an endoscope, as well as instillation of topical 4% formalin, which has demonstrated successful cessation of bleeding in up to 70–90%.[182,183] Finally, resistant bleeding or ulcerations may require hyperbaric oxygen therapy, which has demonstrated good clinical results in small case series of refractory disease.[184] The protocol commonly employed treats the whole body for 60 min at two atmospheres of 100% O_2 for 30 days. Prostaglandin E_1 can be co-administered for its vasodilatory properties.

TABLE 34-2. Acute and late complications according to the RTOG and RTOG/EORTC morbidity scales for radiation toxicity

	Grade 2	Grade 3	Grade 4
Acute GI toxicity	Diarrhea requiring medications, rectal pain requiring analgesics, *rectal bleeding requiring topical medications*	Diarrhea requiring parenteral support, severe mucous, or bloody discharge requiring pads, abdominal distension, *bleeding requiring multiple cauteries, or surgery*	Obstruction, fistula, or perforation. Abdominal pain or tenesmus requiring decompression or diversion
Late GI toxicity (>12 weeks)	Moderate diarrhea, intermittent, severe cramping; bowel movements >5 per day. Frequent bleeding, requiring single cautery treatment and/or transfusion	Watery diarrhea, obstruction requiring surgery; bleeding requiring surgery or ≥2 cauteries and/or transfusions	Necrosis, perforation, abdominal pain or tenesmus requiring decompression or diversion

RTOG Radiation Therapy Oncology Group, *EORTC* European Organization for the Research and Treatment of Cancer, *GI* gastrointestinal.
Modifications in italics.
Adapted from Peeters ST, et al. Int J Rad Biol Phys. 2005;61(4):1019–34.

Patients with significant diarrhea may undergo a trial of antimotility agents such as loperamide or octreotide, as well as be encouraged to take in a low residual diet.[185] Focus is also on prevention of injury, with some evidence suggesting both 5-aminosalicylates and probiotics may be effective; though reduction of radiation dose and size of the field remains the most important factor in this effort.[186] In addition, cessation of radiation, even if temporarily, will often allow most patients to resolve the acute changes. For those with extensive bowel disease in which oral intake is severely limited, nutrition therapy via total parental nutrition may be required for support or in preparation for surgery.

In general, operative indications for radiation-induced toxicities fall into one of a few categories: refractory disease (i.e., bleeding, nonhealing ulcer), septic complications (i.e., fistula, perineal sepsis), bowel obstruction or stricture, and secondary malignancies. A study of 5,719 patients undergoing EBRT or BT found a 0.2% incidence of surgical therapy for late recto-urethral fistulae and intractable bleeding.[178] Other series have reported a much higher rate of surgical therapy at 1–6%, with the vast majority of these secondary to small bowel obstruction from small bowel radiation.[187] Fistulizing complications are best managed conservatively, when possible. When not possible, the type of surgery will depend on fistula origin (i.e., proximal vs. distal) as well as the secondarily involved organ. Rectovaginal fistulas have been reported in up to 18% at 3 years following radiation therapy for advanced gynecological malignancy and often require diversion or nonirradiated tissue flaps (i.e., gracillus or Martius).[187]

Embarking on surgical therapy should not be taken lightly, as simply entering the abdomen following radiation may be wrought with hazard. Surgeons must balance limited adhesiolysis in the face of matted bowel loops with that of adequate exposure of the offending source. Though not ideal, proximal diversion for more distal lesions plays a prominent role. In the case of radiation-induced intestinal stenosis or obstruction, the same surgical considerations apply. Where feasible, resection and anastomosis to normal appearing bowel is preferred. Meticulous technique must be emphasized as operative management of small bowel radiation injury has mortality rates of 5–38%, with approximately one-third of patients developing postoperative complications such as recurrent obstruction, fistula, and anastomotic leak.[188–190] Other radiation-induced complications have a much lower rate of surgical therapy requirement. In general, only rarely will RTOG acute grade 3 or higher toxicity result in recalcitrant bleeding that requires operative evaluation for control. Though limited data, good results have been reported in small series for pull-through operations for severe proctitis.[191] Nonhealing ulcers may require resection, diversion, or biopsy for diagnosis. Finally, secondary malignancies need to have appropriate evaluation and staging with standard oncological resection performed in the absence of widely metastatic disease.

Microscopic Colitis: Collagenous and Lymphocytic Colitis

Distinct from other forms of more overt colitis, microscopic colitis is an inflammatory condition of the colon that is responsible for up to 20% of patients referred for colonoscopy with nonbloody chronic diarrhea.[192] Though clinically similar, microscopic colitis encompasses both lymphocytic and collagenous colitis, with roughly half of patients in each group.[193] Also shared by these two subtypes is the lack of a known underlying etiology, despite an estimated incidence of 4–10 per 100,000 people.[194,195] The hallmark of each, however, is the characteristic histological changes identified in the setting of normal colonic mucosa on endoscopy within the context of what can be profound chronic diarrhea.

The majority of patients are older than 50 years of age at disease onset, with a female predominance (especially in collagenous colitis).[195–197] Common associations include bile acid malabsorption, underlying autoimmune conditions, smoking, and a postulated infectious etiology – largely in part to its improvement following treatment with antibiotics.[197–200] In addition, several medications have been described as having a frequent association with microscopic colitis including acarbose, acetylsalicylic acid, lansoprazole, chronic nonsteroidal anti-inflammatory drugs (NSAIDs) use, ranitidine, sertraline, and ticlopidine, among others.[201] Yet, despite it being a described entity since Lindstrom[202] and several common associations, no identifiable underlying cause has been identified.

Like many of these "benign" colorectal diseases, patients may present across a spectrum of courses, from mild abdominal pain and diarrhea, to severe volume depletion, electrolyte abnormalities and protein-losing enteropathy. The vast majority of patients experience crampy abdominal pain, 3–20 loose bowel movements per day, and weight loss. Although described, fever, vomiting, and gastrointestinal bleeding suggest an alternative diagnosis such as infectious or inflammatory bowel disease, and should be evaluated appropriately.

In addition to a thorough history and physical examination, the mainstay of diagnosis is endoscopy with multiple colonic mucosal biopsies. Clinically the mucosa of the colon appears normal, thus random biopsies are required for diagnosis. Focal directed biopsies are taken of any specific abnormalities, though more indicative of concomitant disease or other pathology. Both collagenous colitis and lymphocytic colitis demonstrate a lymphocytic proliferation and infiltration of the lamina propria and epithelium of the bowel wall. In fact, the histologic criteria for lymphocytic colitis require more than 10 lymphocytes per 100 epithelial cells in the colon, with a normal colon having less than 5 per 100 cells (Figure 34-12). What distinguishes collagenous colitis is the presence of marked thickening of subepithelial collagen layer (Figure 34-13).[203] In addition, while lymphocytic colitis tends to occur evenly throughout the colon and

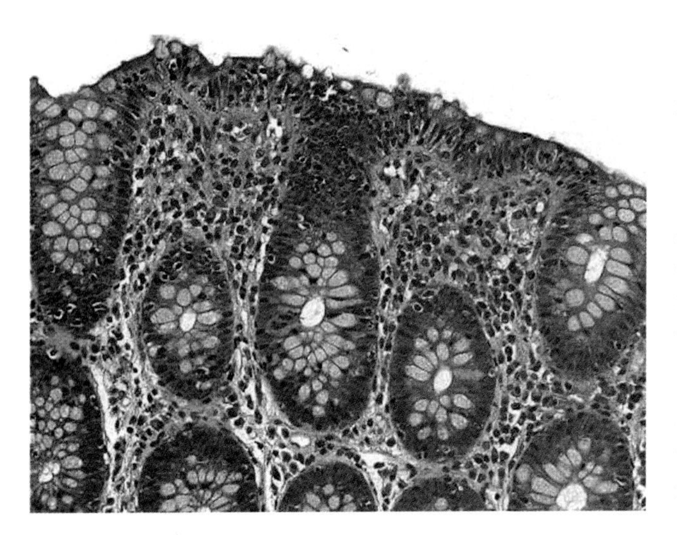

FIGURE 34-12. Lymphocytic colitis. A significant increase in the intraepithelial lymphocyte is present particularly in the surface epithelium.

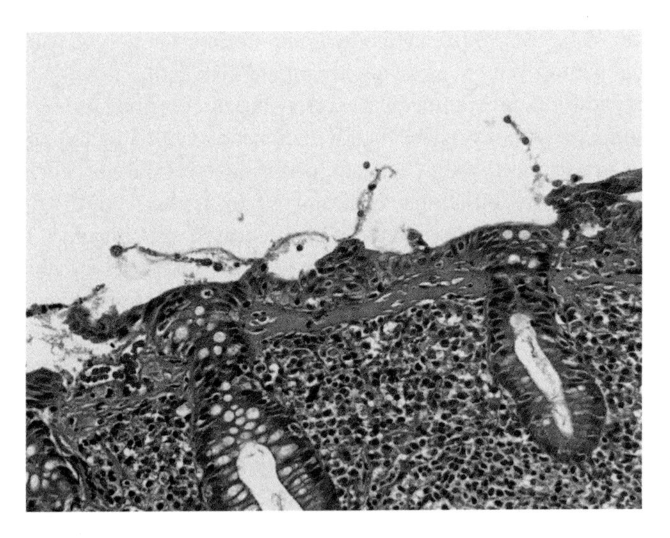

FIGURE 34-13. Collagenous colitis. Note the thick band of pink collagen beneath the surface epithelium (H and E stain).

rectum, collagenous colitis is characterized more in a random patchy distribution microscopically.[204] Although the vast majority (>95%) of patients have disease in the left colon, up to 10% will have isolated right-sided disease; therefore, full colonoscopy with multiple random biopsies is generally recommended.[198,205]

Because the disease is still relatively unknown and uncommon, treatment options are based on a paucity of high-quality evidence. As such, therapy is often empiric, directed at controlling symptoms, attempting to decrease inflammation, and individualized. A thorough medication history is imperative, as a simple trial of stopping the more commonly associated medications (especially NSAIDs), where possible, may result in improved symptoms. In addition, dietary modifications with elimination of caffeine, dairy, alcohol, and artificial sweeteners may also provide significant improvements in symptom control. Chronic loose stools are the hallmark for each of these diseases, thus antidiarrheal therapy with loperamide and diphenoxylate/atropine are effective first-line therapeutic agents. Although there is only a small number of series to support their use, their high safety profile, inexpensiveness, and effectiveness make these excellent initial choices for patients with mild or moderate diarrhea.[200,206] Similarly, in a small study of 12 patients, bismuth subsalicylate has been reported to cause resolution of diarrhea in 92% of patients and histological improvement in 75% following an 8-week course of eight tablets per day, and is often used for patients with more mild disease.[207] With the known association of bile-acid malabsorption, bile-acid binding agents such as cholesytramine have shown response rates of 59–92%, and are particularly useful in those patients in whom symptoms of microscopic colitis arise after cholecystectomy.[197,208] Budesonide has the best evidence to support its use for these patients. With its decreased systemic absorption, dosages of 9 mg daily for 6 weeks have demonstrated clinical and histological improvement and resolution in the majority of patients with collagenous colitis.[209] It is generally recommended that budesonide is used for patients with more severe or resistant disease, and may be effective in helping with initial remission prior to changing to one of the less toxic medications above for long-term therapy. In patients with recalcitrant disease, medications ranging from immunomodulator and anti-inflammatory drugs such as 5-aminosalicylic acid products, steroids, azathioprine, 6-mercaptopurine, and methotrexate to probiotics and even octreotide have been described with each demonstrating some success.[201] Surgery has been described mostly in case reports for severe disease when all medical options have failed. The most common described surgical option is a diverting ileostomy with excellent control of symptoms.[210,211] Unfortunately, the vast majority of patients develop recurrence of disease following stoma closure. In extreme settings, colectomy with or without restoration of continence has been described,[212,213] although the paucity of evidence precludes definitive recommendations for this approach – especially in light of the response rates to medical therapy.

Eosinophilic Colitis

Rarer than the two subtypes of microscopic colitis, eosinophilic gastrointestinal disease (EGD) was described much earlier by Kaijser.[214] Eosinophilic colitis, one component of EGD, is the least commonly affected site. All subtypes of EGD are characterized by eosinophilic infiltration of the involved tissues and elevated eosinophil counts in peripheral blood.[215] Unlike its more proximal counterparts that tend to mainly affect pediatric aged population, eosinophilic colitis has a bimodal age distribution affecting neonates as well as young adults, with equal gender distribution.[215] Patients most frequently present with nonspecific symptoms include abdominal pain, nausea, vomiting, diarrhea, and weight loss. Depending on the degree of colon wall involvement, symptoms can range from diarrhea, malabsorption, and protein-losing enteropathy with mucosal disease to bowel thickening and obstruction with involvement of the deeper layers of the bowel wall. In extreme form, serosal involvement leads to an eosinophilic ascites that may detect eosinophils in up to 90% on paracentesis.[216] Similar to microscopic colitis, the underlying etiology is largely unknown. Several authors have suggested a connection with food allergies with cow's milk and soy protein being the most common, as well as a history of allergies or atopy in 75%.[215] The diagnosis of eosinophilic colitis is generally made by the trilogy of peripheral eosinophilia (5–35%), gastrointestinal symptoms, and greater than 20 eosinophils per high power field on histological examination of endoscopic biopsies – all with no other defined source for the eosinophiliic manifestations.[217] Colonoscopic findings may range from normal in appearance to diffuse edema, but commonly demonstrates patchy areas of edema and punctate erythema.[218] The differential diagnosis includes infectious etiologies such as tuberculosis or parasite infestations, allergic enteropathies, collagen vascular disorders, and Crohn's colitis. Multiple medications have also been associated with this condition to include gold, NSAIDs, rifampin, and tacrolimus.[219–221] Not surprisingly, the majority of treatment recommendations are based on case reports and anecdotal experience. Most importantly, a thorough history and physical examination should be performed to identify potential other sources for the clinical picture (i.e., parasitic or drug-induced). That aside, corticosteroids are the first-line therapy for eosinophilic colitis, with up to 90% of patients demonstrating some response within 2 weeks.[222,223] Surgery has a role only for management of complications, such as intussusception, obstruction, hemorrhage, or perforation, or in difficult cases where a diagnosis is in question.[224,225]

Gastrointestinal Manifestations of Vasculitis and Connective Tissue Disorders

Although rare, vasculitis can also involve the gastrointestinal tract, commonly resulting in mesenteric ischemia. Patients generally present with abdominal pain, nausea, vomiting, diarrhea, and gastrointestinal bleeding. Symptoms can present acutely with bowel necrosis, massive bleeding, perforation, or chronically with stricture-related obstruction.

Polyarteritis Nodosa

Polyarteritis nodosa (PAN) is a focal segmental vasculitis that affects small and medium-sized arteries. Antigen–antibody complexes are deposited in the vessel walls, causing local inflammation and eventual necrosis ("fibroid necrosis") that result in stenosis, thrombosis, aneurismal dilatation, and rupture. The organs supplied by these vessels may have impaired perfusion, resulting in ulcerations, infarcts, or ischemic atrophy.[226] It is felt to be associated with hepatitis B virus (HBV) in approximately 7% of cases. Overall, gastrointestinal involvement occurs in 14–65% of patients with PAN, and is a major cause of morbidity and mortality in this cohort.[227] Most patients have concomitant systemic symptoms, such as hypertension, renal insufficiency, neurological dysfunction, myalgias, and cutaneous disease. The small bowel and gallbladder are the most commonly affected areas in the GI tract, although liver, biliary tract, pancreas, and colonic ischemia may occur as well. Clinical presentation depends on whether ischemia is transmural, varying from postprandial abdominal pain and weight loss or superficial ulcerations to perforation with peritonitis. The Churg–Strauss syndrome is a variant of PAN, where GI involvement caused by eosinophilic infiltration causes abdominal pain, bloody stools, and diarrhea. Arteriography is a primary modality used to diagnose PAN, revealing focal and segmental saccular aneurysms or stenosis, particularly at areas of bifurcation. Tissue biopsy may confirm the diagnosis, and common biopsy sites include sural nerve, muscle, and skin lesions that may be present. The mainstay of treatment is 1 year of corticosteroid therapy, resulting in remission in 50% of cases. Cyclophosphamide for 6 months of duration can be added to improve response rates and to reduce the incidence of relapse. Untreated, the prognosis in PAN is poor, mostly secondary to renal failure and mesenteric, cardiac, or cerebral infarction. One-year and 5-year survival rates in this setting are approximately 50 and 13%, respectively.[228] While gastrointestinal involvement portends a poor overall prognosis, aggressive treatment has improved survival to approximately 80% at 5 years.[229]

Henoch-Schonlein Purpura

Henoch-Schönlein purpura (HSP), the most common systemic vasculitis in childhood, is a small vessel inflammatory disease that classically results in lower extremity purpura, arthritis, and hematuria. The gastrointestinal tract is affected in up to 50% of patients.[230] Although a variety of infectious and chemical triggers have been proposed, the underlying cause of HSP remains unknown. IgA deposits in the arterial wall result in extravasation of erythrocytes and infiltration of tissue with neutrophils, creating the picture of leukocytoclastic vasculitis. In the small intestinal villi, this eventually leads to necrosis. Abdominal pain, associated with nausea, vomiting, or bleeding, occurs in 51–74% of patients.[231] While the small intestine is the most frequently involved site in the GI tract, the colon can also demonstrate petechiae, hyperemia, ecchymotic lesions resembling the rash, and aphthoid ulcers. Intussusception, typically due to a lead point of intramural hemorrhage, is the most common surgical complication of HSP in childhood.[232] In adults, advanced presentation can include GI hemorrhage, necrosis, and stricture/obstruction. Diagnostic tools include ultrasound, CT scan, upper and lower endoscopy, and video capsule endoscopy. The ideal method of diagnosis is to identify leukocytoclastic vasculitis with IgA on tissue biopsy (whether from the skin, kidney, or GI tract) coupled with classic clinical manifestations. The natural history of the disease is spontaneous resolution, and as such, the role of medical treatment remains unclear. Analgesics (acetaminophen or NSAIDs) and H2-blockers appear to help with symptoms, while the use of corticosteroids is controversial. Over 80% of patients recover within 2 weeks; however, a generally milder and shorter recurrence takes place in one-third of patients most often within 4 months of the initial presentation.

Systemic Lupus Erythematosis

Systemic lupus erythematosis (SLE) is a chronic multisystem inflammatory disease of unknown cause that can affect any organ system of the body, following a relapsing and remitting course. Disturbances within the immune system result in the formation of immune complexes in the microvasculature leading to complement activation and inflammation. Patients with SLE can develop a small- and medium-sized vessel vasculitis that involves the GI tract in approximately 25–40% of patients.[233] Similar to Crohn's disease, SLE can affect any portion of the GI tract. Confusing the situation, abdominal pain may be secondary to any of the concomitant disorders that are associated with lupus such as infection, peritonitis, peptic ulcer disease, mesenteric vasculitis with intestinal infarction, and pancreatitis. The development of abdominal pain is often intermittent and insidious in onset, typically associated with nausea, vomiting, fever, and diarrhea. However, patients may also present acutely with mesenteric vasculitis and infarction in a septic picture. Diagnosis generally involves CT scan, though arteriography may prove helpful. More invasive testing including endoscopy or laparoscopy may be employed. Treatment options include broad-spectrum intravenous antibiotics and systemic corticosteroids, with the possible addition of other immunosuppressives. As steroids may mask the physical examination findings of evolving peritonitis and visceral perforation, surgeons should maintain a high index of suspicion for other signs or worsening physiology. Surgical intervention is indicated for failure to respond to aggressive resuscitation or signs of perforation.

Patients with SLE peritoneal inflammation can also present with an acute abdomen with abdominal ascites. When paracentesis reveals a transudate (excluding infection) a trial of steroids may be considered, though often require operative exploration. SLE-related intestinal pseudo-obstruction may occur as a result of impaired intestinal motility, likely due to a dysfunction of the visceral smooth muscle or the enteric nervous system.[234] Early treatment with high-dose corticosteroids is efficacious, while other treatment options include immunosuppressive medications (azathioprine, cyclosporin A, and cyclophosphamide) along with promotility agents. Finally, while rare, patients with lupus may develop a protein-losing enteropathy, which responds well to steroids.

Behcet's Disease

Behcet's disease is a chronic, relapsing, inflammatory disease mainly affecting young men in the Middle East and women in Japan and Korea.[235] Classically, it causes painful oral and genital apthous ulcerations, uveitis, arthritis, and skin lesions. Yet, 15–60% may also experience gastrointestinal manifestations, with 10–20% developing neurological changes, and up to one-third acquiring vascular abnormalities. This vasculitis is unique as it involves blood vessels of all sizes – small, medium, and large – and affects both the arterial and venous systems. Behcet's disease typically has a waxing and waning course characterized by exacerbations and remissions. From a GI perspective, patients present with anorexia, nausea, abdominal pain, diarrhea, and bleeding. Ulcerations may be superficial or transmural, and are most often seen in the terminal ileum, cecum, and ascending colon. Endoscopically, these ulcerations appear round and deep with discrete margins. When located in the ileocecal location (96%), they are often single (67%), and tend to be larger than 1 cm (76%).[236] It is often difficult to distinguish between Bechet's and inflammatory bowel disease, due to the similarity in intestinal symptoms including GI ulcerations, inflammatory masses, anorectal pathology, and rectovaginal fistulas. In addition, both have extra-intestinal symptoms such as oral ulceration, erythema nodosum, uveitis, and arthritis. While nonspecific serum markers of inflammation may be elevated, there are no pathognomonic laboratory tests in Behcet's disease. Therefore, the diagnosis is often one of the exclusion, and made purely on the basis of the clinical spectrum. Treatment is dictated both by the type of organ system involved and by the severity of disease. Due to a paucity of reliable data, medical options remain controversial, though most often include corticosteroids and a variety of immunosuppressive medications. For those patients with GI involvement, treatment typically involves corticosteroids plus azathioprine, while several reports have demonstrated success with infliximab.[237] Surgery is generally reserved for the management of complications. There is some controversy on the proper resection margins on the bowel, with some authors advocating wide surgical margins, while others recommending removal of only the grossly involved disease.[238] Intestinal anastomosis is normally discouraged as anastomotic leaks, reperforation, and fistulization are common.[239] Long-term, the rate of recurrence after surgery has been reported to be 40–56%, and typically occurs at the anastomotic site.[240]

Scleroderma

Systemic sclerosis (scleroderma) is a multisystem fibrotic disease secondary to alterations of the microvasculature, the autonomic nervous system, and the immune system. Neurohumoral mediators, cytokines, and physical agents such as cold temperature and trauma mediate these alterations in small vessel function. Ultimately, this results in smooth muscle atrophy and gut wall fibrosis. Nearly 90% of patients with systemic sclerosis have GI involvement. While the entire GI tract can be affected, esophageal disease is the most common site.[241] In the small bowel, mucosal villous structure is normal, but collagen deposits around Brunner's glands, leading to periglandular sclerosis. Patients develop malabsorption as a result of intestinal stasis, bowel dilation, and bacterial overgrowth – often resulting in malnutrition. More rare complications include pseudo-obstruction, small bowel perforation, pneumatosis intestinalis, and small bowel volvulus. Bacterial overgrowth can be treated with yogurt and cyclical, chronic oral antibiotics. Pseudo-obstruction and small bowel dysmotility are challenging to treat. Typically, prokinetic agents are not helpful, though daily balanced electrolyte solutions containing polyethylene glycol (PEG) may be beneficial. Octreotide therapy (50 μg/day, subcutaneously), by inducing phase III-like migrating motor complexes, may offer some improvement, although experience of this treatment is still limited.[242] Patients with advanced intestinal failure require total parenteral nutrition, either on a temporary or long-term basis. Surgical resection is rarely beneficial due to the diffuse nature of GI involvement and risk for short bowel syndrome with extended resections. Dietary changes including lactose and fiber avoidance, intake of medium chain triglycerides, and supplementation with vitamins, calcium, and iron have all demonstrated varying results. Anorectal and colonic disease occur in 10–50% of patients with systemic sclerosis. Collagen is deposited in the mucosa and submucosa, while the muscularis externa undergoes atrophy. Wide-mouthed diverticuli can be visible protruding through the weakened wall on the antimesenteric border. Clinically, both constipation, due to dysmotility and pseudo-obstruction, and fecal incontinence are common problems. Disordered defecation often results in fecal incontinence as a consequence of decreased internal anal sphincter pressures, reduced rectal compliance, and an absent or diminished rectoanal inhibitory reflex.[243] Constipation can be managed with bulking agents or PEG, although this may paradoxically worsen proximal dysmotility. For patients with fecal incontinence, treatment options include sphincter muscle training by biofeedback, sacral nerve stimulation, and proximal diversion with a stoma.[244]

Miscellaneous Colitis

As depicted, inflammation of the colon and rectum can result from a vast number of underlying pathologic processes, but also may occur following iatrogenic and rare sources. Included in this mixed bag are colitides from diversion, immunosuppression, medications, toxins, and autoimmune conditions. In this final section, we briefly review a few of the more unusual, though not entirely uncommon, causes of colitis.

Diversion Colitis

Fecal diversion is performed for a variety of reasons, with the ultimate purpose to prevent the fecal stream from reaching the distal segment of large intestine to prevent complications including perineal infection, fecal incontinence, fistula, stricture, or anastomotic protection/leak. Yet, while diversion in these situations is often critically important, it may result in clinically evident disease, particularly following extended periods in which the colorectal mucosa is devoid of fecal matter. The defunctionalized colon and rectum develops a nonspecific inflammation that is felt to be secondary to a lack of short chain fatty acids – the primary colonocyte nutrient.[245] While this is the leading theory, the lack of consistent findings on endoscopy and histological examination has led to alternative hypotheses including infection and ischemia.[246,247] Patients most often present with symptoms of abdominal and/or pelvic pain, tenesmus, bright red blood per rectum, and mucus discharge. Endoscopy commonly reveals erythema, friable mucosa, contact bleeding, and mucus plugs (Figure 34-14). In extreme cases, severe bleeding occurs due to gross ulceration.[248] It is often difficult to differentiate the clinical appearance from inflammatory bowel disease.[249] While the temporal relationship with stoma construction may help with the diagnosis, symptoms normally occur months, and in rare reported cases, 17 years following diversion.[246] Most often patients are asymptomatic and do not require treatment. For those patients with a temporary stoma, resolution of symptoms is the norm once intestinal continuity is restored, while failure to improve should prompt an evaluation for other underlying pathology.[250,251] In symptomatic patients in whom the diversion is permanent or not ready for stomal reversal, treatment regimens including 5-aminosalicylate, sucralfate, and steroid enemas have demonstrated moderate success for symptom control.[252] In addition, there is good evidence that twice-daily irrigation of short-chain fatty acid enemas for 2–4 weeks or even longer will lead to resolution of symptoms.[253,254] It is also critically important for even asymptomatic patients

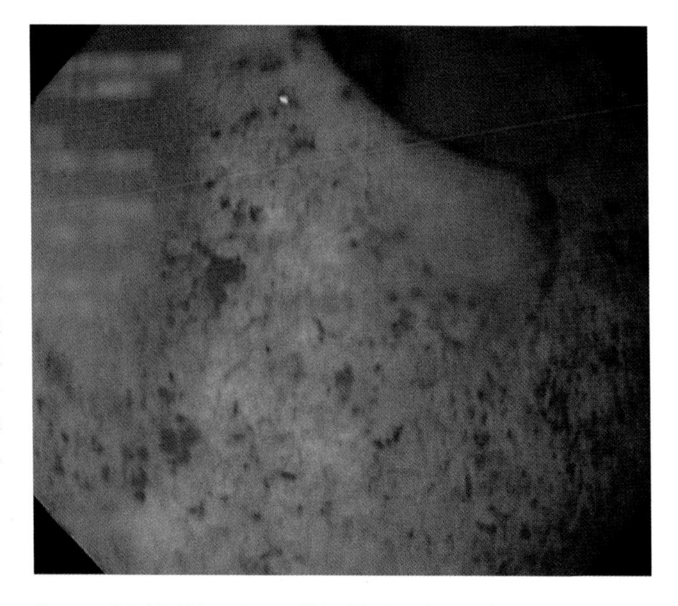

FIGURE 34-14. Diversion colitis. Notice the erythematous, friable mucosa.

with long-term diversion to undergo periodic endoscopic and digital examination for screening and surveillance of colorectal cancer and polyps.

Neutropenic Enterocolitis

Neutropenic enteroclotis, or typhlitis, is a potentially fatal complication of cytotoxic chemotherapy for malignancy, most commonly seen with leukemia or lymphoma.[255] Additionally, immunosuppressed patients from other causes such as following transplantation, aplastic anemia, or AIDS may present with a similar clinical picture. While the exact pathogenesis is unknown, leading proposed mechanisms include alterations of normal bowel flora, weakened immunologic defenses, mucosal injury, and development of more virulent GI pathogens.[256] One consistent factor is the presence of neutropenia, with most patients having absolute neutrophil counts less than 500/mm^3. The process has a predilection for the terminal ileum and cecum, although any segment of the bowel can be involved. During the course of chemotherapy, patients often present with watery diarrhea, vomiting, fever, and abdominal pain, while more severe forms result in perforation and sepsis.[257] Computed tomography is the most widely used method of diagnosis, with characteristic right-sided colonic and ileal wall thickening with or without adjacent fat stranding and free fluid.[258] Pneumatosis has been reported in up to 21% of patients.[259] Due to the patients' underlying condition, the mainstay of therapy remains nothing per os, intravenous fluid resuscitation, broad-spectrum antibiotics, and continued supportive care. Consideration may be given for parenteral nutrition, although in most cases the clinical condition improves as the neutropenia resolves. Patients should be frequently examined for signs of worsening examination or peritonitis. Surgical therapy is generally reserved for patients with signs of nonviable bowel, perforation, or sepsis.[260–262] When surgery is required, consideration is normally given for resection of the involved bowel with the formation of a proximal stoma (i.e., ileostomy).

Disinfectant Colitis

With the prominent role that endoscopy possesses in gastrointestinal screening and treatment, the potential for development of significant contact irritation and subsequent colitis exists. Endoscopic disinfectants commonly use hydrogen peroxide bases or glutaraldehyde formulations for cleaning in part due to their broad spectrum of action against acid and alcohol resistant bacilli, hydrophilic viruses, and spores. While the scopes are thoroughly rinsed and cleansed as a part of the sterilization process, residual formulation or response analogous to contact dermatitis may provoke a change in the mucosa that has been referred to as pseudolipomatosis.[263] This remains somewhat of a controversial topic, as the exact mechanism of this is unknown, as well as whether the irritation results from the bowel preparation, mechanical trauma from the scope itself, or another source. The lesion plaque resembling pseudomembranous colitis, and often appears on withdrawal of the scope in regions which appeared relatively normal on introduction. Patients may have a variety of nonspecific complaints ranging from mild cramping abdominal pain to fever, bloody diarrhea, and significant tenderness starting approximately 24–48 h following endoscopy. The vast majority of patients will have complete symptom resolution without need for therapy, though a paucity of data exists pertaining to this topic, owing to its relatively rare entity.[264] Consideration should be given to appropriate evaluation that often includes history and physical examination, as well as laboratory evaluation to include stool studies to exclude other sources of colitis. In more advanced cases, radiographic evaluation with plain films and CT scan to exclude perforation, and/or repeat endoscopy to determine severity and extent of the process as well as biopsy with histological examination may be required. Most importantly, prevention of this entity may be aided with diligent rinsing and forced-air drying of the endoscopes, along with proper maintenance and routine use of automatic disinfecting machines whenever possible.[265]

Corrosive Colitis

Specific formulations, such as previously described glutaraldehyde and formalin preparations that are used in a variety of medical capacities may result in an iatrogenic corrosive colitis. In addition, self-induced agents per rectum such as household bleach, coffee enemas, colas, and other potentially hazardous liquids and gels may result in varying degrees of bowel wall injury. In the former, changes may occur in the setting of mucosal contact with residual cleaning solutions during endoscopy or rectal instillation to treat diffuse bleeding from radiation proctitis. In the latter, underlying motives such as autoeroticism or attempts at "cleaning" the rectum have been described.[266] Similar to disinfectant colitis, most patients develop a self-limiting symptom complex of abdominal pain, mucous discharge, diarrhea, and rectal bleeding within hours to a few days depending on the extent of exposure and chemical composition of the offending corrosive agent. Treatment typically remains supportive with bowel rest, intravenous fluids, and occasional topical medications (i.e., mesalamine, steroids) as needed, though anecdotal reports of full thickness rectal injury and need for diversion and/or proctectomy with severe cases.[264,267–269] Depending on the degree of injury, patients may also develop symptoms of tenesmus, chronic rectal pain, and even stricture formation long-term that may require therapy.[266]

NSAIDs and Salicylate-Induced Colitis

Many nonsteroidal and salicylate derivatives are used in various ways for the treatment of a number of disease processes. As in the setting of peptic ulcer disease, chronic (or even short-term) NSAID use has been postulated to play a role in the pathogenesis of chronic colitis or colonic ulcer formation.[270] The degree to which they play a role remains undetermined. This is especially interesting in light of the information regarding a potential chemoprotective effect of long-term use of NSAIDS against development of colorectal neoplasia.[271] These drugs have also been associated with causing a reactivation of previously quiescent inflammatory bowel disease (especially ulcerative colitis) via lowering levels of prostaglandins by dual inhibition of the cyclooxygenase (COX) enzymes.[272,273] Relapse may occur in up to 30% of patients and commonly occurs within 10–14 days of NSAID consumption.[274] However, the available data remains very mixed on this topic. Presenting symptoms are often diarrhea, rectal bleeding, and abdominal pain, coupled with a history of NSAID usage. Endoscopic findings include patchy erythema, ulcerations, and in many cases the colonic mucosa appearance will mimic inflammatory or idiopathic colitis. Treatment involves discontinuing NSAID and salicylate use as well as administering topical or steroid preparations – especially in those patients with underlying IBD. Though most patients will have resolution of the symptoms, recurrence is frequent and chronic colitis may require surgery.[275]

Toxic Epidermal Necrolysis

Toxic epidermal necrolysis (TEN), also known as Stevens–Johnson syndrome, is a severe dermatological disease that is characterized by extensive epidermal and mucocutaneous necrosis and exfoliation. Whereas the primary manifestation is the appearance of an erythematous confluent eruption that rapidly evolves into necrosis and exfoliation of the skin at the dermal–epidermal junction, it is also been occasionally associated with disseminated mucosal erosions throughout the gastrointestinal tract.[276] Although this has an unknown etiology, this process appears to be immune-complex mediated and often occurs as an idiosyncratic reaction to a drug or chemical agent. The disease has an extremely high mortality rate and manifests with sepsis, gastrointestinal hemorrhage, diarrhea, high fevers, leukopenia, fluid/electrolyte imbalance, and renal insufficiency.[277,278] The ulceration is not limited to the colon, with diffuse ulceration anywhere from mouth to anus. Radiographically, the colon may appear stenotic or even "lead-pipe" like, similar to chronic ulcerative colitis. Endoscopically, the colon may resemble severe ulcerative or pseudomembranous colitis, however, biopsies show extensive necrosis and lymphocytic infiltration without crypt abscesses or neutrophils and pathologically the muscular layers remain intact. The mucosal sloughing of the bowel may result in melena or intestinal perforation.[70] Patients are critically ill and require aggressive surgical resection along with multisystem intensive care support including extensive skin care that is often only available in burn units.

Conclusion

The wide array of pathology affecting the colon and rectum presents some of the most challenging diagnostic and therapeutic situations. Though each is unique in their own way, varying in extent, severity, and outcome, they share many common bonds. Clinicians should stay abreast of these conditions and possess a well thought out algorithm to evaluate patients presenting with these similar constellation of symptoms.

Acknowledgments. This chapter was authored by Walter E. Longo and Gregory C. Oliver in the previous edition of this textbook.

References

1. Daly JS, Porter KA, Chong FK, et al. Disseminated, non-meningeal gastrointestinal infection in an HIV-negative patient. Am J Gastroenterol. 1990;85:1421–4.
2. Glandt M, Adachi JA, Mathewson JJ, et al. Enteroaggregative *Escherichia coli* as a cause of traveler's diarrhea: clinical response to ciprofloxacin. Clin Infect Dis. 1999;29:335–8.
3. Ashida H, Ogawa M. Shigella infection of intestinal epithelium and circumvention of the host innate defense system. Curr Top Microbiol Immunol. 2009;337:231–55.
4. Ina K, Kusugami K, Ohta M. Bacterial hemorrhagic enterocolitis. J Gastroenterol. 2003;38:111–20.
5. Goldsweig CD, Pacheco PA. Infectious colitis excluding *E. coli* O 157:H7 and *C. difficile*. Gastroenterol Clin North Am. 2001;30:709–33.
6. Bennish ML. Potentially lethal complications of shigellosis. Rev Infect Dis. 1991;13 Suppl 4:S319–24.
7. Bennish ML, Azad AK, Yousefzadeh D. Intestinal obstruction during shigellosis: incidence, clinical features, risk factors and outcome. Gastroenterology. 1991;101:626–34.
8. Christopher PR, David KV, John SM, Sankarapandian V. Antibiotic therapy for *Shigella* dysentery. Cochrane Database Syst Rev. 2010;1:CD006784.
9. Smith T. The hog-cholera group of bacteria. US Bur Anim Ind Bull. 1894;6:6–40.
10. Preliminary FoodNet data on the incidence of infection with pathogens transmitted commonly through food – 10 States, United States, 2005. MMWR Morb Mortal Wkly Rep 2006;55:392.
11. Voetsch AC, Van Gilder TJ, Angulo FJ, et al. FoodNet estimate of the burden of illness caused by nontyphoidal Salmonella infections in the United States. Clin Infect Dis. 2004;38 Suppl 3:S127–34.
12. Infectious disease. In: Beers MH, Berkow R, editors. The Merck Manual. 17th ed. White House Station: Merck Research Laboratories; 1999. p. 1147–209.
13. Mandal BK, Brennand J. Bacteraemia in salmonellosis: a 15 year retrospective study from a regional infectious diseases unit. BMJ. 1988;297:1242–3.
14. Cohen JI, Bartlett JA, Corey GR. Extra-intestinal manifestations of Salmonella infections. Medicine (Baltimore). 1987;66: 349–88.

15. Sirinavin S, Garner P. Antibiotics for treating Salmonella gut infections. Cochrane Database Syst Rev. 2000;Suppl 2:CD001167.
16. Scott DA. Vaccines against *Campylobacter jejuni*. J Infect Dis. 1997;176 Suppl 2:S183–8.
17. Bereswill S, Kist M. Recent developments in *Campylobacter* pathogenesis. Curr Opin Infect Dis. 2003;16:487–91.
18. Blaser MJ, Reller LB. Campylobacter enteritis. N Engl J Med. 1981;305:1444–52.
19. Cover TL, Aber RC. Yersinia enterocolitica. N Engl J Med. 1989;321:16–24.
20. Ostroff SM, Kapperud G, Lassen J, et al. Clinical features of sporadic *Yersinia enterocolitica* infections in Norway. J Infect Dis. 1992;166:812–7.
21. Guth AA, Kim U. The reappearance of abdominal tuberculosis. Surg Gynecol Obstet. 1991;172:432–6.
22. Hamer DH, Gorbach SL. Tuberculosis of the intestinal tract. In: Felman M, Scharschmidt BF, Sleisenger MH, editors. Sleisenger and Fordtrans's gastrointestinal and liver disease. Pathophysiology, diagnosis, management. 6th ed. Philadelphia: WB Saunders; 1998. p. 1622–4. Vol 2.
23. Almadi MA, Ghosh S, Aljebreen AM. Differentiating intestinal tuberculosis from Crohn's disease: a diagnostic challenge. Am J Gastroenterol. 2009;104:1003–12.
24. Chong VH, Lim KS. Gastrointestinal tuberculosis. Singapore Med J. 2009;50:638–45.
25. Krishnan P, Vayoth SO, Dhar P, Surendran S, Ponnambathayil S. Laparoscopy in suspected abdominal tuberculosis is useful as an early diagnostic method. ANZ J Surg. 2008;78:987–9.
26. Kim SH, Cho OH, Park SJ, et al. Diagnosis of abdominal tuberculosis by T-cell-based assays on peripheral blood and peritoneal fluid mononuclear cells. J Infect. 2009;59(6):409–15.
27. Muneef MA, Memish Z, Mahmoud SA, et al. Tuberculosis in the belly: a review of forty-six cases involving the gastrointestinal tract and peritoneum. Scand J Gastroenterol. 2001;36(5):528–32.
28. Choudhury B, Risley CL, Ghani AC, et al. Identification of individuals with gonorrhoea within sexual networks: a population-based study. Lancet. 2006;368:139–46.
29. Hamlyn E, Taylor C. Sexually transmitted proctitis. Postgrad Med J. 2006;82:733–6.
30. McMillan A, Young H. Clinical correlates of rectal gonococcal and chlamydial infections. Int J STD AIDS. 2006;17: 387–90.
31. Wang SA, Harvey AB, Conner SM, et al. Antimicrobial resistance for Neisseria gonorrhoeae in the United States, 1988 to 2003: the spread of fluoroquinolone resistance. Ann Intern Med. 2007;147:81–8.
32. Nieuwenhuis RF, Ossewaarde JM, Gotz HM, et al. Resurgence of lymphogranuloma venereum in Western Europe: an outbreak of Chlamydia trachomatis serovar L2 proctitis in the Netherlands among men who have sex with men. Clin Infect Dis. 2004;39:996–1003.
33. Richardson D, Goldmeier D. Lymphogranuloma venereum: an emerging cause of proctitis in men who have sex with men. Int J STD AIDS. 2007;18:11–5.
34. Van der Bij AK, Spaargaren J, Morre SA, et al. Diagnostic and clinical implications of anorectal lymphogranuloma venereum in men who have sex with men: a retrospective case-control study. Clin Infect Dis. 2006;42:186–94.
35. Kaplan JE, Benson C, Holmes KH, et al. Guidelines for prevention and treatment of opportunistic infections in HIV-infected adults and adolescents: recommendations from CDC, the National Institutes of Health, and the HIV Medicine Association of the Infectious Diseases Society of America. MMWR Recomm Rep. 2009;58(RR-4):1–207.
36. Centers for Disease Control and Prevention, Workowski KA, Berman SM. Sexually transmitted diseases treatment guidelines. MMWR Recomm Rep. 2006;55(RR-11):1–94.
37. Skalsky K, Yahav D, Bishara J, et al. Treatment of human brucellosis: systematic review and meta-analysis of randomised controlled trials. BMJ. 2008;336:701–4.
38. Uddin MJ, Sanyal SC, Mustafa AS, et al. The role of aggressive medical therapy along with early surgical intervention in the cure of Brucella endocarditis. Ann Thorac Cardiovasc Surg. 1998;4:209–13.
39. Cintron JR, Del Pino A, Duarte B, Wood D. Abdominal actinomycosis. Dis Colon Rectum. 1996;39:105–8.
40. Yang SH, Li AF, Lin JK. Colonoscopy in abdominal actinomycosis. Gastrointest Endosc. 2000;51:236–8.
41. Garner JP, Macdonald M, Kumar PK. Abdominal actinomycosis. Int J Surg. 2007;5:441–8.
42. Staras SA, Dollard SC, Radford KW, Flanders WD, Pass RF, Cannon MJ. Seroprevalence of cytomegalovirus infection in the United States, 1988–1994. Clin Infect Dis. 2006;43:1143–51.
43. Rafailidis PI, Mourtzoukou EG, Varbobitis IC, Falagas ME. Severe cytomegalovirus infection in apparently immunocompetent patients: a systematic review. Virol J. 2008;5:47.
44. Solomon L, Cannon MJ, Reyes M, et al. Epidemiology of recurrent genital herpes simplex virus types 1 and 2. Sex Transm Infect. 2003;79:456–9.
45. Schacker T, Hu HL, Koelle DM, et al. Famciclovir for the suppression of symptomatic and asymptomatic herpes simplex virus reactivation in HIV-infected persons. A double-blind, placebo-controlled trial. Ann Intern Med. 1998;128:21–8.
46. Li E, Stanley Jr SL. Protozoa. Amebiasis. Gastroenterol Clin North Am. 1996;25:471–92.
47. Petri WA, Singh U. Enteric amebiasis. In: Guerrant R, Walker DH, Weller PF, editors. Tropical infectious diseases: principles, pathogens, and practice. 2nd ed. Philadelphia: Elsevier; 2006. p. 967.
48. Aristizábal H, Acevedo J, Botero M. Fulminant amebic colitis. World J Surg. 1991;15:216–21.
49. Stanley Jr SL. Amoebiasis. Lancet. 2003;361:1025–34.
50. Schuster FL, Ramirez-Avila L. Current world status of *Balantidium coli*. Clin Microbiol Rev. 2008;21:626–38.
51. Knight R. Giardiasis, isosporiasis, and balantidiasis. Clin Gastroenterol. 1978;7:31–47.
52. Castro J, Vasquez-Iglesias JL, Arnal-Monreal F. Dysentery caused by *Balantidium coli*. Endoscopy. 1983;15:272–4.
53. Chen XM, Keithly JS, Paya CV, LaRusso NF. Cryptosporidiosis. N Engl J Med. 2002;346:1723–31.
54. Framm SR, Soave R. Agents of diarrhea. Med Clin North Am. 1997;81:427–47.
55. Jokipii L, Jokipii AM. Timing of symptoms and oocyst excretion in human cryptosporidiosis. N Engl J Med. 1986;315:1643–7.
56. Gross TL, Wheat J, Bartlett M, O'Connor KW. AIDS and multiple system involvement with cryptosporidium. Am J Gastroenterol. 1986;81:456–8.

57. Rossignol JF, Kabil SM, El-Gohary Y, Younis AM. Effect of nitazoxanide in diarrhea and enteritis caused by cryptosporidium species. Clin Gastroenterol Hepatol. 2006;4:320–4.
58. Rossignol JF, Ayoub A, Ayers MS. Treatment of diarrhea caused by *Cryptosporidium parvum*: a prospective randomized, double-blind, placebo-controlled study of nitazoxanide. J Infect Dis. 2001;184:103–6.
59. Blanshard C, Jackson AM, Shanson DC, et al. Cryptosporidiosis in HIV-seropositive patients. Q J Med. 1992;85: 813–23.
60. Chute CG, Smith RP, Baron JA. Risk factors for endemic giardiasis. Am J Public Health. 1987;77:585–7.
61. Nash TE, Herrington DA, Losonsky GA, et al. Experimental human infections with *Giardia lamblia*. J Infect Dis. 1987;156:974–84.
62. Hill DR, Nash TE. Intestinal flagellate and ciliate infections. In: Guerrant RL, Walker DA, Weller PF, editors. Tropical infectious diseases: principles, pathogens and practice. Philadelphia: WB Saunders; 1999.
63. Hiatt RA, Markell EK, Ng E. How many stool examinations are necessary to detect pathogenic intestinal protozoa? Am J Trop Med Hyg. 1995;53:36–9.
64. Dias JC. The indeterminate form of human chronic Chagas' disease. A clinical epidemiological study. Rev Soc Bras Med Trop. 1989;22:147–56.
65. Chagas C. The discovery of *Trypanosoma cruzi* and of American Trypanosomiasis. Mem Inst Oswaldo Cruz. 1922;15:1.
66. de Oliveira RB, Troncon LE, Dantas RO, Menghelli UG. Gastrointestinal manifestations of Chagas' disease. Am J Gastroenterol. 1998;93:884–9.
67. Braga MS, Lauria-Pires L, Arganaraz ER, Nascimento RJ. Persistent infections in chronic Chagas' disease patients treated with anti-*Trypanosoma cruzi* nitroderivatives. Rev Inst Med Trop São Paulo. 2000;42:157–61.
68. Khuroo MS. Ascariasis. Gastroenterol Clin North Am. 1996;25:553–77.
69. Teneza-Mora NC, Lavery EA, Chun HM. Partial small bowel obstruction in a traveler. Clin Infect Dis. 2006;43(214):256–8.
70. Weller PF. Eosinophilia in travelers. Med Clin North Am. 1992;76:1413–32.
71. Norhayati M, Oothuman P, Azizi O, Fatmah MS. Efficacy of single dose albendazole on the prevalence and intensity of infection of soil-transmitted helminths in Orang Asli children in Malaysia. Southeast Asian J Trop Med Public Health. 1997;28:563–9.
72. Keating JH, Wilson RA, Skelly PJ. No overt cellular inflammation around intravascular schistosomes in vivo. J Parasitol. 2006;92:1365–9.
73. Cheever AW, Hoffmann KF, Wynn TA. Immunopathology of schistosomiasis mansoni in mice and men. Immunol Today. 2000;21:465–6.
74. Strickland GT. Gastrointestinal manifestations of schistosomiasis. Gut. 1994;35:1334–7.
75. Lucey DR, Maguire JH. Schistosomiasis. Infect Dis Clin North Am. 1993;7:635–53.
76. Brinkmann UK, Werler C, Traore M, et al. Experiences with mass chemotherapy in the control of schistosomiasis in Mali. Trop Med Parasitol. 1988;39:167–74.
77. Shekhar KC. Schistosomiasis drug therapy and treatment considerations. Drugs. 1991;42:379–405.
78. Siddiqui AA, Genta RM, Berk SL. Strongyloidiasis (Chap. 111). In: Guerrant RL, Walker DH, Weller PF, editors. Tropical infectious diseases – principles, practices and pathogens. Philadelphia: Churchhill-Livingstone Elsevier; 2006. p. 1274.
79. Longworth DL, Weller PF. Hyperinfection syndrome with strongyloidiasis. In: Remington JS, Swartz MN, editors. Current clinical topics in infectious diseases. New York: McGraw-Hill; 1986. p. 1.
80. Muennig P, Pallin D, Challah C, Khan K. The cost-effectiveness of ivermectin vs. albendazole in the presumptive treatment of strongyloidiasis in immigrants to the United States. Epidemiol Infect. 2004;132:1055–63.
81. Cooper E. Trichuriasis. In: Guerrant R, Walker DH, Weller PF, editors. Tropical infectious diseases: principles, pathogens and practice, vol 2. 2nd ed. Philadelphia: Churchill Livingstone; 2006. p. 1252.
82. Albonico M, Smith PG, Hall A, et al. A randomized controlled trial comparing mebendazole and albendazole against Ascaris, Trichuris and hookworm infections. Trans R Soc Trop Med Hyg. 1994;88:585–9.
83. Liu LX, Chi J, Upton MP, Ash LR. Eosinophilic colitis associated with larvae of the pinworm *Enterobius vermicularis*. Lancet. 1995;346:410–2.
84. Burkhart CN, Burkhart CG. Assessment of frequency, transmission, and genitourinary complications of enterobiasis (pinworms). Int J Dermatol. 2005;44:837–40.
85. Grencis RK, Cooper ES. Enterobius, trichuris, capillaria, and hookworm including ancylostoma caninum. Gastroenterol Clin North Am. 1996;25:579–97.
86. Lopez-Serrano MC, Gomez AA, Daschner A, et al. Gastroallergic anisakiasis: findings in 22 patients. J Gastroenterol Hepatol. 2000;15:503–6.
87. Hidalgo JA, Vazquez JA. Candidiasis. 2002. http://www.emedicine.com. Accessed Nov 2009.
88. Bodey GP. Candidiasis: pathogenesis, diagnosis, and treatment. New York: Raven Press; 1993.
89. Clarkston WK, Bonacini M, Peterson I. Colitis due to *Histoplasma capsulatum* in the acquired immunodeficiency syndrome. Am J Gastroenterol. 1991;86:913–6.
90. Weber R, Ledergerber B, Zbinden R, et al. Enteric infections and diarrhea in human immunodeficiency virus-infected persons: prospective community-based cohort study. Swiss HIV Cohort Study. Arch Intern Med. 1999;159:1473–80.
91. Mayer HB, Wanke CA. Diagnostic strategies in HIV infected patients with diarrhea. AIDS. 1994;8:1639–48.
92. Cello JP, Day LW. Idiopathic AIDS enteropathy and treatment of gastrointestinal opportunistic pathogens. Gastroenterology. 2009;136:1952–65.
93. Aslam S, Musher D. An update on diagnosis, treatment, and prevention of *Clostridium difficile*-associated disease. Gastroenterol Clin North Am. 2006;35:315–35.
94. Johnson S, Clabots CR, Linn FV, et al. Nosocomial *Clostridium difficile* colonization and disease. Lancet. 1990;336: 97–100.
95. Kyne L, Sougioultzis S, McFarland LV, et al. Underlying disease severity as a major risk factor for nosocomial *Clostridium difficile* diarrhea. Infect Control Hosp Epidemiol. 2002;23: 653–9.
96. Senior K. Concern over *Clostridium difficile* in the USA. Lancet Infect Dis. 2008;8:777–84.

97. Yee J, Dixon CM, Mclean AP, Meakins JL. *Clostridium difficile* disease in a department of surgery. The significance of prophylactic antibiotics. Arch Surg. 1991;126:241–6.
98. Gerding DN, Muto CA, Owens RC. Treatment of *Clostridium difficile* infection. Clin Infect Dis. 2008;46:S32–42.
99. Warny M, Pepin J, Fang A, et al. Toxin production by an emerging strain of *Clostridium difficile* associated with outbreaks of severe disease in North America and Europe. Lancet. 2005;366:1079–84.
100. Efron PA, Mazuski JE. *Clostridium difficile* colitis. Surg Clin North Am. 2009;89:489–500.
101. Schwaber MJ, Simhon A, Block C, et al. Risk factors for *Clostridium difficile* carriage and *C. difficile*-associated disease on the adult wards of an urban tertiary care hospital. Eur J Clin Microbiol Infect Dis. 2000;19:9–15.
102. Bartlett JG, Onderdonk AB, Cisneros RL, Kasper DL. Clindamycin-associated colitis due to a toxin-producing species of Clostridium in hamsters. J Infect Dis. 1977;136:701–5.
103. Bartlett J, Moon N, Chang TW, Taylor N, Onderdonk AB. Role of *Clostridium difficile* in antibiotic-associated pseudomembranous colitis. Gastroenterology. 1978;75:778–82.
104. Garey KW, Sethi S, Yadav Y, DuPont HL. Meta-analysis to assess risk factors for recurrent *Clostridium difficile* infection. J Hosp Infect. 2008;70:298–304.
105. Bignardi G. Risk factors for *Clostridium difficile* infection. J Hosp Infect. 1998;40:1–15.
106. Kim H, Rhee SH, Pothoulakis C, Lamont JT. Inflammation and apoptosis in *Clostridium difficile* enteritis is mediated by PGE2 up-regulation of Fas ligand. Gastroenterology. 2007;133:875–86.
107. Bartlett JG, Chang TW, Gurwith M, Gorbach SL, Onderdonk AB. Antibiotic-associated pseudomembranous colitis due to toxin producing clostridia. N Engl J Med. 1978;298:531–4.
108. Surawicz CM, McFarland LV. Psuedomembranous colitis: causes and cures. Digestion. 1999;60:91–100.
109. Fekety R. Guidelines for the diagnosis and management of *Clostridium difficile*-associated diarrhea and colitis. Am J Gastroenterol. 1997;92:739–50.
110. Kelly CP, Pothoularis C, LaMont JT. *Clostridium difficile* colitis. N Engl J Med. 1994;330:257–61.
111. Byrn JC, Maun DC, Gingold DS, et al. Predictors of mortality after colectomy for fulminant *Clostridium difficile* colitis. Arch Surg. 2008;143:150–4.
112. Hall JF, Berger D. Outcome of colectomy for *Clostridium difficile* colitits: a plea for early surgical management. Am J Surg. 2008;196:384–8.
113. Koo HL, Koo DC, Musher DM, et al. Antimotility agents for the treatment of *Clostridium difficile* diarrhea and colitis. Clin Infect Dis. 2009;48:598–605.
114. Zar F, Bakkanagari SR, Moorthi KM, Davis MB. A comparison of vancomycin and metronidazole for the treatment of *Clostridium difficile*-associated diarrhea, stratified by disease severity. Clin Infect Dis. 2007;45:302–7.
115. Wenisch C, Parschalk B, Hasenhündl M, Hirschl AM, Graninger W. Comparison of vancomycin, teicoplanin, metronidazole, and fusidic acid for the treatment of *Clostridium difficile*-associated diarrhea. Clin Infect Dis. 1996;22:813–8.
116. Follmar KE, Condron SA, Turner II, Nathan JD, Ludwig KA. Treatment of metronidazole-refractory *Clostridium difficile* enteritis with vancomycin. Surg Infect (Larchmt). 2008;9:195–200.
117. Fekety R, Silva J, Kauffman C, Buggy B, Deery HG. Treatment of antibiotic-associated *Clostridium difficile* colitis with oral vancomycin: comparison of two dosage regimens. Am J Med. 1989;86:15–9.
118. Mylonakis E, Ryan ET, Calderwood SB. *Clostridium difficile*-associated diarrhea. Arch Intern Med. 2001;161: 525–33.
119. Klinger PJ, Metzger PP, Seelig MH, et al. *Clostridium difficile* infection: risk factors, medical and surgical management. Dig Dis. 2000;18:147–50.
120. Kyne L, Warny M, Qamar A, Kelly CP. Asymptomatic carriage of *Clostridium difficile* and serum levels of IgG antibody against toxin A. N Engl J Med. 2000;342:390–7.
121. Seder C, Villalba M, Robbins J, et al. Early colectomy may be associated with improved survival in fulminant *Clostridium difficile* colitis: an 8-year experience. Am J Surg. 2009;197:302–7.
122. Jaber MR, Olafsson S, Fung WL, et al. Clinical review of the management of fulminant *Clostridium difficile* infection. Am J Gastroenterol. 2008;103:3195–203.
123. Miller AT, Tabrizian P, Greenstein AJ. Long-term follow-up of patients with fulminant *Clostridium difficile* colitis. J Gastrointest Surg. 2009;13:956–9.
124. Sailhamer EA, Carson K, Chang Y, et al. Fulminant *Clostridium difficile* colitis: patterns of care and predictors of mortality. Arch Surg. 2009;144:433–9.
125. Musher DM, Aslam S, Logan N, et al. Relatively poor outcome after treatment of *Clostridium difficile* colitis with metronidazole. Clin Infect Dis. 2005;40:1586–90.
126. Johnson S. Recurrent *Clostridium difficile* infection: a review of risk factors, treatments, and outcomes. J Infect. 2009;58:403–10.
127. Bauer MP, van Dissel JT, Kuijper EJ. *Clostridium difficile*: controversies and approaches to management. Curr Opin Infect Dis. 2009;22:510–24.
128. Mazuki JE, Longo WE. *Clostridium difficile* colitis. Probl Gen Surg. 2002;19:121–32.
129. Ricciardi R, Rothenberger DA, Madoff RD, et al. Increasing prevalence and severity of *Clostridium difficile* colitis in hospitalized patients in the United States. Arch Surg. 2007;142:1524–31.
130. Mazeh H, Samet Y, Abu-Wasel B, et al. Application of a novel grading system for surgical complications after colorectal resection. J Am Coll Surg. 2009;208:355–61.
131. Shaw RS, Green Jr TH. Massive mesenteric infarction following inferior mesenteric artery ligation in resection of the colon for carcinoma. N Engl J Med. 1953;248:890–1.
132. Smith RF, Szilagyi DE. Ischemia of the colon as a complication in the surgery of the abdominal aorta. Arch Surg. 1960;80:806–21.
133. Boley SJ, Schwartz S, Lash J, Sternhill V. Reversible vascular occlusion of the colon. Surg Gynecol Obstet. 1963;116:53–60.
134. Marston A, Pheils MT, Thomas ML, Morson BC. Ischemic colitis. Gut. 1966;7:1–15.
135. Brandt LJ, Boley SJ. Colonic ischemia. Surg Clin North Am. 1992;72:203–29.
136. Macdonald PH. Ischaemic colitis. Best Pract Res Clin Gastroenterol. 2002;16:51–61.
137. Bower TC. Ischemic colitis. Surg Clin North Am. 1993;73: 1037–53.

138. Hagihara PF, Ernst CB, Griffen Jr WO. Incidence of ischemic colitis following abdominal aortic reconstruction. Surg Gynecol Obstet. 1979;149:571–3.
139. Sandison AJ, Panayiotopoulos Y, Edmondson RC, Tyrrell MR, Taylor PR. A 4-year prospective audit of the cause of death after infrarenal aortic aneurysm surgery. Br J Surg. 1996;83:1386–9.
140. Israeli D, Dardik H, Wolodiger F, Silvestri F, Scherl B, Chessler R. Pelvic radiation therapy as a risk factor for ischemic colitis complicating abdominal aortic reconstruction. J Vasc Surg. 1996;23:706–9.
141. Longo WE, Lee TC, Barnett MG, et al. Ischemic colitis complicating abdominal aortic aneurysm surgery in the U.S. veteran. J Surg Res. 1996;60:351–4.
142. Gandhi SK, Hanson MM, Vernava AM, Kaminski DL, Longo WE. Ischemic colitis. Dis Colon Rectum. 1996;39:88–100.
143. Yamazaki T, Shirai Y, Tada T, Sasaki M, Sakai Y, Hatakeyama K. Ischemic colitis arising in watershed areas of the colonic blood supply: a report of two cases. Surg Today. 1997;27:460–2.
144. Longo WE, Ballantyne GH, Gusberg RJ. Ischemic colitis: patterns and prognosis. Dis Colon Rectum. 1992;35:726–30.
145. Assadian A, Assadian O, Senekowitsch C, et al. Plasma D-lactate as a potential early marker for colon ischaemia after open aortic reconstruction. Eur J Vasc Endovasc Surg. 2006;31:470–4.
146. Murray MJ, Gonze MD, Nowak LR, Cobb CF. Serum D-lactate levels as an aid to diagnosing acute intestinal ischemia. Am J Surg. 1994;167:575–8.
147. Poeze M, Froon AHM, Greve JWM, Ramsay G. D-Lactate as an early marker of intestinal ischemia after ruptured abdominal aortic aneurysm repair. Br J Surg. 1998;85:1221–4.
148. Scherpenisse J, van Hees PAM. The endoscopic spectrum of colonic mucosal injury following aortic aneurysm resection. Endoscopy. 1989;21:174–6.
149. Forde KA, Lebwohl O, Wolff M, Voorhees AB. Reversible ischemic colitis: correlation of colonoscopic and pathologic changes. Am J Gastroenterol. 1979;72:182–5.
150. Wolf EA, Sprayregen S, Bakel CW, et al. Radiology in intestinal ischemia: plain film contrast, and other imaging studies. Surg Clin North Am. 1992;72:107–24.
151. Wiesner W, Mortele KJ, Glickman JN, Ji H, Khurana B, Ros PR. CT findings in isolated ischemic proctosigmoiditis. Eur Radiol. 2002;12:1762–7.
152. Balthazar EJ, Yen BC, Gordon RB. Ischemic colitis: CT evaluation of 54 cases. Radiology. 1999;211:381–8.
153. Teefey SA, Roarke MC, Brink JA, et al. Bowel wall thickening: differentiation of inflammation from ischemia with color Doppler and duplex US. Radiology. 1996;198:547–51.
154. Fitzgerald SF, Kaminski DL. Ischemic colitis. Semin Colon Rectal Surg. 1993;4:222–8.
155. van Saene HK, Percival A. Bowel microorganisms – a target for selective antimicrobial control. J Hosp Infect. 1991;19(Suppl C):19–41.
156. Poth EJ, McClure JN. Intestinal obstruction: protective action of sulfasuxidine and sulfathalidine to ileum following vascular damage. Ann Surg. 1950;131:159–63.
157. Sarnoff SJ, Fine J. Effect of chemotherapy on ileum subjected to vascular injury. Ann Surg. 1945;121:74–8.
158. Scharff JR, Longo WE, Vartanian SM, et al. Ischemic colitis: spectrum of disease and outcome. Surgery. 2003;134:624–30.
159. Kaminsky O, Yampolski I, Aranovich D, Gnessin E, Greif F. Does a second-look operation improve survival in patients with peritonitis due to acute mesenteric ischemia? A five-year retrospective experience. World J Surg. 2005;29:645–8.
160. Schneider DB, Nelken NA, Messina LM, Ehrenfeld WK. Isolated inferior mesenteric artery revascularization for chronic visceral ischemia. J Vasc Surg. 1999;30:51–8.
161. Rapp JH, Reilly LM, Qvarfordt PG, Goldstone J, Ehrenfeld WK, Stoney RJ. Durability of endarterectomy and antegrade grafts in the treatment of chronic visceral ischemia. J Vasc Surg. 1986;3:799–806.
162. Bailey JA, Jacobs DL, Bahadursingh A, Longo WE. Endovascular treatment of segmental ischemic colitis. Dig Dis Sci. 2005;50:774–9.
163. Cappell MS. Intestinal (mesenteric) vasculopathy III. Ischemic colitis and chronic mesenteric ischemia. Gastroenterol Clin North Am. 1998;27:827–60.
164. Bharucha AE, Tremaine WJ, Johnson CD, Batts KP. Ischemic proctosigmoiditis. Am J Gastroenterol. 1996;91:2305–9.
165. Peeters ST, Heemsbergen WD, van Putten WL, et al. Acute and late complications after radiotherapy for prostate cancer: results of a multicenter randomized trial comparing 68 Gy to 78 Gy. Int J Radiat Oncol Biol Phys. 2005;61:1019–34.
166. Michalski JM, Winter K, Purdy JA, et al. Toxicity after three-dimensional radiotherapy for prostate cancer on RTOG 9406 dose. Level V. Int J Radiat Oncol Biol Phys. 2005;62:706–13.
167. Baker DG. The response of the microvascular system to radiation: a review. Cancer Invest. 1989;7:287–94.
168. Novak JM, Collins JT, Donowitz M, et al. Effects of radiation on the human gastrointestinal tract. J Clin Gastroenterol. 1979;1:9–39.
169. Pinkawa M, Piroth MD, Fischedick K, et al. Self-assessed bowel toxicity after external beam radiotherapy for prostate cancer-predictive factors on irritative symptoms, incontinence and rectal bleeding. Radiat Oncol. 2009;4:36.
170. Leupin N, Curschmann J, Kransbuhler H, et al. Acute radiation colitis in patients treated with short-term preoperative radiotherapy for rectal cancer. Am J Surg Pathol. 2002;26:498–504.
171. Nussbaum ML, Campana TJ, Weese JL. Radiation-induced intestinal injury. Clin Plast Surg. 1993;20:573–80.
172. van Lin EN, Kristinsson J, Philippens ME, et al. Reduced late rectal mucosal changes after prostate three-dimensional conformal radiotherapy with endorectal balloon as observed in repeated endoscopy. Int J Radiat Oncol Biol Phys. 2007;67:799–811.
173. Chism DB, Horwitz EM, Hanlon AL, et al. Late morbidity profiles in prostate cancer patients treated to 74-84 Gy by a simple four-field coplanar beam arrangement. Int J Radiat Biol Phys. 2003;55:71–7.
174. Zeitman AL, DeSilvio ML, Slater JD, et al. Comparison of conventional-dose vs high-dose conformal radiation therapy in clinically localized adenocarcinoma of the prostate. JAMA. 2005;294:1233–9.
175. Shah SA, Cima RR, Benoit E, et al. Rectal complications after prostate brachytherapy. Dis Colon Rectum. 2004;47:1487–92.
176. Stone NN, Stock RG. Long-term urinary, sexual, and rectal morbidity in patients treated with Iodine-125 prostate brachytherapy followed up for a minimum of 5 years. Urology. 2007;69:338–42.

177. Talcott JA, Clark JA, Stark PC, Mitchell SP. Long term treatment related complications of brachytherapy for early prostate cancer: a survey of patients previously treated. J Urol. 2001;166:494–9.
178. Larson DW, Chrouser K, Young-Fadok T, Nelson H. Rectal complications after modern radiation for prostate cancer: a colorectal surgical challenge. J Gastrointest Surg. 2005;9:461–6.
179. Kjorstadt RJ, Halligan JB, Steele SR. Colorectal complications of external beam radiation versus brachytherapy for prostate cancer. Am J Surg. 2008;195:616–20.
180. Goldstein F, Khoury J, Thornton JJ. Treatment of chronic radiation enteritis and colitis with salicylazosulfapyridine and systemic corticosteroids. A pilot study. Am J Gastroenterol. 1976;65:201–8.
181. Denton A, Forbes A, Andreyev J, Maher EJ. Non surgical interventions for late radiation proctitis in patients who have received radical radiotherapy to the pelvis. Cochrane Database Syst Rev. 2002;Suppl 1:CD003455.
182. Luna-Pérez P, Rodríguez-Ramírez SE. Formalin instillation for refractory radiation-induced hemorrhagic proctitis. J Surg Oncol. 2002;80:41–4.
183. de Parades V, Etienney I, Bauer P, et al. Formalin application in the treatment of chronic radiation-induced hemorrhagic proctitis – an effective but not risk-free procedure: a prospective study of 33 patients. Dis Colon Rectum. 2005;48:1535–41.
184. Jones K, Evans AW, Bristow RG, Levin W. Treatment of radiation proctitis with hyperbaric oxygen. Radiother Oncol. 2006;78:91–4.
185. Zimmerer T, Böcker U, Wenz F, Singer MV. Medical prevention and treatment of acute and chronic radiation induced enteritis – is there any proven therapy? A short review. Z Gastroenterol. 2008;46:441–8.
186. Jahraus CD, Bettenhausen D, Malik U, Sellitti M, St Clair WH. Prevention of acute radiation-induced proctosigmoiditis by balsalazide: a randomized, double-blind, placebo controlled trial in prostate cancer patients. Int J Radiat Oncol Biol Phys. 2005;63:1483–7.
187. Kasibhatla M, Clough RW, Montana GS, et al. Predictors of severe gastrointestinal toxicity after external beam radiotherapy and interstitial brachytherapy for advanced or recurrent gynecologic malignancies. Int J Radiat Oncol Biol Phys. 2006;65:398–403.
188. Regimbeau JM, Panis Y, Gouzi JL. French University Association for surgical research. Operative and long term results after surgery for chronic radiation enteritis. Am J Surg. 2001;182:237–42.
189. Russell JC, Welsh JP. Operative management of radiation injuries of the intestinal tract. Am J Surg. 1979;137:433–42.
190. Meissner K. Late radiogenic small bowel damage: guidelines for the general surgeon. Dig Surg. 1999;16:169–74.
191. Onodera H, Nagayama S, Mori A, Fujimoto A, Tachibana T, Yonenaga Y. Reappraisal of surgical treatment for radiation enteritis. World J Surg. 2005;29:459–63.
192. Freeman HJ, Weinstein WM, Shnitka TK, et al. Watery diarrhea syndrome associated with a lesion of the colonic basement membrane-lamina propria interface. Ann R Coll Physicians Surg Can. 1976;9:45.
193. Pardi DS, Loftus EVJ, Smyrk TC, et al. The epidemiology of microscopic colitis: a population-based study in Olmsted County, Minnesota. Gut. 2007;56:504–8.
194. Olesen M, Eriksson S, Bohr J, et al. Lymphocytic colitis: a retrospective clinical study of 199 Swedish patients. Gut. 2004;53:536–41.
195. Fernandez-Banares F, Salas A, Forne M, et al. Incidence of collagenous and lymphocytic colitis: a 5-year population-based study. Am J Gastroenterol. 1999;94:418–23.
196. Bohr J, Tysk C, Eriksson S, et al. Collagenous colitis in Orebro, Sweden, an epidemiological study 1984–1993. Gut. 1995;37:394–7.
197. Bohr J, Tysk C, Eriksson S, et al. Collagenous colitis: a retrospective study of clinical presentation and treatment in 163 patients. Gut. 1996;39:846–51.
198. Tanaka M, Mazzoleni G, Riddell RH. Distribution of collagenous colitis: utility of flexible sigmoidoscopy. Gut. 1992;33:65–70.
199. Fernandez-Banares F, Esteve M, Salas A, et al. Bile acid malabsorption in microscopic colitis and in previously unexplained functional chronic diarrhea. Dig Dis Sci. 2001;46:2231–8.
200. Bohr J, Tysk C, Yang P, et al. Autoantibodies and immunoglobulins in collagenous colitis. Gut. 1996;39:73–6.
201. Data I, Brar SS, Andrews CN, Dupre M, Ball CG, Buie WD, et al. Microscopic colitis: a review for the surgical endoscopist. Can J Surg. 2009;52:E167–72.
202. Lindstrom CG. "Collagenous colitis" with watery diarrhoea – a new entity? Pathol Eur. 1976;11:87–9.
203. Abdo AA, Urbanski SJ, Beck PL. Lymphocytic and collagenous colitis: the emerging entity of microscopic colitis. An update on pathophysiology, diagnosis and management. Can J Gastroenterol. 2003;17:425–32.
204. Pardi DS, Smyrk TC, Tremaine WJ, et al. Microscopic colitis: a review. Am J Gastroenterol. 2002;97:794–802.
205. Fine KD, Seidel RH, Do K. The prevalence, anatomic distribution, and diagnosis of colonic causes of chronic diarrhea. Gastrointest Endosc. 2000;51:318–26.
206. Zins BJ, Tremaine WJ, Carpenter HA. Collagenous colitis: mucosal biopsies and association with fecal leukocytes. Mayo Clin Proc. 1995;70:430–3.
207. Fine KD, Lee EL. Efficacy of open-label bismuth subsalicylate for the treatment of microscopic colitis. Gastroenterology. 1998;114:29–36.
208. Ung KA, Gillberg R, Kilander A, et al. Role of bile acids and bile acid binding agents in patients with collagenous colitis. Gut. 2000;46:170–5.
209. Chande N, McDonald JW, MacDonald JK. Interventions for treating collagenous colitis. Cochrane Database Syst Rev 2006;Suppl 4:CD003575.
210. Jarnerot G, Tysk C, Bohr J, et al. Collagenous colitis and fecal stream diversion. Gastroenterology. 1995;109:449–55.
211. Munch A, Soderholm JD, Wallon C, et al. Dynamics of mucosal permeability and inflammation in collagenous colitis before, during, and after loop ileostomy. Gut. 2005;54:1126–8.
212. Riaz AA, Pitt J, Stirling RW, et al. Restorative proctocolectomy for collagenous colitis. J R Soc Med. 2000;93:261.
213. Varghese L, Galandiuk S, Tremaine WJ, et al. Lymphocytic colitis treated with proctocolectomy and ileal J-pouch-anal anastomosis: report of a case. Dis Colon Rectum. 2002;45:123–6.
214. Kaijser R. Zur Kenntnis der allergischen affektionen des verdauungs kanals vom standput des chirurgen aus. Arch Klin Chir. 1937;188:36–64.

215. Rothenberg ME. Eosinophilic gastrointestinal disorders (EGID). J Allergy Clin Immunol. 2004;113:11–28.
216. Kravis LP, South MA, Rosenlund ML. Eosinophilic gastroenteritis in the pediatric patient. Clin Pediatr (Phila). 1982;21:713–7.
217. Yan BM, Shaffer EA. Primary eosinophilic disorders of the gastrointestinal tract. Gut. 2009;58:721–32.
218. Okpara N, Aswad B, Baffy G. Eosinophilic colitis. World J Gastroenterol. 2009;15:2975–9.
219. Lange P, Oun H, Fuller S, Turney JH. Eosinophilic colitis due to rifampicin. Lancet. 1994;344:1296–7.
220. Bridges AJ, Marshall JB, Diaz-Arias AA. Acute eosinophilic colitis and hypersensitivity reaction associated with naproxen therapy. Am J Med. 1990;89:526–7.
221. Jimenez-Saenz M, Gonzalez-Campora R, Linares-Santiago E, Herrerias-Gutierrez JM. Bleeding colonic ulcer and eosinophilic colitis: a rare complication of nonsteroidal anti-inflammatory drugs. J Clin Gastroenterol. 2006;40:84–5.
222. Chen MJ, Chu CH, Lin SC, Shih SC, Wang TE. Eosinophilic gastroenteritis: clinical experience with 15 patients. World J Gastroenterol. 2003;9:2813–6.
223. Khan S. Eosinophilic gastroenteritis. Best Pract Res Clin Gastroenterol. 2005;19:177–98.
224. Shin WG, Park CH, Lee YS, et al. Eosinophilic enteritis presenting as intussusception in an adult. Korean J Intern Med. 2007;22:13–7.
225. Fraile G, Rodriguez-Garcia JL, Beni-Perez R, Redondo C. Localized eosinophilic gastroenteritis with necrotizing granulomas presenting as acute abdomen. Postgrad Med J. 1994;70:510–2.
226. Ebert EC, Hagspiel KD, Nagar M, et al. Polyarteritis nodosa and extrahepatic manifestations of HBV infection: the case against autoimmune intervention in pathogenesis. J Autoimmun. 2001;16:269–74.
227. Levine SM, Hellmann DB, Stone JH. Gastrointestinal involvement in polyarteritis nodosa (1986–2000): presentation and outcomes in 24 patients. Am J Med. 2002;112:386–91.
228. Frohnert PP, Sheps SG. Long-term follow-up study of periarteritis nodosa. Am J Med. 1967;43:8–14.
229. Gayraud M, Guillevin L, le Toumelin P, et al. Long-term follow up of polyarteritis nodosa, microscopic polyangiitis, and Churg-Strauss syndrome. Arthritis Rheum. 2001;44:666–75.
230. Goldman LP, Lindenberg RL. Henoch-Schonlein purpura. Gastrointestinal manifestations with endoscopic correlation. Am J Gastroenterol. 1981;75:357–60.
231. Ebert EC. Gastrointestinal manifestations of Henoch-Schonlein purpura. Dig Dis Sci. 2008;53:2011–9.
232. Trapani S, Micheli A, Grisolia F, et al. Henoch Schonlein purpura in childhood: epidemiological and clinical analysis of 150 cases over a 5-year period and review of literature. Semin Arthritis Rheum. 2005;35:143–53.
233. Jovaisas A, Kraag G. Acute gastrointestinal manifestations of systemic lupus erythematosus. Can J Surg. 1987;30:185–8.
234. Perlemuter G, Chaussade S, Wechsler B, et al. Chronic intestinal pseudo-obstruction in systemic lupus erythematosus. Gut. 1998;43:117–22.
235. Sakane T, Takeno M, Suzuki N, Inaba G. Behcet's disease. N Engl J Med. 1999;341:1284–91.
236. Lee CR, Kim WH, Cho YS, et al. Colonoscopic findings in intestinal Behçet's disease. Inflamm Bowel Dis. 2001;7:243–9.
237. Naganuma M, Sakuraba A, Hisamatsu T, et al. Efficacy of infliximab for induction and maintenance of remission in intestinal Behçet's disease. Inflamm Bowel Dis. 2008;14:1259–64.
238. Ebert EC. Gastrointestinal manifestations of Behçet's disease. Dig Dis Sci. 2009;54:201–7.
239. Matsumoto T, Uekusa T, Fukuda Y. Vasculo-Behcet's disease: a pathologic study of eight cases. Hum Pathol. 1991;22:45–51.
240. Kasahara Y, Tanaka S, Nishino M, Umemura H, Shiraha S, Kuyama T. Intestinal involvement in Behcet's disease: review of 136 surgical cases in the Japanese literature. Dis Colon Rectum. 1981;24:103–6.
241. Forbes A, Marie I. Gastrointestinal complications: the most frequent internal complications of systemic sclerosis. Rheumatol Oxf. 2009;48 Suppl 3:iii36–9.
242. Soudah HC, Hasler WL, Owyang C. Effect of octreotide on intestinal motility and bacterial overgrowth in scleroderma. N Engl J Med. 1991;325:1461–7.
243. deSouza NM, Williams AD, Wilson HJ, et al. Fecal incontinence in scleroderma: assessment of the anal sphincter with thin-section endoanal MR imaging. Radiology. 1998;208:529.
244. Kenefick NJ, Vaizey CJ, Nicholls RJ, Cohen R, Kamm MA. Sacral nerve stimulation for faecal incontinence due to systemic sclerosis. Gut. 2002;51:881–3.
245. Murray FE, O'Brien M, Birkett DH, Kennedy SM, LaMont JT. Diversion colitis: pathologic findings in a resected sigmoid colon and rectum. Gastroenterology. 1987;93:1404–8.
246. Geraghty JM, Talbot IC. Diversion colitis: histological features in the colon and rectum after defunctiong colostomy. Gut. 1991;32:1020–3.
247. Villanacci V, Talbot IC, Rossi E, Bassotti G. Ischaemia: a pathogenetic clue in diversion colitis? Colorectal Dis. 2007;9:601–5.
248. Ferguson CM, Siegel RJ. A prospective evaluation of diversion colitis. Am Surg. 1991;57:46–9.
249. Glotzer DJ, Glick ME, Goldman H. Proctitis and colitis following diversion of the fecal streatm. Gastroenterology. 1981;80:438–41.
250. Roediger WE. The starved colon – diminished mucosal nutrition, diminished absorption and colitis. Dis Colon Rectum. 1990;33:856–62.
251. Orsay CP, Kim DO, Pearl RK, Abcarian H. Diversion colitis in patients scheduled for colostomy closure. Dis Colon Rectum. 1993;36:366–7.
252. Szczepkowski M, Kobus A, Borycka K. How to treat diversion colitis? – current state of medical knowledge, own research and experience. Acta Chir Iugosl. 2008;55:77–81.
253. Harig JM, Soergel KH, Komorowski RA, Wood CM. Treatment of diversion colitis with short-chain-fatty acid irrigation. N Engl J Med. 1989;320:23–8.
254. Guillemot F, Colombel JF, Neut C, et al. Treatment of diversion colitis by short chain fatty acids. Prospective double blind study. Dis Colon Rectum. 1991;34:861–4.
255. Davila ML. Neutropenic enterocolitis. Curr Opin Gastroenterol. 2006;22:44–7.
256. Cappell MS. Colonic toxicity of administered drugs and chemicals. Am J Gastroenterol. 2004;99:1175–90.
257. Cardona AF, Combariza JF, Reveiz L, et al. Clinical and microbiological characteristics of neutropenic enterocolitis in adults with blood cancer in the National Cancer Institute of Bogota D.C. Enferm Infecc Microbiol Clín. 2004;22:462–6.

258. Thoeni RF, Cello JP. CT imaging of colitis. Radiology. 2006; 240:623–38.
259. Kirkpatrick ID, Greenberg HM. Gastrointestinal complications in the neutropenic patient: characterization and differentiation with abdominal CT. Radiology. 2003;226:668–74.
260. Bavaro MF. Neutropenic enterocolitis. Curr Gastroenterol Rep. 2002;4:297–301.
261. Moir CR, Scudamore CH, Benny WB. Typhlitis: selective surgical management. Am J Surg. 1986;151:563–6.
262. Keidan RD, Fanning J, Gatenby RA, Weese JL. Recurrent typhlitis. A disease resulting from aggressive chemotherapy. Dis Colon Rectum. 1989;32:206–9.
263. Jonas G, Mahoney A, Murray J, Gertler S. Chemical colitis due to endoscope cleaning solutions: a mimic of pseudomembranous colitis. Gastroenterology. 1988;95:1403–8.
264. Stein BL, Lamoureux E, Miller M, Vasilevsky CA, Julien L, Gordon PH. Glutaraldehyde-induced colitis. Can J Surg. 2001;44:113–6.
265. Ryan CK, Potter GD. Disifectant colitis: rinse as well as you wash. J Clin Gastroenterol. 1995;21:6–9.
266. Sheibani S, Gerson LB. Chemical colitis. J Clin Gastroenterol. 2008;42:115–21.
267. Gan SI, Price IM. Waiting list induced proctitis: the hydrogen peroxide enema. Can J Gastroenterol. 2003;17:727–9.
268. Cappell MS, Simon T. Fulminant acute colitis following a self-administered hydrofluoric acid enema. Am J Gastroenterol. 1993;88:122–6.
269. Ahishali E, Uygur-Bayramicli O, Dolapcioglu C, et al. Chemical colitis due to glutaraldehyde: case series and review of the literature. Dig Dis Sci. 2009;54:2541–5.
270. Shibuya T, Ohkusa T, Yokoyama T, et al. Colonic mucosal lesions associated with long-term or short-term administration of nonsteroidal anti-inflammatory drugs. Colorectal Dis. 2009;12:1113–21.
271. Grau MV, Sandler RS, McKeown-Eyssen G, et al. Nonsteroidal anti-inflammatory drug use after 3 years of aspirin use and colorectal adenoma risk: observational follow-up of a randomized study. J Natl Cancer Inst. 2009;101:267–76.
272. Hawkey CJ. NSAIDs, coxibs, and the intestine. J Cardiovasc Pharmacol. 2006;47 Suppl 1:S72–5.
273. Kefalakes H, Stylianides TJ, Amanakis G, Kolios G. Exacerbation of inflammatory bowel diseases associated with the use of nonsteroidal anti-inflammatory drugs: myth or reality? Eur J Clin Pharmacol. 2009;65:963–70.
274. Takeuchi K, Smale S, Premchand P, et al. Prevalence and mechanism of nonsteroidal anti-inflammatory drug-induced clinical relapse in patients with inflammatory bowel disease. Clin Gastroenterol Hepatol. 2006;4:196–202.
275. Gleeson MH, Davis AJM. Non-steroidal anti-inflammatory drugs, aspirin and newly diagnosed colitis: a case controlled study. Aliment Pharmacol Ther. 2003;17:817–25.
276. Jäckel R, Fuchs M, Raff T. Wiedemann B [Drug-induced toxic epidermal necrolysis with involvement of the intestinal and respiratory tract. A case report]. Anaesthesist. 2002;51:815–9.
277. Otomi M, Yano M, Aoki H, et al. A case of toxic epidermal necrolysis with severe intestinal manifestation. Nippon Shokakibyo Gakkai Zasshi. 2008;105:1353–61.
278. Carter FM, Mitchell CK. Toxic epidermal necrolysis – an unusual cause of colonic perforation. Report of a case. Dis Colon Rectum. 1993;36:773–7.

35 Advanced Laparoscopic Colorectal Surgery

Tonia Young-Fadok

Introduction

Since the first edition of this textbook, advances in laparoscopic colorectal surgery have been made in the arenas of education, research, and practice. In education, the vast majority of, if not all, trainees now finishing colorectal surgery fellowships have learned laparoscopic techniques. All laparoscopic colorectal procedures continue to be considered advanced procedures and are considered as such in this chapter. In the research arena, a multicenter randomized controlled trial is in progress evaluating the safety and other outcomes of laparoscopic resection of rectal cancer. In clinical practice, single-incision laparoscopic surgery has sparked interest in making these procedures even less invasive, and there is at least intellectual and experimental interest in natural orifice transluminal endoscopic surgery (NOTES) even though this approach has not yet made its way into practice. This chapter will review these issues and provide an assessment of the use of laparoscopic techniques for the common disease processes seen by colorectal surgeons.

Learning Curve

There continues to be relatively slow adoption of laparoscopic colectomy into the surgeon's practice. Laparoscopic colorectal surgery faces certain challenges which distinguish it from other minimally invasive procedures. In comparison to laparoscopic cholecystectomy, the performance of laparoscopic colectomy requires working in multiple quadrants of the abdomen. This requires a better understanding of depth perception and proprioception. A coordinated team consisting of a surgeon, an assistant, and often a cameraperson is required. All three must work together along with the nursing and anesthesia teams. All of these add to the complexity of the procedure and this results in the need to perform a number of cases before the surgeon and surgical team become proficient. Numerous previous studies have evaluated the "learning curve" of laparoscopic colectomy, although the actual definition of learning curve remains somewhat nebulous.[1–3]

Although earlier studies estimated the learning curve for laparoscopic colectomy to be at least 20 cases, several publications have suggested the learning curve is greater than this.[4] The initial randomized trials of laparoscopic resection for colon cancer demonstrate this, with a fall in conversion rates over the course of the trials. In a prospective randomized study of colorectal cancer in the United Kingdom, the "CLASICC" trial, surgeons had to perform at least 20 laparoscopic resections before they were allowed to enter the study.[5] The study began in July 1996 and was completed in July 2002. Despite the surgeon's prior experience, the rate of conversion dropped from 38 to 16% over the course of the study, suggesting that a minimum of 20 cases may not be enough to reach the plateau of the "learning curve." In the COLOR trial from Europe,[6] a prospective randomized study for colon cancer that required a prerequisite experience in laparoscopic colon resection before surgeons could enter patients in to the study, surgeon and hospital volume were directly related to a number of operative and postoperative outcomes. The median operative time for high-volume (>10 cases/year) hospitals was 188 min compared to 241 min for low volume (<5 cases/year) hospitals, and likewise conversion rates were 9% vs. 24% for the two groups. High-volume groups also had more lymph nodes in the resected specimens, fewer complications, and shortened hospital stay. These studies suggest that the learning curve is clearly greater than 20 cases and surgeons need to perform a minimum yearly number of procedures to maintain their skills.

A major achievement has been the introduction of laparoscopic training into most, if not all, of the accredited colorectal fellowships, so that graduates of these programs have laparoscopic skills. There are three groups of surgeons among whom laparoscopic approaches remain slow to permeate: colorectal surgeons who finished training prior to the introduction of laparoscopic cholecystectomy; general surgeons who perform few colorectal procedures; and residents graduating from general surgery programs with no

D.E. Beck et al. (eds.), *The ASCRS Textbook of Colon and Rectal Surgery: Second Edition*,
DOI 10.1007/978-1-4419-1584-9_35, © Springer Science+Business Media, LLC 2011

laparoscopic colorectal training. Regarding the first group, it is challenging for established colorectal surgeons to assimilate laparoscopic procedures into their practice, when they are not familiar with the basics of laparoscopy. This is reflected in the data obtained from board-certified colorectal surgeons who are taking recertification examinations: only 30% perform laparoscopy which indicates that less than 30% of cases being performed by recertifying colorectal surgeons are being performed by this approach as even experienced laparoscopic colorectal surgeons acknowledge that some cases must be performed open.

For general surgeons, the difficulty with the broad application of laparoscopic colectomy is that most general surgeons perform far fewer than 50 segmental colon resections per year. In a review of 2,434 general surgeons who were taking the recertification examination of the American Board of Surgery, all of whom supplied their operative lists from the previous year, most surgeons performed fewer than 20 colon resections in 1 year.[7] In fact, the mean number of colon resections performed was 11. Even at the 90th percentile, only 23 colectomies were performed in a single year. If the average surgeon performs 11 resections and approximately half are eligible for a laparoscopic approach, assuming a learning curve of even just 20 cases, it would take a surgeon 4 years to feel comfortable performing laparoscopic colectomy, and many would argue that so few cases per year is not sufficient to build up one's skill level. Most surgeons (and their patients!) cannot afford to go through such a learning curve. Either the learning curve will need to be shortened, as some have suggested may be possible by the use of hand-assisted laparoscopic techniques, or the performance of laparoscopic colectomy may be limited to surgeons who perform a greater number of colon resections per year.

Conversion

Rates of conversion vary widely in the literature, from 0% to as high as 48%, depending on multiple factors such as date of publication, disease process, patient factors and of course, surgeon experience and ability. Most series report the need to convert in 5–25% of cases. While surgical proficiency would likely decrease the need to convert, this is counterbalanced by the surgeon's desire to perform more complex cases.[2] Several patient and disease-related factors such as obesity, prior abdominal surgery (a marker for adhesions), acuity of inflammation (i.e., abscess and fistula formation), tumor bulk or contiguous involvement, and disease location, may also affect the rate of conversion. Obesity, defined as a body mass index greater than 30 kg/m^2, was once considered a relative contraindication to a laparoscopic approach. For a surgeon early in his/her learning curve, it should remain a relative contraindication. However, once more experience is gained by the surgeon, several reports have demonstrated that obesity itself is not a contraindication to a minimally invasive approach.[8–10] For inflammatory conditions such as Crohn's disease and diverticulitis, the presence of an abscess or fistula may result in the need for conversion in up to 50% of cases,[11,12] with reports from experienced centers suggesting a conversion rate of 25–35% for enteric fistulae.[13–15] The presence of a fistula or small abscess is not a contraindication to a minimally invasive approach but should alert the surgeon to consider a variation in operative approach if obstacles cannot be overcome. Conversion from a laparoscopic to open resection should *not* be viewed as a failure of the surgeon but as a sign of mature surgical judgment. Based on preoperative studies, it is difficult to predict which cases cannot be completed laparoscopically.

More crucial than the rate of conversion may be the time spent prior to conversion. Delayed conversion, occurring only after a complication has occurred, may in some cases reflect poor judgment or little experience. An initial laparoscopic survey may quickly identify a complex process, allowing a speedy alteration in the operative plan. If the approach is expeditiously changed, additional time and costs may be avoided. Early reports suggested worse outcomes for patients who required conversion, but later studies suggest that if conversion is made early, the outcome of converted cases is similar to patients undergoing conventional surgery.[16,17] The goal is to perform a preemptive conversion; once it is determined the case cannot be completed laparoscopically, rather than a reactive conversion to a complication which occurred due to adverse conditions which the surgeon could have avoided.

Outcomes

This section is an overview and summary of the types of outcomes measured for laparoscopic colectomy; disease-specific outcomes are provided in the next section and in the accompanying tables. In comparison with conventional colectomy, benefits of laparoscopic colectomy may include shorter duration of postoperative ileus, less postoperative pain and concomitant reduction in the need for analgesics, earlier tolerance of diet, shortened hospital stay, earlier resumption of normal activities, improved cosmetic results, and possibly preservation of immune function. This is offset by a prolongation in operative time, the cost of laparoscopic equipment, and the learning curve of these technically challenging procedures. When reporting the outcomes of laparoscopic colectomy, there is, however, a natural selection bias when comparing conventional and laparoscopic cases. More complex cases are generally not suitable for a laparoscopic approach and therefore are performed "open." Also, in many series the results of the successfully completed laparoscopic cases are compared to both conventional cases and the cases converted from a laparoscopic to conventional procedure. Few studies, with the exception of the larger prospective randomized studies, leave the "converted" cases in the laparoscopic group as part of the "intention to treat" laparoscopic group. This clearly introduces selection bias.

The vast majority of studies reporting outcomes of laparoscopic vs. open colectomy are retrospective case–control studies or even just case series. Although some postoperative outcomes are available from randomized trials, most of the well-performed randomized trials are designed to answer important oncologic issues such as safety and survival in cancer patients, and postoperative outcomes have been of secondary interest. Conclusions regarding outcomes, therefore, often come from the repetitiveness of the results rather than the superiority of study design. For any one study, the evidence is weak, but collectively, due to the reproducibility of results by a large number of institutions, even with different operative techniques and postoperative management parameters, the preponderance of evidence favors a minimally invasive approach with respect to postoperative outcomes. Also, the prospective randomized studies which are available corroborate the findings demonstrated in nonrandomized studies.

Operative Time

Most comparative studies provide information regarding operative times. The definition of the operative time may vary with each series, and there may be different groups of surgeons performing the laparoscopic and conventional procedures. Most studies demonstrate a longer operative time associated with a laparoscopic procedure. In prospective randomized trials, the procedure was roughly 40–60 min longer in the laparoscopic groups. As the surgeon and team gain experience with laparoscopic colectomy, operating times do reliably fall, but rarely does it return to the comparable time for a conventional approach.

Return of Bowel Activity and Resumption of Diet

Reduction in postoperative ileus is one of the proposed major advantages of minimally invasive surgery. Most studies comparing open and laparoscopic colectomy have shown a statistically significant reduction in the time to passage of flatus and stool. Most series demonstrate a 1–2-day advantage for the laparoscopic group. Whether the reduction of ileus relates to less bowel manipulation, or less intestinal exposure to air and desiccation, or some other factor during minimally invasive surgery, remains unknown.

In clinical studies, it is difficult to eliminate the biases of the physician and the higher expectations of the patient undergoing laparoscopic surgery. Psychological conditioning of the patient preoperatively may interfere with an objective assessment of bowel activity postoperatively. To answer this question formally, both human and animal studies have evaluated the return of gastrointestinal motility. Both canine and porcine models have confirmed an earlier return of intestinal myoelectric activity following laparoscopic resection.[18,19] A study in dogs demonstrated an earlier return to preoperative motility, utilizing radionucleotide techniques in animals subjected to laparoscopic resection.[20] These studies clearly demonstrate a more rapid return of bowel activity without the subjective bias which may be introduced in clinical studies.

With shorter postoperative ileus, tolerance of both liquids and solid food is sooner following laparoscopic resection. The time to resumption of diet varies from 2 to 7 days (depending, interestingly, on the country in which the study was performed, reflecting accepted local practices), but in the majority of comparative studies this is 1–2 days sooner than in patients undergoing conventional surgery. Again, the physician and patient are usually not blinded, which may alter patient expectations. The overwhelming reproducible data reported in both retrospective and prospective studies of laparoscopic procedures, however, does favor a shorter period of postoperative ileus and earlier tolerance of liquid and solid diet.

Postoperative Pain and Recover of Pulmonary Function

A variety of assessments have demonstrated a significant reduction in pain following minimally invasive surgery: some studies utilize an analog pain scale, while others measure narcotic requirements. Physician bias and psychological conditioning of the patients may interfere with the evaluation of postoperative pain. There are also cultural variations in the response to pain. Three of the early prospective randomized trials evaluated pain postoperatively and all three found a reduction in narcotic requirements in patients undergoing laparoscopic colectomy.[21–23] In the COST study,[24,25] the need both for intravenous and oral analgesics was less in patients undergoing laparoscopic resection. Numerous other nonrandomized studies have shown a reduction in postoperative pain and narcotic usage.

Closely related to the severity and duration of postoperative pain is the return of pulmonary function. Adequate pain management allows the patient to inspire more deeply. Following conventional abdominal surgery, suppression of pulmonary function is a well-known sequela. Several studies of laparoscopic colectomy have evaluated the return of pulmonary function. In a randomized trial of patients undergoing surgery for colon cancer from the Cleveland Clinic, preoperative and postoperative spirometry was performed every 12 h in 55 patients in the laparoscopic group and 54 patients in the conventional group.[21] An 80% recovery of baseline forced vital capacity (FVC) and forced expiratory volume in 1 s (FEV_1) was measured in each patient. The median recovery for the laparoscopic group was 3 days which was half the recovery (6 days) seen in the conventional group. A similarly designed study by Schwenk et al.[23] confirmed these results. Although subject to bias, the results of comparative studies suggest a quicker recovery of pulmonary function and reduction in postoperative pain in patients subjected to laparoscopic colectomy.

Length of Stay

More rapid resolution of ileus, earlier resumption of diet and reduced postoperative pain results in a shortened length of stay after laparoscopic resection compared with traditional procedures. Recovery after open operation has also been shortened by fast-track practices, but this is not consistent throughout the literature. In the absence of minimally invasive techniques, it would seem unlikely that the length of stay could be further reduced. In most studies, the length of hospitalization is 1–6 days less for the laparoscopic group. In an attempt to minimize the differences between a conventional midline incision and a laparoscopic incision, Fleshman et al.[25] compared the outcomes of 35 patients whose surgery was performed through a minilaparotomy (12 cm, mean incision length) to 54 laparoscopic patients. Outcome was similar for both groups with a mean day of discharge of 6.9 days (range 3–15 days) for the minilaparotomy group and 6.0 days for the laparoscopic group (range 1–15 days). However, when the results of successfully completed laparoscopic cases (75%) where compared, the results favored the laparoscopic group (5.3 days, range 1–14 days). Therefore, despite an attempt to minimize the incision, the overall length of stay was still longer in the minilaparotomy group.

While psychological conditioning of the patient cannot be avoided and likely has a desirable effect, the benefits of minimally invasive procedures on the overall length of stay cannot be discounted. The benefit, however, is more likely a 1–2-day advantage only. The more recent introduction of fast-track clinical pathways in conventional and laparoscopic surgery has also narrowed the gap, but laparoscopy still appears to confer advantages.[26,27]

Quality of Life and Return to Work

If laparoscopic colectomy results in less postoperative pain and earlier return to normal activities, one would anticipate that quality of life after a laparoscopic procedure should be improved compared with conventional procedures. Few studies, however, have objectively examined the patient's assessment of recovery. In a nonrandomized study, Psaila et al.[28] evaluated the recovery of hand grip strength and quality of life utilizing an SF-36 symptom score 2 and 4 months postoperatively. Hand grip strength, as a measure of protein loss, recovered more rapidly after laparoscopic surgery. In six of eight areas the SF-36 questionnaire showed less impairment of health following laparoscopic colectomy. By 4 months postoperatively, this trend persisted but to a lesser degree. In the COST study, quality of life was evaluated by three complementary viewpoints: patient self-reported symptoms, patient self-reported functional status, and a third more objective measurement scale of compliance to treatment referred to as Q-TWiST (quality-adjusted time without symptoms of disease and toxicity of treatment).[24,29] Due to a high conversion rate of 25% in the initial study report, and the "intention to treat" design of the study, there were no significant differences between the conventional and laparoscopic groups with the exception of a global rating score at 2 weeks. In every category, however, patients who had a laparoscopically completed procedure were improved compared with open procedures and with laparoscopic patients who required a conversion to open surgery, although this did not achieve significance. The results of the CLASICC trial found similar results.[5]

Few studies have assessed the ability of patients undergoing laparoscopic colectomy to return to work. With less postoperative pain and reduced narcotic usage one would presume that patients undergoing a minimally invasive approach would return more quickly to normal activities and employment compared with patients undergoing conventional resection. In a nonrandomized study, patients undergoing laparoscopy returned to full activities and work sooner than matched patients undergoing conventional resection (mean – 4.2 weeks vs. 10.5 weeks, 3.8 weeks vs. 7.5 weeks, respectively ($P<0.01$ for all)).[30]

Hospital Costs

A theoretical disadvantage of laparoscopy is higher operative costs related to longer operative times and disposable equipment. Whether the total cost of the hospitalization (operative and hospital costs) is higher following laparoscopic colectomy is debatable. A case control study from the Mayo Clinic looked at total costs following laparoscopic and open ileocolic resection for Crohn's disease.[31] Sixty-six patients underwent laparoscopic ($n=33$) or conventional ($n=33$) ileocolic resection during the same time period (10/95 to 7/99) and were well matched. Patients in the laparoscopic group had less postoperative pain, tolerated a regular diet sooner by 1–2 days and had a shorter length of stay (4.0 days vs. 7.0 days). In their cost analysis, despite higher operative cost, the overall mean costs were $3,273 less in the laparoscopic group. The procedures were performed by different groups of surgeons at the institution, and while the surgeon may have introduced bias, this study was undertaken during the current era of cost containment. Other studies by Dupree et al.[32] and Shore et al.[33] have confirmed these findings with a mean reduction of $438 in costs and $7,465 in hospital charges, respectively, in patients undergoing laparoscopic compared to conventional ileocolic resection. The results are similar for elective sigmoid diverticular resection with a mean cost savings of $700–$800[34,35] (and there are additional examples in the disease-specific section). Increased operative times and equipment expenditures appear to be offset by a shorter hospital stay.

Disease-Specific Outcomes

Crohn's Disease

Laparoscopy in the setting of inflammatory bowel disease has its own unique challenges. In Crohn's disease, there may be inflammatory changes, difficulty in assessing bowel involvement, and associated abscess and fistulous disease.[11] In the patient with Crohn's colitis, the challenges are also technical owing to the difficulty in performing laparoscopic total colectomy.

Crohn's disease of the terminal ileum seems an ideal model for a minimally invasive approach. The disease is usually limited to one area of the abdomen and only mobilization and vascular pedicle ligation are required laparoscopically, with resection and anastomosis performed extracorporeally. Patients with Crohn's are typically young and interested in a procedure that minimizes scars. Additionally, since many of these patients require reoperation over their lifetime, a minimally invasive approach is appealing. Early reports of laparoscopic ileocolic resection showed it to be feasible and safe but were typically small nonrandomized uncontrolled studies. More recent studies (Table 35-1) demonstrate a more extensive experience.[36–55] The majority of studies, however, are retrospective case control series. Most series report the rate of conversion from 10 to 20% with the mix of complex cases (abscess, fistula, or reoperative surgery) ranging from 40 to 50%.

As expected, outcomes of laparoscopic ileocolic resection for Crohn's disease mirror those seen in other studies of laparoscopic colectomy for benign and malignant disease. In comparative studies (Table 35-1), laparoscopic ileocolic resection is associated with earlier return of bowel function and tolerance of oral diet. The quicker resolution of ileus, earlier resumption of diet, and reduced postoperative pain results in a shorter length of stay for patients after laparoscopic resection compared with traditional procedures. Milsom et al.[43] reported a prospective randomized trial comparing conventional and laparoscopic ileocolic resection for refractory Crohn's disease. Sixty patients were randomized to either conventional or laparoscopic resection after an initial diagnostic laparoscopy to assess feasibility of a laparoscopic resection. The results favor a laparoscopic approach with regards to pulmonary function, morbidity, and length of stay. There were no apparent short-term disadvantages. All patients had oral intake withheld for 3 days to evaluate nutritional parameters. This impacted on the timing of dietary intake and was likely responsible for a delay in discharge in some patients. The total length of stay in this randomized study was 1 day shorter in the laparoscopic group (5 days vs. 6 days) but did not reach statistical significance. Had dietary intake not been withheld, a shortened length of stay of the laparoscopic group might have achieved significance.

Without tactile sensation, one of the concerns of laparoscopic surgery in the patient with Crohn's is missing an isolated proximal ileal lesion. Many patients following ileocolic resection, whether open or laparoscopic, will develop a symptomatic recurrence proximal to the ileocolic anastomosis, but whether patients undergoing a laparoscopic procedure will present more frequently as a result of unrecognized proximal disease remains unclear. There are, however, several studies that have reported recurrence rates following laparoscopic ileocolic resection. In one study, the long-term follow-up results (mean 39 months) of 32 patients over 7 years who underwent a laparoscopic ileocolic resection were compared to 29 patients undergoing open resection.[46] The rate of Crohn's recurrence was high but similar in both groups (48% laparoscopic, 44% conventional) as was the disease-free interval (24 months). In another review of long-term outcome, Bergamaschi et al.[47] reported the results of 39 laparoscopic and 53 conventional ileocolic resections with a 5-year follow-up. Recurrent disease was determined by patient symptoms and confirmed both radiographically and endoscopically in 27% of patients undergoing a laparoscopic procedure and in 29% of patients with a conventional resection. Interestingly, the incidence of small bowel obstruction was significantly less in the laparoscopic group (11% vs. 35%, $P=0.02$). This was thought to be due to less adhesion formation following a laparoscopic procedure. Laparoscopic ileocolic resection does not appear to offer any advantage over conventional resection with regard to symptomatic recurrence, but it also did not lead to a higher rate of recurrence or discovery of a missed lesion. There are two options for evaluating the small bowel to evaluate for proximal lesions: the bowel can be run from ligament of Treitz to the ileocecal valve using a "hand-over-hand" instrument evaluation; alternatively, if a specimen is being removed, the small bowel can be evaluated manually as it can usually be exteriorized through a small periumbilical incision.

Laparoscopic ileocolic resection for Crohn's disease appears to be safe and feasible and offers the advantages seen in other reports of laparoscopic colorectal procedures. For the inexperienced laparoscopist, the initial uncomplicated terminal ileal resection is an ideal procedure in which to gain laparoscopic experience. An initial laparoscopic survey should be performed, with a low threshold to convert to open if a complex case beyond the skill of the surgeon is encountered.

Ulcerative Colitis

There are a few small prospective randomized studies of laparoscopic proctocolectomy for ulcerative colitis[56,57] but the vast majority of reports are prospective and retrospective case control studies and noncomparative reports (Tables 35-2A and 35-2B).[58–76] Several reasons likely account for the slow adoption of laparoscopic proctocolectomy including the steep learning curve for even segmental colectomy, the technical challenges of transverse colon resection, and unfavorable early reports of laparoscopic total colectomy. The

TABLE 35-1. Studies of laparoscopic resection for Crohn's disease: ileocolic resection

Author	Year	No. of patients		OP time (min)		LOS (day)		Morbidity (%)		Comment
		LAP	OPEN	LAP	OPEN	LAP	OPEN	LAP	OPEN	
Bauer et al.[11]	1996	25	14	–	–	6.5	8.5	–	–	High conversion if mass and fistula
Wu et al.[36]	1997	46	70	144	202	4.5	7.9	10	21	52% complex or redo cases
Dunker et al.[37]	1998	11	11	–	–	5.5	9.9	9	9	Improved cosmesis
Wong et al.[38]	1999	55		150		6.0		5		46% complex cases
Canin-Endres et al.[39]	1999	70		183		4.2		14		41 with fistulae, 1 conversion
Alabaz et al.[40]	2000	26	48	150	90	7.0	9.6	–	–	Favorable results
Bemelman et al.[41]	2000	30	48	138	104	5.7	10.2	15	10	Different hospitals for each group
Young-Fadok et al.[31]	2001	33	33	147	124	4.0	7.0	–	–	Laparoscopy less expensive
Schmidt et al.[42]	2001	46		207		5.7				Safe and effective, high conversion rate
Milsom et al.[43]	2001	31	29	140	85	5.0	6.0	16	28	Prospective, randomized trial
Evans et al.[44]	2002	84		145		5.6		11		Results improve with experience
Dupree et al.[32]	2002	21	24	75	98	3.0	5.0	14	16	Laparoscopy less expensive
Shore et al.[33]	2003	20	20	145	133	4.3	8.2	–	–	Laparoscopy less expensive
Benoist et al.[45]	2003	24	32	179	198	7.7	8.0	20	10	Similar operative times, 17% converted
Bergamaschi et al.[47]	2003	39	53	185	105	5.6	11.2	9	10	Long-term obstruction less, 11% vs. 35%
Huilgol et al.[49]	2004	21	19	136	120	6.4	8.2	19	16	
Rosman et al.[50]	2005			26.8 min longer		2.62 days less		OR 0.62		Meta-analysis, SBO reduced in LAP cases
Tilney et al.[51]	2006	338	445	29.6 min longer						Meta-analysis, conversion 6.8%
Tan et al.[52]	2007			26 min longer		1.82 days less		12.8	20.2	Meta-analysis, conversion 11.2%
Lesperance et al.[53]	2009	2,826 (6%)	46,783			6.0	9.0	8	16	Nationwide Inpatient Sample
Soop et al.[54]	2009	109		150		4.0		11		Conversion 6%
Nguyen et al.[55]	2009	335		177		5.0		13		Largest series, conversion rate 2%

OP operative, *LOS* length of stay, *LAP* laparoscopic, *CON* conventional, *SBO* small bowel obstruction.

TABLE 35-2A. Early descriptive studies of laparoscopic colectomy for ulcerative colitis

Author	Year	No. of patients	Comment
Meijerink et al.[48]	1999	10	Feasible, 7 for acute colitis
Marcello et al.[58]	2000	13	Restorative proctocolectomy, favorable results
Seshadri et al.[59]	2001	37	25% morbidity
Hamel et al.[60]	2001	21	Compared with ileocolic resection, similar morbidity and LOS
Marcello et al.[61]	2001	16	For acute colitis, comparative study, favorable results
Brown et al.[62]	2001	25	Longer op time in LAP group
Dunker et al.[63]	2001	35	Better cosmesis
Ky et al.[64]	2002	32	Single-stage procedure, good results
Bell and Seymour[65]	2002	18	Total colectomy for acute colitis, seems safe
Rivadeneira et al.[66]	2004	23	Hand-assisted procedure reduced operative time
Kienle et al.[67]	2003	59	Large study, laparoscopic colon mobilization only
Nakajima et al.[68]	2004	16	Hand-assisted technique, favorable results

IPAA ileal pouch-anal anastomosis, *EBL* estimated blood loss, *LOS* length of stay.

TABLE 35-2B. Comparative studies of laparoscopic resection for ulcerative colitis

		No. of patients		OP time (min)		LOS (day)		Morbidity (%)		
Author	Year	LAP	OPEN	LAP	OPEN	LAP	OPEN	LAP	OPEN	Comment
Maartense et al.[70]	2004	30	30	210	133	10	11	20	17	SF-36 and GIQLI scores similar
Larson et al.[71]	2006	100	200	333	230	4	7	33	37	LAP faster than hand-assist (320 min vs. 372 min)
Zhang et al.[72]	2007	21	25	325	220	9	11	25	28	
Benavente-Chenhalls[73]	2008	16	16	500	382	25	44	5.3	9.9	UC and primary sclerosing cholangitis
Ahmed Ali et al.[74]	2009	253	354	91 min longer		2.7 days less		38–47	42–53	Cochrane review
Fichera et al.[75]	2009	73	106	335	322	8.3	7.4			Incisional hernia repair 7.8% open vs. 0% LAP
Chung et al.[76]	2009	37	44	223	140	4.9	8.5	9/37	21/44	1st of 3 stage procedure, 2nd stage earlier in LAP

earliest attempts at laparoscopic proctocolectomy showed longer operative time, higher blood loss, and longer hospital stay than matched open procedures, with no apparent benefit, thus discouraging this approach.[77,78] However, with advances in technology and experience gained with segmental resection, many groups have re-evaluated the role of laparoscopic total colectomy and proctocolectomy for inflammatory bowel disease.

Recent reports demonstrate that laparoscopic total colectomy and proctocolectomy with and without ileal pouch-anal anastomosis is technically feasible and shares the same advantages as seen with segmental colonic resection. Laparoscopic proctocolectomy has been performed in the elective setting, but several groups have performed laparoscopic total colectomy on an urgent basis for the patient with non-resolving acute colitis. These procedures, however, are still not recommended for the patient with toxic colitis.

One important potential benefit of a laparoscopic approach in this group of patients is a reduction in adhesions. A large multicenter randomized trial of an adhesion barrier (glycerol hyaluronate/carboxymethylcellulose bioresorbable (GHA/CMC) adhesion barrier) used the two-stage operation model in ulcerative colitis to evaluate adhesions.[79] At the second stage, i.e., ileostomy closure, laparoscopic evaluation of abdominal adhesions was performed. In the control group, without the use of the barrier, 90% of patients had adhesions to the anterior abdominal wall, compared with 67% in the study arm. Indar et al.[80] showed in a series of 34 patients (21 female) that after a laparoscopic approach to the first stage, only 32% of patients had adhesions to the anterior abdominal wall, and these were all flimsy, i.e., no dense adhesions. Also, in the 21 female patients, 15 (71%) had no adhesions to the adnexae, and in the six patients with pelvic adhesions, none had both adnexae affected. This has potential significance in the maintenance of fertility in young female patients, for whom pelvic adhesions are considered to be the most likely cause of reduced fecundity after operative intervention for ulcerative colitis.

Diverticulitis

Laparoscopic sigmoid resection remains the leading indication for minimally invasive colon resection for benign disease. The surgery is hampered by both the fibrotic changes associated with elective resection of recurrent disease and the inflammatory changes associated with acute disease. As surgeons acquire their laparoscopic skills, more complex cases involving abscess and fistulous communications have been successfully completed laparoscopically. There are now a large number of studies evaluating laparoscopic surgery for diverticulitis (Tables 35-3A and 35-3B).[81–98] These are both large case series and nonrandomized comparative studies with open resection. Most series report an operative time of 2–3 h with a conversion rate of 10–20% for larger series. The largest series of diverticular resection comes from a German multi-institutional study of 1,545 patients accumulated over 7 years at 52 institutions.[87] The study demonstrated a low morbidity and mortality with an overall conversion rate of 6.1%. As experience increased the percentage of complex cases increased without significantly altering the morbidity or rate of conversion. High-volume centers performed more of the complex cases with a similar conversion rate to the low volume centers which performed less complex cases.

Nearly all comparative studies of laparoscopic to open sigmoid resection demonstrate a benefit for the laparoscopic approach including a shorter duration of ileus, shortened length of stay, but as in other studies, with a longer operative time. Early reports suggested a higher overall cost associated with a laparoscopic approach for diverticular resection; however, more recent studies have demonstrated a cost saving with the laparoscopic approach. This cost reduction has been noted not only in the USA, but also in European countries. It should be noted that these are generally the elective uncomplicated cases with fewer patients presenting with abscess or fistula formation. For more complex cases, where the operative times are longer and the rate of conversion is higher, the cost savings benefit of a laparoscopic approach may be lost. This highlights the importance of case selection when considering a laparoscopic approach. Less experienced surgeons should consider an early conversion of complicated diverticular resection or potentially an alteration in the approach to a hybrid approach where the difficult pelvic dissection can be guided by the hand laparoscopically or by conventional means through the open wound.[99,100]

One of the more recent areas of interest – and concomitant controversy – involves the use of laparoscopic lavage and placement of drains for purulent peritonitis secondary to perforated diverticulitis. Following early sporadic reports, one of the earliest large series was from Winters' group in Dublin. Myers et al.[101] reported the results of a prospective multi-institutional study of 100 patients. Patients with perforated diverticulitis causing generalized peritonitis underwent attempted laparoscopic peritoneal lavage. The Hinchey grading system was used to record the degree of peritonitis. The median age was 62.5 years, with a male:female ratio of 2:1. Eight patients with grade 4 (feculent) diverticulitis were converted to open Hartmann's procedure. Laparoscopic lavage was performed in the other 92 patients, with morbidity and mortality rates of 4 and 3%, respectively. Two patients developed a pelvic abscess postoperatively, requiring intervention. Only two patients presented with recurrent diverticulitis at a median follow-up of 36 months. The authors concluded that laparoscopic management of perforated diverticulitis with generalized (purulent) peritonitis is feasible, with a low recurrence risk in the short term.

Franklin et al.[102] reported 40 patients undergoing laparoscopic lavage and placement of drains in complicated diverticulitis and diverticulitis without fecal peritonitis. The average operative time was 62 min and there were no conversions. Just over 50% underwent elective interval sigmoid colectomy, and none of the remaining patients required surgical intervention after 96 months follow-up. The authors note that this approach avoids a colostomy, allows elective interval sigmoidectomy, and was associated with minimal morbidity. They went as far as to state that the approach should be considered the standard of care. Alamili et al.[103]

TABLE 35-3A. Descriptive series of laparoscopic resection for diverticulitis

Study	Year	N	Mortality (%)	Morbidity (%)	Conversion (%)	OR time (min)[a]	Resume diet (day)[a]	Flatus/BM (day)[a]	LOS (day)[a]
Eijsbouts et al.[81]	1997	41	0	18	15	195	NA	NA	6.5
Stevenson et al.[82]	1998	100	0	21	8	180	2	2	4
Tuech et al.[83]	2000	77	0	17	14	NA	NA	NA	NA
Trebuchet et al.[84]	2002	170	0	8.2	4.1	141	3.4	NA	8.5
Bouillot et al.[85]	2002	179	0	15	14	223	3.3	2.5	9.3
Pugliese et al.[86]	2004	103	0	8	3	190	NA	4	9.7
Schneidbach et al.[87]	2004	1,545	0.4	17	6.1	169	NA	NA	NA
Pessaux et al.[88]	2004	582	1.2	25	NA	NA	NA	NA	NA
Schwandner et al.[89]	2005	363	0.6	22	6.6	192	2.8	4.0	11.8
Jones et al.[90]	2008	500	0.2	11	8–1.5	120	NA	NA	4

OR operating room, *BM* bowel movement, *LOS* length of stay, *NA* not available.
[a]Median or mean values listed.

TABLE 35-3B. Case–control studies of laparoscopic resection for diverticulitis

Study	Year	No. of patients		Mortality (%)		Morbidity (%)		Convert (%)	OR time (min)[a]		Resume diet (day)		Flatus/BM (day)		LOS (day)		Total costs[a]	
		CON	LAP	CON	LAP	CON	LAP		CON	LAP	CON	LAP	CON	LAP	CON	LAP	CON	LAP
Diverticulitis																		
Liberman et al.[91]	1996	14	14	0	0	14	14	0	182	192	6.1	2.9[b]	NA		9.2	6.3[b]	P 13,400	11,500
Bruce et al.[92]	1996	17	25	0	0	23	16	12	115	397[b]	5.7	3.2[b]	NA		6.8	4.2[b]	$7,068	10,230[b]
Kohler et al.[93]	1998	34	27	0	0	61	15	7	121	165[b]	5.8	4.1[b]	5.3	3.7[b]	14.3	7.9[b]	DM 8,975	7,185[b]
Senagore et al.[34]	2002	71	61	0	1.6	30	8[b]	7	101	107	NA		NA	6.8		3.1[b]	$4,321	3,458[b]
Dwivedi et al.[35]	2002	88	66	0	0	24	18	20	143	212[b]	4.9	2.9[b]	NA		8.8	4.8[b]	$14,863	13,953[b]
Lawrence et a1.[94]	2003	215	56	1.6	1	27	9[b]	7	140	170[b]	NA		NA		9.1	4.1[b]	$25,700	17,414[b]
Gonzalez et al. [95c]	2004	80	95	4	1	31	19[b]	NA	156	170	NA		3.7	2.8	12	7[b]	NA	
Alves et al.[96]	2005	169	163			31.4	16.0	15.3										
Lee et al.[97]	2006	21	21						171	197					18	10		
Shapiro et al.[98]	2008	166	80	0	0	7.8	6.3	12.5	153	185					4	8		

OR operating room, *BM* bowel movement, *LOS* length of stay, *CON* conventional surgery, *LAP* laparoscopic surgery, *NA* not available, *P* pounds, *DM* Deutsch Marks.
[a]Median or mean values listed.
[b]Statistically significant difference.
[c]Results of nonconverted laparoscopic cases given.
[d]*Minilaparotomy.*

performed a review of the literature which included eight studies, none randomized, reporting 213 patients with acute complicated diverticulitis managed by laparoscopic lavage. Mean age was 59 years and most patients had Hinchey stage III disease. Conversion to laparotomy occurred on 6 patients (3%) and the complication rate was 10%. Mean hospital stay was 9 days. After mean follow-up of 38 months, 38% underwent elective sigmoid resection. Potential benefits were acknowledged, but larger studies were recommended.

Rectal Prolapse

Full-thickness rectal prolapse repaired by an abdominal fixation procedure is potentially an ideal procedure for a laparoscopic approach since there is no specimen to remove or anastomosis to create. Early reports were primarily technical descriptions of the procedure.[104–109] A large number of studies have evaluated not only laparoscopic fixation procedures but also the combination of sigmoid resection and rectopexy for the treatment of rectal prolapse (Table 35-4).[110–125] The magnified view into the pelvis with the laparoscope provides unparalleled visualization of the pelvic floor and the relative laxity of the rectal fixation to the presacral area is beneficial to performance of a laparoscopic procedure. This likely is the reason for the relatively low rate of conversion (<10%) for a laparoscopic rectopexy or resection and rectopexy in comparison to other laparoscopic colorectal procedures. The mobilization of the rectum for rectal prolapse is an ideal procedure in which to learn the laparoscopic technique of rectal mobilization which may then be applied to other procedures such as laparoscopic proctocolectomy or total mesorectal excision for rectal cancer.

In addition to case series results there have been several nonrandomized comparative studies of laparoscopic vs. conventional rectopexy and resection rectopexy.[114,115,121] These studies showed a longer operative time of 45–60 min with the laparoscopic procedures but with a shortened length of stay of 2–3 days. Functional results following surgery were similar in laparoscopic and conventional groups, with the majority of patients reporting an improvement in incontinence and constipation. Solomon also reported a prospective randomized study of 40 patients with full-thickness rectal prolapse.[120] This was a well-designed study with the use of blinded observers, and a standardized clinical pathway for both groups. As expected, the mean surgical time was 153 min in the laparoscopic group compared to 102 min in the open group ($P<0.01$). In the laparoscopic group, however, 75% of patients followed the clinical pathways as compared to only 37% of patients in the conventional group. The mean length of stay was also less (3.9 days vs. 6.6 days, $P<0.01$) with 19/20 patients in the laparoscopic group discharged by postoperative day 5 as compared to 9/19 patients in the conventional group. There were no differences in postoperative pain scores but total intravenous narcotic usage was less in the laparoscopic group. Functional outcomes of surgery were equivalent, and there were no recurrences of prolapse in either group with a short mean follow-up of 24 months. While the study is small in size, the outcomes mirror the results of other prospective randomized studies of laparoscopic surgery for other diseases and procedures. A later cost analysis of this study demonstrated an overall mean cost savings of £357 per patient in the laparoscopic group.[126]

One of the major issues when discussing surgery for rectal prolapse is the rate of recurrent prolapse. For an abdominal approach the risk of recurrence should be less than 5–10% over 5 years. Unfortunately, the majority of reports on laparoscopic surgery for rectal prolapse have limited follow-up (less than 3 years). The reported rate of recurrence ranges from 0 to 6% in these studies (Table 35-4). Recently, however, there have been two studies with a mean follow-up of 5 years.[122,124] In a study of 42 patients by D'Hoore et al.,[122] with a mean follow-up of 61 months, the rate of recurrent prolapse was 4.8%. In the largest study of laparoscopic surgery for rectal prolapse by Ashari et al.[124], with 117 patients over a 10 year period and a mean follow-up of 62 months, the rate of recurrent full-thickness prolapse was only 2.5%. The study, however, noted an 18% rate of mucosal prolapse, which is somewhat concerning. Further long-term follow-up of these patients is needed to ensure that the rate of recurrence remains acceptable. If the rate of recurrent prolapse is confirmed to occur at a rate equal to conventional surgery, a minimally invasive approach to rectal prolapse appears to be an ideal operation for surgeons with laparoscopic skills.

One of the concerns regarding rates of recurrent prolapse is reflected in a study comparing three techniques for rectopexy: open (OR), laparoscopic (LR), and robotic rectopexy (RR).[127] All consecutive patients who underwent a rectopexy over a 7-year period were enrolled in the study. Eighty-two patients (71 females, mean age 56.4 years) underwent a rectopexy for rectal prolapse. Nine patients (11%) had a recurrence; one (2%) after OR, four (27%) after LR, and four (20%) after RR. RR showed significantly higher recurrence rates when controlled for age and follow-up time compared to OR ($P=0.027$), while LR showed near-significant higher rates ($P=0.059$). It was concluded that LR and RR were adequate procedures but have a higher risk of recurrence. A RCT was proposed to assess the definitive role of robotic assistance in laparoscopic surgery in rectopexy. This study raises concerns regarding the completeness of rectal mobilization whether performed laparoscopically or with robotic assistance. While there is much interest in utilizing the rather spectacular technical abilities of the robot, the device does not compensate for lack of advanced laparoscopic surgical skills.

Colorectal Cancer

It is estimated that more than 106,100 new cases of colon cancer (52,010 in males and 54,090 in females) and 40,870 new cases of rectal cancer (23,580 males, 17,290 females)

TABLE 35-4. Laparoscopy for rectal prolapse

Study	Year	No. of patients	Follow-up (month)	Procedure	Operative time (min) LR/LRR	LOS (day)	Recurrence (%)	Comment
Poen et al.[110]	1996	12	19	LR	195	10	0	Improved continence
Himpens et al.[111]	1999	37	6–48	LR	130	7	0	3% conversion
Stevenson et al.[112]	1998	34	18	LR/LRR	185	5	0	7% mucosal prolapse, no recurrence
Bruch et al.[113]	1999	57	30	LR/LRR	227/257	15	0	Constipation improved in 76%
Boccasanta et al.[114]	1999	10						Compared with open – longer op time, lower cost, shorter LOS
Xynos et al.[115]	1999	10	NS	LRR	130	4.7	NS	Compared with open – longer op time, shorter LOS
Kessler et al.[116]	1999	32	33	LR/LRR	150	5	FT 6.2	10% developed bowel obstruction
Heah et al.[117]	2000	25	26	LR	96	7	0	16% conversion
Kellokumpu et al.[118]	2000	34	24	LR/LRR	150/255	5	7	Constipation improved in 70%
Benoist et al.[119]	2001	48	20–47	LR/LRR	–	–	MP 8	Suture rectopexy preferred to mesh
Solomon et al.[120]	2002	20	24	LR	153	3.9	0	Prospective, randomized study
Kairaluoma et al.[121]	2003	53	12	LR/LRR	127/210	5	6	Compared with open – longer op time, shorter LOS
D'Hoore et al.[122]	2004	42	61	LR	NS	NS	FT 4.8	Constipation improved in 84%
Lechaux et al.[123]	2005	48	36	LR/LRR	193	4–7	MP 4.2	Constipation worsened in 23%
Ashari et al.[124]	2005	117	62	LRR	110–180	5	FT 2.5; MP 18	Large study with long-term follow-up
Heemskerk et al.[125]	2007	33		LR	39 min longer			OR time longer for robotic vs. LAP, more expensive

RR resection rectopexy, *PFR* pelvic floor repair, *AR* anterior resection, *FRM* full rectal mobilization without fixation, *LRR* laparoscopic resection rectopexy, *LR* laparoscopic rectopexy, *FT* full thickness, *MP* mucosal prolapse, *NS* not specified. (Adapted from: Heemskerk J, de Hoog DE, van Gemert WG, Baeten CG, Greve JW, Bouvy ND. Robot-assisted vs. conventional laparoscopic rectopexy for rectal prolapse: a comparative study on costs and time. Dis Colon Rectum 2007;50:1825–30.)[125]

were diagnosed in the USA in 2009.[128] Despite the fact that colon and rectal cancer together comprise the second most frequent cause of cancer death, the commonest source of cancer statistics[128] does not break out the mortality rates for each cancer type, resulting in 49,920 deaths for the combined groups (25,240 males, 24,680 females).

Prior to 2004, fewer than 5% of resections for colon and rectal cancer were being performed laparoscopically. There are no good sources for estimating current figures although approximately 30% of candidates for recertification for the American Board of Colon and Rectal Surgery (ABCRS) denote that they perform "some" laparoscopy. Early in the history of laparoscopic resection of colorectal cancer there was controversy related to the phenomenon of cancer implants at incision sites. Data from randomized controlled trials, however, have laid to rest these controversial aspects of the minimally invasive approach. The percentage of colon cancer cases performed laparoscopically is expected to increase, as more surgeons become familiar with these techniques, and especially as young surgeons graduate from colorectal fellowships with advanced laparoscopic skills. The issue of laparoscopic resection for rectal cancer is still unresolved. The American College of Surgeons Oncology Group (ACSOG) is sponsoring the ongoing study of laparoscopic vs. open resection for rectal cancer for advanced rectal neoplasms requiring preoperative chemoradiation.

Outcomes for Colon Cancer

After the initial success of minimally invasive techniques for cholecystectomy, reports of laparoscopic colon resections soon appeared.[129] Sadly, the specter of wound implants, or recurrence of cancer in the laparoscopic incisions, followed shortly thereafter.[130] In retrospect, it appears that as surgeons attempted to bring the benefits of minimally invasive techniques to their patients, some were performing operations for colon cancer that did not fulfill accepted oncologic principles, i.e., short-cuts were being taken with the extent of resection. Subsequent larger series by experienced surgeons showed that wound implants were not an inevitable accompaniment of the laparoscopic approach,[131] but the damage was done. From 1994 to 2004, there was essentially a moratorium on laparoscopic resection for colon cancer, with national surgical societies, such as The American Society of Colon and Rectal Surgeons (ASCRS) and the Society of American Gastrointestinal and Endoscopic Surgeons (SAGES) calling for these procedures to be performed only under the auspices of randomized controlled trials or with other means of careful prospective data collection.[132] These concerns prompted an unprecedented number of randomized controlled trials[5,6,21–24,133–136] and a new field of tumor and immunology investigation as they pertain to the pneumoperitoneum.

Lacy and colleagues[134] published the first large single-center randomized controlled trial in 2002. With median follow-up of 39 months, he and his colleagues reported higher cancer-related survival for the laparoscopic arm. Specifically, he showed no difference between arms for stage II cancers, but an improved survival for the laparoscopic approach in stage III cancers where the outcome was similar to that of stage II patients.

This was followed in 2004 by the results of the large multicenter COST study group.[29] With almost 900 patients randomized either to the open or the laparoscopic arm of the study, no differences were found in overall survival nor disease-free survival. Further reassurance was provided in finding that there were only two wound recurrences in the laparoscopic group, and one in the open arm.

The "CLASICC" trial from the United Kingdom included both colon and rectal cancers. The findings were similar, except for a rather spectacularly high rate of conversion, at 29%.[5] Those results were updated more recently in 2007.[135] Concerning issues from that trial were the very high conversion rate, the rate of positive radial margins in patients undergoing resection for rectal cancer (in both the laparoscopic *and* the open arms), and the 20% reduction in survival in patients undergoing abdominoperineal resection compared with low anterior resection. This raises very realistic concerns regarding technical issues.

The COLOR (COlon cancer Laparoscopic or Open Resection) trial was performed as a multicenter randomized trial at 37 centers throughout Europe.[6] The study accrued patients from 1997 to 2003 and there were several interim reports regarding accrual and outcomes compared with operative volumes, but the long-term oncologic outcomes were not reported until 2009, and even then only 3 year outcomes were reported.[136]

The results of these four trials are summarized in Table 35-5. Interestingly, all four studies reported the overall survival rates and disease-free survival rates for the entire study, but none actually reported the stage-specific rates. The values in the table have been obtained manually by extracting the data from graphs presented within the manuscript, and thus may have an error of 1–3% depending on the accuracy of reproduction and the thickness of the lines used within the graph.

The results of these trials (Table 35-5) have demonstrated that similar oncologic resections can be achieved by experienced surgeons performing laparoscopic colon resections. After publication of the COST study results, ASCRS and SAGES co-published an approved statement, that laparoscopic colectomy for cancer appeared to produce similar oncologic outcomes, but emphasized that these procedures should only be attempted by surgeons experienced with laparoscopic techniques.[137]

Outcomes for Rectal Cancer

Surgical resection of rectal cancer has the potential to achieve a curative result. Total mesorectal excision (TME) is currently the standard of care, minimizing the risk of local recurrence and providing accurate information regarding

TABLE 35-5. Prospective, randomized trials comparing laparoscopic and conventional surgery for colorectal cancer

	Lacy et al. 2002[134]	COST 2004[29]	CLASICC 2005[135]		COLOR 2009[136]
Baseline characteristics	LAP vs. OPEN	LAP vs. OPEN	LAP vs. OPEN		LAP vs. OPEN
No. assigned	111:108	435:437	526:268		627:621
No. completed (dead or no data)	105:101	435:428	452:231 (74:37)		534:542 (83:70)
Age	68:71	70:69	69:69		71:71
Gender (F)	55:58	49%:51%	44%:46%		48%:47%
Previous surgery	40:47	43%:46%			38%:38%
BMI					24.5:24.9
Operative findings					
Procedure					
Right	49:49	54%:54%	24%:24%		48%:47%
Left	4:1	7%:7%	7%:9%		11%:11%
Sigmoid	52:46	38%:38%	13%:12%		38%:39%
AR/LAR	3:9		37%:36%		
			12%:13%		
Other	3:3		4%:3%		4%:4%
TNM stage					
0		5%:8%	Not given		
I	27:18	35%:26%			24%:25%
II	42:48	31%:34%			43%:41%
III	37:36	26%:28%			33%:34%
IV	5:6	4%:2%			
No. lymph nodes	11.1:11.1	12:12	12:13.5		
Conversion	12 (11%):N/A	21%:N/A	29%:N/A		19%:N/A
OR time (min)	142:118[a]	150:95[a]	180:135 (anesthesia time)		
Incision length (cm)		6:18[a]	10:22		
Short-term outcomes					
Oral intake (h)	54:85[a]				
(day)			6:6		
Hospital stay (day)	5.2:7.9[a]	5:6[a]	9:11		
30-Day mortality		<1%:1%	4%:5%		
Postoperative complications	12:31[a]	19%:19%	33%:32%		21%:20%
			Colon	Rectum	
Wound infection	8:18		5%:5%	13%:12%	4%:3%
Pneumonia	0:0		7%:4%	10%:4%	1%:2%
Ileus	3:9				
Leak	0:2		2%:0%	10%:7%	3%:2%
Duration of oral analgesics (day)		1:2[a]			
Duration of parenteral analgesics (day)		3:4[a]			
Cancer outcomes					
Tumor recurrence	18:28	76:84			
Distant	7:9				56:54
Locoregional	7:14				26:26
Peritoneal seedling	3:5				
Port site	1:0	2:1	9 (2.5%):1 (0.6%)		7 (1.3%):2 (0.4%)
5-Year overall survival[b]	82%:74%	79%:78%	3-Year reported 68.4%:66.7%		3-Year reported 81.8%:84.2%
I	85%:94%	84%:94%	No graphs by TNM stage		84%:82%
II	75%:77%	78%:81%	No graphs by TNM stage		78%:82%
III	72%:45%	60%:63%	No graphs by TNM stage		62%:57%
5-Year disease-free survival[b]		78%:80%	3-Year reported 66.3%:67.7%		3-Year reported 74.2%:76.2%
I	90%:88%	92%:96%	No graphs by TNM stage		80%:77%
II	80%:76%	82%:88%	No graphs by TNM stage		70%:75%
III	70%:45%	62%:60%	No graphs by TNM stage		58%:55%
Cancer-related survival[b]	91%:79%[a]				
I	100%:99%				
II	88%:85%				
III	84%:50%[a]				

[a] Statistically significant difference.
[b] Extrapolated from graphs in manuscript.

staging, that affects prognosis and subsequent therapy. The surgical integrity and pathologic staging of the resection is the most important prognostic factor in preventing recurrent rectal cancer. Laparoscopic resection of rectal cancer must achieve at least equivalent oncologic results in comparison with open laparotomy and TME prior to becoming an established means of resection.

Early prospective studies, from experienced surgeons, suggested that laparoscopic resection did not worsen survival or disease control in patients with rectal cancer compared with open resection.[138–141] There were limited early data available from randomized controlled trials. An early study by Leung et al.[142] evaluated laparoscopic vs. open resection for rectosigmoid cancer, so this was not a trial of TME. A total of 403 patients were accrued between 1993 and 2002, 203 in the laparoscopic arm and 200 open. The probability of survival at 5 years for the laparoscopic and open resection groups were 76.1 and 72.9%, respectively. Five-year disease-free survival rates were 75.3 and 78.3%, respectively. The operative time for the laparoscopic group was significantly longer, whereas postoperative recovery was significantly better than for the open resection group. These benefits, however, were at the expense of higher direct cost. Reassuringly, the distal margin, the number of lymph nodes found in the resected specimen, overall morbidity, and operative mortality did not differ between groups.

The first randomized trial to provide outcomes for rectal cancer was not reassuring at all.[4,135] The CLASICC randomized controlled trial in the UK differed from its contemporaneous trials (COST, COLOR) in that patients with both colon cancer and rectal cancer were included. The study enrolled 268 patients to the open arm, of which 128 (48%) had rectal cancer, and 526 patients to the laparoscopic arm, of whom 253 (48%) had rectal cancer. The conversion rate for the study overall was 29%, with a 25% conversion rate for colon cancer and 34% for rectal cancer. The conversion rate dropped by year of the study, from 38% in year 1 to 16% in year 6 of the study. Operative time was longer for the laparoscopic rectal resections (180 min vs. 135 min), time to bowel movement shorter (5 days vs. 6 days), time to regular diet the same (6 days), and hospital stay shorter (11 days vs. 13 days). It was noted that the rate of positive circumferential resection margins (CRM) was the same between the two groups, but a closer look at the data is very disturbing. The CRM was positive in 14% of open patients and 16% of laparoscopic patients ($P=0.8$). Admittedly, these are not significantly different but the fact they are not different is not reassuring as the rate in the open group is hardly acceptable! In the low anterior resection group, it was noted that there was a nonsignificant trend toward a higher positive CRM rate in the laparoscopic group (12% vs. 6%, $P=0.19$). It was noted that no difference was seen in CRM positivity in the abdominoperineal group, but again the actual figures are far from reassuring with a 20% (10/49) positive rate in the open group vs. 26% (7/27) in the laparoscopic group.

Thus although the reports of the randomized controlled trials for colon cancer were reassuring, the CLASICC trial raised concerns regarding the application of laparoscopic techniques for rectal cancer. The fact that there were also high rates of CRM positivity in the open cases raised the issue of technical competence in the CLASICC trial, and deflected some of the attention away from the laparoscopic technique itself. Fortunately, overall, there were no differences in the long-term outcomes in the follow-up report of oncologic outcomes.[135] There was no statistically significant difference in 3-year overall survival for patients undergoing anterior resection (AR) or abdominal perineal resection (APR) in either technique group (AR-open 66.7%, laparoscopic 74.6%; APR-open 57.7%, laparoscopic 65.2%.) The higher positivity of the circumferential resection margin reported after laparoscopic anterior resection did not translate into an increased incidence of local recurrence. There was no difference in 3-year local recurrence rates after anterior resection of rectal cancer (7% open, 7.8% laparoscopic) or abdominoperineal resection of rectal cancer (21% open, 15% laparoscopic).

Numerous single-institution prospective case series have since supported the safety and efficacy of laparoscopic resection of rectal cancer in experienced centers and experienced hands.[143–147] Ng et al.[148] reported short-term outcomes and long-term survival in a large single-institution series of 579 patients undergoing laparoscopic resection for rectosigmoid and rectal cancer. Rectosigmoid and upper rectal cancers (12–18 cm from the anal verge), both undergoing low anterior resection, were grouped together for the subsequent analysis. Patients with tumors in the mid-rectum (7–12 cm from the anal verge) underwent sphincter-preserving TME. Patients with low-rectal tumors (<7 cm from the anal verge) underwent either TME or APR. Over a 15-year period, there were 316 laparoscopic anterior resections, 152 sphincter-preserving TME, and 92 laparoscopic APRs. Median follow-up was 56 months. Overall, early and late operative morbidity rates were 18.8 and 9.7%, respectively. The anastomotic leak rate was 3.5% ($n=20$). Conversion occurred in 31 patients (5.4%). Port site recurrence was seen in 0.4% of patients (1 laparoscopic anterior resection, 1 laparoscopic TME) and locoregional recurrence in 7.4% of patients. Microscopic resection margin involvement was identified in 6 laparoscopic TME and in 2 laparoscopic APR. Overall 5- and 10-year survival rates were 70 and 45.5%, and cancer-specific 5- and 10-year survival rates were 75 and 56%, respectively. Of note, patients in the anterior resection group were not stratified by tumor location, so the number of patients with rectosigmoid vs. upper rectal cancer is unclear. The authors concluded that laparoscopic resection for rectal cancer is safe and offers long-term oncologic outcomes equivalent to those of open resection.

In a retrospective study of 421 patients comparing outcome between open (310 patients) and laparoscopic (111) resection for stage II and stage III rectal cancer, Law et al.[149]

reported 5-year actuarial survival rates of 71.1% vs. 59.3% in the laparoscopic vs. open arms, respectively ($P=0.029$), after a median follow-up of 34 months. There was no difference in local recurrence. Laparoscopic resection was associated with decreased blood loss (200 ml vs. 350 ml, $P<0.001$) and shorter hospital stay (7 days vs. 9 days, $P<0.001$). The conversion rate was 12.5%. On multivariate analysis, laparoscopic resection was an independent factor associated with improved survival ($P=0.03$, hazards ratio 0.558 [95% confidence interval, 0.339–0.969]). There was, however, no breakdown of the number of stage II vs. stage III rectal cancer patients. The study concluded that compared to open resection, laparoscopic resection for locally advanced rectal cancer is associated with more favorable overall survival.

Thus in these large retrospective and prospective single-institution studies, the data consistently demonstrate improved early postoperative outcomes with no negative impact on oncologic outcomes, and even improved oncologic outcomes in some series. Interestingly, the potential for improved TME specimens has been demonstrated in an elegant study by Gouvas et al. [150] in 39 open and 33 laparoscopic proctectomies.

A more recent single-institution randomized controlled trial was reported by Lujan et al. [151] After neoadjuvant chemoradiation, 204 patients with mid- and low-rectal cancer were randomized to open (103) or laparoscopic resection (101). Sphincter preservation rates were not different, 78.6 and 76.2% in the open and laparoscopic group, respectively. Complication rates and involvement of CRM rates were similar, but the lymph node retrieval rates were greater in the laparoscopic group (mean 13.6 vs. 11.6). There were no differences in oncologic outcomes in terms of local recurrence, disease-free, or overall survival.

Concerns still remained regarding the applicability of laparoscopic techniques for rectal cancer outside highly specialized, high-volume institutions. For this reason, there are several multicenter randomized trials in various stages of accrual. In the USA, a prospective, multicenter randomized trial was established to determine the feasibility, reproducibility, and oncologic applicability of minimally invasive techniques in the resection of rectal cancer. [152] This study is currently accruing patients under the auspices of the ACOSOG Study AZ6051.[153] The primary objective of the trial is to test the hypothesis that laparoscopic resection of rectal cancer is not inferior to open resection. Outcomes being measured are based on a composite primary endpoint of oncologic factors which are considered to indicate a safe and feasible operation. These parameters are circumferential margin >1 mm; distal resected margin >2 cm (or >1 cm with clear frozen section in the low rectum); and completeness of TME, defined by careful evaluation by an experienced pathologist. Secondary objectives are to assess patient-related benefit of laparoscopic-assisted vs. open rectal resection (blood loss, length of stay, pain medicine utilization); to assess disease-free survival and local pelvic recurrence at 2 years; and to assess quality of life, sexual function, bowel and stoma function.

The UK MRC CLASICC trial [5,135] is close to reporting its mature 5-year data. The Japan Clinical Oncology Group Study JCOG 0404, [154] which has been evaluating laparoscopic surgery for colorectal cancer, was activated in October 2004 and is also close to reporting its long-term data. At present, the European Colon Cancer Laparoscopic or Open Resection (COLOR) II trial COLOR II is a randomized, international, multicenter study comparing the outcomes of laparoscopic and conventional resection of rectal carcinoma with curative intent. [155] Prior to its start, a feasibility study is to be performed with the objective of controlling for quality of laparoscopic TME. The primary endpoint is locoregional recurrence at 3 years. Secondary endpoints are recurrence-free and overall survival at 3, 5, and 7 years, rate of distant metastases, port site and wound site recurrences, microscopic evaluation of the resected specimen, 8 week morbidity and mortality, quality of life, and cost.

Given limited prospective data, laparoscopic resection for rectal cancer remains investigational in the USA. [156] Although it is performed in some specialist centers by experienced surgeons, open surgical resection is still the standard of care in most hands, and the role of laparoscopy is yet to be confirmed. Studies consistently show improved short-term outcomes, such as quicker recovery times, shorter hospital stays, and reduced analgesic requirements, but these are at the price of longer operative times and higher overall costs. Careful patient and tumor selection are essential. Mature 5-year data are pending from the MRC CLASICC and the JCOG 0404 trials. The European COLOR II trial and the ACOSOG-Z6051 trial, specifically comparing outcomes of laparoscopic-assisted and open resection for rectal cancer, are under way but far from reporting results.

Laparoscopic Resection of Colon and Rectal Cancer

The following description regarding the safe performance of laparoscopic resection for curable colon and rectal cancer is based on current literature and experience. The attention to technical detail is in response to the early concerns regarding oncologic outcomes. It is predicated on the understanding that patients with curable colon and rectal cancer are treated by experienced surgeons whose minimally invasive skills fulfill the Credentialing Recommendations endorsed jointly by ASCRS and SAGES. [137]

General Considerations

Following detection of a colon or rectal cancer, routine evaluation incorporates preoperative staging, assessment of resectability, and determination of the patient's operative risk. As part of this assessment, a laparoscopic approach may be contemplated. There are several factors to consider, primarily in terms of gauging the difficulty of the procedure and the likelihood of being able to perform it laparoscopically. The site of the tumor is important, as right and sigmoid colectomy are generally less technically demanding than, for example, low anterior resection. Documented extensive adhesions may preclude a minimally invasive approach, although laparoscopic resection is frequently possible in patients who have had prior abdominal operations. Obesity, and particularly the distribution of abdominal fat, may preclude laparoscopic resection, especially in the case of a rectal cancer in an obese male patient with a narrow pelvis. The patient should be informed of both laparoscopic and open alternatives, and the possible need for conversion. Above all, the surgeon must have adequate experience prior to embarking on resection for a potentially curable malignancy. Patients are increasingly sophisticated regarding their health care, and the surgeon must be prepared to answer questions about experience with the procedure.

Tumor Localization

The entire colon and rectum should be evaluated to eliminate synchronous lesions.[157,158] This is usually achieved with colonoscopy, but this has limitations in terms of localization, particularly if a minimally invasive approach is being considered. Colonoscopy is most accurate for localization of a tumor in the rectum and cecum only. Lesions elsewhere in the colon may be inaccurately localized by colonoscopy in up to 14% of cases.[159] A laparoscopic approach requires accurate localization of the tumor to a specific segment of the colon, as even a known cancer may not be visualized from the serosal aspect of the bowel during laparoscopy. The wrong segment of colon may be removed if accurate localization has not been performed.[160]

A variety of other options are available to localize a lesion including, preoperative colonoscopic marking with ink tattoo or metallic clips, barium enema, or intraoperative endoscopy. The area adjacent to a cancer or polyp may be marked either by endoscopic clips or submucosal India ink injection. If clips are placed, immediate abdominal X-rays films should be taken; otherwise, intraoperative imaging with laparoscopic ultrasound or fluoroscopy is necessary to localize the clip's location. This procedure is not commonly employed since it requires an experienced radiologist and/or endoscopist. Preoperative endoscopic tattooing is a common method of tumor localization.[161,162] India ink is a nonabsorbable marker which has been reported in more than 600 cases for tumor localization since 1975. The ink is injected into the submucosa in three or four quadrants around the lesion, or 2 cm distal to the lesion if the tumor is in the distal colon and distal margins are potentially an issue (typically, 0.5 cc per site). During diagnostic laparoscopy the ink marking can be identified even at the flexures or transverse colon. India ink injection appears to be safe with few reported complications. Intraoperative endoscopy is hampered by persistent bowel distention, prolongation of operative times, and need for equipment and endoscopist intraoperatively. More recent studies have evaluated CO_2 colonoscopy which allows for more rapid absorption of the intracolonic gas which may facilitate its use during laparoscopic procedures.[163]

Preoperative Staging

Guidelines are available for standard practices in preoperative assessment for open resection of colon or rectal cancer.[164,165] There are additional considerations with a laparoscopic approach to ensure accurate staging of the liver. In patients with colorectal cancer the liver should be thoroughly evaluated either using computed tomography with intravenous contrast, ultrasound, or magnetic resonance imaging. Due to limitation in tactile sensation associated with laparoscopy, these studies should be performed preoperatively. Alternatively, intraoperative laparoscopic ultrasonography offers the ability to fully evaluate the liver at the time of colorectal resection. Several studies have confirmed the feasibility and efficacy of laparoscopic ultrasound in the evaluation of liver metastasis from colorectal cancer.[166–168] Preoperative CT or US was a requirement of the COST randomized controlled trial.[29] No excess of stage IV disease was noted in the laparoscopic arm, suggesting that routine preoperative evaluation of the liver was equivalent in terms of oncologic outcome to palpation of the liver intraoperatively in the open arm of the study.

These considerations do not apply to rectal cancer, where staging CT scan and transanal rectal US should be routine.[165,169] Preoperative CT of the abdomen and pelvis or hepatic US are routinely utilized in planning resection of rectal cancer, as the results may markedly alter the need for neoadjuvant therapy and the timing of the operative approach.

Perioperative Preparation

Perioperative guidelines address the use of outpatient bowel preparation, prophylactic antibiotics, blood cross matching and thromboembolism prophylaxis.[164] None of these aspects of patient care are affected by a laparoscopic approach, although some surgeons prefer to modify the bowel preparation. Despite lack of clear evidence of benefit from meta-analysis[170] and randomized controlled trials,[171–175] a mechanical bowel preparation is commonly used in North America. Aside from the aesthetic aspects, an empty colon facilitates manipulation of the bowel with laparoscopic instruments. Use of large volume mechanical bowel preparations may occasionally leave fluid-filled loops of small bowel that are more difficult to handle with laparoscopic instruments. A smaller volume preparation may be used or the large volume preparation may be followed by use of laxatives such as bisacodyl to reduce the volume of residual fluid. Some surgeons use 2- to 3-day periods of preparation rather than the usual 24 h, especially if a completely laparoscopic approach and intracorporeal anastomosis is contemplated.[176]

Operative Issues

Certain operative principles pertain specifically either to the colon or to the rectum. Other issues are relevant to both.

Operative Techniques: Colon

Oncologic principles must not be compromised by a laparoscopic resection for colon cancer. Guidelines for colon cancer surgery outline recommendations for: proximal and distal resection margins (based upon the area supplied by the named feeding arterial vessel); mesenteric lymphadenectomy containing a minimum of 12 lymph nodes; and ligation of the primary feeding vessel at its base.[177] The randomized trials of laparoscopic colectomy adhered to these standard principles[5,29,134,136] and showed no significant difference in bowel margins, lymph nodes harvested, and, in the COST study, perpendicular length of the mesentery (a guide to the length of the vascular pedicle).[29] Inability to achieve these aims laparoscopically should prompt conversion to an open procedure.

These principles guide which steps of a procedure performed for cancer may be completed intracorporeally or extracorporeally. In the individual with a normal body mass index (BMI) undergoing right colectomy, it may be possible to divide the origin of the ileocolic pedicle extracorporeally using a small periumbilical extraction incision which overlies the base of the pedicle, and achieve an oncologically correct proximal ligation; intracorporeal ligation is obviously also an acceptable approach. In patients with BMI > 25, this ligation should be performed intracorporeally to ensure the base of the pedicle is ligated. Intracorporeal ligation is required for proximal division of all other vessels unless a larger incision such as used for hand-assisted devices permits access via the incision to the origin of the vascular pedicle.

Operative Techniques: Rectum

Similar guidelines exist for oncologically appropriate open rectal cancer surgery, with levels of evidence and grades of recommendation.[165,169] These include a distal margin of 1–2 cm, removal of the blood supply and lymphatics up to the origin of the superior rectal artery (or inferior mesenteric artery if indicated), and appropriate mesorectal excision with radial clearance. Again, these principles of adequate clearance of the primary tumor and supporting tissues should not be compromised by a laparoscopic approach.

There is little data from randomized trials evaluating laparoscopic resection of rectal cancer.[5,142,151] Current opinion among laparoscopic experts is that the principles outlined apply equally to laparoscopic as to open procedures. Prospective and retrospective case series[138–141,143–149,178–181] indicate that laparoscopic rectal resection is possible in selected patients. Compared with colonic resection, additional technical challenges are associated with operating within the confines of the pelvis. Multiple factors affect feasibility of an oncologically adequate laparoscopic resection for rectal cancer: tumor factors such as bulkiness, proximal or distal location; and patient factors, e.g., width of the pelvis, obesity, presence of a bulky uterus, and obscuration of tissue planes by prior radiation. Inability to perform an appropriate resection should prompt conversion.

Contiguous Organ Attachment

En bloc resection is recommended for locally advanced adherent colorectal tumors.[177] A bulky tumor invasive into an adjacent organ may be detected by preoperative imaging, such as CT scan, and guide the recommendation for an open resection. A known T4 colonic cancer will prompt an open approach in the vast majority of cases,[177] although some experienced surgeons may complete en bloc resection of involved small bowel or abdominal wall laparoscopically. If a T4 lesion is discovered intraoperatively, conversion is indicated unless the surgeon is capable of performing en bloc resection.

Prevention of Wound Implants

Port site recurrences, or wound implants, have been reported at both extraction site and trocar site incisions.[130,182] This unanticipated phenomenon has prompted extensive investigation. Current consensus is that wound implants should be kept at a rate less than 1% by correct oncologic technique and experience.

In vitro and in vivo animal models, not clinical practice, have generated most recommendations for avoidance of wound implants. Avoidance of the pneumoperitoneum and alternative gases has been evaluated. Gasless laparoscopy has shown decrease in port site metastases,[183,184] and no effect.[185,186] Tumor growth may be proportional to insufflation pressure.[187] Carbon dioxide is associated with increased tumor implantation and growth,[188] but is clinically the safest and most widely used gas. Helium decreases tumor implants but is not easily adapted to the clinical setting.[189–191] Wound excision may either decrease[192] or increase[193] the rate of tumor implants.

Some experimental results are easily adapted to the clinical setting. The significance of aerosolization of tumor implants is controverisal,[194,195] but as evacuation of the pneumoperitoneum via the ports rather than via the incision is easily performed; some experts advocate this practice.[196] Gas leakage along loosely fixed trocars (the "chimney effect") may be associated with increased cancer wound implantation[197] so some surgeons fix the trocars to prevent slippage. Irrigation of the abdominal cavity and/or trocar site incisions with a variety of substances (e.g., povidone-iodine, heparin, methotrexate, cyclophosphamide, taurolidine, and 5-fluoro-uracil) has decreased wound implants in animal models.[68,186,190,198–212]

An expert panel convened by the European Association of Endoscopic Surgery (EAES) reported that half the members irrigated the port sites and all members protected the extraction site and/or extracted the specimen in a bag.[196]

The most important development in the issue of wound implants is experience and the refinement of laparoscopic techniques and equipment that permit a true oncologic resection to be performed. Early reports of implant rates of 2–21%[130,182] have not been reproduced in large retrospective series by experienced surgeons, who reported rates of 1% or less.[131] This is similar to the incisional recurrence rate for open colorectal cancer resection.[204] The multicenter randomized trial from the COST study group reported tumor recurrence in the surgical wounds in 2 of 435 laparoscopic cases (0.5%) and in 1 of 428 patients in the open colectomy group (0.2%, $P=0.50$).[29] Lacy, in a single-center randomized trial, reported 1 implant in 111 patients for a rate of 0.9%.[134] The COST study required all surgeons to have performed at least 20 colorectal resections prior to participation in the trial.[29] The member surgeons at Lacy's institution had extensive experience. In the clinical setting, the experience of the surgeon is considered the most important factor in the prevention of implants.

Training and Credentialing in Laparoscopic Colorectal Surgery

In terms of technical complexity, laparoscopic colon and especially rectal operations are considered toward the higher end of the spectrum. Adequate resection mandates mobilization of a large structure, arranging ports to facilitate dissection in several quadrants of the abdomen, ligation of large blood vessels, extraction of a bulky specimen, and creation of a safe anastomosis. Oncologic resections have the additional requirements of adequate distal and proximal margins, wide lymphadenectomy, ligation of the origin of the primary feeding vessel, and safe handling of the bowel.

Early studies estimated the learning curve for laparoscopic colectomy to be 20–50 cases.[1–3] The randomized, controlled multicenter COST study on laparoscopic vs. open colectomy for colon cancer required each participating surgeon to have performed 20 cases.[24] This was also seen in the CLASICC trial.[5] This figure became the basis of the Approved Statement from the ASCRS and endorsed by SAGES following the publication of the results of the COST study.[137] Since the results of this trial showed that the oncologic outcomes for laparoscopic colectomy were equivalent to those of open colectomy, the statement took the unusual step of defining a specific number of cases based on the study entry criteria. The following is the approved statement:

> Laparoscopic colectomy for curable cancer results in equivalent cancer related survival to open colectomy when performed by experienced surgeons. Adherence to standard cancer resection techniques including but not limited to complete exploration of the abdomen, adequate proximal and distal margins, ligation of the major vessels at their respective origins, containment and careful tissue handling, and en bloc resection with negative tumor margins using the laparoscopic approach will result in acceptable outcomes. Based upon the COST trial,[29] prerequisite experience should include at least 20 laparoscopic colorectal resections with anastomosis for benign disease or metastatic colon cancer before using the technique to treat curable cancer. Hospitals may base credentialing for laparoscopic colectomy for cancer on experience gained by formal graduate medical educational training or advanced laparoscopic experience, participation in hands-on training courses and outcomes.[137]

The issue of defining numbers for credentialing purposes is a source of considerable controversy.[205] National surgical societies have traditionally avoided specifying required case numbers in credentialing guidelines, trying to balance the needs of their member surgeons with the safety of patients. The learning curve for laparoscopic colectomy likely varies depending on the actual procedure (as the term "laparoscopic colectomy" in this case encompasses a wide variety of procedures, from simple right colectomy to advanced proctocolectomy and J-pouch), the underlying pathologic diagnosis, and the prior laparoscopic experience of the surgeon coupled with innate skill. The COST study, however, provides a basis for specifying a minimum experience. For perspective, a resident completing a General Surgery Residency Program in 2003 and entering practice had performed a mean of 120 cases on the large intestine (mode 106, Residency Review Committee for Surgery, Reporting Period 2002–2003). Of these, an average of 50 cases required resection and anastomosis. Thus the guideline for 20 laparoscopic cases is not excessive or unreasonable in terms of attaining comparable experience prior to independent practice.

Alternative Approaches

Hand-Assisted Laparoscopy

Hand-assisted laparoscopic colectomy has been advocated as an alternative to straight laparoscopic techniques. The reintroduction of the hand back into the abdomen during laparoscopy may overcome some of the technical challenges associated with laparoscopic colectomy. Since an extraction site is required for specimen removal, supporters of a hand-assisted approach believe the hand should be placed through that wound to facilitate dissection and mobilization of the colon. Current hand-assist devices provide for hand exchanges without loss of pneumoperitoneum, allowing surgeons to perform procedures without disruption, unlike earlier versions. Opponents point out that the incision required for the hand-assist device, although smaller than for laparotomy, is still approximately twice the length of the incision required for a straight laparoscopic procedure.

There have been a number of randomized and nonrandomized studies which have evaluated hand-assisted laparoscopic colectomy.[68,206–215] In 1995, Ou[206] reported his initial experience in 12 patients undergoing colectomy by hand-assisted methods and compared it to 12 patients undergoing a conventional open method. He demonstrated that the hand-assisted procedures required on average 135 min as compared to 100 min for the standard open method. Length of stay was reduced in the hand-assisted group with an average of 5.6 days as compared to 8.3 days for open patients. Randomized trials by the HALS Study Group[209,210] and Targarona[211] have demonstrated that hand-assisted colectomy provides similar functional results to straight laparoscopic resection with fewer conversions. In a randomized study by Kang et al.[213], comparing hand-assisted vs. open colon resection, the hand-assisted approach resulted in shortened postoperative ileus, shortened length of stay, and smaller incision size with no difference in operative time or complications. Differing results were seen in another randomized study by Maartense et al.[214], which compared the results of open proctocolectomy with ileoanal pouch construction to a hand-assisted approach. In this study, there was no difference in length of stay (>10 days) and longer operative times in the hand-assisted group. The majority of patients, however, were not diverted at the time of procedure which likely impacted the results of the operation. In a study of straight laparoscopic proctocolectomy with ileoanal pouch, patients who were not diverted had a prolonged hospitalization in comparison to those who were diverted.[58] The long length of stay in the Maartense[214] study may relate to the avoidance of proximal fecal diversion and likely influenced their results and conclusions.

Nonrandomized studies have shown benefit to the hand-assisted approach in comparison to a straight laparoscopic technique, but most have a limited number of any single procedure. A study by Chang, however, did report on a large series of laparoscopic and hand-assisted sigmoid resection.[99] The results of 85 straight laparoscopic sigmoid resections were compared to 66 hand-assisted procedures. The patients shared similar demographics including a mean body mass index of 29 kg/m^2. The rate of conversion was significantly less in the hand-assisted group (0% vs. 13%, $P<0.01$) with a shortened mean operative time (189 min vs. 205 min). The mean size of the extraction was larger in the hand-assisted group (8 cm vs. 6 cm, $P<0.01$) but there was no difference in return of bowel function (mean, 2.5 days vs. 2.8 days) or the median length of stay (4 days).

One of the more challenging colorectal procedures is proctocolectomy and ileal pouch-anal anastomosis. While a few groups perform this procedure routinely, the procedures remain technically challenging with operative times in the 3–5 h range. In an effort to reduce operative times, hand-assisted techniques have been evaluated.[56,66,68] In a small comparative study, Rivadeneira et al.[66] compared the effectiveness of hand-assisted laparoscopic approach to a conventional laparoscopic method in patients undergoing laparoscopic proctocolectomy. Both groups (10 hand-assisted [HAL] vs. 13 standard laparoscopy [SL]) were well matched, with no differences in age, sex, ASA level, operative indication, steroid usage, or diagnosis. The results demonstrated no differences in incision size (mean 8 cm), operative blood loss, rate of conversion (HAL 10% vs. SL 0%), or complications (HAL 40% vs. SL 31%). The operative times progressively decreased in the hand-assisted group (mean 247 min) while remaining constant in the laparoscopic group (mean 300 min, $P<0.05$) over the period of study. This reduction in operative times has also been demonstrated in a multicenter randomized study of laparoscopic vs. hand-assisted sigmoid and total colectomy, with significantly shorter operative times in the hand-assisted group (175 min vs. 208 min in the sigmoid colectomy group, and 127 min vs. 184 min for total colectomy).[56] Another recent study by Nakajima showed similar advantages of hand-assisted total colectomy for ulcerative colitis.[68] Interestingly, the opposite was found in a case–control study from Mayo Clinic comparing 100 laparoscopic IPAA with 200 open cases.[71] Operative time for the laparoscopic group as a whole was 333 min vs. 230 min in the open group. Within the laparoscopic group, however, 75 cases were performed with a true laparoscopic approach primarily by one surgeon, and compared with 25 hand-assisted cases performed by four surgeons. The hand-assisted cases actually took longer, 372 min vs. 320 min in the true laparoscopic group, and hospital stay was a day longer (5 days vs. 4 days).

Proponents of the hand-assisted approach suggest that by returning the hand back to the abdomen, one of the potential advantages is that surgeons with less advanced laparoscopic skills may be able to perform these complex procedures more easily. In the study by Chang et al.,[99] colorectal surgeons without a large laparoscopic experience participated in 27% of hand-assisted resections compared to only 16% ($P<0.05$) of the straight laparoscopic procedures. In a similar study, comparing 85 straight laparoscopic total colectomy procedures to 45 hand-assisted operations, less experienced surgeons were able to perform 22.2% of the hand-assisted procedures and only 10.6% of the straight laparoscopic operations.[215] One interpretation is that a hand-assisted laparoscopic colectomy may be easier to adopt than a straight laparoscopic approach; an alternative interpretation is that these rates of adoption are unacceptable even with the device and perhaps such surgeons should not be attempting laparoscopic procedures.

Robotic Colorectal Surgery

The robotic device allows for precise control of movement, restoration of all the "degrees of freedom" provided by the human wrist, magnification and three-dimensional images. The most convincing application to date has been in the field of urology, where the device has allowed for intracorporeal suturing of the bladder to urethra anastomosis. Even this has been challenged recently.[216]

In the field of colorectal surgery, the use of the device remains controversial. It is hard to justify its use in colectomies. Even those who have used it for right and left colectomy have demonstrated increased operative times and increased costs.[217] It may potentially have a greater role in the resection of rectal cancer. Baik et al.[218] reported a series of 56 robotic vs. 57 laparoscopic low anterior resections for rectal cancer. The operative times were similar (190 min vs. 191 min). One benefit of the robotic approach was a reduced risk of conversion (0 in the robotic group vs. 10.5% in the laparoscopic group, $P=0.013$). The quality of the TME specimen was acceptable in both groups, but there were more complete specimens in the robotic group: the mesorectal grade was complete ($n=52$) and nearly complete ($n=4$) in the robotic group and complete ($n=43$), nearly complete ($n=12$), and incomplete ($n=2$) in the laparoscopic group ($P=0.033$). Choi et al.[219] in a series of 50 patients undergoing a standardized step-by-step approach, demonstrated a positive circumferential radial margin in only 1 of 50 patients (2%).

Patriti et al.[220] evaluated 66 patients with rectal cancer. Twenty-nine patients underwent robotic anterior resection (RAR) and 37 laparoscopic anterior resection (LAR). Groups were matched for age, BMI, sex ratio, ASA status, and TNM stage and were followed up for a mean time of 12 months. RAR resulted in shorter operative times when a total mesorectal excision was performed (166 min vs. 210 min; $P<0.05$). The conversion rate was significantly lower for RAR, with 19% conversion to open rate in the LAR group, and in the robotic group only two patients were "converted" to a laparoscopic approach but with no conversions to an open approach ($P<0.05$). Postoperative morbidity was comparable between groups. Overall survival and disease-free survival were comparable between groups; although a trend toward better disease-free survival in the RAR group was observed, the follow-up period was short. The authors concluded that RAR was a safe and feasible procedure that facilitates laparoscopic total mesorectal excision, but randomized clinical trials and longer follow-up are needed to evaluate a possible influence of the robotic approach on patient survival.

Consensus has not been reached on this approach. It is salutary to read the editorial of Cadeddu et al.[216] on robotic prostatectomy. He reflects upon the issue that marketing of the robotic device has reached such heights that opinion has "reached the level of surgical dogma among patients and physicians at the expense of objective data." The robotic device fascinates surgeons and patients alike. It is a wonderful tool. But it remains just that – a tool. Many surgeons who are currently performing advanced laparoscopic colorectal procedures have skills such that they do not require a robot. The robot may facilitate dissection in the pelvis for rectal cancer, especially for surgeons who might not otherwise be able to complete a pelvic dissection laparoscopically, but it remains to be seen if the current economic climate will continue to support expensive technology to support lack of acquisition of operative skills.

Single-Incision Colectomy

This development of single-incision colectomy is still in its seminal stages. Initial publications are primarily case reports, or press releases.[221–224] At the time of writing, there is considerable interest amongst laparoscopic aficionados regarding the potential for improved outcomes with this approach. As interest in the approach has grown, new single-port devices have been developed and several are available for use, each with their pros and cons. Reports have expanded from the original cholecystectomy,[225] to include appendectomy, sleeve gastrectomy, adrenalectomy, and colectomy. A multicenter prospective comparative study is underway to compare early results of single-incision colectomy with laparoscopic procedures. Given the difficulty of demonstrating benefits of the laparoscopic approach with laparotomy, any incremental benefits may be very difficult to confirm with current methodology, but an initial impression is that surgeons involved in this development are motivated regarding the potential benefits for their patients.

NOTES Colectomy

Natural orifice transluminal endoscopic surgery (NOTES) became a focus of intellectual and surgical creativity after the pairing of a surgeon and a gastroenterologist in India led to the release of a video of an appendectomy performed via a gastrotomy with flexible endoscopic instruments, with extraction of the specimen transorally.[226] It is now 5 years and millions of dollars of research and development money later, yet the approach is still seeking what Jeff Ponsky has referred to as the "Killer App" or the application that transcends obstacles to its use (personal communication). Although surgeons see this approach as potentially being the same quantum leap in surgical technique that laparoscopy was compared with laparotomy, there are different barriers.

There are basically three different areas of research that pertain to colorectal surgery. First, the rectum has been highlighted as a means of access to upper abdominal organs. Early procedures focused on cholecystectomy, as a common procedure, requiring limited dissection, control of a single duct and artery, and no requirement for any form of re-establishment of gastrointestinal continuity. The transgastric approach is hampered by the need for retroflexion to visualize and work on the gallbladder, need to close a gastrotomy far from the "working port" (the mouth) and limitations of the diameter of the esophagus in terms of extracting a bulky specimen. Hence, attention was redirected to using transrectal and transvaginal approaches which would permit forward-focusing of the flexible endoscopic instruments and extraction of a larger specimen. The transvaginal approach has been used primarily, as the majority of patients requiring cholecystectomy are female, and this approach affords greater confidence in the quality of the preparation. The transrectal approach does have its merits, however, and transrectal endoscopic microsurgery (TEMS) has illustrated that this path of access can be adequately prepped.

Second, and likely least pertinent, the rectum has been used as a means of obtaining access to the peritoneal cavity with a flexible instrument that is then used to perform dissection and resection of a segment of colon. Transgastric, and bidirectional approaches with both transgastric and transrectal approaches have been described. These are *tour-de-forces* of technique but not immediately relevant to clinical practice.

The third area of research has focused on use of the TEMS device as a means of access. This makes sense that the planned anastomotic site becomes the means of access to the abdominal cavity and has implications for sigmoidorectal surgery (and also for bariatric surgery with upper endoscopy using the planned anastomotic site). Several groups have described using the TEMS device to make a circumferential incision in the rectum at the planned level of anastomosis, and then continuing the dissection in the presacral space and the left retroperitoneum[227–230] The technique does not reliably allow for mobilization of the splenic flexure, so again, applications are limited at this point with current instrumentation.

Future Considerations

It is actually quite fascinating to see how slowly laparoscopic techniques for colorectal surgery have been adopted. The procedures are likely similar in terms of technical difficulty to bariatric procedures, yet the vast majority of bariatric procedures are performed laparoscopically as opposed to less than 30% of colorectal procedures. One wonders if market forces are implicated, as many bariatric procedures are not covered by insurance and the patient pays out of pocket. Over the next few years, the field of colorectal surgery may become quite divergent, especially within the subspecialist field of minimally invasive procedures. Surgeons who have adopted hand-assisted techniques may not be able to adopt single-incision techniques, if the latter prove to have benefits. The realm of NOTES is still undetermined but there will likely be considerable cross-fertilization with the techniques and instrumentation used for single-incision procedures. Bemelman[231] phrased this upcoming period best: when fast-track protocols make it difficult to differentiate laparoscopic from open approaches, then the long-term implications of a laparoscopic approach carry far more weight than such short-term benefits as time to bowel function and time in the hospital. More important are long-term outcomes such as rates of bowel obstruction and preservation of fertility. This is an exciting time for this field, not least for our patients who will hopefully continue to benefit from the extensive efforts being expended in making these major procedures less invasive.

References

1. Simons AJ, Anthone GJ, Ortega AE, et al. Laparoscopic assisted colectomy learning curve. Dis Colon Rectum. 1995;38:600–3.
2. Senagore AJ, Luchtefeld MA, Mackeigan JM. What is the learning curve for laparoscopic colectomy? Am Surg. 1995;61:681–5.
3. Wishner JD, Baker JWJ, Hoffman GC, et al. Laparoscopic assisted colectomy. The learning curve. Surg Endosc. 1995;9:1179–83.
4. Park IJ, Choi GS, Lim KH, Kang BM, Jun SH. Multidimensional analysis of the learning curve for laparoscopic colorectal surgery: lessons from 1,000 cases of laparoscopic colorectal surgery. Surg Endosc. 2009;23:839–46.
5. Guillou PJ, Quirke P, Thorpe H, et al. Short-term endpoints of conventional vs. laparoscopic-assisted surgery in patients with colorectal cancer (MRC-CLASICC trial): multicenter, randomized controlled trial. Lancet. 2005;365:1718–26.
6. The COLOR Study Group. Impact of hospital case volume on short-term outcome after laparoscopic operation for colonic cancer. Surg Endosc. 2005;19:687–92.
7. Hyman N. How much colorectal surgery do general surgeons do? J Am Coll Surg. 2002;194:37–9.
8. Tuech JJ, Regenet N, Hennekinne S, et al. Laparoscopic colectomy for sigmoid diverticulitis in obese and nonobese patients: a prospective comparative study. Surg Endosc. 2001; 15:1427–30.
9. Stern LE, Chang YJ, Marcello PW, et al. Is obesity a contraindication to laparoscopic colectomy? A case control study. Dis Colon Rectum. 2004;47:583.
10. Delaney CP, Pokala N, Senagore AJ, et al. Is laparoscopic colectomy applicable to patients with body mass index >30? A case-matched comparative study with open colectomy. Dis Colon Rectum. 2005;48:975–81.
11. Bauer JJ, Harris MT, Grumbach NM, et al. Laparoscopic assisted intestinal resection for Crohn's disease. Which patients are good candidates? J Clin Gastroenterol. 1996;23:44–6.
12. Sher ME, Agachan F, Bortul JJ, et al. Laparoscopic surgery for diverticulitis. Surg Endosc. 1997;11:264–7.
13. Pokala N, Delaney CP, Brady KM, Senagore AJ. Elective laparoscopic surgery for benign internal enteric fistulas: a review of 43 cases. Surg Endosc. 2005;19:222–5.
14. Bartus CM, Lipof T, Sarwar S, et al. Colovesical fistula: not a contraindication to elective laparoscopic colectomy. Dis Colon Rectum. 2005;48:233–6.
15. Regan JP, Salky BA. Laparoscopic treatment of enteric fistulas. Surg Endosc. 2004;18:252–4.
16. Young-Fadok TM, COST Study Group. Conversion does not adversely affect oncologic outcomes after laparoscopic colectomy for colon cancer: results from a multicenter prospective randomized study [abstract]. Dis Colon Rectum. 2005;48:637–8.
17. Casillas S, Delaney CP, Senagore AJ, et al. Does conversion of a laparoscopic colectomy adversely affect patient outcome? Dis Colon Rectum. 2004;47:1680–5.
18. Bohm B, Milsom JW, Fazio VW. Postoperative intestinal motility following conventional and laparoscopic intestinal surgery. Arch Surg. 1995;130:415–9.
19. Bessler M, Whelan RL, Halverson A, et al. Controlled trial of laparoscopic-assisted vs open colon resection in a porcine model. Surg Endosc. 1996;10:732–5.

20. Hotokezaka M, Combs MJ, Schirmer BD. Recovery of gastrointestinal motility following open versus laparoscopic colon resection in dogs. Dig Dis Sci. 1996;41:705–10.
21. Milsom JW, Bohm B, Hammerhofer KA, et al. A prospective, randomized trial comparing laparoscopic versus conventional techniques in colorectal cancer surgery: a preliminary report. J Am Coll Surg. 1998;187:46–54.
22. Stage JG, Schulze S, Moller P, et al. Prospective randomized study of laparoscopic versus open colonic resection for adenocarcinoma. Br J Surg. 1997;84:391–6.
23. Schwenk W, Böhm W, Müller JM. Postoperative pain and fatigue after laparoscopic or conventional colorectal resections: a prospective randomized trial. Surg Endosc. 1998;12:1131–6.
24. Weeks JC, Nelson H, Gelber S, et al. Short-term quality-of-life outcomes following laparoscopic-assisted colectomy vs open colectomy for colon cancer: a randomized trial. JAMA. 2002;287:321–8.
25. Fleshman JW, Fry RD, Birnbaum EH, et al. Laparoscopic assisted and minilaparotomy approaches to colorectal diseases are similar in early outcome. Dis Colon Rectum. 1996;39:15–22.
26. Senagore AJ, Duepree HJ, Delaney CP, et al. Results of a standardized technique and postoperative care plan for laparoscopic sigmoid colectomy. Dis Colon Rectum. 2003;46:503–9.
27. Raue W, Haase O, Junghans T, et al. "Fast-track" multimodal rehabilitation program improves outcome after laparoscopic sigmoidectomy. Surg Endosc. 2004;18:1463–8.
28. Psaila J, Bulley SH, Ewings P, et al. Outcome following laparoscopic resection for colorectal cancer. Br J Surg. 1998;85:662–4.
29. Nelson H, The Clinical Outcomes of Surgical Therapy Study Group. A comparison of laparoscopically assisted and open colectomy for colon cancer. N Engl J Med. 2004;350:2050–9.
30. Chen HH, Wexner SD, Weiss EG, et al. Laparoscopic colectomy for benign colorectal disease is associated with a significant reduction in disability as compared with laparotomy. Surg Endosc. 1998;12:1397–400.
31. Young-Fadok TM, Hall Long K, McConnell EJ, et al. Advantages of laparoscopic resection for ileocolic Crohn's disease. Improved outcomes and reduced costs. Surg Endosc. 2001;15:450–4.
32. Dupree HJ, Senagore AJ, Delaney CP, et al. Advantages of laparoscopic resection for ileocecal Crohn's disease. Dis Colon Rectum. 2002;45:605–10.
33. Shore G, Gonzalez QH, Bondora A, et al. Laparoscopic vs. conventional ileocolectomy for primary Crohn's disease. Arch Surg. 2003;138:76–9.
34. Senagore AJ, Duepree HJ, Delaney CP, et al. Cost structure of laparoscopic and open sigmoid colectomy for diverticular disease: similarities and differences. Dis Colon Rectum. 2002;45:485–90.
35. Dwivedi A, Chachin F, Agrawal S, et al. Laparoscopic colectomy vs. open colectomy for sigmoid diverticular disease. Dis Colon Rectum. 2002;45:1309–15.
36. Wu JS, Birnbaum EH, Kodner IJ, et al. Laparoscopic-assisted ileocolic resections in patients with Crohn's disease: are abscesses, phlegmons, or recurrent disease contraindications? Surgery. 1997;122:682–8.
37. Dunker MS, Stiggelbout AM, van Hogezand RA, et al. Cosmesis and body image after laparoscopic-assisted and open ileocolic resection for Crohn's disease. Surg Endosc. 1998;12:1334–40.
38. Wong SK, Marcello PW, Hammerhoffer KA, et al. Laparoscopic surgery for Crohn's disease: an analysis of 92 cases. Surg Endosc. 1999;13:S4.
39. Canin-Endres J, Salky B, Gattorno F, et al. Laparoscopic assisted intestinal resection in 88 patients with Crohn's disease. Surg Endosc. 1999;13:595–9.
40. Alabaz O, Irotulam AJ, Nessim A, et al. Comparison of laparoscopically assisted and conventional ileocolic resection for Crohn's disease. Eur J Surg. 2000;166:213–7.
41. Bemelman WA, Slors JFM, Dunker MS, et al. Laparoscopic assisted vs open ileocolic resection for Crohn's disease: a comparative study. Surg Endosc. 2000;14:721–5.
42. Schmidt M, Talamini MA, Kaufman HS, et al. Laparoscopic surgery for Crohn's disease: a single institution experience. Ann Surg. 2001;233:733–9.
43. Milsom JW, Hammerhofer KA, Bohm B, et al. A prospective, randomized trial comparing laparoscopic versus conventional surgery for refractory ileocolic Crohn's disease. Dis Colon Rectum. 2001;44:1–9.
44. Evans J, Poritz L, MacRae H. Influence of experience on laparoscopic ileocolic resection for Crohn's disease. Dis Colon Rectum. 2002;45:1595–600.
45. Benoist S, Panis Y, Beaufour A, et al. Laparoscopic ileocecal resection in Crohn's disease: a case-matched comparison with open resection. Surg Endosc. 2003;17:814–8.
46. Tabet J, Hong D, Kim CW, et al. Recurrence after laparoscopic bowel resection for Crohn's disease: comparison to open technique. Can J Gastroenterol. 2001;15:237–42.
47. Bergamaschi R, Pessaux P, Arneaud JP. Comparison of conventional and laparoscopic ileocolic resection for Crohn's disease. Dis Colon Rectum. 2003;46:1129–33.
48. Meijerink WJH, Eijsbouts QAJ, Cuesta MA, et al. Laparoscopically assisted bowel surgery for inflammatory bowel disease. Surg Endosc. 1999;13:882–6.
49. Huilgol RL, Wright CM, Solomon MJ. Laparoscopic versus open ileocolic resection for Crohn's disease. J Laparoendosc Adv Surg Tech A. 2004;14:61–5.
50. Rosman AS, Melis M, Fichera A. Metaanalysis of trials comparing laparoscopic and open surgery for Crohn's disease. Surg Endosc. 2005;19:1549–55.
51. Tilney HS, Constantinides VA, Heriot AG, Nicolaou M, Athanasiou T, Ziprin P, et al. Comparison of laparoscopic and open ileocecal resection for Crohn's disease: a metaanalysis. Surg Endosc. 2006;20:1036–44.
52. Tan JJ, Tjandra JJ. Laparoscopic surgery for Crohn's disease: a meta-analysis. Dis Colon Rectum. 2007;50:576–85.
53. Lesperance K, Martin MJ, Lehmann R, Brounts L, Steele SR. National trends and outcomes for the surgical therapy of ileocolonic Crohn's disease: a population-based analysis of laparoscopic vs. open approaches. J Gastrointest Surg. 2009;13:1251–9.
54. Soop M, Larson DW, Malireddy K, Cima RR, Young-Fadok TM, Dozois EJ. Safety, feasibility, and short-term outcomes of laparoscopically assisted primary ileocolic resection for Crohn's disease. Surg Endosc. 2009;23:1876–81.
55. Nguyen SQ, Teitelbaum E, Sabnis AA, Bonaccorso A, Tabrizian P, Salky B. Laparoscopic resection for Crohn's disease: an experience with 335 cases. Surg Endosc. 2009;23:2380–4.
56. Marcello PW, Fleshman JW, Milsom JW, Read TE, Arnell TD, Birnbaum EH, et al. Hand-assisted laparoscopic vs. laparoscopic

colorectal surgery: a multicenter, prospective, randomized trial. Dis Colon Rectum. 2008;51:818–26. discussion 826–8.
57. Polle SW, Dunker MS, Slors JF, Sprangers MA, Cuesta MA, Gouma DJ, et al. Body image, cosmesis, quality of life, and functional outcome of hand-assisted laparoscopic versus open restorative proctocolectomy: long-term results of a randomized trial. Surg Endosc. 2007;21:1301–7.
58. Marcello PW, Milsom JW, Wong SK, et al. Laparoscopic restorative proctocolectomy: a case-matched comparative study with open restorative proctocolectomy. Dis Colon Rectum. 2000;43:604–8.
59. Seshadri PA, Poulin EC, Schlachta CM, et al. Laparoscopic total colectomy and proctocolectomy: short and long term results. Surg Endosc. 2001;15:837–42.
60. Hamel C, Hilderbrandt U, Weiss E, et al. Laparoscopic surgery for inflammatory bowel disease: ileocolic resection versus subtotal colectomy. Surg Endosc. 2001;15:642–5.
61. Marcello PW, Milsom JW, Wong SK, et al. Laparoscopic total colectomy for acute colitis: a case control study. Dis Colon Rectum. 2001;44:1441–5.
62. Brown SR, Eu KW, Seow-Choen F. Consecutive series of laparoscopic-assisted vs. minilaparotomy restorative proctocolectomies. Dis Colon Rectum. 2001;44:397–400.
63. Dunker MS, Bemelman WA, Slors JF, et al. Functional outcome, quality of life, body image, and cosmesis in patients after laparoscopic-assisted and conventional restorative proctocolectomy: a comparative study. Dis Colon Rectum. 2001;44:1800–7.
64. Ky AJ, Sonoda T, Milsom JW. One-stage laparoscopic restorative proctocolectomy: an alternative to the conventional approach? Dis Colon Rectum. 2002;45:207–11.
65. Bell RL, Seymour NE. Laparoscopic treatment of fulminant ulcerative colitis. Surg Endosc. 2002;16:1778–82.
66. Rivadeneira DE, Marcello PW, Roberts PL, et al. Benefits of hand-assisted laparoscopic restorative proctocolectomy: a comparative study. Dis Colon Rectum. 2004;47:1371–6.
67. Kienle P, Weitz J, Benner A, et al. Laparoscopically assisted colectomy and ileoanal pouch procedure with and without protective ileostomy. Surg Endosc. 2003;17:716–20.
68. Nakajima K, Lee SW, Cocilovo C, et al. Hand assisted laparoscopic colorectal surgery using Gelport: initial experience with a new hand access device. Surg Endosc. 2004;18:102–5.
69. Schmitt SL, Cohen SM, Wexner SD, et al. Does laparoscopic assisted ileal pouch anal anastomosis reduce the length of hospitalization? Int J Colorectal Dis. 1994;9:134–7.
70. Maartense S, Dunker MS, Slors JF, Cuesta MA, Gouma DJ, van Deventer SJ, et al. Hand-assisted laparoscopic versus open restorative proctocolectomy with ileal pouch anal anastomosis: a randomized trial. Ann Surg. 2004;240:984–91.
71. Larson DW, Cima RR, Dozois EJ, Davies M, Piotrowicz K, Barnes SA, et al. Safety, feasibility, and short-term outcomes of laparoscopic ileal-pouch-anal anastomosis: a single institutional case-matched experience. Ann Surg. 2006;243:667–70. discussion 670–2.
72. Zhang H, Hu S, Zhang G, Wang K, Chen B, Li B, et al. Laparoscopic versus open proctocolectomy with ileal pouch-anal anastomosis. Minim Invasive Ther Allied Technol. 2007;16:187–91.
73. Benavente-Chenhalls L, Mathis KL, Dozois EJ, Cima RR, Pemberton JH, Larson DW. Laparoscopic ileal pouch-anal anastomosis in patients with chronic ulcerative colitis and primary sclerosing cholangitis: a case-matched study. Dis Colon Rectum. 2008;51:549–53.
74. Ahmed Ali U, Keus F, Heikens JT, Bemelman WA, Berdah SV, Gooszen HG, van Laarhoven CJ. Open versus laparoscopic (assisted) ileo pouch anal anastomosis for ulcerative colitis and familial adenomatous polyposis. Cochrane Database Syst Rev 2009;(1):CD006267.
75. Fichera A, Silvestri MT, Hurst RD, Rubin MA, Michelassi F. Laparoscopic restorative proctocolectomy with ileal pouch anal anastomosis: a comparative observational study on long-term functional results. J Gastrointest Surg. 2009;13:526–32.
76. Chung TP, Fleshman JW, Birnbaum EH, Hunt SR, Dietz DW, Read TE, et al. Laparoscopic vs. open total abdominal colectomy for severe colitis: impact on recovery and subsequent completion restorative proctectomy. Dis Colon Rectum. 2009;52:4–10.
77. Wexner SD, Johansen OB, Nogueras JJ, Jagelman DG. Laparoscopic total abdominal colectomy. A prospective trial. Dis Colon Rectum. 1992;35:651–5.
78. Reissman P, Salky BA, Pfeifer J, et al. Laparoscopic surgery in the management of inflammatory bowel disease. Am J Surg. 1996;171:47–50.
79. Cohen Z, Senagore AJ, Dayton MT, Koruda MJ, Beck DE, Wolff BG, et al. Prevention of postoperative abdominal adhesions by a novel, glycerol/sodium hyaluronate/carboxymethylcellulose-based bioresorbable membrane: a prospective, randomized, evaluator-blinded multicenter study. Dis Colon Rectum. 2005;48:1130–9.
80. Indar AA, Efron JE, Young-Fadok TM. Laparoscopic ileal pouch-anal anastomosis reduces abdominal and pelvic adhesions. Surg Endosc. 2009;23:174–7.
81. Eijsbouts QA, Cuesta MA, de Brauw LM, et al. Elective laparoscopic-assisted sigmoid resection for diverticular disease. Surg Endosc. 1997;11:750–3.
82. Stevenson AR, Stitz RW, Lumley JW, et al. Laparoscopically assisted anterior resection for diverticular disease: follow-up of 100 consecutive patients. Ann Surg. 1998;227:335–42.
83. Tuech JJ, Pessaux P, Rouge C, et al. Laparoscopic vs open colectomy for sigmoid diverticulitis: a prospective comparative study in the elderly. Surg Endosc. 2000;14:1031–3.
84. Trebuchet G, Lechaux D, Leclave JL. Laparoscopic left colon resection for diverticular disease: results of 170 consecutive cases. Surg Endosc. 2002;16:18–21.
85. Bouillot JL, Berthou JC, Champault G, et al. Elective laparoscopic colonic resection for diverticular disease. Surg Endosc. 2002;16:1320–3.
86. Pugliese R, Di Lernia S, Sansonna F, et al. Laparoscopic treatment of sigmoid diverticulitis: a retrospective review of 103 cases. Surg Endosc. 2004;18:1344–8.
87. Schneidbach H, Schneider C, Rose J, et al. Laparoscopic approach to treatment of sigmoid diverticulitis: changes in the spectrum of indications and results of a prospective, multicenter study on 1545 patients. Dis Colon Rectum. 2004;47:1883–8.
88. Pessaux P, Muscari F, Ouellet JF, et al. Risk factors for mortality and morbidity after elective sigmoid resection for diverticulitis: prospective multicenter multivariate analysis of 582 patients. World J Surg. 2004;28:92–6.
89. Schwandner O, Farke S, Bruch HP. Laparoscopic colectomy for diverticulitis is not associated with increased morbidity

when compared with nondiverticular disease. Int J Colorectal Dis. 2005;20:165–72.
90. Jones OM, Stevenson AR, Clark D, Stitz RW, Lumley JW. Laparoscopic resection for diverticular disease: follow-up of 500 consecutive patients. Ann Surg. 2008;248:1092–7.
91. Liberman MA, Phillips EH, Carroll BJ, et al. Laparoscopic colectomy vs traditional colectomy for diverticulitis. Outcome and costs. Surg Endosc. 1996;10:15–8.
92. Bruce CJ, Coller JA, Murray JJ, et al. Laparoscopic resection for diverticular disease. Dis Colon Rectum. 1996;39:S1–6.
93. Kohler L, Rixen D, Troidl H. Laparoscopic colorectal resection for diverticulitis. Int J Colorectal Dis. 1998;13:43–7.
94. Lawrence DM, Pasquale MD, Wasser TE. Laparoscopic versus open sigmoid colectomy for diverticulitis. Am Surg. 2003;69:499–504.
95. Gonzalez R, Smith CD, Mattar SG, et al. Laparoscopic vs open resection for the treatment of diverticular disease. Surg Endosc. 2004;18:276–80.
96. Alves A, Panis Y, Slim K, Heyd B, Kwiatkowski F, MAntion G. Association Francais de Chirurgie. French multicentre prospective observational study of laparoscopic versus open colectomy for sigmoid diverticular disease. Br J Surg. 2005;92:1520–5.
97. Lee SW, Yoo J, Dujovny N, Sonoda T, Milsom JW. Laparoscopic vs. hand-assisted laparoscopic sigmoidectomy for diverticulitis. Dis Colon Rectum. 2006;49:464–9.
98. Shapiro SB, Lambert PJ, Mathiason MA. A comparison of open and laparoscopic techniques in elective resection for diverticular disease. WMJ. 2008;107:287–91.
99. Chang YJ, Marcello PW, Rusin LC, et al. Hand assisted laparoscopic colectomy: a helping hand or hindrance? Surg Endosc. 2005;19:656–61.
100. Rink AD, John-Enzenauer K, Haaf F, Straub E, Nagelschmidt M, Vestweber KH. Laparoscopic-assisted or laparoscopic-facilitated sigmoidectomy for diverticular disease? A prospective randomized trial on postoperative pain and analgesic consumption. Dis Colon Rectum. 2009;52:1738–45.
101. Myers E, Hurley M, O'Sullivan GC, Kavanagh D, Wilson I, Winter DC. Laparoscopic peritoneal lavage for generalized peritonitis due to perforated diverticulitis. Br J Surg. 2008;95:97–101.
102. Franklin Jr ME, Portillo G, Trevino JM, Gonzalez JJ, Glass JL. Long-term experience with the laparoscopic approach to perforated diverticulitis plus generalized peritonitis. World J Surg. 2008;32:1507–11.
103. Alamili M, Gogenur I, Rosenberg J. Acute complicated diverticulitis managed by laparoscopic lavage. Dis Colon Rectum. 2009;52:1345–9.
104. Berman IR. Sutureless laparoscopic rectopexy for procidentia: technique and implications. Dis Colon Rectum. 1992;35:689–93.
105. Kwok SP, Carey DP, Lau WY, Li AK. Laparoscopic rectopexy. Dis Colon Rectum. 1994;37:947–8.
106. Cuschieri A, Shimi SM, Vander Velpen G, et al. Laparoscopic prosthesis fixation rectopexy for rectal prolapse. Br J Surg. 1994;81:38–9.
107. Graf W, Stefanson T, Arvidson D, Pahlmann L. Laparoscopic suture rectopexy. Dis Colon Rectum. 1995;38:211–2.
108. Darzi A, Henery MM, Guillou PJ, et al. Stapled laparoscopic rectopexy for rectal prolapse. Surg Endosc. 1995;9:301–3.
109. Solomon MJ, Eyers AA. Laparoscopic rectopexy using mesh fixation with a spiked chromium staple. Dis Colon Rectum. 1996;39:279–84.
110. Poen AC, de Brauw M, Felt-Bersma RJ, et al. Laparoscopic rectopexy for complete rectal prolapse. Clinical outcome and anorectal function tests. Surg Endosc. 1996;10:904–8.
111. Himpens J, Cadiere GB, Brutns J, Vertruyen M. Laparoscopic rectopexy according to Wells. Surg Endosc. 1999;13:139–41.
112. Stevenson AR, Stitz RW, Lumley JW. Laparoscopic-assisted resection rectopexy for rectal prolapse: early and medium follow-up. Dis Colon Rectum. 1998;41:46–54.
113. Bruch HP, Herold A, Schiedeck T, Schwandner O. Laparoscopic surgery for rectal prolapse and outlet obstruction. Dis Colon Rectum. 1999;42:1189–94.
114. Boccasanta P, Venturi M, Reitano MC, et al. Laparotomic vs. laparoscopic rectopexy in complete rectal prolapse. Dig Surg. 1999;16:415–9.
115. Xynos E, Chrysos E, Tsiaoussis J, et al. Resection rectopexy for rectal prolapse: the laparoscopic approach. Surg Endosc. 1999;13:862–4.
116. Kessler H, Jerby BL, Milsom JW. Successful treatment of rectal prolapse by laparoscopic suture rectopexy. Surg Endosc. 1999;13:858–61.
117. Heah SM, Hartley JE, Hurley J, et al. Laparoscopic suture rectopexy without resection is effective treatment for full thickness rectal prolapse. Dis Colon Rectum. 2000;43:638–43.
118. Kellokumpu IH, Vironen J, Scheinin T. Laparoscopic repair of rectal prolapse: a prospective study evaluating surgical outcome and changes in symptoms and bowel function. Surg Endosc. 2000;14:634–40.
119. Benoist S, Taffinder N, Gould S, et al. Functional results two years after laparoscopic rectopexy. Am J Surg. 2001;182:168–73.
120. Solomon MJ, Young CJ, Eyers AA, Roberts RA. Randomized clinical trial of laparoscopic versus open abdominal rectopexy for rectal prolapse. Br J Surg. 2002;89:35–9.
121. Kairaluoma MV, Viljakka MT, Kellokumpu IH. Open vs. laparoscopic surgery for rectal prolapse: a case-controlled study assessing short-term outcomes. Dis Colon Rectum. 2003;46:353–60.
122. D'Hoore A, Cadoni R, Penninckx F. Long-term outcome of ventral rectopexy for total rectal prolapse. Br J Surg. 2004;91:1500–5.
123. Lechaux D, Trebuchet G, Siproudhis L, Campion JP. Laparoscopic rectopexy for full-thickness rectal prolapse: a single-institution retrospective study evaluating surgical outcome. Surg Endosc. 2005;19:514–8.
124. Ashari LH, Lumley JW, Stevenson ARL, Stitz RW. Laparoscopically-assisted resection rectopexy for rectal prolapse: ten years' experience. Dis Colon Rectum. 2005;48:982–7.
125. Heemskerk J, de Hoog DE, van Gemert WG, Baeten CG, Greve JW, Bouvy ND. Robot-assisted vs. conventional laparoscopic rectopexy for rectal prolapse: a comparative study on costs and time. Dis Colon Rectum. 2007;50:1825–30.
126. Salkeld G, Bagia M, Solomon M. Economic impact of laparoscopic versus open abdominal rectopexy. Br J Surg. 2004;91:1188–91.
127. de Hoog DE, Heemskerk J, Nieman FH, van Gemert WG, Baeten CG, Bouvy ND. Recurrence and functional results after open versus conventional laparoscopic versus robot-assisted laparoscopic rectopexy for rectal prolapse: a case–control study. Int J Colorectal Dis. 2009;24:1201–6.

128. Jemal A, Siegel R, Ward E, et al. Cancer statistics, 2009. CA Cancer J Clin. 2009;59:225–49.
129. Jacobs M, Verdeja JC, Goldstein HS. Minimally invasive colon resection (laparoscopic colectomy). Surg Laparosc Endosc. 1991;1:144–50.
130. Johnstone PAS, Rohde DC, Swartz SE, Fetter JE, Wexner SD. Port site recurrences after laparoscopic and thoracoscopic procedures in malignancy. J Clin Oncol. 1996;14:1950–6.
131. Fleshman JW, Nelson H, Peters WR, Kim HC, Larach S, Boorse RR, et al. Early results of laparoscopic surgery for colorectal cancer. Retrospective analysis of 372 patients treated by Clinical Outcomes of Surgical Therapy (COST) Study Group. Dis Colon Rectum. 1996;39(10 Suppl):53–8.
132. American Society of Colon and Rectal Surgeons. Approved statement on laparoscopic colectomy. Dis Colon Rectum. 1994;37:638.
133. Stocchi L, Nelson H. Laparoscopic colectomy for colon cancer: trial update. J Surg Oncol. 1998;68:255–67.
134. Lacy AM, García-Valdecasas JC, Delgado S, et al. Laparoscopy-assisted colectomy versus open colectomy for treatment of non-metastatic colon cancer: a randomised trial. Lancet. 2002;359:2224–9.
135. Jayne DG, Guillou PJ, Thorpe H, Quirke P, Copeland J, Smith AM, et al. CLASICC Trial Group. Randomized trial of laparoscopic-assisted resection of colorectal carcinoma: 3-year results of the UK MRC CLASICC Trial Group. J Clin Oncol. 2007;25:3061–8.
136. Colon Cancer Laparoscopic or Open Resection Study Group, Buunen M, Veldkamp R, Hop WC, Kuhry E, Jeekel J, et al. Survival after laparoscopic surgery versus open surgery for colon cancer: long-term outcome of a randomised clinical trial. Lancet Oncol. 2009;10:44–52.
137. The American Society of Colon and Rectal Surgeons. Approved statement: laparoscopic colectomy for curable cancer. Dis Colon Rectum. 2004;47(8):A1.
138. Fleshman JW, Wexner SD, Anvari M, LaTulippe J-F, et al. Laparoscopic vs. open abdominoperineal resection for cancer. Dis Colon Rectum. 1999;42:930–9.
139. Kockerling F, Scheidbach H, Schneider C, Barlehner E, The Laparoscopic Colorectal Surgery Study Group, et al. Laparoscopic abdominoperineal resection: early postoperative results of a prospective study involving 116 patients. Dis Colon Rectum. 2000;43:1503–11.
140. Feliciotti F, Guerrieri M, Paganini AM, DeSanctis A, et al. Long term results of laparoscopic vs open resections for rectal cancer for 124 unselected patients. Surg Endosc. 2003;17:1530–5.
141. Morino M, Parini U, Giraudo G, et al. Laparoscopic total mesorectal excision: a consecutive series of 100 patients. Ann Surg. 2003;237:335–42.
142. Leung KL, Kwok SP, Lam SC, Lee JF, Yiu RY, Ng SS, et al. Laparoscopic resection of rectosigmoid carcinoma: prospective randomised trial. Lancet. 2004;363:1187–92.
143. Fukunaga Y, Higashino M, Tanimura S, Takemura M, Fujiwara Y. Laparoscopic rectal surgery for middle and lower rectal cancer. Surg Endosc. 2010;24:145–51.
144. Biondo S, Ortiz H, Lujan J, Codina-Cazador A, Espin E, Garcia-Granero E, et al. Quality of mesorectum after laparoscopic resection for rectal cancer – results of an audited teaching programme in Spain. Colorectal Dis. 2010;12:24–31. Comment in: Colorectal Dis 2010;12:31–2.
145. Bege T, Lelong B, Esterni B, Turrini O, Guiramand J, Francon D, et al. The learning curve for the laparoscopic approach to conservative mesorectal excision for rectal cancer: lessons drawn from a single institution's experience. Ann Surg. 2010;251:249–53.
146. Kim JG, Heo YJ, Son GM, Lee YS, Lee IK, Suh YJ, et al. Impact of laparoscopic surgery on the long-term outcomes for patients with rectal cancer. ANZ J Surg. 2009;79:817–23.
147. Laurent C, Leblanc F, Wutrich P, Scheffler M, Rullier E. Laparoscopic versus open surgery for rectal cancer: long-term oncologic results. Ann Surg. 2009;250:54–61.
148. Ng KH, Ng DC, Cheung HY, et al. Laparoscopic resection for rectal cancers: lessons learned from 579 cases. Ann Surg. 2009;249:82–6.
149. Law WL, Poon JT, Fan JK, et al. Comparison of outcome of open and laparoscopic resection for stage II and stage III rectal cancer. Ann Surg Oncol. 2009;16:1488–93.
150. Gouvas N, Tsiaoussis J, Pechlivanides G, Tzortzinis A, Dervenis C, Avgerinos C, et al. Quality of surgery for rectal carcinoma: comparison between open and laparoscopic approaches. Am J Surg. 2009;198:702–8.
151. Lujan J, Valero G, Hernandez Q, Sanchez A, Frutos MD, Parrilla P. Randomized clinical trial comparing laparoscopic and open surgery in patients with rectal cancer. Br J Surg. 2009;96:982–9.
152. Fleshman J. American College of Surgeons Oncology Group (ACOSOG)-Z6051. A phase III prospective randomized trial comparing laparoscopic-assisted resection versus open resection for rectal cancer. http://clinicaltrials.gov/ct2/show/NCT00726622.
153. https://www.acosog.org/studies/gastrointestinal-cancer-studies-pancreas-rectum.
154. Kitano S, Inomata M, Sato A, et al. Randomized controlled trial to evaluate laparoscopic surgery for colorectal cancer: Japan Clinical Oncology Group Study JCOG 0404. Jpn J Clin Oncol. 2005;35:475–7.
155. COLOR II. A randomized clinical trial comparing laparoscopic and open surgery for rectal cancer. http://clinicaltrials.gov/ct2/show/NCT00297791?term=color+II&rank=1.
156. Row D, Weiser MR. An update on laparoscopic resection for rectal cancer. Cancer Control. 2010;17:16–24.
157. Simmang CL, Senatore P, Lowry A, et al. Practice parameters for detection of colorectal neoplasms. Dis Colon Rectum. 1999;42:1123–9.
158. Winawer S, Fletcher R, Rex D, et al. Colorectal cancer screening and surveillance: clinical guidelines and rationale – update based on new evidence. Gastroenterology. 2003;124:544–60.
159. Vignati P, Welch JP, Cohen JL. Endoscopic localization of colon cancers. Surg Endosc. 1994;8:1085–7.
160. Larach SW, Patankar SK, Ferrara A, et al. Complications of laparoscopic colorectal surgery: analysis and comparison of early vs latter experience. Dis Colon Rectum. 1997;40:592–6.
161. Kim SH, Milsom JW, Church JM, et al. Perioperative tumor localization for laparoscopic colorectal surgery. Surg Endosc. 1997;11:1013–6.
162. McArthur CS, Roayaie S, Waye JD. Safety of preoperation endoscopic tattoo with India ink for identification of colonic lesions. Surg Endosc. 1999;13:397–400.
163. Nakajima K, Lee SW, Sonoda T, Milsom JW. Intraoperative carbon dioxide colonoscopy: a safe insufflation alternative

for locating colonic lesions during laparoscopic surgery. Surg Endosc. 2005;19:321–5.
164. Otchy D, Hyman NH, Simmang C, et al. Practice parameters for colon cancer. Dis Colon Rectum. 2004;47:1269–84.
165. The Standards Practice Task Force, ASCRS, Tjandra JJ, Kilkenny JW, Buie WD, et al. Practice parameters for the management of rectal cancer (revised). Dis Colon Rectum. 2005;48:411–23.
166. Goletti O, Celona G, Galatioto C, et al. Is laparoscopic sonography a reliable and sensitive procedure for staging of colorectal cancer? A comparative study. Surg Endosc. 1998;12:1236–41.
167. Milsom J, Jerby BL, Kessler H, et al. Prospective blinded comparison of laparoscopic ultrasonography versus contrast enhanced computerized tomography for liver assessment in patients undergoing colorectal carcinoma surgery. Dis Colon Rectum. 2000;43:44–9.
168. Kumar H, Hartley J, Heer K, et al. Efficacy of laparoscopic ultrasound scanning (USS) in detection of colorectal liver metastases during surgery. Dis Colon Rectum. 2000;43:320–5.
169. Abel ME, Rosen L, Kodner IJ, et al. Practice parameters for the treatment of rectal carcinoma. Dis Colon Rectum. 1993;36:989–1006.
170. Platell C, Hall J. What is the role of mechanical bowel preparation in patients undergoing colorectal surgery? Dis Colon Rectum. 1998;41:875–82.
171. Brownson P, Jenkins SA, Nott D, et al. Mechanical bowel preparation before colorectal surgery: results of a prospective, randomized trial. Br J Surg. 1992;79:461–2.
172. Burke P, Mealy K, Gillen P, et al. Requirement for bowel preparation in colorectal surgery. Br J Surg. 1994;81:580–1.
173. Santos JC, Batista J, Sirimarco MT, et al. Prospective randomized trial of mechanical bowel preparation in patients undergoing elective colorectal surgery. Br J Surg. 1994;81:1673–6.
174. Miettinen RP, Laitinen ST, Makela JT, Paakkonen ME. Bowel preparation with oral polyethylene glycol electrolyte solution vs. no preparation in elective open colorectal surgery: prospective, randomized study. Dis Colon Rectum. 2000;43:669–77.
175. Zmora O, Mahajn A, Barak B, et al. Colon and rectal surgery without mechanical bowel preparation: randomized prospective trial. Ann Surg. 2003;237:363–7.
176. Franklin ME, Rosenthal D, Abrego-Medina D, et al. Prospective comparison of open vs. laparoscopic colon surgery for carcinoma. Five-year results. Dis Colon Rectum. 1996;39:S35–46.
177. Nelson H, Petrelli N, Carlin A, et al. Guidelines 2000 for colon and rectal cancer surgery. J Natl Cancer Inst. 2001;93:583–96.
178. Wu WX, Sun YM, Hua YB, Shen LZ. Laparoscopic versus conventional open resection of rectal carcinoma: a clinical comparative study. World J Gastroenterol. 2004;10:1167–70.
179. Tsang WW, Chung CC, Li MK. Prospective evaluation of laparoscopic total mesorectal excision with colonic J-pouch reconstruction for mid and low rectal cancers. Br J Surg. 2003;90:867–71.
180. Leroy J, Jamali F, Forbes L, et al. Laparoscopic total mesorectal excision (TME) for rectal cancer surgery: long-term outcomes. Surg Endosc. 2004;18:281–9.
181. Anthuber M, Fuerst A, Elser F, et al. Outcome of laparoscopic surgery for rectal cancer in 101 patients. Dis Colon Rectum. 2003;46:1047–53.
182. Berends FJ, Kazemier G, Bonjer HJ, Lange JF. Subcutaneous metastases after laparoscopic colectomy. Lancet. 1994;344:58.
183. Bouvy ND, Marquet RL, Jeekel H, et al. Impact of gas(less) laparoscopy and laparotomy on peritoneal tumor growth and abdominal wall metastases. Ann Surg. 1996;224:694–700.
184. Watson DI, Mathew G, Ellis T, et al. Gasless laparoscopy may reduce the risk of port-site metastases following laparoscopic tumor surgery. Arch Surg. 1997;132:166–8.
185. Gutt CN, Riemer V, Kim ZG, et al. Impact of laparoscopic colonic resection on tumour growth and spread in an experimental model. Br J Surg. 1999;86:1180–4.
186. Iwanaka T, Arya G, Ziegler MM. Mechanism and prevention of port-site tumor recurrence after laparoscopy in a murine model. J Pediatr Surg. 1998;33:457–61.
187. Wittich P, Steyerberg EW, Simons SH, et al. Intraperitoneal tumor growth is influenced by pressure of carbon dioxide pneumoperitoneum. Surg Endosc. 2000;14:817–9.
188. Jacobi CA, Sterzel A, Braumann C, et al. The impact of conventional and laparoscopic colon resection (CO_2 or helium) on intraperitoneal adhesion formation in a rat peritonitis model. Surg Endosc. 2001;15:380–6.
189. Neuhaus SJ, Ellis T, Rofe AM, et al. Tumor implantation following laparoscopy using different insufflation gases. Surg Endosc. 1998;12:1300–2.
190. Jacobi CA, Sterzel A, Braumann C, et al. Influence of different gases and intraperitoneal instillation of antiadherent or cytotoxic agents on peritoneal tumor cell growth and implantation with laparoscopic surgery in a rat model. Surg Endosc. 1999;13:1021–5.
191. Bouvy ND, Giuffrida MC, Tseng LN, et al. Effects of carbon dioxide pneumoperitoneum, air pneumoperitoneum, and gasless laparoscopy on body weight and tumor growth. Arch Surg. 1998;133:652–6.
192. Wu JS, Guo LW, Ruiz MB, et al. Excision of trocar sites reduces tumor implantation in an animal model. Dis Colon Rectum. 1998;41:1107–11.
193. Watson DI, Ellis T, Leeder PC, et al. Excision of laparoscopic port sites increases the likelihood of wound metastases in an experimental model. Surg Endosc. 2003;17:83–5.
194. Wittich P, Marquet RL, Kazemier G, et al. Port-site metastases after CO(2) laparoscopy: is aerosolization of tumor cells a pivotal factor? Surg Endosc. 2000;14:189–92.
195. Whelan RL, Sellers GJ, Allendorf JD, et al. Trocar site recurrence is unlikely to result from aerosolization of tumor cells. Dis Colon Rectum. 1996;39:S7–13.
196. Veldkamp R, Gholghesaei M, HJ B, et al. Laparoscopic resection of colon cancer. Consensus of the European Association of Endoscopic Surgery. Surg Endosc. 2004;18:1163–85.
197. Tseng LN, Berends FJ, Wittich P, et al. Port-site metastases: impact of local tissue trauma and gas leakage. Surg Endosc. 1998;12:1377–80.
198. Neuhaus SJ, Watson DI, Ellis T, et al. Influence of cytotoxic agents on intraperitoneal tumor implantation after laparoscopy. Dis Colon Rectum. 1999;42:10–5.
199. Lee SW, Gleason NR, Bessler M, et al. Peritoneal irrigation with povidone-iodine solution after laparoscopic-assisted splenectomy significantly decreases port-tumor recurrence in a murine model. Dis Colon Rectum. 1999;42:319–26.
200. Neuhaus SJ, Ellis T, Jamieson GG, et al. Experimental study of the effect of intraperitoneal heparin on tumour implantation following laparoscopy. Br J Surg. 1999;86:400–4.

201. Braumann C, Ordemann J, Wildbrett P, et al. Influence of intraperitoneal and systemic application of taurolidine and taurolidine/heparin during laparoscopy on intraperitoneal and subcutaneous tumour growth in rats. Clin Exp Metastasis. 2001;8:547–52.
202. Jacobi CA, Peter FJ, Wenger FA, et al. New therapeutic strategies to avoid intra- and extraperitoneal metastases during laparoscopy: results of a tumor model in the rat. Dig Surg. 1999;16:393–9.
203. Eshraghi N, Swanstrom LL, Bax T, et al. Topical treatments of laparoscopic port sites can decrease the incidence of incision metastasis. Surg Endosc. 1999;13:1121–4.
204. Reilly WT, Nelson H, Schroeder G, et al. Wound recurrence following conventional treatment of colorectal cancer: a rare but perhaps underestimated problem. Dis Colon Rectum. 1996;39:200–7.
205. Young-Fadok TM, Fanelli RD, Price RR, Earle DB. Laparoscopic resection of curable colon and rectal cancer: an evidence-based review. Surg Endosc. 2007;21:1063–8.
206. Ou H. Laparoscopic-assisted mini laparotomy with colectomy. Dis Colon Rectum. 1995;38:324–6.
207. Mooney MJ, Elliott PL, Galapon DB, et al. Hand-assisted laparoscopic sigmoidectomy for diverticulitis. Dis Colon Rectum. 1998;41:630–5.
208. Southern Surgeons' Club Study Group. Handoscopic surgery: a prospective multicenter trial of minimally invasive technique for complex abdominal surgery. Arch Surg. 1999;134:477–86.
209. HALS Study Group. Hand-assisted laparoscopic surgery vs standard laparoscopic surgery for colorectal disease: a prospective randomized trial. Surg Endosc. 2000;14:896–901.
210. Litwin D, Darzi A, Jakimowicz J, et al. Hand-assisted laparoscopic surgery (HALS) with the HandPort system: initial experience with 68 patients. Ann Surg. 2000;231:715–23.
211. Targarona EM, Gracia E, Garriga J, et al. Prospective randomized trial comparing conventional laparoscopic colectomy with hand-assisted laparoscopic colectomy. Surg Endosc. 2002;16:234–9.
212. Cobb WS, Lokey JS, Schwab DP, et al. Hand-assisted laparoscopic colectomy: a single-institution experience. Am Surg. 2003;69:578–80.
213. Kang JC, Chung MH, Yeh CC, et al. Hand-assisted laparoscopic colectomy vs open colectomy: a prospective randomized study. Surg Endosc. 2004;18:577–81.
214. Maartense S, Dunker MS, Slors JF, et al. Hand-assisted laparoscopic versus open proctocolectomy with ileal pouch anal anastomosis: a randomized trial. Ann Surg. 2004;240:984–92.
215. Boushey RP, Marcello PW, Martel G, Rusin LC, Roberts PL, Schoetz Jr DJ. Laparoscopic total colectomy: an evolutionary experience. Dis Colon Rectum. 2007;50:1512–9.
216. Cadeddu JA, Gautam G, Shalhav AL. Robotic prostatectomy. J Urol. 2010;183:858–61.
217. Rawlings AL, Woodland JH, Vegunta RK, Crawford DL. Robotic versus laparoscopic colectomy. Surg Endosc. 2007;21:1701–8.
218. Baik SH, Kwon HY, Kim JS, Hur H, Sohn SK, Cho CH, et al. Robotic versus laparoscopic low anterior resection of rectal cancer: short-term outcome of a prospective comparative study. Ann Surg Oncol. 2009;16:1480–7.
219. Choi DJ, Kim SH, Lee PJ, Kim J, Woo SU. Single-stage totally robotic dissection for rectal cancer surgery: technique and short-term outcome in 50 consecutive patients. Dis Colon Rectum. 2009;52:1824–30.
220. Patriti A, Ceccarelli G, Bartoli A, Spaziani A, Biancafarina A, Casciola L. Short- and medium-term outcome of robot-assisted and traditional laparoscopic rectal resection. JSLS. 2009;13:176–83.
221. Merchant AM, Lin E. Single-incision laparoscopic right hemicolectomy for a colon mass. Dis Colon Rectum. 2009;52:1021–4.
222. http://www.mayoclinic.org/news2009-sct/5326.html.
223. Law WL, Fan JK, Poon JT. Single-incision laparoscopic colectomy: early experience. Dis Colon Rectum. 2010;53:284–8.
224. Ostrowitz MB, Eschete D, Zemon H, DeNoto G. Robotic-assisted single-incision right colectomy: early experience. Int J Med Robot. 2009;5(4):465–70.
225. Piskun G, Rajpal S. Transumbilical laparoscopic cholecystectomy utilizes no incisions outside the umbilicus. J Laparoendosc Adv Surg Tech A. 1999;9:361–4.
226. Palanivelu C, Rajan P, Rangarajan M, Parthasarathi R, Senthilnathan P, Prasad M. Transvaginal endoscopic appendectomy in humans: a unique approach to NOTES-world's first report. Surg Endosc. 2008;22:1343–7.
227. Denk PM, Swanstrom LL, Whiteford MH. Transanal endoscopic microsurgical platform for natural orifice surgery. Gastrointest Endosc. 2008;68(5):954–9.
228. Whiteford MH, Spaun GO. A colorectal surgeons viewpoint on natural orifice translumenal endoscopic surgery. Minerva Chir. 2008;63(5):385–8.
229. Leroy J, Cahill RA, Perretta S, Forgione A, Dallemagne B, Marescaux J. Natural orifice translumenal endoscopic surgery (NOTES) applied totally to sigmoidectomy: an original technique with survival in a porcine model. Surg Endosc. 2009;23:24–30.
230. Ramamoorthy SL, Fischer LJ, Jacobsen G, Thompson K, Wong B, Spivack A, et al. Transrectal endoscopic retrorectal access (TERA): a novel NOTES approach to the peritoneal cavity. J Laparoendosc Adv Surg Tech A. 2009;19:603–6.
231. Bemelman WA. Laparoscopic ileoanal pouch surgery. Br J Surg. 2010;97(1):2–3.

36 Polyps

Paul E. Wise

Polyps are defined as pathologic epithelial elevations of the aerodigestive and genitourinary tracts. This term serves to describe any of the types of abnormal growths identified on or involving the colonic mucosa that protrude into the bowel lumen. Polyps are of concern to clinicians due to their malignant potential depending on the histologic type of the polyp identified. The primary histologic colonic polyp types include the following: adenomas, serrated polyps (including hyperplastic polyps and sessile serrated adenomas (SSAs)), hamartomas, and inflammatory polyps. Because some of these polyps are neoplastic, they are the target of screening modalities (including colonoscopy, computed tomography (CT) colonography, etc.) to remove them prior to their malignant degeneration. Other polyp-like lesions, usually submucosal rather than mucosal in nature, such as carcinoids, leiomyomas, and lipomas will be described and discussed in Chap. 49.

Adenomas

Definition and Pathology

Adenomas are the most common neoplastic polyps identified in the colon (50–67% of all polyps) and are thought to be the precursor lesion to the majority of colorectal cancers (and therefore the target of screening programs).[1] They are by definition a low grade dysplastic lesion with the potential for progression of the dysplasia to an invasive malignancy. Grossly, these lesions can be pedunculated (mushroom-like on a stalk of submucosa lined by normal mucosa, Figure 36-1) or sessile with a broader base (Figure 36-2), can occur singly or as multiple lesions, and can vary greatly in size and extent.

Adenomas are classified as tubular, villous, or tubulovillous. The former lesions comprise approximately 75–87% of all adenomas identified in the colon and contain uniform-sized tubules and glands. As the tubules become more elongated with less stroma between glands, they assume a more villous character. For pathologists, tubular adenomas (Figure 36-3) can consist of up to 20–25% villous features and still be considered a "tubular adenoma" while villous adenomas (5–10% of all adenomas) contain more than 50–75% villous features, making tubulovillous adenomas (8–15% of all adenomas, Figure 36-4) those polyps in between.[2,3] While the likelihood of a polyp to harbor malignancy may be impacted by this classification, the treatment for the three classes of adenomas remains the same and thus has little true clinical significance.

Adenomas are differentiated from hyperplastic polyps in that they display cellular atypia with lack of differentiation into specialized cell types. The epithelial lining will show increasing mitoses and some degree of hyperchromasia (darker hematoxylin and eosin staining) depending on the degree of dysplasia. In adenomas, because cellular proliferation is not limited to the lower half of the tubule as in normal colonic epithelium, the normal process of cellular maturation and differentiation from the base of the crypt to the surface does not occur.

Adenomas can be graded by the degree to which epithelial growth is disturbed. Mild or low grade dysplasia is characterized by tubules which are lined from top to bottom by epithelium which is morphologically similar to the normal basal proliferative zone. The nuclei are enlarged, oval, hyperchromatic, and have normal orientation. There is a slight excess of mitotic figures but the architecture is not disrupted. By definition, all adenomas show at least low grade dysplasia. In moderate dysplasia, the nuclear features are more advanced, cellular polarity is less preserved, there is nuclear stratification, and the glands are more crowded. In severe or high grade dysplasia, there are large vesicular nuclei, irregular and conspicuous nucleoli, scalloped nuclear membranes, and increased nuclear to cytoplasmic ratio. Nuclear polarity is disrupted and marked cellular pleomorphism and both numerous and aberrant mitoses are present. Structural alterations include budding and branching tubules, back-to-back arrangement of glands, and cribriform growth of epithelial cells in clusters and sheets. The terms "carcinoma *in situ*" and "intramucosal carcinoma" are often used to describe these high grade dysplastic adenomas, but these terms are potentially misleading as these lesions do not have metastatic potential.[4,5]

D.E. Beck et al. (eds.), *The ASCRS Textbook of Colon and Rectal Surgery: Second Edition*,
DOI 10.1007/978-1-4419-1584-9_36, © Springer Science+Business Media, LLC 2011

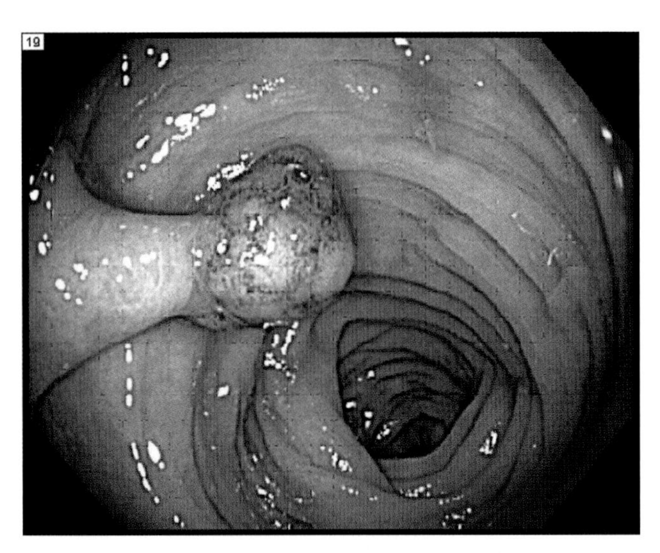

FIGURE 36-1. Endoscopic appearance of a pedunculated adenoma.

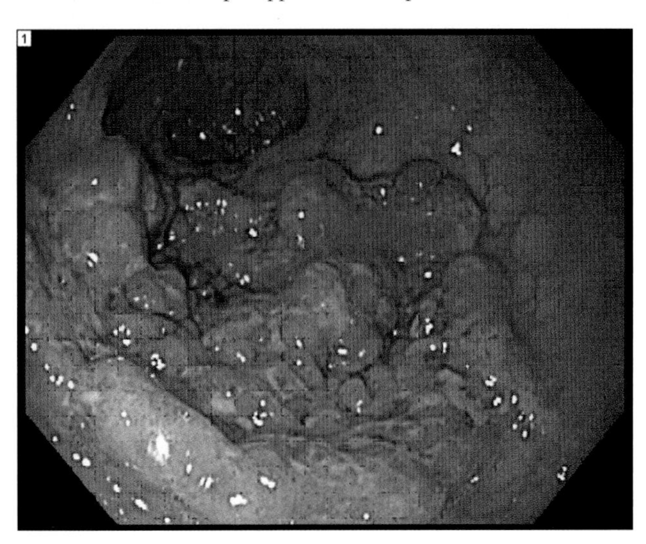

FIGURE 36-2. Endoscopic appearance of a sessile adenoma (Courtesy of Roberta L. Muldoon).

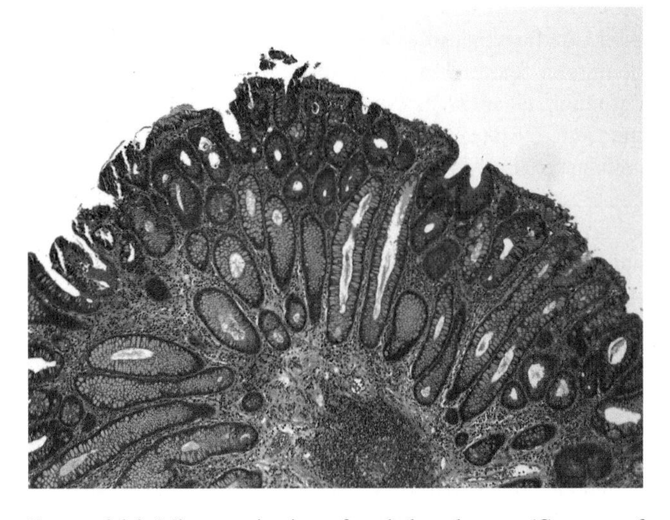

FIGURE 36-3. Microscopic view of a tubular adenoma (Courtesy of William Chopp, MD).

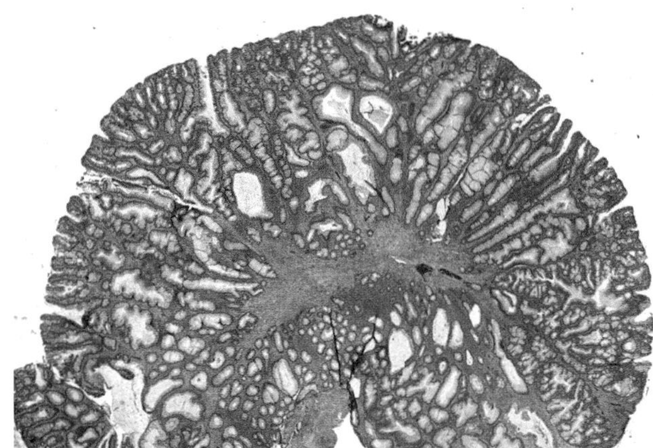

FIGURE 36-4. Microscopic view of a tubulovillous adenoma (Courtesy of M. Kay Washington, MD, PhD).

Presentation and Diagnosis

Most adenomas are asymptomatic and are therefore found with screening studies or incidentally diagnosed through investigations of symptoms unrelated to the adenoma. Larger adenomas may display overt hematochezia or anemia secondary to occult or overt blood loss. Adenomas in the rectum may cause rectal bleeding, mucoid discharge, tenesmus, and/or fecal urgency. Very large adenomas may rarely cause electrolyte abnormalities or diarrhea or may lead to intussusception of the colon or prolapse through the anus.

Adenomas are often multifocal and can be identified anywhere in the colon and rectum but tend to be more prevalent distally. In one large prospective study (U.S. National Polyp Study), the distribution of adenomas was as follows: cecum 8%, ascending colon 9%, hepatic flexure 5%, transverse colon 10%, splenic flexure 4%, descending colon 14%, sigmoid 43%, and rectum 8%.[3] Other studies have also documented that 24–31% of adenomas are proximal to the splenic flexure in colonoscopies in higher-risk or symptomatic patients.[3,6] In addition, when a sporadic adenoma is identified in the colon or rectum, the likelihood of a synchronous adenoma elsewhere in the colon ranges from 31 to 40%.[6,7] Therefore, when a distal adenoma is found, a complete colonic assessment is necessary because of this high rate of synchronous neoplasms.[8,9] The features of the adenomas may dictate the likelihood of synchronous lesions being found, however. Most, but not all,[10] studies of screening flexible sigmoidoscopy suggest that patients with no distal polyps, distal hyperplastic polyps, or a single small tubular adenoma have a low risk of proximal advanced adenomas (0–4%). Multiple other studies, however, support the recommendation that villous adenomas (regardless of size) and any adenoma >1 cm are important markers for the presence of advanced adenomas and even carcinoma in the proximal colon.[11]

The fact that adenomas are often asymptomatic precursor neoplasms justifies the use of screening to identify and remove these lesions before they become clinically recognizable, thus halting the adenoma to carcinoma sequence (discussed below). In general, colorectal cancer screening has been shown to reduce mortality and be cost-effective. Screening timing and frequency is usually based on risk factors with higher-risk individuals having personal or family history of colorectal neoplasia, high-risk hereditary colorectal cancer syndromes, and/or the presence of inflammatory bowel disease (see Chap. 39).

Colonoscopy is the most accurate test for polyps, especially when compared to double contrast barium enema (DCBE) as shown by the U.S. National Polyp Study.[12] DCBE alone has been repeatedly shown to be less sensitive than colonoscopy (even for polyps >10 mm with a miss rate of 52%), offers no therapeutic benefit, and has not been shown to reduce cancer incidence or mortality. Colonoscopy, on the other hand, decreases the risk of colorectal cancer incidence by 76–90% and has been indirectly shown to reduce cancer mortality.[13] Flexible sigmoidoscopy has also been shown to lead to a decrease in distal colon cancer mortality as much as 80% (45% for all colorectal cancers) but does not show a reduction in deaths from more proximal cancers.[14] More recently, CT colonography or "virtual colonoscopy" has been supported as a potential screening modality.[1] Three meta-analyses (between 1,300 and 6,400 patients in each analysis) have shown sensitivities and specificities for detecting polyps ≥10 mm to be in the 85–95% and 95–97% ranges, respectively. Medium-sized polyps (6–9 mm) had lower sensitivities and specificities of 70–86% and 86–93%, respectively.[15,16] Newer screening modalities such as chromoendoscopy or dye-spray endoscopy, narrow band imaging, magnification endoscopy, and pill colonoscopy have not been established as effective means for surveillance or screening for all patients and are not equivalent in the hands of all providers. They are only considered adjunctive at this time by most surgical and medical societies and warrant further study. Further discussion of screening modalities and their effectiveness can be found in Chap. 39.

Epidemiology

Adenoma prevalence, the percentage of the population with one or more colorectal adenomas at a given point in time, is primarily a function of age, gender, and family history.[17] Colonoscopy-determined prevalence rates in asymptomatic, average-risk individuals ≥50 years range from 24 to 50%,[18–22] with the prevalence of advanced adenomas (≥1 cm in size, with villous features, and/or with high grade dysplasia)[23] varying from 3.4 to 9.5% depending on age and gender.[9,10,24] Prevalence rates have been shown to increase with age, even doubling between ages 50 and 60.[9,24] Higher adenoma prevalence rates have been identified in men, with a relative risk of 1.5 to 2.0 compared to age-matched women.[18,19,21,24] Interestingly, however, in one study of screening colonoscopies performed on 1,463 asymptomatic women ≥40 years old, 20.4% were diagnosed with an adenoma and 4.9% with an advanced adenoma. When these women were compared to a matched group of men (8.6% of whom had advanced adenomas on screening colonoscopy), almost 65% had their advanced adenomas in the proximal colon versus 34% of the men, suggesting that gender differences may lead to changes in adenoma location as well as overall prevalence.[8] In terms of family history risk, a multicenter screening colonoscopy study examining the risk of colorectal adenomas in a cohort of individuals with one affected first-degree relative with sporadic colorectal cancer found the odds ratio to be 1.5 for adenomas, 2.5 for large adenomas, 1.2 for small adenomas, and 2.6 for high-risk adenomas (see below).[25] The prevalence of adenomas and advanced adenomas is higher in relatives of individuals with colorectal cancer or adenoma at a young age, and in individuals with multiple relatives with cancer or adenomas.[26,27] Adenoma prevalence rates determined by colonoscopy are roughly double the rates determined by flexible sigmoidoscopy.[10,17] The prevalence of a proximal synchronous adenoma in a patient with a distal adenoma (or even hyperplastic polyps in some studies)[10] is such that proximal colonic assessment is warranted if a distal lesion is found on screening.[8,9]

The incidence of adenomas is the rate at which individuals develop colorectal adenomas over a specified time interval.[17] The incidence of adenomas at intervals ranging from 6 months to 5 years in post-polypectomy surveillance colonoscopy studies varies from 20 to 50%.[28–32] Most incident polyps are small, and a higher incidence has been associated with multiple adenomas at the index colonoscopy, larger size of the index adenoma, older age, and a family history of a parent with colorectal cancer.[13,28,33–36] The incidence rate of colorectal adenomas after a clearing colonoscopy is actually the sum of the true incidence rate of new adenoma formation plus the miss rate at the initial colonoscopy plus the recurrence rate of incompletely removed polyps.[17] Judging by repeat endoscopy, including studies with same day back-to-back colonoscopies, the miss rate for adenomas ≥1 cm is approximately 5%, for adenomas 6–9 mm it is approximately 10%, and for adenomas ≤5 mm it approaches 30%.[37–40] These high miss rates for small lesions suggest that many adenomas detected on surveillance colonoscopy are actually lesions that were missed during the index examination. Incident polyps are distributed more proximally, consistent with the observation that miss rates for adenomas are higher in the proximal colon.[37]

More important than the overall incidence rate of adenomas is the incidence rate for advanced adenomas and cancers, especially in the context of the above-described screening miss rates. The incidence rate for advanced adenomas ranges from 6 to 9%[23] and is closely related to the findings at initial colonoscopy.[41] Based on a pooled analysis of more than 9,000 patients in North America, of which 11.2% had advanced neoplasia (adenoma or cancer) on subsequent colonoscopy, a greater number of adenomas at initial colonoscopy, histologic features (villous architecture) of the excised adenoma, larger adenoma size, proximal adenoma location (odds ratio

[OR] 1.68; 95% confidence interval [CI], 1.43–1.98), and male gender (OR 1.40; 95% CI, 1.19–1.65) were all attributed to increased risk of development of advanced neoplasia.[32] Three or more polyps at the initial colonoscopy has been shown to increase the risk of subsequent advanced adenomas, and in the U.S. National Polyp Study, age >60 years plus a family history of a parent with colorectal cancer was also a predictor of incident advanced adenomas.[36,42] The cumulative incidence of advanced adenomas at 3 and 6 years of follow-up in the U.S. National Polyp Study in the highest risk group (three or more adenomas at baseline, or age ≥60 years plus a parent with colorectal cancer) were 10 and 20%, respectively.[42] The lowest risk group (only one adenoma and age <60 years at baseline) had an incidence of advanced adenomas of <1% at both 3 and 6 years of follow-up. The 5-year incidence of advanced adenomas in individuals with a previously negative colonoscopy is also <1%.[43] Similarly, post-polypectomy surveillance studies have shown that cancer incidence is also low, and in the U.S. National Polyp Study, colonoscopic surveillance was associated with a 76–90% reduction in the cancer incidence compared to reference populations.[36] The rare appearance of incident cancers at short intervals in patients who have had a clearing colonoscopy suggests that either the neoplasm was initially missed or incompletely treated (27–31% of incident cancers may be due to "ineffective" polypectomy)[44] or the cancer developed rapidly. Based on long-term follow-up from the Polyp Prevention Trial, these interval cancers are even more common in those patients with a previous history of advanced adenoma.[45] Despite the initial colonoscopy miss rates, however, modeling shows that >90% of the reduced incidence of colorectal cancer over the first 5–6 years after screening colonoscopy is the result of the initial polypectomy rather than removal of adenomas at subsequent surveillance.[46] Long-term follow-up studies are ongoing.

Adenoma to Carcinoma Sequence

The idea that an adenoma would progress into a carcinoma has been based primarily on observational epidemiologic studies, clinical studies, pathologic findings, and molecular genetic studies, and therefore the evidence, while extensive, is truly circumstantial. Given the high prevalence of sporadic adenomas in the general population but the relatively low lifetime risk of developing colorectal cancer in Western countries (6% by age 85), it appears that only a few adenomas become adenocarcinomas. While not all adenomas develop into colorectal cancer, it appears that most sporadic colorectal cancers (80–85%) develop from adenomas, although there is evidence for rare *de novo* colorectal cancer development as well as other less-rare carcinoma sequences. Adenoma size seems to be important in the likelihood for malignant degeneration, and the likelihood that a diminutive tubular adenoma will progress to become an adenocarcinoma is likely very low. In a study that analyzed 7,590 adenomatous polyps to determine risk factors for high grade dysplasia or invasion, size was the strongest predictor.[5] The percent of adenomas with high grade dysplasia or invasive cancer based on the size of the polyp was: <5 mm – 3.4%, 5–10 mm – 13.5%, and >10 mm – 38.5%. No invasive cancer was found in polyps ≤5 mm. Villous change, left-sided lesions, and age ≥60 years were also associated with advanced histologic features.[5]

One longitudinal study showed that over a 3–5-year period only 4% of 213 adenomas measuring 2–15 mm increased in size.[47] A mathematical model suggested that it takes 2–3 years for an adenoma ≤5 mm to grow to 1 cm, and another 2–5 years for the 1 cm adenoma to progress to cancer.[48] For a lesion ≥1 cm, the cancer probability is 3, 8, and 24% after 5, 10, and 20 years, respectively.[49] This supports that the transformation of adenomas to cancer is a slow process, also supported by the fact that the mean age of adenoma patients precedes the mean age of cancer patients by 7 years. Overall, the yearly rate of conversion from adenoma to carcinoma has been estimated to be 0.25%, but the risk is higher depending on size and histologic factors such as the conversion rate for polyps >1 cm (3%), for villous adenomas (17%), and for adenomas with high grade dysplasia (37%).[50] Gender does not appear to affect the rate of transition from advanced adenoma to carcinoma, but age clearly impacts malignant degeneration (ranging from 2.6% at age <60 to >5% annually at age >80 years for both men and women).[51]

On a molecular level, the "traditional" pathway from adenoma to adenocarcinoma (also known as the "loss of heterozygosity" (LOH) or "chromosomal instability" (CIN) pathway), thought to account for the development of 80–85% of sporadic colorectal cancers, was elucidated from studies on patients with familial adenomatous polyposis (FAP). The process starts with a single colorectal epithelial cell undergoing a series of genetic alterations leading to the inactivation of both copies of the tumor suppressor adenomatous polyposis coli (*APC*) gene on chromosome 5q that regulates cell growth and apoptosis.[52,53] This appears to occur very early in the process of the normal epithelial cell transitioning into adenomatous tissue or low grade dysplasia by leading to increased cell proliferation. The next alteration in the pathway is thought to occur with *k-ras*, an oncogene involved in signal transduction from the cell membrane to the nucleus. Mutation of this gene (seen in 50% of colorectal cancers) in the setting of the *APC* mutation appears to lead to exophytic growth and transition to an "intermediate" adenoma. Important to the transition from intermediate to advanced adenoma is mutation of the deleted in colon cancer (*DCC*) gene that is important for encoding an adhesion molecule and facilitating apoptosis and therefore tumor suppression.[54] The final step to the development of invasive adenocarcinoma (found in 75% of colorectal adenocarcinomas) is a mutation in the p53 gene which regulates the cell cycle after DNA injury to allow for DNA repair.[53] The accumulation of some or all of these molecular abnormalities is therefore associated with the development of invasive colorectal cancer. As noted, however, not all colorectal cancers develop via this sequence, and alternate pathways to colorectal cancer are being increasingly recognized including pathways that may involve other polypoid lesions such as serrated polyps known as the "serrated neoplasia" pathway (see below), thought to account for the other 10–15% of sporadic colorectal cancers. This pathway is characterized by cancers showing microsatellite instability (MSI), likely due to hypermethylation of the *hMLH1* mismatch repair gene promoter leading to its inactivation, likely occurring after *BRAF* (a serine-threonine kinase involved in the *k-ras* pathway) gene mutations. These cancers are morphologically and pathologically similar to the MSI cancers that are associated with the germline mismatch repair gene mutations seen in hereditary nonpolyposis colorectal cancer (HNPCC)/Lynch syndrome (see Chap. 37).[55–57] While these cancers do appear to develop through an adenoma-carcinoma sequence, the adenomas are not considered the traditional adenomas seen in the *APC* adenoma-carcinoma sequence and are more likely the SSAs discussed below. See Chap. 38 for a more detailed review on the molecular basis of carcinogenesis.

Management

All adenomas or apparent adenomas should be completely removed for confirmation of the diagnosis and to exclude a concurrent malignancy and the potential need for further intervention. The majority of adenomas are able to be endoscopically removed by various means including "cold" (without electrocautery) or "hot" (with electrocautery) biopsy forceps or loops/snares. Removal also precludes malignant degeneration. Complications of polypectomy, primarily bleeding and perforation can be limited through the appropriate use of these standard techniques. Electrocautery is frequently used during endoscopy, but the amount of thermal injury must be balanced with the need for vascular control, as a full thickness injury to the colon wall can easily occur given that it ranges from only 1.7 to 2.2 mm in thickness.[58] Prospective assessments are lacking as to how best to approach small polyps, and therefore preferences vary between endoscopists. Because of the concern for perforations related to the use of cautery, recommendations include limiting the use of hot forceps to small polyps (<5 mm) while tenting the mucosa and somewhat deflating the colon. The majority of these smaller polyps are usually amenable to single-bite or piecemeal excision with cold forceps that will eliminate the cautery risks.[44]

Large pedunculated polyps can often be removed with snare cautery techniques (although bleeding is uncommon after removal of these). The important aspect of removal of these types of polyps is to ensure that the blood supply through a thick stalk (>1 cm), which may contain substantial vasculature, is controlled prior to the polypectomy. This maneuver is facilitated by gently closing the snare and cauterizing the base of the stalk followed by firmer closure and cutting through the stalk with cautery above the initial cauterized base. Alternatively, metal clips or endoloops can be placed at the base, or the stalk can be injected with epinephrine to provide hemostasis. The base of the stalk may be tattooed with ink or carbon agents to allow for subsequent identification (endoscopically or surgically) if the polyp has a concerning appearance for malignancy. At times, piecemeal resection of the polyp head is necessary before a large snare can even get around the polyp to reach the stalk.[44]

Larger sessile polyps (>15–20 mm) will usually require piecemeal resection with a large snare cautery. Care must be taken to ensure only inclusion of the polyp and its surrounding mucosa in the snare as accidental inclusion of adjacent folds or mucosa can potentially lead to perforation. Safe polypectomy while avoiding injury to surrounding normal tissues may also be facilitated by saline lift as described below. When performing a standard piecemeal polypectomy, starting on the proximal aspect of the polyp with or without using a spike-tip snare (allows the snare to be anchored so that pushing the sheath causes the snare loop to widen for more effective placement around the polyp) will allow for easier and more complete polyp resection. While the piecemeal technique is an effective means of removal, it requires meticulous removal of the entire polyp and capture of the pieces. This technique ensures that pathologic examination of the polyp will be complete, although the margins will be unclear when the specimen is resected in this fashion. Larger pieces might require basket retrieval, division of the larger pieces with the cold snare, or may necessitate multiple insertions and withdrawals of the colonoscope to remove them.[59] Careful coagulation of the base and edge of the polypectomy defect with the argon plasma coagulator or other electrocautery device has been shown to decrease the incidence of residual polyp.[60] It is also advisable to utilize endoscopic tattooing techniques to identify the area again for subsequent examinations of the site as well as potential surgical resection if invasive cancer is identified.[44] Both the resection area itself and the opposing colonic walls should be injected to ensure identification of the area surgically if necessary. Retroflexion can also facilitate visualization and resection of difficult polyps, primarily in the rectum and right colon. Any remaining polyp tissue should be treated with argon plasma coagulation or other coagulation techniques as noted above and has been shown to be effective in decreasing recurrence of the polyp. It has been repeatedly shown in retrospective studies that endoscopic resection of large polyps can be performed safely with low risk of perforation (rare and often treatable nonoperatively, although 5% can be fatal)[44] or bleeding (2–24%, treatable medically or endoscopically).[59] If a polyp is too large for a safe polypectomy (piecemeal or otherwise) to be performed, a conventional oncologic surgical resection should be done.

Submucosal injection of various agents has been utilized to elevate and more safely facilitate endoscopic resection of large sessile polyps in the colon and rectum by elevating the submucosa and thus increasing the distance between the mucosa and the muscularis propria.[59] This operation not only decreases the risk of perforation but also increases the potential for complete excision. Agents that are useful include saline with or without methylene blue (to distinguish the layers) and with or without epinephrine. Other agents used to slow absorption of the fluid and prolong the elevation effect during the polypectomy include 0.5% sodium hyaluronate and 0.83% hydroxypropyl methylcellulose. Carbon/ink solutions can also be used to both tattoo the area for subsequent identification as well as elevate the polyp. The volume of the agent to use is not standardized, but injection of 1–4 mL at a time to create swelling of the submucosa, and up to 20–30 mL or greater may be needed for larger polyps. Injection distal to a polyp (along the front edge on retrograde view) may obscure the view and make polypectomy more difficult. Therefore, starting with proximal injections (far edge of the polyp) may facilitate the lateral and distal injections and thus the ability to view the polyp and allow for its subsequent removal. Failure of the polyp to elevate at the time of submucosal injection despite appropriate swelling of the submucosa ("nonlifting sign") is concerning for invasion of the polyp into the submucosa or deeper and should therefore indicate need for surgical resection.[59,61] The nonlifting sign may be falsely positive if a previous biopsy of the polyp has caused scarring in the area.

The greatest concern, of course, is whether the polyp harbors a malignancy. There are no prospective studies on how to visually identify a malignancy in a polyp, but most endoscopists seem to agree that ulceration, friability, or induration in addition to tactile clues with a biopsy forceps such as fixation or being firm suggest that there is likely an underlying malignancy and surgical resection should be favored. Biopsies may be helpful but may suffer from sampling bias. In situations where a large polyp is identified incidentally on a screening colonoscopy, a simple biopsy rather than more aggressive resection may be warranted as the patient and/or endoscopist may not be prepared for the increased complications associated with a complex polypectomy. A repeat endoscopy after further discussion and informed consent is then appropriate. If a complex polypectomy is to be performed, the patient must understand that repeat procedures may be necessary to completely remove the polyp. Of note, polyps that occupy greater than one-third the circumference of the colon, encompass two or more haustral folds, or involve a diverticulum or the base of the appendix are rarely able to be endoscopically removed.[44]

At the time of surgical resection for an endoscopically challenging polyp, intraoperative colonoscopy is a technique useful for localizing nonpalpable or softer polyps which have not been preoperatively tattooed. This technically can complicate a surgical resection, however, due to insufflation of the colon and potentially the small bowel. Use of carbon dioxide insufflation rather than room air can help in this regard based on its quick resorption and resulting colonic decompression. It has been shown to be safe even in patients with pulmonary disease.[62] Intraoperatively maneuvering the colonoscope can also be a challenge without having the advantage of compressing the abdominal wall to provide counter pressure and limit the colon's mobility. However, the surgeon can frequently telescope the bowel over the scope itself to an area known to be proximal to the lesion and then the mass can be found during withdrawal while desufflating the colon.

Hybrid minimally invasive and endoscopic procedures have been shown to be safe with long-term success in removing large colonic polyps.[63–65] This technique utilizes intraoperative colonoscopic polypectomy in conjunction with laparoscopic confirmation of complete polypectomy while assessing for colonic perforation or uses endoscopic assistance with a laparoscopic wedge resection of the polyp. These procedures are also best performed in combination with the use of carbon dioxide as the endoscopic gas. While the endoscopist identifies the mass, the surgeon performs diagnostic laparoscopy to examine the affected area of the colon as well as the remainder of the abdomen for other pathology. Other trocars may be placed to allow for manipulation of the bowel at the same time. As the polyp is excised endoscopically (with or without lift techniques), the exterior of the bowel can be observed for perforation or near-perforation. If this occurs, or there is an area of concern, this can be repaired or oversewn laparoscopically while the polyp is removed and examined with frozen section. Any invasive cancer or concerning features may warrant immediate laparoscopic colectomy, which would be discussed with preoperatively and consented to by the patient. This may necessitate unwarranted reservation of surgical block time if a resection is not needed but would require only one general anesthetic for the patient. Rare inaccuracy of the frozen section (if the initial pathology was benign but permanent sections showed cancer or other concerning features) might necessitate a subsequent operation. Alternatively, the diagnostic laparoscopy with or without bowel repair can be completed and the final permanent (rather than frozen section) pathologic examination performed – usually taking 2–3 days – after which the patient can undergo resection if needed. An additional hybrid option involves using laparoscopic techniques to divide intrabdominal adhesions, usually in the sigmoid colon, that prevent passage of a colonoscope to the cecum.

Surveillance

Improvements in colorectal cancer incidence and mortality rates are attributed to prevention through adenoma removal with screening and surveillance endoscopy, as well as risk factor modifications and improved therapies.[1] Patients with adenomas are at increased risk for metachronous adenomas and have been shown to have a decreased incidence of subsequent cancer with follow-up surveillance. Surveillance recommendations after colonoscopic polypectomy, therefore, are based on the estimated risk of metachronous neoplasia.[66,67] After polypectomy of large (≥1 cm) or multiple adenomas (three or more) or advanced adenomas, cancer risk is increased three- to five-fold.[68] The risk of subsequent cancer is not measurably increased in patients with only one or two small tubular adenomas.[33,69] The U.S. National Polyp Study determined that colonoscopy performed 3 years after initial polypectomy protects patients just as well as more frequent examinations.[13] Currently, no other modalities other than colonoscopy are advocated for post-polypectomy surveillance (although CT colonography has had some support as a surveillance option for patients with <1 cm adenomas who refuse or are not candidates for colonoscopy).[1] In fact, utilizing other surveillance modalities such as fecal occult blood testing (positive predictive value in surveillance of <30%) has been ineffective at best and is currently discouraged for those patients having undergone screening colonoscopy.[46]

Current recommendations for colonoscopic surveillance based on the ASCRS Practice Parameters[70] and the joint guidelines from the American Cancer Society, the U.S. Multi-Society Task Force on Colorectal Cancer, and the American College of Radiology[1,46] are as follows (see also Table 36-1): Patients with one to two <1 cm tubular adenomas should have a repeat in 5–10 years, depending on personal and family history. Patients with advanced adenomas or cancer in a completely resected polyp or patients with 3–10 adenomas all completely removed should have a repeat colonoscopy in 3 years, assuming a complete colonoscopy in a well-prepared colon. If they have more than ten polyps, or an incomplete or poorly prepared colon, they should have a repeat in <3 years. After the follow-up colonoscopy for these conditions is clear, a repeat examination every 5 years is warranted if the repeat is normal and well-prepared. Due to a high recurrence rate after endoscopic polypectomy, patients with large, sessile adenomas that are resected piecemeal should undergo repeat in 2–6 months to verify complete removal. Even when the endoscopist believes that a large polyp has been completely removed, follow-up examinations reveal residual or recurrent polyp in approximately 14–55% of patients.[44] Once complete removal is confirmed, there should be close follow-up of these patients with the frequency based on clinical judgment (usually within 1 year). Most patients with hyperplastic polyps, except those with hyperplastic polyposis, are considered average risk depending on family and personal history otherwise and should continue routine screening. Patients with a strong family history of colorectal cancer concerning for a hereditary predisposition (e.g., HNPCC/Lynch syndrome, familial polyposis, etc.) warrant more frequent surveillance (see Chap. 37). Overall surveillance recommendations after polypectomy should be individualized based on patient age and comorbidity (e.g., after removal of a small tubular adenoma, no follow-up may be indicated in elderly patients or for those with significant comorbidity).[1]

Adenoma Prevention

Because the majority of colorectal cancers are thought to develop from adenomas, prevention of the development of adenomas has been at the center of an extensive body of work trying to prevent the development of colorectal cancer. Observational studies looking at the affect of diet initially suggested that excess dietary fat and limited dietary fiber lead to increased incidence of colorectal cancer, but prospective trials on fiber supplements (e.g., Nurses Health Study) as well as dietary fat intake did not show any decrease in adenoma development. Certain foods, especially certain fruit and vegetable types, have been shown in case–controlled trials to decrease colorectal cancer risk between 13 and 40%, but long-term follow-up in large prospective trials such as the Polyp Prevention Trial and the Women's Health Initiative have shown no difference in colon cancer incidence with dietary alterations.[22] Increased body mass index, decreased physical activity levels, red meat intake,[71] smoking, and alcohol intake have all been lifestyle issues that have been associated with increased colorectal cancer risk, but alterations in these factors have not been studied in relation to the possible improvement in adenoma or colorectal cancer development.[22,57] Folate was thought to be an effective colorectal cancer preventative agent in observational trials, but prospective trials have shown weaker effects leading to

Table 36-1. Colonoscopy surveillance guidelines[a]

Screening colonoscopy finding	Recommended follow-up	Comments
No polyps	10 year colonoscopy or standard screening recommendations	Assumes no familial colorectal cancer history
Small distal hyperplastic polyps	10 year colonoscopy or standard screening recommendations	Assumes no hyperplastic polyposis or familial colorectal cancer history
≤2 small (<1 cm) tubular adenomas	5–10 year colonoscopy	Timing based on clinical factors (e.g., family history, patient preference, physician judgment)
3–10 adenomas or 1 adenoma >1 cm or any adenoma with villous features or high grade dysplasia	3 year colonoscopy	All lesions completely removed. If follow-up scope shows only 1–2 small tubular adenomas, repeat colonoscopy in 5 years
>10 adenomas	<3 years colonoscopy	Consider polyp syndrome
Sessile adenoma(s) removed piecemeal	2–6 months colonoscopy to ensure complete excision	Once complete removal confirmed, subsequent follow up is based on clinical factors as above

[a]Assumes a full colonoscopy to the cecum in a well-prepared colon by an experienced endoscopist with a withdrawal time of 6–10 min from the cecum. (Adopted from Winawer SJ, Fletcher RH, Miller L, et al. Colorectal cancer screening: clinical guidelines and rationale. Gastroenterology. 1997;112:594–642.)

low enthusiasm for its use as a chemoprevention agent.[10,22] Chemoprevention methods that have been shown repetitively to lead to decreased adenoma development, however, include the intake of aspirin (relative risk between 0.65 and 0.96 for adenoma formation compared to that of controls), calcium (15% decline in adenoma risk), selenium, and cyclooxygenase-2 (cox-2) inhibitors (e.g., celecoxib).[22] Given the variable efficacy of these agents for preventing colon cancer, not all are recommended for institution as standard chemoprevention.[72] Of course, the cox-2 inhibitors have been the subject of controversy due to their association with cardiovascular toxicity that was identified during adenoma prevention trials. These agents were shown conclusively to decrease the development of advanced adenomas in high-risk individuals between 28 and 66% after 3 years of use, but the longevity of these affects was variable once the agents were discontinued due to the concerns about the cardiovascular side effects.[73,74] Further studies are ongoing to assess means to ameliorate the cardiovascular risks while preserving the chemoprevention advantages of these agents.

Special Adenomas

Rectal Adenomas

Rectal adenomas often create a more complex situation in terms of assessment and management than do colonic adenomas. When larger adenomas are encountered in the rectum, they may not be amenable to endoscopic polypectomy and therefore transanal excision or transabdominal radical resection may be necessary to ensure complete extirpation of the polyp as well as accurate pathologic assessment. For lesions in the lower half of the rectum, transanal excision is generally performed and can be facilitated with submucosal injection of saline or epinephrine under the lesion and use of any of the multitude of hemostasis devices that are available. Patient positioning and polyp exposure with appropriate retraction instruments and/or operative anoscopes can greatly facilitate removal of these sometime complex lesions. Other operative options include transsacral (Kraske or York-Mason) or transperineal approaches. For more proximal rectal lesions, transanal endoscopic microsurgery (TEM) may be appropriate. Larger lesions that extend too proximally for transanal excision will usually be best managed by anterior resection. If the lesion extends into the anal canal, anterior resection with anal mucosectomy and hand sewn coloanal anastomosis may be needed in order to maintain intestinal continuity and avoid the need for an abdominoperineal resection for a benign lesion. The technical aspects of TEM and the other noted procedures are discussed in more detail in Chap. 43.

Resection of difficult sessile rectal polyps (lower and middle third of the rectum, primarily) is best performed after full evaluation/staging for underlying malignancy using endorectal ultrasound or other staging procedure (e.g., MRI with endorectal coil). Endorectal ultrasound may offer some guidance for therapy after endoscopic polypectomy of a malignant polyp.[75] In general, however, endorectal ultrasound of these lesions is notoriously inaccurate after polypectomy due to the postprocedure inflammatory response of the local site and local lymph nodes, making accurate determination of the polyp stage difficult prior to neoadjuvant therapy or resection.[76] These staging evaluations are unnecessary if the patient is not even a candidate for radical resection or chemoradiation if an underlying malignancy were to be found.[77]

Malignant Polyps

Malignant polyps are defined as pedunculated or sessile polyps with cancer cells penetrating the lamina propria and muscularis mucosa into the submucosa. These polyps (T_1 lesions by definition) account for 2–12% of polyps in colonoscopic polypectomy series.[78–81] They may appear benign on gross endoscopic appearance and are therefore usually noted to harbor an invasive malignancy only once they are excised and examined histologically. These differ from polyps with high grade dysplasia (also called carcinoma *in situ*) in that dysplastic polyps have their malignant component superficial to the lamina propria and muscularis mucosa and therefore have no chance of metastatic spread. Dysplastic polyps require the same follow up as benign polyps as long as they are completely excised. Malignant polyps also differ from more deeply invasive cancers or larger T_1 lesions in that malignant polyps are excisable endoscopically while the more extensive lesions would require surgical resection for cure. The risk of a malignant polyp increases with patient age, degree of dysplasia noted in the polyp, and polyp size. One study noted the risk of cancer in an adenoma to be 1.3% in polyps <1 cm, 9.5% in polyps between 1 and 2 cm, and 46% in polyps ≥2 cm.[79] The risk of malignancy in another series was 2% for adenomas 0.6–1.5 cm; 19% for polyps 1.6–2.5 cm; 43% for polyps 2.6–3.5 cm; and 76% for polyps >3.5 cm.[78]

The clinical decision to proceed with further treatment after polypectomy for a malignant polyp, such as surgical resection or local excision, depends on the patient's general condition and the depth of invasion of the cancer (which offers a surrogate for the estimated risk of lymph node metastasis).[82] Haggitt's classification system of malignant polyps[83] is based on the level of invasion into the stalk of a pedunculated polyp (or the submucosa underlying a sessile polyp) (Figure 36-5):

Level 0 – noninvasive (high grade dysplasia)
Level 1 – cancer invading through the muscularis mucosa but limited to the head of a pedunculated polyp
Level 2 – cancer invading the neck of a pedunculated polyp
Level 3 – cancer invading the stalk of a pedunculated polyp
Level 4 – cancer invading into the submucosa of the bowel wall below the stalk of a pedunculated polyp. All sessile polyps with invasive cancer are level 4.

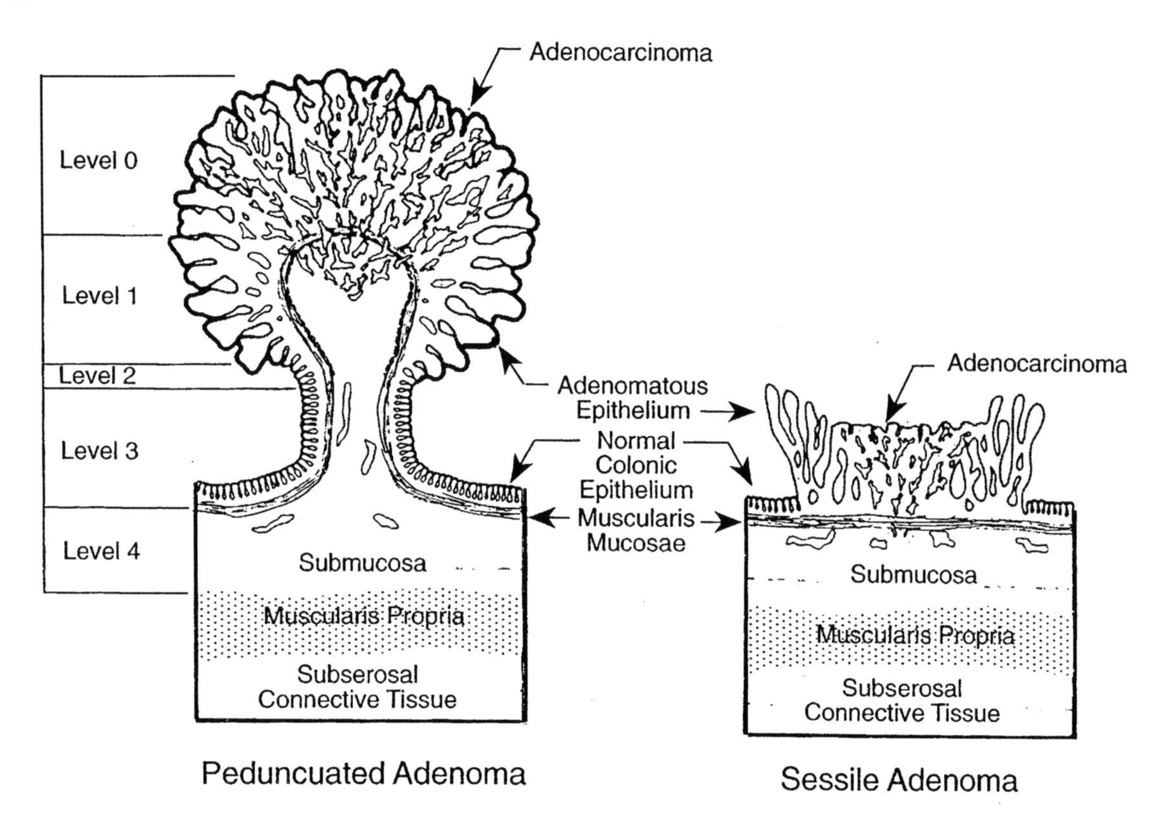

FIGURE 36-5. Anatomic landmarks of pedunculated and sessile malignant polyps. (Reprinted from Haggitt RC, Glotzbach RE, Soffer EE, et al. Prognostic factors in colorectal carcinomas arising in adenomas: implications for lesions removed by endoscopic polypectomy. Gastroenterology. 1985;89:328–36. With permission from the American Gastroenterological Society).

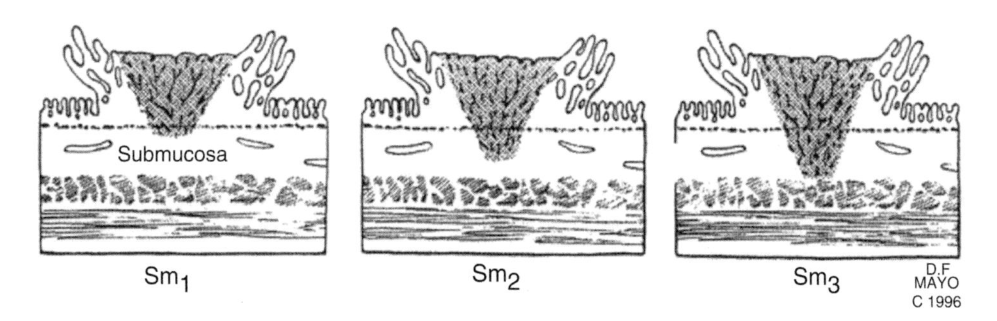

FIGURE 36-6. Depth of submucosal invasion in sessile malignant polyps; Sm_1: invasion into the upper third; Sm_2: invasion into the middle third; Sm_3: invasion into the lower third. (Reprinted with permission from Nivatvongs S. Surgical management of early colorectal cancer. Surg Clin North Am. 2000;8:1052–5).

The stalk of a pedunculated polyp is covered by normal mucosa and has a central core of submucosa. A line drawn at the junction of normal and adenomatous epithelium is the transition between the stalk and the head of the polyp, also called the neck (level 2). The risk of lymph node metastasis is <1% for pedunculated polyps with Haggitt level 1, 2, or 3 invasion.[79,83–85] The risk of lymph node metastasis for Haggitt level 4 lesions, pedunculated or sessile, ranges from 12 to 25%.[79,86–88] In order to better estimate the likelihood of nodal metastasis for a sessile malignant polyp (Haggitt level 4), Kudo[89] further stratified the depth of submucosal invasion into three levels (Figure 36-6):

SM_1 – invasion into the upper third of the submucosa
SM_2 – invasion into the middle third of the submucosa
SM_3 – invasion into the lower third of the submucosa

Haggitt levels 1, 2, and 3 are all considered equivalent to SM_1 while Haggitt level 4 may be SM_1, SM_2, or SM_3.

SM_3 level of invasion seems to have the greatest impact on likelihood of nodal metastases relative to SM_1 or SM_2.[81,82,86,90]

Other factors reported to be associated with an increased risk of lymph node metastases include lymphovascular invasion (LVI),[79,87,91] poor differentiation,[79,91–93] gender,[94] extensive budding, microacinar structure,[94] and flat or depressed lesions.[93] In a series of 353 T_1 sessile colorectal cancers, the risk factors for lymph node metastasis that were statistically significant on multivariate analysis included SM_3 level of invasion, LVI, and location in the lower third of the rectum.[86] In another study, only SM_3 invasion was an independent risk factor for lymph node metastases.[90] A positive polypectomy margin, regarded as inadequate treatment for a malignant polyp, has not been shown to be associated with increased nodal metastasis in some but not all studies,[95] but it is associated with increased local recurrence, distant metastases, and cancer-related death.[79] A distance of 2 mm beyond the deepest level of invasion is needed to consider the margin of polyp resection clear,[82] although there is debate as to how to define a positive margin.[95,96]

The rate of lymph node metastases from rectal lesions is not different from that of colon lesions. However, T_1 lesions in the distal third of the rectum have been found to have a higher risk of lymph node metastases than more proximal rectal lesions.[79,86] This finding is consistent with the high local recurrence rates, in the range of 5–28%, which have been observed following full thickness local excision of T_1 lesions of the distal rectum.[91,92,97,98] Controversy does exist, however, with some authors suggesting that malignant polyps in this location can actually be effectively treated endoscopically. Current NCCN guidelines for the treatment of rectal cancer recommend at least full thickness transanal excision of T_1 rectal cancers.[96]

In view of the very low risk of lymph node metastases with pedunculated polyps with invasion to Haggitt levels 1–3, these can be safely treated by margin-negative snare polypectomy. Level 4 pedunculated lesions are treated as sessile adenomas. Sessile lesions that are snared in one piece and have a margin of at least 2 mm are considered adequately treated.[82] This excision may be facilitated by endoscopic mucosal resection or other techniques described in above. If a piecemeal polypectomy was performed, margins can be difficult to assess adequately and therefore further endoscopic or surgical treatment is necessary to ensure complete removal of the polyp, staging, and cure. High-risk sessile lesions, such as those with SM_3, a resection margin of <2 mm, LVI, and/or poor differentiation should undergo appropriate oncologic resection.[79] For rectal lesions that are well- to moderately differentiated, <3 cm in size, <30% of the circumference of the bowel wall, mobile, and nonfixed, within 8 cm of the anal verge, without LVI or perineural invasion, and without evidence of nodal metastases on preoperative imaging, full thickness transanal excision with or without consideration of the use of TEM is acceptable based on NCCN guidelines.[96] Otherwise, transabdominal resection is recommended. Transanal excision of these lesions with adjuvant chemoradiation is an alternative approach but not considered the standard of care. See also *Rectal Adenomas* above.

Close endoscopic follow-up is required after polypectomy for a malignant polyp due to the concern for local recurrence of these lesions. A reasonable schedule is to examine the polypectomy site in 2–3 months and then every 6–12 months for the first 2 years with a complete colonoscopy done in the third year, and then at 3–5 year intervals depending on other findings and family history. For further discussion about the management of colorectal malignancies, see Chaps. 41 and 43.

Flat and Depressed Adenomas

Some adenomas display a flat or depressed growth pattern and are therefore not considered "true" polyps since they are not elevated above the mucosal surface.[99] They are defined in some classification systems as being elevated <2.5 mm off the surface of the colon ("flat" or "nonpolypoid") or depressed into the surface <2.5 mm ("depressed").[41,100] These are concerning in that they have a greater tendency to grow laterally or, in the case of the depressed lesions especially, into the wall of the colon rather than into the lumen. This makes their identification and potential for harboring malignancy concerning (between 27 and 36% of depressed cancers invade the submucosa versus <3% of cancers in polypoid lesions).[41] These lesions are recognized macroscopically by color and textural changes and by interruption of the capillary network pattern of the colonic wall.[41,99,101] They are most readily identified by chromoendoscopy with indigo carmine or other dye-spray techniques.[102] The pathogenesis of these lesions is thought to arise through different mechanisms than the traditional adenoma-carcinoma sequence, with a low level of *k-ras* and *APC* mutations in these lesions, a higher level of p53 mutations, and greater prevalence of MSI noted. In addition, these lesions appear to be more frequently associated with *de novo* adenocarcinomas, thus apparently bypassing the adenoma-carcinoma sequence entirely.[41]

The prevalence of flat and depressed adenomas in three Western population studies was approximately 20%, and these lesions contained cancer more often than polypoid adenomas.[103–105] One U.S. series showed <2% of lesions were depressed,[100] and reassessment of the original U.S. National Polyp Study polyp classification showed that 31.4% of the polyps in the original study would have been considered "flat."[41] Large Japanese series have also shown up to 42% of the all identified lesions to be of the nonpolypoid variety with <5% being depressed.[100] In a large UK study of 1,000 patients in which chromoendoscopy was used to search for small flat lesions, 36% of the 321 detected adenomas were flat or depressed.[103] The overall risk of a polypoid lesion containing early cancer was 8% but was 14% for the flat lesions. Flat or depressed lesions that were >1 cm were about twice as likely as polypoid lesions of a similar size to contain high grade dysplasia or cancer. Twenty nine percent of flat lesions >1 cm contained either high grade dysplasia or cancer. The average size of advanced flat and depressed adenomas is smaller than that of their polypoid counterparts.

Because of the risk of cancer, these lesions (except in rare cases with a normal overlying mucosal pattern in a <1 cm nonpolypoid lesions) should be removed, either by endoscopic polypectomy or by operative resection. It has been suggested that using special dyes and magnifying colonoscopy should be incorporated into general endoscopic practice to better identify these lesions.[99]

Serrated Polyps

Serrated polyps are a group of morphologically related lesions of the colon and rectum that differ in terms of their molecular etiology and malignant potential. Initially, these polyps were all categorized as hyperplastic polyps, but further research and closer histologic assessment revealed subsets of serrated polyps distinct from the benign hyperplastic polyps.[55,57,106] Serrated polyps include at least hyperplastic polyps and SSAs. Debate continues over the semantics and pathologic features of other subtypes of these polyps such as "sessile adenomas," "traditional sessile adenomas," and "sessile serrated polyps" (with interobserver variability as high as 40% among "expert" pathologists).[56] Concern about the nomenclature is mainly due to the use of "adenoma" in the names of these lesions and its implications for the malignant potential of these polyps and the need for further surveillance once these lesions are identified and treated. For the purpose of this review, the term "sessile serrated adenoma" will be used to describe those sessile polyps that are dysplastic and are clearly distinct from nondysplastic hyperplastic polyps. More important than the semantics debate is how the research into these lesions has lead to the discovery of the serrated neoplastic pathway, critical to the development of some sporadic and hereditary colorectal cancers with further implications for their treatment.

Hyperplastic Polyps

Hyperplastic polyps are considered metaplastic, nonneoplastic epithelial elevations with well-formed glands and crypts with frequent goblet cells (unlike adenomas with few goblet cells), although mucin-poor and microvesicular variants exist.[41,56] Because of the goblet cells, hyperplastic polyps are frequently coated with a layer of mucous (again, unlike adenomas), and they don't show the papillary infoldings or more prominent vasculature of adenomas, so this can facilitate their gross identification endoscopically. Although hyperplastic and adenomatous polyps have characteristic appearances, biopsy is needed to confirm the diagnosis, especially with smaller lesions. These polyps develop when epithelial cells from the base of the crypts differentiate and mature normally, but the cells accumulate on the mucosal surface leading to crowding of the epithelium and infoldings of the mucosa giving them a saw-toothed appearance histologically without dysplasia (Figure 36-7). This crowding is thought to be due to delayed shedding of the epithelial cells on the surface of the polyp and a failure of programmed cell death.[52,107–109]

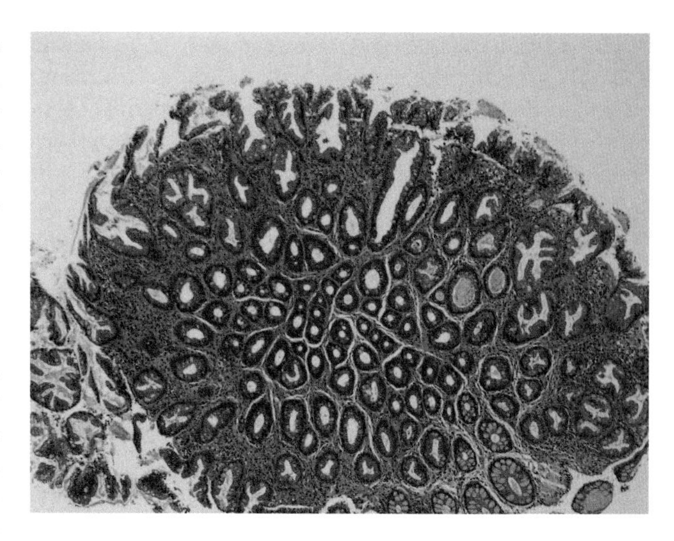

FIGURE 36-7. Microscopic view of a hyperplastic polyp (Courtesy of William Chopp, MD).

Endoscopic diagnosis based on visual appearance alone with standard colonoscopy has a sensitivity of 80% and specificity of 71%.[109] Chromoendoscopy can improve the ability to distinguish hyperplastic from adenomatous polyps. Hyperplastic polyps have a characteristic star-like pit pattern when stained with indigo carmine and assessed with magnifying colonoscopy. The sensitivity and specificity of this technique in discriminating between adenomatous and nonadenomatous polyps was found to be 93 and 95%, respectively.[57,111]

Hyperplastic polyps have a prevalence of 10–15% in adults in Western populations and represent 25% of all endoscopically excised polyps. They are usually small (<5 mm), sessile, and often are present in multiples. They are found primarily in the distal colon and rectum, although larger or more proximal lesions are described.[44,56] They are rarely symptomatic regardless of location. Because of their predominantly distal location, hyperplastic polyps are commonly found on flexible sigmoidoscopy. In a study of 1964 diminutive (≤5 mm) polyps on sigmoidoscopy, 41% were adenomas, 37% hyperplastic polyps, and 18% nonneoplastic.[11] Hyperplastic polyps are found more commonly in patients who smoke, consume alcohol, and have low dietary folate intake.[56]

Data conflict as to whether hyperplastic polyps found on a screening examination represent an increased risk of synchronous or metachronous neoplasia. While some authors have suggested that left-sided hyperplastic polyps are predictors of proximal adenomas, the U.S. National Polyp Study found no association between left-sided hyperplastic polyps and synchronous adenomas.[36] A report using data from two large chemoprevention studies demonstrated that hyperplastic polyps were not predictive of an increased risk of developing adenomatous polyps on follow-up colonoscopy.[112] Multiple professional societies state that hyperplastic polyps found on flexible sigmoidoscopy are not an indication for colonoscopy and that small, distal hyperplastic polyps on colonoscopy do not warrant more frequent surveillance.[1,113]

The risk of cancer developing in small, distal hyperplastic polyps is so small that these lesions do not warrant treatment, but lesions >1 cm and those identified in the proximal colon should be excised.[41] While the majority of hyperplastic polyps are thought to be nonneoplastic, these lesions have been implicated in the pathogenesis of some MSI-related and sporadic colorectal cancers. Their malignant degeneration is thought to occur through the serrated neoplasia pathway described below, but this is more likely due to misclassification of a SSA as a hyperplastic polyp.

The rare hereditary syndrome of hyperplastic polyposis facilitated the identification of the serrated neoplasia pathway once it was appreciated that this syndrome was not without cancer risk. This syndrome is characterized by either ≥30 hyperplastic polyps regardless of size or location or by five large (at least one or two being >1 cm) proximal hyperplastic polyps or by any number of hyperplastic polyps with a positive family history of hyperplastic polyposis. The more diffuse variety is thought to have a low malignant potential and be associated with *k-ras* mutations while the type with larger more proximal lesions (more likely SSAs than true hyplerplastic polyps) are thought to have greater malignant potential through the *BRAF*/MSI-related serrated neoplasia pathway.[56,57] The actual genotypic and phenotypic definitions of this syndrome remain under debate. Reports of patients with hyperplastic polyposis syndrome showed an average age of 52 years, >100 polyps in half the cases, an average polyp diameter of 16 mm (range 5–45 mm), and more than half of the patients had a cancer present (half of these in the right colon).[103,108] Management of this syndrome includes endoscopic removal of all polyps >5 mm and consideration of total abdominal colectomy and ileorectal anastomosis (lifelong distal endoscopy still required) for those patients who wish to avoid repeat colonoscopy or if their lesions are not endoscopically treatable due to polyp size, number, or presence of malignancy. Genetic counseling and familial assessment is recommended despite the lack of a clear gene for testing. Surveillance colonoscopy is recommended every 1–2 years with consideration for the use of chromoendoscopy to facilitate identification of the polyps.[57]

Sessile Serrated Adenomas

SSAs are uncommon polyps accounting for approximately 0.2–9% (usually <2%) of colorectal polyps, depending on the definition used.[56,114,115] Initially, these were described as hyperplastic polyps that contained adenomatous features but were later delineated as intermediate polyps. The SSA has exaggerated serrated crypts that are longer and broader than in hyperplastic polyps but still has a similar serrated or sawtooth epithelial appearance.[57] The SSA crypts contain cells with slight cytologic atypia like enlarged hyperchromatic and stratified nuclei (as in adenomas) as well as cells with normally arranged, small, basal nuclei (as in hyperplastic polyps).[103,108] They are also characterized by dilated crypts and crypt branching as well as hypermucinous epithelium (Figure 36-8).[56,57] Endoscopically, many SSAs grossly appear like hyperplastic polyps with pale, slightly protruding lesions, and most are in the range of 0.2–7.5 mm in diameter (Figure 36-9). Some SSAs are larger, however, and may resemble villous adenomas grossly. Unlike hyperplastic polyps, SSAs are more often found in the proximal colon and cecum. It is unclear whether SSAs develop in association with hyperplastic polyps or develop *de novo*, but it appears that the former is more likely based on molecular and pathologic studies.[57]

The relationship between SSAs and cancer has evolved since their initial description in the early 1990s and has

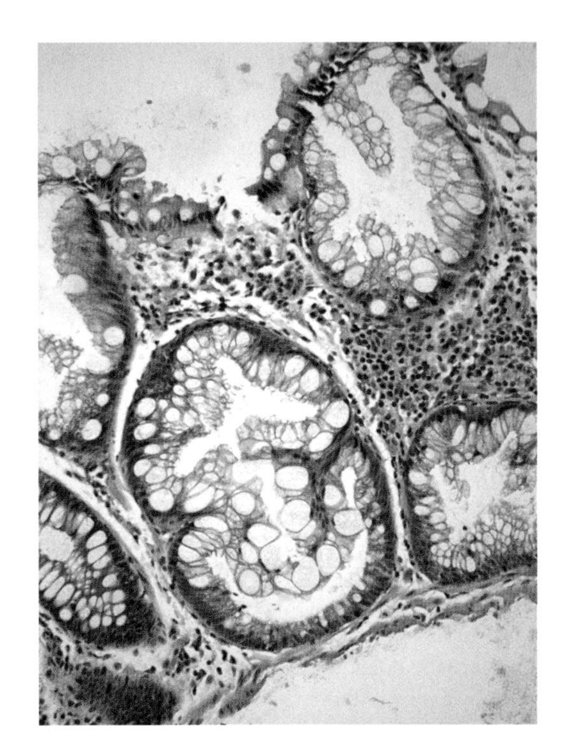

FIGURE 36-8. Microscopic view of a sessile serrated adenoma (Courtesy of M. Kay Washington, MD, PhD).

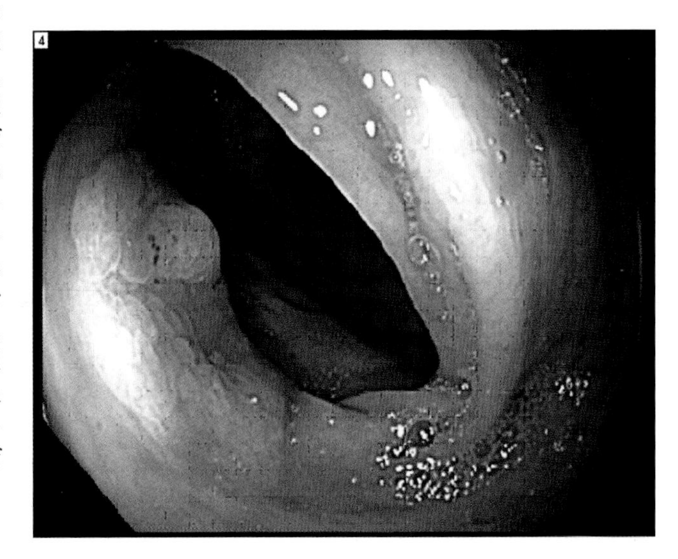

FIGURE 36-9. Endoscopic appearance of a sessile serrated adenoma.

elucidated the serrated neoplasia pathway. In one report, 5.8% of colorectal cancers were associated with an adjacent SSA and up to 37% of SSAs harbored dysplasia.[56,57,110,115] One review concluded that the risk of high grade dysplasia was the same in SSAs as in the more common adenomatous phenotypes.[115] In addition, the association of cancer with hyperplastic polyposis syndrome (when the syndrome is characterized by the SSA-predominant type of polyps) seems to make the link between SSAs and cancer development more conclusive. The relative rarity of SSAs being identified at the time of malignant transformation may be due to a rapid transition from dysplasia to malignancy in these lesions. This may be similar to the quick malignant transformation in HNPCC-associated cancers due to germline mismatch repair deficiency. The serrated neoplasia pathway is believed to be characterized by initial loss of *BRAF* with subsequent hypermethylation of promoter regions of a number of genes including the *hMLH1* mismatch repair gene leading to MSI phenotype cancers. When SSAs are found concomitantly with a cancer, their molecular characteristics are often similar, including loss of the *hMLH1* protein, further supporting the serrated neoplasia theory.[55] Individuals with sporadic colorectal cancer with high level MSI (MSI-H) cancers are four times more likely to harbor at least one serrated polyp than individuals with low MSI cancers.[103] Sporadic adenocarcinomas arising through the serrated neoplasia pathway occur in older patients (>70 years), have a female gender bias, and are predominantly located in the right colon, similar to SSAs. Because the rate of malignant degeneration of SSAs and their recurrence rate have not been determined, current recommendations support management and surveillance similar to traditional adenomas.[55,56] Initial detection and treatment of SSAs is also facilitated by the techniques useful in identifying hyperplastic polyps including chromoendoscopy and magnification colonoscopy.[57]

Hamartomas

The term hamartoma was originally coined by Albrecht in 1904 to refer to abnormally arranged but nondysplastic architecture of any of the layers of the normal lining of the colon (or other tissues).[116] These polyps are usually considered nonneoplastic except when associated with rare hereditary disorders that have been linked to an increased risk of colorectal cancer and include the following: familial juvenile polyposis syndrome (JPS), Peutz–Jeghers syndrome (PJS), PTEN hamartoma tumor syndrome (PHTS), multiple endocrine neoplasia syndrome 2B, hereditary mixed polyposis syndrome, Cronkhite–Canada syndrome, basal cell nevus syndrome, and neurofibromatosis 1 (some of which are discussed in Chap. 37). These conditions represent the etiology of <1% of all gastrointestinal malignancies.[117]

Whether part of a syndrome or when occurring as a sporadic hamartomatous polyp, there are two primary hamartoma types described in the colon: juvenile (or retention) polyps and Peutz–Jegher type polyps. The former term was introduced in the late 1950s by Horrilleno after a review of pediatric colorectal polyps, but they are named based on their histology and not the age of presentation as they can occur at any age.[118] Juvenile polyps are characterized by three classic histologic features including dilated mucous-filled glands/retention cysts lined by columnar epithelium, an expanded and abundant lamina propria, and infiltration of inflammatory cells, often eosinophils.[118,119] The muscularis is not usually part of the structure of these polyps. They are usually round with a smooth, often shiny appearance and are frequently pedunculated. Juvenile polyps can reach several centimeters in diameter.[119] These are differentiated from the Peutz–Jegher type polyp which are grossly more red and lobulated with their histology characterized by arborizing smooth muscle proliferation from the muscularis mucosa that is then lined by normal colonic epithelium with extensive goblet cells (Figure 36-10). Neither of these polyp types is characterized by abnormal mucosal lining or increase in mitoses to suggest premalignancy.[117]

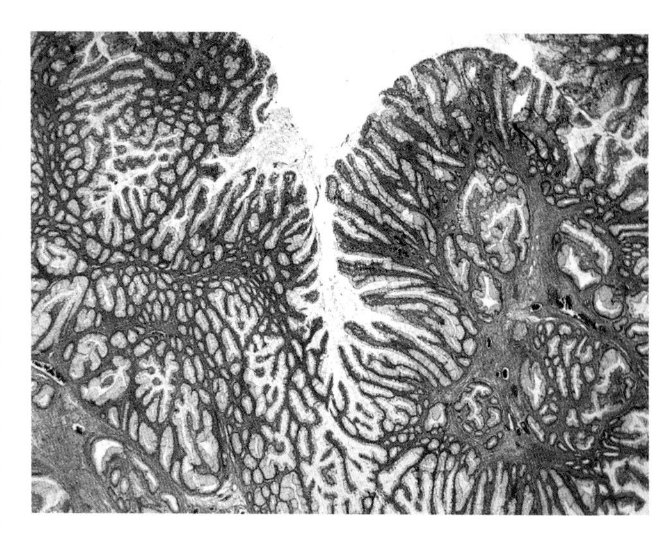

FIGURE 36-10. Microscopic view of a hamartomatous Peutz–Jegher polyp (Courtesy of Tonia Zuluaga Toro, MD).

The majority of isolated colorectal hamartomas present as juvenile polyps before the age of 10 with a peak presentation around the age of 5 years and are diagnosed with endoscopic assessment and biopsy/excision. Sporadic hamartomas represent <1% of polyps identified in adults, are usually larger than 1 cm and pedunculated at the time of diagnosis.[120] The majority of these isolated polyps in adults and children are found in the sigmoid colon and rectum and present with symptoms of rectal bleeding and/or polyp prolapse, but patients may present with anemia, diarrhea, and/or mucoid stools. Colonic intussusception is rarely associated with more proximal polyps. These polyps can autoamputate when they become larger due to their long stalks, and they can therefore be passed in the stool. Treatment of hamartomas is usually endoscopic but may require resection if the polyp is too large to be removed endoscopically or if there is evidence of malignancy within the polyp.

Malignant degeneration of solitary colorectal hamartomas appears to be a very rare phenomenon, so much so that some authors feel that this is purely "coincidental."[119] The malignant degeneration of these polyps in the hamartomatous polyposis syndromes is not well understood. Theories have been based on histologic findings of hamartoma-related adenomas and cancers as well as genetic studies in hamartomatous polyposis syndrome patients. These theories include a mechanism whereby changes affecting the lamina propria may lead directly to epithelial cancers and/or alterations in cell polarity (due to *STK11* mutations) combined with colonic stem cell expansion leading to cancers (hamartoma to carcinoma sequence),[118,119] a hamartoma to adenoma to carcinoma sequence mechanism,[119,121] or simply "traditional" degeneration of sporadic adenomas in the setting of hamartomatous polyps.[119] More specific theories of malignant degeneration of these polyps suggests that it is related to aberrations in the TGF-β pathway that has been associated with colorectal cancers in Lynch syndrome/HNPCC as well as in some sporadic microsatellite unstable cancers, perhaps due to *SMAD4* mutations (a tumor suppressor gene associated with some hamartomatous polyposis syndromes). Further studies are ongoing to elucidate the likely multifactorial mechanisms associated with the degeneration of these polyps.

Inflammatory Polyps

Inflammatory polyps are islands or elevations of normal or near-normal colonic mucosa and submucosa surrounded by denuded or abnormal colonic lining and therefore are not considered true "polyps" (Figure 36-11). They are usually associated with a chronic inflammatory process of the colon, especially with inflammatory colitis (Crohn's and ulcerative colitis) but can also be due to regeneration of the colonic lining in inflammatory, infectious, or ischemic conditions.[122] Symptoms from the polyps including bleeding and diarrhea can be difficult to differentiate from the symptoms of the underlying condition leading to the development of these polyps.[123] Rarely, obstruction or intussusception can occur if the inflammatory polyps become very large ("giant inflammatory polyposis").[124] Treatment is focused on the underlying disease causing the chronic inflammation or ischemia. Inflammatory polyps are not neoplastic but can make screening for neoplasia in chronic inflammatory conditions of the colon difficult due to their concerning appearance with endoscopic surveillance and their potential to mask an underlying malignancy.[125]

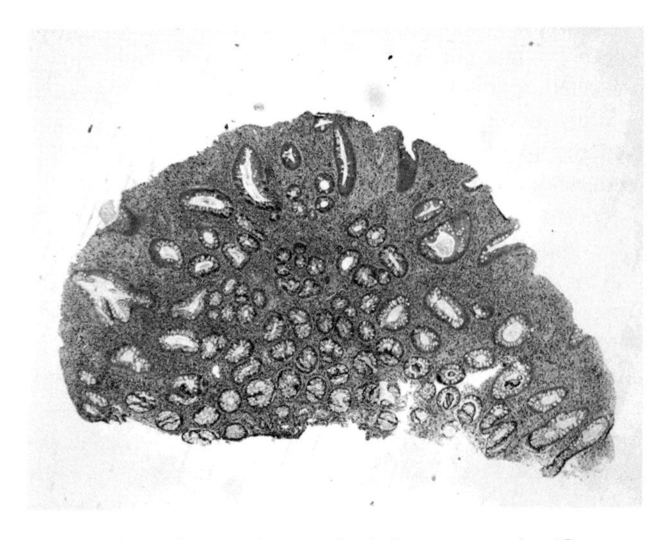

FIGURE 36-11. Microscopic view of an inflammatory polyp (Courtesy of Tania Zuluaga Toro, MD).

References

1. Levin B, Lieberman DA, McFarland B, et al. Screening and surveillance for the early detection of colorectal cancer and adenomatous polyps, 2008: a joint guideline from the American Cancer Society, the US Multi-Society Task Force on Colorectal Cancer, and the American College of Radiology. CA Cancer J Clin. 2008;58(3):130–60.
2. Turner JR. The gastrointestinal tract. In: Kumar V, Abbase AK, Fausto N, Aster JC, editors. Robbins and Cotran pathologic basis of disease, Professional edition. 8th ed. Philadelphia, PA: Saunders Elsevier; 2009.
3. Winawer SJ, Fletcher RH, Miller L, et al. Colorectal cancer screening: clinical guidelines and rationale. Gastroenterology. 1997;112:594–642.
4. Simons BD, Morrison AS, Lev R, et al. Relationship of polyps to cancer of the large intestine. J Natl Cancer Inst. 1992;84:962–6.
5. Gschwantler M, Kriwanek S, Langner E, et al. High-grade dysplasia and invasive carcinoma in colorectal adenomas; a multivariate analysis of the impact of adenoma and patient characteristics. Eur J Gastroenterol Hepatol. 2002;14:183–8.
6. Patel K, Hoffman NE. The anatomical distribution of colorectal polyps at colonoscopy. J Clin Gastroenterol. 2001;33(3):222–5.
7. Bond JH. Polyp guideline: diagnosis, treatment, and surveillance for patients with nonfamilial colorectal polyps. The Practice Parameters Committee of the American College of Gastroenterology. Ann Intern Med. 1993;119:836–43.
8. Schoenfeld P, Cash B, Flood A, et al. Colonoscopic screening of average-risk women for colorectal neoplasia. N Engl J Med. 2005;352(20):2061–8.
9. Boursi B, Halak A, Umansky M, et al. Colonoscopic screening of an average-risk population for colorectal neoplasia. Endoscopy. 2009;41(6):516–21.
10. Giacosa A, Frascio F, Munizzi F. Epidemiology of colorectal polyps. Tech Coloproctol. 2004;8 Suppl 2:s243–7.
11. Farraye FA, Wallace M. Clinical significance of small polyps found during screening with flexible sigmoidoscopy. Gastrointest Endosc Clin North Am. 2002;12:41–51.
12. Winawer SJ, Stewart ET, Zauber AG, et al. A comparison of colonoscopy and double-contrast barium enema for surveillance after polypectomy. National Polyp Study Work Group. N Engl J Med. 2000;342:1766–72.
13. Winawer SJ, Zauber AG, Ho MN, et al. Prevention of colorectal cancer by colonoscopic polypectomy. The National Polyp Study Workgroup. N Engl J Med. 1993;329:1977–81.
14. Davila RE et al. ASGE guideline: colorectal cancer screening and surveillance. Gastrointest Endosc. 2006;63:546–57.
15. Blachar A, Sosna J. CT colonography (virtual colonoscopy): technique, indications, and performance. Digestion. 2007; 76:34–41.

16. Landeras LA, Aslam R, Yee J. Virtual colonoscopy: technique and accuracy. Radiol Clin North Am. 2007;45:333–45.
17. Villavicencio RT, Rex DK. Colonic adenomas: prevalence and incidence rates, growth rates, and miss rates at colonoscopy. Semin Gastrointest Dis. 2000;11:185–93.
18. Lieberman DS, Smith FW. Screening for colon malignancy with colonoscopy. Am J Gastroenterol. 1991;86:946–51.
19. Foutch PG, Mai H, Pardy K, et al. Flexible sigmoidoscopy may be ineffective for secondary prevention of colorectal cancer in asymptomatic, average-risk men. Dig Dis Sci. 1991;36:924–8.
20. Johnson DA, Gurney MS, Volpe RJ, et al. A prospective study of the prevalence of colonoscopic neoplasms in asymptomatic patients with an age-related risk. Am J Gastroenterol. 1990;85:969–74.
21. Rex DK, Lehman GA, Ulbright TM, et al. Colonic neoplasia in asymptomatic persons with negative fecal occult blood tests: influence of age, gender and family history. Am J Gastroenterol. 1993;88:825–31.
22. Marshall JR. Prevention of colorectal cancer: diet, chemoprevention, and lifestyle. Gastroenterol Clin North Am. 2008; 37:73–82.
23. Leiberman DA, Weiss DG, Bond JH, et al. Use of colonoscopy to screen asymptomatic adults for colorectal cancer. Veterans Affairs Cooperative Study Group 380. N Engl J Med. 2000;343:162–8.
24. Brenner H, Hoffmeister M, Stegmaier C, et al. Risk of progression of advanced adenomas to colorectal cancer by age and sex: estimates based on 840, 149 screening colonoscopies. Gut. 2007;56:1585–9.
25. Pariente A, Milan C, Lafon J, et al. Colonoscopic screening in first-degree relatives of patients with "sporadic" colorectal cancer: a case-control study. The Association Nationale des Gastroenterologues des Hopitaux and Registre Bourguinon des Cancers Digestifs (INSERM CRI 9505). Gastroenterology. 1998;115:7–12.
26. Gaglia P, Atkin WS, Whitelaw S, et al. Variables associated with the risk of colorectal adenomas in asymptomatic patients with a family history of colorectal cancer. Gut. 1995;36:385–90.
27. Menges M, Fischinger J, Gärtner B, et al. Screening colonoscopy in 40- to 50-year-old first-degree relatives of patients with colorectal cancer is efficient: a controlled multicentre study. Int J Colorectal Dis. 2006;21(4):301–7.
28. Rex DK. Colonoscopy: a review of its yield for cancers and adenomas by indication. Am J Gastroenterol. 1995;90: 353–65.
29. Schatzkin A, Lanza E, Corle D, et al. Lack of effect of a low-fat, high-fiber diet on the recurrence of colorectal adenomas. Polyp Prevention Trial Study Group. N Engl J Med. 2000;342: 1149–55.
30. Triantafyllou K, Papatheodoridis GV, Paspatis GA, et al. Predictors of the early development of advanced metachronous colon adenomas. Hepatogastroenterology. 1997;44:533–8.
31. Alberts DS, Martinez ME, Roe DJ, et al. Lack of effect of a high-fiber cereal supplement on the recurrence of colorectal adenomas. Phoenix Colon Cancer Prevention Physicians' Network. N Engl J Med. 2000;342:1156–62.
32. Martínez ME, Baron JA, Lieberman DA, et al. A pooled analysis of advanced colorectal neoplasia diagnoses after colonoscopic polypectomy. Gastroenterology. 2009;136(3):832–41.
33. Noshirwani KC, van Stolk RU, Rybicki LA, et al. Adenoma size and number are predictive of adenoma recurrence: implications for surveillance colonoscopy. Gastrointest Endosc. 2000;51(4 Pt 1):433–7.
34. Holtzman R, Poulard JB, Bank S, et al. Repeat colonoscopy after endoscopic polypectomy. Dis Colon Rectum. 1987;30:185–8.
35. Woolfson IK, Eckholdt GJ, Wetzel CR, et al. Usefulness of performing colonoscopy one year after endoscopic polypectomy. Dis Colon Rectum. 1990;33:389–93.
36. Winawer SJ, Zauber AG, Fletcher RH, et al. Guidelines for colonoscopy surveillance after polypectomy: a consensus update by the US Multi-Society Task Force on Colorectal Cancer and the American Cancer Society. Gastroenterology. 2006;130:1872–85.
37. Rex DK, Cutler CS, Lemmel GT, et al. Colonoscopic miss rates of adenomas determined by back-to-back colonoscopies. Gastroenterology. 1997;112:24–8.
38. Hoff G, Vatn M. Epidemiology of polyps of the rectum and sigmoid colon. Endoscopic evaluation of size and localization of polyps. Scand J Gastroenterol. 1985;20:356–60.
39. Kronborg O, Hage E, Deichgraeber E. A prospective, partly randomized study of the effectiveness of repeated examination of the colon after polypectomy and radical surgery for cancer. Scan J Gastroenterol. 1981;16:879–84.
40. Hixson LS, Fennerty MB, Sampliner RE, et al. Prospective study of the frequency and size distribution of polyps missed by colonoscopy. J Natl Cancer Inst. 1990;82:1769–72.
41. Kudo S, Lambert R, Allen JI, et al. Nonpolypoid neoplastic lesions of the colorectal mucosa. Gastrointest Endosc. 2008;68(4 Suppl):S3–47.
42. Winawer SJ. Appropriate intervals for surveillance. Gastrointest Endosc. 1999;49(3 Pt 2):S63–6.
43. Rex DK, Cummings OW, Helper DJ, et al. Five-year incidence of adenomas after negative colonoscopy in asymptomatic average-risk persons. Gastroenterology. 1996;111:1178–81.
44. Tolliver KA, Rex DK. Colonoscopic polypectomy. Gastroenterol Clin North Am. 2008;37(1):229–51.
45. Leung K, Pinsky P, Laiyemo AO, et al. Ongoing colorectal cancer risk despite surveillance colonoscopy: the Polyp Prevention Trial Continued Follow-up Study. Gastrointest Endosc. 2010;71(1):111–7.
46. Winawer SJ et al. Guidelines for colonoscopy surveillance after polypectomy: a consensus update by the US Multi-Society Task Force on Colorectal Cancer and the American Cancer Society. CA Cancer J Clin. 2006;56:143–59.
47. Knoernschild HE. Growth rate and malignant potential of colonic polyps: early results. Surg Forum. 1963;14:137–8.
48. Carroll RLA, Klein M. How often should patients be sigmoidoscoped? A mathematical perspective. Prev Med. 1980;9:741–6.
49. Stryker SJ, Wolff BG, Culp CE, et al. Natural history of untreated colonic polyps. Gastroenterology. 1987;93:1009–13.
50. Eide TJ. Risk of colorectal cancer in adenoma-bearing individuals within a defined population. Int J Cancer. 1986;38:173–6.
51. Brenner H, Hoffmeister M, Stegmaier C, et al. Risk of progression of advanced adenomas to colorectal cancer by age and sex: estimates based on 840, 149 screening colonoscopies. Gut. 2007;56:1585–9.
52. Lamlum H, Papadopoulou A, Ilyas M, et al. APC mutations are sufficient for the growth of early colorectal adenomas. Proc Natl Acad Sci USA. 2000;97:2225–8.

53. Cappell MS. Pathophysiology, clinical presentation, and management of colon cancer. Gastroenterol Clin North Am. 2008;37(1):1–24. v.
54. Konishi M, Kikuchi-Yanoshita R, Tanaka K, et al. Molecular nature of colon tumors in hereditary nonpolyposis colon cancer, familial polyposis, and sporadic colon cancer. Gastroenterology. 1996;111:307–17.
55. Harvey NT, Ruszkiewicz A. Serrated neoplasia of the colorectum. World J Gastroenterol. 2007;13(28):3792–8.
56. Vakiani E, Yantiss RK. Pathologic features and biologic importance of colorectal serrated polyps. Adv Anat Pathol. 2009;16(2):79–91.
57. East JE, Saunders BP, Jass JR. Sporadic and syndromic hyperplastic polyps and serrated adenomas of the colon: classification, molecular genetics, natural history, and clinical management. Gastroenterol Clin North Am. 2008;37(1):25–46. v.
58. Tsuga K, Haruma K, Fujimura J, et al. Evaluation of the colorectal wall in normal subjects and patients with ulcerative colitis using an ultrasonic catheter probe. Gastrointest Endosc. 1998;48:477–84.
59. Waye JD. Endoscopic mucosal resection of colonic polyps. Gastrointest Endosc Clin North Am. 2001;11:537–48. vii.
60. Zlatanic J, Waye JD, Kim PS, et al. Large sessile colonic adenomas: use of argon plasma coagulator to supplement piecemeal snare polypectomy. Gastrointest Endosc. 1999;49: 731–5.
61. Uno Y, Munakata A. The non-lifting sign of invasive colon cancer. Gastrointest Endosc. 1994;40:485–9.
62. Dellon ES, Hawk JS, Grimm IS, Shaheen NJ. The use of carbon dioxide for insufflation during GI endoscopy: a systematic review. Gastrointest Endosc. 2009;69(4):843–9.
63. Winter H, Lang RA, Spelsberg FW, et al. Laparoscopic colonoscopic rendezvous procedures for the treatment of polyps and early stage carcinomas of the colon. Int J Colorectal Dis. 2007;22(11):1377–81.
64. Franklin Jr ME, Portillo G. Laparoscopic monitored colonoscopic polypectomy: long-term follow-up. World J Surg. 2009;33(6):1306–9.
65. Wilhelm D, von Delius S, Weber L, et al. Combined laparoscopic-endoscopic resections of colorectal polyps: 10-year experience and follow-up. Surg Endosc. 2009;23(4):688–93.
66. Bond JH. Colorectal cancer update. Prevention, screening, treatment and surveillance for high-risk groups. Med Clin North Am. 2000;84:1163–82. viii.
67. Bond JH. Colon polyps and cancer. Endoscopy. 2003;35: 27–35.
68. Atkin WS, Morson BC, Cuzick J. Long-term risk of colorectal cancer after excision of rectosigmoid adenomas. N Engl J Med. 1992;326:658–62.
69. Spencer RJ, Melton III LJ, Ready RL, et al. Treatment of small colorectal polyps: a population based study of risks of subsequent carcinoma. Mayo Clin Proc. 1984;59:305–10.
70. Ko C, Hyman NH. Practice parameter for the detection of colorectal neoplasms: an interim report (revised). Dis Colon Rectum. 2006;49:299–301.
71. Ferrucci LM, Sinha R, Graubard BI, et al. Dietary meat intake in relation to colorectal adenoma in asymptomatic women. Am J Gastroenterol. 2009;104(5):1231–40.
72. Weingarten MA, Zalmanovici A, Yaphe J. Dietary calcium supplementation for preventing colorectal cancer and adenomatous polyps. Cochrane Database Syst Rev. 2008;(1):CD003548.
73. Bertagnolli MM, Eagle CJ, Zauber AG, et al. Five year efficacy and safety analysis of the adenoma prevention with celecoxib (APC) trial. Cancer Prev Res. 2009;2(4):310–21.
74. Dubois R. New, long-term insights from the adenoma prevention with celecoxib trial on a promising but troubled class of drugs. Cancer Prev Res. 2009;2(4):285–7.
75. Kruskal JB, Sentovich SM, Kane RA. Staging of rectal cancer after polypectomy: usefulness of endorectal US. Radiology. 1999;211(1):31–5.
76. García-Aguilar J, Hernández de Anda E, Rothenberger DA, et al. Endorectal ultrasound in the management of patients with malignant rectal polyps. Dis Colon Rectum. 2005;48(5):910–6. discussion 916–7.
77. Nivatvongs S, Nicholson JD, Rothenberger DA, et al. Villous adenomas of the rectum: the accuracy of clinical assessment. Surgery. 1980;87:549–51.
78. Nusko G, Mansmann U, Partzsch U, et al. Invasive carcinoma in colorectal adenomas: multivariate analysis of patient and adenoma characteristics. Endoscopy. 1997;29:626–31.
79. Ramirez M, Schierling S, Papaconstantinou HT, Scott Thomas J.Management of the malignant polyp. Clin Colon Rectal Surg. 2008;21(4):286–90.
80. Nivatvongs S. Complications in colonoscopic polypectomy: an experience with 1, 555 polypectomies. Dis Colon Rectum. 1986;29:825–30.
81. Seitz U, Bohnacker S, Seewald S, et al. Is endoscopic polypectomy an adequate therapy for malignant colorectal adenomas? Presentation of 114 patients and review of the literature. Dis Colon Rectum. 2004;47(11):1789–96.
82. Nivatvongs S. Surgical management of malignant colorectal polyps. Surg Clin North Am. 2002;82:959–66.
83. Haggitt RC, Glotzbach RE, Soffer EE, et al. Prognostic factors in colorectal carcinomas arising in adenomas: implications for lesions removed by endoscopic polypectomy. Gastroenterology. 1985;89:328–36.
84. Kyzer S, Begin LR, Gordon PH, et al. The care of patients with colorectal polyps that contain invasive adenocarcinoma: endoscopic polypectomy or colectomy. Cancer. 1992;70:2044–50.
85. Nivatvongs S, Rojanasakul A, Reiman ME, et al. The risk of lymph node metastases in colorectal polyps with invasive adnenocarcinoma. Dis Colon Rectum. 1991;34:323–8.
86. Nascimbeni R, Burgart LG, Nivatvongs S, et al. Risk of lymph node metastases in T1 carcinoma of colon and rectum. Dis Colon Rectum. 2002;45:200–6.
87. Cooper HS, Deppisch LM, Gourley WK, et al. Endoscopically removed malignant colorectal polyps: clinical pathologic correlations. Gastroenterology. 1995;108:1657–65.
88. Coverlizza S, Risio M, Ferrari A, et al. Colorectal adenomas containing invasive carcinoma: pathologic assessment of lymph node metastatic potential. Cancer. 1989;64:1937–47.
89. Kudo S. Endoscopic mucosal resection of flat and depressed types of early colorectal cancer. Endoscopy. 1993;25:455–61.
90. Kikuchi R, Takano M, Takagi K, et al. Management of early invasive colorectal cancer: risk of recurrence and clinical guidelines. Dis Colon Rectum. 1995;38:1286–95.
91. Blumberg D, Paty PB, Guillem JG, et al. All patients with small intramural rectal cancers are at risk for lymph node metastases. Dis Colon Rectum. 1999;42:881–5.
92. Brodsky JT, Richard GK, Cohen AM, et al. Variables correlated with the risk of lymph node metastases in early rectal cancer. Cancer. 1992;69:322–6.

93. Tanaka S, Harouma K, Teixeira CR, et al. Endoscopic treatment of submucosal invasive colorectal carcinoma with special reference to risk factors for lymph node metastases. J Gastroenterol. 1995;30:710–7.
94. Goldstein NS, Hart J. Histologic features associated with lymph node metastases in stage T1 and superficial T2 rectal adenocarcinomas in abdominoperineal resection specimens. Identifying a subset of patients for whom treatment with adjuvant therapy or completion abdominoperineal resection should be considered after local excision. Am J Clin Pathol. 1999;111:51–8.
95. Boenicke L, Fein M, Sailer M. The concurrence of histologically positive resection margins and sessile morphology is an important risk factor for lymph node metastasis after complete endoscopic removal of malignant colorectal polyps. Int J Colorectal Dis. 2010;25(4):433–8.
96. The National Comprehensive Cancer Network (NCCN) clinical practice guidelines in oncology, colon cancer and rectal cancer, v.1.2010. www.nccn.org. Accessed 8 Feb 2010.
97. Garcia-Aguilar J, Mellgren A, Sirivongs P, et al. Local excision of rectal cancer without adjuvant therapy: a word of caution. Ann Surg. 2000;231:345–51.
98. Chakravarti A, Compton CC, Shellito PC, et al. Long-term follow-up of patients with rectal cancer managed by local excision with and without adjuvant irradiation. Ann Surg. 1999;230:49–54.
99. Reinacher-Schick A, Schmiegel W. Surveillance strategies in patients after polypectomy. Dig Dis. 2002;20:61–9.
100. Lambert R, Kudo SE, Vieth M, et al. Pragmatic classification of superficial neoplastic colorectal lesions. Gastrointest Endosc. 2009;70(6):1182–99.
101. Muto T, Kamiya J, Sawada T, et al. Small "flat adenoma" of the large bowel with special reference to its clinicopathologic features. Dis Colon Rectum. 1985;28:847–51.
102. Jaramillo E, Watanabe M, Slezak P, et al. Flat neoplastic lesions of the colon and rectum detected by high-resolution video endoscopy and chromoscopy. Gastrointest Endosc. 1995;42:114–22.
103. Rembacken BJ, Fujii T, Cairns A, et al. Flat and depressed colonic neoplasms: a prospective study of 1000 colonoscopies in the UK. Lancet. 2000;355:1211–4.
104. Saitoh Y, Waxman I, West AB, et al. Prevalence and distinctive biologic features of flat colorectal adenomas in the North American population. Gastroenterology. 2001;120:1657–65.
105. Smith GA, Oien KA, O'Dwyer PJ. Frequency of early colorectal cancer in patients undergoing colonoscopy. Br J Surg. 1999;86:1328–31.
106. Estrada RG, Spjut HJ. Hyperplastic polyps of the large bowel. Am J Surg Pathol. 1980;4(2):127–33.
107. Jass JR. Pathogenesis of colorectal cancer. Surg Clin North Am. 2002;82:891–904.
108. Hawkins NJ, Bariol C, Ward RL. The serrated neoplasia pathway. Pathology. 2002;34:548–55.
109. Rembacken BJ, Trecca A, Fujii T. Serrated adenomas. Dig Liver Dis. 2001;33:305–12.
110. Norfleet RG, Ryan ME, Wyman JB. Adenomatous and hyperplastic polyps cannot be reliably distinguished by their appearance through the fiberoptic sigmoidoscope. Dig Dis Sci. 1988;33:1175–7.
111. Axelrad AM, Fleischer DE, Geller AJ, et al. High resolution chromoendoscopy for the diagnosis of diminutive colon polyps: implications for colon cancer screening. Gastroenterology. 1996;110:1253–8.
112. Bensen SP, Cole BF, Mott LA, et al. Colorectal hyperplastic polyps and risk of recurrence of adenomas and hyperplastic polyps. Polyp Prevention Study (Letter). Lancet. 1999;354:1873–4.
113. Bond JH. Polyp guidelines: diagnosis, treatment, and surveillance for patients with colorectal polyps: Practice Parameters Committee of the American College of Gastroenterology. Am J Gastroenterol. 2000;95:3053–63.
114. Longacre TA, Fenoglio-Preiser CM. Mixed hyperplastic adenomatous polyps/serrated adenomas. A distinct form of co1orectal neoplasia. Am J Surg Pathol. 1990;14:524–37.
115. Matsumoto T, Mizuno M, Shimizu M, et al. Clinicopathological features of serrated adenoma of the colorectum: comparison with traditional adenoma. J Clin Pathol. 1999;52:513–6.
116. Ober WB. Selected items from the history of pathology: Eugen Albrecht, MD (1872-1908): hamartoma and choristoma. Am J Pathol. 1978;91(3):606.
117. Chen HM, Fang JY. Genetics of the hamartomatous polyposis syndromes: a molecular review. Int J Colorectal Dis. 2009;24:865–74.
118. Calva D, Howe JR. Hamartomatous polyposis syndromes. Surg Clin North Am. 2008;88(4):779–817.
119. Zbuk KM, Eng C. Hamartomatous polyposis syndromes. Nat Clin Pract Gastroenterol Hepatol. 2007;4(9):492–502.
120. Mesiya S, Ancha HB, Ancha H, Lightfoot S, Kida M, Guild R, et al. Sporadic colonic hamartomas in adults: a retrospective study. Gastrointest Endosc. 2005;62(6):886–91.
121. Brahim EB, Jouini R, Khayat O, et al. Adenomatous transformation in hamartomatous polyps cases of two patients with Peutz–Jeghers Syndrome. Int J Colorectal Dis. 2009;24:1361–3.
122. Pidala MJ, Slezak FA, Hlivko TJ. Delayed presentation of an inflammatory polyp following colonic ischemia. Am Surg. 1993;59(5):315–8.
123. Kosugi I, Tada T, Tsutsui Y, Sato Y, Mitsui T, Itazu I. Giant inflammatory polyposis of the descending colon associated with a Crohn's disease-like colitis. Pathol Int. 2002;52(4):318–21.
124. Esaki M, Matsumoto T, Fuyuno Y, Maehata Y, Kochi S, Hirahashi M, et al. Giant inflammatory polyposis of the cecum with repeated intussusception in ulcerative colitis: report of a case. Am J Gastroenterol. 2009;104(11):2873–4.
125. Buck JL, Dachman AH, Sobin LH. Polypoid and pseudopolypoid manifestations of inflammatory bowel disease. Radiographics. 1991;11(2):293–304.

37 Hereditary Colorectal Cancer

James Church

Colorectal cancer is both a genetic and epigenetic disease. It arises because of an accumulation of genetic and epigenetic abnormalities that perturb gene expression and lead to carcinogenesis within the colorectal mucosa. The classes of genes primarily involved are largely those concerned with regulation of cell growth: tumor suppressor genes and proto-oncogenes, and the average sporadic colorectal cancer has accumulated 90 different mutations.[1] Most mutations occur because of the environment. However, about one third of colorectal cancers have a hereditary component. Hereditary colorectal cancer is important because members of affected families can be identified as high risk and be advised to have early, intensive surveillance or even prophylactic surgery, because of the complex, multidisciplinary care the families need, and because of what it teaches about the biology of sporadic colorectal cancer. In this chapter, the syndromes of hereditary colorectal cancer are reviewed.

Hereditary colorectal cancer can be broadly divided into non-syndromic and syndromic conditions (Figure 37-1). Non-syndromic hereditary colorectal cancer refers to familial clustering that does not fit criteria for the definition of a syndrome. It is associated with a significantly increased risk of colorectal cancer but finding a germ line mutation in a tumor suppressor gene is unlikely. However, because the criteria used to define hereditary colorectal cancer syndromes are not completely sensitive, some of these families may turn out to be "syndromes in disguise." They may also represent inheritance of one or more polymorphisms that confer an altered risk for colorectal cancer, a particularly strong, shared environmental factor, or they may just be unlucky families. Syndromic hereditary colorectal cancer is more important, however, because of the extremely high level of risk associated with it and because it is relatively easier to identify.

Syndromic Hereditary Colorectal Cancer

A syndrome is a condition characterized by a constellation of symptoms, signs, and associations that go together so that the presence of one feature may alert the clinician to the presence of others. Hereditary colorectal cancer syndromes can be broadly separated into those that are associated with multiple polyps (the hereditary polyposis syndromes) and those that are not (hereditary non-polyposis colorectal cancer (HNPCC)). These syndromes and their definitions are listed in Table 37-1. All of them confer an enhanced risk of colorectal and extracolonic cancers on affected patients, and demand a sophisticated knowledge of genetics, medical, and surgical treatment from caregivers.

The Polyposis Syndromes

Multiple colorectal polyps occur in a number of conditions, and include lymphoid follicles, so common and so prominent in young patients, the inflammatory and pseudo-polyps of colitis, intestinal lipomatosis, and neurofibromatosis. Usually, these can all be identified histopathologically, and are not discussed further in this chapter. However, biopsy of a sampling of polyps is always essential in diagnosing polyposis syndromes.

The Adenomatous Polyposes

Familial Adenomatous Polyposis

Familial adenomatous polyposis (FAP) is an autosomal, dominantly inherited condition due to a germ line mutation of *APC*, which occurs with a frequency of about 1:10,000 live births.[2] About 22% of germ line *APC* mutations occur

D.E. Beck et al. (eds.), *The ASCRS Textbook of Colon and Rectal Surgery: Second Edition*,
DOI 10.1007/978-1-4419-1584-9_37, © Springer Science+Business Media, LLC 2011

"de novo," meaning that there is no family history of the syndrome.[3] Inactivating mutations of this tumor suppressor gene result in a generalized disorder of growth regulation with a range of clinical manifestations, principally the formation of multiple gastrointestinal adenomas and carcinomas. FAP is thought to account for between 0.05% and 1% of all colorectal cancers. Patients with a diagnosis of FAP and their family should be referred to a polyposis registry.

Polyposis Registries

The aim of polyposis registries is to provide counseling, support, and clinical services for families with FAP.[4] This includes thorough pedigree analysis and identification of at-risk family members, who are offered genetic testing and clinical surveillance. Those shown to be affected can be offered prophylactic surgery. Some registries also coordinate postoperative surveillance and provide a focal point for education, audit, and research.

Observational studies suggest that the introduction of registries, together with the use of prophylactic surgery, has led to increased life expectancy and a dramatic reduction in the incidence of colorectal cancer in FAP.[5]

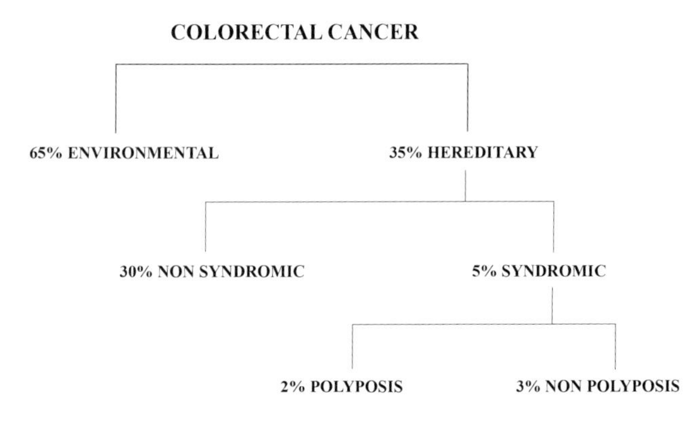

FIGURE 37-1. Colorectal cancer viewed broadly.

Features of FAP

The Large Bowel. The cardinal manifestation of FAP is the development of over 100 colorectal adenomatous polyps, one or more of which inevitably progress to carcinoma if not removed (Figure 37-2). Polyps usually appear in adolescence, with colorectal cancer diagnosed at an average age of about 40 years. The severity of the colorectal polyposis is an important determinant of treatment and is used to define the pattern of FAP. Patients with less than 100 adenomas are classified as having attenuated FAP and this phenotype overlaps significantly that of MYH-associated polyposis (MAP). Patients with 100–1,000 adenomas have classical FAP while those with >1,000 adenomas have profuse FAP. Polyposis severity is partly a reflection of the location of the *APC* mutation[6] and partly due to unidentified modifying factors.

TABLE 37-1. Hereditary colorectal cancer syndromes

Polyposis syndromes	Phenotypic definition	Genotype
Familial adenomatous polyposis	Attenuated: <100 synchronous adenomas Mild: <1,000 synchronous adenomas Severe/Profuse: >1,000 synchronous adenomas	Dominant inheritance of germ line mutation in *APC*
MYH-associated polyposis	Attenuated/mild polyposis	Recessive inheritance: biallelic mutations of *hMUTYH*
Hyperplastic polyposis	>30 hyperplastic polyps of any size or location >10 hyperplastic polyps proximal to sigmoid, 2 >10 mm Any number of hyperplastic polyps with a family history of hyperplastic polyposis	Unknown
Hamartomatous polyposes	Two of the following criteria:	
1. Peutz–Jeghers syndrome	Mucocutaneous pigmentation Gastrointestinal Peutz–Jegher's polyps Family history of Peutz–Jegher's polyposis	Dominant inheritance of germ line mutation in *STK11*
2. Juvenile polyposis coli	>4 Juvenile polyps in the colorectum Any number of juvenile polyps and a family history of juvenile polyposis	Dominant inheritance of germ line mutation in *SMAD4* or *BMPR1*
3. PTEN tumor-hamartoma syndromes		Dominant inheritance of a germ line mutation in *PTEN*
(a) Cowdens syndrome	International Cowden Consortium Criteria	
(b) Bannayan Ruvalcaba Riley syndrome		
(c) Proteus syndrome		
Non-polyposis colorectal cancer		
Lynch syndrome	Dominant family history, microsatellite unstable (high) colorectal cancer, young age of onset	Dominantly inherited germ line mutation of DNA mismatch repair gene*: hMLH1*, *hMSH2*, *hPMS2*, *hMSH6*
Familial Colorectal Cancer Type X	Dominant family history, microsatellite stable tumor	Unknown

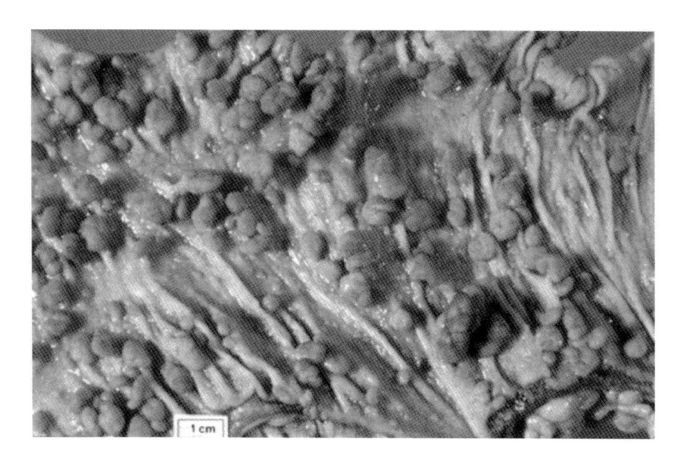

FIGURE 37-2. The large bowel in classical familial adenomatous polyposis.

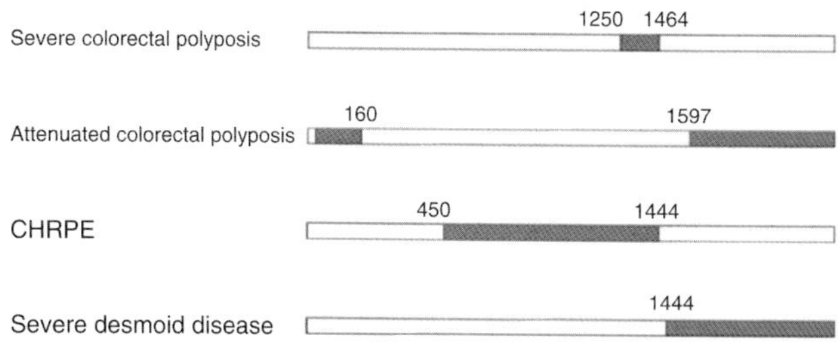

FIGURE 37-3. Schematic representation of the APC gene showing genotype–phenotype correlations.

TABLE 37-2. Extracolonic features of familial adenomatous polyposis[23]

System	Feature	Frequency (%)
Upper gastrointestinal tract	Upper gastrointestinal adenomas	95
	Upper gastrointestinal carcinoma	5
	Fundic gland polyps	40
Connective tissue	Osteomas (especially jaw)	80
	Desmoids	15
Dental	Unerupted and supernumerary teeth	17
Cutaneous	Epidermoid cysts	50
Endocrine	Adrenocortical adenomas	5
	Papillary thyroid carcinoma	1
Hepatobiliary	Biliary tract carcinoma	<1
	Hepatoblastoma	<1
Central nervous system[24]	Congenital Hypertrophy of the Retinal Pigmented Epithelium (CHRPE)	75
	Tumors (especially medulloblastoma)	<1

The "hotspot" mutation at *APC* codon 1309 is reliably associated with profuse polyposis.[7]

Genetics

The APC Gene. *APC* is a large gene on chromosome 5q21 (q = the long arm). It is a key (gatekeeper) gene in colorectal carcinogenesis and is mutated in a majority of sporadic colorectal cancers.[8] Over 820 different germ line *APC* mutations causing FAP have been identified, almost all resulting in truncation of the APC protein.[9] Mutations have been found between codons 168 (exon 4) and 2839 (exon 15), but most are between codons 168 and 1640 (exon 15) in the 5′ half of the coding region, with a particular concentration at two "hotspots," codons 1061 and 1309.

The APC Protein. *APC* is expressed in all organs, but the mRNA is found at particularly high levels in normal colonic mucosa.[10] In many epithelia, APC is only found when cell replication has ceased and terminal differentiation is established.[11]

The 300 kDa APC protein is found in the cytoplasm and has sites of interaction with a range of other proteins, including β-catenin and the cytoskeleton. It plays a central role in the highly conserved Wnt signaling pathway, which is involved in the normal development of three-dimensional structures and is abnormally activated in some malignancies. APC binds and downregulates cytoplasmic β-catenin, preventing its translocation to the nucleus. Abnormal APC fails to do this so that β-catenin is free to enter the nucleus and form a complex which results in specific transcription of cell cycle stimulating DNA sequences, and hence cell proliferation.[12]

Genotype–Phenotype Correlation in FAP. There is evidence of correlation between the position of the germ line *APC* mutation (genotype) and some aspects of phenotype (Figure 37-3). Mutation at codon 1309 is associated with profuse polyposis,[6,7,13] and between codon 1250 and 1464 with earlier onset of, and death from, colorectal cancer. Mutations located 5′ of codon 160 and 3′ of codon 1597 are associated with mild or attenuated colonic polyposis,[14] accounting for about 10% of those affected.

Some extracolonic manifestations have also been associated with mutations at certain sites, although not for upper gastrointestinal polyposis.[6,15] Congenital hypertrophy of the retinal pigmented epithelium (CHRPE) occurs only with mutations between codons 450 (exon 9) and 1444.[16] The association of desmoid disease with germ line *APC* mutations 3′ of codon 1444 can be clinically important,[17] although identical *APC* mutations may be associated with diverse phenotypes, suggesting that other genetic modifiers are involved.[18] The environment probably has some influence.

Clinical Variations of FAP

Extracolonic Manifestations. The extracolonic manifestations of FAP are shown in Table 37-2. Two of these, duodenal cancer and desmoid disease, are major sources of morbidity and mortality (Figure 37-3).[19] Other features may be a useful clue in diagnosis. CHRPE are hyper- or hypo-pigmented spots seen on retinal examination. They have no effect on vision but act as markers of FAP in the 66% of families that have four or more in both eyes.[20]

Attenuated Familial Adenomatous Polyposis. A group of patients have been described who develop fewer than 100 colorectal adenomas (oligopolyposis) at a greater age (34–44 years) than in "classical" FAP, but who are at high risk of colorectal cancer, may exhibit extracolonic manifestations and carry a germ line *APC* mutation.[21] The colorectal cancers have a later age of onset than with classical or profuse FAP (mean age 56 years). The polyps have a rather different distribution, being more frequently found proximal to the splenic flexure, and their number varies significantly between family members, some of whom may have hundreds of adenomas.

The genotype of this group of patients may be one of the three: germ line *APC* mutation, biallelic *MYH* mutations, and germ line DNA mismatch repair (MMR) gene mutations. *APC* mutations associated with attenuated familial adenomatous polyposis (AFAP) are at either end of the gene: exons 3 and 4, at the 5′ end of the gene, and also at the 3′ end of exon 15. Fundic gland polyps (FGP) and duodenal adenomas are frequent, but CHRPEs are not found in this group. Desmoid disease is rare in those with a 5′ mutation but families with 3′ mutations (beyond about codon 1444) have a high risk of desmoid disease together with attenuated polyposis. The missense *APC* mutation I1307K has been identified in Ashkenazi Jews with multiple adenomas and E1317Q [[22]] has also been found in association with AFAP. When *APC* is normal, up to 30% of patients with oligopolyposis have biallelic *MYH* mutations.[22]

It is can be difficult to recognize AFAP clinically, leading to the clinical situation of an obstructing transverse colon cancer where right-sided polyposis is only found when the specimen is opened.

Because the polyps in AFAP are predominantly right-sided, screening and work-up must include a full colonoscopy. Genetic testing for germ line *APC* and *MYH* mutations has a relatively low yield, partially because of technical difficulties in detection of abnormalities that may be present and partly because gene expression may be lost for reasons other than a mutation. A careful search (including upper gastrointestinal endoscopy) for extracolonic features of FAP, dye-spray colonoscopy to confirm polyp number, and testing of tumor or polyp tissue for microsatellite instability (MSI) and MMR immunohistochemistry (IHC) (to exclude Lynch syndrome) may be helpful. Genetic testing for a germ line *APC/MYH* mutation should be pursued in patients with a total of ten or more colorectal adenomas, especially if there is a positive family history for colorectal adenomas or cancers. A positive result has implication for family screening, but the patient is managed in the same way regardless of the result. If the polyps are controllable endoscopically, then yearly colonoscopy is reasonable. If the adenoma burden is uncontrollable or dangerous, colectomy with ileorectal anastomosis (IRA) should be performed.

Gardner's Syndrome. Gardner described the association between FAP and epidermoid cysts, osteomas and "fibromas" (later found to be desmoid tumors) in 1953. The term "Gardner's syndrome" was later used to describe colorectal adenomatous polyposis occurring with these extracolonic manifestations. However, Gardner's syndrome is genetically the same as FAP, and systematic examination[23] has revealed that most patients with FAP have at least one extra-intestinal feature. Though it is of historical interest, the term "Gardner's syndrome" is no longer considered a genetic or clinically useful entity and should be regarded as obsolete.

Turcot's Syndrome. This is the association between colorectal adenomatous polyposis and central nervous system tumors. Recent molecular genetic investigation[24] has shown that about two thirds of families have mutations in *APC*, with cerebellar medulloblastoma as the predominant brain tumor. Most of the other third, including Turcot's original family, appear to be variants of HNPCC with glioblastoma as the predominant brain tumor, and multiple (but fewer than 100) colorectal adenomas.

Presentation

Patients with FAP present either with or without symptoms (on screening). There is a significant difference in cancer incidence between these two groups, with over 60% of unscreened, symptomatic patients having colorectal cancer at presentation.[25]

Screening

Clinical FAP screening begins at puberty because the risk of colorectal cancer under the age of 12 years is very small. Genetic testing of at-risk family members in a family with a known mutation usually starts when endoscopic surveillance would start, at ages 12–14. Earlier testing may be requested in a family where a relative has had hepatoblastoma but this is unusual. When a relative is identified as a mutation carrier, full colonoscopy is performed. EGD screening usually begins at age 20 years. Thyroid screening with ultrasound should also start then.

If genetic testing is uninformative or cannot be done in a family with classical FAP, endoscopic screening starts at age 12–14 with flexible sigmoidoscopy. An alternative would be to do retinal examinations for CHRPE or look for other extracolonic examinations with a skull X-ray or panorex examination of the jaw. If a marker of FAP is found, full colonoscopy follows. The polyp burden is documented endoscopically and histologically and a decision made regarding the timing and type of surgery.

Symptoms

About 22% of FAP patients have no family history. While this may be because of adoption, non-paternity, ignorance or alienation from the family, most of the cases are due to a de novo mutation (occurring at conception).[3] The first thing that the patient knows of the lurking danger in their colon is the rectal bleeding, abdominal pain or diarrhea caused by the neoplasia. Symptomatic patients need expeditious surgery after a diagnostic colonoscopy and EGD. Their parents and siblings are usually unaffected although family screening should be done either genetically or endoscopically. Their children are at the usual 50% risk of inheriting the disease.

Diagnosis

Genetic Testing. Genetic testing should be preceded by counseling, ideally from a Genetic Counselor. Counseling includes the provision of written information about the process and its consequences, after which informed consent is documented. The implications of genetic testing with respect to confidentiality, employment, insurance, and other financial issues vary from country to country, but must be discussed prior to testing. In the USA, the Genetic Information Nondiscrimination Act (GINA) that became law in 2008 offers protection against genetic discrimination in Health and Life insurance. Posttest counseling deals with the implications of the genetic test results, and may include psychological help to deal with emotional reactions, such as guilt (in an unaffected person), anxiety (in an affected person), and the effect of the results on family relationships.

DNA from an individual with FAP is sequenced to identify a mutation in *APC*, a process which is successful in about 80% of cases. Failure to detect an *APC* mutation does not exclude a diagnosis of FAP, and may occur for a variety of reasons, including the presence of large deletions or missense mutations. Such results have been misinterpreted as ruling out the diagnosis of FAP,[26] with potentially serious consequences.

If a deleterious mutation is found in an affected family member, at-risk family members can be offered predictive testing with a high degree of accuracy. This is generally done between the ages of 12 and 15 years, when the individual is old enough to take part in genetic counseling. There is no need for testing to be done earlier, as the disease does not usually become clinically manifest and treatment is rarely indicated before the mid-teens. When an individual does not carry the family mutation, that person can be discharged from further surveillance and be reassured that they do not have FAP. This removes the costs and risks of endoscopic surveillance, as well as the anxiety of living with a potential diagnosis of FAP. A positive test result allows surveillance and prophylaxis to be targeted to those who need it, and knowledge of the site of mutation can aid decision making with regard to prophylactic surgery.

If no mutation can be found in an affected patient, then the family must be managed without genetic testing. The negative result does not mean that the family does not have FAP; it means that the genetic cause of the FAP has not been found. Under these circumstances, a negative result in an at-risk relative is unhelpful. In such kindreds, at-risk individuals should be offered regular clinical surveillance with flexible endoscopy. This starts at the age of 12–14 years, when adenomas would be expected to develop. While there have been reports of polyps and even cancers occurring earlier than this, they are very rare. Clearly, anyone at risk of FAP should undergo full colonoscopy if they become symptomatic.

Management of the Large Bowel

Aims of Treatment. While the prevention of cancer remains an important priority in the management of patients with hereditary colorectal cancer, maintaining the quality of life is also important. This is especially the case in young, asymptomatic patients who have been diagnosed by screening. Where options exist for the timing and type of surgery, those with the least impact on social, academic, and vocational activities should be chosen. After all, surgery will not cure FAP.

Prophylactic Surgery. Patients with FAP, if untreated, are almost guaranteed to develop colorectal cancer. Prevention of cancer by endoscopic control of the polyposis is not possible and so colectomy or proctocolectomy is necessary to prevent cancer. Newly diagnosed patients are generally referred to a surgeon soon after diagnosis, and if the diagnosis is certain, then surgery is inevitable. The two questions that the surgeon must answer concern the timing and the type of surgery.

Timing. Patients with severe polyposis (over 1,000 colonic or over 20 rectal polyps), or those who are symptomatic, should have surgery as soon as possible. In asymptomatic patients with mild disease (100–1,000 adenomas, all <1 cm, none with severe dysplasia), surgery can usually be delayed until the patient reaches appropriate physical and intellectual maturity. An important reason for delay is the concern for the development of desmoid disease. Affected women with a family history of desmoid disease, extracolonic manifestations of Gardner's syndrome and a 3′ *APC* mutation are at highest risk.[27] As long as surgery is delayed, annual colonoscopy is recommended to monitor the polyps. Most patients with classical polyposis have surgery between the ages of 16 and 20, which is well before cancer usually develops.

Choice of Operation. The colorectal surgical options for the management of FAP are proctocolectomy with end ileostomy (with or without Koch pouch), colectomy with IRA or proctocolectomy with ileoanal pouch (IPAA). Few patients desire a permanent ileostomy, and so proctocolectomy with ileostomy is rarely done. It remains an option which may be necessary if a low rectal cancer invades the anus, if ileoanal pouch formation is impossible (e.g., because of mesenteric desmoid) or ill advised (e.g., in the presence of poor sphincter function). In most cases, however, the choice of surgery is between the latter two options, and is a matter of considerable ongoing debate, the essence of which is the balance between functional results and morbidity of surgery on the one hand and prevention of cancer on the other. Both procedures can be performed with laparoscopic mobilization of the colon so that a long midline incision is not essential. Minimally invasive technique offers the advantages of less pain and quicker recovery, advantages that are especially important in the context of familial disease in teenagers.

IRA is more straightforward to perform than IPAA, and requires only one procedure, with a shorter hospital stay and fewer complications.[28] The risks of erectile and ejaculatory dysfunction caused by nerve damage during pelvic dissection are minimized, as is the significant reduction in fecundity observed in women after IPAA.[29] In addition, bowel frequency and soiling are less,[30] and no temporary stoma is necessary. In a teenager facing prophylactic surgery, these factors are important, particularly when most cancer risk is a few decades away and later conversion to a pouch is usually possible.

The critical aspect of cancer control in patients with an IRA is correct selection of which rectum to keep. Polyp counts are a reliable way to identify a low-risk rectum,[31] but patients still need yearly surveillance proctoscopy. Any polyps over 5 mm should be removed and polyps with high-grade dysplasia are relative indications for completion proctectomy. Occasionally, a patient with severe rectal polyposis has an IRA as the index surgery in FAP. This rectum is at high risk of progressive polyposis and cancer.[32]

Compared to an IRA, IPAA has the advantage of removing the entire colon and rectum. Although complication rates and functional results have improved with experience, they are still worse than those associated with IRA. There has been controversy over the need for mucosectomy to remove the anorectal transition zone, which theoretically prevents cuff neoplasia, but causes more complications and perhaps poorer function. Dysplasia in the transition zone occurs after both double-stapled and mucosectomy techniques and the latter is probably only indicated in individuals with severe low rectal polyposis.[33] The indications and contraindications, advantages and disadvantages of each surgical option are summarized in Table 37-3.

In summary, IRA is reasonable and safe in mildly affected patients, particularly if there are fewer than five rectal polyps. Most individuals presenting with severe polyposis or those known to carry a mutation in codon 1309 should be advised to undergo IPAA. But there are other issues. Pouch surgery in young men has an approximately 1% risk of damage to erection, ejaculation, and bladder function; in women, fertility is compromised. Pouch surgery is difficult and a diverting stoma may be impossible in obese patients. In some of these cases, the concept of a "staged pouch" may be applied. Here, an initial IRA is done despite the severity of the polyposis warranting a pouch. The patient is kept under close surveillance with the realization that a proctectomy and pouch will be required some years later. Hopefully by that time circumstances for the surgery will be more propitious. This strategy should not be applied in patients at high risk of desmoid disease.

Postoperative Surveillance. After IRA the retained rectum should be examined using a flexible sigmoidoscope, with a basic interval of 12 months or shorter, depending on the severity of disease. In about two thirds of patients, rectal adenoma regression is seen in the first few years after IRA.[34] Polyps over 5 mm should be removed cleanly with a snare. Repeated polyp fulguration can result in rectal scarring, making future surveillance difficult and unreliable. In patients with chronically scarred rectal mucosa, random biopsy is recommended to detect invisible dysplasia. If severe dysplasia or uncontrolled polyposis develops, completion proctectomy with or without ileoanal pouch formation is indicated.

Surveillance of ileoanal pouches at several centers has shown adenomas in up to 53%[35,36] and even some cancers.[37] IPAA has been available for about 30 years, and has only been performed frequently for FAP in the last 15, so the natural history of pouch adenomatosis will not be clear for some time. However, the cases reported to date confirm that neoplasia occurs in these pouches, and careful follow-up is

Table 37-3. Surgical options for familial adenomatous polyposis

Surgical option	Indication	Advantages	Disadvantages
Colectomy and Ileorectal anastomosis (leave 15 cm rectum)	<20 rectal adenomas	Low complication rate No stoma Close to normal bowel function	Risk of rectal cancer
Proctocolectomy and ileal pouch anal anastomosis (stapled)	>20 rectal adenomas Large rectal adenoma Rectal adenoma with severe dysplasia Sparing of low rectum	Minimizes risk of rectal cancer Avoids permanent stoma Bowel function better than with mucosectomy and hand sewn anastomosis	Complex surgery Often needs stoma Bowel function unpredictable but may be quite abnormal Risk of damage to pelvic nerves and decreased the ability of women to conceive Risk of pouch and anal transitional adenomas and cancer
Proctocolectomy and ileal pouch anal anastomosis (hand sewn)	As above but with adenomas to dentate line	Minimizes risk of rectal cancer Avoids permanent stoma	As above but bowel function is worse than with stapled anastomosis
Proctocolectomy with end ileostomy	Low rectal cancer Poor anal sphincters	Simple operation with lower complication rate and minimal chance of reoperation	Permanent stoma

essential. Flexible pouchoscopy after one or two enemas usually gives a good view. Not all pouch polyps are adenomas. Prominent lymphoid follicles are common, especially in children or teenagers. Isolated pouch ulcers are also common, especially over suture lines and at the opening of the afferent limb. These have no clinical significance. Representative polyps are biopsied. Treatment of pouch adenomas depends on their number and size. Polyps over 5 mm should be removed by snare excision while multiple small polyps respond to sulindac (150 mg by mouth twice daily).

Anal transition zone (ATZ) adenomas occur commonly after both stapled and handsewn IPAA, although they are twice as common in the former as the latter. Several case reports of cancer in the ATZ underline the difficulty in following this critical area.[37] In particular, a handsewn anastomosis is often stenotic, the perianal skin excoriated, and patients do not tolerate examination well. Under these circumstances, endoscopy may be possible in the office using xylocaine jelly as lubricant and a pediatric gastro scope. Otherwise, examination under anesthesia is needed. Adenomas in the ATZ can be excised individually (under anesthesia), or the entire ATZ can be stripped. If stripping is chosen because of the extent of the polyposis, the procedure should be performed in two stages to avoid stenosis.

Adenoma Chemoprevention. A range of chemopreventive agents have been studied in FAP, in part because of the problems of managing the retained rectum after IRA, but also because this disease provides a useful experimental model of colorectal carcinogenesis. In placebo controlled trials, both the nonsteroidal anti-inflammatory drugs (NSAIDs) sulindac[38] and the COX-2 inhibitor celecoxib[39] have reduced the number and size of colorectal adenomas. Chemoprevention, however, is not an alternative to prophylactic surgery, as no benefit in terms of cancer reduction has been demonstrated, and there have been reports of rectal carcinoma occurring in patients on sulindac despite reduction in polyp number and size.[40,41] The whole philosophy of artificial manipulation of polyp number, size, and shape, when polyps are the main marker guiding the decision for surgery, is troubling. However, there are circumstances when the use of chemoprevention has a definite place; for example, when completion proctectomy is impossible because of desmoid disease, while awaiting surgery which must otherwise unavoidably be delayed, in patients with a very high family risk of desmoid disease, or in treating pouch polyposis.

Upper Gastrointestinal Polyposis

Fundic gland polyps (FGP), made up of areas of cystic hyperplasia,[42] are found in the stomach of about 80–90% of individuals with FAP. These are benign but a recent prospective survey showed that low-grade dysplasia was present in FGP in 41% of patients.[43] Three percent of patients had high-grade dysplasia in FGP. This is concerning as some patients have profuse FGP, impossible to survey. Current practice is to biopsy representative FGPs during regular surveillance, but not to try and treat all. Gastric adenomas can be found, usually in the antrum, in 10% of patients in western series. It is likely that these give rise to the very rare gastric cancers in western patients.[44] The incidence of gastric cancers in FAP patients in Japan is seven times that in the West, and for Korea, three times.[45] An excess of gall bladder and bile duct adenomas and carcinoma has also been reported.[46,47]

Prospective studies have demonstrated that over 95% of individuals with FAP have duodenal adenomas,[48] which tend to occur about 15 years later than large bowel polyps.[49] Duodenal cancers are the second most common cause of death in patients with FAP because although they are relatively rare (5%), they are highly lethal. Average age at diagnosis is 50 years.

The highest density of adenomas is on and around the Ampulla of Vater, testimony to the tumorigenic effect of bile. Patients with ampullary adenomas are predisposed to pancreatitis, either spontaneous or after endoscopic biopsy. Fifty percent of normal-appearing ampullas are dysplastic on biopsy.

Adenomas can also be found throughout the small intestine, and early studies of capsule endoscopy show that incidence of jejunal and ileal adenomas is higher in patients with severe duodenal polyposis (Spigelman Stages III and IV).[50] Occasional cases of small bowel adenocarcinoma occur, but routine small bowel screening is not recommended.

Surveillance of the Duodenum. Duodenal adenomas are flat, white mucosal patches, completely different in appearance to colorectal adenomas. There may be clearly defined polyps or more confluent areas, and biopsies of macroscopically normal mucosa may reveal microadenomas. The Spigelman staging system allows an objective assessment of the severity of duodenal polyposis in FAP (Table 37-4).[51] A prospective 10 year follow-up of Spigelman's original cohort has identified a 36% risk of developing invasive carcinoma in those with stage IV disease at the start of the study, and a 2% risk in those with stage II or III disease. Several carcinomas were missed on endoscopy, and all of those who developed cancer died as a result, despite surgery.[52]

Regular endoscopic surveillance of the stomach and duodenum is recommended so that individuals at high risk of developing carcinoma can be identified and offered intervention (although there is currently no evidence that this approach decreases the rate of invasive disease).[53] Examination of the duodenum using both forward and side viewing scopes starts at the age of 25 years. Table 37-5 shows

TABLE 37-4. Scoring of polyp features in Spigelman staging for duodenal adenomas

Points allocated	Number of polyps	Size of polyps (mm)	Histology	Dysplasia
1	1–4	1–4	Tubular	Mild
2	5–20	5–10	Tubulovillous	Moderate
3	>20	>10	Villous	Severe

TABLE 37-5. Derivation of Spigelman stage from scores

Total points	Spigelman stage	Suggested interval to next duodenoscopy (years)
0	0	5
1–4	I	3–5
5–6	II	3
7–8	III	1
9–12	IV	Consider duodenectomy. If not, rescope in 6 months

recommended surveillance intervals according to the severity of duodenal polyposis. Duodenal polyps are sampled for histology and even a normal appearing Ampulla is biopsied.

Management. Management of severe duodenal polyposis is difficult, but once invasive carcinoma has developed the outcome is poor. Duodenectomy and open polypectomy is associated with 100% recurrence a year after surgery.[54] Endoscopic mucosal resection seems a more attractive option, but is made difficult by the frequently plaque-like morphology of the polyps and involvement of the ampulla. Even simple biopsy of the ampulla can result in acute pancreatitis,[55] and repeated diathermy in this region can lead to scarring and stricturing. Argon plasma coagulation is of some use. Photodynamic therapy has been tried, but photosensitization and the need for multiple treatments[56] mean that it is not currently a practical option.

The use of chemoprevention to prevent progression of earlier stage disease has attracted great interest. Calcium, starch, vitamin C, and ranitidine have been tried with no effect. Sulindac can result in regression of small polyps,[57] but has little effect on larger ones. A randomized trial of the COX-2 inhibitor celecoxib showed significant improvement in the Spigelman stage for those with mild to moderate disease.[58]

Duodenectomy, whether by classical Whipple's procedure or using pylorus or pancreas preserving techniques, has been considered a last resort because of its significant morbidity and mortality. However, given the very poor prognosis once neoplasia becomes frankly invasive preemptive duodenectomy should be seriously considered for Spigelman IV disease. Pancreas preserving duodenectomy provides satisfactory control with reasonably low morbidity.[59] When cancer is suspected a Whipple's procedure is the better choice, but carries a high rate of complications.

Desmoid Disease

Desmoids are locally invasive, non-metastasizing clonal proliferations of myofibroblasts that are rare in the general population but can be found in 30% of patients with FAP.[60] Their etiology, pathogenesis, and natural history are not clearly understood. Desmoid disease is the third most common cause of death in FAP patients overall, after colorectal cancer and duodenal cancer.[19] Overall desmoid-related mortality ranges from 10 to 50%[61] and desmoids can also contribute to death from other causes by making surgery for rectal or upper gastrointestinal malignancy difficult or even impossible.[62,63]

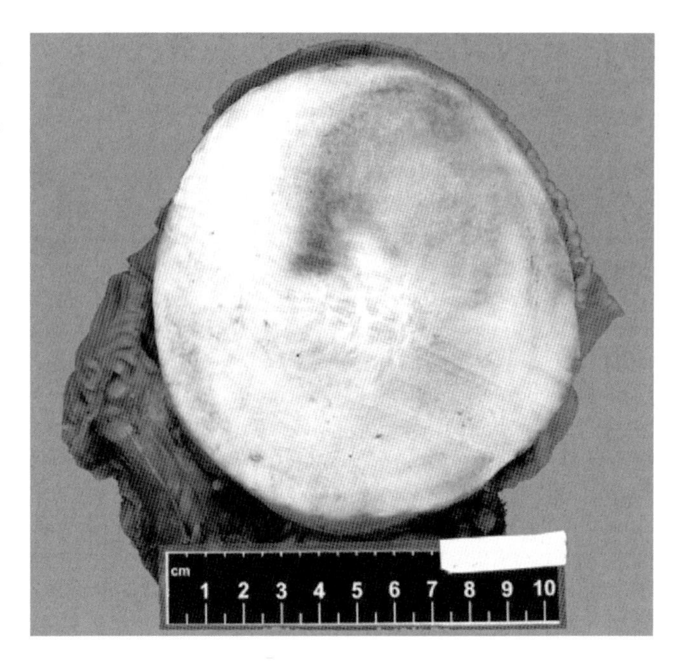

FIGURE 37-4. Desmoid tumor arising in the small bowel mesentery.

Desmoid disease is a spectrum from white, sheet-like plaques to large rapidly growing tumors. When found within the abdomen, desmoid disease can be seen to pucker and distort adjacent tissues, causing obstruction in tubular organs.

Ten to fifteen percent of patients with FAP develop desmoid tumors while another 15% develop the plaques.[60] The peak incidence is around 30 years of age, 2–3 years after surgery. While sporadic desmoids are considerably more common in females than males, this difference is less marked in the setting of FAP.

Clinical Features. Desmoids occurring in association with FAP typically arise within the abdomen (50%), especially in the small bowel mesentery, and in the abdominal wall (45%), although many extra-abdominal sites have been described. Mesenteric desmoids (Figure 37-4) encase or compress mesenteric blood vessels. Rarely, this can result in ischemia and perforation of the bowel, but it always makes resection hazardous.

Trauma (particularly in the form of surgery) and estrogens have both been identified as causes of desmoids, although they can occur spontaneously. There is evidence for some degree of genotype–phenotype correlation in that desmoids have been reported to occur more frequently in patients with 3′ germ line *APC* mutations.[6] Some mutations in this region are associated with severe desmoid disease inherited with high penetrance, but individuals with such mutations do not always develop this manifestation. However, many patients with desmoid have mutations in the 5′ half of the gene so modifier genes may well also play a part. Recent publication of a "desmoid risk factor" score underlines the importance of female gender, the presence of extracolonic manifestations (especially Gardner's syndrome) and most importantly a family history of desmoids, in alerting surgeons to the likelihood of desmoid disease in their patients.[27] Abdominal surgery in patients at high risk of desmoid disease should be delayed as long as possible, and when performed, should preferably be a laparoscopic ileorectal anastomosis.

Presentation

Asymptomatic desmoid disease can be found incidentally, on physical examination, on CT scan or at laparotomy. Desmoids found in this way are generally small and often plaque-like. Symptomatic desmoids cause pain, bowel or ureteric obstruction, or are apparent as a mass.

Investigation. CT or MRI scans are the mainstays of investigation and follow-up (Figure 37-5), allowing imaging and measurement of the desmoid itself, as well as demonstrating the relationship to other structures, such as the ureter and bowel. Early mesenteric fibrosis appears as ill-defined soft tissue infiltration of the mesenteric fat, with a characteristic, whorled appearance.[64] There is some evidence that MRI, T2 weighted signal intensity correlates with subsequent growth.[65] As only a small proportion of desmoids grow and cause significant clinical problems, the ability to predict such progression might be very useful.

Management. The treatment of desmoids is controversial, often empirical and difficult. The natural history of desmoid disease in FAP is variable, with about 10% resolving spontaneously, 10% growing rapidly and relentlessly and the remainder either showing cycles of growth and resolution or remaining stable.[66] A desmoid staging system has been proposed that allows separation of desmoid tumors by prognosis and sets the stage for a more rational approach to treatment.[67,68]

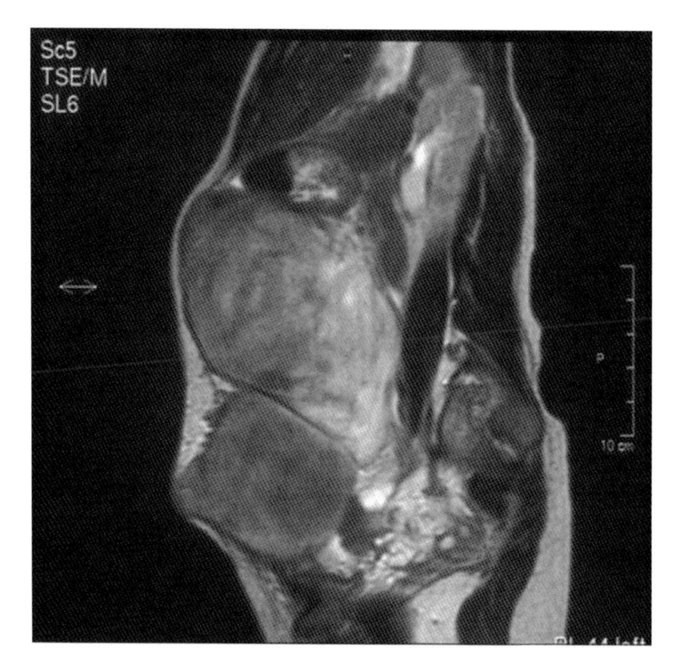

Figure 37-5. MRI scan showing intra-abdominal desmoid tumor.

Surgery is widely accepted as the first-line treatment for troublesome extra-abdominal and abdominal wall desmoids. Recurrence is common (20–50%), but complications are few. Within the abdomen the situation is very different, as the majority of desmoids develop in the small bowel mesentery. When the tumors are at the root of the mesentery, encasing the mesenteric vessels, surgery is a last resort and may mean small bowel transplant. Sometimes, intra-abdominal tumors are more distal in the mesentery, or are elsewhere in the abdomen away from the mesentery. Under these circumstances resection is often possible, sacrificing a minimum of small bowel. Preoperative CT scan and abdominal examination are keys in deciding which abdominal tumors are resectable. Even after R0 resections, however, recurrence rates are in the order of 50%.[69] Attempts at resection of desmoids in the mesenteric root may lead to high perioperative mortality rate (usually from hemorrhage)[70] and substantial morbidity, particularly due to extensive loss of small bowel.

Ureteric obstruction is best managed with stents, although even stents may be poorly tolerated due to pain or sepsis. Ureterolysis is rarely effective and may lead to nephrectomy. Renal autotransplant has proven effective, however, when medical treatments do not resolve the ureteric obstruction.[71]

Nonresective surgery may be needed to treat the complications of desmoid disease. Bowel obstruction can be managed by lysis of adhesions although this is tricky as multiple attachments of the small bowel to a retroperitoneal desmoid occur on the mesenteric border, lysis risks perforation, hemorrhage, and devascularization of the bowel. Bypass is safer and as effective. Sometimes, a stoma is necessary if there is no opportunity to bypass to a downstream loop. Enterocutaneous fistulas in the context of desmoid disease are difficult problems and may be unrepairable, committing the patient to lifetime nutritional support or small bowel transplant. However, some fistulas can be repaired, or at least bypassed.

Various medical treatments for desmoid disease have been reported, the most widely used being NSAIDs (particularly sulindac) and antiestrogens (raloxifene, tamoxifen, or toremifene). There have been no prospective controlled trials, and particularly in view of the unpredictable and variable behavior of desmoids, the small retrospective series are difficult to interpret. Cytotoxic chemotherapy has been used in irresectable or aggressive desmoid disease, and objective remissions have been noted with a variety of different agents. There have been a number of encouraging reports of an anti-sarcoma regimen consisting of doxorubicin and dacarbazine

Table 37-6. Staging system for abdominal desmoid tumors

Stage	Definition
I	Size <10 cm, not growing, asymptomatic
II	Size <10 cm, mildly symptomatic, slow growing[a]
III	Size 10–20 cm, moderate symptoms (bowel obstruction, ureteric obstruction), slow growing
IV	Size >20 cm, or rapid growth[b] or severe symptoms (abscess, fistula, hemorrhage)

[a] Slow growth = <50% increase in maximum diameter in 6 months.
[b] Rapid growth = >50% increase in maximum diameter in 6 months.

in the treatment of life-threatening intra-abdominal desmoid disease[72,73] and more recently the better tolerated liposomal doxorubicin has shown benefit. A less toxic combination of vinblastine and methotrexate has also produced some responses.[74]

A treatment regimen can be proposed that uses the staging system outlined in Table 37-6. Stage I tumors may receive either no treatment or sulindac, 150–200 mg twice daily. Stage II tumors are treated with sulindac and an estrogen modifying agent (tamoxifen or raloxifene 120 mg per day). Stages III and IV require chemotherapy. Liposomal doxorubicin is a reasonable agent to use, with methotrexate/vinorelbine as an alternative.[75] If a septic complication precludes chemotherapy, or if the maximum safe dose of adriamycin has been reached, agents such as gleevac, bevacizumab, or erbitux can be tried.

MYH-Associated Polyposis

MAP is an autosomal recessive form of familial adenomatous polyposis, due to mutations in the human MutY homolog (*hMUTYH*) gene. It was originally described in 2003.[76] While many of the individuals identified with biallelic *hMUTYH* mutations have fewer than 100 polyps, some have many hundreds, and thus appear as if they are a genuine clinical case of FAP. Colonic microadenomas and duodenal adenomas, desmoids and fundic gland polyps, sessile serrated polyps, and a variety of extracolonic cancers have also been reported in this group.[77,78] In fact, MAP can mimic many of the other hereditary forms of colorectal cancer, from sporadic cancer to FAP, from Lynch syndrome to hyperplastic polyposis (HPP). This is because the polyp phenotype can vary in number and histology, and the family history can also vary from dominant inheritance to no family history at all.

MAP has major implications for genetic counseling as, for the first time, an autosomal recessive form of FAP has been identified. This diagnosis should be considered in patients where no *APC* mutation has been identified, the mode of inheritance is not clearly autosomal dominant, or polyp numbers are low.

Genetics. Base excision repair corrects the sequelae of oxidative damage to the DNA. Oxidation changes the pattern of guanine coupling from G=C to G°=T. In subsequent cell division, an uncorrected G°=T becomes A=T, creating a "G=C to A=T transversion." This change, when uncorrected, produces mutations in several genes, including *APC* and *KRAS*. The effect on APC is enough to produce adenomatous polyposis, and serrated polyps harboring similar mutations in *KRAS* have been reported in patients with MAP.[79]

The locations of the pathogenic *hMUTYH* mutations vary according to ethnicity.[80] The common mutations in the USA are Y179C and G396D, and these are screened for in Caucasian patients. If this screen is negative or if the patient is not Caucasian, whole gene sequencing can also be performed. There is some evidence that the Y179C mutation is associated with a more severe phenotype.[81]

Clinical. Patients usually present with oligopolyposis (<100 adenomas), although some cases with hundreds of polyps have been reported. Prior to awareness of these syndromes, patients with MAP were sometimes diagnosed as having attenuated FAP. Although some affected individuals have a very few adenomas, the presence of ten or more synchronous adenomas should trigger a referral for genetic counseling and testing, regardless of family history of colorectal neoplasia. The presence of serrated polyps with multiple adenomas should also stimulate a referral for genetic testing.

Once the genotype of MAP is confirmed, full colonoscopy and EGD are performed. The syndrome has not been known for long enough to have an accurate list of all extracolonic manifestations.

Treatment of the large bowel depends on whether the adenomas can be controlled endoscopically. If this can be done, surgery may be avoided. However, surgery is often necessary, usually colectomy with ileorectal anastomosis. Remaining large intestine is surveyed yearly. If a patient presents with cancer at a young age with either no family history or a weak history, and there is no evidence of Lynch syndrome, testing for MAP should be considered.

Genetic Testing. MAP generally follows an autosomal recessive pattern of inheritance, although monoalleic mutations (carriers) have a mildly increased risk of colorectal cancer. There has been a report of MAP with a dominant pattern of inheritance.[82] However, recessive inheritance means that both parents of a proband are likely to be unaffected carriers, with the risk to siblings being 25%. Genetic testing of a family therefore begins with the affected proband and if mutations are found continues with the spouse. This determines the risks to the children. A negative spouse means that children are carriers and can be counseled accordingly. Carriers should have enhanced colonoscopic surveillance, beginning 10 years before any cancer in the family and continuing at least 5 yearly. If the spouse is a carrier, then the inheritance pattern within that family becomes dominant, with each child at 50% risk of having MAP. In addition, antecedents on both sides of the family must be alerted to the possibility that they are carriers or affected.

In a study screening 9,268 colorectal cancer patients for the two commonly mutated alleles, Lubbe et al. found biallelic *hMutYH* mutations in 0.3% of cases. This conferred a 28-fold increase in colorectal cancer risk, and was associated with proximal tumors and synchronous adenomas. Monoallelic mutations were not associated with an increase in colorectal cancer risk.[83]

The Hamartomatous Polyposes

Peutz–Jeghers Syndrome

Peutz–Jegher's syndrome (PJS) is a dominantly inherited cancer syndrome defined by the presence of two of the following three characteristics: perioral, buccal, and occasionally genital melanin pigmentation; gastrointestinal hamartomatous (Peutz–Jegher's) polyposis; a family history of PJS. The pigmentation can also be seen on the lips and sometimes on the eyelids, hands, and feet, or be absent altogether. It usually appears in early childhood and tends to fade in the late 20s. The polyps occur predominantly in the small intestine (78%), but are also found in the stomach (38%), colon (42%), and rectum (28%).[84] They are hamartomas with a characteristic branching morphology, containing smooth muscle in the submucosa. Adenomatous change with dysplasia and progression to invasive adenocarcinoma has been observed.[85] PJS has an incidence of 1 in 200,000.

Inheritance

Peutz–Jegher's polyposis is autosomal, dominantly inherited with high penetrance, and is caused by mutation of *LKB1* (also known as *STK11*) on chromosome 19 p13.3. The gene encodes a serine–threonine kinase. Mutation of *LKB1* is only found in about 60–70% of cases, and has been formally excluded in some,[86] suggesting that either other genes are responsible, or *LKB1* may be inactivated by epigenetic mechanisms. While a family history is common, de novo mutations are responsible for a significant number of cases.

Clinical Issues

Polyp-Related Complications. The most common clinical problems in PJS are anemia due to chronic blood loss from large polyps and small bowel obstruction due to intussusception with a polyp at the apex. Repeated emergency bowel resections can lead to increasing operative difficulty and even short-bowel syndrome.

Risk of Malignancy. Follow-up studies have shown that individuals with this syndrome are at increased risk of developing a range of malignancies at a particularly young age.[87] Indeed, by the age of 57 years approximately half of all patients in one series had died of cancer, of which about half were gastrointestinal. The lifetime risk of any cancer in affected patients is over 90%. It is estimated that there is a 50-fold excess of gastrointestinal cancer in Peutz–Jegher's syndrome, resulting in a lifetime risk of approximately 20% of colorectal cancer and about 5% of gastric cancer, as well as breast, pancreatic (30% lifetime risk), ovarian sex-cord tumors (10% of females), feminizing Sertoli cell testicular tumors in prepubertal boys, pulmonary and cervical malignancies.

Management

Probands usually present at a young age with complications of their small bowel polyposis. This often involves laparotomy for intussusception or bleeding. A symptom-focused approach predisposes to frequent laparotomies as untreated polyps enlarge to cause a new set of symptoms. The technique of laparotomy with intra-operative enteroscopy was introduced to reduce the number of repeat emergency laparotomies and small bowel resections.[88] During laparotomy a colonoscope is passed from below through the colon, and, with the assistance of the surgeon, into the small bowel for as far as it will go. The most proximal site of insertion is marked with a suture or tape. Then, the colonoscope is withdrawn in a darkened operating room and the sites of polyps marked as it is withdrawn. The procedure is repeated with an enteroscope inserted through the stomach and encouraged to pass distally. The mucosa between the limits of endoscopy can usually be examined through an enterotomy. In most patients, the intussusception is obvious and even if it is reduced a serosal dimple can be seen at the site of the polyp. The bowel is palpated and at the site of palpable polyp an enterotomy is made. The polyps are removed and the bowel intussuscepted through the incision up and down as far as possible. All visible lesions are either removed or cauterized. The enterotomies are closed. Polypectomy is best done by ligating the stalk and excising the polyp with cautery distal to the tie. Otherwise, the stalk may bleed copiously. The fourth part of the duodenum and proximal jejunum is typically a difficult part of the bowel to palpate and to operate.

Using this "clean sweep" technique, the entire small bowel is cleared of all macroscopic lesions, minimizing the number of laparotomies in subsequent years.[88] The recent availability of capsule endoscopy and double/single balloon enteroscopy offers the potential for endoscopic diagnosis and treatment of the polyps; however, the vascularity of the polyps makes endoscopic treatment in the mid small bowel worrisome. There is a role for capsule endoscopy, however, in surveillance of asymptomatic patients. Colonic polyps can usually be controlled colonoscopically.[89]

Gastrointestinal Surveillance. Surveillance intervals depend on polyp number, size, histology, and location. A near normal examination can be followed 2 or 3 years later by repeat EGD, capsule endoscopy, and colonoscopy. Hemoglobin should be checked annually. Small bowel polyps causing symptoms or anemia, or measuring over 1.5 cm, should be removed, either endoscopically or at laparotomy with intra-operative enteroscopy.

Extra-intestinal Surveillance. Mammography in premenopausal woman lacks sensitivity, but there is little evidence to support ultrasound or MRI as alternatives. Testicular tumors tend to occur in prepubertal boys, and it would seem sensible to encourage regular examination. Women should undergo standard cervical and breast screening according to nationally agreed protocols.[90] While in some centers regular ultrasound scanning of the pancreas and ovaries are performed, there is no evidence that such measures have any impact on prognosis. It is important that clinicians caring for these patients are aware of the high cancer risk, and maintain a low index of suspicion.

Juvenile Polyposis

Juvenile polyps are hamartomas which lack smooth muscle histologically, having poor anchorage to the bowel wall. They may become detached and are then passed through the anus. Solitary juvenile polyps are the commonest colorectal lesion in children, being found in up to 2%. They have little or no malignant potential.[91] Juvenile polyposis (JPS) is defined as the presence of five or more juvenile polyps in the large bowel, or any number of juvenile polyps in a patient with a family history of JPS. Although the colorectum is always affected, the stomach (and perhaps small intestine) is also affected in about 50%.[91–94] Most affected individuals develop 50–200 polyps, but some have very few.

JPS is rare with a frequency of about 1 per 100,000. It presents with rectal bleeding, anemia, or polyp prolapse, at an average age of about 9 years. The polyps are hamartomas, with a characteristic hyperplastic stroma, abundant lamina propria, cystic glands, and inflammation. They are sometimes reported as inflammatory polyps. Adenomatous dysplasia occurs in up to half, which may then progress to adenocarcinoma.

Other morphologic abnormalities, including macrocephaly, mental retardation, cleft lip or palate, congenital heart disease, genitourinary malformations, and malrotations, are found in 10–20%.[95] Some patients with JPS have a familial pattern of disease, while in others there is no family history. In those with familial disease, the chances of finding a causative mutation are relatively high (>60%).

Genetics

This syndrome is genetically heterogeneous, with three separate genes currently implicated. Mutations in *SMAD4* have been identified in affected individuals. *SMAD4* is a tumor suppressor gene on chromosome 18q21 and is implicated in sporadic colorectal carcinogenesis. It codes for a protein involved in the TGFβ signaling pathway, and germ line mutations have been found in 35–60% of juvenile polyposis patients in the USA, but rather fewer (3–28%) in Europe.[94] Germ line mutations in a second gene, *BMPR1A* on 10q22, have been found in a further 15% of cases.[95] *BMPR1A* encodes a protein involved in the same signaling pathway. *PTEN* mutations have also been reported in the so-called juvenile polyposis,[96] but it is as yet unclear whether these cases have Cowden's syndrome, or whether they represent is simply a variant of juvenile polyposis.[97]

Patients with JPS due to a *SMAD4* mutation have a high likelihood of also having Hereditary Hemmorhagic Telangiectasia (HHT). This manifests as multiple vascular anomalies that may be in the brain, lungs, mediastinum, and bowels. Patients with a SMAD4 mutation need a vascular assessment to diagnose or exclude this potentially dangerous condition.[94,98]

Cancer Risk and Management

The cumulative risk of colorectal cancer in patients with JPS has been estimated at 30–50%, and that of upper gastrointestinal cancer at 10–20%.[93,99] First degree relatives of affected individuals should be screened by colonoscopy from around the age of 12 years if asymptomatic[100] and, if normal, 5 yearly thereafter. In many cases, the polyps can be controlled by regular endoscopic polypectomy, with both upper gastrointestinal endoscopy and colonoscopy recommended at least every 2 years. In cases where polyps are either too numerous or too large to be managed in this way, or when patients are symptomatic with diarrhea, mucus, bleeding and cramps, colectomy and IRA or restorative proctocolectomy is advised.[101] Cleveland Clinic experience showed a high rate of secondary proctectomy after initial ileorectal anastomosis.[102] Aggressive polyposis is also possible in ileal pouches but can be controlled by sulindac.

It is not clear whether endoscopic surveillance and polypectomy is adequate to prevent malignancy, but there are insufficient data to justify purely prophylactic colectomy. Affected individuals should also undergo upper gastrointestinal surveillance from the age of 25 years.

PTEN Tumor Hamartoma Syndromes

Three very rare dominantly inherited conditions have been described in which hamartomatous colorectal polyps occur together with multiple craniofacial, skeletal, and dermatological phenotypic features. They share a common genetic origin, namely, germ line mutations of *PTEN*. *PTEN* is an important tumor suppressor gene with key roles in the mTOR/AKT pathway.[103]

Cowden's Syndrome

This autosomal dominantly inherited syndrome is characterized by macrocephaly (30%), trichilemmomas (which are considered pathognomonic) and both benign and malignant neoplasms of the thyroid, breast, uterus, and skin. Hamartomas occur in the mouth as well as other parts of the gastrointestinal tract, resulting in a nodular appearance of the buccal mucosa. The International Cowden's Syndrome Group has described a set of major and minor criteria by which to diagnose the syndrome.[104]

In CS patients, the colon is affected with a variety of polyps, the histology of which includes hamartomas, lipomas, fibromas, neurofibromas, ganglioneuromas, and adenomas. Although CS has not been considered a high risk for colorectal cancer, recent data seems to suggest otherwise.[105] Certainly, it is safe to start colonoscopic screening when patients are in their 30s and to continue it at least every 3 years, or more often if findings indicate. Prophylactic colectomy is indicated when polyposis cannot be controlled endoscopically.

Bannayan–Riley–Ruvalcaba Syndrome

Here, the colorectal hamartomas (50%) are associated with characteristic pigmented penile macules, macrocephaly, mental retardation (50%), lipomatosis and hemangiomas.[106] It seems likely that as Cowden and Bannayan–Riley–Ruvalcaba syndromes are caused by mutation of the same gene, they are slightly different forms of the same disorder,[95] and families have been identified in which both phenotypes are evident.[107] There is no evidence to suggest an increased risk of colorectal cancer in this syndrome.

Serrated Polyposis

Serrated polyps are non-neoplastic lesions of the large bowel that were until recently thought to have no premalignant potential. Over the last 5 years, however, the true significance of these lesions has begun to be appreciated. They are part of a class of lesions termed serrated polyps because the overcrowded hyperplastic glands in the epithelium are thrown into a saw-toothed or serrated pattern. A new nomenclature has arisen wherein serrated polyps with abnormal proliferation are termed sessile serrated polyps (or sessile-serrated adenomas), and are now known to be potential premalignant precursors in a serrated polyp to cancer pathway.[108] This pathway is linked genetically to BRAF mutations and DNA hypermethylation, particularly when it leads to loss of expression of *hMLH1*.[109] While sporadic serrated polyps are common, and mostly of the hyperplastic type, some patients have multiple lesions and are at high risk of developing colorectal cancer. The WHO definition for serrated polyposis is any one of the following: 30 or more serrated polyps of any size and location; more than 10 serrated polyps proximal to the splenic flexure of which 2 are larger than 10 mm; any number or size of serrated polyps with a family history of SPP.[110] There is reason to believe that these criteria are overly restrictive and that high risk families are being missed.

No germ line mutation has been identified as causing serrated polyposis and the pattern of inheritance is still not clear. Many patients with SPP have no family history at all. The presence of multiple synchronous-serrated polyps has, however, been shown to confer a very high risk of colorectal cancer, approaching 50%.[111]

Treatment

Treatment of patients with SPP is either endoscopic or surgical. Colonoscopy must be careful as serrated polyps can be difficult to recognize and are likely to be easier to miss than adenomas. Yearly, colonoscopy is necessary to prevent cancer. If the polyps are not controllable endoscopically, colectomy, and IRA is indicated. First degree relatives of patients with SPP are candidates for early screening colonoscopy (10 years prior to the earliest age at diagnosis of a neoplastic lesion in the family). If a colon cancer is detected, or if the polyposis is progressive and not able to be controlled, colectomy and IRA is indicated.

Hereditary Non-polyposis Colorectal Cancer

Introduction

HNPCC refers to a dominant pattern of inheritance of colorectal cancer predisposition without an association with unusual numbers of colorectal polyps. This lack of an easily identifiable colonic phenotype makes clinical diagnosis difficult and can affect treatment as surgeons seem reluctant to remove an endoscopically normal colon for prophylaxis. Multiple diagnostic criteria have been proposed for the identification of HNPCC families. The most widely used are the Amsterdam I and II criteria, originally proposed to facilitate research but almost immediately adapted for clinical use (see Table 37-7).[112,113] Subsequent research has shown that Amsterdam I patients can be divided into two broad

TABLE 37-7. Amsterdam criteria

Amsterdam criteria
- At least 3 family members with colorectal cancer, one of whom is first-degree relative of the other 2.
- At least 2 generations with colorectal cancer.
- At least 1 individual <50 years at diagnosis of colorectal cancer.

Amsterdam criteria II
- At least 3 family members with HNPCC-related cancer, one of whom is first-degree relative of the other 2.
- At least 2 generations with HNPCC-related cancer.
- At least 1 individual <50 years at diagnosis of HNPCC-related cancer.

Modified Amsterdam criteria
- 2 first-degree relatives with CRC involving 2 generations.
- At least one case diagnosed before 55 years OR
- 2 first-degree relatives with CRC and a third relative with endometrial cancer or another HNPCC-related cancer.

Modified from Chung DC, Rustgi AK. The hereditary nonpolyposis colorectal cancer syndrome: genetics and clinical implications. Ann Intern Med. 2003;138:560–70.

subgroups: those whose tumors are microsatellite unstable (Lynch syndrome) and those whose tumors are microsatellite stable (Familial Colorectal Cancer Type X).[114] Type X families are likely to be a heterogeneous group of colorectal cancer predisposition states, sharing an apparent dominant inheritance but with different genetic abnormalities. Some may have underlying MAP, some SPP, some Lynch syndrome due to *hMSH6* mutations, and some may have genetic abnormalities yet to be discovered. Type X families have a significantly lower risk of colorectal cancer than that found with Lynch syndrome, and they do not have the same array of extracolonic cancers. Lynch syndrome, or hereditary mismatch repair (MMR) deficiency, is a better defined syndrome and is the main topic of this section.

Lynch Syndrome

Definition

Lynch syndrome is hereditary DNA MMR deficiency associated with the early onset of colorectal and other cancers (mean age for colorectal cancer, 45 years). Multiple generations are affected with a pattern suggesting dominant inheritance. Colorectal cancers tend to be proximal to the splenic flexure, and there is an increased frequency of synchronous and metachronous cancers. There is also a high risk of extracolonic cancers, including endometrial, ovarian, gastric, small bowel, hepatobiliary, and transitional cell carcinomas. The lifetime risk of cancer is up to 80%, with colon cancer being the most commonly diagnosed.[115]

History

Aldred Warthin, a pathologist at the University of Michigan, first described a family with inherited intestinal cancer in 1895. Detailed descriptions of this family, (known as "Family G" because they came from Germany) as well as other families, were published in 1913. Gastric cancer was the predominant cancer but colorectal and uterine cancers also featured.[116] Nearly 50 years later, a medical oncologist named Henry Lynch published the pedigrees of two large midwestern families ("Family N" from Nebraska and "Family M" from Michigan). He commented on the wide spectrum of cancers and the probability of a heritable mutation.[117] By the mid-1980s, two patterns of disease became apparent; Lynch I (colorectal cancer only) and Lynch II (colorectal and other malignancies). Concurrent observations showed that the number of colorectal adenomas in these patients was no greater than that in the general population, and that there was considerable overlap between Lynch I and II syndromes. The syndrome became known as HNPCC. Terminology has now come full circle with Lynch Syndrome now a genetic diagnosis, referring to families with a germ line mutation in a MMR gene.

In order to promote research collaborative studies, an International Collaborative Group on HNPCC met in Amsterdam in 1990.[112] A set of diagnostic guidelines was agreed upon that would allow researchers to gather homogeneous populations to be studied (*Amsterdam I criteria*, see Table 37-7). Once HNPCC was clinically defined, rapid progress was made finding the genetic defects as well as in diagnosis and treatment of the disease. The DNA of colorectal tumors in some Amsterdam positive families was found to have multiple mismatched nucleotides. This unique genetic abnormality was termed replication error phenotype or RER+. Most of the mismatched bases were in areas of the gene called "microsatellites," so the term "microsatellite instability" is now preferred.[118] Extensive research in yeast and *Escherichia coli* had identified a group of genes referred to as MMR genes. Using linkage studies, the first human homolog, *hMSH2*, was identified in 1993 by Fishel[119] and germ line mutations in *hMSH2* were found in families with HNPCC. Other MMR genes were found and associated with HNPCC.

Genetics

DNA Microsatellites

DNA is a very long molecule that is replicated during each cell division. Microsatellites are short, tandem repeating base sequences, usually mononucleotide or dinucleotide base repeats, most often found in the non-coding or intronic portions of DNA. However, microsatellites can occur anywhere within genes, and when they do, mutations within microsatellites can cause changes in gene expression. The length of each microsatellite marker is normally constant within any particular patient, so that when the number of repeats in a microsatellite sequence in a cancer cell is different from the surrounding normal tissue, this is termed "microsatellite instability (MSI)."

DNA Mismatch Repair

When a cell divides, DNA is replicated. The parent strands separate, and are reconstituted by DNA polymerase into two new double-stranded molecules. DNA mismatches occur when one strand slips on the other as the new DNA molecule is reconstituted. This is especially likely to happen in DNA microsatellites that can be thought of as "slippery" parts of the DNA. Unrepaired mismatches are seen as MSI. The system of DNA MMR in humans involves at least six genes. Their protein products act in pairs to recognize mismatches and excise them, allowing DNA polymerase to restore normal DNA. (Figure 37-6). The genes are *hMLH1*, *hPMS1*, *hPMS2*, *hMSH2*, *hMSH3*, and *hMSH6*. MSH2 acts as a "scout" and identifies the mismatches in the new DNA strand. It then complexes with MSH6 to form the MutSα complex that identifies single nucleotide mismatches. Alternatively, MSH2 can complex with hMSH3 forming MutSβ complex that repairs insertion and deletion loops (IDL) with up to 10 base pairs. Both MSH3 and MSH6 must be

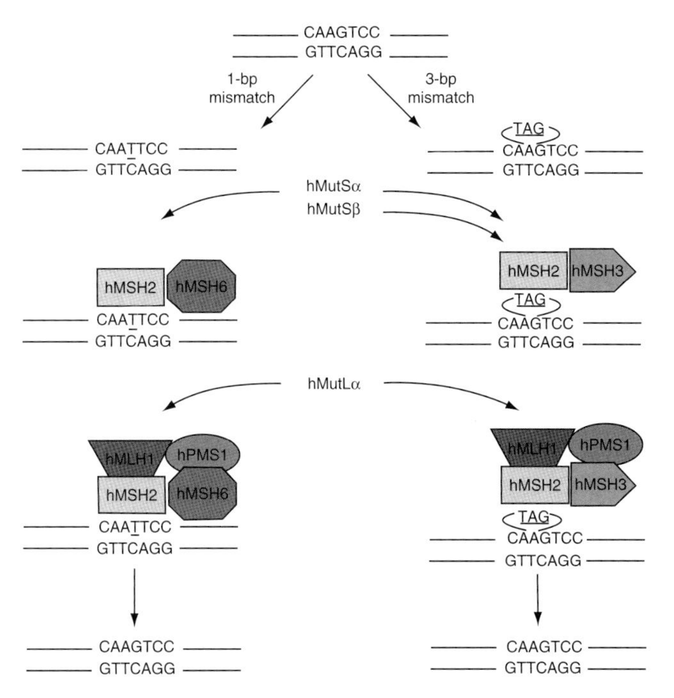

FIGURE 37-6. The DNA mismatch repair system can correct either single base-pair mismatches or larger loops of mismatched DNA. hMSH2 serves as the "scout" that recognizes mismatched DNA. It forms a complex with either hMSH6 or hMSH3, depending on the number of mismatched nucleotides. A second heterodimeric complex (hMLH1/hPMSI) is then recruited to excise the mispaired nucleotides. hMUTSα = hMSH2/hMSH6; hMuTSβ = hMSH2/hMSH3; hMutLα = hMLH1/hPMS1. *bp* base pair. (Reprinted with permission from Chung DC, Rustgi AK. The hereditary non-polyposis colorectal cancer syndrome: genetics and clinical implications. Ann Intern Med. 2003;138:560–70).

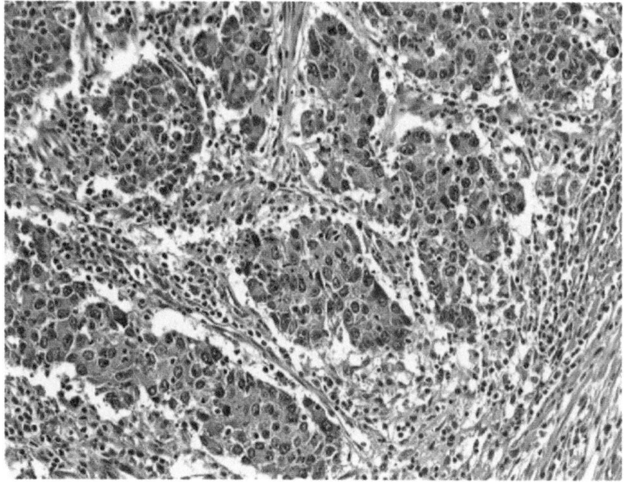

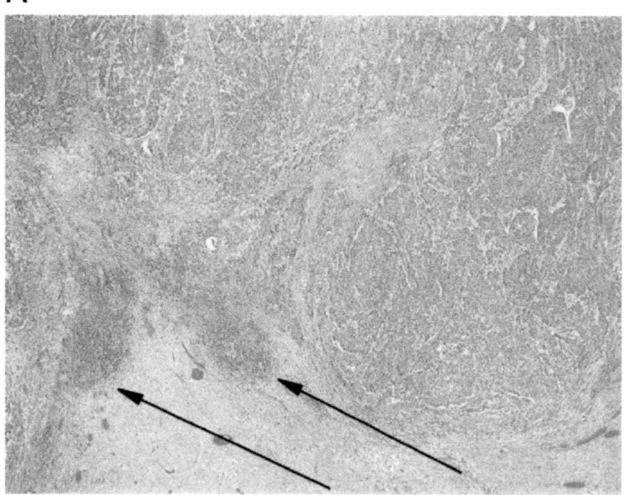

FIGURE 37-7. **A** Medullary carcinoma type pattern with peritumoral lymphocytic infiltrate, **B** MSI-H cancer with marked peritumoral lymphocytic infiltrate (Crohn's-like reaction), ×20 magnification. (Courtesy of Robert E. Petras, MD, National Director Gastrointestinal Pathology Services, Ameripath Inc., Oakwood Village, OH and Associate Professor of Pathology, Northeastern Ohio University College of Medicine).

abnormal to have complete loss of hMSH2-dependent mismatch repair.[120]

MLH1 and PMS2 bind to form a second heteroduplex that interacts with the MutS duplex, stimulating excision and resynthesis. When an inactivating mutation silences expression of an MMR gene, the microsatellite mismatches go unrepaired and are propagated into lines of daughter cells as mutations. This so-called mutator phenotype of Lynch syndrome is characterized by an increased genome-wide mutation rate. When tumor suppressor genes contain a microsatellite, they are vulnerable to loss of expression in the mutator phenotype. Examples of such genes are *MSH3*, *MSH6*, *TCF4*, *BLM*,[121] *Caspase-5*,[122] *TGFβRII*, *IGFRII*, *BAX*, *PTEN*, and *APC*,[123] many of which are involved in control of colonocyte growth.

The most commonly mutated genes in Lynch syndrome families are *MLH1* (33% of families) and *MLH2* (31%).[124] Of the mutations identified, 90% occur in *MLH1* and *MSH2*.[125] Recently, a meta-analysis of index families fulfilling the Amsterdam criteria revealed that a mutation in *MLH1* is found in 25.5–29.6% of families, and *MSH2* is found in 14.8–21.6% of the families.

Pathology

Some pathologic features can be seen in tumors associated with the mutator phenotype and MSI. These include mucinous differentiation with signet ring cells, the presence of tumor infiltrating lymphocytes (Figure 37-7A), a Crohn's like reaction (Figure 37-7B), and the absence of dirty necrosis.[126,127] Despite what appears to be unfavorable histology, the incidence of metastatic tumor in lymph nodes is less than that found with sporadic colon cancer.[128]

Flow cytometry has shown that most Lynch syndrome tumors are diploid. This contrasts with the frequent aneuploidy of sporadic colon cancer, where tumorigenesis is related to sporadic mutations and loss of heterozygosity (LOH).[129]

Clinical Features

Patients with Lynch syndrome have an increased lifetime risk of colon cancer and other extracolonic cancers (see Table 37-8). Colon cancer is the most frequently diagnosed cancer (80%) and endometrial cancer is the most frequent extracolonic cancer (50–60%).[130] Colorectal cancers in Lynch syndrome are usually proximal to the splenic flexure (68% vs. 49% of sporadic cancers), more likely to have associated synchronous cancers (7% vs. 1% sporadic colon cancer), and have increased metachronous cancers at 10 years (29% vs. 5% sporadic cancers).[131] Similarly, women with Lynch syndrome-related endometrial cancer have a 75% risk of a second cancer during a 26-year follow-up. The median age of onset of colon cancer is 42 years and for endometrial cancer it is 49 years.[115]

In Lynch syndrome, an adenoma is the precursor lesion for cancer. In a Danish surveillance study, 70% of mutation carriers developed adenoma by age 60 as opposed to 37% in the control group. The adenomas in the mutation carrier group were larger and had a higher proportion of villous components and high-grade dysplasia. Adenomas were located in the proximal colon and 70% of the polyps had an absent MMR protein on immunohistochemistry.[132] One cancer is prevented for every 2.8 polyps removed in HNPCC patients[133] compared to one cancer being prevented for every 41–119 polypectomies in the general population.[134] It is estimated that malignant transformation occurs in 3 years in HNPCC as opposed to 10 years in sporadic colon cancer.

Two other types of polyps – the flat adenoma and serrated adenoma – have been implicated as possible precursors of Lynch syndrome cancers. Flat adenomas are found proximally in up to 50% of Lynch syndrome patients (Figure 37-8A and B).[135] About 20% of flat adenomas show MSI-H and have a mutation in the *TGFβRII* gene.[136] These polyps are difficult to detect during colonoscopy and flat adenomas with advanced histology (high-grade dysplasia or cancer) are significantly smaller (10.7 mm) than comparable polypoid lesions (20 mm).[137]

Genotype/Phenotype Relationships

Few studies evaluate phenotype–genotype correlations in Lynch syndrome. One study of 35 families found the *MSH2* mutation to be associated with a later age of onset of rectal cancer and more extracolonic cancers than in the *MLH1* mutation-positive group.[138] Another study confirmed the association of *MSH2* mutations and extracolonic cancers.[139] Germ line *MSH6* mutations are uncommon, and associated with a particularly high risk of uterine cancer, which is more common than colon cancer in affected women. Colorectal cancer occurs at a later age of onset in these families than in those with the more common *MLH1* and *MSH2* genotypes. In 91 patients with familial colorectal cancer, 6 (7.0%) were found to have *MSH6* mutations, their tumors were microsatellite low (MSI-L), had a median onset of 61 years, and the families did not fulfill Amsterdam I criteria.[140] The International Collaborative Group has collected over 30 potentially

TABLE 37-8. Lifetime risks for cancer associated with the hereditary non-polyposis colorectal cancer syndrome

Type of cancer	Persons with HNPCC	General population
Colorectal	80–82	5–6
Endometrial	50–60	2–3
Gastric	13	1
Ovarian	12	1–2
Small bowel	1–4	0.01
Bladder	4	1–3
Brain	4	0.6
Kidney, renal, pelvis	3	1
Biliary tract	2	0.6

Adapted from Chung DC, Rustgi AK. The hereditary nonpolyposis colorectal cancer syndrome: genetics and clinical implications. Ann Intern Med. 2003; 138:560–70.

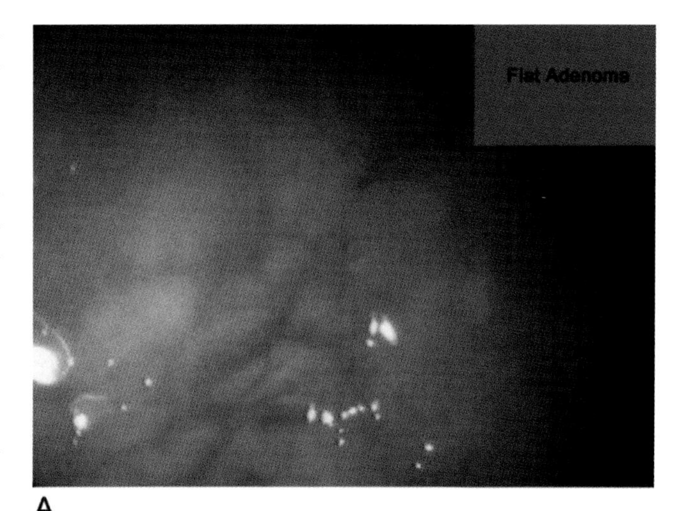

A

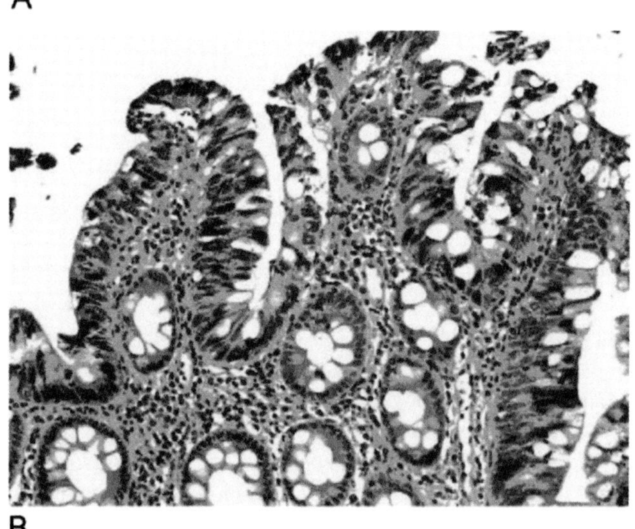

B

FIGURE 37-8. **A** Colonoscopic view of a flat adenoma in the cecum that could easily be overlooked. Such polyps are more easily seen using dye-spraying techniques, **B** Microscopic view of same polyp following endoscopic removal, showing severe dysplasia, ×100 magnification. (Courtesy of Dr. Robert E. Petras, MD, National Director Gastrointestinal Pathology Services, Ameripath Inc., Oakwood Village, OH and Associate Professor of Pathology, Northeastern Ohio University College of Medicine).

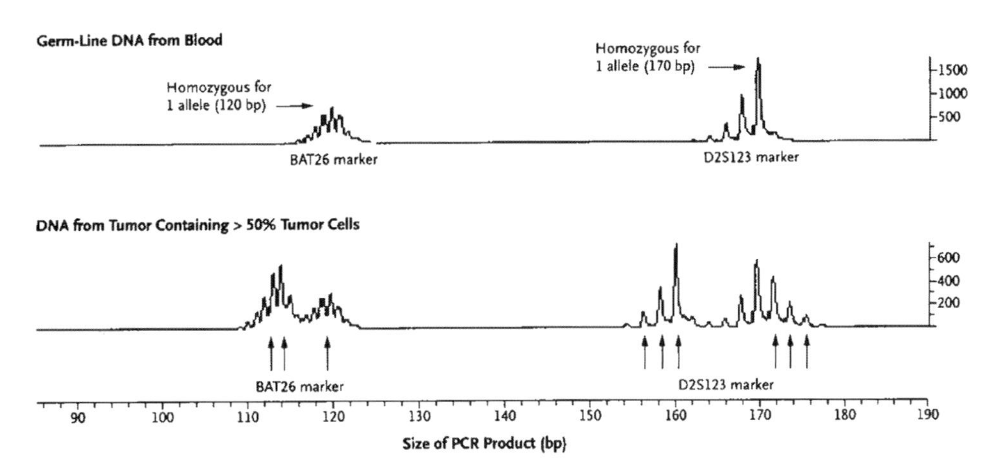

FIGURE 37-9. Detection of microsatellite instability with the use of fluorescent labeling of polymerase chain reaction (PCR) products analyzed in an automatic sequencer. Two markers are analyzed in the same track: the mononucleotide repeat marker BAT26 is shown on the *left*, and the dinucleotide marker D2S123 is shown on the *right*. The upper tracking is from germ line DNA from blood. The lower tracing is from DNA extracted from a histologic section of a tumor containing more than 50% tumor cells. For marker BAT26, germ line DNA shows a *single peak*, indicating that the patient is homozygous for this marker (*arrow*). Tumor DNA shows, in addition to the normal allele (*single arrow*), a new allele (*double arrows*) that has lost approximately five nucleotides. This constitutes microsatellite stability. For marker D2S123, germ line DNA is homozygous, whereas tumor DNA shows two new alleles (*triple arrows*), one with a loss of approximately 10 nucleotides (*left*) and one with a gain of two nucleotides (*right*). Thus, the tumor shows microsatellite instability with both markers. All peaks display "stutter" – that is, small amounts of material with a gain or a loss of one or a few nucleotides. This is a normal phenomenon. (Reprinted with permission from Lynch HT, De la Chapelle A. Hereditary colorectal cancer. N Engl J Med. 2003;348:919–32. Copyright © 2003 Massachusetts Medicine Society. All rights reserved).

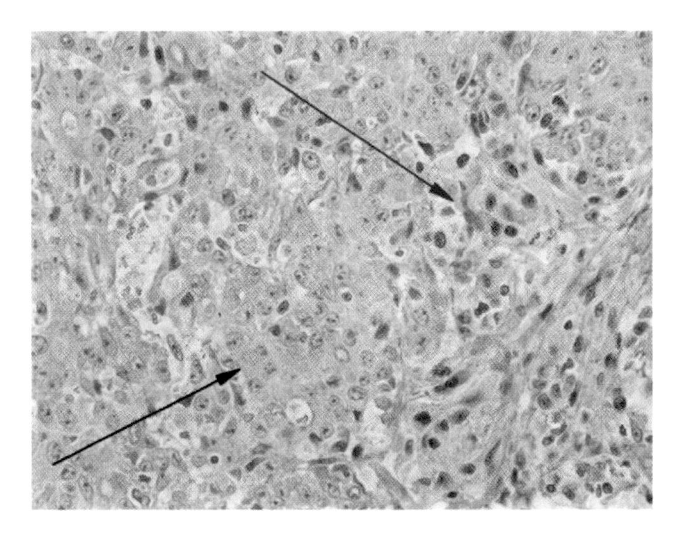

FIGURE 37-10. hMLH1 immunohistochemistry. *Blue arrow* indicates positive nuclear staining for the presence of hMLH1 protein within an inflammatory cell. *Black arrow* demonstrates the absence of protein within cancer cells, ×400 magnification. (Courtesy of Robert E. Petras, MD, National Director Gastrointestinal Pathology Services, Ameripath Inc., Oakwood Village, OH, and Associate Professor of Pathology, Northeastern Ohio University College of Medicine).

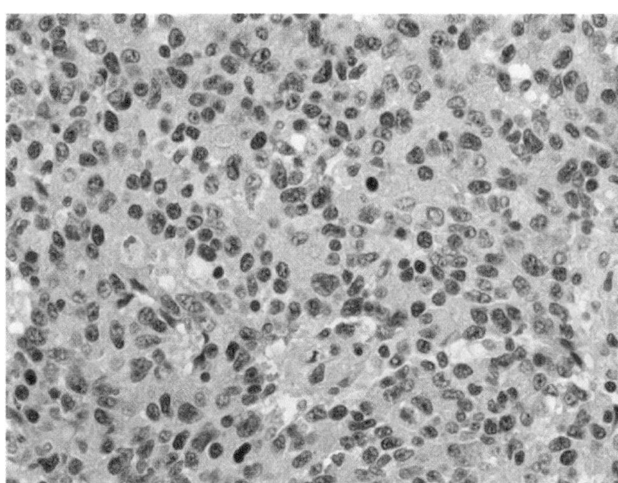

FIGURE 37-11. hMSH2 immunohistochemistry. Positive nuclear staining demonstrates the normal presence of hMSH2 protein, ×400 magnification. (Courtesy of Robert E. Petras, MD, National Director Gastrointestinal Pathology Services, Ameripath Inc., Oakwood Village, OH, and Associate Professor of Pathology, Northeastern Ohio University College of Medicine).

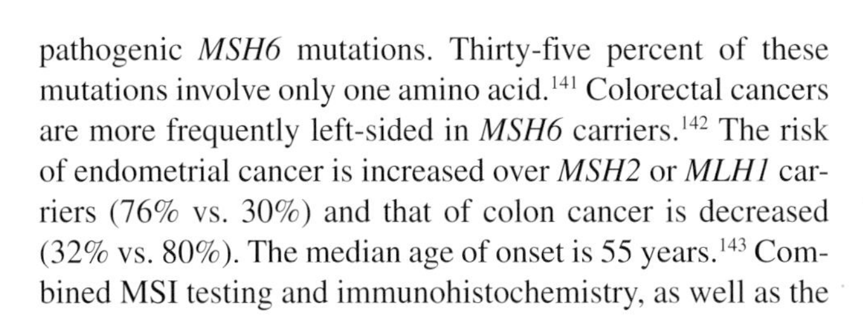

pathogenic *MSH6* mutations. Thirty-five percent of these mutations involve only one amino acid.[141] Colorectal cancers are more frequently left-sided in *MSH6* carriers.[142] The risk of endometrial cancer is increased over *MSH2* or *MLH1* carriers (76% vs. 30%) and that of colon cancer is decreased (32% vs. 80%). The median age of onset is 55 years.[143] Combined MSI testing and immunohistochemistry, as well as the distinctive phenotype are used to select families for *MSH6* mutation analysis (Figures 37-9–37-11).

Muir–Torre Syndrome

The Muir–Torre syndrome is the combination of Lynch syndrome and sebaceous adenomas, sebaceous carcinomas, and keratoacanthomas. Colorectal cancers are most commonly found (51%) and are often proximal to the splenic flexure (60%). Although only 25% of Muir–Torre patients develop a polyp, 90% of patients who develop polyps develop colon cancer. The second most frequent tumors are genitourinary (24%).[144,145] Germ line mutations in *MLH1* and *MSH2* [[145]] have been identified, and many of the tumors exhibit MSI. The visceral tumors are often low-grade and prolonged survival in the presence of metastatic disease has been reported. The median age of diagnosis is 55 years and only 60% has a positive family history.[144]

Diagnosis

1. Amsterdam Criteria
   The key to the diagnosis of Lynch syndrome is a high index of suspicion and an awareness of some of the subtle phenotypic clues. The easiest clue to detect is a strong family history of colorectal and Lynch syndrome cancers. The first Amsterdam criteria (I) (Table 37-7) were created to identify patients with a high probability of having HNPCC. However, the Amsterdam I criteria were faulted for not including extracolonic cancers, and so Amsterdam II criteria were published to correct this (Table 37-7). A third set of Amsterdam Criteria (Amsterdam-like) have been used, where an advanced adenoma is allowed to qualify one of the three affected individuals, accounting for the phenotype attenuation caused by increasingly widespread screening. However Hampel et al. have shown that when Lynch syndrome was diagnosed by MSI-directed mutational testing, 22% of families did not meet Amsterdam criteria and 10/23 probands were older than 50 years.[146] Therefore, although Amsterdam criteria are still useful, on their own they have a high false negative rate. The "false positive" rate of Amsterdam criteria for MMR gene mutation carriers (Lynch syndrome) represents Familial Colorectal Cancer Type X.
2. Bethesda Criteria
   In 1996, a National Cancer Institute workshop on MSI produced a set of criteria to identify patients who's cancers are likely to be microsatellite unstable. These Bethesda criteria and their revision (Table 37-9).[147,148]

Table 37-9. Modified Bethesda guidelines

- Patient with 2 HNPCC-related tumors.
- Patient with CRC with first-degree relative with HNPCC-related cancer; one of the cancers at <50 years or adenoma at <40 years.
- Patient with CRC or endometrial cancer at <50 years.
- Patient with right-sided, undifferentiated CRC at <50 years.
- Patient with signet ring CRC at <50 years.
- Patient with adenoma at <40 years.

Modified from Rodriguez-Bigas MA, Boland CR, Hamilton SR, Henson DE, Jass JR, Khan PM, Lynch H, Perucho M, Smyrk T, Sobin L, Srivastava S. A National Cancer Institute Workshop on hereditary nonpolyposis colorectal cancer syndrome: meeting highlights and Bethesda guidelines. J Natl Cancer Inst. 1997;89:1758–62.

   include family history as well as tumor characteristics, such as histology and site. The Bethesda criteria are a useful screen for triaging colorectal cancers for MSI testing but were never intended as diagnostic criteria for Lynch syndrome.
3. Tumor testing with MSI and Immunohistochemistry
   MSI testing is being used as a screening test to detect Lynch syndrome although 15% of sporadic colorectal cancers are unstable due to promoter methylation of *hMLH1*. Thus, in screening colorectal cancers for Lynch syndrome, an MSH-High tumor may be further tested with IHC to detect lack of expression of an MMR protein. If hMSH2 is not expressed, this is good evidence for Lynch syndrome. If hMLH1 is not expressed, the clinical situation (i.e., family history, age and site of the cancer) may give a clue as to the existence of Lynch syndrome. The tumor can also be tested for a *BRAF* mutation which, if present, suggests a sporadic, hypermethylated cancer rather than Lynch. After tumor triage by MSI and IHC testing, patients can be selected for genetic testing for a germ line mutation.
4. Histology
   Pathologists may recognize cancers that have arisen due to the mutator phenotype by the presence of tumor infiltrating lymphocytes, a Crohn's-like reaction, mucinous differentiation, signet ring cells, and the absence of dirty necrosis.[149] A tumor with any of these features is a candidate for MSI or IHC testing. Several institutions now routinely perform either MSI or IHC on every colorectal cancer, which minimizes the importance of a pathologist's suspicion.
5. Predictive models
   At least three predictive scores have been created to predict the presence of MMR deficiency in a patient or tumor. MSPath was constructed by Jenkins et al. using tumor-infiltrating lymphocytes, tumor location (proximal vs. distal), mucinous histology, poor differentiation, Crohn's-like reaction, and diagnosis before age 50 years.[149] It had a sensitivity of 93% and a specificity of 55% for MSI-High. MMRpro was devised by Chen et al. to predict the probability that a patient carries a deleterious mutation of *MLH1*, *MSH2*, or *MSH6*, and the chances of developing colorectal or endometrial cancer in the future.[150] It includes family history, endometrial cancer status, and current age or age at last follow-up (in years) if unaffected. Results of MSI testing or IHC are used if available as is the result of previous germ line testing of *MLH1*, *MSH2*, or *MSH6* (positive or not found). The formula had a concordance index of 0.83 and a ratio of observed to predicted cases of 0.94. It is available online at http://www4.utsouthwestern.edu/breasthealth/cagene/ Barnetson et al.[151] produced a predictive formula to calculate the risk of carrying a germ line MMR gene mutation. It is: $Pr/(1-Pr)=1.39\times 0.89$ age at

diagnosis × 2.57 gender (male = 1, female = 0.57) × 4.45 (site of tumor, proximal = 1, distal = 0) × 9.53 synchronous or metachronous tumor (yes = 1, no = 0) × 46.26 family history of colorectal cancer (youngest < 50) × 7.04 family history of colorectal cancer (youngest > 50 years of age) (yes = 1, no = 0) × 59.36 family history of endometrial cancer <50 years of age(yes = 1, no = 0). This model provided a subset of patients in whom preoperative tumor biopsies could be subjected to IHC, and the combination has a positive predictive value of 80% for mutation carriers.

Genetic Testing for a Germ line MMR Gene Mutation

Indications

Patients whose families fulfill Amsterdam I, II and like criteria, patients fulfilling revised Bethesda criteria, patients with MSI-high tumors with wild type *BRAF* or loss of expression of an MMR protein are candidates for genetic testing (Table 37-10).

Procedure

Genetic counseling is routine. Patients and family members must understand the advantages and potential disadvantages of testing. The significance and implications of genetic testing in general, and in Lynch syndrome in particular, are discussed, as they apply to the patient and their family. This includes the remote possibility of genetic discrimination and the protection afforded by the recently enacted GINA. Financial concerns are addressed. After all this, informed consent is obtained.

Sequencing of *MSH2*, *MLH1*, *PMS2* and *hMSH6* is now commercially available. The cost of this testing is usually covered by the patient's health insurance. Once the pathologic mutation in the family has been found, screening of at-risk relatives is considerably cheaper. The mutations themselves include a broad spectrum of truncating, frameshift, and missense mutations. A missense mutation results in the substitution of a single amino acid, and the effect on protein function may be negligible. This type of missense mutation is often reported as a variant of unknown significance. About 31% of *MLH1* mutations are this type and further testing by a specialized center is required to determine its clinical significance and usefulness. A data bank of known mutations is kept by the International Society for Gastrointestinal Hereditary Tumors (InSiGHT).[152] Some affected families do not have a point mutation but may have a large gene deletion or an intronic mutation that is not detected by sequencing. Such false negative testing is minimized by other molecular techniques, such as Southern Blotting or Conversion analysis.[153]

TABLE 37-10. Direct mutation finding ($n = 70$)

Category	Sensitivity (%)	Specificity (%)
Amsterdam [$n = 28$]	61	67
Amsterdam II [$n = 34$]	78	61
Bethesda [$n = 56$]	94	25
Bethesda (1–3) [$n = 44$]	94	49

Adapted and reproduced from Syngal S, Fox EA, Eng C, Kolodner RD, Garber JE. Sensitivity and specificity of clinical criteria for hereditary non-polyposis colorectal cancer associated mutations in MSH2 and MLH1. J Med Genet. 2000;37:641–45.

Strategy of Genetic Testing

Testing should begin with an affected individual (in whom a Lynch syndrome cancer has been diagnosed). When the proband has a negative or a noninformative test (including variant of unknown significance), genetic testing of at-risk family members is not helpful and all at-risk family members require intensive surveillance. When the proband has a pathologic mutation, at-risk family members can be offered genetic screening. Those that carry the mutation need intensive surveillance and/or prophylactic surgery. At-risk family members who are mutation negative are at average population risk of colorectal cancer.

Surveillance

Colorectal cancers in Lynch syndrome can occur in very young patients and develop within 2 years of a negative colonoscopy.[154,155] Adenomas occur earlier and are more likely to be villous. The adenoma to carcinoma transition occurs early and small cancers can be missed.[156] Screening colonoscopy must therefore be thorough and uncompromising with excellent preparation. Most guidelines suggest beginning colonoscopy at age 21, or 10 years younger than the youngest affected relative's age at diagnosis (whichever is younger). Colonoscopies continue every 2 years until age 40 when they are every year. If an adenoma is found, colonoscopy is every year thereafter.

The value of screening colonoscopy in Lynch syndrome was demonstrated by Jārvinen and colleagues who studied a group of 252 individuals belonging to 22 HNPCC families.[155] Of these, 137 participated in screening colonoscopy every 3 years, while the remainder refused such evaluation. Colorectal cancer developed in 8% of the screened family members, compared to 16% of those who refused screening. In those individuals who were known to have a DNA MMR gene mutation (Lynch syndrome), the rate of colorectal cancer in those who underwent screening was 18% compared to 41% in those who did not undergo screening. All cancers that developed in the screened group were either Dukes' A or B lesions, with no attributable deaths, compared to more advanced lesions in the unscreened group and nine deaths due to cancer (8%).

Due to the high risk of endometrial cancer in women, annual pelvic ultrasound to examine the endometrium is recommended beginning between ages 25 and 35 years as the increased risk for gynecological cancer in these patients begins at age 25.[157,158] Endometrial biopsy is done if the ultrasound is abnormal. There are no data demonstrating the efficacy of this type of screening.[159] Should a Lynch syndrome patient be diagnosed with endometrial cancer, they should undergo surveillance colonoscopy prior to hysterectomy in the event that colonic pathology is present and colonic resection required at the same surgery. Similarly, when a Lynch syndrome patient develops colorectal cancer, prophylactic hysterectomy should be considered at the same time as the bowel resection.

Prophylactic colectomy and hysterectomy is the most effective way to prevent cancer in Lynch syndrome patients. Although prophylactic colectomy is not commonly performed in unaffected mutation carriers, its benefits must be discussed.

Treatment

Surgery

The surgical options for colon cancer in a Lynch syndrome patient are a standard right, left, or sigmoid colectomy, or a colectomy and ileorectal anastomosis. For a rectal cancer, the options are a standard anterior proctosigmoidectomy and colorectal or coloanal anastomosis, or abdominal perineal resection with end colostomy, versus a total proctocolectomy with ileal pouch anal anastomosis or end ileostomy. The aim of the more extensive option in either case is to remove at risk mucosa and prevent metachronous cancer, in the way that is routinely done for classical FAP. Oncologically, IRA is the operation of choice for colon cancer. It minimizes cancer risk, preserves anal sphincter function, and retains the reservoir capacity of the rectum.[160,161] This operation eliminates the need for annual surveillance colonoscopy, since only rigid or fiberoptic examination of the rectum is required. The estimated risk of rectal cancer after colectomy and IRA is 12% at 12 years.[162] However, colectomy and IRA may not be the ideal operation for patients with impaired anal sphincter function due to either obstetrical injury or age, for patients with comorbidities, or for those with decreased mobility. It may also predispose some patients to diarrhea and poor functional results. In these patients, a lesser resection may be preferable. It is essential, however, that both the patient and physician recognize the need for ongoing annual colonoscopy, since the risk for a metachronous colon cancer in HNPCC is 45%.[131]

In cases of rectal cancer not involving the sphincters, either anterior resection, coloanal anastomosis or colectomy and ileal pouch anal anastomosis can be considered. In the event that the last option is chosen, preoperative endorectal ultrasound or MRI staging is desirable. In uT3 or uN1 cancers, preoperative chemoradiation should be given since ileal pouches tolerate radiation poorly.

In women undergoing colectomy, strong consideration should be given to performing a hysterectomy and bilateral salpingo-oophorectomy if their family is complete, due to the increased risk of both endometrial and ovarian carcinoma.

There is controversy as to whether surgical treatment or continued surveillance should be offered to the asymptomatic patient who has a mutation identified by genetic testing, but an as yet "normal" colon. Several studies have examined this question using decision analysis methods; however, factors such as patient compliance must be taken into account.[163,164]

Prognosis

The survival rate in Lynch syndrome patients with colorectal cancer is better than that of patients with sporadic colorectal cancer when matched for stage and age of onset.[165,166] There is also evidence that patients with stage II or III microsatellite unstable colorectal cancers do not benefit from 5-fluorouracil-based adjuvant therapy, and may even do worse with it.[167,168]

Chemoprevention

While data exist to support the efficacy of NSAIDs in reducing the risk of colorectal cancer in the general population, such data are lacking for Lynch syndrome.[169,170] The recent CAPP II trial was a controlled, randomized trial of colorectal polyp and cancer prevention using aspirin and resistant starch in carriers of a germ line MMR gene mutation. Its first report described no impact of this chemoprevention on the development of adenomas or carcinomas,[171] although extended follow-up suggests that there may be a benefit in reduced cancer incidence (J. Burn, personal communication).

Calcium and vitamin D intake have been associated with a decreased risk of sporadic colorectal cancer.[172] A trial of supplemental calcium in HNPCC families did not demonstrate a decrease in epithelial proliferation, although the sample size was small and the study was conducted before genetic testing was available.[173]

Familial Colorectal Cancer Type X

This collection of families, where the history of colorectal cancer is strong enough to comply with Amsterdam Criteria but where tumors are microsatellite stable, is poorly defined. The original report that separated these families from Lynch syndrome found a moderate increase in risk of colorectal cancer but no risk of the usual Lynch spectrum of extracolonic cancers. Genetically, the Type X families may include Lynch syndrome due to *hMSH6* mutations (unlikely as a predominance of uterine cancer would be expected), MAP, SPP, and other as yet unknown genotypes. Until FCC Type X is better defined genetically, intensive colonoscopic surveillance for all related family members is all that can be advised.

Our knowledge about Lynch syndrome continues to grow. This disorder is associated with a germ line mutation in one of several MMR genes. Genetic testing is currently available for mutations in *hMLH1*, *hMHS2*, *hMSH6*, and *hPMS2*.

Suspicion of this disorder in a given patient is raised by a family history of early age onset cancer, an increased number of first-degree relatives with colorectal cancer, or a Lynch syndrome-related cancer. Endometrial cancer is the most common extracolonic cancer. While there is debate regarding the frequency and beginning of screening, most clinicians believe that colonic examinations yearly or every 2 years should be performed beginning in the early 20s, or 10 years younger than the youngest affected relative (whichever is first). Prophylactic colectomy may be offered to known mutation carriers as well as members of at-risk families who develop advanced adenomas. Removal of all of the colon and IRA is suitable for patients with a colon cancer while total proctocolectomy and ileal pouch anal anastomosis should be considered for patients with rectal cancer. Continued surveillance of residual colon, rectum, and pouch is mandatory. With careful surveillance and management, colorectal cancer can be prevented in these patients and the mortality rate decreased. In those who develop colorectal carcinoma, the overall survival rate is more favorable than that of patients with sporadic colorectal cancer.

Registries for Patients with Hereditary Colorectal Cancer and Their Families

Treatment of patients with hereditary colorectal cancer requires a thorough understanding of the role that genetics plays in the origin of the syndromes and their inheritance in the families. Care of affected individuals and their families involves clinical recognition, genetic diagnosis, and clinical management. Ongoing care requires careful follow-up and integration of multiple medical specialties. This sort of sophisticated care is best delivered through a Center or Registry dedicated to hereditary colorectal cancer. Such a Center is ideally positioned to conduct meaningful research on their often illuminating cases and families. This chapter assumes that patients and families have access to doctors with suitable knowledge, experience, and support to deliver the kind of care that is needed.

Registries

Once a diagnosis of HNPCC is suspected, a referral to a registry for inherited colorectal cancer or to a cancer center with a high-risk clinic is important. A registry has a database or list of families and their members who have a high frequency of colorectal cancer. Personnel at the registry may include a coordinator, a genetic counselor and a physician director. The mission of registries is to prevent death from hereditary cancer, and to preserve quality of life for the patients and their families. This is accomplished through expert patient care, careful education of patients and other healthcare providers, and innovative research. Care of families with hereditary colorectal cancer is complex and needs to be multidisciplinary. The registry functions to coordinate care between specialties and between the family doctor and the specialist unit. Registry personnel provide further support for myriad problems, such as family stress, health insurance difficulties, and job discrimination. A local registry can be found by accessing the Collaborative Group of the Americas on Inherited Colorectal Cancer at http://www.cgaicc.com.

Acknowledgment. This chapter was previously authored by Robin K.S. Phillips and Susann K. Clark (separate chapter) and Lawrence C. Rusin and Susan Galandiuk (separate chapter) in the first edition. The two chapters were merged for this second edition.

References

1. Wood LD, Parsons DW, Jones S, Lin J, Sjöblom T, et al. The genomic landscapes of human breast and colorectal cancers. Science. 2007;318(5853):1108–13.
2. Bisgaard ML, Fenger K, Bulow S, et al. Familial adenomatous polyposis (FAP): frequency, penetrance and mutation rate. Hum Mutat. 1994;3:121–5.
3. Ripa R, Bisgaard ML, Bulow S, Nielsen FC. De novo mutations in familial adenomatous polyposis (FAP). Eur J Hum Genet. 2002;10:631–7.
4. Church JM, McGannon E. A polyposis registry; how to set one up and make it work. Semin Colon Rectal Surg. 1995;6: 48–54.
5. Bulow S. Results of national registration of familial adenomatous polyposis. Gut. 2003;52:742–6.
6. Church JM. Anatomy of a gene: functional correlations of APC mutation. Semin Colon Rectal Surg. 1998;9(1):49–52.
7. Wu JS, Paul P, McGannon EA, Church JM. Polyp number and surgical options in familial adenomatous polyposis. Ann Surg. 1998;227(1):57–62.
8. Nakamura Y, Nishisho I, Kinzler KW, Vogelstein B, Miyoshi Y, Miki Y, et al. Mutations of the adenomatous polyposis coli gene in familial polyposis coli patients and sporadic colorectal tumors. Princess Takamatsu Symp. 1991;22:285–92. Review.
9. Van der Luijt RB, Khan PM, Vasen HFA, et al. Molecular analysis of the APC gene in 105 Dutch kindreds with familial adenomatous polyposis. Hum Mutat. 1997;9:7–16.
10. Schnitzler M, Dwight T, Marsh DJ, et al. Quantitation of APC messenger RNA in human tissues. Biochem Biophys Res Commun. 1995;217:385–92.
11. Midgley CA, White S, Howitt R, et al. APC expression in normal human tissues. J Pathol. 1997;181:426–33.
12. Fodde R. The APC gene in colorectal cancer. Eur J Cancer. 2002;20:905–11.
13. Nugent KP, Phillips RKS, Hodgson SV, et al. Phenotypic expression in familial adenomatous polyposis: partial prediction by mutation analysis. Gut. 1994;35:1622–3.
14. Friedl W, Caspari R, Senteller M, et al. Can APC mutation analysis contribute to therapeutic decisions in familial adenomatous polyposis? Experience in 680 FAP families. Gut. 2001;48:515–21.
15. Gómez García EB, Knoers NV. Gardner's syndrome (familial adenomatous polyposis): a cilia-related disorder. Lancet Oncol. 2009;10(7):727–35.

16. Caspari R, Olschwang S, Friedl W, et al. Familial adenomatous polyposis: desmoid tumours and lack of ophthalmic lesions (CHRPE) associated with APC mutations beyond codon 1444. Hum Mol Genet. 1995;4:337–40.
17. Eccles DM, van der Luijt R, Breukel C, et al. Hereditary desmoid disease due to a frameshift mutation at codon 1924 of the APC gene. Am J Hum Genet. 1996;59:1193–201.
18. Crabtree MD, Tomlinson IPM, Hodgson SV, et al. Explaining variation in familial adenomatous polyposis: relationship between genotype and phenotype and evidence for modifier genes. Gut. 2002;51:420–3.
19. Arvanitis ML, Jagelman DG, Fazio VW, Lavery IC, McGannon E. Mortality in patients with familial adenomatous polyposis. Dis Colon Rectum. 1990;33(8):639–42.
20. Heyen F, Jagelman DG, Romania A, Zakov ZN, Lavery IC, Fazio VW, et al. Predictive value of congenital hypertrophy of the retinal pigment epithelium as a clinical marker for familial adenomatous polyposis. Dis Colon Rectum. 1990;33(12):1003–8.
21. Hernegger GS, Moore HG, Guillem JG. Attenuated familial adenomatous polyposis: an evolving and poorly understood entity. Dis Colon Rectum. 2002;45:127–34.
22. Sieber OM, Lipton L, Crabtree M, et al. Multiple colorectal adenomas, classic adenomatous polyposis and germ-line mutations in MYH. N Engl J Med. 2003;348:791–9.
23. Parks TG. Extracolonic manifestations associated with familial adenomatous polyposis. Ann R Coll Surg Engl. 1990;72:181–4.
24. Paraf F, Jothy S, Van Meir EG. Brain tumour–polyposis syndrome: two genetic diseases? J Clin Oncol. 1997;15: 2744–58.
25. Bülow S, Bülow C, Nielsen TF, Karlsen L, Moesgaard F. Centralized registration, prophylactic examination, and treatment results in improved prognosis in familial adenomatous polyposis. Results from the Danish Polyposis Register. Scand J Gastroenterol. 1995;30(10):989–93.
26. Giardiello FM, Brensinger JD, Petersen GM, et al. The use and interpretation of commercial APC gene testing for familial adenomatous polyposis. N Engl J Med. 1997;336:823–7.
27. Elayi E, Manilich E, Church J. Polishing the crystal ball: knowing genotype improves ability to predict desmoid disease in patients with familial adenomatous polyposis. Dis Colon Rectum. 2009;52:1623–9.
28. van Duijvendijk P, Slors JF, Taat CW, Oosterveld P, Vasen HF. Functional outcome after colectomy and ileorectal anastomosis compared with proctocolectomy and ileal pouch-anal anastomosis in familial adenomatous polyposis. Ann Surg. 1999;230(5):648–54.
29. Olsen KØ, Juul S, Bülow S, Järvinen HJ, Bakka A, Björk J, et al. Female fecundity before and after operation for familial adenomatous polyposis. Br J Surg. 2003;90(2):227–31.
30. Bülow C, Vasen H, Järvinen H, Björk J, Bisgaard ML, Bülow S. Ileorectal anastomosis is appropriate for a subset of patients with familial adenomatous polyposis. Gastroenterology. 2000; 119(6):1454–60.
31. Church J, Burke C, McGannon E, Pastean O, Clark B. Predicting polyposis severity by proctoscopy: how reliable is it? Dis Colon Rectum. 2001;44(9):1249–54.
32. Nugent KP, Phillips RKS. Rectal cancer risk in older patients with familial adenomatous polyposis and an ileorectal anastomosis: a cause for concern. Br J Surg. 1992;79:1204–6.
33. Remzi FH, Church JM, Bast J, Lavery IC, Strong SA, Hull TL, et al. Mucosectomy vs. stapled ileal pouch-anal anastomosis in patients with familial adenomatous polyposis: functional outcome and neoplasia control. Dis Colon Rectum. 2001;44(11):1590–6.
34. Feinberg SM, Jagelman DG, Sarre RG, McGannon E, Fazio VW, Lavery IC, et al. Spontaneous resolution of rectal polyps in patients with familial polyposis following abdominal colectomy and ileorectal anastomosis. Dis Colon Rectum. 1988;31(3):169–75.
35. Groves CJ, Beveridge IG, Swain DJ, et al. Adenoma prevalence and ileal mucosa in pouch vs. neoterminal ileum. Gut. 2002;50 Suppl 2:A22–3.
36. Parc YR, Olschwang S, Desaint B, et al. Familial adenomatous polyposis: prevalence of adenomas in the ileal pouch after restorative proctocolectomy. Ann Surg. 2001;233:360–4.
37. Church J. Ileoanal pouch neoplasia in familial adenomatous polyposis: an underestimated threat. Dis Colon Rectum. 2005;48(9):1708–13.
38. Giardello FM, Hamilton SR, Krush AJ, et al. Treatment of colonic and rectal adenomas with sulindac in familial adenomatous polyposis. N Engl J Med. 1993;328:1313–6.
39. Steinbach LT, Lynch P, Phillips RKS, et al. The effect of Celecoxib, a cyclo-oxygenase inhibitor, in familial adenomatous polyposis. N Engl J Med. 2000;342:1946–58.
40. Lynch HT, Thorson AG, Smyrk T. Rectal cancer after prolonged sulindac chemoprevention. A case report. Cancer. 1995;75(4):936–8.
41. Niv Y, Fraser GM. Adenocarcinoma in the rectal segment in familial polyposis coli is not prevented by sulindac therapy. Gastroenterology. 1994;107(3):854–7.
42. Wallace MH, Phillips RKS. Upper gastrointestinal disease in patients with familial adenomatous polyposis. Br J Surg. 1998;85:742–50.
43. Bianchi LK, Burke CA, Bennett AE, Lopez R, Hasson H, Church JM. Fundic gland polyp dysplasia is common in familial adenomatous polyposis. Clin Gastroenterol Hepatol. 2008;6(2):180–5.
44. Zwik A, Munir M, Ryan CK, et al. Gastric adenocarcinoma and dysplasia in fundic gland polyps of a patient with attenuated adenomatous polyposis coli. Gastroenterology. 1997;113:659–63.
45. Iwama T, Mishima Y, Utsonomiya J. The impact of familial adenomatous polyposis on the tumorigenesis and mortality at the several organs. Ann Surg. 1993;217:101–8.
46. Nugent KP, Spigelman AD, Talbot IC, et al. Gallbladder dysplasia in patients with familial adenomatous polyposis. Br J Surg. 1994;81:291–2.
47. Jarvinen HJ, Nyberg M, Peltokallio P. Biliary involvement in familial polyposis coli. Dis Colon Rectum. 1983;26:525–8.
48. Heiskanen I, Kellokumpu I, Jarvinen H. Management of duodenal adenomas in 98 patients with familial adenomatous polyposis. Endoscopy. 1999;31:412–6.
49. Sanabria JR, Croxford R, Berk TC, et al. Familial segregation in the occurrence and severity of periampullary neoplasms in familial adenomatous polyposis. Am J Surg. 1996;171: 136–40.
50. Burke CA, Santisi J, Church J, Levinthal G. The utility of capsule endoscopy small bowel surveillance in patients with polyposis. Am J Gastroenterol. 2005;100(7):1498–502.

51. Spigelman AD, Williams CB, Talbot IC, et al. Upper gastrointestinal cancer in patients with familial adenomatous polyposis. Lancet. 1989;2:783–5.
52. Groves CJ, Saunders BP, Spigelman AD, Phillips RKS. Duodenal cancer in patients with familial adenomatous polyposis (FAP): results of a 10 year prospective study. Gut. 2002;50:636–41.
53. Burke CA, Beck GJ, Church JM, van Stolk RU. The natural history of untreated duodenal and ampullary adenomas in patients with familial adenomatous polyposis followed in an endoscopic surveillance program. Gastrointest Endosc. 1999;49:358–64.
54. Penna C, Bataille N, Balladur P, et al. Surgical treatment of severe duodenal polyposis in familial adenomatous polyposis. Br J Surg. 1998;85:665–8.
55. Nugent KP, Spigelman AD, Williams CB, et al. Iatrogenic pancreatitis in familial adenomatous polyposis. Gut. 1993;34:1269–70.
56. Mlkvy P, Messman H, Debinsky H, et al. Photodynamic therapy for polyps in familial adenomatous polyposis – a pilot study. Int J Colorectal Dis. 1995;31A:1160–5.
57. Wallace MH, Phillips RK. Preventative strategies for periampullary tumours in FAP. Ann Oncol. 1999;10 Suppl 4: 201–3.
58. Phillips RKS, Wallace MH, Lynch PM, et al. A randomised, double blind, placebo controlled study of celecoxib, a selective cyclooxygenase 2 inhibitor, on duodenal polyposis in familial adenomatous polyposis. Gut. 2002;50:857–60.
59. Mackey R, Walsh RM, Chung R, Brown N, Smith A, Church J, et al. Pancreas-sparing duodenectomy is effective management for familial adenomatous polyposis. J Gastrointest Surg. 2005;9(8):1088–93.
60. Hartley JE, Church JM, Gupta S, McGannon E, Fazio VW. Significance of incidental desmoids identified during surgery for familial adenomatous polyposis. Dis Colon Rectum. 2004;47(3):334–40.
61. Clark SK, Phillips RKS. Desmoids in familial adenomatous polyposis. Br J Surg. 1996;83:1494–504.
62. Penna C, Kartheuser A, Parc R, et al. Secondary proctectomy and ileal pouch-anal anastomosis after ileorectal anastomosis for familial adenomatous polyposis. Br J Surg. 1993;80: 1621–3.
63. Mao C, Huang Y, Howard JM. Carcinoma of the ampulla of Vater and mesenteric fibromatosis (desmoid tumour) associated with Gardner's syndrome: problems in management. Pancreas. 1995;10:239–45.
64. Brooks AP, Reznek RH, Nugent KP, et al. CT appearances of desmoid tumours in familial adenomatous polyposis: further observations. Clin Radiol. 1994;49:601–7.
65. Healy JC, Reznek RH, Clark SK, et al. MR a pearances of desmoid tumours in familial adenomatous polyposis. AJR Am J Roentgenol. 1997;169:465–72.
66. Church JM. Desmoid tumors in patients with familial adenomatous polyposis. Semin Colon Rectal Surg. 1995;6(1):29–32.
67. Church J, Berk T, Boman BM, Guillem J, Lynch C, Lynch P, et al. Staging intra-abdominal desmoid tumors in familial adenomatous polyposis: a search for a uniform approach to a troubling disease. Dis Colon Rectum. 2005;48(8):1528–34.
68. Church J, Lynch C, Neary P, LaGuardia L, Elayi E. A desmoid tumor-staging system separates patients with intra-abdominal, familial adenomatous polyposis-associated desmoid disease by behavior and prognosis. Dis Colon Rectum. 2008;51(6): 897–901.
69. Latchford AR, Sturt NJ, Neale K, Rogers PA, Phillips RK. A 10-year review of surgery for desmoid disease associated with familial adenomatous polyposis. Br J Surg. 2006;93: 1258–64.
70. Clark SK, Neale KF, Landgrebe JC, Phillips RKS. Desmoid tumours complicating familial adenomatous polyposis. Br J Surg. 1999;86:1185–9.
71. Mignanelli E, Joyce M, Church J. Ureteric obstruction in FAP associated desmoid disease. Dis Colon Rectum. 2009;52:811.
72. Lynch HT, Fitzgibbons Jr R, Chong S, et al. Use of doxorubicin and dacarbazine for the management of unresectable intra-abdominal desmoid tumours in Gardner's syndrome. Dis Colon Rectum. 1994;37:260–7.
73. Poritz LS, Blackstein M, Berk T, Gallinger S, McLeod RS, Cohen Z. Extended follow-up of patients treated with cytotoxic chemotherapy for intra-abdominal desmoid tumors. Dis Colon Rectum. 2001;44:1268–73.
74. Azzarelli A, Gronchi A, Bertulli R, et al. Low-dose chemotherapy with methotrexate and vinblastine for patients with advanced aggressive fibromatosis. Cancer. 2001;92:1259–64.
75. Bertagnolli MM, Morgan JA, Fletcher CD, Rant CP, Dileo P, Gill RR, et al. Multimodality treatment for mesenteric desmoid tumors. Eur J Cancer. 2008;44:2404–10.
76. Al-Tassan N, Chmiel NH, Maynard J, Fleming N, Livingston AL, Williams GT, et al. Inherited variants of MYH associated with somatic G:C→T:A mutations in colorectal tumors. Nat Genet. 2002;30(2):227–32.
77. Terdiman JP. MYH-associated disease: attenuated adenomatous polyposis of the colon is only part of the story. Gastroenterology. 2009;137(6):1883–6.
78. de Ferro SM, Suspiro A, Fidalgo P, Lage P, Rodrigues P, Fragoso S, et al. Aggressive phenotype of MYH-associated polyposis with jejunal cancer and intra-abdominal desmoid tumor: report of a case. Dis Colon Rectum. 2009;52(4):742–5.
79. Boparai KS, Dekker E, Van Eeden S, Polak MM, Bartelsman JF, Mathus-Vliegen EM, et al. Hyperplastic polyps and sessile serrated adenomas as a phenotypic expression of MYH-associated polyposis. Gastroenterology. 2008;135(6):2014–8.
80. Gismondi V, Meta M, Bonelli L, Radice P, Sala P, Bertario L, et al. Prevalence of the Y165C, G382D and 1395delGGA germline mutations of the MYH gene in Italian patients with adenomatous polyposis coli and colorectal adenomas. Int J Cancer. 2004;109(5):680–4.
81. Poulsen ML, Bisgaard ML. MUTYH associated polyposis (MAP). Curr Genomics. 2008;9(6):420–35.
82. Olschwang S, Blanché H, de Moncuit C, Thomas G. Similar colorectal cancer risk in patients with monoallelic and biallelic mutations in the MYH gene identified in a population with adenomatous polyposis. Genet Test. 2007;11(3):315–20.
83. Lubbe SJ, Di Bernardo MC, Chandler IP, Houlston RS. Clinical implications of the colorectal cancer risk associated with MUTYH mutation. J Clin Oncol. 2009;27(24):3975–80.
84. McGarrity TJ, Kulin HE, Zaino RJ. Peutz–Jeghers syndrome. Am J Gastroenterol. 2000;95:596–604.
85. Gruber SB, Entius EM, Petersen GM, et al. Pathogenesis of adenocarcinoma in Peutz–Jeghers syndrome. Cancer Res. 1998;58:5267–70.

86. Boardman LA, Couch FJ, Burgart LJ, et al. Genetic heterogeneity in Peutz–Jeghers syndrome. Hum Mutat. 2000; 16:23–30.
87. Giardello FM, Bresinger JD, Tersmette AC, et al. Very high risk of cancer in familial Peutz–Jeghers syndrome. Gastroenterology. 2000;119:1447–53.
88. Remzi FH, Church JM, Connor JT, Fazio VW. Benefits of 'clean sweep' in Peutz–Jeghers patients. Colorectal Dis. 2004;6(5):332–5.
89. Ewards DP, Khosraviani K, Stafferton R, et al. Long-term results of polyp clearance by intraoperative enteroscopy in the Peutz–Jeghers syndrome. Dis Colon Rectum. 2003;46:48–50.
90. van Lier MG, Wagner A, Mathus-Vliegen EM, Kuipers EJ, Steyerberg EW, van Leerdam ME. High cancer risk in Peutz–Jeghers syndrome: a systematic review and surveillance recommendations. Am J Gastroenterol. 2010. 2011;60:141–7.
91. Nugent KP, Talbot IC, Hodgson SV, et al. Solitary juvenile polyps: not a marker for subsequent malignancy. Gastroenterology. 1993;105:698–700.
92. Desai DC, Murday V, Phillips RKS, et al. A survey of phenotypic features in juvenile polyposis. J Med Genet. 1998;35:476–81.
93. Howe JR, Mitros FA, Summers RW. The risk of gastrointestinal carcinoma in familial juvenile polyposis. Ann Surg Oncol. 1998;5:751–6.
94. Gallione C, Aylsworth AS, Beis J, Berk T, Bernhardt B, et al. Overlapping spectra of SMAD4 mutations in juvenile polyposis (JP) and JP-HHT syndrome. Am J Med Genet A. 2010;152A(2):333–9.
95. Zhou XP, Woodford-Richens K, Lehtonen R, et al. Germline mutations in BMPR1A/ALK3 cause a subset of juvenile polyposis syndrome and of Cowden and Bannayan–Riley–Ruvalcaba syndrome. Am J Hum Genet. 2001;69:704–11.
96. Olschwang S, Serova-Sinilnikova AM, Lenoir GM, et al. PTEN germ-line mutations in juvenile polyposis coli. Nat Genet. 1998;18:1214.
97. Lynch ED, Ostermeyer EA, Lee MK, et al. Inherited mutations in PTEN that are associated with breast cancer, Cowden disease and juvenile polyposis. Am J Hum Genet. 1997;61:1254–60.
98. Poletto ED, Trinh AM, Levin TL, Loizides AM. Hereditary hemorrhagic telangiectasia and juvenile polyposis: an overlap of syndromes. Pediatr Radiol. 2009;40(7):1274–7.
99. Calva D, Howe JR. Hamartomatous polyposis syndromes. Surg Clin North Am. 2008;88(4):779–817.
100. Hoffenberg EJ, Sauaia A, Malttzman T, et al. Symptomatic colonic polyps in childhood: not so benign. J Pediatr Gastroenterol Nutr. 1999;28:175–81.
101. Jarvinen H. Juvenile gastrointestinal polyposis. Probl Gen Surg. 1993;10:749–57.
102. Oncel M, Church JM, Remzi FH, Fazio VW. Colonic surgery in patients with juvenile polyposis syndrome: a case series. Dis Colon Rectum. 2005;48:49–55.
103. Murday V, Slack J. Inherited disorder associated CRC. Cancer. 1989;8:139–57.
104. Eng C. Will the real Cowden syndrome please stand up? Revised diagnostic criteria. J Med Genet. 2000;37:828–30.
105. Leach B. personal communication.
106. Marsh DJ, Coulon V, Lunetta KL, et al. Mutation spectrum and genotype–phenotype analyses in Cowden disease and Bannayan–Zonana syndrome, two hamartoma syndromes with germline PTEN mutation. Hum Mol Genet. 1998;7:507–15.
107. Zori RT, March DJ, Graham GE, et al. Germline PTEN mutation in a family with Cowden syndrome and Bannayan–Riley–Ruvalcaba syndrome. Am J Med Genet. 1998;80:399–402.
108. Young J, Jenkins M, Parry S, Young B, Nancarrow D, English D, et al. Serrated pathway colorectal cancer in the population: genetic consideration. Gut. 2007;56(10):1453–9.
109. East JE, Saunders BP, Jass JR. Sporadic and syndromic hyperplastic polyps and serrated adenomas of the colon: classification, molecular genetics, natural history, and clinical management. Gastroenterol Clin North Am. 2008;37(1):25–46.
110. Ferrández A, Samowitz W, DiSario JA, Burt RW. Phenotypic characteristics and risk of cancer development in hyperplastic polyposis: case series and literature review. Am J Gastroenterol. 2004;99(10):2012–8.
111. Rubio CA, Stemme S, Jaramillo E, Lindblom A. Hyperplastic polyposis coli syndrome and colorectal carcinomas. Endoscopy. 2006;38:266–70.
112. Vasen HF, Mecklin JP, Khan PM, Lynch HT. The International Collaborative Group on Hereditary Non-Polyposis Colorectal Cancer (ICG-HNPCC). Dis Colon Rectum. 1991;34:424–5.
113. Vasen HF, Watson P, Mecklin JP, Lynch HT. New clinical criteria for hereditary nonpolyposis colorectal cancer (HNPCC, Lynch syndrome) proposed by the International Collaborative group on HNPCC. Gastroenterology. 1999;116:1453–6.
114. Lindor NM, Rabe K, Petersen GM, Haile R, Casey G, Baron J, et al. Lower cancer incidence in Amsterdam-I criteria families without mismatch repair deficiency: familial colorectal cancer type X. JAMA. 2005;293:1979–85.
115. Aarnio M, Mecklin JP, Aaltonen LA, Nystrom-Lahte M, Jarvinen HJ, et al. Life time risk of different cancers in hereditary nonpolyposis colorectal cancer. Int J Cancer. 1995;64:430–3.
116. Warthin A. Hereditary with reference to carcinoma. Arch Intern Med. 1913;12:546–55.
117. Lynch HT, Shaw MW, Magnuson CW, et al. Hereditary factors in cancer. Study of two large midwestern kindreds. Arch Intern Med. 1966;117:206–12.
118. Ionov Y, Punado MA, Malklosyan S, et al. Ubiquitous somatic mutations in simple repeated sequences reveal a new mechanism for colonic carcinogenesis. Nature. 1993;363:558–61.
119. Fishel R, Lesco MK, Roa MR, et al. The human mutator gene homolog MSH2 and its association with hereditary nonpolyposis colon cancer. Cell. 1993;75:1027–38.
120. Gyapuy G, Morissette J, Vignal A, et al. The 1993–94 genethon genetic linkage map. Nat Genet. 1994;7:246–339.
121. Charames GS, Bapat B. Genomic instability and cancer. Curr Mol Med. 2003;3:589–96.
122. Jacob S, Praz F. DNA mismatch repair defects: role in carcinogenesis. Biochimie. 2002;84:27–47.
123. Johnson R, Korovali G, Prakash L, et al. Requirement of the yeast MSH3 and MSH6 genes for MSH2 genomic stability. J Biol Chem. 1996;271:7285–8.
124. Liu B, Parsons R, Papadoupolos N, et al. Analysis of mismatch repair genes in hereditary nonpolyposis colorectal cancer patients. Nat Med. 1996;2:169–74.
125. Mitchell J, Farrington S, Dunlop M, et al. Mismatch repair genes in MLHI and in MSH2 and colorectal cancer: a HUGE review. Am J Epidemiol. 2002;156:885–902.

126. Mecklin JP, Sipponen P, Jarvinen HJ, et al. Histopathology of colorectal carcinomas in cancer family syndrome. Dis Colon Rectum. 1986;29:849–53.
127. Jass JR. Pathology of hereditary nonpolypsis colorectal cancer. Ann NY Acad Sci. 2000;910:62–73.
128. Guillem JG, Pueg-LaCalle Jr J, Cellini C, et al. Varying features of early age-onset colon cancer. Dis Colon Rectum. 1999;42:36–42.
129. Chung D, Rustgi A. The hereditary nonpolyposis colorectal cancer syndrome: genetics and clinical implications. Ann Intern Med. 2003;138:560–70.
130. Aarino M, Mecklin JP, Aaltonen LA, et al. Life-time risk of different cancers in HNPCC. Int J Cancer. 1995;64:430–3.
131. Fitzsimmons Jr RJ, Lynch HT, Stanislav GV, et al. Recognition and treatment of patients with hereditary nonpolyposis colon cancer (Lynch syndromes I and II). Ann Surg. 1987;206: 289–94.
132. DeJong A, Morreau H, Van Puijenbroek M, et al. The role of mismatch repair gene defects in the development of adenomas in patients with HNPCC. Gastroenterology. 2004; 126:42–8.
133. Jarvinen HJ, Mecklin JP, Sistonen P. Screening reduces colorectal cancer rate in families with hereditary nonpolyposes colon cancer. Gastroenterology. 1995;108:1405–11.
134. Winawer SJ, Zauber AG, Ho MN, et al. Prevention of colorectal cancer by colonoscopic polypectomy: The National Polyp Study Workgroup. N Engl J Med. 1993;329:1977–81.
135. Lanspa ST, Lynch HT, Smyrk TC, et al. Colorectal adenomas in the Lynch syndromes: results of a colonoscopy screening program. Gastroenterology. 1990;98(5 Pt. 1):1117–22.
136. Olschwang S, Slezak P, Roze M, et al. Somatically acquired genetic alterations in flat colorectal neoplasias. Int J Cancer. 1998;77:366–9.
137. Saitoh Y, Waxman I, West AB, et al. Prevalence and distinctive biologic features of flat colorectal adenomas in a North American population. Gastroenterology. 2001;120:1657–65.
138. Weber TK, Conlon W, Pitrelli NJ, et al. Genomic DNA-based h MSH2 and h MLH1 mutation screening in 35 eastern United States hereditary nonpolyposis colorectal cancer pedigrees. Cancer Res. 1997;57:3798–803.
139. Vasen HF, Winjen JT, Menko FH, et al. Cancer risk in families with hereditary nonpolyposis colorectal cancer diagnosed by mutation analysis. Gastroenterology. 1996;110:1020–7.
140. Kolodner RD, Tytell JD, Schmeits JL, et al. Germ-line MSH6 mutations in colorectal cancer families. Cancer Res. 1999;59:5068–74.
141. Karrola R, Raevaara TE, Lonnqvist KE, et al. Functional analysis of MSH6 mutations linked to kindreds with putative HNPCC. Hum Mol Genet. 2002;11:1303–10.
142. Berends MJW, Wu Y, Sijmons RH, et al. Molecular and clinical characteristics of MSH6 of 25 index cases. Am J Hum Genet. 2002;70:26–37.
143. Wagner A, Hendricks Y, Meijers-Heyboer EJ, et al. MSH6 germline mutations; analysis of a large Dutch pedigree. J Med Genet. 2001;58:318–22.
144. Schwartz RA, Torre DP. The Muir–Torre syndrome: 25 year retrospective. J Am Acad Dermatol. 1995;33:90–104.
145. Kruse R, Lamerti C, Wang Y, et al. Is the mismatch repair deficient type of Muir–Torre syndrome confined to mutations in the MSH2 gene? Hum Genet. 1996;98:747–50.
146. Hampel H, Frankel WL, Martin E, Arnold M, Khanduja K, Kuebler P, et al. Screening for the Lynch syndrome (hereditary nonpolyposis colorectal cancer). N Engl J Med. 2005; 352:1851–60.
147. Rodriguez-Bigas M, Boland CR, Hamilton SR, et al. A National Cancer Institute Workshop on HNPCC: meeting highlights and Bethesda guidelines. J Natl Cancer Inst. 1997; 89:1758–62.
148. Syngal S, Fox EA, Eng C, et al. Sensitivity and specificity of clinical criteria for HNPCC associated mutations in MSH2 and MSL1. J Med Genet. 2000;37:641–5.
149. Jenkins MA, Hayashi S, O'Shea AM, Burgart LJ, Smyrk TC, Shimizu D, et al. Pathology features in Bethesda guidelines predict colorectal cancer microsatellite instability: a population-based study. Gastroenterology. 2007;133:48–56.
150. Chen S, Wang W, Lee S, Nafa K, Lee J, Romans K, et al. Prediction of germline mutations and cancer risk in the Lynch syndrome. JAMA. 2006;296:1479–87.
151. Barnetson RA, Tenesa A, Farrington SM, Nicholl ID, Cetnarskyj R, Porteous ME, et al. Identification and survival of carriers of mutations in DNA mismatch-repair genes in colon cancer. N Engl J Med. 2006;354:2751–63.
152. Peltomaki P, Vasen HF. Mutations predisposing to hereditary nonpolyposis colorectal cancer: database and results of a collaborative study. International Collaborative Group on HNPCC. Gastroenterology. 1997;113:1146–58.
153. Casey G, Lindor NM, Papadopoulos N, Thibodeau SN, Moskow J, Steelman S. Conversion analysis for mutation detection in MLH1 and MSH2 in patients with colorectal cancer. JAMA. 2005;293(7):799–809.
154. Vasen HF, Nagengast FM, Khan PM. Interval cancers in hereditary nonpolyposis colorectal cancer. Lancet. 1995;345:1183–4.
155. Jārvinen HJ, Aarnio M, Mustonen H, et al. Controlled 15-year trial on screening for colorectal cancer in families with hereditary nonpolyposis colorectal cancer. Gastroenterology. 2000;118:829–34.
156. Church J. Hereditary colon cancers can be tiny: a cautionary case report of the results of colonoscopic surveillance. Am J Gastroenterol. 1998;93(11):2289–90.
157. Brown GJ, St. John DJ, Macrae FA, et al. Cancer risk in young women at risk of hereditary nonpolyposis colorectal cancer: implications for gynecologic surveillance. Gynecol Oncol. 2001;80:346–9.
158. Lynch P. If aggressive surveillance in hereditary nonpolyposis colorectal cancer is now state of the art, are there any challenges left? Gastroenterology. 2000;118:969–71.
159. Dove-Edwin I, Boks D, Goff S, et al. The outcome of endometrial carcinoma surveillance by ultrasound scans in women at risk of hereditary nonpolyposis colorectal carcinoma and familial colorectal carcinoma. Cancer. 2002;94:1708–12.
160. Natarajan N, Watson P, Silva-Lopez E, Lynch HT. Comparison of extended colectomy and limited resection in patients with Lynch syndrome. Dis Colon Rectum. 2010;53:77–82.
161. Church J. Prevention of metachronous colorectal cancer in patients with Lynch syndrome. Dis Colon Rectum. 2010;53(1):1–2.
162. Rodriguez-Bigas MA, Vasen HF, Pekka-Mecklin J, et al. Rectal cancer risk in hereditary nonpolyposis colorectal cancer after abdominal colectomy. International Collaborative Group on HNPCC. Ann Surg. 1997;225:202–7.

163. Syngal S, Weeks JC, Schrag D, et al. Benefits of colonoscopic surveillance and prophylactic colectomy in patients with hereditary nonpolyposis colorectal cancer. Ann Intern Med. 1998;129:787–96.
164. Vasen HF, Buskens E, et al. A cost-effectiveness analysis of colorectal screening of hereditary nonpolyposis colorectal carcinoma gene carriers. Cancer. 1998;82:1632–7.
165. Watson P, Lin K, Rodriguez-Bigas MA, et al. Colorectal carcinoma survival among hereditary non-polyposis colorectal cancer family members. Cancer. 1998;83:259–66.
166. Sankila R, Aaltonen LA, Jarvinen HA, et al. Better survival rates in patients with MLH1 associated hereditary nonpolyposis colorectal cancer. Gastroenterology. 1996;110: 682–7.
167. Ribic CM, Sargent DJ, Moore MJ, et al. Tumor microsatellite-instabilitystatus as a predictor of benefit from fluorouracil-based adjuvant chemotherapyfor colon cancer. N Engl J Med. 2003;349:247–57.
168. Elsaleh H, Joseph D, Grieu F, et al. Association of tumour site and sex with survival benefit from adjuvant chemotherapy in colorectal cancer. Lancet. 2000;355:1745–50.
169. Giovannucci E, Rimm EB, Meir J, et al. Aspirin use and the risk for colorectal cancer and adenoma in male health professionals. Ann Intern Med. 1994;121:241–6.
170. Thun MJ, Namboodiri MM, Calle EE, et al. Aspirin use and risk of fatal cancer. Cancer Res. 1993;53:1322–7.
171. Burn J, Bishop DT, Mecklin JP, Macrae F, Möslein G, et al. Effect of aspirin or resistant starch on colorectal neoplasia in the Lynch syndrome. N Engl J Med. 2008;359(24):2567–78.
172. Garland C, Shekelle RB, Barret-Connor E, et al. Dietary vitamin D and calcium and risk of colorectal cancer. A 19-year prospective study in men. Lancet. 1985;1:307–9.
173. Cats A, Kleibeuker JH, Van der Meer R, et al. Randomized, double-blinded, placebo-controlled intervention study with supplemental calcium in families with hereditary nonpolyposis colorectal cancer. J Natl Cancer Inst. 1995;87:598–603.

38 Colorectal Cancer: Epidemiology, Etiology, and Molecular Basis

Harvey G. Moore, Nancy N. Baxter, and Jose G. Guillem

Epidemiology

Colorectal cancer (CRC) is a disease with a major worldwide burden. It is the fourth most frequently diagnosed malignancy in men and third most common in women, with almost one million people developing CRC annually.[1] In the world, CRC is the third most common cause of cancer death, responsible for 639,000 deaths annually.[2] In the USA, CRC is the third most common cancer in men and women and the second most common cause of cancer death overall, accounting for 11% of cancers diagnosed.[3] It was estimated that 147,000 cases were diagnosed in the USA in 2009 and that there were 50,000 deaths from the disease.[3]

The worldwide incidence of CRC is increasing; in 1975, the worldwide incidence of CRC was only 500,000.[4] In western countries, some of the increase is due to the aging of the population; however, in countries with a low baseline rate of CRC, the incidence is increasing even after age-adjustment. Prior to 1985, the age-adjusted incidence of CRC in the USA also increased; however, since this time the rates have declined an average of −1.6% per year. In the time period 1998–2005, the rate of decline accelerated; −2.8% per year in men and −2.3% per year in women (Figure 38-1).[3] This reduction has been mainly confined to those of white race and is largely limited to a decrease in the incidence of distal cancers. Although the cause of the decrease in incidence is unknown, and may have been influenced by many factors, it is likely that much may be attributable to screening by sigmoidoscopy and colonoscopy.[5] In contrast, the incidence of proximal cancers has remained relatively stable over the same time period.[5] Currently, the overall probability of an individual developing CRC in the USA over a lifetime is 5.5% in men and 5.1% in women.[6]

From a population perspective, age is the most important risk factor for CRC. CRC is predominantly a disease of older individuals; 90% of cases are diagnosed over the age of 50.[6] The risk of CRC continues to increase with age (Figure 38-2). The incidence per 100,000 people age 80–84 is over seven times the incidence in people age 50–54. However, CRC can occur at any age and the incidence of CRC occurring before age 40 may be increasing.[7]

In the USA, the risk of CRC differs by sex. The age-adjusted incidence of CRC is over 40% higher in men than women. Overall, the incidence of CRC in men is 61 per 100,000 males as compared to 45 per 100,000 females.[6] In addition, the ratio of colon to rectal cancer differs by sex; the ratio of colon to rectal cases for women is 3:1 as compared to 2:1 for males.[6]

Race and ethnicity influence CRC risk. Ashkenazi Jewish individuals appear to be at a slightly increased risk of CRC. At least part of this increased incidence may be due to a higher prevalence of the *I1307K* mutation of the adenomatous polyposis gene (*APC*), a mutation that confers an increased risk of CRC development (18–30% lifetime risk). The *I1307K* mutation is found in 6.1% of unselected Ashkenazi Jewish individuals and 28% of Jewish individuals with CRC[8], while the mutation is rare in other populations. In the USA, the incidence of CRC is higher in African Americans of either sex as compared to white Americans. Asian American/Pacific Islanders, Native Americans, and Hispanic Americans experience a lower incidence of CRC than Caucasians (Table 38-1).[3,6] African Americans have not experienced the substantial reduction in incidence of CRC found to have occurred in whites; prior to 1980 incidence in African Americans was actually lower than in white Americans. In African Americans, the increased rate of cancer is predominantly due to a higher rate of proximal cancers.[9,10]

According to the American Cancer Society, between 1996 and 2004 for all patients diagnosed with CRC, 40% of patients were diagnosed with localized disease, 36% with regional disease and 19% with metastatic disease. Five percent of patients were unstaged. As a proportion of total cases, African Americans were more likely to present with advanced disease; 24% of African Americans have metastatic disease at presentation (Table 38-2).[3] Rates of metastatic disease have fallen overtime, most notably for CRC of the distal colon and rectum in whites.[10]

D.E. Beck et al. (eds.), *The ASCRS Textbook of Colon and Rectal Surgery: Second Edition*,
DOI 10.1007/978-1-4419-1584-9_38, © Springer Science+Business Media, LLC 2011

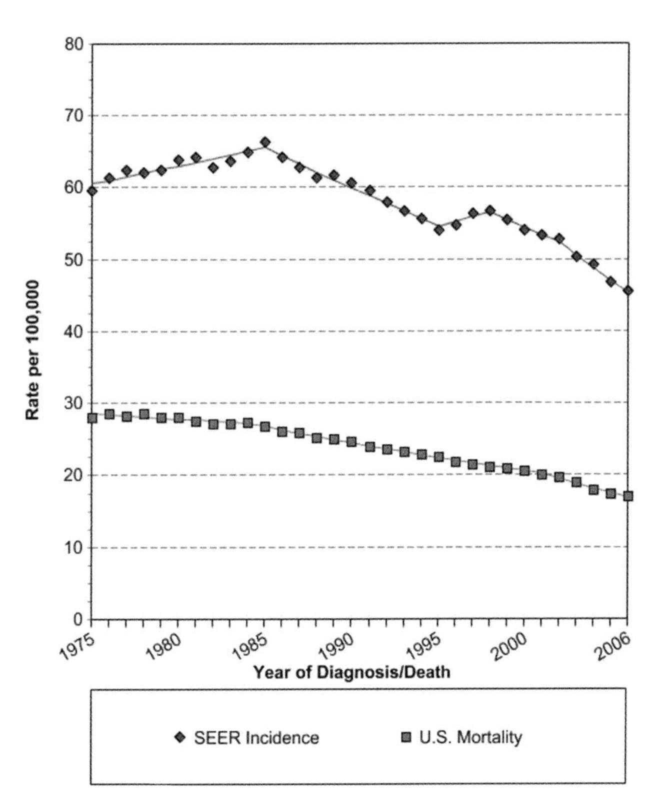

FIGURE 38-1. Age-adjusted colorectal cancer incidence and death rates in the United States 1975–2006.

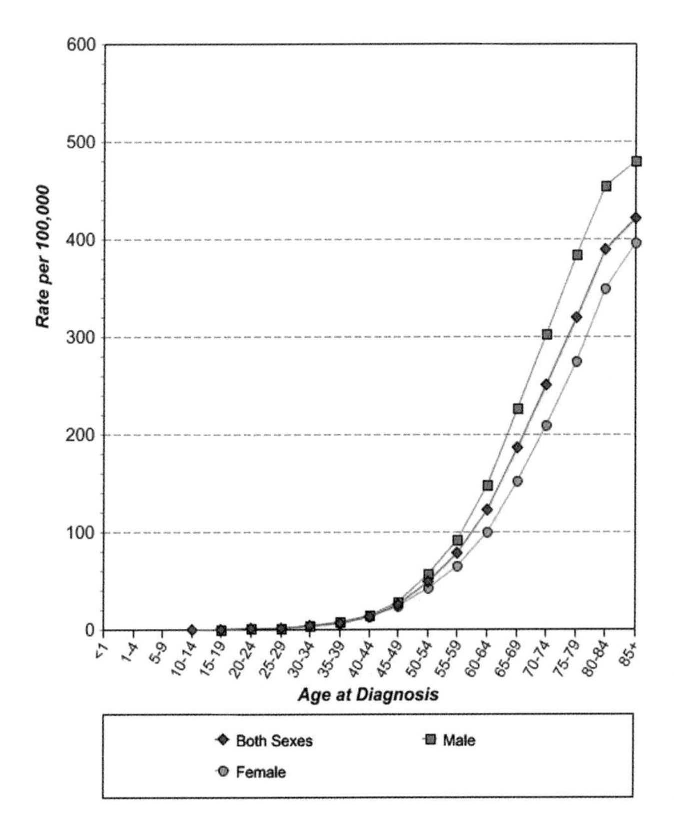

FIGURE 38-2. Age-specific SEER incidence rates in the United States 1992–2006.

There is substantial geographic variation in the incidence of CRC, with relatively high rates in North America, Western Europe, and Australia and relatively low rates in Africa and Asia (Figure 38-3).[11] Such observations led to Burkitt's hypothesis; that dietary differences, specifically fiber and fat intake, between populations were responsible for the marked variation in rates of CRC found around the world.[12] Burkitt observed that populations in low-risk areas of the third world had greater stool bulk, a faster colonic transit time, and higher dietary fiber intake than populations in high-risk, westernized regions. Although such ecological studies are confounded by numerous factors (for example, variations in average life expectancy, cancer detection methods, etc.), environmental factors (most prominently dietary factors) are still considered to have a major role in this disease. This is supported by studies of migrants from low prevalence areas to high prevalence areas. Such studies generally demonstrate that the incidence of CRC in the migrants increases rapidly to become similar and in some cases to exceed the incidence of the high-risk area.[13] Interestingly, there is less variation in the incidence of rectal cancer between countries as compared to the incidence of colon cancer.[14]

Mortality from CRC is declining in the USA (Figure 38-1). Age-adjusted CRC death rates peaked in the 1940s at 35 per 100,000. In women, rates steadily declined since this time, and between 2001 and 2005 the CRC death rate in white and African American women was 15.3 and 22.4 per 100,000, respectively. In men, death rates changed little until the 1980s and 1990s, then declined significantly; between 2001 and 2005 the CRC death rate in white and African American men was 22.1 and 31.8 per 100,000, respectively (Table 38-1).[3] Improvements in surgical and medical treatments likely explain some of the change, particularly improvements before 1985. More recently, the reduced mortality rate is likely secondary to the reduced incidence of CRC. However, for those who develop CRC, no improvement in case-fatality has been identified since 1986[15] indicating that the trends in mortality are likely complex. African Americans suffer the highest mortality rate from CRC in the USA (Table 38-1).[3] The reasons for the higher mortality rate are likely multifactorial, including the higher incidence of CRC, and the differences in stage distribution. However, African Americans had worse 5-year survival for all stages of disease, and the difference in 5-year survival rates between white and African Americans has actually increased over time, from an absolute difference of 5% in the 1970s (51% vs. 46%) to an absolute difference of 13% in 1990s (63% vs. 53%).[16] Between 1996 and 2004, 5-year survival for colon cancer in Caucasians and African Americans was 66% and 55%, respectively; for rectal cancer 67% and 59%, respectively.[3] Differences in incidence, stage distribution and survival of CRC between white and African Americans are in part due to differences in socioeconomic status, screening rates and treatment;[17] however, the differences may also be due to genetic and environmental factors that have yet to be elucidated.

TABLE 38-1. Incidence and mortality rates* for CRC by site, race and ethnicity, US 2001–2005

		White	African American	Asian American and Pacific Islander	American Indian/ Alaska Native	Hispanic/Latino
Incidence	Male	58.9	71.2	48.0	46.0	47.3
	Female	43.2	54.5	35.4	41.2	32.8
Mortality	Male	22.1	31.8	14.4	20.5	16.5
	Female	15.3	22.4	10.2	14.2	10.8

*per 100,000 age-adjusted to the 2000 US standard population

Adapted from Jemal A, Siegal R, Ward E, Hao Y, Xu J, Ward E, and Thun MJ; American Cancer Society. Cancer statistics, 2009. CA Cancer J Clin. 2009;59:225–249. Table 11. Incidence and mortality rates for by site, race and ethnicity, United States, 2001–2005. Pg 242.

TABLE 38-2. Stage at diagnosis (United States 1996–2004)

	Whites	African Americans
Localized	40	35
Regional	36	34
Distant	19	24
Unstaged	5	7

Numbers are percentages

Adapted from Jemal A, Siegal R, Ward E, Hao Y, Xu J, Ward E, and Thun MJ; American Cancer Society. Cancer statistics, 2009. CA Cancer J Clin. 2009;59:225–249. Figure 9. Incidence and mortality rates for by site, race and ethnicity, United States, 2001–2005. Pg 246.

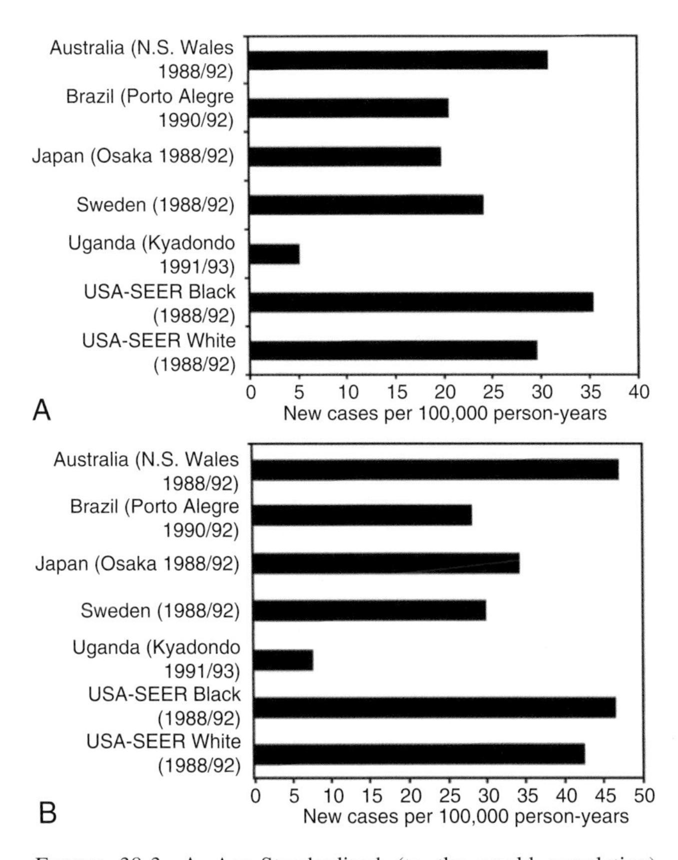

FIGURE 38-3. **A** Age-Standardized (to the world population) incidence rates of cancer of the large bowel among females, **B** Age-standardized (to the world population) incidence rates of cancer of the large bowel among males.

Because CRC is a survivable cancer, with a 5-year survival rates adjusted for life expectancy of 64%,[6] the prevalence of people living with a diagnosis of CRC in the population is substantial. In total, over one million Americans alive in 2006 have had a diagnosis of CRC.[18]

Etiology

Dietary Constituents and Supplements

The colon is constantly exposed to the substances we ingest and the by-products of ingestion. Thus, the role of diet in the pathogenesis of CRC has long been speculated. However, the relationship between diet and CRC risk is at best unclear. Studies in this area are difficult to conduct, as exposures tend to be multifactorial and change, with our diet, over time. In addition, because colorectal carcinogenesis is a multistep process, a number or combination of exposures may be necessary, and genetic susceptibility is likely to play a role. In addition, in most cases randomized trials are not feasible, and therefore studies must be observational in nature. When intervention studies are possible, follow-up is relatively short term (compared to the long-term exposure that may be necessary for cancer development), and single dietary components are generally selected for evaluation although the influence of diet may depend on complex interactions between dietary constituents. In addition, to reduce sample size some studies are conducted on patients with a previous history of adenomatous polyps. Some interventions in these patients may not be effective, as such patients may have already acquired numerous genetic alterations in normal appearing colonic mucosa. Some interventions may need to be instituted prior to the development of polyps. Although it can be stated that an individual with no other risk factors for CRC who ingests a diet that is high in fiber, fruits, vegetables, and low in animal fat and red meat is on average at lower risk of CRC than an individual who eats a diet low in fiber, fruits, and vegetables and high in animal fat and red meat, it is difficult to determine with certainty which dietary components or combinations are responsible for the decreased risk.

Dietary Fat

Dietary fat, particularly saturated animal fat, has been implicated in carcinogenesis of the colon and rectum. Early research using animal models demonstrated a carcinogenic effect of dietary fat on colonic mucosa,[19,20] and epidemiologic studies found parallels between CRC rates and dietary fat consumption. Countries with populations eating a high fat diet had higher CRC rates than countries with populations eating a lower fat diet.[21] However, dietary fat consumption is related to a number of other factors that may influence cancer risk, including other dietary factors such as dietary fiber and micronutrient consumption, as well as life-style factors, such as exercise and alcohol consumption. Therefore, ecological comparisons between countries are subject to a substantial risk of confounding.[22]

Over 13 case-control studies have been conducted to evaluate the relationship between dietary fat intake and the risk of CRC. These have been quantitatively summarized by Howe et al.[23] and include 5,287 cases with CRC and 10,470 controls. Although positive associations were identified for total energy intake and CRC in almost all of the studies, there was no energy-independent relationship between dietary fat intake and CRC risk. After controlling for total energy intake, the odds of development of CRC in subjects with the highest dietary fat intake as compared to those with the lowest intake was 0.90 (95% CI, 0.72–1.13). Overall, there was no evidence for any association of total dietary fat intake and development of CRC.

In addition, at least six cohort studies have been conducted to evaluate the relationship between dietary fat and CRC.[24–27] Only one of these studies[25] identified an association between dietary animal fat and development of CRC, with a twofold increase of CRC in the highest consumers of animal fat compared to the lowest consumers. In a randomized, controlled clinical trial, 48,835 women were randomized to either dietary modification (aimed at reducing dietary fat and increasing consumption of fruits, vegetables, and grains) or to the control group (no dietary modification). At a mean follow-up of 8.1 years, there was no difference in the incidence of CRC between those in the dietary modification group and controls (RR = 1.08; 95% CI, 0.91–1.29). Of note, the amount of reduction of dietary fat achieved by patients in the dietary modification group was only 70% of the target reduction described in the original study design, and it is possible that better compliance might have resulted in a positive finding.[28] However, taken together, the preponderance of evidence does not support an increased risk of CRC with increasing consumption of dietary fat.

Red Meat

There are a number of potential carcinogenic mechanisms unrelated to fat content that may result in a causal relationship between red meat ingestion and CRC. Red meat is high in iron, a prooxidant. Dietary iron may increase free radical production in the colon, and these free radicals may cause chronic mucosal damage or promote other carcinogens. In humans, red meat ingestion stimulates the production of N-nitroso compounds in a dose-response fashion.[29] As many N-nitroso compounds are known carcinogens, this is a potential mechanism for an association between red meat and CRC. Formation of heterocyclic amines and polycyclic aromatic hydrocarbons in meat by cooking over an open flame or cooking until well done may be an important factor as these compounds are carcinogenic in animal models.[30] Alternatively, dietary heme, present in red meat, may have a cytotoxic effect on colonic surface epithelium, resulting in rebound inhibition of apoptosis and crypt hyperplasia.[31]

A large number of epidemiologic studies have been conducted to determine the effect of ingestion of red meat on CRC risk. Three meta-analyses have been published,[32–34] one combining the results of 13 cohort studies,[33] the second combining 21 case-control studies and six cohort studies,[34], and the third involving 17 prospective cohort studies and two case-control studies.[32] In the three meta-analyses, the pooled estimate for the increase in the risk of CRC due to red meat consumption was similar; odds of development of CRC in the highest meat consuming groups as compared to the lowest was 1.14–1.28. A daily increase of 100 g of red meat (3.5 oz) was associated with a 12–17% increased risk of CRC (RR = 1.24–1.28). The risk was substantially higher with the ingestion of processed meat in two studies (49–54%),[33,34] but was slightly less for red meat in the most recent analysis.[32] Of note, individuals that consume diets high in red meat generally consume diets low in other dietary factors, such as antioxidants that may themselves be important in colorectal carcinogenesis. It is therefore difficult to rule out the possibility that the apparent effect of red meat on the development of CRC may be confounded or modified by other dietary or lifestyle factors. Genetics may also play a role. In the Fukuoka Colorectal Cancer Study, colon cancer risk was increased in relation to red meat intake only in individuals with a specific polymorphism of Cytochrome P450 2E1 (CYP2E1).[35]

Fruit and Vegetable Intake

The effect of dietary intake of fruit and vegetables on CRC risk has been evaluated extensively. Fruits and vegetables are a source of antioxidants, including carotenoids and ascorbate. Other bioactive constituents in fruits and vegetables that may protect against carcinogenesis include the indoles and isothiocyanates. Previous research, including results from 22 case-control studies and four prospective cohort studies, has provided substantial support for the hypothesis that vegetable intake reduces the risk of CRC, while intake of fruit did not seem to have an effect.[36] Other studies, however, did not demonstrate a convincing link between vegetable or fruit intake and a reduced risk of CRC. In four large prospective cohort studies (the Nurse's Health Study of 121,700 women, the Health Professionals Follow-up Study of 51,529 men, the Netherlands Cohort Study on Diet and Cancer including 120,852 men and women, and the Cancer Prevention Study II Nutrition Cohort, including 133,163 men and women),[37–39] fruit and vegetable intake was not statistically significantly associated with a reduced risk of CRC.

More recent studies have reported conflicting results. A pooled analysis of 14 cohort studies, including 756,217 men and women followed between 6 and 20 years also did not find a significantly reduced risk of CRC in the highest consumers of total fruits and vegetables, total vegetables, or total fruits. However, when examined by colon site, high total fruit and vegetable intake was inversely correlated with the risk of CRC of the distal colon (RR=0.74; 95% CI, 0.57–0.95) but not for the proximal colon.[40] Finally, the recently reported European Prospective Investigation into Cancer and Nutrition (EPIC) study, involving a cohort of 452,755 men and women followed an average of 8.8 years, reported a significant inverse relationship between total fruit and vegetable consumption and the risk of colon cancer (RR=0.76; 95% CI, 0.63–0.91).[41]

The influence of fruit and vegetable consumption on the development of colorectal adenomas has also been investigated. The Polyp Prevention Trial randomized 2,079 people with a history of colorectal adenomas to either intensive dietary counseling with assignment to a diet low in fat and high in fruits, vegetables, and fiber, or to a control group (no dietary change).[42] No difference in adenoma recurrence rate was found in the intervention group as compared to the control group. However, follow-up of 34,467 women participating in the Nurses' Health Study found an inverse relationship for total consumption of fruit, but not vegetables, on the risk of colorectal adenomas. Women who consumed five or more servings of fruit daily had a relative risk of 0.60 (95% CI, 0.44–0.81) for developing adenomas in the distal colon or rectum (<60 cm from the anal verge) compared to women who consumed one or fewer servings.[43] A nested case-control study compared 3,057 men and women with at least one adenoma detected during participation in the Prostate, Lung, Colorectal, and Ovarian (PLCO) Cancer Screening trial to 29,413 control subjects. Similar to the Nurses' Health Study, total fruit consumption was associated with a significantly reduced risk of distal adenoma (odds ratio (OR)=0.75; 95% CI, 0.66–0.86), whereas total vegetable consumption was not. However, high intake of certain vegetable groups, specifically deep-yellow vegetables, onions, and garlic was associated with a lower risk of adenoma development.[44]

Overall, the evidence for an association between fruit and vegetable intake and the risk of CRC is inconsistent. Given this, it is unlikely that a large number of cases of CRC can be attributed directly to a lack of intake of fruits or vegetables, or that major additional interventions to increase consumption would lead to a substantial reduction in the incidence of CRC.

Fiber

Dietary fiber was one of the first dietary components thought to have a protective role in carcinogenesis. An association of a high fiber diet with a decreased risk of CRC was first theorized in 1969 by Burkitt;[12] however, the data regarding the association between fiber and CRC risk are conflicting. A number of mechanisms have been proposed for the protective effects of fiber; fiber may increase intestinal transit and therefore reduce the length of exposure of the colon to carcinogens, or fiber may dilute or absorb various potential carcinogens, particularly bile salts. In addition, products of fiber degradation and fermentation in the colon (such as butyrate) may also play a role.[45] Surprisingly, two large American cohort studies, the Nurses' Health study[46] and the Health Professionals' Follow-up Study[24] found no evidence of benefit of fiber on CRC risk.

However, more recent studies have reopened the debate. In the PLCO Cancer Screening Trial,[47] a nested case control study of over 37,508 people undergoing flexible sigmoidoscopy was performed using food frequency questionnaires. People who reported the highest amounts of fiber in their diets had the lowest risk of colorectal adenomas; 27% risk reduction compared to people who ate the least amount of fiber. The strongest association was found for fiber from grains, cereals, and fruits but not for fiber from legumes and vegetables. When colonic and rectal adenomas were evaluated separately, the effect of fiber was seen only in colonic adenoma. In a second prospective cohort study, comparing the diet of over 500,000 people in 10 European countries, investigators[48,49] found that people who consumed the most fiber had a 25% lower incidence of CRC than those who consumed the least fiber. Again, the protective effect was greater for the colon than for the rectum. These discordant results prompted a meta-analysis in which the data from 13 prospective cohort studies were reanalyzed. Although dietary fiber intake was inversely associated with the risk of CRC in age-adjusted analyses, this association did not hold when adjusted for other dietary risk factors.[50] More recent cohort studies have produced conflicting results.[51,52]

Dietary interventions to increase fiber intake have proven unsuccessful in reducing the risk of colorectal neoplasia. A meta-analysis has evaluated the effect of five intervention trials.[53] These studies randomized a total of 4,349 individuals to some form of fiber supplementation or high fiber dietary intervention. When the data were combined, there was no difference between the intervention and control groups for the number of subjects developing at least one adenoma (RR=1.04; 95% CI, 0.95–1.13). The authors concluded that there is currently no evidence from randomized studies to suggest that increased dietary fiber intake reduces the incidence or recurrence of adenomatous polyps within a 2–4-year period. However, recently data from the US Polyp Prevention trial revealed that although there was no protective effect of fiber in those assigned to fiber therapy, in the subgroup of those most adherent to dietary changes (high-fiber, high-fruit and -vegetables, low-fat), defined as "super compliers," there was a 35% reduced incidence of recurrent adenomas (RR = 0.65; 95% CI, 0.47–0.92).[54]

Currently, there is no single accepted definition of fiber. Many different types of fiber exist (soluble/non-soluble; polysaccharides/non-polysaccharides) and these differences may influence CRC risk. Several studies suggest that fiber from whole grains may be protective against CRC.[51,55] In addition, fiber intake itself may not be protective but may be correlated with other healthy lifestyle choices as well as other components of a healthy diet (for example, high vegetable, low fat, and low meat). The lack of effect found in randomized trials as compared to observational studies indicates this may be the case. However, the intervention trials may have been too short in duration to demonstrate an effect.

Calcium and Vitamin D

Substantial epidemiologic and experimental evidence exists to support the beneficial effect of calcium for the prevention of colorectal neoplasia. Calcium has the capacity to bind and precipitate bile acids and may directly influence mucosal cell proliferation. Most, although not all, of the observational studies evaluating the influence of dietary calcium have demonstrated a protective effect of calcium on the risk of CRC. Two randomized, double-blind, placebo-controlled intervention trials of calcium for the prevention of adenoma recurrence that included a total of 1,346 subjects[56,57] have demonstrated that the use of calcium supplementation (1,200 mg daily for a mean duration of 4 years or 2,000 mg daily for a mean duration of 3 years) was associated with a reduction in the recurrence of colorectal adenoma, although only one study[56] achieved statistical significance. In a meta-analysis of the two studies, the relative risk of developing recurrent adenomas was 0.74 for patients randomized to receive calcium as compared to placebo.[58]

The effect of calcium on a non-high-risk cohort is less clear. A meta-analysis of available studies conducted in 1996[59] concluded that the evidence to support the benefit of calcium intake on reduction of colorectal neoplasia was not consistent with a substantial effect. A more recent pooled analysis of ten cohort studies, including 534,536 individuals[60] published in 2004 evaluating the influence of dairy foods and calcium on CRC demonstrated a consistently decreased risk of CRC for those with the highest intake of dietary calcium as compared to those with the lowest intake (RR = 0.86; 95% CI, 0.78–0.95). Several subsequent large cohort studies have reported an inverse relationship between calcium intake and CRC incidence, with relative risks between 0.68 and 0.84 in men and 0.64 and 0.70 in women.[61–64] However, a randomized, placebo-controlled trial of calcium plus vitamin D supplementation involving 36,282 postmenopausal women produced conflicting results. Women randomized to 1,000 mg daily of elemental calcium plus 400 IU vitamin D for an average of 7 years had a relative risk of CRC of 1.08 (95% CI, 0.86–1.34) compared to women who received placebo.[65] This trial has been criticized for having an insufficient follow-up period, too small a dose of daily calcium, and many potential nutritional confounders.[66]

Vitamin D alone may also have a chemopreventive effect via modulation of calcium absorption and gene expression.[67] Observational data provided the first suggestion of a link between vitamin D concentrations and CRC risk.[68] Preclinical investigation revealed several possible mechanisms by which Vitamin D exerts a chemopreventive effect on CRC, including inhibition of β-catenin[69] or other antiproliferative effects.[70,71] A large epidemiological study found a 29% reduction in CRC risk in individuals with the highest Vitamin D intake.[39] In a case control study nested within the Multiethnic Cohort Study, plasma 25 (OH) D levels were measured using a chemiluminescence assay in 229 patients with CRC and 434 matched controls. An inverse trend was observed between Vitamin D level and the risk of CRC (OR, per doubling of 25(OH)D = 0.68; 95% CI, 0.51–0.92).[72] A recent meta-analysis investigated the relationship between circulating 25(OH)D levels and Vitamin D intake on the incidence of colorectal adenomas. Circulating 25(OH)D was inversely correlated with the incidence of adenomas (OR = 0.70; 95% CI, 0.56–0.87) for the high versus low circulating 25(OH) D groups. A similar finding was noted for high versus low Vitamin D intake (OR = 0.89; 95% CI, 0.78–1.02).[73] However, two recent meta-analyses addressing the relationship between Vitamin D and CRC incidence have produced conflicting results.[74,75] In a meta-analysis of eight longitudinal studies addressing the relationship between serum 25(OH) D levels and CRC incidence, in patients with an increase of 25(OH)D by 20 ng/ml the OR for CRC incidence was 0.57 (95% CI, 0.43–0.76).[74] However, a meta-analysis of ten cohort studies involving 2,813 cancer cases reported that Vitamin D intake was associated with only a nonsignificant 6% reduction on CRC risk (RR = 0.94; 95% CI, 0.83–1.06).[75]

Folate

Folate, a B vitamin, is important for normal DNA methylation. Methylation is important in the regulation of cellular gene expression. Folate deficiency may lead to cancer through disruption of DNA synthesis and repair, or loss of control of proto-oncogene activity.[76] In 15 retrospective epidemiologic studies evaluating the association between folate and CRC risk, most demonstrate a statistically significant or trend toward a significant relationship between higher intake of folate and a reduced risk of CRC or adenoma formation. In an unpublished meta-analysis of 11 prior prospective studies, a 20% reduction in the risk of CRC was found in those with the highest folate ingestion as compared to those with the lowest level of ingestion.[77]

However, recently results of two randomized, double-blind, placebo-controlled intervention trials have been published that do not support a protective effect of folate supplementation.[78,79] In the first study, patients with a prior history of colorectal adenomas randomized to 1 mg of folic acid daily had a 44.1% incidence of at least one adenoma during follow-up, versus 42.4% in the placebo group. Patients on folate had a trend toward a higher incidence of advanced adenoma (11.4% vs. 8.6%, RR = 1.32; 95% CI, 0.90–1.32), as well as a higher incidence of ≥3 adenomas (9.9% vs. 4.3%, RR = 2.32; 95% CI, 1.23–4.35).[79] In the second study, 0.5 mg/day of folate was found to have no effect on adenoma recurrence (RR = 1.07; 95% CI, 0.43–0.91). No increase in advanced adenoma for folate users was observed in that study.[78] Taken together, these studies demonstrate that folate supplementation is unlikely to be of benefit as secondary prevention in patients with a history of colorectal adenomas, and may actually be detrimental. One hypothesis to explain these results is that folate plays a "dual-modulator" role. There may be a protective influence of moderate dietary increases initiated before the establishment of neoplastic foci, but a promoter effect on preestablished, clinically occult neoplastic foci. Early prevention is likely due to the protection against DNA damage by maintaining adequate methyl groups for DNA methylation and nucleotide synthesis. A possible mechanism underlying enhanced tumor growth is an increased provision of nucleotide precursors to rapidly replicating neoplastic cells.[80,81]

Consistent with this data, one recent observation suggests folate supplementation may actually increase the risk of CRC. Since 1996 and 1997, the US Food and Drug Administration (FDA) has required folate fortification of all flour and cereal grain products in the USA and Canada, respectively,[82] in an effort to reduce the incidence of neural tube defects. Concurrent with this mandate, a downward trend in CRC incidence seen in the USA and Canada during the early 1990s began to reverse with marked increases seen between 1997 and 1998.[83] While this observation clearly does not establish a causal relationship, it is a provocative finding and underscores the fact that the relationship between folate and CRC deserves further study.

Alcohol

Alcohol ingestion has a possible role in colorectal carcinogenesis. Alcohol may alter folate absorption, increasing CRC through the reduction of folate bioavailability. Acetaldehyde, a product of alcohol metabolism may have a role, and alcohol may also contribute to abnormal DNA methylation directly. A meta-analysis of five follow-up studies and 22 case-control studies published in 1990[84] demonstrated only a weak association between alcohol and CRC, although the effect was stronger when only rectal cancer was considered. Two more recent meta-analyses of 16[85] and 5 cohort studies[86] demonstrate a strong association between alcohol consumption and development of CRC. In the first, high alcohol intake was significantly associated with an increased risk of colon (RR = 1.50; 95% CI, 1.25–1.79) and rectal cancer (RR = 1.63; 95% CI, 1.35–1.97), corresponding to a 15% increase of colon or rectal cancer for an increase of 100 g of alcohol intake per week.[85] In the second, increasing consumption of alcohol was significantly correlated with an increased risk of CRC in men and women (RR = 2.96; 95% CI, 2.27–3.86 for consumption ≥92 g/day in men).[86] The EPIC trial, a prospective cohort trial involving 478,732 subjects, looked at both baseline and lifetime intake of alcohol as risk factors. Lifetime alcohol intake was significantly correlated with increased CRC risk (RR = 1.08; 95% CI, 1.04–1.12 for 15 g/day increase). Similar results were obtained when only baseline alcohol consumption was considered.[87]

The findings of an association with alcohol intake are consistent, and there are no studies that demonstrate a protective effect of higher alcohol consumption. Thus, the totality of the evidence indicates that a high level of alcohol intake (two or more drinks per day) is associated with an increased risk of CRC.

Of note, higher intake of a Western-style diet (high intake of meat, fat, refined grains, and dessert) versus a prudent diet (high intake of fruits and vegetables, poultry, and fish) has been associated with an increased risk of recurrence and mortality in patients with Stage III colon cancer treated with surgery and adjuvant chemotherapy.[88] In a prospective cohort study involving 1,009 Stage III CRC patients enrolled in a randomized adjuvant chemotherapy trial, food frequency questionnaires were administered during and for 6 months after adjuvant chemotherapy. At a median follow-up of 5.3 years, patients in the highest quintile of Western dietary intake had a significantly worse disease-free (adjusted hazard ratio (AHR) 3.25; 95% CI, 2.04–5.19) and overall survival (AHR 2.32; 95% CI, 1.36–3.96) compared to those in the lowest quintile of Western dietary pattern.

Aspirin and Nonsteroidal Anti-inflammatory Drugs

There is considerable observational evidence that the use of aspirin or other nonsteroidal anti-inflammatory drugs (NSAIDs) has protective effects at all stages of colorectal carcinogenesis (aberrant crypt foci, adenoma, carcinoma, and death from CRC).[67] The mechanism of antineoplastic action of NSAIDs is incompletely understood, but it is believed that both cyclooxygenase (COX)-dependent and COX-independent pathways may be involved.

At least 30 observational studies have been conducted to evaluate the influence of NSAID (primarily aspirin) use on the development of CRC and colorectal adenoma. A consistent reduction in the risk of colorectal neoplasia in NSAID users is identified in these studies of various design.[67] In a pooled analysis of studies evaluating the effect on colorectal adenoma, the summary risk ratio for colorectal adenoma in aspirin users was 0.7 and in NSAID users was 0.6, indicating a statistically significant reduction of the risk in aspirin and NSAID users.[89] In the pooled analysis of the effect of aspirin and NSAIDs on CRC risk, the results were virtually the same.[90] Overall, the data evaluating the effect of nonaspirin NSAIDs is more limited than that for aspirin.

A number of intervention studies have been conducted, and a Cochrane review of the results of the randomized, controlled intervention trials has been published.[91] The authors of this meta-analysis reviewed one population-based prevention trial (including 22,071 people),[92] three secondary prevention trials in patients with sporadic polyps (including 2,028 patients),[93–95] and four trials in 150 patients with familial adenomatous polyposis.[96–99] The authors conclude based on data from these high quality trials that there is some evidence for the effectiveness of intervention strategies using NSAIDs for the prevention of colorectal adenoma. However, the single primary prevention trial reviewed[92] did not demonstrate a decreased incidence of CRC in the intervention group. Subsequent primary prevention trials also did not demonstrate efficacy,[100,101] leading to a recommendation by the US Preventive Services Task Force against aspirin/NSAID use for primary CRC prevention in average-risk individuals.[102] However, a recent pooled analysis of two large randomized trials from the UK with over 20 years of follow-up revealed a statistically significant reduction in CRC incidence in aspirin users (RR = 0.63; 95% CI, 0.47–0.85, $P = 0.002$, if allocated to aspirin for 5 years or more), but only after a latency period of 10 years or longer.[103]

NSAIDs and aspirin may play an important role in secondary chemoprevention of colorectal adenomas and cancer. Recently, Logan et al.[78] reported a randomized, double-blind trial of aspirin and folate in the prevention of recurrent colorectal adenomas. Patients randomized to aspirin 300 mg/day had a significantly reduced risk of recurrent adenoma compared to the placebo group (RR = 0.79; 95% CI, 0.63–0.99).[7] Baron et al.[104] randomized 2,587 to either the COX-2 inhibitor rofecoxib 25 mg/day versus placebo. Adenoma recurrence was less frequent for rofecoxib subjects than for those randomized to placebo (41% vs. 55%; $P < 0.0001$; RR = 0.76; 95% CI, 0.69–0.83).[104] Other recent studies have evaluated the role of COX-2 inhibitors in the prevention of CRC.[105,106]

Prolonged use of NSAIDs may have additional benefits. Long-term follow-up of the Aspirin/Folate Polyp Prevention Study revealed that patients who used regular NSAIDs in the four years following the study intervention (3 years of 81 mg aspirin/day) had a persistent reduction in the development of adenoma versus patients who were infrequent poststudy NSAID users (RR = 0.62; 95% CI, 0.39–0.98).[107] In addition, regular aspirin use may result in lower cancer-specific mortality in patients with a history of CRC. In a prospective cohort study involving 1,279 patients previously treated for Stage I–III colorectal cancer, regular aspirin users had a significantly reduced risk of CRC-specific mortality versus nonusers (RR = 0.71; 95% CI, 0.53–0.95).[108]

Because chemopreventive agents must be used in the general population to substantially reduce the burden of disease, the risks of chemoprophylaxis with aspirin or NSAIDs may outweigh the benefits. Serious GI complications occur in regular users of aspirin and NSAIDs. Although events are rare, hospitalizations for gastrointestinal complications occur in 7–13 per 1,000 chronic users of NSAIDS per year.[109] In addition, there are potential cardiotoxic effects of COX-2 inhibitors and thus their use in chemoprevention cannot be supported.[110] A number of authors have evaluated the cost-effectiveness of chemoprevention of CRC with NSAIDs[111] or COX-2 inhibitors[112] and found that chemoprophylaxis with these compounds is not cost-effective.

Hormone Replacement Therapy

Observational studies have demonstrated an association between hormone replacement therapy (HRT) in women and a reduction in both incidence and mortality from CRC. Possible mechanisms for the effect of HRT include a reduction in bile acid secretion (a potential promoter or initiator of CRC), as well as estrogen effects on colonic epithelium, both directly and through alterations in insulin-like growth factor with the use of estrogens. A meta-analysis of 18 observational studies of postmenopausal HRT demonstrated a 20% reduction in incidence of CRC in women who had taken HRT as compared to those that had never taken HRT.[113] The Women's Health Initiative was a randomized trial of estrogen plus progestin in 16,608 postmenopausal women. The study was discontinued early, as after a mean of 5.2 years of follow-up, it was determined that the relative risk of breast cancer in the treatment group exceeded the predefined stopping boundary and the overall risk of adverse outcomes exceeded the benefits.[114] At that time, there appeared to be a protective effect of HRT on the incidence of CRC. With further follow-up, a total of 122 cases of CRC developed in this cohort[115] 43 cases in the group receiving HRT and 72 cases in the group receiving placebo, indicating that relatively short-term HRT was associated with a significantly decreased risk of CRC. In a recent case-control study of 2,648 patients with CRC and 2,566 controls self-reported the use of HRT was associated with a 63% relative reduction in the risk of CRC (RR = 0.67; 95% CI, 0.51–0.89). Similar to prior studies,[116] a significant effect was seen only in women who used combined estrogen–progestin combinations, and not in users of estrogen-only preparations.[117] Others, however, have reported a protective effect of HRT regardless of the preparation used.[118] Postmenopausal HRT has also been associated with a decreased incidence of colorectal adenomas[119] and improved colorectal cancer-specific and overall survival (with the initiation of estrogen therapy within 5 years of diagnosis of CRC).[120]

Overall, there appears to be a consistent reduction in the risk of CRC with the use of HRT. However, given the potential adverse effect of HRT, this should not be used as a primary preventive strategy for CRC.[121]

Obesity

Obesity appears to increase the risk of colon cancer in men and premenopausal women. Case-control studies[122,123] and cohort studies[124–126] have demonstrated a strong association between a high body mass index (BMI) and incidence of CRC, with an up to twofold increased risk of CRC found in the obese. A more accurate predictor than BMI may be the waist-hip ratio, a measure of abdominal obesity. A recent meta-analysis of 30 prospective studies revealed an increasing risk of colon cancer with increasing waist-hip ratio (per 0.1 unit) in men (RR = 1.43; 95% CI, 1.19–1.71) and women (RR = 1.20; 95% CI, 1.08–1.33).[127] One of the proposed mechanisms for the association is the relative insulin resistance found in many obese patients. Insulin resistance results in hyperinsulinemia and increased activity of Insulin Growth Factor (IGF) peptides. High IGF-1 levels are associated with cell proliferation[124] and may increase the risk of colonic neoplasia. In the past, most studies have demonstrated a stronger association between obesity and CRC risk in men than in women.[127,128] More recent evidence has demonstrated that in women, the association between obesity and CRC risk may be modified by estrogen. A number of observational studies have demonstrated an increased risk of CRC in obese women; however, the association was limited to premenopausal women.[125,129] In postmenopausal women, the increased estrogen production associated with obesity was thought to mitigate the risk. Of note, not all studies have confirmed this relationship.[124,130,131]

Obesity is also a risk factor for the development of colorectal adenomas, although like the risk of CRC, the effect appears to be stronger in men than in women.[132,133] In a pooled analysis of six prospective trials involving 8,213 participants, obesity was statistically significantly associated with the risk of metachronous adenoma in men (OR = 1.36; 95% CI, 1.17–1.58) but not in women (OR = 1.10; 95% CI, 0.89–1.37).[133] In men, obesity may also be associated with a shortened interval for the development of metachronous adenomas, as well as a higher incidence of advanced adenomas, particularly with a positive family history.[134]

Physical Activity

Over 50 studies have been conducted to evaluate the influence of physical activity on CRC risk. Overall, the literature is relatively consistent with respect to the effect: Greater physical activity (occupational, recreational, or total activity) is associated with a reduced risk of CRC. The effect is relatively small; the estimated increased risk of colon cancer in the sedentary ranges from 1.6 to 2.0. (Of note, this compares to the increased risk of heart disease due to a sedentary lifestyle of 1.3–1.4).[135] The effect of physical activity on colon cancer is consistent in both case-control studies and cohort studies.[136] A meta-analysis of 19 cohort studies and 28 case-control studies revealed a protective effect against colon cancer in physically active males (RR = 0.78; 95% CI, 0.68–0.91) and females (RR = 0.71, 95% CI, 0.57–0.88).[137] A recent prospective cohort study involving 488,720 participants revealed that men who participated in exercise/sports five or more times a week, compared to rarely or never, had a relative risk of colon cancer of 0.79 (95% CI, 0.68–0.91, $P = 0.001$), corresponding to a 21% risk reduction. In women, there was a trend toward a protective effect (RR = 0.85, $P = 00.376$).[135] Sedentary behavior (time spent watching television/videos, ≥9 h/day) was positively correlated with colon cancer (RR = 1.61, 95% CI, 1.14–2.27, $P < 0.001$) in men.[135] The effect of physical activity on the risk of rectal cancer is somewhat less consistent; some studies demonstrate no effect,[137,138] and in studies that do demonstrate an effect, it is weaker.[135] In the NIH-AARP study, there was a nonsignificant trend toward protection from rectal cancer in men (RR = 0.76, $P = 0.07$), but no protective effect in women (RR = 0.95, $P = 0.23$).[135] The amount of physical activity required to have an effect is substantial – risk reduction is estimated to occur with 3.5–4 h of vigorous activity (running) per week but requires 7–35 h of moderate activity (walking at a brisk pace) per week.[135,136]

The biological mechanisms that explain the relationship between physical activity and CRC risk are unclear. Increased physical activity leads to changes in insulin sensitivity and IGF levels, and both insulin and IGF are potentially involved with colorectal carcinogenesis.[139,140] Additional proposed mechanisms include effects of physical activity on prostaglandin synthesis, effects on antitumor immune defenses, and the reduction in percent body fat associated with exercise.[141] The mechanism is almost certainly multifactorial. Nonetheless, for a host of health-related reasons, frequent moderate to vigorous physical activity can be recommended to most patients without hesitation.

Smoking

Consistent with a 35–40 year time lag between exposure and induction of cancer, early studies did not demonstrate an association between cigarette smoking and colorectal neoplasia. More recent studies are more consistently positive. In a review of the literature conducted in 2001,[142] 21 of 22 studies evaluating the relationship between cigarette smoking and colorectal adenoma were positive, smokers demonstrating a two to threefold elevation of adenoma risk as compared with nonsmokers. Twenty-seven epidemiologic studies that demonstrate an association between tobacco and the risk of CRC have been conducted.[142] Of studies in the USA conducted after 1970 in men, and 1990 in women (studies with adequate induction time – 35 to 40 years after smoking became common), most demonstrate an association between heavy smoking and increased CRC risk. The majority of studies demonstrate an effect at relatively high levels of smoking (20 or more cigarettes per day). A recently reported pooled analysis of the Women's Health Initiative study involving 146,877 women revealed a significant association between cigarette smoking and the risk of CRC overall, but this association was found only for rectal cancer (RR = 1.95; 95% CI, 1.10–3.47) and not colon cancer (RR = 1.03; 95% CI, 0.77–1.38).[143] A meta-analysis of 106 studies revealed a positive dose-response relationship between increasing cigarette consumption and CRC risk. The risk increased by 7.8% for every additional 10 cigarettes per day or by 4.4% for every additional 10 pack-years. The incidence of CRC was 65.5 per 100,000 in smokers and 54.7 per 100,000 in nonsmokers.[144]

Smoking may modify the effect of micronutrients on CRC risk. A recent case-control study revealed a strong protective effect of several dietary carotenoids found in fruits and vegetables, including beta-carotene, on the development of CRC. However, this protective effect was attenuated, or in some cases reversed, in heavy smokers.[145] Similarly, the inverse association found between fruit and vegetable consumption and CRC risk in the EPIC trial for never and former smokers was reversed in current smokers.[41] Another case-control study utilizing a case-unaffected sibling design involving 2,248 siblings did not reveal a positive association between cigarette smoking and CRC overall, but an association between increasing duration of smoking and microsatellite instability-high (MSI-H) tumors was observed (RR = 1.94; 95% CI, 1.09–3.46 for smoking >30 years vs. nonsmokers).[146] There are a number of possible explanations for these findings; cigarette smoke may generate replication errors, overwhelming the DNA mismatch repair (MMR) mechanism, or may affect MMR directly.

Cholecystectomy

Abnormal bile acid metabolism may predispose both to CRC and cholelithiasis. After cholecystectomy, increased quantities of secondary bile acids have been detected in the feces and may have a role in colonic carcinogenesis. Studies in this area are difficult, as dietary and lifestyle factors related to cholelithiasis may confound the relationship between gallbladder disease and CRC risk. A meta-analysis of studies evaluating the effect of cholecystectomy on CRC risk published in 1993[147] demonstrated conflicting results. Analysis of the 33 case-control studies generated a pooled relative risk of CRC after cholecystectomy of 1.34 (95% CI, 1.14–1.57), limited to the proximal colon. However, no significant effect was found when the results of six cohort studies were evaluated.

In a long-term follow-up study of 278,460 patients after cholecystectomy followed for up to 33 years,[148] a significantly increased risk of small bowel malignancies and proximal colonic malignancies was found as compared to the general population. No association was found with more distal bowel cancer. In another study using data from the Nurses' Health Study, a significant positive association between cholecystectomy and the risk of CRC was found (RR = 1.21; 95% CI, 1.01–1.46 after adjusting for important CRC risk factors, including diet, family history, calcium intake, BMI, and the use of HRT). In this study, the risk of CRC after cholecystectomy was elevated both for proximal bowel and rectal cancers.[149] A more recent retrospective cohort study comparing 55,960 cholecystectomy patients to 574,668 control patients found an increased risk of colon cancer (RR = 1.51) but not rectal cancer (RR = 1.00) following cholecystectomy.[150] Other large studies have found no association between cholecystectomy and CRC.[151,152]

Prior cholecystectomy does not seem to affect the risk of adenoma formation. In the Nurses' Health Study,[149] no elevation in the risk of colorectal adenoma was identified in those patients having had a cholecystectomy. Similarly, in a study involving data from three large randomized adenoma chemoprevention trials, no increased risk for adenomas was observed for patients who had undergone cholecystectomy (RR = 1.02; 95% CI, 0.88–1.18).[153] In summary, prior cholecystectomy does not appear to be a risk factor for adenoma formation. The association with CRC is inconsistent, but seems to be strongest for cancer of the proximal colon.

Inflammatory Bowel Disease

Patients with long-standing inflammatory bowel disease (IBD) are known to be at an elevated risk of CRC, although it is difficult to precisely estimate the risk. The magnitude of the risk has been studied extensively in ulcerative colitis (UC); however, rates vary between studies, particularly those performed in referral centers versus population-based studies. In addition, treatment and surveillance may influence the risk and thus more recent studies may have a lower risk than studies conducted before surveillance was common. A meta-analysis of 116 studies evaluating the risk of CRC in UC patients found the overall prevalence of CRC in UC patients was 3.7% (95% CI, 3.2–4.2%). In 19 of the studies reviewed, the duration of colitis was reported by decade. In the first 10 years, after the onset of colitis the incidence rate of CRC was 2/1,000 per year of disease, for the second decade the incidence rate of CRC was estimated to be 7/1,000 per year of disease, and in the third decade the incidence rate of CRC was 12/1,000 per year of disease. This corresponds to a cumulative probability of CRC of 2% after 10 years of disease, 8% after 20 years, and 18% after 30 years. The risk of CRC varied geographically and was higher in studies conducted in the USA. The meta-analysis did not evaluate the extent of disease (pancolitis vs. left-sided disease vs. proctitis).[154]

These findings are not universal; however, two recent population-based studies from Denmark and the Mayo Clinic failed to demonstrate any increased risk of CRC in ulcerative colitis patients.[155,156] In the Mayo Clinic study, based on 378 ulcerative colitis patients from Olmsted County, Minnesota, six cases of CRC were observed versus 5.38 expected based on SEER data (standardized incidence ratio (SIR) = 1.1; 95%

CI, 0.4–2.4). However, the risk of CRC was increased in the subset of patients with extensive colitis (SIR = 2.4; 95% CI, 0.6–6.0). Similar results were found in a cohort of 1,160 ulcerative colitis patients in Copenhagen, Denmark followed a median of 19 years. The observed number of CRC cases was almost identical to the expected number (13 vs. 12.42, SIR = 1.05; 95% CI, 0.56–1.79).

The extent of disease does appear to have a significant influence on CRC risk in UC. In a Swedish population-based cohort of 3,117 patients with UC,[157] less extensive disease was associated with a lesser risk of CRC. As a ratio of the observed to expected incidence, the increased risk of CRC in this cohort was 1.7 for those with ulcerative proctitis (95% CI, 0.8–3.2); 2.8 for those with left-sided colitis (95% CI, 1.6–4.4); and 14.8 for those with pancolitis (95% CI, 11.4–18.9). Other studies have supported these findings.[158]

Other factors that may modify the risk of CRC in patients with UC include the coexistence of primary sclerosing colangitis (PSC),[159] presence of inflammatory pseudopolyps,[160] and severity of inflammation.[161] For patients with long-standing, extensive UC, colectomy is an effective strategy for the prevention of CRC. Other strategies include endoscopic surveillance for dysplasia and/or the use of chemopreventive agents. Although the efficacy of endoscopic surveillance has not been definitively proven in a randomized trial, a recent Cochrane review found that although there was no direct evidence of prolonged survival, patients with UC in surveillance programs tended to have cancers diagnosed earlier with a correspondingly improved prognosis.[162] Despite a lack of definitive evidence, endoscopic surveillance is commonly performed in patients with pancolitis for more than 10 years duration who wish to avoid colectomy. There is some evidence that chemoprevention of CRC in patients with UC may be possible. 5-ASA products may decrease the rate of dysplasia in patients with UC.[163] Other agents include folate, calcium, and in patients with primary sclerosing cholangitis, Ursodiol.[163]

The relationship between Crohn's disease and the development of CRC has been less consistently demonstrated. In studies using data from referral-based practices, the risk of development of CRC appears to be significantly increased in patients with extensive Crohn's colitis.[158] The magnitude of increased risk appears similar to that of UC.[164] However, in population-based studies, particularly those more recently published, a less dramatic effect is seen. In a Canadian population-based cohort study, the risk of CRC in 2,857 patients with Crohn's disease was compared to a randomly selected group of controls matched 10:1 for age, sex, and geographic location. Patients with Crohn's disease were found to have an elevated risk of colon cancer (incidence rate ratio (IRR) = 2.6; 95% CI, 1.69–4.12) but not rectal cancer (IRR = 1.08; 95% CI, 0.43–2.70). Patients with Crohn's disease also had an elevated risk of cancer of the small intestine (IRR = 17.4; 95% CI, 4.16–72.9), and lymphoma (IRR = 2.40; 95% CI, 1.17–4.97). Some of these results are similar to those from a population-based study in Denmark of 2,645 patients hospitalized for Crohn's disease[165] and followed for up to 17 years. The rate of CRC in this group was not substantially higher than the expected rate of CRC in the Danish population; the SIR for CRC was 1.1 (95% CI, 0.6–1.9). However, similar to the Canadian study, the risk of small intestinal cancer was increased 18-fold in the Crohn's disease group. In a more recently reported population-based study from Olmsted County, Minnesota, a moderately increased risk of CRC SIR = 1.9; 95% CI, 0.7–4.1) was reported for patients with Crohn's disease. Similar to the other studies, patients with Crohn's disease had a 40-fold increased risk for small intestinal cancer.[155] In summary, it appears that the risk of CRC in patients with Crohn's disease is elevated, but the exact magnitude of increased risk remains unclear and requires further investigation.

Family History

Individuals with a family history of CRC are at an increased risk of themselves developing CRC. In a recent meta-analysis involving 59 studies, the relative risk of developing CRC with one affected first-degree relative was 2.24 (95% CI, 2.06–2.43) and 3.97 if more than two first-degree relatives were affected.[166] This corresponds to a pooled lifetime risk of a 50-year-old of 1.8% with no family history, 3.4% with one affected first-degree relative, and 6.9% with two or more first-degree relatives. The clustering of risk in families may be attributed to an inherited susceptibility, common environmental exposures, or a combination of both. The influence of a more distant family history of CRC on individual risk has not been determined with certainty.

Some of the increased risk attributed to family history is due to inheritance of known susceptibility genes, such as mutations in the *APC* gene, *p53* gene, or in MMR genes, particularly *MSH2*, *MLH1*, and *MSH6*;[167] these are discussed in detail elsewhere in this text. Importantly, the majority of cases of CRC cannot be attributed to known genetic defects even when associated with a family history of CRC as recognized genetic syndromes account for only a small proportion of all cases of CRC. Additional autosomal dominant genetic defects conferring a high risk of CRC almost certainly is found; however, at least some of the increased risk of CRC associated with a family history is likely attributable to other genetic factors, such as recessive susceptibility genes, autosomal dominant genes with low penetrance, or complex interactions between an individual's genetic makeup and environmental factors.

Despite the importance of family history on the risk of CRC, up to 25% of individuals with a first-degree relative with confirmed CRC do not report having such a family history,[168] and even those that do report a history may not be aware of the increased risk associated with this.[169] This has important implications for the assessment of family history as well as patient and family counseling.

Other Risk Factors

Radiation

Cases of rectal carcinoma have been reported in individuals who have undergone radiation for pelvic malignancies, primarily cervical cancer[170] and prostate cancer.[171] Close observation may be required for survivors of childhood pelvic tumors treated with radiation therapy, as secondary colorectal malignancies may develop decades later.[172] Because rectal cancer is relatively common, these cases may represent sporadic rectal cancers developing after long-term survival from other pelvic malignancies. However, the cancers occur in the radiated field, tend to be associated with radiation changes to the adjacent rectal mucosa and are more likely to be of mucinous histology[173] than typical sporadic cancers, thereby strengthening the likelihood of a causal association. Nevertheless, the vast majority of individuals undergoing radiation for pelvic malignancies do not develop rectal cancer.

Ureterosigmoidostomy

Formation of a ureterosigmoidostomy has been associated with an increased risk of carcinoma in the area of the ureter-sigmoid anastomosis. It is difficult to estimate the increase in the risk of colon cancer due to ureterosigmoidostomy – many were fashioned for malignant diseases that may themselves be associated with an increased risk of colon cancer, nevertheless the risk appears to be high. The estimated increase ranges from 100 to 7,000 times the risk in the normal population[174] and up to 24% of patients with a ureterosigmoidostomy develops neoplasia at the anastomosis.[175] The average latency period from the formation of the ureterosigmoidostomy to the development of malignancy is 26 years.[175] Patients who have undergone conversion to another form of urinary diversion remain at the risk of neoplasia if the ureterosigmoid anastomoses were not resected in their entirety. Although the cause of this dramatic increased risk in not known, it appears to require the exposure of colonic mucosa to the mixture of urine and feces[174] with conversion of urinary nitrates into N-nitroso compounds by colonic bacteria.

Fortunately, with a number of options for urinary diversion, this procedure is now rarely performed. Those living with a functional ureterosigmoidostomy should be counseled regarding their heightened risk and undergo regular sigmoidoscopic or colonoscopic surveillance.[174,175]

Acromegaly

Acromegaly, a rare endocrine syndrome resulting from the secretion of excess growth hormone from a pituitary neoplasm has been found to be associated with an increased risk of CRC in a number of studies.[176,177] The magnitude of the risk is unclear, with reports ranging from nonsignificant increases in the risk to a relative risk of 18.3.[177–179] In a population-based cohort study performed in Sweden and Denmark, the standardized incidence ratio of colon cancer in patients with acromegaly as compared to the general population was 2.6 (95% CI, 1.6–2.7).[176] In a more recent meta-analysis, the pooled odds ratio for the development of colon cancer was 4.35 (95% CI, 1.5–12.4)[179] Patients treated with growth hormone have been shown to have an increased incidence of and mortality from CRC.[180] Furthermore, patients with acromegaly have elevated levels of circulating IGF-1, and this may be partly responsible for the increased risk of colorectal neoplasia identified in these patients.[181] Patients with acromegaly also have an increased incidence of adenomatous polyps.[178,182]

Molecular Basis

All cancer has a genetic basis. Carcinogenesis is a multistep process, requiring an accumulation of inherited and acquired genetic alterations. With this succession of genetic alterations, cells acquire a growth advantage over surrounding cells, and in a Darwinian-type process normal cells evolve into cancer cells.[183] In normal cells, growth and replication is a highly regulated process, and disruption of this regulation at multiple levels is required for clinically relevant cancer to develop. Defects in genes that code for important proteins in the regulation of the cell cycle appear to be critical for carcinogenesis. Hanahan and Wienberg[183] have described the following six alterations in regulatory mechanisms that appear constant in most cancers from the several hundred genetic mutations that have been identified in cancer cells Figure 38-4.

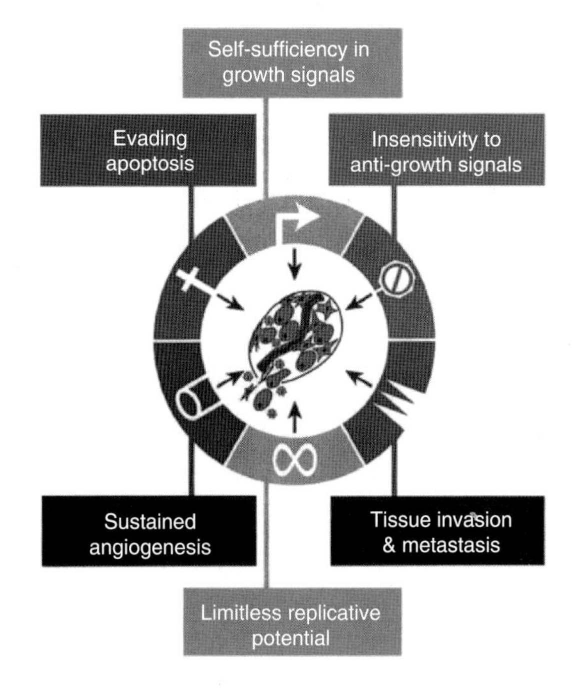

FIGURE 38-4. Alterations in regulatory mechanisms important for carcinogenesis.

Self-Sufficiency in Growth Signals

Ordinarily, cells must receive growth signals to actively proliferate, assuring that cellular proliferation occurs only when necessary to maintain homeostasis. To proliferate autonomously, cancer cells must lose this need for exogenous growth signal.

1. Insensitivity to antigrowth signals.
   Normally, there are numerous growth-inhibitory signals that function within a cell to maintain the cell in a quiescent and/or differentiated state. Cells with neoplastic potential must develop mechanisms to evade these antigrowth signals, enabling proliferation and dedifferentiation.

2. Evading Apoptosis
   Development of cancer requires not only a loss of control over cellular proliferation, but also a loss of control over programed cell death (apoptosis). Apoptosis normally occurs in response to the cellular environment and is likely a major mechanism whereby cells that have acquired significant genetic mutations are destroyed. Tumor cells must circumvent apoptosis (either at a regulatory level or at an effector level) to continue to develop and proliferate.

3. Limitless Replicative Potential
   Many cells are able to replicate only a finite number of times, thereby preventing clonal expansion of any given cell. Even after acquiring independence from normal signals for cellular growth and death to develop into clinically significant cancer, cancer cells must gain unlimited capacity for replication. Intrinsic limits to proliferation must be evaded.

4. Sustained Angiogenesis
   Virtually, all cells must reside within 100 μm of a capillary capable of delivering to the cell oxygen and nutrients required for functioning. Angiogenesis in normal tissue is closely regulated, and balancing of inducers and inhibitors of angiogenesis is an essential component of homeostasis. For neoplastic cells to develop into clinically significant cancer, they must develop the ability to circumvent these homeostatic mechanisms and provide an adequate blood supply required for ongoing growth.

5. Development of Ability to Invade and Metastasize
   For cancer cells to develop the ability to invade other tissue and metastasize, a number of changes must occur. Normally, cells in tissue adhere to each other. A loss of this normal cell to cell adhesion must occur in the cancer microenvironment to permit metastasis to occur. In addition, the cancer cells must develop methods of modifying new environments to support continued growth.

Although all six alterations in cell regulation are required for the development of clinically significant cancer, the sequence of events and mechanisms are variable. The sequence of genetic mutations (or alterations) is less important than the accumulation of mutations, although some mutations tend to occur early in the neoplastic process and are termed initiators, where as others tend to occur later and are termed promoters. In addition, certain genetic mutations (somatic or inherited) may be particularly critical and affect cell regulation in a number of important ways. Many such critical genes belong to two broad categories of genes involved in carcinogenesis; oncogenes and tumor suppressor genes. Additionally, caretaker genes that function to prevent the accumulation of somatic mutations are also critical to colorectal carcinogenesis. Abnormalities in caretaker genes greatly increase the risk of cancer development, independent of environmental influence. Of note, although the role of genes in carcinogenesis is described, in reality it is the protein products of the genes that are directly involved in changes in cell regulation.

Mutations in oncogenes result in an abnormal gain or excess of a particular protein function. An oncogene product when expressed in a given cell (or when the product is expressed at the wrong time in the cell cycle, expressed with an enhanced function, or expressed in larger quantities than normally present) contributes to the development of critical alterations in the mechanisms of cell regulation. Mutations causing such expression behave in a dominant fashion, i.e., mutation of only one of the two alleles present is required to produce activation and phenotypic expression and promote carcinogenesis.

The *ras* oncogene is the most frequently mutated oncogene identified in colorectal cancers. The *K-ras* proto-oncogene, located on the short arm of chromosome 12 (12p) is mutated in approximately half of all CRC.[184] The *K-ras* gene product appears to be involved in the transduction of exogenous growth signals. Point mutations in the *K-ras* gene lead to a function gain, conferring a growth advantage to the cells. Patients with mutant K-*ras* may have a poor response to the chemotherapeutic agent erbitiux.[185] Other oncogenes that are frequently identified in sporadic CRC include c-*myc* and *c-erbB2*.[186]

Tumor suppressor genes normally inhibit cellular proliferation or promote apoptosis. When gene expression is lost, there is a loss of this normal inhibitory control of the cell cycle. In general, gene expression is lost only when both alleles of the gene are inactivated (Knudson's 2-hit theory of carcinogenesis,[187] Figure 38-5) either through inherited mutation, somatic mutations or both. There are a number of tumor suppressor genes that have been found to play an important role in CRC carcinogenesis, including the *APC*, *DCC*, *p53*, and *MCC* genes.

The *APC* gene, located on the long arm of chromosome 5 (5q), is considered a gatekeeper gene of colorectal carcinogenesis, as mutations in the *APC* gene appear to be initiators of disease. Mutations in the *APC* gene have been found in 50% of sporadic adenomas and in 75% of sporadic cases of CRC.[184] Familial Adenomatous Polyposis (FAP), discussed in detail elsewhere in this text, results from inheritance of a germ line mutation in the *APC* gene. Mutations involve base-pair mutations, insertions, or deletions that result in the

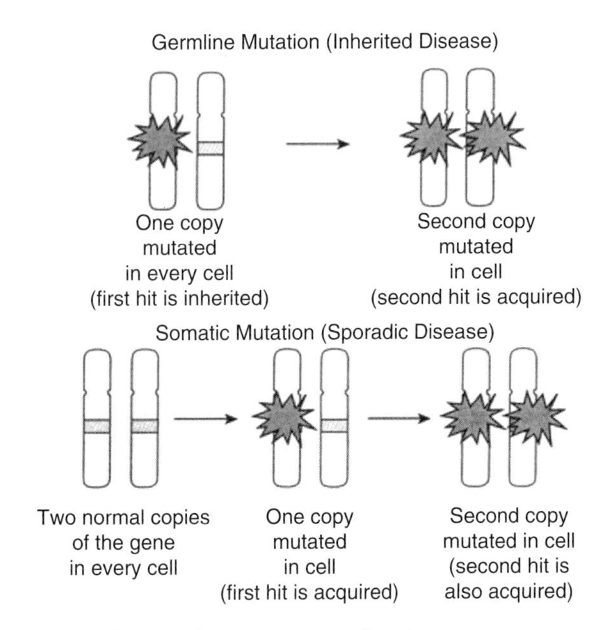

FIGURE 38-5. Loss of suppressor-gene function.

formation of a stop codon, halting protein synthesis leading to the formation of a truncated or shortened protein product that affects the function of the protein. The location of the germ-line mutation in the *APC* gene varies between families with FAP, and results in the varying phenotypic expression of FAP found between families. Although only a single abnormal allele is inherited in FAP, sporadic mutations are always acquired resulting in the formation of hundreds to thousands of colonic adenomas and ultimately carcinoma. The *APC* protein normally regulates the *Wnt* (wingless signaling pathway), an important pathway in cell regulation and development, through modulation of beta-catenin – a critical protein in the *Wnt* pathway. Normally, the protein product of the *APC* gene binds beta-catenin intracellularly forming a multiprotein complex that inhibits beta-catenin function. The increased functional levels of beta-catenin that result from alterations in *APC* protein product function leads to cell proliferation, and enhances cell-to-cell adhesion, limiting cell migration. Thus, hyperproliferating cells accumulate and result in aberrant crypt foci, the earliest phase of colorectal neoplasia.[188]

The *p53* gene, located on the short arm of chromosome 17 (17p) is an important gatekeeper gene for carcinogenesis – it is the most commonly mutated gene in human cancers.[189] Normally, by slowing the cell cycle, *p53* facilitates DNA repair during replication and when repair is not feasible, *p53* induces apoptosis. Inactivation of *p53* is found in up to 75% of sporadic colorectal tumors,[186] however, the mutation appears to occur late in the tumorigenic sequence. Thus, *p53* gene mutations do not appear to be initiators of carcinogenesis but act as key limiting factors for malignant transformation. This is supported by the finding that patients with Li Fraumeni syndrome (an inherited defect in p53) do not have an increased risk of CRC.[190] In addition, *p53* expression may be an independent prognostic marker in patients with CRC.[191,192] Most studies demonstrate a lower survival rate in patients with advanced cancers that are *p53* negative as compared to those whose tumors express *p53* gene product, particularly in those who receive chemotherapy.[193]

The "deleted in colorectal cancer" (*DCC*) gene was identified on the long arm of chromosome 18 (18q) in 1989.[194] Mutations in this gene have been found in the majority of CRC. The gene product of *DCC* is a transmembrane protein that is important in cell–cell adhesion, and therefore inactivation of *DCC* may enhance the metastatic potential of CRC through changes in adhesion. Similar to *p53*, patients who have *DCC*-positive tumors may have a better prognosis than those with *DCC*-negative (mutated) tumors.[195]

Located in close proximity to the *DCC* gene, mutations in a group of genes terms *SMAD*s (*SMAD2* and *SMAD4*) have been reported in colorectal cancers. The protein products of these genes are components of the transforming growth factor-β (*TGF-β*) signaling pathway, which mediates growth inhibitory signals from cell surface to nucleus.

Because millions of base-pairs must be replicated during mitosis, errors in DNA replication occur and must be corrected by caretaker genes. The MMR system has a critical function in the detection and correction of errors in DNA replication, maintaining DNA integrity. MMR genes function as spell checkers – base-pair mismatches are identified, excised, and the correct sequence is synthesized and replaced.[196] Lack of MMR function results in an accumulation of errors in DNA replication, increasing the probability that a mutation in an important gene in cell regulation occurs and carcinogenesis is thus initiated or promoted. Defects in the MMR system are identified by the detection of microsatellite instability. Microsatellites are small regions of DNA located throughout the genome that do not code for individual genes. They consist of small base sequences that are repeated in a highly polymorphic fashion – the number of repeats may range from dozens to hundreds and the number of repeats varies from allele to allele, and from individual to individual. Microsatellites are particularly susceptible to MMR gene defects, thus in cases of CRC due to MMR gene mutations, microsatellite replication errors accumulate, leading to detectable differences in the pattern of microsatellites in the tumor and in normal tissue – this is termed microsatellite instability (MSI). When testing CRC for MSI, laboratories evaluate a number of microsatellite loci. The National Cancer Institute recommends the testing of five microsatellite sequences[197] to determine the MSI status of a tumor. If two or more of the five sequences demonstrate MSI, the tumor is designated MSI-high (MSI-H). If only one of the five sequences demonstrates changes in tumor microsatellite markers, the tumor is designated MSI-low (MSI-L). If no markers are changed, the tumor is microsatellite stable. Approximately 15% of CRC demonstrate MSI.[197] MSI-H tumors are more likely to be high-grade, right-sided,[198]

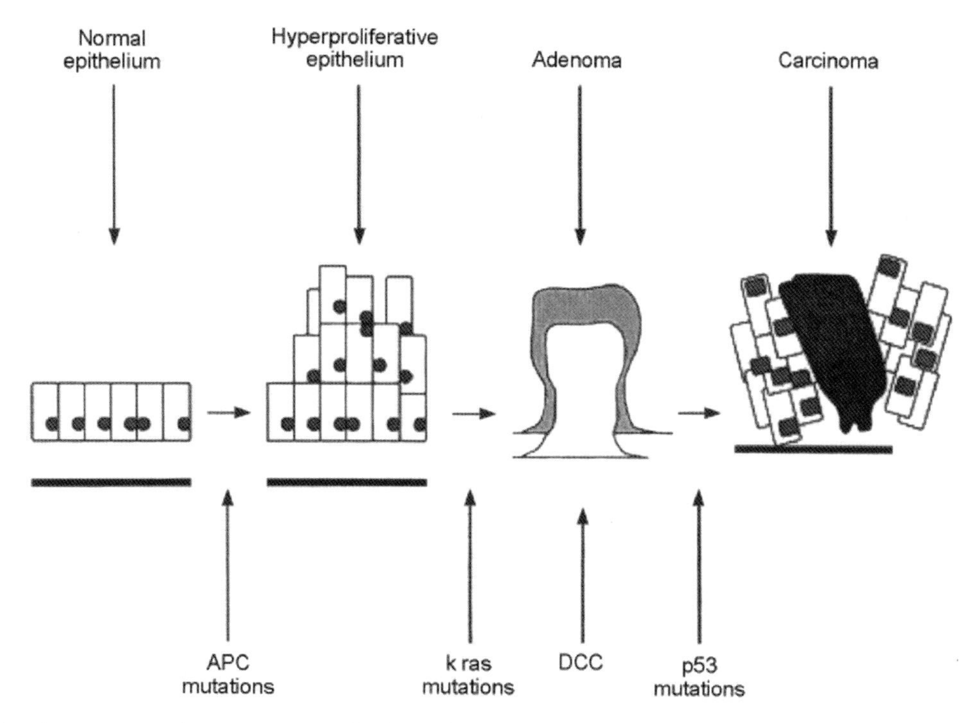

FIGURE 38-6. The adenoma to carcinoma sequence of colorectal carcinogenesis.

mucinous, and have tumor infiltrating lymphocytes.[199,200] In addition, MSI tumors may have a better prognosis than microsatellite stable tumors,[201] but may be less responsive to chemotherapy.[202]

A number of MMR genes (*MLH1*, *MSH2*, *MSH3*, *MSH6*, and *PMS1*) have been identified. Germ line mutations in the *MLH1* and *MSH2* genes are responsible for the majority (>90%)[203,204] of cases of the Hereditary Nonpolyposis Colorectal Cancer (HNPCC) (discussed elsewhere in the text), while approximately 5–10% of HNPCC cases are due to mutations in the *MSH6* gene. Germ line mutations in other MMR genes are rare. Similar to tumor suppressor genes, both alleles of an MMR gene must be mutated or inactivated for MMR function to be lost. These tumors are diploid and tend not to demonstrate gross chromosomal abnormalities. MMR defects in these tumors lead to genetic mutations in key cell regulator genes, particularly the *TGF-β* pathway. Sporadic tumors that demonstrate an MSI-H phenotype generally have a loss of *MLH1* function, not due to mutation but due to aberrant methylation of the promoter region of the *MLH1* gene (see below).[205]

MYH is an additional DNA repair gene specifically active for adenine–guanine mismatches.[206] This gene has been found to be responsible for some cases of *APC* mutation-negative FAP. This defect is inherited in an autosomal recessive fashion, i.e., defects must be inherited from both parents to result in phenotypic expression of the disease.[207] Biallelic carriers have a 53-fold increased risk of CRC with a cumulative risk by age 70 of 80%.[208] Monoallelic carriers may also be at increased risk to develop CRC; relative risk estimates for monoallelic carriers have ranged between 1.4 to 3.0.[208–211]

In their landmark article, Vogelstein and Fearon[212] (Figure 38-6) described the pathogenesis of colon cancer as one that follows a predictable sequence of events, from adenoma to carcinoma, with histological changes developing as genetic mutations are acquired over time. Initially, a mutation in a gatekeeper gene such as *APC* occurs resulting in proliferation of the colorectal mucosa and the initial histologically detectable event, the aberrant crypt focus. In aberrant crypt foci, the crypts have larger diameters than normal, stain more darkly with methylene blue,[188] and can be detected in rats as soon as 2 weeks after carcinogen exposure.[213] With additional genetic changes, cells within the aberrant crypt become dysplastic and an adenoma forms. Further genetic alterations are acquired, resulting in an increase in the size of the adenoma. However, the majority of adenomas do not develop into carcinoma. Therefore, additional genetic alterations are required before the severity of dysplasia increases, and eventually, particularly with mutations in tumor promoters, such as *p53*, carcinoma develops. This pathway to carcinogenesis is termed the chromosomal instability pathway. Tumors forming through this pathway demonstrate extensive cytogenetic abnormalities, such as aneuploidy, and visible chromosomal losses and gains.[214] CRC most commonly demonstrates chromosomal instability, indicating this is the most common genetic cause of colorectal carcinogenesis.[215]

Although MSI-H tumors may arise from adenomas, there is increasing evidence that sporadic MSI-H tumors also arise from serrated lesions (hyperplastic polyps, serrated adenomas, and sessile serrated adenomas).[216–220] As only 70% of colorectal carcinomas are believed to arise from classic adenomas, serrated lesions may be the precursor lesion for a substantial number of cancers.[221] However, the risk associated with serrated lesions, in terms of progression to cancer, is unclear; it has been suggested that serrated polyps progress to cancer faster than do adenomas.[222] This recently described pathway of colorectal carcinogenesis is believed to be initiated by hypermethylation of the promoter region of various genes and is associated with increasing age.[223] Methylation of cytosines in cytosine–guanosine dinucleotide repeats (termed CpG islands) results in the silencing of transcription, without an actual change in the nucleotide sequence of the gene.[224] Tumors exhibiting this phenomenon are referred to as CpG island methylator phenotype (CIMP).[225] Although the *MLH1* gene is often involved (resulting in sporadic, MSI-H CRC), it need not be, and thus approximately 50% of CIMP tumors do not exhibit microsatellite instability. Accumulating evidence indicates that activating somatic mutations in the *BRAF* gene may be responsible for promoter methylation.[216,226] The *MCC* gene may also play a key role in this pathway.[227,228]

Hyperplastic polyposis (HPP) syndrome is characterized by multiple hyperplastic polyps and other serrated lesions and may be familial.[229] There may be an autosomal recessive pattern of inheritance, and the familial HPP-serrated lesions show a similar frequency of CIMP and *BRAF* mutations compared to sporadic serrated polyps.[230] Similarly, the "serrated pathway syndrome" may arise from as of yet unrecognized inherited mutations and shares phenotypic features with HNPCC.[231]

A relatively recent theory of carcinogenesis contends that subpopulations of CRC stem cells are primarily responsible for driving tumor growth.[232] This hypothesis purports that not all cells within a tumor have the same proliferative or tumorigenic capabilities; nonstem cancer cells can neither self-renew nor propagate the tumor. Successful treatment of tumors, therefore, may depend on complete eradication of these "cancer-initiating" stem cells. Colon cancer stem cells may be more resistant to chemotherapy[233] and radiotherapy.[234] A number of mechanisms may be responsible for this survival advantage, among them an ATP-binding cassette drug transporter that results in the extrusion of chemotherapy agents from the cell.[233] A number of markers have been described that may identify CRC stem cells, including CD133,[235,236] Lgr5,[237] Bmil,[238], and CD44.[239] It is likely that colon cancer stem cells arise from normal stem cells that have acquired mutations, (e.g., *APC* gene)[240] and have lost their regulation of self-renewal. The existence of these colon cancer stem cells would have significant implications for the management of CRC, including screening, surgical therapy, delivery of chemotherapy and radiotherapy, and targeted therapy such as gene therapy.[239]

References

1. Center MM, Jemal A, Smith RA, Ward E. Worldwide variations in colorectal cancer. CA Cancer J Clin. 2009;59:366–78.
2. World Health Organization Mortality Datebase. World Health Organization. (Accessed 9 Dec 2009, at http://www-dep.iarc.fr/.)
3. Jemal A, Siegel R, Ward E, Hao Y, Xu J, Thun MJ. Cancer statistics, 2009. CA Cancer J Clin. 2009;59:225–49.
4. Boyle P, Langman JS. ABC of colorectal cancer: epidemiology. BMJ. 2000;321:805–8.
5. Rabeneck L, Davila JA, El-Serag HB. Is there a true "shift" to the right colon in the incidence of colorectal cancer? Am J Gastroenterol. 2003;98:1400–9.
6. American Cancer Society Website Cancer Facts and Figures. http://www.cancer.org/downloads/STT/500809web.pdf. Accessed 16 Dec 2009.
7. O'Connell JB, Maggard MA, Liu JH, Etzioni DA, Livingston EH, Ko CY. Rates of colon and rectal cancers are increasing in young adults. Am Surg. 2003;69:866–72.
8. Laken SJ, Petersen GM, Gruber SB, et al. Familial colorectal cancer in Ashkenazim due to a hypermutable tract in APC. Nat Genet. 1997;17:79–83.
9. Cheng X, Chen VW, Steele B, et al. Subsite-specific incidence rate and stage of disease in colorectal cancer by race, gender, and age group in the United States, 1992–1997. Cancer. 2001;92:2547–54.
10. Troisi RJ, Freedman AN, Devesa SS. Incidence of colorectal carcinoma in the U.S.: an update of trends by gender, race, age, subsite, and stage, 1975–1994. Cancer. 1999;85:1670–6.
11. Lagiou P, Adami HO. Burden of cancer. In: Adami HO, Hunter D, Trichopoulos D, editors. Textbook of cancer epidemiology. Oxford: Oxford University Press; 2002. p. 3–28.
12. Burkitt DP. Related disease–related cause? Lancet. 1969;2: 1229–31.
13. Flood DM, Weiss NS, Cook LS, Emerson JC, Schwartz SM, Potter JD. Colorectal cancer incidence in Asian migrants to the United States and their descendants. Cancer Causes Control. 2000;11:403–11.
14. Wingo PA, Cardinez CJ, Landis SH, et al. Long-term trends in cancer mortality in the United States, 1930–1998. Cancer. 2003;97:3133–275.
15. Rabeneck L, El-Serag HB, Davila JA, Sandler RS. Outcomes of colorectal cancer in the United States: no change in survival (1986–1997). Am J Gastroenterol. 2003;98:471–7.
16. Anderson WF, Umar A, Brawley OW. Colorectal carcinoma in black and white race. Cancer Metastasis Rev. 2003;22: 67–82.
17. Morris AM, Billingsley KG, Baxter NN, Baldwin LM. Racial disparities in rectal cancer treatment: a population-based analysis. Arch Surg. 2004;139:151–5. discussion 6.
18. National Cancer Society Cancer Control and Population Sciences Estimated US Cancer Prevalence. http://cancercontrol.cancer.gov/ocs/prevalence. Accessed 16 Dec 2009.
19. Nigro ND, Singh DV, Campbell RL, Sook M. Effect of dietary beef fat on intestinal tumor formation by azoxymethane in rats. J Natl Cancer Inst. 1975;54:439–42.
20. Reddy BS, Narisawa T, Vukusich D, Weisburger JH, Wynder EL. Effect of quality and quantity of dietary fat and dimethylhydrazine in colon carcinogenesis in rats. Proc Soc Exp Biol Med. 1976;151:237–9.
21. Hursting SD, Thornquist M, Henderson MM. Types of dietary fat and the incidence of cancer at five sites. Prev Med. 1990;19:242–53.
22. Willett WC. Dietary fat intake and cancer risk: a controversial and instructive story. Semin Cancer Biol. 1998;8:245–53.
23. Howe GR, Aronson KJ, Benito E, et al. The relationship between dietary fat intake and risk of colorectal cancer: evidence

from the combined analysis of 13 case-control studies. Cancer Causes Control. 1997;8:215–28.

24. Giovannucci E, Rimm EB, Stampfer MJ, Colditz GA, Ascherio A, Willett WC. Intake of fat, meat, and fiber in relation to risk of colon cancer in men. Cancer Res. 1994;54: 2390–7.
25. Willett WC, Stampfer MJ, Colditz GA, Rosner BA, Speizer FE. Relation of meat, fat, and fiber intake to the risk of colon cancer in a prospective study among women. N Engl J Med. 1990;323:1664–72.
26. Flood A, Velie EM, Sinha R, et al. Meat, fat, and their subtypes as risk factors for colorectal cancer in a prospective cohort of women. Am J Epidemiol. 2003;158:59–68.
27. Weijenberg MP, Luchtenborg M, de Goeij AF, et al. Dietary fat and risk of colon and rectal cancer with aberrant MLH1 expression, APC or KRAS genes. Cancer Causes Control. 2007;18:865–79.
28. Beresford SA, Johnson KC, Ritenbaugh C, et al. Low-fat dietary pattern and risk of colorectal cancer: the Women's Health Initiative Randomized Controlled Dietary Modification Trial. JAMA. 2006;295:643–54.
29. Bingham SA, Pignatelli B, Pollock JR, et al. Does increased endogenous formation of N-nitroso compounds in the human colon explain the association between red meat and colon cancer? Carcinogenesis. 1996;17:515–23.
30. de Kok TM, van Maanen JM. Evaluation of fecal mutagenicity and colorectal cancer risk. Mutat Res. 2000;463:53–101.
31. de Vogel J, van-Eck WB, Sesink AL, Jonker-Termont DS, Kleibeuker J, van der Meer R. Dietary heme injures surface epithelium resulting in hyperproliferation, inhibition of apoptosis and crypt hyperplasia in rat colon. Carcinogenesis. 2008;29:398–403.
32. Larsson SC, Wolk A. Meat consumption and risk of colorectal cancer: a meta-analysis of prospective studies. Int J Cancer. 2006;119:2657–64.
33. Sandhu MS, White IR, McPherson K. Systematic review of the prospective cohort studies on meat consumption and colorectal cancer risk: a meta-analytical approach. Cancer Epidemiol Biomarkers Prev. 2001;10:439–46.
34. Norat T, Lukanova A, Ferrari P, Riboli E. Meat consumption and colorectal cancer risk: dose-response meta-analysis of epidemiological studies. Int J Cancer. 2002;98:241–56.
35. Morita M, Le Marchand L, Kono S, et al. Genetic polymorphisms of CYP2E1 and risk of colorectal cancer: the Fukuoka Colorectal Cancer Study. Cancer Epidemiol Biomarkers Prev. 2009;18:235–41.
36. World. Cancer Research Fund/American Institute for Cancer Research. Food, nutrition and the prevention of cancer: a global perspective. In: 1997 Washington DC: American Institute for Cancer Research 1997.
37. Michels KB, Edward G, Joshipura KJ, et al. Prospective study of fruit and vegetable consumption and incidence of colon and rectal cancers. J Natl Cancer Inst. 2000;92:1740–52.
38. Voorrips LE, Goldbohm RA, van Poppel G, Sturmans F, Hermus RJ, van den Brandt PA. Vegetable and fruit consumption and risks of colon and rectal cancer in a prospective cohort study: The Netherlands Cohort Study on Diet and Cancer. Am J Epidemiol. 2000;152:1081–92.
39. McCullough ML, Robertson AS, Chao A, et al. A prospective study of whole grains, fruits, vegetables and colon cancer risk. Cancer Causes Control. 2003;14:959–70.
40. Koushik A, Hunter DJ, Spiegelman D, et al. Fruits, vegetables, and colon cancer risk in a pooled analysis of 14 cohort studies. J Natl Cancer Inst. 2007;99:1471–83.
41. van Duijnhoven FJ, Bueno-De-Mesquita HB, Ferrari P, et al. Fruit, vegetables, and colorectal cancer risk: the European Prospective Investigation into Cancer and Nutrition. Am J Clin Nutr. 2009;89:1441–52.
42. Schatzkin A, Lanza E, Corle D, et al. Lack of effect of a low-fat, high-fiber diet on the recurrence of colorectal adenomas. Polyp Prevention Trial Study Group. N Engl J Med. 2000;342: 1149–55.
43. Michels KB, Giovannucci E, Chan AT, Singhania R, Fuchs CS, Willett WC. Fruit and vegetable consumption and colorectal adenomas in the Nurses' Health Study. Cancer Res. 2006;66:3942–53.
44. Millen AE, Subar AF, Graubard BI, et al. Fruit and vegetable intake and prevalence of colorectal adenoma in a cancer screening trial. Am J Clin Nutr. 2007;86:1754–64.
45. Sengupta S, Tjandra JJ, Gibson PR. Dietary fiber and colorectal neoplasia. Dis Colon Rectum. 2001;44:1016–33.
46. Fuchs CS, Giovannucci EL, Colditz GA, et al. Dietary fiber and the risk of colorectal cancer and adenoma in women. N Engl J Med. 1999;340:169–76.
47. Peters U, Sinha R, Chatterjee N, et al. Dietary fibre and colorectal adenoma in a colorectal cancer early detection programme. Lancet. 2003;361:1491–5.
48. Bingham SA, Day NE, Luben R, et al. Dietary fibre in food and protection against colorectal cancer in the European Prospective Investigation into Cancer and Nutrition (EPIC): an observational study. Lancet. 2003;361:1496–501.
49. Bingham SA, Norat T, Moskal A, et al. Is the association with fiber from foods in colorectal cancer confounded by folate intake? Cancer Epidemiol Biomarkers Prev. 2005;14: 1552–6.
50. Park Y, Hunter DJ, Spiegelman D, et al. Dietary fiber intake and risk of colorectal cancer: a pooled analysis of prospective cohort studies. JAMA. 2005;294:2849–57.
51. Schatzkin A, Mouw T, Park Y, et al. Dietary fiber and whole-grain consumption in relation to colorectal cancer in the NIH-AARP Diet and Health Study. Am J Clin Nutr. 2007;85:1353–60.
52. Wakai K, Date C, Fukui M, et al. Dietary fiber and risk of colorectal cancer in the Japan collaborative cohort study. Cancer Epidemiol Biomarkers Prev. 2007;16:668–75.
53. Asano T, McLeod RS. Dietary fibre for the prevention of colorectal adenomas and carcinomas. Cochrane Database Syst Rev. 2002:CD003430.
54. Sansbury LB, Wanke K, Albert PS, Kahle L, Schatzkin A, Lanza E. The effect of strict adherence to a high-fiber, high-fruit and -vegetable, and low-fat eating pattern on adenoma recurrence. Am J Epidemiol. 2009;170:576–84.
55. Larsson SC, Giovannucci E, Bergkvist L, Wolk A. Whole grain consumption and risk of colorectal cancer: a population-based cohort of 60,000 women. Br J Cancer. 2005;92:1803–7.
56. Baron JA, Beach M, Mandel JS, et al. Calcium supplements for the prevention of colorectal adenomas. Calcium Polyp Prevention Study Group. N Engl J Med. 1999;340:101–7.
57. Bonithon-Kopp C, Kronborg O, Giacosa A, Rath U, Faivre J. Calcium and fibre supplementation in prevention of colorectal adenoma recurrence: a randomised intervention trial. European Cancer Prevention Organisation Study Group. Lancet. 2000;356:1300–6.

58. Weingarten MA, Zalmanovici A, Yaphe J. Dietary calcium supplementation for preventing colorectal cancer and adenomatous polyps. Cochrane Database Syst Rev. 2008:CD003548.
59. Bergsma-Kadijk JA, van't Veer P, Kampman E, Burema J. Calcium does not protect against colorectal neoplasia. Epidemiology. 1996;7:590–7.
60. Cho E, Smith-Warner SA, Spiegelman D, et al. Dairy foods, calcium, and colorectal cancer: a pooled analysis of 10 cohort studies. J Natl Cancer Inst. 2004;96:1015–22.
61. Ishihara J, Inoue M, Iwasaki M, Sasazuki S, Tsugane S. Dietary calcium, vitamin D, and the risk of colorectal cancer. Am J Clin Nutr. 2008;88:1576–83.
62. Larsson SC, Bergkvist L, Rutegard J, Giovannucci E, Wolk A. Calcium and dairy food intakes are inversely associated with colorectal cancer risk in the Cohort of Swedish Men. Am J Clin Nutr. 2006;83:667–73. quiz 728–9.
63. Park Y, Leitzmann MF, Subar AF, Hollenbeck A, Schatzkin A. Dairy food, calcium, and risk of cancer in the NIH-AARP Diet and Health Study. Arch Intern Med. 2009;169:391–401.
64. Park SY, Murphy SP, Wilkens LR, Nomura AM, Henderson BE, Kolonel LN. Calcium and vitamin D intake and risk of colorectal cancer: the Multiethnic Cohort Study. Am J Epidemiol. 2007;165:784–93.
65. Wactawski-Wende J, Kotchen JM, Anderson GL, et al. Calcium plus vitamin D supplementation and the risk of colorectal cancer. N Engl J Med. 2006;354:684–96.
66. Forman MR, Levin B. Calcium plus vitamin D3 supplementation and colorectal cancer in women. N Engl J Med. 2006;354:752–4.
67. Hawk ET, Umar A, Viner JL. Colorectal cancer chemoprevention – an overview of the science. Gastroenterology. 2004;126:1423–47.
68. Garland CF, Garland FC, Gorham ED. Calcium and vitamin D. Their potential roles in colon and breast cancer prevention. Ann NY Acad Sci. 1999;889:107–19.
69. Palmer HG, Gonzalez-Sancho JM, Espada J, et al. Vitamin D(3) promotes the differentiation of colon carcinoma cells by the induction of E-cadherin and the inhibition of beta-catenin signaling. J Cell Biol. 2001;154:369–87.
70. Gaschott T, Steinmeyer A, Steinhilber D, Stein J. ZK 156718, a low calcemic, antiproliferative, and prodifferentiating vitamin D analog. Biochem Biophys Res Commun. 2002;290:504–9.
71. Holt PR, Arber N, Halmos B, et al. Colonic epithelial cell proliferation decreases with increasing levels of serum 25-hydroxy vitamin D. Cancer Epidemiol Biomarkers Prev. 2002;11:113–9.
72. Woolcott CG, Wilkens LR, Nomura AM, et al. Plasma 25-hydroxyvitamin D levels and the risk of colorectal cancer: the multiethnic cohort study. Cancer Epidemiol Biomarkers Prev. 2010;19:130–4.
73. Wei MY, Garland CF, Gorham ED, Mohr SB, Giovannucci E. Vitamin D and prevention of colorectal adenoma: a meta-analysis. Cancer Epidemiol Biomarkers Prev. 2008;17:2958–69.
74. Yin L, Grandi N, Raum E, Haug U, Arndt V, Brenner H. Meta-analysis: longitudinal studies of serum vitamin D and colorectal cancer risk. Aliment Pharmacol Ther. 2009;30:113–25.
75. Huncharek M, Muscat J, Kupelnick B. Colorectal cancer risk and dietary intake of calcium, vitamin D, and dairy products: a meta-analysis of 26,335 cases from 60 observational studies. Nutr Cancer. 2009;61:47–69.
76. Kim YI. Folate, colorectal carcinogenesis, and DNA methylation: lessons from animal studies. Environ Mol Mutagen. 2004;44:10–25.
77. Hunter DJ. In: Environmental Mutagen Society Colon Cancer Conference; 2003 May 14–16, 2003; Miami Florida; 2003.
78. Logan RF, Grainge MJ, Shepherd VC, Armitage NC, Muir KR. Aspirin and folic acid for the prevention of recurrent colorectal adenomas. Gastroenterology. 2008;134:29–38.
79. Cole BF, Baron JA, Sandler RS, et al. Folic acid for the prevention of colorectal adenomas: a randomized clinical trial. JAMA. 2007;297:2351–9.
80. Ulrich CM, Potter JD. Folate and cancer – timing is everything. JAMA. 2007;297:2408–9.
81. Luebeck EG, Moolgavkar SH, Liu AY, Boynton A, Ulrich CM. Does folic acid supplementation prevent or promote colorectal cancer? Results from model-based predictions. Cancer Epidemiol Biomarkers Prev. 2008;17:1360–7.
82. U.S. Food and Drug Adminstration. Food standards: amendment of standards of identity for enriched grain products to require addition of folic acid. Final rule. 21 DFR Parts 136, 137, and 139. Fed. Regsit. 1996; 61:8781–807. In; 1996.
83. Mason JB, Dickstein A, Jacques PF, et al. A temporal association between folic acid fortification and an increase in colorectal cancer rates may be illuminating important biological principles: a hypothesis. Cancer Epidemiol Biomarkers Prev. 2007;16:1325–9.
84. Longnecker MP, Orza MJ, Adams ME, Vioque J, Chalmers TC. A meta-analysis of alcoholic beverage consumption in relation to risk of colorectal cancer. Cancer Causes Control. 1990;1:59–68.
85. Moskal A, Norat T, Ferrari P, Riboli E. Alcohol intake and colorectal cancer risk: a dose-response meta-analysis of published cohort studies. Int J Cancer. 2007;120:664–71.
86. Mizoue T, Inoue M, Wakai K, et al. Alcohol drinking and colorectal cancer in Japanese: a pooled analysis of results from five cohort studies. Am J Epidemiol. 2008;167:1397–406.
87. Ferrari P, Jenab M, Norat T, et al. Lifetime and baseline alcohol intake and risk of colon and rectal cancers in the European prospective investigation into cancer and nutrition (EPIC). Int J Cancer. 2007;121:2065–72.
88. Meyerhardt JA, Niedzwiecki D, Hollis D, et al. Association of dietary patterns with cancer recurrence and survival in patients with stage III colon cancer. JAMA. 2007;298:754–64.
89. Garcia Rodriguez LA, Huerta-Alvarez C. Reduced incidence of colorectal adenoma among long-term users of nonsteroidal antiinflammatory drugs: a pooled analysis of published studies and a new population-based study. Epidemiology. 2000;11:376–81.
90. Garcia Rodriguez LA, Huerta-Alvarez C. Reduced risk of colorectal cancer among long-term users of aspirin and nonaspirin nonsteroidal antiinflammatory drugs. Epidemiology. 2001;12:88–93.
91. Asano TK, McLeod RS. Non steroidal anti-inflammatory drugs (NSAID) and Aspirin for preventing colorectal adenomas and carcinomas. Cochrane Database Syst Rev. 2004: CD004079.
92. Gann PH, Manson JE, Glynn RJ, Buring JE, Hennekens CH. Low-dose aspirin and incidence of colorectal tumors in a randomized trial. J Natl Cancer Inst. 1993;85:1220–4.
93. Baron JA, Cole BF, Sandler RS, et al. A randomized trial of aspirin to prevent colorectal adenomas. N Engl J Med. 2003;348:891–9.
94. Sandler RS, Halabi S, Baron JA, et al. A randomized trial of aspirin to prevent colorectal adenomas in patients with previous colorectal cancer. N Engl J Med. 2003;348:883–90.

95. Benamouzig R, Deyra J, Martin A, et al. Daily soluble aspirin and prevention of colorectal adenoma recurrence: one-year results of the APACC trial. Gastroenterology. 2003;125:328–36.
96. Giardiello FM, Hamilton SR, Krush AJ, et al. Treatment of colonic and rectal adenomas with sulindac in familial adenomatous polyposis. N Engl J Med. 1993;328:1313–6.
97. Giardiello FM, Yang VW, Hylind LM, et al. Primary chemoprevention of familial adenomatous polyposis with sulindac. N Engl J Med. 2002;346:1054–9.
98. Labayle D, Fischer D, Vielh P, et al. Sulindac causes regression of rectal polyps in familial adenomatous polyposis. Gastroenterology. 1991;101:635–9.
99. Steinbach G, Lynch PM, Phillips RK, et al. The effect of celecoxib, a cyclooxygenase-2 inhibitor, in familial adenomatous polyposis. N Engl J Med. 2000;342:1946–52.
100. Cook NR, Lee IM, Gaziano JM, et al. Low-dose aspirin in the primary prevention of cancer: the Women's Health Study: a randomized controlled trial. JAMA. 2005;294:47–55.
101. Sturmer T, Glynn RJ, Lee IM, Manson JE, Buring JE, Hennekens CH. Aspirin use and colorectal cancer: post-trial follow-up data from the Physicians' Health Study. Ann Intern Med. 1998;128:713–20.
102. Dube C, Rostom A, Lewin G, et al. The use of aspirin for primary prevention of colorectal cancer: a systematic review prepared for the U.S. Preventive Services Task Force. Ann Intern Med. 2007;146:365–75.
103. Flossmann E, Rothwell PM. Effect of aspirin on long-term risk of colorectal cancer: consistent evidence from randomised and observational studies. Lancet. 2007;369:1603–13.
104. Baron JA, Sandler RS, Bresalier RS, et al. A randomized trial of rofecoxib for the chemoprevention of colorectal adenomas. Gastroenterology. 2006;131:1674–82.
105. Rahme E, Barkun AN, Toubouti Y, Bardou M. The cyclooxygenase-2-selective inhibitors rofecoxib and celecoxib prevent colorectal neoplasia occurrence and recurrence. Gastroenterology. 2003;125:404–12.
106. Gupta RA, Dubois RN. Colorectal cancer prevention and treatment by inhibition of cyclooxygenase-2. Nat Rev Cancer. 2001;1:11–21.
107. Grau MV, Sandler RS, McKeown-Eyssen G, et al. Nonsteroidal anti-inflammatory drug use after 3 years of aspirin use and colorectal adenoma risk: observational follow-up of a randomized study. J Natl Cancer Inst. 2009;101:267–76.
108. Chan AT, Ogino S, Fuchs CS. Aspirin use and survival after diagnosis of colorectal cancer. JAMA. 2009;302:649–58.
109. Wolfe MM, Lichtenstein DR, Singh G. Gastrointestinal toxicity of nonsteroidal antiinflammatory drugs. N Engl J Med. 1999;340:1888–99.
110. Bresalier RS, Sandler RS, Quan H, et al. Cardiovascular events associated with rofecoxib in a colorectal adenoma chemoprevention trial. N Engl J Med. 2005;352(11):1092–102.
111. Suleiman S, Rex DK, Sonnenberg A. Chemoprevention of colorectal cancer by aspirin: a cost-effectiveness analysis. Gastroenterology. 2002;122:78–84.
112. Hur C, Simon LS, Gazelle GS. The cost-effectiveness of aspirin versus cyclooxygenase-2-selective inhibitors for colorectal carcinoma chemoprevention in healthy individuals. Cancer. 2004;101:189–97.
113. Grodstein F, Newcomb PA, Stampfer MJ. Postmenopausal hormone therapy and the risk of colorectal cancer: a review and meta-analysis. Am J Med. 1999;106:574–82.
114. Rossouw JE, Anderson GL, Prentice RL, et al. Risks and benefits of estrogen plus progestin in healthy postmenopausal women: principal results From the Women's Health Initiative randomized controlled trial. JAMA. 2002;288: 321–33.
115. Chlebowski RT, Wactawski-Wende J, Ritenbaugh C, et al. Estrogen plus progestin and colorectal cancer in postmenopausal women. N Engl J Med. 2004;350:991–1004.
116. Newcomb PA, Zheng Y, Chia VM, et al. Estrogen plus progestin use, microsatellite instability, and the risk of colorectal cancer in women. Cancer Res. 2007;67:7534–9.
117. Rennert G, Rennert HS, Pinchev M, Lavie O, Gruber SB. Use of hormone replacement therapy and the risk of colorectal cancer. J Clin Oncol. 2009;27:4542–7.
118. Hoffmeister M, Raum E, Krtschil A, Chang-Claude J, Brenner H. No evidence for variation in colorectal cancer risk associated with different types of postmenopausal hormone therapy. Clin Pharmacol Ther. 2009;86:416–24.
119. Purdue MP, Mink PJ, Hartge P, Huang WY, Buys S, Hayes RB. Hormone replacement therapy, reproductive history, and colorectal adenomas: data from the Prostate, Lung, Colorectal and Ovarian (PLCO) Cancer Screening Trial (United States). Cancer Causes Control. 2005;16:965–73.
120. Chan JA, Meyerhardt JA, Chan AT, Giovannucci EL, Colditz GA, Fuchs CS. Hormone replacement therapy and survival after colorectal cancer diagnosis. J Clin Oncol. 2006;24: 5680–6.
121. Rymer J, Wilson R, Ballard K. Making decisions about hormone replacement therapy. BMJ. 2003;326:322–6.
122. Caan BJ, Coates AO, Slattery ML, Potter JD, Quesenberry Jr CP, Edwards SM. Body size and the risk of colon cancer in a large case-control study. Int J Obes Relat Metab Disord. 1998;22:178–84.
123. Kune GA, Kune S, Watson LF. Body weight and physical activity as predictors of colorectal cancer risk. Nutr Cancer. 1990;13:9–17.
124. Lin J, Zhang SM, Cook NR, Rexrode KM, Lee IM, Buring JE. Body mass index and risk of colorectal cancer in women (United States). Cancer Causes Control. 2004;15:581–9.
125. Reeves GK, Pirie K, Beral V, Green J, Spencer E, Bull D. Cancer incidence and mortality in relation to body mass index in the Million Women Study: cohort study. BMJ. 2007; 335:1134.
126. Sturmer T, Buring JE, Lee IM, Gaziano JM, Glynn RJ. Metabolic abnormalities and risk for colorectal cancer in the physicians' health study. Cancer Epidemiol Biomarkers Prev. 2006;15:2391–7.
127. Larsson SC, Wolk A. Obesity and colon and rectal cancer risk: a meta-analysis of prospective studies. Am J Clin Nutr. 2007;86:556–65.
128. Moghaddam AA, Woodward M, Huxley R. Obesity and risk of colorectal cancer: a meta-analysis of 31 studies with 70,000 events. Cancer Epidemiol Biomarkers Prev. 2007;16:2533–47.
129. Slattery ML, Ballard-Barbash R, Edwards S, Caan BJ, Potter JD. Body mass index and colon cancer: an evaluation of the modifying effects of estrogen (United States). Cancer Causes Control. 2003;14:75–84.
130. Wang Y, Jacobs EJ, Teras LR, et al. Lack of evidence for effect modification by estrogen of association between body mass index and colorectal cancer risk among postmenopausal women. Cancer Causes Control. 2007;18:793–9.

131. Hoffmeister M, Raum E, Winter J, Chang-Claude J, Brenner H. Hormone replacement therapy, body mass, and the risk of colorectal cancer among postmenopausal women from Germany. Br J Cancer. 2007;97:1486–92.
132. Kim Y, Kim Y, Lee S. An association between colonic adenoma and abdominal obesity: a cross-sectional study. BMC Gastroenterol. 2009;9:4.
133. Jacobs ET, Ahnen DJ, Ashbeck EL, et al. Association between body mass index and colorectal neoplasia at follow-up colonoscopy: a pooling study. Am J Epidemiol. 2009;169:657–66.
134. Jacobs ET, Martinez ME, Alberts DS, et al. Association between body size and colorectal adenoma recurrence. Clin Gastroenterol Hepatol. 2007;5:982–90.
135. Howard RA, Freedman DM, Park Y, Hollenbeck A, Schatzkin A, Leitzmann MF. Physical activity, sedentary behavior, and the risk of colon and rectal cancer in the NIH-AARP Diet and Health Study. Cancer Causes Control. 2008;19:939–53.
136. Slattery ML. Physical activity and colorectal cancer. Sports Med. 2004;34:239–52.
137. Samad AK, Taylor RS, Marshall T, Chapman MA. A meta-analysis of the association of physical activity with reduced risk of colorectal cancer. Colorectal Dis. 2005;7:204–13.
138. Harriss DJ, Atkinson G, Batterham A, et al. Lifestyle factors and colorectal cancer risk (2): a systematic review and meta-analysis of associations with leisure-time physical activity. Colorectal Dis. 2009;11:689–701.
139. Woodson K, Flood A, Green L, et al. Loss of insulin-like growth factor-II imprinting and the presence of screen-detected colorectal adenomas in women. J Natl Cancer Inst. 2004;96:407–10.
140. Haydon AM, Macinnis RJ, English DR, Morris H, Giles GG. Physical activity, insulin-like growth factor 1, insulin-like growth factor binding protein 3, and survival from colorectal cancer. Gut. 2006;55:689–94.
141. Friedenreich CM, Orenstein MR. Physical activity and cancer prevention: etiologic evidence and biological mechanisms. J Nutr. 2002;132:3456S–64.
142. Giovannucci E. An updated review of the epidemiological evidence that cigarette smoking increases risk of colorectal cancer. Cancer Epidemiol Biomarkers Prev. 2001;10:725–31.
143. Paskett ED, Reeves KW, Rohan TE, et al. Association between cigarette smoking and colorectal cancer in the Women's Health Initiative. J Natl Cancer Inst. 2007;99:1729–35.
144. Botteri E, Iodice S, Bagnardi V, Raimondi S, Lowenfels AB, Maisonneuve P. Smoking and colorectal cancer: a meta-analysis. JAMA. 2008;300:2765–78.
145. Chaiter Y, Gruber SB, Ben-Amotz A, et al. Smoking attenuates the negative association between carotenoids consumption and colorectal cancer risk. Cancer Causes Control. 2009;20(8):1327–38.
146. Poynter JN, Haile RW, Siegmund KD, et al. Associations between smoking, alcohol consumption, and colorectal cancer, overall and by tumor microsatellite instability status. Cancer Epidemiol Biomarkers Prev. 2009;18:2745–50.
147. Giovannucci E, Colditz GA, Stampfer MJ. A meta-analysis of cholecystectomy and risk of colorectal cancer. Gastroenterology. 1993;105:130–41.
148. Lagergren J, Ye W, Ekbom A. Intestinal cancer after cholecystectomy: is bile involved in carcinogenesis? Gastroenterology. 2001;121:542–7.
149. Schernhammer ES, Leitzmann MF, Michaud DS, et al. Cholecystectomy and the risk for developing colorectal cancer and distal colorectal adenomas. Br J Cancer. 2003;88:79–83.
150. Shao T, Yang YX. Cholecystectomy and the risk of colorectal cancer. Am J Gastroenterol. 2005;100:1813–20.
151. Goldacre MJ, Abisgold JD, Seagroatt V, Yeates D. Cancer after cholecystectomy: record-linkage cohort study. Br J Cancer. 2005;92:1307–9.
152. Lieberman DA, Prindiville S, Weiss DG, Willett W. Risk factors for advanced colonic neoplasia and hyperplastic polyps in asymptomatic individuals. JAMA. 2003;290:2959–67.
153. Vinikoor LC, Robertson DJ, Baron JA, Silverman WB, Sandler RS. Cholecystectomy and the risk of recurrent colorectal adenomas. Cancer Epidemiol Biomarkers Prev. 2007;16:1523–5.
154. Eaden JA, Abrams KR, Mayberry JF. The risk of colorectal cancer in ulcerative colitis: a meta-analysis. Gut. 2001;48:526–35.
155. Jess T, Loftus Jr EV, Velayos FS, et al. Risk of intestinal cancer in inflammatory bowel disease: a population-based study from olmsted county, Minnesota. Gastroenterology. 2006;130:1039–46.
156. Winther KV, Jess T, Langholz E, Munkholm P, Binder V. Long-term risk of cancer in ulcerative colitis: a population-based cohort study from Copenhagen County. Clin Gastroenterol Hepatol. 2004;2:1088–95.
157. Ekbom A, Helmick C, Zack M, Adami HO. Ulcerative colitis and colorectal cancer. A population-based study. N Engl J Med. 1990;323:1228–33.
158. Sharan R, Schoen RE. Cancer in inflammatory bowel disease. An evidence-based analysis and guide for physicians and patients. Gastroenterol Clin North Am. 2002;31:237–54.
159. Soetikno RM, Lin OS, Heidenreich PA, Young HS, Blackstone MO. Increased risk of colorectal neoplasia in patients with primary sclerosing cholangitis and ulcerative colitis: a meta-analysis. Gastrointest Endosc. 2002;56:48–54.
160. Velayos FS, Loftus Jr EV, Jess T, et al. Predictive and protective factors associated with colorectal cancer in ulcerative colitis: a case-control study. Gastroenterology. 2006;130:1941–9.
161. Rutter M, Saunders B, Wilkinson K, et al. Severity of inflammation is a risk factor for colorectal neoplasia in ulcerative colitis. Gastroenterology. 2004;126:451–9.
162. Collins PD, Mpofu C, Watson AJ, Rhodes JM. Strategies for detecting colon cancer and/or dysplasia in patients with inflammatory bowel disease. Cochrane Database Syst Rev. 2006:CD000279.
163. Croog VJ, Ullman TA, Itzkowitz SH. Chemoprevention of colorectal cancer in ulcerative colitis. Int J Colorectal Dis. 2003;18:392–400.
164. Gillen CD, Walmsley RS, Prior P, Andrews HA, Allan RN. Ulcerative colitis and Crohn's disease: a comparison of the colorectal cancer risk in extensive colitis. Gut. 1994;35:1590–2.
165. Mellemkjaer L, Johansen C, Gridley G, Linet MS, Kjaer SK, Olsen JH. Crohn's disease and cancer risk (Denmark). Cancer Causes Control. 2000;11:145–50.
166. Butterworth AS, Higgins JP, Pharoah P. Relative and absolute risk of colorectal cancer for individuals with a family history: a meta-analysis. Eur J Cancer. 2006;42:216–27.
167. Lynch HT, de la Chapelle A. Hereditary colorectal cancer. N Engl J Med. 2003;348:919–32.

168. Glanz K, Grove J, Le Marchand L, Gotay C. Underreporting of family history of colon cancer: correlates and implications. Cancer Epidemiol Biomarkers Prev. 1999;8:635–9.
169. Rubin DT, Gandhi RK, Hetzel JT, et al. Do colorectal cancer patients understand that their family is at risk? Dig Dis Sci. 2009;54:2473–83.
170. Tamai O, Nozato E, Miyazato H, et al. Radiation-associated rectal cancer: report of four cases. Dig Surg. 1999;16:238–43.
171. Brenner DJ, Curtis RE, Hall EJ, Ron E. Second malignancies in prostate carcinoma patients after radiotherapy compared with surgery. Cancer. 2000;88:398–406.
172. Park SS, Kim BK, Kim CJ, et al. Colorectal adenocarcinoma as a second malignant neoplasm following rhabdomyosarcoma of the urinary bladder: a case report. J Korean Med Sci. 2000;15:475–7.
173. Shirouzu K, Isomoto H, Morodomi T, Ogata Y, Araki Y, Kakegawa T. Clinicopathologic characteristics of large bowel cancer developing after radiotherapy for uterine cervical cancer. Dis Colon Rectum. 1994;37:1245–9.
174. Woodhouse CR. Guidelines for monitoring of patients with ureterosigmoidostomy. Gut. 2002;51 Suppl 5:V15–6.
175. Azimuddin K, Khubchandani IT, Stasik JJ, Rosen L, Riether RD. Neoplasia after ureterosigmoidostomy. Dis Colon Rectum. 1999;42:1632–8.
176. Baris D, Gridley G, Ron E, et al. Acromegaly and cancer risk: a cohort study in Sweden and Denmark. Cancer Causes Control. 2002;13:395–400.
177. Jenkins PJ, Besser M. Clinical perspective: acromegaly and cancer: a problem. J Clin Endocrinol Metab. 2001;86: 2935–41.
178. Terzolo M, Reimondo G, Gasperi M, et al. Colonoscopic screening and follow-up in patients with acromegaly: a multicenter study in Italy. J Clin Endocrinol Metab. 2005;90:84–90.
179. Rokkas T, Pistiolas D, Sechopoulos P, Margantinis G, Koukoulis G. Risk of colorectal neoplasm in patients with acromegaly: a meta-analysis. World J Gastroenterol. 2008;14: 3484–9.
180. Swerdlow AJ, Higgins CD, Adlard P, Preece MA. Risk of cancer in patients treated with human pituitary growth hormone in the UK, 1959–85: a cohort study. Lancet. 2002;360:273–7.
181. Jenkins PJ, Frajese V, Jones AM, et al. Insulin-like growth factor I and the development of colorectal neoplasia in acromegaly. J Clin Endocrinol Metab. 2000;85:3218–21.
182. Bogazzi F, Cosci C, Sardella C, et al. Identification of acromegalic patients at risk of developing colonic adenomas. J Clin Endocrinol Metab. 2006;91:1351–6.
183. Hanahan D, Weinberg RA. The hallmarks of cancer. Cell. 2000;100:57–70.
184. Robbins DH, Itzkowitz SH. The molecular and genetic basis of colon cancer. Med Clin North Am. 2002;86:1467–95.
185. Karapetis CS, Khambata-Ford S, Jonker DJ, et al. K-ras mutations and benefit from cetuximab in advanced colorectal cancer. N Engl J Med. 2008;359:1757–65.
186. Calvert PM, Frucht H. The genetics of colorectal cancer. Ann Intern Med. 2002;137:603–12.
187. Knudson Jr AG. Mutation and cancer: statistical study of retinoblastoma. Proc Natl Acad Sci USA. 1971;68:820–3.
188. Takayama T, Katsuki S, Takahashi Y, et al. Aberrant crypt foci of the colon as precursors of adenoma and cancer. N Engl J Med. 1998;339:1277–84.
189. Kirsch DG, Kastan MB. Tumor-suppressor p53: implications for tumor development and prognosis. J Clin Oncol. 1998;16:3158–68.
190. Birch JM, Blair V, Kelsey AM, et al. Cancer phenotype correlates with constitutional TP53 genotype in families with the Li-Fraumeni syndrome. Oncogene. 1998;17:1061–8.
191. Rosati G, Chiacchio R, Reggiardo G, De Sanctis D, Manzione L. Thymidylate synthase expression, p53, bcl-2, Ki-67 and p27 in colorectal cancer: relationships with tumor recurrence and survival. Tumour Biol. 2004;25:258–63.
192. Resnick MB, Routhier J, Konkin T, Sabo E, Pricolo VE. Epidermal growth factor receptor, c-MET, beta-catenin, and p53 expression as prognostic indicators in stage II colon cancer: a tissue microarray study. Clin Cancer Res. 2004;10:3069–75.
193. Iacopetta B. TP53 mutation in colorectal cancer. Hum Mutat. 2003;21:271–6.
194. Fearon ER, Cho KR, Nigro JM, et al. Identification of a chromosome 18q gene that is altered in colorectal cancers. Science. 1990;247:49–56.
195. Shibata D, Reale MA, Lavin P, et al. The DCC protein and prognosis in colorectal cancer. N Engl J Med. 1996;335:1727–32.
196. Potter JD. Colorectal cancer: molecules and populations. J Natl Cancer Inst. 1999;91:916–32.
197. Umar A, Boland CR, Terdiman JP, et al. Revised Bethesda Guidelines for hereditary nonpolyposis colorectal cancer (Lynch syndrome) and microsatellite instability. J Natl Cancer Inst. 2004;96:261–8.
198. Ward R, Meagher A, Tomlinson I, et al. Microsatellite instability and the clinicopathological features of sporadic colorectal cancer. Gut. 2001;48:821–9.
199. Smyrk TC, Watson P, Kaul K, Lynch HT. Tumor-infiltrating lymphocytes are a marker for microsatellite instability in colorectal carcinoma. Cancer. 2001;91:2417–22.
200. Jass JR, Do KA, Simms LA, et al. Morphology of sporadic colorectal cancer with DNA replication errors. Gut. 1998;42: 673–9.
201. Gryfe R, Kim H, Hsieh ET, et al. Tumor microsatellite instability and clinical outcome in young patients with colorectal cancer. N Engl J Med. 2000;342:69–77.
202. Ribic CM, Sargent DJ, Moore MJ, et al. Tumor microsatellite-instability status as a predictor of benefit from fluorouracil-based adjuvant chemotherapy for colon cancer. N Engl J Med. 2003;349:247–57.
203. Peltomaki P. Deficient DNA mismatch repair: a common etiologic factor for colon cancer. Hum Mol Genet. 2001;10:735–40.
204. Lynch HT, de la Chapelle A. Genetic susceptibility to non-polyposis colorectal cancer. J Med Genet. 1999;36:801–18.
205. Cunningham JM, Christensen ER, Tester DJ, et al. Hypermethylation of the hMLH1 promoter in colon cancer with microsatellite instability. Cancer Res. 1998;58:3455–60.
206. Al-Tassan N, Chmiel NH, Maynard J, et al. Inherited variants of MYH associated with somatic G:C → T:A mutations in colorectal tumors. Nat Genet. 2002;30:227–32.
207. Sieber OM, Lipton L, Crabtree M, et al. Multiple colorectal adenomas, classic adenomatous polyposis, and germ-line mutations in MYH. N Engl J Med. 2003;348:791–9.
208. Jenkins MA, Croitoru ME, Monga N, et al. Risk of colorectal cancer in monoallelic and biallelic carriers of MYH mutations: a population-based case-family study. Cancer Epidemiol Biomarkers Prev. 2006;15:312–4.

209. Peterlongo P, Mitra N, Sanchez de Abajo A, et al. Increased frequency of disease-causing MYH mutations in colon cancer families. Carcinogenesis. 2006;27:2243–9.
210. Croitoru ME, Cleary SP, Di Nicola N, et al. Association between biallelic and monoallelic germline MYH gene mutations and colorectal cancer risk. J Natl Cancer Inst. 2004; 96:1631–4.
211. Balaguer F, Castellvi-Bel S, Castells A, et al. Identification of MYH mutation carriers in colorectal cancer: a multicenter, case-control, population-based study. Clin Gastroenterol Hepatol. 2007;5:379–87.
212. Vogelstein B, Fearon ER, Hamilton SR, et al. Genetic alterations during colorectal-tumor development. N Engl J Med. 1988;319:525–32.
213. Bird RP, Good CK. The significance of aberrant crypt foci in understanding the pathogenesis of colon cancer. Toxicol Lett. 2000;112–113:395–402.
214. Lengauer C, Kinzler KW, Vogelstein B. Genetic instability in colorectal cancers. Nature. 1997;386:623–7.
215. Grady WM. Genomic instability and colon cancer. Cancer Metastasis Rev. 2004;23:11–27.
216. Rosenberg DW, Yang S, Pleau DC, et al. Mutations in BRAF and KRAS differentially distinguish serrated versus non-serrated hyperplastic aberrant crypt foci in humans. Cancer Res. 2007;67:3551–4.
217. Messick CA, Church J, Casey G, Kalady MF. Identification of the methylator (serrated) colorectal cancer phenotype through precursor serrated polyps. Dis Colon Rectum. 2009;52:1535–41.
218. Higuchi T, Jass JR. My approach to serrated polyps of the colorectum. J Clin Pathol. 2004;57:682–6.
219. Yang S, Farraye FA, Mack C, Posnik O, O'Brien MJ. BRAF and KRAS Mutations in hyperplastic polyps and serrated adenomas of the colorectum: relationship to histology and CpG island methylation status. Am J Surg Pathol. 2004;28:1452–9.
220. Young J, Jenkins M, Parry S, et al. Serrated pathway colorectal cancer in the population: genetic consideration. Gut. 2007;56:1453–9.
221. Jass JR. Pathogenesis of colorectal cancer. Surg Clin North Am. 2002;82:891–904.
222. Jass JR. Serrated route to colorectal cancer: back street or super highway? J Pathol. 2001;193:283–5.
223. Kakar S, Burgart LJ, Thibodeau SN, et al. Frequency of loss of hMLH1 expression in colorectal carcinoma increases with advancing age. Cancer. 2003;97:1421–7.
224. Toyota M, Ohe-Toyota M, Ahuja N, Issa JP. Distinct genetic profiles in colorectal tumors with or without the CpG island methylator phenotype. Proc Natl Acad Sci USA. 2000;97:710–5.
225. Weisenberger DJ, Siegmund KD, Campan M, et al. CpG island methylator phenotype underlies sporadic microsatellite instability and is tightly associated with BRAF mutation in colorectal cancer. Nat Genet. 2006;38:787–93.
226. Kambara T, Simms LA, Whitehall VL, et al. BRAF mutation is associated with DNA methylation in serrated polyps and cancers of the colorectum. Gut. 2004;53:1137–44.
227. Fukuyama R, Niculaita R, Ng KP, et al. Mutated in colorectal cancer, a putative tumor suppressor for serrated colorectal cancer, selectively represses beta-catenin-dependent transcription. Oncogene. 2008;27:6044–55.
228. Kohonen-Corish MR, Sigglekow ND, Susanto J, et al. Promoter methylation of the mutated in colorectal cancer gene is a frequent early event in colorectal cancer. Oncogene. 2007;26:4435–41.
229. Burt J, Jass J. Hyperplastic polyposis. In: Hamilton S, Aaltonen L, editors. World Health Organisation classification of tumors Pathology and Genetics Tumors of the digestive system. Lyon: IARC Press; 2000.
230. Beach R, Chan AO, Wu TT, et al. BRAF mutations in aberrant crypt foci and hyperplastic polyposis. Am J Pathol. 2005;166:1069–75.
231. Young J, Barker MA, Simms LA, et al. Evidence for BRAF mutation and variable levels of microsatellite instability in a syndrome of familial colorectal cancer. Clin Gastroenterol Hepatol. 2005;3:254–63.
232. Yeung TM, Mortensen NJ. Colorectal cancer stem cells. Dis Colon Rectum. 2009;52:1788–96.
233. Lou H, Dean M. Targeted therapy for cancer stem cells: the patched pathway and ABC transporters. Oncogene. 2007;26:1357–60.
234. Rich JN. Cancer stem cells in radiation resistance. Cancer Res. 2007;67:8980–4.
235. O'Brien CA, Pollett A, Gallinger S, Dick JE. A human colon cancer cell capable of initiating tumour growth in immunodeficient mice. Nature. 2007;445:106–10.
236. Ricci-Vitiani L, Lombardi DG, Pilozzi E, et al. Identification and expansion of human colon-cancer-initiating cells. Nature. 2007;445:111–5.
237. Barker N, van Es JH, Kuipers J, et al. Identification of stem cells in small intestine and colon by marker gene Lgr5. Nature. 2007;449:1003–7.
238. Sangiorgi E, Capecchi MR. Bmi1 is expressed in vivo in intestinal stem cells. Nat Genet. 2008;40:915–20.
239. Subramaniam V, Vincent IR, Gilakjan M, Jothy S. Suppression of human colon cancer tumors in nude mice by siRNA CD44 gene therapy. Exp Mol Pathol. 2007;83:332–40.
240. Barker N, Ridgway RA, van Es JH, et al. Crypt stem cells as the cells-of-origin of intestinal cancer. Nature. 2009;457:608–11.

39 Colorectal Cancer: Screening

Jason F. Hall and Thomas E. Read

Cancer of the colon and rectum is the second leading cause of cancer-related death in the USA. In 2009, it was estimated that 147,000 Americans will be diagnosed with colorectal cancer and 50,000 will die from this disease.[1] Without undergoing screening or preventive action, approximately 1 in every 17 people in this country will develop colorectal cancer at some point in life. There is clear evidence that colorectal adenocarcinoma can be prevented by detecting and removing adenomatous polyps and that detecting early stage cancers reduces mortality from the disease.[2–9] Both polyps and early stage cancers are usually asymptomatic; cancers that have grown large enough to cause symptoms have a much worse prognosis. This contrast highlights the need for screening in asymptomatic persons.

The effectiveness of screening for colorectal cancer has been a subject of controversy. In 1995, the US Preventive Task Force reversed earlier position statements and endorsed screening of asymptomatic average-risk persons, using fecal occult blood testing and sigmoidoscopy.[10,11] In 1996, the federal Agency for Health Care Policy and Research (AHCPR) convened a collaborative group of experts representing the American College of Gastroenterology, American Gastroenterological Association, American Society of Colon and Rectal Surgeons, American Society for Gastrointestinal Endoscopy, and Society of American Gastrointestinal Endoscopic Surgeons to critically evaluate the available evidence on colorectal cancer screening and to develop appropriate clinical practice guidelines.[12] The panel studied 3,500 peer-reviewed publications to assess the performance, effectiveness, acceptability to patients, cost-effectiveness, and outcome of different screening examinations. The AHCPR guidelines[13] were, in essence, endorsed by the American Cancer Society[14] and were used to create the Practice Parameters for the Detection of Colorectal Neoplasms published by the Standards Committee of the American Society of Colon and Rectal Surgeons.[15,16] The AHCPR guidelines provided the framework for colorectal cancer screening guidelines in the USA since they were published. The guidelines have been revised by various groups, including the US Preventive Task Force,[9] based on new data, new technology and evolving expert opinion.

Most people will be of average risk and require screening for colorectal cancer and polyps beginning at age 50. A substantial number of people are at increased risk because of an inherited predisposition to the disease and need screening or treatment as early as puberty. By virtue of their practice, colon and rectal surgeons, gastroenterologists, and medical oncologists have contact with a large number of patients with colorectal carcinoma as well as at-risk family members. These specialists have the opportunity to guide the evaluation of at-risk persons and be advocates for appropriate screening examinations.

Classification of Risk and Screening Recommendations

Making appropriate recommendations for screening of individuals depends on determining a patient's risk of future development of colorectal cancer. The cornerstone of determining a patient's risk for developing colorectal cancer is the family history. Failure to properly investigate a patient's family history of colorectal neoplasia can lead to inappropriate and inadequate treatment of both the patient and at-risk family members.

Average Risk

The majority of patients who develop colorectal cancer have no identifiable risk factors (Table 39-1). Persons considered to be at average risk for colorectal cancer do not fit any of the higher-risk categories. Specifically, average-risk persons have no symptoms associated with colorectal cancer, no personal history of colorectal cancer or adenomatous polyps, no family history of colorectal neoplasia, no inflammatory bowel disease, and no unexplained anemia.

In October 2008, the US Preventive Task Force recommended that average-risk persons should undergo one of

D.E. Beck et al. (eds.), *The ASCRS Textbook of Colon and Rectal Surgery: Second Edition*,
DOI 10.1007/978-1-4419-1584-9_39,

TABLE 39-1. Patients with colorectal cancer

75%	Average risk (sporadic)
15–20%	Family history of colorectal cancer
3–8%	Hereditary nonpolyposis colorectal cancer
1%	Familial adenomatous polyposis
1%	Ulcerative colitis

TABLE 39-2. Screening for colorectal cancer and polyps

Risk category	Screening method	Age to begin screening
Average risk	Choose one of the following: 1. High-sensitivity FOBT annually[a] 2. Flexible sigmoidoscopy every 5 years combined with high-sensitivity FOBT every 3 years[a] 3. Colonoscopy every 10 years	50 years
Family history	Choose one of the following: 1. Colonoscopy every 10 years 2. Colonoscopy every 5 years if diagnosis of colorectal cancer was made before age 60 3. Air contrast barium enema every 5 years[b]	40 or 10 years prior to diagnosis of the youngest affected family member, whichever is earliest
Lynch syndrome	Colonoscopy every 1–3 years Genetic counseling Consider genetic testing	21 years
Familial adenomatous polyposis	Flexible sigmoidoscopy or colonoscopy every 1–2 years Genetic counseling Consider genetic testing	Puberty
Inflammatory bowel disease (ulcerative colitis and Crohn's colitis)	Colonoscopy with random biopsies for dysplasia every 1–2 years	7–8 years after the onset of pancolitis; 12–15 years after the onset of left-sided colitis

FOBT fecal occult blood test.
[a]The American Cancer Society recommends the combination of yearly FOBT and flexible sigmoidoscopy is preferable to either examination alone.
[b]Proctoscopy is recommended as an adjunctive examination to allow adequate visualization of the distal rectum. Furthermore, flexible sigmoidoscopy may be necessary to more completely evaluate a tortuous or spastic sigmoid colon.

the following screening regimens, beginning at age 50 and continuing until age 75[9] (Table 39-2):

1. High-sensitivity fecal occult blood testing (FOBT) annually.
2. Flexible sigmoidoscopy every 5 years with high-sensitivity FOBT every 3 years.
3. Colonoscopy every 10 years.

Additionally, the taskforce recommended against routine screening in adults age 76–85, leaving the decision to continuing screening in this age range to the patient and primary care physician. The US Preventive Task Force specifically recommended against screening for colorectal cancer in patients greater than 85 years. Although the panel stated that all of the screening strategies are acceptable, they emphasized that each technique has unique strengths and weaknesses.[9]

The American Cancer Society, the US Multi-Society Task Force on Colorectal Cancer, and the American College of Radiology also recommended screening average-risk persons beginning at age 50. However, these groups did not recommend against routine screening in persons older than 76 years. Screening recommendations included several options[7,17]:

1. High-sensitivity FOBT or fecal immunochemical testing annually
2. Flexible sigmoidoscopy every 5 years
3. Double-contrast barium enema every 5 years
4. CT colonography every 5 years
5. Colonoscopy every 10 years
6. Fecal DNA testing (No interval specified).

In 2000, the American College of Gastroenterology proposed guidelines that outlined a "preferred" strategy for colorectal cancer screening. These were updated in 2008.[18] This approach was proposed based on evidence that patient compliance increased when there is a "preferred" strategy rather than a "menu" of options.[19] Preferred screening recommendations for average-risk persons beginning at age 50 included (screening should begin at age 45 in black patients):

1. Colonoscopy every 10 years
2. Annual fecal immunochemical test (FIT) for blood.

Alternative prevention tests

1. Flexible sigmoidoscopy every 5–10 years
2. CT colonography every 5 years.

Alterative cancer detection tests

1. Annual Hemoccult Sensa
2. Fecal DNA testing every 3 years.

Fecal Screening Tests

There are two types of fecal occult blood tests. The most common is a guaiac-based test for peroxidase activity that is nonspecific and will fail to detect many small cancers and precancerous lesions.[20] Nevertheless, several large randomized controlled trials as well as high-quality systematic reviews have shown that annual or biannual testing for fecal occult blood, with complete diagnostic evaluation of the colon (primarily with colonoscopy) for patients with a positive FOBT, reduces mortality from colorectal cancer.[3,21–24] More sensitive guaiac testing (Hemoccult Sensa, Beckman Coulter) is associated with a slightly higher sensitivity for detecting colorectal cancer. Testing of three samples is more sensitive than testing of a single sample. An alternative method of FOBT is the fecal immunochemical test. This exam employs antibodies specific to blood components.

A major drawback to using stool testing as a screening technique is poor compliance. Only 38–60% of the patients in prospective trials completed all the planned FOBT tests,[3,21,22] and use of FOBT in the general population is estimated to be lower than that in the research environment.[25] The steps necessary for adequate sample collection, combined with dietary restrictions to avoid agents that can cause false-positive and false-negative results may also hinder compliance with FOBT. Proper performance of FOBT involves the sampling of atraumatically obtained stool from three consecutive bowel movements in a patient who has not ingested red meat, aspirin, nonsteroidal inflammatory medications, turnips, melons, salmon, sardines, horseradish, or vitamin C for the 2 days preceding the test and throughout the test period.[13,26] The restriction of commonly ingested foods and medications, combined with the natural aversion to stool sampling, makes annual FOBT unappealing to many persons.

FOBT should not be confused with random stool guaiac testing, which is the analysis of stool found on digital rectal exam for blood. The lack of adequate diet and medication restriction prior to the test, potential for trauma to the anal canal during digital rectal examination, and the inability to reliably obtain stool from the distal rectum make the test unreliable.[27] To date, random stool guaiac examination has not been demonstrated to have benefit in screening for colorectal cancer.

In some settings, FOBT test slides are rehydrated, which contributes to the high incidence of false-positive tests and is not recommended by the manufacturer. Hemoccult Sensa, which appears to be at least as sensitive as the original hemoccult test, is the guaiac technique currently recommended for use.[28]

In the future, immunochemical techniques or genetic analysis of cellular material in stool may prove to be more effective than current FOBT technology in detecting occult colorectal neoplasms via stool sampling.[29,30] Colonic cells are constantly shed by colonic epithelium, DNA material can isolate from these cells and analyzed. Because there is variation in the genotypes of tumors, the ideal test would screen for a large panel of genetic mutations.[31] In 2004, the Colorectal Cancer Study Group compared Hemoccult II with fecal DNA testing (21 mutations) in 5,486 patients who subsequently underwent a colonoscopy.[32] The sensitivity of the fecal DNA test for advanced neoplasms (cancer, adenomas with villous or dysplastic histology, adenomas ≥ 10 mm) was 18% in comparison to Hemoccult II, which was 11%. The specificities were 94 and 95%, respectively. Another recent large study compared two different fecal DNA tests with Hemoccult II testing in patients who subsequently underwent colonoscopy.[33] The commercially available fecal DNA test, which examines 21 standard mutations including K-ras, APC, p53, BAT-26, and long DNA, provided no advantage over Hemoccult in the detection of dysplastic neoplasms or cancer. Sensitivity for "screen-relevant neoplasms" was modest: 20% by the DNA test, 11% by Hemoccult, and 21% by Hemoccult Sensa. A second novel fecal DNA test using three tumor-specific markers (K-ras mutations, APC mutator cluster regions, and vimentin methylation) was more sensitive than the commercial DNA test, Hemoccult, or Hemoccult Sensa in the detection of colorectal cancer and large adenomas but less specific. It remains unclear whether there are adequate data to support widespread use of fecal DNA tests as a viable colorectal cancer screening strategy.

Sigmoidoscopy

The effectiveness of sigmoidoscopy as a screening tool depends on its ability to detect cancers and adenomatous polyps in the distal colon. If adenomatous polyps are found at flexible sigmoidoscopy, colonoscopy should be strongly considered because almost one-third of such patients will have neoplastic lesions in the proximal colon.[34] The effectiveness of sigmoidoscopy in reducing mortality from colorectal cancer has never been proven by a randomized controlled trial, although case–control studies have shown a benefit.[2,6,35] There was only a trend toward limited benefit of one-time screening sigmoidoscopy, followed by colonoscopy for patients found to have polyps, in the Telemark study from Norway.[36,37] The Prostate, Lung, Colon, and Ovary Trial supported by the National Cancer Institute is evaluating flexible sigmoidoscopy in a randomized, controlled setting, but mortality data are not available at this time.[13] In this trial, wide variability in polyp detection rate was observed between endoscopists,[38] which raises concern regarding adequacy of the examination in the hands of inexperienced endoscopists. A multicenter prospective trial examining the potential benefit of one-time screening flexible sigmoidoscopy at age 60 is currently underway in the UK and Italy.[39] In this trial, it was noted that women who have undergone hysterectomy had fewer polyps detected at sigmoidoscopy and more pain than other patients, suggesting that these patients have less complete examinations.[40] A large randomized study in Norway could not demonstrate a decreased incidence of colorectal cancer or mortality when comparing one-time flexible sigmoidoscopy to no screening.[41]

Flexible sigmoidoscopy alone will fail to detect neoplasms in the proximal colon unless adenomatous polyps or cancer are found in the distal colon that prompt colonoscopy. For this reason, The American Cancer Society recommends combining flexible sigmoidoscopy every 5 years with annual FOBT, rather than utilizing flexible sigmoidoscopy alone as a screening method.[7,14] Although this combined approach may detect more proximal neoplasms than flexible sigmoidoscopy alone, 15–30% of patients with negative flexible sigmoidoscopy and negative FOBT will have neoplastic lesions in the proximal colon at colonoscopy, calling the rationale for this approach into question.[42–48] Given all the limitations of flexible sigmoidoscopy, it is unlikely that it will be the screening examination of choice in societies that can afford other screening methods that have greater efficacy and less patient discomfort.

Contrast Enema

The efficacy of barium enema in preventing colorectal cancer mortality has never been evaluated in a controlled trial, but can be inferred from the fact that detecting polyps and early stage cancers by other methods reduce the incidence and mortality from colorectal cancer. Air contrast barium enema will detect 50–80% of polyps < 1 cm, 70–90% of polyps > 1 cm, and 50–80% of Stage I and II adenocarcinomas.[49–52] Single column barium enema is less sensitive and should be combined with flexible sigmoidoscopy, if used as a screening tool.[13] Proctoscopy should be considered as an adjunct exam because the balloon on the enema catheter often prevents adequate imaging of the distal rectum. Another major limitation of barium enema as a screening method is that patients usually require colonoscopy, if lesions are detected.

Colonoscopy

Colonoscopy is the only screening technique that allows the detection and removal of premalignant lesions throughout the colon and rectum and is the final common pathway for any positive screening test. Although its effectiveness depends on the skill and experience of the endoscopist to both reach the cecum and identify small lesions, it remains the gold standard to evaluate the colonic mucosa.[13] The ability of colonoscopy to reduce colorectal cancer mortality has been demonstrated indirectly through studies showing that detecting and removing polyps reduces the incidence of colorectal cancer and that detecting early cancers lowers the mortality from the disease.[2–6] Compliance with screening colonoscopy may be superior to that of other methods because no confirmatory exams are required, and thus, patients are subjected to a single cathartic bowel preparation.

CT Colonography

CT colonography (virtual colonoscopy) was developed in an attempt to increase compliance with colorectal cancer screening, based on the impression that people would be more inclined to have a "scan" that a "scope." The technique involves thin-section computed tomography (CT) with three dimensional computer reconstructions to examine the colonic mucosa (Figure 39-1A and B).[53,54] Although the technique has the advantages of being considered "noninvasive" and not requiring sedation, a vigorous oral cathartic laxative preparation is required, because adherent stool cannot be reliably differentiated from neoplasia on CT. In

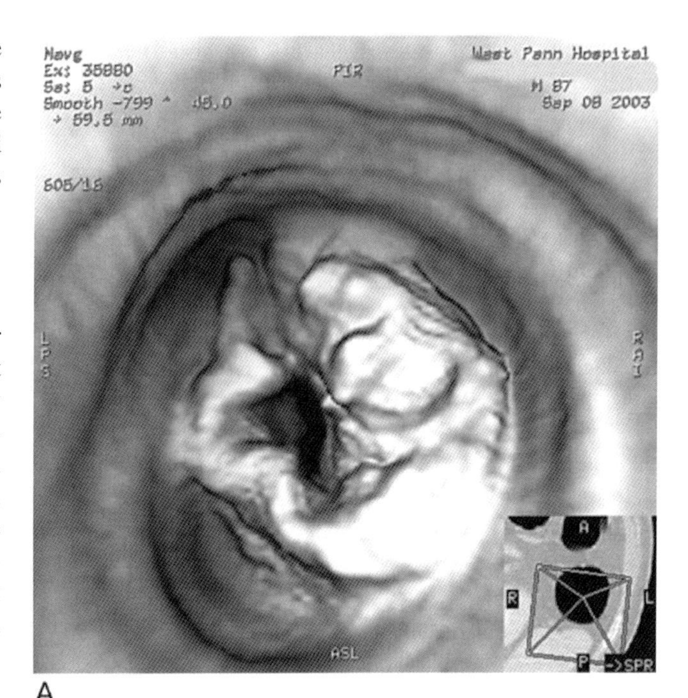

A

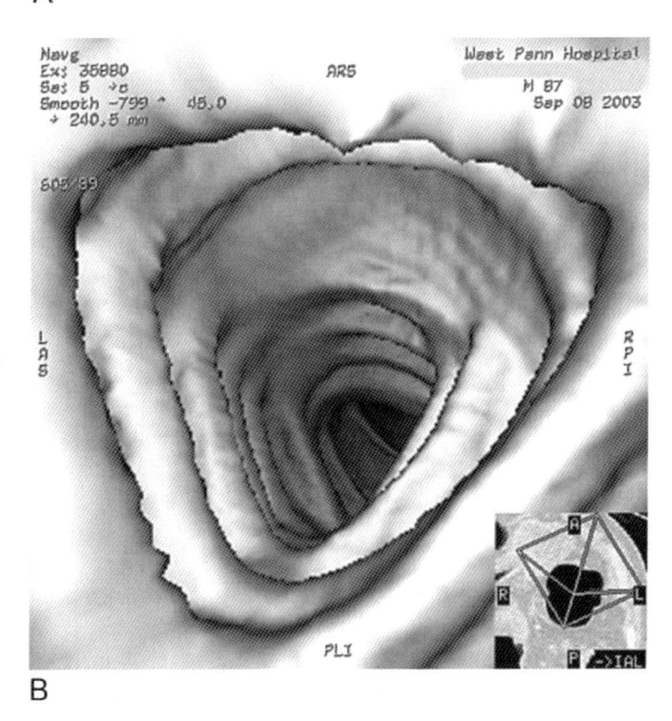

B

FIGURE 39-1. **A** CT colonography of an 87-year-old patient with a large tumor of the splenic flexure who could not undergo colonoscopy. The circumferential cancer can be seen occupying the lumen of the colon. **B** CT colonography of an 87-year-old patient with a large tumor of the splenic flexure who could not undergo colonoscopy. This image is of the transverse colon proximal to the cancer.

addition, a rectal catheter and air insufflation is utilized to distend the colon. CT colonography cannot be assumed to be more appealing to all patients who are reluctant to undergo colonoscopy, because many patients are deterred more by the laxative preparation beforehand than by the endoscopic procedure itself and find rectal air insufflation in the absence of sedation uncomfortable.[55] Initial trials demonstrated that CT colonography was not as sensitive as colonoscopy in the detection of small polyps.[56] Recent improvements in technology and experience with interpretation have resulted in improved performance of the test. The sensitivity for the detection of polyps 10 mm or larger can be up to 90% with a specificity of 86% in the hands of interested radiologists.[57] Polyps that are 6 mm or larger have detection rate of up to 78% with a specificity of 88%.[7,57–60] CT colonography is both less sensitive and less specific in the detection of polyps less than 6 mm in size.

Controversy exists regarding the size of polyp detected at CT colonography that should prompt optical colonoscopy. If the polyp size cutoff is small, then the number of patients that are referred for colonoscopy will be large and the cost of the program high. If the polyp size cutoff is larger, then the number of patients that are referred for colonoscopy will be smaller and the cost of the program will be lower, although there is an increased risk of leaving neoplastic polyps in situ. If 6 mm is chosen as a cutoff size, it is estimated that 15–25% of patient undergoing screening CT colonography would be referred for colonoscopy.[59,61,62] Even at this small polyp cutoff size, there is controversy regarding the practice of leaving polyps in situ because the natural history of small polyps (<6 mm) is unknown.[59,63] Regardless of its accuracy, CT colonography suffers (as does contrast enema) from the disadvantage that biopsies cannot be obtained and positive findings require endoscopic confirmation. Other disadvantages include radiation exposure and the cost of managing extracolonic findings. It is estimated that 27–69% of patients who have CT colonography will have at least one potentially pathologic finding in an organ outside of the colon.[7–9]

For all these reasons, CT colonography is not utilized at most centers as the preferred initial screening test. CT colonography is an excellent choice, however, for the evaluation of a patient who has just had an incomplete colonoscopy. The colon is already prepared and it is distended by air. Ultimately, if stool labeling technology improves to the point where cathartic bowel preparation and transanal gas insufflation of the colon are no longer necessary, then CT colonography could gain traction as the preferred initial screening test for colorectal cancer.

Cost and Reimbursement

The Office of Technology Assessment of the US Congress found that FOBT, flexible sigmoidoscopy, air contrast barium enema, and colonoscopy are equally cost-effective as screening strategies, with an estimated cost of less than $20,000 per year of life saved (assuming screening begins at age 50 and is discontinued at age 85).[13,64,65] Although cost–benefit analyses such as these are exceedingly complex, this estimate is well within the acceptable range of cost-effectiveness by US health standards and compares favorably to screening mammography for women over age 50. As of January 1, 1998, the Centers for Medicare and Medicaid Services (CMS) has reimbursed screening examinations for colorectal cancer in average-risk persons over the age of 50.[66] In 2001, CMS authorized reimbursement for screening colonoscopy for average-risk persons. As of January 2010, the CMS guidelines for reimbursement for colorectal cancer screening are as follows (excerpted from their website, http://www.cms.hhs.gov/ColorectalCancerScreening).

- Fecal occult blood test (FOBT) – once every year.
- Flexible sigmoidoscopy – once every 4 years.
- Colonoscopy – once every 2 years, if the patient is at high risk for colon cancer; and once every 10 years (but not within 47 months of a screening sigmoidoscopy), if the patient is not at high risk for colon cancer.
- Double-contrast barium enema – physician can decide to use instead of a sigmoidoscopy or colonoscopy.

At present, the choice of screening strategy for average-risk persons is made with influence from primary care physicians, patients, and third-party payors. Several of the recommended strategies depend on compliance with yearly FOBT, which has been extremely difficult to achieve even in the setting of controlled trials. Only air contrast barium enema and colonoscopy provide total colonic evaluation, and contrast enema suffers from the necessity of performing colonoscopy if a lesion is detected. The American College of Gastroenterology suggested that screening colonoscopy every 10 years beginning at age 50 is the preferred method of screening average-risk persons for colorectal cancer.[18]

Personal History of Adenomatous Polyps or Adenocarcinoma

A personal history of adenomatous polyps or colorectal adenocarcinoma places a person at higher than average risk for the development of metachronous neoplasms. Patients who undergo curative resection of colorectal adenocarcinoma should undergo regular surveillance colonoscopy to detect new metachronous primary neoplasms. The recommendation of the Standards Task Committee of the American Society of Colon and Rectal Surgeons is for initial postresection colonoscopy at 1 year, followed by colonoscopy every 3–5 years thereafter, depending on the pathology found at the preceding colonoscopic examination. The US Multi-Society Task Force on Colorectal Cancer and the American Cancer Society outlined guidelines for colonoscopy after polypectomy and colorectal cancer resection in 2008.[67] This panel recommended that patients with hyperplastic polyps should be considered average risk and therefore screened every 10 years. Patients with an adenomatous polyp greater than 1 cm should have a repeat colonoscopy in 3 years. Patients who have adenomas with villous features or high-grade dysplasia are also recommended to have a surveillance colonoscopy in 3 years. Patients with fewer than three small adenomas may be surveyed every 5–10 years. After resection of colorectal cancers, the panel recommended that patients undergo a colonoscopy at 1 year.

Clearly, these recommendations can be altered given the specific details of the clinical situation. A rational surveillance strategy should take into account the patient's age, comorbid conditions, life expectancy, completeness of prior examinations, pattern of neoplastic growth, family history, and histologic features of previously resected neoplasms. For example, a patient in good health who is found to have adenomas that are multiple, large, sessile, dysplastic, or removed in a piecemeal fashion on initial screening colonoscopy should be considered for colonoscopy at an earlier interval, such as 6–12 months. However, a 90-year-old patient with severe comorbidities and limited life expectancy may not benefit from surveillance examinations, because removal of premalignant lesions will probably not alter lifespan or quality of life.

Family History of Colorectal Cancer or Adenomatous Polyps

A family history of colorectal cancer or adenomatous polyps increases the risk of developing colorectal cancer. In general, closer familial relationships to affected relatives, younger age of onset, and larger numbers of affected relatives increase the risk.[13,68,69] A careful family history should always be obtained to exclude one of the better-defined inherited colorectal cancer syndromes, such as Lynch syndrome or familial adenomatous polyposis (FAP).

As a greater understanding of the molecular genetics of colorectal cancer is gained, many patients with familial colorectal cancer may eventually be categorized as having distinct inherited syndromes. For example, a germline mutation of the adenomatous polyposis coli gene (I1307K variant) was identified in persons of Ashkenazi Jewish descent that predisposes to the development of colorectal adenomas and carcinoma.[12,70–75]The mutation causes hypermutability of the adenomatous polyposis coli gene and is thought to contribute to carcinogenesis independent of mismatch repair deficiency.[72] In the future, genetic testing for this mutation in at-risk persons may have clinical utility.

Screening Recommendations

The AHCPR panel recommended that patients with first-degree relatives with colorectal cancer or adenomatous polyps begin screening for colorectal neoplasia at age 40, or 10 years prior to the age at diagnosis of the affected relative, whichever is earliest.[13] Those patients whose first-degree relatives developed colorectal cancer prior to age 50 may be at higher risk, and complete colonic evaluation with colonoscopy should be strongly considered.[13] Patients with a second-degree relative with colorectal cancer, or relative with adenomatous polyps diagnosed over age 60, may be screened as an average-risk person.[13]

More recently, the American College of Gastroenterology recommended that patients with a single first-degree relative (<60 years) with colorectal cancer or an adenoma > 1 cm or an adenoma with villous features or high-grade dysplasia begin screening at age 40 or 10 years before the diagnosis in the youngest affected relative. Surveillance should be repeated every 5 years. If the initial diagnosis of colorectal cancer was made after age 60, then surveillance can be carried out every 10 years. This recommendation emphasizes that an increased level of screening is not recommended for a history of adenomas without adverse features in a first-degree relative.[18]

Lynch Syndrome

Lynch syndrome (formerly hereditary nonpolyposis colorectal cancer syndrome) is an inherited disorder that predisposes patients to the development of colorectal cancer, with up to 75% of patients developing colorectal cancer by age 65.[76–79] Lynch syndrome is inherited in an autosomal dominant fashion and is thought to be the result of germline mutations in mismatch repair genes (genes that code for proteins responsible for correcting errors during DNA replication). Patients with Lynch syndrome typically develop cancer between age 40 and 50 and most tumors occur proximal to the splenic flexure. "Nonpolyposis" in the term "hereditary nonpolyposis colorectal cancer" refers to the distinction between Lynch syndrome and FAP (in which patients have hundreds of polyps), but is somewhat misleading as patients with Lynch syndrome will develop adenomatous polyps. The major distinction is that progression from adenoma to carcinoma appears to be accelerated in Lynch syndrome patients as compared to patients with sporadic cancers and FAP, and there is a tendency to develop multiple colorectal cancers in Lynch syndrome.[76,80–82] Patients with Lynch syndrome have germline mutations and are also at high risk for the development of other cancers including endometrial, ovarian, gastric, transitional cell, small bowel, and hepatobiliary neoplasms.

The ability to conclusively identify gene carriers is not yet fully developed, thus the penetrance of colorectal cancer in gene carriers can only be estimated (about 90%). In addition, some patients in Lynch syndrome families who do not have identifiable germline mismatch repair gene mutations will develop colorectal cancer.[83] For these reasons, the diagnosis of Lynch syndrome in a family remains clinical. The Amsterdam I criteria (colorectal cancer in three or more family members, two generations affected, one affected person a first-degree relative of another, and one cancer diagnosed prior to age 50) are the most stringent criteria and have the highest concordance with known mismatch repair gene mutations.[83] These criteria were originally developed for research purposes, to standardize the definition of Lynch syndrome. However, they fail to identify patients who may be affected with Lynch syndrome but do not fit the strict criteria because of unknown or abbreviated family histories, as well as patients with a personal or family history of extracolonic malignancies associated with Lynch syndrome. The Bethesda criteria were developed to acknowledge the shortcomings of the Amsterdam I criteria as clinical guidelines and to expand the clinical suspicion of Lynch syndrome to a broader range of patients.[79,84] Other groups have also published revised criteria for Lynch syndrome because of the above reasons. It is thus of paramount importance that persons being interviewed to determine their risk for colorectal cancer be questioned regarding a family history of the most common Lynch syndrome-related cancers.

Microsatellite instability has been reported in 85–90% of Lynch syndrome colorectal cancers.[77] Detection of this phenotype has been proposed as a screening method to trigger germline mutational analysis in kindreds with uncertain family histories.[79] However, microsatellite instability is also found in approximately 15% of sporadic cancers and has not been universally found to be predictive of familial cancer.[83,85] Patients who satisfy the Bethesda criteria should have immunohistochemistry staining for mismatch repair proteins or microsatellite testing of their, or an afflicted family member's, neoplasm. Germline mutational analysis can then be performed. If a proband tests positive, the appropriate family members can be offered screening. Clinically, the absence of microsatellite instability or mismatch repair gene mutation does not negate a family history that suggests an autosomal dominant predisposition to developing colorectal cancer. At-risk family members still require aggressive screening.

Screening Recommendations

The American College of Gastroenterology recommends that persons who are members of a family that fits clinical criteria for Lynch syndrome undergo colonoscopy at age 20–25 and repeat colonoscopy every 2 years until age 40. The panel recommends that patients should have annual colonoscopies after age 40.[18] The short-time interval between colonoscopies results from the accelerated adenoma to carcinoma progression thought to occur in Lynch syndrome. Patients and at-risk family members should be referred for genetic counseling. A number of authors have recommended that patients with Lynch syndrome may have increased polyp detection rates, if they are screened with chromoendoscopy or narrow band imaging.[86–89] It is not known whether these techniques may allow longer screening intervals in the future.

Familial Adenomatous Polyposis

Familial adenomatous polyposis (FAP) is caused by a germline defect in the adenomatous polyposis coli gene, which is inherited in autosomal dominant fashion.[90] Patients with FAP develop hundreds of adenomatous polyps as early as puberty and will ultimately develop colorectal cancer usually by age 40.[91,92] Patients with FAP are also prone to develop a variety of extracolonic tumors, notably duodenal adenomas and carcinomas, and desmoid tumors.[91] FAP mutations do occur spontaneously, accounting for patients who are diagnosed with the disease without a family history of FAP.[93] Attenuated FAP is a rare variant of the disease, with polyps and cancers developing later in life.[94]

In the past, a commonly used genetic test for FAP was an assay for a truncated protein product of the mutated adenomatous polyposis coli gene. Because only about 80% of families with FAP will have a mutation that produces a truncated protein, the predictive value of testing at-risk family members is greatest if the proband (affected relative) has a positive test.[95] At present, germline mutational analysis is the preferred method of confirmation of the disease. If patients suspected of having FAP are not found to have an APC mutation, then MYH polyposis should be considered.

Screening Recommendations

Patients with a family history of FAP should undergo flexible sigmoidoscopy or colonoscopy at puberty.[13,96] Lower endoscopy should be repeated every 1–2 years. Patients with FAP are also at risk for the development of gastric, periampullary, and duodenal adenomas. Patients with FAP should undergo upper endoscopic surveillance every 1–3 years.[18,97] Genetic testing should be considered, especially in large pedigrees where genotyping might be more cost-effective than repeated endoscopy.[96] If the proband has a positive genetic assay, at-risk relatives who test negative may be screened as average-risk persons.[96]

Because of the socioeconomic, medicolegal, and emotional issues surrounding genetic testing, it cannot be emphasized enough that genetic testing for FAP should be done after genetic counseling and informed consent.[95] Trained genetic counselors can guide patients through the testing process and help interpret results. Lest physicians think that they do not need assistance in this regard, they should look at the work of Giardiello et al. who found that 32% of physicians ordering genetic tests for FAP misinterpreted the results of the test and that less than 20% of patients tested had received pretest genetic counseling or written informed consent.[95] These numbers are sobering when one considers that FAP has 100% mortality if left untreated. Patients should also undergo screening upper endoscopy for duodenal adenomas.[98]

Inflammatory Bowel Disease

Patients with ulcerative colitis have an increased risk of developing colorectal cancer, probably because of the chronic effects of inflammation on the mucosa, leading to malignant degeneration. However, because of the altered appearance of the mucosa, carcinomas are sometimes difficult to identify endoscopically. Frequent colonoscopy with random biopsy is recommended, in an attempt to identify early stage carcinomas or premalignant change (dysplasia) that would predict the presence of occult carcinoma or predict the subsequent development of carcinoma. Proctocolectomy could then be performed for cure or prophylaxis. The risk of colorectal cancer in patients with Crohn's disease is now considered to be similar to that of patients with ulcerative colitis and therefore they should be screened in similar fashion.[97,99]

Screening Recommendations

It is now common practice for patients with inflammatory bowel disease to undergo screening colonoscopy with multiple random biopsies looking for dysplasia every 1–2 years, beginning 7–8 years after disease onset in patients with pancolitis, and 12–15 years after disease onset in patients with left-sided colitis.[13,100,101] Mucosal biopsies are taken every 10 cm from normal appearing mucosa. Abnormal appearing lesions should also be biopsied.[97] Random biopsies should be avoided in areas of acute colitis. Despite the consensus recommendation to perform surveillance colonoscopy with random biopsy, definitive evidence that surveillance reduces mortality, or is better than timing a colectomy according to extent and duration of disease, is lacking.[13,100,101]

Future Directions

It is troubling that so much energy and expense is devoted to the cure of advanced or recurrent colorectal cancer in the USA, while so little is devoted to screening for polyps and early stage cancers. It is estimated that only 50% of adults over the age of 50 in this country underwent FOBT or endoscopy for colorectal cancer screening in 2005.[102] Although this represents a substantial increase from screening rates of the past, it is still woefully inadequate given that colorectal cancer is the second leading cause of cancer-related death and is largely preventable by adequate screening. In a report issued in 2002, the US General Accounting Office found that colorectal cancer screening is the least utilized preventive health benefit available to Medicare beneficiaries (General Accounting Office, Medicare – Beneficiary Use of Clinical Preventive Services, Report No. GAO-22-422; April 2002). As is the case in the general population, only 25% of Medicare beneficiaries are screened each year with FOBT, compared with much higher rates for other regular cancer screening tests such as mammography (75%) or Pap smear testing (66%). More recent data suggest that among Medicare beneficiaries aged 65–80, colonoscopy rates have increased while FOBT rates decreased.[103] Both health care professionals and the public need to become more aware of the potential benefits of colorectal cancer screening.

As the genetics of inherited colorectal cancer syndromes become better understood, it will be possible to conclusively identify high-risk populations. It is of paramount importance that screening efforts be directed toward these populations. Genetic counselors are invaluable resources, both to counsel family members and to help direct genetic testing.

References

1. Jemal A, Siegel R, Ward E, Hao Y, Xu J, Thun MJ. Cancer statistics, 2009. CA Cancer J Clin. 2009;59:225–49.
2. Newcomb P, Norfleet R, Storer B, Surawicz T, Marcus P. Screening sigmoidoscopy and colorectal cancer mortality. J Natl Cancer Inst. 1992;84:1572–5.
3. Kronborg O, Fenger C, Olsen J, Jorgensen OD, Sondergaard O. Randomised study of screening for colorectal cancer with faecal-occult-blood test. Lancet. 1996;348:1467–71.
4. Winawer SJ, Flehinger BJ, Schottenfeld D, Miller DG. Screening for colorectal cancer with fecal occult blood testing and sigmoidoscopy. J Natl Cancer Inst. 1993;85:1311–8.
5. Winawer SJ, Zauber AG, Ho MN, et al. Prevention of colorectal cancer by colonoscopic polypectomy. The National Polyp Study Workgroup. N Engl J Med. 1993;329:1977–81.
6. Muller AD, Sonnenberg A. Protection by endoscopy against death from colorectal cancer. A case-control study among veterans. Arch Intern Med. 1995;155:1741–8.
7. Levin B, Lieberman DA, McFarland B, et al. Screening and surveillance for the early detection of colorectal cancer and adenomatous polyps, 2008: a joint guideline from the American Cancer Society, the US Multi-Society Task Force on Colorectal Cancer, and the American College of Radiology. Gastroenterology. 2008;134:1570–95.
8. Whitlock EP, Lin JS, Liles E, Beil TL, Fu R. Screening for colorectal cancer: a targeted, updated systematic review for the U.S. Preventive Services Task Force. Ann Intern Med. 2008;149:638–58.
9. U.S. Preventive Services Task Force. Screening for colorectal cancer: U.S. Preventive Services Task Force recommendation statement. Ann Intern Med. 2008;149:627–37.
10. Frame PS, Berg AO, Woolf S. U.S. Preventive Services Task Force: highlights of the 1996 report. Am Fam Physician. 1997;55:567–76. 581–2.
11. Levin B, Bond JH. Colorectal cancer screening: recommendations of the U.S. Preventive Services Task Force. American Gastroenterological Association. Gastroenterology. 1996;111:1381–4.
12. Laken SJ, Petersen GM, Gruber SB, et al. Familial colorectal cancer in Ashkenazim due to a hypermutable tract in APC. Nat Genet. 1997;17:79–83.
13. Winawer SJ, Fletcher RH, Miller L, et al. Colorectal cancer screening: clinical guidelines and rationale. Gastroenterology. 1997;112:594–642.

14. Byers T, Levin B, Rothenberger D, Dodd GD, Smith RA. American Cancer Society guidelines for screening and surveillance for early detection of colorectal polyps and cancer: update 1997. American Cancer Society Detection and Treatment Advisory Group on Colorectal Cancer. CA Cancer J Clin. 1997;47:154–60.
15. Simmang CL, Senatore P, Lowry A, et al. Practice parameters for detection of colorectal neoplasms. The Standards Committee, The American Society of Colon and Rectal Surgeons. Dis Colon Rectum. 1999;42:1123–9.
16. Ko C, Hyman NH. Practice parameter for the detection of colorectal neoplasms: an interim report (revised). Dis Colon Rectum. 2006;49:299–301.
17. Levin B, Lieberman DA, McFarland B, et al. Screening and surveillance for the early detection of colorectal cancer and adenomatous polyps, 2008: a joint guideline from the American Cancer Society, the US Multi-Society Task Force on Colorectal Cancer, and the American College of Radiology. CA Cancer J Clin. 2008;58:130–60.
18. Rex DK, Johnson DA, Anderson JC, Schoenfeld PS, Burke CA, Inadomi JM. American College of Gastroenterology guidelines for colorectal cancer screening 2009 [corrected]. Am J Gastroenterol. 2009;104:739–50.
19. Inadomi J, Kuhn L, Vijan S, et al. Adherence to competing colorectal cancer screening strategies. Am J Gastroenterol. 2005;100:S387–8.
20. Rockey DC, Koch J, Cello JP, Sanders LL, McQuaid K. Relative frequency of upper gastrointestinal and colonic lesions in patients with positive fecal occult-blood tests. N Engl J Med. 1998;339:153–9.
21. Hardcastle JD, Chamberlain JO, Robinson MH, et al. Randomised controlled trial of faecal-occult-blood screening for colorectal cancer. Lancet. 1996;348:1472–7.
22. Mandel JS, Bond JH, Church TR, et al. Reducing mortality from colorectal cancer by screening for fecal occult blood. Minnesota Colon Cancer Control Study. N Engl J Med. 1993;328:1365–71.
23. Hewitson P, Glasziou P, Irwig L, Towler B, Watson E. Screening for colorectal cancer using the faecal occult blood test, Hemoccult. Cochrane Database Syst Rev. 2007. CD001216.
24. Jorgensen OD, Kronborg O, Fenger C. A randomised study of screening for colorectal cancer using faecal occult blood testing: results after 13 years and seven biennial screening rounds. Gut. 2002;50:29–32.
25. Anderson LM, May DS. Has the use of cervical, breast, and colorectal cancer screening increased in the United States? Am J Public Health. 1995;85:840–2.
26. Ransohoff DF, Lang CA. Screening for colorectal cancer with the fecal occult blood test: a background paper. American College of Physicians. Ann Intern Med. 1997;126:811–22.
27. Nakama H, Fattah AS, Zhang B, Kamijo N. Digital rectal examination sampling of stool is less predictive of significant colorectal pathology than stool passed spontaneously. Eur J Gastroenterol Hepatol. 2000;12:1235–8.
28. Colorectal Cancer Screening. Clinical practice guidelines in oncology. J Natl Compr Canc Netw. 2003;1:72–93.
29. Traverso G, Shuber A, Levin B, et al. Detection of APC mutations in fecal DNA from patients with colorectal tumors. N Engl J Med. 2002;346:311–20.
30. Limburg PJ, Devens ME, Harrington JJ, Diehl NN, Mahoney DW, Ahlquist DA. Prospective evaluation of fecal calprotectin as a screening biomarker for colorectal neoplasia. Am J Gastroenterol. 2003;98:2299–305.
31. An SW, Kim NK, Chung HC. Genetic and epigenetic marker-based DNA test of stool is a promising approach for colorectal cancer screening. Yonsei Med J. 2009;50:331–4.
32. Imperiale TF, Ransohoff DF, Itzkowitz SH, Turnbull BA, Ross ME. Fecal DNA versus fecal occult blood for colorectal-cancer screening in an average-risk population. N Engl J Med. 2004;351:2704–14.
33. Ahlquist DA, Sargent DJ, Loprinzi CL, et al. Stool DNA and occult blood testing for screen detection of colorectal neoplasia. Ann Intern Med. 2008;149:441–50. W481.
34. Read TE, Read JD, Butterly LF. Importance of adenomas 5 mm or less in diameter that are detected by sigmoidoscopy. N Engl J Med. 1997;336:8–12.
35. Selby J, Friedman G, Quesenberry C, Weiss N. A case-control study of screening sigmoidoscopy and mortality from colorectal cancer. N Engl J Med. 1992;326:653–7.
36. Thiis-Evensen E, Hoff GS, Sauar J, Langmark F, Majak BM, Vatn MH. Population-based surveillance by colonoscopy: effect on the incidence of colorectal cancer. Telemark Polyp Study I. Scand J Gastroenterol. 1999;34:414–20.
37. Thiis-Evensen E, Hoff GS, Sauar J, Majak BM, Vatn MH. The effect of attending a flexible sigmoidoscopic screening program on the prevalence of colorectal adenomas at 13-year follow-up. Am J Gastroenterol. 2001;96:1901–7.
38. Pinsky PF, Schoen RE, Weissfeld JL, Kramer B, Hayes RB, Yokochi L. Variability in flexible sigmoidoscopy performance among examiners in a screening trial. Clin Gastroenterol Hepatol. 2005;3:792–7.
39. Atkin WS, Edwards R, Wardle J, et al. Design of a multicentre randomised trial to evaluate flexible sigmoidoscopy in colorectal cancer screening. J Med Screen. 2001;8:137–44.
40. Adams C, Cardwell C, Cook C, Edwards R, Atkin WS, Morton DG. Effect of hysterectomy status on polyp detection rates at screening flexible sigmoidoscopy. Gastrointest Endosc. 2003;57:848–53.
41. Hoff G, Grotmol T, Skovlund E, Bretthauer M. Risk of colorectal cancer seven years after flexible sigmoidoscopy screening: randomised controlled trial. BMJ. 2009;338:b1846.
42. Lieberman D, Smith F. Screening for colon malignancy with colonoscopy. Am J Gastroenterol. 1991;86:946–51.
43. Achkar E, Carey W. Small polyps found during fiberoptic sigmoidoscopy in asymptomatic patients. Ann Intern Med. 1988;109:880–3.
44. Brady PG, Straker RJ, McClave SA, Nord HJ, Pinkas M, Robinson BE. Are hyperplastic rectosigmoid polyps associated with an increased risk of proximal colonic neoplasms? Gastrointest Endosc. 1993;39:481–5.
45. Rex DK, Smith JJ, Ulbright TM, Lehman GA. Distal colonic hyperplastic polyps do not predict proximal adenomas in asymptomatic average-risk subjects. Gastroenterology. 1992;102:317–9.
46. Mehran A, Jaffe P, Efron J, Vernavay A, Liberman A. Screening colonoscopy in the asymptomatic 50- to 59-year-old population. Surg Endosc. 2003;17:1974–7.
47. Lieberman DA, Weiss DG, Bond JH, Ahnen DJ, Garewal H, Chejfec G. Use of colonoscopy to screen asymptomatic adults

for colorectal cancer. Veterans Affairs Cooperative Study Group 380. N Engl J Med. 2000;343:162–8.
48. Imperiale TF, Wagner DR, Lin CY, Larkin GN, Rogge JD, Ransohoff DF. Risk of advanced proximal neoplasms in asymptomatic adults according to the distal colorectal findings. N Engl J Med. 2000;343:169–74.
49. Steine S, Stordahl A, Lunde OC, Loken K, Laerum E. Double-contrast barium enema versus colonoscopy in the diagnosis of neoplastic disorders: aspects of decision-making in general practice. Fam Pract. 1993;10:288–91.
50. Hixson LJ, Fennerty MB, Sampliner RE, McGee D, Garewal H. Prospective study of the frequency and size distribution of polyps missed by colonoscopy. J Natl Cancer Inst. 1990;82:1769–72.
51. Hixson LJ, Fennerty MB, Sampliner RE, Garewal HS. Prospective blinded trial of the colonoscopic miss-rate of large colorectal polyps. Gastrointest Endosc. 1991;37:125–7.
52. Fork FT. Double contrast enema and colonoscopy in polyp detection. Gut. 1981;22:971–7.
53. Fenlon HM, Nunes DP, Clarke PD, Ferrucci JT. Colorectal neoplasm detection using virtual colonoscopy: a feasibility study. Gut. 1998;43:806–11.
54. Rex DK. CT and MR colography (virtual colonoscopy): status report. J Clin Gastroenterol. 1998;27:199–203.
55. Akerkar GA, Yee J, Hung R, McQuaid K. Patient experience and preferences toward colon cancer screening: a comparison of virtual colonoscopy and conventional colonoscopy. Gastrointest Endosc. 2001;54:310–5.
56. Fenlon HM, Nunes DP, Schroy 3rd PC, Barish MA, Clarke PD, Ferrucci JT. A comparison of virtual and conventional colonoscopy for the detection of colorectal polyps. N Engl J Med. 1999;341:1496–503.
57. Johnson CD, Chen MH, Toledano AY, et al. Accuracy of CT colonography for detection of large adenomas and cancers. N Engl J Med. 2008;359:1207–17.
58. Gluecker TM, Johnson CD, Harmsen WS, et al. Colorectal cancer screening with CT colonography, colonoscopy, and double-contrast barium enema examination: prospective assessment of patient perceptions and preferences. Radiology. 2003;227:378–84.
59. Lieberman D, Moravec M, Holub J, Michaels L, Eisen G. Polyp size and advanced histology in patients undergoing colonoscopy screening: implications for CT colonography. Gastroenterology. 2008;135:1100–5.
60. Rex DK, Imperiale TF. CT colonography versus colonoscopy for the detection of advanced neoplasia. N Engl J Med. 2008;358:88. author reply 90.
61. Cotton PB, Durkalski VL, Pineau BC, et al. Computed tomographic colonography (virtual colonoscopy): a multicenter comparison with standard colonoscopy for detection of colorectal neoplasia. JAMA. 2004;291:1713–9.
62. Rockey DC, Paulson E, Niedzwiecki D, et al. Analysis of air contrast barium enema, computed tomographic colonography, and colonoscopy: prospective comparison. Lancet. 2005;365:305–11.
63. Butterly LF, Chase MP, Pohl H, Fiarman GS. Prevalence of clinically important histology in small adenomas. Clin Gastroenterol Hepatol. 2006;4:343–8.
64. Wagner JL. Cost-effectiveness of screening for common cancers. Cancer Metastasis Rev. 1997;16:281–94.
65. Wagner J, The Congressional Office of Technology Assessment. JAMA. 1990;264:2732.
66. Sheldon GF. Professionalism, managed care and the human rights movement. Bull Am Coll Surg. 1998;83:13–33.
67. Brooks DD, Winawer SJ, Rex DK, et al. Colonoscopy surveillance after polypectomy and colorectal cancer resection. Am Fam Physician. 2008;77:995–1002.
68. Winawer SJ, Zauber AG, Gerdes H, et al. Risk of colorectal cancer in the families of patients with adenomatous polyps. National Polyp Study Workgroup. N Engl J Med. 1996;334:82–7.
69. Fuchs CS, Giovannucci EL, Colditz GA, Hunter DJ, Speizer FE, Willett WC. A prospective study of family history and the risk of colorectal cancer. N Engl J Med. 1994;331:1669–74.
70. Frayling IM, Beck NE, Ilyas M, et al. The APC variants I1307K and E1317Q are associated with colorectal tumors, but not always with a family history. Proc Natl Acad Sci USA. 1998;95:10722–7.
71. Gryfe R, Di NN, Lal G, Gallinger S, Redston M. Inherited colorectal polyposis and cancer risk of the APC I1307K polymorphism. Am J Hum Genet. 1999;64:378–84.
72. Prior TW, Chadwick RB, Papp AC, et al. The I1307K polymorphism of the APC gene in colorectal cancer. Gastroenterology. 1999;116:58–63.
73. Rozen P, Shomrat R, Strul H, et al. Prevalence of the I1307K APC gene variant in Israeli Jews of differing ethnic origin and risk for colorectal cancer. Gastroenterology. 1999;116:54–7.
74. Woodage T, King SM, Wacholder S, et al. The APCI1307K allele and cancer risk in a community-based study of Ashkenazi Jews. Nat Genet. 1998;20:62–5.
75. Gryfe R, Di NN, Gallinger S, Redston M. Somatic instability of the APC I1307K allele in colorectal neoplasia. Cancer Res. 1998;58:4040–3.
76. Burke W, Petersen G, Lynch P, et al. Recommendations for follow-up care of individuals with an inherited predisposition to cancer. I. Hereditary nonpolyposis colon cancer. Cancer Genetics Studies Consortium. JAMA. 1997;277:915–9.
77. Lynch HT, Smyrk T. Hereditary nonpolyposis colorectal cancer (Lynch syndrome). An updated review. Cancer. 1996;78:1149–67.
78. Myrhoj T, Bisgaard ML, Bernstein I, Svendsen LB, Sondergaard JO, Bulow S. Hereditary non-polyposis colorectal cancer: clinical features and survival. Results from the Danish HNPCC register. Scand J Gastroenterol. 1997;32:572–6.
79. Rodriguez-Bigas MA, Boland CR, Hamilton SR, et al. A National Cancer Institute workshop on hereditary nonpolyposis colorectal cancer syndrome: meeting highlights and Bethesda guidelines. J Natl Cancer Inst. 1997;89:1758–62.
80. Box JC, Rodriguez-Bigas MA, Weber TK, Petrelli NJ. Clinical implications of multiple colorectal carcinomas in hereditary nonpolyposis colorectal carcinoma. Dis Colon Rectum. 1999;42:717–21.
81. Fitzgibbons Jr RJ, Lynch HT, Stanislav GV, et al. Recognition and treatment of patients with hereditary nonpolyposis colon cancer (Lynch syndromes I and II). Ann Surg. 1987;206:289–95.
82. Watson P, Lin KM, Rodriguez-Bigas MA, et al. Colorectal carcinoma survival among hereditary nonpolyposis colorectal carcinoma family members. Cancer. 1998;83:259–66.
83. Park JG, Vasen HF, Park KJ, et al. Suspected hereditary nonpolyposis colorectal cancer: International Collaborative

Group on Hereditary Non-Polyposis Colorectal Cancer (ICG-HNPCC) criteria and results of genetic diagnosis. Dis Colon Rectum. 1999;42:710–5.

84. Umar A, Boland CR, Terdiman JP, et al. Revised Bethesda Guidelines for hereditary nonpolyposis colorectal cancer (Lynch syndrome) and microsatellite instability. J Natl Cancer Inst. 2004;96:261–8.
85. Samowitz WS, Slattery ML, Kerber RA. Microsatellite instability in human colonic cancer is not a useful clinical indicator of familial colorectal cancer. Gastroenterology. 1995;109:1765–71.
86. East JE, Suzuki N, Stavrinidis M, Guenther T, Thomas HJ, Saunders BP. Narrow band imaging for colonoscopic surveillance in hereditary non-polyposis colorectal cancer. Gut. 2008;57:65–70.
87. Lecomte T, Cellier C, Meatchi T, et al. Chromoendoscopic colonoscopy for detecting preneoplastic lesions in hereditary nonpolyposis colorectal cancer syndrome. Clin Gastroenterol Hepatol. 2005;3:897–902.
88. Stoffel EM, Turgeon DK, Stockwell DH, et al. Chromoendoscopy detects more adenomas than colonoscopy using intensive inspection without dye spraying. Cancer Prev Res (Phila). 2008;1:507–13.
89. Stoffel EM, Turgeon DK, Stockwell DH, et al. Missed adenomas during colonoscopic surveillance in individuals with Lynch Syndrome (hereditary nonpolyposis colorectal cancer). Cancer Prev Res (Phila). 2008;1:470–5.
90. Leppert M, Dobbs M, Scambler P, et al. The gene for familial polyposis coli maps to the long arm of chromosome 5. Science. 1987;238:1411–3.
91. Arvanitis ML, Jagelman DG, Fazio VW, Lavery IC, McGannon E. Mortality in patients with familial adenomatous polyposis. Dis Colon Rectum. 1990;33:639–42.
92. Vasen HF, Griffioen G, Offerhaus GJ, et al. The value of screening and central registration of families with familial adenomatous polyposis. A study of 82 families in The Netherlands. Dis Colon Rectum. 1990;33:227–30.
93. Rustin RB, Jagelman DG, McGannon E, Fazio VW, Lavery IC, Weakley FL. Spontaneous mutation in familial adenomatous polyposis. Dis Colon Rectum. 1990;33:52–5.
94. Spirio L, Olschwang S, Groden J, et al. Alleles of the APC gene: an attenuated form of familial polyposis. Cell. 1993;75:951–7.
95. Giardiello FM, Brensinger JD, Petersen GM, et al. The use and interpretation of commercial APC gene testing for familial adenomatous polyposis. N Engl J Med. 1997;336:823–7.
96. Cromwell DM, Moore RD, Brensinger JD, Petersen GM, Bass EB, Giardiello FM. Cost analysis of alternative approaches to colorectal screening in familial adenomatous polyposis. Gastroenterology. 1998;114:893–901.
97. Winawer SJ. Screening of colorectal cancer. Surg Oncol Clin N Am. 2005;14:699–722.
98. Marcello PW, Asbun HJ, Veidenheimer MC, et al. Gastroduodenal polyps in familial adenomatous polyposis. Surg Endosc. 1996;10:418–21.
99. Ahmadi AA, Polyak S. Endoscopy/surveillance in inflammatory bowel disease. Surg Clin North Am. 2007;87:743–62.
100. Provenzale D, Kowdley KV, Arora S, Wong JB. Prophylactic colectomy or surveillance for chronic ulcerative colitis? A decision analysis. Gastroenterology. 1995;109:1188–96.
101. Lennard JJ, Melville DM, Morson BC, Ritchie JK, Williams CB. Precancer and cancer in extensive ulcerative colitis: findings among 401 patients over 22 years. Gut. 1990;31:800–6.
102. Shapiro JA, Seeff LC, Thompson TD, Nadel MR, Klabunde CN, Vernon SW. Colorectal cancer test use from the 2005 National Health Interview Survey. Cancer Epidemiol Biomarkers Prev. 2008;17:1623–30.
103. Doubeni CA, Laiyemo AO, Reed G, Field TS, Fletcher RH. Socioeconomic and racial patterns of colorectal cancer screening among Medicare enrollees in 2000 to 2005. Cancer Epidemiol Biomarkers Prev. 2009;18:2170–5.

40
Colon Cancer Evaluation and Staging

Eric G. Weiss

Introduction

Colorectal cancer is the third most common cancer affecting persons in the USA. In 2008, there were an estimated 148,810 new cases of colon and rectal cancer with colon cancer making up the majority of new cases at 107,143 and the remaining 28% arising in the rectum.[1] Overall, approximately 33.6% of newly diagnosed patients with colorectal cancer in the USA will die of their disease.

Clinical Presentation

His beneficial that colon cancers are diagnosed when patients are asymptomatic, who undergo surveillance, or who are investigated for problems such as anemia. This underscores the importance of colorectal cancer screening in the asymptomatic patient based on age, and also any other associated risk factors that would increase the risk and require earlier screening. Currently the most common screening test is standard colonoscopy, but combinations of DRE, FOBT, FFS, and BE are still acceptable. In symptomatic patients, the most common presenting symptoms are abdominal pain, change in bowel habits, rectal bleeding, and occult blood in the stool.[2] These symptoms are more frequently associated with a tumor that is more advanced than in asymptomatic patients.

Abdominal pain is the most common presenting symptom of colon cancer. The pain can vary in type, location, and intensity. In the early phases or stages of colon cancer without evidence of obstructive symptoms, the pain can be vague, dull, and poorly localized. The pain is often in the lower abdomen, but may also occur periumbilically or elsewhere. With progression of the disease and a larger mass or a mass causing obstruction, symptoms of intestinal obstruction will eventually occur. This type of pain is characterized by crampy, colicky pain, often associated with meals, and occurring after meals. The location of the pain is often periumbilical or midabdominal, but can be located at the site of obstruction.

A change in bowel habits is the second most common symptom of colon cancer. The changes seen can be very subtle or very significant. In early lesions the change may be minor, with only a change in stool frequency. There can be changes in size, shape, and/or consistency of bowel movements. Characteristic changes include narrowing of the stool, irregular shape, and typically looser or diarrheal stool. The symptoms will depend on the location of the tumor. Right-sided tumors occur where the bowel lumen is larger and the stool is liquid. Symptoms occur later, but on the left side where the stool is more solid and the lumen narrower symptoms occur at an earlier stage.

Rectal bleeding may be present in as many as 25% of patients with colon cancer.[3,4] The bleeding may be of varying intensity and color. Bright red rectal bleeding is more consistent with a more distal location of a cancer. The mistake of attributing rectal bleeding to hemorrhoids even in a young population can lead to serious and at times fatal delays in the diagnosis of a colon cancer. Almost all patients regardless of age who present with rectal bleeding should undergo colonoscopic evaluation or a minimum flexible sigmoidoscopy depending on patient age and characteristics of the bleeding. In a series of 570 patients, 50 years of age or younger with rectal bleeding who underwent endoscopic evaluation, there was a 17.5% incidence of colorectal neoplasm.[5]

Patients undergoing stool guaiac tests for occult blood in the stool for routine screening with a positive result have a 5.1% chance of having an invasive cancer and a 24% chance of having a benign polyp.[6] Newer tests of either blood or DNA in the stool may be more sensitive than standard guaiac and lead to increased yields. The fecal immunohistochemical test (FIT) uses a monoclonal antibody to human hemoglobin and is more specific to colorectal cancer or advanced adenomas.[7]

As mentioned previously some of the symptoms that occur may be early or late based on the distribution of cancer

D.E. Beck et al. (eds.), *The ASCRS Textbook of Colon and Rectal Surgery: Second Edition*,
DOI 10.1007/978-1-4419-1584-9_40, © Springer Science+Business Media, LLC 2011

within the colon. There has been an overall more proximal shift of colon cancers with more tumors being in the proximal colon. The Lahey Clinic reported a 10-year representative anatomical site distribution in which the cancer was located in the right colon in 18%, the transverse colon in 9%, the descending colon in 5%, the sigmoid colon in 25%, and the rectum in 43%.[8]

Staging and Prognostic Factors

Evolution of Staging Systems

The original staging system for colorectal cancer was reported by Cuthbert Dukes' in 1930 and then revised by him in 1932.[9] This classification had three stages, A, B, and C. Stage A had the cancer limited to the bowel wall, Stage B had cancer that spread by direct extension to extrarectal tissues, and Stage C had cancer with regional lymph node metastasis. Dukes' further revised the classification in 1944 to subdivide the Stage C group into those with positive regional lymph nodes below a ligature (C1) and at a ligature (C2). In addition, a more advanced stage, Stage D was added for distant metastases.

Others have subsequently modified the Dukes' staging system in an attempt to further stratify, prognosticate, and treat patients with a more useful system. Kirklin first modified this system by subdividing Dukes' B into B1 and B2 based on invasion of the submucosa and muscularis propria versus full thickness invasion.[10] The most common modification is known as the Astler–Coller Modification.[11] In this modification, the Dukes' B and Dukes' C tumors are subdivided into two groups, depending on depth of tumor invasion Stage B, tumors penetrate partially into the muscularis propria, Stage B2 penetrate full thickness; both lack lymph node metastases. Stage C, and C2 parallel B1 and B2 but have lymph node metastases. Although both the Dukes' and Modified Dukes' staging systems are still utilized, the TMN staging system is the preferred method of colorectal cancer staging.

Current Staging Systems

The TNM classification is the system developed by the American Joint Committee on Cancer (AJCC) and the International Union Against Cancer (UICC). It utilizes three descriptors based on each letter in the name, T for tumor depth, N for nodal involvement, and M for metastases. Based on a combination of T, N, and M for any given tumor, an overall stage from Stage I to IV can be determined. The most recent AJCC/UICC definitions were published in 2010.[12]

The T stage can be divided into seven possible categories based on the depth of invasion. Tis, carcinoma in situ represents a nonmalignant tumor; T1 has invasion into the submucosa; T2 has invasion into the muscularis propria; T3 has invasion into the subserosa or nonperitonealized pericolonic or rectal tissue (through the bowel wall); and T4 has invasion of other organs or structures. The T3 category can be further subdivided by the depth of penetration into the muscularis propria. The N stage can be divided into three categories. N0, with no lymph node involvement; N1, with one to three lymph nodes involved; and N2 with four or more lymph nodes involved. The M stage is only divided into two categories, either no metastases (M0) or distant metastases (M1).

Typically, the combination of T, N, and M will lead to one of the four stages based on the combination of findings. Stage 0 is Tis, N0, and M0. Stage 1 is T1 or T2, N0, M0. Stage 2 is T3 or T4, N0, M0. Stage 3 is Any T, N1 or N2, and M0. Stage 4 is Any T, Any N and M1. In the most recent AJCC/UICC definitions, Stage II and III are further subdivided, Stage IIA (T3, N0, and M0) and Stage IIB (T4, N0, and M0); and three Stage III categories, Stage IIIA (T1 or T2, N1, and M0), Stage IIIB (T3 or T4, N1, and M0), and Stage IIIC (Any T, N2, and M0).

In the seventh Edition of the AJCC Staging Manual, Stage II and Stage III colon cancers were reclassified based on the Hindgut Taskforce recommendations.[13] Based on SEER population based data compared to NCDB data the reclassification occurred. T4bN0 was reclassified from IIB to IIC, T1-2N2a from IIIC to IIIB, T1-2N2b from IIIC to IIIB as well as T3N2a. T4bN1a and T4bN1b both were reclassified from IIIB to IIIC.

The importance of staging is for treatment planning and prognosis.

Clinical Prognostic Factors

Age

As with many cancers, colon cancer incidence increases with increasing age. Most series report a mean age in the sixth decade for nonhereditary colon cancer. Patients with familial adenomatous polyposis (FAP) will present with colon cancer in their mid to late 30s if colectomy is not performed prior to this age. Patients with HNPCC can present at any age, but tend to have colon cancer between the ages of 40 and 60, significantly younger than individuals with nonhereditary colon cancers.

It has been reported that younger patients present with worse tumors of more advanced stage and grade. However, recent studies refute this claim. O'Connell et al. recently reported (using SEER data) a comparison of two groups of patients with colon cancer.[14] The SEER database is a prospectively entered database of the National Cancer Institute in the USA and stands for Surveillance, Epidemiology, and End Results. They compared outcome in patients 20–40 years of age to those 40–60 years of age. Although there was an increased incidence of higher stage tumors, stage for stage they had an equivalent or improved 5-year survival.

Symptoms

Obstruction and perforation are poor prognostic signs often associated with advanced disease. In addition, because patients are operated on in an urgent fashion, their operative morbidity and mortality is increased. Chen et al. reported outcome in patients with obstructing and/or perforated colon cancer.[15] Perforated cancers had a 9% operative mortality compared to obstructed cancers of 5%. Overall 5-year survival was 33% in each group, much lower than the expected rate based on similar stages in noncomplicated cases.

Blood Transfusion

Blood transfusions can cause immunosuppression in the postoperative period, which may allow for an inability to combat tumor cells shed at the time of surgery and theoretically lead to a worse prognosis. Sibbering et al. reported on 266 patients with colon cancer some of who received blood transfusions and others who did not.[16] There was no difference in survival when comparing the two groups. However, Chung et al. reviewed 20 papers, representing 5,236 patients supporting the hypothesis that perioperative blood transfusions are associated with an increased recurrence and death from colon carcinoma.[17]

Adjacent Organ Involvement

Local extension of colon carcinoma can involve any structure or organ adjacent to the primary tumor. It occurs in 5–12% of colorectal cancers. All tumors with local extension would be considered T4. For right colon cancers the most commonly involved structures are the liver, duodenum, pancreas, and abdominal wall. Kama et al. reported a 75% disease-free survival of 14–41 months following en bloc pancreaticoduodenectomy and right colectomy.[18] Similarly Izbicki et al. reported on 83 patients with colorectal cancer undergoing extended en bloc resections.[19] Comparing extended to nonextended resections, mean survival of both groups was around 45 months conferring the benefit of extended resections when necessary to achieve R0 resections. These data were supported by Kroneman et al. where 4-year survival was 33 % following en bloc resection compared to those receiving noncurable resections, of 6 months.[20]

Histologic/Biochemical/Genetic Factors

Histologic Grade

Broders described classifying adenocarinomas by the degree of differentiation. He described four grades based on how much of the tumor had differentiated cells within it. Today, three grades are used and include Grade 1 with well-differentiated features, Grade 2 moderately differentiated, and Grade 3 poorly differentiated. The vast majority of colon cancers are moderately differentiated (Grade 2) with preservation of gland forming architecture. However, the amount of preservation of this architecture is variable and when absent leads to sheets of invasive cells classified as poorly differentiated. The degree of differentiation corresponds to prognosis. Poorly differentiated tumors have a worse prognosis stage for stage compared to better differentiated tumors.[21]

Tumor Budding

Tumor budding is now recognized and reported by pathologists and represents an undifferentiated portion of tumors at the leading invasive edge. There is a transition from the glandular structures to single cells or clusters of cells at the invasive margin. Also known as dedifferentiation and first described by Morodomi et al. in 1989[22], it is recognized by less than five cells of single infiltrating cancer cells at the invasive edge. Tumor budding is associated with a high risk of recurrence.[23] In addition, it has been associated as an independent risk factor for local spread, lymph node and distant metastases, and worse survival.[24]

Mucin Production and MSI

The most common pathway for the development of colorectal cancer is via the mechanism of chromosomal instability pathway (microsatellite stable or MSS). This pathway is responsible for an estimated 75–85% of all colorectal cancers. The remaining 15–20% of colorectal cancers occur via a different pathway associated with a high frequency of MSI.

Microsatellite Instability known as MSI is associated with HNPCC. MSI is an alteration in mismatch repair genes, which are important to repairing errors in replication. When altered, they can lead to colorectal cancer. Since there is loss of one of the two alleles in HNPCC, these patients tend to present earlier in life, with multiple colonic and extracolonic cancers. Many HNPCC cancers are mucin producing, which when present have a better prognosis compared to non-mucin producing tumors in these patients.

Signet-Cell Histology

Signet-ring or signet-cell tumors have a worse prognosis in many intestinal cancers. Signet-cell tumors tend to be of a more advanced stage when discovered. In a comparison between signet-ring and nonsignet ring colon cancers, it was noted that patients with signet-ring cancers were younger, had more advanced stages, and an increased incidence of liver metastases.[25] In addition, the rate of curative resection was lower at 35% compared to 79%. This rate was similar to poorly differentiated tumors at 46% at 5 years. In another study, the risk of peritoneal seeding was higher in signet-cell tumors leading to a high incidence of palliative resections and a mean survival of 16 months.[26]

Venous Invasion

Blood vessel invasion has been linked with poor prognosis both independently as well as with its association with lymph node metastasis. Blood vessel invasion can occur intramurally within the wall of the colon itself or in the surrounding tissue. Although arterial invasion occurs, most series define and describe vascular invasion based on venous invasion. Venous invasion in colon cancer occurs in 42% of patients and increases with increasing grade and stage.[27] Patients with blood vessel invasion had a 74% survival compared to those without it at 85%. In those patients with both intramural and extramural vascular invasion the prognosis was even worse at 32%.

Perineural Invasion

The growth of tumor along perineural spaces is known as perineural invasion and like venous invasion it increases with increasing grade and stage of the tumor. It occurs in 14–32% of colorectal cancers and can extend to as far away as 10 cm from the primary tumor. Numerous studies have confirmed poorer prognosis when perineural invasion is noted.[28,29]

Lymph Node Involvement

Lymph node metastasis has been long understood to be one of if not the most important prognostic factor in colon cancer outcome. All currently utilized staging systems as described above for colon cancer employ and rely on the presence or absence of lymph node metastases. It is therefore important to adequately remove the lymph node bearing tissue associated with the underlying colon cancer. It has been reported by Scott and Grace that if 13 lymph nodes are not recovered, adequate staging cannot be performed.[30] The main determinant for an adequate lymph node harvest is surgical, but a variety of means to enhance the yield have been developed and include fat clearance with xylene, other chemicals, and PCR techniques.[31–33] Using these techniques more lymph nodes or lymph nodes not found by standard techniques can be discovered, thus improving the accuracy of staging and allowing for better prognosis and application of adjuvant treatment. The ability to find occult metastases in otherwise H&E negative lymph nodes may improve survival by upstaging patients to a Stage 3, which would then lead to a recommendation for adjuvant chemotherapy. Cytokeratin immunohistochemistry can convert 25–30% of otherwise H&E negative lymph nodes in patients with colorectal cancer.[34]

Carcinoembryonic Antigen

Carcinoembryonic antigen (CEA), a glycoprotein absent in normal colonic mucosa, but present in 97% of patients with colon cancer was discovered in 1965.[35] CEA elevation correlates with either disease that has metastasized to the liver or with very large tumors. Patients with disease confined to the colonic mucosa or submucosa will have elevated CEA in 30–40% of cases. It is therefore not useful for screening, but can be used to follow patients with colon cancer. In patients with elevated CEA preoperatively and localized disease that is expectable, the CEA should fall following surgery. If the CEA level does not fall then occult metastases may be present and may be an indication for adjuvant therapy. The absolute level of CEA is also important. A CEA of greater than 15 mg/ml predicts an increased risk of metastases in an otherwise apparently curable colon cancer.[36] A normal preoperative CEA may become elevated with metastatic disease. Controversy exists as to the utility of following CEA postoperatively as it may not allow any advantage to salvage or treatment when compared to symptomatic recurrences[37] despite the fact that routine periodic CEA measurement is endorsed by the American Society of Colon and Rectal Surgeons in their practice parameters.[38]

Sentinel Node

The idea of a sentinel lymph node being present and if identified be able to predict lymph node metastases has become standard of care in breast cancer and melanoma. Its application to colon cancer is in its infancy and may be less important in colon cancer than the others. The idea that the lymphatic drainage can be mapped, and the first node identified, has significance in oncologic surgery. In colon cancer, resecting the associated lymphovascular pedicle with the primary cancer is considered paramount to performing an adequate operation; this adds little to no morbidity unlike excising level 3 nodes in breast cancer patients. In an attempt to validate the sentinel lymph node theory in colon cancer, Paramo et al. reported on their experience with 45 patients who underwent intraoperative sentinel lymph node mapping using isosulfan blue dye.[39] Sentinel lymph nodes were identified 82% of the time and predicted regional metastases in 98% of cases, with only a single case of a false-negative sentinel lymph node. Others have agreed that its utility may be marginal in colon cancer.[40]

DNA Ploidy

Normal cells are made up of diploid cells. Tumors can maintain normal diploid cells or can be aneuploid. Numerous studies show that nondiploid tumors have a worse prognosis and correlate with more advanced Dukes' stage.[41]

Spreading Patterns

Colon cancer can spread via a variety of pathways. Spread can be local or distant based on these pathways.

Intramural Spread

Intramural spread is tumor spreading along the bowel wall either proximally or distally in one of the bowel wall layers. Like rectal cancers, colon cancer rarely spreads this way. In a study of 42 colorectal cancers of which 64% were colonic, the maximum extent of intramural spread was 2 cm.[42] This supports the practice of excising 5 cm or more of colon on either side of a tumor to decrease the risk of anastomotic recurrence.[43]

Transmural Spread

As they become more advanced, colon cancers invade the colonic wall. Almost all colon cancers start as a mucosal lesion and then penetrate a variable degree into deeper layers of the colonic wall. This colonic wall invasion is the basis of many of the currently used staging systems including the Dukes' and TNM. Transmural spread is the mechanism that produces T4 tumors. T4 tumors penetrate full thickness into the colonic wall and then by direct extension or adherence, invade into other structures in proximity to the primary tumor. When present, en bloc resection is mandatory for an R0 resection. Preoperative evaluation can sometimes predict adjacent organ involvement, but often it is an intraoperative finding.

Margins

The acceptable bowel wall margins are dictated by three issues: First, thickness of penetration of the bowel wall margin and the risk based on the distance of local tumor spread intramurally. As described above, colon cancer rarely invades proximally or distally along the bowel wall for more than 2 cm. Convention has led to the recommendation that proximal and distal margins be a minimum of 5 cm. It has been stated that the "ideal extent of a bowel resection is defined by removing the blood supply and the lymphatics at the level of the origin of the primary feeding arterial vessel.[43]" These other two factors may modify the length of the proximal and/or distal margins as further resections may be required due to these issues.

Radial Margins

The circumferential margins are important to both colon and rectal cancer, but most series and studies have been confined to rectal cancers. It has been shown that positive circumferential margins in rectal cancer are associated with local recurrence rates as high as 85%.[44] In colon cancer the radial margins are less important with the exception of T4 tumors where en bloc resection is required. Typically for colon cancer the only radial margin which may be involved in a tumor less then T4 are those tumors with serosal involvement. In 279 patients with colon cancer, serosal involvement was not associated with a poorer outcome, and outcome was related only to tumor stage.[45]

Transperitoneal/Implantation

Tumors with serosal involvement can shed viable tumor cells which can spread throughout the peritoneal cavity and implant on a variety of structures. Most commonly tumors will implant on the ovaries, omentum, serosal or peritoneal surfaces. When widespread, this is known as carcinomatosis. When localized to the ovaries, which occurs in 3–5% of patients, bilateral oophorectomy should be performed. In a recent series, 86% of patients with ovarian metastases had transmural extension of the primary colon cancers.[46]

Lymphatic

Lymphatic invasion is the most common mechanism leading to metastatic disease. Lymphatics exist within the colonic wall and lymphatic invasion correlates with the depth of penetration of colon cancers. T1 tumors have a risk of lymph node involvement up to 9%, T2 up to 25% and T3 up to 45%. Most currently used staging systems assign increased stage to increasing T stage and lymph node involvement and prognosis correlates with the overall stage. The lymphatic drainage goes along the venous drainage of the colon, ultimately coursing through the portal vein and into the liver. Metastatic liver disease is felt to occur typically due to lymphatic spread.

Hematogenous

Hematogenous spread of colon cancer is less common than lymphatic spread. Hematogenous spread will bypass the liver and allow tumor cells to go peripherally into the systemic circulation. This is thought to be the mechanism for the development of pulmonary metastases.

Metastatic Evaluation

Once diagnosed with colon carcinoma, a search for metastatic disease is often performed. This assessment includes a variety of imaging studies, laboratory tests, and endoscopic procedures.

Detection and Management of Synchronous Lesions

Synchronous polyps and cancers occur in patients with colon cancer. Most colon cancers are diagnosed by colonoscopy and the remainder of the colon is evaluated at the same time by colonoscopy. However, if an obstructing lesion is noted that will not allow a colonoscope to pass, evaluation of the more proximal colon may be jeopardized. Alternatives to evaluating the remainder of the colon in these instances include contrast enemas, CT colonoscopy, or intraoperative colonoscopy at the time of resection. In a series of 158 patients with incomplete colonoscopies, barium enema was used to examine the remainder of the colon. Six lesions greater than 1 cm were identified with five of six being proximal cancers or advanced adenomas.[47] CT colonoscopy was used in 34 patients suspected of colon cancer with incomplete colonoscopies. CT colonoscopy identified all primary and three synchronous tumors proximal to the primary tumor.[48]

More recently, the combination of PET/CT colonography was used to evaluate the colon proximal to obstructive colon cancer in 13 patients previously diagnosed with colorectal cancer by standard colonoscopy. PET/CT colonography was performed to evaluate both the proximal colon as well as to identify metastatic disease. PET/CT Colonography identified the 13 primary tumors, two synchronous tumors proximal to the obstructions, and metastatic lung and liver disease in two and four patients respectively.[49]

When a colon cancer is diagnosed by colonoscopy, synchronous cancers occur in 6% or less of patients. When present, it should raise the suspicion of HNPCC which is associated with synchronous colon cancer. When synchronous colon cancer is diagnosed, the treatment should include a subtotal colectomy.

Distant Metastatic Disease

Distant metastatic disease associated with colon cancer is almost always either liver or lung metastases. Although bone, brain, and other organ involvement can occur, it is rare and therefore the search for these metastases in an asymptomatic patient is unwarranted. The search for liver and lung metastases can be accomplished by a variety of imaging studies including; ultrasound, CT scan, MRI, CXR, and PET scans. Each test has different abilities, availabilities, and costs.

Liver Metastases

An easily available test for the evaluation of the liver for metastases is surface ultrasound. Surface ultrasound is available in almost all institutions, however, its accuracy compared to newer modalities is lower in studies comparing it to CT and liver scans.[50,51]

CT scan is the most commonly employed method to preoperatively and postoperatively determine the presence or absence of liver metastases associated with colon cancer. There are numerous advantages to cross sectional imaging such as CT over US and include the ability to find abdominal wall or contiguous organ invasion as well as liver metastases. Standard CT scan is 64% sensitive in identifying liver lesions greater than 1 cm. MRI of the liver has been poorly studied and is not typically utilized in the evaluation of liver metastases.

Lung Metastases

Lung metastases occur in 3.5% of patients with colon cancer[52]; there are limited data on the utility of plain chest radiographs or CT scans in the initial evaluation of the lungs for metastatic disease. CT scan clearly has advantages over plain radiographs and can identify and characterize lung pathology better than plain X-rays. Given that most patients will undergo CT imaging of the abdomen prior to surgical intervention, the addition of imaging of the chest via CT seems reasonable. One must be careful about the amount of intravenous contrast when simultaneously scanning multiple regions such as chest, abdomen, and pelvis.

PET Scans

PET scans were initially approved only for patients with suspected metastatic disease and not for the use in primary staging of colon cancer. More recently with increased experience as well as the combination of PET & CT scans as well as further combinations with CT colonography, their roles in determining if any metastatic disease exists at the time of initial diagnosis are increasing.

Most commonly, PET scans involve the IV administration of a glucose analog, ^{18}F-flourodeoxyglucose (FDG). This glucose analog is preferentially taken up and trapped by tumor cells making those areas with trapped FDG show up brightly on PET scanning. Due to the lack of spatial resolution, the specific anatomic locations of the lesion(s) are difficult. Therefore combinations of PET with CT allow for precise spatial correlation and location with abnormally identified areas on PET. There are few publications supporting PET or PET/CT for initial staging of colon cancer, but there are initial rectal cancer for staging.

A recent meta-analysis was reported in 2005 using 61 published studies comparing CT, MR, and PET for the diagnosis of liver metastases in colorectal cancer.[53] Comparisons of nonhelical and helical CT, 1.5 T MR and FDG-PET showed sensitivities of 60.2, 64.7, 75.8, and 94.6%. FDG-PET had a significantly higher sensitivity compared to the other studies.

Response to Potential Chemotherapy

Recent publications and clinical trials have shown that patients with metastatic colorectal cancer benefit from treatment with monoclonal antibodies to EGFR. Monoclonal antibodies to EGFR include cetuximab, panitumumab, and the more commonly used bevacizumab. Patients with KRAS mutations at codon 12 or 13 do not appear to benefit from this therapy. It is therefore important to determine if patients have KRAS mutations so that expensive therapy and ineffective therapy is not given. Patients without KRAS mutations are known as wild type KRAS whereas those with mutations are considered abnormal. Multiple methods exist to determine KRAS mutations including PCR and Direct Sequencing. A recent Provisional Clinical Opinion by the American Society of Clinical Oncology about testing for KRAS gene mutations was published in 2009.[52]

Other markers that may predict the response to anti EGFR therapy include mutations of BRAF, PIK3CA, or loss of PTEN expression.[54]

Thymidylate synthase (TS), an enzyme required for DNA synthesis and targeted by competitive inhibition by 5FU based chemotherapy can now be measured. It is measured by either IHC or RT-PCR, but it is unclear as to which is the more reliable method. Elevated levels of TS in tumor cells are associated with resistance to 5FU based chemotherapy.[55]

References

1. Colorectal Cancer Facts and Figures 2008–10. American Cancer Society.
2. Beart RW, Steele GD, Merck HR, et al. Management and survival of patients with adenocarcinoma of the colon and rectum; a national survey of the Commission on Cancer. J Am Coll Surg. 1995;181:225–36.
3. Ferraris R, Senore C, Fracchia M, et al. Predictive value of rectal bleeding for distal colonic neoplastic lesions in a screened population. Eur J Cancer. 2004;40:245–52.
4. Helfand M, Marton KI, Zimmer-Gembeck MJ, et al. History of visible rectal bleeding in a primary care population: initial assessment and 10-year follow-up. JAMA. 1997;277:44–8.
5. Lewis JD, Shih CE, Blecker D. Endoscopy for hematochezia in patients under 50 years of age. Dig Dis Sci. 2001;46:2660–5.
6. Gilbertsen VA, Williams SE, Schuman L, et al. Paper presentation at the International Symposium on Colorectal Cancer, New York, March 1979.
7. Cole SR, Young GP, Esterman A, Cadd A, Morcom J. A randomised trial of the impact of new faecal haemoglobin test technologies on population participation in screening for colorectal cancer. J Med Screen. 2003;10:117–22.
8. Corman ML, Veidenheimer MC, Coller JA. Colorectal carcinoma: a decade of experience at the Lahey Clinic. Dis Colon Rectum. 1979;22:477–9.
9. Duke CE. The spread of cancer of the rectum. Br J Surg. 1930;17:643–8.
10. Kirklin JW, Dockerty MB, Waugh JM. The role of retroperitoneal reflection in the prognosis of carcinoma of the rectum and sigmoid colon. Surg Gynecol Obstet. 1949;88:326–31.
11. Astler VB, Coller FA. Prognostic significance of direct extension of carcinoma of the colon and rectum. Ann Surg. 1954;139:846.
12. Edge SB, Byrd DR, Compton CC, Fritz AG, Green FL, Trotti A. AJCC staging manual. 7th ed. New York: Springer; 2010.
13. Gunderson LL, Jessup JM, Sargent DJ, Greene FL, et al. Revised TN categorization for colon cancer based on national survival outcomes data. J Clin Oncol. 2009;28:264–71.
14. O'Connell JB, Maggard MA, Liu JH, Etzioni DA, et al. Do young colon cancer patients have worse outcomes? World J Surg. 2004;28:558–62.
15. Chen HS, Sheen-Chen SM. Obstruction and perforation in colorectal adenocarcinoma: an analysis of prognosis and current trends. Surgery. 2000;127:370–6.
16. Sibbering DM, Locker AP, Hardcastle JD, et al. Blood transfusion and survival in colorectal cancer. Dis Colon Rectum. 1994;37:358–63.
17. Chung M, Steinmetz OK, Gordon PH. Perioperative blood transfusion and outcome after resection for colorectal carcinoma. Br J Surg. 1993;80:427–32.
18. Kama NA, Reis E, Doganay M, et al. Radical surgery of colon cancers directly invading the duodenum, pancreas and liver. Hepatogastroenterology. 2001;48:114–7.
19. Izbicki JR, Hosch SB, Knoefel WT, et al. Extended resections are beneficial for patients with locally advanced colorectal cancer. Dis Colon Rectum. 1995;38:1251–6.
20. Kroneman H, Castelein A, Jeekel J. En bloc resection of colon carcinoma adherent to other oragans: an efficacious treatment? Dis Colon Rectum. 1991;34:780–3.
21. Cooper HS, Slemmer JR. Surgical pathology of carcinoma of the colon and rectum. Semin Oncol. 1991;18:367–80.
22. Morodomi T, Isomoto H, Shirouzo K, et al. An index for estimating the probability of lymph node metastases in rectal cancer. Lymph node metastasis and histopathology of actively invasive regions of cancer. Cancer. 1989;63(3): 539–43.
23. Park K-J, Choi H-J, Roh M-S, et al. Intensity of tumor budding and its prognostic implications in invasive colon carcinoma. Dis Colon Retum. 2005;48(8):1597–602.
24. Nakamura T, Mitomi H, Kikuchi S, et al. Evaluation of usefulness of tumor budding on the prediction of metastases to the lung and liver after curative excision of colorectal cancer. Hepatogastroenterology. 2005;52:1432–5.
25. Bittorf B, Merkel S, Matzel KE, et al. Primary signet-ring cell carcinoma of the colorectum. Langenbecks Arch Surg. 2004;389:178–83.
26. Psathakis D, Schiedick TH, Krug F, et al. Ordinary colorectal adenocarcinoma vs primary colorectal signet-ring cell carcinoma: study matched for age, gender, grade and stage. Dis Colon Rectum. 1999;42:1618–25.
27. Minsky BD, Mies C, Recht A, et al. Resectable adenocarcinoma of the rectosigmoid and rectum: II. The influence of blood vessel invasion. Cancer. 1988;61:1417–24.
28. Knudsen JB, Nilsson T, Sprechler M, et al. Venous and nerve invasion as prognostic factors in postoperative survival of patients with respectable cancer of the rectum. Dis Colon Rectum. 1983;26:613–7.
29. Compton CC. Pathology report in colon cancer: what is prognostically important. Dig Dis. 1999;17:67–79.
30. Scott KW, Grace RH. Detection of lymph node metastases in colorectal carcinoma before and after fat clearance. Br J Surg. 1989;76:1165–7.
31. Herrera L, Luna P, Villarreal JR. Lymph-node clearance techniques. Dis Colon Rectum. 1991;34:513–4.
32. Koren R, Seigal A, Klein B, Halpern M, et al. Lymph node revealing solution: simple new method for detecting minute lymph nodes in colon cancer. Dis Colon Rectum. 1997; 40:407–10.
33. Gold P, Freedman SO. Demonstration of tumor-specific antigens in human colonic carcinomata by immunological tolerance and absorption techniques. J Exp Med. 1965;121:439.
34. Rosenberg R, Friederichs J, Gertler R, et al. Prognostic evaluation and review of immunohistochemically detected disseminated tumor cells in peritumoral lymph nodes of patients with pNo colorectal cancer. Int J Colorectal Dis. 2004;19(5):430–7.
35. Wiratkapun S, Kraemer M, Seow-Choen F, et al. High pre-operative serum cancinoembryonic antigen predicts metastatic recurrence in potentially curative colonic cancer: results of a five-year study. Dis Colon Rectum. 2001; 44:231–5.

36. Moertel CG, Fleming TR, Mac Donald JS, et al. An evaluation of the carcinoembryonic antigen (CEA) for monitoring patients with resected colon cancer. JAMA. 1993;270:943–7.
37. The Standards Practice Task Force, The American Society of Colon and Rectal Surgeons. Practice parameters for the surveillance and follow up of patients with colon and rectal cancer. Dis Colon Rectum. 2004;47:807–17.
38. Paramo JC, Summerall J, Poppiti R, Mesko TW. Validation of sentinel node mapping in patients with colon cancer. Ann Surg Oncol. 2002;9:550–4.
39. Fazio VW, Kirian RP. Surgical treatment of colon cancer: does sentinel node technology have a role? Adv Surg. 2003;37:71–94.
40. Scott NA, Rainwater LM, Weiand HS, et al. The relative prognostic value of flow cytometric DNA analysis and conventional clinicopathologic criteria in patients with operable cancer. Dis Colon Rectum. 1987;30:513–20.
41. Hughes TG, Jenevein EP, Poulos E. Intramural spread of colon carcinoma. A pathologic study. Am J Surg. 1983;146:697–9.
42. Nelson H, Petrelli N, Carlin A, et al. Guidelines 2000 for colon and rectal cancer surgery. J Natl Cancer Inst. 2001;93:583–96.
43. de Haas-kock DF, Baeten CG, Jager JJ, et al. Prognostic significance of radial margins of clearance in rectal cancer. Br J Surg. 1996;83:781–5.
44. Tominaga T, Sakabe T, Koyama Y, et al. Prognostic factors for patients with colon or rectal carcinoma treated with resection only. Five-year follow-up report. Cancer. 1996;78:403–8.
45. Wright JD, Powell MA, Mutch DG, et al. Synchronous ovarian metastases at the time of laparotomy for colon cancer. Gynecol Oncol. 2004;92:851–5.
46. Chong A, Shah JN, Levine MS, et al. Diagnostic yield of barium enema examination after incomplete colonoscopy. Radiology. 2002;223:620–4.
47. Neri E, Giusti P, Battolla L, et al. Colorectal cancer: role of CT colonography in the preoperative evaluation after incomplete colonoscopy. Radiology. 2002;223:615–9.
48. Alderson PO, Adams DF, McNeil BJ, et al. Computed tomography, ultrasound, and scintigraphy of the liver in patients with colon or breast carcinoma: a prospective comparison. Radiology. 1983;149:225–30.
49. Nagata K, Ota Y, Okawa T, Endo S, et al. PET/CT colonography for the preoperative evaluation of the colon proximal to the obstructive colorectal cancer. Dis Colon Rectum. 2008;51(6):882–90.
50. Glover C, Douse P, Kane P, et al. Accuracy of investigations for asymptomatic colorectal liver metastases. Dis Colon Rectum. 2002;45:476–84.
51. Pihl E, Hughes ES, McDermott FT, et al. Lung recurrence after curative surgery for colorectal cancer. Dis Colon Rectum. 1987;30:417–9.
52. Allegra CJ, Jessup M, Somerfield MR, Hamilton SR, et al. American Society of Clinical Oncology provisional clinical opinion: testing for KRAS gene mutations in patients with metastatic colorectal carcinoma to predict response to anti-epidermal growth factor receptor monoclonal antibody therapy. J Clin Oncol. 2009;27(12):2091–96.
53. Bipat S, van Leeuwen MS, Comans EFI, Pilil ME, et al. Colorectal liver metastases A: CT, MR imaging, and PET for diagnosis – meta-analysis. Radiology. 2005;237(1):123–31.
54. Siena S, Sartore-Bianchi A, Di Nicolantonio F, Balfour J, et al. Review: biomarkers predicting clinical outcome of epidermal growth factor receptor-targeted therapy in metastatic colorectal cancer. J Natl Cancer Inst. 2009;101(19):1308–24.
55. Mutch MG. Molecular profiling and risk stratification of adenocarcinoma of the colon. J Surg Oncol. 2007;96(8):693–703.

41 Surgical Management of Colon Cancer

Matthew Mutch and Christina Cellini

Introduction

All colorectal cancer develops from a single transformed cell which ultimately grows large enough to present as a macroscopic lesion involving the lumen of the bowel. The staging of colorectal cancer is most dependent upon the depth of penetration of the bowel wall and the involvement of regional lymph nodes. An increasingly wide variety of putative molecular markers for aggressiveness and metastatic potential have been analyzed; however, the two most important prognostic indicators remain the degree of bowel wall invasion and status of the lymph nodes. This fact has lead to the continued importance of adequate locoregional oncological principles when performing curative resections of colon cancer. The purpose of this chapter is to primarily address issues directly related to the safe and oncologically sound methods of performing a curative resection of a colonic carcinoma. Important and related issues, such as clinicopathologic staging systems, the role of adjuvant or neoadjuvant treatments, and molecular markers are addressed in detail in other sections of this text.

Preoperative Preparation

Effective preparation of the patient requiring a colonic resection for colon cancer requires knowledge of the patient's physiologic status, tumor location, and clinical stage.

A variety of scoring systems are available for grading operative risk of surgical patients. The most widely applied scoring system is the American Society of Anesthesia (ASA) score;[1–4] however, this tool only provides information regarding the risk of an anesthesia complication given a certain physiologic status.[1,2] An alternative tool is the POSSUM and the modified p-POSSUM which include the additional risks related to underlying nutritional status and the performance of a colectomy.[3–5] Recent studies have found that POSSUM and P-POSSUM overpredict mortality in colorectal cancer patients undergoing elective surgery and underpredict mortality in the elderly patients and those undergoing emergency cases.[6] This has led to the development of a colorectal specific POSSUM (CR-POSSUM) score.[7] CR-POSSUM differs from the previous scoring systems in terms of number and type of physiologic and operative measures. Multicenter and single center analyses have shown that CR-POSSUM is an accurate predictor of mortality in colorectal cancer surgery in the UK and the USA.[8–11] These tools, while of limited specificity for the individual patient, do provide an estimation of the relative risks for both the patient and the entire surgical team. Additional discussions are presented in Chap. 8.

Localization of the tumor and its histopathology are important in selecting an operative plan and the optimal resection margins. The presence of a lesion at watershed areas of vascular supply may require a more extensive resection of the colon. In addition, information consistent with the Hereditary Non-Polyposis Colon Cancer Syndrome [(HNPCC) – right-sided lesion, Crohn's like inflammatory response, young patient, family history] would support resection of the entire abdominal colon rather than a segment. This diagnosis may also be supported by special stains of the biopsy specimen which demonstrate microsatellite instability, the hallmark of the disease.

Colonoscopy is widely used today and represents the optimal means of detecting a cancer, identifying its location, providing histopathologic material, and tattooing for intraoperative localization when required. Precise localization of the lesion with ink tattooing is paramount in the era of laparoscopy since manual palpation is not possible. The lesion should be inked in three separate areas around the circumference of the colon wall distal to the lesion. A second option is to place endoscopic mucosal clips distal to the lesion and obtain an abdominal radiograph in the recovery area. The clips can be seen on the X-ray and anatomically localize the lesion. Contrast enema is another means of localizing the lesion anatomically. Computer tomography (CT) allows the localization of larger lesions, identification of local organ invasion, and provides important staging information regarding the presence of extracolonic disease, particularly liver involvement.

D.E. Beck et al. (eds.), *The ASCRS Textbook of Colon and Rectal Surgery: Second Edition*,
DOI 10.1007/978-1-4419-1584-9_41, © Springer Science+Business Media, LLC 2011

The preoperative detection of distant metastasis can influence the initial management of a colorectal cancer patient. Computed tomography is the most widely used imaging modality to screen for liver metastasis because of its availability and relative low cost compared to positron emission tomography (PET). However, combined PET/CT imaging appears to provide the most accurate detection of liver metastasis (PET alone 93%, CT alone 92%, and PET/CT combined 97%).[12] It is unknown at this time if this increased accuracy has any impact on the management of those patients. The PET scan has a role in detecting recurrent disease or extrahepatic disease when evaluating a patient for surgical resection of the local recurrence or liver metastasis.

Bowel preparation has historically been considered an essential component of the preoperative preparation of the patient. Mechanical cleansing combined with oral antibiotics reduces the concentration of aerobic and anaerobic bacteria within the colon and decreases the incidence of wound infection from 35 to 9%.[13–15] However, more recent prospective randomized studies have questioned the additional benefit of luminal preparation, compared to the use of appropriate intravenous antibiotics administered in a timely manner. A meta-analysis by Bucher et al.[16] reviewed 565 patients with a mechanical bowel preparation versus 579 without a preparation. Interestingly, all but one study demonstrated a higher anastomotic leak rate in the mechanical prep group with an odds ratio of 1.8.[17,18] Other surgical site infectious complications were also more frequent in the mechanical preparation group. More recently, Slim et al.[19] reported an updated review and meta-analysis of randomized controlled trials of patients. They found no difference between the groups for anastomotic leak rate or the incidence of pelvic or abdominal abscess. There was a slightly higher risk of deep abdominal abscess with no bowel preparation; however, given that the number needed to have a complication was greater than 300 patients, they concluded that this risk did not seem to be clinically relevant. The study did not confirm the harmful effect of mechanical bowel preparation suggested in the previous studies.[16,20,21] While there is not enough data to make recommendations for the use of bowel preparation in rectal surgery with low anastomosis, the authors conclude that the routine use of mechanical bowel preparation should be abandoned.

Surgical Technique

Surgery remains the mainstay for the treatment of colon cancer. The 2000 National Cancer Institute issued guidelines for the surgical management of colon cancer.[22] They stated that the principles of an oncologic resection were a wide mesenteric resection achieved by ligating the feeding artery at its origin with adequate distal and proximal margins. They recommend that a minimum of 12 lymph nodes should be examined. There are several studies that support a survival benefit for patients who have 12 or more lymph nodes examined after surgical resection. This benefit most likely occurs for two reasons. First, the greater number of lymph nodes examined increases the accuracy of the final pathologic staging, a phenomenon known as stage migration.[23] Second, there is clearly an oncologic benefit to a radical mesenteric resection, where all involved lymph nodes are resected.[24]

Right Colectomy

The patient is placed supine on the operating table. If laparotomy rather than a minimally invasive technique is chosen, a vertical midline incision is made sufficiently long to allow complete visualization of the operative field. A self-retaining retractor should be placed so as to allow the entire surgical team free hands to conduct the surgical procedure. After the incision is fashioned, a thorough examination of the abdominal and pelvic contents should be performed. Particular attention should be paid to potential metastatic sites, especially the liver. The increasing access and familiarity with intraoperative ultrasound has demonstrated the superiority of liver assessment with this modality compared to clinical exam or CT.[25] In the female patient, the ovaries should be examined not only for metastatic deposits, but also for primary neoplasms. The resectability of the tumor should be assessed with minimal manipulation of the lesion. It is important to determine if disease is adherent to adjacent viscera which should then be included as an en bloc resection. It is rare that a right-sided tumor is unresectable, however, extensive involvement of the vena cava, superior mesenteric artery, or the pancreas may dictate a palliative resection or bypass procedure.

The key to an oncologically safe and effective resection of a colon cancer requires clear lateral margins, resection of the locoregional lymph node bearing mesentery for both cure and staging, and performance of an accurate and well-vascularized anastomosis.

A right-sided hemicolectomy begins by gaining access to the retroperitoneum. This maneuver can be accomplished via four different approaches. First, there is the traditional lateral to medial mobilization begun by incising the lateral peritoneal attachments of the colon. Second, a posterior approach (Figure 41-1) enters the retroperitoneum by reflecting the small bowel to the right upper quadrant and incising the peritoneum under the small bowel mesentery from the fourth portion of the duodenum to the cecum. Third, the superior approach enters the retroperitoneum by opening the lesser sac and incising the peritoneum at the hepatic flexure. Finally, with the medial to lateral approach, the ileocolic pedicle is grasped and elevated. The peritoneum on the caudal side of the pedicle is incised and the retroperitoneum is entered. Regardless of how the retroperitoneum is accessed, the principles of the resection are the same. The right colon mesentery is elevated off the retroperitoneum and the duodenum is identified. The lateral attachments are incised and the hepatic flexure is fully mobilized. For cancer operations, it is best to resect the omentum with the specimen, so when entering the lesser sac, the lesser omentum or gastrocolic attachments are divided. The ileocolic (Figure 41-2)

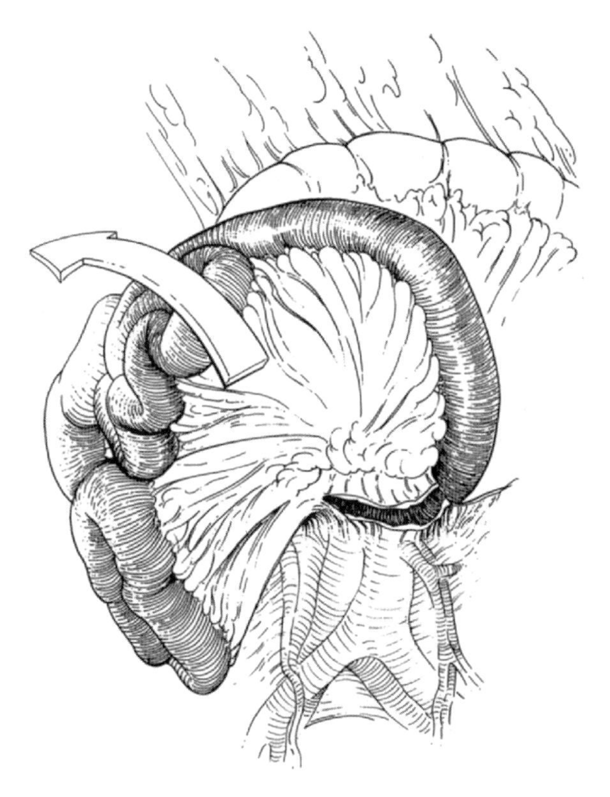

FIGURE 41-1. The drawing demonstrates the incision made at the root of the right colon mesentery just caudal to the third portion of the duodenum to the right of the superior mesenteric artery.

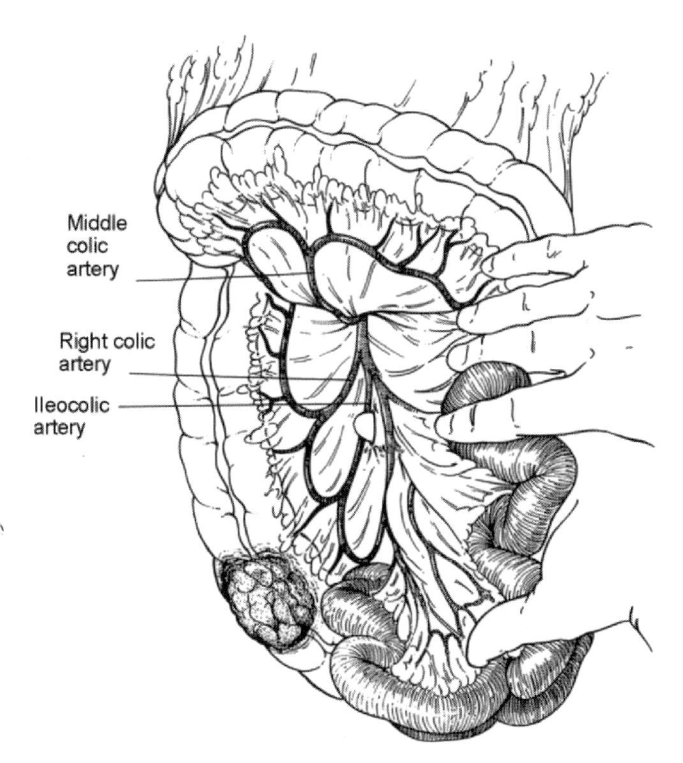

FIGURE 41-2 The vessel(s) is elevated off the retroperitoneum and a proximal ligation is performed at the origin of the superior mesenteric artery. The surgeon's finger is used to demonstrate the vascular origin for accurate placement of the ligation.

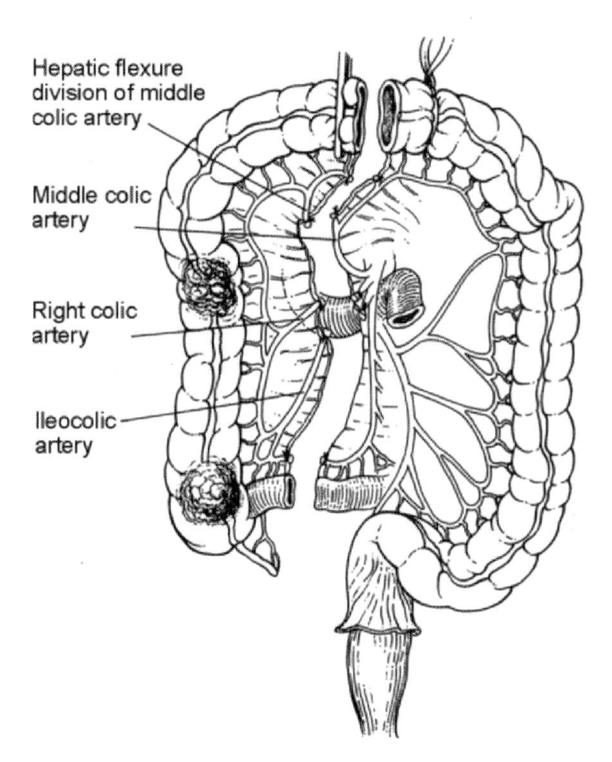

FIGURE 41-3. The drawing demonstrates the appropriate levels for vascular ligation and colonic transition for a right hemicolectomy. Notably, the transverse colon is divided just to the right of the main trunk of the MCA, although the right branch of the MCA may be taken, if required. The middle colic vessels are demonstrated and may be ligated during the performance of an extended right hemicolectomy. This leaves the descending colon in place supported by the left colic artery.

and right or hepatic branch of the middle colic vessels are ligated at their origins. The terminal ileum should be divided 10–15 cm proximal to the ileocecal valve to allow for good vascular supply (see Figure 41-3 for extent of resection). The transverse colon is divided just to the right of the main trunk of the middle colic artery. The ileocolic anastomosis can be fashioned according to the desire of the operating surgeon. The authors prefer to divide the ileum and colon with linear staplers and perform a functional end-to-end anastomosis by anastomosing the antimesenteric surfaces of the bowel segments with a linear stapler and closing the remaining colostomy with a linear stapler or sutures.

Extended Right Colectomy

An extended right colectomy should usually be performed for any lesion involving the transverse colon. This procedure once again should achieve complete resection, lymph node clearance, and most importantly two optimally vascularized bowel segments for anastomosis.

The operation proceeds in similar fashion as the right colectomy described above. However, rather than proceeding through the transverse colon mesentery to ligate and divide the right branch of the middle colic artery, dissection continues in the retroperitoneal plane to identify the main middle colic arterial trunk anterior to the pancreas. This vessel is ligated and divided. The right colon is then mobilized medially as before, and the lesser omentum is divided along the entire transverse colon. The splenic flexure is released and the bowel with its mesentery is divided just proximal to the left colic artery which is preserved for right-sided lesions. The left colic may be sacrificed for left transverse colon lesions, where a more distal colonic anastomosis is desired. The ileocolic anastomosis is then constructed based upon surgeon preference.

Left Colectomy

The left colon can be mobilized in either a lateral to medial or medial to lateral approach. For the lateral to medial approach, the small bowel is packed to the right upper quadrant. The lateral peritoneum from the sigmoid colon to the splenic flexure is incised. The left colon mesentery is elevated off the retroperitoneum, so the left ureter is exposed and the colon and its mesentery are brought to the midline. This allows the inferior mesenteric artery to be ligated at its origin at the aorta and the inferior mesenteric vein to be ligated near the ligament of Treitz and the inferior border of the pancreas. For the medial to lateral approach, the small bowel mesentery is mobilized to the right upper quadrant to expose the origin of the inferior mesenteric artery located just caudal to the third portion of the duodenum. The superior rectal artery is grasped at the level of the sacral promontory, the peritoneum is incised, and the retroperitoneum is entered. The left ureter is reflected into the retroperitoneum and the IMA is traced up to its origin. A window is then created on the cephalad side of the artery, medial to the IMV, and the artery is then ligated. The inferior mesenteric vein is ligated at the base of the pancreas. The mesentery is elevated off the retroperitoneum toward the abdominal wall and the lateral attachments are then incised (Figure 41-4). For either approach, the splenic flexure is mobilized by separating the omentum from the transverse colon. This completely opens the lesser sac and allows the posterior attachments to the inferior border of the pancreas to be divided. The bowel is transected with at least a 5 cm proximal margin and the distal site of resection on the top of the rectum.

The authors' preference is to perform an end-to-end circular stapled anastomosis, after dividing the rectosigmoid junction with a linear stapler or purse-string suture. A leak test with air insufflation of a submerged anastomotic segment should be performed in all cases.

Resection of proximal left colon lesions may require division of the middle colic artery to allow the right transverse colon to reach the rectal stump for an anastomosis. However, an extended right colectomy and ileosigmoid

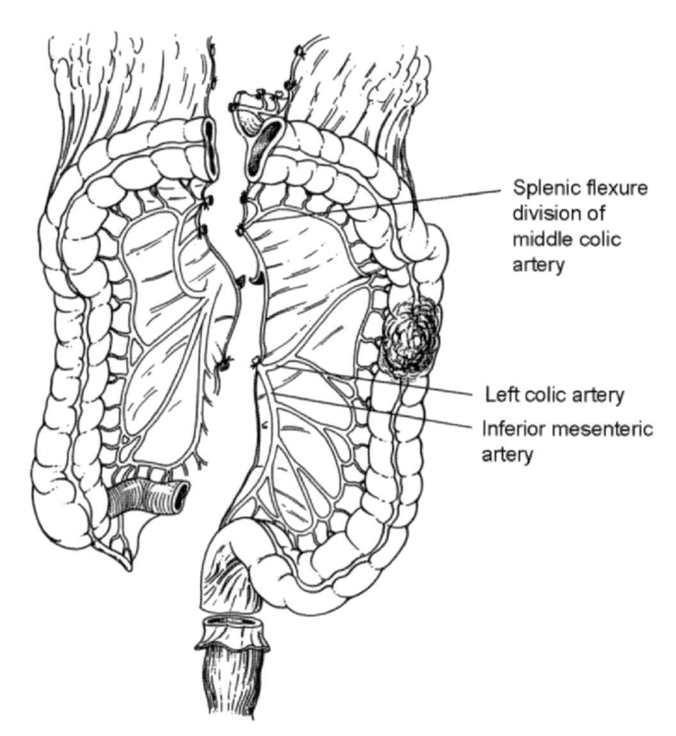

FIGURE 41-4. The small bowel mesentery is mobilized to the right upper quadrant to expose the origin of the IMA located just caudal to the third portion of the duodenum (see figure). An incision running along the base of the left colic and sigmoid mesentery from the sacral promontory to the ligament of Treitz, exposes the aorta, bifurcation of the common iliac arteries, and IMA vein. The IMA is ligated and divided proximal to the take-off of the left colic artery. The left branch of the middle colic vessels requires ligation and division for a formal left colectomy.

or ileorectal anastomosis may be preferable if there is any concern related to the blood supply. Another alternative is to perform a retroileal right colon to rectum anastomosis if maintenance of the right colon is desired (Figure 41-5). Once again the type of anastomosis is left to the discretion of the surgeon.

Total Abdominal Colectomy with Ileorectal Anastomosis

This procedure should be applied to circumstances, where the patient has been diagnosed with HNPCC, attenuated Familial Adenomatous Polyposis, metachronous cancers in separate colon segments, and frequently in acute malignant distal colon obstructions with unknown status of the proximal bowel. The access to vascular supply and mesenteric dissection has been described above. The terminal ileum should be sufficiently mobilized to allow easy reach to the rectum. The authors prefer a circular stapled end-to-end anastomotic technique.

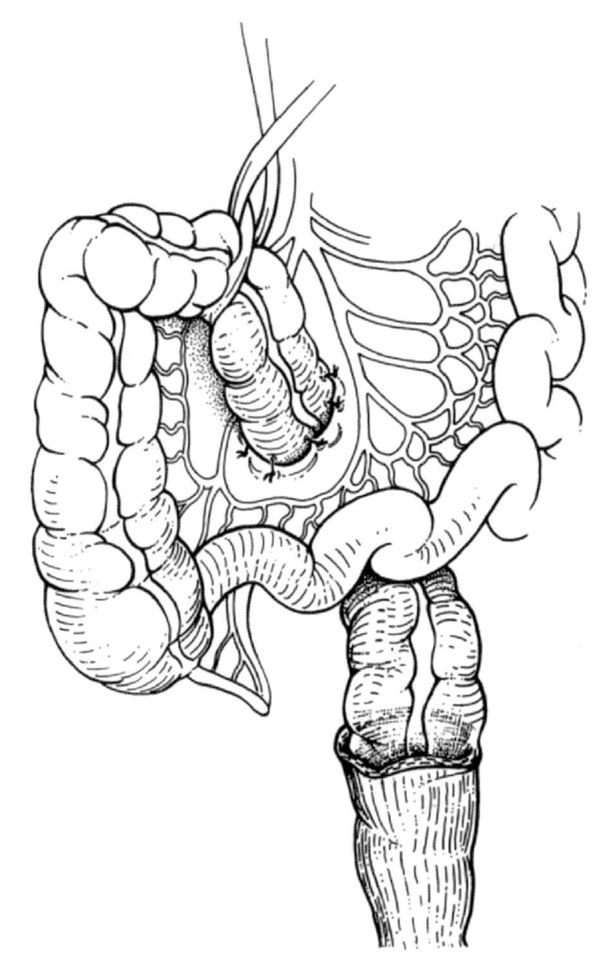

FIGURE 41-5. An alternative method of reconstruction that preserves the right colon is a retroileal right colon to rectum anastomosis. This is performed by swinging the fully mobilized colon in a counter-clockwise direction down into the pelvis to place the cut edge of the right colon mesentery across the pelvic brim.

Special Circumstances

Laparoscopic Colon Resection for Cancer

The application of laparoscopic techniques has been used in colorectal surgery for more than 15 years. However, it is only since the publication of the multicenter prospective randomized COST trial results in 2004 that it has been widely applied to the management of colorectal cancer.[26] The first publication from the COST trial focused on the quality of life.[27] It demonstrated many of the short-term benefits of laparoscopy, such as faster return of bowel function, shorter length of stay, and less narcotic use, but there was minimal short-term quality of life benefit with laparoscopy. In 2004, the 3-year oncologic results were published.[26] The study was designed as a noninferiority study and was not designed to demonstrate that laparoscopy was better. The overall survival was equivalent between the laparoscopic and open groups. Additionally, there was no difference in survival or recurrence for any stage of cancer. Port site recurrences were not an issue in this study, which has put this controversial issue to rest. These results have held up through the 5-year follow-up period.[28] Furthermore, it was demonstrated that conversion did not have a negative impact on the oncologic outcome of these patients.

The findings of the COST trial have been confirmed by at least two additional international, multicenter, prospective randomized trials on laparoscopy versus open colectomy for cancer. In 2007 and 2009, the 3-year follow-up results from the UK CLASICC and the European COLOR trials were published.[29,30] Both studies reported equivalent survival and recurrence rates stage for stage for laparoscopic and open colectomy for colon cancer. The CLASICC trial included the quality of life measures and once again found no difference between laparoscopic and open colectomy. Both trials demonstrated that a significant learning curve is associated with laparoscopic colectomy. The CLASICC trial saw the conversion rate fall from 38% in year 1 to 16% in year 6 of the study.[31] Similarly, the COLOR trial found that case volume impacted many of the parameters of the study. High volume centers (>20 cases/year) had shorter operative times, fewer conversions, and fewer complications than medium volume (10–20 cases/year) and low volume (<10 cases/year) centers.[30] Therefore, with adequate experience, laparoscopic colectomy for right- or left-sided colon cancers is safe and provides similar outcomes to open colectomy. There currently is no data regarding laparoscopic resection of transverse colon cancers.

Acute Obstruction

Acute colonic obstruction produces dilated bowel with a large amount of fecal loading proximal to the blockage. The associated bacterial overgrowth coupled with possible impairment of blood flow in the proximal bowel has been the primary factors that have classically dictated resection and proximal diversion. Lee et al.[32–36] compared left- and right-sided resections managed by primary anastomosis and found similar leak rates (left-6.9% vs. right-5.2%) or mortality rates (left-8.9% vs. right-7.3%). On-table colonic lavage has been advocated as an alternative means of dealing with the obstructed colon. A number of cohort studies have demonstrated the safety and efficacy of this approach for avoiding a colostomy without increasing leak rates (<5%) or sepsis.[34–36] Another approach to protect at-risk anastomoses has been omental wrapping. A large prospective randomized trial by Merad et al.[37] did not demonstrate any significant difference in anastomotic leak rates or the sequelae of those leaks. The success of managing these patients without a need for colostomy depends upon the amount of colonic and small bowel distention and the physiologic state of the patient.

More recently, endoscopically placed self expanding metal stents have been used to manage patients with malignant large bowel obstruction. Emergency surgery is associated with operative mortalities as high as 23% and a reduced quality of life.[38–40] Colonic stenting can serve as a bridge to elective surgery converting an emergency procedure into an elective one in patients with operable cancers.[41] Recent large reviews have reported technical and clinical success rates of over 90% for stenting.[42,43] Complications of the procedure include stent migration, blockage, and perforation although migration and blockage is not as big a concern if elective surgery is to follow shortly after the resolution of obstruction and optimization of medical comorbidities. Nonrandomized trials have shown that stenting used as a bridge to surgery helps reduce postanastomotic leak rates, reduces wound infection rate, decreases in-hospital length of stay and has comparable survival rates to emergency resections.[44–46] Other advantages include opportunity for preoperative visualization of the entire colon prior to surgery as well as avoidance of stoma creation as the majority of patients do not achieve stoma closure after a Hartmann's procedure.[47] Stenting has been used largely for left-sided lesions; however, some studies have shown success with stenting lesions proximal to the splenic flexure with better postoperative outcomes when compared to emergency surgeries.[48] Stenting is therefore feasible over the entire colon except the lower rectum because of pain and tenesmus. The presence of a stent does not seem to compromise a laparoscopic approach.[39,41,49,50] The wider application of this treatment option warrants further studies.

Prophylactic Oophorectomy

The debate continues regarding the relative risks and benefits of a prophylactic bilateral oophorectomy in women with colon cancer. The potential benefits are the removal of an ovary seeded by colon cancer cells which manifests as a delayed metastatic site and the reduction in the risk of primary ovarian cancer in this age group. The data are limited for both issues. The risk of micrometastatic implants in the ovary increases with tumor stage and approaches 10%.[51,52] A comparison of cohorts of women with and without prophylactic oophorectomy could not demonstrate a survival advantage, but a 3.2 vs. 0% risk of primary ovarian cancer in survivors with ovaries not resected was noted.[53]

Colon Cancer and Abdominal Aortic Aneurysm

This is a frequently employed line of questioning in board examinations; however, the best answer is not available based upon incontrovertible evidence. In fact, a survey of general surgery program directors revealed that the vascular surgeons preferred to repair the aneurysm first, whereas the nonvascular surgeons preferred colectomy.[54] The primary risk is that performing either operation first may cause complications that significantly delay the second procedure. The risk of performing a colectomy synchronously with the placement of graft material is a graft infection; however, this risk does not appear excessive based upon the small data sets available.[55–57] Probably, the best guidance suggests that any aneurysm >6 cm should be repaired first or synchronously with the removal of a colon cancer to avoid the risk of rupture.[58] The advent of endovascular repairs, when feasible, has greatly impacted the management of synchronous colon neoplasms and abdominal aortic aneurysms. The aneurysm and cancer can be addressed in either a staged fashion (endovascular repair followed by colectomy within the next couple of days) or synchronously under a single anesthetic, and this is being increasingly supported by the literature.[59,60]

Management of Colon Cancer and Liver Metastases

The potential benefit of simultaneous colectomy and hepatectomy is the avoidance of two laparotomies and possible reduction in operative risk. Conversely, delayed management of colonic hepatic metastases offers the ability to accurately stage patients and avoid the risk of hepatectomy in a group of patients who prove to have more widely metastatic disease in several months. The risks of simultaneous colectomy and hepatectomy do not appear to be excessive in select patients operated by expert groups[61–63] and long-term survival rates seem to be similar.[64] However, the risks may be less with smaller nonanatomic liver resections coupled with right colectomy. In the situation where liver metastases are unresectable, recent studies suggest that upfront chemotherapy without prophylactic resection of the primary tumor is appropriate.[65] In addition, up to 16% of previously unresectable patients can be downstaged and eventually undergo curative resection with as high as 40% 5-year survival.[66,67]

The role of resection of the primary tumor in patients with unresectable liver metastases is debatable. About 70% of patients diagnosed with Stage IV colorectal cancer in the USA during the last two decades underwent primary tumor resection as their initial treatment.[68] Studies have shown that resection of with primary lesions is safe, provides good local control, and allows the patient to proceed to adjuvant therapy in a timely fashion.[69–71] In addition, some retrospective data suggest that noncurative resection of asymptomatic colorectal primary tumors may prolong survival when compared to nonresected patients.[72–74] Median survival in these studies ranged from 11 to 16 months in resected groups versus 2–9 months in the unresected groups. Other studies, however, have not reported a survival benefit.[75,76] Local complications caused by primary tumors left in situ may prompt surgeons to opt for preemptive resection. In a recent study, Poultsides et al.[65] retrospectively studied 233 patients with synchronous stage IV colorectal cancer who received up front chemotherapy. They found that only 7% of these patients required surgical palliation for their intact primary tumor. Previous studies have noted a 9–29% need for operative intervention due to tumor-related complications.[72,77–79] In the era of improved chemotherapeutic agents and multimodality treatment, patients with metastatic rectal cancer are achieving significant improvements in outcomes and can now be approached with curative intent. When metastatic disease is not resectable, upfront chemotherapy without resection of the primary lesion may be a reasonable approach although as patients live longer with disease, the need for palliative surgical intervention may increase.

Sentinel Node Assessment

Sentinel node assessment was first described as a means of improving staging and treatment for melanoma patients and is currently considered the standard of care for breast cancer patients.[80,81] Saha[82] described the application of sentinel node identification for colorectal cancer patients with the proposed benefit of a high rate of node identification and pathologic upstaging. The technique involves either in vivo injection of 0.5–1 cc of isosulfan blue dye subserosally at the periphery of the tumor (node visualization within 30–60 s), or ex vivo injection of 1–2 cc in a similar fashion after the bowel has been resected.[83] Subsequent evaluation of the technique, including some modifications, has demonstrated a false negative rate approaching 60%, and limitations have been noted in rectal cancers.[84–86]

There are several concerns which restrict routine implementation of sentinel node assessment in colorectal cancer. First, there is no consensus of opinion regarding the prognostic significance of micrometastatic lymph nodes in colorectal cancer, particularly those identified by immunohistochemistry or PCR.[87–90] Second, the relatively high false negative rates and/or lack of node visualization mentioned previously, limit the confidence in restricting microsectioning and the use of special stains to the group with stained nodes. Finally, there is limited data that the technique is sufficiently accurate to alter the extent of surgical resection in a reasonable number of patients. Before sentinel node assessment can be routinely recommended, two hurdles must be overcome: (1) provision of incontrovertible evidence that micrometastatic disease identified by any technique correlates with survival; and (2) that the survival rates can be favorably impacted by an adjuvant chemotherapy regimen.

Outcome of Colectomy for Colon Cancer

In general, the operative outcome and long-term survival following colon cancer resections parallels the American Joint Committee on Cancer staging system (I: well above 90%; II: 65–90%; III: 45–75%) which may be modulated by adjuvant chemotherapy.[91–93] The risk of locoregional recurrence following colectomy is a rare occurrence and should be below 5%.[94,95] However, the impact of the surgeon's experience and the expertise of the institution have recently been found to have a profound effect on outcome. High volume surgeons, particularly those at high volume institutions have demonstrated significantly lower perioperative complications and improved survival after colectomy for colon cancer.[96–98]

In addition to experience, the overall surgical approach to the management of margins and extent of resection has a significant effect on outcome after colon cancer resection. Although not clearly defined, it is generally agreed that 5 cm proximal and distal bowel margins are sufficient to allow resection of mural tumor spread. Grinnell originally evaluated the patterns of mural spread of tumor in the colon via lymphatics and found no instance of spread greater than 4 cm in the most advanced cases.[99] More recent data would suggest that mural tumor migration is rarely greater than 2 cm either proximal or distal to the palpable tumor edge.[100] Similarly, there is no need to resect any specific amount of terminal ileum, other than defined by vascular supply as mural spread to the ileum is a very rare event. Vascular ligation is generally performed at the origin of the primary feeder vessel to a colonic segment. For resection of the right colon and transverse colon, the debate is relatively moot due to the constraints of the arterial origin of the right colic and middle colic arteries. Ligation for left-sided resections has been debated, primarily in sigmoid or anterior resections as ligation of the inferior mesenteric artery may be performed at the aorta, or just distal to the left colic artery takeoff. A report from St. Marks assessed this issue in 1,370 patients and found that survival was equivalent for all stages for the ligation options except for the most advanced node positive cases who fared worse with ligation at the aorta.[101] This counter-intuitive finding was more likely related to the higher stage of patients identified by the wider lymphatic resection. A comparison of left hemicolectomy and segmental colectomy (ligation of the IMA vs. more distal) by the French Association for Surgical Research could not discern either a different survival rate or pattern based upon the ligation or resection performed.[102] Jagoditsch et al.[92] demonstrated the benefits of careful surgical technique which resulted in a complete resection of all tumor (R0). Their data demonstrated an operative mortality of 1.3% and a 5-year survival rate of 71.8% for curative operations in Stage I–III disease.

Summary

Surgery for colonic cancer has been increasingly better defined and the data clearly support the benefits of wide mesenteric resection, clear radial margins, and resection of adherent adjacent organs. The mesenteric resection is obtained by ligating the feeding vessel at its origin. This maximizes the chances that 12 or more lymph nodes are examined to allow for accurate staging. Attentions to surgical detail, coupled with improved perioperative care strategies, are essential to minimize operative morbidity and mortality.

Acknowledgment. This chapter was written by Robert Fry and Anthony Senagore in the previous version of this textbook.

References

1. Menke H, Klein A, John KD, et al. Predictive value of ASA classification for the assessment of the perioperative risk. Int Surg. 1993;78:266–70.
2. Keats AS. The ASA classification of physical status – a recapitulation. Anesthesiology. 1978;49:233–6.
3. Copeland GP, Jones D, Walters M. POSSUM: a scoring system for surgical audit. Br J Surg. 1991;78:355–60.
4. Jones DR, Copeland GP, de Cossart L. Comparison of POSSUM with APACHE II for prediction of outcome from a surgical high-dependency unit. Br J Surg. 1992;79:1293–6.
5. Prytherch DR, Whiteley MS, Higgins B, et al. POSSUM and Portsmouth POSSUM for predicting mortality. Physiological and Operative Severity Score for the enUmeration of Mortality and morbidity. Br J Surg. 1998;85:1217–20.
6. Tekkis PP, Kocher HM, Bentley AJ, et al. Operative mortality rates among surgeons: comparison of POSSUM and p-POSSUM scoring systems in gastrointestinal surgery. Dis Colon Rectum. 2000;43:1528–32. discusssion 1532–24.
7. Tekkis PP, Prytherch DR, Kocher HM, et al. Development of a dedicated risk-adjustment scoring system for colorectal surgery (colorectal POSSUM). Br J Surg. 2004;91:1174–82.
8. Senagore AJ, Warmuth AJ, Delaney CP, et al. POSSUM, p-POSSUM, and Cr-POSSUM: implementation issues in a United States health care system for prediction of outcome for colon cancer resection. Dis Colon Rectum. 2004;47:1435–41.
9. Bromage SJ, Cunliffe WJ. Validation of the CR-POSSUM risk-adjusted scoring system for major colorectal cancer surgery in a single center. Dis Colon Rectum. 2007;50:192–6.
10. Al-Homoud S, Purkayastha S, Aziz O, et al. Evaluating operative risk in colorectal cancer surgery: ASA and POSSUM-based predictive models. Surg Oncol. 2004;13:83–92.
11. Ramkumar T, Ng V, Fowler L, et al. A comparison of POSSUM, P-POSSUM and colorectal POSSUM for the prediction of postoperative mortality in patients undergoing colorectal resection. Dis Colon Rectum. 2006;49:330–5.
12. Orlacchio A, Schillaci O, Fusco N, et al. Role of PET/CT in the detection of liver metastases from colorectal cancer. Radiol Med. 2009;114:571–85.
13. Matheson DM, Arabi Y, Baxter-Smith D, et al. Randomized multicentre trial of oral bowel preparation and antimicrobials for elective colorectal operations. Br J Surg. 1978;65:597–600.
14. Clarke JS, Condon RE, Bartlett JG, et al. Preoperative oral antibiotics reduce septic complications of colon operations: results of prospective, randomized, double-blind clinical study. Ann Surg. 1977;186:251–9.
15. Solla JA, Rothenberger DA. Preoperative bowel preparation. A survey of colon and rectal surgeons. Dis Colon Rectum. 1990;33:154–9.
16. Bucher P, Mermillod B, Morel P, et al. Does mechanical bowel preparation have a role in preventing postoperative complications in elective colorectal surgery? Swiss Med Wkly. 2004;134:69–74.
17. Guenaga KF, Matos D, Castro AA, et al. Mechanical bowel preparation for elective colorectal surgery. Cochrane Database Syst Rev. 2003:CD001544.
18. Zmora O, Mahajna A, Bar-Zakai B, et al. Colon and rectal surgery without mechanical bowel preparation: a randomized prospective trial. Ann Surg. 2003;237:363–7.
19. Slim K, Vicaut E, Launay-Savary MV, et al. Updated systematic review and meta-analysis of randomized clinical trials on the role of mechanical bowel preparation before colorectal surgery. Ann Surg. 2009;249:203–9.
20. Slim K, Vicaut E, Panis Y, et al. Meta-analysis of randomized clinical trials of colorectal surgery with or without mechanical bowel preparation. Br J Surg. 2004;91:1125–30.
21. Guenaga KF, Matos D, Castro AA, et al. Mechanical bowel preparation for elective colorectal surgery. Cochrane Database Syst Rev. 2005:CD001544.
22. Nelson H, Petrelli N, Carlin A, et al. Guidelines 2000 for colon and rectal cancer surgery. J Natl Cancer Inst. 2001;93:583–96.
23. Wright FC, Law CH, Last L, et al. Lymph node retrieval and assessment in stage II colorectal cancer: a population-based study. Ann Surg Oncol. 2003;10:903–9.
24. Tsai HL, Lu CY, Hsieh JS, et al. The prognostic significance of total lymph node harvest in patients with T2-4N0M0 colorectal cancer. J Gastrointest Surg. 2007;11:660–5.
25. Leen E, Ceccotti P, Moug SJ, et al. Potential value of contrast-enhanced intraoperative ultrasonography during partial hepatectomy for metastases: an essential investigation before resection? Ann Surg. 2006;24:236–40.
26. Nelson H. A comparison of laparoscopically assisted and open colectomy for colon cancer. N Engl J Med. 2004;350:2050–9.
27. Weeks JC, Nelson H, Gelber S, et al. Short-term quality-of-life outcomes following laparoscopic-assisted colectomy vs open colectomy for colon cancer: a randomized trial. Jama. 2002; 287:321–8.
28. Fleshman J, Sargent DJ, Green E, et al. Laparoscopic colectomy for cancer is not inferior to open surgery based on 5-year data from the COST Study Group trial. Ann Surg. 2007;246:655–62. discussion 662–54.
29. Jayne DG, Guillou PJ, Thorpe H, et al. Randomized trial of laparoscopic-assisted resection of colorectal carcinoma: 3-year results of the UK MRC CLASICC Trial Group. J Clin Oncol. 2007;25:3061–8.
30. Buunen M, Veldkamp R, Hop WC, et al. Survival after laparoscopic surgery versus open surgery for colon cancer: long-term outcome of a randomised clinical trial. Lancet Oncol. 2009;10:44–52.
31. Guillou PJ, Quirke P, Thorpe H, et al. Short-term endpoints of conventional versus laparoscopic-assisted surgery in patients with colorectal cancer (MRC CLASICC trial): multicentre, randomised controlled trial. Lancet. 2005;365:1718–26.
32. Lee YM, Law WL, Chu KW, et al. Emergency surgery for obstructing colorectal cancers: a comparison between right-sided and left-sided lesions. J Am Coll Surg. 2001;192:719–25.
33. Murray JJ, Schoetz Jr DJ, Coller JA, et al. Intraoperative colonic lavage and primary anastomosis in nonelective colon resection. Dis Colon Rectum. 1991;34:527–31.
34. Kressner U, Antonsson J, Ejerblad S, et al. Intraoperative colonic lavage and primary anastomosis – an alternative to Hartmann procedure in emergency surgery of the left colon. Eur J Surg. 1994;160:287–92.
35. Biondo S, Jaurrieta E, Jorba R, et al. Intraoperative colonic lavage and primary anastomosis in peritonitis and obstruction. Br J Surg. 1997;84:222–5.

36. Torralba JA, Robles R, Parrilla P, et al. Subtotal colectomy vs. intraoperative colonic irrigation in the management of obstructed left colon carcinoma. Dis Colon Rectum. 1998;41:18–22.
37. Merad F, Hay JM, Fingerhut A, et al. Omentoplasty in the prevention of anastomotic leakage after colonic or rectal resection: a prospective randomized study in 712 patients. French Associations for Surgical Research. Ann Surg. 1998;227:179–86.
38. Soto S, Lopez-Roses L, Gonzalez-Ramirez A, et al. Endoscopic treatment of acute colorectal obstruction with self-expandable metallic stents: experience in a community hospital. Surg Endosc. 2006;20:1072–6.
39. Morino M, Bertello A, Garbarini A, et al. Malignant colonic obstruction managed by endoscopic stent decompression followed by laparoscopic resections. Surg Endosc. 2002;16: 1483–7.
40. Mauro MA, Koehler RE, Baron TH. Advances in gastrointestinal intervention: the treatment of gastroduodenal and colorectal obstructions with metallic stents. Radiology. 2000;215:659–69.
41. Stipa F, Pigazzi A, Bascone B, et al. Management of obstructive colorectal cancer with endoscopic stenting followed by single-stage surgery: open or laparoscopic resection? Surg Endosc. 2008;22:1477–81.
42. Sebastian S, Johnston S, Geoghegan T, et al. Pooled analysis of the efficacy and safety of self-expanding metal stenting in malignant colorectal obstruction. Am J Gastroenterol. 2004;99:2051–7.
43. Khot UP, Lang AW, Murali K, et al. Systematic review of the efficacy and safety of colorectal stents. Br J Surg. 2002;89:1096–102.
44. Finan PJ, Campbell S, Verma R, et al. The management of malignant large bowel obstruction: ACPGBI position statement. Colorectal Dis. 2007;9 Suppl 4:1–17.
45. Saida Y, Sumiyama Y, Nagao J, et al. Long-term prognosis of preoperative "bridge to surgery" expandable metallic stent insertion for obstructive colorectal cancer: comparison with emergency operation. Dis Colon Rectum. 2003;46:S44–9.
46. Ng KC, Law WL, Lee YM, et al. Self-expanding metallic stent as a bridge to surgery versus emergency resection for obstructing left-sided colorectal cancer: a case-matched study. J Gastrointest Surg. 2006;10:798–803.
47. Deans GT, Krukowski ZH, Irwin ST. Malignant obstruction of the left colon. Br J Surg. 1994;81:1270–6.
48. Dronamraju SS, Ramamurthy S, Kelly SB, et al. Role of self-expanding metallic stents in the management of malignant obstruction of the proximal colon. Dis Colon Rectum. 2009;52:1657–61.
49. Dulucq JL, Wintringer P, Beyssac R, et al. One-stage laparoscopic colorectal resection after placement of self-expanding metallic stents for colorectal obstruction: a prospective study. Dig Dis Sci. 2006;51:2365–71.
50. Chung TS, Lim SB, Sohn DK, et al. Feasibility of single-stage laparoscopic resection after placement of a self-expandable metallic stent for obstructive left colorectal cancer. World J Surg. 2008;32:2275–80.
51. MacKeigan JM, Ferguson JA. Prophylactic oophorectomy and colorectal cancer in premenopausal patients. Dis Colon Rectum. 1979;22:401–5.
52. Graffner HO, Alm PO, Oscarson JE. Prophylactic oophorectomy in colorectal carcinoma. Am J Surg. 1983;146:233–5.
53. Schofield A, Pitt J, Biring G, et al. Oophorectomy in primary colorectal cancer. Ann R Coll Surg Engl. 2001;83:81–4.
54. Lobbato VJ, Rothenberg RE, LaRaja RD, et al. Coexistence of abdominal aortic aneurysm and carcinoma of the colon: a dilemma. J Vasc Surg. 1985;2:724–6.
55. Bachoo P, Cooper G, Engeset J, et al. Management of synchronous infrarenal aortic disease and large bowel cancer: a North-east of Scotland experience. Eur J Vasc Endovasc Surg. 2000;19:614–8.
56. Tilney HS, Trickett JP, Scott RA. Abdominal aortic aneurysm and gastrointestinal disease: should synchronous surgery be considered? Ann R Coll Surg Engl. 2002;84:414–7.
57. Luebke T, Wolters U, Gawenda M, et al. Simultaneous gastrointestinal surgery in patients with elective abdominal aortic reconstruction: an additional risk factor? Arch Surg. 2002;137:143–7. discussion 148.
58. Robinson G, Hughes W, Lippey E. Abdominal aortic aneurysm and associated colorectal carcinoma: a management problem. Aust N Z J Surg. 1994;64:475–8.
59. Veraldi GF, Minicozzi AM, Leopardi F, et al. Treatment of abdominal aortic aneurysm associated with colorectal cancer: presentation of 14 cases and literature review. Int J Colorectal Dis. 2008;23:425–30.
60. Veraldi GF, Minicozzi A, Genco B, et al. Endovascular treatment (EVAR) in patients with abdominal aortic aneurysms and synchronous neoplasms. Chir Ital. 2008;60:23–31.
61. Weber JC, Bachellier P, Oussoultzoglou E, et al. Simultaneous resection of colorectal primary tumour and synchronous liver metastases. Br J Surg. 2003;90:956–62.
62. Martin R, Paty P, Fong Y, et al. Simultaneous liver and colorectal resections are safe for synchronous colorectal liver metastasis. J Am Coll Surg. 2003;197:233–41. discussion 241–32.
63. de Santibanes E, Lassalle FB, McCormack L, et al. Simultaneous colorectal and hepatic resections for colorectal cancer: postoperative and longterm outcomes. J Am Coll Surg. 2002;195:196–202.
64. Thelen A, Jonas S, Benckert C, et al. Simultaneous versus staged liver resection of synchronous liver metastases from colorectal cancer. Int J Colorectal Dis. 2007;22:1269–76.
65. Poultsides GA, Servais EL, Saltz LB, et al. Outcome of primary tumor in patients with synchronous stage IV colorectal cancer receiving combination chemotherapy without surgery as initial treatment. J Clin Oncol. 2009;27:3379–84.
66. Adam R, Delvart V, Pascal G, et al. Rescue surgery for unresectable colorectal liver metastases downstaged by chemotherapy: a model to predict long-term survival. Ann Surg. 2004;240:644–57. discussion 657–48.
67. Bismuth H, Adam R. Reduction of nonresectable liver metastasis from colorectal cancer after oxaliplatin chemotherapy. Semin Oncol. 1998;25:40–6.
68. Eisenberger A, Whelan RL, Neugut AI. Survival and symptomatic benefit from palliative primary tumor resection in patients with metastatic colorectal cancer: a review. Int J Colorectal Dis. 2008;23:559–68.
69. Nash GM, Saltz LB, Kemeny NE, et al. Radical resection of rectal cancer primary tumor provides effective local therapy in patients with stage IV disease. Ann Surg Oncol. 2002;9: 954–60.
70. Al-Sanea N, Isbister WH. Is palliative resection of the primary tumour, in the presence of advanced rectal cancer, a safe and useful technique for symptom control? ANZ J Surg. 2004;74:229–32.

71. Law WL, Chu KW. Outcomes of resection of stage IV rectal cancer with mesorectal excision. J Surg Oncol. 2006;93: 523–8.
72. Ruo L, Gougoutas C, Paty PB, et al. Elective bowel resection for incurable stage IV colorectal cancer: prognostic variables for asymptomatic patients. J Am Coll Surg. 2003;196:722–8.
73. Cook AD, Single R, McCahill LE. Surgical resection of primary tumors in patients who present with stage IV colorectal cancer: an analysis of surveillance, epidemiology, and end results data, 1988 to 2000. Ann Surg Oncol. 2005;12:637–45.
74. Konyalian VR, Rosing DK, Haukoos JS, et al. The role of primary tumour resection in patients with stage IV colorectal cancer. Colorectal Dis. 2007;9:430–7.
75. Scoggins CR, Meszoely IM, Blanke CD, et al. Nonoperative management of primary colorectal cancer in patients with stage IV disease. Ann Surg Oncol. 1999;6:651–7.
76. Scheer MG, Sloots CE, van der Wilt GJ, et al. Management of patients with asymptomatic colorectal cancer and synchronous irresectable metastases. Ann Oncol. 2008;19:1829–35.
77. Sarela AI, Guthrie JA, Seymour MT, et al. Non-operative management of the primary tumour in patients with incurable stage IV colorectal cancer. Br J Surg. 2001;88:1352–6.
78. Scoggins CR, Campbell ML, Landry CS, et al. Preoperative chemotherapy does not increase morbidity or mortality of hepatic resection for colorectal cancer metastases. Ann Surg Oncol. 2009;16:35–41.
79. Michel P, Roque I, Di Fiore F, et al. Colorectal cancer with nonresectable synchronous metastases: should the primary tumor be resected? Gastroenterol Clin Biol. 2004;28:434–7.
80. Morton DL, Wen DR, Wong JH, et al. Technical details of intraoperative lymphatic mapping for early stage melanoma. Arch Surg. 1992;127:392–9.
81. Giuliano AE, Jones RC, Brennan M, et al. Sentinel lymphadenectomy in breast cancer. J Clin Oncol. 1997;15:2345–50.
82. Saha S, Wiese D, Badin J, et al. Technical details of sentinel lymph node mapping in colorectal cancer and its impact on staging. Ann Surg Oncol. 2000;7:120–4.
83. Wood TF, Saha S, Morton DL, et al. Validation of lymphatic mapping in colorectal cancer: in vivo, ex vivo, and laparoscopic techniques. Ann Surg Oncol. 2001;8:150–7.
84. Joosten JJ, Strobbe LJ, Wauters CA, et al. Intraoperative lymphatic mapping and the sentinel node concept in colorectal carcinoma. Br J Surg. 1999;86:482–6.
85. Feig BW, Curley S, Lucci A, et al. A caution regarding lymphatic mapping in patients with colon cancer. Am J Surg. 2001;182:707–12.
86. Broderick-Villa G, Ko A, O'Connell TX, et al. Does tumor burden limit the accuracy of lymphatic mapping and sentinel lymph node biopsy in colorectal cancer? Cancer J. 2002;8: 445–50.
87. Cutait R, Alves VA, Lopes LC, et al. Restaging of colorectal cancer based on the identification of lymph node micrometastases through immunoperoxidase staining of CEA and cytokeratins. Dis Colon Rectum. 1991;34:917–20.
88. Jeffers MD, O'Dowd GM, Mulcahy H, et al. The prognostic significance of immunohistochemically detected lymph node micrometastases in colorectal carcinoma. J Pathol. 1994;172: 183–7.
89. Hayashi N, Ito I, Yanagisawa A, et al. Genetic diagnosis of lymph-node metastasis in colorectal cancer. Lancet. 1995;345:1257–9.
90. Greenson JK, Isenhart CE, Rice R, et al. Identification of occult micrometastases in pericolic lymph nodes of Duke's B colorectal cancer patients using monoclonal antibodies against cytokeratin and CC49. Correlation with long-term survival. Cancer. 1994;73:563–9.
91. Read TE, Mutch MG, Chang BW, et al. Locoregional recurrence and survival after curative resection of adenocarcinoma of the colon. J Am Coll Surg. 2002;195:33–40.
92. Jagoditsch M, Lisborg PH, Jatzko GR, et al. Long-term prognosis for colon cancer related to consistent radical surgery: multivariate analysis of clinical, surgical, and pathologic variables. World J Surg. 2000;24:1264–70.
93. McDermott FT, Hughes ES, Pihl E, et al. Comparative results of surgical management of single carcinomas of the colon and rectum: a series of 1939 patients managed by one surgeon. Br J Surg. 1981;68:850–5.
94. Chapuis PH, Dent OF, Fisher R, et al. A multivariate analysis of clinical and pathological variables in prognosis after resection of large bowel cancer. Br J Surg. 1985;72:698–702.
95. Steinberg SM, Barkin JS, Kaplan RS, et al. Prognostic indicators of colon tumors. The Gastrointestinal Tumor Study Group experience. Cancer. 1986;57:1866–70.
96. Karanicolas PJ, Dubois L, Colquhoun PH, et al. The more the better?: the impact of surgeon and hospital volume on in-hospital mortality following colorectal resection. Ann Surg. 2009;249:954–9.
97. Birkmeyer NJ, Goodney PP, Stukel TA, et al. Do cancer centers designated by the National Cancer Institute have better surgical outcomes? Cancer. 2005;103:435–41.
98. Paulson EC, Mitra N, Sonnad S, et al. National Cancer Institute designation predicts improved outcomes in colorectal cancer surgery. Ann Surg. 2008;248:675–86.
99. Grinnell RS. Distal intramural spread of carcinoma of the rectum and rectosigmoid. Surg Gynecol Obstet. 1954;99: 421–30.
100. Quirke P, Durdey P, Dixon MF, et al. Local recurrence of rectal adenocarcinoma due to inadequate surgical resection. Histopathological study of lateral tumour spread and surgical excision. Lancet. 1986;2:996–9.
101. Pezim ME, Nicholls RJ. Survival after high or low ligation of the inferior mesenteric artery during curative surgery for rectal cancer. Ann Surg. 1984;200:729–33.
102. Rouffet F, Hay JM, Vacher B, et al. Curative resection for left colonic carcinoma: hemicolectomy vs. segmental colectomy. A prospective, controlled, multicenter trial. French Association for Surgical Research. Dis Colon Rectum. 1994;37: 651–9.

42 The Preoperative Staging of Rectal Cancer

Susan L. Gearhart and Jonathan E. Efron

Introduction

The classification of a newly diagnosed cancer of the rectum into a staging system with both therapeutic and prognostic applications has been the goal of pathologists and clinicians for the greater part of the last century. Most staging systems rely on the examination of the pathological specimen as well as information gained during surgery. Thus, they are useful only in the postoperative setting and have little use for the purpose of preoperative therapy. Cuthberg Dukes declared in 1932 "If it would be possible to decide the category of the case before operating, this would be very useful information."[1] As the therapeutic options available for the treatment of rectal cancer increase, the ability to accurately stage a rectal tumor preoperatively takes on greater importance. Accurate and reproducible preoperative staging provides uniformity among numerous investigative centers; specifically, those involved in adjuvant preoperative therapy trials.

The effective evaluation of a newly diagnosed rectal cancer should result in a determination of the need for neoadjuvant therapy, the potential for sphincter preservation, and the expected quality of life following treatment. Furthermore, the ability to stage the tumor preoperatively permits the physician to convey more accurate information to the patient and the family with regards to therapeutic options and expected overall prognosis. However, the ability of the treating physician to make these determinants is based on the methods of assessment currently available. The accuracy of these methods is variable and is discussed in this chapter. The currently used system proposed by American Joint Committee on Cancer (AJCC) Staging of Squamous Cell Carcinoma (SCC) for staging colorectal cancer is listed in Table 20-1.

The tumor-related factors of prognostic significance which may be evaluated prior to the treatment of rectal cancer include the depth of penetration of the tumor through the rectal wall, the presence or absence of metastases to the regional and pelvic lymph nodes, and the presence of distant metastases. Clinicians have a variety of diagnostic tools at their disposal that can aid in delineating these aforementioned factors. The most commonly used modalities for the preoperative staging of rectal tumors available today are digital rectal examination, computed tomography (CT), endorectal ultrasonography (ERUS), magnetic resonance imaging (MRI), and positron emission tomography combined with computerized tomography (PET/CT).

Local and Regional Staging

Digital Rectal Examination

Careful digital exam of rectal tumor may yield valuable information regarding the location and degree of fixation of the tumor to the sphincter muscles. Table 42-1 lists some of the important parameters that should be recorded during the DRE of a tumor. A clinical staging system based on tumor mobility was first established by York-Mason in 1976[2] and subsequently modified in 1982.[3] In this clinical staging system, tumor mobility is correlated with the level of tumor penetration in the different layers of the rectal wall. Nicholls et al.[3] evaluated this clinical staging system and discovered that senior examiners had an 80% accuracy in distinguishing superficial tumors from deep tumors and was more accurate with more advanced lesions, but only a 50% accuracy in detecting lymph node metastasis. Therefore, the accuracy of DRE in staging rectal cancer was considered not dependable and directly proportional to the experience of the examiner. The use of DRE alone in the staging of rectal cancer is considered inadequate.

Endorectal Ultrasound

Endorectal ultrasound (EUS) is an outpatient procedure requiring only enema preparation and often no sedation or

D.E. Beck et al. (eds.), *The ASCRS Textbook of Colon and Rectal Surgery: Second Edition*,
DOI 10.1007/978-1-4419-1584-9_42,

anesthesia. Endoscopic assessment can occur with a rigid or flexible ultrasound probe. The frequency of the ultrasound transducer determines its focal range and ultrasonographic resolution. Complete circular imaging of the rectal wall can be obtained with the 360-degree rotating endorectal probe. Most investigators use a two-dimensional (2D) 7.0 or a 10 mHz transducer which provides a five layer anatomic model of the rectal wall with three hyperechoic circles and two hypoechoic concentric circles (Figure 42-1A and B).[4] A multiplanar three-dimensional (3D) ERUS with coronal, sagittal, and transverse images has more recently been employed to increase the accuracy of the 2D ERUS.

The accuracy of ERUS in the initial evaluation of rectal cancer is user dependent and variable. Mor et al.[5] surveyed 100 members of the American Society of Colon and Rectal Surgery (ASCRS) who were experienced in EUS. The survey asked members to review and stage 26 ultrasound images. The overall accuracy was 39–60% with 15% of tumors overstaged and 23% understaged. The Minnesota series is one of the largest series published in 2002 by Garcia-Aguilar et al.[6] These investigators reported their experience with 1,184 patients with rectal carcinoma or villous adenoma that underwent ERUS. Histopathologic correlation was available for the 545 patients who had no prior radiotherapy. The accuracy of ERUS in assessing the level of penetration was only 69%, with 18% overstaged and 13% understaged. The accuracy was notably higher for benign lesions and for full thickness lesions. Lower accuracy rates occurred for T1 and T2 lesions. For nodal involvement, the accuracy in the 238 patients who had radical surgery was poor, 64% with 25% overstaged and 11% understaged. However, a recent meta-analysis suggests that the sensitivity and specificity for nodal staging in rectal cancer is 75%.[7]

TABLE 42-1. Tumor characteristics to assess on digital examination

Location
Morphology
Number of quadrants involved
Degree of fixation
Mobility
Extrarectal growths
Direct continuity with other structures (vagina)

Early studies by Hunerbein et al.[8] using 3D ultrasound in the initial staging of rectal cancer demonstrated no significant benefit between conventional ERUS or 3D ERUS. However, the investigators did suggested that the multiplanar effect of 3D imaging may be useful in planning surgery. More recently, Kim et al.[9] demonstrated in 86 patients that the accuracy of 3D ERUS was 10% improved over conventional ERUS. This study also demonstrated that conical protrusions along the deep tumor border seen best on 3D images correlated closely with tumor infiltration, advanced T-stage, and lymph node metastasis.

There are several limitations to the use of ERUS. There is a significant learning curve associated with the interpretation of the endorectal ultrasound image. Orrom and Wong et al.[10] at the University of Minnesota demonstrated an accuracy of 75% at determining bowel wall invasion; however, during the last 6 months of the study, the authors showed improvement with a 95% accuracy. Rafalesen et al.[11] reported that the reader experience had a significant effect of the assessment of penetration of the bowel wall by tumor. When comparing more experienced with less experienced radiologist, the accuracy for bowel wall penetration was 90% vs. 66%, respectively.

Overstaging tumor is common in many reported series because of the inability of ultrasound to differentiate perirectal inflammation from tumor infiltration in the perirectal fat. Furthermore, the differentiation between inflammatory or neoplastic nodes is difficult with ERUS. Morphologic criteria suggestive of metastatic involvement within the

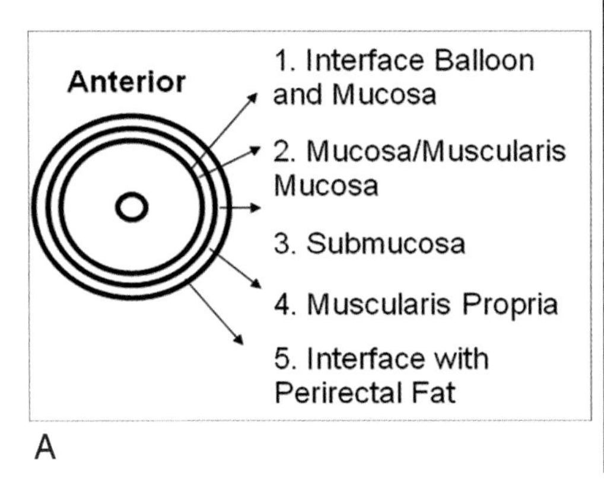

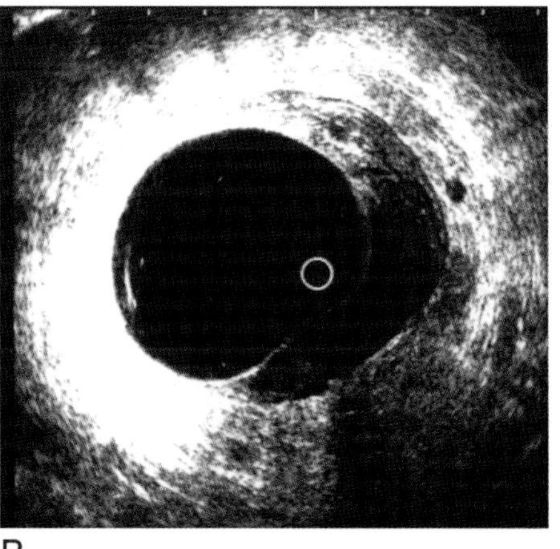

FIGURE 42-1. **A** EUS demonstrating the five layers of the rectum. **B** Standard EUS of rectal tumor.

lymph node are listed in Table 42-2. Methods to differentiate include further characterization of the node with ERUS or ERUS-guided biopsy. Hildebrandt et al.[12] determined that hypoechoic lymph nodes represented tumor metastases, whereas hyperechoic lymph nodes represented inflammatory changes. They reported an overall accuracy rate of 78%. Errors in ERUS lymph node staging were attributed to micrometastases, mixed lymph nodes, and changing echo patterns within inflammatory nodes. The impact of ERUS-guided fine-needle aspiration of perirectal nodes has been investigated by Harewood et al.[13] ERUS-guided biopsy was utilized in the preoperative staging of 80 consecutive patients with rectal cancer.[13] In this series, FNA did not significantly improve nodal staging over ERUS alone. Based on these results and the potential risk of spreading cancer cells into the mesorectum, ultrasound-guided biopsy of enlarged perirectal nodes is not routinely used in clinical practice.

ERUS is difficult to perform in near obstructing lesions and those higher up in the rectum. Early studies by Sentovich et al.[14] and Senesse et al.[15] reported significantly better result in determining the depth of invasion of a rectal tumor that was within 6 cm of the anal verge as compared to those >6 cm from the anal verge. One suggested method to improve placement of the ultrasound probe to accurately evaluate higher tumors is by insertion of the probe with the assistance of a proctoscope.[5] Using this method, Santoro et al. was able to demonstrate staging with pathological correlation to an accuracy of 78.9% for tumors of the upper rectum.[16]

TABLE 42-2. Morphologic lymph node characteristics on EUS suggestive of possible malignancy

Hyperechoic appearance
Round shape
Peritumoral location
>5 mm

Magnetic Resonance Imaging

Accuracy rates for MRI in the preoperative staging of rectal cancer have varied according to technique. Initial experience with using body-coil MRI was poor. However, with the introduction of dedicated phase array coils, high-resolution imaging of the anorectum is possible without an intraluminal coil. The main concept in the use of MRI to stage rectal cancer is to obtain high-resolution images within small field-of-view thin sections with fast/turbo spin echo (FSE/TSE) T-2 weighted axial and coronal views of the rectum (Figure 42-2A and B).[17] This method provides inherent contrast between the hypointense extramural component of the tumor and the bright signal of the mesorectal fat. Acquiring images that are directly parallel or perpendicular to the tumor and distending the rectum with gel increase the accuracy of MRI on determining the depth of bowel wall invasion.

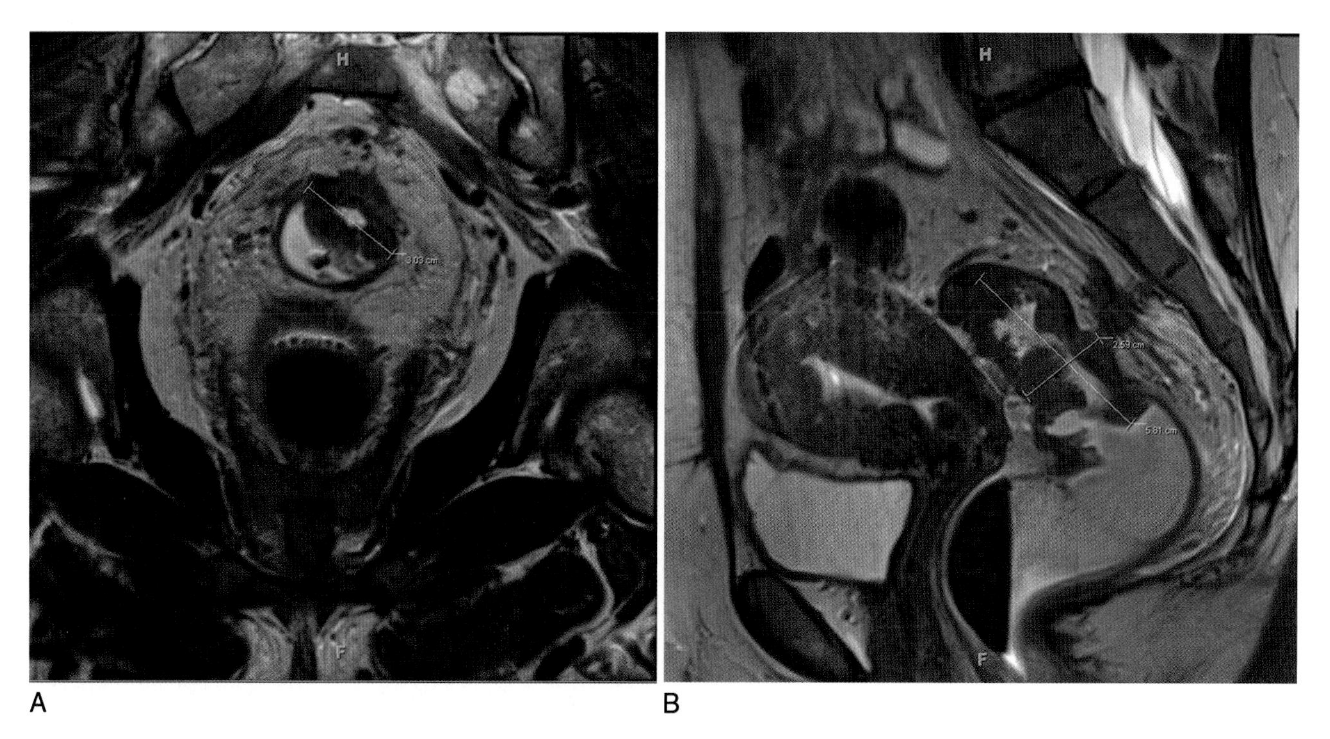

FIGURE 42-2. **A** and **B** The main concept in the use of MRI to stage rectal cancer is to obtain high-resolution images within small field-of-view thin sections with fast/turbo spin echo (FSE/TSE) T-2 weighted axial and coronal views of the rectum.

Since its original description in 1986, multiple studies have evaluated the accuracy of MRI in staging rectal cancer. Kim et al.[18] in the largest published trial to date examining the accuracy of MRI staging of rectal cancer, compared the histopathological staging with the preoperative staging in 217 patients. The accuracy for the depth of invasion was 81% and for regional lymph node metastasis was 63%. Similar to staging of bowel wall infiltration on EUS, MRI T staging has been defined by Brown et al.[19] (Table 42-3).

MRI identification of metastatic lymph node involvement has not been standardized. According to Brown et al.[20] criteria that are most predictable for determining lymph node metastasis are signal heterogeneity and an irregular border. Size criteria are not adequate. It is important to remember that in patients with rectal cancer, approximately 15% of lymph nodes smaller than 5 mm are positive for metastasis. With the use of ultrasmall superparamagnetic iron oxide (UPSIO)-enhanced MRI, recent advances have been made in the evaluation of lymph nodes. The iron oxide nanoparticle is given intravenously and is transported to the lymphatic system where it is picked by macrophages. The nanoparticle causes a decrease in signal intensity, and therefore, inflammatory lymph nodes exhibit less signal intensity. Initial results using this technique demonstrate up to a 93% sensitivity and 96% specificity for perirectal lymph node metastasis.[21] However, larger prospective trials are needed to validate initial findings.

In recent years, tumor involvement of the circumferential resection margin (CRM) has been identified as an important predictor of locoregional recurrence in rectal cancer patients undergoing a radical proctectomy with total mesorectal excision (TME).[22–25] Postoperative radiation is not effective in reducing the risk of local recurrence in patients with a positive CRM,[26] and a curative operation in these patients requires either tumor downstaging by preoperative chemoradiation, an extended resection, or both. Consequently, the preoperative assessment of the relationship of the tumor with the fascia propria of the rectum, the CRM in patients treated with TME, has become upmost importance in deciding the type of neoadjuvant therapy and planning the surgical resection. The fascia propria of the rectum is well visualized by phased-array coil MRI, and several studies have suggested that MRI can predict with high degree of accuracy the distance of the tumor to the fascia propria of the rectum (Figure 42-3).[27,28] Furthermore, due to its multiplanar capabilities, MRI is the most accurate imaging technique in assessing the relationship of the tumor with the levator plate and the sphincter complex. This information may be useful in selecting patients with low rectal cancer for a sphincter saving procedure.

In 2004, Bipat et al.[29] reported their findings on a meta-analysis looking at the assessment of local staging for rectal cancer by ERUS, MRI, and CT. Their findings demonstrated that ERUS proved to be the most accurate modality overall. However, the sensitivity and specificity of each method varied greatly dependent on the depth of tumor invasion or the presence of lymph node metastasis (Table 42-4). The authors concluded from their findings suggest that MRI may result in overstaging of early lesions. Furthermore, this analysis did not show any difference in the known MR technique that was used in imaging (body coil alone, body coil and additional coil, unenhanced, enhance with gadolinium, low vs. high magnetic field). Newer studies using phase-array MR techniques have only shown a marginal benefit with the detection of lymph node metastasis (Table 42-5).[30] Figure 42-3 demonstrates a small pelvic lymph node detected on phase-array MR.

TABLE 42-3. MRI T staging as proposed by Brown et al[19]

MRI T stage
T1: Low signal in the submucosal layer or replacement of the submucosal layer by abnormal signal not extending into circular muscle layer.
T2: Intermediate signal intensity within muscularis propria. Outer muscle coat replaced by tumor of intermediate signal intensity that does not extend beyond the outer rectal muscle into perirectal fat.
T3: Broad-based bulge or nodular projection (not fine speculation) of intermediate signal intensity projecting beyond outer muscle coat.
T4: Extension of abnormal signal into adjacent organ, extension of tumor signal through the peritoneal reflection.

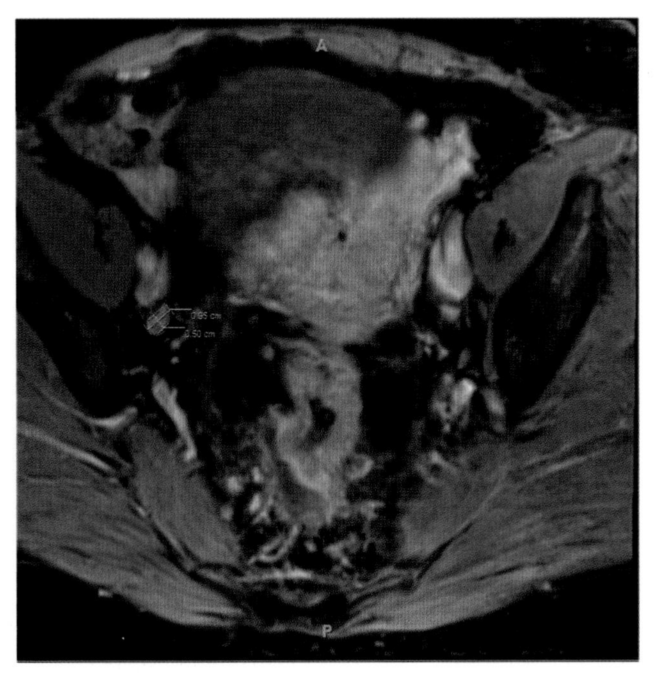

FIGURE 42-3. High resolution MRI image demonstrating an enlarged right pelvic side wall lymph node.

Table 42-4. Sensitivity and specificity for EUS, CT, and MRI in the preoperative staging of rectal cancer

Stage	Imaging modality	Sensitivity % (95% CI)	Specificity % (95% CI)
T2	EUS	94 (90–97)	86 (80–90)
	MRI	94 (89–97)	69 (52–82)*
	CT	–	–
T3	EUS	90 (88–92)	75 (69–81)
	MRI	82 (74–87)*	76 (65–84)
	CT	79 (74–84)*	78 (73–83)
T4	EUS	70 (62–77)	97 (96–98)
	MRI	74 (63–83)	96 (95–97)
	CT	72 (64–79)	96 (95–97)
Node Positive	EUS	67 (60–73)	78 (71–84)
	MRI	66 (54–76)	76 (59–87)
	CT	55 (43–67)	74 (67–80)

Modified from Bipat S, van Leeuwen M, Comans E, Pijil M, Bossuyt P, Zwinderman A, Stoker J. Colorectal liver metastases: CT, MR Imaging, and PET for diagnosis – meta-analysis. Radiology. 2005:237;123–31.[29]
EUS endorectal ultrasound, *CT* computed tomography, *MRI* magnetic resonance imaging, *CI* confidence interval.
*$p<0.05$ EUS to other.

Table 42-5. Accuracy of nodal staging in preoperative evaluation of rectal cancer with MRI pelvic-phased array coil

References	No. of patients	Accuracy (%)
Ferri (2005)	29	59
Matsuoka (2003)	19	89.5
Brown (2003)	60	85
Gagliardi (2002)	26	69
Blomqvist (2000)	47	47
Kim (2000)	217	63
Hadfield (1997)	28	76

Modified from Skandarajah A and Tjandra J. Preoperative loco-regional imaging in rectal cancer. ANZ J Surg. 2006;76:497–504.[30]
MRI magnetic resonance imaging.

Distant Metastases

Computed Tomography

The detection of distant metastasis is of prime importance for the accurate staging of rectal cancer. The most common sites of distant metastasis include the liver and lung. The common imaging modalities used today to detect liver metastasis preoperatively is computerized tomography; however, MRI and PET/CT are being used more frequently. Even after preoperative imaging, up to one-third of colorectal cancer patients are found at the time of surgery to have unsuspected additional liver lesions or extrahepatic metastases. A recent meta-analysis reported by Bipat et al.[31] evaluated the use of CT, MRI, or PET for the diagnosis of colorectal liver metastatsis. The investigators found that 18-fluorodeoxyglucose positron emission tomography (FDG-PET) was the more accurate method to detect liver metastasis on a per-patient basis. When evaluating different lesions, MR imaging at 1.5T and FDG-PET were comparable and significantly more accurate than CT. Sensitivity estimates for all imaging modalities studied for lesions less than 1 cm, where much less than for lesions ≥1 cm (11.6–29.3% vs. 65.7–90.2%).

CT is universally available which makes it appealing as a method for local regional staging. However, CT has not proven to be very accurate in determining the depth of penetration of the tumor through rectal wall or assessing involved perirectal lymph nodes metastasis. The reported accuracy rate of CT in determining tumor penetration through the rectal wall is 52–100% and in determining lymph node involvement is 35–70%.[32–39] Newer technology, such as the multidetector-row computed tomography (MDRCT), may significantly improve the ability of CT scans to accurately determine the depth of invasion and lymph node metastasis in rectal cancer. MDRCT utilizes four detectors which result in a much higher resolution and better multiplanar reformation of the images. Matsuoka et al.[40] compared 21 patients who had MDRCT to 21 patients that had MRI evaluations of the pelvis for rectal cancer. They reported an accuracy rate of 95% on the depth of invasion for MDRCT vs. 100% for MRI, whereas lymph node accuracy was 70% vs. 61% for MDRCT and MRI, respectively.

18-Fluorodeoxyglucose Positron Emission Tomography

At the present time, FDG-PET is primarily used for the diagnosis of local and distant recurrence after curative surgery for colorectal cancer. It is also being used with increased frequency to detect distant metastasis of the time of the primary diagnosis of rectal cancer. FDG-PET has been shown to have higher sensitivity and specificity in detecting recurrent rectal cancer than both CT and MRI.[41,42] While sensitivity and specificity for diagnosing tumor recurrence are higher for

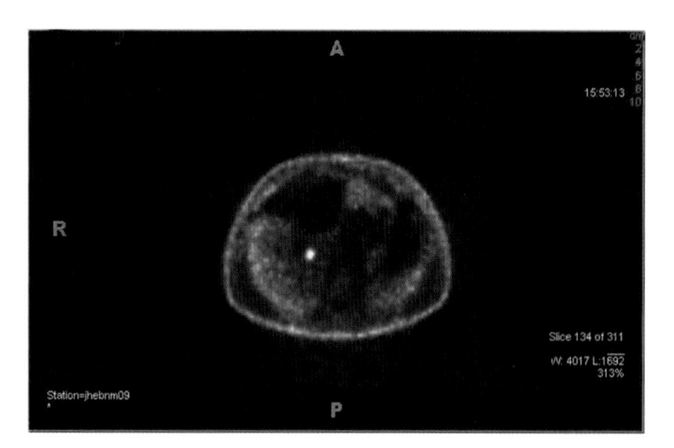

Figure 42-4. PET scan.

FDG-PET, its specificity for the tumor location is not very accurate, and therefore other studies, such as MRI and/or CT scans are required to define the precise location of the tumor to important anatomical landmarks. To enhance the image, current scanners that fuse CT or MR images with the FDG-PET images are available. When comparing FDG-PET scan and PET/CT images in a series of 45 patients with colorectal cancer, the overall staging accuracy increased from 78 to 89% with PET/CT.[43]

The impact of FDG-PET and FDG-PET/CT in the preoperative staging and management of rectal cancer patients has been studied by Heriot et al.[44] in a series of 46 patients who were assessed with FDG-PET scans at the time of their initial diagnosis. The surgical management was changed in 17% of the patients because of positive FDG-PET scan findings that upstaged the disease. Furthermore, Gearhart et al. demonstrated in 37 patients that FDG-PET/CT was able to demonstrate additional significant findings in 38% of patients with a known primary rectal cancer resulting in an alteration in the treatment planning for 27% of patients.[45] These changes in management included canceling surgery and changing the field of administered radiation.

Radiographic Assessment of Response to Neoadjuvant Therapy

Preoperative radiation of rectal cancer causes various degrees of tumor regression resulting in scarring and fibrosis that impairs accurate imaging. Napoleon et al.[46] demonstrated that EUS was not accurate at determining bowel wall invasion following radiation. The depth of wall invasion was correctly determined in 86% of patients without radiotherapy, but in only 47% in those patients in whom previous radiotherapy had been administered. The use of EUS in restaging rectal cancer following radiation is limited.

The limitation of MRI imaging in rectal cancer has been its inherent inability to differentiate fibrosis from residual tumor following treatment. For this reason, conventional MRI has not been shown to be useful in determining response to therapy. However, functional MR imaging, has been demonstrated to be useful in the evaluation of the response of rectal cancer to neoadjuvant therapy. Functional MR techniques provide in vivo physiologic and metabolic information about a tumor over time. The components of functional MR include spectroscopy, diffusion, and contrast enhancement. Spectroscopy provides assessment of the concentration of several metabolites and is useful as a noninvasive technique as a means of studying the biochemistry of a lesion relative to normal tissue. Diffusion-weighted MR measures the apparent diffusion coefficient (ADC) which detects thermally induced motion of water molecules and cellular integrity. Viable tumors have intact cell membranes limiting the mobility of water molecules that is reflected as a low ADC value. If there is cellular necrosis, there is enhanced cell membrane permeability which allows for increased motion of water molecules and results in a rise in the ADV value. Kim et al.[47] demonstrated that the diagnostic accuracy of diffusion-weighted MR was significantly improved over conventional MR at predicting a complete response to neoadjuvant therapy. Finally, Dynamic Contrast-enhanced MRI (DCE-MRI) measures the degree of extracellular contrast enhancement which reflects vascular integrity. A decrease in contrast enhancement of a lesion is expected after locoregional therapy and may predict the extent of tumor necrosis. Further studies to validate these findings are necessary.

The use of serial FDG-PET/CT in predicting response to neoadjuvant therapy has been evaluated by several investigators.[48–57] Melton et al.[48] demonstrated that serial FDG-PET/CT is more effective at discerning the presence of minimal or microscopic disease and less effective at identifying lymph node metastasis when correlated with histological findings at the time of surgery (Figure 42-4). The reported specificity for predicting a near complete or complete pathological response to therapy with serial FDG-PET/CT is 60–95% (Table 42-6).[49–51] The timing of serial FDG-PET appears to be important in that FDG-PET/CT after 2 weeks of treatment can predict pathological response with similar specificity to FDG-PET/CT performed at the end of treatment.[52] This earlier time period may be advantageous for determining if the neoadjuvant regimen should be modified in patients that appear not to be responding.

Currently, the use of a newer modality, 3′-deoxy-3′ (^{18}F) fluorothymidine (FLT) in PET scanning has been utilized in the assessment of malignant tumors because of its potential to noninvasively monitor cellular proliferation. The appeal of monitoring thymidine activity is the importance of thymidine in DNA synthesis and cell proliferation. Cell uptake studies have demonstrated that FLT accumulates in cancer cells and tumors in proportion to their rate of cellular proliferation. Furthermore, several studies have indicated that early changes in FLT uptake, measured soon after treatment begins, may be able to predict a tumors response to chemoradiation.[53–55] The use of this modality in monitoring response to therapy in colorectal cancer has not been formally evaluated.

TABLE 42-6. Specificity of FDG-PET to predict near complete or complete pathologic response following chemoradiation for primary rectal cancer

Author	Year	*N*	Specificity (%)	Parameter	Endpoint
Guillem	2004	10	80	VRS	pCR (TRG 1)
Amthauer	2004	20	86	RI	R1
Capirci	2004	78	76	VRS	TRG 1–2
Chessin	2005	21	95	VRS	Response
Deneke	2005	23	60	RI	Major response
Melton	2007	21	81	RI	TRG 1–2
Cascini	2006	33	87	RI	TRG 1–2
Caprici	2009	81	80	RI	TRG 1–2

Modified from Capirci C, Rubello D, Pasini F, et al. The role of dual-time combined 18-fluoridedoexyglucose positron emission tomography and computed tomography in the staging and restaging workup of locally advanced rectal cancer, treated with preoperative chemoradiation therapy and radical surgery. Int J Radiation Oncology Biol Phys. 2009;74:1461–69.[51]
VRS visual response score, *RI* response index, *TRG* tumor regression grade.

Finally, perfusion CT has emerged as a noninvasive method to assess the microvascular status of tumor tissue. Regression of tumor microvasculature is considered an important surrogate marker for response to treatment. Sequential imaging using CT perfusion techniques is thought to provide a better method for the determination of response of the tumor to chemoradiation.[56] However, perfusion techniques in DCE-MRI have demonstrated superiority in gauging response with MRI.[57]

Conclusion

The accurate preoperative tumor staging is essential to select the best therapy for the rectal cancer patient. Presently, the depth of invasion and evidence of perirectal lymph nodes involvement is best assessed with high-resolution MRI. Whole-body CT scanning or abdominal MRI is also important to detect extrarectal tumor. The role of serial imaging modalities to determine clinical response is currently under investigation.

References

1. Dukes C. The classification of cancer of the rectum. J Pathol Bacteriol. 1932;35:323–32.
2. York-Mason A. Rectal cancer. The spectrum of selective surgery. Proc R Soc Med. 1976;69:237–44.
3. Nicholls RJ, York-Mason A, Morson BC, et al. The clinical staging of rectal cancer. Br J Surg. 1982;69:404–9.
4. Nogueras JJ. Endorectal ultrasonography: technique, image interpretation, and expanding indications in 1995. Semin Colon Rectal Surg. 1995;6:70–7.
5. Mor I, Hull T, Hammel J, Zutshi M. Rectal endosonography: just how good are we at its interpretation? Int J Colorectal Dis. 2010;25:87–90.
6. Garcia-Aguilar J, Pollack J, Lee SH, et al. Accuracy of endorectal ultrasonography in preoperative staging of rectal tumors. Dis Colon Rectum. 2002;45:10–5.
7. Puli S, Reddy J, Bechtold M, Choudhary A, Antillon M, Brugge W. Accuracy of endoscopic ultrasound to diagnose nodal invasion by rectal cancer: meta-analysis and systematic review. Ann Surg Onc. 2009;16:1255–65.
8. Hunerbein M, Pegios W, Rau B, Vogl TJ, Felix R, Schlag PM. Prospective comparison of endorectal ultrasound, 3-D endorectal ultrasound, and endorectal MRI in the preoperative evaluation of rectal tumors. Preliminary results. Surg Endosc. 2000;14:1005–9.
9. Kim JC, Cho YK, Kim SY, et al. Comparison study of three-dimensional and conventional endorectal ultrasounography used in rectal cancer staging. Surg Endosc. 2002;16(9):1280–5.
10. Orrom WJ, Wong WD, Rothenberger DA, et al. Endorectal ultrasound in the preoperative staging of rectal tumors: a learning experience. Dis Colon Rectum. 1990;33:654–9.
11. Rafaelsen S, Sorensen T, Jakobsen A, Bisgaard C, Lindebjerg J. Transrectal ultrasonography and magnetic resonance imaging in the staging of rectal cancer. Effect of experience. Scan J Gastroenterol. 2008;43:440–6.
12. Hildebrandt U, Klein T, Fiefel G, et al. Endosonography of pararectal lymph nodes: in vitro and in vivo evaluation. Dis Colon Rectum. 1990;33:863–8.
13. Harewood GC, Wiersema MJ, Nelson H, et al. A prospective, blinded assessment of the impact of preoperative staging on the management of rectal cancer. Gastroenterology. 2002;123:24–32.
14. Sentovich S, Blatchford G, Falk F, Thorson A, Christensen M. Transrectal US of rectal tumors. Am J Surg. 1993;166:638–41.
15. Senesse P, Khemissa F, Lemar S, et al. Contribution of EUS in the preoperative evaluation of low rectal cancer. Gastroentérol Clin Biol. 2001;25:24–8.
16. Santoro G, D'Ella A, Battistella G, Di Falco G. The use of dedicated rectosigmoidoscope for US staging of tumors of the upper and middle third of the rectum. Colorectal Dis. 2007;9:61–6.
17. Jhaveri K, Sdaf A. Role of MRI for staging of rectal cancer. Expert Rev Anticancer Ther. 2009;9:469–81.
18. Kim NK, Kim MJ, Park JK, Park SIL, Min JS. Preoperative staging of rectal cancer with MRI: accuracy and clinical usefulness. Ann Surg Oncol. 2000;7(10):732–7.
19. Brown G, Daniels IR. Preoperative staging of rectal cancer: the MERCURY research project. Recent Results Cancer Res. 2005;165:58–74.
20. Brown G, Richard CJ, Williams GT, et al. Morphological predictors of lymph node status in rectal cancer using high spatial

resolution magnetic resonance imaging with histopathological comparison. Radiology. 2003;90(3):355–64.
21. Lahaye M, Engelen S, Kessels A, et al. USPIO-enhanced MR imaging for nodal staging in patients with primary rectal cancer: predictive criteria. Radiology. 2008;246:804–11.
22. Quirke P, Durdey P, et al. Local recurrence of rectal adenocarcinoma due to inadequate surgical resection: histopathological study of lateral tumor spread and surgical excision. Lancet. 1986;2:996–9.
23. Adam IJ, Mohamdee MO, et al. Role of circumferential margin involvement in the local recurrence of rectal cancer. Lancet. 1994;344:707–11.
24. Hall NR, Finan PJ, et al. Circumferential margin involvement after mesorectal excision of rectal cancer with curative intent: predictor of survival but not local recurrence? Dis Colon Rectum. 1998;41(8):979–83.
25. Nagtegaal ID, Marijnen CA, et al. Circumferential margin involvement is still an important predictor of local recurrence in rectal carcinoma: not one millimeter but two millimeters is the limit. Am J Surg Pathol. 2002;26(3):350–7.
26. Marijnen CA, Nagtegaal ID, et al. Radiotherapy does not compensate for positive resection margins in rectal cancer patients: report of a multicenter randomized trial. Int J Radiat Oncol Biol Phys. 2003;55(5):1311–20.
27. Beets-Tan RG. MRI in rectal cancer: the T stage and circumferential resection margin. Colorectal Dis. 2003;5(5):392–5.
28. Branagan G, Chave H, et al. Can magnetic resonance imaging predict circumferential margins and TNM stage in rectal cancer? Dis Colon Rectum. 2004;47(8):1317–22.
29. Bipat S, Las A, Slors F, Zwinderman A, Bossuyt P, Stoker J. Rectal cancer: local staging and assessment of lymph node involvement with endoluminal US, CT, and MRI imaging – a meta-analysis. Radiology. 2004;232:773–83.
30. Skandarajah A, Tjandra J. Preoperative loco-regional imaging in rectal cancer. ANZ J Surg. 2006;76:497–504.
31. Bipat S, van Leeuwen M, Comans E, Pijil M, Bossuyt P, Zwinderman A, et al. Colorectal liver metastases: CT, MR imaging, and PET for diagnosis – meta-analysis. Radiology. 2005;237:123–31.
32. Dixon AK, Frye IK, Morson BC, et al. Pre-operative computed tomography of carcinoma of the rectum. Br J Radiol. 1981;54:655–9.
33. Thompson WM, Halvorsen RA, Foster Jr WL, et al. Pre-operative and post-operative CT staging of rectosigmoid carcinoma. AJR. 1986;146:703–10.
34. Freeny PC, Marks WM, Tyan JA, et al. Colorectal carcinoma evaluation with CT: pre-operative staging and detection of post-operative recurrence. Radiology. 1986;158:347–53.
35. Holdsworth PJ, Johnston D, Chalmers AG, et al. Endoluminal ultrasound and computed tomography in the staging of rectal cancer. Br J Surg. 1988;75:1019–22.
36. Goldman S, Arvidsson H, Norming U, et al. Transrectal ultrasound and computed tomography in preoperative staging of lower rectal adenocarcinoma. Gastrointest Radiol. 1991;16:259–63.
37. Zerhouni EA, Rutter C, Hamilton SR, et al. CT and MR imaging in the staging of colorectal carcinoma: report of the Radiology Diagnostics Oncology Group II. Radiology. 1996;200:443–51.
38. Matsuoka H, Nakamura A, Masaki T, et al. Preoperative staging by multidetector-row computed tomography in patients with rectal carcinoma. Am J Surg. 2002;184:131–5.
39. Chiesura-Corona M, Muzzio PC, Giust G, et al. Rectal cancer: CT local staging with histopathologic correlation. Abdom Imaging. 2001;26:134–8.
40. Matsuoka H, Nakamura A, Masaki T, et al. A prospective comparison between multidetector-row computed tomography and magnetic resonance imaging in the preoperative evaluation of rectal carcinoma. Am J Surg. 2003;185(6):556–9.
41. Whiteford MH, Whiteford HM, Yee LF, et al. Usefulness of FDG-PET scan in the assessment of suspected metastatic or recurrent adenocarcinoma of the colon and rectum. Dis Colon Rectum. 2000;43(6):759–67.
42. Cohade C, Osman MM, Leal J, Wahl RL. Direct comparison of (18)F-FDG PET and PET/CT in patients with colorectal carcinoma. J Nucl Med. 2003;44(11):1804–5.
43. Cohade C, Osman M, Leal J, Wahl RL. Direct comparison of (18)F-FDG PET and PET/CT in patients with colorectal carcinoma. J Nucl Med. 2003;44(11):1797–803.
44. Heriot AG, Hicks RJ, Drummond EGP, et al. Does positron emission tomography change management in primary rectal cancer? A prospective assessment. Dis Colon Rectum. 2004; 47(4):451–8.
45. Gearhart SL, Frassica D, Rossen R, Choti M, Schulick R, Wahl R. Improved staging with pre-treatment PET/CT in low rectal cancer. J Surg Oncol. 2006;13(3):397–404.
46. Napoleon B, Pujol B, Berger F, et al. Accuracy of endosonography in the staging of rectal cancer treated by radiotherapy. Br J Surg. 1991;78:785–8.
47. Kim SH, Lee JM, Hong SH, et al. Locally advanced rectal cancer: added value of diffusion-weighted MR imaging in the evaluation of tumor response to neoadjuvant chemoradiotherapy. Radiology. 2009;253(1):116–25.
48. Melton G, Lavely W, Jacene H, Schulick R, Choti M, Wahl R, et al. Efficacy of preoperative combined 18-fluorodeoscyglucose positron emission tomography and computed tomography for assessing primary rectal cancer response to neoadjuvant therapy. J Gastrointest Surg. 2007;11(8):961–9.
49. Guillem JG, Puig-La Calle Jr J, Akurst T. Prospective assessment of primary rectal cancer response to preoperative radiation and chemotherapy using 18-flourodeoxyglucose positron emission tomography. Dis Colon Rectum. 2000;43(1):18–24.
50. Delrio P, Lastoria S, Avallone A, et al. Early evaluation using PET-FDG of the efficiency of neoadjuvant radiochemotherapy treatment in locally advanced neoplasia of the lower rectum. Tumori. 2003;89(4 Suppl):50–3.
51. Capirci C, Rubello D, Pasini F, et al. The role of dual-time combined 18-Fluoridedoexyglucose positron emission tomography and computed tomography in the staging and restaging workup of locally advanced rectal cancer, treated with preoperative chemoradiation therapy and radical surgery. Int J Radiat Oncol Biol Phys. 2009;74:1461–9.
52. Janssen M, Ollers M, Riedel R, et al. Accurate prediction of pathological rectal tumor response after 2 weeks of preoperative radiochemotherapy using ^{18}fluorodeoxyglucose-positron emission tomography-computed tomography imaging. Int J Radiat Oncol Biol Phys. 2009;4:1–8.

53. Wieder H, Geinitz H, Rosenberg R, et al. PET imaging with 18-F-3-doxy-3-fluorothympidine for prediction of response to neoadjuvant treatment in patients with rectal cancer. Eur J Nucl Med Mol Imaging. 2007;34:878–83.
54. Amthauer H, Deneke T, Rau N. Response prediction by FDG-PET after neoadjuvant radiochemotherapy and combined hyperthermia of rectal cancer. Eur J Nulc Med Mol Imaging. 2004;31:811–9.
55. Chessin B, Akhurst T, Yeung H. Positron emission tomography during preoperative combined modality therapy for rectal cancer may predict ultimate pathologic response: a prospective analysis. J Clin Oncol. 2005;16:3612.
56. Denke T, Rau N, Hoffmann K. Comparison of CT, MRI, and FDG-PET in response prediction of patients with locally advanced rectal cancer after multimodal preoperative therapy; is there a benefit in using functional imaging? Eur Radiol. 2005;15:1658–66.
57. Kim S, Lee J, Hong S, Kim G, Lee J, Han J, et al. Locally advanced rectal cancer: added value of diffusion-weighted MR imaging in the evaluation of tumor response to neoadjuvant chemo-radiation therapy. Radiology. 2009;1:116–25.

43
Local Excision of Rectal Cancer

Peter A. Cataldo

The earliest surgery for rectal cancer involved local excision. Due to limitations in anesthesia, surgical instruments, operative techniques, and blood transfusions, transabdominal, radical resections were thought to be too risky. Local excision, however safe, was associated with high local recurrence rates and poor overall survival, perhaps due to patient selection and inability to remove peritumoral lymph nodes containing regional metastases. For these reasons, Sir Earnest Miles expanded the indications for abdominal–perineal resection[1] (APR), originally described by Faget for perianal sepsis[2] for the treatment of rectal cancer. He believed that excision of regional lymph nodes would improve overall cure rates. Miles theories were correct, but not without consequences, as seven of his original nine patients died from complications of surgery.[1] Complication concerns following APR continue today with mortality rates ranging from 0 to 6.3%[3,4] and complication rates as high as 61%.[5] In addition, APR is associated with a high rate of sexual dysfunction (67%) and stoma related problems (66%).[6] Finally, despite these complications and long-term functional consequences, some early rectal cancers recur despite radical surgery. The 5-year survival for Stage I rectal cancer following radical surgery is 73% as reported by the National Cancer Data Base.[7]

For these reasons, many surgeons have sought alternative treatment options for early rectal cancer. These include chemoradiotherapy alone, and local excision with or without adjuvant treatment. Appropriate treatment always begins with appropriate patient selection, and in the case of cancer therapy, proper patient selection is dependent upon accurate (preoperative) tumor staging. This is the major challenge for local excision of rectal cancer.

In the case of rectal cancer, staging can be divided into local and distant (or systemic) staging. Staging of distant disease is straightforward and well-established. Computed tomography (CT), magnetic resonance imaging (MRI), and positron emission tomography (PET) scanning have very high accuracy rates when detecting distant disease and are discussed in Chap. 40. Local staging represents a much more difficult and important challenge in rectal cancer. Tumor staging must include the depth of penetration of the rectal wall (T-Stage) and evaluation of adjacent lymph nodes (N-Stage). The impact of this information helps identify which patients are candidates for local excision (T1), prompt surgery (T2), or who require neoadjuvant chemoradiotherapy (T3). The presence or absence of lymphadenopathy has great impact as patients with metastatic regional lymph nodes (N+) are not candidates for any type of curative local excision.

Unfortunately, the accuracy of local staging with both pelvic MRI (with or without endorectal coil) and endorectal ultrasound is variable at best. Accuracy rates range from 71 to 90% for T-Stage assessment by ultrasound[8] and 54 to 81% for MRI, respectively.[9,10] Similarly, the accuracy for lymph nodes staging remains poor 61–80% for EUS[8] and 41–55% for MRI.[11] Perhaps more importantly, the accuracy of these techniques is not improving and is unlikely to improve in the near future. Andreola et al. evaluated lymph node metastases in 101 patients with distal rectal cancer. Forty-five percent of all metastatic lymph nodes were smaller than 5 mm. Fourteen percent of Stage III patients (only) had lymph nodes <5 mm, and 43% of these patients eventually developed metastatic disease.[12] Small metastatic lymph nodes are common and clinically significant, and it is unlikely that our current staging techniques identify these lymph nodes. MRI with tumor injection of ultra-small magnetic particles has shown some promise, but is not clinically available at this time.

Treatment Algorithm

With the aforementioned caveats, rectal cancer should be staged as accurately as possible, both locally and systemically, and patients considered for local excision if appropriate. Any stage patient may be a candidate for *palliative* local excision provided the lesion is accessible and safe excision (and rectal closure) is technically possible. However, the criteria for "*curative*" transanal excision (TAE) are much stricter. Opinions and practice patterns vary widely as do published oncologic results. A reasonable patient selection guide and

D.E. Beck et al. (eds.), *The ASCRS Textbook of Colon and Rectal Surgery: Second Edition*,
DOI 10.1007/978-1-4419-1584-9_43, © Springer Science+Business Media, LLC 2011

treatment algorithm is as follows: For T_1N_0, lesions without adverse histologic features (lymphovascular invasion or poor differentiation) local excision alone without adjuvant therapy is adequate. For T_1N_0, lesions with adverse histologic features, local excision must be combined with postoperative chemoradiotherapy (histologic features are rarely available on preoperative, endoscopic biopsy). For T_2N_0 tumors, local excision should be combined with preoperative or postoperative chemoradiotherapy. T_3N_0 patients are candidates for local excision only if major comorbidities preclude radical surgery or patients refuse a radical approach. Node positive patients (N_1 or N_2) are not candidates for curative local excision as mesorectal lymph nodes cannot be reliably removed transanally.

Traditional criteria for local excision (<10 cm from dentate line, <4 cm in diameter, <40% of rectal circumference) no longer apply due to more sophisticated, yet imperfect, staging and more advanced surgical techniques, such as Transanal Endoscopic Microsurgery (TEM).

Transanal Techniques

Once the decision to perform local excision has been made, traditional surgical principles apply as they do in all surgery. The goals are very straightforward, (1) remove the tumor with negative resection margins, (2) restore normal anatomy to the fullest extent possible, (3) minimize morbidity and mortality, and (4) minimize any impact on long-term function. Once a patient has been selected for local excision, one cannot change the tumor characteristics or stage; one can only affect the quality of surgical resection. Positive resection margins result from inadequate surgical technique and dramatically increase the risk of local recurrence and treatment failure. In order to perform a successful local excision, there must be good exposure and access, visualization must be optimum, and surgical technique precise. In addition, these must be accomplished with minimal impact on postoperative function. Four techniques are described in the ensuing paragraphs, TAE, Kraske technique, York–Mason or transsphincteric, and TEM. Traditional TAE creates minimal disruption to local anatomic structures, but is applicable only to the very distal rectum, and exposure, visualization, and precision are limited. The Kraske, or transcoccygeal, approach provides better exposure, but is more destructive (i.e., coccygectomy) and has a high fecal fistula rate.[13–15] The York–Mason, or transsphincteric technique, again provides better exposure than TAE, but by definition, disrupts the anal sphincters, and is as associated with high rates of postoperative fecal incontinence. TEM is currently gaining popularity; it provides excellent exposure and visualization throughout the rectum, and offers a precise surgical excision and wound closure. It does, however, require specialized equipment, specialized training, and an adequate volume of cases to become adept.

Transanal Excision

Local excision can be accomplished via a transanal approach for the majority of low rectal cancers. In a prospective study of 48 local excisions for rectal cancer, 33 were performed using a transanal approach.[13] Prior to local excision, all patients should receive a full mechanical and antibiotic bowel preparation. After the induction of anesthesia, the patient is flipped over and placed in the prone-jackknife position, with the buttocks taped apart. A pudendal nerve block should then be administered, which aids in postoperative pain control and more importantly relaxes the sphincter complex. An anal retractor in combination alone or in combination with a retractor with self-retaining hooks is then used to dilate the anus and expose the lesion. Once adequate visualization has been obtained, traction sutures are often placed 1–2 cm distal to the tumor, and the line of dissection is marked on the mucosa using electrocautery. This line of dissection should be approximately 1–2 cm from the border of the tumor circumferentially (Figure 43-1A). If visualization is not initially adequate, serial traction sutures should be used to prolapse the lesion into the field of view. Next, the electrocautery is used to make a full-thickness incision along the previously marked mucosa (Figure 43-1B). The specimen is then oriented accurately for the pathologist (Figure 43-1C). Upon completion of this incision, the perirectal fat should be visible beneath the lesion to confirm a full-thickness excision. For anterior lesions, care must be taken not to injure the back wall of the vagina in females, or the prostate or membranous urethra in males. The lesion is then excised leaving visible perirectal fat at the base of the lesion. The defect in the bowel

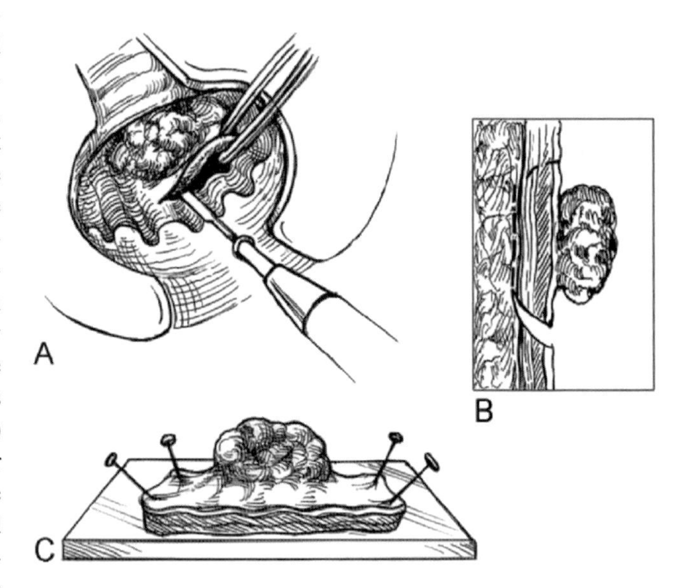

FIGURE 43-1. **A–C** Transanal excision. **A** A transanal excision is performed by marking out a 1 cm or greater margin around the tumor. **B** A full-thickness excision is then performed to obtain adequate radial as well as lateral margins. **C** The specimen is then oriented accurately for the pathologist.

wall is then closed transversely using interrupted 3–0 polyglycolic sutures.

The complications most closely associated with transanal excisions include urinary retention, urinary tract infections, delayed hemorrhage, infections of the perirectal and ischiorectal space, and fecal impactions. However, the overall incidence of these complications is quite low, and the mortality rate is 0% in most series.

Transcoccygeal Exision

The transcoccygeal approach was used historically over the transanal approach for larger, more proximal lesions. It was originally popularized by Kraske who found it beneficial when operating on lesions within the middle or distal third of the rectum. This approach is especially useful for lesions on the posterior wall of the rectum, but can certainly be used for anterior or lateral lesions as well. In this series, the transcoccygeal approach was used, when the distal margin was approximately 4.8 cm from the dentate line as compared to 3.0 cm for the transanal approach.[13]

All patients should undergo a full antibiotic and mechanical bowel preparation the day prior to surgery. The patient is again placed in the prone-jackknife position with the buttocks taped apart after the induction of general anesthesia. The tape is released for closure in order to facilitate the approximation of the subcutaneous tissues and skin. Unlike the transanal approach, a pudendal block is not required, as the sphincters do not require relaxation. The patient is prepped and draped in a sterile fashion with povidone–iodine solution, and an incision is made in the posterior midline adjacent to the sacrum and coccyx down to the upper border of the posterior aspect of the external sphincter. The coccyx, which along with the anal coccygeal ligament lies immediately deep to the skin and subcutaneous tissue, is removed to improve exposure. In order to do so, the anal coccygeal ligaments and other attachments are cauterized from each side and from the lower edge of the coccyx. The dissection then proceeds along the undersurface, anterior edge, of the coccyx until a cutting wire can pass through the sacral coccygeal joint. The coccyx is then removed with occasional bleeding from an extension of the middle sacral artery, which is easily controlled with electrocautery. The levator ani muscles are now visible at the base of the wound and should be separated in the midline, exposing a membrane that resides just outside of the perirectal fat. Division of this membrane allows for complete mobilization of the rectum within the intraperitoneal pelvis.

For posterior based lesions, the distal margin of the tumor can be palpated via a rectal examination, and then the mesorectum and rectum are transected at a point 1–1.5 cm distal to the tumor (Figure 43-2). The excision is then completed with a 1 cm margin surrounding the lesion. For posterior lesions, the transcoccygeal approach allows for the removal of perirectal nodes that lie in the surrounding mesorectal tissue. For anterior lesions, a posterior proctotomy is made, and then the lesion is approached under direct vision, again excising the lesion down to the perirectal fat with a 1 cm margin (Figure 43-3). Following removal, the specimen is reoriented for the pathologist and all the rectal incisions are closed in either a longitudinal or transverse manner in order to avoid narrowing of the rectum, using an absorbable suture. An air test should be performed, filling the operative field with sterile saline, and insufflating air in the rectum in order to check for air leaks in the suture line. Once these air leaks are controlled, the levator ani is reapproximated in the midline, and the anal coccygeal ligament is reattached to the sacrum. The operation is completed with the closure of the skin and subcutaneous tissue.

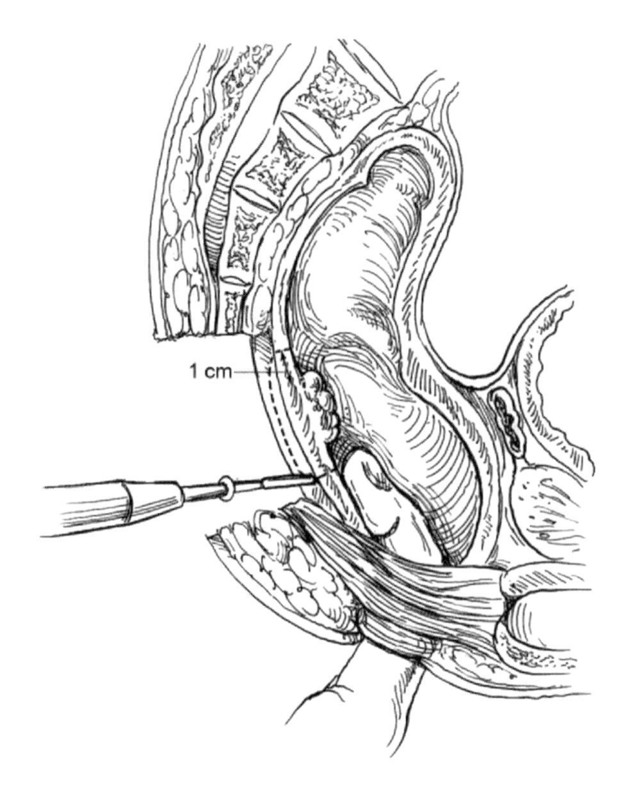

FIGURE 43-2. Transcoccygeal excision. For posterior lesions using a transcoccygeal or "Kraske" approach, one can palpate the lower border of the tumor to ensure an adequate distal margin.

An unfortunate complication of this procedure is the development of a fecal fistula that extends from the rectum to the posterior midline incision. The incidence of this complication ranges from 5 to 20%,[13–15] and most heal after temporary diversion of the fecal stream via a loop ileostomy or colostomy. For this reason, the Kraske approach is used much less frequently than other methods for local treatment.

Transsphincteric Excision

The transsphincteric approach developed by York and Mason involves the complete division of the sphincters and the posterior wall of the rectum. Patients undergo an antibiotic and

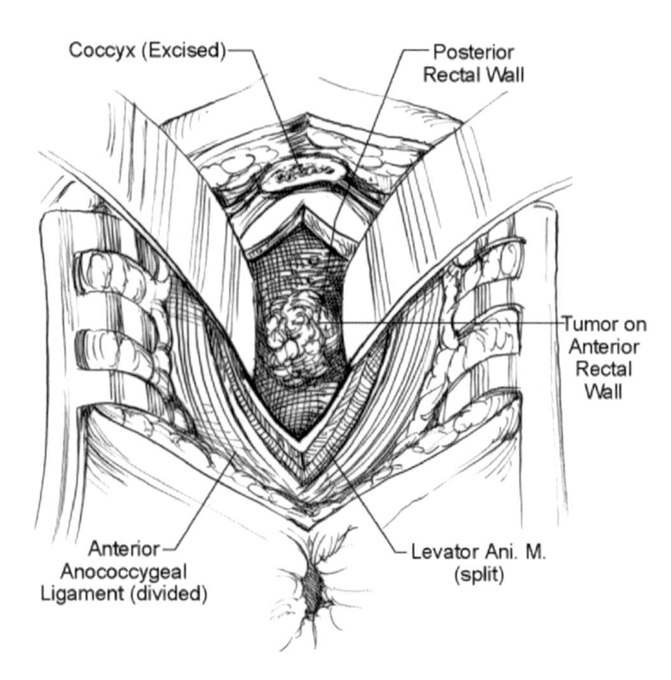

FIGURE 43-3. Transcoccygeal excision. Anterior lesions need to be approached by first making a posterior proctotomy and then excising the lesion through the rectum. The anterior and posterior walls of the rectum then need to be repaired, usually in a transverse manner in order to maintain the lumen diameter.

mechanical bowel preparation on the day before surgery. General anesthesia is chosen for the operation. The procedure starts similarly to the Kraske transcoccygeal approach; except the levator ani and the external sphincter muscles are divided in the midline. These muscles are carefully tagged, so matching sutures can be reapproximated exactly at the end of the procedure. Care must be taken to remain in the midline in order to avoid the nerve supply to the sphincters that lie in a posterolateral position bilaterally. Once the lesion is removed, the rectum, sphincters, and overlying musculature are closed in a careful stepwise manner. This procedure has an increased risk of incontinence secondary to sphincter dysfunction. Since the exposure provided from this approach is similar to that from the Kraske procedure, which carries less of a risk of incontinence, there are very few indications for this technique.

Transanal Endoscopic Microsurgery

TEM was developed by Gerhard Buess and the Richard Wolf Medical Instruments Company in 1983 in Germany. Originally designed for the removal of large rectal polyps beyond the reach of traditional transanal excision, its indications eventually expanded to include the excision of early stage rectal cancers.

TEM is essentially the earliest natural orifice transluminal endoscopic surgery (NOTES). It utilizes endoluminal insufflation to create rectal distension and exposure. Access is obtained via a proctoscope 4 cm in diameter and either 12 or 20 cm in length, which allows for resection of lesions anywhere in the rectum. Visualization is provided by a special binocular optic passed through the proctoscope which creates three-dimensional viewing. In addition, a laparoscopic camera can be attached to a separate optic with the image being viewed on a standard video monitor.

TEM is a closed system and a faceplate on the end of the proctoscope maintains an airtight seal. Instruments are passed through three-gasket ports, similar to laparoscopy. All instruments are 5 mm in diameter, and >30 cm in length, and include graspers, cautery, needle holders, suction, scissors, and clip appliers.

With TEM, it is possible to resect large lesions throughout the entire rectum and to meticulously suture the ensuing defects closed. Complete sleeve resection of the mid portion of the rectum with primary endoluminal anastomosis is possible and has been done in many instances.

Briefly, the technique is as follows. The lesion and its location are precisely identified and the patient is positioned on the operating room table with the lesion oriented toward the floor. (i.e., prone for anterior lesions, lithotomy for posterior lesions, etc.) This is important as the TEM equipment is designed to operate from "the top down." The proctoscope is inserted, the lesion is located, and the proctoscope is then fixed in place by attaching it to the "Martin Arm," a three-elbowed gadget that attaches to the OR table, locks in place, and keeps the TEM scope fixed (Figure 43-4A, B). Lidocaine with epinephrine is instilled underneath the lesion and 1 cm margins (5 mm for benign lesions) are marked with electrocautery surrounding the lesion. Using cautery, the lesion is then excised circumferentially in the full-thickness plane until it has been completely detached from the surrounding rectal wall (Figure 43-5). Following this, the deep dissection, often to include a significant portion of perirectal fat, is completed and the lesion removed through the open faceplate of the proctoscope. The specimen is pinned on a corkboard to facilitate microscopic evaluation. The defect is then closed transversely to prevent rectal stenosis. The mid-point of the proximal and distal edges of the defect are identified and approximated with a single suture to insure correct orientation and to facilitate transverse closure. The remaining defect is closed from each corner to the middle. Silver clips or "bbs" are used at the beginning and end of all sutures (usually running) in lieu of tying knots as this is tedious in the small operative field (Figure 43-6). Alternatively small, distal rectal, extra-peritoneal defects can be left open, although this is not commonly recommended as it is important to master suturing skills as some defects may be "intra-peritoneal" where failure to close accurately can lead to peritonitis.

Postoperative recovery is usually uneventful, with most patients being discharged directly from the recovery room. Patients experience pelvic pressure and irregular bowel movements for 1 or 2 weeks following surgery, but little pain

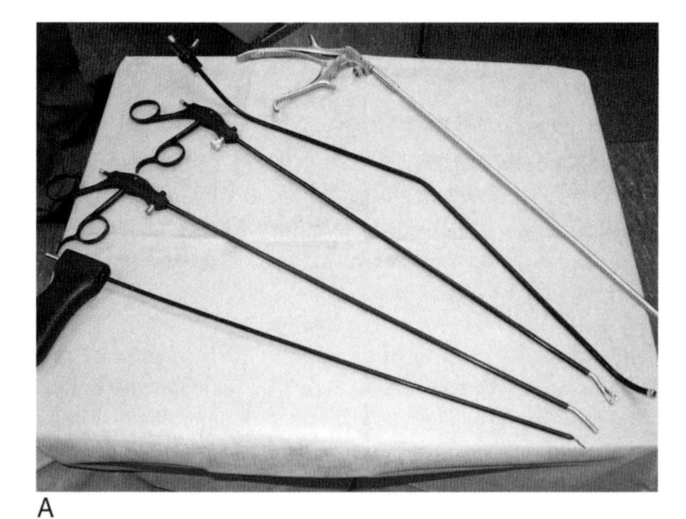

A

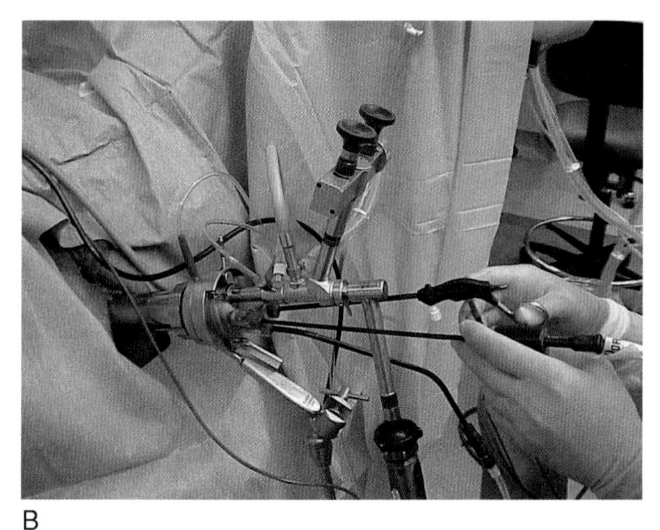

B

FIGURE 43-4. **A** Five mm TEM instruments, including needle cautery, graspers, suction, and needle holder. **B** External view of assembled TEM equipment in use.

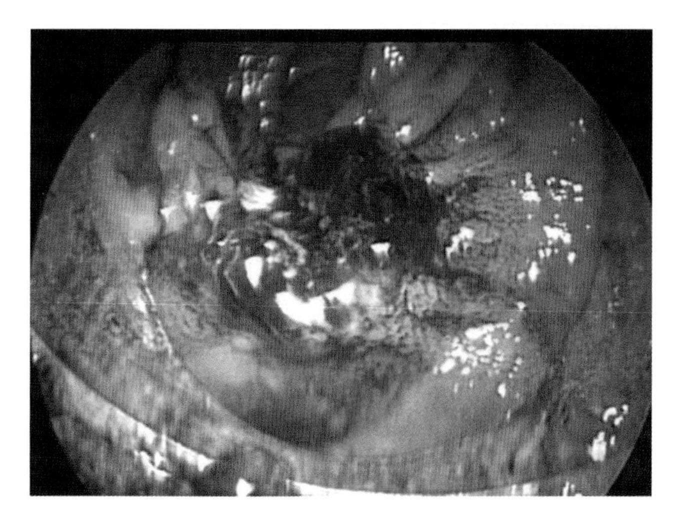

FIGURE 43-5. Lesion properly positioned for TEM.

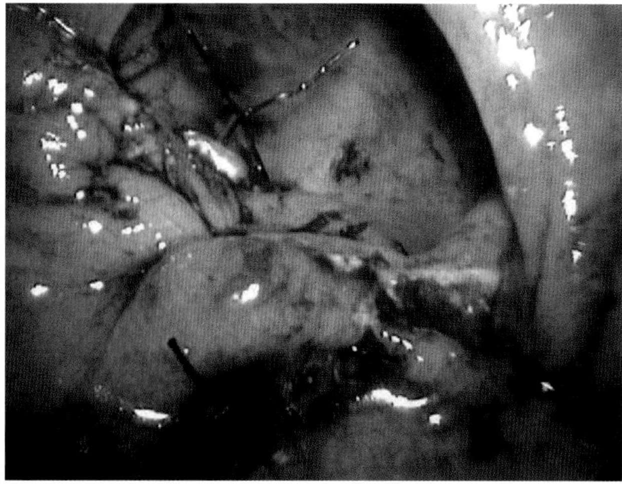

FIGURE 43-6. Defect closed in transverse fashion in order to prevent stenosis. Silver "bbs" are used in lieu of tying knots.

unless the resection involves the distal rectum adjacent to the dentate line, which is innervated by the somatically controlled inferior hemorrhoidal nerve.

Complications of TEM are rare, but include transient urinary retention, dehiscence of the operative closure, hemorrhage, perirectal or intraperitoneal infection, and rectovaginal fistulae. Rarely reoperation and even temporary fecal diversion are necessary to treat severe complications.

Follow-up after resection for rectal cancer is essential as local recurrence, if identified early, can be cured with radical resection. History and physical exam and CEA are performed every 3 months for 2 years, and every 6 months for the following 3 years. Flexible sigmoidoscopy is performed at 3 and 9 months following surgery and yearly thereafter. Colonoscopy is scheduled at 1 year and every 3 years regularly. CT scans begin at 1 year postoperatively and are then performed yearly. Long-term, vigilant follow-up is important, particularly after adjuvant radiation, as recurrence may develop up to 10 years postoperatively.

Results

When evaluating results following various treatments for rectal cancer, local recurrence and survival are naturally most important. It is important to also consider surgical morbidity and mortality, functional consequences, and the quality of life. Various local excision techniques can be compared to each other, and/or compared to traditional, radical resection.

Survival following radical resection for rectal cancer as reported by the National Cancer Database is 73% for Stage I; 56% for Stage II; 47% for Stage III, and 6% for Stage IV[7]. As we evaluate survival following local excision, it is essential to remember that not all patients with early stage rectal cancer are cured by radical resection. If a patient undergoes a well-performed, oncologically sound radical resection and then recurs, it is traditionally blamed on tumor biology. If recurrence develops after local excision, we assume that recurrence is due to inadequate surgery. While that may sometimes be the case, it is certainly not always the case as judged by the survival data following radical resection.

Many local failures following local excision are thought to arise in undiagnosed metastatic lymph nodes in the mesorectum. If this is in fact the case, then these are truly Stage III rectal cancers which have been under-staged, not Stage I rectal cancers that have recurred. In this situation, the problem lies with under-staging, and subsequent inadequate treatment. This only occurs following local excision (as lymph nodes are excised and evaluated with radical resection) and therefore artificially increases local recurrence rates and lowers overall survival following local excision of "early stage" rectal cancers.

You et al.[16] performed the most extensive study evaluating local excision of early rectal cancers with data obtained from the National Cancer Database. They compared standard resection (SR) (abdominoperineal and low anterior resection) to local excision (LE) and looked at operative mortality, local recurrence, disease specific survival (DSS) and overall survival (OS) for both groups for T_1 and T_2 rectal cancers. A total of 2,124 patients treated between 1994 and 1996 were included; LE 765 (T_1 601, T_2 164) SR 1359 (T_1 493, T_2 866). Overall operative mortality was lower for LE (0.5% vs. 1.8%). Thirty-day mortality was also lower for LE (5.6% vs. 14.6%). For T_1 tumors, overall survival was similar at 8 years (LE 61.7% vs. SR 66.3%, $p=0.09$). However, local recurrence was significantly higher for LE compared with SR (14.3% vs. 8.5%, $p=0.007$) at 8 years. Similarly, DSS was worse for LE (93.2% vs. 97.2%, $p=0.004$). For T_2 tumors, local recurrence again was higher for LE (22.1% vs. 15.1%, $p=0.01$) but DSS was similar for LE and SR (90.2% vs. 91.7%, $p=0.95$). OS was worse for LE (67.6% vs. 76.5%, $p=0.01$) at 5 years.

These data suggest that LE is clearly safer than SR, but at the cost of inferior oncologic outcomes. Yet, when overall survival is evaluated both groups are essentially similar. Despite being a large, exhaustive project, this study has several shortcomings. (1) Many patients included in the LE group did not have R_0 excisions, which would clearly increase the LR rate and decrease the overall survival. In addition, any patient who received adjuvant therapy (chemotherapy or radiation) was excluded from the analysis. Many surgeons would consider chemoradiation a standard component of treatment for any T_2 tumor and selected T_1 tumors treated by LE. Also, the authors did not evaluate the type of LE performed (TAE vs. TEM vs. Kraske vs. York Mason). Finally, no mention is made of the "stage shift" phenomenon, where a small but significant number of T_1 and T_2 tumor treated by LE (but not by SR) were truly Stage III cancers, and had undocumented disease in unresected perirectal lymph nodes.

Ptok et al.[17] compared local and radical resection for low risk T_1 rectal cancer. Similar to the large database study by You, morbidity was lower with LE (9.2% vs. 22.8%, $p=0.001$), but local recurrence was higher (6% vs. 2%, $p=0.049$). However, 5-year tumor free survival was similar for both groups. Although the authors divided the LE group into TAE and TEM for demographic purposes, they did not analyze the groups separately when looking at local recurrence or survival.

Garcia-Aguilar et al.[18] reviewed the University of Minnesota experience with local excision of early stage, low-risk rectal cancers. Their series included 82 patients who underwent TAE for T_1 or T_2 rectal cancers with favorable histology (moderately or well differentiated and with no lymphovascular invasion). All included patients had negative resection margins. Recurrence was identified in 18% of T_1 tumors (nine local, one distant, one local and distant recurrence) and 37% for T_2 tumors (eight local, two combined local and distant). Salvage surgery was performed when appropriate. One patient in the T_1 group and two patients in the T_2 died as a result of cancer recurrence. Mean follow-up was 54 months. The authors concluded that local recurrence rates were high, but salvage was often possible with radical resection. Cancer free survival was high for both groups, but long-term outcomes were inconclusive. Interestingly, preoperative staging with endorectal ultrasound, which should ideally improve staging and patient selection, had no effect on outcomes.

Paty et al.[19] at Memorial Sloan-Kettering Cancer Center, evaluated long term follow-up in 125 patients with T_1 and T_2 rectal cancers undergoing local excision. Median follow-up was 6.7 years, local recurrence was 17% for T_1, and 28% for T_2 tumors. Ten-year survival was 74% and 72%, respectively. Positive resection margins were found in 10% (11 of 125) patients. Adjuvant radiotherapy with or without chemotherapy did not influence local recurrence or overall survival, but radiation was used selectively in high-risk patients. Radiation did, however, seem to delay recurrence; 28% of all cancer deaths occurred more than 5 years after initial treatment.

In evaluating multiple studies of traditional local excision for early rectal cancer, several patterns arise. (1) Morbidity, mortality, and functional outcomes are better with local excision. (2) Local recurrence rates are higher following local excision when compared with radical resection. (3) Salvage radical surgery is possible in 30–50% of patients developing local recurrence after local excision. (4) Disease free survival and overall survival are similar following local excision and radical resection for T_1 and T_2 rectal cancers.

Transanal Endoscopic Microsurgery

TEM has been in use since the early 1980s, but only in select centers, particularly in Europe. Over the past 10 years, its role has expanded significantly and its use is now widespread in Europe, Great Britain, and more recently the USA. It has been advocated as technically superior to TAE, and oncologically favorable results have been reported. Few studies, however, directly compare TEM to traditional techniques. Yet, the limited data is encouraging.

Lin et al.[20] compared TEM to the York–Mason approach in 82 patients with benign and malignant rectal masses. Postoperative pain, hospital stay, and complication rates were significantly higher for the York–Mason approach. With short-term median follow-up of 30 months recurrence was 0% for the TEM group and 3.9% for the controls. This is a small study, but clearly shows the technical superiority of TEM. Christforidis et al.[21] at the University of Minnesota retrospectively compared TEM to traditional TAE in 171 patients (42 TEM, 129 TAE). Negative resection margins were obtained in 98% of the TEM group compared with 84% of the TAE group. Disease free survival at 5 years was slightly better for the TEM group (84% vs. 76%), but did not reach statistical significance. Multivariate analysis identified T-stage, resection margin status, the use of adjuvant therapy, and distance from the anal verge (lower = worse prognosis), but not surgical technique (TEM vs. TAE) as predictive of local recurrence. Moore et al.[22] evaluated 171 patients subject to TEM (82) or TAE (89) at the University of Vermont for rectal adenomas and carcinomas. In the group of patients undergoing resection for cancer, TEM, when compared to TAE, provided an intact, nonfragmented specimen more often (100% vs. 63%), achieved negative resection margins (98% vs. 78%, $p = 0.01$) and was associated with a lower recurrence rate (8% vs. 24%). When only curative resections were considered, recurrence rate for TEM was 3% compared with 22% for TAE. In this study, TEM was clearly technically and oncologically superior to TAE.

Many other studies have reported individual institution's experience with TEM with some comparisons to historical controls. Whitehouse et al.[23] reported on 42 patients undergoing TEM for rectal cancer. Resection margins were positive in 8%. Adjuvant chemoradiation was used at the surgeon's discretion. Local recurrence rates were as follows, T_1 20% (6/23); T_2 22% (2/9); T_3 0% (0/4). Conclusions indicated TEM to be safe but recurrence rates were high.

In a much larger series Guerrieri et al.[24] reviewed 196 patients (51 T_1, 84 T_2, 61 T_3) treated with TEM for rectal cancer. All patients with T_2 or T_3 lesions underwent preoperative radiotherapy, combined with chemotherapy in some instances. All patients achieved negative resection margins (real time frozen section analysis was used when necessary). Follow-up ranged from 12 to 178 months and local recurrence rates were 0% for T_1, 6% for T_2, and 5% for T_3 lesions. Disease free survival was 100% for T_1, 90% for T_2, and 77% for T_3 lesions. Downsizing and downstaging were good prognostic indicators and the authors only found local recurrence in patients with lesions deemed "non-responders" to radiation therapy.

Zacharakis et al.[25] reviewed the St. Mary's experience with TEM for benign and malignant rectal masses. Specifically regarding malignant masses, positive resection margins were found in 3.7% (1/28). No patient received chemoradiotherapy either before or after surgery. Recurrence occurred in 7.1% of T_1, 42% of T_2, and 66.6% of T_3 lesions. TEM alone seemed adequate treatment for T_1, but not for T_2 or T_3 rectal cancers.

Floyd and Saclarides[26] followed 53 patients with T_1 rectal cancer after curative TEM. None had chemotherapy or radiotherapy. Mean follow-up was 2.84 years. Four patients developed recurrence (7.5%). All patients with recurrence were treated with surgical resection, and at the time of publication were disease free.

Maslekar et al.[27] reported their experience with TEM on 52 patients with rectal cancer. T_1 cancers received TEM alone. While TEM was combined with postoperative chemoradiation for select T_2 and T_3 lesions, recurrence rate was 0% for T_1 (0/27), 20% for T_2 (4/22), and 33% for T_3 (1/3); overall recurrence 14%.

Two prospective, randomized trials have compared TEM to radical surgery for early rectal cancer. Winde et al.[28] randomized 53 patients with ultrasound-staged T_1 rectal cancer to TEM vs. anterior resection (TEM 25; LAR 28). Complication rates were significantly higher for radical resection while 5-year survival was similar for both groups at 96%.

Lezoch et al.[29] published 5-year follow-up data from a prospective randomized trial for the treatment of early rectal cancer. Patients with UT_2N_0 biopsy proven, low-grade rectal cancer underwent preoperative chemoradiotherapy (5,040 rads with continuous infusion of 5-FU) and were then randomized to TEM vs. laparoscopic radical resection (APR vs. LAR). Median follow-up was 84 months. Local recurrence following TEM was 5.7% (2/35) and 2.8% after radical resection (1/35). One patient developed distant metastases in each group. The 5-year disease free survival was 94% for both groups. The authors concluded that TEM provided equivalent oncologic results to radical resection.

Experience and outcomes vary significantly from center to center and country to country with regard to TEM in the treatment of early rectal cancer. Several clear points emerge from a cloudy picture. TEM appears to be technically superior to traditional TAE in its ability to produce a nonfragmented specimen with tumor free margins. It is clearly associated with lower morbidity and mortality than radical resection. Patient selection and preoperative staging are essential. TEM alone may be justified for select T_1 rectal cancers, but recurrence rates are prohibitive without adjuvant chemoradiotherapy for T_2 (and T_3) tumors. When compared to radical resection in a prospective, randomized fashion, TEM, in limited data, compares well to radical resection for T_1 cancers. In addition TEM, combined with preoperative adjuvant therapy, again compares well to radical resection with T_2 rectal cancers.

In the USA, a multicenter prospective phase II trial ACOSOG Z-6041 has been evaluating local excision (TAE and TEM) for UT_2N_0 rectal cancer following 5040 gray combined with 5 FU and oxaliplatin.[30] Accrual is currently complete but data is not yet available. The results of this study may help clarify the role of local excision and adjuvant therapy for Stage I rectal cancer.

Predicting Lymph Node Metastases

The reasons for local recurrence following local excision of rectal cancer are likely multifactorial, but remain obscure. Clearly, leaving tumor behind at the site of resection (i.e., positive margins) increases the risk of recurrence, and is responsible for many treatment failures. However, many patients with clear margins ultimately develop local recurrence. The current thinking is that these failures may be the result of undiagnosed and untreated metastatic lymph nodes in the mesorectum.

The incidence of lymph node positivity is directly related to T-stage, and is well documented in the literature.[31–33] Interestingly, local recurrence rates following local excision for rectal cancer seem to parallel the likelihood of lymph node positivity stage for stage. Unfortunately, endorectal ultrasound is inadequate to diagnose some patients with positive lymph nodes. MRI is no better.

Metastatic lymph nodes are found in 5–10% of T_1 tumors, 10–20% of T_2 tumors, and 30–50% of T_3 tumors.[32] However, many of these lymph nodes are very small making ultrasound or MRI detection difficult. Andreola et al.[12] looked at metastatic lymph nodes in cancer of the distal third of the rectum following radical resection in 101 patients. Forty-five percent of all metastatic lymph nodes were smaller than 5 mm in diameter. Fourteen percent of all lymph node positive patients had only lymph nodes smaller than 5 mm. Forty-three percent of patients with metastatic lymph nodes less than 5 mm developed systemic recurrence. Clearly small, metastatic lymph nodes are common, are poorly detected by current staging methods, and are important factors in the development of metastatic disease.

Many individuals have looked at multiple factors in an attempt to predict the presence or absence of occult lymph node metastases and local recurrence following local excision of rectal tumors. In an insightful study, Read et al. used residual T-stage following chemoradiation in 644 patients as a predictor for the presence of mesenteric lymph nodes containing tumor.[34] Patients were staged and selected for neoadjuvant therapy with or without chemotherapy. All patients then underwent radical resection with excision of the mesorectum. Postradiation T-stage was determined and then correlated with the presence or absence of metastatic lymph nodes. For postradiation T_0 lesions, the risk of positive nodes was 2%, for T_1 4%, for T_2 23%, and for T_3 47%. These data may be useful in identifying patients with residual lymph node metastases who fail local excision, and hence should undergo radical resection. Further confirmation of the "response to radiation" as a predictor of successful outcomes is provided by the multicenter study authored by Capirci et al.[35] As part of the Gastro-Intestinal Working Group in the Italian Association of Radiation Oncology, data was gathered on 566 patients with complete clinical response following preoperative chemoradiotherapy. Patients underwent low anterior resection (73%) abdominoperineal resection (22%) and TEM (5%). Complete pathologic response following neoadjuvant therapy was associated with a 1.6% local recurrence rate, disease free survival of 85%, overall survival of 90%, and cancer specific survival of 94%.

Perez et al.[36] in Sao Paolo, Brazil evaluated postneoadjuvant chemoradiation staging as a predictor of lymphatic involvement and recurrence. Only patients with an incomplete clinical response were included for evaluation ($n=289$). All patients underwent radical resection. Eighty-eight patients had ypT_2 tumors. Lymph node metastases were identified in 19% of this group. The presence of perineural invasion, vascular invasion, and decreased interval between chemoradiation and surgery (12 vs. 18 weeks) were associated with lymph node metastases and tumor recurrence. The presence of tumor in mesorectal lymph nodes was associated with decreased disease-free survival (30% vs. 49%) even after radical surgery. These authors recommended radial resection for all patients with ypT_2 tumors following chemoradiation. The important clinical implication of this data is any patient undergoing local excision following chemoradiation found to have ypT_2 disease, is at high risk for recurrence and should be considered for subsequent radical surgery.

While response to neoadjuvant treatment has been advocated as a predictor of lymph node involvement by some, others have advocated identifying histopathologic factors present in the primary tumor to predict the presence of metastatic lymph nodes in the mesorectum.

Kikuchi et al.[37] evaluated the depth of submucosal tumor spread (sm level) as a predictor of lymphatic metastases and adverse outcome following endoscopic polypectomy in 182 patients. They identified polyp configuration (pedunculated vs. sessile), polyp location (rectum vs. colon) and sm level as predictors of adverse outcome. Conversely, Rasheed et al.[38] failed to find sm level predictive of lymph node involvement in 55 T_1 rectal cancers.

Park et al.[39] analyzed 90 patients with early colorectal cancer and found lymph node metastases in 8.9%. Lymph node metastases were associated with deep sm invasion, lymphovascular invasion, vessel configuration, absence of a residual adenomatous component, and unfavorable histologic grade. Similarly, Choi et al.[40] evaluated 168 patients with early colorectal cancer who underwent curative bowel resection. They again identified sm 3 invasion and poor differentiation as predictive of lymph node metastases. They, however, also identified tumor cell dissociation (TCD), solid cancer cell clusters and groups of dissociated cancer cells at the tumor front, as predictive of lymph node metastases. (TCD appears to be similar to tumor budding).

Tominaga et al.[41] at the National Cancer Hospital in Tokyo, Japan evaluated 155 submucosal colorectal cancers looking for histopathologic factors associated with lymph node metastases. Twelve percent of patients were found to have lymph nodes containing cancer. On multivariate analysis, lymphatic invasion and high-grade focal dedifferentiation at the submucosal front were predictive of lymph node metastases. No patients with minimal submucosal involvement (<1.3 mm) had cancer in regional nodes. Sakuragi et al.[42] in evaluating 278 early rectal cancers, found the depth of submucosal invasion and lymphatic invasion predictive of lymph node metastases.

In a slightly different approach, Masaki et al.[43] evaluated tumor budding (single cells or clusters of cells at the invasive margin) grade, lymphovascular invasion, tumor dedifferentiation at the invasive margin, residual adenomatous tissue, and depth and width of submucosal invasion in 76 patients with T_1 colon and rectal cancer. Multivariate analysis found only tumor budding to be associated with nodal disease. The authors created a formula to predict the likelihood of lymph node metastases. $Z=0.07\times(\#\text{ budding units})-3.726$, where the probability of positive lymph nodes $=1/1+e^{-z}$. This formula, in theory, can be used to determine if the risk of radical surgery is greater than the risk of residual lymphatic disease.

In yet another study evaluating risk factors for mesenteric lymph node positively, Yasuda et al.[44] analyzed 86 patients undergoing resection for colorectal carcinoma. Multivariate analysis once again identified vascular invasion and tumor budding to be independent predictors of lymph node involvement. In addition, no patients with submucosal invasion ≤1,000 μm had lymph node metastases.

In a large cooperative British and Irish study, reported by Bach et al.[45] 424 patients undergoing TEM for localized rectal cancer were evaluated for risk factors associated with recurrence. Local recurrence rates were 18.6% for T_1 lesions, 29.3% for T_2 lesions, and 47% for T_3 lesions at 5 years. Recurrence rates were relatively high, but incomplete resection (positive margins) was found in 11% of T_1, 22.5% of T_2, and 42% of T_3 lesions. The authors identified increasing tumor size, the presence of lymphatic invasion, and increasing depth of penetration (as measured by sm levels and T-stage) as independent predictors of recurrence. Surprisingly R_1 resection was not found to be predictive for recurrence.

In summarizing the data from the above series, it appears that several factors consistently put patients at risk for untreated regional lymph node disease following local excision for early rectal cancer. The presence of lymphovascular invasion, increasing sm levels of tumor invasion, tumor budding at the invasive tumor margin, and poor differentiation are relatively consistent predictors of adverse outcome. These histologic criteria should clearly be evaluated and thoughtfully considered when assessing the oncologic adequacy of local excision for early rectal cancers. In the future, perhaps a predictive "histologic score" will be developed to accurately identify patients at significant risk for lymph node metastases. These individuals may benefit from radical resection or more aggressive adjuvant chemoradiation.

Conclusions

Local excision will likely continue to play a significant role in the treatment of selected patients with early stage rectal cancer. TEM is utilized much more commonly due to its ability to access the entire rectum, its superior visualization, and its precise surgical technique. Early results indicate lower local recurrence rates and higher overall survival when compared to traditional techniques of transanal excision. In order to improve cure rates and decrease local recurrence, local staging must improve. Considering the significance of very small metastatic lymph nodes, it is unlikely that ultrasound will continue as the primary staging tool. Perhaps a "functional study" which utilizes tumor metabolism will provide more accurate staging. In addition, a "scoring system" based on anatomic tumor factors (i.e., TNM) combined with histopathologic and genetic factors may be developed to help predict success and failure of local excision.

The future of local therapy for rectal cancer may evolve similar to that of breast cancer treatment. Patients will be staged based on anatomic, histologic, and genetic data, then treated with neoadjuvant chemotherapy and radiation. Local excision, likely TEM, will follow neoadjuvant treatment, and will act as a "staging biopsy." If response to neoadjuvant treatment is deemed adequate, no further therapy will be necessary. However, tumors with a lesser response to therapy will receive radical resection. In this way, major surgery and its associated morbidity and mortality will be reserved for patients who truly require it. The above algorithm is by no means the current standard of care, but many unanswered questions remain and treatment recommendations are in flux. No progress can be made unless we honestly evaluate past treatments, let go of traditional prejudices, and embrace sound scientific research, and be willing to change based on new information.

Acknowledgment. A previous version of this chapter was authored by Ronald Bleday and Julio Garcia-Aguilar.

References

1. Miles WE. A method of performing abdominoperineal excision for carcinoma of the rectum and terminal portion of the pelvic colon. Lancet. 1908;2:1812–3.
2. Meade RH. An introduction to the history of general surgery. Philadelphia: Saunders; 1968. p. 277–314.
3. Wallengrenn NO, Holtas S, Andren-Sandberg A, et al. Rectal carcinoma: double-contrast MR imaging for preoperative staging. Radiology. 2000;215(1):108–14.

4. Wong CS, Sten H, Cummings BJ. Local excision and postoperative radiation therapy for rectal carcinoma. Int J Radiat Oncol Biol Phys. 1993;25(4):669–75.
5. Rosen L, Veidenheimer MC, Coller JA, Corman ML. Mortality and morbidity, and patterns of recurrence after abdomino-perineal resection for cancer of the rectum. Dis Colon Rectum. 1982;25(3):202–8.
6. Williams NS, Johnston D. The quality of life after rectal excision for low rectal cancer. Br J Surg. 1983;70(8):460–2.
7. Wang SJ, Fuller CD, Emery R, et al. Conditional survival in rectal cancer: a seer database analysis. Gastrointest Cancer Res. 2007;1(3):84–9.
8. Massari M, De Simone M, Cioffi U, et al. Value and limits endorectal ultrasonography for preoperative staging of rectal carcinoma. Surg Laparosc Endosc. 1998;8(6):438–44.
9. Hünerbein M, Pegios W, Rau B, et al. Prospective comparison of endorectal ultrasound, three-dimensional endorectal ultrasound, and endorectal MRI in the preoperative evaluation of rectal tumors. Surg Endosc. 2000;14:1005–9.
10. Kim KN, Kim MJ, Park JK, et al. Preoperative staging of rectal cancer with MRI: accuracy and clinical usefulness. Ann Surg Oncol. 2000;7(10):732–7.
11. Blomqvist L, Machado M, Rubio C, et al. Rectal tumour staging: MR imaging using pelvic phased-array and endorectal coils vs endoscopic ultrasonography. Eur Radiol. 2000;10:653–60.
12. Andreola S, Leo E, Belli F, et al. Adenocarcinoma of the lower third of the rectum: metastases in lymph nodes smaller than 5 mm and occult micrometastases; preliminary results on early tumor recurrence. Ann Surg Oncol. 2001;8(5):413–7.
13. Bleday R, Breen E, Jessup JM, et al. Prospective evaluation of local excision for small rectal cancers. Dis Colon Rectum. 1997;40(4):388–92.
14. Killingback M. Local excision of carcinoma of the rectum: indications. World J Surg. 1992;16(3):437–46.
15. Christiansen J. Excision of mid-rectal lesions by the Kraske sacral approach. Br J Surg. 1980;67(9):651–2.
16. You YN, Baxter NN, Steward A, et al. Is the increasing rate of local excision for stage I rectal cancer in the United States justified? A nationwide cohort study from the National Cancer Database. Ann Surg. 2007;245(7):726–33.
17. Ptok H, Marusch F, Meyer F, et al. Oncological outcome of local vs radical resection of low-risk pT1 cancer. Arch Surg. 2007;142(7):649–56.
18. Garcia-Aguilar J, Mellgre A, Sirivongs P, et al. Local excision of rectal cancer without adjuvant therapy. Ann Surg. 2000;231(3):345–51.
19. Paty PH, Nash GM, Baron P, et al. Long-term results of local excision for rectal cancer. Ann Surg. 2002;236(4):522–30.
20. Lin GL, Meng WCS, Lau PYY, et al. Local resection for early rectal tumours: comparative study of transanal endoscopic microsurgery (TEM) versus posterior trans-sphincteric approach (Mason's Operation). Asian J Surg. 2006;29(4):227–32.
21. Christoforidis D, Cho HM, Dixon MR, et al. Transanal endoscopic microsurgery versus conventional transanal excision for patients with early rectal cancer. Ann Surg. 2009;249(5):776–82.
22. Moore JS, Cataldo P, Osler T, et al. Transanal endoscopic microsurgery is more effective than traditional transanal excision for resection of rectal masses. Dis Colon Rectum. 2008;51:1026–31.
23. Whitehouse PA, Armitage JN, Tilney HS, et al. Transanal endoscopic microsurgery: local recurrence rate following resection of rectal cancer. Colorectal Dis. 2007;10:187–93.
24. Guerrieri M, Baldarelli M, Organetti L, et al. Transanal endoscopic microsurgery for the treatment of selected patients with distal rectal cancer: 15 years experience. Surg Endosc. 2008;22:2030–5.
25. Zacharakis E, Freilich S, Rekhraj S, et al. Transanal endoscopic microsurgery for rectal tumors: the St. Mary's experience. Am J Surg. 2007;194:694–8.
26. Floyd ND, Saclarides TJ. Transanal endoscopic microsurgical resection of pT1 rectal tumors. Dis Col Rectum. 2005;49(2):164–8.
27. Maslekar S, Pillinger SH, Monson JRT. Transanal endoscopic microsurgery for carcinoma of the rectum. Surg Endosc. 2007;21:97–102.
28. Winde G, Schmid KW, Reers B, et al. Prospective randomized comparison of transanal endoscopic microsurgery (TEM) with perianal local excision or anterior resection for rectal adenomas and superficial carcinomas. Langenbecks Arch Chir Suppl Kongressbd. 1996;113:265–68.
29. Lezoch G, Baldarelli M, Paganini MAM, et al. A prospective randomized study with a 5-year minimum follow-up evaluation of transanal endoscopic microsurgery verus laparoscopic total mesorectal excision after neoadjuvant therapy. Surg Endosc. 2008;22:352–8.
30. Ota DM. ACOSOG Group Co-Chairs. Local excision of rectal cancer revisited: ACOSOG protocol Z6041. Ann Surg Oncol. 2007;14(2):271.
31. Nascimbeni R, Burgart LJ, Nivatvongs S, et al. Risk of lymph node metastasis in T1 carcinoma of the colon and rectum. Dis Colon Rectum. 2002;45:200–6.
32. Morson BC. Factors influencing the prognosis of early cancer of the rectum. Proc R Soc Med. 1966;59:607–8.
33. Brodsky JT, Richard GK, Cohen AM, et al. Variables correlated with the risk of lymph node metastasis in early rectal cancer. Cancer. 1992;69:322–26.
34. Read TE, Andujar JE, Caushaj PF, et al. Neoadjuvant therapy for rectal cancer histologic response of the primary tumor predicts nodal status. Dis Colon Rectum. 2004;47(6):825–31.
35. Capirci C, Valentini V, Cionini L, et al. Prognostic value of pathologic complete response after neoadjuvant therapy in locally advanced rectal cancer: long-term analysis of 566 ypCR patients. Int J Radiat Oncol Biol Phys. 2008;72(1):99–107.
36. Perez RO, Habr-Gama A, Proscurshim I, et al. Local excision for ypT2 rectal cancer – much ado-about something. J Gastrointest Surg. 2007;11:1431–40.
37. Kikuchi R, Takano M, Takagi K, et al. Management of early invasive colorectal cancer. Dis Colon Rectum. 1995;38(12):1286–95.
38. Rasheed S, Bowley DM, Aziz O, et al. Can depth of tumour invasion predict lymph node positivity in patients undergoing resection for early rectal cancer? A comparative study between T1 and T2 cancers. Colorectal Dis. 2008;10:231–7.
39. Park YJ, Kim WH, Paeng SS, et al. Histoclinical analysis of early colorectal cancer. World J Surg. 2000;24(9):1029–35.
40. Choi PW, Yu CS, Jang SJ, et al. Risk factors for lymph node metastasis in submucosal invasive colorectal cancer. World J Surg. 2008;32:2089–94.

41. Tominaga K, Nakanishi Y, Nimura S, et al. Predictive histopathologic factors for lymph node metastasis in patients with nonpedunculated submucosal invasive colorectal carcinoma. Dis Colon Rectum. 2005;48(1):92–100.
42. Sakuragi M, Togashi K, Konishi F, et al. Predictive factors for lymph nodes metastasis in T1 stage colorectal carcinomas. Dis Colon Rectum. 2003;46(12):1626–32.
43. Masaki T, Matsuoka H, Sugiyama M, et al. Actual number of tumor budding as a new tool for the individualization of treatment of T1 colorectal carcinomas. J Gastroenterol Hepatol. 2006;21:115–1121.
44. Yasuda K, Inomata M, Shiromizu A, et al. Risk factors for occult lymph node metastasis of colorectal cancer invading the submucosa and indications for endoscopic mucosal resection. Dis Colon Rectum. 2007;50(9):1370–6.
45. Bach SP, Hill J, Monson JRT, et al. A predictive model for local recurrence after transanal endoscopic microsurgery for rectal cancer. Br J Surg. 2009;96:280–90.

44 Surgical Treatment of Rectal Cancer

Ronald Bleday and Nelya Brindzei

Approximately 42,000 patients each year are diagnosed with rectal cancer in the USA. Approximately 8,500 die of this disease. Despite remarkable recent advances in new oncologic agents for the treatment of colon and rectal cancer, cure is almost never achieved without surgical resection. However, the current management of rectal cancer is now more varied and complex because of the new approaches with multimodality therapy and the refinements in surgical techniques. For example, small distal rectal cancers with minimal invasion can be treated with a local excision with or without adjuvant therapy. More proximal or more invasive tumors require a "radical" resection. The two most common procedures are the low anterior resection (LAR) and the abdominoperineal resection (APR). Extended resections are occasionally required for patients with cancers that invade or adhere to adjoining structures such as the sacrum, pelvic sidewalls, prostate, or bladder.

This chapter discusses the surgical management of rectal cancer including a basic review of the preoperative evaluation and how it pertains to surgical planning, the preoperative preparation, the surgical procedures, the biology of rectal cancer as it relates to surgery, the issue of margins, and the technical nuances that need to be appreciated for a successful resection.

Evaluation of the Patient with Rectal Cancer

History

The patient with rectal cancer usually presents to the surgeon after a definitive endoscopic diagnosis. The patient's initial complaint may be rectal bleeding, a change in bowel habits, or a sense of rectal pressure. However, with the increase in surveillance colonoscopy, many patients are completely asymptomatic on presentation. During the initial history, the surgeon should ask about certain symptoms because it will aid in selecting the best therapy for the patient. For example, tenesmus (the constant sensation of needing to move the bowels) is often indicative of a large cancer. Constant anal pain or pain with defecation suggests invasion of the anal sphincters or pelvic floor. Preemptive procedures such as a diverting colostomy may be required in patients with these distal painful cancers. Also, cancers growing into the anal sphincter are not candidates for a sphincter-sparing procedure. Questions concerning a patient's fecal continence should also be discussed before any therapy. Sphincter-sparing procedures can put a tremendous stress on even the most normal of pelvic floors and anal sphincters. A history of significant continence problems should prompt a discussion with the patient concerning quality-of-life issues. Sphincter-sparing surgery in these patients, even if technically possible, often leads to significant fecal soiling, and the patient may be better served with a resection and permanent colostomy.

Physical Examination and Rigid Sigmoidoscopic Examination

A digital rectal examination (DRE) and a rigid sigmoidoscopy are essential to the surgical decision-making process. Both a proper examination and rigid sigmoidoscopy should be performed on the initial patient visit unless the patient has a painful invasive lesion. On DRE, fixation of the lesion to the anal sphincter, its relationship to the anorectal ring (the collection of muscles that make up the sphincters), and possible fixation to both the rectal wall and the pelvic wall can be evaluated. For mid rectal or upper rectal lesions, the DRE and rigid sigmoidoscopy can help determine how much normal rectum lies distal to the lower border of the tumor. With the combination of DRE and sigmoidoscopy at the initial visit, the surgeon can often determine whether a patient is a candidate for sphincter-sparing surgery, whether a temporary diverting ostomy is likely, and what anorectal function will be like posttreatment.

D.E. Beck et al. (eds.), *The ASCRS Textbook of Colon and Rectal Surgery: Second Edition*,
DOI 10.1007/978-1-4419-1584-9_44, © Springer Science+Business Media, LLC 2011

Colonoscopy

A colonoscopy should be performed before surgical resection of a rectal cancer. Colonoscopy allows for confirmation of a malignancy through biopsy and the diagnosis and possible removal of synchronous colonic lesions. Synchronous benign polyps have been reported in 13–62% of cases,m and synchronous cancers have been reported in 2–8% of cases.[1–6] Even if a colonoscopy has been recently performed on a patient, the surgeon should still perform a rigid sigmoidoscopy because estimates of the location of the lesion are often misleading. For example, because of the flexibility of the colonoscope, a lesion that is described as 15 cm from the anal verge can sometimes be a close as 5 cm from the anal verge when evaluated with the rigid scope. Finally, both with a colonoscope and rigid sigmoidoscope, one should describe the distance from the lower border of the lesion to a standard distal landmark. The National Cancer Institute (NCI) consensus group recommends the use of the "anal verge" as the starting point for measuring distance; however, this anatomic landmark is variable. An alternative is to use the dentate line as the zero point and measure the distance from the lower border of the lesion to the proximal border of the anorectal ring. This distance is essentially a measure of the maximal amount of rectum that one can resect before considering an APR.

Preoperative Staging

Preoperative staging of a patient with a rectal cancer is becoming essential in the decision-making process as adjuvant modalities become increasingly used preoperatively. Also, the range of surgical procedures that can be offered to a patient is in part dependent on the preoperative imaging. For a basic evaluation, all patients should receive a chest X-ray or chest computed tomography (CT) scan to exclude pulmonary metastases. One can obtain a carcinoembryonic antigen (CEA) level. If increased preoperatively, the CEA level should decrease to the normal range after treatment. CEA can then be followed postoperatively to detect a recurrence. Most other laboratory evaluations obtained preoperatively are useful for determining pertinent medical problems, but are not very helpful in staging. By far, the most useful staging for rectal cancer is abdominal/pelvic imaging with CT, magnetic resonance imaging (MRI), or ultrasound (US)

Imaging for Rectal Cancer

Pretreatment abdominal and pelvic imaging of the patient with rectal cancer is necessary in this era because of the increasing value of preoperative adjuvant therapies. Therapy differs depending on stage, depth of invasion into the rectal wall within a stage, size of lesion, and location of the tumor. In particular, distal and mid rectal cancer treatment management will differ depending on the preoperative staging and imaging. For upper rectal cancers, imaging to determine stage will often not influence the treatment plan. Many of these patients with upper rectal tumors will benefit from an LAR regardless of the stage and may not require neoadjuvant therapy as often as low and mid rectal cancers.

Computed Tomography Scan

Differing opinions exist as to whether a CT scan is a useful routine assessment modality in a patient diagnosed with a rectal cancer. Some would argue that for routine, uncomplicated malignancies, a CT scan is generally not necessary, since the information obtained will not usually affect the treatment plan. This concept is probably more applicable to patients with colon cancers versus patients with rectal cancers. For rectal cancer, there may be some merit to a baseline preoperative CT scan for advanced lesions. CT scanning is quite accurate in assessing rectal tumors that have invaded adjacent organs. However, for assessment of small primary lesions, CT scanning has many limitations. CT scans do not effectively visualize the layers of the rectal wall and so do not help in evaluating the extent of rectal wall invasion of an early cancer. The overall accuracy of CT scanning in determining depth of invasion is approximately 70%. Additionally, CT scanning is limited in its ability to determine the presence or absence of lymph node metastases. Overall accuracy with CT scanning for assessing lymph nodes in rectal cancer is only 45%.[7–11]

The most current CT scanning, especially with dynamic contrast infusion, has a high accuracy rate in detecting liver metastases. However, abdominal US, similar to CT scan, can also detect occult liver metastases and should be used when the information obtained would alter therapeutic decisions.[12] MRI is also very useful in evaluating the liver before resection.

Endoluminal Imaging

Endoluminal imaging in the form of endoluminal US and endoluminal MRI has become extremely useful in the accurate preoperative staging of a rectal cancer. These modalities allow for more precise determination of the depth of invasion and the presence or absence of mesorectal lymph node metastasis. The knowledge of these factors is critical in determining the sequence and type of therapy for any given rectal cancer.

Endoscopic US is performed with a probe that is inserted into the rectum via the anus. The patient usually takes a small preparation to clear the rectum of stool prior to the US. A water-filled balloon is inflated and pressed against the rectal lesion. A 7.0- to 10.0-MHz transducer is then used to delineate the layers of the bowel wall into five distinct lines. Localized cancers involving only the mucosa and submucosa can therefore be distinguished from those tumors that penetrate the muscularis propria or extend through the rectal wall into the perirectal fat.[13] A modified TNM classification has been proposed,[14,15] in which a US stage T1 lesion (uT1) denotes a malignancy confined to the mucosa and submucosa, a uT2 lesion implies penetration of the muscularis propria, but confinement to the rectal wall, a uT3 lesion indicates invasion into the perirectal fat, and a uT4 lesion denotes a primary rectal malignancy that invades an adjacent organ. Studies have compared endorectal US (ERUS)[16,17] to DRE[17] and have found the US much more accurate. A recent meta-analysis evaluating all ERUS studies from 1980 to 2008 showed that accuracy was high (88–95%). The sensitivity and specificity of ERUS to diagnose stage T1 cancer were 87.8 and 98.3%, respectively. For stage T2, ERUS had a sensitivity and specificity of 80.5 and 95.6%. For stage T3, ERUS had a sensitivity and specificity of 96.4 and 90.6%, respectively. In diagnosing stage T4 cancer, ERUS had a sensitivity of 95.4% and a specificity of 98.3%.[18]

ERUS is less useful in predicting lymph node metastases with a sensitivity of 73.2% and a specificity of 75.8%.[19]

Endosonographically identified malignant lymph nodes are generally more hypoechoic in perirectal tissues.[20] However, these results are only seen with experienced operators. The disadvantage of ERUS is that it is operator dependent and is less accurate for bulky disease or advanced rectal cancer due to depth of penetration.

Two methods of MRI can be used for the evaluation of rectal cancer. One can use the endorectal coil (ecMRI) or the surface coil MRI. The use of the MRI, either the endorectal or the surface coil, may offer some advantages compared with ERUS. First, it permits a larger field of view. Second, it may be less operator and technique dependent. And third, using the MRI may allow for the study of stenotic tumors.[21–24] Similar to ERUS, endorectal MRI (eMRI) can stage small-volume nodal disease and subtle transmural invasion. In general, eMRI has been more helpful in the assessment of perirectal nodal involvement than T stage. One reason is that MRI can identify involved nodes on the basis of characteristics other than size.[25] Reported accuracy rates of MRI for nodal staging range from 50 to 95%.[24–27]

Several series have compared the preoperative staging accuracy of ecMRI to ERUS in patients with rectal cancer.[24,26–28] In a report of 89 patients, the overall accuracy for T staging was similar (81%) for ecMRI and ERUS compared with only 65% for CT.[29] The accuracy for N staging was equally poor among the three modalities (63, 64, and 57% for ecMRI, ERUS, and CT, respectively). Somewhat similar results were noted in a series of 49 patients.[28] Transmural penetration was predicted by ecMRI with equal sensitivity (89%), but higher specificity (65 versus 33%) than ERUS. With both techniques, the predicted N stage had a relatively low correlation with pathologic N stage (45 versus 53%). In one report of 21 patients, ERUS seemed to be superior to ecMRI for determination of pathologic T stage (accuracy 83 versus 40%) because of better differentiation between T1 and T2 tumors. The accuracy for detecting perirectal tumor infiltration was 80% for ecMRI versus 100% for ERUS.[27]

The ecMRI is less operator dependent, and in answering the critical question of whether a patient has Stage I versus Stage II or Stage III disease, ecMRI was 88% accurate. Those patients who were not staged correctly were usually overstaged and not understaged.

Double-contrast MRI may permit more accurate T staging of rectal cancer by allowing better distinction among mucosa, muscularis, and perirectal tissues.[30,31] The specificity and sensitivity of ecMRI to predict infiltration of the anal sphincter was 100 and 90%, respectively. However, *N* staging was not improved with this approach; the sensitivity and specificity for nodal disease was 68 and 24%, respectively.

Phased-array surface coil MRI may prove to be the option of choice for staging of more advanced rectal cancers. The technique has been useful in predicting the likelihood of a tumor-free resection margin by visualizing tumor involvement of the mesorectal fascia.[32] However, it is less accurate for prediction of the correct T stage. Currently, we use this MRI technique along with CT scan of the abdomen and pelvis as our baseline imaging for all rectal cancers.

Preparation of the Rectal Cancer Patient for Surgery

After the diagnosis and staging of a rectal cancer, a decision needs to be made regarding optimal method of treatment. The surgical approach is dependent on the location of the tumor, its depth of invasion, and whether, in the preoperative evaluation, metastases have been discovered. If the patient is a candidate for a local excision or for a radical resection, the patient needs to be prepared for the procedure and the anesthetic so as to minimize perioperative and postoperative complications. Particular attention needs to be given to the patient's medical comorbidities. Unique to colon and rectal surgery is the use of a bowel preparation.

Bowel Preparation

There were multiple studies questioning the benefit of a bowel preparation in colorectal surgery. The rationale for a bowel preparation is that it improves visualization of luminal surfaces and reduces fecal flora, which possibly translates into reduction of anastomotic and infectious complications. Cochrane database review study published in 2005 showed no difference in terms of mortality, wound infection rates, extraabdominal complications, and reoperations in bowel preparation group versus nonbowel preparation group. It did, however, show statistically significant increased incidence of anastomotic leak in bowel preparation group (6.2 versus 3.2%, $p=0.003$). The difference was not statistically significant upon stratification of the groups based on the site of the surgery.[33] More recent RCTs published in 2007 did not show a difference in anastomotic leaks (4.8 versus 5.4%) or other complications.[34,35] The most recent meta-analysis study published by Pineda et al.[36] showed no difference in terms of anastomotic leak (4.2 versus 3.5%) or wound complications (9.9 versus 8.8%). Despite these studies, bowel preparation is still widely practiced by many surgeons.

Currently, there are several methods used to mechanically cleanse the large intestine. These methods include a diet of clear liquids 1–3 days before surgery combined with one of the following: laxatives, enemas, whole-gut irrigation with saline via a nasogastric tube, mannitol solutions, polyethylene glycol (PEG) electrolyte lavage solutions, or PEG-based tablets. In a 1990 survey of colon and rectal surgeons, almost two-thirds preferred the PEG solutions for their patients because of the reliability of the cleansing results.[37] Many surgeons today continue to use these PEG solutions as a bowel preparation. Despite these recent studies, we would still recommend some type of colonic cleansing before surgery because it is easier to manipulate the bowel if it is not filled with stool. It should be emphasized that one should not force a preparation on a patient because the benefits may be minimal. Furthermore, the choice of preparation should be selected depending on the individual. For instance, large-volume lavage solutions should not be used in patients with gastric emptying problems such as gastroparesis caused by diabetes. Saline laxatives are often phosphate- or magnesium-based and should not be used in patients with renal failure.

Antibiotic Prophylaxis

Antibiotic prophylaxis is used to decrease the incidence of postoperative septic complications, as mechanical cleansing decreases the total volume of stool in the colon but does not affect the concentration of bacteria per milliliter of effluent.[38] Traditional prophylaxis uses an oral regimen known as the Nichols/Condon preparation. This regimen consists of neomycin 1 g and erythromycin base 1 g by mouth at 1:00 p.m., 2:00 p.m., and 11:00 p.m. on the day before surgery.[39] Many surgeons have substituted metronidazole 500 mg for the erythromycin base because it is bacteriocidal against a greater percentage of gut anaerobes.

Most surgeons use perioperative systemic antibiotics instead of oral antibiotics for antibiotic prophylaxis. Regimens need to include coverage for both aerobic and anaerobic gut bacteria. For long procedures, redosing should be considered depending on the serum half-life of the antibiotics used. Some have argued that double prophylaxis with both oral and intravenous antibiotics is of benefit in immunocompromised patients or in patients in whom the dissection is below the peritoneal reflection.

Other Perioperative Issues

Besides the mechanical and antibiotic preparation of the bowel, all patients are prepared in the usual manner for major surgery. Blood loss is usually quite minimal for most elective colorectal surgery, and typically patients are not asked to donate autologous blood. Cardiac, pulmonary, and nutritional evaluations are performed when necessary. Perioperative systemic antibiotic coverage is expanded in patients with high-risk cardiac lesions such as prosthetic heart valves, a history of endocarditis, or a surgically constructed systemic-pulmonary shunt, and with intermediate-risk cardiac lesions such as mitral valve prolapse, valvular heart disease, or idiopathic hypertrophic subaortic stenosis.[38] Intravenous ampicillin 2 g and gentamicin 1.5 mg/kg are given 1/2–1 h before the procedure and for at least one postoperative dose. Oral anticoagulation is stopped and patients are placed on intravenous anticoagulation or on Lovenox® approximately 5 days before surgery. The heparin or Lovenox® is then stopped at the appropriate time before surgery (8 or 12 h, respectively). Depending on the individual risk of the patient and the extent of the operative dissection, anticoagulation is restarted as early as 8 h after surgery, but without a bolus. Careful monitoring of the patient's hematocrit and partial thromboplastin time is necessary if early reheparinization is instituted.

Anatomic and Biologic Issues

Surgical Anatomy

The type of operation that can be offered to a patient with rectal cancer depends not only on the tumor's stage but also on its location as this may determine resectability and sphincter preservation or sacrifice. The NCI consensus on rectal cancer recommended localizing the tumor relative to the anal verge, which is defined as starting at the intersphincteric groove. Another important landmark defining the upper limit of the anal canal is the anorectal ring. From the surgeon's perspective, the top of the anorectal ring is the lower limit of a distal resection margin. A large, full-thickness cancer needs to be located high enough above the top of the anorectal ring to allow for an adequate distal margin if sphincter preservation is contemplated. If the dissection is to be carried lower toward the dentate line, then the tumor must be confined to the mucosa, submucosa, and superficial layer of the internal sphincter.

Biologic Issues

It is important to understand the clinical biology of rectal cancer. "Clinical" biology means the typical pattern of growth and natural history of the spread of the disease. Studies have shown that colon cancer frequently arises in adenomatous polyps of the colon or rectum. Also, there is a 13–62% incidence of polyps in patients with carcinoma of the colon or rectum.[40–43] The variation observed in the incidence of coexisting adenomas with carcinoma of the colon or rectum depends in part on the method of study.[1,2] Whatever method used to study the issue, one can clearly say that the vast majority of carcinomas arise in preexisting adenomas.[44–46] In preparing a patient for surgery, the surgeon should have the colon completely evaluated preoperatively so as to be able to operatively treat any synchronous disease that cannot be endoscopically removed.

The biology of lymph node metastases with invasive rectal cancer is important to note and is somewhat different from that of other solid tumors such as breast cancer. Gabriel et al.[47] reported in 1935 that colorectal cancers tend not to have "skip" metastases. Rectal cancers usually proceeded in an orderly sequence from the adjacent mesorectal nodes up the lymphatic chain to the upper extent of the mesentery along the inferior mesenteric artery (IMA) and vein systems. From the surgeon's perspective, this usually predictable progression means that early intervention along with proper locoregional resection will cure most cancers. As part of a multimodality team that now treats most solid tumors, it must be emphasized to our medical colleagues that a rectal cancer is not a systemic disease from the first abnormal cell division. Aggressive local therapy in the form of an adequate resection is still the "anchor" to any therapy.

Surgical therapy may need to be customized in patients with certain polyposis syndromes or in cancers associated with inflammatory bowel disease. With both of these conditions, a total proctocolectomy needs to be performed. Sphincter preservation can be considered in certain patients; however, it should be recognized that any mucosa left intact is at an increased risk of developing cancer. The anal transitional zone needs to be biopsied to identify dysplasia. If dysplasia is present, then a proctocolectomy with end ileostomy needs to be performed.

Surgical Procedures: Principles

Resection of the bowel with primary anastomosis was not a common phenomenon until the late 1940s. Before that time, surgery of the colon and rectum usually meant a permanent stoma.[48] Recent advances have been made in the surgical techniques for rectal cancer. The result is that primary resection and anastomosis without a colostomy or ileostomy are now the rule rather than the exception.

Palliation should be the goal in a patient for whom curative resection is not possible. If the patient is a reasonable operative risk and the extent of metastatic disease is minimal, then complete but palliative resection of the primary tumor leads to a better quality of life and prevents many of the distressing symptoms of an advanced primary lesion such as obstruction, bleeding, and pain. If the primary lesion is not resectable, then diversion of the fecal stream can significantly improve the patient's immediate status. However, nonoperative therapy should be considered when there is significant metastatic disease and the primary tumor is relatively small and uncomplicated. In these cases, a colonic stent can be used if the patient needs to be relieved of an significant partial obstruction. Placement of a stent, however, is just a temporizing maneuver. If the patient responds to chemotherapy after a stent is placed, then a more definitive diversion or resection can be reconsidered in the otherwise healthy patient. As highlighted in a study from Memorial Sloan-Kettering, resection of a primary tumor in a patient with metastatic disease did not prolong overall survival. However, one has to individualize the therapy to each situation. Further, greater response to chemotherapy or the ability of new chemotherapy regimens to stop progression of disease will force us to reevaluate this clinical scenario on an ongoing basis.

Variability in Outcome Based on Surgeon and Hospital Volume

The cancer resection margin in the extraperitoneal rectum is limited by the bony confines of the pelvis, as well as by the proximity of adjacent anterior organs. In some cases, locoregional recurrence may be inevitable. However, locoregional failure may also result from incomplete surgery. There is accumulating evidence of variability among surgeons in local recurrence rates for stage-matched rectal cancers. McArdle and Hole[49] presented a review of 645 patients undergoing colorectal cancer resection at the Royal Infirmary in Glasgow. They observed significant variability in patients' postoperative morbidity, mortality, and ultimate survival, depending on the surgeon. The proportion of patients undergoing a curative resection varied from 40 to 76%, operative mortality from 8 to 30%, local recurrence from 0 to 21%, and anastomotic leak rates from 0 to 25%.

Hospital volume can also have an impact on colostomy rates, postoperative mortality, and overall survival as shown in a series of 7,257 patients diagnosed with Stage I–III rectal cancer between 1994 and 1997.[50] When hospitals with the highest quartile of volume (more than 20 procedures annually) were compared with those with volumes in the lowest quartile (fewer than seven procedures annually), there were statistically significant differences in colostomy rates (29.5 versus 36.6%), 30-day postoperative mortality (1.6 versus 4.8%), and overall 2-year survival (83.7 versus 76.6%).

The ability to perform sphincter-sparing surgery is also affected by hospital volume. In the USA Intergroup 0114 trial of 1,330 patients with Stage II or III rectal cancer participating in an adjuvant treatment trial, APR rates were significantly higher in low-volume hospitals (46 versus 32% at lowest and highest volume hospitals, respectively).[51] Low hospital surgical volume was only an important predictor of inferior overall or recurrence-free survival in patients who did not complete their planned adjuvant chemoradiotherapy.

Total Mesorectal Excision

Total mesorectal excision in conjunction with an LAR or an abdominal perineal resection involves precise sharp dissection and removal of the entire rectal mesentery, including that distal to the tumor, as an intact unit.[52] Unlike conventional blunt dissection, the rectal mesentery is removed sharply under direct visualization emphasizing autonomic nerve preservation, complete hemostasis, and avoidance of violation of the mesorectal envelope. Its rationale is underscored by the hypothesis that the field of rectal cancer spread is limited to this envelope and its total removal encompasses virtually every tumor satellite. The reduction of positive radial margins can be reduced from 25% in conventional surgery to 7% in cases resected by TME. Furthermore, Adam et al.[53] showed that patients with positive radial margins were three times more likely to die and 12 times more likely to have local recurrence than patients without radial margin involvement.

Conventional surgery violates the circumference of the mesorectum during the blunt dissection along undefined planes. This leaves residual mesorectum in the pelvis. The higher rate of pelvic recurrence in conventional surgery is a reflection of inadequate resection and residual viable tumor burden within the pelvis. Several surgical teams using the TME technique have reported local failure rates ranging from 5 to 7% for Stage II and Stage III cancers.[52–56] By contrast, the North Central Cancer Treatment Group, NCCTG, control arm consisting of surgery plus radiotherapy had a local failure rate of 25%, and the addition of chemotherapy only decreased the local failure rate to half of that value.[57]

Fortunately, improved local control seems to be translatable into improved overall survival. Survival ranges from 68 to 78% are observed among large published series when this technique is applied.

The meticulous dissection, however, is not without consequence. Prolonged operative time and increased anastomotic leak rates are noted. Anastomoses 3–6 cm from the anal verge have led up to 17% leak rates such that many centers routinely fashion a protective diverting stoma.

Conventional rectal surgery is associated with a significant incidence of sexual and urinary dysfunction. Presumably, this problem is related to damage to the pelvic autonomic parasympathetic and sympathetic nerves by blunt dissection forces.[58] Postoperative impotence and retrograde ejaculation or both have been observed in 25–75% of cases particularly if lateral-wall lymphadenectomy and splanchnic nerve resection are performed. By contrast, after TME with its careful nerve-sparing dissection, impotence has been reported in only 10–29% of cases. A recent prospective study has confirmed that autonomic nerve preservation yields good results in terms of morbidity and functional outcome.[59]

There are well-recognized points during the rectal dissection where nerve injury can occur. The most proximal is the sympathetic nerve plexus surrounding the aorta. These sympathetic nerve trunks are also prone to injury near the pelvic brim as the bifurcate to each side of the pelvis. Intact nerves should look like a "wishbone" near the sacral promontory after a proper dissection. The clinical consequence of an isolated sympathetic nerve injury is retrograde ejaculation. If one proceeds with a dissection beneath the presacral or pelvic fascia from the sacral promontory around to the lateral pelvic sidewall, then one can injure both parasympathetic and sympathetic nerves, which can result in impotence and bladder dysfunction. In the lower part of the mid rectum, the hypogastric plexus and nervi erigentes can be injured in the anterolateral pelvis. A radial dissection well outside the lymphovascular bundle, which lies adjacent to the nerve and nerve plexus, can also lead to a mixed parasympathetic and sympathetic injury. This bundle and the nerve structure are typically located just lateral to the seminal vesicles in a man or the cardinal ligaments in a woman. Finally, a dissection anterior to both layers of Denonvillier's fascia in a man can also put at risk the nerve and nerve plexus.

To date, all data are from prospectively gathered series and comparisons with historical controls. There are no randomized control data clearly showing benefits in terms of disease-specific and overall survival in patients undergoing TME as opposed to more conventional resection.

Adjuvant therapy has recently been shown to improve the results of TME surgery. In a two-arm, randomized study comparing TME with or without preoperative radiotherapy for resectable rectal cancer, patients receiving the combined therapy had a lower rate of local recurrence at 2 years. Subset analysis showed the most significant benefit in node-positive cancers.[60] The "completeness" of the TME also correlated with prognosis.[61] Adjuvant therapy should therefore be considered in patients undergoing TME surgery with Stage II and Stage III disease.

Figure 44-1 demonstrates schematically how the dissection should proceed. Figure 44-2 shows a cross-section of the rectum, the mesorectal fat, and the associated fascia.

Distal Margins and Radial Margins

The extent of resection margins in rectal cancer remains controversial. Although the first line of rectal cancer spread is upward along the lymphatic course, tumors below the peritoneal reflection also spread distally by intramural or extramural lymphatic and vascular routes. When distal intramural spread occurs, it is usually within 2.0 cm of the tumor, unless the lesion is poorly differentiated or widely metastatic.[62–64] Williams et al.[65] in 1983 reported distal intramural spread in 12 of 50 resected rectal cancer surgical patients. It was observed that 10 of the 12 had Stage III lesions. Only 6% had distal intramural spread greater than 2 cm. They concluded a "wet" margin of 2.5 cm was adequate in 94% of the patients. They noted that only five patients (10%) had tumors beyond a 1.5-cm margin, and all five of these patients had poorly differentiated, node-positive cancers. Also, the mortality in this group of patients was attributable to distant metastases, not local recurrence. All of these patients had undergone an APR and had distal margins of greater than 5 cm. Grinnell[62] reported five cases of extramural retrograde lymphatic spread within 1.5 cm in 93 rectal cancers. He also reviewed 28 patients with atypical retrograde lymphatic dissemination all of whom died within 5 years. He concluded that retrograde lymphatic spread was a poor

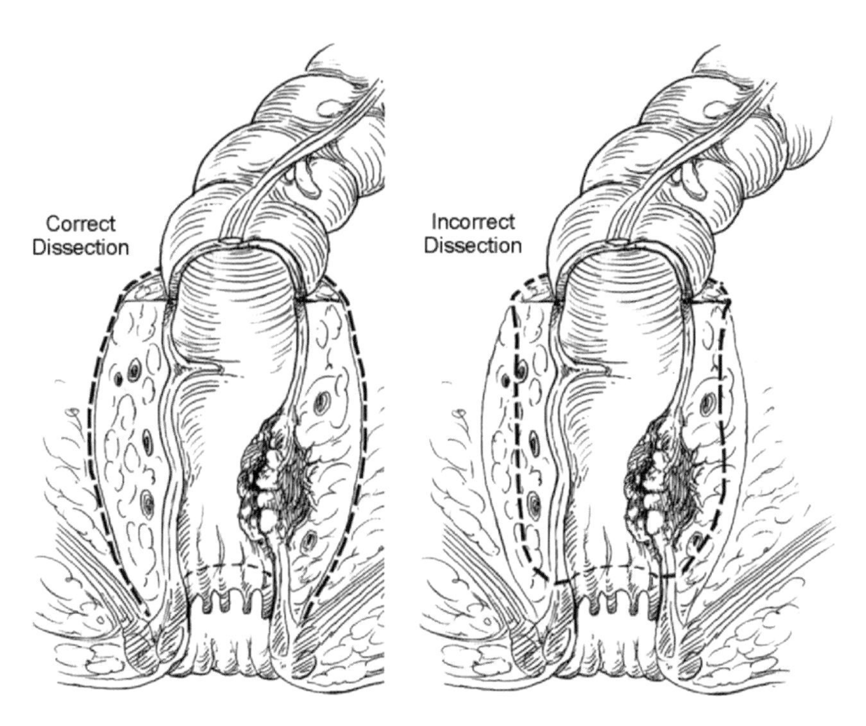

FIGURE 44-1. Schematic representation of the correct TME dissection versus an incorrect dissection. The dissection should proceed between the mesorectal fascia and the pelvic wall fascia to ensure a "complete" TME.

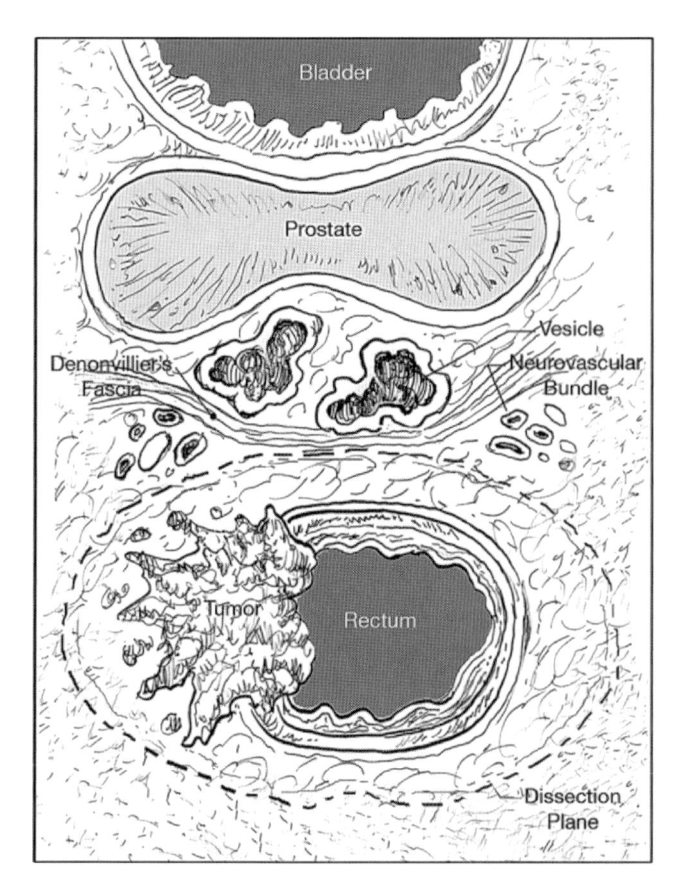

FIGURE 44-2. Transverse diagram of the structures of the mid rectum. The proper dissection proceeds just outside the mesorectal fat and fascia but with sparing of the neurovascular bundle and hypogastric plexus that is located anterolaterally along the pelvic sidewall. One or both layers of Denonvillier's fascia should be included in males and the equivalent fascial dissection along the back of the vagina in females.

prognostic sign and that more radical operations were not advantageous. Pollett and Nicholls[66] observed no difference in local recurrence rates whether distal margins of <2 cm, 2–5 cm, or >5 cm were achieved. Finally, in two early studies from the British literature, surgical pathology of rectal and rectosigmoid cancer demonstrated the clinical biology of extramural lymphatic spread. In the series by Goligher et al.[67] from 1951, only 6.5% of patients had metastatic glands below the primary tumor, whereas 93.5% had no retrograde spread. Approximately two-thirds of patients with retrograde spread had metastasis limited to within 6 mm of the distal tumor edge, and only 2% had metastasis beyond 2 cm. Dukes[68] published similar results in a study of more than 1,500 patients who had undergone APR.

Further data from a randomized, prospective trial conducted by the National Surgical Adjuvant Breast and Bowel Project demonstrated no significant differences in survival or local recurrence when comparing distal rectal margins of <2 cm, 2–2.9 cm, and >3 cm.[69] As a result, a 2-cm distal margin has become acceptable for resection of rectal carcinoma, although a 5-cm proximal margin is still recommended.[70] The radial margin is more critical for local control.

Based upon these extensive data, a 2-cm distal margin can is generally justifiable over a 5-cm distal margin. Even smaller distal margins may be acceptable in certain patients for whom there is no other option for sphincter preservation. In these cases, a frozen section analysis of the distal margin must be performed to confirm a cancer-free margin.

The discussion concerning the distal margin should not be confused with the issues regarding a TME and the radial margin. It is now clear that the status of the radial margin is perhaps the most critical in determining prognosis. Quirke et al.[71]

in 1986 demonstrated tumor spread to the radial margins of 14 of 52 rectal cancers on whole mount specimens (27%). Twelve of these 14 patients subsequently developed local recurrence, suggesting that local recurrence is largely a result of radial spread. Cawthorn et al.[55] also documented that tumor involvement of the lateral resection margin correlated with poor prognosis; however, it seemed to correlate more with distant spread, and it was not a useful indicator of local recurrence.

Lateral Lymph Node Dissection

A complete clearance of lateral lymph nodes or extended lateral lymph node dissection (ELD) for low-lying rectal cancers with suspected or high risk for lateral lymph node metastasis has become a routine practice in Japan. The practice is based on the existence of lateral lymphatic drainage of the rectum, which TME does not encompass. Lateral lymphatic flow passes from the lower rectum and through lateral ligaments beyond mesorectum and ascends along internal iliac arteries and inside the obturator spaces. The recent study from Japan showed that the incidence of lateral lymph node involvement for low-lying rectal cancer is 16.4%.[72]. A recent study from The Netherlands compared the treatment of rectal cancer between Japan and The Netherlands and showed 5-year local recurrence rates of 6.9% for the Japanese ELD group, 5.8% in the Dutch RT+TME group, and 12.1% in the Dutch TME group.[73]

ELD is associated with a much higher rate of urinary and sexual dysfunctions as compared to standard TME. Another study from Japan showed that degree of urinary and sexual dysfunction depended not only on the extent of autonomic nerve resection but also on the extent of ELD in independent fashion.[74]

ELD is a controversial topic, and more studies need to be done on its effectiveness and the benefits versus increased morbidity before it can be recommended as a standard of care. However, in some patients where there are palpable nodes along the pelvic sidewall and along the iliacs, a patient may benefit from this extended dissection.

Selection of Appropriate Therapy for Rectal Cancer

The management of rectal cancer has become increasingly complex. Presently, a surgeon has three major curative options: local excision, sphincter-saving abdominal surgery, and APR. Ideal candidates for local therapy that preserves anal sphincter anatomy and function include small T1 lesions (invasion only into the submucosa) and T2 lesions (invasion into the muscularis propria). As will be discussed, patients with T2 lesions probably should not have surgery alone. Recurrence is high. Preoperative or postoperative adjuvant chemoradiation is of benefit. At present, patients with T3 lesions (invasion into the perirectal fat) are not suitable candidates for local therapy and should be treated with an appropriate major resection as well as adjuvant therapy in most cases.

Certain clinical features also may have an impact on decisions about the appropriate therapy. Patients with physical handicaps may have significant difficulty in managing a stoma. Body habitus and patient gender influence the surgeon's ability to perform a sphincter-saving operation because of pelvic anatomy. Whereas a sphincter-saving procedure in a multiparous thin female can be straightforward, performing a low anastomosis in an obese male with a narrow pelvis can be extremely difficult. A history of pelvic irradiation or nonrectal pelvic malignancy can make a rectal resection and sphincter preservation more difficult.

In summary, each patient with rectal cancer should be individually evaluated, and a technical plan for their resection is customized to their stage, gender, age, and body habitus (Figure 44-3). With these issues in mind, the technical choices for a radical resection are discussed below. In all of these resections, a TME should be performed. Local treatments are then described in detail.

Techniques of Rectal Excision

Abdominoperineal Resection

The APR was the first radical resection described by Miles in 1908 (reprinted in 1971).[75] Miles set out several principles to be achieved with any radical resection. These principles included:

- Removal of the whole pelvic mesocolon
- Removal of the "zone of upward spread" in the rectal mesentery
- Wide perineal dissection
- An abdominal anus
- Removal of the lymph nodes along the iliacs.

Four of five of these principles are the anchor of our technique even today (the dissection along the iliacs is not routinely done).

Candidates for an APR include patients whose tumors are either into the anal sphincter or are so close to the anal sphincter that a safe distal margin cannot be obtained. Also, there is a small subset of patients with mid rectal tumors but with poor continence who may benefit from an APR, even though they are technically sphincter-preservation candidates. There have been recent reports that obturator/pelvic sidewall lymph nodes are more often involved in patients with very low rectal cancers. It has been suggested that these patients should undergo an extrafascial TME dissection.[72] Although there is some merit to this concept, we describe herein two approaches to APR with TME, excision of the sphincter and levators, and creation of a permanent colostomy. Traditionally, the APR has been done in lithotomy position. Recently, there have been reports of oncologic superiority of

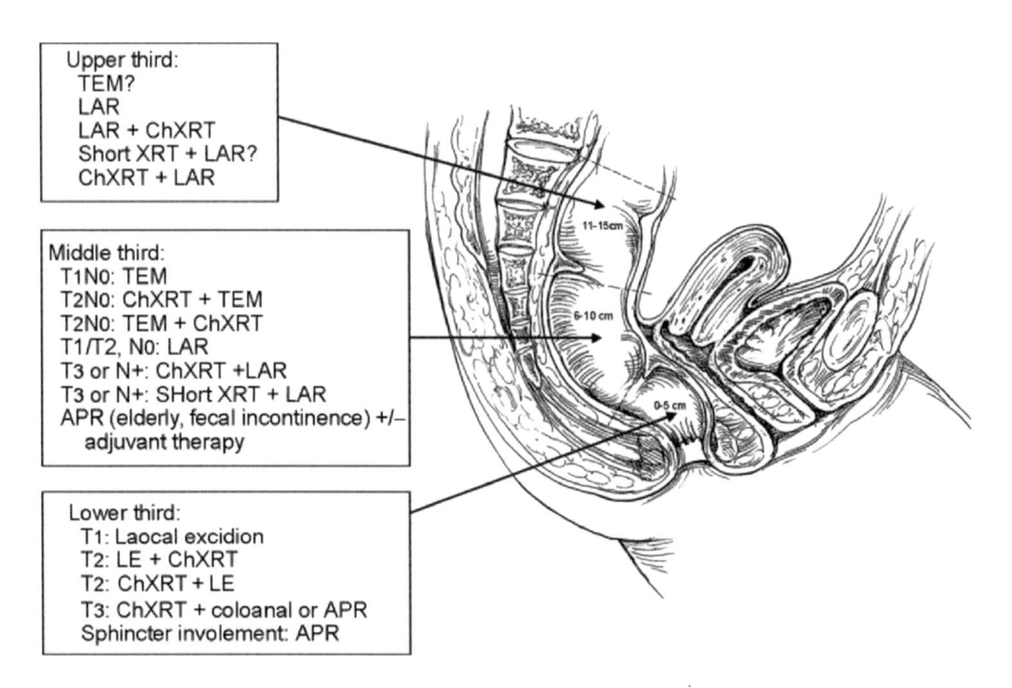

FIGURE 44-3. Treatment options for rectal cancer depending on stage and location. Stage I (T1N0, T2N0 – the cancer is confined to the rectal wall, and no nodes are involved). Distal rectal cancers: T1 (invasion into the submucosa only): Local excision; Radical resection, often an APR; Adjuvant therapy is usually not recommended. Distal rectal cancers: T2 (invasion into the muscularis propria): Local excision with preoperative or postoperative adjuvant therapy; Radical resection without adjuvant therapy, often an APR. Mid rectal cancer: T1: TEM (transanal endoscopic microsurgery); Radical resection, usually an LAR with low anastomosis. A temporary proximal diverting ostomy is often required; Adjuvant therapy is usually not recommended. Mid rectal cancer: T2: TEM with either preoperative or postoperative adjuvant therapy; Radical resection similar to a T1 cancer; Adjuvant therapy is not recommended if a radical resection is performed but is recommended before or after a TEM resection. Upper rectal cancers: T1 and T2: LAR; TEM? Stage II and Stage III cancers [Stage II cancers have invasion into the mesorectal fat (T3) but no involved mesorectal lymph nodes. Stage III cancers are any rectal cancer (T1, T2, or T3) but with involved lymph nodes.] Distal rectal cancers: Preoperative adjuvant therapy is most often recommended followed by a radical resection, usually an APR; If preoperative imaging does not clearly define the stage of the cancer, resection can be done first followed by postoperative adjuvant therapy. Mid rectal cancers: Same as above for distal rectal cancers except an LAR is usually performed instead of an APR. Upper rectal cancers: LAR, with either preoperative or postoperative adjuvant therapy. Stage IV cancers: Treatment for any cancer is dependent on the extent of metastasis. With better surgical and medical treatments for metastatic disease, locoregional control of the primary should be aggressive and similar to the above recommendations except in the most advanced cases. Key: *LE* local excision, *short XRT* short-course radiation therapy given two times a day for 5 days in larger fractions, *ChXRT* long-course therapy given in 30 smaller fractions over 6 weeks in combination with chemotherapy.

cylindrical APR that is performed in prone position.[76] The cylindrical approach closely resembles the original Miles APR.[75,77] The recent paper of West et al. showed that cylindrical APR results in more cylindrical specimen (hence the name) and removes more tissue in the distal rectum and leads to lower radial margin involvement (14.8 versus 40.6%) and intraoperative rectal perforations (3.7 versus 22.8%).[76] The experience in our center shows that cylindrical APR leads to fewer wound complications likely due to better visualization and better skin preparation; operative time remains the same.

Position

For traditional APR, the patient is placed in the lithotomy position. We often elevate the mid and upper sacrum off the bed with a blanket or a towel so that the coccyx is away from the bed and therefore able to be more easily prepped into the field. For cylindrical APR, the patient is placed supine for TME portion of the operation and stoma creation and rotated to prone for perineal dissection. We usually have the second OR table ready with appropriate padding for all the pressure points so that the patient can be easily moved to prone position.

Incision and Exploration

The abdomen is usually entered through a midline incision. In thin patients, the incision can often be kept below the umbilicus. Low transverse incisions can also be performed as long as the ostomy site is not compromised. The APR is also a good application of laparoscopic surgery, as the abdominal portion of the procedure can be performed using laparoscopic techniques with extraction of the specimen through the perineum.

The exploration of the abdomen and pelvis should be the first step after accessing the abdomen. The liver, aortic lymph nodes, superior hemorrhoidal lymph nodes, iliac lymph nodes, and the pelvis should all be examined. A large tumor burden, particularly multiple peritoneal implants, should lead to a reassessment of the need for resection, and perhaps only a colostomy should be performed.

Mobilization

The sigmoid colon and left colon need to be mobilize to excise the whole pelvic mesocolon and "zone of upward spread." The mobilization begins along the left pelvic brim. The gonadal vessels, ureter, and iliacs are reflected toward the retroperitoneum, and the colon and mesocolon are pulled toward the midline. The left colon is mobilized, but the splenic flexure rarely needs to be taken down. The dissection then is started on the right pelvic brim. Often, one can identify the sympathetic nerve trunks behind the superior hemorrhoidal artery (SHA) as one mobilizes the rectal mesocolon away from the sacral promontory.

Resection and Ligation

After mobilization of the mesentery, the bowel is divided near the sigmoid colon/left colon junction at right angles to the blood supply (Figure 44-4). Because a high ligation of the SHA or of the IMA is planned, the blood supply to most of the sigmoid colon will be compromised. For most cases, a ligation of the SHA flush with the left colic artery should be performed. A higher ligation of the IMA should be performed if there is any question of lymph node involvement outside the pelvis (e.g., palpable nodes along the SHA up to or above the left colic artery). The IMA should be ligated flush with the aorta, and the inferior mesenteric vein should be ligated near the ligament of Treitz. A high ligation may also be required for additional colonic mobilization.

After dividing the bowel, sequential clamps of the sigmoid vessels are placed and the mesentery is ligated and divided. A high ligation is performed of the SHA with care being taken to not injure the ureters, and also to make sure that the sympathetic nerve trunks are preserved.

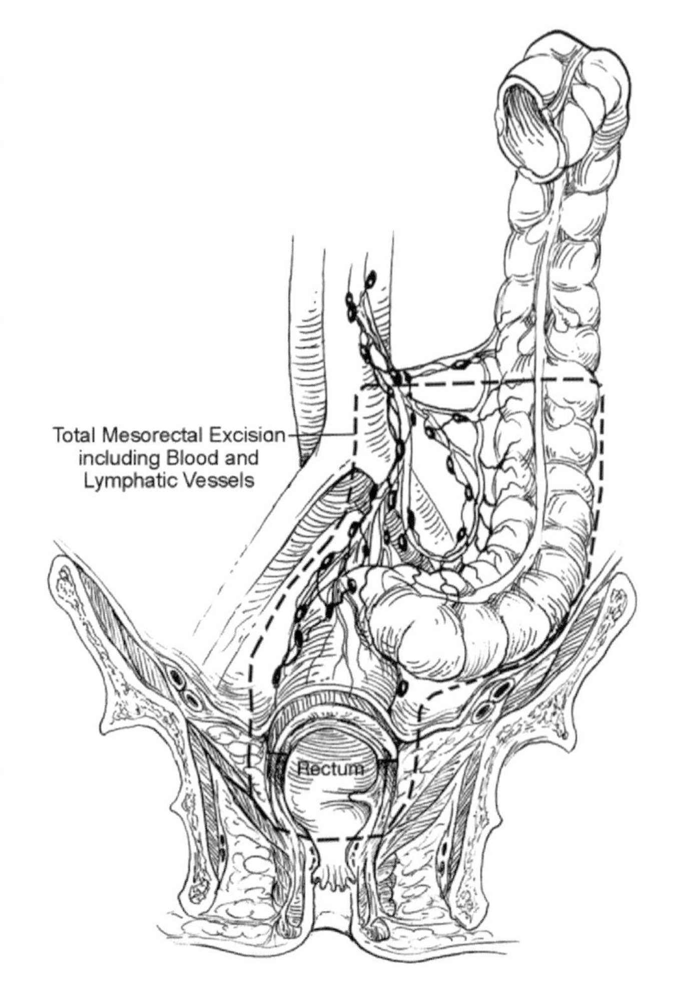

FIGURE 44-4. The vascular supply of the sigmoid and rectum. A typical ligation is performed at the junction of the SHA and left colic artery. In patients with a clinical suspicion of positive nodes at the level of the IMA, or if vascular mobilization is needed for the left and transverse colon, a ligation of the IMA is performed at the aorta.

Total Mesorectal Excision

A successful total mesorectal excision (TME) starts with the proper ligation of the SHA or IMA. As one dissects down toward the sacral promontory, the sympathetic nerve trunks are identified. The dissection plane is just anterior or medial to these nerves. Using the cautery or scissors, the nerves are reflected toward the pelvic sidewall, while the mesorectal fascia surrounding the mesorectal fat is kept as an intact unit. The dissection starts posteriorly and then at each level proceeds laterally and then anteriorly. In the mid rectal area along the lateral sidewalls, one can sometimes see the parasympathetic nerves tracing anteriorly toward the hypogastric plexus. The plexus is usually on the anterolateral sidewall of the pelvis, just lateral to the seminal vesicles in the man and the cardinal ligaments in the woman. There is often a tough "ligament" that traverses the mesorectum at this point. It theoretically contains the middle rectal artery. However, in a study by Jones et al.[78], this artery is only present to any significance about 20% of the time.

The anterior dissection is perhaps the most difficult. In men, one should try to include the two layers of Denonvillier's fascia. This fascia is composed of peritoneum that has been entrapped between the seminal vesicles and prostate anterior and the rectum posterior (Figure 44-5). In woman, the peritoneum at the base of the pouch of Douglas is incised, and the rectovaginal septum is then separated.

If properly done, the mesorectum begins to appear as a bulky bilobed structure. As one progresses distally beyond the mid rectum, the mesorectal fat begins to attenuate. At the pelvic floor, there is often only a thin layer of mesorectal fat around the bowel.

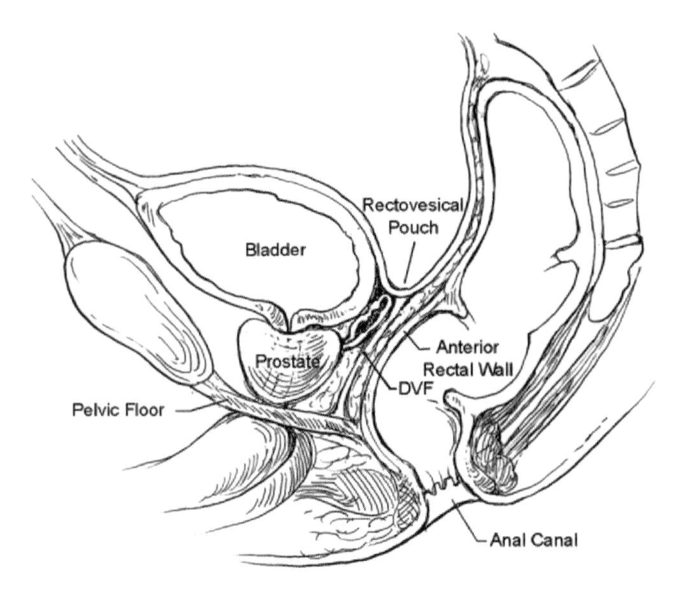

FIGURE 44-5. Sagittal view of the rectum, bladder, Denonvillier's fascia, and the prostate. The dissection should proceed anterior to one or both layers of Denonvillier's fascia.

Perineal Dissection

In traditional APR, as the abdominal procedure proceeds distally, the perineal dissection can commence. Before the preparation and draping of the patient, the position of the perineum is ensured so as to allow a wide elliptical incision around the anus. The rectum is usually cleared of any stool or residual preparation, and the anus is sewn closed. The incision for the perineal dissection starts anteriorly at the perineal body, goes laterally to the ischiorectal spines, and then finishes posteriorly at the tip of the coccyx. After incising the skin and subcutaneous ischiorectal membrane and fat, the levators are then encountered. The perineal surgeon then coordinates their dissection with the abdominal team in the posterior precoccygeal plane. A pair of long scissors or an electrocautery can be used to divide the ligaments in the posterior midline behind the rectum. Once a connection has been opened, the perineal surgeon places their finger above the levators and "hooks" them down toward the perineal field. The levators are then divided with the cautery. The dissection starts posteriorly and then proceeds laterally and anteriorly. Often, it is best to complete the anterior dissection after the proximal portion of the specimen has been everted out to the perineal surgeon. The remaining attachments in the anterior plane are then divided with the cautery. Once the specimen is removed, hemostasis is ensured with the cautery or absorbable figure-of-8 sutures. Typically, there are vessels that need to be ligated in the crease between the lateral prostate and the pelvic floor.

If a cylindrical APR is planned, the patient needs to be changed to prone position after TME is complete and permanent colostomy is created. The pelvis is elevated on a pillow, and the buttocks are taped apart. The skin incision is marked in elliptical fashion to extend from coccyx to ischial tuberosities to perineal body. The incision is made with knife through the skin and extended down through subcutaneous tissues with electrocautery. At this point, two Gelpi retractors or a Lone Star retractor (Lone Star Medical Products Inc., Stafford, TX) facilitate the dissection. Similar to traditional approach, anococcygeal ligament is broken through with a pair of large scissors or an elctrocautery and which are retracted wide open to create enough space for surgeon's finger to hook the levators, thus facilitating the lateral dissection of the rectum. Care is taken to dissect the levators of pelvic sidewall. After lateral attachments are taken down, the rectum is everted onto the field and by holding the rectum up anterior dissection is complete. Sometimes coccyx can be removed as well in continuity with the main specimen.

After irrigating the pelvis, one reapproximates the residual levators with absorbable sutures, and then the subcutaneous fat, ischiorectal fat, and skin are closed in several layers. Drains in the pelvis can be brought out through the pelvis or via the abdomen.

Ostomy

Ideally, the patient has been preoperatively marked by a certified ostomy therapist. The end of the colon is carefully cleaned of any fat. The skin is divided in a circular shape at the ostomy site. The subcutaneous tissues are split and the fascia is divided in a vertical or cruciate manner. The muscle is split but not divided, and then the peritoneum is incised. The hole is made wide enough to accommodate the bowel and the accompanying mesentery. The bowel should then be brought up through the opening so that it is 1–3 cm higher than the skin and the ostomy is matured.

LAR with Sphincter Preservation

Sphincter-sparing procedures for resection of mid and some distal rectal cancers have become increasingly prevalent as their safety and efficacy have been established. The advent of circular stapling devices is largely responsible for their increasing popularity and utilization. An LAR involves dissection and anastomosis below the peritoneal reflection with ligation of the superior and middle hemorrhoidal arteries. An extended LAR indicates complete mobilization of the rectum down to the pelvic floor with division of the lateral ligaments and posterior mobilization through Waldeyer's fascia to the tip of the coccyx. Additionally, there is dissection of the plane between the anterior rectal wall and the vagina in a female patient and dissection of the plane between the rectum and the prostate in a male patient to a level distal to the inferior margin of the prostate gland. As long as the surgeon can obtain a distal margin of at least 2 cm, an anastomosis can be considered appropriate if technically feasible. Body habitus, adequacy of the anal sphincter, encroachment of the tumor on the anal sphincters, and adequacy of the distal margin are all factors in determining the applicability of a sphincter-sparing operation.

Coloanal Anastomosis

The ultimate procedure in sphincter-saving operations is the ultra-LAR with coloanal anastomosis. This operation preserves the sphincter mechanism in patients with very low-lying rectal cancer in whom the distal margin is at the minimally acceptable level yet adequate for cancer clearance. These operations are reserved for patients who have a distal rectal cancer that does not invade the sphincter musculature and in whom a standard extended LAR is technically not possible. After an adequate distal margin is achieved, the rectum is transected at the level of the pelvic floor musculature. The remaining anal mucosa between the dentate line and the level of transection of the pelvic floor can then be "stripped," and an anastomosis between the colon and the anus is performed to restore continuity. Alternatively, the procedure can be started at the dentate line with a tubular mobilization of the distal rectum in the intersphincteric groove. This perineal resection can proceed up to the superior margin of the puborectalis muscle before dissecting into the pelvis and connecting with the pelvic and abdominal dissection. The procedure usually requires full mobilization of the splenic flexure, such that the vascular supply of the left colon now based on the middle colic vessels can reach the distal pelvis. The coloanal anastomosis can also be undertaken with a colonic J pouch. Because of the larger capacity of the J pouch construction, anorectal function is thought to be improved, especially early after the surgery. The J pouch is created by folding the distal end of the colon back on itself approximately 5–8 cm and then creating a common channel (Figure 44-6). The actual anastomosis to the anus is then done from the apex of the J in side-to-end manner. An alternative to the colonic J pouch is the coloplasty. This technique is similar in concept to a stricturoplasty. The distal colon is divided in a longitudinal direction for 8–10 cm starting 4–6 cm from the distal edge of the pedicle. The longitudinal incision is then approximated transversely, making a larger reservoir capacity (Figure 44-7). The technique can decrease frequency in the early postoperative period, but it has been associated with an increased number of anastomotic leaks. A proximal diverting stoma is advisable because of the potential for an anastomotic leak or vascular compromise of the left colon. Contraindications to the procedure include the following: baseline fecal incontinence from deteriorated anal sphincter muscles, tumor invasion of the anal sphincter musculature or rectovaginal septum, tenesmus, and technical factors such as body habitus, tumor location, and tumor size. An end rectum to side colonic anastomosis is another option to the commonly used colonic J pouch.

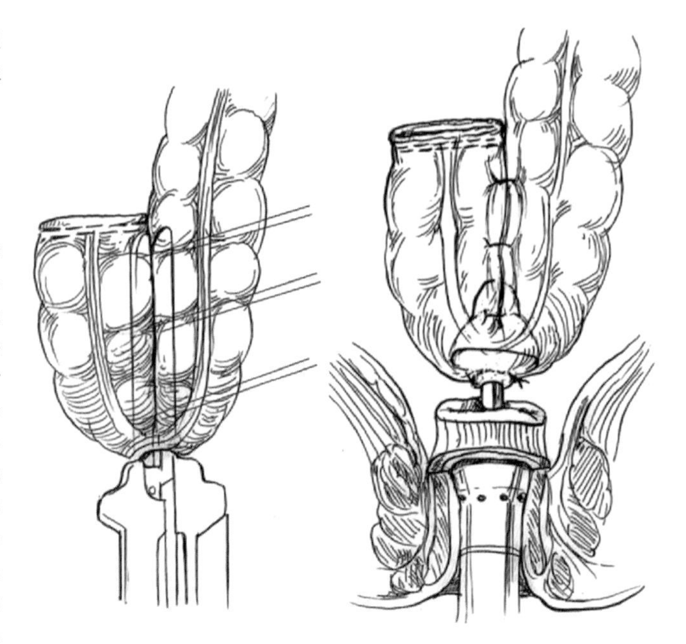

FIGURE 44-6. Construction of a colonic J pouch after an ultra LAR. The distal colon pedicle is folded back on itself to make a "J." A common channel is then created using a stapling device that will staple and divide. A larger reservoir is then created. The J pouch is then anastomosed to the anus using a circular stapler or in a hand-sewn manner.

Laparoscopically Assisted Resections for Rectal Cancer

The application of laparoscopy for the treatment of intraabdominal malignancies including proctectomy for rectal cancer is now being performed. In these operations, part of the procedure is done using the laparoscope, and completion of the procedure is in the traditional manner. In particular, exploration and mobilization of the colon and rectum can be done with the laparoscope and laparoscopic instruments.[79] Ligation of the vascular pedicle is performed with laparoscopic clips, vascular stapling devices, or radiofrequency coagulation devices. The improved optics of laparoscopy can provide a much better view in the pelvis, thus facilitating rectal dissection. In the recent years, there has been an increased use of laparoscopic resection for rectal cancer. Most often, however, the actual resection of the bowel and an anastomosis are still more easily performed in an extracorporeal manner.

The main questions about laparoscopic-assisted proctectomy for colorectal cancer are whether it provides the same TME specimen as traditional open techniques, and whether there is any other unique biologic alteration in the laparoscopic procedure that leads to a change in survival or in recurrence patterns. Concerning the latter point, there have been several reports of unusual wound recurrences at trocar sites in patients undergoing laparoscopic-assisted colectomy. It is of paramount importance that laparoscopic resection follows

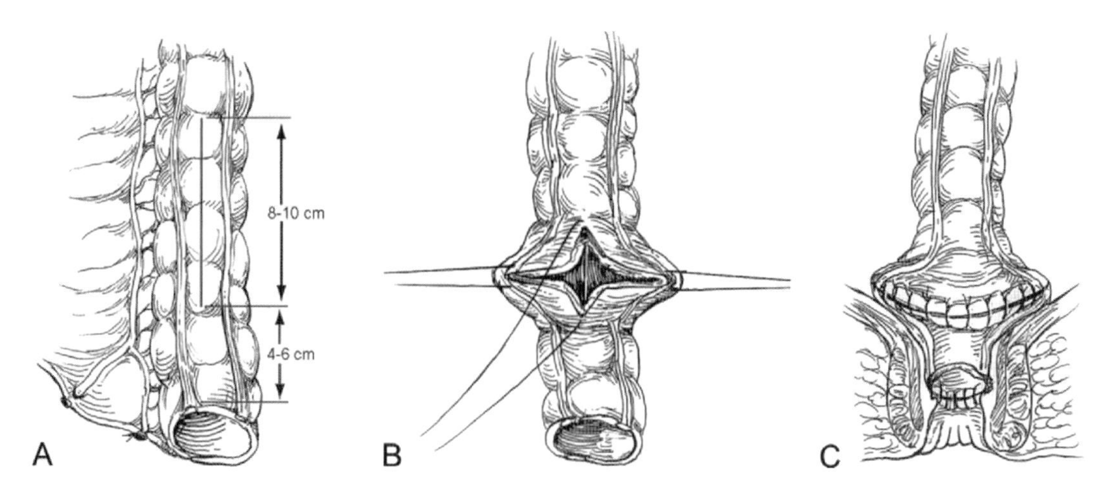

FIGURE 44-7. Construction of a coloplasty. The bowel is divided in a longitudinal manner as shown and resutured transversely to create a larger reservoir capacity.

the same oncologic principle as open surgery including precise TME. The recent studies have indicated that there is no difference between laparoscopic and open surgery as far as 3 and 5-year survival,[80,81] radial margin involvement [81], and local recurrence rate.[81,82]

The mean operative time for laparoscopic rectal surgery ranges from 180 to 260 min[80,82], although some studies report similar times to open surgery.[79] The blood loss is usually less. Most of the studies report earlier return of bowel function, decreased hospital stay, and reduction in pain.

The rate of anastomotic leak in sphincter sparing rectal surgery is comparable between two approaches and is approximately 10% and can be as high as 17%.[81] Also, there have been two reports of an increase in erectile dysfunction with the laparoscopic rectal resection versus open surgery.

One of the indicators of feasibility of laparoscopic rectal surgery is the conversion rate, which is found to be between 6 and 15%. It was also noted the conversion is associated with higher operative mortality, higher complication rate, and higher local recurrence rate.

The recommendation from ASCRS is that laparoscopic rectal cancer resection be practiced by expert, trained surgeons in an environment where the outcomes can be meaningfully evaluated. Ultimately, the question may be answered with the current American College of Surgeons Oncology Group (ACOSOG) Trial comparing laparoscopic versus open resection of rectal cancers.

Local Excision Versus Radical Resection

Although the LAR and the APR are the mainstays of therapy for many distal rectal cancers, the radical resection is associated with significant morbidity and mortality. A review of the literature showed that mortality rates for the APR range from 0 to 6.3%,[79,83,86] with some studies having a 61% incidence of postoperative complications.[84] The majority of these complications are urinary dysfunction and perineal wound infections, with rates as high as 50 and 16%, respectively.[85] In our experience, the incidence of major wound complications was 10%.[87] Radical surgery, especially the APR, leads to a significant change in body image and social habits. In a patient survey performed in 1983 by Williams and Johnston,[88] 66% of patients complained of significant leaks from their stoma appliances, 67% experienced sexual dysfunction, and only 40% of patients who were working preoperatively returned to their jobs after their operation. Unfortunately, radical surgery does not guarantee a recurrence-free survival; the 5-year survival rate in the National Cancer Data Base for Stage I disease is 78%.[89] The complication rates, the change in body image with a colostomy, and the improvements in patient selection secondary to innovations in preoperative imaging modalities have led to a renewed interest in local excision of rectal cancers. This topic is discussed in another chapter in the book. The Colorectal surgeon should be well versed in all techniques to remove and resect a rectal cancer either through a radical resection (TME) or via a local excision to give the patient the best options for treatment.

Survival After Rectal Cancer Excision

Overall 5-year survival rates for colorectal cancer have shown improvement over recent decades with the combination of better surgery and adjuvant therapy. Reports from 20 years previous have assured us that a sphincter-sparing surgical approach does not sacrifice survival in selected patients where an adequate margin can be achieved.[90–92] Overall 5-year survival rates after major surgery for rectal cancer are as follows: Stage I, 85–100%; Stage II, 60–80%; and Stage III, 30–50%.[57,66,90,93–99]

Local excision of cancers confined to the rectal wall without lymphatic or distant spread (T1 and T2N0) can achieve cure rates of 80–100%; however, the results published in retrospective trials are extremely unreliable because many studies span decades and have no standard entrance criteria and standard adjuvant therapy policy. In some retrospective studies, local recurrence seemed high, but overall survival was not different than a comparative group of patients who underwent radical resection.[100] Future emphasis on earlier diagnosis, accurate preoperative staging, and appropriate choice of resection procedure, combined with improved adjuvant therapy, should influence favorably overall survival using this conservative technique.

Synchronous Cancers

Synchronous cancers of the large intestine occur with an incidence of approximately 3.5%. Also, synchronous polyps are common with a primary cancer. If one finds two cancers within the colon and rectum, then one must plan an approach to the surgical resection that depends on the location of the two lesions. Certainly, two resections and two primary anastomoses can be performed in large bowel surgery with a complication rate that is similar to that of just one anastomosis.[101] If a patient has a small rectal cancer that is amenable to local excision along with a synchronous cancer of the colon, one can consider a local excision of the rectal lesion followed by primary resection of the colon lesion. It is important, however, to realize that surveillance after local excision of a rectal cancer needs to be more aggressive in monitoring for local recurrence and metachronous cancers or precancers than after resection of single bowel cancer.

Extended Resection for Locally Advanced Colon or Rectal Cancer

Carcinoma of the colon and rectum will sometimes invade adjacent organs or the abdominal wall. Even when such invasion occurs, extended resection of the cancer along with the tissue or organ to which it has adhered can lead to a 5-year survival rate of >50%, provided the surgical margins are tumor free.[102,103] Patients with inflammatory adhesions to contiguous organs have a slightly higher survival rate than patients with malignant infiltration, but the distinction between malignant and inflammatory contiguity often cannot be made until after en bloc resection. The organs that are usually involved with adhesions from colon or rectal cancer include the uterus, small bowel, urinary bladder, and abdominal wall. In general, approximately 5% of patients will present with locally advanced lesions.[103]

Surgical Treatment of Recurrent Colorectal Carcinoma

Recurrent colorectal cancer affects between 12 and 50% of patients with Dukes B or C (T2N0 through T3N1) disease. Although adjuvant treatment has some effect on survival, surgery remains the mainstay in treatment of recurrent disease. Most often, the intent of surgery for recurrent disease is not curative, but to improve survival or to palliate symptoms.

There are three main patterns of recurrence after resection of a primary colorectal cancer. The most common site of recurrence is the liver. However, isolated recurrences can also be seen locoregionally or in the lung. Although 60–70% of patients who die of colorectal cancer have liver metastasis, the liver is an isolated site of recurrence in <20% of patients. Of the latter group, only 5–10% will be candidates for curative hepatic resection.[104]

Locoregional recurrence of rectal cancer has been decreasing over the past two decades. With the use of adjuvant therapy and the wider application of TME, local failure has been reported as low as 3%. However, when a patient develops a local recurrence, it is often not just a suture line recurrence, but a regional recurrence. The workup of these patients requires extensive imaging to identify features of the tumor that would make it unresectable.

Wanebo et al.[105] demonstrated a 25% actuarial 5-year survival after abdominal sacral resection for recurrent colorectal cancer. They concluded that patients presenting after a long disease-free interval could benefit from such a large procedure. Noncurative surgery has only a small role in the treatment of symptomatic pelvic recurrence, particularly with sacral involvement. Newer approaches such as cryoablation of perineal recurrences may replace heroic procedures and may be useful in symptomatic relief of nonresectable pelvic recurrence.

ASCRS guidelines

The American Society of Colon and Rectal Surgeons has published practice parameters for the management of rectal cancer.[106]

References

1. Floyd CE, Stirling CT, Cohn Jr I. Cancer of the colon, rectum and anus: review of 1,687 cases. Ann Surg. 1966;163(6): 829–37.
2. Reilly JC, Rusin LC, Theuerkauf Jr FJ. Colonoscopy: its role in cancer of the colon and rectum. Dis Colon Rectum. 1982;25(6): 532–8.
3. Travieso Jr CR, Knoepp Jr LF, Hanley PH. Multiple adenocarcinomas of the colon and rectum. Dis Colon Rectum. 1972;15(1):1–6.

4. Heald RJ, Bussey HJ. Clinical experiences at St. Mark's Hospital with multiple synchronous cancers of the colon and rectum. Dis Colon Rectum. 1975;18(1):6–10.
5. Langevin JM, Nivatvongs S. The true incidence of synchronous cancer of the large bowel. A prospective study. Am J Surg. 1984;147(3):330–3.
6. Brahme F, Ekelund GR, Norden JG, Wenckert A. Metachronous colorectal polyps: comparison of development of colorectal polyps and carcinomas in persons with and without histories of polyps. Dis Colon Rectum. 1974;17(2):166–71.
7. Dixon AK, Fry IK, Morson BC, et al. Pre-operative computed tomography of carcinoma of the rectum. Br J Radiol. 1981;54(644):655–9.
8. Grabbe E, Lierse W, Winkler R. The perirectal fascia: morphology and use in staging of rectal carcinoma. Radiology. 1983;149(1):241–6.
9. Adalsteinsson B, Glimelius B, Graffman S, et al. Computed tomography in staging of rectal carcinoma. Acta Radiol Diagn (Stockh). 1985;26(1):45–55.
10. Freeny PC, Marks WM, Ryan JA, Bolen JW. Colorectal carcinoma evaluation with CT: preoperative staging and detection of postoperative recurrence. Radiology. 1986;158(2):347–53.
11. Thompson WM, Halvorsen RA, Foster Jr WL, et al. Preoperative and postoperative CT staging of rectosigmoid carcinoma. AJR Am J Roentgenol. 1986;146(4):703–10.
12. Kane R. The accuracy of CT, MRI, and ultrasound in the detection of hepatic metastatic disease from colon cancer. Abstract. Proceedings of the 76th Scientific Assembly and Annual Meeting of the Radiological Society of North America. Chicago, IL; 1990.
13. Beynon J, Foy DM, Roe AM, et al. Endoluminal ultrasound in the assessment of local invasion in rectal cancer. Br J Surg. 1986;73(6):474–7.
14. Hildebrandt U, Feifel G. Preoperative staging of rectal cancer by intrarectal ultrasound. Dis Colon Rectum. 1985;28(1):42–6.
15. Hildebrandt U, Feifel G, Schwarz HP, Scherr O. Endorectal ultrasound: instrumentation and clinical aspects. Int J Colorectal Dis. 1986;1(4):203–7.
16. Rifkin MD, Wechsler RJ. A comparison of computed tomography and endorectal ultrasound in staging rectal cancer. Int J Colorectal Dis. 1986;1(4):219–23.
17. Beynon J, Roe AM, Foy DM, et al. Preoperative staging of local invasion in rectal cancer using endoluminal ultrasound. J R Soc Med. 1987;80(1):23–4.
18. Puli SR, Bechtold ML, Reddy JB, Choudhary A, Antillon MR, Brugge WR. How good is endoscopic ultrasound in differentiating various T stages of rectal cancer? Meta-analysis and systematic review. Ann Surg Oncol. 2009;16:254–65.
19. Puli SR, Reddy JB, Bechtold ML, Choudhary A, Antillon MR, Brugge WR. Accuracy of endoscopic ultrasound to diagnose nodal invasion by rectal cancers: a meta-analysis and systematic review. Ann Surg Oncol. 2009;16:1255–65.
20. Beynon J. An evaluation of the role of rectal endosonography in rectal cancer. Ann R Coll Surg Engl. 1989;71(2):131–9.
21. Hulsmans FJ, Tio TL, Fockens P, et al. Assessment of tumor infiltration depth in rectal cancer with transrectal sonography: caution is necessary. Radiology. 1994;190(3):715–20.
22. Orrom WJ, Wong WD, Rothenberger DA, et al. Endorectal ultrasound in the preoperative staging of rectal tumors. A learning experience. Dis Colon Rectum. 1990;33(8):654–9.
23. Ng A, Recht A, Busse PM. Sphincter preservation therapy for distal rectal cancer: a review. Cancer. 1997;79:671.
24. Gualdi GF, Casciani E, Guadalaxara A, et al. Local staging of rectal cancer with transrectal ultrasound and endorectal magnetic resonance imaging: comparison with histologic findings. Dis Colon Rectum. 2000;43(3):338–45.
25. Brown G, Richards CJ, Bourne MW, et al. Morphologic predictors of lymph node status in rectal cancer with use of high-spatial-resolution MR imaging with histopathologic comparison. Radiology. 2003;227:371–7.
26. Kim NK, Kim MJ, Yun SH, et al. Comparative study of transrectal ultrasonography, pelvic computerized tomography, and magnetic resonance imaging in preoperative staging of rectal cancer. Dis Colon Rectum. 1999;42(6):770–5.
27. Meyenberger C, Huch Boni RA, Bertschinger P, et al. Endoscopic ultrasound and endorectal magnetic resonance imaging: a prospective, comparative study for preoperative staging and follow-up of rectal cancer. Endoscopy. 1995;27(7):469–79.
28. Blomqvist L, Machado M, Rubio C, et al. Rectal tumour staging: MR imaging using pelvic phased-array and endorectal coils vs endoscopic ultrasonography. Eur Radiol. 2000;10(4):653–60.
29. Gastrointestinal Tumor Study Group. Adjuvant therapy of colon cancer: results of a prospectively randomized trial. N Engl J Med. 1984;310(12):737–43.
30. Wallengren NO, Holtas S, Andren-Sandberg A, et al. Rectal carcinoma: double-contrast MR imaging for preoperative staging. Radiology. 2000;215(1):108–14.
31. Urban M, Rosen HR, Holbling N, et al. MR imaging for the preoperative planning of sphincter-saving surgery for tumors of the lower third of the rectum: use of intravenous and endorectal contrast materials. Radiology. 2000;214(2):503–8.
32. Beets-Tan RG, Beets GL, Vliegen RF, et al. Accuracy of magnetic resonance imaging in prediction of tumour-free resection margin in rectal cancer surgery. Lancet. 2001;357(9255):497–504.
33. Guenaga KF, Matos D, Castro AA, Atallah AN, Wille-Jorgensen P. Mechanical bowel preparation for elective colorectal surgery. Cochrane Database Syst. Rev. 2005;25(1):CD001544. Update 2009;(1):CD001544.
34. Jung B, Pahlman L, Nystrom P, Nilsson E. Multicentre randomized clinical trial of mechanical bowel preparation in elective colonic resection. Br J Surg. 2007;94:689–95.
35. Contant CM, Hop WC, van't Sant HP, et al. Mechanical bowel preparation for elective colorectal surgery: a multicentre randomised trial. Lancet. 2007;370:2112–7.
36. Pineda CE, Shelton AA, Hernandez-Boussard T, Morton JM, Welton ML. Mechanical bowel preparation in intestinal surgery: a meta-analysis and review of the literature. J Gastrointest Surg. 2008;12(11):2037–44.
37. Solla JA, Rothenberger DA. Preoperative bowel preparation. A survey of colon and rectal surgeons. Dis Colon Rectum. 1990;33(2):154–9.
38. Morotomi M, Guillem JG, Pocsidio J, et al. Effect of polyethylene glycol-electrolyte lavage solution on intestinal microflora. Appl Environ Microbiol. 1989;55(4):1026–8.
39. Nichols RL, Broido P, Condon RE, et al. Effect of preoperative neomycin–erythromycin intestinal preparation on the incidence of infectious complications following colon surgery. Ann Surg. 1973;178(4):453–62.

40. Muto T, Bussey HJ, Morson BC. The evolution of cancer of the colon and rectum. Cancer. 1975;36(6):2251–70.
41. Morson BC. Factors influencing the prognosis of early cancer of the rectum. Proc R Soc Med. 1966;59(7):607–8.
42. Morson B. President's address. The polyp-cancer sequence in the large bowel. Proc R Soc Med. 1974;67(6):451–7.
43. Tierney RP, Ballantyne GH, Modlin IM. The adenoma to carcinoma sequence. Surg Gynecol Obstet. 1990;171(1):81–94.
44. Dukes CE. Simple tumors of the large intestine and their relationship to cancer. Br J Surg. 1925;13:720.
45. Helwig EB. The evolution of adenomas of the large intestine and their relationship to carcinoma. Surg Gynecol Obstet. 1947;84:36–49.
46. Jass JR. Do all colorectal carcinomas arise in preexisting adenomas? World J Surg. 1989;13(1):45–51.
47. Gabriel WB, Dukes CE, Bussey HJ. Lymphatic spread in cancer of the rectum. Br J Surg. 1935;25:395–413.
48. Corman ML. Principles of surgical technique in the treatment of carcinoma of the large bowel. World J Surg. 1991;15(5):592–6.
49. McArdle CS, Hole D. Impact of variability among surgeons on postoperative morbidity and mortality and ultimate survival. BMJ. 1991;302(6791):1501–5.
50. Hodgson DC, Zhang W, Zaslavsky AM, et al. Relation of hospital volume to colostomy rates and survival for patients with rectal cancer. J Natl Cancer Inst. 2003;95(10):708–16.
51. Meyerhardt JA, Tepper JE, Niedzwiecki D, et al. Impact of hospital procedure volume on surgical operation and long-term outcomes in high-risk curatively resected rectal cancer: findings from the Intergroup 0114 Study. J Clin Oncol. 2004;22(1):166–74.
52. Heald RJ. The 'Holy Plane' of rectal surgery. J R Soc Med. 1988;81(9):503–8.
53. Adam IJ, Mohamdee MO, Martin IG, et al. Role of circumferential margin involvement in the local recurrence of rectal cancer. Lancet. 1994;344(8924):707–11.
54. Havenga K, DeRuiter MC, Enker WE, Welvaart K. Anatomical basis of autonomic nerve-preserving total mesorectal excision for rectal cancer. Br J Surg. 1996;83(3):384–8.
55. Cawthorn SJ, Parums DV, Gibbs NM, et al. Extent of mesorectal spread and involvement of lateral resection margin as prognostic factors after surgery for rectal cancer. Lancet. 1990;335(8697):1055–9.
56. Enker WE, Thaler HT, Cranor ML, Polyak T. Total mesorectal excision in the operative treatment of carcinoma of the rectum. J Am Coll Surg. 1995;181(4):335–46.
57. Krook JE, Moertel CG, Gunderson LL, et al. Effective surgical adjuvant therapy for high-risk rectal carcinoma. N Engl J Med. 1991;324(11):709–15.
58. Heald RJ. Rectal cancer: anterior resection and local recurrence – a personal view. Perspect Colon Rectal Surg. 1988;1(2):1–26.
59. Masui H, Ike H, Yamaguchi S, et al. Male sexual function after autonomic nerve-preserving operation for rectal cancer. Dis Colon Rectum. 1996;39(10):1140–5.
60. Kapiteijn E, Marijnen CA, Nagtegaal ID, et al. Preoperative radiotherapy combined with total mesorectal excision for resectable rectal cancer. N Engl J Med. 2001;345(9):638–46.
61. Nagtegaal ID, van de Velde CJ, van der Worp E, et al. Macroscopic evaluation of rectal cancer resection specimen: clinical significance of the pathologist in quality control. J Clin Oncol. 2002;20(7):1729–34.
62. Grinnell RS. Distal intramural spread of carcinoma of the rectum and rectosigmoid. Surg Gynecol Obstet. 1954;99(4):421–30.
63. Black WA, Waugh JM. The intramural extension of carcinoma of the descending colon, sigmoid, and rectosigmoid: a pathologic study. Surg Gynecol Obstet. 1948;87:457.
64. Quer EA, Dahlin DC, Mayo CW. Retrograde intramural spread of carcinoma of the rectum and rectosigmoid: a microscopic study. Surg Gynecol Obstet. 1953;96(1):24–30.
65. Williams NS, Dixon MF, Johnston D. Reappraisal of the 5 centimetre rule of distal excision for carcinoma of the rectum: a study of distal intramural spread and of patients' survival. Br J Surg. 1983;70(3):150–4.
66. Pollett WG, Nicholls RJ. The relationship between the extent of distal clearance and survival and local recurrence rates after curative anterior resection for carcinoma of the rectum. Ann Surg. 1983;198(2):159–63.
67. Goligher JC, Dukes CE, Bussey HJ. Local recurrences after sphincter saving excisions for carcinoma of the rectum and rectosigmoid. Br J Surg. 1951;39(155):199–211.
68. Dukes CE. The surgical pathology of rectal cancer. Proc R Soc Med. 1943;37:131.
69. Wolmark N, Fisher B, Wieand HS. The prognostic value of the modifications of the Dukes' C class of colorectal cancer. An analysis of the NSABP clinical trials. Ann Surg. 1986;203(2):115–22.
70. Nelson H, Petrelli N, Carlin A, et al. Guidelines 2000 for colon and rectal cancer surgery. J Natl Cancer Inst. 2001;93(8): 583–96.
71. Quirke P, Durdey P, Dixon MF, Williams NS. Local recurrence of rectal adenocarcinoma due to inadequate surgical resection. Histopathological study of lateral tumour spread and surgical excision. Lancet. 1986;2(8514):996–9.
72. Takahashi T, Ueno M, Azekura K, Ohta H. Lateral node dissection and total mesorectal excision for rectal cancer. Dis Colon Rectum. 2000;43(10 Suppl):S59–68. Review.
73. Kusters M, Beets GL, van de Velde CJ, Beets-Tan RG, Marijnen CA, Rutten HJ, et al. A comparison between the treatment of low rectal cancer in Japan and the Netherlands, focusing on the patterns of local recurrence. Ann Surg. 2009;249(2): 229–35.
74. Akasu T, Sugihara K, Moriya Y. Male urinary and sexual functions after mesorectal excision alone or in combination with extended lateral pelvic lymph node dissection for rectal cancer. Ann Surg Oncol. 2009;16(10):2779–86.
75. Miles WE. A method of performing abdomino-perineal excision for carcinoma of the rectum and of the terminal portion of the pelvic colon (1908). CA Cancer J Clin. 1971;21(6):361–4.
76. West NP, Finan PJ, Anderin C, Lindholm J, Holm T, Quirke P. Evidence of the oncologic superiority of cylindrical abdominoperineal excision for low rectal cancer. J Clin Oncol. 2008;26(21):3517–22.
77. Holm T, Ljung A, Häggmark T, Jurell G, Lagergren J. Extended abdominoperineal resection with gluteus maximus flap reconstruction of the pelvic floor for rectal cancer. Br J Surg. 2007;94(2):232–8.
78. Jones OM, Smeulders N, Wiseman O, Miller R. Lateral ligaments of the rectum: an anatomical study. Br J Surg. 1999;86(4):487–9.
79. Braga M, Frasson M, Vignali A, Zuliani W, Capretti G, Di Carlo V. Laparoscopic resection in rectal cancer patients:

outcome and cost-benefit analysis. Dis Colon Rectum. 2007;50(4):464–71.
80. Guillou PJ, Quirke P, Thorpe H, Walker J, Jayne DG, Smith AM, et al. Short-term endpoints of conventional versus laparoscopic-assisted surgery in patients with colorectal cancer (MRC CLASICC trial): multicentre, randomised controlled trial. Lancet. 2005;365(9472):1718–26.
81. Jayne DG, Guillou PJ, Thorpe H, Quirke P, Copeland J, Smith AM, et al. Randomized trial of laparoscopic-assisted resection of colorectal carcinoma: 3-year results of the UK MRC CLASICC Trial Group. J Clin Oncol. 2007;25(21):3061–8.
82. Zhou ZG, Hu M, Li Y, Lei WZ, Yu YY, Cheng Z, et al. Laparoscopic versus open total mesorectal excision with anal sphincter preservation for low rectal cancer. Surg Endosc. 2004;18(8):1211–5.
83. Rothenberger DA, Wong WD. Abdominoperineal resection for adenocarcinoma of the low rectum. World J Surg. 1992;16(3):478–85.
84. Wong CS, Stern H, Cummings BJ. Local excision and postoperative radiation therapy for rectal carcinoma. Int J Radiat Oncol Biol Phys. 1993;25(4):669–75.
85. Rosen L, Veidenheimer MC, Coller JA, Corman ML. Mortality, morbidity, and patterns of recurrence after abdominoperineal resection for cancer of the rectum. Dis Colon Rectum. 1982;25(3):202–8.
86. Pollard CW, Nivatvongs S, Rojanasakul A, Ilstrup DM. Carcinoma of the rectum. Profiles of intraoperative and early postoperative complications. Dis Colon Rectum. 1994;37(9):866–74.
87. Christian CK, Kwaan MR, Betensky RA, et al. Risk factors for perineal wound complications following abdominoperineal resection. Dis Colon Rectum. 2005;48(1):43–8.
88. Williams NS, Johnston D. The quality of life after rectal excision for low rectal cancer. Br J Surg. 1983;70(8):460–2.
89. Steele Jr GD, Herndon JE, Bleday R, et al. Sphincter-sparing treatment for distal rectal adenocarcinoma. Ann Surg Oncol. 1999;6(5):433–41.
90. Papillon J, Berard P. Endocavitary irradiation in the conservative treatment of adenocarcinoma of the low rectum. World J Surg. 1992;16(3):451–7.
91. Slanetz Jr CA, Herter FP, Grinnell RS. Anterior resection versus abdominoperineal resection for cancer of the rectum and rectosigmoid. An analysis of 524 cases. Am J Surg. 1972;123(1):110–7.
92. McDermott F, Hughes E, Pihl E, et al. Long term results of restorative resection and total excision for carcinoma of the middle third of the rectum. Surg Gynecol Obstet. 1982;154(6):833–7.
93. Jones PF, Thomson HJ. Long term results of a consistent policy of sphincter preservation in the treatment of carcinoma of the rectum. Br J Surg. 1982;69(10):564–8.
94. Manson PN, Corman ML, Coller JA, Veidenheimer MC. Anterior resection for adenocarcinoma. Lahey Clinic experience from 1963 through 1969. Am J Surg. 1976;131(4):434–41.
95. Strauss RJ, Friedman M, Platt N, Wise L. Surgical treatment of rectal carcinoma: results of anterior resection vs. abdominoperineal resection at a community hospital. Dis Colon Rectum. 1978;21(4):269–76.
96. Sauer R, Becker H, Hohenberger W, et al. Preoperative versus postoperative chemoradiotherapy for rectal cancer. N Engl J Med. 2004;351(17):1731–40.
97. Heberer G, Denecke H, Pratschke E, Teichmann R. Anterior and low anterior resection. World J Surg. 1982;6(5):517–24.
98. Localio SA, Eng K, Coppa GF. Abdominosacral resection for midrectal cancer. A fifteen-year experience. Ann Surg. 1983;198(3):320–4.
99. Wilson SM, Beahrs OH. The curative treatment of carcinoma of the sigmoid, rectosigmoid, and rectum. Ann Surg. 1976;183(5):556–65.
100. Heald RJ. Synchronous and metachronous carcinoma of the colon and rectum. Ann R Coll Surg Engl. 1990;72(3):172–4.
101. Whelan RL, Wong WD, Goldberg SM, Rothenberger DA. Synchronous bowel anastomoses. Dis Colon Rectum. 1989;32(5):365–8.
102. Curley SA, Carlson GW, Shumate CR, et al. Extended resection for locally advanced colorectal carcinoma. Am J Surg. 1992;163(6):553–9.
103. Gall FP, Tonak J, Altendorf A. Multivisceral resections in colorectal cancer. Dis Colon Rectum. 1987;30(5):337–41.
104. Steele Jr G, Ravikumar TS. Resection of hepatic metastases from colorectal cancer. Biologic perspective. Ann Surg. 1989;210(2):127–38.
105. Wanebo HJ, Gaker DL, Whitehill R, et al. Pelvic recurrence of rectal cancer. Options for curative resection. Ann Surg. 1987;205(5):482–95.
106. Tjandra JJ, Kilkenny JW, Buie WD, et al. Practice parameters for the management of rectal cancer (revised). Dis Colon Rectum. 2005;48:411–23.

45
Rectal Cancer: Locally Advanced and Recurrent

Robert R. Cima

Introduction

Of patients with newly diagnosed colorectal cancer who will undergo surgery with curative intent as part of their treatment, approximately 5–12% will have tumors that have spread beyond the anatomic landmarks of a standard resection and have invaded adjacent organs or structures.[1–3] The goal of surgery in such cases is a wide, en bloc resection of the tumor and any involved adjacent organ or structure. Of patients who undergo resection with curative intent and receive adjuvant therapy, between 7 and 33% develop isolated local or regional recurrences.[4,5] In up to 20% of these recurrences, resection can be curative.[4,6,7]

Although tumor biology must influence the rate and location of recurrence, no tumor-specific characteristics have been clearly associated with local recurrence. The most important factor that influences tumor recurrence is the stage of disease at presentation.[8] Other factors include obstruction or perforation at presentation, adjacent organ involvement, tumor aneuploidy, increased tumor grade, mucin production, or evidence of venous or perineural invasion. Over the last decade, the adequacy of surgical resection and the use of preoperative chemoradiation have been shown to influence the rate of pelvic recurrence.[9–12] Detailed discussion of these aspects of rectal cancer treatment is addressed elsewhere in the textbook. The focus of this chapter is to discuss the evaluation, operative management, and multimodality treatment of patients with locally advanced rectal cancer. Since the preoperative evaluation, operative approach, and often the perioperative oncologic therapy are similar for primary locally advanced and recurrent rectal cancer, they are discussed together. The outcomes for the different approaches are evaluated later in the chapter.

Locally advanced primary rectal cancers include tumors that are T4 N1-2 MX at the time of initial presentation. They are often associated with a higher rate of metastatic disease at the time of diagnosis and have a poorer overall prognosis than earlier stage disease.[8] T4 tumors are found to be fixed by physical examination or to be invading adjacent organs or structures by diagnostic imaging studies. For T4 tumors, standard surgery alone offers a limited chance of significant local tumor control and/or long-term survival. In cases where an extended en bloc resection cannot be performed to achieve complete resection, patient survival is dismal: after no treatment or after palliative surgery, mean survival time is less than 1 year.[13]

Multimodality therapy incorporating radiation, chemotherapy, and surgery should be used to achieve local tumor control and to prevent or control systemic tumor dissemination, thereby improving patient survival for patients with locally advanced primary or recurrent colorectal cancers. To achieve these goals, appropriate surgery is combined with external-beam radiation (EBRT), and, under ideal circumstances, intraoperative radiation therapy (IORT) and adjuvant or neoadjuvant chemotherapy.

Patients with isolated hepatic or pulmonary metastasis from a rectal cancer are known to have reasonable survival after surgical treatment; however, survival with an isolated, untreated, locoregional, rectal cancer recurrence is quite poor.[14,15] Most of these patients develop disabling complications, including severe pain from bony or nervous tissue involvement, urinary obstruction, fecal obstruction or incontinence, or persistent bleeding. Nearly 90% of rectal cancer recurrences after surgery alone occur in the central or posterior pelvis, and 19% occur at the anastomosis.[16] Stage T4 primary tumors are significantly associated with relapse in the anterior pelvic region.[16] External-beam radiation alone or combined with systemic chemotherapy may result in temporary improvement of symptoms, but the 5-year survival rate is less than 5%.[14,15] Surgical palliation without the addition of systemic chemotherapy and radiation therapy adds little to the overall survival. For these patients, length of survival is perhaps less important than quality of life.

A patient who presents with a locally advanced primary or recurrent rectal cancer must be thoroughly evaluated for the presence of extrapelvic disease. If extensive extrapelvic disease is found, the degree and scope of surgical resection should be changed from one of curative intent to palliation.

D.E. Beck et al. (eds.), *The ASCRS Textbook of Colon and Rectal Surgery: Second Edition*,
DOI 10.1007/978-1-4419-1584-9_45,

An exception may be considered in younger patients with no significant comorbidities in whom a single, isolated, resectable hepatic metastasis is found. However, if a patient has multiple sites of spread or significant comorbidities, extensive surgery involving multiple structures is not warranted, as the chance for cure is quite small. Whether a patient is a candidate for surgery is influenced by a number of factors, including the patient's overall physical condition and comorbid diseases and the extent of spread and fixation of the tumor outside of the rectum.

Preoperative Evaluation and Patient Selection

Complete resection of a locally advanced primary or recurrent rectal cancer is a significant undertaking. Complete resection may be technically possible in some patients, but if their overall physical condition does not make them an appropriate candidate, surgical palliation combined with chemoradiation is the more prudent course of action. To be considered for a complete resection, the patient should be in generally good health. Any significant cardiac or respiratory conditions should be thoroughly evaluated and treated. Patients who are in poor health, or who will not be able to tolerate multimodality therapy combined with complete surgical resection, or have an ASA classifications of IV–V are not considered acceptable surgical candidates. Nearly as important as their physical condition is consideration of the patient's motivation and emotional preparedness for undergoing this extensive treatment. They should be thoroughly informed about and accepting of the short-term and long-term risks associated with the surgery, as well as possible subsequent surgeries or interventions required for postoperative complications.

If the patient is deemed an acceptable candidate for surgery, the next step is evaluation for the extent of local spread and the possibility of extrapelvic spread. A detailed history should be obtained. Symptoms that may suggest metastatic disease, such as back or bone pain outside of the pelvis, new respiratory symptoms, or headaches need to be carefully examined. A thorough physical exam, with particular attention placed on the rectal and vaginal exam, needs to be performed, and any fixation of the tumor to rigid pelvic structures needs to be assessed. Complete endoscopic evaluation of the colon needs to be performed, if technically possible, to rule out the presence of a synchronous lesion. Endoluminal ultrasound of the rectum may be combined with this evaluation in cases of recurrent disease to determine if there is a discrete mass adjacent to the intestine that might be amenable to endoscopic biopsy. Imaging should be repeated before surgery is considered and compared to similar previous studies to give some reassurance that there has been no progression or spread of the disease that might change or preclude any surgical intervention. The abdomen and pelvis need to be evaluated with a double-contrast (intravenous and oral) computed tomography (CT) scan to exclude extrapelvic spread and to assess the extent of possible resection. CT scans are generally reliable for identifying the extent of disease and adjacent organ involvement but are less discriminating for predicting local tumor resectability.[17] Any suspicious hepatic lesion should be examined with ultrasound. If the lesion is worrisome for metastatic disease, it should be biopsied. Questionable findings on the chest X-ray film should be further investigated. Any worrisome lesion that is technically accessible should be biopsied percutaneously.

Although the above tests are the standard evaluation for diagnosing recurrence and excluding extrapelvic spread of the tumor, other more tumor-specific tests have been proposed as adjuncts. Magnetic resonance imaging (MRI) might be more accurate than conventional CT scanning for detecting recurrences in the pelvis or elsewhere in the abdomen because of better image resolution. However, similar to CT scans, MR images provide only anatomic details and may not be any better at distinguishing tumor recurrence from scar in a postoperative field, particularly after pelvic irradiation. To overcome this limitation, a metabolic-based imaging modality such at positron emission tomography (PET) has been studied.[18–22] Colorectal cancer is known to rapidly metabolize fluorine-18 fluorodeoxyglucose (FDG), which therefore can be used as a metabolic label to detect tumor deposits, not only in the pelvis, but also throughout the entire body. Numerous nonrandomized studies have shown that FDG-PET imaging for recurrent colorectal cancer has a significantly higher sensitivity and specificity than CT scanning. When CT scanning was compared with FDG-PET imaging in postoperative patients with colorectal locoregional recurrences, the sensitivity of FDG-PET was significantly higher than CT plus colonoscopy (90 vs. 71%, respectively), although the specificities were similar (92 vs. 85%, respectively).[23] FDG-PET imaging has been shown to maintain this high sensitivity and specificity, 84 and 88%, respectively, even in the setting of the previously irradiated and postoperative pelvis.[18] Thus, FDG-PET might be a useful tool in the postoperative patient in whom there is a suspicion of recurrence but equivocal CT findings, and in whom extensive reoperative surgery might be of extremely high risk.

Even the combination of physical examination and radiographic studies may not be able to prove that there is a pelvic recurrence of a rectal cancer, especially if the patient has undergone a previous pelvic operation or pelvic irradiation. We generally accept three ways of differentiating postoperative changes from tumor. The first is to document a change in the lesion, such as increase in size over time; the second is invasion of the adjacent organs; the third is histological evidence obtained from endoscopic, CT-, or ultrasound-guided biopsies of the suspicious tissue. However, occasionally, pelvic disease is suspected from a rising CEA or development of symptoms without any definable anatomic change on exam. In such situations, histologic proof should be vigorously sought.

Exploratory pelvic surgery should be strongly discouraged, as it poses an extreme risk to the patient and makes future evaluation of the pelvis even more difficult.

Determining Tumor Resectability

Locally advanced primary or locoregional recurrences of rectal cancers can extend to involve any of the pelvic organs or rigid bony structures of the pelvis. Resectability is based upon the anatomic location and what other structures are fixed to the lesion. Although there are other schemes for assessing resectability, we use the following one to classify our patients who are being considered for possible resection. The tumor is classified as F0 when it is not fixed to any pelvic organ or structure, FR when the tumor is fixed but resectable, and FNR when the tumor is fixed and not resectable. FR is further subdivided by noting the anatomical extent of the fixation (anterior, posterior, and lateral).[24] The anatomic extent of the tumor determines the scope of the required resection. For example, anterior fixed lesions may require a hysterectomy, vaginectomy, a partial or complete cystectomy, or prostatectomy, whereas lesions that are fixed posteriorly may require a sacrectomy (Figures 45-1–45-3).

Although we have found this classification scheme to be extremely useful, it does not reliably predict resectability before surgery because new findings may be discovered at operation. However, in our experience, some factors are clearly associated with an unresectable tumor (Table 45-1). Any circumferential tumor that extends to the pelvic sidewall is considered unresectable. Evidence of bilateral ureteral obstruction is a very worrisome finding. Unless there is focal infiltration of the bladder trigone causing bilateral ureteral obstruction, this finding usually indicates that a bulky tumor has invaded both lateral pelvic sidewalls. This means that the disease is present at the level of the pelvic inlet, making complete resection impossible. Finally, S1 and S2 nerve root involvement or evidence of invasion of the sacral bone at the level of S1 and S2 indicates an unresectable tumor. A sacrectomy proximal to S2 results in sacroiliac joint instability and although internal fixation is possible, it is not warranted for cases of locally recurrent rectal cancer. Pain from nerve root involvement with tumor occasionally needs to be differentiated from sciatic nerve compression. Nerve compression symptoms may completely resolve after pelvic irradiation and chemotherapy. On the other hand, persistent buttock and perineal pain usually resulting from tumor expansion and in growth is a more ominous symptom.

Multimodality Therapy for Advanced or Locally Recurrent Rectal Cancer

Surgery with curative intent is the mainstay of treatment for advanced or locally recurrent rectal cancer. However, surgery alone results in a high rate of local and distant failure.[13] To improve outcomes, surgery is combined with multimodality therapy, radiation, and chemotherapy. Radiotherapy is used to improve local control and systemic chemotherapy is used to treat possible disseminated disease.

Although EBRT may relieve symptoms and pain resulting from a large primary or recurrent rectal tumor, it alone does not offer a significant chance of cure.[25] However, when it is combined with sensitizing chemotherapy, the probability of achieving a resection with negative margins and the rate of local tumor control increases.[26–33] In the setting of a locally advanced or recurrent rectal cancer, centers have combined multimodality therapy with intraoperative radiotherapy – either as electron-beam radiation therapy, high-dose rate brachytherapy, or traditional perioperative brachytherapy to further improve patient outcomes.[34–41] These forms of locally directed radiation reduce toxicity by limiting normal tissue exposure and deliver a high biologically equivalent dose to the localized area of the tumor.

In general, patients who never received prior pelvic radiation therapy, a full course of external-beam radiation (5,040 cGy) is administered with concurrent 5-fluorouracil chemotherapy. Often, patients with recurrent rectal cancer have previously received a full course of pelvic external-beam radiation. We treat such patients with an additional course of 2,000 cGy of external-beam radiation combined with additional 5-fluorouracil chemotherapy before repeating pelvic surgery. A recent multicenter study has shown that hyperfractionated preoperative chemoradiation can be safely administered in recurrent rectal cancer patients who have previously received pelvic radiation.[42] The overall tumor response rate was 44.1%. Furthermore, there was no increase in postoperative complications as compared to patients who did not receive the hyperfractionated therapy. Therapeutic synergy between external-beam and intraoperative radiation reaches its peak within 8 weeks of completion of external-beam therapy. The disease is restaged both clinically and radiographically 4 weeks after completion of the external beam and chemotherapy course. If there is no evidence of disease progression in the pelvis or extrapelvic metastasis, the patient is scheduled for surgery within the next 4 weeks.

Surgery

Before surgery, the magnitude of the operation and the possible complications are discussed in depth with the patient and family members. In cases of large locally advanced primary rectal cancers, the sphincter mechanism is preserved. In recurrent cancers, there is little role for an attempt at sphincter preservation, as the risk of complications or poor functional outcomes is quite high. Therefore, the patient must be accepting of a permanent colostomy. In addition, the resection of adjacent structures or organs and the functional implications and reconstruction alternatives, such as an ileal

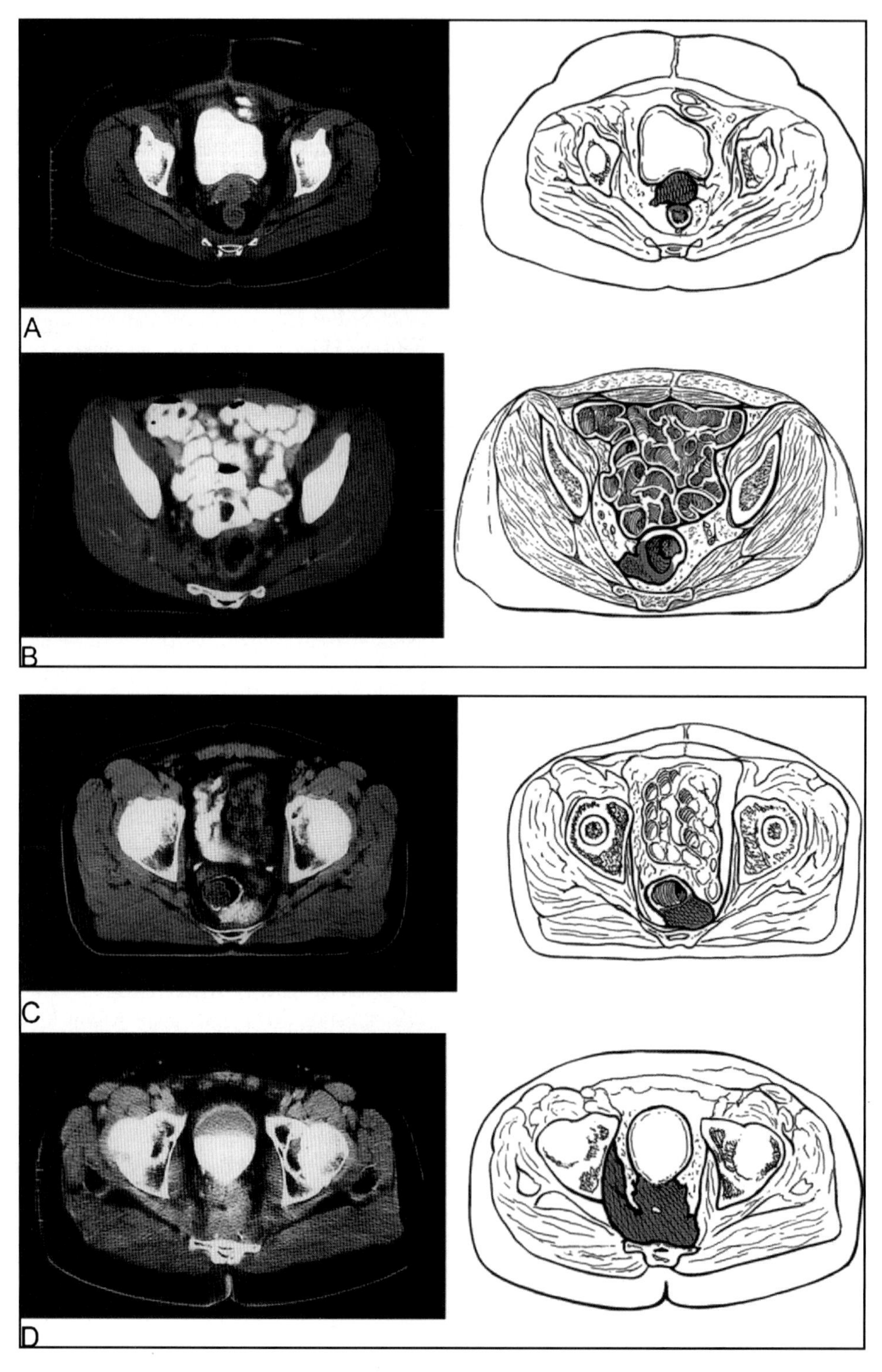

FIGURE 45-1. **A** A primary T3N0M0 rectal cancer treated with a lower anterior resection without adjuvant therapy. The anterior recurrent tumor fixed at the base of the bladder was treated with preoperative chemoradiation and then resected with IORT. **B** After a primary low anterior resection for T2N0M0 rectal cancer without adjuvant therapy, this patient developed a lateral pelvic recurrence. After preoperative chemoradiation, the patient underwent an abdominal resection with negative margins. **C** A recurrence after a T3N0M0 lesion treated with postoperative chemoradiation therapy was found to invade the sacrum. After additional EBRT and chemotherapy, IORT combined with an en bloc resection of the tumor and distal sacrum was performed with negative margins. **D** A massive recurrent cancer found in the pelvis after an abdominal perineal resection and postoperative chemoradiation. The tumor was fixed to vital pelvic structures and was deemed unresectable (with permission from Nicholls RJ, Dozois RR, editors. Surgery of the colon and rectum. New York: Churchill Livingston; 1997).

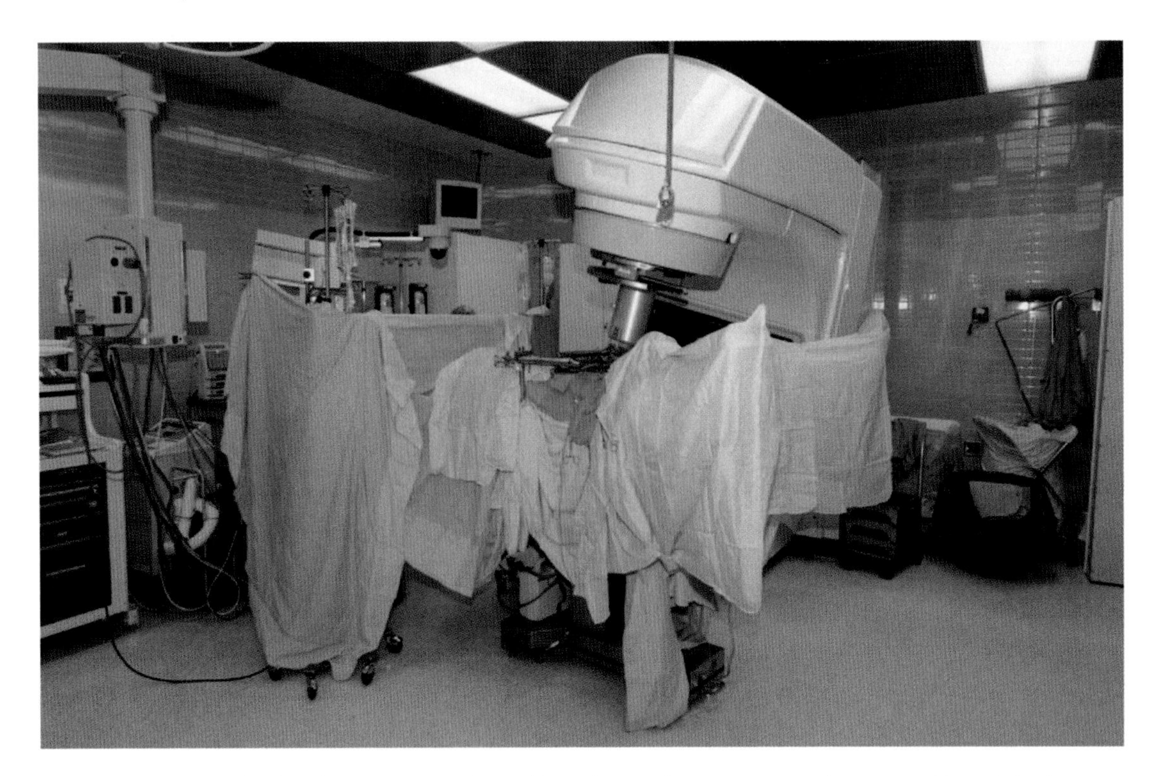

FIGURE 45-2. The IORT suite, showing the equipment, the position of the patient on the operating room table, and the linear accelerator.

conduit, need to be discussed. All patients visit with and are marked for multiple ostomies by an enterostomal therapist.

Depending upon the patient's medical condition, they may need admission at the night prior to surgery, although the majority of patients can be admitted on the day of surgery. While the need for a mechanical bowel preparation in a routine colectomy is under debate, we routinely prepare these patients to minimize the potential for contamination. At our institution, all cases of locally advanced or recurrent rectal cancers are scheduled in a dedicated IORT suite. This suite within the OR complex houses the standard operating room equipment, a linear accelerator, and special anesthetic equipment that permits the anesthetized patient to be moved from operating to irradiating positions (Figure 45-2). In addition, remote controls are used to monitor the patient outside the suite while radiation is given. The patient is placed in the lithotomy position with both arms tucked and the legs supported in Allen stirrups. Special care is taken to ensure that the arms are well padded and in a neutral position to avoid any nerve injury. The calves are positioned and padded to avoid any pressure from directly resting on the stirrups, since the lengthy operation may result in compartment syndrome and/or venous thrombosis.[43] Bilateral ureteral stents are inserted cystoscopically preoperatively in all patients.

A midline incision is usually made. Transverse abdominal incisions should be avoided, as they compromise the placement of any stomas and may injure the inferior epigastric vessels, the primary blood supply of the rectus muscle. Preservation of the rectus muscle is important in case a transpelvic rectus abdominis flap is required to reconstruct the pelvic floor. If the patient has had prior abdominal surgery, all adhesions need to be lysed. If any of the small bowel is adhered into the pelvis or in a region that might be indicative of tumor, a sample should be sent for intraoperative biopsy. If the bowel is involved with tumor, then that portion of the small bowel needs to be resected with the rectal tumor en bloc. Once all adhesions have been lysed, the entire abdomen needs to be thoroughly explored for evidence of extrapelvic tumor deposits. The liver, omentum, retroperitoneum, peritoneal lining, and the area of any prior surgical incision should be carefully examined for metastatic disease. Any suspicious finding should be biopsied and analyzed by frozen section. The presence of extrapelvic disease would be a contraindication to radical resection. Very rarely, exceptions may be made in a young patient who has limited pelvic and liver disease; in such cases, the pelvic recurrence and secondary liver tumor are resected simultaneously.

A self-retaining retractor is placed and the small bowel is packed into the upper abdomen to facilitate pelvic exposure. As pelvic irradiation or prior pelvic surgery would have induced significant fibrosis in the tissues of the pelvis, we begin the dissection at the level of the aortic bifurcation. Starting at this level allows us to enter a virgin fascial plane, which aids in the posterior dissection to the level of the pelvic floor. Similarly, the ureters are identified before they enter the pelvis and are then mobilized along their length along the pelvic sidewall and into the bladder. Identifying the ureters all the way to their insertion into the bladder is important

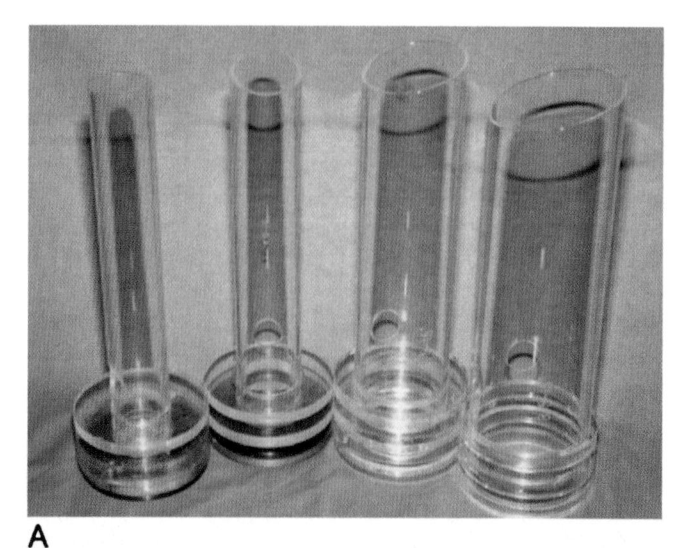

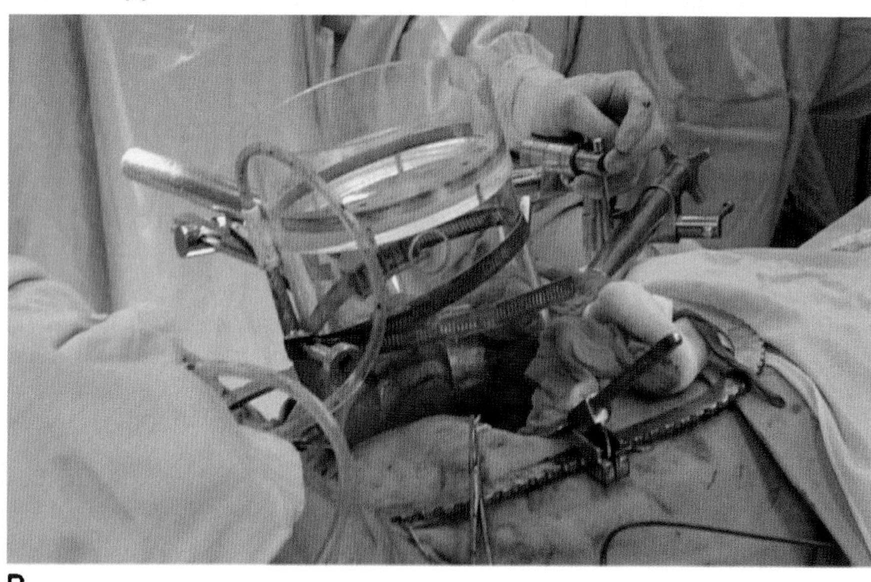

FIGURE 45-3. **A** The assortment of the Lucite tubes used to direct the electron beam to a fixed site in the operating field to deliver the IOT. **B** Place of a large Lucite tube to deliver the IORT into the pelvis. The tube is fixed in place by securing it to an external support apparatus attached to the operating table.

TABLE 45-1. Symptoms or findings suggestive of an unresectable tumor for cure

Sciatic pain
Bilateral ureteral obstruction
Multiple points of tumor fixation to the pelvic sidewall
Circumferential involvement of the pelvic sidewall
S1 or S2 bony or neural involvement
Extrapelvic disease

to ensure adequate length if an ileal conduit is required for urinary tract reconstruction.

For rectal cancer recurrences that are not fixed to any pelvic structure (F0), a completion abdominoperineal resection (APR) is required. The scope of the resection is similar to a standard APR, but the pelvic fibrosis induced by any prior surgery would have distorted or eliminated the ideal, relatively bloodless plane between the mesorectum and sacral fascia. The distinction between fibrosis and tumor infiltration into adjacent tissue can be very difficult to discern at the time of the operation. If there is any question about the nature of the tissue, particularly when it occurs outside the realm of planned resection, for example, at the level of the sacral promontory or at the lateral pelvic walls, a frozen section should be analyzed. If tumor cells are seen, a complete resection with negative margins is not feasible. As discussed later, it is in this setting that the use of IORT improves clinical outcomes.

When the tumor is fixed, either anteriorly or posteriorly, the scope of the operation is much larger than for the nonfixed lesion (F0). If the fixed tumor is considered resectable, we classify it as a FR (fixed, resectable) lesion. For anteriorly fixed tumors, there are different operations that need to be considered, whereas for a primary or recurrent posteriorly fixed tumor, our operation of choice is an en bloc distal sacrectomy.

For the anteriorly fixed lesion, the choice of operation is influenced somewhat by the sex of the patient. In a woman, depending on the level and extent of the tumor, the resection may require only an en bloc excision of the posterior wall of the vagina, with immediate reconstruction. When the upper vagina or lower uterus is involved more extensively, en bloc hysterectomy and posterior vaginectomy would be necessary. A woman who has her uterus in situ usually does not need a cystectomy. However, a man with an anteriorly fixed tumor commonly needs a cystectomy or cystoprostatectomy. A partial cystectomy with a wide margin may be an option for an upper rectal lesion, but the functional results may be poor due to a decrease in bladder size and radiation-induced injury to the bladder. In such patients, an ileal conduit at the time of resection may be preferred to subjecting the patient to a second surgery.

Posteriorly fixed lesions require an en bloc distal sacrectomy. The proximal extent of the resection is to S2-3. A more proximal resection would require internal fixation of the sacroiliac joints to stabilize the pelvis. We consider a resection of this magnitude too extensive for primary or recurrent rectal cancer. Furthermore, when the resection is limited to the S2-3 level, it is generally possible to preserve one S3 root, which is usually sufficient to preserve bladder function. The sacrectomy proceeds through four distinct steps: (1) the anterior resection, (2) the posterior resection, (3) the use of IORT if required, and (4) the reconstruction of the pelvic tissue defect. The abdominal dissection is begun as described previously. The dissection in the posterior plane in carried out to the level of proximal tumor extent along the sacrum. This permits reevaluation to insure that the tumor does not extend above the S2-3 level. If it does, then the rectum is dissected free in the anterior and lateral planes, leaving the point of sacral fixation as the only point of attachment. A sacrectomy that needs to include a resection proximal to S3-4 requires bilateral ligation of the internal iliac arteries and veins. This is done to decrease blood loss during the sacrectomy. Once the rectum is completely freed anteriorly and laterally, all required abdominal wall stomas are created, and an omental or rectus abdominis flap is mobilized and placed into the pelvis, to be used for later reconstruction. Then, the abdominal incision is closed, and the patient is repositioned in the prone-jackknife position. A posterior midline incision is made from the region of the last lumbar vertebrae to the coccyx. The gluteal muscles are dissected free of the sacrum and the proposed site of transection is identified. The important nervous structures to the lower pelvis and extremities, the pudendal and sciatic nerves, respectively, are identified and preserved. With the assistance of our orthopedic or neurosurgical colleagues, the sacrum is transected and the dural sac is closed. The defect is closed either over an omental flap or over the mobilized rectus abdominis flap. As the resulting tissue defect can be quite sizable, local muscle flaps may need to be mobilized to close the defect. Multiple closed suction drains should be used, as any pelvic fluid collection can easily become infected and lead to wound breakdown. The wound complications and breakdown in this heavily irradiated field are not uncommon and occur in as many as 65% of patients who undergo radical resection with concurrent IORT.[44] These postoperative wounds often require transfer of nonirradiated, well-vascularized tissue-like muscle flaps to heal if that transfer was not done at the initial operation.

Postoperatively, these patients are managed quite conservatively as prolonged ileus and urinary retention is quite common. Given the high risk of venous thromboembolism, these patients are given unfractionated heparin three times a day, and use of mechanical compression devices and mandatory early ambulation are enforced.

Use of Intraoperative Radiation Therapy

In cases of close margins, known microscopically positive margins, or minimal gross unresectable disease in the pelvis or after the sacrectomy, our policy is to use intraoperative electron-beam radiation therapy (IORT). To give IORT, a Lucite cylinder is positioned in the pelvis to target the at-risk area. The patient is then positioned under the linear accelerator. One thousand to 2,000 cGy is delivered, depending on the extent of margin involvement. A dose of 1,000 cGy is recommended for minimal residual disease; 1,500 cGy is given for gross residual disease less than 2 cm, and 2,000 cGy is reserved for unresectable or gross residual disease more than 2 cm. The IORT dose that can be given should take into account the total of any prior external-beam radiation that has been administered.

Although we only have experience with electron-beam radiation therapy, other institutions have used other ways of delivering intraoperative or prolonged local radiation therapy. At Memorial Sloan-Kettering, a combined-modality treatment protocol uses high-dose intraoperative brachytherapy (HDR-IORT).[34] The radiation is delivered via an array of catheters that are imbedded in a flexible rubber pad. This pad is then sutured to the area of concern and other normal tissues are packed away and protected. The catheters are connected to a high-dose rate ^{192}Ir source. After the total dose is delivered, the pad is removed and the operation proceeds. Another approach is to use perioperative brachytherapy as a way to combine local delivery of radiation with extended surgery.[35–38] With this method, brachytherapy catheters are loosely secured to a mesh material that is then secured to the region of interest. The operation is completed and the ends of the catheters are brought out through separate skin incisions and secured to the skin. Then, usually between postoperative day 3 and 5, removable radioactive elements are placed into the brachytherapy catheters. Once the desired total dose is delivered, the catheters are removed at the bedside without the need for sedation or anesthesia. These techniques do not require a dedicated OR with a linear accelerator to administer radiation regionally and may therefore expand where this type of surgery can be performed. One possible disadvantage with the use of the postoperative brachytherapy catheters is that it is difficult to protect normal tissue, particularly the small intestine, once the operation is complete. However, these alternative methods for delivering local radiation therapy, when combined with extended surgery and chemotherapy, seem to result in morbidity and survival outcomes that are comparable to our experience with intraoperative electron-beam radiation therapy.

Results of Multimodality Treatment for Advanced Primary or Locally Recurrent Rectal Cancer

Disease recurrence and survival in patients with rectal cancer is highly dependent upon the stage of disease and the mode of treatment. In recent reports, the combination of preoperative external-beam radiation and total mesorectal excision surgery for resectable rectal cancer resulted in a recurrence-free rate of 94% for Stage II and 85% for Stage III tumors.[45] However, more locally advanced rectal cancers often have a higher recurrence rate.[46] Although the cause of death in these patients is commonly due to systemic disease, a mortality rate of 16–44% has been attributed to isolated local failure.[47,48] Also, advanced primary disease and recurrences in the pelvis are associated with significant pain, bleeding, and urinary or neurologic complications that often dominate the clinical picture and affect the patient's quality of life.[14] Traditionally, palliative pelvic radiation has been used, but it often only provides short-term palliation of symptoms or of local disease progression.[14,49] To better address the significant symptoms associated with advanced primary or recurrent rectal cancer and to perhaps improve survival, a number of institutions have used multimodality therapy, including preoperative chemoradiation, extensive surgery, and intraoperative-directed local radiation therapy.

For patients with advanced primary rectal cancer, studies have shown the benefit of combined preoperative chemoradiation followed by radical surgery. In a retrospective review of 60 patients with primary locally advanced rectal cancers, 81% were able to undergo curative resection.[28] Their overall 2-year survival was 91%, and their local regional recurrence rate was 7.5%. In another study, preoperative chemoradiation with extensive surgery improved overall survival and control of pelvic disease compared to preoperative radiation therapy alone.[39] In that study, the use of IORT improved local control in patients with microscopic residual disease or clinically fixed tumors. None of the patients treated with IORT developed local failure in the pelvis. Similar findings of improved local control and survival were reported in a series of patients with primary advanced rectal cancers who were given high-dose-rate intraoperative radiation therapy (HDR-IORT).[40] These 22 patients with primary unresectable rectal cancer underwent multimodality therapy including preoperative chemotherapy, external-beam irradiation, and extensive surgery with intraoperative brachytherapy, which led to actuarial 2-year local control of 81%. Local tumor control was 92% for patients who underwent resection with negative margins vs. 38% for those with microscopic positive margins. The overall 2-year actuarial disease-free survival rates were 77% for patients with negative margins and 38% for patients with positive margins. In summary, a number of reports of patients with locally advanced primary rectal cancer who were treated with intraoperative radiation and surgery have shown an overall improvement in local control compared to historical controls.

Surgery alone has been used to treat recurrent rectal cancers. In Garcia-Aguilar and colleagues reported a series of 87 patients with recurrent rectal cancer.[50] Sixty-four patients underwent surgical exploration, and only 42 were able to undergo resection with curative intent. The estimated 5-year survival rate for patients who had curative-intent surgery was significantly better than that for patients who had only palliative or no surgery (35 vs. 7%). In most series, recurrence and survival rates for patients with recurrent rectal cancer treated with surgery alone are less than those for patients with primary advanced rectal cancer, but are still better than historical data for patients treated with palliative therapies. In general, patients treated with multimodality therapy including preoperative or intraoperative radiation therapy experience 3-year local control rates ranging from 25 to 78%, and long-term survival has been reported to be between 25 and 40%.[30–33,51–58] The most consistent findings from all of these reports is that the most predictive factor associated with a better outcome, decreased local recurrence, cancer-specific and overall survival is an R0 resection. The presence of microscopic positive or grossly positive margins markedly reduces survival.

The institution with the largest reported experience using multimodality therapy including IORT for recurrent rectal cancer is the Mayo Clinic. Between 1981 and 1996, 394 patients were treated, 90 of whom had unresectable local or extrapelvic disease at the time of surgical exploration.[51] Although 304 patients underwent resection of the recurrent tumor, only 138 (45%) underwent a histologically confirmed curative resection. The 166 remaining patients had a palliative operation because of either gross ($n=139$) or microscopic ($n=27$) residual cancer in the pelvis. Nine percent of the patients who had surgery with curative intent underwent extended resections (i.e., sacrectomy, pelvic exenteration, cystectomy with ileal conduit) due to the advanced nature of the tumor. These patients were prospectively monitored to determine long-term survival and the factors influencing survival.

The 1-year, 3-year, and 5-year survival rates for the 304 patients were 84, 43, and 25%. The median survival time was 31 months. The 5-year survival rate was greater after curative surgery (i.e., negative histologic margins) than after palliative surgery (37 vs. 16%, $P<0.001$). The presence of gross residual disease in patients who underwent nonpalliative resections resulted in decreased survival compared to those patients with microscopic residual disease. However, survival for patients who had extended resections was not significantly different than that for patients who had a limited resection (28 vs. 21%, $P=0.11$, respectively). Logistic regression analysis found several independent factors that contributed to the ability to perform a curative resection. On univariate analysis, an initial surgery with end colostomy or painful recurrence was associated with having palliative surgery. On multivariate analysis, increasing number of tumor fixation sites was associated with a palliative resection. These factors also affected overall survival; patients with pain and more than one site of fixation had significantly lower survival rates. The best 5-year survival rates were in patients who had nonfixed tumors (41%) or asymptomatic recurrences (41%). Other institutions that have used a multimodality approach that included some form of intraoperative radiation have reported similar improvements in local recurrence and survival.[55–58]

Patients whose tumors can be resected with negative margins often have better outcomes. Because of this, some investigators have questioned the routine use of the intraoperative, locally directed radiation therapy.[59] Recently, Wiig and colleagues[60] have reported a nonrandomized prospective study evaluating the value of IORT in reoperative surgery for recurrent rectal cancer. The estimated overall 5-year survival was 30%. However, patients who had an R0 resection had a 60% survival compared to 25 and 0% for R1 and R2, respectively. The use of IORT did not improve survival or local recurrence when controlling for R-stage resection. However, other reports indicate that IORT improves local control and survival even in patients with R1 resections when compared to most control series of patients.[52] In addition, many series report that pelvic recurrences after multimodality therapy that included IORT occur outside the intraoperative radiation field. In the most recent study to look specifically at the rate of local recurrence after the use of high-dose-rate brachytherapy, significantly more recurrences occurred outside of the IORT field than within the radiation field.[58] In that series, the time to pelvic recurrence was 16 months in patients who had a pelvic recurrence outside the radiation field, and 31 months in patients who had a pelvic recurrence within the radiation field; however, the difference was not statistically significantly ($P=0.07$). To specifically address the benefit of adding IORT to the combined multimodality treatment of patients with advanced primary or recurrent rectal cancer, a prospective randomized trial would be required. However, this would be a difficult undertaking given the relatively few institutions capable of delivering this complex therapy, the variations in different intraoperative radiation techniques, and the relatively limited number of patients for whom this therapy is appropriate. For now, most studies, although retrospective and often based on single institutions, suggest that combined multimodality therapy that includes IORT provides the best chance for cure for patients with locally advanced or recurrent rectal cancer.

Perioperatively related mortality was very low in patients who undergo this multimodality treatment (0.3%).[51] Unfortunately, the treatment-related morbidity is relatively high. In one series of 304 patients who underwent surgery with curative intent, 96 (32%) required prolonged hospitalizations, 78 (26%) of whom required readmissions and/or additional surgical procedures. The most frequent complications included pelvic abscesses (6.6%), bowel obstructions (5.3%), enteric fistulas (4.3%), and perineal wound complications (4.6%).[51] The complication rate was significantly higher in patients who underwent extended surgical resections and in patients who had recurrences fixed in more than two sites in the pelvis. These findings underscore the need for thorough preoperative patient selection to ensure that the patient is fit enough to tolerate the surgery and the potential complications and that there is no evidence of disease outside of the region of resection.

Palliative Care for Advanced or Recurrent Rectal Cancer

Patients who present with locally advanced or recurrent rectal cancer must first be evaluated with the intent to cure. An equally important consideration is palliation of symptoms if a cure does not seem to be achievable. The local effect within the pelvis of an advanced or recurrent rectal cancer drives the need to address control of symptoms. These symptoms often include rectal bleeding, rectal obstruction, urinary obstruction due to local invasion, and severe pain related to invasion of the pelvic sidewall or direct invasion of pelvic nerves. Over the past decade, the choice of palliative options has expanded, and the choice of option requires careful consideration of the presenting symptoms, possible future symptoms, extent of local and distant spread of the disease, and the overall physical condition of the patient.

Palliative interventions may be broadly classified as noninvasive, minimally invasive, and surgical. The primary noninvasive palliative option is radiotherapy. In patients who have never received pelvic radiation, a full course of external beam irradiation may be a very effective treatment for bleeding, pelvic pain, and near obstruction. The use of external-beam radiotherapy may result in palliation of severe pelvic pain in 50–90% of patients.[61,62] However, virtually all patients will experience progression of the tumor and recurrent symptoms before they die. Lingareddy and colleagues[49] have shown that there is a significant use for palliative reirradiation in treating recurrent rectal cancers. In their study of 52 patients with recurrent rectal cancer, pelvic reirradiation resulted in complete palliation of bleeding, pain, and mass effect in 100, 65, and 24% of cases, respectively. The median initial radiation dose to the pelvis was 50 cGy; the median reirradiation dose was 30 cGy. Most patients had palliation of their symptoms until their deaths. Grade 3 and 4 toxicities were seen in 23 and 10% of patients, respectively. The 2-year overall actuarial survival was 25%.

Minimally invasive approaches to palliation usually involve mechanical means to reduce symptoms related to pelvic tumors. These include ureteral stents to alleviate urinary obstruction and expandable metal colonic wall stents or the use of lasers to relieve rectal obstruction. Self-expanding metal stents (SEMS) are useful for the nonsurgical management of rectal obstructions, bleeding, and malignant fistulas.[63] In a review of the literature, palliation with SEMS was achieved in 90% of patients.[64] In the largest series to report on SEMS for malignant rectal obstructions, stents could be deployed successfully in 36/37 patients with rectal obstructions,[65] and 28 had good long-term results with no need for subsequent intervention.[65]

Endoscopic lasers are an alternative to SEMS. The neodymium yttrium argon garnet (Nd:YAG) laser is the most commonly used. Endoscopic laser treatments remove the tissue from the lumen by coagulative necrosis or immediate tissue vaporization, depending on the amount of energy applied. Palliation of symptoms and marked improvement in quality of life is achieved after repeated laser sessions (usually 2–5) in 80–90% of patients.[66,67] Unfortunately, laser therapy does not appear to be a durable treatment. Effective palliation declines as patients survive longer; successful palliation at 1 year was only 42%.[68]

There is no data on the use of palliative resections in patients with locally advanced or recurrent rectal cancer. However, a report from Memorial Sloan-Kettering has evaluated the role of palliative resection in 80 patients with Stage IV rectal cancer.[69] Twenty-four percent had clinical evidence of obstruction and 94% had either T3 or T4 lesions. None had received prior surgery or radiation therapy. They underwent radical resection of the primary lesion and surgical treatment of solitary hepatic metastasis, if present. There was one death, a 15% postoperative morbidity, and a 20% colostomy rate. The overall local recurrence rate was 6%, the actuarial local control at 2 years was 94%, and the median survival was 25 months. This study shows that in appropriately selected patients with stage IV disease and complicated or advanced rectal cancer, surgical resection of the primary tumors can achieve very reasonable oncologic results and provide good palliation of symptoms related to the tumor.

Summary

For patients with advanced primary or recurrent rectal cancers, the only hope of cure requires a coordinated multidisciplinary approach to treatment. In general, EBRT, chemotherapy, extensive surgery, and the use of directed IORT appears to improve local control and survival. Surgery in these patients carries a higher morbidity rate than surgery for primary rectal cancer but one that is acceptable in appropriately selected patients. Before proceeding with multimodality therapy, patients should be thoroughly evaluated for the presence of disseminated extrapelvic or metastatic disease, which would, in most instances, preclude a curative operation. Experience indicates that isolated anterior or posterior fixation of the tumor does not preclude a curative resection. In these cases, en bloc resection of involved organs or bony structures can result in resection with negative margins. However, tumors fixed to the lateral pelvic sidewall, fixed at multiple points, or fixed circumferentially are often unresectable or incurable. Available data from many institutions indicate that multimodality therapy for advanced primary or recurrent rectal cancer results in better local control and higher survival rates than palliative therapy.

References

1. Curly SA, Carlson GW, Shumate CR, et al. Extended resection for locally advanced colorectal carcinoma. Am J Surg. 1992;163:553–9.
2. Polk Jr HC. Extended resection for selected adenocarcinomas of the large bowel. Ann Surg. 1972;175:892–9.
3. Bonfanti G, Bozzetti F, Doci R, et al. Results of extended surgery for cancer of the rectum and sigmoid. Br J Surg. 1982;69:305–7.
4. McDermott FT, Hughes ES, Pihl E, et al. Local recurrence after potentially curative resection for rectal cancer in a series of 1008 patients. Br J Surg. 1985;72:34–7.
5. Wanebo HJ, Koness RJ, Vezeridas MP. Pelvic resection of recurrent rectal cancer. Ann Surg. 1994;220:586–97.
6. Philipshen SJ, Heilweil M, Quan SHQ, et al. Patterns of pelvic recurrence following definitive resections of rectal cancer. Cancer. 1984;53:1354–62.
7. Rich T, Gunderson LL, Lew R, et al. Patterns of recurrence of rectal cancer after potentially curative surgery. Cancer. 1983;52:1317–29.
8. Gunderson LJ, Sargent DJ, Tepper JE, et al. Impact of T and N substage on survival and disease relapse in adjuvant rectal cancer: a pooled analysis. Int J Radiat Oncol Biol Phys. 2002;54:386–96.
9. Heald RJ, Ryall RD. Recurrence and survival after total mesorectal excision for rectal cancer. Lancet. 1986;1:1479–82.
10. MacFarlane JK, Ryall RD, Heald RJ. Mesorectal excision for rectal cancer. Lancet. 1993;341:457–60.
11. Swedish Rectal Cancer Trial. Improved survival with preoperative radiotherapy in respectable rectal cancer. N Engl J Med. 1997;336:980–7.
12. Camma C, Giunta M, Fiorica F, et al. Preoperative radiotherapy for respectable rectal cancer: a meta-analysis. J Am Med Assoc. 2000;284:1008–15.
13. Kramer T, Share R, Kiel K, et al. Intraoperative radiation therapy of colorectal cancer. In: Abe M, editor. Intraoperative radiation therapy. New York: Pergamon; 1991. p. 308–10.
14. Wong CS, Cummings BJ, Brierley JD, et al. Treatment of locally recurrent rectal carcinoma-results and prognostic factors. Int J Radiat Oncol Biol Phys. 1998;40:427–35.

15. Knol HP, Hanssens PE, Rutten HJ, et al. Effects of radiation therapy alone or in combination with surgery and/or chemotherapy on tumor and symptom control of recurrent rectal cancer. Strahlenther Onkol. 1997;173:43–9.
16. Hruby G, Barton M, Miles S, et al. Site of local recurrence after surgery, with or without chemotherapy, for rectal cancer: implications for radiotherapy field design. Int J Radiat Oncol Biol Phys. 2003;55:138–43.
17. Farouk R, Nelson H, Radice E, et al. Accuracy of computed tomography in determining resectability for locally advanced primary or recurrent colorectal cancers. Am J Surg. 1998;175:283–7.
18. Moore HG, Akhurst T, Larson SM, et al. A case-controlled study of 18-fluorodeoxyglucose positron emission tomography in the detection of pelvic recurrence in previously irradiated rectal cancer patients. J Am Coll Surg. 2003;197:22–8.
19. Ogunbiyi OA, Flanagan FL, Dehdashti F, et al. Detection of recurrent and metastatic colorectal cancer: comparison of positron emission tomography and computed tomography. Ann Surg Oncol. 1997;4:613–20.
20. Miller E, Lerman H, Gutman M, et al. The clinical impact of camera-based positron emission tomography imaging in patients with recurrent colorectal cancer. Invest Radiol. 2004; 39:8–12.
21. Valk PE, Abella-Columna E, Haseman MK, et al. Whole-body PET imaging with [^{18}F] fluorodeoxyglucose in management of recurrent colorectal cancer. Arch Surg. 1999;134:503–11.
22. Arulampalam T, Costa D, Visvikis D, et al. The impact of FDG-PET on the management algorithm for recurrent colorectal cancer. Eur J Nucl Med. 2001;28:1758–65.
23. Whiteford MH, Whiteford HM, Yee LF, et al. Usefulness of FDG-PET scan in the assessment of suspected metastatic or recurrent adenocarcinoma of the colon and rectum. Dis Colon Rectum. 2000;53:759–70.
24. Suzuki K, Dozois RR, Devine RM, et al. Curative reoperations for locally recurrent rectal cancer. Dis Colon Rectum. 1996;39:730–6.
25. Guiney MJ, Smith JG, Worotniuk V, et al. Radiotherapy treatment for isolated loco-regional recurrence of rectosigmoid cancer following definitive surgery: Peter Maccallum Cancer Institute experience, 1981-1990. Int J Radiat Oncol Biol Phys. 1997;38:1019–25.
26. Aleksic M, Hennes N, Ulrich B. Surgical treatment of locally advanced rectal cancer. Options and strategies. Dig Surg. 1998;15:342–6.
27. Rau B, Hohenberger P, Gellermann J, et al. T4 rectal carcinoma. Surgical and multimodal therapy. Chirug. 2002;73:147–1453.
28. Platell C, Cassidy B, Heywood J, et al. Use of adjuvant, preoperative chemo-radiotherapy in patients with locally advanced rectal cancer. ANZ J Surg. 2002;72:639–42.
29. Gohl J, Merkel S, Rodel C, et al. Can neoadjuvant radiochemotherapy improve the results of multivisceral resections in the advanced rectal carcinoma (cT4a). Colorectal Dis. 2003;5: 436–41.
30. Pacelli F, Tortorelli AP, Rosa F, et al. Locally recurrent rectal cancer: prognostic factors and long-term outcomes of multimodal therapy. Ann Surg Oncol. 2010;17(1):152–62.
31. Hansen MH, Balteskard L, Dørum LM, Eriksen MT, et al. Locally recurrent rectal cancer in Norway. Br J Surg. 2009;96:1176–82.
32. Heriot AG, Byrne CM, Lee P, et al. Extended radical resection: the choice for locally recurrent rectal cancer. Dis Colon Rectum. 2008;51:284–91.
33. Ferenschild FTJ, Vermaas M, Verhoef C, et al. Abdominosacral resection for locally advanced and recurrent rectal cancer. Br J Surg. 2009;96:1341–7.
34. Alektiar KM, Zelefsky MJ, Paty PB, et al. High-dose-rate intraoperative brachytherapy for recurrent colorectal cancer. Int J Radiat Oncol Biol Phys. 2000;48:219–26.
35. Keuhne J, Kleisli T, Biernacki P, et al. Use of high-dose-rate brachytherapy in the management of locally recurrent rectal cancer. Dis Colon Rectum. 2003;46:895–9.
36. Martinez-Monge R, Nag S, Martin EW. ^{125}Iodine brachytherapy for colorectal adenocarcinoma recurrent in the pelvis and paraortics. Int J Radiat Oncol Biol Phys. 1998;42:545–50.
37. Goes RN, Beart RW, Simons AJ, et al. Use of brachytherapy in management of locally recurrent rectal cancer. Dis Colon Rectum. 1997;40:1177–9.
38. Martinez-Monge R, Nag S, Martin EW. Three different intraoperative radiation modalities (electron beam, high-dose-rate brachytherapy, and iodine-125 brachytherapy) in the adjuvant treatment of patient with recurrent colorectal adenocarcinoma. Cancer. 1999;86:236–47.
39. Weinstein GD, Rich TA, Shumate CR, et al. Preoperative infusional chemoradiation and surgery with or without an electron beam intraoperative boost for advanced primary rectal cancer. Int J Radiat Oncol Biol Phys. 1995;32:197–204.
40. Harrison LB, Minsky BD, Enker WE, et al. High dose rate intraoperative radiation therapy (HDR-IORT) as part of the management strategy for locally advanced and recurrent rectal cancer. Int J Radiat Oncol Biol Phys. 1998;42:325–30.
41. Willett CG, Shellito PC, Tepper JE, et al. Intraoperative electron beam radiation therapy for recurrent locally advanced rectal or rectosigmoid carcinoma. Cancer. 1991;67:1504–8.
42. Valentini V, Morganti AG, Gambacorta MA, et al. Preoperative hyper-fractionated chemoradiation for locally recurrent rectal cancer in patients previously irradiated to the pelvis: a multicentric phase II study. Int J Radiat Oncol Biol Phys. 2006;64:1129–39.
43. Neagle CE, Schaffer JL, Heppenstall RB. Compartment syndrome complicating prolonged use of the lithotomy position. Surgery. 1991;110:566–9.
44. Kim HK, Jessup JM, Beard CJ, et al. Locally advanced rectal carcinoma: pelvic control and morbidity following preoperative radiation therapy, resection and intraoperative radiation therapy. Int J Radiat Oncol Biol Phys. 1997;38:777–83.
45. Kapiteijin E, Marijnen CAM, Nagtegaal ID, et al. Preoperative radiotherapy combined with total mesorectal excision for resectable rectal cancer. N Engl J Med. 2001;345:638–46.
46. Tepper JE, O'Connell M, Niedzwiecki D, et al. Adjuvant therapy in rectal cancer: analysis of stage, sex, and local control – final report of intergroup 0114. J Clin Oncol. 2002;20:1744–50.
47. Lindel K, Willett CG, Shellito PC, et al. Intraoperative radiation therapy for locally advanced recurrent rectal or rectosigmoid cancer. Radiother Oncol. 2001;58:83–7.
48. Hashiguchi Y, Sekine T, Sakamoto H, et al. Intraoperative irradiation after surgery for locally recurrent rectal cancer. Dis Colon Rectum. 1999;42:886–93.
49. Lingareddy V, Ahmad NR, Mohiuddin M. Palliative reirradiation for recurrent rectal cancer. Int J Radiat Oncol Biol Phys. 1997;38:785–90.

50. Garcia-Aguilar J, Cromwell JW, Marra C, et al. Treatment of locally recurrent rectal cancer. Dis Colon Rectum. 2001;44: 1743–8.
51. Hahnloser D, Nelson H, Gunderson LL, et al. Curative potential of multimodality therapy for locally recurrent rectal cancer. Ann Surg. 2003;237:502–8.
52. Mannaerts G, Rutten HJT, Martijin H, et al. Comparison of intraoperative radiation therapy-containing multimodality treatment with historical treatment modalities for locally recurrent rectal cancer. Dis Colon Rectum. 2001;44:1749–58.
53. Mannaerts G, Martijin H, Crommelin MA, et al. Feasibility and first results of multimodality treatment, combining EBRT, extensive surgery, and IOERT in locally advanced primary rectal cancer. Int J Radiat Oncol Biol Phys. 2000;47:425–33.
54. Haddock MG, Gunderson LL, Nelson H, et al. Intraoperative irradiation for locally recurrent colorectal cancer in previously irradiated patients. Int J Radiat Oncol Biol Phys. 2001;49: 1267–74.
55. Calvo FA, Gomez-Espi M, Diaz-Gonzalez JA, et al. Intraoperative presacral electron boost following preoperative chemoradiation in $T_{3-4}N_x$ rectal cancer: initial local effects and clinical outcomes analysis. Radiother Oncol. 2002;62:201–6.
56. Bussieres E, Gilly FN, Rouanet P, et al. Recurrences of rectal cancers: results of a multimodal approach with intraoperative radiation therapy. Int J Radiat Oncol Biol Phys. 1996;34:49–56.
57. Shoup M, Guillem JG, Alektiar KM, et al. Predictors of survival in recurrent rectal cancer after resection and intraoperative radiotherapy. Dis Colon Rectum. 2002;45:585–92.
58. Nuyttens JJ, Kolkman-Deurloo IK, Vermaas M, et al. High dose-rate intraoperative radiotherapy for close or positive margins in patients with locally advanced or recurrent rectal cancer. Int J Radiat Oncol Biol Phys. 2004;58:106–12.
59. Wiig JN, Poulsen JP, Tveit KM, Olsen DR, Giercksky KE. Intraoperative irradiation (IORT) for primary advanced and recurrent rectal cancer: a need for randomised studies. Eur J Cancer. 2000;36:868–74.
60. Wiig JN, Tveit KM, Poulsen JP, Olsen DR, Giercksky KE. Preoperative irradiation and surgery for recurrent rectal cancer. Will intraoperative radiotherapy (IORT) be of additional benefit? A prospective study. Radiother Oncol. 2002;62:207–13.
61. Allum WH, Mack P, Priestman TJ, et al. Radiotherapy for pain relief in locally recurrent colorectal cancer. Ann R Coll Surg Engl. 1987;69:220–1.
62. Whiteley Jr HW, Stearns Jr MW, Leaming RH, et al. Palliative radiation therapy in patients with cancer of the colon and rectum. Cancer. 1970;25:343–6.
63. Baron TH. Indications and results of endoscopic rectal stenting. J Gastrointest Surg. 2004;8:266–9.
64. Khot UP, Lang AW, Murali K, et al. Systematic review of the efficacy and safety of colorectal stents. Br J Surg. 2002;89: 1096–102.
65. Spinelli P, Mancini A. Use of self-expanding emtal stents for palliation of rectosigmoid cancer. Gastrointest Endosc. 2001;53: 203–6.
66. Kimmey MB. Endoscopic methods (other than stents) for palliation of rectal carcinoma. J Gastrointest Surg. 2004;8:270–3.
67. McGowan I, Barr H, Krasner N. Palliative laser therapy for inoperable rectal cancer-does it work. Cancer. 1989;63:967–9.
68. Cutsem EV, Boonen A, Geboes K, et al. Risk factors which determine the long-term outcome of Neodymium-YAG laser palliation of colorectal carcinoma. Int J Colorectal Dis. 1989;4:9–11.
69. Nash GM, Saltz LB, Kemeny NE, et al. Radical resection of rectal cancer primary tumor provides effective local therapy in patients with stage IV disease. Ann Surg Oncol. 2002;9:954–60.

46 Colorectal Cancer: Adjuvant Therapy

Kelli Bullard Dunn and Judith L. Trudel

Colon Cancer

The stage of disease at presentation is the most important predictor of outcome for colon cancer patients. Stage I (T1-2N0M0) disease carries an excellent prognosis of up to 95% 5-year survival rate after resection, and surgical treatment alone is considered sufficient; adjuvant treatment is not indicated.[1] Patients with stage II disease (T3-4N0M0) also have excellent 5-year survival, averaging 70–80%, but a subset of high-risk patients have poorer prognosis.[1] As such, it has been suggested that some stage II patients may benefit from adjuvant therapy, but the role of treatment in this patient population remains controversial. In contrast, adjuvant treatment repeatedly has been shown to improve survival for stage III (TanyN1-2M0) disease.

Adjuvant Chemotherapy for Stage II and III Colon Cancer

Nodal status is the single most important prognostic factor in colon cancer. Overall 5-year survival after curative surgery for stage III colon cancer ranges from approximately 40–60%.[2] Recurrences are often systemic, hence the need for adjuvant treatment in these high-risk patients. Because the outlook for patients with stage II disease is considerably better, oncologists have been hesitant to offer adjuvant therapy to these patients. Nevertheless, some stage II patients will develop systemic recurrence, and a number of trials have attempted to address whether adjuvant chemotherapy is appropriate in these patients.

The efficacy of 5-fluorouracil (5-FU)/leucovorin (LV)-based adjuvant chemotherapy for stage III disease has long been well established and is now considered to be the standard of care in the USA.[3] Historically, single-agent chemotherapeutic agents such as thiotepa or fluoropyrimidines did not prove helpful as adjuvant treatment for colon cancer. Progressively, several combination trials of chemotherapy and immune modulators helped refine the recommendations made for adjuvant treatment. In 1988, the NSABP (National Surgical Adjuvant Breast and Bowel Project) CO-1 trial documented 8% improvement in overall 5-year survival for both stage II and stage III disease when adjuvant chemotherapy with MOF (semustine, vincristine, and 5-FU) was used.[4] In 1989, the NCCTG (North Central Cancer Treatment Group) compared surgical resection alone to levamisole and to 5-FU plus levamisole. 5-FU plus levamisole significantly decreased recurrence rates and improved overall survival, particularly in Dukes' C (stage III) patients.[5] The 1990 Intergroup Trial INT-0035 study subsequently confirmed the efficacy of 5-FU plus levamisole in Dukes' stage C cancer.[6] As a result of these trials, the National Institutes of Health published a consensus statement in 1990 establishing 5-FU plus levamisole as the standard adjuvant therapy for stage III colon cancer.[7]

While the usefulness of 5-FU/levamisole in stage III disease was being confirmed, leucovorin emerged as a beneficial agent for the treatment of metastatic disease. Its applicability to stage II and stage III disease was confirmed by the IMPACT (International Multicenter Pooled Analyses of Colon Cancer Trials) study in 1995; 3-year disease-free survival increased from 62 to 71% ($p=0.0001$) while overall survival increased from 78 to 83% ($p=0.029$) in the 5-FU/leucovorin group.[8] The NSAPB C-03 randomized trial of stage II and stage III patients comparing MOF to 5-FU/leucovorin had documented a similar advantage of 5-FU/leucovorin, with a 3-year disease-free survival increased from 64 to 73% ($p=0.0004$) and an overall survival increased from 77 to 84% ($p=0.003$) in the 5-FU/leucovorin group compared to MOF.[9]

The relative merits of levamisole and leucovorin as modulators of 5-FU-based adjuvant chemotherapy, and the optimal duration of treatment have been documented in several studies between 1998 and 2000. The NCCTG/NCIC (National Cancer Institute of Canada)[10] study of 915 patients compared 6 months 5-FU/leucovorin; 6 months 5-FU/leucovorin/levamisole; 1 year 5-FU/levamisole; and 1 year 5-FU/leucovorin/

D.E. Beck et al. (eds.), *The ASCRS Textbook of Colon and Rectal Surgery: Second Edition*,
DOI 10.1007/978-1-4419-1584-9_46, © Springer Science+Business Media, LLC 2011

levamisole. Triple therapy for 6 months was as effective as 12 months; and 6-month triple therapy provided superior 5-year overall survival and disease-free survival compared to 5-FU/levamisole. The Intergroup Trial INT-0089 of 3,759 patients compared 1 year 5-FU/levamisole; 5-FU/high-dose leucovorin for 32 weeks; 5-FU/low-dose leucovorin for 6 cycles; and 5-FU/low-dose leucovorin/levamisole for 6 cycles.[11] There were no differences between the four treatment arms with regards to 5-year disease-free and overall survival. The NSABP CO-4 study essentially confirmed these results.[12] The QUASAR Collaborative Group study[13] confirmed the survival advantage provided by leucovorin modulation over levamisole. Based on the results of these studies, the new standard for treatment was changed to 6 months of adjuvant chemotherapy with 5-FU/leucovorin for stage III disease.

While the efficacy and benefits of adjuvant chemotherapy for stage III node-positive disease is unequivocally documented through numerous randomized trials, the role of adjuvant chemotherapy for stage II node-negative disease is still controversial. The data from the early studies which prompted the NIH recommendation for adjuvant treatment in stage III disease did not support a similar recommendation for stage II disease.[5,6] Recent meta-analyses have yielded conflicting results. The IMPACT-B_2 (International Multicenter Pooled Analysis of B_2 colon Cancer Trials) Group published a pooled analysis of five trials conducted from 1982 to 1989 and regrouping 1,016 patients with stage B_2 colon cancer.[14] Relapse rates, all-cause death rates, 5-year event-free survival and overall survival were similar with adjuvant 5-FU/leucovorin compared to controls. Increasing age and poor tumor differentiation were indicators of poor prognosis.[14] A SEER-Medicare cohort analysis of 3,700 patients with resected stage II colon cancer did not reveal any change in 5-year survival in patients having received adjuvant chemotherapy (74% vs. 72%).[15] In contrast, the NSABP concluded that all Dukes' B colon cancers should be offered adjuvant chemotherapy[16] after reviewing data from four very different trials (CO-1, CO-2, CO-3 and CO-4) regrouping 1,565 patients with Dukes' B disease, 2,255 patients with Dukes' C disease, and with widely different treatment and control arms. The authors calculated a 30% relative reduction in mortality for stage II patients having received adjuvant chemotherapy. That meta-analysis has since been widely criticized for its methodological flaws, and the controversy rages on. The likelihood of reaching a resolution on this subject is remote: in order to detect a significant survival benefit among stage II colon cancer patients (who have an estimated 5-year survival of 80%), an adjuvant trial with a no-treatment control arm would require a sample size of 5,000–8,000 patients.[17] At this time, the use of adjuvant chemotherapy for stage II disease remains an unanswered question, mainly because the prognosis for stage II node-negative disease is good overall, and many patients would face unnecessary treatment. For the time being, high-risk patients might be considered for adjuvant treatment on an individual basis or might be entered in a clinical trial.

The observation that the newer chemotherapy agents irinotecan and oxaliplatin are effective in treating stage IV (metastatic) colorectal cancer led to postulation that these agents might further improve survival in stage II and III disease. To assess the efficacy of irinotecan in the adjuvant setting, the PETACC-3 trial randomized over 2,000 patients with stage III colon cancer to 5-FU/LV plus irinotecan or 5-FU alone. In contrast to stage IV disease, no survival advantage was achieved by adding irinotecan to 5-FU (5-year survival was 74% vs. 71%) and toxicity (gastrointestinal and hematologic) was increased.[18] Results for oxaliplatin, on the other hand, are more promising. Recent data from the multicenter international randomized MOSAIC Trial have confirmed that the addition of oxaliplatin to 5-FU/leucovorin (FOLFOX) further decreases the risk of recurrence in stage II and stage III disease by 23%, resulting in a significant improvement in 3-year disease-free survival.[19] This improvement in survival has proven durable in stage III disease and 6-year overall survival recently has been reported to be 73% in the FOLFOX group compared to 69% in the 5-FU group. Toxicity also proved to be acceptable, with fewer than 1.5% of patients experiencing grade 3 peripheral sensory neuropathy.[20] Although initial reports suggested that this benefit would also extend to stage II patients,[21] longer-term follow-up has once again muddied the waters. For stage II patients, the addition of oxaliplatin offered no survival advantage over 5-FU alone. As a result of these recent studies, FOLFOX is now recommended for adjuvant therapy in stage III colon cancer. This regimen may also be useful in select stage II patients, especially those with high-risk features such as T4 tumors, vascular invasion, or poor differentiation, but definitive recommendations must await additional trials.[22]

Targeted Biologic Therapy

Over the past several years, monoclonal antibodies targeting specific tumor proteins have proven useful in treating selected patients with metastatic colorectal cancer. This utility has raised the possibility that these agents may prove efficacious in the adjuvant setting. Antibodies against epidermal growth factor receptor (cetuximab) and vascular endothelial growth factor (bevacizumab) are of greatest interest and several trials are currently accruing patients. The AVANT trial and NSABP C-08 trial both compare standard 5-FU and oxaliplatin-based therapy to standard therapy plus bevacizumab. NSABP C-08 recently has released safety data showing that the addition of bevacizumab is well tolerated.[23] The Eastern Cooperative Oncology Group 5202 is stratifying stage II colon cancer patients based upon loss of heterozygosity and microsatellite instability to test the efficacy of FOLFOX plus bevacizumab. Finally, PETACC-8 and INT No 147 are comparing FOLFOX to FOLFOX plus cetuximab in stage III colon cancer.[22,24] The results of these trials are anxiously awaited.

Radiotherapy

Local recurrence of rectal cancer after surgery with curative intent has always been recognized as a significant clinical problem. Combined chemoradiotherapy has been shown to increase both local control and survival for patients with locally advanced and node-positive rectal cancer (see below).[25] In contrast, although local failure and recurrence after surgery for colon cancer had been described, there long existed an unwritten consensus that treatment failures in colon cancer surgery were primarily systemic rather than local. Thus, no prospective randomized study was devised to provide data on the role of external beam radiotherapy in preventing local recurrence or improving survival after colon surgery. The recognition that selected individuals with colon cancer were at a high risk for local recurrence eventually came from retrospective reviews of patterns of failure after surgery with curative intent. Two large retrospective reviews helped define the risk factors for local recurrence after surgery for colon cancer.[26,27] Loco-regional failure was identified in 19%[26] to 46%[27] of patients overall; at least half of local recurrences were in the original tumor bed. Only 13% of the local recurrences were salvageable surgically.[26] The most important risk factors for local recurrence were (1) pathological staging, with local recurrence rates of 35% in modified Astler–Coller stages B3, C2, or C3 vs. 7% in stages A, B1, and C1[26]; (2) primary tumor localization in a fixed, nonperitonealized segment of the colon, with the highest failure rates in the cecum, descending colon, hepatic or splenic flexures, and sigmoid colon[26,27]; (3) colon carcinoma complicated by perforation or obstruction, with a two- to threefold increase in local recurrence for any given pathological stage.[26]

Identification of individuals at high risk for local recurrence after curative surgery for colon cancer triggered a number of studies on the role of external beam radiotherapy in preventing local recurrence or improving survival after colon surgery. Several disparate single-institutional retrospective studies suggested an improvement in local failure and recurrence rates with adjuvant radiotherapy compared to historical controls.[28–30] Wide variations in radiation techniques and doses, concurrent use and choice of chemotherapy, and patient selection criteria make comparison between studies difficult. Overall, local control rates ranged from 60 to 88%, a significant improvement over controls treated by surgery alone. A single randomized prospective study initiated jointly by the NCCTG and RTOG, comparing chemotherapy alone with F-FU/levamisole vs. combined chemotherapy/radiotherapy closed prematurely because of poor accrual; although no differences were observed in overall survival between treatment arms, the study lacked sufficient statistical power to draw valid conclusions.[31]

At this time, the precise role of adjuvant radiotherapy in the treatment of colon cancer remains undefined. There is no data to support a systematic recommendation for therapy or a well-recognized adjuvant regimen. The potential risks of adjuvant radiotherapy for colon cancer, particularly radiation damage to surrounding organs (e.g., small bowel) are significant. Treatment for individuals deemed at high-risk for local recurrence after curative surgery for colon cancer should be individualized.

Rectal Cancer

Although surgery remains the central treatment of rectal cancer, the overall approach to treatment has changed dramatically over the last three decades. Surgical technique has been refined to become more focused and precise, with specific attention given to a locally more aggressive and meticulous technique. Optimal treatment requires precise local staging as well as evaluation of potential disease spread to distant organs. The modern multimodal therapy approach individualizes rectal cancer care, thus offering the best and most appropriate treatment to every patient. Local and distant staging orients the decision for adjuvant radiotherapy and/or chemoradiotherapy and for available surgical approaches, such as local excision or an abdominal procedure.

Adjuvant/Neoadjuvant Therapy for Stage I Rectal Cancer

Like stage I colon cancer, 5-year survival after curative intent surgery (radical resection) for stage I rectal cancer exceeds 90%.[32] For this reason, adjuvant or neoadjuvant therapy is not recommended for patients who undergo radical resection of T1 or T2N0 tumors.

The morbidity of radical surgery has led some surgeons to consider local (transanal) excision for these early lesions. Advantages of local excision include sphincter preservation in some cases and the avoidance of an abdominal procedure in patients who are medically compromised. Despite these advantages, concern increasingly has arisen as to the oncologic efficacy of local excision. Recurrence after local resection of T1 tumors ranges from 4 to 18%; for T2 tumors recurrence ranges from 27 to 67%.[33–35] For this reason, adjuvant radiation and/or chemoradiation therapy after local (transanal) excision have been suggested as an adjunct to surgery to improve local control and prolong survival. Uncontrolled studies suggest that the addition of adjuvant therapy improves outcome.[34–40] ACOSOG Z6041 currently is accruing patients with T2 rectal cancers in an attempt to determine if preoperative chemoradiation followed by transanal excision will result in disease-free survival equivalent to that seen after radical surgery.[41] For patients in whom medical comorbidities preclude an abdominal procedure, adjuvant or neoadjuvant chemoradiation therapy may be appropriate to improve local control.[42]

Adjuvant/Neoadjuvant Therapy for Stage II and III Rectal Cancer

Combined modality chemotherapy and radiation have long been used as adjuvant therapy for locally advanced (stage II and III) rectal cancer. Several studies demonstrated both improved local control and prolonged survival, and resulted in the 1990 NIH consensus conference recommendation for postoperative chemoradiation therapy in these patients.[7] There is little controversy regarding adjuvant or neoadjuvant therapy for stage III (TanyN1M0) disease. However, advances in surgical technique, such as total mesorectal excision (TME), for locally advanced node-negative cancers (T3-4, N0, M0; stage II) have improved local control with surgery alone, prompting some surgeons to abandon adjuvant therapy in these patients.[43,44] Although the data from these studies are intriguing, other reports have shown that chemoradiation improves local control and survival even in patients who undergo TME.[45] Adjuvant or neoadjuvant therapy is still recommended for all patients with stage III disease and the majority of patients with stage II disease. In well-selected patients with T3 tumors, favorable histology, and negative radial margins, chemoradiation may not be necessary, but larger prospective studies are required before this approach can be recommended.

Radiation Therapy

Initial neoadjuvant radiation has long been considered an important adjunct in the treatment of rectal cancer. A short preoperative course, 20–30 Gy given over 1 week (most commonly used) is biologically equivalent to the traditional postoperative course of 45–55 Gy given over 5–6 weeks. It was long held that neoadjuvant radiation alone only improved local control but did not improve survival. In 1993, the randomized Swedish Rectal Cancer Trial (SRCT) demonstrated that a biologically equivalent short course (25 Gy) of preoperative radiotherapy with surgery within the next week significantly reduced local recurrence from 27 to 12%, and improved 5-year survival rates from 48 to 58% when compared to surgery alone.[46] The main objection to all trials showing improvement in local recurrence and survival rates with radiotherapy, including the SRCT, is that surgical technique was not optimal. The average local recurrence rate in the "surgery alone" arm in all trials discussed in the meta-analyses was 29–30%.[47–49] Although the undisputed major benefits of preoperative radiotherapy remain loco-regional tumor control and decreased local recurrence, several reports have shown that lower local recurrence rates have been achieved in specialized centers using a more meticulous surgical technique.[50–52] Several reports from different countries have confirmed that surgical skill is of utmost importance, thus opening for discussion the real role of radiotherapy when surgical technique is optimized.[53–56]

Those concerns prompted the reexamination of short-course neoadjuvant radiotherapy followed by surgery within 1 week vs. surgery alone in the Dutch trial. All participating surgeons had adopted the technical "gold standard" of total mesorectal excision (TME) before entering patients. In this randomized multicenter study of 1,861 patients with rectal cancer, 2-year local recurrence rates were significantly improved from 8.2 to 2.4% when preoperative radiation was given prior to TME.[52] Five years figures confirm a reduction in local recurrence rates from 11.4% after TME alone vs. 5.6% for preoperative radiotherapy followed by TME but this does not translate into an improvement in 5-year survival rates (van de Velde, personal communication). Thus it seems that neoadjuvant radiotherapy still has a place in the treatment of rectal cancer, even when surgical technique is optimized.[57]

The advisability of adding chemotherapy to preoperative radiation (and therefore to use neoadjuvant combined chemoradiotherapy) is undergoing intense scrutiny. Additional 5-FU-based chemotherapy may theoretically act as a radio-sensitizer at the high cost of increased hematologic and gastrointestinal toxicity. Neoadjuvant chemoradiotherapy is recommended for advanced disease (T4, N0-2), but until recently there was no randomized phase III study comparing neoadjuvant radiotherapy vs. neoadjuvant chemoradiotherapy in resectable rectal cancer (T2-3, N0-2). The EORTC 22921 trial initially reported that the addition of chemotherapy (either pre- or postoperatively) did not substantially improve survival in resectable rectal cancer; however, the survival curves began to diverge several years into the study, suggesting that a subgroup of patients might benefit from chemotherapy.[58] A recent update confirms that chemotherapy in addition to radiation therapy is beneficial for patients who respond well (ypT0-2) vs. those who respond poorly (ypT3-4).[59] Because it is difficult, if not impossible, to predict tumor response to neoadjuvant therapy, most oncologists currently recommend combination chemoradiation therapy.

Adjuvant vs. Neoadjuvant Therapy

Although combination chemotherapy and radiation have been shown to decrease local recurrence and improve survival for patients with stage III rectal cancer and many with stage II rectal cancer, the optimal timing of therapy has been controversial. Preoperative chemoradiation has been advocated based on tumor shrinkage/downstaging, improved resectability, and the possibility of performing a sphincter sparing operation in some patients. In addition, the absence of small bowel adhesions in the pelvis may decrease toxicity.[60–70] However, preoperative radiation therapy may increase operative complications and impairs wound healing.[71–75] Although preoperative endorectal ultrasound and MRI have improved our ability to stage rectal cancer, clinical "overstaging" can be problematic and neoadjuvant therapy may therefore overtreat patients with pT1-2, N0 tumors. Advocates of postoperative radiation therapy cite more accurate pathologic staging and fewer operative/postoperative complications. However, large, bulky tumors may be unresectable or require a more extensive operation (APR, pelvic exenteration) without preoperative therapy. In addition, postoperative pelvic radiation may compromise function of the neorectum.[76]

According to three recently published meta-analyses, there is no doubt that neoadjuvant treatment is superior to adjuvant treatment with regards to reduction in local failure rates and cancer-specific survival.[47–49] The results of two out of three other trials that specifically studied preoperative vs. postoperative radiotherapy support the conclusions from the meta-analyses. The first report was the Uppsala trial in which short-course preoperative radiotherapy in all patients was compared with postoperative prolonged course only in patients with advanced cancers (stage II and III).[77] The other two trials compare neoadjuvant chemoradiotherapy with adjuvant chemoradiotherapy with same schedules and doses. The results from the NSABP R-03 trial, which closed prematurely because of poor accrual, showed that 44% of patients having undergone preoperative chemoradiation were disease-free at 1 year, compared with 34% of patients who had received postoperative chemoradiation. Results from the German CAO/ARO/AIO-94 trial address the issue of toxicity, postoperative complications, and oncologic outcome. This study randomized 823 patients with T3-4 and/or node-positive rectal cancer to either pre- or postoperative chemoradiation (5-FU-based chemotherapy + 5,040 cGy radiation). An initial report showed equivalent toxicity (11–12%), equivalent postoperative complications (12%), and equivalent anastomotic leak rate (3%).[78] A subsequent report noted that preoperative chemoradiation improved local control (local recurrence = 6% in the preoperative chemoradiation group vs. 13% in the postoperative chemoradiation group). Long-term survival was equivalent in both groups (76% vs. 74%). Interestingly, both short and long-term toxicity were significantly lower in the preoperative chemoradiation group.[79] As such, preoperative chemoradiation is now recommended for all patients with clinical stage III disease and most with clinical stage II disease.

Chemotherapeutic Agents

Like colon cancer, adjuvant and neoadjuvant therapy for rectal cancer has long utilized 5-FU-based regimens. Infusional 5-FU and, increasingly, oral 5-FU (capecitabine) have used as radio-sensitizing agents. Because additional agents such as oxaliplatin have shown synergistic efficacy in the metastatic setting, the addition of this agent to neoadjuvant regimens has been suggested. Two recent phase II studies of oxaliplatin in combination with capecitabine and radiation demonstrated good complete pathologic responses (16 and 24%) with acceptable toxicity (grade 3–4 toxicity in only 12 and 20% of patients).[80,81] Prospective randomized phase III trials (PETACC-6 and NSABP R-04) are currently underway to assess the efficacy of this approach.[24]

Radiation Dose and Timing of Surgery After Completion of Treatment

Controversy also exists as to the optimal radiation dose and timing of posttreatment surgery. Current regimens in the USA typically give a total of 45–54 Gy of radiation over 4–6 weeks. Surgery is then performed 6 weeks later. Many European centers, in contrast, favor a short course of radiation consisting of five fractions of 500 cGY (total dose = 25 Gy) without chemotherapy followed by surgery within 1–2 weeks. Advocates of the short course of radiotherapy suggest that the lower dose of pelvic radiation will result in fewer complications while maintaining efficacy in tumor control. Earlier surgery theoretically may prevent tumor progression. Detractors counter that the lower dose may not be as efficacious and that immediate surgery does not allow enough time for maximal tumor shrinkage.[82] The Swedish Rectal Cancer Trial has shown that short-course radiotherapy improves local control and long-term survival compared to surgery alone.[83] Similarly, the Dutch Colorectal Cancer Group has shown that short-course preoperative radiotherapy decreases local recurrence and increases survival compared to total mesorectal excision alone.[45] However, there are no studies to date that compare short-course vs. long-course chemoradiation and the majority of radiation oncologists in the USA continue to offer standard 45–54 Gy treatment.

The European experience with short-course chemotherapy followed by early surgery has also led to questions about optimal timing for surgery following preoperative chemoradiation. It has been suggested that delaying resection may improve the clinical response to chemoradiation and lead to a larger proportion of patients having a pathologic complete response (pCR).[84] For this reason, several centers have begun to study the timing of surgery following neoadjuvant treatment. Stein et al.[85] performed a retrospective review of 40 patients who underwent chemoradiation for low rectal cancer followed by resection from 28 to 97 days later. These authors found no difference in tumor response based upon the timing of resection. Moreover, no difference could be detected in peri-operative morbidity. However, definitive conclusions await larger studies.

Chemotherapy Alone

In contrast to colon cancer, chemotherapy alone as adjuvant treatment in rectal cancer remains questionable. Early 1980s underpowered US radiotherapy trials concluded that chemotherapy improved survival compared to surgery alone. Two large randomized trials comprising more than 4,000 patients have studied the value of chemotherapy vs. surgery alone in colorectal cancer. Rectal cancer patients were included in both studies. Combination 5-FU/levamisole and 5-FU/leucovorin were found to improve survival in colon cancer patients but showed no benefit in rectal cancer patients.[86,87] These results underscore the difference in chemotherapy effectiveness for rectal cancer and colon cancer. The reasons for this are unclear: different tumor profiles or lack of proper surgical technique at the time of these trials may partly explain the results. At this time, adjuvant chemotherapy alone for stage III rectal cancer is not acceptable.

Neoadjuvant Therapy in Unresectable Rectal Cancer

Based on the literature, it is obvious that there is no uniform definition of a nonresectable rectal cancer. For the purpose of this section we will define a nonresectable rectal cancer as a tumor which cannot be resected without a very high risk of local recurrence. These tumors are clinically tethered or fixed, but it is difficult to know whether or not the fixity is due to cancer overgrowth or fibrosis. Such tumors probably involve the rectal fascia, and resection carries a high likelihood of involvement of the circumferential resection margin. Based on available data, patients with such large tumors benefit from long-course preoperative radiotherapy (45–55 Gy over 5–6 weeks) with the aim of downsizing the tumor. Approximately 10–15% of all patients with rectal cancer have an advanced cancer which could be considered nonresectable; half of those patients have no metastases, indicating that there is potential for a curative procedure.[88] Based on tumor characteristics, surgery alone is unlikely to be curative and it is indicated to offer radiotherapy to those patients.

The role of additional chemotherapy has been unclear in this context. There is very little solid evidence from randomized trials using chemoradiotherapy. One older trial from 1969 reports positive results from chemoradiotherapy in locally unresectable rectal cancer.[89] Two other negative trials, published in the late 1980s reported increased toxicity.[90,91] One recent underpowered Swedish trial (2001) showed improved local recurrence rate and overall survival in patients randomized to chemoradiotherapy vs. radiotherapy alone followed by surgery.[92] Several phase II trials have reported a reduction in local recurrence rates and impressive data regarding survival;[93,94] problems with interpretation of case-mix and definition of "nonresectability" make the results of those trials difficult to interpret. One study including 106 patients with unresectable rectal cancer has shown improved local control and survival in patients who receive aggressive multimodality therapy (preoperative chemoradiation, surgery, and intraoperative radiation).[95] Despite the lack of strong evidence, this approach is probably reasonable in selected patients who will tolerate such an aggressive approach. Newer chemotherapeutic agents currently in use or under study for treatment of locally advanced and metastatic colon cancer (especially oxaliplatin) will doubtlessly be evaluated for their usefulness in neoadjuvant and adjuvant treatment of rectal cancer in the near future. Their efficacy and usefulness is unknown at this time.[96]

Neoadjuvant Therapy and Sphincter Preservation

Several series claim that preoperative radiotherapy (and preferably chemoradiotherapy) downsizes tumors to the extent that it is possible to increase the number of patients in whom the sphincters can be preserved.[97–101] There is even a report showing complete response to chemoradiotherapy in some patients with T4 tumors; some of these patients were not operated upon and reportedly remain alive and well.[84]

Caution must be exercised when reading these studies. First, rates of sphincter preservation do not tell the entire story; second, the main criticism of these studies is that modern therapies are compared to historical controls. The dramatic recent changes in surgical technique (TME, staplers) and the modern approach to rectal cancer treatment may partially explain the increased rate of sphincter preservation. We now accept a 5–10 mm distal margin as curative procedure if a stapled anastomosis is done.[102,103] Modern randomized trials must be done to verify the sturdiness of the conclusions. In the French R9001 trial, patients with T2 and T3 tumors received preoperative 39 Gy (13×3 Gy) and were randomized to immediate surgery or surgery 5 weeks after irradiation. Surgeons were asked before any treatment to evaluate the possibility to preserve the sphincters. Delaying surgery for 5 weeks after the end of radiation only slightly increased the rate of sphincter preservation.[104] This small trial indicates that there might be a downstaging and downsizing effect, which in turn might increase the rate of sphincter preservation. Of note, the overall recurrence rate in the trial was 9%, which is considered a high figure; more crucially, the local recurrence rate was 12% among the patients in whom the surgeon had originally planned an APR but changed intraoperatively to a sphincter-preserving procedure because of the downsizing effect of radiotherapy.[104] The German trial (CAO/ARO/AIO) trial had a more positive result. Among 194 patients initially determined to require APR, neoadjuvant therapy allowed sphincter preservation in 39% compared to 19% in the postop adjuvant-treated group.[79] Nevertheless, long-term outcome in the patients who underwent sphincter preservation have not yet been compared to patients who underwent APR.

An important consequence of increased sphincter preservation is poor function. Poor quality of life may be the price to pay for intact sphincters: up to 20% of all patients who undergo a low anterior resection are incontinent of solid stool.[105] This contrasts with reports that patients with a stoma had a better quality of life compared to those with an anterior resection.[86] This must be considered when selecting surgical options for individual patients.

Immunotherapy, Tumor Vaccines, and Gene Therapy

The goal of cancer immunotherapy treatments is to stimulate the body's immune system in order to improve host defense mechanisms against growing tumors. Colorectal cancer immunotherapy strategies have evolved dramatically over the past 30 years. Nonspecific immune stimulation with bacterial cell products (e.g., BCG) and cytokines (e.g., IL-2) has recently been superseded by more specific immune stimulation targeted against colorectal tumor-expressed antigens. While some tumor antigens are present in normal tissues but overexpressed in cancer, other tumor antigens are restricted to cancer tissues. Vaccines stimulate the immune system to recognize and act specifically against these tumor-expressed antigens, through either the humoral or cellular pathway.

Over 25 phase I and phase II studies have explored a variety of vaccines based on whole colorectal tumor cells, virus-modified tumor cells, gene-modified tumor cells, tumor antigen-derived peptides, tumor cell lysates, proteins or carbohydrates, monoclonal antibodies, plasmid or viral vectors encoding tumor antigens, and dendritic cell-based vaccines. Promising results were observed in some animal models and phase I and II studies, prompting ongoing research efforts.

A few phase III studies have also yielded promising results.[106] Three large studies have looked at the effect of immune stimulation with autologous irradiated tumor vaccine plus BCG in colorectal cancer patients. Hoover et al.[107] randomized 98 patients with colon or rectal cancer to surgical resection alone or surgical resection followed by vaccination with autologous irradiated tumor plus BCG. There was no difference in disease-free or overall survival in 80 eligible patients, but subset analysis showed a significant improvement in disease-free survival for colon cancer patients. The Eastern Cooperative Oncology Group (ECOG) randomized stage II and stage III colon cancer patients to either observation or vaccination with autologous irradiated tumor plus BCG. There was no survival difference between groups, but patients with a marked delayed cutaneous hypersensitivity showed a trend toward better disease-free and overall survival, suggesting that survival correlated with the patient's immune response to vaccination.[108] Vermorken et al.[109] randomized 254 patients operated for colon cancer to either observation or vaccination with autologous irradiated tumor plus BCG immediately post-op, followed by a vaccine booster 6 months post-op. The overall risk for recurrence was decreased by 44% in all vaccinated patients, with a 61% reduction in stage II patients. Vaccination significantly increased recurrence-free survival, and there was a trend toward improved overall survival.[109]

Gene therapy is based on the concept of transferring genetic material into target cells, which would allow for correction of genetic defects in tumor suppressor genes, inactivation of oncogenes, or insertion of treatment-sensitizing genes (such as drug-converting enzymes) or "suicide genes" into the colorectal cells. Correction of p53 mutations, inactivation of k-ras gene product p21, delivery of pro-drug-converting enzymes are currently being studied. The long-term potential for clinical usefulness of these techniques remains to be defined.

Molecular Profiling and Chemoresistance

Increasingly, tumor characteristics are found to influence response to chemotherapy and "personalized" treatment based upon molecular profiling shows increasing promise for increasing response to therapy while decreasing toxicity. Microsatellite instability (MSI) and rates of phenotypic expression of DNA synthesis-associated enzymes recently have been found to predict chemoresistance to 5-FU and irinotecan.[110,111] For example, microsatellite instability appears to confer not only better prognosis but may also predict poor response to chemotherapy, suggesting that patients with MSI-high tumors may not benefit from adjuvant therapy.[112] Similarly, polymorphisms in the enzymes that synthesize and metabolize folate may affect both efficacy and toxicity of 5-FU-based therapy.[113,114] Finally, the observation that k-ras status predicts response to EGFR-targeted therapy in metastatic colorectal cancer has implications for adjuvant therapy.[115,116] This is an area of research which is evolving rapidly, and our increasing knowledge on the impact of molecular characteristics will certainly change the recommendations for adjuvant treatment in the future.

References

1. Parkin DM et al. Global cancer statistics, 2002. CA Cancer J Clin. 2005;55(2):74–108.
2. Jemal A et al. Cancer statistics, 2002. CA Cancer J Clin. 2002;52(1):23–47.
3. NCCNetwork. Clinical practice guidelines in oncology. J Natl Compr Canc Netw. 2003;1:40–53.
4. Wolmark N et al. Postoperative adjuvant chemotherapy or BCG for colon cancer: results from NSABP protocol C-01. J Natl Cancer Inst. 1988;80(1):30–6.
5. Laurie JA et al. Surgical adjuvant therapy of large-bowel carcinoma: an evaluation of levamisole and the combination of levamisole and fluorouracil. The North Central Cancer Treatment Group and the Mayo Clinic. J Clin Oncol. 1989;7(10):1447–56.
6. Moertel CG et al. Levamisole and fluorouracil for adjuvant therapy of resected colon carcinoma. N Engl J Med. 1990;322(6):352–8.
7. Conference NC. Adjuvant therapy for patients with colon and rectal cancer. JAMA. 1990;264:1444–50.
8. Efficacy of adjuvant fluorouracil and folinic acid in colon cancer. International Multicentre Pooled Analysis of Colon Cancer Trials (IMPACT) investigators. Lancet. 1995;345(8955):939–44.
9. Wolmark N et al. The benefit of leucovorin-modulated fluorouracil as postoperative adjuvant therapy for primary colon cancer: results from National Surgical Adjuvant Breast and Bowel Project protocol C-03. J Clin Oncol. 1993;11(10):1879–87.

10. O'Connell MJ et al. Prospectively randomized trial of postoperative adjuvant chemotherapy in patients with high-risk colon cancer. J Clin Oncol. 1998;16(1):295–300.
11. Haller DG, Catalano PJ, MacDonald JS, et al. Fluorouracil (FU), leucovorin (LV) and levamisole (LEV) adjuvant therapy for colon cancer: five-year final report of INT-0089. Proc Am Soc Clin Oncol. 1998;17:256.
12. Wolmark N et al. Clinical trial to assess the relative efficacy of fluorouracil and leucovorin, fluorouracil and levamisole, and fluorouracil, leucovorin, and levamisole in patients with Dukes' B and C carcinoma of the colon: results from National Surgical Adjuvant Breast and Bowel Project C-04. J Clin Oncol. 1999;17(11):3553–9.
13. Comparison of fluorouracil with additional levamisole, higher-dose folinic acid, or both, as adjuvant chemotherapy for colorectal cancer: a randomised trial. QUASAR Collaborative Group. Lancet. 2000;355(9215):1588–96.
14. Efficacy of adjuvant fluorouracil and folinic acid in B2 colon cancer. International Multicentre Pooled Analysis of B2 Colon Cancer Trials (IMPACT B2) Investigators. J Clin Oncol. 1999;17(5):1356–63.
15. Schrag D, Gelfand S, Bach P, et al. Adjuvant chemotherapy for stage II colon cancer: insight from a SEER-Medicare cohort. Proc Am Soc Clin Oncol. 2001;20:488.
16. Mamounas E et al. Comparative efficacy of adjuvant chemotherapy in patients with Dukes' B versus Dukes' C colon cancer: results from four National Surgical Adjuvant Breast and Bowel Project adjuvant studies (C-01, C-02, C-03, and C-04). J Clin Oncol. 1999;17(5):1349–55.
17. Buyse M, Piedbois P. Should Dukes' B patients receive adjuvant therapy? A statistical perspective. Semin Oncol. 2001;28(1 Suppl 1):20–4.
18. Van Cutsem E et al. Randomized phase III trial comparing biweekly infusional fluorouracil/leucovorin alone or with irinotecan in the adjuvant treatment of stage III colon cancer: PETACC-3. J Clin Oncol. 2009;27(19):3117–25.
19. Topham C, Boni C, Navarro M, et al. Multicenter international randomized study of oxaliplatin/5FU/LV (FOLFOX) in stage II and III colon cancer (MOSAIC trial): final results. Eur J Cancer. 2003;1 Suppl 5:S324–5. abstract 1085.
20. Andre T et al. Improved overall survival with oxaliplatin, fluorouracil, and leucovorin as adjuvant treatment in stage II or III colon cancer in the MOSAIC trial. J Clin Oncol. 2009;27(19):3109–16.
21. Andre T et al. Oxaliplatin, fluorouracil, and leucovorin as adjuvant treatment for colon cancer. N Engl J Med. 2004;350(23):2343–51.
22. O'Connell MJ. Oxaliplatin or irinotecan as adjuvant therapy for colon cancer: the results are in. J Clin Oncol. 2009;27(19):3082–4.
23. Allegra CJ et al. Initial safety report of NSABP C-08: a randomized phase III study of modified FOLFOX6 with or without bevacizumab for the adjuvant treatment of patients with stage II or III colon cancer. J Clin Oncol. 2009;27(20):3385–90.
24. Carrato A. Adjuvant treatment of colorectal cancer. Gastrointest Cancer Res. 2008;2(4 Suppl):S42–6.
25. Krook JE et al. Effective surgical adjuvant therapy for high-risk rectal carcinoma. N Engl J Med. 1991;324(11):709–15.
26. Willett C et al. Local failure following curative resection of colonic adenocarcinoma. Int J Radiat Oncol Biol Phys. 1984;10(5):645–51.
27. Gunderson LL, Sosin H, Levitt S. Extrapelvic colon – areas of failure in a reoperation series: implications for adjuvant therapy. Int J Radiat Oncol Biol Phys. 1985;11(4):731–41.
28. Willett CG et al. Postoperative radiation therapy for high-risk colon carcinoma. J Clin Oncol. 1993;11(6):1112–7.
29. Schild SE et al. The treatment of locally advanced colon cancer. Int J Radiat Oncol Biol Phys. 1997;37(1):51–8.
30. Amos EH et al. Postoperative radiotherapy for locally advanced colon cancer. Ann Surg Oncol. 1996;3(5):431–6.
31. Martenson J, Willett C, Sargent D, et al. A phase III study of adjuvant radiation therapy (RT), 5-fluorouracil (5-FU), and levamisole (LEV) vs. 5-FU and LEV in selected patients with resected, high-risk colon cancer: initial results of INT 0130. Proc Am Soc Clin Oncol. 1999;18:235. abstract.
32. Gunderson LL et al. Impact of T and N substage on survival and disease relapse in adjuvant rectal cancer: a pooled analysis. Int J Radiat Oncol Biol Phys. 2002;54(2):386–96.
33. Schultz I et al. Longterm results and functional outcome after Ripstein rectopexy. Dis Colon Rectum. 2000;43(1):35–43.
34. Shibata D et al. Immediate reconstruction of the perineal wound with gracilis muscle flaps following abdominoperineal resection and intraoperative radiation therapy for recurrent carcinoma of the rectum. Ann Surg Oncol. 1999;6(1):33–7.
35. Paty P et al. Long-term results of local excision for rectal cancer. Ann Surg. 2002;236:522–9.
36. Russell A et al. Anal sphincter conservation for patients with adenocarcinoma of the distal rectum: long-term results of radiation therapy oncology group protocol 89-02. Int J Radiat Oncol Biol Phys. 2000;46:313–22.
37. Chakravarti A et al. Long-term follow-up of patients with rectal cancer managed by local excision with and without adjuvant irradiation. Ann Surg. 1999;230:49–54.
38. Mendenhall W et al. Local excision and postoperative radiation therapy for rectal adenocarcinoma. Int J Cancer. 2001;96:89–96.
39. Hight D et al. Linear cauterization for the treatment of rectal prolapse in infants and children. Surg Gynecol Obstet. 1982;154:400–2.
40. Gimbel M, Paty P. A current perspective on local excision of rectal cancer. Clin Colorectal Cancer. 2004;4(1):26–35.
41. Ota DM, Nelson H. Local excision of rectal cancer revisited: ACOSOG protocol Z6041. Ann Surg Oncol. 2007;14(2):271.
42. Bullard Dunn K. Adjuvant and neoadjuvant therapy for rectal cancer. Access MedicineUpdate, Schwartz's principles of surgery. 8th ed. doi: http://www.accessmedicine.com/updates-Content.aspx?aid=1000693.
43. Heald R, Husband E, Ryall R. The mesorectum in rectal cancer surgery: the clue to pelvic recurrence? Br J Surg. 1982;69:613–6.
44. Heald R et al. Rectal cancer: the Basingstoke experience of total mesorectal excision, 1978–1997. Arch Surg. 1998;133:894–9.
45. Kapeteijn E et al. Preoperative radiotherapy combined with total mesorectal excision for resectable rectal cancer. N Engl J Med. 2001;345:638–46.
46. Initial report from a Swedish multicentre study examining the role of preoperative irradiation in the treatment of patients with

resectable rectal carcinoma. Swedish Rectal Cancer Trial. Br J Surg. 1993;80(10):1333–6.
47. Camma C et al. Preoperative radiotherapy for resectable rectal cancer: a meta-analysis. JAMA. 2000;284(8):1008–15.
48. Colorectal Cancer Collaborative Group. Adjuvant radiotherapy for rectal cancer: a systematic overview of 8,507 patients from 22 randomised trials. Lancet. 2001;358(9290):1291–304.
49. Glimelius B et al. A systematic overview of radiation therapy effects in rectal cancer. Acta Oncol. 2003;42(5–6):476–92.
50. Moriya Y et al. Significance of lateral node dissection for advanced rectal carcinoma at or below the peritoneal reflection. Dis Colon Rectum. 1989;32(4):307–15.
51. Heald RJ, Karanjia ND. Results of radical surgery for rectal cancer. World J Surg. 1992;16(5):848–57.
52. Enker WE. Potency, cure, and local control in the operative treatment of rectal cancer. Arch Surg. 1992;127(12):1396–401. discussion 1402.
53. Wibe A et al. Prognostic significance of the circumferential resection margin following total mesorectal excision for rectal cancer. Br J Surg. 2002;89(3):327–34.
54. Dahlberg M, Glimelius B, Pahlman L. Changing strategy for rectal cancer is associated with improved outcome. Br J Surg. 1999;86(3):379–84.
55. Martling AL et al. Effect of a surgical training programme on outcome of rectal cancer in the County of Stockholm. Stockholm Colorectal Cancer Study Group, Basingstoke Bowel Cancer Research Project. Lancet. 2000;356(9224):93–6.
56. Swedish Rectal Cancer Register. http://www.SOS.se/mars/kvaflik.htm.
57. Kapiteijn E et al. Preoperative radiotherapy combined with total mesorectal excision for resectable rectal cancer. N Engl J Med. 2001;345(9):638–46.
58. Bosset JF et al. Chemotherapy with preoperative radiotherapy in rectal cancer. N Engl J Med. 2006;355(11):1114–23.
59. Collette L et al. Patients with curative resection of cT3-4 rectal cancer after preoperative radiotherapy or radiochemotherapy: does anybody benefit from adjuvant fluorouracil-based chemotherapy? A trial of the European Organisation for Research and Treatment of Cancer Radiation Oncology Group. J Clin Oncol. 2007;25(28):4379–86.
60. Garcia-Aguilar J et al. A pathologic complete response to preoperative chemoradiation is associated with lower local recurrence and improved survival in rectal cancer patients treated by mesorectal excision. Dis Colon Rectum. 2003;46(3):298–304.
61. Chen E et al. Downstaging of advanced rectal cancer following combined preoperative chemotherapy and high dose radiation. Int J Radiat Oncol Biol Phys. 1994;30:169–75.
62. Minsky B et al. Enhancement of radiation-induced downstaging of rectal cancer by fluorouracil and high-dose leucovorin chemotherapy. J Clin Oncol. 1992;10(1):79–84.
63. Minsky B et al. Sphincter preservation with preoperative radiation therapy and coloanal anastomosis. Int J Radiat Oncol Biol Phys. 1995;31:553–9.
64. Minsky B et al. Preoperative 5-FU, low-dose leucovorin, and radiation therapy for locally advanced and unresectable rectal cancer. Int J Radiat Oncol Biol Phys. 1997;37:289–95.
65. Rouanet P et al. Conservative surgery for low rectal carcinoma after high-dose radiation. Functional and oncologic results. Ann Surg. 1995;221(1):67–73.
66. Janjan N et al. Tumor downstaging and sphincter preservation with preoperative chemoradiation in locally advanced rectal cancer: the M. D. Anderson Cancer Center experience. Int J Radiat Oncol Biol Phys. 1999;44(5):1027–38.
67. Kaminsky-Forrett M et al. Prognostic implications of downstaging following preoperative radiation therapy for operable T3–T4 rectal cancer. Int J Radiat Oncol Biol Phys. 1998;42:935–41.
68. Chan A et al. Preoperative chemotherapy and pelvic radiation for tethered or fixed rectal cancer: a phase II dose escalation study. Int J Radiat Oncol Biol Phys. 2000;48:843–56.
69. Theodoropoulos G et al. T-level downstaging and complete pathologic response after preoperative chemoradiation for advanced rectal cancer result in decreased recurrence and improved disease-free survival. Dis Colon Rectum. 2002;45:895–903.
70. Moore H et al. Rate of pathologic complete response with increased interval between preoperative combined modality therapy and rectal cancer resection. Dis Colon Rectum. 2004;47(3):279–86.
71. Bullard KM et al. Primary perineal wound closure after APR: doomed to fail? Dis Colon Rectum. 2005;48(3):438–443.
72. Nissan A et al. Abdominoperineal resection for rectal cancer at a specialty center. Dis Colon Rectum. 2001;44(1):27–36.
73. Luna-Perez P et al. Morbidity and mortality following abdominoperineal resection for low rectal adenocarcinoma. Rev Invest Clin. 2001;53(5):388–95.
74. Papacontantinou H et al. Salvage APR after failed Nigro protocol: modest success, major morbidity. Dis Colon Rectum. 2003;46(5):A63.
75. Janjan N et al. Locally advanced rectal cancer: surgical complications after infusional chemotherapy and radiation therapy. Radioology. 1998;206(1):131–6.
76. Temple L, Wong W, Minsky B. The impact of radiation on functional outcomes in patients with rectal cancer and sphincter preservation. Semin Rad Oncol. 2003;13(4):469–77.
77. Pahlman L, Glimelius B. Pre- or postoperative radiotherapy in rectal and rectosigmoid carcinoma. Report from a randomized multicenter trial. Ann Surg. 1990;211(2):187–95.
78. Sauer R et al. Adjuvant vs. neoadjuvant radiochemotherapy for locally advanced rectal cancer: the German rectal cancer trial. Colorectal Dis. 2003;5:406–15.
79. Sauer R et al. Preoperative versus postoperative chemoradiation for rectal cancer. N Engl J Med. 2004;351(17):1731–40.
80. Fakih MG et al. Phase II study of weekly intravenous oxaliplatin combined with oral daily capecitabine and radiotherapy with biologic correlates in neoadjuvant treatment of rectal adenocarcinoma. Int J Radiat Oncol Biol Phys. 2008;72(3):650–7.
81. Rodel C et al. Multicenter phase II trial of chemoradiation with oxaliplatin for rectal cancer. J Clin Oncol. 2007;25(1):110–7.
82. Bamberger P, Otchy D. Ileoanal pouch in the active duty population: effect on military career. Dis Colon Rectum. 1997;40(1):60–6.
83. Swedish Rectal Cancer Trial. Improved survival with preoperative radiotherapy for resectable rectal cancer. N Engl J Med. 1997;336:980–7.
84. Habr-Gama A et al. Low rectal cancer: impact of radiation and chemotherapy on surgical treatment. Dis Colon Rectum. 1998;41(9):1087–96.

85. Stein D et al. Longer time interval between completion of neoadjuvant chemoradiation and surgical resection does not improve downstaging of rectal cancer. Dis Colon Rectum. 2003;46(4):448–53.
86. Frigell A et al. Quality of life of patients treated with abdominoperineal resection or anterior resection for rectal carcinoma. Ann Chir Gynaecol. 1990;79(1):26–30.
87. Taal BG, Van Tinteren H, Zoetmulder FA. Adjuvant 5FU plus levamisole in colonic or rectal cancer: improved survival in stage II and III. Br J Cancer. 2001;85(10):1437–43.
88. Pahlman L, Glimelius B, Enblad P. Clinical characteristics and their relation to surgical curability in adenocarcinoma of the rectum and rectosigmoid. A population-based study on 279 consecutive patients. Acta Chir Scand. 1985;151(8): 685–93.
89. Moertel CG et al. Combined 5-fluorouracil and supervoltage radiation therapy of locally unresectable gastrointestinal cancer. Lancet. 1969;2(7626):865–7.
90. Overgaard M, Berthelsen K, Dahlmark M, Gadeberg CG, van der Maase H, Overgaard J, et al. A randomized trial of radiotherapy alone or combined with 5-FU in the treatment of locally advanced colorectal carcinoma. ECCO 5, meeting abstract;1989:0-0626.
91. Wassif SB. The role of pre-operative adjuvant therapy in the management of borderline operability rectal cancer. Clin Radiol. 1982;33(3):353–8.
92. Frykholm GJ, Pahlman L, Glimelius B. Combined chemo- and radiotherapy vs. radiotherapy alone in the treatment of primary, nonresectable adenocarcinoma of the rectum. Int J Radiat Oncol Biol Phys. 2001;50(2):427–34.
93. Janjan NA et al. Prognostic implications of response to preoperative infusional chemoradiation in locally advanced rectal cancer. Radiother Oncol. 1999;51(2):153–60.
94. Bouzourene H et al. Importance of tumor regression assessment in predicting the outcome in patients with locally advanced rectal carcinoma who are treated with preoperative radiotherapy. Cancer. 2002;94(4):1121–30.
95. Mathis KL et al. Unresectable colorectal cancer can be cured with multimodality therapy. Ann Surg. 2008;248(4):592–8.
96. Glynne-Jones R, Sebag-Montefiore D. Chemoradiation schedules – what radiotherapy? Eur J Cancer. 2002;38(2):258–69.
97. Valentini V et al. Preoperative chemoradiation with cisplatin and 5-fluorouracil for extraperitoneal T3 rectal cancer: acute toxicity, tumor response, sphincter preservation. Int J Radiat Oncol Biol Phys. 1999;45(5):1175–84.
98. Grann A et al. Preliminary results of preoperative 5-fluorouracil, low-dose leucovorin, and concurrent radiation therapy for clinically resectable T3 rectal cancer. Dis Colon Rectum. 1997;40(5):515–22.
99. Hyams DM et al. A clinical trial to evaluate the worth of preoperative multimodality therapy in patients with operable carcinoma of the rectum: a progress report of National Surgical Breast and Bowel Project Protocol R-03. Dis Colon Rectum. 1997;40(2):131–9.
100. Rouanet P et al. Restorative and nonrestorative surgery for low rectal cancer after high-dose radiation: long-term oncologic and functional results. Dis Colon Rectum. 2002;45(3): 305–13. discussion 313–5.
101. Mohiuddin M et al. High-dose preoperative radiation and the challenge of sphincter-preservation surgery for cancer of the distal 2 cm of the rectum. Int J Radiat Oncol Biol Phys. 1998;40(3):569–74.
102. Moore HG et al. Adequacy of 1-cm distal margin after restorative rectal cancer resection with sharp mesorectal excision and preoperative combined-modality therapy. Ann Surg Oncol. 2003;10(1):80–5.
103. Karnjia ND, Schache DJ, North WR, Heald RJ. "Close shave" in anterior resection. Br J Surg. 1990;63:673–7.
104. Francois Y et al. Influence of the interval between preoperative radiation therapy and surgery on downstaging and on the rate of sphincter-sparing surgery for rectal cancer: the Lyon R90-01 randomized trial. J Clin Oncol. 1999;17(8):2396.
105. Bujko K, Nowacki MP, Nasierowska-Guttmejer A, et al. Sphincter preservation following preoperative radiotherapy for rectal cancer: report of a randomised trial comparing short-term radiotherapy vs. conventionally fractionated radiochemotherapy. Radiother Oncol. 2004;72:15–24.
106. Hanna Jr MG et al. Adjuvant active specific immunotherapy of stage II and stage III colon cancer with an autologous tumor cell vaccine: first randomized phase III trials show promise. Vaccine. 2001;19(17–19):2576.
107. Hoover Jr HC et al. Adjuvant active specific immunotherapy for human colorectal cancer: 6.5-year median follow-up of a phase III prospectively randomized trial. J Clin Oncol. 1993;11(3):390–9.
108. Harris JE et al. Adjuvant active specific immunotherapy for stage II and III colon cancer with an autologous tumor cell vaccine: Eastern Cooperative Oncology Group Study E5283. J Clin Oncol. 2000;18(1):148–57.
109. Vermorken JB et al. Active specific immunotherapy for stage II and stage III human colon cancer: a randomised trial. Lancet. 1999;353(9150):345–50.
110. Fallik D et al. Microsatellite instability is a predictive factor of the tumor response to irinotecan in patients with advanced colorectal cancer. Cancer Res. 2003;63(18):5738–44.
111. Barratt PL et al. DNA markers predicting benefit from adjuvant fluorouracil in patients with colon cancer: a molecular study. Lancet. 2002;360(9343):1381–91.
112. Des Guetz G et al. Does microsatellite instability predict the efficacy of adjuvant chemotherapy in colorectal cancer? A systematic review with meta-analysis. Eur J Cancer. 2009;45(10):1890–6.
113. Gusella M et al. Predictors of survival and toxicity in patients on adjuvant therapy with 5-fluorouracil for colorectal cancer. Br J Cancer. 2009;100(10):1549–57.
114. Afzal S et al. MTHFR polymorphisms and 5-FU-based adjuvant chemotherapy in colorectal cancer. Ann Oncol. 2009;20(10):1660–6.
115. Khambata-Ford S et al. Expression of epiregulin and amphiregulin and K-ras mutation status predict disease control in metastatic colorectal cancer patients treated with cetuximab. J Clin Oncol. 2007;25(22):3230–7.
116. Freeman DJ et al. Association of K-ras mutational status and clinical outcomes in patients with metastatic colorectal cancer receiving panitumumab alone. Clin Colorectal Cancer. 2008;7(3):184–90.

47
Colorectal Cancer: Metastatic (Palliation)

Elisabeth C. McLemore and Sonia Ramamoorthy

Introduction

Approximately 20% of colorectal cancer patients present with established distant metastases.[1] Metastases are often detectable with noninvasive imaging such as CT scan and MRI that are performed for staging of cancer. A diagnosis of stage IV disease then allows for appropriate operative and oncologic planning. Among these patients there is enormous heterogeneity with respect to sites of disease, extent of disease, symptoms, performance status, and comorbidities. The clinical spectrum at the time of diagnosis ranges from the asymptomatic patient with a single metastatic lesion to the rapidly deteriorating patient with colon obstruction and advanced, multiorgan metastases. While treatment algorithms may exist for some forms of metastatic disease such as a solitary liver lesion, others are still being defined.

Despite considerable progress in the treatment of advanced colorectal cancer, the vast majority of stage IV patients are not curable by current treatment protocols. A recent analysis of data from the SEER population-based database estimates that the 5-year survival rate for stage IV patients diagnosed between 1991 and 2000 was 8%.[2] Despite a low overall cure rate treatment options are available to extend survival and enhance quality of life. Systemic chemotherapy, endoscopic treatments to palliate obstruction, surgical diversion, and surgical resection all have important roles in treatment of stage IV patients. Treatment approaches must be individualized based on the extent and resectability of local and distant disease, the presence or absence of bowel obstruction, performance status, and co-morbidities. For patients with good performance status and minimal symptoms from their primary cancers, standard treatment is systemic chemotherapy, which is well documented to increase survival and quality of life.[3,4] Surgical resection of the primary tumor and if indicated, of the metastatic lesions can provide excellent palliation, and in some cases can provide lasting cure.

First-line therapy with either FOLFOX or FOLFIRI now yields major responses in up to 50% of previously untreated patients, and achieves minor responses or stable disease in an additional 20% of patients.[5] Multiple effective drug combinations are available as well, and second-line chemotherapy has become more effective and more likely to impact survival. Over the past 10 years, the median survival for patients with metastatic disease who are treated with chemotherapy has improved from 12–14 to 21 months.[6] Although cure from chemotherapy alone remains extremely rare, effective chemotherapy combined with aggressive surgery may be increasing the overall cure rate. In this setting, the care of patients with advanced disease has become quite complex. The goal of this chapter is to provide a reference source for surgeons managing patients who present with metastatic stage IV colorectal cancer.

Biology of Metastatic Disease

Metastasis is defined as the spread of malignant cells from a primary tumor to a distant organ. It is estimated that 90% of all cancer deaths are a result of metastasis.[7] The biologic process of metastasis is poorly understood. Numerous clinical and laboratory studies have attempted to define the complex process of metastasis formation. The process relies on properties of the tumors cells, as well as the microenvironment of the primary and secondary sites.[8,9] A series of major events must occur (Figure 47-1).

The first step is tumorigenesis, which occurs after the initial malignant transformation. The tumor proliferates into a small mass of heterogeneous cells that are of varying metastatic or malignant potential. These tumor cells undergo multiple and sequential genetic changes, characterized by the appearance of oncogenes and a decrease in tumor suppressor genes. As the tumor grows beyond 1 mm in diameter and becomes relatively hypoxic, angiogenesis is initiated. The process of tumor angiogenesis is tightly regulated by pro- and anti-angiogenic factors secreted by both the tumor and its environment. As tumors successfully grow, suppressors of angiogenesis are inhibited and pro-angiogenic factors predominate, resulting in neovascularity and further growth of

D.E. Beck et al. (eds.), *The ASCRS Textbook of Colon and Rectal Surgery: Second Edition*,
DOI 10.1007/978-1-4419-1584-9_47,

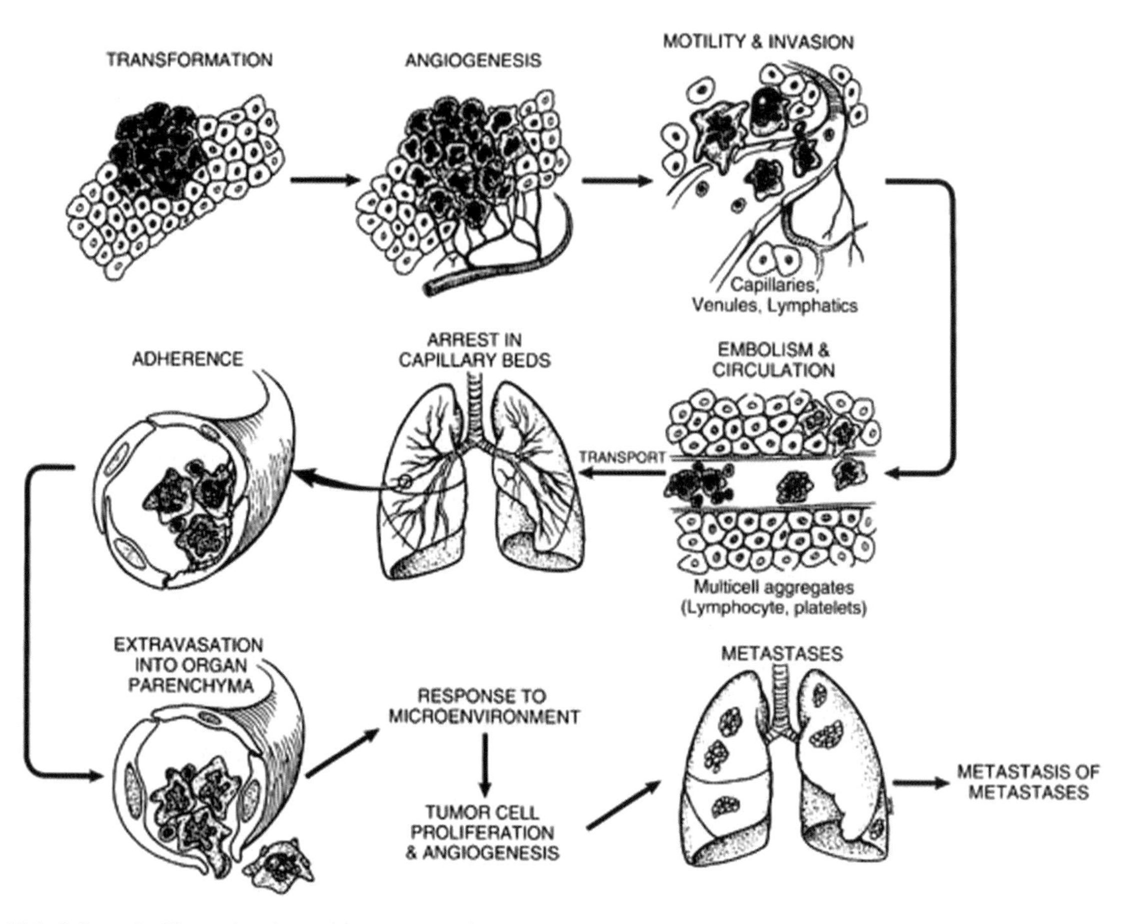

FIGURE 47-1. Schematic illustrating the multistep process involved in the development of metastasis. (With permission from DeVita VT Jr., Hellman S, Rosenberg SA. Cancer: Principles and Practice of Oncology, 6th ed., Lippincott Williams and Wilkins, copyright 2001).

the tumor.[10] Some tumors may grow by utilizing other existing blood vessels in nearby tissues.

In the next step, some cells will develop an invasive phenotype. Most researchers believe that there is a selection process resulting in the clonal expansion of certain cell subpopulations with growth advantages and invasive properties. Whether this process represents a property of the whole tumor cell mass or true clonal selection of more invasive cell sub-populations is not known, and it is a subject of intense research.[11] Malignant invasion is characterized by down-regulation of cell adhesion, resulting in detachment of the cell from the primary tumor mass and the extracellular matrix. Stromal invasion is accomplished through interactions with the basement membrane, including adhesion, proteolysis, and migration, ultimately resulting in detachment and invasion through the basement membrane. This invasive phenotype also enables these cells to enter thin-walled lymphatics and vasculature, allowing access to systemic circulation.[12,13]

Once inside the vascular system, cells or cell clumps (emboli) are circulated, and must survive hemodynamic filtering as well as immune surveillance. They must then arrest in a distant organ. There is likely a complex interaction between the malignant cell and the endothelium or exposed basement membrane, allowing cell arrest. Once arrested in a tissue bed, the cells extravasate into the tissue, enabling formation of a metastatic focus. These metastatic cells can become dormant or proliferate; what determines this fate is not fully understood. Growth in the distant organ after deposition is a major limiting factor in the formation of metastasis. Some metastatic cells can remain dormant while others proliferate, and must again go through tumorigenesis, angiogenesis, and evasion of the immune system. This complex multistep process of metastasis formation is related to multiple genetic changes among malignant cells. Recent studies have shown differences in the genetic fingerprints of matched primary tumors and their lymph node metastasis suggesting that tumors may undergo continual mutagenesis. The metastatic tumor cells may genetically look very different from its parent primary tumor cells.[14] This finding appears to confirm that there are genes specific to tumorigenesis, invasion, angiogenesis and other steps. A number of genes have been identified that suppress metastatic potential and, by their down-regulation, affect a cell's ability to metastasize without affecting tumorigenicity.[14]

These discoveries provide a sense of the future challenge in elucidating the multiple, step-wise and specific changes that regulate a cell's ability to metastasize. Advances in this field will have obvious and profound implications for the treatment of cancer.

Diagnosis/Staging

Initial staging evaluation should include colonoscopy with biopsy, and imaging of the primary tumor, liver, and lungs. When feasible, endorectal ultrasound or MRI is recommended for rectal cancers to document the initial T and N stage. Spiral CT scanning of the chest/abdomen/pelvis is a highly accurate and efficient method of detecting metastases. PET scanning detects occult disease not seen on CT scan in 20% of stage IV patients and should be considered if such findings might affect patient management.[15] Increasingly, more patients are undergoing combination CT/PET scans to evaluate both the primary and metastatic lesions as this combined modality allows for better localization of tumor deposits and can assist with operative planning as well as radiation-based therapy.[16]

Once the extent of disease workup is complete and distant metastases have been documented, the surgeon must make three important judgments. First is whether the patient is fit for aggressive treatment. Patients with poor performance status or serious co-morbidities may not tolerate chemotherapy or major surgery. Second is whether the primary tumor presents a clinically significant risk of bowel obstruction. Symptoms, radiographic findings, and endoscopic findings are important considerations. If the proximal colon is not dilated on radiographic studies and a colonoscope can traverse the tumor, it is generally safe to begin treatment with chemotherapy. The third determination is whether the patient's metastases are surgically resectable, and the patient can be treated with curative intent. If complete resection of all disease can be expected, then surgical intervention should be attempted.

Multidisciplinary Evaluation

Management of patients with advanced disease is complex, and multidisciplinary evaluation can be helpful in determining initial therapy. The multidisciplinary team or "tumor board" ideally involves a surgeon, medical oncologist, radiation oncologist, pathologist, radiologist, and gastroenterologist. As treatment plans become increasingly complex and we enter an era of targeted therapies for specific gene mutations, patients are best served in a center where the goals, priorities, and expected course of treatment, as well as opportunities for enrollment into clinical trials are reviewed and vetted through a multidisciplinary group of experts.

Palliative Management of the Primary Cancer: Laser, Fulguration, and Stents

Incidence and Presentation

Approximately 8–29% of patients with colorectal cancer initially present with symptoms of partial or complete bowel obstruction.[17] In a review of 713 obstructing carcinomas, 77% were left-sided and 23% were right-sided cases.[18] The majority of patients with obstructing colorectal carcinomas have either stage III or stage IV disease.[19] Acute malignant colon or rectal obstruction is an indication for emergent surgical intervention. However, these emergency operations are associated with a mortality rate of 15–34% and a morbidity rate of 32–64% despite advances in perioperative care.[19,20] Therefore, alternative palliative endoluminal strategies aimed at relieving obstruction have gained increasing popularity over the past decades.

The initial symptoms of bowel obstruction include mild discomfort and a change in bowel habits. With disease progression and luminal narrowing, the symptoms may worsen ranging from crampy abdominal pain, abdominal distension, nausea, abdominal tenderness, and obstipation. Vomiting is a late symptom unless there is an associated small bowel obstruction. Leukocytosis is a concerning finding and may indicate a near or complete obstruction. Without treatment, the process can progress to complete obstruction, ischemia, and perforation. The risk of cecal perforation is greatest in patients who have a competent ileocecal valve which does not allow decompression of the large intestine into the proximal small intestine.

In the setting of metastatic cancer, the clinician must first answer the following critical question, "is the colon or rectal obstruction a contraindication for systemic chemotherapy or radiotherapy?" The degree of obstructive symptoms, endoscopic, and radiographic findings are key elements to consider when answering this question. If the patient has minimal symptoms, the cancer can be traversed endoscopically, and there is no radiographic evidence of high grade obstruction, many patients with partially obstructing colon and rectal cancers will tolerate aggressive chemotherapy. In those patients with partially obstructing rectal cancers, the addition of radiation therapy is also well tolerated and can be highly effective. Patients must be instructed to monitor their symptoms closely, and to report any signs of worsening obstruction immediately. A liquid diet or pureed diet with adequate protein and calorie intake taken in small portions may help reduce obstructive symptoms. For patients with advanced obstruction, nonsurgical palliative options include laser therapy, fulguration, and colonic self-expanding metal stents. If less invasive endoluminal strategies are not successful in patients with nonresectable malignant obstruction of the colon and rectum, surgical creation of a palliative proximal diverting stoma or intestinal bypass should be performed.

Laser Therapy and Fulguration

Laser therapy has been utilized for palliation of obstructing rectal cancers.[21–24] In a large series of 272 patients who underwent palliative laser therapy for rectosigmoid cancers, the immediate success rate in treating obstructive symptoms was 85%.[25] Other studies have shown similar success rates, in the range of 80–90%.[23,24] However, laser therapy is practical only for treating cancers of the distal colon and rectum and is rarely used to treat proximal lesions. In addition, multiple sessions are often required in order to achieve lasting relief of symptoms. Serious complications like bleeding, perforation, and severe pain have been reported in 5–15% of patients, especially those undergoing multiple treatment sessions.[22,24–26]

Surgical fulguration of rectal cancers is another method of opening the rectal lumen and relieving obstruction.[27,28] Fulguration, in combination with endoluminal debulking, can remove a large volume of tumor. However, unlike laser therapy, fulguration and debulking requires hospital admission and regional or general anesthesia.

Self-Expanding Metal Stents

Since their introduction in 1991, colonic stents have become an effective method of palliation for obstruction in colorectal cancer patients, especially those with unresectable metastatic disease. These self-expanding metallic stents can potentially dilate the lumen to a near-normal diameter, providing quick relief of symptoms. Stents can be placed in patients using minimal sedation and allow endoscopic assessment of the proximal colon. Moreover, these stents can be placed across relatively long lesions by overlapping stents in a "stent-within-stent" fashion. Laser therapy has also been used in certain situations, in conjunction with colonic stents, to recanalize and decompress large bowel.

A systematic review from 1990 to 2000 of the published data on stenting of colorectal obstruction included 29 case series in the analysis.[29] The review evaluated technical and clinical success, complications, and reobstruction. Cases involving stent placement for palliation and stent placement as a "bridge to surgery" were both assessed. Stent insertion was attempted in 598 cases. Stent deployment was technically feasible in 551 (92%) cases and clinically successful in relieving obstruction in 525 (88%) cases. Palliation of obstruction was achieved in 302 (90%) of 336 cases. Stent placement as a "bridge to surgery" was successful in 223 (88%) of 262 insertions of which 95% had a one-stage surgical procedure. There were three deaths (1%). Perforation occurred in 22 cases (4%). Stent migration was reported in 54 (1%) of the 551 technically successful cases. Stent reobstruction occurred in 52 (10%) of the 525 clinically successful cases and trended toward a higher incidence of reobstruction in the palliative treatment group. The reviewers concluded that "stent usage can avoid the need for a stoma and is associated with low rates of mortality and morbidity."[29] A series of 52 patients with malignant obstruction secondary to either primary or recurrent colon or rectal carcinoma, who underwent stent placement by colorectal surgeons reported that 50 out of 52 were successfully palliated.[30] One patient had a perforation, and in another patient obstruction was not relieved because of multiple sites of obstruction. The overall complication rate in this series was 25%. Stent migration was the most common complication (15%), followed by reobstruction secondary to tumor ingrowth (4%), perforation (2%), colovesical fistula (2%), and severe tenesmus (2%). Surgical intervention was required in 17% of cases due primarily to one of the above complications or recurrent obstruction.

A large series of 102 colorectal stents placed over a 5-year period predominantly for palliative intent reported success in 87 patients (85%).[31] The procedure was performed as a palliative procedure in 90 of these patients. Stent placement location was primarily in the rectum, rectosigmoid, and sigmoid colon ($n=75$). The location of the remaining stents were descending colon ($n=15$), splenic flexure ($n=3$), and transverse colon ($n=3$). Perforation occurred in four patients. Late complications occurred in 9%, and included five stent migrations, two blocked stents, and one colovesical fistula. Ninety percent ($n=76$) of the successful cases needed no further radiological or surgical intervention.[31]

There is limited data evaluating stent placement proximal to the splenic flexure. In a recent publication, colonic stenting was attempted in 97 patients with malignant large-bowel obstruction.[32] Sixteen (17%) patients had lesions proximal to the splenic flexure (eight ascending, eight transverse colon). Stenting was successful in relieving obstruction in 14 (88%) of these patients. Stenting was performed for definitive palliation in nine of these patients, and as a bridge to elective surgery in the other seven patients. One patient developed gastrointestinal bleeding that was managed conservatively. No perforations or stent migrations were reported.[32]

Complications reported in the literature for colonic and rectal stents include stent malpositioning, stent migration, tumor ingrowth (through the stent interstices), tumor overgrowth (beyond the ends of a stent), perforation, stool impaction, bleeding, tenesmus, and postprocedure pain. Stenting of cancers in the mid to low rectum may result in urgency, pain, and incontinence. While the complications associated with stents and other less invasive endoluminal strategies should not be taken lightly, one must keep in mind that emergency operations for malignant colon and rectal obstruction have a mortality rate of 15–34% and a morbidity rate of 32–64%. As more experience is gained, these endoluminal palliative strategies provide increasingly effective and durable relief for patients with malignant obstruction.

Surgical Management of the Primary Cancer: To Resect or Not to Resect?

The role of surgical resection of the primary colon or rectal cancer in patients with unresectable metastases is controversial. It is important to recognize that there are no randomized controlled trials demonstrating a survival benefit for bowel resection in stage IV patients. However, palliative resection of the primary tumor does provide durable local control, is generally well tolerated, and can benefit select stage IV patients.[33] Randomized trials of 5FU-based chemotherapy vs. best supportive care, conducted in the 1990s, have shown that stage IV patients receiving systemic chemotherapy have increased length and quality of life.[34] Moreover, with modern multidrug regimens and monoclonal antibody therapy options, the beneficial impact of chemotherapy continues to increase. At this time, standard management for patients with unresectable metastatic colorectal cancer is systemic chemotherapy.

The proper use of elective colon and rectal resections in nonobstructed patients is a source of continuing debate. Loss of performance status, risk of surgical complications, and delay in chemotherapy are potential downsides to palliative surgical resection. On the other hand, elective operations have a far lower morbidity than emergency surgery. In addition, there are increased risks and potential complications associated with operations performed on patients who develop large-bowel obstruction while receiving chemotherapy or who present with more advanced disease after multiple cycles of ineffective chemotherapy.

Table 47-1 lists six retrospective studies comparing operative and nonoperative management of the primary cancer in patients with stage IV colon and rectal cancer.[34–38] The data is predominantly from the 1990s, when 5-flourouracil-based chemotherapy was the standard systemic therapy. In all of these studies, the majority of patients were treated by initial resection of the primary cancer. Patients who did not undergo surgical resection were more likely to have rectal cancers, to have more extensive metastatic disease, and to be older. The operative mortality for patients undergoing initial bowel resection ranged from 1.6 to 11%. Patients who did not undergo bowel resection underwent a subsequent colorectal operation in 9.3–32% of cases, although the indications for subsequent operation were often not specified and "colorectal operation" included palliative stoma creation and intestinal bypass. From these limited data, it is clear that initial colon resection is frequently practiced, particularly for patients with colon primaries and with less extensive metastatic disease. However, it is difficult to assess the impact of colon and rectal resection on symptom control, tolerance to subsequent chemotherapy, quality of life, or survival from these studies.

A recent meta-analysis evaluating patients with stage IV colorectal cancer treated with chemotherapy combined with and without surgical resection revealed prolonged survival in patients undergoing palliative surgical resection and chemotherapy when compared to chemotherapy alone.[39] Chemotherapy regimens included 5-flourouracil, oxaliplatin, and irinotecan. Eight retrospective studies with a sum total of 1,062 patients met the inclusion criteria for this study. The median survival for palliative surgical resection

TABLE 47-1. Retrospective analysis of bowel resection for patients with unresectable stage IV colorectal cancer: 5-flourouracil-based chemotherapy

Study	Publication year	Surgical group	n	Group features	Operative mortality (%)	Subsequent colon surgery (%)	Median surveillance (months)
Cleveland Clinic[37]	1997	Resection	57	Colon cancer	11	–	10.6
		No resection	5	Colon cancer	–	NR	2
Vanderbilt[36]	1999	Resection	66	Proximal cancers	4.6	–	14.5
		No resection	23	Rectal cancers	–	9	16.6
MSKCC[35]	2003	Resection	127	Proximal cancers fewer metastases	1.6	–	16
			103	Rectal cancers more metastases	–	29	9
Medicare[163]	2004	Resection	6,469	Proximal cancers younger age	9		10
		No resection	2,542	Rectal cancers		32	3
SEER[34]	2005	Resection[a]	17,658	Proximal cancers younger age	NR		Colon 11, rectum 16
		No resection	9,096	Rectal primary older age		NR	Colon 2, rectum 6
Harbor UCLA/UCI[38]	2006	Resection	62	NR	4.8	–	12.5[b]
		No resection	47	NR	–	36	4.6[b]

NR not reported.
[a]Resection group includes both initial and delayed bowel resection.
[b]Significant difference in median survival ($p<0.0001$).

combined with chemotherapy ranged from 14 to 22 months (data extracted from studies with 100% patient participation in systemic chemotherapy). The median survival for chemotherapy alone was 6–15 months. The estimated standardized median difference in survival was 6.0 months in favor of palliative surgical resection (standardized difference 0.55; 95% CI 0.29, 0.82; $p<0.001$). In addition, patients managed with chemotherapy alone were more likely to experience a complication related to the primary tumor (95% CI 1.7, 34.4; $p=0.008$). There was no difference in the incidence of metastatic disease tumor burden becoming more favorable and amenable to curative resection after systemic chemotherapy in either group (0.85; 95% CI 0.40, 1.8; $p=0.662$). There are obvious limitations of this meta-analysis given the retrospective nature of the studies available for review as well as the chemotherapy regimens utilized in these studies not being equivalent to current regimens. The group acknowledged these limitations and concluded that palliative resection of the primary tumor in asymptomatic or minimally symptomatic patients with stage IV colorectal cancer is associated with prolonged survival. In addition, palliative resection of the primary tumor is associated with a reduced incidence of complications from the primary tumor and the need for emergency procedures.[39]

There is little published data evaluating the effectiveness of radiotherapy in palliative management of stage IV rectal cancer. Crane and colleagues reported 55 patients who received chemoradiotherapy and 25 patients who received chemoradiotherapy followed by surgery. The majority of both groups received systemic therapy (78% of patients).[40] Pelvic symptom control was high (81%) in the chemoradiotherapy group but not as high as in the chemoradiotherapy combined with surgical resection group (91%). There was limited data on the durability of symptom control over time.

To summarize the treatment options for stage IV patients with unresectable metastases, treatment algorithms are shown for patients with stage IV colon cancer (Figure 47-2) and stage IV rectal cancer (Figure 47-3). The algorithms show multiple treatment options, reflecting the heterogeneity

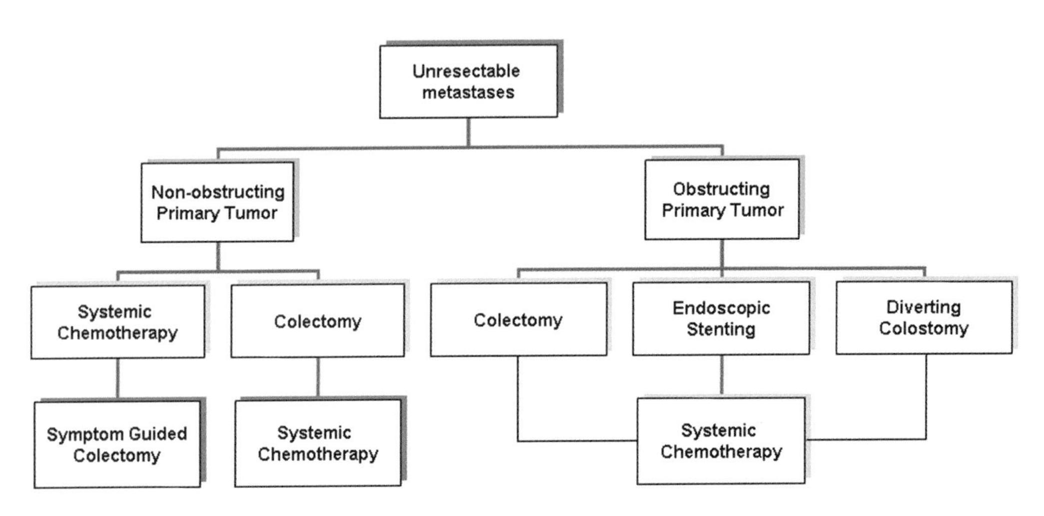

FIGURE 47-2. Treatment algorithm for patients with stage IV colon cancer: use of palliative colon resection.

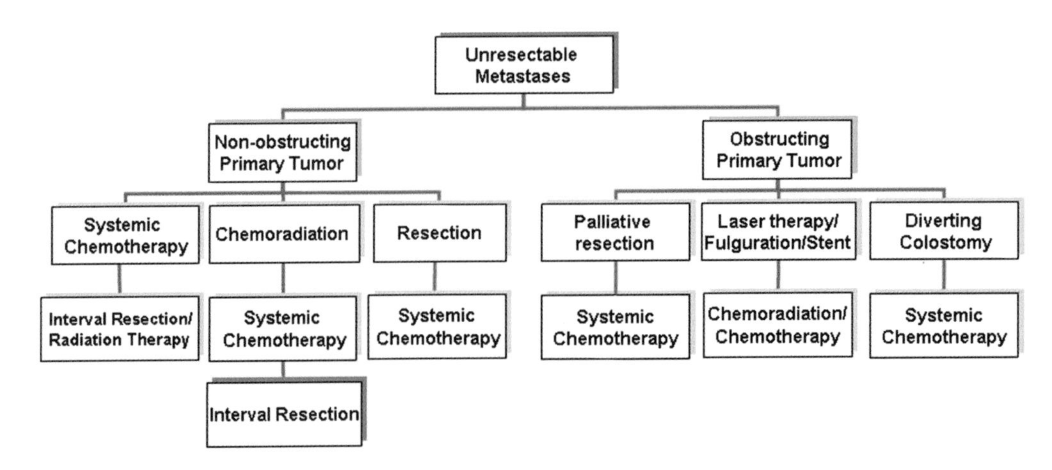

FIGURE 47-3. Treatment algorithm for patients with stage IV rectal cancer: use of palliative rectal resection.

of disease presentation. The major variables to consider are location of the primary tumor, degree of colon and/or rectal obstruction, extent of metastatic disease, and fitness of the patient for surgery. For patients with nonobstructing primary tumors, initial treatment with systemic chemotherapy is favored because, in this era of increasingly effective chemotherapy, it is important that patients be given the full benefit of aggressive systemic therapy. However, it should be remembered that the goal of therapy is effective palliation, and surgical resection remains the most effective and durable local treatment option.

Liver Metastasis

Of the 150,000 new cases of primary colorectal cancer diagnosed in the USA each year, approximately 60% of these patients will develop liver metastases and about one-third will have disease limited to the liver.[1] Liver resection and tumor ablation are currently the only available curative treatments for metastatic colorectal cancer with 5-year survival ranging from 28 to 45%.[41] Overall, it is been estimated that about 10% of all patients with colorectal liver metastases are candidates for potentially curative hepatic surgery.[42] Of those able to undergo complete hepatic resection, 25–35% achieve long-term survival.[43] The remaining majority of patients receive palliative therapy. This underscores the importance of patient selection in determining optimal treatment. These statistics also highlight the fact that the majority of patients with liver metastases have unresectable disease and require evaluation for chemotherapy or supportive care. It should be noted, however, that with improvements in chemotherapy, surgical technique, and ablative techniques, the number of patients eligible for hepatic surgery is on the rise.[44,45]

Natural History of Untreated Liver Metastases

In order to understand the impact of any therapy on outcome for patients with hepatic colorectal metastases, the natural history of untreated disease must be reviewed. This is especially relevant in understanding the impact of surgery for hepatic metastases, as there has never been a randomized trial comparing any therapy to surgery (nor is there ever likely to be). Prior to the 1980s, most hepatic metastases were left untreated. Several investigators have retrospectively studied untreated patients, documenting median survivals of 5–10 months; long-term survival was rarely seen.[46] The majority of these patients, however, had extensive disease, and most had their primary tumor in place, making comparison to modern surgical series irrelevant. Nonetheless, some investigators retrospectively identified patients with isolated, potentially resectable hepatic metastases who were left untreated. In these patients with limited metastases isolated to the liver, who would otherwise be potential candidates for surgery, 3-year survival was 14–23% and 5-year survival was 2–8%.[46–48] While these studies were instrumental in demonstrating the relationship between bulk of disease and survival, they also clearly showed that, even in the best of circumstances, 5-year survival of patients with untreated liver metastases is distinctly uncommon.

Diagnosis

Once a diagnosis of colorectal cancer is made a careful evaluation is made to accurately stage the patient with appropriate imaging. Complete cross-sectional imaging of the abdomen and pelvis with triple phase CT and or MRI is essential to rule out extrahepatic disease. The additional advantage of routine chest CT is low compared to that of a plain chest X-ray but should be considered in high-risk cases.[49, 18] F-FDG positron emission tomography (PET) scanning is routinely performed because of early prospective data documenting its utility. The information obtained from PET scanning changes management decisions in patients with recurrent colorectal carcinoma 20–50% of the time. The major strength of PET scanning appears to be the detection of occult extrahepatic disease.[18] In many centers, the combination of PET/CT imaging allows for operative planning and accurate tumor localization. Once the issue of extrahepatic disease has been addressed, high-quality imaging of the liver is essential in determining bulk of disease and resectability. CT scans are the most common modality used to address liver disease and, with modern dynamic helical scanning techniques, this remains the mainstay of hepatic imaging. Routine CT scans can now evaluate the liver in combination with CT angiography or triphasic imaging of the parenchyma through various phases of intravenous contrast circulation.

Ultrasound and magnetic resonance imaging (MRI) are additional imaging techniques that can be useful in specific circumstances. Ultrasound is not an accurate method for addressing extrahepatic disease and, indeed, often cannot visualize the entire liver. However, in experienced hands ultrasound is excellent at distinguishing neoplastic tumors from benign lesions such as cysts, focal nodular hyperplasia or hemangiomata. Additionally, ultrasound can specifically evaluate the relationship of specific lesions to major vascular structures and the biliary tree. It can be of particular utility when performing intraoperative ablative procedures. MRI is an excellent method for characterizing liver lesions. Particularly if there are multiple hepatic lesions, not all of which are suspected to be metastatic tumors, MRI can help distinguish malignant lesions from cysts, hemangiomata, and other benign lesions. MRI is also an excellent modality for evaluating relationships of tumor to the biliary tree (via magnetic resonance cholangiopancreatography – MRCP) and to hepatic vasculature. High-quality MRI and triple phase CT are probably equivalent for evaluating extent of liver disease, and as aids in surgical planning.[50–52] In any patient being considered for hepatic resection, a complete medical workup should be performed to assess the patient's fitness for undergoing a major abdominal operation.

Any potential for liver dysfunction, such as alcohol abuse or chronic hepatitis, must be carefully evaluated.

Treatment Options

In the patient who presents with liver metastases, the first consideration must be whether the liver disease is curable. The second consideration is whether the patient's disease if initially unresectable can be made amenable to surgery or ablative procedures with the addition of systemic chemotherapy.

Chemotherapy

Until recently, chemotherapy was considered largely ineffective as treatment of unresectable metastatic colorectal cancer. However, with the development of irinotecan, oxaliplatin, hepatic arterial infusional chemotherapy with FUDR, and newer molecular-based therapies, there are now more effective chemotherapeutic options for these patients. For nearly 50 years, 5-fluoruracil (5FU) was the only effective chemotherapeutic regimen for metastatic colorectal cancer. Despite many attempts to modify 5FU with other agents, response rates generally ranged from 15 to 20%, and survival beyond 1 year was uncommon. The addition of leucovorin (5FU/LV) and the use of infusional dosing techniques are associated with an increased response rate, and are commonly utilized despite no improvement in survival.[53,54]

Irinotecan (CPT-11) in conjunction with 5FU/LV has been recently shown to be more effective than 5FU/LV alone for treatment of metastatic colorectal cancer. Two randomized trials established the superiority of single-agent irinotecan over 5FU/LV alone or best supportive care as second-line therapy.[55,56] Additionally, two randomized trials utilizing combined irinotecan/5FU/LV (FOLFIRI) as first-line chemotherapy have shown response rates of 40%, with modestly improved survival (median 15–17 months vs. 12–14 months).[57,58] The addition of oxaliplatin has been particularly exciting because of the in vitro sensitivity seen in cisplatin-resistant cell lines, as well as its synergy with 5FU.[58,59] In a trial comparing oxaliplatin/5FU/LV (FOLFOX) to 5FU/LV, response rates for FOLFOX were in excess of 50% (compared to 22% for 5FU/LV). There was no difference in survival, but this is likely due to a 37% crossover from 5FU/LV to FOLFOX during the trial.[60] Early analyses of comparisons of irinotecan/5FU/LV to FOLFOX have so far shown FOLFOX to yield superior response rates.[61] Ongoing trials continue to define optimal timing, dosing, and sequence of various combination regimens.

Biomarker Targeted Therapy

Monoclonal antibodies that target epidermal growth factor receptor (EGFR) have increased the treatment options for patients with metastatic colorectal cancer. The detection of positive EGFR immunostaining of the primary tumor is not a reliable predictor of response to therapy and as a result biomarker assays for *Kras* mutation are used to determine potential response to treatment.[62] Epidermal growth factor receptor is a member of the tyrosine kinase family and its activation stimulates many cancer-related processes such as proliferation, angiogenesis, invasion, and metastasis.[62] Overexpression of EGFR is found in a number of tumor types and in most cases is associated with poorer outcomes.[63] Several studies have found an association between a *Kras* mutation and a lack of response to EGFR-directed therapy. The importance of defining the KRAS status of the primary tumor has provided oncologists with important information about response to treatment. Early results from studies on patients with metastatic colorectal cancer show that the addition of cetuximab to FOLFIRI, improved overall survival (OS) by 3.5 months in *KRAS* wild-type patients. The response rate was 57.3% for the addition of cetuximab compared with 39.7%. As these trials mature, and modern systemic chemotherapy regimens are refined, we are now seeing median survivals in excess of 20 months.[59,62] More recent data from the CAIRO (capecitabine, irinotecan, and oxaliplatin)-2 study found the addition of an EGFR inhibitor had no effect on progression-free interval among those with wild-type *Kras* expression but was deleterious to those patients whose had *Kras* mutations in the tumor.[64] Similar data has been shown with the BRAF mutation as well.[65] Interestingly, it has been shown that the multikinase inhibitor sorafenib may restore sensitivity to EGFR inhibitors in BRAF-mutated colorectal cancer cell line.[65,66] As a result, studies are underway to determine the significance of this in human trials. As the understanding of molecular pathways in colorectal cancer continue to be elucidated, parallel developments are occurring in the fields of drug discovery and biomarker assay.

Hepatic Arterial Infusion

Regional hepatic therapy via hepatic artery infusional chemotherapy (HAI) has been studied since the 1970s. Hepatic metastases derive their blood supply largely from the hepatic arterial branches compared with mixed arterial and portal blood supply of the surrounding parenchyma.[41,67] This has an advantage over systemically delivered chemotherapy as the drugs used in HAI have a higher therapeutic index due to high first-pass hepatic extraction and high systemic clearance. Conversely, when regional therapy is given in the form of HAI, less is delivered to the systemic blood supply and therefore fewer systemic side effects are experienced. The most commonly used agent for HAI is fluorodeoxyuridine (FUDR), which has a 90% hepatic extraction ratio, while this is beneficial for isolated hepatic disease it limits treatment of occult extrahepatic disease. This can be addressed by giving additional systemic agents, or by using 5FU via the hepatic artery with a higher "spill-over" effect into the systemic circulation.

Early phase II trials of HAI FUDR or 5FU for unresectable colorectal hepatic metastases demonstrated remarkable

TABLE 47-2. 2010 Meta-analysis of survival of patients with stage IV colorectal cancer managed with surgical resection vs. chemotherapy alone

Study	Tumor burden					
	% Right sided	>25% Liver involvement	% Extrahepatic	PS 0–1 (%)	Received chemotherapy (%)	Median survival (months)
A. Palliative surgical resection and chemotherapy[39]						
Scoggins et al.	47	32	15	–	0	15
Michel et al.	90[a]	36[b]	58	81	97	21
Ruo et al.	46	41	44	–	0	16*
Tebbutt et al.	67[a]	–	20	80	100	14
Benoist et al.	28	84	6	41[c]	94	23
Kaufman et al.	–	–	–	–	100	22
Galizia et al.	29	62	10	74	100	15*
Bajwa et al.	47	–	0	67	100	14*
B. Palliative chemotherapy alone[39]						
Scoggins et al.	26	40	39	–	96	17
Michel et al.	65[a]	39[b]	13	91	100	14
Ruo et al.	28	55	59	–	83	9*
Tebbutt et al.	54[a]	–	13	62	100	8
Benoist et al.	33	89	7	30[c]	100	22
Kaufman et al.	–	–	–	–	100	15
Galizia et al.	26	61	0	74	100	12*
Bajwa et al.	29	–	0	34	100	6*

Data from Table 34-2.[39]
* ≤0.005.
[a] % Colon.
[b] 5 or more liver metastases.
[c] % WHO performance status score of 0.

response rates ranging from 29 to 88%.[68–71] Subsequently 10 randomized phase III trials comparing HAI chemotherapy to systemic chemotherapy have been completed (Table 47-2). From 1987 through 1990, five trials were done comparing HAI FUDR to intravenous FUDR or intravenous 5FU/LV. All of these trials showed significantly increased response rates, but only trials comparing HAI chemotherapy to best supportive care showed improved survival. Most of these trials were underpowered and most allowed crossover, making conclusions about survival difficult. Two meta-analyses of the first seven trials have been performed on the assumption that each was underpowered, in an attempt to detect significant survival differences.[72,73] Both clearly confirmed the increased response rates, and both showed a modest survival benefit. A CALGB trial comparing HAI FUDR to systemic 5FU/LV without crossover found response rates to be significantly higher with HAI FUDR (48% vs. 25%), as was overall survival (22.7 months vs. 19.8 months).[74] Finally, a meta-analysis of FUDR-HAI vs. systemic chemotherapy for unresectable liver metastases from colorectal cancer that included results from ten RCT has shown a greater tumor response rate with FUDR-HAI when compared with systemic therapy; however, this did not translate to a survival advantage over 5FU-based systemic therapy.[75]

One explanation for the lack of survival advantage is while control of hepatic disease was excellent with HAI, there was significant extrahepatic failure. FUDR while an effective agent for treating liver metastases can have liver-related complications including biliary sclerosis (18–29%).[41] Finally, the placement of the HAI catheter is an invasive procedure and technical complications including primary catheter failure, catheter-related thrombosis, and infection.[41]

Currently, with the explosion of new active systemic agents, a new paradigm has developed in the treatment of hepatic colorectal metastases. Many phase I and II trials are now evaluating combinations of HAI FUDR or oxaliplatin with systemically administrated 5FU/LV with irinotecan and/or oxaliplatin. Even in pre-treated patients, impressive response rates in excess of 80% are being seen.[72] The combination of HAI and systemic 5FU/LV has further improved transformation rates of previously isolated unresectable colorectal liver mets into resectable lesions in as many as 26% of cases.[41] While recent advances in cytotoxic chemotherapy for colorectal cancer over the last decade have been very exciting, the development of targeted molecular-based therapy provides even greater hope for more effective systemic treatments. Results of current clinical trials are anxiously awaited to see where these molecular-based targeted therapies will ultimately fit in among the armamentarium of systemic therapy for colorectal cancer.

Resection

As described above, it is clear that patients with untreated hepatic colorectal metastases have poor survival. Although response rates to chemotherapeutic regimens are improving, the only therapy ever shown to be potentially curative for hepatic colorectal metastases is complete resection. Traditional principles that govern surgical intervention reserved hepatic resection of colorectal metastases for those would had unilobar disease, less than four lesions, lesions that were less than 5 cm in greatest dimension and those without extrahepatic disease.[66] However, in modern times with the addition of more effective systemic therapies, ablative techniques and treatment modalities aimed at "downstaging" the liver disease, more patients can be made amenable to resection. Mortality rates for hepatectomy for metastatic colorectal cancer are uniformly 5% or less (Table 47-3). Nonetheless, morbidity for these operations remains substantial and is usually reported between 20 and 50%. Fortunately, this morbidity does not generally translate into long hospital stays, intensive care unit stays, long-term disability, or early mortality. The most ominous complications, such as liver failure and significant hemorrhage, are now distinctly uncommon, thanks to better surgical technique and postoperative care. A recent review of more than 1,800 liver resections (57% of a lobe or greater) over the last decade, the median hospital stay was 8 days, morbidity was 45% and mortality was 3%. Furthermore, of the 1,245 hepatectomies performed for metastatic disease, mortality was 2.4%.[76]

Major institutional and multi-institutional reviews have now clearly documented the 5-year survival of patients undergoing hepatectomy for metastatic colorectal cancer ranges from 25 to 40%, 10-year survival ranges from 20 to 26%, and median survivals range from 24 to 46 months (Table 47-3). These results obviously compare favorably to the results of no treatment (median survival 5–10 months) and to those of chemotherapy (median survival 10–14 months). Despite recent improvements in chemotherapy resulting in median survivals as high as 20 months, complete resection still provides the best outcomes. True long-term cure from chemotherapy is extraordinarily rare, while at least half of the long-term survivors after liver resection are disease-free and presumably cured.[77] For these reasons, no trial has ever compared hepatectomy to no treatment or chemotherapy alone. Liver resection for resectable hepatic colorectal metastases is the treatment of choice.

TABLE 47-3. Outcome of patients undergoing pulmonary metastasectomy for colorectal cancer

Study	*n*	Operative mortality (%)	5-yr survival (%)	Significant risk factors
Mori et al.[164]	35	–	38	None found
McCormack et al.[165]	144	0	44	Margin
McAfee et al.[97]	139	1	31	Number of lesions, CEA
Yano et al.[166]	27	–	41	Number of lesions
Saclarides et al.[167]	23	–	16	Number of lesions
van Halteren et al.[168]	38	–	43	DFI
Shirouzu et al.[169]	22	–	37	Number of lesions, size
Girard et al.[170]	86	1	24	CEA, margin
Okumura et al.[171]	159	2	41	Number of lesions, LN status
Zanella et al.[172]	22	0	62	None found
Zink[173]	110	0	33	Size, CEA
Dahabre et al.[95]	52	–	33	None found

n number of patients, yr year, LN lymph nodes, DFI disease-free interval.
Source: Adapted from Rizk et al.[100]

Patient Selection

Many studies of patients undergoing liver resection for isolated hepatic metastases have evaluated prognostic factors to help select those patients most likely to benefit from hepatectomy and, conversely, to identify those unlikely to benefit. The two most consistent negative prognostic factors are the presence of extrahepatic disease and the inability to resect all tumor; these two factors remain contraindications to hepatectomy. The exception to this rule is the patient with limited pulmonary metastases or colonic anastomotic recurrence, who may undergo combined resections with some success.[42] Although there are many inconsistencies in the major reported series, a list of other poor prognostic factors exist; these include lymph nodes involved by the primary colorectal tumor, synchronous presentation (or shorter disease-free interval), larger number of tumors, bilobar involvement, CEA elevation greater than 200 ng/ml, and involved histologic margins.[78–82] While it appears to be true that the stage of the primary tumor, the interval in which metastatic disease has developed, and the bulk of tumor in the liver (measured by size, number, and/or CEA level) can provide prognostic information on outcome after hepatectomy, none of these findings in and of themselves preclude the potential for long-term survival. Fong et al. conducted a multivariate analysis of 1,001 patients who underwent potentially curative hepatectomy, and identified five factors as having the most influence on outcome.[83,84] These included size greater than 5 cm, disease-free interval of less than 1 year, more than one tumor, lymph node-positive primary, and CEA greater than 200 ng/ml (Table 47-3). A clinical risk score (CRS) was created using regression analysis may be used preoperatively as a prognostic indicator of long-term outcome and hence aid in patient selection.

Margin Status

The importance of obtaining negative margins with hepatectomy has been demonstrated in multiple studies showing improved disease-free and overall survival. By comparison a recent study demonstrated a survival benefit of 46 months for those patients who underwent resection with negative margins vs. 24 months for those with positive margins.[85] Wide resection margins with >1 cm clearance is desirable; however, a consensus statement from the Society of Surgical Oncology concluded that while wide margins of >1 cm are desirable and should be sought, anticipation of a close margin should not preclude a resection.[86] As a result, a more recent study examined the difference in outcomes between those patients with R0 resections vs. R1 resections. When coupled with SCT, the R1 resection group has similar 5-year overall survival rates to the R0 resection group (57% vs. 60%, $p=0.12$). Intrahepatic recurrence demonstrated a higher recurrence of 28% for the R1 resection group vs. 17% for the R0 resection ($p=0.004$) group.[87] One can surmise again from this study that an R1 resection.

Recurrence

Recurrence following hepatectomy for colorectal metastases is common, occurring in more than two-thirds of patients. In fact, long-term survival does not necessarily imply that there has been no recurrence. In a study of 96 actual 5-year survivors, nearly half had experienced a recurrence at some point and received further therapy.[87] In patients who do recur, the liver is the most common site of recurrence and is involved approximately 45% of the time. Most of these recurrences are isolated to the liver. Other common sites are lung, bone, and various intra-abdominal sites.[88] Since many recurrences are isolated to the liver, repeat liver resection has been attempted by several surgeons with some success. Unfortunately, only 5–10% of patients are candidates for a second liver resection, underscoring the importance of patient selection. Currently, at least 14 series reporting on more than 700 patients have documented that repeat hepatectomy for metastatic colorectal cancer is safe and effective in well-selected patients. Mortality is less than 5%, median survival from the time of the second liver resection ranges from 23 to 46 months, and 5-year survival ranges from 30 to 41%.[88] The factors most commonly associated with a poor outcome following repeat hepatectomy are size and number of tumors, as well as short disease-free interval. Because of the potential for further effective therapeutic interventions after primary liver resection, patients eligible for such treatment should be followed with serial CEA and imaging studies to detect recurrences at an early and potentially treatable phase.

Since recurrence after hepatectomy for metastatic colorectal cancer is common, there is a sound rationale for use of adjuvant therapy. Indeed, adjuvant 5FU-based systemic chemotherapy after liver resection was often given, but its use was not supported by prospective trials. A number of retrospective comparisons have been performed, but no definitive published data support the routine use of adjuvant postoperative 5FU-based systemic chemotherapy. The effect of newer, more effective chemotherapeutic regimens on long-term survival following hepatectomy is not known but is promising.

Since hepatic metastases derive their blood supply from the hepatic artery and the most common site of recurrence after hepatectomy is within the remnant liver, there is a strong argument for the use of HAI chemotherapy. Three randomized trials have addressed the efficacy of adjuvant HAI chemotherapy. In the German Cooperative multicenter study, HAI 5FU/LV was compared to no treatment after hepatectomy. No significant differences in outcome were found; however, many patients in the HAI arm did not receive therapy, and 5FU is not considered the optimal therapeutic for HAI chemotherapy.[89]

In the recently published Intergroup study, adjuvant HAI FUDR combined with systemic 5FU was compared to no treatment. A significant improvement in survival (46% vs. 25% 4-year survival, $p=0.04$) was demonstrated only when analyzed by actual treatment received. There was no significant difference in outcome when analyzed in an intent-to-treat manner.[90] The third trial, performed at MSKCC, compared systemic 5FU/LV to systemic 5FU/LV combined with HAI FUDR. Ninety-two percent of patients received therapy as assigned, and there was a significant improvement in 2-year survival (the primary endpoint) favoring the addition of HAI FUDR (86% vs. 72%).[91]

Given the growing number of chemotherapeutic options for patients with metastatic colorectal cancer, there are many options for the patient who has had all of his or her liver metastases resected. Since HAI FUDR combined with systemic 5FU/LV is the only therapy ever shown to improve survival in this setting, there is a strong argument for the use of this modality; however, the surgeon and medical oncologist need to have experience with pump implantation and management. With the advent of more effective systemic chemotherapy such as irinotecan and oxaliplatin, as well as molecular targeted agents, new trials are needed to assess optimal adjuvant therapy.

Because the large majority of patients with hepatic colorectal metastases are technically unresectable, the development of more effective chemotherapy has inspired many oncologists to employ a "neoadjuvant" chemotherapy strategy in an attempt to render patients resectable. In a series from France, 701 patients with unresectable liver metastases received chronomodulated 5FU/LV and oxaliplatin. Ninety-five (14%) of these patients became resectable, secondary to chemotherapeutic response, and underwent staged resection. The resections employed techniques such as portal vein embolization and intraoperative ablation to extirpate all tumor, and achieved an actuarial 5-year survival rate of 35%.[44] Another study analyzed 23 previously treated patients with unresectable liver metastases. HAI FUDR was administered, and six patients (26%) were ultimately able to undergo an R0 resection.[45] These early studies suggest that patients with unresectable liver metastases should be treated aggressively with chemotherapy and reevaluated at intervals for the possibility of resection.

Ablative Procedures

While resection has become the gold standard for treatment of liver metastases it is curative in a minority of patients, therefore other methods of tumor destruction utilizing thermal ablation techniques have also been developed to treat and palliate those tumors that are not amenable to resection.

Cryotherapy has been used for decades and employs the use of probes to freeze tumors and surrounding normal hepatic parenchyma. Cryotherapy generally requires a laparotomy, and complications such as bleeding, liver cracking, and a cryoshock phenomena characterized by thrombocytopenia and disseminated intravascular coagulation can occur.

Radiofrequency ablation (RFA) and microwave ablation (MWA) probes have been developed that can heat liver tumors and a surrounding margin of tissue to create coagulation necrosis. RFA and MWA can be employed percutaneously, laparoscopically, and at laparotomy under ultrasound, CT, or MRI guidance. Furthermore, RFA has low morbidity that generally ranges around 10% and is rarely serious.[91–93] While RFA can be used near blood vessels, as the heat-sink effect of blood flow protects the endothelium, major bile ducts can be seriously injured, limiting the use of RFA in central tumors situated near major bile ducts. Local recurrence following RFA is a significant problem, and appears to be strongly correlated with tumor size. Generally, recurrence is more common in tumors greater than 4 or 5 cm in diameter and in tumors abutting major blood vessels. With improvements in localization and monitoring of thermal application, however, these therapies are very promising alternatives to surgery. Perhaps the greatest application of ablative techniques will be in their use as additions to resection in patients with multiple bilobar tumors.

Yttrium-90 microspheres is a way of delivering a pure beta emitting form of radiation to an unresectable liver lesion without suffering the locoregional side effects of external beam radiation. The microspheres are most often administered via a angiographic guided catheter placement. The procedure first requires accessible feeding vessels that allows for treatment of the lesions, but it is imperative that healthy liver and lungs are excluded and therefore appropriate treatment dosing is critical. The first study to combine radioembolization (REB) with systemic chemotherapy (SCT) randomly assigned patients to either treatment arm with REB plus The overall median survival was 29.4 months in the study arm vs. 12.8 months in the SCT alone arm.[94] This trial and others show promising results in patients with metastatic colorectal cancer. Currently, radioembolization is undergoing multicenter trials that include simultaneous and sandwiched systemic chemotherapy as for both treatment and radiosenstization. The results from these trials will ultimately determine whether REB has a role in the management of unresectable metastatsis from colorectal cancer.

Lung Metastasis

Approximately 10% of patients with colorectal cancer develop pulmonary metastasis. The vast majority of patients with metastatic colorectal cancer to the lung have advanced disease, and are therefore treated with systemic chemotherapy or best supportive care. Approximately 11% of these individuals will have isolated pulmonary metastases.[95] Patients with isolated or limited pulmonary may be considered candidates for pulmonary metastasectomy.[96]

Due to the retrospective nature of the reported information in the literature, clinical outcome data after metastasectomy for colorectal lung metastases must be interpreted with caution. Improved clinical outcome and survival data is more likely due to ideal patient selection and tumor biology rather than the surgical intervention in and of itself. In addition, there are no adequate control groups in these reports; therefore, survival statistics are difficult to interpret. However, there are patients who undergo pulmonary metastasectomy with no evidence of disease after long-term follow-up.[95] In addition, long-term survival without complete resection is very rare, suggesting that select patients do occasionally benefit from pulmonary metastasectomy.

Modern series of lung resection for metastatic colorectal cancer report operative mortalities of less than 2% (Table 47-3). Five-year survival rates range from 16 to 64%, but generally cluster around 30% to 40%. Most studies evaluate factors associated with outcome; however, given the limited number of cases, the statistical power of these studies to detect significant factors is limited. In general, the pathology of the primary tumor (grade, location, stage) has not been shown to impact clinical outcome. The most commonly cited significant factors associated with adverse outcomes include the number and size of pulmonary metastasis, short disease-free interval (DFI), elevated CEA, and incomplete resection.

While the majority of series evaluate metastatic disease limited to the lungs, several series have evaluated patients with both liver and lung metastases. Some authors advocate resection of synchronous limited extrapulmonary disease[97]; however, the majority of studies that have analyzed synchronous liver and lung metastases report a uniformly poor outcome following combined resections. Long-term survival is very uncommon in this situation.[98,99] In the setting of isolated pulmonary recurrence after partial hepatectomy, pulmonary metastasectomy appears to have more favorable outcomes similar to those for the initial hepatectomy.[98–100]

The surgical approach to patients who are potential candidates for pulmonary metastasectomy has been somewhat controversial. Based on older studies reported in the 1980s citing a 38% yield of contralateral thoracotomy in finding radiographically occult disease, routine bilateral thoracotomy had been advocated.[101] With modern day imaging, routine bilateral thoracotomy is no longer justified. The use of video-assisted thoracoscopic surgery (VATS) has increased significantly and is often used in metastasectomy when a minimal parenchymal resection is necessary. Initially, VATS was deemed substandard to thoracotomy due to the inability to palpate the lung parenchyma; a prospective study evaluating confirmatory thoracotomy after VATS showed that 22% of lesions were missed.[101,102] However, with improvements in modern imaging and VATS technique, a minimally invasive approach can be justified.

Radiation therapy for colorectal cancer pulmonary metastasis has been of limited utility in the past due to radiation-induced pneumonitis, rib and spinal fractures, and skin toxicities. However, these toxicities can be minimized with the advent of robotic assisted Gamma Knife radiotherapy or "cyberknife."[103] Initial reports appear to have minimal toxicity associated with single-session lung radiotherapy using robotic image-guided real-time respiratory and tumor tracking. This is an exciting field of research and may become an additional therapeutic modality in the future. However, the outcome and efficacy data is limited at this time and the associated cost of robotic image-guided radiotherapy will be a limiting factor in widespread availability.

Peritoneal Metastasis

Peritoneal carcinomatosis represents one of the most challenging aspects of metastatic colorectal cancer. The peritoneal surface is involved in approximately 10–15% of colorectal cancer patients at time of initial presentation (synchronous metastases) and in 20–50% of patients who develop recurrence (metachronous metastases).[104–106] As a site of colorectal cancer metastasis, the peritoneal surface ranks second only to the liver. It is characterized by intraperitoneal spread of metastatic nodules. Peritoneal metastasis occurs by direct implantation of cancer cells via one of four mechanisms (1) spontaneous intraperitoneal seeding from a T4 colorectal cancer that has penetrated the serosal surface of the colon; (2) extravasation of tumor cells at the time of colon perforation from an obstructing cancer; (3) iatrogenic tumor perforation through an area of serosal injury or enterotomy at the time of colon resection; and (4) leakage of tumor cells from transected lymphatics or veins at the time of colon resection.[105] The risk of peritoneal metastasis is therefore highest in the setting of locally advanced cancers.

Peritoneal metastases are clinically important because of their frequent progression to malignant ascites and/or malignant bowel obstruction.[106–110] Synchronous peritoneal carcinomatosis was found in 58.5% of the patients with colorectal cancer. The most frequent symptoms were ascites (29.7%) and bowel obstruction (19.5%).

Preoperative detection of peritoneal metastases is not reliable. Noninvasive imaging frequently misses small peritoneal lesions, even when these are widely disseminated. The sensitivity of CT scanning for lesions smaller than 5 mm is only 28%, as compared to 70% for lesions 2 cm or greater.[111] Thus, indirect signs such as bulky primary tumor, ascites, or bowel obstruction are important clues. The utility of MRI in diagnosis of peritoneal carcinomatosis beyond that of CT is largely unknown and PET scans are of limited value. Unfortunately, in the majority of cases, diagnosis is made at the time of primary resection.[112]

The extent of carcinomatosis is a major prognostic factor and is best assessed by either laparoscopic or open exploration. Two different peritoneal carcinomatosis staging systems (Gilly's classification and Peritoneal Cancer Index of Sugarbaker) can be used to assess the extent of carcinomatosis.[113,114] These staging systems have both shown utility in determining the prognosis and treatment of patients with peritoneal carcinomatosis. By Gilly's classification, carcinomatosis is classified principally by the dimensions of the peritoneal tumor implants: stage I, tumor nodules less than 5 mm in diameter localized in one part of the abdomen; stage II, tumor nodules less than 5 mm disseminated widely through the abdomen; stage III, tumor nodules 5–2 cm in diameter; and stage IV, tumor nodules greater than 2 cm. The Peritoneal Cancer Index scores the extent of carcinomatosis on the basis of tumor size and location within 13 regions of the abdomen and pelvis. The lesion with the largest size in each abdominopelvic region is scored on a scale of 0–3 (0, no tumor; 1, tumor up to 0.5 cm; 2, tumor up to 5.0 cm; 3, >5 cm or confluence). The total score of the Peritoneal Cancer Index can vary from 0 to 39. The Peritoneal Cancer Index is shown to correlate with survival. Median survival and 5-year survival after surgical debulking and intraperitoneal chemotherapy were 48 months and 50% for peritoneal index <10, compared to 12 months and 0% for index >20.

Standard management of patients known to have peritoneal metastases at initial presentation is systemic chemotherapy. Colon resection plays an important role for patients with obstructing primary cancers, and also for patients with occult metastases that are first detected in the operating room. Historically, the median survival for patients with unresected peritoneal metastasis treated with 5-fluorouracil-based systemic chemotherapy was very poor (6–8 months).[115,117] However, patient survival is highly variable, depending on the extent of metastatic disease and response to chemotherapy.[116,117] Contemporary combination chemotherapy regimens have significantly greater efficacy and can produce long periods of disease control in certain patients.

Despite the grim prognosis for patients with peritoneal carcinomatosis from colorectal cancer, a subset of patients once thought unsalvageable are now being considered for surgery with curative intent. Pioneered by Sugarbaker, the goal of cytoreductive surgery and intraperitoneal (IP) chemotherapy is to remove all macroscopic disease with peritonectomy procedures and visceral resections followed by perioperative IP chemotherapy to destroy residual microscopic disease. IP delivery offers a pharmacokinetic advantage over standard intravenous delivery by producing high regional concentrations of drug while simultaneously minimizing systemic toxicities.[118–120] The most widely reported method of IP chemotherapy is intraoperative delivery of mitomycin in a hyperthermic (41C) circuit for 90 min. An alternative approach is postoperative infusion of 5-fluoro-2′-deoxyuridine (FUDR) via an implanted intraperitoneal catheter.[120]

Despite early skepticism, in carefully selected cases there appears to be a survival benefit. Multiple phase II and one phase III study establish superiority over conventional palliative surgery or systemic chemotherapy[121] Several phase II studies show 5-year survival rates ranging between 19 and 28%.[122] The most consistent and important prognostic factor in these studies is the ability to achieve complete resection of all gross disease. Five-year survival rates reported for patients with completely resected disease range from 27 to 54%.[122–124]

A phase III study conducted by the Netherlands Cancer Institute randomized 105 colorectal cancer patients with peritoneal carcinomatosis to either standard treatment (systemic 5-fluorouracil/leucovorin with or without palliative colectomy) or experimental therapy (aggressive cytoreductive surgery, hyperthermic IP mitomycin, and systemic 5-fluorouracil/leucovorin).[123–125] In the experimental arm, median operation time was 585 min, treatment toxicity was high, and treatment-related mortality was 8%. After a median follow-up of 22 months, median survival was 12.6 months in the standard therapy arm and 22.3 months in the experimental therapy arm. It is not known if the survival benefit observed in the experimental therapy arm is due to surgical debulking, IP chemotherapy, or both.

In summary, the standard therapy for patients with peritoneal metastases is systemic chemotherapy. However, there is evidence that aggressive surgical cytoreduction and IP chemotherapy will benefit patients with limited peritoneal tumor burden. Additional clinical trials are needed to define optimal use of this aggressive treatment approach.

Ovarian Metastasis

Approximately 4–30% of ovarian neoplasms are metastatic cancers, the most common being colorectal and breast cancer.[126] Between 6 and 14% of all women dying with colorectal cancer are found to have ovarian metastases at the time of autopsy.[127] The risk of developing ovarian metastasis is substantially higher in woman with stage IV disease and approaches 90% in women with established peritoneal metastases. In addition, women with adenocarcinoma of the vermiform appendix have a very high risk of ovarian metastasis. Thus, in a woman with recent diagnosis of advanced colorectal cancer, any ovarian mass should be considered a metastasis from colorectal cancer until proven otherwise.

The pathogenesis of colorectal cancer ovarian metastasis is variable. Metastatic spread occurs primarily through the peritoneum but can also occur via the blood stream, through lymphatic vessels, or by direct extension. Careful intraoperative assessment of the ovaries at the time of colon cancer surgery is essential. Synchronous metastases occur in 0–8.6% of patients in various clinical studies,[128–132] while metachronous metastases develop in 1.4–6.8% of colorectal cancer cases,[126,127,133,134] usually within 2 years after the primary resection.[129–136] Most often these metastatic lesions are large, and at least half of the cases have bilateral ovarian involvement.[137,138] Approximately 40% of these patients also have associated extraovarian pelvic metastasis.[137] Distinguishing a metastatic colorectal cancer from primary ovarian tumor is difficult by gross assessment alone, but a correct diagnosis can generally be determined through integration of clinicopathologic, immunohistochemical, and cytogenetic features. Most metastatic colorectal lesions are $CK20^+/CEA^+/CK7^-$ on staining, while primary ovarian neoplasms are $CK20^-/CEA^-/CK7^+$.[138–141]

Primary en bloc resection of CRC with direct extension to the ovary (T4) or resection of macroscopic metastatic disease to the ovary with prophylactic bilateral resection has been suggested to offer survival benefit and should be performed with curative intent in the absence of other significant metastatic disease. However, the removal of macroscopically normal ovaries, prophylactic oophorectomy, in women with colorectal cancer is the subject of much debate. Proponents of resection argue that removal improves the cure rate by removing potential microscopic "undetectable" synchronous disease, eliminates the risk of ovarian cancer and removes the risk of future metachronous ovarian metastatic disease.[127] Others argue that the low incidence of ovarian metastasis, paucity of supportive data and few clinical correlations with predictive value make this additional intervention unnecessary.[127] Clinical studies attempting to document the benefit of ovarian metastasectomy in patients with colorectal cancer are small and retrospective.[128,142,143] The majority of studies to date, however, fail to show any survival benefit for prophylactic oophorectomy and most studies demonstrate that when ovarian metastatsis is present it is a poor prognostic sign.[127] Based on the available data, it is reasonable to offer prophylactic oophorectomy to all postmenopausal patients, in particular to those women who have undergone pelvic radiation as part of their treatment for rectal cancer. For premenopausal patients, only those with established peritoneal metastases, those with a clearly increased risk of developing ovarian carcinoma [strong family history, known carriers of breast cancer (BRCA) or hereditary nonpolyposis colorectal cancer (HNPCC) mutation], or those who have already completed their families should be considered for prophylactic oophorectomy.

Most ovarian metastases are asymptomatic and are only detected at the time of surgery; however, large metastatic ovarian lesions can compress or invade adjacent organs (ureter, bladder, bowel), rupture, and on rare occasions bleed. Survival of women with synchronous ovarian colorectal metastases is significantly worse than that of patients without such metastases.[126,144] Ovarian metastases are frequently resistant to systemic chemotherapy even when other sites of metastatic disease are responding, and therefore, resection of synchronous ovarian metastases should be performed when noted intraoperatively.[145–148] Bilateral oophorectomy and complete resection of gross disease is recommended. Reoperation for metachronous metastases should be considered in selected patients with good performance status and limited tumor burden elsewhere. To prevent local tumor progression, an aggressive surgical approach should be undertaken to achieve complete resection. The survival benefit of removing ovarian metastases has never been well documented, although complete metastasectomy is associated with significantly better outcome when compared to palliative debulking, especially in the setting of metastatic disease confined to the pelvis.[149,150] It should be noted that complete resection is only possible in 50% of these cases. The median postresection survival for women with isolated ovarian metastases is 18 months.[145] Women with other sites of disease have shorter survival, however, and 5-year survival after resection of established ovarian metastases is rare.[146,147] In these cases, systemic chemotherapy should be strongly considered, particularly when residual disease is present. With the availability of stronger chemotherapeutic regimens containing oxaliplatin, irinotecan, and/or bevacizumab, better survival can be expected.[151–154]

Bone and Brain Metastases

Bone metastases from colorectal cancer reportedly occur in 7–9% of cases, and most often present in the context of widespread metastatic disease.[155–158] Routine diagnostic bone imaging is not indicated in colorectal cancer patients, however, unless there are specific bone-related symptoms. There are no curative modalities, but palliation of pain, fractures, or spinal cord involvement are important issues for these patients. Symptomatic relief from bony metastases can usually be accomplished with radiation and medical therapy. However, pathologic fractures are best treated by operative internal fixation. The systemic issues related to bone metastases are serious and include debilitation, immobility, hypercalcemia, and thromboembolic disease.

Cerebral metastases from colorectal cancer are uncommon, occurring in 1–4% of colorectal cancer cases.[155–157] Colorectal tumors account for approximately 3% of all metastatic brain tumors.[158] These are generally found in the context of widespread metastases to multiple organ sites, but on rare occasion can present as an isolated brain metastasis. There is no role for routine brain imaging at primary presentation or at presentation with metastases elsewhere, unless there are specific neurologic symptoms. Once brain metastases occur, symptoms are common; palliative therapies include steroids to decrease swelling and anticonvulsants to control seizures. Definitive therapy of colorectal brain metastases usually involves surgery, radiation, or a combination of the two. For isolated, single brain metastases, resection can result in survival beyond 1–2 years.[157–160] As with pulmonary metastasis, there is increasing interest and data in the literature regarding Gamma Knife and Cyber Knife radiotherapy for bone and brain metastasis.[161] The outcome and efficacy data is limited at this time and the associated cost of robotic real-time image-guided radiotherapy may be a limiting factor in widespread applicability.

References

1. Jemal A, Murray T, Ward E, et al. Cancer statistics, 2005. CA Cancer J Clin. 2005;55(1):10–30.
2. O'Connell JB, Maggard MA, Ko CY. Colon cancer survival rates with the new American Joint Committee on Cancer sixth edition staging. J Natl Cancer Inst. 2004;96(19): 1420–5.
3. Nordic Gastrointestinal Tumor Adjuvant Therapy Group. Expectancy or primary chemotherapy in patients with advanced asymptomatic colorectal cancer: a randomized trial. J Clin Oncol. 1992;10(6):904–11.
4. Scheithauer W, Rosen H, Kornek GV, Sebesta C, Depisch D. Randomised comparison of combination chemotherapy plus supportive care with supportive care alone in patients with metastatic colorectal cancer. BMJ. 1993;306(6880):752–5.
5. Tournigand C, Andre T, Achille E, et al. FOLFIRI followed by FOLFOX6 or the reverse sequence in advanced colorectal cancer: a randomized GERCOR study. J Clin Oncol. 2004;22(2):229–37.
6. Hurwitz H, Fehrenbacher L, Novotny W, et al. Bevacizumab plus irinotecan, fluorouracil, and leucovorin for metastatic colorectal cancer. N Engl J Med. 2004;350(23):2335–42.
7. Hanahan D, Weinberg RA. The hallmarks of cancer. Cell. 2000;100(1):57–70.
8. Woodhouse EC, Chuaqui RF, Liotta LA. General mechanisms of metastasis. Cancer. 1997;80(8 Suppl):1529–37.
9. Fidler IJ. Critical factors in the biology of human cancer metastasis: twenty-eighth G.H.A. Clowes memorial award lecture. Cancer Res. 1990;50(19):6130–8.
10. Folkman J. How is blood vessel growth regulated in normal and neoplastic tissue? G.H.A. Clowes memorial Award lecture. Cancer Res. 1986;46(2):467–73.
11. Hynes RO. Metastatic potential: generic predisposition of the primary tumor or rare, metastatic variants – or both? Cell. 2003;113(7):821–3.
12. Bogenrieder T, Herlyn M. Axis of evil: molecular mechanisms of cancer metastasis. Oncogene. 2003;22(42):6524–36.
13. Chambers AF, Groom AC, MacDonald IC. Dissemination and growth of cancer cells in metastatic sites. Nat Rev Cancer. 2002;2(8):563–72.
14. Messick CA, Church JM, Liu X, Ting AH, Kalady MF. Stage III colorectal cancer: molecular disparity between primary cancers and lymph node metastates. Ann Surg Oncol. 2010;17(2):425–31.
15. Shevde LA, Welch DR. Metastasis suppressor pathways – an evolving paradigm. Cancer Lett. 2003;198(1):1–20.
16. Chin BB, Wahl RL. 18F-Fluoro-2-deoxyglucose positron emission tomography in the evaluation of gastrointestinal malignancies. Gut. 2003;52 Suppl 4:iv23–9.

17. Deans GT, Krukowski ZH, Irwin ST. Malignant obstruction of the left colon. Br J Surg. 1994;81(9):1270–6.
18. Phillips RK, Hittinger R, Fry JS, Fielding LP. Malignant large bowel obstruction. Br J Surg. 1985;72(4):296–302.
19. Van Hooft JE, Bemelman WA, Fockens P. A study of the value of colonic stenting as a bridge to elective surgery for the management of acute left-sided malignant colonic obstruction: the STENT-IN 2 study. Ned Tijdschr Geneeskd. 2007;151: 1249–51.
20. Vemulapalli R, Lara LF, Sreenarasimhaiah J, Harford WV, Siddiqui AA. A comparison of palliative stenting or emergent surgery for obstructing incurable colon cancer. Dig Dis Sci. 2010;55(6):1732–7.
21. Gandrup P, Lund L, Balslev I. Surgical treatment of acute malignant large bowel obstruction. Eur J Surg. 1992;158(8):427–30.
22. Loizou LA, Grigg D, Boulos PB, Bown SG. Endoscopic Nd:YAG laser treatment of rectosigmoid cancer. Gut. 1990;31(7):812–6.
23. Daneker Jr GW, Carlson GW, Hohn DC, Lynch P, Roubein L, Levin B. Endoscopic laser recanalization is effective for prevention and treatment of obstruction in sigmoid and rectal cancer. Arch Surg. 1991;126(11):1348–52.
24. Mandava N, Petrelli N, Herrera L, Nava H. Laser palliation for colorectal carcinoma. Am J Surg. 1991;162(3):212–4;discussion 5.
25. Brunetaud JM, Maunoury V, Cochelard D. Lasers in rectosigmoid tumors. Semin Surg Oncol. 1995;11(4):319–27.
26. Gevers AM, Macken E, Hiele M, Rutgeerts P. Endoscopic laser therapy for palliation of patients with distal colorectal carcinoma: analysis of factors influencing long-term outcome. Gastrointest Endosc. 2000;51(5):580–5.
27. Salvati EP, Rubin RJ, Eisenstat TE, Siemons GO, Mangione JS. Electrocoagulation of selected carcinoma of the rectum. Surg Gynecol Obstet. 1988;166(5):393–6.
28. Eisenstat TE, Oliver GC. Electrocoagulation for adenocarcinoma of the low rectum. World J Surg. 1992;16(3):458–62.
29. Khot UP, Lang AW, Murali K, Parker MC. Systematic review of the efficacy and safety of colorectal stents. Br J Surg. 2002;89(9):1096–102.
30. Law WL, Choi HK, Lee YM, Chu KW. Palliation for advanced malignant colorectal obstruction by self-expanding metallic stents: prospective evaluation of outcomes. Dis Colon Rectum. 2004;47(1):39–43.
31. Athreya S, Moss J, Urquhart G, Edwards R, Downie A, Poon FW. Colorectal stenting for colonic obstruction: the indications, complications, effectiveness and outcome – 5-year review. Eur J Radiol. 2006;60(1):91–4.
32. Dronamraju SS, Ramamurthy S, Kelly SB, Hayat M. Role of self-expanding metallic stents in the management of malignant obstruction of the proximal colon. Dis Colon Rectum. 2009;52(9):1657–61.
33. Rosen SA, Buell JF, Yoshida A, et al. Initial presentation with stage IV colorectal cancer: how aggressive should we be? Arch Surg. 2000;135(5):530–4;discussion 4–5.
34. Cook AD, Single R, McCahill LE. Surgical resection of primary tumors in patients who present with stage IV colorectal cancer: an analysis of surveillance, epidemiology, and end results data, 1988 to 2000. Ann Surg Oncol. 2005;12(8): 637–45.
35. Ruo L, Gougoutas C, Paty PB, Guillem JG, Cohen AM, Wong WD. Elective bowel resection for incurable stage IV colorectal cancer: prognostic variables for asymptomatic patients. J Am Coll Surg. 2003;196(5):722–8.
36. Scoggins CR, Meszoely IM, Blanke CD, Beauchamp RD, Leach SD. Nonoperative management of primary colorectal cancer in patients with stage IV disease. Ann Surg Oncol. 1999;6(7):651–7.
37. Liu SK, Church JM, Lavery IC, Fazio VW. Operation in patients with incurable colon cancer – is it worthwhile? Dis Colon Rectum. 1997;40(1):11–4.
38. Konyalian VR, Rosing DK, Haukoos JS, Dixon MR, Sinow R, Bhaheetharan S, et al. The role of primary tumour resection in patients with stage IV colorectal cancer. Colorectal Dis. 2006;9:430–7.
39. Stillwell AP, Buettner PG, Ho YH. Meta-analysis of survival of patients with stage IV colorectal cancer managed with surgical resection versus chemotherapy alone. World J Surg. 2010;34(4):797–807.
40. Crane CH, Janjan NA, Abbruzzese JL, et al. Effective pelvic symptom control using initial chemoradiation without colostomy in metastatic rectal cancer. Int J Radiat Oncol Biol Phys. 2001;49(1):107–16.
41. Goere D, Deshaies I, De Baere T, et al. Prolonged survival of initially unresectable hepatic colorectal cancer patients treated with hepatic arterial infusion of oxaliplatin followed by radical surgery of metastases. Ann Surg. 2010;251(4):686–91.
42. McCarter MD, Fong Y. Metastatic liver tumors. Semin Surg Oncol. 2000;19(2):177–88.
43. Fong Y. Surgical therapy of hepatic colorectal metastasis. CA Cancer J Clin. 1999;49(4):231–55.
44. Adam R, Avisar E, Ariche A, et al. Five-year survival following hepatic resection after neoadjuvant therapy for nonresectable colorectal. Ann Surg Oncol. 2001;8(4):347–53.
45. Clavien PA, Selzner N, Morse M, Selzner M, Paulson E. Downstaging of hepatocellular carcinoma and liver metastases from colorectal cancer by selective intra-arterial chemotherapy. Surgery. 2002;131(4):433–42.
46. Blumgart LH, Fong Y. Surgical options in the treatment of hepatic metastasis from colorectal cancer. Curr Probl Surg. 1995;32(5):333–421.
47. Wagner JS, Adson MA, Van Heerden JA, Adson MH, Ilstrup DM. The natural history of hepatic metastases from colorectal cancer. A comparison with resective treatment. Ann Surg. 1984;199(5):502–8.
48. Wood CB, Gillis CR, Blumgart LH. A retrospective study of the natural history of patients with liver metastases from colorectal cancer. Clin Oncol. 1976;2(3):285–8.
49. Kronawitter U, Kemeny NE, Heelan R, Fata F, Fong Y. Evaluation of chest computed tomography in the staging of patients with potentially resectable liver metastases from colorectal carcinoma. Cancer. 1999;86(2):229–35.
50. Kim HC, Kim TK, Sung KB, et al. CT during hepatic arteriography and portography: an illustrative review. Radiographics. 2002;22(5):1041–51.
51. Poyanli A, Sencer S. Computed tomography scan of the liver. Eur J Radiol. 1999;32(1):15–20.
52. Hann LE, Winston CB, Brown KT, Akhurst T. Diagnostic imaging approaches and relationship to hepatobiliary cancer staging and therapy. Semin Surg Oncol. 2000;19(2):94–115.
53. Fong Y, Blumgart LH, Fortner JG, Brennan MF. Pancreatic or liver resection for malignancy is safe and effective for the elderly. Ann Surg. 1995;222(4):426–34;discussion 34–7.

54. D'Angelica MI, Shoup MC, Nissan A. Randomized clinical trials in advanced and metastatic colorectal carcinoma. Surg Oncol Clin N Am. 2002;11(1):173–91.
55. Rougier P, Van Cutsem E, Bajetta E, et al. Randomised trial of irinotecan versus fluorouracil by continuous infusion after fluorouracil failure in patients with metastatic colorectal cancer. Lancet. 1998;352(9138):1407–12.
56. Cunningham D, Pyrhonen S, James RD, et al. Randomised trial of irinotecan plus supportive care versus supportive care alone after fluorouracil failure for patients with metastatic colorectal cancer. Lancet. 1998;352(9138):1413–8.
57. Saltz LB, Cox JV, Blanke C, et al. Irinotecan plus fluorouracil and leucovorin for metastatic colorectal cancer. Irinotecan Study Group. N Engl J Med. 2000;343(13):905–14.
58. Douillard JY, Cunningham D, Roth AD, et al. Irinotecan combined with fluorouracil compared with fluorouracil alone as first-line treatment for metastatic colorectal cancer: a multicentre randomised trial. Lancet. 2000;355(9209):1041–7.
59. Kuebler JP, de Gramont A. Recent experience with oxaliplatin or irinotecan combined with 5-fluorouracil and leucovorin in the treatment of colorectal cancer. Semin Oncol. 2003;30 (4 Suppl 15):40–6.
60. de Gramont A, Figer A, Seymour M, et al. Leucovorin and fluorouracil with or without oxaliplatin as first-line treatment in advanced colorectal cancer. J Clin Oncol. 2000;18(16):2938–47.
61. Goldberg RM, Morton RF, Sargent DJ, et al. N9741: oxaliplatin (oxal) or CPT-11 + 5-fluorouracil (5FU)/leucovorin (LV) or oxal + CPT-11 in advanced colorectal cancer (CRC). Initial toxicity and response data from a GI Intergroup study. Proc Am Soc Clin Oncol. 2002;21:128a;abstract 511.
62. Siena S, Sartore-Bianchi A, Di Nicolantonio F, et al. Biomarkers predicting clinical outcomes of epidermal growth factor receptor-targeted therapy in metastatic colorectal cancer. J Natl Cancer Inst. 2009;101(19):1308–24.
63. Nicholson RI, Gee JM, Harper ME. EGFR and cancer prognosis. Eur J Cancer. 2001;37 Suppl 4:S9–15.
64. Tol J, Koopman M, Cats A, et al. Chemotherapy, bevacizumab, and cetuximab in metastatic colorectal cancer. N Engl J Med. 2009;360(6):563–72.
65. Di Nicolantonio F, Martini M, Molinari F, et al. Wild-type BRAF is required for response to panitumumab or cetuximab in metastatic colorectal cancer. J Clin Oncol. 2008;26(35): 5705–12.
66. Abdel-Misih SR, Schmidt CR, Bloomston PM. Update and review of the multidiciplinary management of stage IV colorectal cancer with liver metastases. World J Surg Oncol. 2009;7(72):2–14.
67. Ackerman NB, Lien WM, Kondi ES, Silverman NA. The blood supply of experimental liver metastases. I. The distribution of hepatic artery and portal vein blood to "small" and "large" tumors. Surgery. 1969;66(6):1067–72.
68. Oberfield RA, McCaffrey JA, Polio J, Clouse ME, Hamilton T. Prolonged and continuous percutaneous intra-arterial hepatic infusion chemotherapy in advanced metastatic liver adenocarcinoma from colorectal primary. Cancer. 1979;44(2):414–23.
69. Weiss GR, Garnick MB, Osteen RT, et al. Long-term hepatic arterial infusion of 5-fluorodeoxyuridine for liver metastases using an implantable infusion pump. J Clin Oncol. 1983;1(5):337–44.
70. Balch CM, Urist MM, Soong SJ, McGregor M. A prospective phase II clinical trial of continuous FUDR regional chemotherapy for colorectal metastases to the liver using a totally implantable drug infusion pump. Ann Surg. 1983;198(5):567–73.
71. Niederhuber JE, Ensminger W, Gyves J, Thrall J, Walker S, Cozzi E. Regional chemotherapy of colorectal cancer metastatic to the liver. Cancer. 1984;53(6):1336–43.
72. Harmantas A, Rotstein LE, Langer B. Regional versus systemic chemotherapy in the treatment of colorectal carcinoma metastatic to the liver. Is there a survival difference? Meta-analysis of the published literature. Cancer. 1996;78(8):1639–45.
73. Meta-Analysis Group in Cancer. Reappraisal of hepatic arterial infusion in the treatment of nonresectable liver metastases from colorectal cancer. J Natl Cancer Inst. 1996;88(5):252–8.
74. Kemeny N, Niedzwiecki D, Hollis DR. Hepatic arterial infusion (HAI) versus systemic therapy for hepatic metastases from colorectal cancer: a CALGB randomized trial of efficacy, quality of life (QOL), cost effectiveness, and molecular markers. Proc Am Soc Clin Oncol. 2003;22:252; abstract 1010.
75. Mocellin S, Pasquali S, Nitti D. Fluoropyrimidine-HAI versus systemic chemotherapy for unresectable liver metastases from colorectal cancer. Cochran Collab. 2009;(3):CD007823.
76. Jarnagin WR, Gonen M, Fong Y, et al. Improvement in perioperative outcome after hepatic resection: analysis of 1,803 consecutive cases over the past decade. Ann Surg. 2002;236(4):397–406;discussion.
77. Silen W. Hepatic resection for metastases from colorectal carcinoma is of dubious value. Arch Surg. 1989;124(9):1021–2.
78. Foster JH. Survival after liver resection for secondary tumors. Am J Surg. 1978;135(3):389–94.
79. D'Angelica M, Brennan MF, Fortner JG, Cohen AM, Blumgart LH, Fong Y. Ninety-six five-year survivors after liver resection for metastatic colorectal cancer. J Am Coll Surg. 1997;185(6):554–9.
80. Scheele J, Stangl R, Altendorf-Hofmann A, Gall FP. Indicators of prognosis after hepatic resection for colorectal secondaries. Surgery. 1991;110(1):13–29.
81. Doci R, Gennari L, Bignami P, Montalto F, Morabito A, Bozzetti F. One hundred patients with hepatic metastases from colorectal cancer treated by resection: analysis of prognostic determinants. Br J Surg. 1991;78(7):797–801.
82. Rosen CB, Nagorney DM, Taswell HF, et al. Perioperative blood transfusion and determinants of survival after liver resection for metastatic colorectal carcinoma. Ann Surg. 1992;216(4):493–504;discussion 5.
83. Fong Y, Fortner J, Sun RL, Brennan MF, Blumgart LH. Clinical score for predicting recurrence after hepatic resection for metastatic colorectal cancer: analysis of 1001 consecutive cases. Ann Surg. 1999;230(3):309–18;discussion 18–21.
84. Fong Y, Cohen AM, Fortner JG, et al. Liver resection for colorectal metastases. J Clin Oncol. 1997;15(3):938–46.
85. Choti MA, Sitzman JV, Tiburi MF, et al. Trends in long-term survival following liver resection of colorectal metastases. Ann Surg. 2002;235:759–66.
86. Charnsangavej C, Clary B, Fong Y, et al. Selection of patients for resection for hepatic colorectal metastases: expert consensus statement. Ann Surg Oncol. 2006;13:1261–8.
87. de Haas RJ, Wicherts DA, Flores E. R1 resection by necessity for colorectal liver metastases: is it still a contraindication to surgery? Ann Surg. 2008;248:626–37.
88. Petrowsky H, Gonen M, Jarnagin W, et al. Second liver resections are safe and effective treatment for recurrent hepatic

metastases from colorectal cancer: a bi-institutional analysis. Ann Surg. 2002;235(6):863–71.
89. Lorenz M, Muller HH, Schramm H, et al. Randomized trial of surgery versus surgery followed by adjuvant hepatic arterial infusion with 5-fluorouracil and folinic acid for liver metastases of colorectal cancer. German Cooperative on Liver Metastases (Arbeitsgruppe Lebermetastasen). Ann Surg. 1998;228(6):756–62.
90. Kemeny MM, Adak S, Gray B, et al. Combined-modality treatment for resectable metastatic colorectal carcinoma to the liver: surgical resection of hepatic metastases in combination with continuous infusion of chemotherapy – an intergroup study. J Clin Oncol. 2002;20(6):1499–505.
91. Kemeny N, Huang Y, Cohen AM, et al. Hepatic arterial infusion of chemotherapy after resection of hepatic metastases from colorectal cancer. N Engl J Med. 1999;341(27): 2039–48.
92. Curley SA. Radiofrequency ablation of malignant liver tumors. Ann Surg Oncol. 2003;10(4):338–47.
93. Nordlinger B, Rougier P. Nonsurgical methods for liver metastases including cryotherapy, radiofrequency ablation, and infusional treatment: what's new in 2001? Curr Opin Oncol. 2002;14(4):420–3.
94. Nicoly NH, Berry DP, Sharma RA. Liver metastases from colorectal cancer: radioembolization with systemic therapy. Nat Rev. 2009;6:687–97.
95. Dahabre J, Vasilaki M, Stathopoulos GP, Kondaxis A, Iliadis K, Papadopoulos G, et al. Surgical management in lung metastases from colorectal cancer. Anticancer Res. 2007;27(6C):4387–90.
96. McCormack PM, Attiyeh FF. Resected pulmonary metastases from colorectal cancer. Dis Colon Rectum. 1979;22(8): 553–6.
97. McAfee MK, Allen MS, Trastek VF, Ilstrup DM, Deschamps C, Pairolero PC. Colorectal lung metastases: results of surgical excision. Ann Thorac Surg. 1992;53(5):780–5;discussion 5–6.
98. Nagakura S, Shirai Y, Yamato Y, Yokoyama N, Suda T, Hatakeyama K. Simultaneous detection of colorectal carcinoma liver and lung metastases does not warrant resection. J Am Coll Surg. 2001;193(2):153–60.
99. Dematteo R, Minnard EA, Kemeny N. Outcome after resection of both liver and lung metastases in patients with colorectal cancer. Proc Am Soc Clin Oncol. 1999;abstract 958.
100. Rizk NP, Downey RJ. Resection of pulmonary metastases from colorectal cancer. Semin Thorac Cardiovasc Surg. 2002;14(1):29–34.
101. Roth JA, Pass HI, Wesley MN, White D, Putnam JB, Seipp C. Comparison of median sternotomy and thoracotomy for resection of pulmonary metastases in patients with adult soft-tissue sarcomas. Ann Thorac Surg. 1986;42(2):134–8.
102. McCormack PM, Bains MS, Begg CB, et al. Role of video-assisted thoracic surgery in the treatment of pulmonary metastases: results of a prospective trial. Ann Thorac Surg. 1996;62(1):213–6;discussion 6–7.
103. Muacevic A, Drexler C, Wowra B, Schweikard A, Schlaefer A, Hoffmann RT, et al. Technical description, phantom accuracy, and clinical feasibility for single-session lung radiosurgery using robotic image-guided real-time respiratory tumor tracking. Technol Cancer Res Treat. 2007;6(4):321–8.
104. Sugarbaker PH, Cunliffe WJ, Belliveau J, et al. Rationale for integrating early postoperative intraperitoneal chemotherapy into the surgical treatment of gastrointestinal cancer. Semin Oncol. 1989;16(4 Suppl 6):83–97.
105. Dawson LE, Russell AH, Tong D, Wisbeck WM. Adenocarcinoma of the sigmoid colon: sites of initial dissemination and clinical patterns of recurrence following surgery alone. J Surg Oncol. 1983;22(2):95–9.
106. Russell AH, Tong D, Dawson LE, et al. Adenocarcinoma of the retroperitoneal ascending and descending colon: sites of initial dissemination and clinical patterns of recurrence following surgery alone. Int J Radiat Oncol Biol Phys. 1983;9(3):361–5.
107. Chu DZ, Lang NP, Thompson C, Osteen PK, Westbrook KC. Peritoneal carcinomatosis in nongynecologic malignancy. A prospective study of prognostic factors. Cancer. 1989;63(2):364–7.
108. Willett CG, Tepper JE, Cohen AM, Orlow E, Welch CE. Failure patterns following curative resection of colonic carcinoma. Ann Surg. 1984;200(6):685–90.
109. Hansen E, Wolff N, Knuechel R, Ruschoff J, Hofstaedter F, Taeger K. Tumor cells in blood shed from the surgical field. Arch Surg. 1995;130(4):387–93.
110. Sadeghi B, Arvieux C, Glehen O, et al. Peritoneal carcinomatosis from non-gynecologic malignancies: results of the EVOCAPE 1 multicentric prospective study. Cancer. 2000;88(2):358–63.
111. Jacquet P, Jelinek JS, Steves MA, Sugarbaker PH. Evaluation of computed tomography in patients with peritoneal carcinomatosis. Cancer. 1993;72(5):1631–6.
112. González-Moreno S, González-Bayón L, Ortega-Pérez G, et al. Imaging of peritoneal carcinomatosis. Cancer J. 2009;15(3):184–9.
113. Gilly FN, Beaujard A, Glehen O, et al. Peritonectomy combined with intraperitoneal chemohyperthermia in abdominal cancer with peritoneal carcinomatosis: phase I–II study. Anticancer Res. 1999;19(3B):2317–21.
114. Jacquet P, Sugarbaker PH. Clinical research methodologies in diagnosis and staging of patients with peritoneal carcinomatosis. Cancer Treat Res. 1996;82:359–74.
115. Pestieau SR, Sugarbaker PH. Treatment of primary colon cancer with peritoneal carcinomatosis: comparison of concomitant vs. delayed management. Dis Colon Rectum. 2000;43(10):1341–6;discussion 7–8.
116. Jayne DG, Fook S, Loi C, Seow-Choen F. Peritoneal carcinomatosis from colorectal cancer. Br J Surg. 2002;89(12): 1545–50.
117. Machover D. A comprehensive review of 5-fluorouracil and leucovorin in patients with metastatic colorectal carcinoma. Cancer. 1997;80(7):1179–87.
118. Sugarbaker PH. Colorectal carcinomatosis: a new oncologic frontier. Curr Opin Oncol. 2005;17(4):397–9.
119. Speyer JL. The rationale behind intraperitoneal chemotherapy in gastrointestinal malignancies. Semin Oncol. 1985;12(3 Suppl 4):23–8.
120. Sugarbaker PH, Graves T, DeBruijn EA, et al. Early postoperative intraperitoneal chemotherapy as an adjuvant therapy to surgery for peritoneal carcinomatosis from gastrointestinal cancer: pharmacological studies. Cancer Res. 1990;50(18):5790–4.

121. Sugarbaker PH, Schellinx ME, Chang D, Koslowe P, von Meyerfeldt M. Peritoneal carcinomatosis from adenocarcinoma of the colon. World J Surg. 1996;20(5):585–91;discussion 92.
122. Verwaal VJ, van Ruth S, Witkamp A, Boot H, van Slooten G, Zoetmulder FA. Long-term survival of peritoneal carcinomatosis of colorectal origin. Ann Surg Oncol. 2005; 12(1):65–71.
123. Verwaal VJ, Bruin S, Boot H, et al. 8-year follow-up of randomized trial: cytoreduction and hyperthermic intraperitoneal chemotherapy versus systemic chemotherapy in patients with peritoneal carcinomatosis of colorectal cancer. Ann Surg Oncol. 2008;15(9):2426–32.
124. Elias D, Blot F, El Otmany A, et al. Curative treatment of peritoneal carcinomatosis arising from colorectal cancer by complete resection and intraperitoneal chemotherapy. Cancer. 2001;92(1):71–6.
125. Verwaal VJ, van Ruth S, de Bree E, et al. Randomized trial of cytoreduction and hyperthermic intraperitoneal chemotherapy versus systemic chemotherapy and palliative surgery in patients with peritoneal carcinomatosis of colorectal cancer. J Clin Oncol. 2003;21(20):3737–43.
126. Ulbright TM, Roth LM, Stehman FB. Secondary ovarian neoplasia. A clinicopathologic study of 35 cases. Cancer. 1984;53(5):1164–74.
127. Omranipour R, Abasahl A. Ovarian metastases in colorectal cancer. Int J Gynecol Cancer. 2009;19(9):1524–8.
128. Webb MJ, Decker DG, Mussey E. Cancer metastatic to the ovary: factors influencing survival. Obstet Gynecol. 1975;45(4):391–6.
129. Barr SS, Valiente MA, Bacon HE. Rationale of bilateral oophorectomy concomitant with resection for carcinoma of the rectum and colon. Dis Colon Rectum. 1962;5:450–2.
130. Blamey S, McDermott F, Pihl E, Price AB, Milne BJ, Hughes E. Ovarian involvement in adenocarcinoma of the colon and rectum. Surg Gynecol Obstet. 1981;153(1):42–4.
131. Morrow M, Enker WE. Late ovarian metastases in carcinoma of the colon and rectum. Arch Surg. 1984;119(12):1385–8.
132. Cutait R, Lesser ML, Enker WE. Prophylactic oophorectomy in surgery for large-bowel cancer. Dis Colon Rectum. 1983;26(1):6–11.
133. Young-Fadok TM, Wolff BG, Nivatvongs S, Metzger PP, Ilstrup DM. Prophylactic oophorectomy in colorectal carcinoma: preliminary results of a randomized, prospective trial. Dis Colon Rectum. 1998;41(3):277–83;discussion 83–5.
134. Burt CA. Carcinoma of the ovaries secondary to cancer of the colon and rectum. Dis Colon Rectum. 1960;3:352–7.
135. Stearns Jr MW, Deddish MR. Five-year results of abdominopelvic lymph node dissection for carcinoma of the rectum. Dis Colon Rectum. 1959;2(2):169–72.
136. Graffner HO, Alm PO, Oscarson JE. Prophylactic oophorectomy in colorectal carcinoma. Am J Surg. 1983;146(2):233–5.
137. Koves I, Vamosi-Nagy I, Besznyak I. Ovarian metastases of colorectal tumours. Eur J Surg Oncol. 1993;19(6):633–5.
138. Harcourt KF, Dennis DL. Laparotomy for "ovarian tumors" in unsuspected carcinoma of the colon. Cancer. 1968;21(6): 1244–6.
139. Lindner V, Gasser B, Debbiche A, Tomb L, Vetter JM, Walter P. Ovarian metastasis of colorectal adenocarcinomas. A clinico-pathological study of 41 cases. Ann Pathol. 1999;19(6):492–8.
140. Rayson D, Bouttell E, Whiston F, Stitt L. Outcome after ovarian/adnexal metastectomy in metastatic colorectal carcinoma. J Surg Oncol. 2000;75(3):186–92.
141. Loy TS, Calaluce RD, Keeney GL. Cytokeratin immunostaining in differentiating primary ovarian carcinoma from metastatic colonic adenocarcinoma. Mod Pathol. 1996;9(11): 1040–4.
142. DeCostanzo DC, Elias JM, Chumas JC. Necrosis in 84 ovarian carcinomas: a morphologic study of primary versus metastatic colonic carcinoma with a selective immunohistochemical analysis of cytokeratin subtypes and carcinoembryonic antigen. Int J Gynecol Pathol. 1997;16(3):245–9.
143. Wauters CC, Smedts F, Gerrits LG, Bosman FT, Ramaekers FC. Keratins 7 and 20 as diagnostic markers of carcinomas metastatic to the ovary. Hum Pathol. 1995;26(8):852–5.
144. Dionigi A, Facco C, Tibiletti MG, Bernasconi B, Riva C, Capella C. Ovarian metastases from colorectal carcinoma. Clinicopathologic profile, immunophenotype, and karyotype analysis. Am J Clin Pathol. 2000;114(1):111–22.
145. Blamey SL, McDermott FT, Pihl E, Hughes ES. Resected ovarian recurrence from colorectal adenocarcinoma: a study of 13 cases. Dis Colon Rectum. 1981;24(4):272–5.
146. Herrera-Ornelas L, Mittelman A. Results of synchronous surgical removal of primary colorectal adenocarcinoma and ovarian metastases. Oncology. 1984;41(2):96–100.
147. Huang PP, Weber TK, Mendoza C, Rodriguez-Bigas MA, Petrelli NJ. Long-term survival in patients with ovarian metastases from colorectal carcinoma. Ann Surg Oncol. 1998; 5(8):695–8.
148. Wright JD, Powell MA, Mutch DG, et al. Synchronous ovarian metastases at the time of laparotomy for colon cancer. Gynecol Oncol. 2004;92(3):851–5.
149. Miller BE, Pittman B, Wan JY, Fleming M. Colon cancer with metastasis to the ovary at time of initial diagnosis. Gynecol Oncol. 1997;66(3):368–71.
150. MacKeigan JM, Ferguson JA. Prophylactic oophorectomy and colorectal cancer in premenopausal patients. Dis Colon Rectum. 1979;22(6):401–5.
151. Ballantyne GH, Reigel MM, Wolff BG, Ilstrup DM. Oophorectomy and colon cancer. Impact on survival. Ann Surg. 1985;202(2):209–14.
152. Sielezneff I, Salle E, Antoine K, Thirion X, Brunet C, Sastre B. Simultaneous bilateral oophorectomy does not improve prognosis of postmenopausal women undergoing colorectal resection for cancer. Dis Colon Rectum. 1997;40(11): 1299–302.
153. Kontoravdis A, Kalogirou D, Antoniou G, Kontoravdis N, Karakitsos P, Zourlas PA. Prophylactic oophorectomy in ovarian cancer prevention. Int J Gynaecol Obstet. 1996;54(3):257–62.
154. Barringer PL, Dockerty MB, Waugh JM, Bargen JA. Carcinoma of the large intestine; a new approach to the study of venous spread. Surg Gynecol Obstet. 1954;98(1):62–72.
155. Besbeas S, Stearns Jr MW. Osseous metastases from carcinomas of the colon and rectum. Dis Colon Rectum. 1978; 21(4):266–8.
156. Buckley N, Peebles Brown DA. Metastatic tumors in the hand from adenocarcinoma of the colon. Dis Colon Rectum. 1987;30(2):141–3.
157. Cascino TL, Leavengood JM, Kemeny N, Posner JB. Brain metastases from colon cancer. J Neurooncol. 1983;1(3):203–9.

158. Rovirosa A, Bodi R, Vicente P, Alastuey I, Giralt J, Salvador L. Cerebral metastases in adenocarcinoma of the colon. Rev Esp Enferm Dig. 1991;79(4):281–3.
159. Zimm S, Wampler GL, Stablein D, Hazra T, Young HF. Intracerebral metastases in solid-tumor patients: natural history and results of treatment. Cancer. 1981;48(2):384–94.
160. Wronski M, Arbit E. Resection of brain metastases from colorectal carcinoma in 73 patients. Cancer. 1999;85(8):1677–85.
161. Ko FC, Liu JM, Chen WS, Chiang JK, Lin TC, Lin JK. Risk and patterns of brain metastases in colorectal cancer: 27-year experience. Dis Colon Rectum. 1999;42(11):1467–71.
162. Wowra B, Muacevic A, Tonn JC. Quality of radiosurgery for single brain metastases with respect to treatment technology: a matched-pair analysis. J Neurooncol. 2009;94(1):69–77.
163. Temple LK, Hsieh L, Wong WD, Saltz L, Schrag D. Use of surgery among elderly patients with stage IV colorectal cancer. J Clin Oncol. 2004;22(17):3475–84.
164. Mori M, Tomoda H, Ishida T, et al. Surgical resection of pulmonary metastases from colorectal adenocarcinoma. Special reference to repeated pulmonary resections. Arch Surg. 1991;126(10):1297–301;discussion 302.
165. McCormack PM, Burt ME, Bains MS, Martini N, Rusch VW, Ginsberg RJ. Lung resection for colorectal metastases. 10-year results. Arch Surg. 1992;127(12):1403–6.
166. Yano T, Hara N, Ichinose Y, Yokoyama H, Miura T, Ohta M. Results of pulmonary resection of metastatic colorectal cancer and its application. J Thorac Cardiovasc Surg. 1993;106(5):875–9.
167. Saclarides TJ, Krueger BL, Szeluga DJ, Warren WH, Faber LP, Economou SG. Thoracotomy for colon and rectal cancer metastases. Dis Colon Rectum. 1993;36(5):425–9.
168. van Halteren HK, van Geel AN, Hart AA, Zoetmulder FA. Pulmonary resection for metastases of colorectal origin. Chest. 1995;107(6):1526–31.
169. Shirouzu K, Isomoto H, Hayashi A, Nagamatsu Y, Kakegawa T. Surgical treatment for patients with pulmonary metastases after resection of primary colorectal carcinoma. Cancer. 1995;76(3):393–8.
170. Girard P, Ducreux M, Baldeyrou P, et al. Surgery for lung metastases from colorectal cancer: analysis of prognostic factors. J Clin Oncol. 1996;14(7):2047–53.
171. Okumura S, Kondo H, Tsuboi M, et al. Pulmonary resection for metastatic colorectal cancer: experiences with 159 patients. J Thorac Cardiovasc Surg. 1996;112(4):867–74.
172. Zanella A, Marchet A, Mainente P, Nitti D, Lise M. Resection of pulmonary metastases from colorectal carcinoma. Eur J Surg Oncol. 1997;23(5):424–7.
173. Zink S, Kayser G, Gabius HJ, Kayser K. Survival, disease-free interval, and associated tumor features in patients with colon/rectal carcinomas and their resected intra-pulmonary metastases. Eur J Cardiothorac Surg. 2001;19(6):908–13.
174. Israel SL, Helsel Jr EV, Hausman DH. The challenge of metastatic ovarian carcinoma. Am J Obstet Gynecol. 1965;93(8):1094–101.
175. Demopoulos RI, Touger L, Dubin N. Secondary ovarian carcinoma: a clinical and pathological evaluation. Int J Gynecol Pathol. 1987;6(2):166–75.

48 Colorectal Cancer: Surveillance

Nadav Dujovny and Jon S. Hourigan

Introduction

The majority of patients with colon and rectal cancer undergo curative resection and become candidates for continuing surveillance. It is well understood that the risk of colorectal cancer recurrence is largely dependent on the stage of disease at initial presentation and the appropriate level of postoperative surveillance should reflect this degree of risk stratification. Therefore, considerable effort has been devoted to the follow-up and surveillance of patients who have undergone curative-intent surgery. Continued surveillance is imperative to detect both metachronous neoplasms and prevent the development of subsequent cancers. In theory, proper surveillance allows subsequent polyps to be removed before malignant transformation occurs and improve survival by early identification of treatable recurrent cancer. Furthermore, surveillance directs family members of patients with hereditary cancers to receive proper screening and genetic counseling.

A dilemma, however, is the lack of agreement on the most effective surveillance program. Although the majority of colorectal surgeons report some degree of patient surveillance after curative resection, frequency of follow-up and surveillance techniques are largely inconsistent. A survey of American Society of Colon and Rectal Surgeons (ASCRS) members indicates that only 50% of practicing colorectal surgeons follow general surveillance guidelines.[1,2] The importance of disease stage is noted, but the risk of recurrence is also influenced by a variety of other factors, including surgical technique (local vs. radical resection, total mesorectal excision, etc.), primary tumor location, disease clearance, and histologic grade. Patient age and comorbidities, in addition to patterns of recurrence, also influence the intensity of surveillance.

In regards to advances in the detection and treatment of cancer recurrence, select patients will be candidates for resection of locoregional and metastatic recurrence. Many patients benefit from the removal of metachronous benign colorectal neoplasms and follow-up is critical for early identification of the subset of patients who benefit from selective treatment of recurrent malignant disease. Recent improvements in chemotherapy, radiation therapy, and surgery have allowed a relative survival advantage for people diagnosed with stages II and III disease. Furthermore, similar advances have extended median survival from 6 to 16 months for patients with stage IV cancer.[3] In addition to improvements in survival, a population-based study by Guyot et al.[4] demonstrated improvements in resectability and management of recurrent disease. The authors of this study showed that the proportion of patients with recurrent disease resected for cure increased from 6.7% (1976–1984) to 23.7%(1994–2003; $p<0.001$) for distant metastases and from 15.9 to 58.1% ($p<0.001$) for local recurrence. Improvements in outcome for metastatic colorectal cancer were demonstrated by Kopetz et al.[5] through the increased use of hepatic resection and advancements in medical therapy. In this study, 5-year survival improved from 9.1 to 19.2% and the median survival improved from 18 to 29.2 months in selected patients with Stage IV disease.

Risk and Timing of Recurrence

In 2009, approximately 147,000 cases of colon and rectal cancer were diagnosed in the USA. Among these newly diagnosed cases, most patients presented with locoregional disease (Stage I–III) and underwent curative intent surgery. The 5-year survival rate in this collective group ranged from 64 to 90% depending primarily on the stage at presentation.[6] Overall, 30–38% of patients who were treated with curative resection for locoregional disease developed a recurrence.[7,8] Patients with Stage IIb and Stage III disease were at the highest risk of recurrence. The risk of recurrence in those high-risk patients with primary colon or rectal cancer was 40 and 52%, respectively.[9] Approximately 20% of patients presented with Stage IV, or metastatic, disease. Most patients with Stage IV colorectal cancer were not candidates for curative

D.E. Beck et al. (eds.), *The ASCRS Textbook of Colon and Rectal Surgery: Second Edition*,
DOI 10.1007/978-1-4419-1584-9_48,

resection and underwent palliative treatment. Surveillance was not applicable for the patients unless their metastatic disease was limited and resected for cure. The majority of recurrences occur within 2 years of a curative resection, and more than 95% of recurrences are evident within 5 years of surgery. Late recurrence, defined as recurrence after 5 years from initial resection, is certainly unusual and typically represents less than 2% of recurrent cancer diagnoses. The longer interval to recurrence in these patients often reflects the use of adjuvant therapy.[9–12]

Hereditary Colorectal Cancer

Hereditary factors play a role in 10–25% of colorectal cancers, and identification of these patients often influences surgical management and surveillance intensity. Patients who are less than 50 years of age, have multiple polyps or synchronous cancers, or have a personal/family history of a malignancy should be recognized and considered for genetic counseling. The important noncolorectal malignancies to consider are those associated with hereditary nonpolyposis colorectal cancer (HNPCC), such as endometrial, ovarian, ureteral, gastric, and others. Obviously, family history plays a substantial role in identifying these patients and needs to be reviewed thoroughly at the initial consultation. Both HNPCC and familial adenomatous polyposis (FAP) are examples of genetic colorectal cancer syndromes that may affect patients and their families. Recognition of affected individuals alters screening and surveillance strategies for both themselves and their family members. This information may also modify surgical management to include a more extensive or prophylactic surgery, and direct surveillance of other potential sites of malignancy.

Surveillance Measures

Intensity of Follow-Up

The first question that must be answered is whether or not routine follow-up should be offered at all to patients based on a proven survival, recurrence, or quality-of-life benefit. At one extreme of comparison, Ohlsson et al.[13] randomized patients to either no follow-up or an intense follow-up program at frequent intervals after curative surgery for colorectal cancer. Of interest, this study demonstrated no significant difference in overall survival (67% vs. 75%), cancer-specific survival (71% vs. 78%), or tumor recurrence (33% vs. 32%) between the control and follow-up groups despite a rigorous surveillance program. This study alone would suggest that there is no benefit to patient follow-up, although it may have been underpowered. A subsequent study with randomization to either risk-adapted follow-up or minimal follow-up by Secco et al.[14] again validated that follow-up, regardless of intensity, had no impact on tumor recurrence. However, in comparison to Ohlsson et al.,[13] improved survival was statistically significant among patients in risk-adapted follow-up programs versus patients with minimal follow-up. The lack of influence on tumor recurrence from these two studies should not be unexpected considering recurrence is primarily determined by the inherent characteristics of the tumor and its stage at presentation. However, the lack of influence on survival by Ohlsson et al.[13] raises the question as to whether the primary goal of improved survival is achieved by surveillance. In a 2007 collaborative review from the Cochrane Database, Jeffery et al.[15] analyzed eight randomized controlled trials to conclude an overall survival benefit in patients followed by a "more intensive" surveillance program after curative colorectal resection. Furthermore, the utilization of more tests in and of itself was significantly associated with improved overall survival. The variation among program strategies did not allow a standardized recommendation regarding timing, frequency, and components of follow-up.[13,16–21]

History and Physical Examination

Various practice guidelines, including those of the ASCRS, American Society of Clinical Oncology (ASCO), and National Cancer Care Network (NCCN), recommend patient history and clinical examination be performed every 3–6 months for the first 2–3 years after curative resection. Subsequent follow-up then occurs for a total of 5 years of surveillance. Additional follow-up after that time may be warranted based on perceived risk of recurrence and is at the physician's discretion.[22–24] Concerning symptoms include coughing, abdominal or pelvic pain, change in bowel habits, rectal bleeding, and fatigue. The physical exam should include wound examination, lymph node palpation, digital rectal exam, and a pelvic examination for female patients. Unfortunately, patients who present with symptomatic recurrences are less likely to be resected for cure. However, posttreatment surveillance also allows for the evaluation of psychosocial distress after colorectal cancer treatment and potential to offer help for other treatment-related sequelae, such as diarrhea, incontinence, and/or stoma care. It also helps to serve as a reminder for patients to check carcinoembryonic antigen (CEA) levels and schedule subsequent colonoscopies. Moreover, it provides patients a teachable moment in regards to genetics/family risk, and for healthy lifestyle choices. Smoking cessation, a healthy body mass index, exercise, and healthy diet have all been associated with improved outcomes in colorectal cancer.[25–27]

Laboratory Evaluation

The only laboratory test recommended for colorectal cancer surveillance is the serum CEA level. CEA is an oncofetal protein, which is elevated in colorectal cancers along with other gastrointestinal malignancies.[28] Preoperative CEA level does have prognostic value in terms of risk of recurrence. A study by Wiratkapun et al.,[29] prospectively followed 261 patients after potentially curative resection and found that those patients with a preoperative CEA level > 5ng/ml had a worse disease free survival (DFS). At 5 years, recurrence was 7.5% compared to 37.2% in patients with normal versus elevated preoperative CEA levels. In addition, failure of elevated preoperative CEA levels to return to normal after potentially curative resection is a poor prognostic indicator[30] and may represent incomplete surgical resection or occult metastases.

After colorectal cancer resection, post-operative CEA levels should be monitored in patients who are medically fit for further treatment if a recurrence were found. The recommended interval of testing varies between societies; however, most recommend checking CEA levels every 3 months for the first 2–3 years and then biannually up to 5 years after resection. Elevated CEA is often the first sign of recurrent disease. CEA often predates other testing modalities in terms of identifying recurrence with a median lead time of 4.5–8 months.[31–34] Of note, sensitivity is much higher in detecting distant metastatic disease than locoregional disease (92% vs. 62%).[35] CEA sensitivity also varies with the site of recurrence, being 78% sensitive for hepatic metastasis, but only 42 and 45% sensitive for pulmonary and local recurrences, respectively.[34] Furthermore, an elevated CEA level should be rechecked prior to searching for recurrent disease because it may be falsely elevated. The false positive rate for CEA levels range from 7 to 16%.[33,34] CEA levels should not be evaluated while the patient is receiving 5-fluorouracil-based chemotherapy because this may falsely elevate the CEA level.[34]

Serum hemoglobin, liver function tests, and fecal occult blood test should not be used as part of a surveillance regimen. In regards to these tests, the ASCRS, ASCO, and NCCN guidelines are in agreement.[22–24]

Chest Surveillance

The incidence of isolated pulmonary metastases is approximately 5–10% and over 20% of patients who develop recurrent disease after curative resection have pulmonary lesions in addition to other areas of metastases. This pattern of recurrence is variable depending on the initial stage and location of the primary malignancy.[36,37] Even though pulmonary recurrence tends to occur more commonly with rectal cancer rather than colon cancer, both groups are followed collectively according to current surveillance recommendations. Plain chest radiograph (CXR) and chest CT scan are the two available options for chest surveillance and their utilization is not mutually exclusive. As with other surveillance measures, the utilization of chest surveillance requires that a patient is medically fit for pulmonary metastasectomy to justify its use. The ability of surveillance CXR to first detect evidence of cancer recurrence is reportedly under 20%, and more realistically less than 10%.[38,39] Graham et al.[40] identified recurrence in 421 of 1,356 (32%) patients who underwent curative resection of a primary colorectal malignancy. Follow-up CXR was the first indication of recurrence in less than 1% of patients. In contrast, routine chest CT has shown an improved ability to primarily detect occult colorectal cancer recurrence within the chest in asymptomatic individuals and is more sensitive than CXR in identifying resectable pulmonary disease.[41,42] Clear evidence indicating which option is superior is not available and various surveillance programs preferentially use routine CXR or chest CT. ASCRS practice parameters neither support nor refute the use of routine chest radiography for surveillance, yet both ASCO and NCCN recommend annual chest CT for the first 3 years following curative resection.[22–24] ASCO and NCCN guidelines seem to be the most reasonable as abnormal findings on surveillance CXR require further imaging with chest CT prior to metastasectomy. Regardless of which method of surveillance is chosen, initial and repeated pulmonary resection for isolated metastatic disease offers an excellent long-term survival advantage with 2- and 5-year survival rates greater than 60 and 40%, respectively.[43–46] Although the majority of patients have multiple pulmonary lesions and may not be candidates for metastasectomy, routine chest imaging for colorectal follow-up is warranted to identify the subset population of patients who benefit from pulmonary resection.[37]

Abdomen/Pelvis Surveillance

There has been continued improvement in both the identification and treatment of metastatic colorectal cancer, and patients now have more options for the treatment of recurrent and advanced stage disease. The detection of abdominal and pelvic recurrence has primarily focused on hepatic imaging because the liver is the most common site of recurrence. Over 30% of patients ultimately develop hepatic metastasis after curative resection.[36] This typically occurs within the first 3 years after surgery. Recommendations regarding the use of routine liver imaging are influenced by the ability of abdominal CT and/or liver ultrasound to identify liver metastasis before clinical symptoms develop or other modalities of surveillance are positive for recurrence. In general, the accuracy of abdominal CT is superior to liver ultrasound for hepatic metastasis. The sensitivity of liver ultrasound is under 60% for the detection of colorectal metastasis, and the ability of ultrasound to identify liver lesions less than 1 cm is truly inadequate.[47] Abdominal CT, on the other hand, is more accurate and able to detect liver metastasis with sensitivity greater than 75%. Some studies suggest that routine liver imaging with both CT and ultrasound should be included in surveillance programs because of improved ability to identify treatable recurrence. For example, Bleeker et al.[48] reported on 42 of 213 patients with recurrence that underwent resection with curative intent and concluded that combined liver imaging was critical in over 30% of patients for identifying curable recurrence before any other method of surveillance.

The most recent Cochrane review suggested an overall survival benefit when routine liver imaging was included as part of intensive surveillance programs.[15] The utilization of routine liver imaging, however, remains controversial because the identification of liver metastases has not historically translated into subsequent resectability or improved survival in either asymptomatic or symptomatic patients.[21] Other topics of debate include the cost-effectiveness of liver imaging and its ability to complement routine surveillance when other measures are normal. Deveney and Way[49] found similar specificity and sensitivity between a less expensive CEA and more costly abdominal CT for routine follow-up. The ability of hepatic imaging to act as the first indicator of recurrence is low and very rarely does it identify recurrence prior to CEA elevation.[17,20] As a result of these concerns, published guidelines for the use of routine hepatic imaging after curative resection are inconsistent.

The most recent ASCRS published guidelines (2004) do not recommend the routine use of hepatic imaging. This is based on the lack of evidence that identification of hepatic recurrence leads to subsequent resection, the overlap of results between elevated CEA measurement and hepatic imaging, and the cost of routine CT imaging.[23] In contrast, both ASCO and NCCN guidelines recommend annual abdominal CT for 3 years after curative resection in patients who are considered to be both high-risk and candidates for subsequent resection if recurrence is found.[22,24] The recommendations for annual imaging focus on a reduction in mortality when imaging strategies are compared to nonimaging strategies for surveillance. Earlier identification of asymptomatic recurrence allows for curative reoperation and improved survival.[22,36]

In conclusion, there is no clear consensus among published guidelines in regards to routine abdominal imaging after curative resection. There is strong evidence that early identification of hepatic recurrence by CT imaging, particularly in asymptomatic patients, improves survival through subsequent curative resection.[41] Otherwise, liver recurrence left untreated carries a very poor prognosis. The survival benefit demonstrated in patients who undergo curative resection, therefore, should prompt serious consideration to imaging strategies in patients at high-risk for recurrence.[50] Clearly, the benefit of liver imaging is best realized when it is used as an adjunct to other modes of surveillance (in-office visit, CEA), and not as a single strategy.

Endoscopic Surveillance

The options for endoscopic evaluation after curative resection include colonoscopy, flexible sigmoidoscopy, and rigid proctoscopy with or without endorectal ultrasound (ERUS). The full benefit of endoscopic surveillance is clearly dependent on clearing the colon and rectum of synchronous neoplasms in the perioperative period. Synchronous colorectal polyps and cancers occur in 30 and 5% of patients, respectively, and their identification at index colonoscopy may change the operative management of a patient.[51,52] Preoperative colonoscopy, or post-operative colonoscopy within 6 months of surgery, is therefore fundamental in the management of patients with a newly diagnosed colorectal cancer. After curative resection, endoscopic surveillance is designed to detect metachronous colorectal neoplasms and early disease recurrence. The timing and frequency of this surveillance is variable among published consensus guidelines and a source of debate.

Metachronous Colon and Rectal Neoplasms

A prior diagnosis of colorectal cancer is a significant risk factor for the subsequent development of polyps and/or cancer. Unlike colorectal cancer recurrence, which typically occurs within 2–3 years after treatment, the risk of developing metachronous colorectal neoplasms is collective over the life of a patient. Metachronous polyps occur in up to 50% of patients and metachronous cancers develop in 2–9% of individuals with a prior colorectal cancer diagnosis.[53,54] A recent systematic review of post-cancer resection surveillance by the US Multi-Society Task Force on Colorectal Cancer described 137 metachronous colorectal cancers among 9,029 patients (approximately 1.5%). Fifty-seven of the 137 malignancies reportedly occurred within 24 months of initial resection. Although some lesions likely may have been missed synchronous lesions, a high incidence of early metachronous cancers were identified. The majority of metachronous lesions were asymptomatic, discovered at an early stage by endoscopic surveillance, and resected for cure. This prompted a joint update by the US Multi-Society Task Force and American Cancer Society to recommend intraluminal surveillance with post-resection colonoscopy 1 year after surgery.[55] Although metachronous cancers were reported within 2 years of surgery, it is understood that they can develop over an extended period of time from the initial diagnosis and patients generally require long-term endoscopic follow-up.[56]

According to their most recent update for colon and rectal cancer surveillance in 2004, the ASCRS Standards Practice Task Force has not endorsed the utility of early (1-year) post-resection colonoscopy. ASCRS practice guidelines indicate that the initial posttreatment colonoscopy should occur 3 years after resection and at subsequent 3-year intervals.[23] Obviously, clinical judgment recognizes that certain risk factors place some patients at greater risk for developing metachronous lesions. This influences the need for endoscopic evaluation with different timing and frequency. Patients who are at risk for hereditary colorectal cancer syndromes should undergo more frequent surveillance endoscopy. The absence of synchronous neoplasms at the initial diagnosis of colorectal cancer confers a lower risk of metachronous lesions.[57] The physician responsible for index colonoscopy should be considered in determining the timing of post-resection colonoscopy, as well. Hyman et al.[58] suggest a lower incidence of high-risk metachronous lesions at 1-year post-resection colonoscopy if the operating surgeon was responsible for the index colonoscopy. Overall, most authors recommend 1-year colonoscopy based on the reported higher risk and incidence of metachronous neoplasms within 2 years and the reality of missed synchronous lesions.[42,59] In consideration of the risk associated with metachronous lesions, colonoscopy is the only option for continued endoscopic surveillance after curative resection. All other options are insufficient.

Locally Recurrent Colon Cancer

In addition to the identification of metachronous lesions, endoscopic surveillance is also utilized to discover local and anastomotic recurrence of colorectal cancer. Unlike metachronous colorectal neoplasms, recurrent colorectal cancer typically occurs within 2–3 years after initial treatment. There is a distinct difference, however, between local recurrence rates of colon cancer and rectal cancer, and their respective patterns of recurrence require different approaches to surveillance. Endoscopic surveillance for recurrent colon cancer has limited utility because of local and anastomotic recurrence is unusual. Distal recurrence is much more typical and not identifiable by endoscopic surveillance. Intraluminal recurrence of colon cancer typically occurs in only 2–4% of patients after resection and the time to recurrence is generally 13–16 months.[60] The low incidence of local recurrence is recognized by ASCRS practice parameters, and periodic evaluation of the colonic anastomosis is not endorsed.[23] Surveillance of metachronous lesions allows for concurrent anastomotic evaluation by the visualization of prior surgery sites and mucosal biopsy as indicated. The incidence of local recurrence is quite low even with poor-risk factors. Harris et al.[61] defined factors predictive of local recurrence to include advanced stage of disease, poor differentiation, perforation, and fistula formation. Nevertheless, routine anastomotic biopsy is not indicated in the absence of mucosal abnormality. Unfortunately, local anastomotic recurrence is frequently associated with unresectable widespread colon cancer recurrence.

Locally Recurrent Rectal Cancer

Locally recurrent rectal cancer is more common than locally recurrent colon cancer; yet, endoscopic visualization remains limited because of the tendency for local rectal cancer recurrence to begin extraluminally. Total mesorectal excision (TME) and chemoradiation therapy have both contributed to improved tumor clearance and locoregional control of rectal cancer. Studies have reported that 5-year local and systemic recurrence rates are 4 and 18%, respectively, with TME.[62] Such improvements translate into patterns of recurrence that make endoscopic follow-up beneficial in only a small percentage of patients because primary anastomotic, or intraluminal, recurrence is low assuming proper surgical technique is employed. ASCO recommends 6-month endoscopic evaluation by flexible sigmoidoscopy or rigid proctoscopy for rectal cancer recurrence in patients who have not received pelvic radiation.[22] Although the exact schedule for surveillance is not defined, periodic anastomotic evaluation is recommended by the most recent ASCRS guidelines. This is despite the fact that intraluminal recurrence is relatively low in comparison to other patterns of recurrence.[26] Local extraluminal recurrence, on the other hand, remains a problem for patients after rectal cancer resection and typically reflects advanced stage disease or incomplete tumor clearance. Circumferential resection margins have been validated as an important prognostic indicator for both local and distant failure.[63,64] Other factors that increase local recurrence and affirm the need for continued endoscopic surveillance include lymphovascular or perineural invasion and lymph node positive disease.[65] As a consequence of extraluminal recurrence, post-resection surveillance not only requires the ability to evaluate the anastomosis, but the ability to look outside the lumen, as well. Visualization of low anastomoses by flexible sigmoidoscopy or rigid proctoscopy is therefore enhanced with other modalities of endoscopic surveillance, such as ERUS.

Practice guidelines for post-resection ERUS have not been firmly established in part because operator dependence and questions regarding the ability of ERUS to differentiate between benign and malignant changes raise concern. Lower sensitivity (65%) is reflective of its inability to differentiate between benign and malignant changes after surgery and/or radiation.[66] Of 44 patients with locally recurrent rectal cancer following local or radical excision, 80% of recurrences were detected on ERUS. Fourteen asymptomatic patients (approximately 30%) were solely diagnosed by ERUS after normal digital examination and endoscopic surveillance.[67] Further studies suggest that ERUS is a useful adjunct to rectal cancer surveillance, however, its position in current guidelines is lacking until further prospective data confirms its impact on survival and changes in patient management.[39]

Positron Emission Tomography

Positron emission tomography (PET) technology uses radiotracers to detect and quantify cellular and biochemical processes noninvasively. ^{18}F-2-fluoro-2-deoxy-D-glucose (FDG) is the most common radiotracer used in oncology. FDG concentrates in malignant tissue because of an increase in glycolysis compared to normal tissue. This modality is frequently combined with CT scans to improve anatomical and functional detail. NCCN guidelines do not recommend routine surveillance with PET scans in detecting recurrences without other evidence of recurrent or metastatic disease.[24]

However, FDG-PET scanning has developed a role in the evaluation of recurrent disease and in the setting of suspected recurrence. For those patients who are asymptomatic with an elevated CEA level, the diagnostic sensitivity and positive predictive value of PET for recurrence is 95.3%.[68] A meta-analysis by Huebner et al., found an overall sensitivity and specificity of 97 and 76%, respectively, for FDG-PET detecting recurrent colorectal cancer. PET imaging changed management in 29% of the patients.[69] Moreover, FDG-PET helps to predict resectability of recurrence and improves the selection of appropriate surgical candidates. A randomized study by Sobhani et al.[70] added PET scan to the surveillance of colorectal cancer patients with a high risk of recurrence. These patients had Stage III or IV disease who had undergone an R0 resection and completed adjuvant chemotherapy. PET scan was performed at 9 and 15 months compared to the conventional group which had a CT scan at those time points. The PET group had a significantly shorter time to recurrence (12.1 vs. 15.4 months, $p=0.01$) and recurrences were more frequently removed for curative intent (R0, $p<0.01$).[70]

Abnormal Results

Abnormal results from surveillance prompt further investigations to detect, confirm, or exclude recurrence. If the CEA level rises after resection, management should include physical exam, colonoscopy and CT of the chest, abdomen, and pelvis. If the work-up is negative, consideration should be given to PET scanning as well. Repeat CT scans should be done every 3 months until recurrent disease is identified or the CEA stabilizes or declines.[24] Abnormalities may require further evaluation, such as biopsies or serial imaging, to confirm lesion stability. If recurrence is identified, PET scan should be performed and consideration given to further resection if possible.

Quality of Life

Surveillance after colorectal cancer resection can be stressful for patients and have a significant impact upon their quality of life. Patients undergo many tests that may lead to further investigations or treatments. Moreover, these tests have a false positive rate and examinations, such as colonoscopy have associated risks. Various studies have looked at the impact of surveillance on the quality of life. A study by Kjeldsen et al.[71] only found marginal benefit to surveillance for health-related quality of life, which did not justify the expense of follow-up. In comparison, Stiggelbout et al.[72] reported a positive attitude toward surveillance in that it reassured the patients. Patients experienced slight nervous anticipation, but expressed a strong preference for follow-up even if it would not lead to earlier detection of a recurrence.

Cost-Effectiveness

When considering an intensive surveillance regimen, expense needs to be considered. Since different societies have disparity among their follow-up regimens, there is a variable cost to the insurers. Using 5-year Medicare allowed charges, the cost between follow-up regimens varied between \$910 and \$26,717 per patient.[73] Another study performed in the UK, found that the adjusted extra cost for each patient was \$4,288 and for each life year gained was \$5,885.[74] Another study performed in France, divided the cost-effectiveness of surveillance between Stage I and II disease compared to Stage III. Only Stage III patients had a favorable cost-effective analysis of 1,058 Euro per quality-adjusted life-years.[75]

Surveillance Effectiveness and Meta-analyses

The effectiveness of surveillance after curative resection is based on its ability to detect recurrent and/or metachronous disease at a point in time when subsequent curative treatment is successful. Of equal importance is a willing patient who is healthy enough to undergo potential therapy. Most surgeons would agree that patients should receive some degree of follow-up after curative resection of colon and rectal cancer. Some studies have shown that intensive follow-up has demonstrated a small but significant survival advantage over minimal or no follow-up after curative resection.[15,36,76] Improved detection of resectable recurrence has been demonstrated with intense surveillance, as well.[13,77] When compared with minimal follow-up, intense surveillance delivers a 5-year improvement in overall survival of 7–10%. The process is most likely multifactorial and is thought to be secondary to earlier detection of both locoregional disease and curable liver metastasis. Earlier palliative chemotherapy and downstaging of pelvic tumors after radiation therapy also play a role.[15,76,78]

Surveillance strategies, however, are limited because the benefits from the independent components of a surveillance program are difficult to validate. Strategies are often classified as "less-intensive" or "more-" or "highly-intensive" and there is considerable variability among intensive-surveillance groups. The literature does not really define what is meant by "more intense follow-up" and this lack of standardization affects the ability to identify which methods of surveillance are truly critical to survival and patient care.[78,79] Although a number of measures are available, the primary components of follow-up include history and physical examination, serial tumor marker measurement, radiographic imaging, and endoscopic evaluation. Still, physicians have multiple options that can be employed at different frequency and intensity.[47]

Different meta-analyses of the available randomized-controlled trials[15,36,76,80] show a significant survival benefit with intensive surveillance compared to nonintensive surveillance. The meta-analysis by Tjandra et al.[76] demonstrated a significant reduction in overall mortality in patients receiving intensive follow-up compared to nonintensive follow-up (21.8 vs. 25.7%; $p=0.01$). CEA surveillance and

TABLE 48-1. Summary of recommended surveillance protocols

Test/procedure	ASCRS [23]	ASCO [22]	NCCN [24]
History and physical	Minimum of 3 times per year for the first 2 years	Every 3–6 months for 3 years, then every 6 months during years 4 and 5, then per physician discretion	Every 3–6 months for 2 years, then every 6 months for 5 years
CEA	Minimum of 3 times per year for the first 2 years	Every 3 months for 3 years or longer, for patients with Stage II or III disease	Every 3–6 months for 2 years, then every 6 months for 5 years for T2 or greater
Flexible sigmoidoscopy or proctoscopy for rectal cancer patients	Periodic anastomotic evaluation is recommended for patients who have undergone resection/ anastomosis or local excision of rectal cancer	Every 6 months for 5 years for patients who have not received pelvic irradiation	Consider proctoscopy every 6 months for 5 years
Colonoscopy	Every 3 years	At 3 years then every 5 years if normal	At 1 year, if advanced adenoma repeat in 1 year, if none repeat in 3 years, then every 5 years
Computed tomography of the chest–abdomen–pelvis	Not recommended	CT chest/abdomen every 1 year for 3 years, consider CT pelvis for rectal cancer patients especially if they have not received radiation therapy	Annually for 3 years, for patients at high risk for recurrence
Fecal occult blood test	Not recommended	Not addressed	Not addressed
Complete blood count	Not recommended	Not recommended	Not addressed
Liver function tests	Not recommended	Not recommended	Not addressed
Chest radiography	Not recommended	Not recommended	Not recommended
Abdominal ultrasound	Not recommended	Not addressed	Not addressed

These are the recommended surveillance protocols for those patients who are candidates for further intervention.

colonoscopy significantly influenced overall mortality, while intensive surveillance detected asymptomatic recurrence earlier and more frequently. Recurrences that were more amenable to curable resection were found more commonly during intensive follow-up. In this study, the cancer-related mortality was not improved and the survival benefit was not related to earlier detection and treatment of recurrent disease. Due to the disparities between the different meta-analyses, it is not possible to say specifically what frequency or combination of surveillance modalities yields the improved survival benefit. Table 48-1 summarizes the recommended surveillance protocols.

Conclusions

Colon and rectal cancer surveillance after curative resection is recommended for patients who can tolerate further surgery or therapy if needed. The optimal surveillance protocol has not been established, however, general agreement supports the use of routine office visits, serum tumor marker measurement, and endoscopic surveillance for post-resection follow-up. Although the timing and frequency of surveillance measures is variable, continued follow-up is recommended based on improved overall survival with intensive surveillance programs.

Acknowledgments. This chapter was authored by Brett T. Gemlo and David A. Rothenberger in the previous version of this textbook.

References

1. Giordano P, Efron J, Vernava 3rd AM, Weiss EG, Nogueras JJ, Wexner SD. Strategies of follow-up for colorectal cancer: a survey of the American Society of Colon and Rectal Surgeons. Tech Coloproctol. 2006;10(3):199–207.
2. Vernava 3rd AM, Longo WE, Virgo KS, Coplin MA, Wade TP, Johnson FE. Current follow-up strategies after resection of colon cancer. Results of a survey of members of the American Society of Colon and Rectal Surgeons. Dis Colon Rectum. 1994;37(6):573–83.
3. Meyerhardt JA, Mayer RJ. Follow-up strategies after curative resection of colorectal cancer. Semin Oncol. 2003;30(3): 349–60.
4. Guyot F, Faivre J, Manfredi S, Meny B, Bonithon-Kopp C, Bouvier AM. Time trends in the treatment and survival of recurrences from colorectal cancer. Ann Oncol. 2005;16(5): 756–61.
5. Kopetz S, Chang GJ, Overman MJ, Eng C, Sargent DJ, Larson DW, et al. Improved survival in metastatic colorectal cancer is associated with adoption of hepatic resection and improved chemotherapy. J Clin Oncol. 2009;27(22):3677–83.
6. Jemal A, Siegel R, Ward E, Hao Y, Xu J, Thun MJ. Cancer statistics, 2009. CA Cancer J Clin. 2009;59(4):225–49.
7. Böhm B, Schwenk W, Hucke HP, Stock W. Does methodic long-term follow-up affect survival after curative resection of colorectal carcinoma? Dis Colon Rectum. 1993;36(3):280–6.
8. Rao AR, Kagan AR, Chan PM, Gilbert HA, Nussbaum H, Hintz BL. Patterns of recurrence following curative resection alone for adenocarcinoma of the rectum and sigmoid colon. Cancer. 1981;48(6):1492–5.
9. Galandiuk S, Wieand HS, Moertel CG, Cha SS, Fitzgibbons Jr RJ, Pemberton JH, et al. Patterns of recurrence after curative

resection of carcinoma of the colon and rectum. Surg Gynecol Obstet. 1992;174(1):27–32.
10. Kobayashi H, Mochizuki H, Sugihara K, Morita T, Kotake K, Teramoto T, et al. Characteristics of recurrence and surveillance tools after curative resection for colorectal cancer: a multicenter study. Surgery. 2007;141(1):67–75.
11. Griffin MR, Bergstralh EJ, Coffey RJ, Beart Jr RW, Melton 3rd LJ. Predictors of survival after curative resection of carcinoma of the colon and rectum. Cancer. 1987;60(9):2318–24.
12. Cho YB, Chun HK, Yun HR, Lee WS, Yun SH, Lee WY. Clinical and pathologic evaluation of patients with recurrence of colorectal cancer five or more years after curative resection. Dis Colon Rectum. 2007;50(8):1204–10.
13. Ohlsson B, Breland U, Ekberg H, Graffner H, Tranberg KG. Follow-up after curative surgery for colorectal carcinoma. Randomized comparison with no follow-up. Dis Colon Rectum. 1995;38(6):619–26.
14. Secco GB, Fardelli R, Gianquinto D, Bonfante P, Baldi E, Ravera G, et al. Efficacy and cost of risk-adapted follow-up in patients after colorectal cancer surgery: a prospective, randomized and controlled trial. Eur J Surg Oncol. 2002;28(4):418–23.
15. Jeffery M, Hickey BE, Hider PN. Follow-up strategies for patients treated for non-metastatic colorectal cancer. Cochrane Database Syst Rev. 2007;(1):CD002200.
16. Kjeldsen BJ, Kronborg O, Fenger C, Jørgensen OD. A prospective randomized study of follow-up after radical surgery for colorectal cancer. Br J Surg. 1997;84(5):666–9.
17. Mäkelä JT, Laitinen SO, Kairaluoma MI. Five-year follow-up after radical surgery for colorectal cancer. Results of a prospective randomized trial. Arch Surg. 1995;130(10):1062–7.
18. Pietra N, Sarli L, Costi R, Ouchemi C, Grattarola M, Peracchia A. Role of follow-up in management of local recurrences of colorectal cancer: a prospective, randomized study. Dis Colon Rectum. 1998;41(9):1127–33.
19. Rodríguez-Moranta F, Saló J, Arcusa A, Boadas J, Piñol V, Bessa X, et al. Postoperative surveillance in patients with colorectal cancer who have undergone curative resection: a prospective, multicenter, randomized, controlled trial. J Clin Oncol. 2006;24(3):386–93.
20. Schoemaker D, Black R, Giles L, Toouli J. Yearly colonoscopy, liver CT, and chest radiography do not influence 5-year survival of colorectal cancer patients. Gastroenterology. 1998; 114(1):7–14.
21. Wattchow DA, Weller DP, Esterman A, Pilotto LS, McGorm K, Hammett Z, et al. General practice vs. surgical-based follow-up for patients with colon cancer: randomised controlled trial. Br J Cancer. 2006;94(8):1116–21.
22. Desch CE, Benson 3rd AB, Somerfield MR, Flynn PJ, Krause C, Loprinzi CL, et al. Colorectal cancer surveillance: 2005 update of an American Society of Clinical Oncology practice guideline. J Clin Oncol. 2005;23(33):8512–9.
23. Anthony T, Simmang C, Hyman N, Buie D, Kim D, Cataldo P, et al. Practice parameters for the surveillance and follow-up of patients with colon and rectal cancer. Dis Colon Rectum. 2004;47(6):807–17.
24. Engstrom PF, Arnoletti JP, Benson AB 3rd, Chen YJ, Choti MA, Cooper HS, et al. NCCN Clinical Practice Guidelines in Oncology: Colon Cancer. J Natl Compr Canc Netw. 2009;7(8): 778–831.
25. Dignam JJ, Polite BN, Yothers G, Raich P, Colangelo L, O'Connell MJ, et al. Body mass index and outcomes in patients who receive adjuvant chemotherapy for colon cancer. J Natl Cancer Inst. 2006;98(22):1647–54.
26. Meyerhardt JA, Heseltine D, Niedzwiecki D, Hollis D, Saltz LB, Mayer RJ, et al. Impact of physical activity on cancer recurrence and survival in patients with Stage III colon cancer: findings from CALGB 89803. J Clin Oncol. 2006;24(22): 3535–41.
27. Meyerhardt JA, Niedzwiecki D, Hollis D, Saltz LB, Hu FB, Mayer RJ, et al. Association of dietary patterns with cancer recurrence and survival in patients with Stage III colon cancer. JAMA. 2007;298(7):754–64.
28. Goldstein MJ, Mitchell EP. Carcinoembryonic antigen in the staging and follow-up of patients with colorectal cancer. Cancer Invest. 2005;23(4):338–51.
29. Wiratkapun S, Kraemer M, Seow-Choen F, Ho YK, Euk W. High preoperative serum CEA predicts metastatic recurrence in potentially curable colon cancer. Dis Colon Rectum. 2001;44(2):231–5.
30. Slentz K, Senagore AJ, Hibbert J, Mazier WP, Talbott TM. Can preoperative and postoperative CEA predict survival after colon cancer resection? Am Surg. 1994;60(7):528–32.
31. Martin EW, Minton JP, Carey LC. CEA-directed second-look surgery in the asymptomatic patient after primary resection of colorectal carcinoma. Ann Surg. 1983;202:310–7.
32. Allen-Mersh TG. Aspects of treatment. Serum CEA in the follow-up of colorectal carcinoma. Experience in a district general hospital. Ann R Coll Surg Eng. 1984;66:751–5.
33. McCall JL, Black RB, Rich CA, et al. The value of serum carcinoembryonic antigen in predicting recurrent disease following curative resection of colorectal cancer. Dis Colon Rectum. 1994;37:875–81.
34. Moertel CG, Fleming TR, Macdonald JS, Haller DG, Lauri JA, Tangen CM. An evaluation of the carcinoembryonic antigen test for monitoring patients with resected colon cancer. JAMA. 1993;270:943–7.
35. Carriquiry L, Pineyro A. Should CEA be used in the management of patients with colorectal cancer? Dis Colon Rectum. 1999;42(7):921–9.
36. Figuerado A, Rumble RB, Maroun J, Earle CC, Cummings B, McLeod R, et al. Follow-up of patients with curatively resected colorectal cancer: a practice guideline. BMC Cancer. 2003;3:26.
37. Fazio VW, Church JM, Delaney CP. Current therapy in colon and rectal surgery. 2nd ed. Philadelphia: Elsevier Mosby Publishing; 2005. Chapter 67, Page 405.
38. Tsikitis VL, Malireddy K, Green EA, Christensen B, Whelan R, Hyder J, et al. Postoperative surveillance recommendations for early stage colon cancer based on results from the clinical outcomes of surgical therapy trial. J Clin Oncol. 2009;27(22):3671–6.
39. Abir F, Alva S, Longo WE, Audiso R, Virgo KS, Johnson FE. The postoperative surveillance of patients with colon cancer and rectal cancer. Am J Surg. 2006;192(1):100–8.
40. Graham RA, Wang S, Catalano PJ, Haller DG. Postsurgical surveillance of colon cancer: preliminary cost analysis of physician examination, carcinoembryonic antigen testing, chest x-ray, and colonoscopy. Ann Surg. 1998;228(1):59–63.

41. Chau I, Allen MJ, Cunningham D, Norman AR, Brown G, Ford HE, et al. The value of routine serum carcino-embryonic antigen measurement and computed tomography in the surveillance of patients after adjuvant chemotherapy for colorectal cancer. J Clin Oncol. 2004;22(8):1420–9.
42. Schwartz RW, McKenzie S. Update on postoperative colorectal cancer surveillance. Curr Surg. 2005;62(5):491–4.
43. Yedibela S, Klein P, Feuchter K, Hoffmann M, Meyer T, Papadopoulos T, et al. Surgical management of pulmonary metastases from colorectal cancer in 153 patients. Ann Surg Oncol. 2006;13(11):1538–44.
44. Rena O, Casadio C, Viano F, Cristofori R, Ruffini E, Filosso PL, et al. Pulmonary resection for metastases from colorectal cancer: factors influencing prognosis. Twenty-year experience. Eur J Cardiothorac Surg. 2002;21(5):906–12.
45. Watanabe K, Nagai K, Kobayashi A, Sugito M, Saito N. Factors influencing survival after complete resection of pulmonary metastases from colorectal cancer. Br J Surg. 2009;96(9): 1058–65.
46. Park JS, Kim HK, Choi YS, Kim K, Shim YM, Jo J, et al. Outcomes after repeated resection for recurrent pulmonary metastases from colorectal cancer. Ann Oncol. 2010;21(6): 1285–9.
47. Longo WE, Johnson FE. The preoperative assessment and postoperative surveillance of patients with colon and rectal cancer. Surg Clin North Am. 2002;82(5):1091–108.
48. Bleeker WA, Mulder NH, Hermans J, Otter R, Plukker JT. Value and cost of follow-up after adjuvant treatment of patients with Dukes' C colonic cancer. Br J Surg. 2001;88(1):101–6.
49. Deveney KE, Way LW. Follow-up of patients with colorectal cancer. Am J Surg. 1984;148(6):717–22.
50. Cummings LC, Payes JD, Cooper GS. Survival after hepatic resection in metastatic colorectal cancer: a population-based study. Cancer. 2007;109(4):718–26.
51. Langevin JM, Nivatvongs S. The true incidence of synchronous cancer of the large bowel. A prospective study. Am J Surg. 1984;147(3):330–3.
52. Piñol V, Andreu M, Castells A, Payá A, Bessa X, Jover R, et al. Synchronous colorectal neoplasms in patients with colorectal cancer: predisposing individual and familial factors. Dis Colon Rectum. 2004;47(7):1192–200.
53. Chen F, Stuart M. Colonoscopic follow-up of colorectal carcinoma. Dis Colon Rectum. 1994;37(6):568–72.
54. Ballesté B, Bessa X, Piñol V, Castellví-Bel S, Castells A, Alenda C, et al. Detection of metachronous neoplasms in colorectal cancer patients: identification of risk factors. Dis Colon Rectum. 2007;50(7):971–80.
55. Rex DK, Kahi CJ, Levin B, Smith RA, Bond JH, Brooks D, et al. Guidelines for colonoscopy surveillance after cancer resection: a consensus update by the American Cancer Society and the US Multi-Society Task Force on Colorectal Cancer. Gastroenterology. 2006;130(6):1865–71.
56. Goldberg RM, Fleming TR, Tangen CM, Moertel CG, Macdonald JS, Haller DG, et al. Surgery for recurrent colon cancer: strategies for identifying resectable recurrence and success rates after resection. Eastern Cooperative Oncology Group, the North Central Cancer Treatment Group, and the Southwest Oncology Group. Ann Intern Med. 1998;129(1):27–35.
57. Rajaratnam SG, Dennett ER. Development of metachronous neoplasms after colorectal cancer resection: absence of synchronous neoplasms predicts a lower risk. N Z Med J. 2009; 122(1294):61–6.
58. Hyman N, Moore J, Cataldo P, Osler T. The high yield of 1-year colonoscopy after resection: is it the handoff? Surg Endosc. 2010;24(3):648–52.
59. Heresbach D, Barrioz T, Lapalus MG, Coumaros D, Bauret P, Potier P, et al. Miss rate for colorectal neoplastic polyps: a prospective multicenter study of back-to-back video colonoscopies. Endoscopy. 2008;40(4):284–90.
60. Obrand DI, Gordon PH. Incidence and patterns of recurrence following curative resection for colorectal carcinoma. Dis Colon Rectum. 1997;40(1):15–24.
61. Harris GJ, Church JM, Senagore AJ, Lavery IC, Hull TL, Strong SA, et al. Factors affecting local recurrence of colonic adenocarcinoma. Dis Colon Rectum. 2002;45(8):1029–34.
62. MacFarlane JK, Ryall RD, Heald RJ. Mesorectal excision for rectal cancer. Lancet. 1993;341(8843):457–60.
63. Nagtegaal ID, Quirke P. What is the role for the circumferential margin in the modern treatment of rectal cancer? J Clin Oncol. 2008;26(2):303–12.
64. Bernstein TE, Endreseth BH, Romundstad P, Wibe A, Norwegian Colorectal Cancer Group. Circumferential resection margin as a prognostic factor in rectal cancer. Br J Surg. 2009;96(11):1348–57.
65. Kim NK, Kim YW, Min BS, Lee KY, Sohn SK, Cho CH. Factors associated with local recurrence after neoadjuvant chemoradiation with total mesorectal excision for rectal cancer. World J Surg. 2009;33(8):1741–9.
66. Romano G, Esercizio L, Santangelo M, Vallone G, Santangelo ML. Impact of computed tomography vs. intrarectal ultrasound on the diagnosis, resectability, and prognosis of locally recurrent rectal cancer. Dis Colon Rectum. 1993;36(3):261–5.
67. de Anda EH, Lee SH, Finne CO, Rothenberger DA, Madoff RD, Garcia-Aguilar J. Endorectal ultrasound in the follow-up of rectal cancer patients treated by local excision or radical surgery. Dis Colon Rectum. 2004;47(6):818–24.
68. Shen YY, Liang JA, Chen YK, Tsai CY, Kao CH. Clinical impact of 18F-FDG-PET in the suspicion of recurrent colorectal cancer based on asymptomatically elevated serum level of carcinoembryonic antigen in Taiwan. Hepatogastroenterology. 2006;53(69):348–50.
69. Huebner RH, Park KC, Shepherd JE, Schwimmer J, Czernin J, Phelps M, et al. A meta-analysis of the literature for whole-body FDG PET detection of recurrent colorectal cancer. J Nucl Med. 2000;41:1177–89.
70. Sobhani I, Tiret E, Lebtahi R, Aparicio T, Itti E, Montravers F, et al. Early detection of recurrence by ^{18}FDG-PET in the follow-up of patients with colorectal cancer. Br J Cancer. 2008;98:875–80.
71. Kjeldsen BJ, Thorsen H, Whalley D, Kronborg O. Influence of follow-up on health-related quality of life after radical surgery for colorectal cancer. Scand J Gastroenterol. 1999;34(5): 509–15.
72. Stiggelbout AM, de Haes JCJM, Vree R, van de Velde CJH, Bruijninckx CMA, van Groninger K, et al. Follow-up of colorectal cancer patients: quality of life and attitudes towards follow-up. Br J Cancer. 1997;75(6):914–20.
73. Virgo KS, Vernava AM, Longo WE, McKirgan LW, Johnson FE. Cost of patient follow-up after potentially

curative colorectal cancer treatment. JAMA. 1995;273(23): 1837–41.
74. Renehan AG, O'Dwyer ST, Whynes DK. Cost effectiveness analysis of intensive versus conventional follow up after curative resection for colorectal cancer. BMJ. 2004; 328(7431):81.
75. Borie F, Combescure C, Daures JP, Tretarre B, Millat B. Cost-effectiveness of two follow-up strategies for curative resection of colorectal cancer: comparative study using a Markov model. World J Surg. 2004;28(6):563–9.
76. Tjandra JJ, Chan MKY. Follow-up after curative resection of colorectal cancer: a meta-analysis. Dis Colon Rectum. 2007;50: 1783–99.
77. Ohlsson B, Pålsson B. Follow-up after colorectal cancer surgery. Acta Oncol. 2003;42(8):816–26.
78. Gan S, Wilson K, Hollington P. Surveillance of patients following surgery with curative intent for colorectal cancer. World J Gastroenterol. 2007;13(28):3816–23.
79. Pfister DG, Benson 3rd AB, Somerfield MR. Clinical practice. Surveillance strategies after curative treatment of colorectal cancer. N Engl J Med. 2004;350(23):2375–82.
80. Renehan AG, Egger M, Saunders MP, O'Dwyer ST. Impact on survival of intensive follow up after curative resection for colorectal cancer: systematic review and meta-analysis of randomized trials. BMJ. 2002;324(7341):813.

49 Miscellaneous Neoplasms

Robin P. Boushey and Husein Moloo

While adenomas and adenocarcinoma account for the majority of colorectal neoplasms, several other less frequent types of malignancy can occur, which can often present as diagnostic and therapeutic challenges to the clinician. These tumors can be classified based on their tissue of origin and include epithelial, mesenchymal, neural, vascular, or lymphoid tumors.

Carcinoid Tumors

The clinical presentation of carcinoid tumors was first described in 1888 by Lubarsch. In 1907, Oberndorfer coined the term carcinoid ("karzinoid") as these tumors were noted to behave differently from adenocarcinoma, acting in a more indolent fashion. Carcinoid tumors are neuroendocrine in origin and originate from Kulchitsky cells in the crypts of Lieberkuhn which represent a type of enterochromaffin cell.[1] They belong to the amine precursor uptake and decarboxylation (APUD) system. These cells are argentaffin positive (silver staining) and usually argyrophilic meaning they are capable of silver staining with the addition of an external reducing agent. These cells use various amine precursors to synthesize various biologically active compounds that exert their biological actions locally and systemically. This includes several hormones, neuropeptides, and neurotransmitters such as serotonin, adrenocorticotrophic hormone, bradykinin, histamine, dopamine, substance P, neurotensin, kallikrein, and prostaglandins E and F.[2] As such, in 1969 Pearse used the term "APUDomas" to describe carcinoid tumors. While neuroendocrine tumors of the gastrointestinal tract are rare, carcinoid tumors are the most common.

Incidence and Classification

Carcinoid tumors can develop in a wide range of organs including the lungs, bronchi, and gastrointestinal tract. Approximately 67% arise within the gastrointestinal tract and about 25% arise within the bronchopulmonary system. The incidence is slightly higher in African Americans and there appears to be a higher incidence in females (as high as 2:1 in some reports). Tumors most commonly occur between the fifth and seventh decade of life.

Several classification schemes have been proposed to categorize carcinoid tumors; however, the most commonly utilized scheme involved classification based on embryological origin. (1) Foregut tumors originating from the lung, bronchus, thymus, stomach, pancreas, and duodenum. (2) Midgut tumors arising from the small intestine, appendix, and right colon. (3) Hidgut tumors arising from the distal colon and rectum.[1]

Within the intestinal tract, midgut carcinoids are most common and account for 62% of all carcinoids, while foregut and hindgut carcinoids account for 7 and 30%, respectively. The greatest density of APUD cells are within the distal small intestine, and as such the most common site for a carcinoid tumor to develop is within the appendix (35%) and small intestine (23%), usually within two feet of the ileocecal valve. Rectal carcinoid tumors account for approximately 20% of all gastrointestinal carcinoids and account for 1% of all rectal tumors. Synchronous carcinoid tumors occur in approximately 25% of patients with foregut and midgut carcinoids while synchronous carcinoid tumors are rare with hind gut tumors. Irrespective of the site of origin, carcinoid tumors are associated with an increased incidence of other malignant tumors that includes gastric, esophageal, colorectal, lung, prostate, and urinary tract tumors. In some series, that estimated incidence to be as high as 50% and is thought to be a result of the trophic effects of the various hormones and peptides secreted by the carcinoid primary including bombesin, gastrin, and cholecystokinin.[1]

Pathology

Grossly, these tumors have a very typical appearance that includes a rounded, well-circumscribed submucosal lesion that are yellow in color on sectioning because of the high lipid content of the tumor. They are often multicentric and <2 cm in size.

D.E. Beck et al. (eds.), *The ASCRS Textbook of Colon and Rectal Surgery: Second Edition*,
DOI 10.1007/978-1-4419-1584-9_49, © Springer Science+Business Media, LLC 2011

Microscopically, carcinoid tumors are composed of small round uniform cells that contain very dense neurosecretory granules that are packed with various secretory peptides. They generally have benign cytoplasmic features and only rare mitotic figures are seen. They have five histologic patterns that include insular, trabecular, glandular, undifferentiated, and mixed. Pathologic analysis alone is rarely able to distinguish a benign from a malignant carcinoid tumor, although increased cellular atypia, high mitotic activity, or necrosis are suggestive of more aggressive tumors and are termed atypical/anaplastic carcinoid tumors.

Traditionally, silver staining has been used to confirm the diagnosis of carcinoid tumors as serotonin is capable of reducing silver salts to metallic silver following carcinoid cell uptake – so-called argentaffin positivity. Tumors capable of uptaking silver salts but not capable of reducing silver unless an external reducing agent is added are termed argyrophilic. Two distinct type of neurosecretory granules have been observed by electron microscopy (EM), a smaller granule associated with argyrophil carcinoids and a larger one with argentaffin tumors although EM is not routinely needed to confirm the diagnosis. Midgut carcinoids are mostly argentaffin positive while hindgut carcinoids are usually mixed with 60–70% being argyrophil and 8–16% being argentaffin positive.

Currently, immunohistochemistry techniques are utilized to diagnose carcinoid tumors and involve antibodies that target various cytoplasmic proteins including chromogranin, synaptophysin, and neuron-specific enolase.[3]

Clinical Presentation

Carcinoid tumors were initially considered indolent tumors with limited metastatic potential when initially described over 100 years ago. However, it is clear that these tumors can lead to significant morbidity and mortality due to local tumor growth, distant metastatic spread or through the production of various bioactive substances acting both locally and distally. Although the carcinoid syndrome is classically described as the hallmark of carcinoid tumors, it occurs in only 10–18% of all patients with carcinoid tumors and in only 50% of individuals with advanced disease. Most patients will be symptomatic for a median duration of 2 years prior to diagnosis. Up to 90% of symptomatic patients will have an advanced tumor often with metastasis.[2]

Approximately 50% of all gastrointestinal carcinoid tumors will be diagnosed following appendectomy. Less than 1% will have the carcinoid syndrome as the initial clinical manifestation. The commonest presentation in patients with midgut carcinoid tumors is abdominal pain and occurs in up to 40% of individuals while hindgut carcinoids are nonsecretory and almost always asymptomatic and discovered incidentally by the pathologist following polypectomy during routine colonic surveillance. Occasionally, larger tumors will present with bleeding, obstructive symptoms, and tenesmus.

The clinical manifestations of the carcinoid syndrome include episodic flushing, wheezing, nonbloody watery diarrhea, abdominal pain, and right-sided heart failure. This can be precipitated by several factors including stress and particular foods including caffeine and alcohol. Serotonin appears to be responsible for many of the gastrointestinal symptoms including abdominal cramping and intestinal hypermotility manifesting as diarrhea and occurs in 80% of patients with the carcinoid syndrome. Kallikrein secretion is thought to account for wheezing and flushing, the latter occurring in 85% of affected patients.[4] Intestinal obstruction leading to possible arterial insufficiency often results from mesenteric fibrosis, although the exact mechanism leading to mesenteric and retroperitoneal fibrosis has yet to be elucidated. Other retroperitoneal structures can be involved including the ureters and Peyronie's disease has been reported (inflammation and scarring of the tunical albuginea). Right-sided heart failure due to severe damage to the tricuspid and pulmonary valves accounts for 50% of the deaths from the carcinoid syndrome. Serotonin and other vasoactive substances have been suspected to be responsible as patients with higher 5-hydroxyindolacetic acid (5-HIAA) levels, a by-product of serotonin metabolism, which correlates with increased valvular damage.[2] The right side of the heart is most commonly affected as the lung will inactivate the humoral substances prior to exposure to the left side of the heart. Attempts at surgical valvular replacement have been associated with high perioperative morbidity and mortality.

Most of the peptide hormones produced and secreted by the carcinoid tumor are metabolized by the liver. Therefore, a patient with the classic carcinoid syndrome must have a tumor with venous drainage into the systemic rather than the portal circulation. Patients often have diarrhea or unexplained abdominal pain with or without the other classic signs of the carcinoid tumor. They are often diagnosed with tumors located in the bronchus (with or without metastasis), primary gastrointestinal tumor with metastasis to the lymph nodes or invasion into the retroperitoneum.[5–7] In contrast, the diagnosis of asymptomatic carcinoid tumors is usually established after the excision of a gastric or colonic polyp that is diagnosed pathologically as a carcinoid tumor, or incidentally at the time of appendectomy or laparotomy.

Midgut tumors are most commonly associated with the carcinoid syndrome as these tumors produce high levels of serotonin.[8] Almost 90% of individuals with the carcinoid syndrome will have a midgut carcinoid tumor. Foregut tumors typically lack the enzyme needed to convert the precursor compound 5-hydroxytryptophan into serotonin. Hindgut tumors rarely produce 5-hydroxytryptophan or serotonin. Therefore, tumors arising from these regions cannot produce the classic carcinoid syndrome even if metastatic lesions are present.

Atypical or variant carcinoid syndrome can occur in patients with gastric carcinoid tumors. Patience will experience patchy cutaneous flushing and pruritis. Diarrhea, bronchospasm, and cardiac lesions are rare. It is thought that the syndrome results from histamine rather than serotonin release.[2]

A life-threatening carcinoid crisis characterized by flushing, severe abdominal pain, diarrhea, hypotension, or hypertension can be precipitated by severe stress including surgery, anesthesia, and adrenergic agents. It is recommended that all patients with carcinoid tumor wear a medical alert bracelet indicating their diagnosis in the event of an accident or the need for emergency surgery. This crisis can often be managed with short-acting octreotide agents.[1]

Diagnostic Tests

Biochemical Tests

The most useful and widely used biochemical test for diagnosing carcinoid tumors in the symptomatic patient is the 24-h urine 5-HIAA measurement with a sensitivity and specificity of 73 and 100%, respectively.[2] 5-HIAA is excreted in the urine after serotonin metabolism and is measured more reliably than serotonin levels, which can vary between persons. Urinary 5-HIAA levels can be falsely elevated if a patient has consumed certain serotonin-rich foods such as bananas, pineapples, nuts, and kiwi fruits or following the ingestion of various medicines affecting urinary 5-HIAA levels. Chromogranin A is a sensitive serum marker but is nonspecific for carcinoid tumors and can be elevated in other types of neuroendocrine tumors. Platelet serotonin levels may be more sensitive than urine or blood tests but is not readily available at many institutions.

Imaging Tests

Computerized tomography (CT) scan of the thorax and abdomen/pelvis should be performed in symptomatic patients to identify the primary tumor and extent of disease. Somatostatin receptor scintigraphy (SRS) scan should be considered in most patients to identify occult metastasis in patients being considered for curative resection and to determine if the patient is likely to respond to octreotide. Approximately 88% of carcinoid tumors express receptors (SSTR 1–3) that possess moderate-to-high affinity for somatostatin and its analogs.[5] The ability of SRS to obtain whole body images, along with its high sensitivity, makes it the imaging modality of choice in patients with carcinoid tumors. However, SRS can fail to detect tumor in approximately 10% of patients who do not express the somatostatin receptor. Whole body positron emission tomography (PET) relies on differential metabolic uptake and is used increasingly but no studies have directly compared SRS and PET scans. 18F-Dopa-PET imaging is more sensitive in identifying the primary tumor and local lymph node involvement, while CT and MRI are more sensitive for identifying distant metastasis. Esophagogastroscopy and colonoscopy should be considered in patients with metastatic disease with an unknown primary. Electrocardiography and echocardiography should be performed in symptomatic and asymptomatic patients to rule out right-sided valvular disease and should be performed prior to elective surgical resection.

Treatment

Small intestinal carcinoids are often multicentric and located in the distal ileum, and associated with the carcinoid syndrome.[9] Most patients will have metastasized to the regional lymph nodes or liver. Size of the tumor correlates poorly with predicting distant metastatic disease as tumors less than 0.5 cm in diameter has been shown to metastasize to the liver. Carcinoid tumors greater than 2 cm diameter and are usually malignant in most locations except in the ileum where nearly all tumors will have metastasized. Small bowel resection including a resection of the mesenteric lymph nodes is indicated even in patients with known metastatic disease to reduce the likelihood of developing small bowel obstruction or mesenteric fibrosis and ischemia. The entire small intestine should be carefully examined at the time of laparotomy to exclude the possibility of a synchronous tumor.

Appendiceal carcinoid tumors represent the most common tumor of the appendix. Approximately 95% of these tumors are less than 2 cm in diameter; nearly 75% of these tumors are located in the distal third of the appendix.[10] These tumors are rarely multicentric and tumor size is the best prognostic indicator, with most tumors less than 2 cm rarely metastasizing to regional lymph nodes or distally. Patients with tumors under 1 cm are usually treated by simple appendectomy, as long as there is no evidence of local tumor spread. In contrast, 30–60% of lesions greater than 2 cm in diameter are associated with nodal or distant metastases and will require formal right hemicolectomy. The treatment of patients with tumor diameter between 1 and 1.9 cm must be individualized based on the risk of recurrence vs. the risk of surgery. The presence of lymphovascular invasion, involvement of the mesoappendix (lymph node involvement or by direct extension), or a positive margin are poor prognostic indicators and usually warrant right hemicolectomy.[11]

Approximately two-thirds of colonic tumors arise in the ascending colon (most in the cecum), and remain asymptomatic until they develop into large tumors with nodal spread or distant metastasis. Most of these patients will require colonic resection and the extent is usually determined by the location of the disease.[12]

Rectal carcinoids are usually asymptomatic and identified at the time of routine endoscopy in approximately 50% of patients. Symptomatic patients usually have rectal bleeding, tenesmus, pain, constipation, and rarely the carcinoid syndrome. Tumor size correlates well with the likelihood of metastasis – tumors less than 1 cm in diameter metastasize in fewer than 5% of patients. Most tumors greater than 2 cm will have metastasized at the time of diagnosis.[13] The majority of rectal carcinoid tumors are smaller than 1 cm and can usually be treated with local endoscopic excision. The management of tumors 1–2 cm in diameter remains controversial. Some authors advocate for more extensive resection in the presence of muscular invasion, symptoms at diagnosis, or ulceration. Tumors with a diameter greater than 2 cm have traditionally been treated by proctectomy.[14,15] This approach has recently been challenged by several retrospective studies that did not demonstrate improved survival beyond that observed with local excision. The correct surgical approach to large rectal carcinoids must be individualized and must consider factors such as patient age and morbid illnesses.

Metastatic Disease

Treatment of liver metastasis is effective in providing long-term palliation of the hormone-related symptoms in patients who do not respond to or tolerate the somatostatin analogs. Tumor debulking can involve hepatic resection, cryotherapy, radiofrequency ablation, hepatic artery embolization, or chemoembolization. Hepatic artery occlusion or chemoembolization can be considered in select patients who are not surgical candidates for hepatic resection. Carcinoid tumors that have metastasized to the liver are extremely vascular and obtain a large proportion of its blood supply from the hepatic artery. Occlusion of the hepatic artery results in less compromise to the hepatocyte which will continue to receive its blood supply from the portal vein. Patients with large tumors or tumors refractory to somatostatin usually experience marked transient symptom improvement. This procedure can be repeated up to four times every 2–3 months in selected patients. Attempts at liver transplantation in patients with metastatic carcinoid tumor have been associated with high perioperative mortality rates and local recurrences, although more recent reports suggest improved survival rates. Carcinoid tumors are slow growing and patients exhibit favorable 5- and 10-year survival rates despite extensive metastasis.

Systemic Therapy

One of the most important advances in the treatment of carcinoid syndrome has been the development of various somatostatin analogs for the diagnosis and treatment of metastatic disease.[16] More than 80% of carcinoid tumors express one of the five subtypes of somatostatin receptors. Although five somatostatin receptors have been identified, the beneficial effects of these somatostatin analogs seems to be mediated by the somatostatin receptor subtype 2.[17] Activation of this receptor results in reduced hormone synthesis and secretion. The 14 amino acid peptide somatostatin has a half-life in the order of minutes, making pharmacological dosing difficult. The somatostatin analog octreotide is an eight-amino acid peptide with a longer half-life and retained specificity for the somatostatin receptor. Octreotide is effective at controlling the hormonal manifestations of the carcinoid syndrome and may halt progression of some of the fibrosing effects, namely cardiac and mesenteric fibrosis. Initial studies using octreotide administered at a dose of 150 μg three times daily improved symptoms in 88% of patients and reduced 5 HIAA urinary excretion in 72%. Some reports in the literature have described a temporary stabilization of tumor growth in as many as 85% of patients, suggesting a role of these analogs in decreasing tumor progression, but no overall improvement in survival rate has been demonstrated.

Long-acting somatostatin analogs, octreotide long-acting repeatable (LAR) and lanreotide prolonged release (PR) are currently available and can be administered as a depot injection.[18] Octreotide LAR can be administered at a dose of 20 mg intramuscularly (IM) monthly and lanreotide PR at a dose of 30 mg IM every 10 days. The most commonly reported adverse effects of these analogs include cholelithiasis in approximately 50% of patients and tachyphylaxis. The effects of these various somatostatin analogs on survival rates in patients with metastatic carcinoid syndrome have not been reported in a large patient series.[19]

Cytotoxic chemotherapy has been ineffective in the treatment of metastatic carcinoid tumors.[20–24] In a trial by the Eastern Cooperative Oncology Group, 118 patients with metastatic carcinoid tumor received streptozocin and cyclophosphamide or streptozocin and 5-fluorouracil (%-FU).[22] Response rates, based on reduced urinary 5-HIAA levels and tumor regression were 26 and 33%, respectively, but were associated with considerable toxicity. The best response to chemotherapy have been in patients with aggressive carcinoid tumors that have been treated in a similar way to small cell lung cancer with cisplatin-based chemotherapeutic regimens. Combined cisplatin and etoposide therapy led to 67% response rate in patients with neuroendocrine tumors but was less effective in the setting of the less aggressive variants of carcinoid tumors.[25] Interferon-alpha has been shown to provide symptom relief in one-third of patients refractory to octreotide treatment. A trial examining the use of interferon-alpha in 111 patients with the carcinoid syndrome demonstrated reduced urinary 5-HIAA levels in 42% and tumor regression in 15% of patients.[25] The routine use of interferon has been limited by the side effect profile which includes fever, weight loss, fatigue, and anorexia.

External beam radiation therapy has not been used extensively in patients with carcinoid tumor, although it has proven to be effective in palliative treatment of bone and central nervous system metastasis.[26,27] However, targeted therapy with radiolabeled somatostatin analogs remains a very exciting development in the treatment of patients with metastatic or inoperable carcinoid tumors. This involves the use of radiolabeled somatostatin analogs for SRS scan positive tumors. Initial results are very encouraging and in the phase IIa MAURITIUS study, 90-yttrium-DOTA-lanreotide in 70 patients with SRS scan positive tumors resulted in stable disease in 35% and regression in 10%.[28]

Neuroendocrine Carcinoma

The neuroendocrine (NE) system is comprised of endocrine cells found throughout the body including the pancreas, thyroid, lung, adrenal gland, as well as the gastrointestinal system amongst other areas. NE tumors occur most commonly in the lung in the form of small cell carcinoma but have been reported less commonly in the colon and rectum. In comparison with carcinoid tumors that are usually slow growing and indolent neuroendocrine tumors, NE tumors of the colon and rectum tend to be poorly differentiated high grade tumors, highly aggressive, and associated with a poor prognosis. In fact, many poorly differentiated adenocarcinomas are probably NE tumors when stained appropriately for the various enteroendocrine cell markers such as chromogranin and synaptophysin. It is important to differentiate these tumors from other small cell cancers such as lymphoma. An extensive metastatic workup is critical to determine an appropriate treatment plan as up to two-third of patients will have metastasis at the time of diagnosis. Multimodality treatment is indicated and involves surgical resection when possible for curative intent, with adjuvant chemotherapy and radiation treatment being utilized. Chemotherapeutic agents used to treat small cell cancer of the lung are often effective in treating these tumors.[29]

Melanoma

Melanomas of the gastrointestinal tract can be divided into (1) metastatic melanoma usually from a cutaneous neoplasm or more rarely (2) a primary GI melanoma.

Metastatic Melanoma

Melanoma is one of the most common cancers to metastasize to the GI tract and studies have documented that the majority of these are to the small intestine (up to 67%), followed by the colon (up to 15%) and stomach (5–7%).[30–34] Although there is a high rate of metastases, less than 5% of patients with melanoma are diagnosed with a GI metastasis, but based on autopsy studies the GI system may be second only to lung in terms of site of spread.[35] Once a melanoma metastasizes, it carries a poor prognosis with usually less than 6 months survival; however, gastrointestinal metastases may be symptomatic and present with bleeding, obstruction, or most commonly pain.[33–35]

Evaluation of a patient with a history of melanoma who presents with obstructive symptoms or anemia may include colonoscopy, upper endoscopy, upper GI series with a small bowel follow through. CT scanning can be useful but sensitivity has been estimated at around 60% – one study identified four patterns of small bowel involvement based on CT including (1) intraluminal mass, (2) mesenteric implants causing compression of the lumen, (3) ulcerating lesions, and (4) diffuse infiltration.[36] PET scanning can also be used to help identify metastatic disease.[37] One study found that only 6% of patients had evidence of GI metastases when CT scanning for staging was routinely used and all of these were thought to be liver metastases.[38] In patients who have already developed metastatic disease, if a patient is not symptomatic, looking for these lesions in the GI tract is likely not going to alter management and therefore probably should not routinely be done.

When patients present with symptoms, intervention in selected patients is likely beneficial even though it will be done for palliative purposes. Studies from various institutions have found that the majority of patients selected for an operation benefit from a surgical intervention with an acceptable morbidity and mortality rate.[33,39–41] Symptom improvement varies between 79 and 97% in published studies. The most common procedure is usually a small bowel resection. The mortality rates in these studies ranged from 1.5 to 3%.[33,39–41] In a multivariate analysis in one study complete resection of all disease as well as a low preoperative serum LDH was predictive of long-term survival – 38% of patients survived to 5 years.[41]

In summary, in terms of lesions metastatic to the GI tract, melanoma is common. However, it is not common to operate on patients with metastatic melanoma to the GI tract. If a patient is symptomatic, even though the resection may be considered palliative, there is improvement in symptoms in the majority of patients who are selected to go to the operating room.

Primary Melanoma

A primary melanoma of the gastrointestinal tract is rare but can occur in the esophagus, small intestine, rectum, and anus.[35,42] Of these, the anus is the most common location. There are very few case reports of primary colonic melanoma.[43,44] Compared to cutaneous melanomas, gastrointestinal lesions carry a worse prognosis – this may be related to the fact that they are discovered at a more advanced stage when they become symptomatic.[45]

The diagnosis of a primary gastrointestinal melanoma is made if after a thorough search there is no cutaneous melanoma identified. In addition, a solitary lesion in the gastrointestinal tract should be present without any metastatic disease to be confident in calling it a primary.

Melanoma affecting the rectum or anus is rare with an estimated incidence of 1–2 cases/million per year.[35,46] Although the rate is low, it ranks third in terms of site of primary melanoma (skin and ocular melanoma being first and second).[46] Cumulatively these represent less than 1% of malignancies discovered in the anus and rectum. In contrast to cutaneous melanomas, there does not appear to be a relationship to sun exposure; women may be at higher risk compared to males and individuals are usually in their seventh decade.[45]

The diagnosis of anorectal melanoma can be difficult – many patients have bleeding which is usually thought to be secondary to hemorrhoids. Other symptoms include pain, tenesmus, and change in bowel habit. Weight loss, decreased energy, and other systemic signs may suggest metastatic disease. Most of these lesions are pigmented; however, up to a third may be a amelanotic.[35] Morphologically, these can present as ulcerated or polypoid lesions and can be mistaken for thrombosed external hemorrhoids. Incidental diagnosis is sometimes made after a routine hemorrhoidectomy is done underscoring the importance of a careful anorectal exam on every patient who presents with issues in this area. Biopsy can be done of any suspicious lesion or ulceration present. The only chance for cure in these patients is early diagnosis and excision.[47] Unfortunately, the prognosis for these patients is poor. Five-year survival is estimated to be 6% and median survival after diagnosis is 12–18 months.[35] Approximately half of these patients will present with metastatic disease and 20% will have gross inguinal lymphadenopathy.[48]

The surgical approach to this disease is made difficult because of the poor prognosis and it does not seem to be based on recent case series that radical excision (APR) results in better survival compared to local excision.[49–51] If a patient has a tumor that is invading into the sphincters and causing intractable pain, then a patient like this may benefit from an APR. In patients who are having only local symptoms, a local excision is a reasonable approach. Again, based on retrospective reviews there does not seem to be a survival advantage with a radical approach.

Chemotherapy thus far has been disappointing. Most of the information regarding the use of chemotherapy is based on the experience with cutaneous melanomas. Dacarbazine, levamisole, and BCG have not yielded survival advantages and two meta-analyses examining the use of interferon-alpha have not demonstrated a consistent advantage with its use.[52,53] Combined use of dacarbazine, nimustine, cisplatin, and tamoxifen plus interferon-beta has been described but not surprisingly can result in significant toxicity to the patient.[54] Molecular-based therapy targeting tyrosine kinase receptors may lead to better survival in the future, but at the present time there is not enough data to support its routine use.[55]

Overall, anorectal melanoma is a "bad actor." It is associated with a poor prognosis and at the present time there is not a good treatment that provides long-term survival. Careful examination of all patients who present to the clinic with any type of anorectal complaint is important and biopsy of suspicious lesions should be done early. In the case of anorectal melanoma, the only chance for cure is an early diagnosis.

Gastrointestinal Stromal Tumor

The concept of "GIST" (gastrointestinal stromal tumor) was first introduced by Mazur and Clark in 1983.[56] They used immunostaining and electron microscopy to show that tumors that had previously been described as leiomyomas or leiomyosarcomas (using light microscopy) actually did not have smooth muscle or Schwann cells. The cell of origin is thought to be the interstitial cell of Cajal. An important article regarding mutations in the protooncogene c-kit in GISTs was written by Hirota et al.[57] This author along with Heinrich et al. described mutations in platelet-derived growth factor receptor a (PDGFRa another tyrosine kinase).[58] Mutations of c-kit and PDGFRa are thought to be two different pathways to the formation of GISTs. Over 90% of GISTs have a mutation in c-kit and up to 10% have a mutation in PDGFRa.[59]

Microscopically, spindle cells are usually seen. CD117 (immunohistochemical marker for KIT) is a very sensitive and specific marker for GISTs. CD34 is seen in approximately 70% of GISTs. If CD117 is negative but the appearance microscopically is consistent with a GIST, the diagnosis can be made if staining for S100, SMA, and desmin are negative.[60]

GISTs represent the most common mesenchymal tumor of the GI tract. They tend to occur in the middle aged and elderly (mean age of 60) with men affected more often.[61] It should be noted that pediatric cases have been reported.[62] The stomach is the most common site followed by the small intestine. GISTs can also be seen in the rectum but rarely in the colon. When considering small intestinal GISTs the jejunum is the most common location followed by the ileum. Duodenal lesions are usually in the second part. Tumors in the stomach have a lower rate of malignancy (20%) compared to lesions in the small and large bowel (40%). It is rare to find a GIST of the esophagus and these are usually leiomyomas.[59,60,63]

Most GISTs occur sporadically but there are some hereditary entities to consider. Carney's triad consists of (1) synchronous or metachronous GISTs, (2) extra-adrenal paraganglionomas, and (3) pulmonary chondromas.[60,63] It is usually seen in women before age 30 and interestingly no mutation in KIT or PDGFRa have been identified.[64,65] Patients affected with neurofibromatosis type I more commonly are affected with GISTs and also present at a younger age than the sporadic cases. These usually present as multiple small intestinal tumors.[66,67] In these patients as well there has been no KIT/PDGFR mutation identified.[60,63]

A recent autopsy series found that one in four patients over the age of 50 had small GISTS located near the gastroesophageal junction. These have been termed "GIST tumorlets" and are thought to be clinically insignificant lesions that would need some additional stimulus to evolve into something that would be clinically significant.[68]

Clinical presentation will depend on the location and size of the tumor.[63,69,70] Symptoms are usually nonspecific and can include dyspepsia, bleeding, and pain. Advanced lesions can present as a palpable mass. Not surprisingly, increased symptoms are associated with increased size. In a study from Sweden, the median size was 8.9 cm in symptomatic patients compared to 2.7 cm in asymptomatic individuals.[63]

Lesions are usually submucosal – as a result imaging is the most important tool in making the presumptive diagnosis. Final diagnosis is usually made once the pathologist has the specimen. Imaging modalities that can be used include CT, MRI, PET, and endoscopic ultrasound. CT and MRI (low intensity on T1, high intensity on T2) scanning are often used.[71] GISTs usually involve the muscularis propria and an intramural mass that is well circumscribed is the characteristic appearance. In tumors that are larger, there can be areas of central necrosis. Percutaneous biopsy with fine or core needle aspiration is not recommended since neovascularisation is associated with these tumors and hemorrhage can occur if they are biopsied. In addition, there is the possibility of tumor rupture and spread.[63] If the tumor is large and extending into the mesentery or other adjacent structures it can be difficult to discern if it is a lymphoma or sarcoma that is the underlying problem. Metastases are most commonly seen in the liver and peritoneum. Lymphatic spread is not common and therefore lymphadenopathy is not usually seen.[72] Lung and bone metastases have seen in advanced cases. CT scan is usually best for staging and for determining if there is potential for surgical resection.[73] PET is not normally required for diagnosis or determining resectability but can be used to see if there has been a response to treatment.[73] Endoscopy as well as endoscopic ultrasound for lesions that are within reach of a scope is likely a good idea to visualize the mass for operative planning as well as biopsy the tumor if possible – this can potentially change treatment if biopsies return with lymphoma. Endoscopic ultrasound-guided fine needle aspirations have a higher rate of diagnosis compared to endoscopy alone but fine needle aspiration with endoscopic ultrasound is controversial because it still carries similar risks to percutaneous biopsy described earlier.[74,75]

The treatment of GIST can be divided into (1) surgical resection and (2) imatinib and sunitinib. Ideal surgical management involves resection of the tumor en bloc with any other associated contiguous involvement with microscopically negative margins.[76,77] In order to attain a microscopically negative margin a gross margin of at least 1 cm is suggested. Even after a complete resection there is a high recurrence rate,[78] and therefore adjuvant therapy with imatinib should be considered.

When rectal GISTs specifically are considered, the symptoms associated are bleeding, pain (abdominal or rectal), or mass found on DRE or with endoscopy. Consistent with other GISTs at other sites, the larger the size, the more symptomatic a patient is. Complete excision is the best treatment including any pseudocapsule that is present. High local recurrence rates exist and are higher with wide local excision when compared to abdominoperineal resection or anterior resection.[79] Another modality that could be used is transanal endoscopic microsurgery as long as the surgeon is confident in being able to perform a complete excision. GISTs do not typically spread lymphatically and therefore a wide excision of the mesentery is not necessary; however, an en bloc resection of the tumor with microscopically negative margins is important.

If a complete resection is not possible due to the size of the tumor there are multiple reports involving the neoadjuvant use of imatinib which have decreased the size of the tumor to a point where surgical resection becomes feasible – at least 50% of patients will have tumor shrinkage.[80–82] CT scan can be used to follow these patients and judge the response to treatment. A trial being done by the RTOG (Radiation Therapy Oncology Group) is looking at this question and patients are given neoadjuvant imatinib therapy for 2–6 months in patients who present with large tumors that would likely require additional organ resection.[82] One additional benefit that is being considered with this neoadjuvant therapy is whether it will decrease the vascularity of the tumor and make the operation safer. It should be remembered that up to 15% of GISTs will be resistant to imatinib, and therefore the lesion could theoretically grow bigger and become unresectable while neoadjuvant therapy is being done. Also, a tissue biopsy in the form of fine needle aspiration usually needs to be done prior to an oncologist agreeing to give neoadjuvant treatment and this can lead to some of the issues that were mentioned earlier in this section.

With respect to prognosis, tumor size and mitotic rate are the most important parameters. A tumor with less than 5 mitoses per 50 high-powered fields is usually benign acting although there are a small number that may metastasize. Lesions with a diameter of less than 2 cm are almost always benign.[60]

When GISTs recur or are metastatic the treatment algorithm is similar. Usually, Imatinib will be used first and then the response to this treatment evaluated radiologically. If patients respond, then lifelong treatment can be used. In patients presenting with metastases, 45% will have a partial response and 30% will have stable disease. Imatinib has had a big impact with respect to survival as median survival with metastatic disease is 5 years; it used to be 15 months after resection of recurrent GIST when imatinib was not available. Imatinib does not offer a cure, and therefore surgery can be attempted. In addition, by utilizing surgery there may be a delay in resistance of the tumor to Imatinib.[59,60,63]

In patients that do not respond to Imatinib one option can be to increase the dose from 400 to 800 mg per day if the patient is only receiving the 400 mg dose. Sunitinib can be used as a second line treatment. In a prospective randomized trial that compared sunitinib to a placebo in patients with imatinib resistance, there was a longer time to tumor progression in the Sunitinib group.[63] These patients also had longer overall survival. With respect to other options, GISTs are considered to be resistant to radiation. Palliative treatment could be considered for rectal GIST. Radiofrequency ablation for lesions in the liver can be attempted. Hepatic artery embolization can also be done for unresectable liver metastases. Other chemotherapy regimens have not been as successful as Imatinib and Sunitinib. Vatalanib and Dasatanib are other tyrosine kinase inhibitors that are being studied.[63]

Leukemia and Neutropenic Enterocolitis

All forms of leukemia can lead to infiltration of the gastrointestinal tract. Most commonly, the ileum, appendix, and colon are affected due to their higher concentrations of lymphatic tissue.[83,84] Involvement can result in diarrhea, pain, obstruction, colitis, or watermelon colon.[83,85] The infiltration can lead to lesions ranging from ulcers to polypoid lesions which can cause obstruction not only from the mass itself but also from intussusception.[86] Anorectal complications include plaques, fistulas, ulcers, fissures, and abscesses.[87] Since there is a high risk of creating infectious complications in patients with leukemia and receiving chemotherapy, instrumentation of the rectum should be avoided if possible.[87]

Neutropenic enterocolitis is a complication that is most frequently seen after the chemotherapy for leukemia. It has been seen in a variety of malignancies – solid and hematologic – secondary to the chemotherapy regimens.[88–93] Numerous agents have been implicated although cytotoxic agents are mainly involved. The small bowel, appendix, and colon can be involved,[94,95] and the organisms involved include Staphylococcus Aureus, Acinetobacter, Enterobacter, Aspergillus, Pseudomonas, Candida, Klebsiella, and Morganella.[96,97] The overall pathogenesis involves a combination of mucosal injury, neutropenia, and decreased defense against gastrointestinal bacteria.[96,97] There has been one systematic review which reported a 5.3% pooled incidence rate in patients who were hospitalized for the treatment of hematologic/solid malignancies or aplastic anemia.[98]

Fever and abdominal pain in the setting of neutropenia (absolute neutrophil count less than 1,500/mm^3) is the triad of findings associated with this diagnosis.[96,97] Other findings can include nausea and vomiting, diarrhea, and distention. Abdominal pain and tenderness can be diffuse but is often localized to the right lower quadrant. CT scanning can show bowel wall thickening, edema/hemorrhage, pneumatosis, free fluid, and free air. Imaging can help decrease the use of nontherapeutic laparotomies and help identify other etiologies for the pain.[96,97] Ultrasound can be used and there are characteristic patterns associated with neutropenic enterocolitis such as "doughnut like hypoechoic, fluid-filled intestinal lumen separated from a thickened bowel wall by a thin mucosal layer."[98] One study demonstrated that using high resolution ultrasonography systematically decreased the time between fever and the diagnosis of neutropenic enterocolitis (3 days vs. 9 days, $p=0.01$).[99] Further, with the use of systematic ultrasound, mortality appeared to be reduced. Ultrasound studies have also shown that bowel wall thickening appears to be related to a longer duration of symptoms and a higher mortality rate compared to patients without this sonographic finding.[99]

There is no high level evidence to guide the treatment of neutropenic enterocolitis.[98] In patients that do not have peritonitis or perforation can likely be managed medically initially. Conservative management consists of hydration, bowel rest, a nasogastric tube if there is a significant ileus, TPN, and broad spectrum antibiotics. Granulocyte colony stimulating factor may be a consideration.[97,98]

If a patient requires exploration, treatment usually consists of a bowel resection and an ostomy since complications have been reported if primary anastomosis is performed on leucopenic patients.[100, 101] In addition, there may be mucosal necrosis even though the serosa may only appear edematous. Based on the systematic review, there is no good evidence to determine the optimal surgical approach.[98]

Overall, there is not good evidence to guide management as a systematic review has shown. In patients who present with fever, abdominal pain, and neutropenia a CT scan or ultrasound should be done as soon as possible. Further treatment depends on the clinical scenario, but broad spectrum antibiotics should be initiated.

Lymphoma

The gastrointestinal tract is the most common site of extranodal lymphoma.[102] Primary colorectal lymphoma is rare accounting for 15–20% of GI lymphomas (stomach 50–60%, small bowel 20–30%).[103] Diffuse large B-cell lymphoma is the most common histologic type seen in the colon with the second most common type being MALT-associated low-grade B-cell lymphoma.[103,104] It should be noted that colorectal lymphomas do not have the association with H. Pylori like their gastric counterpart. As a result, they cannot be treated with H. Pylori eradication therapy.[102] In terms of staging, the modified Ann Arbor staging system is usually used. HIV, EBV, prolonged steroid therapy, and inflammatory bowel disease have been suggested as possible risk factors.[105] Dawson's criteria has been used for the diagnosis of primary colorectal lymphoma.[106]

Patients are usually between the ages of 50 and 70 with a slight male predominance (1.5:1). Weight loss and abdominal pain are the most common symptoms at presentation and many patients present with a palpable mass as these tumors often progress without symptoms until reaching a large size. Interestingly, although reaching a large size, they rarely cause obstruction or perforate. Gastrointestinal bleeding can also be seen in 20–30% of cases.[102,107,108]

Most colonic lesions are found in the cecum and ascending colon with 70% of colorectal lymphomas occurring proximal to the hepatic flexure likely because of the increased lymphoid tissue in this area of the bowel.[104, 109–111] Treatment involves a multidisciplinary approach using surgery and chemotherapy. Surgical excision still appears to the main treatment for this disease as it provides staging information as well as the chance for cure (with or without chemotherapy). It also helps avoid possible complications such as bleeding or obstruction.[104,112,113]

The role of chemotherapy as the initial treatment has not been studied except for some series in which there have been patients included in whom surgery was contraindicated.[104,112,113] In these patients, there was no benefit shown compared to the patients in groups receiving surgical therapy or combined therapy. Radiation therapy is used in selected cases. Five-year survival rates range between 27 and 55%.[100–102,104] While one study suggested that patients with tumors larger than 5 cm or are lymph node positive have the worst prognosis.[114]

Acknowledgments. This chapter was authored by Richard Devine and Marc Brand in the previous edition of this textbook.

References

1. Kulke MH, Mayer RJ. Carcinoid tumours. N Engl J Med. 1999;340:858–68.
2. Ganim RB, Norton JA. Recent advances in carcinoid pathogenesis, diagnosis and management. Surg Oncol. 2000;9:173–9.
3. Eriksson B, Oberg K, Stridsberg M. Tumour markers in neuroendocrine tumours. Digestion. 2000;62:33–8.
4. Lucas KJ, Feldman JM. Flushing in the carcinoid syndrome and plasma kallikrein. Cancer. 1986;58:2290–3.
5. Reubi JC, Laissue J, Waser B. Expression of somatostatin receptors in normal, inflamed, and neoplastic human gastrointestinal tissues. Ann N Y Acad Sci. 1994;733:122–37.
6. Rea F, Binda R, Spreafico G. Bronchial carcinoids: a review of 60 patients. Ann Thorac Surg. 1989;47:412–4.
7. Schreurs AJ, Westermann CJ, van den Bosch JM. A twenty-five-year follow-up of ninety-three resected typical carcinoid tumours of the lung. J Thorac Cardiovasc Surg. 1992; 104:1470–5.
8. Barclay TH, Schapira DV. Malignant tumours of the small intestine. Cancer. 1983;51:878–81.
9. Makridis C, Oberg K, Juhlin C. Surgical treatment of mid-gut carcinoid tumors. World J Surg. 1990;14:377–83.
10. Moertel CG, Dockerty MB, Judd ES. Carcinoid tumors of the vermiform appendix. Cancer. 1968;21:270–8.
11. Moertel CG, Weiland LH, Nagorney DM, Dockerty MB. Carcinoid tumor of the appendix: treatment and prognosis. N Engl J Med. 1987;317:1699–701.
12. Berardi RS. Carcinoid tumors of the colon (exclusive of the rectum): review of the literature. Dis Colon Rectum. 1972; 15:383–91.
13. Jetmore AB, Ray JE, Gathright Jr JB. Rectal carcinoids: the most frequent carcinoid tumor. Dis Colon Rectum. 1992; 35:717–25.
14. Naunheim KS, Zeitels J, Kaplan EL. Rectal carcinoid tumors – treatment and prognosis. Surgery. 1983;94:670–6.
15. Burke M, Shepherd N, Mann CV. Carcinoid tumours of the rectum and anus. Br J Surg. 1987;74:358–61.
16. Eriksson B, Oberg K. Summing up 15 years of somatostatin analog therapy in neuroendocrine tumors: future outlook. Ann Oncol. 1999;10:S31–8.
17. Kubota A, Yamada Y, Kagimoto S. Identification of somatostatin receptor subtypes and an implication for the efficacy of somatostatin analogue SMS 201-995 in the treatment of human endocrine tumors. J Clin Invest. 1994;93:1321–5.
18. Kvols LK, Moertel CG, O'Connell MJ. Treatment of the malignant carcinoid syndrome: evaluation of a long-acting somatostatin analogue. N Engl J Med. 1986;315:663–6.
19. Tomassetti P, Migliori M, Corinaldesi R, Gullo L. Treatment of gastroenteropancreatic neuroendocrine tumours with octreotide LAR. Aliment Pharmacol Ther. 2000;14:557–60.
20. O'Toole D, Ducreux M, Bommelaer G, Wemeau JL, Bouché O, Catus F, et al. Treatment of carcinoid syndrome: a prospective crossover evaluation of lanreotide versus octreotide in terms of efficacy, patient acceptability, and tolerance. Cancer. 2000;88:770–6.
21. Rubin J, Ajani J, Schirmer W, Venook AP, Bukowski R, Pommier R, et al. Octreotide acetate long-acting formulation versus open-label subcutaneous octreotide acetate in malignant carcinoid syndrome. J Clin Oncol. 1999;17:600–6.
22. Moertel CG, Hanley JA. Combination chemotherapy trials in metastatic carcinoid tumor and the malignant carcinoid syndrome. Cancer Clin Trials. 1979;2(4):327–34.
23. Engstrom PF, Lavin PT, Moertel CG, Folsch E, Douglass Jr HO. Streptozocin plus fluorouracil versus doxorubicin therapy for metastatic carcinoid tumor. J Clin Oncol. 1984;2(11):1255–9.
24. Bukowski RM, Johnson KG, Peterson RF, Stephens RL, Rivkin SE, Neilan B, et al. A phase II trial of combination chemotherapy in patients with metastatic carcinoid tumors. A Southwest Oncology Group Study. Cancer. 1987;60(12):2891–5.
25. Moertel CG, Kvols LK, O'Connell MJ, Rubin J. Treatment of neuroendocrine carcinomas with combined etoposide and cisplatin. Evidence of major therapeutic activity in the anaplastic variants of these neoplasms. Cancer. 1991;68(2):227–32.
26. Moertel CG, Johnson CM, McKusick MA, Martin Jr JK, Nagorney DM, Kvols LK, et al. The management of patients with advanced carcinoid tumors and islet cell carcinomas. Ann Intern Med. 1994;120(4):302–9.
27. Schupak KD, Wallner KE. The role of radiation therapy in the treatment of locally unresectable or metastatic carcinoid tumors. Int J Radiat Oncol Biol Phys. 1991;20(3):489–95.
28. Virgolini I, Britton K, Buscombe J, Moncayo R, Paganelli G, Riva P. In- and Y-DOTA-lanreotide: results and implications of the MAURITIUS trial. Semin Nucl Med. 2002;32(2):148–55.
29. Barakat MT, Meeran K, Bloom SR. Neuroendocrine tumours. Endocr Relat Cancer. 2004;11(1):1–18.
30. Rengtgen DS, Thompson W, Garbutt J, Seigler HF. Radiologic, endoscopic and surgical considerations of melanoma metastatic to the GI tract. Surgery. 1984;95:635–9.
31. Malik A, Hull TL, Floruta C. What is the best surgical treatment for anorectal melanoma? Int J Colorectal Dis. 2004;19(2):121–3.
32. Tessier DJ, McConnell EJ, Young-Fadok T, Wolff BG. Melanoma metastatic to the colon: case series and review of the literature with outcome analysis. Dis Colon Rectum. 2003;46(4):441–7.
33. Ollila DW, Essner R, Wanek LA, Morton DL. Surgical resection for melanoma metastatic to the gastrointestinal tract. Arch Surg. 1996;131:975–9.
34. Allen PJ, Cott DG. The surgical management of metastatic melanoma. Ann Surg Oncol. 2002;9(8):762–70.
35. Schuchter LM, Green R, Fraker D. Primary and metastatic diseases in malignant melanoma of the gastrointestinal tract. Curr Opin Oncol. 2000;12:181–5.
36. Kawashima A, Fishman EK, Kuhlman JE, Schuchter LM. CT of malignant melanoma: patterns of small bowel and mesenteric involvement. J Comput Assist Tomogr. 1991;15:570–1.
37. Damian DL, Fulham MJ, Thompson E, Thompson JF. Positron emission tomography in the detection and management of metastatic melanoma. Melanoma Res. 1996;6:325–9.
38. Buzaid AC, Sandler AB, Mani S, Curtis AM, Poo WJ, Bolognia JL, et al. Role of computed tomography in the staging of primary melanoma. J Clin Oncol. 1993;11:638–43.
39. Agrawal S, Yao TJ, Coit DG. Surgery for melanoma metastatic to the gastrointestinal tract. Ann Surg Oncol. 1999;6:636–44.
40. Khadra MH, Thompson JF, Milton GW, McCarthy WH. The justification for surgical treatment of metastatic melanoma of the gastrointestinal tract. Surg Gynecol Obstet. 1990;171:413–6.
41. Ricaniadis N, Konstandoulakis MM, Walsh D, Karakousis CP. Gastrointestinal metastases from malignant melanoma. Surg Oncol. 1995;4:105–10.

42. Clemmensen OJ, Fenger C. Melanoctyes in the anal canal epithelium. Histopathology. 1991;18:237–41.
43. Avital S, Romaguera RL, Sands L, Marchetti F, Hellinger MD. Primary malignant melanoma of the right colon. Am Surg. 2004;70:649–51.
44. Sarah P, MaNiff JF, Madison MD, Wen-Jen Poo H, Bayar S, Sallem RR. Colonic melanoma, primary or regressed primary. J Clinic Gastroenterol. 2000;30:440–4.
45. Gervasoni Jr JE, Wanebo HJ. Cancers of the anal canal and anal margin. Cancer Invest. 2003;21(3):452–64.
46. Blecker D, Abraham S, Furth EE, Kochman ML. Melanoma of the gastrointestinal tract. Am J Gastroenterol. 1999; 94(12):3427–33.
47. Wanebo HJ, Woodruff JM, Farr GH, Quan SH. Anorectal melanomas. Cancer. 1981;47:1891–5.
48. Brady MS, Kavolius JP, Quan SH. Anorectal melanoma. A 64-year experience at Memorial Sloan-Kettering Cancer Center. Dis Colon Rectum. 1995;38(2):146–51.
49. Billingsley KG, Stern LE, Lowy AM, Kahlenberg MS, Thomas Jr CR. Uncommon anal neoplasms. Surg Oncol Clin N Am. 2004;13(2):375–88.
50. Yeh JJ, Shia J, Hwu WJ, Busam KJ, Paty PB, Guillem JG, et al. The role of abdominoperineal resection as surgical therapy for anorectal melanoma. Ann Surg. 2006;244(6):1012–7.
51. Belli F, Gallino GF, Lo Vullo S, Mariani L, Poiasina E, Leo E. Melanoma of the anorectal region. The experience of the National Cancer Institute of Milano. Eur J Surg Oncol. 2009;35(7):757–62.
52. Lens MB, Dawes M. Interferon alfa therapy for malignant melanoma: a systematic review of randomized controlled trials. J Clin Oncol. 2002;20(7):1818–25.
53. Verma S, Quirt I, McCready D, Bak K, Charette M, Iscoe N. Systematic review of systemic adjuvant therapy for patients at high risk for recurrent melanoma. Cancer. 2006;106(7):1431–42.
54. Kawano N, Tashiro M, Taguchi M, Kihara Y, Yoshikawa I, Syukuwa K, et al. Combined treatment with dacarbazine, nimustine, cisplatin, and tamoxifen plus interferon-beta in a patient with advanced anorectal malignant melanoma. Nippon Shokakibyo Gakkai Zasshi. 2008;105(11):1627–33.
55. Quintas-Cardama A, Lazar AJ, Woodman SE, Kim K, Ross M, Hwu P, et al. Complete response of stage IV anal mucosal melanoma expressing KIT Val560Asp to the multikinase inhibitor sorafenib. Nat Clin Pract Oncol. 2008;5(12):737–40.
56. Mazur MT, Clark HB. Gastric Stromal tumors: reappraisal of histogenesis. Am J Surg Pathol. 1983;7:507–19.
57. Hirota S, Isozaki K, Moriyama Y, Hashimoto K, Nishida T, Ishiguro S, et al. Gain of function mutations of c-kit in human gastrointestinal stromal tumors. Science. 1998;279:577–80.
58. Heinrich MC, Corless CL, Duensing A, McGreevey L, Chen CJ, Joseph N, et al. PDGFRA activating mutations in gastrointestinal stromal tumors. Science. 2003;299(5607):708–10.
59. Biasco G, Velo D, Angriman I, Astorino M, Baldan A, Baseggio M, et al. Gastrointestinal stromal tumors: report of an audit and review of the literature. Eur J Cancer Prev. 2009;18(2):106–16.
60. Steigen SE, Eide TJ. Gastrointestinal stromal tumors (GISTs): a review. APMIS. 2009;117:73–86.
61. Tryggvason G, Gisalason HG, Magnusson MK, Jonasson JG. Gastrointestinal stromal tumors in Iceland, 1990–2003: the Icelandic GIST study, a population based incidence and pathologic risk stratification study. Int J Cancer. 2005;117:289–93.
62. Miettinen M, Lasota J, Sobin LH. Gastrointestinal stromal tumors of the stomach in children and young adults: a clinicopathologic, immunohistochemical, and molecular genetic study of 44 cases with long term follow up and review of the literature. Am J Surg Pathol. 2005;29:1373–81.
63. Kingham TP, DeMatteo RP. Multidisciplinary treatment of gastrointestinal stromal tumors. Surg Clin N Am. 2009;89:217–33.
64. Diment J, Tamborini E, Casali P, Gronchi A, Carney JA, Colecchia M. Carney triad: case report and molecular analysis of gastric tumor. Hum Pathol. 2005;36:112–6.
65. Matyakhina L, Bei TA, McWhinney SR, Pasini B, Cameron S, Gunawan B, et al. Genetics of Carney triad: recurrent losses at chromosome 1 but lack of germline mutations in genes associated with paragangliomas and gastrointestinal stromal tumors. J Clin Endocrinol Metab. 2007;92:3728–32.
66. Miettinen M, Fetsch JF, Sobin LH, Lasota J. Gastrointestinal stromal tumors in patients with neurofibromatosis 1: a clinicopathologic and molecular genetic study of 45 cases. Am J Surg Pathol. 2006;30(1):90–6.
67. Takazawa Y, Sakurai S, Sakuma Y, Ikeda T, Yamaguchi J, Hashizume Y, et al. Gastrointestinal stromal tumors of neurofibromatosis type I (von Recklinghausen's disease). Am J Surg Pathol. 2005;29(6):755–63.
68. Agaimy A, Wünsch PH, Hofstaedter F, Blaszyk H, Rümmele P, Gaumann A, et al. Minute gastric sclerosing stromal tumors (GIST tumorlets) are common in adults and frequently show c-KIT mutations. Am J Surg Pathol. 2007;31(1):113–20.
69. Nilsson B, Bümming P, Meis-Kindblom JM, Odén A, Dortok A, Gustavsson B, et al. Gastrointestinal stromal tumors: the incidence, prevalence, clinical course, and prognostication in the preimatinib mesylate era – a population-based study in western Sweden. Cancer. 2005;103(4):821–9.
70. Ueyama T, Guo KJ, Hashimoto H, Daimaru Y, Enjoji M. A clinicopathologic and immunohistochemical study of gastrointestinal stromal tumors. Cancer. 1992;69:947–55.
71. Sandrasegaran K, Rajesh A, Rushing DA, Rydberg J, Akisik FM, Henley JD. Gastrointestinal stromal tumors: CT and MRI findings. Eur Radiol. 2005;15(7):1407–14.
72. Miettinen M, Lasota J. Gastrointestinal stromal tumors: review on morphology, molecular pathology, prognosis, and differential diagnosis. Arch Pathol Lab Med. 2006;130(10):1466–78.
73. Goerres GW, Stupp R, Barghouth G, Hany TF, Pestalozzi B, Dizendorf E, et al. The value of PET, CT and in-line PET/CT in patients with gastrointestinal stromal tumours: long-term outcome of treatment with imatinib mesylate. Eur J Nucl Med Mol Imaging. 2005;32(2):153–62.
74. Rader AE, Avery A, Wait CL, McGreevey LS, Faigel D, Heinrich MC. Fine-needle aspiration biopsy diagnosis of gastrointestinal stromal tumors using morphology, immunocytochemistry, and mutational analysis of c-kit. Cancer. 2001;93:269–75.
75. Stelow EB, Stanley MW, Mallery S, Lai R, Linzie BM, Bardales RH. Endoscopic ultrasound guided fine needle aspiration findings of gastrointestinal leiomyomas and gastrointestinal stromal tumors. Am J Clin Pathol. 2003;119:703–8.
76. DeMatteo RP, Lewis JJ, Leung D, Mudan SS, Woodruff JM, Brennan MF. Two hundred gastrointestinal stromal tumors: recurrence patterns and prognostic factors for survival. Ann Surg. 2000;231:51–8.
77. Novitsky YW, Kercher KW, Sing RF, Heniford BT. Long-term outcomes of laparoscopic resection of gastric gastrointestinal stromal tumors. Ann Surg. 2006;243:738–45.

78. Eisenberg BL, Judson I. Surgery and imatinib in the management of GIST: emerging approaches to adjuvant and neoadjuvant therapy. Ann Surg Oncol. 2004;11:465–75.
79. Yeh C, Chen H, Tang R, Tasi W, Lin P, Wang J. Surgical outcome after surgical resection of rectal leiomyosarcoma. Dis Colon Rectum. 2000;43:1517–21.
80. van Oosterom AT, Judson I, Verweij J, Stroobants S, Donato di Paola E, Dimitrijevic S, et al. Safety and efficacy of imatinib (STI571) in metastatic gastrointestinal stromal tumours: a phase I study. Lancet. 2001;358(9291):1421–3.
81. Gold JS, DeMatteo RP. Combined surgical and molecular therapy: the gastrointestinal stromal tumor model. Ann Surg. 2006;244:176–84.
82. dos Santos Fernandes G, Blanke CD, Freitas D, Guedes R, Hoff PM. Perioperative treatment of gastrointestinal stromal tumors. Oncology. 2009;23(1):54–61.
83. Malhotra P, Singh M, Kochhar R, Nada R, Wig JD, Varma N, et al. Leukemia infiltration of bowel in chronic lymphocytic leukemia. Gastrointest Endosc. 2005;62(4):614–5.
84. Heiberg E, Wolverson M, Sandaram M, Sheilds JB. CT findings in leukemia. AJR Am J Roentgenol. 1984;143:1317–23.
85. Salek J, Sideridis K, White S. Chronic lymphocytic leukemia of the intestinal tract. Gastrointest Endosc. 2006;63(7):1072–3.
86. Hunter T, Bjelland JC. Gastrointestinal complications of leukemia and its treatment. AJR Am J Roentgenol. 1984;142:513–8.
87. Gavan DR, Hendry GM. Colonic complications of acute lymphoblastic leukemia. Br J Radiol. 1994;67:449–52.
88. Sloas MM, Flynn PM, Kaste SC, Patrick CC. Typhlitis in children with cancer: a 30 year experience. Clin Infect Dis. 1993;17:484–90.
89. Hayes Jr D, Leonardo JM. Neutropenic enterocolitis in a woman treated with 5-fluorouracil and leucovorin for colon carcinoma. NC Med J. 2002;63:132–4.
90. Avigan D, Richardson P, Elias A, Demetri G, Shapiro M, Schnipper L, et al. Neutropenic enterocolitis as a complication of high dose chemotherapy with stem cell rescue in patients with solid tumors: a case series with a review of the literature. Cancer. 1998;83(3):409–14.
91. Pestalozzi BC, Sotos GA, Choyke PL, Fisherman JS, Cowan KH, O'Shaughnessy JA. Typhlitis resulting from treatment with taxol and doxorubicin in patients with metastatic breast cancer. Cancer. 1993;71(5):1797–800.
92. Paulino AF, Kenney R, Forman EN, Medeiros LJ. Typhlitis in a patient with acute lymphoblastic leukemia prior to the administration of chemotherapy. Am J Pediatr Hematol Oncol. 1994;16:348–51.
93. Cunningham SC, Fakhry K, Bass BL, Napolitano LM. Neutropenic enterocolitis in adults: case series and review of the literature. Dig Dis Sci. 2005;50:215–20.
94. Kulaylat M, Doerr R, Ambrus J. A case presentation and review of neutropenic enterocolitis. J Med. 1997;28:1–19.
95. Hsu TF, Huang HH, Yen DH. ED presentation of neutropenic enterocolitis in adult patients with acute leukemia. Am J Emerg Med. 2004;22:276–9.
96. Ullery BW, Pieracci FM, Rodney JRM, Barie PS. Neutropenic enterocolitis. Surg Infect. 2009;10(3):307–14.
97. Davila ML. Neutropenic enterocolitis. Curr Opin Gastroenterol. 2006;22:44–7.
98. Gorshluter M, Ulrich M, Strehl J, Ziske C, Schepke M, Schmidt-Wolf IGH, et al. Neutropenic enterocolitis in adults: systematic analysis of evidence quality. Eur J Hematol. 2005;75:1–13.
99. Picardi M, Camera A, Pane F, Rotoli B. Improved management of neutropenic enterocolitis using early ultrasound scan and vigorous medical treatment. Clin Infect Dis. 2007;45:403–7.
100. Villar HV, Warneke JA, Peck MD, Durie B, Bjelland JC, Hunter TB. Role of surgical treatment in the management of complications of the gastrointestinal tract in patients with leukemia. Surg Gynecol Obstet. 1987;165(3):217–22.
101. Glenn J, Funkhouser WK, Schneider PS. Acute illnesses necessitating urgent abdominal surgery in neutropenic cancer patients: description of 14 cases and review of the literature. Surgery. 1989;105:778–9.
102. Quayle FJ, Lowney JK. Colorectal lymphoma. Clin Colon Rectal Surg. 2006;19:49–53.
103. Koch P, del Valle F, Berdel WE, Willich NA, Reers B, Hiddemann W, et al. Primary gastrointestinal non-Hodgkin's lymphoma: I. Anatomic and histologic distribution, clinical features, and survival data of 371 patients registered in the German Multicenter Study GIT NHL 01/92. J Clin Oncol. 2001;19(18):3861–73.
104. Zighelboim J, Larson MV. Primary colonic lymphoma, clinical presentation, histopathologic features and outcome with combination chemotherapy. J Clin Gastroenterol. 1994;18:291–7.
105. Dionigi G, Annoni M, Rovera F, Boni L, Villa F, Castano P, et al. Primary colorectal lymphomas: review of the literature. Surg Oncol. 2007;16 Suppl 1:S169–71.
106. Dawson IM, Cornes JS, Morson BC. Primary malignant lymphoid tumours of the gastrointestinal tract. Br J Surg. 1961;49:80–9.
107. Musallam K, Hatoum H, Barada K, Taher A, Salem ME, Malek EM, et al. Primary colorectal lymphoma. Med Oncol. 2010;27(2):249–54.
108. Wong MTC, Eu KW. Primary colorectal lymphomas. Colorectal Dis. 2006;8:586–91.
109. Lewin KJ, Ranchod M, Dorfmann RF. Lymphomas of the gastrointestinal tract – a study of 119 cases presenting with gastrointestinal disease. Cancer. 1978;43:693–707.
110. Contreary K, Nance FC, Becker WF. Primary lymphoma of the gastrointestinal tract. Ann Surg. 1980;191:593–8.
111. Wychulis AR, Bears OH, Woolner LB. Malignant lymphoma of the colon – a study of 69 cases. Arch Surg. 1966;93:215–25.
112. Fan CW, Changchien CR, Wang JY, Chen JS, Hsu KC, Tang R, et al. Primary colorectal lymphoma. Dis Colon Rectum. 2000;43(9):1277–82.
113. Azab MB, Henry-Amar M, Rougier P, Bognel C, Theodore C, Carde P, et al. Prognostic factors in primary gastrointestinal non-Hodgkin's lymphoma. A multivariate analysis, report of 106 cases, and review of the literature. Cancer. 1989;64(6):1208–17.
114. Jinnai D, Iwasa Z, Watanuki T. Malignant lymphoma of the large intestine – operative results in Japan. Surg Today. 1983;13:331–6.

50
Pediatric Colorectal Disorders

Marc A. Levitt and Alberto Peña

Hirschsprung's Disease

Hirschsprung's disease (congenital megacolon) is an anomaly characterized by functional partial colonic obstruction due to the absence of ganglion cells. It occurs in approximately 1 in 5,000 births. Boys are more frequently affected than girls and it is more common in caucasians.[1] The functional disturbances in this condition are attributed to the absence of ganglion cells from the Auerbach's myenteric plexus (located between the circular and longitudinal layers of smooth muscle of the intestine), the Henle's plexus (located in the submucosa), and the Meissner's plexus (in the superficial submucosa). The absence of these cells most probably produces uncoordinated contractions of the affected colon, which translates into a lack of relaxation of the colon that result in partial colonic obstruction.

The length of the aganglionic colonic segment varies. In the most common type, it includes the rectum and most of the sigmoid colon. Nearly 80% of all patients suffer from this type. In approximately 10% of the patients, the aganglionosis extends to the area of the splenic flexure or the upper descending colon. Total colonic aganglionosis occurs in another 8–10% of the patients. In those cases, the absent ganglion cells sometimes extend to the distal terminal ileum. In the rather controversial condition of "ultrashort" aganglionosis, the ganglion cells supposedly are lacking for only a few centimeters above the pectinate line. Very rarely, one can see patients who suffer from universal aganglionosis, meaning that ganglion cells are absent in the entire gastrointestinal tract, which is a lethal condition, unless the patient undergoes intestinal transplantation.

The clinical manifestations are those of a partial colonic obstruction. In addition, these patients suffer from a poorly characterized immunologic mucosal defect that may explain why they can get an inflammatory process called enterocolitis, which is the main cause of death. In addition, fecal stasis seems to promote the proliferation of abnormal colonic flora as well as production of endotoxins that contribute to the aggravation of the clinical condition.

Usually the patient becomes symptomatic during the first 24–48 h of life. Delayed passage of meconium (more than 24 h), abdominal distention, and vomiting are the most common symptoms. A rectal examination may produce explosive passage of liquid bowel movements and gas, which dramatically improves the baby's condition. This clinical improvement only lasts for a few hours, following which, the symptoms recur. If the colon is not decompressed, the infant usually suffers from sepsis, hypovolemia, and endotoxic shock. Cecal perforation may occur. About 25–30% of these babies die when unrecognized or not treated. Patients that do survive unrecognized and without treatment, ultimately develop the classic clinical picture initially described for this condition. They suffer from severe constipation, a huge megacolon, and an enormously distended abdomen, a clinical situation that is extremely rare nowadays in developed countries. Occasionally, these patients are misdiagnosed as suffering from idiopathic chronic constipation. In the latter condition, the patients are not seriously ill, and it is very common for them to suffer from overflow pseudoincontinence (encopresis). A rectal examination discloses a rectum full of fecal matter. Patients with Hirschsprung's disease on the other hand usually suffer from malnutrition, and a lack of normal development. They usually have an empty, aganglionic, and narrow rectum, and they do not suffer from soiling.

The presence of distention, vomiting, and delayed passage of meconium in a newborn must alert the clinician to the diagnosis of Hirschsprung's disease. An abdominal film shows massive dilatation of small bowel and colon. A contrast enema is used to clarify the diagnosis. The catheter for the study should be introduced only a few centimeters into the rectum in order to be able to visualize the nondilated aganglionic segment of the rectosigmoid, followed by a transitional zone and then a proximal dilatation. These typical changes are often not obvious during the neonatal period. The older the patient, the more obvious the size difference between normal and aganglionic segment. In patients with total colonic aganglionosis, the entire colon is not distended; the dilatation affects the small bowel only.

D.E. Beck et al. (eds.), *The ASCRS Textbook of Colon and Rectal Surgery: Second Edition*,
DOI 10.1007/978-1-4419-1584-9_50, © Springer Science+Business Media, LLC 2011

The definitive diagnosis by a rectal biopsy is based on both the histological absence of ganglion cells, and the presence of hypertrophic nerves. Acetylcholinesterase staining used by some centers is also abnormal. The biopsy can be taken full-thickness under direct vision, or a suction biopsy can be performed. The specimen, however, must include mucosa and submucosa.

Medical Management

Colonic decompression and irrigation with saline solution is the most valuable tool for the emergency management of newborns. This maneuver may dramatically improve a very ill neonate. Irrigations should not be confused with enemas. An enema is a procedure in which an amount of fluid is instilled into the colon. In a normal patient, it is expected that this fluid will be spontaneously expelled. However, patients with Hirschsprung's disease are incapable of expelling this fluid and, therefore, enemas are contraindicated. A colonic irrigation, on the other hand, promotes the expelling of the rectocolonic contents through the lumen of a large rubber tube, which is cleared with small amounts of saline solution. Rectocolonic irrigations may save the baby's life but of course are not the ideal long-term form of treatment. Once the histologic diagnosis has been established, the irrigations must continue in preparation for the surgical treatment.

Surgical Treatment

The basis of the surgical treatment consists in the resection of the aganglionic segment and pull-through of a normoganglionic segment to be anastomosed just above the anal canal, immediately above the pectinate line. This should guarantee the preservation of bowel control as the anal canal and sphincters are preserved. There are several ways to achieve these basic goals. The surgical treatment has evolved significantly since 1948 when the first surgical technique was described.[1]

Originally, these patients were subjected to a staged approach. The first stage consisted in the opening of a diverting colostomy, usually in the transverse colon. The second stage included the resection of the aganglionic segment and pull-through of the normoganglionic bowel, and the third stage was the colostomy closure. Subsequently, surgeons adopted a two-stage modality that included the opening of the colostomy during the newborn period at the level of the ganglion cells. The second stage consisted in the pull-through, leaving the patient without a colostomy.

More recently, the treatment most commonly used consists in a neonatal primary procedure without a protective colostomy.[2,3] This approach is less invasive and avoids the morbidity of a stoma and multiple surgeries. This can be done with a transanal approach alone (Figure 50-1).[4,5] or with the addition of laparoscopy to the transanal approach.[6] However, approaches may vary from country-to-country and with the surgeon's experience. In addition, a primary procedure, without a protective colostomy requires the presence of an experienced clinical pathologist, familiar with the interpretation of frozen sections. Also, in the case of a very ill, low-birth weight newborn, or a very sick baby, with enterocolitis unresponsive to the irrigations, a colostomy is still the optimal way to protect the patient. If a two-stage approach is chosen, in the presence of an experienced pathologist, the colostomy must be opened in a normoganglionic portion of the colon. In the absence of an experienced pathologist, the surgeon must open the colostomy, proximal to the transition zone in the right transverse colon or with an ileostomy. In the event of a colon that is not dilated, the patient should receive an ileostomy.

The definitive procedure (resection of the aganglionic segment and pull-through of the normal ganglionic colon) can be done in different ways. Swenson and Bill[1] described their operation consisting in an intra-abdominal resection of the aganglionic segment including a part of the normoganglionic dilated colon, and pull-through of a normoganglionic bowel, with a coloanal anastomosis of the normoganglionic bowel to the rectum, above the pectinate line. Nowadays, this can be done transanally.

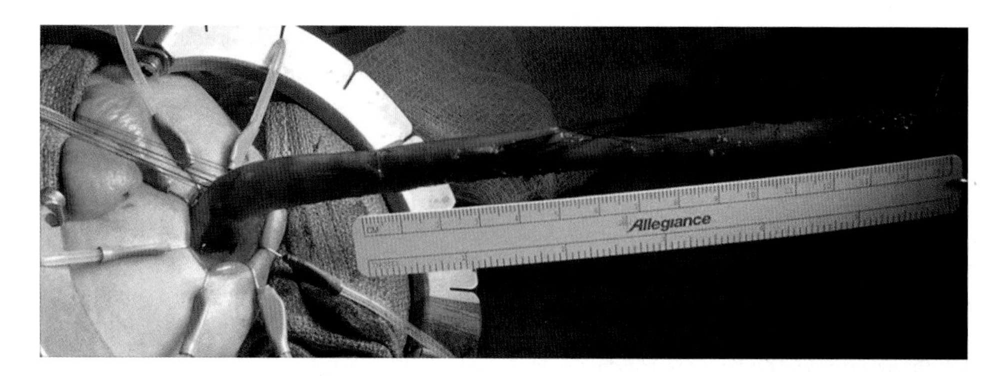

FIGURE 50-1. Transanal procedure.

Duhamel[7] described an operation designed to avoid pelvic dissection and potential nerve damage. He proposed to preserve the aganglionic rectum, dividing the colon at the peritoneal reflection. The normoganglionic colon is then pulled through a presacral space, created by blunt dissection and anastomosed to the rectal wall above the pectinate line.

Soave[8] designed a procedure consisting in an endorectal (submucosal) dissection of the aganglionic colon, leaving a seromuscular cuff. He carried this dissection down to the rectum above the pectinate line. The normally innervated colon is passed through the muscular cuff and anastomosed to the rectum. The purpose of this operation, again, was to avoid the perirectal dissection and its potential negative effects due to denervation of pelvic organs. This is now done transanally[4,5] sometimes with laparoscopy[6] and is the most commonly chosen technique worldwide.

The original Soave procedure was performed in two stages. During the first stage, the colon was pulled down but was not anastomosed to the rectum. It was left protruding outside the rectum. In the second stage, a week later, the protruded bowel was resected and the anastomosis was performed. Subsequently, Boley[9] proposed a primary anastomosis.

The abdominal portion of all of these operations can be done laparoscopically.[6,10,11] The technique of a seromuscular biopsy done laparoscopically has an important limitation in that it may avoid sampling the submucosa. We advocate for a full-thickness biopsy which includes submucosa.[12] It is possible to have ganglion cells in the muscularis but have hypertrophic nerves in the submucosa. Thus the wrong position for the pull-through could be selected.

In 1998, de la Torre and Ortega[4] and subsequently in 1999 Langer et al.[5] reported the novel transanal approach for the management of this condition. They demonstrated that the whole procedure can be done transanally provided the transition zone is in the sigmoid. If not, laparoscopy can be added for splenic flexure mobilization. A special retractor (Lone Star Retractor, Lone Star Medical Products®, Stafford, TX, USA) is very helpful to expose the dentate line and anal canal.

We recommend the use of multiple fine sutures taking the rectal mucosa 1 cm above the pectinate line, taking great care to preserve it. These allow the surgeon to exert a uniform traction on the rectal mucosa (Figure 50-2). Peripheral to this series of silk stitches, an incision is performed with cautery and a circumferential dissection of the rectum is performed applying uniform traction (Figure 50-3). The dissection can be performed submucosally (Soave-like) or full-thickness (Swenson-like) and is carried up through the peritoneal reflection. As the surgeon progresses in the dissection, full-thickness biopsies are taken to determine the place where the normoganglionic portion of the colon is reached. If laparoscopy was used to start the case, the ganglionic level is already known. The peritoneal reflection is soon found. The normoganglionic bowel is transanally anastomosed to the anal canal, 1 cm above the pectinate line.

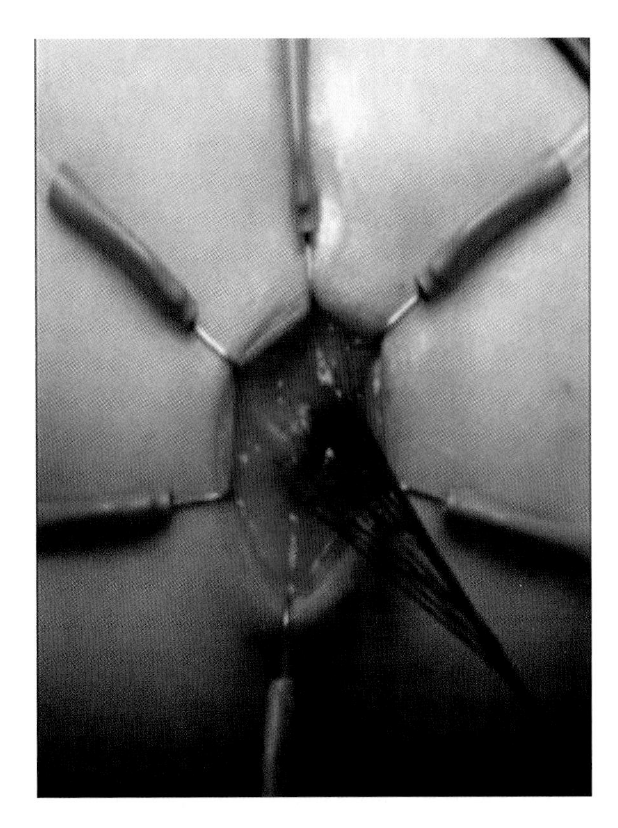

FIGURE 50-2. Multiple fine sutures taking the rectal mucosa 1 cm above the pectinate line, allowing the surgeon to apply uniform traction on the rectal mucosa.

Since the majority of patients have a transition zone in the sigmoid colon, it is possible to repair the entire defect using this technique, without a laparotomy or laparoscopy.[4,5] When the transition zone is located higher, the surgeon determines when he or she needs a laparoscopic-assisted procedure or a laparotomy. We specifically recommend resecting not only the aganglionic segment of the colon but also the very dilated part of the colon since a very dilated colon also has very poor peristalsis.

Complications and postoperative sequelae can be divided into two categories: preventable and nonpreventable. An algorithm to the approach to post pull-through Hirschsprung's patients with problems is shown in Figure 50-4. Preventable complication should not occur since they are due to technical errors. A feared preventable sequela is fecal incontinence. This is most likely related to injury to the continence mechanism.[13] All these procedures were originally designed to prevent this from happening, providing they are performed correctly. The key factors are preservation of the dentate line and not overstretching the sphincters. Dehiscence, retraction, stricture, abscess, and fistula are all considered preventable since they are usually due to technical errors (Table 50-1).[14] During the pull-through, the surgeon must be familiar with the manipulation of the blood supply and the arcades of the colon in order to guarantee a good blood supply in the

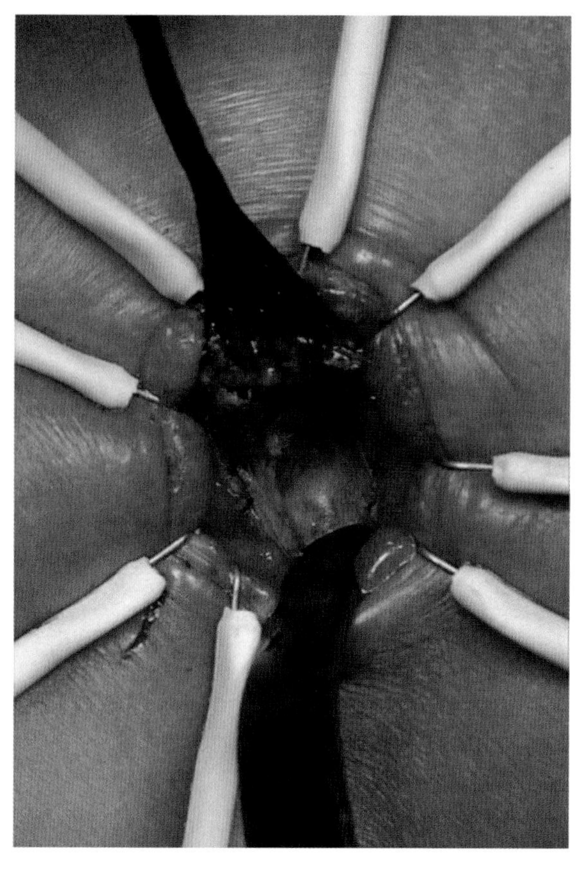

Figure 50-3. Peripheral to this series of silk stitches, an incision is performed with cautery and a circumferential dissection of the rectum is performed applying uniform traction.

pulled-through colon. The anastomosis should be done without tension.

A relatively nonpreventable complication is enterocolitis unless there is an anatomic explanation, such as a stricture causing stasis. This is also an unpredictable, and a rather mysterious condition. Despite receiving a technically adequate operation, patients may suffer from enterocolitis. The frequency of this condition varies[15] and its etiology is unknown. Fecal stasis is the most important predisposing factor. If this occurs in the colon in a normal individual it produces constipation; in patients with Hirschsprung's disease, stasis frequently results in proliferation of abnormal bacteria, ulcerations of the colon, absorption of endotoxins, shock, and sometimes perforation. These patients respond to colonic irrigations, and on rare occasion require a colostomy. In a patient with recurrent episodes of enterocolitis there may be an anatomic cause and a secondary pull-through may be curative.[12]

Constipation may also occur after these procedures. It is more common in patients in whom the aganglionic segment was resected, but a dilated portion of the colon was pulled down.[12] This is a partially preventable condition. Most cases of constipation can be avoided by resecting not only the aganglionic segment but also the dilated portion of the colon. In addition, a Duhamel pouch that is too large can compress the ganglionic pull-through causing obstructive symptoms. Many of the issues can present years after the pull-through, even in adulthood, and the adult surgeon caring for a Hirschsprung's patient must understand these anatomic issues.

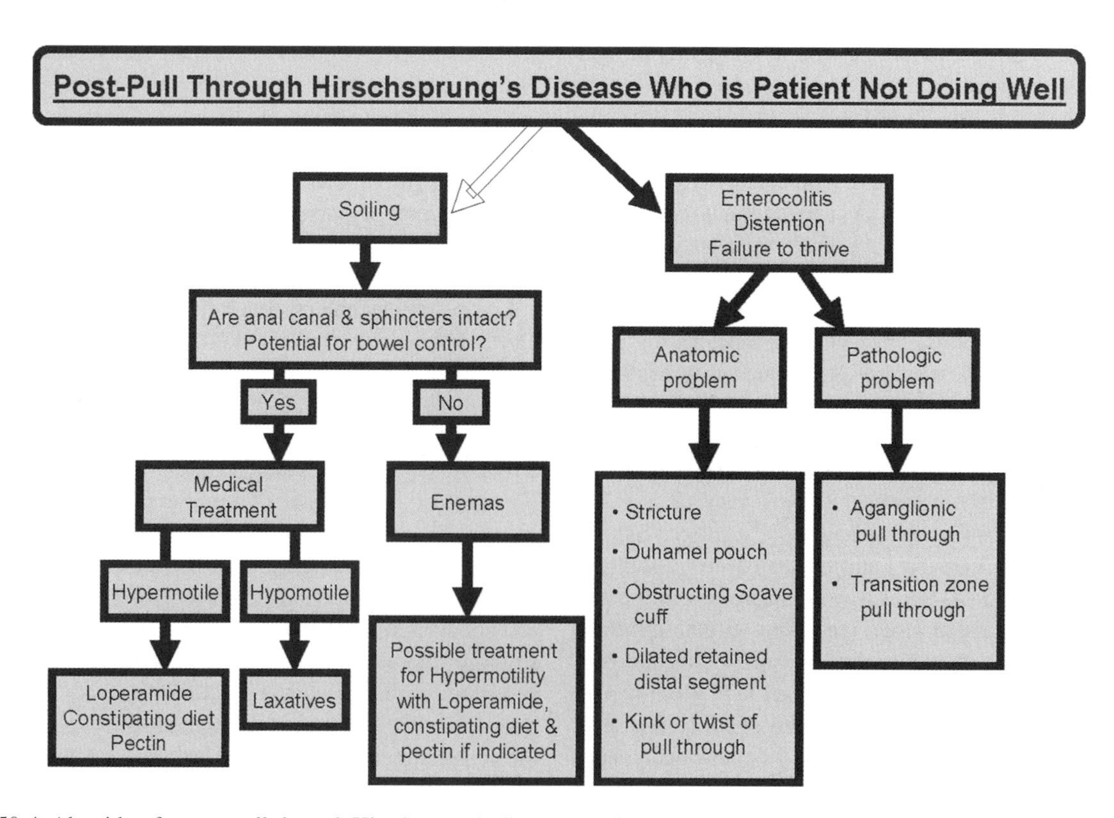

Figure 50-4. Algorithm for post-pull-through Hirschpsrung's disease who is not doing well.

TABLE 50-1. Indications for Hirschsprung's disease reoperations

Reoperations for Hirschsprung's disease (75 patients[a,b])	
Mechanical indications	
Stricture	29
Megarectal pouch (post-Duhamel)	22
Obstructing Soave cuff	11
Dilated segment	5
Pathological indications	
Aganglionosis	15
Transition zone	8
Other indications	
Fistulae (rectocutaneous, rectourethral, rectovaginal)	12
Recurrent pelvic abscess	7

[a] Several patients may have more than one indication for surgery.
[b] The first 51 patients have been reported in Peña, Elicevik, Levitt.[14]

Each one of the techniques described has its own advocates. The analysis of different series shows that the most important factor that affects the clinical results is the experience and familiarity of the surgeon with their chosen procedure. Some surgeons claim that the Swenson operation exposes the patient to nerve damage that may provoke urinary and sexual disturbances. We as well as Dr. Swenson have not found this to be true. The Duhamel procedure is commonly followed by severe problems of constipation and dilatation of the aganglionic piece of colon left in place.[16] In the Soave operation, patients may suffer from fecal incontinence,[13] as well as perianal fistulas and abscesses due to the presence of islets of mucosa left behind during the endorectal dissection, much like the known complication of this sort following a mucosectomy for ulcerative colitis.

Advocates of a transanal approach site the decreased morbidity and enhanced recovery as a consequence of a procedure without the intra-abdominal dissection.[17–19] In addition, this approach permits early postoperative feeding, shorter length of stay, faster recovery, and possibly less chance for postoperative adhesions.

Surgical Management of Total Colonic Aganglionosis

The current treatment of this condition consists in a newborn ileostomy and then at age 1–3 years resection of the entire aganglionic colon and pull-through of the normal ganglionic terminal ileum that is anastomosed just above the anal canal. In order to avoid fluid losses and in an attempt to decrease the number of bowel movements per day, as well as to promote water absorption, Martin[20] proposed to leave a part of the rectosigmoid and descending aganglionic segment in place, and anastomose the normoganglionic terminal ileum to this colon and connect it to the posterior aspect of the rectum like in the Duhamel procedure. Kimura et al.[21] proposed the use of a right colon patch with the hope of creating a reservoir for water absorption. The use of a pouch can cause stasis of stool in the small bowel which is why many surgeons choose an ileo-Duhamel[22]; however, this stasis can produce bacterial proliferation and enterocolitis. Rather than absorbing water, very often the intestine secretes fluid into the lumen, producing a secretory diarrhea. It is therefore our opinion, as well as others,[23] that a straight ileorectal anastomosis is the preferred option.

They, as all patients with a surgically resected colon, suffer from multiple stools. Treatment of this with loperamide, pectin, and a constipating diet helps. We also like to wait until the child can sit on a potty and is toilet trained for urine as the avoidance of stool in a diaper dramatically reduces the problem of a perineal rash.

Surgical Treatment of Ultrashort Hirschsprung's

The surgical treatment of the ultrashort-segment aganglionosis is as controversial as the existence of this condition. Normal individuals have an area of aganglionosis above the pectinate line, but the length of this aganglionic area has not been accurately or scientifically determined. This is the reason why the diagnosis of ultrashort Hirschsprung is so controversial. Some surgeons propose an operation called a myectomy, consisting in the resection of a strip of smooth muscle from the anal verge up to the area where ganglion cells are found. The results of this procedure, again, are highly controversial and there is no scientific basis to explain why this may improve the condition. More scientifically conducted studies are required to clarify this issue.

Most cases of Hirschsprung's disease are diagnosed early in life, but a few patients reach their late teens and even adulthood before a diagnosis is made. Hirschsprung's disease in adults must be distinguished from other causes of mega colon such as Chagas disease, sigmoid volvulus, colonic inertia, Oglvie's syndrome, and other disorders of the central nervous system. Typically, Hirschsprung's in adults is of the short segment variety. Many such patients are confused with Hirschsprung's and in fact have idiopathic constipation which responds to laxative therapy.

Neuronal Intestinal Dysplasia

Neuronal intestinal dysplasia (NID) refers to a histologic condition that includes hypertrophy of ganglion cells, immature ganglia, hypoganglionosis, hyperplasia of the submucosal and myenteric plexus, giant ganglion cells as well as hypoplasia or aplasia of the sympathetic innervations of the myenteric plexus. These histologic abnormalities have been described as occurring in a localized or disseminated manner,[24] but even the existence of this condition can be questioned.[25] We suspect that most cases described as NID are in fact a sampled areas of colon that is actually transition zone bowel in a Hirschsprung's patient.

Anorectal Malformations (Imperforate Anus)

Anorectal malformations represent a spectrum of defects characterized by the absence of an external anal orifice. The overwhelming majority of the patients have an abnormal communication between the rectum and the perineum (perineal fistula), the vestibule (vestibular fistula), or the vagina (vaginal fistula), in the female. In some female patients, rectum, vagina, and urethra are fused together forming a common channel (cloacal malformation) and open into a single external orifice. In the male, the communication is with the urethra (rectourethral fistula), or the bladder (rectobladder neck fistula). Only 5% of the entire spectrum of patients are born with no fistula and the rectum is blind-ending. Anorectal malformations occur in about one in every 5,000 newborns. Males seem to suffer from this condition slightly more frequently than females. The most common type of defects seen in boys is a rectourethral fistula and the most common type in girls is vestibular fistula. Table 50-2 shows the anatomic classification.

Associated Anomalies

Urogenital abnormalities occur in about 50% of all patients with anorectal malformations. The higher and more complex the anorectal malformation, the higher the incidence of associated urologic defects. Urologic malformations are a common source of morbidity in these patients. About 90% of patients with a rectobladder neck fistula in males as well as in cases of cloacas with a common channel longer than 3 cm, have an associated urological problem. Unilateral renal agenesis is the most common urologic anomaly, followed by vesicoureteral reflux. Other important abnormalities include cryptorchidism, hypospadias, renal ectopia, and hydronephrosis.

Table 50-2. Current classification of anorectal malformations

Male
Perineal fistula
Rectourethral fistula
Bulbar
Prostatic
Rectobladder neck fistula
Imperforate anus without fistula
Rectal atresia and stenosis
Female
Perineal fistula
Vestibular fistula
Imperforate anus without fistula
Rectal atresia and stenosis
Cloaca
Complex malformations

Sacral and spinal abnormalities are also very common in patients with anorectal malformations. The sacrum is frequently abnormal. The sacral abnormalities also represent a spectrum that varies from a completely absent sacrum to a completely normal one, including different degrees of hypo development. There seems to be a direct relationship between the degree of sacral abnormality and the final functional prognosis. These patients also suffer from hemivertebrae and as a consequence different degrees of scoliosis. The presence of hemivertebrae also seems to be related to a poorer functional prognosis.

Twenty-five percent of patients with anorectal malformations suffer from a defect called tethered cord.[26] In this condition, the cord is abnormally attached (tethered) to the spine. During the baby's natural growth, it is believed that the spine grows faster than the cord, producing traction on the nerve fibers that may produce functional disturbances in the motion of the lower extremities and may contribute to sphincter problems particularly impacting bladder emptying.

Hemi sacrum is sometimes associated with an anorectal malformation and there can be a mass located in the area of the sacral defect. An anorectal malformation with hemisacrum and a presacral mass is known as the Currarino triad. The most common sacral masses in these patients are a dermoid, teratoma, lipoma, anterior meningocele, or a combination of all these. These patients also have a poor functional prognosis.

Approximately 8% of all patients with anorectal malformations suffer from esophageal atresia. About 30% have some sort of cardiovascular congenital anomaly. Most commonly seen are patent ductus arteriosus, atrial septal defect, ventricular septal defect, tetralogy of Fallot, as well as other more complex malformations. Only 10% of patients have a cardiovascular malformation with significant hemodynamic repercussions that requires surgical treatment.

The main concern in a patient with anorectal malformation is whether or not the child will have bowel control, urinary control, and sexual function in the future. The higher the malformation, the worse the functional prognosis will be. The higher the anorectal defect, the more likely the child will suffer from fecal incontinence, but the less the chance of suffering from constipation. Conversely, the lower the malformation, the higher the incidence of constipation but the lower the incidence of fecal incontinence.

Description of Specific Defects

Males

Perineal Fistula

This is the simplest of all defects. The rectum opens anterior to the center of the sphincter mechanism in the perineum. The rectal orifice is usually too narrow to allow normal passage of stool. Sometimes, the end of the rectum lies immediately below a very thin layer of epithelium with an external opening located at the base of the scrotum or sometimes at the base of the penis. The meconium or mucous sometimes can be seen below that very thin layer of epithelium giving an impression of a black or white ribbon. The overwhelming majority of these patients have a normal sacrum, less than 10% of them have associated defects. The final functional prognosis is excellent,[27] provided these patients receive adequate treatment. These patients can be operated on during the newborn period, with an operation that consists in moving the anal orifice back to the center of the sphincter creating a normal-sized anus.

Rectouretheral Fistula

In this group of malformations, the rectum connects to the urethra. In the most common subtype, the rectum opens into the lower part of the posterior urethra known as the bulbar urethra, and, therefore, the defect is called rectourethral bulbar fistula (Figure 50-5A). The rectum passes through a funnel-like striated sphincter mechanism to reach the lowest part of the posterior urethra. Eighty-five percent of these patients achieve bowel control when treated properly.[27] Approximately 30% of them have other associated defects.[27]

In the second subtype, the rectum opens into the upper part of the posterior urethra (prostatic), and, therefore, it is called rectoprostatic fistula (Figure 50-5B). Only 60% of these patients achieve bowel control later in life. Sixty percent of them have significant associated defects.[27] Most of these patients (rectourethral fistula) require a colostomy at birth and subsequently (usually 1–2 months later) they receive the definitive repair of the malformation.

The perineum of patients with anorectal malformations, have characteristic features that must be recognized. The higher the malformation, the more likely the patient will have a flat bottom, meaning that the natural midline groove is absent and there is no distinguishable anal dimple. The lower the malformation, the more prominent the midline groove and the anal dimple. In patients with rectourethral bulbar fistula, there is a recognizable midline groove as well as an anal dimple and in patients with rectoprostatic fistula, there is a tendency for the perineum to be flat. Also, the anal dimple tends to be closer to the scrotum the higher the malformation. One can also frequently see a bifid scrotum in cases of prostatic fistula.

Rectobladder Neck Fistula

This is the highest of all defects in male patients (Figure 50-5C). The rectum is connected to the bladder neck. Ninety percent of these patients have significant associated defects. The perineum is frequently flat. These patients are the only ones that require a laparotomy or laparoscopy in addition to the posterior sagittal approach to be repaired. Only 15% of these patients achieve bowel control later in life.[27]

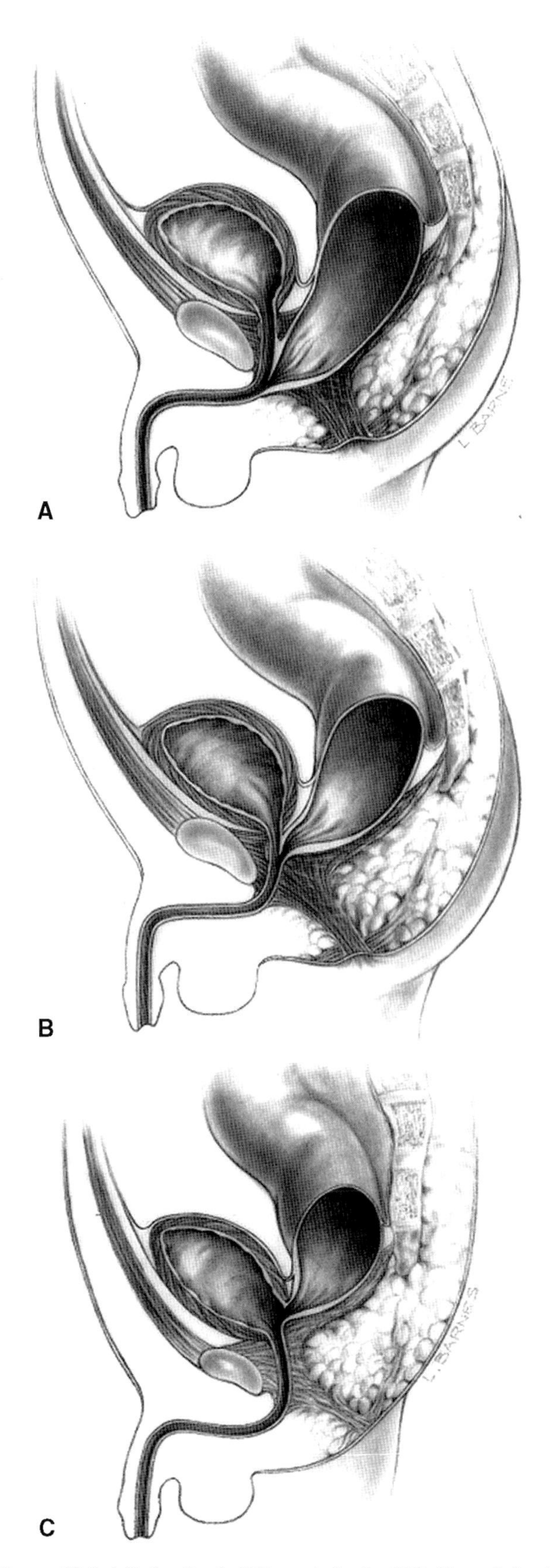

FIGURE 50-5. **A** Bulbar fistula, **B** Prostatic fistula, **C** Bladderneck fistula. (Reprinted with permission from Pena A. Atlas of surgical management of anorectal malformations. New York: Springer Verlag; 1989).

Imperforate Anus Without Fistula

This is a rather unusual anomaly that occurs in 5% of all children with anorectal malformations. Half of them also suffer from Down's syndrome. More than 90% of all patients with Down's syndrome who suffer from an anorectal malformation have this specific type of defect, clearly pointing to a genetic influence.[28] Eighty percent of the babies with Down's syndrome and this malformation will eventually have bowel control when they receive an adequate operation. Approximately 90% of patients with this defect and without Down's syndrome have bowel control,[29] and patients usually have a good sphincter mechanism and a good sacrum.

Rectal Atresia or Stenosis

This malformation occurs in only 1% of all cases. It consists of a complete or partial interruption of the rectal lumen located between the anal canal and the rectum. The external appearance of the perineum is normal and the anal canal is normal or appears like a funnel with a long skin lined canal. The malformation is usually discovered when a nurse tries to take the newborn's rectal temperature. The sacrum is normal as is the sphincter mechanism. Some patients have a hemisacrum and a presacral mass which must be screened for. All of these patients (100%) will have bowel control after a correctly performed operation.[27]

Female Defects

Perineal Fistula

In these female newborns, the rectum opens in what is called the perineal body between the normal location of the anus and the female genitalia. All that was described about this defect in males is true for females. These patients can be repaired at birth without a colostomy. The prognosis is excellent.[27]

Vestibular Fistula

This is by far the most common defect seen in female patients (Figure 50-6). The rectum opens in the vestibule of the female genitalia just outside the hymen. The rectum and vagina share a very thin common wall. About 30% of these babies have associated defects; 95% of these babies will have bowel control when properly treated.[27] The sacrum is usually normal. Vestibular fistula is frequently misdiagnosed as a rectovaginal fistula.[30] Vaginal fistula is an extremely unusual defect, representing less than 1% of all the female defects. In those unusual cases of vaginal fistula, the rectum opens into the posterior vaginal wall deeper to the hymen.

Most of the vestibular fistula cases are successfully operated on at birth without a colostomy. However, those undiverted patients can suffer from dehiscence and retraction, when the surgical technique employed is not adequate so diversion is a safe approach. A secondary operation in these cases does not render the same good result as in cases of a well-done primary procedure.

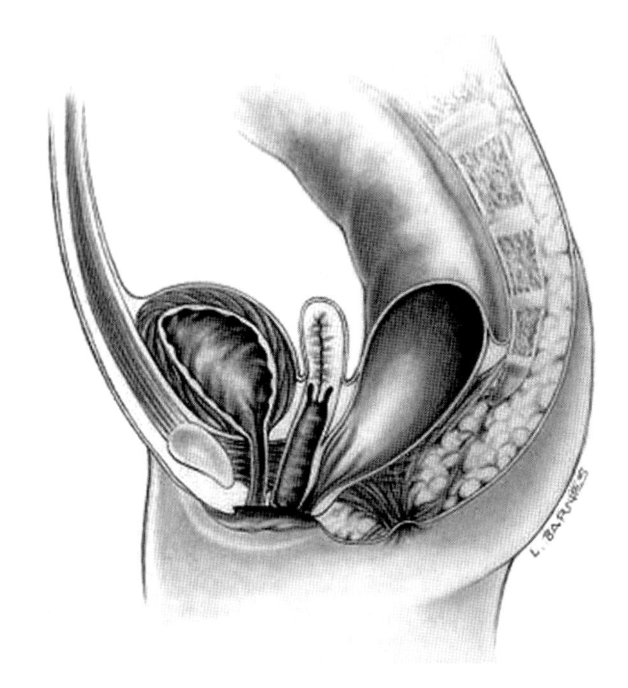

FIGURE 50-6. Vestibular fistula. (Reprinted with permission from Pena A. Atlas of surgical management of anorectal malformations. New York: Springer Verlag; 1989).

Imperforate Anus Without Fistula

It is uncommon to see this type of defect in females. All that was mentioned about this defect in males is true about this defect in females, except of course that the distal rectum is adjacent to the posterior vagina rather than to the urethra.

Rectal Atresia or Stenosis

This condition does not differ from the defect described in males. Again, the patient must be screened for a presacral mass.

Cloaca

A cloaca is defined as a malformation in which the rectum, vagina, and urinary tract are fused together forming a common channel (Figure 50-7). This single channel opens where the normal urethra is located in females. Externally, these babies have rather small-looking genitalia. Separation of the small labia allows the observer to see a single orifice, which confirms the clinical diagnosis of a cloaca. Cloacas represents another spectrum of defects. The length of the common channel varies from 1 to 7 or even 10 cm, and is directly related to the final functional prognosis for bowel and urinary control. Patients with a common channel shorter than 3 cm can be repaired posterior sagittally without opening the abdomen and the prognosis for bowel and urinary control is good.

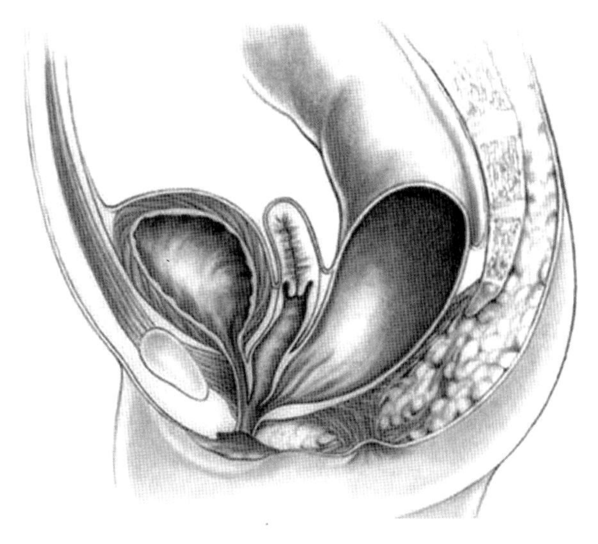

FIGURE 50-7. Cloaca. (Reprinted with permission from Pena A. Atlas of surgical management of anorectal malformations. New York: Springer Verlag; 1989).

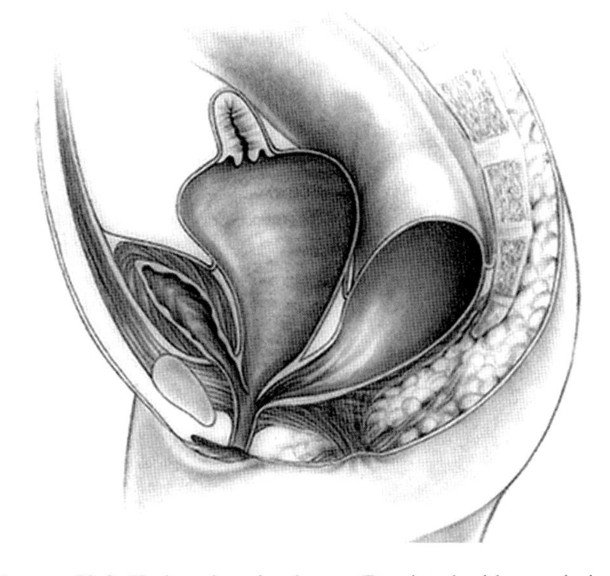

FIGURE 50-8. Hydrocolpos in cloaca. (Reprinted with permission from Pena A. Atlas of surgical management of anorectal malformations. New York: Springer Verlag; 1989).

On the other hand, cloacas with a common channel longer than 3 cm represent a serious technical challenge, whereby the operation frequently requires not only a posterior sagittal approach but also a laparotomy and a creative vaginoplasty or a vaginal replacement. The repair of these complex defects requires experience with pediatric urology. The final functional prognosis is not very good in cases with a long common channel.[27] Associated defects occur in about 90% of all patients with a common channel longer than 3 cm.

About 40% of patient with cloaca suffer from hydrocolpos (a very dilated vagina full of fluid). The dilated vagina compresses the trigone and may produce ureterovesical obstruction, megaureters, and hydronephrosis (Figure 50-8).

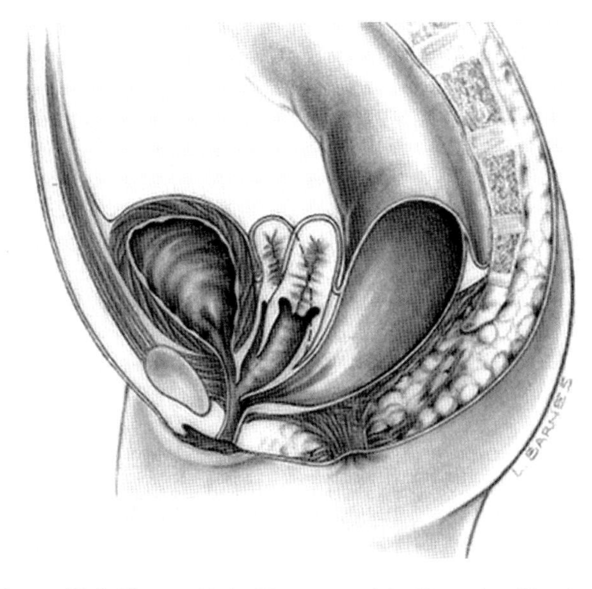

FIGURE 50-9. Cloaca with double uterus and double vagina. (Reprinted with permission from Pena A. Atlas of surgical management of anorectal malformations. New York: Springer Verlag; 1989).

Approximately 40% of the patients with cloaca also have different degrees of septation of the vagina and the uterus (Figure 50-9) which have important future implications, impacting menses as well as obstetric potential.[31]

Initial Management

Male Newborns

Perineal inspection and urinalysis allows the clinician to determine the type of malformation that the baby has in about 90% of cases.

The presence of a perineal orifice, by definition makes the diagnosis of a perineal fistula. This is also true when the baby has an external defect called a "bucket-handle" malformation that is a skin bridge in the midline in the area of the anal dimple. If a patient has a good midline groove, an anal dimple, and meconium in the urine, that is consistent with a prostatic or rectourethral fistula. A flat bottom and bifid scrotum are signs of a very high malformation, high prostatic or bladderneck fistula.

Diagnostic studies should be done after 24 h of life, but not later than 36 h. The reason for this is that is necessary to wait until the most distal part of the rectum is distended in order for it to be seen by any diagnostic modalities. An MRI, ultrasound, CAT scan, or simple X-ray film done prior to 24 h will not show the most distal part of the rectum, because it is collapsed by compression of the sphincteric funnel. In order for meconium to be forced through a tiny distal fistula, it is necessary to wait until the intraluminal pressure is high enough to overcome the tone of the striated muscle

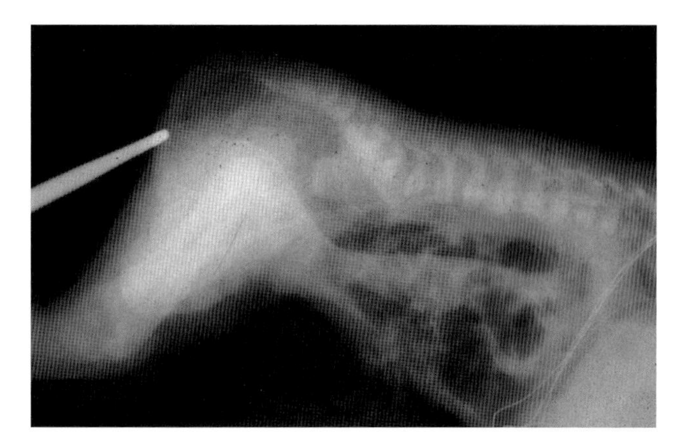

FIGURE 50-10. Cross-table lateral X-ray. (Reprinted with permission from Levitt MA, Peña A. Imperforate anus and claocal malformations. In: Ashcraft's pediatric surgery. 5th ed.; 2010 with permission from Elsevier).

that surrounds the distal rectum, which usually happens after 24 h. During the first 24 h, the clinician must try to answer two very important questions:

1. Does the baby have an associated defect that threatens his/her life?
2. Does the baby need a primary repair or a colostomy?

The baby should be examined to rule out the presence of cardiovascular defects. The patient will remain with nothing by mouth, and insertion of a nasogastric tube is recommended to avoid vomiting and potential risk of aspiration. Passage of this tube also rules out an associated esophageal atresia. An ultrasound of the abdomen is indicated to rule out the presence of hydronephrosis. An ultrasound of the spine is also useful to evaluate for the presence of tethered cord. An X-ray film of the lumbar spine and the sacrum will assess for the presence of hemi vertebrae and sacral abnormalities. A very abnormal sacrum is usually associated with a very high defect. If after 24 h, the surgeon is still not sure as to the type of defect that the baby has, a cross-table lateral film with the baby in prone position and the pelvis elevated should be performed. This will show the location of gas inside a distended rectum (Figure 50-10). If the rectum is visualized below the coccyx and the surgeons have experience with the neonatal repair of this malformation, the patient can be approached primarily. Conversely, if the rectum is located higher than the coccyx, or the surgeons have no experience with these neonatal operations, it is better to perform a diverting colostomy and to postpone the main repair for a later date.

Female Newborns

It is also true in females that simple inspection of the perineum will allow for a correct diagnosis during the neonatal period in most cases. The presence of a small opening in the perineum anterior to the sphincter mechanism makes the diagnosis of perineal fistula. Sometimes, it is difficult to see the opening of the rectum in the vestibule because the female genitalia are swollen at birth due to the effect of the maternal hormones. The presence of a fistula in the vestibule establishes the diagnosis of a rectovestibular fistula (Figure 50-6). In order to make the diagnosis of a rectovaginal fistula (extremely unusual defect) one would have to see meconium coming from inside the vagina, deeper than the hymen. The presence of a single perineal orifice makes the diagnosis of a cloaca (Figure 50-7).

If none of these signs are present after 24 h, the baby should have a cross-table lateral film in prone position (Figure 50-10). Most likely the baby has an imperforated anus with no fistula – which represent 5% of all cases.

During the first 24 h of life, the baby should be subjected to the same tests described for the male patient. If the baby has a cloaca, an ultrasound of the abdomen should be performed not only in the upper abdomen to rule out hydronephrosis but also in the lower abdomen to rule out the presence of hydrocolpos (Figure 50-8). Most babies with a cloaca need a diverting colostomy. These babies should not be taken to the operating room unless the surgeon has already ruled out the presence of hydrocolpos. The hydrocolpos must be drained at birth, usually with a tube at the time of colostomy opening, particularly when the baby suffers from hydronephrosis. Prior to trying other procedures for the treatment of a hydronephrosis and megaureter, the hydrocolpos must be drained, which most of the time will decompress the urinary system.

Colostomy

Colostomies in babies with anorectal malformation should be totally diverting. Loop colostomies are contraindicated as they may allow the passing of stool from the proximal into the distal colon, producing direct fecal contamination of the urinary tract. The ideal colostomy should be created in the descending colon, with separated stomas (Figure 50-11). Both stomas should be separated enough as to allow the placement of a stoma bag over the proximal stoma. Distal to the mucus fistula, the baby should have enough length of colon to allow a comfortable pull-through at the time of the main repair.

In cases of cloaca, the surgeon must also drain the hydrocolpos through the abdomen. When the vagina is so distended that it reaches the upper abdomen, it can be drained with a vaginostomy, suturing the vaginal wall directly to the abdominal wall. When the vagina is not that large, it can be drained with a tube that is exteriorized through a separate hole in the abdominal wall.

Two to four weeks after the colostomy, a high-pressure distal colostogram should be performed. This involves injection of hydrosoluble contrast material through the distal limb of the colostomy to delineate the anatomy of the distal colon and to establish an accurate anatomic diagnosis (Figure 50-12). This is, by far, the most important diagnostic study in anorectal malformations. Trying to repair these malformations without a good distal colostogram exposes the babies to serious injuries of the urinary tract, particularly in males.[32] For cloacas, a constrast study should be done to delineate all three systems; urologic, gynecologic, and colorectal (Figure 50-13). We do not do contrast studies for perineal or vestibular fistulas as their anatomy is known by clinical inspection alone.

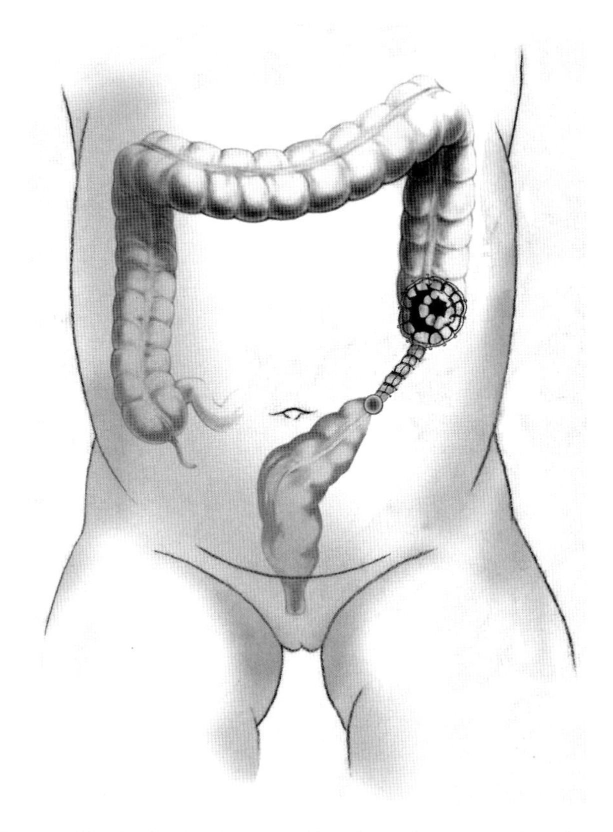

FIGURE 50-11. Ideal colostomy. (Reprinted from Pena A. Atlas of surgical management of anorectal malformations with permission from Springer; 1986).

Main Repair

Males

Perineal fistulas can be repaired performing a minimal posterior sagittal anoplasty. The baby is placed in prone position with the pelvis elevated. Multiple stitches are placed at the mucocutaneous junction of the fistula orifice. An incision dividing the sphincter mechanism, posterior to the anal orifice, is performed, and the rectum is carefully dissected to be moved back and relocated within the limits of the sphincter. During the dissection of the anterior rectal wall, special care must be taken to avoid injury to the posterior urethra, which is the most common and feared complication in these operations.[32] The babies must have a Foley catheter in the urethra. A useful alternative in a very sick baby or when the surgeon does not have enough experience is simply to subject the patient to dilatations of the fistula, with a plan for a future definitive repair.

In cases of rectourethral fistulas, after their newborn colostomy, the patients undergo a posterior sagittal anorectoplasty (PSARP). The baby is placed in prone position with the pelvis elevated and with a Foley catheter in place. A posterior sagittal incision is performed between both buttocks running from the lower portion of the sacrum to the base of the scrotum. The entire sphincter mechanism is divided exactly in the midline, making sure to leave an equal amount of sphincter muscle on both sides.

The posterior rectal wall is identified and is opened in the midline. The fistula is visualized and multiple fine silk stitches are placed taking the rectal mucosa immediately above the fistula in order to exert uniform traction to facilitate the dissection and separation of the rectum from the urethra. A submucosal plane is established in the anterior rectal wall to avoid damage to the urinary tract. About 1 cm above the fistula site, the dissection is continued full-thickness until

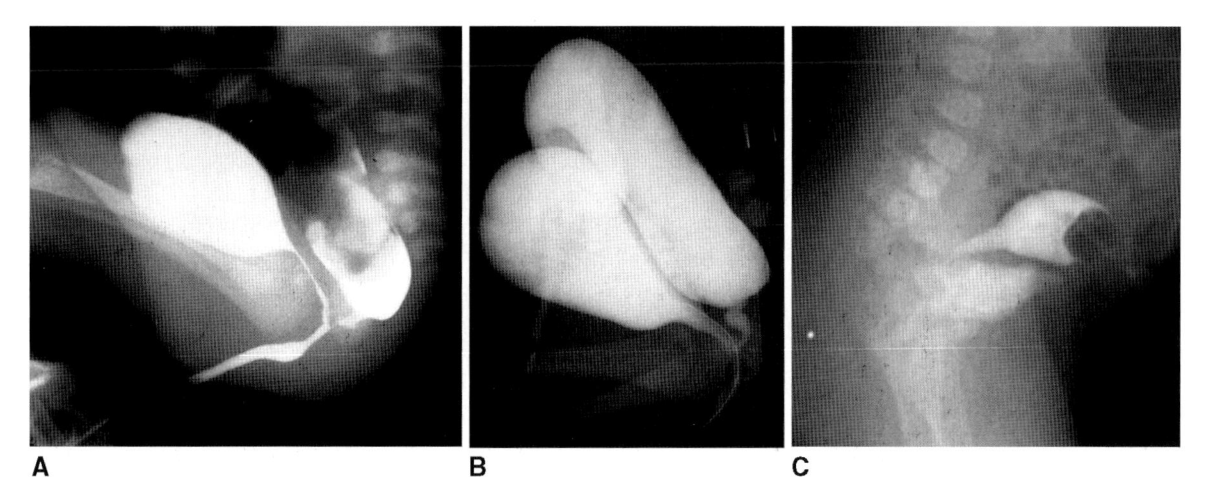

FIGURE 50-12. **A** Colostogram showing bulbar fistula. (Reprinted from Levitt MA, Peña A. Imperforate anus and claocal malformations In: Ashcraft's pediatric surgery. 5th ed.; 2010 with permission from Elsevier.) **B** Colostogram showing prostatic fistula. **C** Colostogram showing Bladderneck fistula.

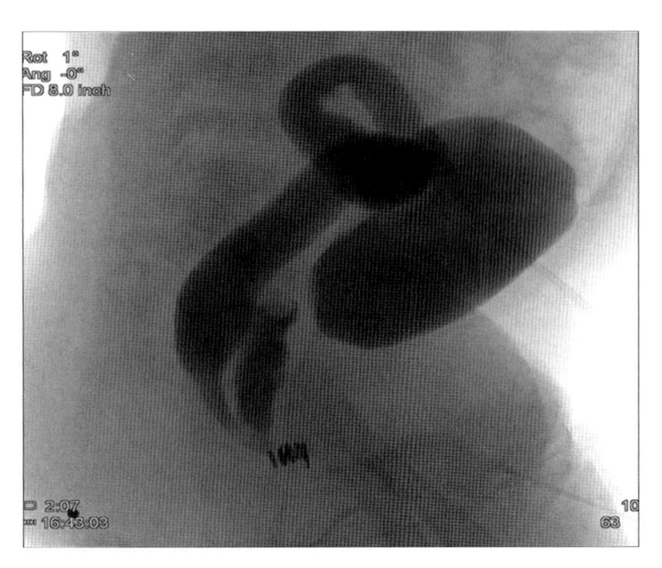

Figure 50-13. 3D cloaca imaging.

the rectum is completely separated from the urinary tract. It is in this plane that one must be extremely meticulous to avoid injuries to the vas deferens, seminal vesicles, and an occasional ectopic ureter. After this, a circumferential dissection with division of extrinsic vessels of the rectum is performed until enough length has been gained to bring the rectum down to the perineum to anastomose it without tension to the skin in the area of the anal sphincter. At this point, the fistula on the posterior urethra is closed with absorbable suture. On rare occasion the rectum is very dilated and cannot be accommodated within the available space of the sphincter mechanism. Under those circumstances, the posterior rectal wall must be tapered. It must be the posterior rectal wall that is tapered, rather than the anterior wall so that a suture line is not opposed to the urethral fistula that was closed. The limits of the sphincter are electrically determined and the rectum is placed within the sphincteric complex. The only difference in the surgical treatment between the rectourethral bulbar fistula and the retroprostatic fistula is that the latter requires a more significant dissection to bring the rectum down.

Rectobladder Neck Fistula

This malformation occurs in only 10% of male patients.[27] This is the only defect that requires a laparotomy or laparoscopic assistance in addition to the posterior sagittal operation. This is because the rectum is located too high to be reached from below. The posterior sagittal incision is performed to create the path through which the rectum should be pulled down and to tack the pull through to the muscle complex. The operation begins with a midline laparotomy or laparoscopy. The rectum is dissected above the peritoneal reflexion. The surgeon must create a plane of dissection as close as possible to the bowel wall but without injuring the rectal wall. One must keep in mind that the ureters and vas deferens run in the same direction toward the bladder neck, and, therefore, those structures must be kept under direct vision during the dissection of the rectum. The bladder neck is located about 2 cm below the peritoneal reflexion, and, therefore, it is very easy to find the end of the rectum and to divide and suture the fistula site. The rectum then must be mobilized to be pulled down through the tract established through the posterior sagittal incision. In such a case, this incistion can be opened with the patient in supine position and the legs lifted up.

Imperforate Anus Without Fistula

In cases of imperforate anus without fistula, the operation is not necessarily easier than in patients with a fistula because the rectum is still intimately attached to the posterior urethra. These patients are approached posterior sagittally, the posterior rectal wall is opened in the midline, and multiple stitches are placed in the edge of the rectal wall to exert uniform traction and to facilitate the separation of the rectum from the urinary tract. Special care must be taken during the dissection of the anterior wall to separate it from the urinary tract.

Rectal Atresia or Stenosis

These patients also require a posterior sagittal approach. The entire sphincter mechanism is divided posterior sagittally. Both rectum and anal canal are opened posteriorly. The dilated proximal rectum is anastomosed to the anal canal and then the sphincter mechanism is meticulously reconstructed in the midline. If a presacral mass is present this is removed through the same posterior sagittal incision.

Female Defects

Perineal Fistulas

The repair of this malformation is the same as that described for male patients, except that the rectum is usually separate from the vagina so there is minimal risk of vaginal injury.

Vestibular Fistulas

The complexity of this malformation should not be underestimated. The patient is placed in prone position with the pelvis elevated. Multiple fine silk stitches are placed at the rectal vestibular orifice. A posterior sagittal incision is performed, dividing the sphincter mechanism to find the posterior rectal wall, which is easy to recognize. The main technical challenge in the repair of this defect is represented by the common wall that exists between the rectum and vagina. There is no plane of separation between these two structures and one must make two walls out of one. This is achieved by a meticulous dissection applying uniform traction with multiple silk stitches into the rectal lumen. The dissection must continue until the rectum has been completely separated from the vagina. Usually the rectum requires very little mobilization because it is located quite low. The limits of the sphincter are electrically determined, the perineal body is reconstructed, and the rectum is placed within the limits of the sphincter.

Rectovaginal Fistula

This is an extremely unusual defect. These malformations can be repaired posterior sagittally. The repair is the same as that described for vestibular fistula, except that these patients require much more mobilization of the rectum in order to move it down and relocate it in the center of the sphincter.

Cloaca

The cloaca repair represents a significant technical challenge, particularly in patients with a long common channel.[33]

Repair of Cloaca with a Common Channel Shorter than 3 cm

These patients are approached posterior sagittally. The entire sphincter mechanism is divided in the midline and the posterior sagittal incision is extended down to the single perineal opening. The common channel is also opened in the midline to expose the anatomy of the defect. The entire defect can be repaired through this incision without opening the abdomen. Once the anatomy has been exposed, the first step is to separate the rectum from the vagina, which is performed in the same manner as was described for a rectovestibular fistula. Once the rectum is separated, it should be mobilized to gain length so that it can be placed within the sphincter mechanism. The next step consists in mobilizing both vagina and urethra together, following a specific technical maneuver called "total urogenital mobilization."[34] Multiple 6-0 silk stitches are placed in the edge of the open common channel as well as the edges of the vagina. These stitches allow the surgeon to exert uniform traction on the entire urogenital structure. The urogenital channel is divided full-thickness approximately 5 mm proximal to the clitoris, creating a plane of dissection, which is very easy to find, between the common channel and the posterior aspect of the pubis. In short order, one can reach the upper portion of the pubis. Conspicuous fascial attachments exist between the vagina, the genitourinary structures and the upper part of the pubis. These fascial attachments are avascular and are known as suspensory ligaments of the vagina and urethra. These are divided and the retropubic fat is identified. By dividing these suspensory ligaments, one can gain approximately 2 cm of mobilization of the urogenital structures. Some extra dissection of the lateral and dorsal walls of the vagina gains another centimeter, and by doing that, one can repair the urethra and the vagina. Over 50% of the patients with cloacas have a common channel shorter than 3 cm, and, therefore, it is possible to repair most of these defects with this reproducible technique.[33,34] The blood supply after this mobilization is excellent. The urethra and vagina are then sutured to the labia in their new position.

The limits of the sphincter are electrically determined and marked with temporary silk stitches. The perineal body is reconstructed with long-term absorbable sutures, the rectum is placed within the limits of the sphincter, and the anoplasty is performed.

Patients with a common channel of less than 3 cm and a good sacrum have over an 80% chance of having bowel control and an 80% chance of having urinary control without bladder intermittent catheterization.[33] After the urethra and vagina have been repaired, the urethral meatus is now located 5 mm deep to the clitoris in a position that makes it perfectly visible which is important if the child needs catheterization. Twenty percent will require intermittent catheterization postoperatively in order to empty the bladder.

Surgical Repair of Patients with Cloaca with a Common Channel Longer than 3 cm

We specifically recommend these patients be referred to specialized centers dedicated to the treatment of complex malformations. The repair of these defects usually requires not only a posterior sagittal approach but also a laparotomy and a series of decision-making steps that require experience and special training in gynecology and urology. The first part of the operation consists in performing a total body preparation so that the patient can be approached through the perineum (posterior sagittally) and through a laparotomy. The posterior sagittal approach and total urogenital mobilization is attempted because occasionally one can achieve a total repair in patients with a common channel up to 4 cm. If this maneuver is not enough to make the vagina comfortably reach the skin of the perineum, one has to go into the abdomen and continue the dissection of the vagina as well as its separation from the urinary tract. This is a difficult and tedious maneuver. The bladder must be opened and the ureters must be catheterized because they run through the common wall that separates the bladder and the vagina. Often the mobilized urogenital complex can be delivered up into the abdomen and further dissected to gain length. If this is inadequate, the vagina must be entirely separated from the urinary tract. At that point, the surgeon evaluates whether or not the vagina will reach the perineum. If that is not possible, then he or she has to make an important decision as to the best way to repair the malformation. In very specific cases, with bilateral hydrocolpos, the surgeon can perform a maneuver called "vaginal switch," consisting in resecting one of the hemiuteri, resecting the vaginal septum, tubularizing both hemivaginas to create a single one and switching down what used to be the dome of one hemivagina to the perineum, taking advantage of the fact that the distance between both hemiuteri is longer than the vertical length of both hemivaginas. This maneuver is only feasible if the patient has two large hydrocolpos.

If this maneuver (vaginal switch) is not feasible, then the surgeon must replace the vagina. The alternatives are first, to replace it with rectum. The distal part of the rectum can be used to replace the vagina, which can be done in two different ways. If the patient has enough length of rectum, one can use the most distal part (preserving its blood supply) to be separated from the fecal stream, mobilized forward, and replacing the distal part of the vagina.

In other cases, if the rectum is very dilated, one can divide it longitudinally. The anterior portion is tubularized and moved forward to form the neovagina preserving the necessary vessels from the inferior mesenteric branches. The posterior aspect will serve as a rectum. The blood supply of the posterior aspect will be provided intramurally from the branches of the inferior mesenteric vessels. This depends on the fact that the rectum has an excellent intramural blood supply. If these maneuvers are not feasible, the next choice is sigmoid or left colon. Sometimes the colostomy site is a useful location for the neovagina. If these maneuvers are not possible, then one can use small bowel.

In cases of extremely high malformations, one may find two little hemivaginas attached to the bladder neck. The rectum also may open in the bladder neck. The separation of these structures is performed through the abdomen. Occasionally the common channel can be left untouched to become the neourethra. The bladder neck needs to be reconstructed. Under those circumstances, the surgeon must have enough experience to decide whether or not the bladder neck can be repaired or whether it is better to permanently close the whole distal part of the bladder and open a vesicostomy, with a plan for a continent diversion later in life. Since these patients have the highest incidence of vesicoureteral reflux, leaving a vesicostomy in such a high cloaca is a safe maneuver with a future ureteral reimplantation and urologic reconstruction performed later in life if necessary.

All patients after cloacal repair are left with a Foley catheter, which stays in place for 2 or 3 weeks. Patients with a common channel longer than 3 cm sometimes require a suprapubic cystostomy or vesicostomy at the end of the operation. Then, 1 month after surgery, a cystogram is performed, the suprapubic tube is clamped, and the patient is observed to see if she is capable of emptying her bladder spontaneously or if she requires intermittent catheterization. Several months after cloacal repair the clinician must be sure that the bladder empties well, checking with a pre- and post-void or cath ultrasound.

The most common sequela from the urinary point of view in babies with cloaca is the incapacity to empty the bladder. These babies do not suffer from the type of neurogenic bladder that is seen in patients suffering from spina bifida and myelomeningocele, but rather have a floppy large bladder that does not empty. Most of the cloaca patients have a competent bladder neck. The combination of a competent bladder neck with a floppy hypotonic bladder, makes them ideal candidates for intermittent catheterization, which allows them to remain completely dry.

Results of Treatment of Anorectal Malformations

About 75% of all patients with anorectal malformations (when subjected to a good operation) have bowel control.[27] The bowel control is not perfect. This becomes evident when the patients suffer from severe constipation, which may produce overflow pseudoincontinence, and soiling. Also, a severe episode of diarrhea may show that the bowel control is not normal. Twenty-five percent of all patients suffer from fecal incontinence and require some form of medical management (Table 50-3).[35]

Since anorectal malformations cover a wide spectrum of defects, the clinical and functional results vary depending on the specific type of malformation. Patients with a cloaca with a common channel longer than 3 cm usually suffer from fecal incontinence and require intermittent catheterization to empty the bladder. Patients with a common channel shorter than 3 cm and a normal sacrum have bowel control 80% of the time and only 20% of them require intermittent catheterization to empty the bladder and remain completely dry. Ninety-five percent of patients with rectovestibular fistulas have bowel control. Babies with perineal fistulas have bowel control 100% of the time. Rectobladder neck fistula patients only have bowel control 15% of the time, with rectoprostatic fistula patients at 60%, and rectourethral bulbar fistula patients at 85%.[27] Patients with imperforate anus with no fistula will have bowel control between 80 and 90% of the time depending on whether or not they suffer from Down's Syndrome.[29]

Constipation is a problem in most patients with anorectal malformations in whom the rectum was preserved during the main repair and should not be underestimated. When not treated properly, the patients develop megacolon and chronic fecal impaction, which may end up producing overflow pseudoincontinence.

TABLE 50-3. Voluntary bowel movement and type of defect

Defect	Cases	Patients with VBMs *n*	%
Atresia or stenosis	11	11	100
Perineal fistula	58	56	97
Vestibular fistula	146	131	90
Imperforate anus without fistula	40	31	78
Bulbar fistula	112	89	79
Cloaca common channel <3 cm	99	65	66
Prostatic fistula	109	71	65
Vaginal fistula	5	3	60
Cloaca common channel >3 cm	69	24	35
Bladderneck fistula	49	10	20
Total	698	491	70

Management of Fecal Incontinence

For the group of patients with anorectal malformations, who suffer from fecal incontinence (25% of cases), a bowel management program that aims to keep those patients completely clean of stool and to make them socially accepted is vital. The basis of this treatment is to teach the family or the patient to clean the colon every day with an enema. Since most patients suffer from constipation, the cleaning of the colon with an enema will prevent the patient from passing stool for 24 or 48 h.[35,36]

Occasionally, however, we find patients who had a different type of repair and lost the rectosigmoid during the main repair or suffer from intractable diarrhea or malabsorption. In those cases, the bowel management is technically more demanding, because it includes not only the cleaning the colon with an enema but also the use of a constipating diet or medications to decrease the colonic motility in order to keep the patient from passing stool for 24 h between the enemas.

The bowel management program is implemented over a period of 1 week by trial and error. Every patient needs a different kind of enema to clean the colon. The cleaning of the colon is monitored, taking X-ray films of the abdomen every day, and adjusting the volume and concentration of the enema by trial and error. The goal is to find the enema that is well tolerated by the patient, is easy to administer, and keeps the patient completely clean. When the patient complains about the rectal enema and feels embarrassed about their parents giving the enema, an operation called the Malone procedure (continent appendicostomy) is an option.[37,38] This consists of creating a connection between the tip of the appendix and the umbilicus. The cecum is plicated around the appendix to create a one-way valve that allows the introduction of a catheter through the umbilicus into the colon and prevents stool from passing through the orifice. The patient is able to sit on the toilet, pass a feeding tube through the umbilicus, administer the enema himself/herself, evacuate the colon, and remain clean the following 24 or 48 h. This allows the patient to become independent. A significant number of patients do not have an appendix. In that case, one can be created with a vascularized flap of the colon (continent neoappendicostomy). Then again, the colon is plicated around the new appendix to make it continent.[38]

Relevant Aspects for Adult Colorectal Surgeons

A large number of adolescent and adult patients may still suffer from fecal incontinence despite successful repair in infancy. Other patients these having undergone surgery for Hirschsprung and patient with spinal anomalies or pelvic trauma may suffer from incontinence. Workup of these patients should include a detailed history and physical exam which includes the type of defect the patient was born with, bowel movement and voiding pattern, type of perineum, location of rectal opening, presence of an anal dimple, and strength of sphincter contraction. A water-soluble enema or defecography, voiding cystourethrogram, sacral films, and an MRI with a rectal coil to assess the location of the rectum are essential. We then classify patients into four groups, as follows.[39]

1. Patients with a poor sacrum, flat perineum, poor muscles, no sensation, and poor bowel movement pattern who are usually incontinent for both urine and stool. These patients are good candidates for a bowel management program.[36] Alternative techniques such as an artificial bowel sphincter or stimulated gracilis muscle flap have been tried with limited success.[40] A permanent stoma is rarely indicated as a properly administered enema program works 95% of the time.[35]
2. Patients with clinical and MRI evidence of a mislocated rectum with a good sacrum and well-developed muscles. These patients may benefit from a secondary pull-through procedure.[41]
3. Patients who suffers from severe constipation but have good potential for bowel control and a contrast enema which shows a severely dilated mega rectosigmoid. These patients need aggressive laxative therapy and possibly a sigmoid resection.[36]
4. Patients who are born with a good prognostic type of malformation and have a well-located rectum, good sacrum, and good muscles but are still incontinent. They may benefit from biofeedback or other behavior modification programs to help them evacuate the rectum at controlled and predictable times.

Some children develop an IBS syndrome as they mature after a successful repair and then have difficulty later in life. They may benefit from regulation of colonic motility with diet, medication or possibly an intestinal pacemaker. We predict that control of rectosigmoid motility and coordination will be easier in the future as techniques develop in improving such patients than any artificial anal sphincter.

Other Pediatric Colorectal Disorders

Idiopathic Constipation

Constipation of unknown origin represents a serious problem in the pediatric population. At least 6% of pediatric consultations are related to this particular problem.[42] We consider this condition to be the result of a colonic hypomotility disorder with different degrees of severity, affecting mainly the rectosigmoid and sometimes the entire colon. The spectrum of colonic hypomotility or colonic inertia varies from mild constipation that can be controlled by dietary measures to severe hypomotility disorders that may fall into the realm of what is called "intestinal pseudoobstruction" and may require intestinal transplantation.[43]

Constipation means an incapacity to empty the colon on a daily basis or the incapacity to empty it completely. As a consequence, the colon stores a large amount of stool and becomes very dilated (megacolon). Megacolon produces constipation and constipation produces more megacolon, creating a vicious cycle. The final result is chronic fecal impaction, which provokes overflow pseudoincontinence (encopresis).

The cause of this condition is unknown. Many authors claim that the origin is a behavior problem, while others believe that it is a consequence of a dietary problem. There are those who think that it is a consequence of a lack of relaxation of the internal sphincter or a consequence of ultrashort segment aganglionosis. None of these theories have been scientifically documented, and that is why we call this condition idiopathic.[43]

The treatments we use for this condition consist in trying to find the amount of laxatives that is capable of producing a bowel movement that empties the colon completely every day.[36] The amount is different in every individual and has to be determined by trial and error. When the laxative requirement is so high that it creates a problem in terms of quality of life, we offer the patient a surgical treatment consisting in the resection of the most dilated portion of the colon (usually the rectosigmoid).[44,45] By doing that, even when we know that we do not cure this mysterious condition, we make the problem more manageable and reduce significantly the amount of laxatives that the patient needs.

Rectal Prolapse

Rectal prolapse occurs in children due to conditions such as myelomeningocele, spina bifida, and malnutrition. The lack of sphincter tone explains the severe prolapse from which these patients may suffer. Also, patients with cystic fibrosis or some patients with inflammatory bowel disease or intestinal parasites may suffer from rectal prolapse. Severe constipation can also cause rectal prolapse.

Most pediatric patients afflicted with this condition are of the idiopathic type. The surgeon must try to identify one of the predisposing conditions already mentioned. If this is not possible, one must try to avoid those factors that exacerbate the problem, such as to treat constipation, and any irritating conditions of the colon, such as milk allergy. If all this fails, the surgeon can offer a surgical treatment.

An old operation designed to treat rectal prolapse includes placement of a nonabsorbable suture around the anus to restrict its caliber. The long-term results of these procedures are not good because eventually the patients develop megacolon and an anal stricture. Other surgeons have tried the injection of sclerosing substances such as hypertonic saline in the perirectal space. This has been followed by severe complications including nerve damage and bowel and urinary incontinence. A posterior sagittal approach has also been used that allows the surgeon to anchor the posterior rectal wall to the cartilage of the coccyx and the sacrum. Some perform an abdominal approach with fixation of the rectum to the presacral fascia, usually with a sigmoid resection. A transanal rectosigmoidectomy (modified Altmier procedure) has emerged as a treatment option in these children mimicking a one-stage pull-through for Hirschsprung's disease, and is our preferred approach.

Perianal Fistula

Perianal abscess and fistula in pediatrics seems to be a completely different condition to that seen in adults. During the first year of life, many babies suffer from perianal abscesses that may be associated with a perianal fistula. The orifice seen externally next to the anus communicates with one of the crypts of the pectinate line. Traditionally, these patients have been subjected to a fistulotomy, consisting in identifying the fistula tract and cutting all the tissue, and mucosa, from inside the rectal lumen leaving the wound open for granulation.

Our experience has been that this is a benign condition that does not require any treatment. If the babies have a perianal abscess, they do not require antibiotics. Very soon, the abscess drains by itself and if not, with a minimal incision and drainage. Following that, for a period of months, it drains intermittently without any discomfort to the patient. The vast majority of fistulas disappear after 1 year of age.[46]

Occasionally, one can see a school-age child with a perianal fistula. This is extremely unusual. In such a case, the surgeon should investigate for inflammatory bowel disease before trying any of the current available surgical techniques used in adults.

Juvenile Polyps

Around the age of 4 years, patients may suffer from polyps in the rectum and in the colon. These polyps are benign. They grow and eventually amputate and disappear. The polyps are mostly located in the posterior rectal wall. A rectal examination makes the diagnosis in most cases. These polyps have a long pedicle. The symptoms in these patients are the presence of blood surrounding the fecal matter. They do not produce any pain. Occasionally, the parents describe the presence of a polyp that prolapses through the anus. The polyps can be easily resected under general anesthesia. Histologically, these are almost always benign inflammatory polyps.

Anal Fissure

Anal fissures in pediatric patients are usually a consequence and not a cause of constipation. The fissure represents a laceration that was produced with the passage of a large hard piece of fecal matter. The patient suffers from painful bowel movements and that contributes to the constipation, and the patient becomes a stool retainer. Stool retention may provoke more constipation and more constipation will make the fissure worse.

The main treatment for this condition is to give enough laxatives as to guarantee that the patient will have soft stool passing through the rectum for several weeks until the fissure heals. No surgical treatment is necessary.

Recently, 0.2% NTG ointment has been used for intractable cases to cause a reversible chemical sphincterotomy.[47] This is a simple alternative treatment since the long-term sequelae of a internal lateral sphincterotomy in children is not known and may be associated with incontinence.

Acknowledgment. This chapter was co-authored by Marc E. Sher in the previous version of this textbook.

References

1. Swenson O, Bill AH. Resection of rectum and rectosigmoid with preservation of the sphincter for benign spastic lesions producing megacolon: an experimental study. Surgery. 1948;24:212.
2. Cilley RE, Statter MB, Hirschl RB, Coran AG. Definitive treatment of Hirschsprung's disease in the newborn with a one-stage procedure. Surgery. 1994;115:551–6.
3. So HB, Schwartz DL, Becher JM, et al. Endorectal pullthrough without preliminary colostomy in patients with Hirschsprung's disease. J Pediatr Surg. 1980;15:470.
4. De la Torre L, Ortega J. Transanal endorectal pullthrough for Hirschsrpung's disease. J Pediatr Surg. 1998;33:1283.
5. Langer JC, Minkes RK, Mazziott MV, et al. Trananal one stage Soave procedure for infants with Hirschsprung's disease. J Pediatr Surg. 1999;34:148.
6. Georgeson KE, Fuenfer MM, Hardin WD. Primary laparoscopic pullthrough for Hirschsprung's disease in infants and children. J Pediatr Surg. 1995;30:1017.
7. Duhamel B. Retrorectal and transanal pull-through procedure for the treatment of Hirschsprung's disease. Dis Colon Rectum. 1964;7:455.
8. Soave F. Hirschsprung's disease – a new surgical technique. Arch Dis Child. 1964;39:116.
9. Boley SJ. A new modification of the surgical treatment of Hirschsprung's disease. Surgery. 1964;56:1015.
10. Georgeson KE, Cohen RD, Hebra A, et al. Primary laparoscopic assisted endorectal colon pullthrough for Hirschsprung's disease: a new gold standard. Ann Surg. 1999;229:678.
11. Curran TJ, Raffensperger JG. The feasibility of laparoscopic swenson pull-through. J Pediatr Surg. 1994;29:1273.
12. Levitt MA, Dickie B, Peña A. Evaluation and treatment of the Hirschsprung's patient who is not doing well after a pull-through procedure. Semin Pediatr Surg. 2010;19(2):146–53.
13. Levitt M, Martin C, Olesevich M, Bauer C, Jackson L, Peña A. Hirschsprung's disease and fecal incontinence: diagnostic and management strategies. J Pediatr Surg. 2009;44:271–7.
14. Peña A, Elicevik M, Levitt MA. Reoperations in Hirschsprung disease. J Pediatr Surg. 2007;42(6):1008–14.
15. Teitelbaum DH, Coran AG. Enterocolitis. Semin Pediatr Surg. 1998;7:162–9.
16. Bax KN. Duhamel lecture: the incurability of Hirschprung's disease. Eur J Pediatr Surg. 2006;16:380–4.
17. Langer JC, Seifert M, Minkes RK. One-stage Soave pull-through for Hirschsprung's disease: a comparison of the transanal and open approaches. J Pediatr Surg. 2000;35(6):820–2.
18. Langer JC, Durrant AC, de la Torre L, Teitebaum D, Minkes RK, et al. One stage tranal Soave pullthrough for Hirschsprung's disease: a multicenter experience with 141 children. Ann Surg. 2003;238(4):569–83.
19. de la Torre L, Langer JC. Transanal pull-through for Hirschsprung disease: technique, controversies, pearls, pitfalls, and an organized approach to the management of postoperative obstructive symptoms. Semin Pediatr Surg. 2010;19:96–106.
20. Martin L. Surgical management of total aganglionosis. Ann Surg. 1972;176:343.
21. Kimura K, Mishijima E, Muraji T. A new surgical approach to extensive aganglionosis. J Pediatr Surg. 1981;16:840.
22. Marquez TT, Acton RD, Hess DJ, Duval S, Saltzman DA. Comprehensive review of procedure for total colonic aganglionosis. J Pediatr Surg. 2009;44:257–65.
23. Wildhaber BE, Teitelbaum DH, Coran AG. Total colonic Hirschsprung's disease: a 28-year experience. J Pediatr Surg. 2005;40:203–7.
24. Meier-Rouge W. Angeborene dysganglionosen des colon. Der Kinderarzt. 1985;16:151.
25. Csury L, Peña A. Intestinal neuronal dysplasia: myth or reality: literature review. Pediatr Surg Int. 1995;10(7):441–6.
26. Levitt MA, Patel M, Rodriguez G, Gaylin DS, Peña A. The tethered spinal cord in patients with anorectal malformations. J Pediatr Surg. 1997;32(3):462–8.
27. Levitt MA, Peña A. Imperforate anus and cloacal malformations. In: Holcomb GW, Murphy JP, editors. Ashcraft's pediatric surgery. 5th ed. Philadelphia: Elsevier; 2010. p. 337–59.
28. Falcone RA, Levitt MA, Peña A, Bates MD. Increased heritability of certain types of anorectal malformations. J Pediatr Surg. 2007;42):124–8.
29. Torres P, Levitt MA, Tovilla JM, Rodriguez G, Peña A. Anorectal malformations and Down's syndrome. J Pediatr Surg. 1998;33(2):1–5.
30. Rosen NG, Hong AR, Soffer SZ, Rodriguez G, Peña A. Rectovaginal fistula: a common diagnostic error with significant consequences in female patients with anorectal malformations. J Pediatr Surg. 2002;37(7):961–5.
31. Breech L. Gynecologic concerns in patients with anorectal malformations. Semin Pediatr Surg. 2010;19(2):139–45.
32. Hong AR, Rosen N, Acuña MF, Peña A, Chaves L, Rodriguez G. Urological injuries associated with the repair of anorectal malformations in male patients. J Pediatr Surg. 2002;37:339–44.
33. Levitt MA, Peña A. Cloacal malformations: lessons learned from 490 cases. Semin Pediatr Surg. 2010;19(2):128–38.
34. Peña A. Total urogenital mobilization-an easier way to repair cloacas. J Pediatr Surg. 1997;32(2):263–8.
35. Bischoff A, Levitt MA, Bauer C, Jackson L, Holder M, Peña A. Treatment of fecal incontinence with a comprehensive bowel management program. J Pediatr Surg. 2009;6(44):1278–84.
36. Levitt MA, Peña A. Update on pediatric fecal incontinence. Eur J Pediatr Surg. 2009;19:1–9.

37. Malone PS, Ransley PG, Kiely EM. Prelim report: the antegrade continence enema. Lancet. 1990;336:1217–8.
38. Levitt MA, Soffer SZ, Peña A. Continent appendicostomy in the bowel management of fecal incontinent children. J Pediatr Surg. 1997;32(11):1630–3.
39. Peña A. Anorectal malformations: new aspects relevant to adult colorectal surgeons. Semin Colon Rectal Surg. 1994;5(2):78–88.
40. da Silva GM, Jorge JM, Belin B, Nogueras JJ, Weiss E, et al. New surgical options for fecal incontinence in patients with imperforate anus. Dis Colon Rectum. 2004;47(2):204–9.
41. Levitt MA, Peña A. Reoperations in anorectal malformations. In: Teich S, Caniano D, editors. Reoperative pediatric surgery. New York, NY: Humana Press; 2008. p. 311–26.
42. Levine MD. Children with encopresis: a descriptive analysis. Pediatrics. 1975;56:412–6.
43. Peña A, Levitt M. Colonic inertia disorders in pediatrics. Curr Probl Surg. 2002;39(7):661–732.
44. Peña A, El-Behery M. Megasigmoid – a source of pseudo-incontinence in children with repaired anorectal malformations. J Pediatr Surg. 1993;28(2):1–5.
45. Levitt MA, Martin CA, Falcone RA, Peña A. Transanal rectosigmoid resection for severe intractable idiopathic constipation. J Pediatr Surg. 2009;44(6):1285–91.
46. Rosen NG, Gibbs DL, Soffer SZ, Hong AR, Sher M, Peña A. The nonoperative management of fistula-in-ano. J Pediatr Surg. 2000;35(6):938–39.
47. Tander B, Guven A, Demirbag S, Ozkan Y, Ozturk H, et al. A prospective randomized double blind trial of glyceryl-trinitrate ointment in the treatment of children with anal fissure. J Pediatr Surg. 1999;34(12):18110–2.

51
Health Care Economics

David A. Margolin and Lester Rosen

"It was the best of times it was the worst of times." How prophetic was Charles Dickens when applied to health care in America today.[1] We are currently experiencing unprecedented technologic and therapeutic advancements; however, these come at a tremendous price. Health care expenditures have increased by double digits for the past decade, physician reimbursement has decreased by over the past 10-years, and hospitals have closed and health care systems have filed for bankruptcy.[2] Furthermore, in 2009, national health care expenditures are projected to have reached $2.5 trillion, an increase of 5.7%, up from the 4.4% increase seen in 2008, while the overall economy, as measured by gross domestic product (GDP) is still in recession, and anticipated to have fallen 1.1% (Table 51-1). From 2009 to 2019 the average annual health care spending growth is projected to grow at a rate of 6.0%, well outpacing the expected average annual growth in the overall economy (4.4%). By 2019, national health spending is expected to reach $4.5 trillion and comprise 19.3% of GDP[3] (Figure 51-1).[4] It is in this environment that President Barak Obama has attempted potentially sweeping changes in the health care landscape. At the time of writing this book, health care reform has passed the democratically controlled congress. However with the republicans regaining control in the 2010 midterm elections renewed partisan opposition to health care reform has occurred.

Multiple interrelated events have led to the current state of health care finance. With the advent of the resource-based relative value scale (RBRVS) physicians have shifted from price setters to price takers. Technology costs, while providing an improvement in patient care, have skyrocketed. While the life expectancy of the population has not increased dramatically over the past decades, the "Baby Boomers" are here and continue to shift the average age of the American population to one that requires increased utilization of health care resources. In 2009, the US census bureau estimated that 46.3 million Americans were without health insurance which was an increase from 45.7 in 2007, leaving 15.4% of Americans with no health insurance, and millions more underinsured, putting a strain on state and federal budgets to provide care.[5] Last but not least is the current professional liability crisis, resulting in increased malpractice rates and driving specialists from specific locations. Despite this, physicians still are able to provide quality care for their patients and receive reasonable compensation. Nonetheless, in the ever-changing face of the socioeconomic landscape, physicians need a solid basis that allows them to function in today's practice environment.

This chapter covers the RBVRS and Medicare reimbursement, the types of contractual agreement between insurers and practitioners and insurers and patients, and what to expect in the future.

The Reimbursement Process

Medicare

The key to begin to understand the business of medicine is to understand the basics of Medicare. While private payors vary in their reimbursement rates and policies, most are tied in some form to the Medicare system. Medicare was created in 1965 by the Federal government as a social insurance program designed to provide all adults over the age of 65 with comprehensive health care coverage at an affordable cost. Medicare is administrated by the Center for Medicare and Medicaid Services (CMS), formerly known as the Health Care Financing Administration (HCFA). When the program began in 1966, 19.1 million persons were enrolled; in 2004 Medicare had over 41 million enrollees and is forecasted to include almost 80 million people by 2030 (Figure 51-2).[6] Medicare is divided into two parts.

Medicare Part A, also known as hospital insurance, helps pay for inpatient hospitalizations, skilled nursing facility (SNF) care, home health and hospice care. Part A is financed primarily through federal payroll taxes (FICA) paid by both employees and employers. In 2010, the current FICA tax was 7.65% of earned income, of which 1.45% went toward Medicare Part A. The maximum tax employees and employers will each pay in 2010 is $6,621.60. Individuals who receive

D.E. Beck et al. (eds.), *The ASCRS Textbook of Colon and Rectal Surgery: Second Edition*,
DOI 10.1007/978-1-4419-1584-9_51, © Springer Science+Business Media, LLC 2011

TABLE 51-1. Selected national economic indicators: 2000–2004

	Calendar year				2001	2001	2001	2002	2002	2002	2002	2003	2003	2003	2003	2004
Indicator	2000	2001	2002	2003	Q2	Q3	Q4	Q1	Q2	Q3	Q4	Q1	Q2	Q3	Q4	Q1
Gross domestic product																
Billions of dollars	9,817	10,101	10,481	10,988	10,088	10,096	10,194	10,329	10,428	10,542	10,624	10,736	10,847	11,107	11,262	11,451
Personal income																
Personal income in billions	8,430	8,713	8,910	9,204	8,690	8,727	8,771	8,804	8,912	8,944	8,981	9,049	9,146	9,256	9,364	9,523
Disposable income in billions	7,194	7,469	7,857	8,213	7,382	7,606	7,528	7,734	7,869	7,891	7,936	8,039	8,146	8,318	8,349	8,531
Prices[a]																
Consumer price index, all items	172	177.1	179.9	184	177.5	177.8	177.3	177.9	179.8	180.6	181.2	183	183.7	184.6	184.6	186.3
All items less medical care	167	171.9	174.3	178.1	172.4	172.5	171.9	172.5	174.3	174.9	175.4	177.2	177.9	178.6	178.6	180.2
Medical care	261	272.8	285.6	297.1	271.6	274.2	276.6	280.9	284	287.2	290.3	293.5	295.5	298.4	300.9	305.7
Annual percent change																
Gross domestic product																
Billions of dollars	5.9	2.9	3.8	4.8	2.7	2.4	2.4	3	3.4	4.4	4.2	3.9	4	5.4	6	6.7
Personal income																
Personal income in billions	8	3.4	2.3	3.3	3.8	2.5	2.4	1.6	2.6	2.5	2.4	2.8	2.6	3.5	4.3	5.2
Prices[a]																
Consumer price index, all items	3.4	2.8	1.6	2.3	3.4	2.7	1.9	1.3	1.3	1.6	2.2	2.9	2.1	2.2	1.9	1.8
All items less medical care	3.3	2.7	1.4	2.2	3.3	2.6	1.7	1	1.1	1.4	2.1	2.7	2	2.1	1.8	1.7
Medical care	4.1	4.6	4.7	4	4.6	4.5	4.7	4.5	4.6	4.8	5	4.5	4	3.9	3.7	4.2

[a]Base period = 1982–1984, unless noted.

Note: Q designates quarter of year. Unlike rows 1–6, quarterly data on GDP, personal income, and disposable personal income, are seasonally adjusted at annual rates.

Adapted from U.S. Department of Commerce, Bureau of Economic Analysis: Survey of Current Business. Washington. U.S. Government Printing Office. Monthly reports for January 1998–October 2003; U.S. Department of Labor, Bureau of Labor and Producer Price Indexes. Washington. U.S. Government Printing Office. Monthly reports for January 1999–March 2004.http://www.cms.hhs.gov/statistics/health-indicators/t7.asp.[19] Accessed 11 Jan 2005.

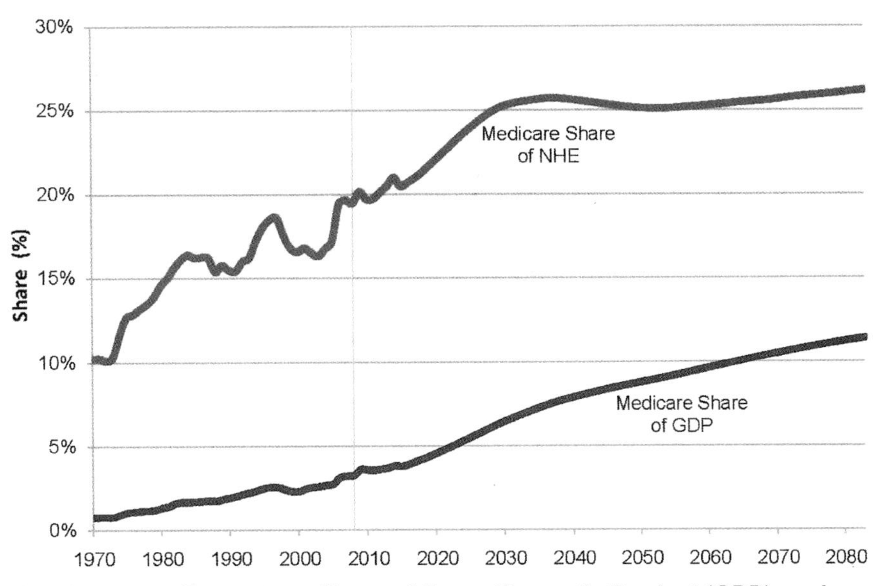

FIGURE 51-1. Health care expenditures (adapted from The Centers for Medicare & Medicaid Services http://www.cms.hhs.gov/Reports TrustFunds/downloads/projectionmethodology.pdf. Accessed 29 Jan 2010.[4]) The *green line* shows the percentage of the gross national product going to national health expenditure. The scale on the left axis measures it. The *purple line*, for gross domestic product (GDP), and the *blue line*, for national health expenditure (NHE), in billions of dollars, measured by the right axis scale. http://hspm.sph.sc.edu/Courses/Econ/Classes/nhe00/.

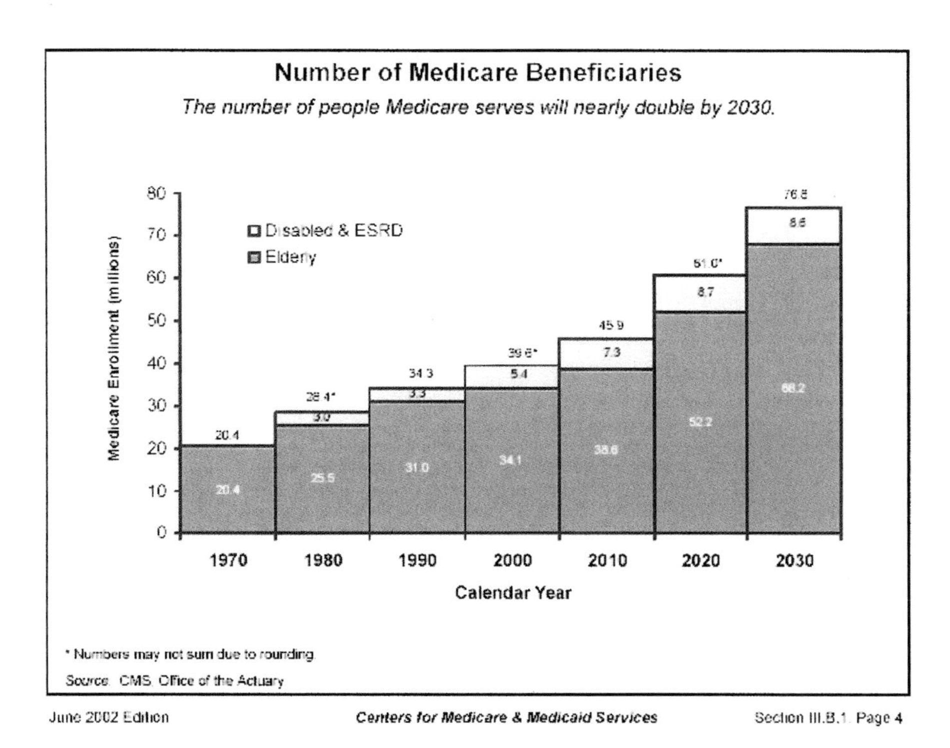

FIGURE 51-2. Expected number of Medicare beneficiaries. (Adapted from The Centers for Medicare & Medicaid Services http://www.cms.hhs.gov/charts/series/sec3-b1-9.pdf. Accessed 5 Jan 2005[6]).

Social Security benefits or Railroad Retirement benefits are automatically enrolled in Part A. Individuals under 65 who receive Social Security disability or those with end-stage renal disease for over 24 months are also eligible for Part A. Despite current misconceptions, Medicare Part A is not free. Although there is no monthly Part A premium for Medicare recipients who have worked 40 quarters of Medicare-covered employment, those who have fewer than 30 quarters of coverage may obtain Part A coverage by paying a monthly premium of $461 per month for 2010. Individuals with 30 to 39 quarters of coverage, will pay a premium of $254 per month in 2010. Medicare enrollees are also responsible for copayments associated with the services provided. In 2010 there is an $1,112 copay for the first hospital stay of the year. For each subsequent hospital stay there is no out-of-pocket expenses for 1–60 days. For any and all hospital stays of 61–90 days there is a cost of $275 per day and after 150 days of inpatient hospitalization all costs were the patient's responsibility. Part A covers the first 20 days of SNF care and costs $139/day for days 21–100. Like the limits for inpatient hospitalization, there was no coverage for SNF after 100 days. It is worth noting that Medicare Part B, also known as Medical Insurance, provides coverage for payments to physicians for services provided. This includes outpatient medical and surgical services, supplies, diagnostic testing and some home health care. Part B is funded by a combination of the federal government's general revenues (75%) and individual monthly premiums (25%). In 2004, Part B did not cover routine physical examinations. However, the federal government has responded to citizens' urging and has instituted a physical examination when one enters into Medicare and covers screening for some specific diseases. Part B covers screening for breast cancer, cervical cancer, prostate cancer, and colorectal cancer. Medicare covers fecal occult blood testing every 24 months, flexible sigmoidoscopy every 48 months, colonoscopy for high-risk individuals once every 24 months or for average-risk individuals every 10 years. Medicare also covers barium enemas (BE) every 24 or 48 months depending on your risk stratification.

Unlike Part A, Medicare Part B has monthly premiums. In 2010, the premium for those who enrolled at the onset of eligibility is between 96.40 and $243.10 per month based on income. If one enrolls at eligibility, this premium is deducted from your Social Security or Railroad Retirement check. You can opt out of Part B. Similar to Part A, Part B enrollees are responsible for copayments and deductibles. For physician services deductible was $155 per calendar year and a 20% copayment of Medicare-approved rates. Copayments for outpatient procedures were charged at a different rate than office services, and the copayment varied based on the procedure performed.

While Part A and B are considered traditional Medicare, Medicare Part C or Medicare Advantage is the government's plan to shift the cost and risks of Medicare patients to the private sector. In Medicare Advantage, private payers receive a monthly payment per covered individual (capitated amount) to provide all of Part A and B services. Private payors then tailor these plans to cover anticipated needs. These plans often provide benefits not seen in traditional Medicare, such as wider prescription drug benefits, routine physicals, preventative care, eyeglasses, and hearing aids. Since these plans are privately administered, individual choice is often severely limited with regards to physicians and hospitals. Nonetheless, these plans are extremely attractive with the Congressional Budget Office (CBO) projecting that, enrollment in Medicare Advantage will grow at an annual average rate of about 7 % over the next 10 years, compared with a growth rate of about 2.5 % for Medicare overall – reaching 21% of total enrollment in 2008 and 26% by 2017. However, according to the CBO the average payment to Medicare Advantage plans is 12% above traditional FFS costs. As such, Reimbursements to private insurers that administer Medicare Advantage plans would fall by as much as 4–4.5% in 2010.[7]

In late 2003, the Federal government instituted another new category of Medicare. Medicare Part D, prescription drug coverage, was signed into law in December 2003. In response to the cost of prescription drugs for seniors the government instituted a program that started in 2006. This program provides for prescription drugs with an initial deductible of $250 and a monthly premium of $35. There is a 75% subsidy for drug cost between $251 and $2,250. The federal government pays for all drugs after a recipient pays $3,600 or $5,100 in total cost. Special assistance will be provided for low-income seniors as well. New to Part D is the institution of means testing. Individuals with incomes $160,000 and above will be subjected to higher Part B and Part D premiums.

Medicare Resources

According to the Office of Management and Budget (OMB), Medicare in 2004 had a budget of $302 billion that increased to $503 billion in 2010.[8] The Medicare budget is determined by legislation and is formula based. It involves the Medicare Economic Index (MEI), a weighted index, and the sustainable growth rate (SGR). The SGR rate compares the cumulative actual spending for physicians' services since 1997 to a cumulative target amount of spending over the same time period. The initial idea was to keep Medicare costs from spiraling out of control. As described by Jacob Goldstein in the Wall Street Journal, "The SGR says essentially that the amount Medicare pays doctors for an average Medicare patient can't grow faster than the economy as a whole. It's fine if total payments to doctors go up because the number of Medicare beneficiaries rises. And it's fine if the average payment per beneficiary rises along with the economy. But if growth in payments per beneficiary grows more than the economy as a whole, the SGR says you have to lower payments to doctors across the board to keep costs under control." [9] Without new federal spending legislation, Medicare spending is not allowed to grow by more than $20 million/year (budget neutrality). However, the government has made exceptions to increases in Medicare spending for new technologies and pilot programs. For more details, the complete Medicare fee schedule can be found in the Federal Register on line at http://www.gpoaccess.gov/fr/index.html.

Hospital (Part A) Reimbursment

Until the mid-1980s the federal government and most private payers reimbursed hospitals retrospectively for all reasonable costs involved in the care of a covered individual. With this form of reimbursement, to compete and remain solvent, hospitals invested in the latest, most-advanced technology. This allowed hospitals to increase patient care volume and expand services; however, it was done without regard to cost or efficiency. Although this methodology had its advantage, it led to a continuing upward spiral in health care costs and a significant duplication of services.

In response to sharply rising hospital costs, the Federal government instituted a prospective payment system. This was modeled after a system developed by Fetter and associates at Yale University that categorized patients based on primary and secondary diagnosis, primary and secondary procedures, age and length of stay, and then set a uniform cost for each category.[10] These diagnostic-related groups (DRGs) set a maximum amount that would be paid for the hospital care of Medicare patients for a specific problem. In 2010, there are 745 DRGs. Each DRG contains a list of specific diagnoses and procedures based on the International Classification of Diseases, Ninth Revision, Clinical Modification (ICD-9-CM).[11] ICD-9 is a coding system that lists specific diseases, diagnosis, and medical acuity. By using this system, Medicare has grouped related ICD-9 codes that utilize similar hospital recourses in specific DRGs.

Private payers have followed Medicare's lead and began utilizing a prospective payment system. It was felt that by utilizing a prospective payment system hospitals would have a true incentive to improve efficiency and keep cost low. While this may have initially slowed the growth of hospital costs and forced improved efficiency in health care delivery, it has not been the panacea that was expected. Hospital costs, while initially controlled, returned to double-digit increases by 2002.[12] Although the reasons for the continued rise in hospital cost are multifactorial, the failure of DRGS to truly control cost can best be summed up: "Hospitals prefer management strategies that are designed to enhance revenues over cost control measures that may be resisted by the physician staff."[13]

Despite the reluctance of physicians to change practice patterns, hospitals have tried to increase their efficiency, and with technologic advances it has been possible to shift procedures from the inpatient setting to outpatient/ambulatory center. While this had some minimal impact in physician reimbursement, it has helped decrease resource utilization. In response to this, to account for this shift in location, Medicare has developed a prospective payment system called the ambulatory payment classification (APC). APCs, like DRGs, are specific reimbursement groupings that Medicare pays to facilities. For these outpatient services Medicare pays a specific rate per procedure determined by the APC in which the procedure is grouped. Specific medical devices and drugs are exempt from this and are reimbursed in addition to the APC fee. These are called pass throughs. Other devices that do not receive pass through are often charged to the patient by private payors. In 2004, 4 APC classifications covered the majority of outpatient anorectal procedures. APCs reimburse facilities between $209 (APC 148, lateral internal anal sphincterotomy) and $1210 (APC 150, hemorrhoidectomy) with a patient copayment between $41 and $437.

With changes in location of services in a constant state of flux, Medicare needed to develop an appropriate and timely methodology to respond to this shift. To add some stability to APC payments and achieve these goals, the Secretary of Health and Human Services (head of CMS) appointed an Advisory Panel on APC Groups. This panel of physicians deals with issues concerning resource use, assigning new current procedural terminology (CPT®) codes to APCs, and reassigning codes to different APCs.

Physician Reimbursement

Currently, physician reimbursement from Medicare is a three-step process: (1) appropriate coding of the service provided by utilizing current procedural terminology (CPT®); (2) the appropriate coding of the diagnosis using ICD-9 code; and (3) CMS determination of the appropriate fee based on the resources-based relative value scale (RBRVS).

CPT® is a uniform coding system that was developed by the American Medical Association (AMA). CPT® originated in 1966 and has undergone yearly updates based on changes in medical and surgical procedures and the development of new technology. CPT® is a proprietary product of the AMA. The CPT® editorial panel is comprised of 16 members in multiple specialties as well as the insurance industry. Advisors from over 90 medical and surgical specialties advise them. They meet four times a year to consider additions and deletions to the code list. A service may be brought before the CPT® editorial panel by any specialty, private physician, insurer, or device manufacture. To receive consideration for a new code, a procedure must meet certain requirements: it must be done by a reasonable number of the specialty that presents the code, be performed at reasonable frequency, be done throughout the country and have peer-reviewed literature supporting its efficacy. The editorial panel allows advisors from other specialties to comment on any proposal. The editorial panel then reviews the clinical description of the procedure or service that describes the typical patient. After assuring that it meets all of the above requirements and that the service should not be coded with a preexisting code, the committee will give the service a unique CPT® code. The code then moves to the Relative Value Update Committee (RUC) where it receives a value relative to other codes (RVU). CPT® also uses a series of modifiers in addition to the original code to better describe the service provided. This allows not only for better data collection regarding the frequency and complexity of services but also for appropriate reimbursement by Medicare.

Medicare implemented the RBRVS in 1992. Previously physicians were reimbursed based on "usual, customary and reasonable charges" (UCR). UCRs were based on the physician's most frequent charge for the service (usual), the average charge for that service in the area (customary), and the actual charge for the service (reasonable).[14] Individuals within the federal government, private insurers, and nonprocedure-based medical specialties felt that this system perpetuated rising health care costs and inequities in medical care. These individuals believed that this system served as an incentive for physicians to inflate charges even in those instances where actual costs were decreasing and to continue the inequities in fees between proceduralists and nonproceduralists. In response to this the federal government instituted the Medicare fee schedule.

The Medicare fee schedule was based on the work of a research team led by William Hsiao, a Harvard economist under contract to CMS.[15–17] The Harvard study ranked procedures and services relative to each other based on the amount of physician work necessary to perform the procedure or service. Work was defined as a combination of the time used to perform the service and the complexity of service (mental effort, knowledge, judgment and diagnostic acumen, technical skill, physical skill, psychological stress, and potential iatrogenic risk).[18] Work was then broken down into three time periods, pre-, intra-, and postservice.

Preservice work for surgical procedures has come to be defined as the physician work provided from the day before, until the time of the operative procedure (i.e., skin incision). This may involve any or all of the following: hospital admission workup; the preoperative evaluation including the procedural workup, review of records, communicating with other professionals, patient and family, and obtaining consent; dressing, scrubbing, and waiting before the operative procedure; preparing patient and needed equipment for the operative procedure; positioning the patient; and other non "skin-to-skin" work done in the operating room prior to incision. Preservice work does not include the consultation or evaluation at which the decision to provide the procedure was made.

Intraservice work includes all "skin-to-skin" work that is a necessary part of the procedure. The time measurement for the intraservice work is from the start of the skin incision until the incision is closed.

Unlike preservice work, postservice work varies depending on the magnitude of the procedure. In an effort to accurately assign the amount of postprocedure work, specific CPT® codes have been assigned specific global periods. There are currently three postprocedural global periods; 0, 10, and 90 days. Routine postprocedure care includes physician work following skin closure that is done on the day of the procedure, including non-"skin-to-skin" work in the OR. This includes patient stabilization in the recovery room, communicating with the patient and other professionals (including written and telephone reports and orders), and patient visits on the day of the procedure. For a surgical service with a global period of 10 or 90 days, the postservice work includes all of the above and, in addition, postoperative hospital care, including the intensive care unit if needed; other in-hospital visits; discharge day management services; and office visits within the assigned global period of 10 or 90 days.[19]

For nonsurgical services such as office evaluation and management (E/M) services, the preservice work includes preparing to see the patient, reviewing records, and communicating with other professionals. The intraservice work includes the work provided while the physician is with the patient and/or family. This includes the time in which the physician obtains the history, performs a physical evaluation and counsels the patient. The postservice work for nonprocedural services includes arranging for further services, reviewing results of studies, and communicating further with the patient, family, and other professionals, including written and telephone reports as well as calls to the patient.

While the study by Hsiao and colleagues[16] initially valued only 200 codes and ranked them according to physician work, the RUC subsequently valued and ranked each CPT® code relative to other codes. New codes were valued using provider surveys to obtain an appropriate work value. These surveys allow for individuals who perform the procedures to value pre-, intra-, and postservice work relative to established codes. According to federal law the relative value of codes is reviewed every 5 years by the RUC allowing for corrections in the relativity of the codes. Currently, physician work is not the only value used to calculate an RVU. While the work RVUs (wRVU) makes up the majority of the total RVUs (tRVU) for a specific CPT® code, RVUs are also calculated for practice expense (peRVU) and malpractice (mRVU) for each code. Similar to wRVUs, peRVUs are calculated based on the amount of resources used in the pre-, intra- and postservice time. This includes not only the nursing and ancillary staff key to the procedure or service but also supplies used during the pre- and postprocedure period. If the procedure is performed in the office, intraservice personnel and supplies are included. For procedures done in a facility, usually a hospital, these costs are reimbursed based on the DRG (Part A) and paid to the health care facility and not to the physician. Malpractice RVUs are calculated from actual malpractice premium data obtained throughout the country. Using previous CMS claims, a value for each CPT®

code is determined based on a risk factor for the dominant specialty that provides service.[20]

Final physician reimbursement by CMS is then multiplied by a geographic practice cost index (GPCI), which is supposed to adjust payments for differences in physician practice costs across geographic areas. For a given service, multiplying the service-specific Physician Work, Practice Expense, and Malpractice Expense RVUs by their respective GPCIs determines the payment amount in a given geographic area. Next, these three products are summed, yielding a geographically adjusted RVU total for the service. This number is then converted to dollars by a conversion factor, which in 2009 was $36.0666 per RVU. Without congressional intervention, adjusting the SGR formula, it could drop as much as 21% in 2010–2011. As an example, in 2009 for CPT® code 44140 (Colectomy, partial; with anastamosis) [(wRVU × wGPCI) + (peRVU × peGPCI) + (mRVU × mGPCI)] × 36.0666 = $CMS reimbursement. As seen the amount paid varies per region:

San Francisco, CA
(22.46 wRVU × 1.059 wGPCI) + (8.69 peRVU × 1.441 peGPCI) + (2.71 mRVU × 0.414 mGPCI) × 36.0666 = $1,349.94.

Boston, MA
(22.46 wRVU × 1.029 wGPCI) + (8.69 peRVU × 1.291 peGPCI) + (2.58 mRVU × 0.764 mGPCI) × 36.0666 = $1,309.29.

New Orleans, LA
(22.46 wRVU × 1.0 wGPCI) + (8.69 peRVU × 1.044 peGPCI) + (2.58 mRVU × 0.956 mGPCI) × 36.0666 = $1,226.22.

Little Rock, AK
(22.46 wRVU × 1.000 wGPCI) + (8.69 peRVU × 0.846 peGPCI) + (2.58 mRVU × 0.446 mGPCI) × 36.0666 = $1,116.70.

While Medicare is an extremely large and at times an unwieldy way to manage health care and health care-related costs, understanding it is key to understanding both hospital and physician reimbursement by private payers. Most private payers today use CPT® codes to identify physician services. While private payer do not have to follow the rules set forth by the Federal government (for instance, they often do not recognize surgical modifiers), they find that CPT® is a well-established and familiar system allowing for correct physician coding. Private payers in noncapitated contracts often set reimbursement based on a percentage of the Medicare fee schedule. The percentage reimbursement will often vary by region. The larger payers have taken this one step further using Medicare to develop their own fee schedule. Again using CPT® terminology, companies will adjust payment based on the individual service provided; for example, paying E&M codes 105% of Medicare, office-based procedures 110% of Medicare and surgical procedures 115%. This is often modified regionally based on the rules of supply and demand. In areas with a paucity of a specific specialty, reimbursement is high as opposed to a saturated market where the insurance company can play one physician or group against another to obtain a favorable contract. Hospital payments are similar. Private payers reimburse hospitals either as a percentage of the DRG or on a per-diem based on the service provided. For outpatient procedures, hospitals are often reimbursed as a percentage of the APC.

Private Payers

While the impact of Medicare on the economic landscape of medicine is clear, the role and type of private payers is more cloudy. Health insurance comes in many forms and has different relations with its customer and its physician providers. Traditionally, there were two types of nongovernmental insurance, individual insurance and group insurance. Individual insurance allows a person to buy health insurance for themselves and their family. However, due to the inability of the insurer to spread the financial risk among many people, individual insurance is becoming prohibitively expensive. The majority of people obtain health insurance through some type of group. This allows for cheaper individual payments as group purchasing allows the insurer to spreads the risk over a larger number of people. Group insurance can be obtained through employers, professional societies (ACS, etc.) or other organizations (AAPR, etc.).

Regardless of how insurance is purchased, the types of insurance plans are distinctly different. The most costly is the fee-for service plan, also known as an indemnity plan in which individuals are free to seek care from any physician or hospital they choose. No preapproval is required. Individuals submit the bills to their carrier and if the deductible has been met, if there is one, the insurance company pays for medical services at the UCR. These plans are often structured so that there is a copayment for all services. The use of copayments and deductibles by insurers is a method of risk sharing. Not only do these costs help defray the cost of providing care for the insurers, but they are designed to make individuals think twice before seeking unnecessary care. In traditional fee-for-service plans, an individual may be responsible for 20% of the bill. Also, they may be responsible for the difference between the UCR and the billed charges.

To help control rising health care costs and stimulate a more efficient use of health care resources, managed care organizations were developed. Since the early 1990s they have evolved into a variety of complex organizational structures. They utilize a variety of tools to manage preauthorization functions, control health care costs, and share the risks associated with group coverage.

Health maintenance organizations (HMOs) were designed to meet these ends. While the HMO model undergoes constant change, they characteristically represent the most restrictive type of health plan. In this model, the HMO restricts patient access in nonemergency incidents to HMO-contracted physicians and hospitals. Out-of-pocket costs for individuals are traditionally low for HMO physicians; however, individuals are responsible for all costs for non-HMO physicians.

Most HMOs initially utilized a "gatekeeper" or primary care physician for specialist referral. Subsequently, HMOs have loosened gatekeeper requirements for specialist referral. This model has propagated the development of health care systems, multispecialty groups that are either owned by or contract with the HMO to provide complete patient care. In these instances, the physicians function as employees of the system. The physician group is then paid a capitated fee (amount per patient per month to provide total care) which is divided among the medical care providers at a rate determined by the medical group administration.

The next iteration of managed care organizations is the preferred provider organization (PPO). Similar to HMOs, PPOs enter into contracts with health care providers and hospitals to provide member care. Often more choice and flexibility are available to the patient than in the traditional HMO model but at the cost of higher beneficiary premiums. Unlike HMOs, PPOs do not own physician practices. To have access to the PPO's beneficiaries and be listed in the "network," physicians often agree to reduce their normal fees. PPOs traditionally do not use a "gatekeeper," thus allowing patients increased access to self-referred specialty care.

The most recent variation in managed care organizations is the development of "Point of Service" plans, a mixture of traditional HMO and PPO plans. In this type of plan, if a patient first sees their primary care physician to receive a referral, much like an HMO the copay, if present, is negligible. Patients are also able to see "network" physicians with minimal financial responsibility. Patients may seek care from someone outside the "network" without a referral. In these instances, the physician is paid a rate less than is characteristically billed, usually the same rate as in network physicians, and the patient is responsible for the difference. This provides increased patient flexibility but at increased cost.

The Future

Despite hopes that managed care would provide cost stability to health care in America, after costs initially slowed they have continued to rise at a rate higher than the consumer price index and personal income (Table 51-1).[21] Is this a failure of managed care or has managed care reached its capacity with regards to improving efficiency and cost containment? The answer is unclear; however, experts now tout a "consumer-centric" or "consumer-driven" health care model as the future of health care delivery. Harvard Professor Regina Herzlinger initially described a system that allows users to become active consumers.[19] Similar to making any large purchases, individuals are given the opportunity to chose from specific benefit packages that will fit their particular need. Aside from having choice, individuals are given information allowing them to make educated and informed choices. Herzlinger and others envision a health care market place similar to a successful industry where individuals are given control, choice, and information. With the rising number of consumers in need of health care resources, these experts see the Internet as a way of rapid dissemination of health care information.[22–25]

While consumer-centric health care and Health Reimbursement Arrangements (HRA) appear to be recreating the way health care is funded, there are potential problems. This model assumes that consumers are sophisticated enough to make sound health care choices, not just those based on cost. As Abramowitz notes, "Choosing based on price is impossible for consumers to do intelligently. The bottom line is that consumers lack the information necessary to use the money wisely. So consumer-driven health care, as it is being discussed today will be a market failure."[26] Another potential problem is that individuals will feel obligated to use all of their HRA or employer contributions, especially as the year-end approaches and individuals run the risk of losing their contributions.

The initial manifestation of a hope to address some of the potential pitfalls of consumer-centric health care is the development of defined contribution plans in which employers provide a set amount to individuals for health care, along with information regarding employer-approved health care choices. Often these are tied to a safety net for catastrophic cost. The idea is to empower individuals and to give them the necessary information to make good choices. Further development of consumer-driven health care is the creation of "health reimbursement arrangements" (HRAs). This IRS plan gives a tax advantage to employers who contribute defined contributions to employee-controlled accounts for health care spending. Any monies not spent during the year are rolled over to help fund the following year's plan. The thought was that this combined with a high deductible plan would lower health care costs. These types of plans also raise some questions: is the unused portion of the plan eligible to be rolled over in an IRA/401K? Can these funds be used for nontraditional health care? What about domestic partners? Are these funds portable? These questions will only be answered by time and possibly federal legislation. Will this next generation of changes significantly help to control health care costs? The answer is unclear; however, one current benefit is the increasing individual awareness and education that these plans foster.

Despite the many and varied attempts to control health care costs, an unacceptably large number of Americans are still unable to obtain adequate health care coverage. This has led to the call in some quarters for the development of universal coverage. The late Senator Edward Kennedy put it best in a 2003 editorial: "Health care is not just another commodity. It is not a gift based on the ability to pay."[27] Proponents of universal coverage envision a system that provides access to quality care when needed and effective preventative care in a cost-effective manner that is delivered and paid for in an equitable way. While these are laudable goals, practical application remains a long way off. As seen from above, the increasing role and complexity of Medicare and Medicaid has not even incrementally achieved these objectives. The current acrimonious debate in Washington shows that these goals are even further than initially thought. Will the government be willing to push forward any health care reform realizing that universal health care will result in the subsequent development of a two-tiered health care system, one for the wealthy and one for the remainder of Americans? Only time will tell.

References

1. Dickens C. A tale of two cities. London: Duncan Baird; 2008.
2. HHS Office of the Inspector General. http://oig.hhs.gov/oei/reports/oei-04-02-00180.pdf(2005). Accessed 5 Jan 2005.
3. The Centers for Medicare & Medicaid Services. http://www.cms.hhs.gov/NationalHealthExpendData/downloads/proj2009.pdf (2010). Accessed 5 Jan 2010.
4. The Centers for Medicare & Medicaid Services http://www.cms.hhs.gov/ReportsTrustFunds/downloads/projection methodology.pdf (2010). Accessed 29 Jan 2010.
5. United States Census Bureau. http://www.census.gov/Press-Release/www/releases/archives/income_wealth/014227.html (2010). Accessed 30 Jan 2010.
6. The Centers for Medicare & Medicaid Services http://www.cms.hhs.gov/charts/series/sec3-b1-9.pdf (2005). Accessed 5 Jan 2005.
7. The Congressional Budget Office http://www.cbo.gov/ftpdocs/82xx/doc8268/06-28-Medicare_Advantage.pdf(2010). Accessed 3 Feb 2010.
8. The Centers for Medicare & Medicaid Services. http://www.cms.hhs.gov/PerformanceBudget/Downloads/CMSFY10CJ.pdf (2010). Accessed 20 Jan 2010.
9. Goldstien J. http://blogs.wsj.com/health/2008/07/10/why-medicare-pay-cuts-for-doctors-will-be-back/ (2010). Accessed 10 Feb 2010.
10. Fetter RB, Thompson JD, Mills RE. A system for cost and reimbursement control in hospitals. Yale J Biol Med. 1976;49:123–36.
11. World Health Organization. Collaborating Center for Classification of Diseases for North America. The International classification of diseases: 9th revision, clinical modification: ICD-9-CM. Washington, DC: Dept. of Health and Human Services, Public Health Service, National Center for Health Statistics; 1986.
12. Hay J, Forrest S, Goetghebeur M. Executive summary hospital costs in the US. www.heartland.org/pdf/14628.pdf (2005). Accessed 10 Jan 2005.
13. Weiner SL, Maxwell JH, Sapolsky HM, et al. Economic incentives and organizational realities: managing hospitals under DRG's. Milbank Q. 1987;65:463–87.
14. Blount LL, Waters JM, Gold RS. Methods of insurance reimbursement, Chicago, IL. In: Mastering the reimbursement process. AMA;2001. p 6–7.
15. Hsiao WC, Braun P, Dunn D, et al. Resource-based relative values. An overview. JAMA. 1988;260:2347–53.
16. Hsiao WC, Couch NP, Causino N, et al. Resource-based relative values for invasive procedures performed by eight surgical specialties. JAMA. 1988;260:2418–24.
17. Hsiao WC, Yntema DB, Braun P, et al. Measurement and analysis of intraservice work. JAMA. 1988;260:2361–70.
18. Hsiao WC, Braun P, Becker ER, et al. The resource-based relative value scale. Toward the development of an alternative physician payment system. JAMA. 1987;258:799–802.
19. Mayberry C. RUC Research Subcommittee. The use of intensity measures in the development of physician work relative value units (RVU's). RUC meeting 14 Jan 2004 (non-published handout).
20. The Centers for Medicare & Medicaid Services. Development of Resource-based Malpractice RVUs. http://www.cms.hhs.gov/physicians/pfs/kpmgrept.asp#_Toc448071075 (2005). Accessed 10 Jan 2005.
21. U.S. Department of Commerce, Bureau of Economic Analysis. http://www.cms.hhs.gov/statistics/health-indicators/t7.asp (2005). Accessed 11 Jan 2005.
22. Herzlinger RE. Market driven health care: who wins, who loses in the transformation of America's largest service industry. Reading, MA: Addison-Wesley; 1997.
23. Gupta AK. The arrival of consumer-centric healthcare. Manag Care Q. 2003;11:20–3.
24. Halterman S, Camero C, Maillet P. The consumer–driven approach: can it pick up where managed care left off? Benefits Q. 2003;19:13–26.
25. Abbott RK, Feltman KE. Consumer driven healthcare and the birth of health reimbursement arrangements. Manag Care Q. 2002;10:4–7.
26. Abramowitz K. Health plan 2009. Consumer-directed health care won't fly. Manag Care. 2004;13:24.
27. Kennedy EM. Quality, affordable healths care for all Americans (editorial). Am J Public Health. 2003;93:14.

52 Ethical and Legal Considerations

Ira J. Kodner, Mark Siegler, Daniel M. Freeman, and William T. Choctaw

Considerations for Surgeons

General Concepts

Defining the Problem

Professional responsibilities have been a concern of surgeons since antiquity; however, the last 25 years have displayed a dramatic growth of both professional and societal attention to moral and ethical issues involved in the delivery of health care. This increased interest in medical ethics has occurred because of factors such as the greater technological power of modern medicine, the assigning of social ills to the responsibility of medicine, the growing sophistication of patients and the information available to them, the efforts to protect the civil rights of the increasing disadvantaged groups in our society, and the continued rapidly escalating cost of health care including medical malpractice costs. All of these factors contribute to the urgency of dealing with ethical and moral issues involved in the delivery of modern surgical care.[1]

The terms *ethics* and *morals* are often used interchangeably to refer to standards regarding right and wrong behavior. *Morals* refer to conduct that conforms to the accepted customs or standards of a people. They vary with time and with the nature of society at that time. *Ethics* is the branch of philosophy that deals with human conduct and can be described as applied morals. *Medical ethics* refers to the ethics of the practice of medicine. *Clinical ethics* refers to the ethics of delivering patient care. The term *bioethics* includes the ethics of all biomedical endeavors and encompasses both medical and clinical ethics.[2] The *law* serves to delineate the *formal rules of society*. It expresses a kind of minimal societal ethical consensus, which society is willing to enforce through civil judgments or criminal sanctions. The law does not always prohibit behavior deemed unethical; however, it usually sets a minimal standard for conduct. Those of us who practice clinical surgery often have trouble differentiating *ethical issues* from *legal issues*. It is the purpose of this chapter to clarify this dichotomy. It should be stated from the outset that it is more important to understand the *process* of dealing with these issues than to assume that anyone can clearly state what is ethically right or wrong in a complex medical/surgical dilemma. The law, on the other hand, can be very explicit and can vary from state to state.

Surgeons live and practice an intense form of applied ethics. We deliver bad news; we guide patients and their families through complicated decisions to arrive at appropriate informed consent; we live a code of truth and trust among ourselves, our patients, and our trainees; we must deal with the end-of-life issues; and we make plans for extended, palliative, and hospice care. Finally, as only we surgeons know, we must go to bed at night knowing that in the morning we will spend hours with someone's life literally in our hands.

In recent decades, although we can technically and scientifically do more for our patients than ever before, our personal, trusting relationship with them has deteriorated to the point where it is sometimes adversarial. We have allowed medicine to become a business, guided in many cases by the financial bottom line, rather than by the uncompromising concern for a sick person. Within this fast-moving corporate system, we see too many patients, do too many surgeries, and do not have time to develop a close mentoring relationship with our chosen role models or with our trainees.[3] The cherished patient–physician relationship has been undermined by our own successful advances. Many of the operations that we do on a routine, daily basis were not even imagined as possible only a few decades ago. Not only can we do more but our patients also have come to expect perfection from us. Our society seems willing to accept flaws from many sources, but not from physicians and medical delivery system. This situation is made even more complicated by a system in which individuals purchase their health-care coverage when they are well and willing to buy the cheapest plan possible but utilize their coverage, especially for surgical problems, when they are sick and want the maximum that the system can deliver, without regard to time and cost. No individual has ever admitted that he purchased a cheaper

D.E. Beck et al. (eds.), *The ASCRS Textbook of Colon and Rectal Surgery: Second Edition*,
DOI 10.1007/978-1-4419-1584-9_52, © Springer Science+Business Media, LLC 2011

plan and, therefore, understood that only limited care should be provided to a loved one who is ill.

Despite these difficulties, we surgeons cannot abandon the needs of our patients and their families. To help them make informed choices, we must communicate completely and compassionately the requisite information about the disease, treatment options, and long-range plans. To do so, we must learn and apply the ethical principle of *truth telling* and the doctrine of *informed consent* for the effective care, which has taken us so long to master. We must also take into account that high-speed communication via the Internet will necessitate reevaluation of issues such as *patient's rights* and *confidentiality*. Surgeons must lead in forging this new era rather than leaving it to bureaucrats, politicians, lawyers, and others who are not intimately involved in patient care.

We cannot rely on intuition or on our own personal value system. Learning the ethical aspects of delivering patient care must become an integral part of the surgical training program, and we must be held accountable for mastering the skillful application of these bioethical principles. After all, the concept of good clinical medicine and surgery implies the best use of scientific, technical, and *ethical* considerations. Just as with medicine and science, bioethics and legal underpinnings of bioethical decision making are evolving all the time. In this chapter, we do not discuss all possible bioethical issues but limit ourselves to those that may be of concern to colon and rectal surgeons and to surgery in general. Important issues relating to matters such as professionalism, research ethics, family, business and financial pressures, genetics, and reproductive considerations are discussed as well.

What Makes the Surgeon Special?

Undergoing major surgery is an extreme experience that changes people's lives. Surgeons are repeatedly involved in these extreme experiences of others. This makes surgeons uniquely placed among health-care professionals to understand the experiences of their patients.

Miles Little explains that there are special ethical considerations for surgeons.[4] These include Rescue, Proximity, Ordeal, Aftermath, and Presence. These terms help to define the ethical relationship between the surgeon and his or her patients. *Rescue*, he describes as the first pillar of surgical ethics. It deals with the fact that surgery conveys power and that power is socially endorsed and may be reinforced by the surgeon's individual charisma; but as with all power, it must be constantly renewed and re-validated. Patients have no choice but to acknowledge surgical power when they consult a surgeon. Surgeons, themselves, sometimes need help and rescue from colleagues when they have trouble with complicated diagnosis, management, or operative procedures. *Proximity* occurs in surgery as in no other act. To operate on persons involves entering their bodies and becoming privy to secrets even denied to the owner of the body. Little states, "To get to my body, my doctor has to get to my character. He has to go to my soul. He doesn't only have to go through my anus." This proximity to the patient can make special ethical demands on the surgeon. This proximity carries with it the penalties of closeness, and particularly the pains of failure. Some surgeons find that distancing themselves from their patients makes failure easier to bear. Understanding the privileges and risks of proximity is critical for the compassionate surgeon. *Ordeals* are periods of extreme experience, capable of disrupting our lives. The author, Little, explains that all medical encounters are ordeals. Patients yield autonomy, acknowledge dependence, place trust, face risk, confront embodiment and mortality, lose control over time and space, experience alienation, pain, fear, discomfort, suffering, and boredom. Surgeons observe and participate in the lives of patients with serious illnesses. A surgeon, who understands the ordeal of the surgical episode, can better help his or her patient through such extreme experiences. *Aftermath* deals with the reality that surgery leaves physical and psychological scars that may persist for life. It is very difficult to communicate the concept of suffering to someone who has not suffered himself. Little describes surgeons as being in a unique position to understand the existential threats that their patients experience, the sense of mortality and bodily frailty they live with, and the difficulty of explaining extreme experience to others. When death approaches our patients, we must remember, not deny, our own mortality. Such an approach takes courage and a sense of personal security, and this does not suit everyone, neither the patient nor the surgeon. *Presence*, as a virtue and a duty, is what the patient desires of the surgeon during all phases of the surgical encounter. Most surgeons have the stamina and cognitive ability to be present for their patients, but not all of us process the personal attributes of charisma, confidence, energy, and empathy, which are necessary to engender *trust* from our patients and our staff. Sometimes, amazingly, our mere presence means more to our patients than defects in the manner with which we deal with them. Even if we cannot teach sensitivity, we can emphasize the importance of surgical presence.

Thus, surgeons are privileged to lead lives of great complexity and moral richness. We can acquire a profound understanding and recognition of patient experience and suffering. Our proximity to patients seeking rescue, facing ordeals, and experiencing the aftermath of surgery presents us with a great challenge.

Unique Problems of Surgery

Surgeons, unlike other members of the health-care team, take on a different level of responsibility as they encounter patients. For the surgeon, the initial contact may just be the beginning of a longer-term relationship. With no previously established doctor–patient relationship, the surgeon and the patient may well be heading to the operating room for sometimes massive and sometimes potentially "futile" surgery. The surgeon and the surgical team take on the continued responsibility of the operative procedure itself, the postoperative care, and usually the long-term follow-up and management of any complications and dilemmas that may result from the initial encounter. This intense relationship is often established very quickly and under frequently adverse circumstances. The family and religion may not be known, and the patient may be unconscious, and certainly will be once the procedure starts.

Arthur R. Derse nicely delineates the array of ethical issues that arise in delivering surgical care. These include *informed consent*, *refusal of treatment*, *determination of decision-making capacity*, *treating patients despite their refusal*, *maintaining confidentiality* while respecting the duty to warn others, *limiting treatment* over issues of "futility," *treating pain* at the end of life, and acting as a *Good Samaritan*. Unlike surgeons, people in most professions have the luxury of time, and the opportunity to redo their work to remedy any mistakes. Attorneys can appeal their cases. Accountants can file an amended return. Movie directors can yell "Cut! Take two!" and reshoot the scene. All doctors understand that they will probably be second-guessed. As everyone who has ever watched a television police drama knows, the first thing a police officer must say to an arrested person is the famous *Miranda* warning. What most people do not realize is that the requirement for those warnings is the result of a Supreme Court decision rendered in June 1966. As a practical matter, the court is telling the arresting police officer, in the heat of making an arrest, that he should have known something, which took the court system 3 years to contemplate and research. The bottom line for surgeons who work under the same kind of time pressures is to do what you think is best. You must use your judgment, based on your medical knowledge and your experience. You are on the front line and you do not have the luxury of waiting for 3 years for the Supreme Court to tell you how to handle a potential situation. However, you also want to be as scrupulous as possible in making sure that bioethical and legal guidelines are followed, both for the benefit of the patient, and, frankly, as protection for yourself.

While it is crucial for the practice of medicine in all fields to be familiar with bioethical concepts, it is unrealistic to be expected to be knowledgeable about the nuances requiring detailed understanding of controversial bioethical dilemmas. However, it is important for surgeons to have a working knowledge of general medical ethical principles and how these principles affect decisions involved with treating patients. Our goal is to distill these general bioethical concepts and their underlying applications to specific situations, which you may face, into a cogent and concise tool for surgeons to use routinely, to include as part of their training, and to have as a reference resource. For specific dilemmas, time permitting, surgeons should obtain an opinion from the hospital ethics consultation service and/or from hospital counsel. By doing so, one can gain the experience and imprimatur of opinions from those who have dealt with such issues and whose training gives them the experience to deal with the issues in a knowledgeable way. It also serves as a cushion of knowledge for the physician when discussing the matter with the patient or the family. Surgeons should do all they can for the patient while at the same time doing what they need to do to protect themselves from personal risk and possibly from negative legal ramifications.

Similarly, doctors have a duty to themselves to avoid situations that violate their own personal beliefs, whether religious or medical. This includes thinking a step or two ahead of the current situation to know what the ramifications of a course of treatment may be. If the anticipated actions may violate a doctor's own personal tenants, he or she should refer the patient to another physician. The most obvious of these situations comes up with regard to religious beliefs. If, for example, a doctor has religious beliefs which would preclude *withdrawal of life support*, the doctor should be very careful about getting into a situation with a patient which might later dictate putting someone on life support. It may, down the line, become bioethically or medically appropriate to *withdraw* life support. If a physician cannot do that, she needs to know that up front and be prepared to withdraw from the case. A similar situation involves doctors who do not believe in *abortion*. They should not get themselves into medical situations where an emergency termination of a pregnancy may become the best medically viable option. You must always be prepared to protect yourself *and* your patients and must recognize your duties, both legal and ethical. You need to be aware of these duties and to avoid situations where they may come into conflict. This may be very difficult at times.

Principles of Bioethics

General Concepts

Philosophical Principles

Two major fundamental theoretical philosophical concepts exist for constructing a theory of ethics: *deontologic* and *consequentialist*. A deontologic theory relies on *rules*, while a consequentialist theory relies on *outcomes*.[2] From these theories are derived *principles of ethics*, such as those delineated by Beauchamp and Childress: respect for *autonomy* (patient self-determination), *beneficence* ("doing good"), *nonmaleficence* ("do no harm"), and *justice* (fairness).[5]

Respect for Autonomy

Adult patients with decision-making capacity have a right to their preferences regarding their own health care. This right is grounded on the legal doctrine of *informed consent*. This means that patients must give their voluntary consent to treatment after receiving all appropriate and relevant information about the nature of their problem, the expected consequences of the recommended treatment, and treatment alternatives.

This is probably the most crucial legal concept in bioethics. It simply means that you as a physician cannot *touch* a person without first getting permission and without telling the individual of the possible ramifications of that "touching." Touching someone without his or her consent is, in legal terms, a "battery," which could result in a lawsuit for damages. Therefore, the principle is that *medical treatment without consent is a battery.* The first major case in this area said "Every human being of adult years and sound mind has a right to determine what shall be done with his own body; and a surgeon who performs an operation without his patient's consent commits an assault, for which he is liable for damages… This is true except in cases of emergency where the patient is unconscious and where it is necessary to operate before consent can be obtained."[6] This case was decided before the concept of *living wills* and *durable powers of attorney* came into being. These documents both facilitate and complicate the consent process because *consent* must be obtained, if time permits, through these documents or via surrogate decision making. Subsequent cases refined the requirements of consent to add to the concept of *informed consent.* The courts now require not only that the patients give *consent* to the procedure, either themselves or through a proper surrogate, but also that sufficient information be given to the patients to help them make an *informed* decision. The courts have held that the quality and quantity of information given to the patient must be sufficient for the reasonable patient to understand, not for the doctor. The law has established the doctrine of the *reasonable man* to be used in deciding what is acceptable in many areas of delivering emergency surgical care.

Doctors are duty-bound to respect the autonomy of each competent patient. The patient is the ultimate decision maker about what he or she wants. The doctor may differ, even vehemently, with the patient's decision; however, the patient has the final say. There are exceptions to this rule also, such as that in the case when a patient demands a certain kind of treatment that the doctor knows will not be efficacious. Permitting *autonomy* to trump *nonmaleficence* poses a serious problem. A simple example of this is a patient who demands antibiotics to treat a viral infection. Giving the requested antibiotic complies with the *autonomy* principle; however, in the long run, it is conceivable that giving an antibiotic in such a case would violate the principle of *nonmaleficence*, would impose the concept of *futility*, and in the long run might enhance the capacity of bacteria to become resistant to certain antibiotics, thus even bringing into play the concept of *justice*. Even this simple example illustrates how medical ethical conundrums are frequently the result of *conflicting duties*.

If the patient is unable to make his or her own decision, the treating surgeon must respect the decision made by a surrogate decision maker, such as one designated in a health-care *durable power of attorney*.

Beneficence

The principle of *beneficence*, simply stated, involves the duty of the physician to act in the best interest of his or her patients. *Beneficence* is *doing good* and is the reason most of us chose to become doctors. Beneficence, or doing good, is probably the universal tenet of the medical profession.

Nonmaleficence

Nonmaleficence is essentially the old philosophical principle, "first, do no harm." It derives from knowing that patient encounters with surgeons can prove harmful as well as helpful. This principle includes not doing harm, preventing harm, and removing harmful conditions. For physicians caring for patients in an emergency environment, it also includes the concept of security, protecting oneself and one's team, as well as the patient, from harm.[7]

This concept also incorporates the principle of *avoiding killing*. This seems very obvious on its face value; however, what is a doctor to do when confronted with a situation where the administration of sufficient medication to alleviate the pain of a patient might have the *secondary effect* of diminishing respiration, and actually hastening the patient's death? This is, of course, the crux of the major debate that is ongoing over *physician-assisted suicide*, if not actual *euthanasia*. There are other situations where avoiding killing must be taken into account. *Abortion* presents another situation which, depending on your personal beliefs, might fall into that same category. This could create a conflict between the duty to respect the autonomy of the patient and the personal religious beliefs of the treating physician. This same conflict has recently, and intensely, come into play over the issue of research and therapeutic utilization of *embryonic stem cells*.

Justice

Justice is *fairness*. It is required to ensure that medical decisions are made with reason and honesty. Selfish or biased influences must be recognized and avoided.[8] For many, the term justice includes the concept of *distributive justice*. This form of *justice* includes the surgeon's obligation not only to an *individual patient* but also to fairness in the allocation of resources for the good of the *broader society*. It is this concept of justice that becomes the basis for society-wide health-care policy determination. *Distributive justice* implies that all individuals and groups should share in society's benefits and burdens. This presents an ethical challenge for the surgeon, dealing with an individual patient, who mistakenly believes that he or she should limit or terminate care based on a need to limit health-care resource expenditures for the *good of society*.[7] It was this temptation to place the good of society before the good of an individual that led the physicians of Europe to fall prey to the fallacious doctrines being promulgated by the Nazi government.[9]

Surgeons should be prepared to respect and seek to understand people from many cultures and from diverse socioeconomic groups. In USA, emergency facilities are obligated to provide necessary care to all patients, regardless of ability to pay. Our current business-based medical delivery system makes it difficult to abide by the principle of having *access* to appropriate inpatient and follow-up medical care dictated by the patient's financial situation. Provision of emergency, and most elective, surgical treatment should not be based on gender, age, race, socioeconomic status, or cultural background. No patient should ever be abused, demeaned, or given substandard care.[1]

Religion and Medical Ethics

In many societies, religion has been looked upon as the determinant of ethical norms. In our American society, we are multicultural with no single religion holding dominance over the entire population. Therefore, a value-based approach to ethical issues depends on the individual patient's values. However, religion still influences bioethical concepts and decisions. Clinical bioethics, in fact, uses many decision-making methods, arguments, and ideals that originated from religion. It is also important for the individual clinician to understand his or her own personal spirituality to relate better to patients and families, representing a broad diversity of religious and ethnic backgrounds. Although religions may appear dissimilar, most are based on some form of the Golden Rule, which holds "do unto others as you would have them do unto you." Problems frequently arise when trying to apply religion-based rules to specific clinical, ethical situations. In so-called modern times, USA began turning away from a reliance on religious principles, relying instead for answers based on more generic secular principles, and the medical/surgical community was no exception. As previously described, we have come to rely instead on the four *ethical principles of autonomy, beneficence, nonmaleficence,* and *fairness*. These are the principles that have guided medical ethical thinking and have become instrumental in forming health-care policies in USA and other Western countries over the past 3 decades.[7]

In a recent survey of physicians' attitudes toward spirituality in clinical practice, 85% said that physicians should be aware of the patients' religious and spiritual beliefs. The survey went on to show that although many physicians believe that they should inquire about their patients' beliefs, fewer than 10% of doctors actually do so, even for their dying patients. There is no hard data to support the benefits of taking a spiritual history, but there is some indirect evidence in support of the practice. It is known that religion is one of the most common ways by which patients cope with medical illness. Religious beliefs are known to be significant influences on medical decisions, especially those made by patients with serious illnesses. In addition, the faith community is a primary source of support for many medically ill patients, and such social support is associated with better adherence to therapy and improved medical outcomes. Several surveys have revealed that from the patient's point of view, satisfaction with the emotional and spiritual aspects of care had one of the *lowest* ratings among all clinical care indicators and was one of the highest areas in need of quality improvement.[10]

The purpose for taking even a brief spiritual or religious history is to learn how patients cope with their illnesses, the kinds of support systems available to them in the community, and to learn of any strongly held beliefs that might influence the delivery of medical care. Venturing into this delicate area is obviously fraught with some hazards. We must be extremely cautious about prescribing religion to nonreligious patients, forcing a spiritual history on patients who are not religious, causing patients to believe our practice and specific ways, attempting to provide spiritual counsel to patients, and arguing with patients over religious matters.[10] It is also imperative for us as surgeons to be comfortable enough with our own beliefs to allow our patients to *pray for us*, according to the faith of their own religion. No comment more than a simple and sincere "thank you" is usually indicated.

Legal Principles

General Concepts

Types of Law

In USA, law is created in one of two systems: *Federal* or *State*, and is made by judges (*common law*), legislatures (*statutory law*), and executive agencies empowered by legislatures (*regulatory law*). The fundamental document that creates and delineates these powers is the Constitution. *Civil law*, including malpractice, is usually enforced by *monetary judgments*. *Criminal law*, including physician-assisted suicide, is usually enforced by *fines* and/or *imprisonment*.[2]

There are three kinds of law, which affect the practice of surgery: *statutes*, *regulations* promulgated by an administrative agency, pursuant to a statute, and *case law*. The legislatures are the designated policy-making entities in our system; *regulations* are written to comply with legislative directives, and the courts are charged with resolving disputes between parties, usually as directed by *statute*, if there is a relevant one. Courts issue written opinions when there is a conflict that results in a lawsuit, especially when the interpretation of a statute or a regulation is in question. The most difficult situations are those where the court is faced with a matter of "first impression," which the legislature has not specifically addressed. The courts, and their written opinions, on this type of case, frequently ask the legislature for guidance in future situations. Until the legislature acts, the written opinion of the court is the only guidance physicians have, and hospital counsel sometimes must interpret this.

Doctors should be generally familiar with *state law*. There are different state laws on many bioethical matters, such as definition of death, competency, organ donation, and now the use of embryonic stem cells, even for research only. Many doctors move from state to state during their careers, and general understanding of state laws governing situations which may confront them in surgical situations is crucial. However, most important legal principles that apply to ethical dilemmas in delivering surgical care are widely accepted among several states. There are some glaring discrepancies in these commonalities, including the neurologic *criteria for death* (a person may be legally dead in one state and not in another) and the legality of *physician-assisted suicide* (punishable as a crime in all states except Oregon, Washington, and Montana).

Statutory Law

Statutory law is made by legislatures and includes such issues as *the statute of limitations*, which defines how long after an adverse event a patient is able to sue a physician for malpractice, and, in some states, statutes on *informed consent*.

The Emergency Medical Treatment and Labor Act (EMTALA) is another example of a *federal statutory law*. It was originally enacted as part of the Consolidated Omnibus Budget Reconciliation Act of 1986. Congress enacted EMTALA as a remedy for "patient dumping." The legislature was particularly concerned about hospitals refusing to render emergency care because of lack of insurance or the economic ability to pay, but it soon came to realize that care was also being refused on the basis of race or other discriminatory criteria. The Act requires that a basic screening examination be provided to all patients seeking care. It therefore became illegal, as well as unethical, to withhold therapy from the poor just because they do not have the ability to pay.[11]

Compilation of statistics from major county hospitals across the country concluded that as many as 650,000 patients were "dumped" annually, and the resulting transfer led to substandard care and/or life-threatening situations in 25–33% of that number. The economic impact of EMTALA on hospitals and physicians has been enormous. Patients without the means to pay for medical care know that they cannot be turned away from the emergency room. Therefore, they use it as their *primary care facility*. That means that hospitals, physicians, and surgeons are carrying the burden of the nation's uninsured, often without adequate compensation. For many health-care facilities, this money lost in the emergency room can mean the difference between bankruptcy and solvency.[12]

Regulatory Law

These administrative laws are created by regulatory agencies including State Medical Boards. Recent examples of regulatory law include not only EMTALA but also the recently implemented Health Insurance Portability and Accountability Act of 1996 (HIPAA). HIPAA, like EMTALA, was intended to protect patients' rights of privacy and to guarantee them continuation of health insurance coverage should they change employers. Also, like EMTALA, HIPAA has taken on many ramifications threatening a huge economic impact on the escalating costs of delivering medical care. Although the good aspects of it are necessary and noble, the burdens of increased costs will cripple some health-care facilities and will probably significantly curtail many clinical research endeavors.

Malpractice

The public and the legal community do not seem to accept that there is an element of uncertainty and unpredictability in a biological system. They seem to understand that eleven men on a playing field cannot score a touchdown on every play, but a surgeon is held to a standard of achieving perfection on every operation. An ethical, as well as legal, consideration is as follows: what to do when we fall short of perfection or, worse, make a blatant error while trying to do the best we can. Several factors come into play. Who is responsible if you did not actually do the damage yourself? What to tell the patient and the family? How to comply with the policies of legal counsel and risk management within your own institution?

Many successful legal actions against surgeons have been based on inadequate information about risks, complications, or adverse outcomes. A surgeon must be able to admit to unwanted events in an honest and compassionate manner. It is clearly possible to accept *responsibility* without admitting *negligence*. It never hurts to admit that you are sorry things had not gone exactly as planned, but that you must go forward, as efficiently as possible, to correct the situation. At this point, a surgeon should never hesitate to seek consultative assistance whenever it might seem helpful. It is never helpful to shift blame to a resident, an assistant, a nurse, a referring physician, or the institution itself. If anyone is to be sued, everyone will be sued, and divisiveness usually damages everyone. Unfortunately, it is also of little help to blame the patient and to invoke the existence of adequate *informed consent*. How nice it would be to tell the morbidly obese person that his postoperative complications should be blamed on his own indiscretions. Even informed consent, including risks based on the patients known status of precarious health, is of little help. A surgeon is not absolved of responsibility and concern by claiming "I told you so!"

Judges, not the legislature, establish the standards that constitute medical malpractice. The familiar elements of medical malpractice include *duty, breach, causation*, and *damages*. Decisions are based on the standard of care, and judges have developed the methods of determining the standards over many years, after the review of many cases. Thus, the courts rule on a specific set of facts that have already occurred. This is extremely frustrating for those practitioners of surgery who need to know what the law *would say* in a particular situation, as it is occurring, not in retrospect.

Unfortunately, resolution of controversy over medical and surgical ethical issues has been the domain of law, not philosophy or medicine. So far, perhaps because of legal constraints, medicine has been unable to "police itself." Because the law has come to champion individual rights and hold physicians liable for malpractice, it has served to condemn medical *paternalism* as it has elevated *patients' rights*. This has had the damaging effect of encouraging many physicians to become more concerned with avoiding litigation then with "doing the right thing." The law has had understandable difficulty in sorting out the complicated *physician–patient relationship*, and thus law does not mandate ethical behavior in these relationships.

A Familiar Case-Management System

Physician-Based Ethics

General Principles

Mark Siegler, a physician, and his co-authors of "Clinical Ethics," the fifth edition, present a technique for using *case analysis* as a practical approach to solving ethical dilemmas in clinical medicine. Contrary to most texts on health-care ethics that are organized around the ethical *principles* of respect for *autonomy*, *beneficence*, *nonmaleficence*, and *fairness*, their publication provides a straightforward *method* for clinicians to use in sorting out the pertinent facts and values of any case into an orderly pattern that facilitates the discussion and resolution of ethical problems.[13] Their technique corresponds to the way in which clinicians usually analyze actual cases. It assimilates the ethical principles and circumstances that comprise a method to facilitate the analysis of cases involving ethical issues.

The *Clinical Ethics* System

Siegler and his colleagues suggest that every clinical case, especially those raising an ethical dilemma, should be analyzed by means of the following four topics: (1) *medical indications*, (2) *patient preferences*, (3) *quality of life*, and (4) *contextual features*, defined as the social, economic, legal, and administrative context in which the case occurs. The authors emphasize that although the facts of each case can differ, these four topics are always relevant. The topics organize the various facts of the particular case and at the same time call attention to the ethical principles appropriate for each case. Their intent is to show clinicians that these four topics provide a systematic method of identifying and analyzing the ethical problems occurring in clinical medicine (Table 52-1).[13]

Examination of the table shows that the authors have clearly related to clinical situations the basic ethical principles previously described. They go on to emphasize that most ethical conflicts can be resolved by falling back on the *medical indications* that represent the medical facts of the case. This information, plus the second category of *patient preferences*, almost always will lead the clinical surgeon to a resolution of the ethical problem. If the ethical dilemma results from conflicts among the patient, the family, the health-care team, or institutional policy, then adequate resolution may become dependent on applying analysis of the additional categories, *quality of life*, and the array of *contextual features*. It is amazing how often reviewing and relying on what the medical facts of the situation actually are can clarify the intensity and emotion of even the most complex situation.

Specific Dilemmas of Colon and Rectal Surgery

Special Considerations for Colon and Rectal Surgeons

We understand that we have chosen a surgical career which includes resolving perplexing problems of anorectal disease, pelvic floor malfunction, and incontinence which cause daily significant discomfort for the patient and have frequently been mismanaged, for a long period of time, by our nonspecialized colleagues. This places us, frequently, in the position of not only having to resolve the technical surgical aspect of the problem but also having to explain the previous misdiagnosis or mismanagement by other physicians, a challenging *ethical dilemma*.

In addition to the seemingly simple anorectal disease, most of our careers also encompass management of some of the most complicated inflammatory bowel disease and cancer. This casts us into a position of having to deal with multiple components of the modern health-care team daily. We know that no one should ever have to die from colorectal cancer because it can be prevented or diagnosed at an early, or even premalignant, stage. Thus, we become actively involved with screening, preventive measures, understanding genetic predisposition to disease, and even the need for what has come to be called *preemptive surgery*. Because of the diseases that we treat, we must understand the science of current genetics as well as the appropriate clinical utilization of genetic testing, including the challenges of respecting *confidentiality* and requesting *genetic counseling* to deal with the long-term aspects involving not only the patient but also the family members who may not wish to be included in the discovery of genetic predisposition to disease. All of these present an intense need for dealing with frequent ethical challenges, especially the need for increasing *preemptive surgery*, subjecting a *well person* to major surgery with significant risk of complications or impact on lifestyle and body image. In fact, because of our experience and expertise in pelvic surgery and the construction and

TABLE 52-1. The four topics: case analysis in clinical ethics

Medical Indications	Patient Preferences
The Principles of Beneficence and Nonmaleficence 1. What is the patient's medical problem? history? diagnosis? prognosis? 2. Is the problem acute? chronic? critical? emergent? reversible? 3. What are the goals of treatment? 4. What are the probabilities of success? 5. What are the plans in case of therapeutic failure? 6. In sum, how can this patient be benefited by medical and nursing care, and how can harm be avoided?	The Principle of Respect for Autonomy 1. Is the patient mentally capable and legally competent? Is there evidence of incapacity? 2. If competent, what is the patient stating about preferences for treatment? 3. Has the patient been informed of benefits and risks, understood this information, and given consent? 4. If incapacitated, who is the appropriate surrogate? Is the surrogate using appropriate standards for decision making? 5. Has the patient expressed prior preferences, e.g., Advance Directives? 6. Is the patient unwilling or unable to cooperate with medical treatment? If so, why? 7. In sum, is the patient's right to choose being respected to the extent possible in ethics and law?
Quality of Life	**Contextual Features**
The Principles of Beneficence and Nonmaleficence and Respect for Autonomy 1. What are the prospects, with or without treatment, for a return to normal life? 2. What physical, mental, and social deficits are the patient likely to experience if treatment succeeds? 3. Are there biases that might prejudice the provider's evaluation of the patient's quality of life? 4. Is the patient's present or future condition such that his or her continued life might be judged undesirable? 5. Is there any plan and rationale to forego treatment? 6. Are there plans for comfort and palliative care?	The Principles of Loyalty and Fairness 1. Are there family issues that might influence treatment decisions? 2. Are there provider (physicians and nurses) issues that might influence treatment decisions? 3. Are there financial and economic factors? 4. Are there religious or cultural factors? 5. Are there limits on confidentiality? 6. Are there problems of allocation of resources? 7. How does the law affect treatment decisions? 8. Is clinical research or teaching involved? 9. Is there any conflict of interest on the part of the providers or the institution?

Source: Reprinted from Jonsen et al.,[13] with permission from McGraw-Hill Companies.

management of intestinal stomas, we are often confronted with such *quality-of-life* issues as body image and impairment of sexual function.

Dealing with our many patients, and their families, who have inflammatory bowel diseases such as Crohn's disease requires us to maintain long-term, perhaps for generations, contact with and care for our patients, much the contrary of our public image of being just "technicians" who do a short-term repair job and then have no other ongoing relationship with our patients.

Because of the complexity of the diseases on which we operate, including those in areas with difficult access and high risk of postoperative complications and recurrence of malignant processes, we often find ourselves on the leading edge of surgical innovation and instrumentation. This creates the ethical challenges of differentiating acceptable surgical *innovation* from truly *investigative* ventures that require research protocols and institutional approval. We must deal with the interpretation and implementation of *autonomy* versus *paternalism* as we guide our patients to the best choices for their care. Sick patients and those suffering from advanced cancer will grasp at straws. They want anything on earth that might help. In such a situation, it is important for the surgeon-scientist to avoid exploiting this universal hope of sick patients by carrying out an operation that is inadequately tested.[14] Because of these challenges of innovation, we are also frequently thrust into the potential conflict of interest between ethical surgery and the pharmaceutical and instrumentation industries.

Needless to say, because of the many things that we have to offer and the need to be concerned with our own long-term financial security in the face of reimbursement and legal challenges, we must walk the narrow line between providing the best care possible for all of our patients and complying with our own personal needs and those of our families. Claude Organ explained that "So much of our orientation today serves to erode our spirit as caregivers." He goes on to say that surgery is under increased public surveillance, and we are consumed by endless paperwork, administrative hassles, ponderous bureaucracy, professional liability concerns, inadequate reimbursement for our work, limited access for our patients, an impersonalized system, and increasingly burdensome documentation. He cites the increasing federal mandates of the Health Insurance Portability and Accountability Act, the Emergency Medical Treatment and Active Labor Act, and the Program for Appropriate Technology in Health audits. He goes on to quote the highly respected surgical mentor, Haile Debas as saying, "professional status is not an inherent right but one granted by society.... This obligates surgeons to put their patients' interests above their own."[15]

Categories of Patient Encounters

Severe Emergency: Life in Immediate Jeopardy

An example would be a critically ill person brought in from a severe motor vehicle accident or one who has suffered a serious gunshot wound. Certainly, there is no preestablished doctor–patient relationship, there is little chance that there will be a reliable surrogate, and many ethicists have questioned if a patient in such dire straits ever has *decision-making capacity*.

Urgent: Serious Problem Needing Surgery

An example would be a patient brought in with peritonitis. The individual may be in hypovolemic shock, is terrified, is in great pain, but is still cognizant of the situation and what is happening. There certainly is no preexisting *doctor–patient relationship*, and no one is absolutely sure of the *decisional capacity*, especially if the patient disagrees with the recommendation of the surgical team. In a case such as this, where there is some but not much time, the presence of a *surrogate* and clearly described *advance directives* would be extremely helpful.

Semi-Elective: Will Probably Need Surgery

An example would be an elderly patient with known extensive intra-abdominal cancer who presents with a significant, unresolving intestinal obstruction. It is clear that the obstruction can only be relieved by surgery, but it is not clear that this will be beneficial to the patient. In this case, determination of *decisional capacity*, the existence of *advance directives*, or the presence of a reliable *surrogate* is very important, and there is enough time to pursue the intended desires of this patient.

Autonomy/Decision-Making Capacity/Competency

General Concepts

Autonomy vs. Paternalism: Trust Is the Bridge

Individual freedom is one of the basic tenets of modern bioethics. This freedom is usually referred to as *autonomy*. This principle implies that a person should be free to make his or her own decisions. It is somewhat the antithesis of the medical profession's long practiced *paternalism* whereby the physician acted on what he or she thought was *good* for the patient, whether or not the patient agreed. The concept of *autonomy* applies to many interpersonal relationships and is essentially a respect for each person as an individual.

It has been difficult for many physicians, perhaps especially surgeons, to accept the principle of *patient autonomy*. This is not difficult to understand because accepting this principle implies a change in the physician's relationship with the patient. The physician must now be a partner in his or her patients' care, and must become an educator, teaching uninformed patients enough about their diseases to make rational decisions, and most distressing, to allow autonomous patients to make foolish choices. For physicians dedicated to helping their patients, allowing them to select what the physician considers a terrible treatment option, or even refusing treatment altogether, is a very frustrating change.[7]

On the other hand, experienced surgeons know that their patients significantly rely on them for guidance through complicated choices, often where life itself is on the line. This is, of course, a form of *paternalism* which our patients request and to which they are entitled. The key to accomplishing this ethically and successfully is based on the principle of *trust*. For surgeons, establishment of this trust must begin at the inception of the relationship and sometimes must be very quickly accomplished. It is sometimes very difficult for our nonsurgical colleagues to understand and accept this element of *paternalism* required in the surgeon–patient relationship.

The crucial issue for the surgeon seeking autonomous informed consent is the *decision-making capacity* or *competence* of the patient involved. Understanding the differences between these terms is important, especially if the patient disagrees with the advice of the surgeon or refuses potentially life-sustaining treatment.

The determination of *decision-making capacity* involves more than just completing a mental status examination and includes the ability of the patient to take in information, to evaluate a decision based on personal values, to make a decision, and to communicate the choice of decision to the physician. The concept of medical *decision-making capacity* is one based on the evaluation by the team providing medical and surgical care. This is distinguishable from a *legal determination* of *incompetence*. A patient is always assumed to be *legally competent* unless a *court* has declared otherwise. For example, patients may not have been declared incompetent by a court but may have lost the capacity to make decisions about their medical care because of their current medical status, including such conditions as intoxication, stroke, hypoxia, blood loss, dementia, or severe trauma. The determination of *decision-making capacity* varies in stringency with the seriousness of the impact of the decision. For example, the more severe the risk posed by the patient's decision, the more stringent should be the standard of determining capacity. This provides an increased protection for patients of questionable capacity when the potential harm from their decision is greater. This reaches the pinnacle of importance when a patient refuses treatment for a potentially life-threatening condition. These decisions are often difficult to make in the emergency environment, and the treating surgeon must sometimes make practical ethical decisions that go beyond the basic law of informed consent.

Refusal of Treatment

Ethical dilemmas usually occur when there is disagreement among the patient, the family, and the health-care team. The clearest example is a patient's refusal to accept the recommended treatment. This is especially critical for the patient who has *decision-making capacity* and refuses potentially life-sustaining treatment. The US Supreme Court, in the *Cruzan case*, upheld the right of persons to refuse lifesaving medical treatment, including resuscitation, ventilators, artificial nutrition and hydration, and lifesaving blood transfusions. The Court based its decision on "the right of every individual to the possession and control of his own person, free from all restraint or interference of others, unless by clear and unquestionable authority of law under the *liberty interest*, protected by the Due Process clause of the Fourteenth Amendment of the Constitution." The courts have, however, identified four *state interests* that override the refusal or termination of medical treatment on behalf of competent and incompetent persons, including the preservation of human life, the protection of the interests of innocent third persons, the prevention of suicide, and the maintenance of the integrity of the medical profession.

In exercising their rights under the autonomy principle, each competent patient has a right to refuse treatment, even if the results of such refusal will be their death. This type of situation comes up most often in the case of religious or cultural beliefs. Jehovah's Witnesses are probably the most familiar example of this type of dilemma. They refuse to accept blood transfusions, based on their religious beliefs. Such refusal, especially where major surgery is indicated, clearly poses the likelihood of avoidable death. Still, the competent patient's *autonomy must rule*. There may be situations where the treating surgeon feels that the competency of the patient refusing treatment may be in doubt. In such a case, if time permits, to protect the doctor and the hospital, it may be appropriate to get a court order permitting the indicated procedure or blood transfusion. The courts will weigh the possible benefits of the treatment against the potential negative effects, risks, and the potential burdens on the patient, and they will issue a ruling. This ruling will insulate the treating physician and the institution from legal liability. There are situations where parents or guardians are involved in refusal to accept and allow treatment on behalf of miners. These are the most common instances where court intervention is sought, and to resolve the problem, the courts must balance the best interests of the child against the desires of the parents.

For sure, *refusal* of a life-sustaining medical treatment should be accompanied by a full assessment of *decision-making capacity* and by an understanding from the patient of the consequences of refusal. If uncertainty prevails, the surgeon on the firing line should still "err on the side of life."

Telling the Truth/Disclosing Errors

General Concepts

Physicians have a duty to tell the truth to their patients. This seems so obvious that it merits no further discussion. However, there may be circumstances where telling the *whole truth* to a patient will have a negative impact on his or her overall well-being. If the physician believes that telling the patient everything about the condition in question, which is a duty, will have a dramatic negative effect on the patient's well-being, the physician must decide which duty is more important in each particular situation.

Truth telling also would apply in situations involving *medical mistakes*, even those mistakes that are minor and arguably have no detrimental effect on the patient. To illustrate this point, let us consider a doctor awakened in the middle of the night who orders 1 mg of a drug, when the appropriate dose is 0.1 mg. The overdose has no detrimental effect on the patient; so, does the doctor still have a duty to reveal the error that he made? Ostensibly, this question would seem to be easy to answer: just tell the truth! However, if informing a patient whose confidence in the medical profession is very low, and his mental stability might be diminished by finding out about a medical error, notwithstanding the fact that the error had no detrimental effect, do doctors still have a duty to tell the truth? In this situation, it might violate the duty of nonmaleficence by doing something that will hurt the patient.

Prognosis: Balance Between Giving False Hope and Removing All Hope

We are all involved in operations whose desired outcomes are not met. Managing these patients through the entire course of their disease, and sometimes death, is an important part of being a good physician and surgeon. This becomes even more important as the population ages and we encounter older patients with multiple comorbidities. Especially in these older, high-risk patients, even what is anticipated to be a fairly straightforward operation may have unexpected, adverse results. It forces us to remember the old adage that not everyone needs to die with an incision. Predicting prognosis, much less conveying it well to the patient and the family, is a difficult skill with little data to help us. We need to communicate with the public the fact that we would welcome the ability to forecast outcomes accurately especially for older patients, with higher risks, and in emergency situations. We truly cannot distinguish which ones may actually do well from such high-risk operations. This necessitates us, as surgeons, to assume an important role in providing *palliative care* even when complete surgical *cure* is no longer a possibility.[16]

Discussing prognosis with our patients and their families is one of the situations, which forces us most carefully to choose our words precisely. Even when we are forced by patients and families to use specific statistics, we must use them in a manner that is helpful and not totally destructive of hope. It helps to explain that statistics are better for 100 people rather than for any given individual. It can be very expeditious for us to use statistics as a form of *truth dumping*, but such an act can be devastating to a terrified, desperate, and inadequately informed patient who is desperately clinging to any possible hope.

Patients with Impaired Decision-Making Capacity

Examples of patients having impaired decision-making capacity include minors, mentally handicapped persons, those with organic brain disease or in toxic states, and those with psychiatric conditions, including suicidal risk. Determining the point at which a "minor" has the capacity to make medical decisions is often very complicated and varies with the laws of an individual state.[17] For example, an "emancipated minor" can make his or her own medical decisions. This includes individuals younger than the age of majority who are living on their own, are married, or are in the military.

Even patients with some forms of dementia cannot be regarded as having lost their *decision-making capacity*. Depending on the severity of their disease, they may well be able to participate in much of the decision-making process. This of course depends on the status of their disease and on the complexity and implications of the decision to be made.

Suicidal Patients

Respect for autonomy has always had its limits. When treating a suicidal patient, the surgeon is faced with a conflict between the ethical principle of *beneficence* and *respect for autonomy*. Sorting out this dilemma is usually based on whether the suicidal patient is currently capable of making a rational, autonomous decision. It also raises the perplexing question "can suicide sometimes be a rational choice?" Generally, surgeons intervene with the suicidal patient based on the assumption that the person is suffering from mental illness and impaired judgment. This assumption is usually correct, with 90% of suicides being found to be associated with mental illness such as depression, substance abuse, or psychosis.[18]

Therefore, relying on the principle of beneficence, surgeons almost always treat the injuries inflicted by suicidal patients despite their expressed intention to die. The conflict arises when the reasons for suicide appear "good," such as in the case of the terminally ill cancer patient with severe, uncontrollable pain. Is the application of lifesaving intervention truly a beneficent act in the patient's best interest? Several studies have shown that physicians rendering care in the emergency department are not likely to recognize treatable depression in their patients. These studies go on to confirm that 80% of patients who attempted suicide subsequently show that they do not continue to wish to die. Thus, although some patients might make a rational decision to commit suicide, in most cases the surgeon delivering care must assume that the person's judgment is impaired and proceed with full indicated, lifesaving measures.[18]

Advance Directives

General Principles: Talking About Death

Facility in routinely addressing end-of-life issues with surgical patients is critical because it allows the surgeon to raise difficult questions with patients during the earlier phases of their disease process. Often, the issues that are most difficult to address when patients near the end of life are those that have not been attended to earlier in the patient's course of treatment. Such early discussion allows the surgeon and the patient to discuss limits on treatment at a time when the patient is able to participate in the process. Usually, we surgeons are intent on cure, and the prospect for death after most of our routine procedures seems very remote. However, these discussions are more important than ever because we now have more options available to prolong life than existed just a few decades ago. In addition, social changes have led to greater participation by patients in the medical decision-making process. With the increasing mobility of our society and the changing allocation of primary care physicians, we as surgeons often do not have the backup of a well-established physician–patient relationship. Add to this the very visible rise in public debate over *euthanasia* and *physician-assisted suicide;* and we can understand the concern the public has over-perceived, or actually, deficiencies in how patients are managed at the end of life.[19]

When a patient does not have the decision-making capacity to give informed consent, or when there is no time to ask the patient or his or her surrogate about treatment preferences, *advance directives* express in written form what the patient's choices would have been if he or she had decision-making capacity. Advance directives include living wills, durable powers of attorneys, and other written documents. In 1991, the federal government passed the Patient Self-determination

Act (PSDA), which required that health-care institutions advise and educate patients regarding advance directives. This affected all institutions participating in the Medicare and Medicaid programs. This law was supposed to increase the use of advanced directives and thus prevent unwanted care. In fact, a major study of advanced directives and seriously ill patients revealed that the PSDA had little impact on health care in USA. This was revealed in the Study to Understand Prognoses and Preferences for Outcomes and Risks of Treatments (SUPPORT), which showed that only 20% of seriously ill patients had advance directives even after the SUPPORT intervention and the PSDA.[20]

Despite these studies, it is still imperative for surgeons to understand the principles involved and the advantages of advocating for appropriate advance directives for our patients and their families. An *advanced directive* is any proactive document stating the patient's wishes in various situations, should they be unable to state their own wishes.

Some states have specific language for each of these documents and provide reciprocity for other states. Both the *living will* and a *durable power of attorney* can be prepared without the benefit of state-approved language as long as the intention of the person executing the document is clear. Such directives provide advanced informed consent for a myriad of courses of treatment, whether it be related to pain medication, "do not resuscitate orders," or management, should the individual enter some level of persistent vegetative state. In a complete set of these documents, the patient has given full thought to all of the possibilities that might occur and has decided what course of treatment would be his or her choice. Unfortunately, most patients have not executed these documents, or they have not given sufficient thought to what their wishes are. Furthermore, many times, when a power of attorney is granted to a surrogate decision maker, the surrogate does not have a full discussion of the wishes of the signatory.

Living Will

The *living will*, which was adopted by many states in 1990, is a document suitable for *terminally ill patients* where the treating physician accepts the patient's wishes regarding withholding of care, including requests restricting heroic resuscitative efforts, in advance. Many state that no life support be used in cases where meaningful recovery will not occur. In a *living will*, the signatory indicates what his or her choices would be for medical treatment in the situation where *death is imminent*, and the individual's wishes are unable to be communicated to the treating physician. Under most state laws, *living wills* indicate the signatory's desire to die a natural death and indicate unwillingness to be kept alive by the so-called heroic measures. This usually amounts to a "Do Not Resuscitate" order. In some states, this also indicates the patient's wishes concerning the level of pain medication, hydration, and nutrition, which the patient would desire if he or she lapses into a nondecisional condition. In most states, the activation of the terms of a living will require an *imminent demise* and a second physician's opinion corroborating that determination. Unfortunately, many people believe that the *living will* is the best form of advanced directive and do not realize that it is intended only for the *terminally ill*.

Durable Power of Attorney

A *durable power of attorney for health care* specifies a surrogate decision maker in the event that the patient no longer has the capacity to make medical decisions. The *durable power of attorney* is a written document that gives the authority to another person, usually a spouse or a relative, to make decisions regarding health care if the patient is incapacitated and unable to make decisions for himself or herself. The reason it is called "durable" is to ensure that the signatory knows that it can be revoked and/or changed at any time. This provides the freedom to change both who the surrogate is and what the patient's stated wishes, if any, are. This is important in situations such as divorce were the person executing the power of attorney may want to change the surrogate before the divorce becomes final or in those family situations where dynamics create a desire to change the surrogate.

Thus, the patient designates a *surrogate decision maker* who should participate in all significant treatment decisions and be kept up to date regarding the patient's health care. The *durable power of attorney* works best when the patient has discussed with a surrogate his or her values and beliefs, as these would apply in making complex decisions regarding health-care issues. If there is no durable power of attorney, surrogate decision makers may be sought based on state laws. There is usually a defined hierarchy regarding surrogate decision makers: spouses, adult children, siblings, and so forth. Such a surrogate decision maker must be acting in the best interest of and according to the wishes and values of the patient. The *durable power of attorney* is a better form of advanced directive than the *living will* because in the former, a surrogate can be educated about the nuances and options regarding each stage of treatment or nontreatment.[20]

Problems

In many situations, the surrogate has the legal authority to make a decision but is not aware of what the patient would want. This is the fault of the patient. All persons, when naming a surrogate decision maker, have a responsibility to fully explain what they would want in certain medical treatment situations. Failure to do so puts the burden on the surrogate to speculate what the patient would do if he or she was able to make the decision.

There are two standards that apply in the situation where the surrogate has not been informed of the patient's wishes. One is the *substitute judgment* standard. When using this standard, the surrogate bases a decision on a prior expressed statement of the patient's preferences or on an in-depth knowledge of the personality of the patient and a willingness to do what the surrogate believes the *patient*, not the surrogate, would want in that specific situation. The second standard is that of the *best interest* of the patient. This is obviously a far more nebulous concept and occurs where the surrogate has not had any specific communication with the patient about the specific type of situation and is not cognizant of any particular patient preferences. In this situation, the surrogate is supposed to do what he believes is in the best interest of the patient. This is an important distinction to make and emphasizes the difference between doing what the patient would want done in a given situation, and having someone else decide what he or she thinks is best.

A further problem with advanced directives that limit full implementation of medical care is the application of such directives in situations for which they were not intended. An example that confronts the colon and rectal surgeon is an elderly patient who is recovering from a complicated colon resection for curable cancer and develops postoperative pneumonia requiring presumed short-term ventilating support. Should such a patient not be intubated because of an advanced directive indicating "do not resuscitate"? In such a case, it would be a serious error to respect the advanced directive and not to treat the patient aggressively. It is clearly probable that the patient would have wanted treatment under these circumstances.

There must also never be confusion when the patient is able to relate his or her preferences to health-care providers. *Verbal communication takes precedence over any written advanced directive*. In addition, when there is any confusion about the advanced directive, disagreement among family members, or concern that it was not meant for the clinical circumstance at hand, *advanced directives limiting treatment should be ignored in favor of prudent medical care*. In general, it is always wise for health-care providers to err on the side of life and to begin standard medical treatment. Treatment options, such as mechanical ventilation and hemodynamic support, can always be withdrawn at a later time once issues are resolved and the family is present. In such situations, the hospital *ethics consultation service* can often prove very helpful.

Perhaps the major problem, at this point in time, is that there is little evidence that advanced directives have made a significant impact on health-care delivery in USA.[20] We, as surgeons, should do all within our power to reverse this situation.

Informed Consent

General Concepts

Studies have revealed that doctors may not adequately inform patients, patients may not understand the information, and such information rarely affects the patient's decision to follow the physician's recommendations. Despite these facts, American courts have long held that a patient's *informed consent* to a medical or surgical procedure or test is *essential*. The physician must give the patient sufficient information to make an intelligent decision before any action is performed. The laws dealing with informed consent require the surgeon to describe to the patient the nature of the procedure, risks, benefits, and alternatives, including no treatment at all. Ethical consensus on just how much disclosure is adequate is still very controversial. What is clear is that permission must be given *voluntarily*, that is, *without coercion* from the physician or anyone else involved in rendering health care or, especially, those participating in the implementation of a *research* project.

The current interpretation of the law requires several elements to constitute *informed consent*. These are the *criteria* that the physician must disseminate to the patient or acting surrogate to meet that standard:

(a) What is the treatment that the doctor wishes to pursue, including a full explanation of the procedure and what it involves, including the necessity for anesthesia and other support functions?
(b) For what reason has the doctor selected this particular treatment, including the doctor's judgment as to why this procedure is chosen to alleviate, cure, or minimize the medical/surgical problem?
(c) What are the risks of the recommended treatment, including an explanation of both the risks of the treatment itself and of any corollary threats to the patient? Surgeons should, in satisfying this requirement, include discussion of their own particular *experience with the procedure* as well as that of the hospital and the medical/surgical colleagues who will be assisting.
(d) What benefits will the patient receive from the proposed treatment? This is similar to the choice of treatment information previously described in that it requires the doctor to explain what the potential benefits will be from the procedure.
(e) What are the chances that the proposed treatment will remedy the problem? This is similar to the information included when describing "benefits and risks" and should also include a description of the *past experience* of the surgeon in performing this specific procedure, as well as the *outcomes* that the surgeon has obtained.
(f) What alternative treatment options exist for the given problem? This is similar to explaining the choice of treatment but emphasizes what other treatment options are available, and why this surgeon has chosen this particular procedure.
(g) What effect will refusal to accept the proposed treatment have on the patient? This must entail a frank discussion of the ramifications of failure to receive the suggested treatment and whether it is life threatening, or of a lesser degree of medical difficulty. This is the part of the discussion where the surgeon must be most sensitive to the patient's religious, cultural, and ethnic background.

Here, the law requires that the sufficiency of the level of information will be judged from the *patient's point of view*, not the doctor's. If a surgeon explains a proposed treatment to the patient in terms that only another surgeon can understand, then the patient is not truly *informed*. This simply boils down to communication skills and the obligation to accurately *record* this discussion in the medical chart prior to performing the recommended surgical treatment. Every profession has its own terms of art or jargon. Physicians must strive to ensure that the language they use is clearly understandable. Achieving acceptable levels of communication may be complicated by language, cultural, and socioeconomic factors. A manager responsible for building a new jetliner was credited with saying, "The main problem with communication is the illusion that it has actually occurred." All too frequently patients and families come away from discussions with surgeons where the surgeon thinks he has effectively communicated and the patient and family seemed to understand, but they did not. Sometimes it just boils down to faith in the doctor, or an individual's unwillingness to reveal his or her lack of comprehension. The physician must use *common sense* in determining whether fully informed consent has truly been granted, taking into account that some cynics claim, "The problem about common sense is that it is not common."

As with every rule of law, there are certain *exceptions* to the requirement for informed consent. When there is an emergency situation that could result in the death of the patient, when time is of the essence, and when there is no surrogate decision maker present, the *consent requirement is waived*. Similarly, when the situation is not an emergency, but the patient is for one reason or another not able to give consent due to unconsciousness, coma, mental disability, or other cause of inadequate decision-making capacity, and when there is no advance directive, or surrogate, informed consent is not necessary. There is also a *therapeutic exception* to the rule. If the physician believes that revelation of the normally required information would have a negative effect on the patient's health, fully informed consent is not necessary. This usually arises in the context of a psychiatric patient. Also, when a competent patient *refuses* to receive information upon which to base a decision, this requirement is waived. There can also be a waiver of the necessity for informed consent when the *government* requires certain medical tests or treatment in the face of possible medical or national security emergencies.

A common misconception among those rendering emergency care is that anyone who presents to an emergency facility falls into the *emergency exception* to informed consent. The *emergency exception* allows a physician to treat a patient without obtaining informed consent. This exception requires the following: the patient must be unconscious or without the capacity to make a decision, and no one else legally authorized to make such a decision is available; time must be of the essence in avoiding risk of serious bodily injury or death; and under the circumstances, the action proposed would be that to which a *reasonable person* would consent. The emergency exception does not apply if the patient has decision-making capacity and is able to communicate a decision about medical care.[2]

Patient–Surgeon Relationship

Siegler explains that the three central ethical aspects of modern surgical practice are (1) clinical competence, (2) respect for patients and their health-care decisions, (3) maintaining the primacy of the patient's needs in the face of external pressures in a changing social, economic, and political climate. Successful clinical practice has always been a unique blend of technical proficiency and ethical sensitivity, which together constitute the art of the physician and surgeon. Once sought out by the patient, the surgeon becomes involved in the patient's problem. He or she is no longer a mere observer. Over the last few decades, the relationship between patients and physicians has been evolving from one of *paternalism*, in which surgeons make choices for their patients, to a more equal and *autonomous* relationship of shared decision making, by which surgeons provide information that allows competent adult patients to make their own choices.[21] For complicated surgical dilemmas, this can never evolve completely because patients depend on the surgeon and their other physicians to guide them to the correct choice.

Sometimes surgical procedures considered "standard of care" by the surgeon are refused, based on the patient's values and beliefs. Such cultural challenges can affect the success of the patient–surgeon relationship and ultimately the health outcome for the patient. Ultimately, the surgeon must learn to take into account the cultural components of the relationship and find ways to respond to them in an ethically and medically responsible manner. In order to deal with these complicated situations, the surgeon is often required to reassess and be secure in his or her own religious and cultural foundations.[22]

As Peter Angelos explains, the relationships that individual patients have with their surgeons are as varied as are the different types of surgical problems with which patients present. Perhaps patients are required to have a great deal of trust in their surgeons because of the nature of surgical intervention itself. This may result in patients frequently feeling a deeper personal bond with their surgeon than with many other physicians who may be involved in their care. Surgeons, as well as their patients, frequently feel the closeness of this bond. Angelos quotes Charles Bosk as explaining

> The specific nature of surgical treatment links the action of the physician and the response of the patient more intimately than in other areas of medicine... When the patient of an internist dies, the natural question his colleagues ask is, "what happened?" When the patient of a surgeon dies his colleagues ask, "What did you do?"

When patients consider the surgeon to be "their doctor," the surgeon must not ever underestimate the importance of maintaining this relationship even, or perhaps especially, as the patient approaches the end of life. The impact of a concerned surgeon on a patient who is dying, or is incurable, can serve to dramatically affirm the appropriateness of comfort care instead of desperate, ineffective, and costly attempts to ward off death.[19]

Communication and the Internet

It seems so easy to be able to respond to a patient's problem or to deliver information to them and their physicians by e-mail. With e-mail delivered via the Internet, there is no problem with timing of the conversation, no recordings, no time on "hold" for the doctor or for the patient. The only limitation seems to be the typing and spelling skills of the surgeon, usually problem enough.

Most of us have learned not to deliver complicated or bad news over telephone, unless we have made a previous agreement with the patient and family to convey such information to save significant travel or other inconveniences that are significant enough to preclude a face-to-face personal communication. Such situations are now increasingly complicated because communication over the Internet is usually not secure, and the information delivered can become a permanent part of the patient's record. A patient's employer and family can usually acquire easy access to the electronic message, potentially to the detriment of the patient, and potentially leaving this sending physician legally liable.

For the medical and medical legal aspect, some of the material we send by e-mail we would never consider sending by "hard copy" unless we had obtained the patient's specific permission to release such information. Currently, there are no guidelines available for the ethical transfer of confidential medical information via the Internet. Until such exists, and it is critical for physicians to participate in the establishment of such principles, all doctors are probably well advised to record in the patient's permanent record that discussions were held and permission was given to communicate *specific* information electronically. Especially with the implementation of HIPAA requirements, until clearer guidelines are defined, surgeons should err on the side of no sensitive information to be delivered by e-mail or telephone.[19]

Of course, the other massive impact of the Internet is the availability of unlimited access to potentially confusing and harmful information to our patients. Remember, there is no quality control for the Internet. Unlike traditional publications with editors, peer-review standards, and vigorous screening, on the Internet, anyone with a computer can be a self-designated author, editor, and publisher. And this can be done anonymously with no attached responsibility. This will continue to have an enormous impact on the patient–physician relationship because "knowledge is power," and our patients and families are making use of that power.[23] Not infrequently patients come to us with confusing and conflicting material from the Internet. A new part of our responsibility, as surgeons, is not only to guide our patients to appropriate and helpful Web sites but also to actively participate in the construction and quality control of electronic information provided by the Internet in our own areas of expertise.

Using Newly Deceased Patients for Teaching Purposes

A unique problem exists for the medical/surgical team caring for patients in the emergency department of a teaching hospital. It involves using the newly dead for teaching purposes. This most commonly involves teaching medical students and residents the techniques of endotracheal intubation. The issue is, of course, do we have the right to perform procedures on this newly deceased person without obtaining permission (informed consent) from the surviving family. The dilemma is complicated by the fact that no better teaching opportunity exists for our trainees who can then go forward, when adequately trained, to save lives and relieve suffering in the future. Clearly, no harm can be done to one who is dead. Furthermore, to our knowledge, there are no state statutes that specifically prohibit the teaching of procedures using newly dead patients, and no court has considered this issue. Although, before death a patient has constitutional protection against nonconsensual invasion of his or her body, it has been established by various state courts that constitutional rights do terminate at the time of death.

Although the law in this situation is very forgiving, compassionate and ethical considerations should supervene. Several medical studies have found that patients and families are likely to consent to such procedures but prefer to be asked permission first. Even the law advises that in this day and age of increasing recognition of personal autonomy, it is probably prudent to approach the next of kin for permission before performing procedures on the newly deceased.[24]

Special Concerns for Participation in Research/Innovation

General Concepts

Surgeons, by our very nature, are innovators. Sometimes, the only way we can complete an operative procedure is by making a deviation from what has been standard procedure in the past. Since we operate on biological systems, we can never predict exactly what will be required for a given procedure. We often use old procedures for new purposes and without much hesitation use new equipment to accomplish old tasks. Thus, we often find ourselves in what McKneally refers to as "the zone of innovation" where it is unclear whether what we are doing is an evolutionary variation on a standard procedure, a unique departure from accepted standards, or the first stage of what should become recognized as a formal surgical research project.[25] When should our deviations be subjected to full evaluation by an Institutional Review Board? How can a surgeon participate, with *equipoise* (the presumption that both arms of a study are equally efficacious) in a prospective randomized trial to evaluate a change that the surgeon has created to be better than the known standard? As Martin McKneally explains, most of the important advances in the history of medicine, such as anesthesia, appendectomy, antibiotics, intensive care, and immunization, were introduced through an informal, unregulated innovative process that has been enormously productive but can easily lead to ratification of an effective or even harmful treatment by well-intended physicians.[25]

Look at the recent challenges facing colon and rectal surgeons. We adopted the construction of ileal and now colonic pouches to improve the quality of life of our patients with inflammatory bowel disease and rectal cancer. The true efficacy of these innovations came significantly later than their description and implementation by many of our colleagues. The use of minimally invasive techniques to accomplish what we were all trained to do via abdominal incisions was clearly initially driven by the new technology and by enthusiastic entrepreneurs who wanted to work on the frontier of innovation. The premature exposure of these new techniques to the lay literature drove the process with even more intensity. Only recently have completed prospectively randomized trials verified the realistic advantages of the new technology. We continue to sort out the appropriate use, for the benefit of our patients and their quality of life, of issues such as circular stapled hemorrhoidectomy, Natural Orifice Translumenal Endoscopic Surgery (NOTES) procedures, and robotic technology. What we need is a process for evaluation of surgical innovation, which provides ethical oversight without the ponderous slow pace inherent in most IRB-approved protocols. Surgical investigators and ethicists are currently crafting such a mechanism, which protects the rights and well-being of our patients without stifling progress and creativity.

Good research is described as that which enhances our ability to prevent illness or injury, to improve the quality or decrease the cost of care, or to improve the lives of our patients. Such research also must protect subjects and patients from harm, preserve their confidentiality, and allow them to enter freely as participants. Subjects and patients must be allowed to make an informed choice to participate, or not, without fear that their treatment might be compromised if they decline the request of the investigator. For a research project to be ethical, it must also be well designed and must investigate an issue of importance for which the answer does not yet exist. Protocols must be scientifically sound and likely to yield meaningful conclusions. Good research is therefore ethical, and bad research is unethical.[26]

In June 1966, Henry Beecher published an analysis of "Ethics and Clinical Research."[27] This benchmark article accelerated the movement that brought human experimentation under rigorous federal and institutional control. Although Beecher was not the first to direct attention to abuses in human experimentation, this presentation of 22 examples of investigators who endangered "the health or the life of their subjects" without informing them of the risks or obtaining their permission was a critical element in reshaping the ideas and practices governing human experimentation.[28]

Special issues for informed consent arise when the surgical patient is asked to participate in a *research project*. The time for decision making is usually short, and the principal investigator of the project may also be the one administering care. This raises the issue not only of adequate informed consent but also of the *risk for coercion* of the patient to participate in the study. The surgeon-researcher should abide by basic principles as outlined by the National Commission for the Protection of Human Subjects of Biomedical and Behavioral Research and by the Declaration of Helsinki. There are also prevailing federal, institutional, and professional guidelines that govern human and animal research. To be ethical, studies must be well designed and worth the risk to patient and society. The institution's review board should approve the study, and the investigator should take the responsibility to assure adequate informed consent, confidentiality, and appropriate protection of the patient's well-being.[1]

All physicians must ensure that trials involving human subjects are of potentially significant value and are conducted ethically. The Nuremberg Code obligates researchers to prepare descriptions of the probability and magnitude of all physical, psychological, social, and economic risks, and to minimize unnecessary pain and suffering. Consent must be voluntary and without any element of force, coercion, or deceit.[11] When discussing the potential *risks* of a proposed procedure, it is essential for the person seeking consent to quantify minimal, low, or high risk using examples from everyday life. Potential benefits from a research project may apply to the individual, to society, or to both. When discussing the benefits of a proposed study, one must distinguish clearly between *therapeutic* and *nontherapeutic research*. Researchers must clearly differentiate, for the patient, the balance between *potential benefit* to the patient and any *potential risks* associated with the protocol. No matter how great the benefit to society, it would not be ethical to expose a subject to anything greater than minimal risk if there is little direct benefit to the patient.[26]

Consent must never be assumed. Many would question the validity of truly "informed" consent rendered by someone who is acutely ill or severely injured. Especially for research, the principle still holds that for consent to be valid, it must be informed, understood, and voluntarily given. Subjects, or their surrogates, must have enough information, in comprehensible form, to enable them to make a proper judgment as to whether or not to participate in the requested study.

Normally, this requires time for reflection before a decision to enroll. This concept is frequently stressed in the emergency situation. In an emergency, the surgeon may be forced to act in the patient's best interests and to presume consent on the basis of necessity. Clearly, this is only appropriate for interventions that will benefit the patient directly; and actual consent should be obtained as soon as possible afterward. In a research context, the intervention must be part of a protocol approved by an independent institutional committee, such as an IRB, and should present no more than minimal risk to the patient.[26]

Placebo Surgery

As investigators sort out the mechanism for insuring that surgical research is carried out ethically and with true *informed consent*, the issue of the use of *placebo surgery* appears based on recently published trials. Horng and Miller, commenting on these trials in the *New England Journal of Medicine*, state that the issue of using *placebo surgery* in clinical trials appears to violate the fundamental ethical principles of *beneficence* and *nonmaleficence*. Specifically, this means that surgeons should not invade the body except for purposes of cure or amelioration of suffering. In evaluating the studies, they emphasize the fact that clinical research always involves the inherent tension between the ethical values of pursuing science and those of protecting subjects from harm. To be considered ethical, overall, they must present a favorable risk–benefit ratio. The burden is on the investigators to justify *placebo surgery* as a warranted means of evaluating the efficacy of a surgical procedure. They conclude that absolute prohibition of *placebo surgery* is not appropriate, but the standard of justification for its use must be extremely high and rigorously enforced.[29]

Conflict of Interest: Industry and Drug Money

Many colon and rectal surgeons interested in research have difficulty obtaining extramural support for their projects and thus turn to private sources, namely, the biomedical and pharmaceutical industry. Industry support for biomedical research now exceeds the financial support from all federal funding sources. The liaison between academic surgery and industry introduces the possibility of remarkable benefits especially to our patients; however, differences between the fundamental goals of physicians and industry can create serious conflicts. Industry strives to complete clinical trials expeditiously and to publish positive results. Conversely, the primary goal of the surgical investigator is to advance and disseminate knowledge by the unimpeded exchange of ideas, despite secondary professional, financial, institutional, and sociopolitical objectives. Critics maintain that the physician–industry relationship will only serve to potentiate bias, and loss of objectivity will fundamentally poison the way research is conducted. Currently, however, the lifeblood of clinical research is external support requiring a productive relationship with the biomedical industry. This potential conflict of interest can only be resolved by scrupulously implementing the principles of integrity, honesty, respect, and equity. Even the mere appearance of a conflict of interest could jeopardize the investigator's integrity and undermine public trust. Surgeon investigators involved with industry-sponsored research should meticulously divorce themselves from any personal or commercial conflict that could compromise patient loyalty or well-being.[11] Ethical recruitment of patients into research protocols is especially challenging for surgeons who, under the current system of financial remuneration, may receive more money by having the patient participate in a study than he/she would receive for doing the surgical procedure indicated for the patient.

A common challenge involves investigators who receive industry-funded materials, discretionary funds, research equipment, and trips to meetings. They must be aware that subsequent restrictions and expectations can create conflicts of interest. These seemingly innocent economic factors become a conflict anytime they influence study design, interpretation of results, or the timing and method by which results are reported. The personal gain of the investigator such as ownership of stock or receipt of funds for testing drugs or devices can introduce bias and compromise objectivity. On the other hand, it is not inappropriate for an investigator to receive economic rewards from a drug or device that is commensurate with his or her efforts involved in the development of the product. It is also acceptable for investigators to receive consultant and lecture fees from companies whose product they are testing, provided that the remuneration is proportionate with his or her efforts and that it is clearly reported, in advance, of all presentations and is clearly stipulated in any publication. It is unethical, however, to sell or purchase stock or have a direct financial interest in the product under investigation until the relationship between the investigator and the company has been terminated, and the results of the research have been published or made public. Although opponents argue that disclosure cannot heal the financial conflicts of interest, it does recognize public concerns, protect the credibility and reputation of investigators, and alerts readers as they access the published report.[11]

The practice of pharmaceutical companies bestowing gifts on physicians is well documented. These gifts, however, cost money, and this cost is ultimately passed on to our patients without their explicit knowledge. The biomedical industry has clearly made outstanding contributions toward the advancement of modern scientific medicine; however, obvious conflict of interest occurs when physicians accept personal gifts that have no benefit to their patients. Acceptance of individual gifts that do not benefit patients, such as trips and subsidies for medical educational conferences in which physicians are not speakers, is strongly discouraged. The acceptance of even small gifts has been shown to affect clinical judgment and to heighten the perception (or reality) of a *conflict of interest*. Until specific guidelines are established, commonsense should always prevail: no gifts should be accepted if suspected *strings are attached*.[11]

Confidentiality

General Principles

Surgeons are bound by the same rules of *confidentiality* as other doctors. Especially with the new restrictions and significant penalties imposed by HIPAA, all health-care personnel must be very cognizant of preserving *confidentiality*. In the hectic morass, which is the waiting area of most big hospitals, it is sometimes difficult to take the time to ensure that doctors convey sensitive and private information to patients, families, or surrogates in a full and complete manner and yet ensure the confidentiality of their information. Certain health information can be very significant in the treatment of a patient, including medication history and psychiatric history. Yet, some patients or families might be reluctant to give such information to the treating physician if the situation is not conducive to confidential communication. Similarly, the families and the patient are most certainly due confidentiality of the information, which the physician is going to impart.

A surgeon's duty to maintain confidentiality regarding information disclosed by the patient has been a long-held medical precept. On occasion, however, the ethical duty to prevent harm to others overrides the duty to keep confidences of a given patient. Although the law generally prevents the divulgence of confidential information, it also *mandates certain exceptions*, such as reporting patients with infectious disease and those who are likely to harm others, the latter being elucidated by the famous 1976 Tarasoff case in which nondisclosure of a patient's homicidal thoughts resulted in the death of the threatened person. This case raises a confusing possibility of preventing harm to others becoming a legal not just an ethical duty. This broadens the concept of mandatory reporting to include more than the currently accepted requirements for reporting child, elder, or domestic abuse. Such legal requirements may force us to compromise the ethical norm of respecting our patient's decisions with regard to confidentiality.[2]

Making and Managing a Genetic Diagnosis

As the results of untangling the mystery of the human genome are translated into clinical considerations, the ethical challenges to the colon and rectal surgeon become significant. Although the presumption is that facility and managing genetically predetermined disease is the lot of the primary care physician, in fact, patients with phenotypic presentation of genetic diseases such as colon and rectal cancer depend on surgeons for final diagnosis, administration of surgical treatment, initiation of long-term follow-up, and clarification of the implications of the genetically predetermined cancer for other family members and other generations. Most commonly, we deal with the autosomal dominant mutations, which cause familial polyposis or hereditary nonpolyposis colorectal cancers.

The ethical hazard involves obtaining the results of a genetic test without adequate counseling of the patient to determine what will be done with the results obtained. Clearly, this should all be determined prior to obtaining the information. Many individuals fear that determination of a genetic abnormality will have adverse effect on their insurability and employability. These risks are supposed to be protected by law, but many members of our society are not willing to take that chance. Because of these fears, many patients and their family members refuse to have genetic testing done in the first place. Once the test is done, a patient may insist on absolute confidentiality to prevent dissemination of the information to others, even those at risk, in the family. Think of the dilemma in which this places the surgeon. You may know that 50% of children and siblings of the patient are at risk for potentially fatal yet preventable cancer. Yet, the patient has forbidden you to inform them. This situation can even ethically and legally justify the physician breaching the patient's confidentiality to save the lives of those potentially at risk. There have even been cases in the courts where the treating physician has been held liable for *not* divulging such risks to family members.

Most of these unpleasant situations can be avoided by appropriate genetic counseling *before* any genetic information is obtained. This should ideally involve the use of professional genetics counselors, since most of us surgeons have not been adequately trained in the skills required to obtain and verify such familial and generational information.

Abuse of the Elderly Patients

It is claimed that approximately two million elderly Americans are mistreated each year, with a significant number falling into the definition of *abandonment*. Although this treatment of elders is a problem that has occurred for centuries, only recently has society become significantly concerned. The problem and concern will increase as does the elderly components of our population. Surgeons are ideally suited to play a significant role in the detection, management, and prevention of elder abuse and neglect. The surgeon may be the only person, outside the family, who sees the older adult and is qualified to intervene in a preventive way. This means we should be aware of risk factors and their detection. It requires an astute clinician to detect abuse based on history alone. Even in the face of injuries, such as fractures at uncommon sites, the elderly patient may continue to conceal the possibility of abuse for fear of embarrassment or abandonment by the abuser. It may well be the surgeon called to see the patient for injury or neglect, who picks up the clues such as evidence of pressure sores, malnutrition, old injuries, or new injuries in unusual locations, such as on the scalp or behind the ears.

The first priority of the physician is to ensure this victim's safety. The surgeon should never hesitate to ask for social service consultation or to report suspicions to the appropriate adult protective services. Such acts are not breaches of confidentiality; they represent implementation of the most sincere duty of the physician.[30]

Futility/Withholding Treatment

General Concepts

Significant, and perhaps inappropriate, concern continues to exist in medicine with regard to the difference between *withholding* and *withdrawing* medical treatment. This has become more of an issue as the potential for resuscitating critically ill patients has become a progressive reality. Depending on the clinical situation, surgeons and other physicians attribute higher legal risk of one procedure over another. Apparently because of this fear of legal retribution, or ridicule and condemnation by professional peers, employing full, almost ritualistic, resuscitation has become the default position of those delivering critical care in cases where no advanced directive exists. In fact, no physician has ever been successfully prosecuted for withholding or withdrawing of medical care from any dying patient in the legal history of USA. This leaves one wondering what actually fuels the fears of legal retribution for making the wrong decision.[31]

The dilemma could of course be alleviated by early meaningful discussion with patients, families, and surrogates with regard to care *options at the end of life* and honest estimates of *prognosis*. Studies have shown, however, that many physicians and surgeons fail to take these opportunities. A disturbing example of this inadequacy can be found in the 1995 Study to Understand Prognoses and Preferences for Outcomes and Risks of Treatment (SUPPORT). This expensive, multi-institutional study demonstrated the physicians' *failure to meet all outcome markers*: failure to include patient and family in pivotal care discussions, failure to provide realistic estimates of outcomes valued by patients, failure to treat pain adequately, and failure to prevent prolonged death in patients with extremely poor prognoses.[31]

Sometimes confusion is created over the venue in which surgical or medical care is delivered. In the usual setting, a decision to *withhold* further medical treatment is done quietly, often without input from the patient or the surrogate decision maker; whereas *withdrawal* of ongoing medical treatment can be more obvious and difficult. Some clinicians and ethicists feel that the *withholding* of medical treatment is more problematic than later *withdrawal* of unwanted or useless interventions. This discrepancy in the urgent situation probably exists because the physicians involved usually lack the vital information about their patients' identities, medical conditions, and expressed wishes. In addition, perhaps because of frequent, but inaccurate, representations on television, society has come to expect only spectacular results in the delivery of surgical care in USA. This concept is in marked contrast to the attitude that those clinicians who *withdrew treatment* (an act leading to death) were more culpable than those who *withheld treatment* (an omission leading to death). This distinction between acts and omissions is now thought to be more of a difference in psychological preference than an ethical norm.[32] For all of these reasons, despite the fact that the law has clearly spoken, the distinction between *withdrawal* and *withholding* of medical treatment will continue to be a challenge.

The surgeon's decision to limit or withhold treatment can be based either on the patient's refusal or on the physician's determination that the treatment would not be of benefit. Although the patient has the ethical and legal right to forego treatment, the physician must be very careful about withholding a treatment that might be beneficial. Such issues are usually intensified by the need for rapid intervention versus the desire to verify the meaning of the patient's current or preexisting desires. The classic example is the patient who is unresponsive, has reversible pulmonary or cardiac disease, and needs cardiopulmonary resuscitation, but is said to have a preexisting DNR (do not resuscitate) order.

Withholding treatment because of a judgment of *futility* is even more of an ethical challenge. *Futility* has been defined as "any effort to achieve a result as *possible*, but that reasoning or experience suggests is *highly improbable*, and cannot be systematically produced." Physicians, as moral agents, should exercise professional judgment in assessing patient's requests. If the request goes beyond well-established criteria of reasonableness, the surgeon ought not feel obliged to provide it. Some ethicists believe that the appropriate *allocation of resources* is another important consideration when one is making decisions regarding invasive, costly, or lengthy procedures. John Lantos even stated that, "given limited resources, it is ethically justifiable to limit access to treatments that are expensive and offer minimal benefit… decisions by doctors to curtail use of those treatments are socially responsible."[33] *Futility* is such a complicated word that it may be of little use in most situations. The classic challenge is the decision not to start resuscitation when a patient with extensive metastatic cancer and cachexia presents in cardiac arrest. The initial emotional inclination is to treat the patient, even if the medical situation, as emphasized by Siegler,[13] leads to a judgment that such a resuscitation will not be beneficial. This requires the difficult objective determination of *ineffectiveness,* rather than any subjective decision based on the worth of the intervention or on the *value* of the patient's continued life.[2] It should be noted that assertions of *futility* come about in two contradictory situations. One is where the patient or surrogate wants the doctor to refrain from a further treatment, which the doctor thinks is not futile, and the other is where the doctor wishes to refrain from treatment which he or she believes to be futile. The only measure of what should be done is the standard of care in a given region for similar cases. Dealing with this concept of *futility* or other *end-of-life* concerns is usually a problem only when disagreement arises among the patient, the family, and the health-care team.

Many ethicists agree that physicians are under no obligation to render treatments that they ascertain to be of little or no benefit to the patient. Many, however, believe that it would be advantageous to abandon the word "futility" and to use instead the construct of "clinically nonbeneficial interventions." We all know that one of the greatest fears of both patients and families is their *abandonment* by the health-care team. It is easy to fall into this trap by declaring that further treatment for a given patient is *futile*. When it is decided that certain interventions should be appropriately withheld, special efforts should be made to maintain effective communication, comfort, support, and counseling for the patient, family, and friends. Although we, as surgeons, may not always proceed with potential technologically advanced nonbeneficial interventions, we always must continue to *care* for the patient and the family.[34]

DNR and the Need for Surgery

There is, and should be, confusion regarding operating on a patient with existing "do not resuscitate" orders. Since there is no universal agreement as to how this situation is to be handled, each surgeon must be aware of specific institutional guidelines. First of all, it is not at all unusual for surgery to be indicated for patients where *cure* is no longer the goal of treatment. Even patients with advanced cancer or severe medical conditions will be offered surgical relief of acute intestinal obstruction or an abscess causing sepsis and pain. The problem usually gets defined when administering anesthesia becomes a consideration because it can be accurately stated that the act of anesthesia is *ongoing resuscitation*. As amazing as it seems, most hospitals have a policy, which allows suspension of the DNR order during the procedure and administration of anesthesia, only to have it resume when the surgery and required anesthesia have been concluded.

Withdrawal of Treatment

General Principles

Taking into account the preceding discussion, an important line of reasoning for the moral and legal equivalents for the two actions of *withholding* or *withdrawing* is the important concept that if a medical intervention will not result in the desired or beneficial results intended for the patient, it makes no difference whether the clinician withholds the intervention before beginning it or discontinues its use after it has been started and found to be not effective.[32]

Special moral issues may arise in the care of *terminally ill patients*. We must be willing to respect a terminally ill patient's wish to forego life-prolonging treatment, as expressed in a living will or through a health-care surrogate appointed via a durable power of attorney for health care. Those of us caring for patients should be willing to honor "do not resuscitate" orders appropriately executed on behalf of terminally ill patients. We should also understand the established criteria for the *determination of death* and should be prepared to assist families in decisions regarding the donation of the patient's organs for transplantation. This involves knowing the specific regulations in our own states and in our own specific institutions, especially the criteria for death and the mechanisms for initiating the conversation relative to organ donation. It is usually not the surgeon, nor any member of the treating team, who first raises the issue with family regarding donation of the dying patient's organs for the purpose of transplantation.

Euthanasia / Physician-Assisted Suicide/Terminal Sedation

The terminology of activities related to the end of life is confusing to the public, has been misused in the press relative to the notorious activities of individuals such as Dr. Kevorkian, and, in fact, is probably not clearly differentiated by many surgeons. The terms all have separate meanings and implications, requiring us to understand them and not use them interchangeably.

First is *euthanasia*, which literally means "good death." Its consideration arises when patients or surrogates claim that the quality of life is so diminished, the pain and suffering is so unbearable, or they have become such a burden on others that they request their physicians to *cause* their deaths quickly and painlessly. Specifically, this implies "mercy killing" of an individual, by a physician, to relieve pain and suffering. Such terms as "voluntary," "nonvoluntary," and "involuntary" have been applied in an attempt to clarify the various ramifications of this process, but, in fact, *euthanasia* is the act of killing by a physician and is *not legal* anywhere in USA.[13]

Physician-assisted suicide, on the other hand, implies a death that a competent person, with decision-making capacity, chooses and *causes* by self-administration of drugs that a physician has prescribed but *did not administer*. Advocates feel that prescription of drugs that a patient can take at will removes the physician from direct participation. The decision and the act of ending life remain in the patient's control. This invokes the important fallback concept for physicians and nurses who deal with patients who are suffering, in an irreversible medical condition, and near the end of life: the distinction between "killing and allowing to die." This distinction is invoked during the process of *terminal sedation* as well as for participation in *physician-assisted suicide*. Currently, the latter is legal only in the states of Oregon, Washington, and Montana.[13]

Terminal sedation, another frequently misunderstood term, is the practice of sedating a patient to unconsciousness to relieve the horrible symptoms, which may occur during the process of dying, including pain, shortness of breath, suffocation, seizures, and delirium. As the sedating medication is administered, other life-sustaining treatments are withdrawn, including ventilatory support, dialysis, artificial nutrition, and hydration. It is critically important to understand that in this frequently employed process, *no lethal doses of opiates or muscle relaxants are administered*. Thus, the intent of the act is to relieve suffering and symptoms by making people unconscious and unable to eat or drink, so that they will die within a short period of time. As in *euthanasia*, *terminal sedation* directly intends the death of the patient.[13] The difference is that, in the latter, the sedating medication is not the agent of death. This differentiation is of utmost importance to avoid the feeling of killing by *double effect* (which will be explained in more detail later) on the part of the health-care team. It invokes the concept of "letting nature take its course" as opposed to the homicidal act of "killing." Cynics claim they are the same, and those of us who claim otherwise are not being honest with ourselves.

Applying the Principles

In order to comply with the principle of *autonomy*, when a competent patient requests, or demands, the withdrawal of further treatment, the treating physician is in a situation analogous to that of the patient who initially refuses treatment. *Autonomy governs*! The surgeon should ensure that the patient is given all the information necessary to allow proper informed consent regarding withdrawal of treatment, but once that is done, it is the ethical duty of the surgeon to withdraw the specified treatment. This is true no matter what the patient requests, whether it be withdrawal of feeding tubes, ventilators, or nutrition and hydration. As long as the patient is fully aware of the consequences, both short term and long term, his or her stated wishes should be respected and acted upon appropriately by the health-care team.

The same principle should be invoked if the patient is not able to understand but has provided, in an advanced directive, an indicated desire with respect to withdrawal of treatment under specified circumstances. It is still the duty of the physician to withdraw the specific treatment because the patient has, in the advance directive, given prior informed consent. The duty of the physician is identical if a designated surrogate requests or demands the withdrawal of treatment. This is the patient speaking through the surrogate, and once again, autonomy governs.

When the surgeon determines that withdrawal of treatment is appropriate and further treatment would be ineffective, consent of the family or surrogate should be sought. In this situation, it is very important and helpful to know what if any *surrogacy laws* exist. These do vary from state to state, and the surgeons faced with potential decision making should know in advance the laws of their state. In states where such laws exist, they can be very helpful in delineating the hierarchy of surrogate designation. In the absence of advanced directives, surgeons have the responsibility to judge what they believe the patient would want, or what is in the best interest of the patient. If no family is available, close friends of the patient may be asked to give their opinions about what the patient would want.

Courts have upheld the principles of *autonomy* and *self-determination*, affirming the right to refuse life-sustaining treatment. The classic illustrations of this include the 1976 ruling by the New Jersey Supreme Court that Karen Ann Quinlan, a woman in a persistent vegetative state, had the right to decide to be removed from a respirator and that this right could be asserted, on her behalf, by her family. This right was extended to include the withdrawal of nutrition by the 1990 Cruzan case in which the US Supreme Court ruled that a life-sustaining feeding tube could be removed from another young woman in a persistent vegetative state.[18]

Should the surgeon have moral or religious beliefs that would preclude her from *withdrawing* treatment, she should remove herself from the case. It is important to recognize this possibility of need for withdrawing treatment at the beginning of the clinical encounter because a physician with such beliefs should extricate herself from the case at the earliest possible stage. As the clinical course evolves, and as the surgeon develops a relationship with the family and the patient, it becomes progressively more difficult for him or her to remove himself or herself from the treatment team.

Palliative Care / Hospice

General Principles

Focusing on making the last months, not minutes, of life meaningful is especially appropriate where death has a significant predictability. Chronic progressive diseases such as cancer, congestive heart failure, and chronic obstructive pulmonary disease account for 50–70% of deaths, compared with the sudden death attributed to stroke, heart attack, trauma, and suicide. In USA, patients' perceptions of human finitude lead them to deny death and to rely on medical achievements that they think will let them live forever. Physicians grapple with their technological power, the imperative to tell the truth about fatal conditions, and despair at denying hope and the promise of cure for their trusting patients. It is probably this mutual self-deception that becomes the central issue in rendering appropriate end-of-life care. It is the management of these intense psychological and spiritual challenges facing terminally ill patients that has come to form the basis of what is called *palliative care*.[31]

A brief definition of *palliative care* is as follows: the act of *total* care of patients whose disease is not responsive to *curative* treatment. Although *palliative care* has been a major focus in Europe for the past 20 years, interest in USA only became significant in the late 1990s with an Institute of Medicine report that evaluated end-of-life care. It revealed significant deficiencies in how we manage end-of-life care. These deficiencies include the management of pain and other symptoms, including nausea and vomiting, dyspnea, depression, and anxiety. Geoffrey Dunn explains that "palliative care is not a concept defined in terms of the amount of time remaining in a patient's life or the terminal nature of his disease. It is defined in terms of the type of need that is being met by the care."[35]

The concept of *palliative surgery* refers to surgery for which the major intent is alleviation of symptoms and improving quality of life, *not necessarily cure*. As the age of our surgical patients increases, we will be progressively involved in performing operations whose desired outcomes are not met. Managing these patients through the entire course of their disease, including death, is an important part of being a good physician and a good surgeon. Surgical emergencies are often the first encounter with older patients, and they often have multiple comorbidities. An example is the 80-year-old person who presents with an acute abdomen. The risk of surgery will be high, the prognosis may be poor, and cure may be impossible. Perhaps, offering surgical treatment would even be inappropriate. Thus we, as surgeons, are immediately thrust into contemplating *palliative care* for the surgical patient, and it becomes clear that surgeons need to be aware of the concepts involved in delivering such care.[35]

Pain Relief and the Doctrine of "Double Effect"

Confusing Principles

When it comes to adequacy of pain control, especially for patients near the end of life, physicians and surgeons have been caught in a complicated dilemma. On the one hand, most of us entered medicine to relieve suffering. On the other hand, we know that administration of excessive doses of pain medication can suppress respiration and run the risk of contributing to the death of patients already near the end of life. At the same time that we are criticized for not giving enough pain medication to our suffering patients, we are also challenged by the law for prescribing medication with the *double effect* of potentially *hastening death*. This doctrine of *double effect* is intended by the courts to recognize the difference between provision of adequate pain treatment that *unintentionally* hastens death and the ordering of medication that *intentionally* causes a patient's death. This concept of *intent* is confusing not only for the courts but also for the physician who is ordering the pain medication.

Double Effect

The application of the principle of *double effect* is controversial because it places significant weight on physician *intent*, which is impossible to prove, and no weight on a patient's right to self-determination. This seems to contradict a paramount principle of American bioethics: *patient autonomy*. Why, when death is on the line, should concern over the physician's *intention* take precedent over the *patient's informed consent*? The physician's fear over misinterpretation of his or her actions often leads to inadequate use of pain medication, leaving patients unjustifiably suffering. It is clearly recognized that opioids should be considered early in the care of the dying patients and in dosages that often exceed the standard range. These analgesics are not only effective in reducing painful sensation but also have an effect in adjusting the sense of well-being, thereby improving the patient's ability to cope with pain. Adjustment of dosage can be aided by using one of the known *pain scales* or by observing patients' objective signs of distress, especially useful in the noncommunicative patient. Despite its significant effect on several components of respiration, respiratory arrest from opioids, in the absence of other central nervous system depressants, is rare. In caring for dying patients, surgeons must acknowledge that they are one part of the often-fragmented medical team. They must accept the goal of providing care where they can, comfort always, consult when necessary, and coordination of the remaining end-of-life issues.[31]

Hastening Death: The "Code"

Since the overwhelming admonition to the physician is "above all do no harm," society has implored the surgeon, in life-threatening situations, to waive informed consent requirements and to act presumptively to save life or limb in situations where the usual consent is impossible to obtain. This leads to our current default in dealing with the critically ill or moribund unknown patient: resuscitating with "a full code" and asking questions later. This practice is probably acceptable as long as the surgeon realizes that *withdrawing life support* is just as acceptable as *withholding life support* initially. The initial full resuscitation may make it possible to assess the patient's end-of-life desires more fully and carefully. If the initial intervention is unsuccessful or is inconsistent with the patient's preference, it can and should be withdrawn, consistent with the patient's identified goals.

What are ethically frowned upon are such deceitful practices as the "slow code," a charade consisting of a halfhearted resuscitation that seems to allow the surgeon to take the moral middle ground by giving the family a false impression of respecting patient autonomy, while knowing full well that the act will not be effective. Experience suggests that this hedge is used fairly commonly. Although no ill is usually intended, the slow code is usually an indication that the surgeon has not realistically communicated with the patient and family to express the medical opinion that resuscitation, in the face of cardiac or respiratory arrest, would be inappropriate.[31]

The concept of "no code" should be clear and is usually instituted at the request of the patient, his advance directive, or an appropriate surrogate. It is ethically inappropriate for the physician to disrespect the patient's autonomous decision even when faced with despairing surrogates requesting interventions over a clear directive to the contrary. The patient with decision-making capacity is, of course, free to change any prior stipulation, even those written in an advance directive. In the absence of any directive, including a decisional patient, the physician must employ *best interest standard*, which requires implementing what a *reasonable patient* would want done in a similar situation.

In order to understand these previously discussed concepts, the surgeon must realize the implications of the three means of accelerating death for patients in USA: *double effect*, *voluntary euthanasia*, and *physician-assisted suicide*. The *rule of double effect*, as previously described, involves the dichotomy of treatment versus side effects, where death is the *unintended* side effect of adequate symptom control. *Voluntary euthanasia*, which is requested by the patient, can be either active or passive. *Passive euthanasia* is the result of withdrawing or withholding life support in situations judged to be medically futile. In USA, this is both ethically and legally acceptable. On the contrary, *active euthanasia* occurs when the physician *intentionally* administers an agent to cause a patient's death. This act is considered *unethical* and *illegal* everywhere in the world except in the Netherlands where it is practiced openly. *Physician-assisted suicide* occurs when a physician supplies a death-causing agent to a patient with the knowledge that the patient intends to use this agent to commit suicide.

In multiple decisions, the courts have emphasized the importance of distinction between "letting a patient die and making that patient die."[18] This, in our opinion, is the most distressing conflict for the physician who must make such decisions. We know full well that when we give high dose opioids or withdraw ventilatory support, we may be hastening the patient's death. The callous ones among us see this as euthanasia and strongly criticize those who claim otherwise. When confronted with this challenge, in a personal communication, Dr. Edmund Pellegrino, one of our most respected medical ethicists, immediately responded with his comforting interpretation of such a situation. In his mind, and in his conscience, he recognizes and acts upon the difference between actively and intentionally hastening a patient's death as opposed to relieving pain and suffering or withdrawing artificial life support, thus "letting nature take its course."

Determination of Death

The attending physician has the discretion and the responsibility to determine death. Statutes in different states use different criteria for death. In some cases, they have not caught up with the science available. Some states use the "irreversible cessation of cardiopulmonary function" criteria, as do some religions. The complete cessation of respiration and circulation constitute "death" under this definition. The concept of *intensive care* has advanced dramatically since these statutes were enacted and have superseded this now antiquated definition. In most states where this is the statutory definition, the courts have now ruled that "brain death" suffices.

Most states use the brain death criteria. There is debate currently about whether the "whole brain" definition of death is no longer valid; and that the appropriate ethical standard for definition of death is cessation of "higher brain" function. Higher brain function includes the cognitive functions or the capacity for consciousness. Once there is irreversible cessation of that capability, a judgment usually made in consultation with a neurologist, then death can be declared. Most neurologists are trained to determine whether death has occurred or whether the patient is in a "permanent vegetative state."

It should be noted that in some states the definition of death includes *either* the *cessation of cardiopulmonary function or irreversible cessation of all brain function*, including the brain stem.

The health-care team, however, should realize that no matter which criterion is being used, it may be appropriate to continue cardiovascular support for the purpose of maintaining perfusion during the eminent birth of a fetus, or to sustain viability of transplantable organs.

Organ Donation

Criteria for organ donation are not always clearly understood. Many patients and families are mistakenly concerned about having death declared prematurely just to facilitate the harvesting of organs for transplantation. Here, the surgeon's bioethical responsibilities are clear. The medical ethical principle of *patient autonomy* dictates that the desires of the patient and the family be respected.

Federal law requires most hospitals to make an inquiry of all patients, during their admission, for any procedure, whether emergency or elective, about their wishes to be a potential *organ donor*. While this can be somewhat of a shock to patients who are coming in for elective surgery, especially a minor procedure, it obviates the need for physicians to make the painful inquiry when a patient is actually facing eminent death. If the admitting personnel ask for this information on a routine basis, the patient is more likely to render a competent decision, and the potential problems of dealing with surrogates, sometimes under difficult circumstances, are alleviated.

However it is obtained, *informed consent* of the *donor* is required. Most states provide organ donor options on driver's licenses, and many people possess other documents such as donor cards, which indicate their desire to become organ donors. In some cases, donors request limits on the organs they wish to donate. For example, some donors have indicated that they do not wish to donate their eyes or some other specific organ. Even though patient autonomy should guide the physician, there are circumstances where the family emphatically wishes to override the clearly stated intention of the donor. These situations are difficult, and while the surgeon's clear ethical duty is to respect the wishes of the donor, the body of the donor, after death, belongs to the family. The treating physician would be well advised to leave the resolution of this situation up to the transplant coordinator. In fact, it is usually inappropriate for anyone on the treating team to initiate the discussion of organ donation. Most hospitals have in place a procedure whereby the discussion of potential organ donation is initiated by a person specifically trained for this purpose. It is often the transplant coordinator, a social worker, or a hospital chaplain.

Insisting on compliance with the donor's clearly stated wishes, in the face of strong family opposition, does not affect the legal position of the surgeon; but it can result in unfortunate lawsuits because of the animosity created with the family. In cases where there are no previously expressed wishes by the potential donor, the family, as custodians of the body, may agree to organ donation. The duty of the physician in this case is to obtain the consent of the family *before* doing anything to preserve the functioning of the organs for potential transplantation.

In cases where there is no surrogate or family, or any evidence of previously stated intention to donate, the ethical position of the doctor is less clear, but absent permission to do something to the body in a situation which is no longer an emergency, assuming that the organs should be harvested for transplantation, would seriously violate the concept of informed consent. While it can be argued the dead person cannot give informed consent, the family whose property the body is, would have to give their consent to have any procedure done at all to the newly dead person. In cases with no directives at all, the best course of action, unfortunately, is to do nothing postmortem.

Ethics/Legal Consultation

Most surgeons work within an institution. Most of these institutions provide a mechanism for obtaining help in sorting out challenging ethical dilemmas. This help usually comes in the form of consultation from the hospital *Ethics Committee* or from in-house *legal consultation*. It is critical to realize that utilization of such resources does not commit the surgeon to accepting an arbitrary decision of what is right and what is wrong in a complicated ethical situation. Consultation is meant to provide a process for most expeditiously sorting out the issues which have arisen and for providing rapid access to the potential mechanisms for solving the problem. Hospital ethics committees are specifically charged to advise physicians, patients, and families who face ethical dilemmas. These situations usually arise when there is *disagreement* among these groups and the health-care team. Consultation from the ethics committee is usually rapidly facilitated through such agencies as the hospital nursing service. Consultation should be available, instantly, 24 h a day. Frequently, it is the hospital chaplain who facilitates the consultation. By bringing in appropriate resources and facilitating meeting with the health-care team, patients, and families, consultation with the ethics committee should help resolve even the most complicated medical ethical challenges. The hospital ethics committee should be charged with what is the right thing to do for the patient. It should have no vested interest in protecting the institution at the risk of embarking on an action, which is ethically unsettled for the good of the patient.

A word of caution, however, is necessary for surgeons working within a given institution. Once *legal counsel* or *risk management* is brought in to deal with a complicated situation, it must be remembered that *they work for the institution.* Their job is to protect the institution, and the advice that they give will be aimed toward that end. This commitment to the institution is important for the physician to realize if there is potential for placing oneself in personal jeopardy. It is also important to realize that legal standards are not always reliable guides to determining what the best ethical and medical decisions are.

Good Samaritan

A Case

The most skilled colon and rectal surgeon in town is out to dinner. At the next table, he sees the local crime boss choking to death over a piece of prime beef. What are the ethical and legal considerations he must consider before performing an emergency tracheotomy? What is he ethically obligated to do? Is the old medical oath binding? Can anyone give consent? Must he identify himself? If he performs the procedure and there is a bad outcome, is it malpractice? What if he is a medical student instead of a famous surgeon? Is a bad outcome here considered battery? What should the surgeon do when the EMT arrives and wants to take the dying crime boss to a known inferior local hospital? What are the obligations and risks for the surgeon?

General Concepts

Good Samaritan acts or deeds are defined as those in which aid is rendered to a person in need, where no fiduciary or legal obligation exists to provide such aid, and neither reward nor remuneration for the aid is anticipated. The aid provided can include a survey of the situation, protection of the victim, notification of other care providers, or personal provision of immediate treatment. The Good Samaritan Ethic is one that is generally endorsed by our culture, which strongly supports assisting an individual who is in danger or in need of help. Surgeons may be regarded as having a greater responsibility to provide Good Samaritan aid than a layperson by reason of the special training and knowledge and commitment to duty for the benefit of individuals and society, which generally drive us to become physicians and surgeons. Clearly, in a situation of sudden medical need, a surgeon will be better able to assess the medical condition of the victim and to render immediate treatment if indicated and feasible. Many feel that the mere status of being a physician entails the duty to use one's skills and knowledge in cases of sudden or emergency need; for some, this duty is an inherent feature of the role and even of the definition of a physician.[38]

Briefly stated, in almost every state, an off-duty surgeon who comes across a person with an emergency medical condition has no *legal duty* to come to the aid of that person. However, a physician's *ethical obligation* inspires him to help in such an emergency. All states in USA have enacted the so-called Good Samaritan statutes, which protect the physician from liability incurred for good-faith efforts to help at the scene of an accident or emergency. The ethical duty should far exceed the legal excuse for inaction.[2]

Generally, Good Samaritan acts include the following principles: (1) There is no legal obligation of doctors to answer or treat emergencies. (2) If the doctor chooses to intervene, the expected standard of care is modified by circumstances of the situation. (3) If aid is given, it needs to be stabilization only and not definitive treatment. (4) Implied consent exists to treat the victim if he or she lacks the capacity to consent. (5) These criteria apply whether or not the physician is paid for his or her services rendered. Despite the establishment of these principles, the extensive coverage in the media of spectacular medical malpractice suits causes many surgeons to develop a strong aversion to the performance of Good Samaritan acts. In order to alleviate this apprehension, Good Samaritan Laws were enacted, the first in California in 1959. Since then, every state has enacted such law. The laws all share the following provisions: there is no legal obligation to provide aid; there is immunity from malpractice suit if aid is provided; there is exception from immunity for gross negligence or lack of "good-faith"; acts are restricted to application outside of hospitals; and there is withdrawal of legal immunity if the doctor accepted payment for aid rendered.[38]

Professionalism and Interpersonal Relations: Working as a Team

General Considerations

There is an ever-increasing challenge to deliver the very best surgical care in the current medical environment which thrives on its speed and frequently impersonal delivery of generic medical care, often at multiple institutions, and without one consistent team of support. Often it becomes difficult to fulfill the responsibility requiring communication, collaboration, respect, and confidentiality as we interact with the components of our health-care team which frequently includes nurses, enterostomal therapists, primary care physicians, consulting physicians, surgical and medical trainees, and the vast array of ancillary services required within our institutions.

Teaching Residents and Fellows

Learning and teaching are critical components in our career choice of medicine, and especially, surgery. At some point in our training, a more senior person turns over to each of us the responsibility to perform the major part of an operative procedure. And then, the converse occurs: each of us, in turn, relinquishes the major part of an operation to one of our trainees. We know how the process works and the importance of a surgical team with "graded" responsibility. The ethical challenge arises when, often the night before surgery, the patient asks "who is going to do my surgery?"[39] The honest answer becomes blurred, especially for those colon and rectal surgeons working in a program with trainees who are senior residents or fellows. We usually fall back on the explanation that we, the attending surgeon will be present and responsible, even when we know that the trainee will be doing the critical part of the procedure. What is the truth? The fellow claims on the training record that he or she did the case, and we charge the payer as if we did the procedure. What is true *informed consent* in such situations?

Previous Suboptimal Care

General Concepts

As colon and rectal surgeons, we are specialists, frequently seeing patients as requested consultation by and referral from other physicians and even other surgeons. It makes the nature of our care, often, "the end of the road." We have no place else to send the patients and frequently find ourselves in the position of correcting or undoing the poor results of the action of another surgeon. This becomes an ethical and personal challenge, especially when the patient or the family asks "Why wasn't that done by the other surgeon, or what did she do wrong?" We can easily become caught up in the dilemma between taking credit for heroic restoration of health and condemnation of the other surgeon, or covering up for incompetent care in an attempt to avoid litigation against another doctor and/or preserving a lucrative source of referrals.

Generally, our surgical and specialty training does not prepare us for the ethical differentiation between "bailing out" and "condemning," responding to patients' pointed questions, communicating with the doctor responsible for the suboptimal care, and certainly not "blowing the whistle" on another surgeon and going to court, when requested, as an "expert witness." Albert Wu suggests that a surgeon who discovers a major error made by another physician has several options, which include the following: waiting for the other doctor to disclose the mistake, advising the other physician to disclose the error, arranging a joint meeting to discuss the mistake, or telling the patient directly. He and his coauthors believe that based on the requirements of the doctor–patient relationship, surgeons have an obligation to facilitate disclosure. Many surgeons are reluctant to say anything because they are not 100% sure of what actually happened, they fear hurting the feelings of colleagues, they wish not to strain professional relationships, or because of the terrifying thought that "there but for the grace of God go I." Wu further suggests that we fulfill our obligation to our patient by advising the doctor who erred to inform the patient; but he goes on to say that if that fails, it is our duty to tell the patient what happened.[40] Each of us must then rely on compassion and tact to tell our patients the truth without unduly condemning the other physicians. We surgeons need to realize that what we take for granted in our weekly *morbidity and mortality* conferences, especially in a teaching hospital, is not the norm for other branches of medicine. We know, and perhaps are obligated to pass on to others, that admitting a mistake may help us to accept responsibility for it and may help to make changes in our practice. Physicians should be able to learn vicariously from mistakes made by others and thus avoid making the same mistake themselves.[40]

"Blowing the Whistle" and Going to Court

The next echelon of concern and potential activity, of course, involves serving as an "expert witness" in medical malpractice litigation. Again, this is an arena of involvement in the medical-care system for which we surgeons are generally ill prepared. Just recently, the American College of Surgeons and the American Society of Colon and Rectal Surgeons has issued some guidelines in an attempt to insure that surgical specialists not abuse the system by offering false testimony or by presenting as "experts" in areas beyond their expertise. Many of our true experts refuse to serve in this capacity when it involves saying something against another surgeon; yet, when any of *us* are involved as the accused, we want only the finest experts available and are repulsed when "hired guns" with little knowledge boldly testify against us. The problem seems to be that many of us do not differentiate *malpractice* with severe damage to a patient from the poor results from proper treatment, which we surgeons all experience in dealing with the complex biological system of the human body. Again, the principle of not stepping up to the plate for fear of the dictum, "There but for the grace of God go I." We should understand that credibility in the medical-legal system should be based on true expertise and on telling the truth, be it for the plaintiff or for the defense of our colleagues, and, in fact, we can be of much greater help to inappropriately accused physicians by establishing such a record of credibility.

Managed Care

All of us, in the current system, participate in some form of managed care, where someone other than the treating physician becomes involved in the mechanism of delivering care to our patients, usually without sharing in the responsibility of rendering the care and the untoward outcome that may be engendered by that care. This presents a true dichotomy for doctors, most of whom have taken an oath or by law are committed to being *advocates* for our patients. It seems an impossible, and perhaps unethical, task to make a decision, which favors the economic advantage of a managed care organization over what we know, medically, is required by an individual patient in need.

Rationing Care/Cutting Corners

Surgeons have a special obligation to deal with these systems because of the loneliness of making the decision and ultimately doing a surgical procedure on another human being. It is a desperate feeling to realize, in the middle of an operation, that our quest for perfection has been compromised by some inadequacy in preoperative management foisted on us by another remote physician hired by a managed care organization to protect the financial interests of a group. We know, as well as others, that medicine, as a system, is in trouble, but the problem is rarely to be solved by rationing or withholding what we know is surgically best for our individual patients. Perhaps it is our job to invoke our "surgical personalities" to become the strongest of all patient advocates and to fully participate in achieving needed improvements in the overall system. We must communicate to others the special understanding and compassion few outside of the field of surgery understand.

Personal Challenges: Competition of Interests

Professionalism

McKneally describes the profession of medicine and surgery as a vocation that requires extensive knowledge and skill. It also requires a high level of discretion and trustworthiness, even in individual practice. The social contract between the profession and the public holds professionals to very high standards of competence and moral responsibility. He goes on to explain that a profession is literally a declaration of a way of life "in which expert knowledge is used not primarily for personal gain, but for the benefit of those who need that knowledge."[19] In our current society, bombarded by endless advertising and hype, many groups call themselves "professionals" sometimes to the point of humor, but for those of us in medicine, and especially surgery, the definition means that when confronted with a choice of what is good for us or what is good for our patient, we choose the latter. This occurs and is expected sometimes to the detriment of our own good and that of our families. Tom Krizek even goes so far as to question if surgery is an "impairing profession."[41] Perhaps it really is an *ethical* concern, which is encouraging us to modify the working hours and conditions for our trainees to offer more of an incentive to enter the surgical specialties. Now that we have appropriately tended to the training programs, it behooves us to explore the same lifestyle improvements for ourselves. It is neither an ethical breach nor a sign of weakness to allocate high priority to our families and to our own well-being.

Family

As financial and professional pressures become more intense, the challenge increases to appropriately prioritize and balance the demands of patient care, family, education, teaching, and research. Mary McGrath presents an all-too-frequent dilemma for the surgeon: choosing between attending a child's graduation or operating on an old patient who requests you instead of your extremely well-trained associate who is currently seeing the patient. How many times have we not chosen wisely? Someone else can competently care for your patient, but only you can be a parent to your child.[19] Time literally flies, and we must often remind ourselves that our lives are not just a "dress rehearsal"!

Among the many considerations of *family* is the issue of caring for, and perhaps even operating on our own family members. What is not only ethical but also what is appropriate for the practice of medicine and surgery with regard to this issue is not as clear as you might, at first, believe. For example, if your spouse cuts her leg while skiing and the only available physician is a psychiatrist who is covering the ER, should you, a trained training surgeon, suture her laceration? On the contrary, if you feel that you are the most experienced colon and rectal surgeon in the community, what should you do when your own mother is found to have a complicated cancer of the low rectum? After all, if you are the "best" why would you deny the best care to your own mother? Many hospitals have dealt with this issue and have a stated policy. The AMA has issued a statement on "Self-Treatment or Treatment of Immediate Family Members." In essence, it speaks against treating family except in emergent situations and for short periods of time. It is, of course, based on the risk of compromise of professional objectivity and influence on medical judgment because of the influence of personal feelings, thus interfering with the care that needs to be delivered.[42]

Competence / Impairment / Insight

Surgical certifying organizations are currently struggling with the definition and determination of *surgical competence*. McKneally stresses that a patient's trust is based on the surgeon's diligent pursuit of competence in both judgment and technical skill. Surgical training programs have diligently attempted to guarantee the competency of individuals completing the process. The board certification process attempts to ensure that the interests of society are represented in these professional processes. Thus, competency is an integral part of the *entry-level*. The problem arises in maintaining a level of competence and assuring that established surgeons who take on new procedures both acquire and maintain competence in these new skills.[15] Perhaps the most obvious recent example for us colon and rectal surgeons has been the advent of laparoscopic, minimally invasive surgical procedures. Now that they are part of all Fellowship training programs, it is less of a problem. But the issue will arise again with the next new wave of technology: how to teach old surgeons new skills.

Related to competence is the issue of *impairment*. Jones emphasizes that drug and alcohol abuse, with the associated functional impairments, are the leading cause of sanction against physicians by professional oversight bodies in USA. More than one in every seven physicians is affected by substance abuse at some time in their careers. He goes on to explain that the surgical patient is potentially at greatest risk in the care of a cognitively or physiologically impaired physician because the surgeon's competence requires simultaneous application of fine neuromuscular, cognitive, and intellectual skills. This is coupled with the emotional composure and critical judgment required to make urgent decisions and the physical endurance of standing for long hours at the operating table. He cites Percival's admonition that the medical profession is a "public trust" that should be relinquished when a physician or surgeon no longer possesses the skills that are essential for clinical care. Unfortunately, most surgeons do not possess or exercise the insight required to know when we are impaired or when it is time to retire.

Jones goes on to quote Verghese's observation on the impaired physician: "the doctors had one common feature – namely, exquisite denial – that allowed them to believe they could still care for patients perfectly well."[43] These observations place great responsibility on those of us who observe *impairment* or *incompetence* in our colleagues who at times may also be close friends. We should never hesitate to request intervention because correction of substance abuse in physicians is highly successful. If we stand by and allow patients to be mismanaged by inadequate physicians, we will not only see the patients suffer but will also allow our colleagues and friends to be destroyed professionally and perhaps devastated emotionally by malpractice suits, condemnation by institutions and colleagues, loss of licensure, and eventually the ravages of substance abuse or personal humiliation.[43] Most state boards of healing arts function best when it comes to providing support for physicians in trouble.

A Final Thought

Perhaps Richard Hayward, who compares a surgeon to the young sea captain in Joseph Conrad's novel, "The Shadow Line," best describes a successful career in surgery. Hayward explains that there are so many variables in the interaction between patient, surgeon, and disease that it is not surprising that the prediction of results becomes uncertain. Even routine procedures can produce complications and can become much more difficult than had been anticipated. As the surgeon crosses Conrad's Shadow Line, energy, enthusiasm, ability to make firm decisions and then act upon them, optimism, self-confidence, and resilience in the face of adversity become necessities without which an individual will have difficulty coping with the pressures of a surgical practice, especially one involving the care of critically ill emergency patients. There becomes a time when a surgeon must learn to come to terms with the inadequacies and, sometimes, downright failures of his or her actions that will be the inevitable companions during a surgical life.[44]

References

1. ACEP Ethics Committee. Code of ethics for emergency physicians. Ann Emerg Med. 1997;30:365–72.
2. Derse AR. Law and ethics in emergency medicine. Emerg Med Clin North Am. 1999;17:307–25.
3. Kodner IJ. Ethics curricula in surgery: needs and approaches. World J Surg. 2003;27:952–6.
4. Little M. Invited commentary: is there a distinctively surgical ethics? Surgery. 2001;129:668–71.
5. Beauchamp TL, Childress JF. Principles of biomedical ethics. 5th ed. Oxford: Oxford University Press; 2001. p. 12–23.
6. Justice Cardoza. Scholendorff v. New York Hospital 105 N.E. 92. New York Court of Appeals 1914.
7. Iserson KV. Principles of biomedical ethics. Emerg Med Clin North Am. 1999;17:283–306.
8. Adams J, Larkin G, Iserson K, et al. Virtue in emergency medicine. Acad Emerg Med. 1996;3:961–6.
9. Alexander L. Medical science under dictatorship. NEJM. 1949;241:39–51.
10. Koenig HG. Taking a spiritual history. JAMA. 2004;291:2881.
11. Weber JE. Conflicts of interest in emergency medicine. Emerg Med Clin North Am. 1999;17:475–90.
12. Buckner F. The Emergency Medical Treatment and Labor Act (EMTALA). Medical Practice Management 2002;Nov/Dec:142–5.
13. Jonsen AR, Siegler M, Winslade WJ. Clinical ethics: a practical approach to ethical decisions in clinical medicine. 5th ed. New York: McGraw-Hill; 2002. p. 41–2.
14. Moore FD. Ethical problems special to surgery: surgical teaching, surgical innovation, and the surgeon in managed care. Arch Surg. 2000;135:14–6.
15. MdKneally MF. Ethical problems in surgery: innovation leading to unforeseen complication. World J Surg. 1999;23:786–8.
16. McCahill LE, Dunn GP, Mosenthal AC, et al. Palliation as a core surgical principle: part I. J Am Coll Surg. 2004;199:149–60.
17. Jacobstein CR, Baren JM. Emergency department treatment of minors. Emerg Med Clin North Am. 1999;17:341–52.
18. Schmidt TA, Zechnich AD. Suicidal patients in the ED: ethical issues. Emerg Med Clin North Am. 1999;17:371–83.
19. Angelos P. End of life issues. American College of Surgeons Ethics Curriculum for Surgical Residents, pp. 91–2.
20. Sander AB. Advance directives. Emerg Med Clin North Am. 1999;17:519–26.
21. Siegler M. Identifying the ethical aspects of clinical practice. Bull Am Coll Surg. 1996;81(11):23–5.
22. Ells C, Caniano DA. The impact of culture on the patient-surgeon relationship. J Am Coll Surg. 2002;195:520–30.
23. Paris JJ, Ferranti J. The changing face of medicine: health care on the Internet. J Perinatol. 2001;21:34–9.
24. Moore GP. Ethics seminars: the practice of medical procedures on newly dead patients – is consent warranted? Acad Emerg Med. 2001;8:389–92.
25. McKneally MF, Daar AS. Introducing new technologies: protecting subjects of surgical innovation and research. World J Surg. 2003;27:930–5.
26. Nee PA, Griffiths RD. Ethical considerations in accident and emergency research. Emerg Med J. 2002;19:423–7.
27. Beecher HK. Ethics and clinical research. NEJM. 1966;274:1354–60.
28. Rothman DJ. Ethics and human experimentation: Henry Beecher revisited. NEJM. 1987;317:1195–9.
29. Horng S, Miller FG. Is placebo surgery unethical? NEJM. 2002;347:137–9.
30. Birrer R, Singh U, Kumar DN. Disability and dementia in the emergency department. Emerg Med Clin North Am. 1999;17:505–17.
31. Schears RM. Emergency physicians' role in end-of-life care. Emerg Med Clin North Am. 1999;17:539–59.
32. Iserson KV. Withholding and withdrawing medical treatment: an emergency medicine perspective. Ann Emerg Med. 1996;28:51–4.
33. Marco CA. Ethical issues of resuscitation. Emerg Med Clin North Am. 1999;17:527–38.
34. Marco CA, Larkin GL. Ethics seminars: case studies in "futility" – challenges for academic emergency medicine. Acad Emerg Med. 2000;7:1147–51.
35. McCahill LE, Dunn GP, Mosenthall AC, et al. Palliation as a core surgical principle: part I. J Am Coll Surg. 2004;199:149–59.
36. The rights of the terminally ill. New York Times 5/28, 2004.

37. Liptak A. Ruling upholds Oregon law authorizing assisted suicide. New York Times 5/27, 2004.
38. Daniels S. Good Samaritan Acts. Emerg Med Clin North Am. 1999;17:491–504.
39. Jones JW, McCullough LB. Consent for residents to perform surgery. J Vasc Surg. 2002;3:655–6.
40. Wu AW, Cavanaugh TA, McPhee SJ, et al. To tell the truth: ethical and practical issues in disclosing medical mistakes to patients. J Gen Intern Med. 1997;12:22–7.
41. Krizek TJ. Ethics and philosophy lecture: surgery…is it an impairing profession? J Am Coll Surg. 2002;194:352–66.
42. Self-treatment or treatment of immediate family members. American Medical Association Policy Number E-8.19.
43. Jones JW, McCullough LB, Richman BW. An impaired surgeon, a conflict of interest, and supervisory responsibilities. Surgery. 2004;135:449–51.
44. Hayward R. The shadow-line in surgery. Lancet. 1987;1 (8529):375–6.

53 Legal Considerations

Michael J. Meehan

Introduction

The dawn of the twenty-first century brought with it many of the same court room challenges for colon and rectal disease practitioners as did the latter half of the twentieth century. The increasing frequency and crushing severity of malpractice claims and lawsuits, data bank reporting, Web-based consumer claims data, new privacy requirements, increasing clinical demands, greater government regulation and enforcement activity, and spiraling malpractice premiums have caused many physicians to leave practice, retire early, or move to more lawsuit-friendly jurisdictions. This chapter addresses many of the causes for these concerns – from communication to documentation, from practice to research – as they relate to colon and rectal surgeons who face these challenges.

Medical Malpractice

Elements of Malpractice

In July 2003, a 12-day trial occurred in Seattle, Washington. The plaintiff, a married 53-year-old computer salesman, presented to his family physician with rectal bleeding and a painful anal lump that looked like a hemorrhoid. When the condition did not improve with treatment, the patient was referred to a general surgeon, who evaluated the condition, thought the patient had a hemorrhoid, and recommended a hemorrhoidectomy. The patient, however, said he thought the condition was improving and declined the procedure. The surgeon told the patient that he should have a hemorrhoidectomy if the condition did not continue to improve and resolve. The patient did not return to the surgeon for 4 months, at which time a hemorrhoidectomy revealed an advanced anal cancer. The patient underwent chemotherapy and radiation, developed impotence, and suffered two recurrences of his cancer. The patient-plaintiff sued both doctors and contended at trial that earlier diagnosis would have resulted in less extensive treatment and a prognosis that he would have survived his cancer (from which he was probably going to die). The defense argued that both the family practitioner and the general surgeon acted appropriately and that an earlier diagnosis would not have made any difference in the treatment or the outcome. Fifteen medical and surgical experts were used in the case. The pre-suit demand of $2.75 million had been met with an offer of $125,000. At trial, the plaintiff asked the jury for $7 million and the defendants requested a defense verdict. The jury awarded no money.[1]

The requisite elements that must be proved by a plaintiff in a medical malpractice case are determined by the laws of the various states. Washington state law governed in this case. Generally speaking, a case for medical malpractice is established when it is shown by a preponderance of the evidence that a patient's injury was caused by the act of a physician or surgeon that would not have been done by a physician or surgeon of ordinary skill, care, and diligence under like or similar conditions or circumstances (or by the omission of an act that a physician or surgeon of ordinary skill, care, and diligence would have done), and that the patient's injury was the direct and proximate result of such act (or omission).[2] What a "physician or surgeon of ordinary skill, care, and diligence would or would not have done under like or similar conditions or circumstances" is called the standard of care. The standard of care for a physician or surgeon in the practice of a board-certified medical or surgical specialty should be that of a reasonable specialist practicing medicine or surgery in that same specialty, regardless of geographical considerations or circumstances.[2]

Family practitioners and surgical specialists, as in the Washington case described above, are usually held to different standards of care, depending on variations in state law. In a case like this, for there to be a plaintiffs' verdict the jury must believe that (1) there was a departure from the standard of care *and* (2) that the departure from the standard of care was the cause of the patient's injury. In order for the defense to prevail, the jury must believe that either (1) or (2) above was not proved by a preponderance of the evidence – or that neither was proved.

D.E. Beck et al. (eds.), *The ASCRS Textbook of Colon and Rectal Surgery: Second Edition*,
DOI 10.1007/978-1-4419-1584-9_53, © Springer Science+Business Media, LLC 2011

Both of these issues were actively debated in the Washington case. (1) The recommendations, treatment, and decision to defer a hemorrhoidectomy were contested by both sides; (2) whether the cancer had metastasized prior to the critical involvement of the doctors was also argued. (If the cancer had metastasized prior to physician mismanagement, if any, then even a timely hemorrhoidectomy would not have changed the outcome or treatment – so physician mismanagement could not have logically been the *cause* of the patient's injuries).

In some cases, the defense attorneys give up on item (1) above, i.e., liability, if they think they cannot prevail on item (1) but if they think they can prevail on item (2), i.e., causation. Such a strategy is challenging at best – consider the following case tried to a Savannah, Georgia jury in November 2001 in which defense attorneys conceded liability and tried to convince a jury that the plaintiff was entitled to receive an award, but that the amount sought by the plaintiff exceeded that to which he should be entitled. The plaintiff had been in an automobile accident and had suffered a rectal tear when thrown from his vehicle. The trauma surgeons who tried to repair the tear negligently stapled the wrong end of his colon. As a result, he suffered a complete obstruction of his digestive tract for 7 days and developed a massive infection, causing the loss of approximately 70% of his abdominal wall. He was left with massive scarring, no abdominal muscles, only a thin layer of skin covering his intestines, and the prospect of constant diarrhea for the remainder of his life. The defendants conceded that the stapling procedure was handled improperly, but disputed the extent of the patient's injuries, including over $1.2 million alleged to represent the present cash value of the patient's future lost income. The jury was not asked whether the trauma surgeons had departed from the standard of care, but rather whether all of the injuries complained of were caused by the negligence (whether too much money was being claimed for the injury). The jury awarded the plaintiff $6.25 million.[3]

Recently, case law has developed expanding the standard care in some instances to include a duty to warn a patient's relatives of their increased genetic risk for colon cancer due to the patient's diagnosis. A New Jersey appellate court has held that a physician not only has a duty to warn the patient of the genetic or hereditary nature of his or her illness and its possible impact on the patient's close relatives, but also may have a duty to inform the patient's immediate family members who may be adversely affected. In that case, the Plaintiff was diagnosed with colon cancer at the age of 36 and sued the estate of a physician who had treated her father for polyposis, some 30 years prior. The woman alleged that the physician had a duty to warn her father's immediate family members of the hereditary nature and risks of polyposis, which may have permitted her to receive earlier detection, prevention, and treatment of polyposis, possibly preventing the development of colon cancer. The court held that ordinarily, a physician's duty to warn of a genetically transferable disease is satisfied by warning the patient, but that a physician must also take reasonable steps to assure that the information actually reaches those likely to be affected or is made available to their benefit.[4] The release of private health information is regulated on the federal level by the Health Insurance Portability and Accountability Act (HIPAA) (discussed below), which authorizes disclosure without consent in the case of a serious and immediate threat to an identifiable third party when the physician has the capability to forestall that harm.

Recurring Malpractice Themes

A study of medical malpractice cases involving colon and rectal disease involved a retrospective review of all cases tried in the federal and state civil court system over a 21-year period from 1971 through 1991[5] and remains instructive today. The study identified 98 malpractice cases over this period of time from a computerized legal data base, involving 103 allegations of negligence. The nature and frequency of allegations were as follows:

- 43% Failure to timely diagnose disease, principally cancer and appendicitis
- 24% Iatrogenic colon injury
- 15% Iatrogenic medical complications during diagnosis or treatment
- 10% Sphincter injury with fecal incontinence from anorectal surgery or midline episiotomy
- 8% Lack of informed consent, usually regarding the extent of procedures or endoscopy

More recent commentators have warned about patients who present with fully developed cancers within 4 years of colonoscopies that apparently cleared the colon of neoplasia. The fear expressed is that the presenting patients may assume their colonoscopies were performed negligently, despite legitimate alternative explanations.[6] A study reviewing 38 malpractice claims against radiologists performing contrast examinations of the colon between 1985 and 1994 revealed the following major allegations: failure to diagnose caused a delay in treatment and death and colon perforation due to improper performance.[7]

Risk management suggestions relevant to colon cancer screening include using authoritative screening guidelines, documenting informed consent and refusals, assessing family histories, recommending that family members of at-risk patients be contacted, repeating sigmoidoscopies and colonoscopies when the preparation is inadequate, and documenting cecal intubation and careful withdrawal techniques.[8]

Lawsuit Stress

Many if not most physicians who are sued experience stress and other normal emotions when their professional care and judgments are criticized in a public lawsuit. The initial stressor typically occurs when the claim letter, summons and complaints, or insurance company notice arrives in the mail. The simple reality is that the profession which you have chosen frequently lends itself to the frustrations and anxiety of litigation. Anger, uncertainty, and even depression are common symptoms among physician defendants, especially those sued for the first time.

Attorneys representing physicians usually advise their clients not to discuss the case with others for fear of losing the protections available through the attorney–client privilege. The tension and vulnerability that you may feel about being sued may be exacerbated by this inability to seek emotional comfort by discussing the case with colleagues and others. It is normal to feel isolated – to assume that colleagues and even subordinates are talking about you and your lawsuit. It is equally important to place your predicament in perspective; many of your colleagues have been in the same situation before you.

If you are involved in a claim or lawsuit and are experiencing any of these normal reactions to litigation or the threat of litigation, you should have a candid conversation with your attorney, risk manager, or insurance company claims representative. Many insurance companies and medical institutions provide resources for defendant physicians that enable them to discuss their lawsuit and their feelings of uncertainty and isolation with counselors or colleagues in a protected fashion. Conversations with psychotherapists should normally be privileged and not admissible in the courtroom as evidence in the case. Remember that your emotional stability is critical to the successful defense of the litigation. You serve yourself best by sharing your feelings with your attorney and asking him or her for a way to receive emotional coaching throughout the stress of the lawsuit and afterward as well.

Informed Consent

The failure of a physician to obtain proper informed consent is often cited as a major component of medical malpractice litigation. In reality, few cases are prosecuted exclusively on the issue of informed consent, and juries do not customarily award damages solely for a lack of informed consent. Nearly every malpractice lawsuit, however, contains a supplementary count that informed consent was not obtained. Properly obtaining and documenting informed consent, therefore, can be critical to the defense of the entire lawsuit. The informed consent discussion is at the heart of physician–patient communication and is usually an important component in the defense of the main medical or surgical issues in every case. You do not have to wait until the day of or the day before the procedure to obtain informed consent. A study involving 60 patients who underwent either colonoscopies or esophagogastroduodenoscopies revealed that patients remember essentially the same information whether consent is obtained immediately prior to a procedure or several days earlier.[9]

Obtaining of Informed Consent

Obtaining informed consent is primarily a physician obligation. Nurses and other nonphysicians cannot normally be blamed for failing to obtain informed consent[10] because they do not have the requisite legal capacity to fully inform patients of issues on which only a physician is licensed to advise. Hospitals, the typical employers of such professionals, do have an obligation to maintain an effective informed consent process within their institutions. Informed consent actions can be successfully brought against hospitals if they breach hospital standards and other duties imposed by law, e.g., where a patient is injured by an experimental procedure without being advised of the experimental study.[11]

Obtaining a patient's informed consent involves more than having the patient sign a form. It is a communication process, in which the physician should disclose and discuss the following information with the patient:[12]

- The patient's diagnosis, if known
- The nature and purpose of the proposed treatment or procedure
- The risks and benefits of a proposed treatment or procedure
- Alternatives (regardless of cost or insurance coverage)
- The risks and benefits of the alternatives
- The risks and benefits of not receiving or undergoing the treatment or procedure

Patients should have the opportunity to ask questions and have their questions answered.

Proving a Case of Lack of Informed Consent

Depending on variations in state laws, plaintiff attorneys typically must prove the following elements to establish a *prima facie* case of lack of informed consent by a physician:

- The physician failed to disclose to the patient and discuss the material risks and dangers inherently and potentially involved with respect to the proposed therapy, if any.
- The unrevealed risks and dangers which should have been disclosed by the physician actually materialize and were the proximate cause of the injury to the patient, and
- A reasonable person in the position of the patient would have decided against the therapy had the material risks and dangers inherent and incidental to the treatment been disclosed to her prior to the therapy.[13]

Whether risks are material or not is normally a jury question,[14] and juries are often instructed that risks are normally considered to be material if a reasonably prudent person would attach significance to the risk in deciding whether or not to accept the treatment. A risk that is either *severe*, like death, or *frequent* are usually risks that are considered material. Some states regulate the information that must be conveyed to patients, while other states leave the determination of materiality to judges and expert witnesses.

You should become familiar with the informed consent laws in the state where you practice. Withholding material risks from patients for cultural, ethnic, or paternalistic reasons is not acceptable.

Documentation of Informed Consent

Informed consent is usually documented with formal consent forms that patients sign. Nearly all hospitals require the use of consent forms for inpatient procedures to comply with applicable law, to abide by the standards of the Joint Commission,[15] and to facilitate patient education of the treatment information. Informed consent is a process and not a form. Forms can be challenged and criticized in the courtroom, and a form with errors or that is incomplete can distract a jury from the real issues involving informed consent.

Claims of lack of informed consent are best defended when a jury is persuaded that the physician had a meaningful conversation with the patient. In addition to a consent form, a chart notation made by the doctor, in the doctor's own words or handwriting, is usually very helpful. A jury that believes that the physician never saw the patient, or had a brief or cursory discussion with the patient, may become more inclined to decide that a surgeon departed from the standard of care in performing the procedure. Producing a diagram that was drawn for the patient can be persuasive for jurors. Similarly, patient information sheets or pamphlets are effective communication devices and serve well in the litigation defense.

Listen carefully to your patients' questions and answer them in a friendly but candid fashion. Chart the presence of any family members who are present for the informed consent discussion. Patients who are minors – usually those under 18 – may not legally consent for themselves unless they are living apart from their parents or are sufficiently mature to provide consent. Regardless of a minor's emancipation or maturity, it is wise to always obtain parental consent for elective procedures performed on minors. Unless parental consent is obtained, there is probably no binding contract enabling you or the hospital to receive payment for services.

Documentation

A patient's medical record is the star witness in any medical malpractice lawsuit. The chart is the one witness whose memory never fades. The medical record can be your best friend when you are sitting on the witness stand, or it can be your worst enemy. Make it your best friend.

Defensive Charting

"If it's not documented, it didn't happen." As a practical matter, this old adage is mostly true, and in any event serves as a good rule of thumb for all caregivers. Defense lawyers like to see professional comprehensive charting because it conveys the appearance of professional and comprehensive care – not only to a jury, but also prior to the suit when a plaintiff's attorney is reviewing records and deciding whether or not to take the case.

Chart notations, as a general rule, need not be cluttered with overwhelming details to be defensible in the courtroom. A good defensive chart notation is written with an eye toward deflecting practical and obvious criticisms that would be made of the healthcare team or the writer of the notation. Examples of concepts to insert, as appropriate, would include the following:

- Descriptions of bedside visits, especially when multiple pages made
- When you were there and what you did, including date, time, and signature
- Your thought process and differential diagnosis
- Presence of family members
- "Spoke with husband at bedside."
- "Patient states that she understands a change in bowel habits should be reported."
- "Patient refuses to comply with treatment recommendations because …"
- "Patient not able to perform fecal occult blood test because …"[16]

Etiology Speculation

The charting of not only the facts, but also speculative opinions can be as damaging as too little charting. It is not uncommon that one member of the medical team may speculate as to the etiology of an adverse event, and that the surmised etiology gets parroted by other members of the healthcare team.

> Example: Physician undertakes a second look laparotomy to rule out recurrence of cancer. During the procedure, the bladder and bowel are perforated, but the perforations are identified and repaired intraoperatively. A bowel leak, however, is detected three days later when the patient is admitted. A second year resident records in the medical chart, "Iatrogenic perforation resulting in sepsis." This reference is repeated by two attendings on other services.

A perforation that is diagnosed within 24 h of an endoscopic procedure may have been iatrogenic, but then again it may have been spontaneous. To assume in the medical chart that a perforation occurred during a procedure, if repeated by others in the medical record, becomes a "reality" that may be insurmountable in the courtroom, even when an expert testifies that the perforation in retrospect was clearly spontaneous.

Everything that is written in the medical chart is critical, and key phrasing is often highlighted or enlarged for juries to see on poster boards. Remember that causation is one of the four elements of medical malpractice, and is frequently the most difficult of the four elements for the plaintiff to prove.

- *ALERT! – Iatrogenic* means "caused by manner or action of physician, not by medical treatment." Do not use the word if you are not absolutely certain that the injury was practitioner-induced.

Also remember that physicians need not always be correct in treating patients. Rather, they must comply with the standard of care. A defensible chart notation reflects a physician's attention, thought process, and a differential diagnosis, even if the working diagnosis turns out to be incorrect in retrospect.

Plaintiff's Pre-claim Review

Because plaintiffs' attorneys are paid on a contingency fee basis, the better plaintiffs' attorneys conduct a review of a new client's medical records before agreeing to take the case and further expending the resources of the law firm. Because nearly all medical malpractice cases are tried before juries (as opposed to judges), attorneys representing patients look for flaws in medical record documentation that juries can understand. For example, a physician's criticism of a colleague in a medical record is easier to showcase before a jury than the related medical facts, which often are too complicated for all jurors to completely understand. While professional differences of opinion are expected, professional conflicts are best resolved verbally. Disagreement with colleagues that appear in the medical records should be kept to a minimum, unless necessary or appropriate to properly document the patient's course of care.

Other items which attorneys and their reviewing physicians look for are missing lab reports, radiology interpretations, or the results of any tests or procedures that were ordered but not present in the chart. Multiple page attempts by the nursing staff that go unanswered are also fertile ground for review and focus.

> Example: Elderly male patient with debilitating back pain underwent spinal surgery. He was on anticoagulation medications due to a mechanical heart valve. Postoperatively he developed a hematoma at the base of the spine. In response to complaints of pain, he was seen three times by a house officer who did perform an appropriate examination but who neither stopped the patient's heparin nor order an MRI. Permanent paralysis and urinary and sexual loss ensued.

A plaintiff's lawyer would be immediately drawn to nursing notes stating that multiple page attempts were made and that no corresponding notes were made by any physician responding to the pages. The attorney immediately assumes that he or she can prove in the courtroom one of the following scenarios: (1) no physician ever responded to the pages; (2) a physician did respond but the response was not timely; or (3) a physician responded but did not conduct a proper examination.

In this example, a comprehensive chart notation by the house officer, reflecting the thought processes and the extent of the examination, may obviate a claim, a verdict, and tens of thousands of dollars in legal fees.

Record Tampering and Deception

Improper altering of the medical record or tampering with the medical record may be grounds for punitive damages and even loss of licensure and should be avoided at all costs. Post-event recording in a medical record should be done with proper disclosure of the timing and reason for the entry and with the advice of risk management or legal counsel if appropriate. You should remember that your medical records are copied for multiple reasons – like insurance, compliance, and quality review – and those copies of any given patient's medical records may exist elsewhere, even at other healthcare facilities. Plaintiffs' attorneys routinely request copies of the same medical records from multiple sources to ensure that all records are gathered, and discrepancies among the various copies may be detected, e.g., a late entry on one copy that does not appear on another copy. When lawyers are suspicious of entries made at different points in time, color copying can be requested and even a handwriting analysis. If a jury were to believe that a physician intentionally altered a medical record to lessen his or her own liability in a malpractice case, the physician would lose credibility with the jury.

Similarly, a surgical error known to the physician but kept from the patient could flame juror anger if it later becomes known to the patient. Surgical needles and other "foreign objects" inadvertently left behind and discovered later by X-ray should be immediately disclosed to patients. The following 2003 Maryland case[17] illustrates this point.

The plaintiff, a 49-year-old married grocer, with a long history of uncontrolled diarrhea and stomach pain diagnosed as ulcerative colitis, presented to a colorectal surgeon for a total proctocolectomy. A temporary ileostomy was performed contemporaneously. The surgeon performed a reanastomosis 90 days later, but the patient experienced a return of her uncontrolled diarrhea and stomach pain. She sought the advice of another physician, who discovered via colonoscopy that one-half of her rectum remained following the proctocolectomy. A second surgeon performed a second proctocolectomy and removed the remaining portion of the rectum, after which she made a full recovery. According to the plaintiff's attorney, the first surgeon's medical notes indicated that he had performed the procedure incorrectly but failed to so inform his patient. The defendant surgeon contended that it was an acceptable practice to leave one-half of the rectum. Her medical expenses had been $51,438. Experts testified on both sides. The jury deliberated one and a half hours and returned a verdict for the woman and her husband in the amount of $591,438. Usually, a jury spends one and a half hours selecting a foreperson and beginning to review the medical records. This jury appears to have been angered by the facts and spent relatively little time deliberating.

Electronic Medical Records

The age of electronic medical records has brought enormous efficiencies and improved medical quality to the health-care delivery system. All patient records, whether paper or electronic, are discoverable and admissible in medical malpractice lawsuits. In addition, the American Recovery and Reinvestment Act of 2009 amended HIPAA privacy regulations to require providers who use or maintain electronic health records with respect to protected health information (PHI) of individuals, to provide to a patient, upon request, an electronic copy of the patient's electronic health records.[18] This change becomes effective on February 17, 2010. Physicians who record entries in computerized medical records must become familiar with how to use electronic medical systems and should understand that danger lurks in these more efficient computerized systems. For example:

- *BEWARE* drop-down menus and checklists
- *BEWARE* prefabricated medical descriptors
- *BEWARE* prefabricated informed consent notations
- *BEWARE* easy click-on techniques

Not all patient evaluations and regimens can be preformatted. There is a natural tendency for caregivers to pick the "closest" option in a menu of options. Physicians should use "free text" whenever appropriate. It is much easier to defend "your own words" than the words of a computer programer who has written a menu of typical patient diagnoses in drop-down menus or other coded formats.

Communication

Adverse Events, Bad News, and Apologies

When an untoward unexpected event occurs involving a patient, several avenues of communication are critical. First and foremost, the patient's medical needs must be promptly addressed. Coordination of ongoing care, including consultation and follow-up if appropriate, is a critical first step in deflecting a lawsuit.

As soon as practical after the event, the patient and family should be informed of the consequences to the patient in a respectful and sympathetic manner. This discussion should be preliminary to a more detailed discussion that should occur once more facts are obtained as discussed below. Without assigning blame or criticism of other practitioners, the patient and family should be informed of the fact that the event occurred, the current and future consequences to the patient, and what steps have been taken to address the patient's medical condition. If the underlying causes for the event are not yet known, which is frequently the case, care should be taken not to speculate about the underlying causes for the complication. This conversation is usually best handled by a physician well known to the patient and family, although differing circumstances may warrant placing others in that role. Questions should be answered honestly and factually. The patient and family should be told that additional information is conveyed to them as it is known, but in any event that a more thorough discussion occurs within a set period of time, ideally 24 h. It is usually advisable to contact the risk manager or legal counsel if applicable, e.g., when the critical incident occurs in an institution, where such personnel are available. Depending on institutional policy, risk managers, or quality management personnel frequently assist in the interactions with patients and family. They also begin any appropriate administrative activity, such as initiating a sentinel event analysis, notifying an insurance carrier, sequestering medical devices or equipment, initiating an equipment analysis, and reporting device failures to the FDA. The administrative staff may also wish to convene a risk management and/or quality management review that would be protected from discovery in a lawsuit under applicable state privilege statutes. It is also advisable for one member of the institutional team to be designated as the spokesperson to the patient and family so that consistent information is being delivered.

When more facts are gathered and a better understanding of the sequence of events is known, but ideally within 24 h, a family meeting is advisable. The spokesperson should lead the discussion and the patient's attending physician, if not the spokesperson, should be present. The anticipated medical consequences and prognosis for the patient should be discussed, as well as the factual circumstances leading to the incident. Physicians and institutions should be willing to express sympathy and perhaps even apologize for what happened.

In recent years, a number of prominent institutions have urged their physicians to say they are sorry for a patient mishap and provide lawsuit-deflecting apologies. A handful of states have even enacted legislation immunizing various forms of apologies from courtroom use.[19] Advice should be sought from institutional or local legal counsel regarding the admissibility of apologetic statements.

At family meetings, the family members should have an opportunity to ask all of their questions, and they should be given the name and contact information of someone to reach if additional questions arise later. The team should anticipate questions about writing off medical bills and the possibility of a malpractice claim. Any questions about malpractice can be deferred at that point with the explanation that institutional legal counsel or an insurance representative contacts the family if desired. Keeping in touch with the patient and family spokesperson is critical during the next several days and weeks.

A senior member of the medical team, perhaps with the assistance of risk management or legal counsel, should be consulted in reviewing the chart and recording the events involving the untoward incident. The sequence of events, the timing, and the identity of personnel should be completely and accurately recorded. All discussions with the patient and family members after the incident should also be clearly described, including the identity of persons present at the family meetings and what was said.

Many patients and family members at this juncture are considering whether to seek the advice of a lawyer, and they may be urged to do so by friends and other family members. Care should be taken by all members of the health care team to provide a courteous, qualitative, and sympathetic continuity of care and interaction with family members. Physicians and other members of the health care team serve themselves and their patients well by using this time to provide as positive and supportive an experience as possible for patients and family members.

Emails

Because of the efficiencies associated with electronic mail communication, many physicians communicate with both patients and other health care providers by using electronic mail (email). Special care should be taken when using email that contains patient identifiable information.

Clinicians may communicate with other clinicians and patients by email. The Federal HIPAA of 1996[20] (discussed later) provides regulation for electronic transmission containing PHI, such as confidential medical information. HIPAA provides that health care providers have in place appropriate administrative, technical, and physical safeguards to protect the privacy of PHI.[21] The HIPAA regulations do not provide a specific regulatory scheme for email communication, but they do require that providers have procedures that limit disclosures of PHI to the amount reasonably necessary to achieve the purposes of PHI disclosures.[22]

The Notice of Privacy Practices that providers give to their patients must explain in a separate statement that the provider may contact the patient to provide appointment reminders or information about treatment alternatives or other health-related benefits or services that may be of interest to the individual.[23] If this is done by email, it is advisable to state that in the Notice of Privacy Practices.

You may wish to inform your patients that email transmission involves privacy and security issues that may be of interest to them. Patients may even be asked whether they wish to communicate by email or not. Email that is sent to a patient's business may be intercepted by the patient's business colleagues, and emails can be inadvertently transmitted to unintended addressees. The Internet is not considered a secure media for transmitting confidential data unless both parties utilize encryption methodology. These types of warnings can be provided to patients who wish to communicate with their physicians by email. Patients may even be asked whether they wish to communicate with you by email or not.

It is advisable for physicians to keep either paper or electronic copies of emails to and from patients that are relevant to patient treatment. These email copies should be maintained in the patient's medical records just as traditional paper correspondence would be.

Physicians may wish to include a Confidentiality Notice that is preprinted at the bottom of email transmissions. A sample Confidentiality Notice appears below:

> Confidentiality Notice: This email message including attachments, if any, is intended only for the person or entity to which it is addressed and may contain confidential and/or privileged material. Any unauthorized review, use, disclosure or distribution is prohibited. If you are not the intended recipient, please contact the sender by reply email and destroy all copies of the original message. If you are the intended recipient, but do not wish to receive communications through this medium, please so advise the sender immediately.

HIPAA

The Federal HIPAA of 1996 provides national privacy protection for patients. Administrative Regulations (The "Federal Privacy Rule")[24] have been promulgated by the US Department of Health and Human Services (HHS) pursuant to HIPAA. The Federal Privacy Rule establishes minimum privacy standards for health care providers, health plans, and health care clearing houses (referred to in HIPAA as "covered entities") to follow when using and disclosing patient-identifiable PHI that they create or maintain. Generally speaking, PHI is any information that is created (or received) and maintained by a covered entity related to the health or health care of a patient (or payment related to the health care) that directly or indirectly identifies the patient.[25]

The Federal Privacy Rule also requires compliance with state laws that afford greater privacy protections than HIPAA. Compliance with the Federal Privacy Rule was required on and after April 14, 2003. All covered entities must have policies and procedures in place that demonstrate compliance with the Federal Privacy Rule.

HIPAA provides that health care providers must make a good faith effort to give each patient a Notice of Privacy Practices that describes the privacy practices of the health care provider. Patients must be asked to acknowledge in writing that they have received this notice. Once a provider makes a good faith effort to provide a Notice of Privacy Practices to a patient and gets the patient's written acknowledgement of receipt of the Notice, the health care provider may use and disclose PHI for reasons related to the treatment of the patient, payment for the patient's health care, and the health care operations of the provider (TPO). Generally, physicians who are independent practitioners of the hospitals of which they practice are part of those hospitals' "organized health care arrangements," enabling the disclosure of PHI between the hospital personnel and the independently practicing physicians. To use or disclose PHI for reasons other than TPO or as otherwise permitted by law, a physician must obtain an additional written permission from the patient called an "authorization."[26] Clinical research, for example, is not considered "treatment" and usually must be separately approved by research subjects by signing an authorization. In many medical centers, authorizations for clinical research are integrated into the consent form approved by the institutional review board. The Federal Privacy Rule requires that authorizations contain certain elements.[27]

HIPAA permits treating physicians to disclose to a patient's family members, other relatives, close personal friends, and others identified by the patient any PHI that is directly relevant to such person's involvement with the patients care or health care payments. Prior to making any of these disclosures, a physician should either obtain the patient's agreement to the disclosure or reasonably infer from the circumstances that the patient does not object.[28]

A physician needs to be aware, however, of the potential for improper disclosures that this situation creates. Prior to the enactment of the American Recovery and Reinvestment Act of 2009, providers had no obligation to notify patients in the event their PHI was improperly disclosed. The amendments made by the Act to HIPAA require that providers notify their patients and HHS when there has been a "breach" of their PHI. The HHS published regulations pertaining to breaches in August 2009 that became effective September 23, 2009. A "breach" is defined as the unauthorized use, acquisition, access, and disclosure of PHI. The definition excludes unintentional or inadvertent acquisitions made by employees or other authorized persons as long as the PHI is not further used or disclosed.[29] In the event of a breach, a provider is required to notify the patient within 60 days. The notice must include a description of what happened, the information involved, the recommended steps the person should take to protect themselves, and a description of any investigation or mitigation efforts made by the provider.[30]

Research and Innovative Surgery

Research Versus Innovative Practice

The emergence of evidence-based medicine has brought new challenges to the academic medical community. Surgeons and other physicians who serve as investigators in clinical trials are very familiar with the review and approval process of institutional review boards – ethics committees established under federal law to oversee the conduct of research. Many disciplines, especially surgery, have evolved historically in an environment of unregulated innovation. It is often not clear when innovative therapy crosses the line into the research arena.

The Belmont Report[31] states that the distinction between research and practice is blurred and that both often occur together. Research is usually described in a formal protocol, and departures from standard practice are not necessarily "research." The Belmont Report also states:

> The fact that a procedure is "experimental," in the sense of new, untested, or different, does not automatically place it in the category of research. Radically new procedures of this description should, however, be made the object of formal research at an early stage in order to determine whether they are safe and effective. Thus, it is the responsibility of medical practice committees, for example, to insist that a major innovation be incorporated into a formal research project.

Regulation of the practice of medicine has historically been the exclusive province of the state medical boards and other state regulatory authorities. When medical practice crosses the line into "research" involving "human subjects" or investigational drugs, devices, or other test articles, however, the activity becomes subject to the regulation of the federal Office for Human Research Protection (OHRP)[32] for the US Food and Drug Administration.[33] "Research," as regulated, is a systematic investigation, including research development, testing and evaluation, designed to develop or contribute to generalizable knowledge.[34] "Human subjects" are living individuals about whom an investigator conducting research obtains data through intervention or interaction with the individual or identifiable private information.[35] Traditional examples of research studies include prospective industry-sponsored trials.

Data Base Registries

In theory physicians who engage in innovative treatment that does not involve a systematic design, a research protocol, a prospective intent to publish, or an investigational item are not regulated by either OHRP or FDA. Over the past decade, however, OHRP has expressed its view that those systematic collections of data performed off-chart, especially if published, carry an implicit prospective intent and are considered research. These may include ongoing patient registries, including outcomes data; tissue banks; static databases, including ad hoc research from closed trials; and even retrospective studies, including chart reviews, if a prospective intent to publish was present.

In recent years, the OHRP has investigated a variety of innovative techniques to determine whether or not the activities should have been prospectively reviewed by an institutional review board as research. Examples are: 14 patients treated with fractionated stereotactic radiosurgery for the treatment of large arteriovenous malformations prior to IRB approval;[36] publication of a retrospective chart review that was conducted without IRB approval;[37] publication describing partial left ventriculectomies performed in the management of patients with dilated cardiomyopathy without IRB approval[38] and fetal surgery procedures.[39] Many if not all of these scenarios involved publications that used research jargon and implied that a prospective research trial had been conducted (without IRB review and approval). In each of these investigations, OHRP suggested that the applicable institution consider the development of "innovative practice committees" or similar institutional vehicles to evaluate major innovative therapies. Physicians, especially surgeons experimenting with minor surgical modifications to accepted techniques, should use care when authoring articles about clinical experiences that did not involve "research" as defined above. When in doubt physicians are encouraged to consult with their local institutional review boards for guidance.

Promotional Prohibitions

Physicians who conduct FDA-regulated research are prohibited from representing in a promotional context that an investigational new drug, device, or other test article is safe or effective (or otherwise beneficial) before it has received regulatory approval.[40] Physicians should carefully review press releases and other promotional disclosures prepared by commercial sponsors or manufacturers before permitting their names to be associated with such test articles prior to approval.

Insider Trading

If you are involved in clinical trials for pharmaceutical companies or medical device companies whose securities are publicly traded, you may have certain obligations to protect the confidentiality of sensitive information you acquire. Your duties may stem from not only being a company officer or holding another fiduciary position, but also from being an investigator or from serving on company advisory committees like scientific advisory boards, clinical trial steering or executive committees, or data safety monitoring boards. The securities laws widely prohibit fraudulent activities of any kind in connection with the offer, purchase, or sale of securities.[41] These provisions are the basis for many types of government enforcement activities, including actions against illegal insider trading. Insider trading is illegal when a person trades a security while in possession of material, nonpublic information, including information from medical research trials, in violation of a duty to withhold the information or refrain from trading in that security. "Tipping" other traders of such information who then trade a security affected by the tip is also illegal as is acting on an illegal tip.

Conclusion

In recent years, the demands and pressures on physicians and surgeons have grown dramatically. Lawyer advertising and malpractice awards and settlements are greater than ever before. Web-based consumer awareness has increased the knowledge base of patients. Government regulation and enforcement activities have become more focused. Greater understanding and awareness of legal and risk management concerns is critical for health care practitioners facing these challenges.

References

1. Farmer v. Minami, 2003 WL 25273762 (SuperCt King Cty 2003).
2. Bruni v. Tatsumi, 346 NE2d 673 (1976).
3. Kniphfer v. Memorial Health University Med Ctr, 2001 WL 35932959 (Ga State Ct Chatham Cty 2001), rev'd in part, 570 S.E.2d 16. (Ga Ct App) (reversing trial court's denial of pre-judgment interest).
4. Safer v. Estate of Pack, 677 A2d 1188 (N.J. App 1996).
5. Kern KA. Medical malpractice involving colon and rectal disease: a 20-year review of United States civil court litigation. Dis Colon Rectum. 1993;36:531–9.
6. Rex DK, Bond JH, Feld AD. Medical-legal risks of incident cancers after clearing colonoscopy. Am J Gastroenterol. 2001;96:952–7.
7. Barloon TJ, Shumway J. Medical malpractice involving radiologic colon examinations; a review of 38 recent cases. AJR Am J Roentgenol. 1995;165:343–6.
8. Feld AD. Medicolegal implications of colon cancer screening. Gastrointest Endosc Clin N Am. 2002;12(1):171–9.
9. Elfant AB, Korn C, Mendez L, Pello MJ, Peiken SR. Recall of informed consent after endoscopic procedures. Dis Colon Rectum. 1995;38(1):1–3.
10. Finney v. Milton S. Hershey Med Ctr of the Pennsylvania State University, 1996 WL 1125142 (Pa Ct Com Pl Dauphin Cty 1996); Ohio Rev Code § 2317.54.
11. Friter v. Iolab Corp, 607 A.2d 1111 (Pa Super 1992).
12. American Medical Association. Informed consent. www.ama-assn.org/ama/pub. Chicago, IL; 2005.
13. Nickell v. Gonzalez, 477 N.E.2d 1145 (Ohio 1985).
14. Dible v. Vagley, 612 A.2d 493 (Pa Super 1992), app denied, 629 A.2d 1380 (1993).
15. The Joint Commission. http://www.jointcommission.org/. Chicago, IL; 2005.
16. Beck DE. Medicolegal aspects of coloproctologic practice. In: Wexner SD, Zbar AP, Pescatori M, editors. Complex anorectal disorders: investigation & management. London: Springer; 2005. p. 767.
17. Yu v. Kim, 2003 WL 25427269 (Md Cir Ct Baltimore Cnty 2003).
18. 42 USC 17935 (2009).
19. Zimmerman R. Medicine means knowing how to say you're sorry. Pittsburgh Post-Gazette (Pa.) May 23, 2004; Ga Code Ann § 24-3-37.1; Ohio Rev Code § 2317.43; 63 Okl St Ann § 1-1708.1H; S.C. Code 1976 § 19-1-190; S.D. Code Laws § 19-12-14.
20. Pub. L. No. 104-191, 110 Stat. 1942 (1996).
21. 45 C.F.R. § 164.530(c).
22. 45 C.F.R. § 164.514(d).
23. 45 C.F.R. § 164.520(b)(iii)(A).
24. 45 C.F.R. § 164.160, 45 C.F.R. § 162, 45 C.F.R. § 164.
25. 45 C.F.R. § 164.501.
26. 45 C.F.R. § 164.508.
27. 45 C.F.R. § 164.508(c) and (d).
28. 45 C.F.R. § 164.510(b).
29. 45 CFR § 164.402.
30. 45 C.F.R. § 164.404.
31. National Institutes of Health, Department of Health and Human Services. Report of the National Commission for the Protection of Human Subjects of Biomedical and Behavioral Research. Bethesda, MD; 1979.

32. 45 C.F.R. § 46.
33. 21 C.F.R. § 50 and 56.
34. 45 C.F.R. § 46.102(d).
35. 45 C.F.R. § 46.102(f).
36. Office for Human Research Protection, Department of Health and Human Services. Compliance Oversight Determination Letter. Rockville, MD; 1 Aug 2001.
37. Office for Human Research Protection, Department of Health and Human Services. Compliance oversight determination letter. Rockville, MD; 8 Jan 2002.
38. Office for Human Research Protection, Department of Health and Human Services. Compliance oversight determination letter. Rockville, MD; 30 Apr 2002.
39. Office for Human Research Protection, Department of Health and Human Services. Compliance oversight determination letter. Rockville, MD; 13 Feb 2003.
40. U.S. Food and Drug Administration, Department of Health and Human Services. www.fda.gov. Rockville, MD.
41. U.S. Securities and Exchange Commission. www.sec.gov. Washington, DC; 2005.

54 Surgical Education

David J. Schoetz

Surgical education is undergoing exciting and challenging major transformational change within the broader context of healthcare reform, physician shortages, and financial uncertainty. Spurred by seemingly diverse forces such as altered lifestyle expectations among residents and attending physicians, the quality/safety movement, and improved recognition of the evolution of effective educational techniques, the training of surgeons has become extraordinarily complex. Pressures on the educators to provide a more nurturing environment for the students while at the same time performing more clinical work to maintain the financial viability of the teaching institution threaten the ability to train the next generation of surgeons adequately. The traditional "see one, do one, teach one" paradigm of bygone years is no longer feasible; patients do not expect a partially trained and sleep-deprived resident to practice on them without supervision.

Traditional "modern" surgical residencies are generally attributed to Halsted, who initiated the competitive pyramidal system at the Johns Hopkins Hospital based on his early observations in Germany. Prior to this, surgeons were trained in a haphazard manner in a strict apprenticeship model. In the Halsted system, residents spent an average of 8 years in training; following gradual assumption of greater responsibility for patient management over the first 6 years, the chief residency experience was 2 years in duration.[1] During these final 2 years, the resident was, in essence, a junior staff with independent operating privileges. Many of the graduates of this particular training program went on to become professors of surgery, and the success of the program prompted other institutions to follow suit.[2]

Objections to the Halsted model revolved around the master/apprentice relationship and thus the total reliance on the master without regard for validation of the qualities of the teacher. The unnecessary interpersonal competition among colleagues within the residency and the extended period of servitude, resulting in loss of a period of potentially great independent productivity, prompted the development of an alternative training plan by Edward Churchill of the Massachusetts General Hospital.[3] Churchill believed that the junior residents were exploited to provide service to the hospital. He was also convinced of the need for flexibility in training, recognizing differing individual resident capabilities. He was strongly supportive of the need for progressive responsibility for the trainee over the course of the training program. Finally, he abolished the pyramid of Halsted and replaced it with a "rectangular" plan; those who wished to pursue academic careers would need to pursue extra experience outside the residency period.

Cognitive Learning

During the first 60 years of the twentieth century, learning was often by osmosis, without a standardized curriculum. Clinical observation, self-study, and independent patient care were the manner of learning, with obvious individual variations for both the teacher and the student. Supplementation of this process might be by independent reading of relatively scarce textbooks and journals. The need to develop and teach a standardized basic body of knowledge was stimulated in part by the Accreditation Council for Graduate Medical Education (ACGME) and the various Residency Review Committees (RRC). In addition, certifying boards were in the process of creating qualifying and certifying examinations that reflected quality patient care as determined by expert practitioners; this also created a standard curriculum.

Definition of a curriculum is an essential step in education, and graduate surgical education is no exception.[4] Curriculum may be "syllabus based," meaning a list of topics that forms the basis of what is being studied. This is convenient, but treats the learner as a passive recipient. "Objectives-based" curricula are predicated on the faculty identifying behavioral objectives and creating learning-based activities and evaluation tools based on these objectives. These two types of "curriculum as product" are relatively simple and are most commonly used for medical education. More complex is "curriculum as process," requiring continuous interaction between teacher and learner. The main advantage of this

D.E. Beck et al. (eds.), *The ASCRS Textbook of Colon and Rectal Surgery: Second Edition*,
DOI 10.1007/978-1-4419-1584-9_54, © Springer Science+Business Media, LLC 2011

latter type of curriculum is the active participation of the learner in the process. However, it is much more challenging for the faculty; moving toward process-based curriculum will necessitate faculty development programs that move the teachers to a more interactive environment.[4]

Current understanding of adult learning theory would suggest that the lecture format, in which the learner is a passive participant in a unilateral process determined solely by the teacher, is grossly inefficient.[5] Rather, the learner should be an active participant who learns best when actively involved in an individualized interactive learning program. Consequently, the traditional lecture formats that are very comfortable for the teacher are becoming progressively less valued by the new generation of learners. Interactive media and case-based discussions are more beneficial.

Academic conferences in surgical programs consist primarily of lectures, case presentations, and Morbidity and Mortality (M&M) conference. Traditional M&M conferences have been ideally used as a platform to teach both process improvement and personal responsibility. Ultimately, the goal is to improve patient care by identifying factors that contributed to the complication and suggesting ways to prevent them in the future. Regular participation in M&M conferences has been shown to cover much of the curriculum of surgery.[6]

Curriculum redesign is being driven in part by the ACGME Outcome Project, introduced in 1999 as the basis for the development and evaluation of a new curriculum for training physicians.[7] Initially, the ACGME endorsed six competencies:

1. Patient care
2. Medical knowledge
3. Professionalism
4. System-based practice
5. Practice-based learning and improvement
6. Interpersonal and communication skills

Since their introduction, all specialties have been stimulated to embrace competency-based curriculum design and evaluation. The American Board of Medical Specialties has also adopted these competencies for primary board certification and maintenance of certification, lending some continuity in concept over the spectrum of postgraduate medical education and subsequent practice.

Within this construct, conferences must be redesigned to reflect these competencies. M&M can be entirely based on the competencies in order to enhance learning and improve the educational content for all participants.[8] In preparation for the conference, participants should identify the competencies that participate in the adverse outcome and take steps to rectify system problems in a collaborative fashion. The same is true for didactic lecture series, which can and should be redesigned to fit within the framework of the Outcome Project.

Evaluation of the quality of the program and of the educational commitment of the institution is also defined by the competencies. Not only are the program goals and objectives centered around them, but the means of evaluating each individual resident is also based on new methods of evaluation within the framework of the competencies. Strategies such as the creation of a self-defined but externally evaluated educational portfolio, 360° evaluations by other care givers and patients, and scheduled formative evaluations with much more constructive feedback to the trainees are an integral part of the ACGME Outcomes project. Consequently, the demands on program directors and institutions are considerably greater than ever before.[9]

Technical Skills

Unique to the education of proceduralists, including surgeons, is the need to provide technical training resulting in sufficient competence to practice independently at the completion of the training period. Debate continues on whether technical skill should be considered part of medical knowledge or a separate seventh competency. Needless to say, technical performance of various procedures is a core curricular requirement for numerous specialties; validated teaching techniques for procedures are perhaps the most challenging aspect of present-day educational programs.

Traditional teaching of technical skills centered around a brief period of observational learning, perhaps with some training in "dog labs." Pressure to "go to the operating room" resulted in a junior level trainee first observing, then assisting, and finally performing actual procedures with variable supervision and input from master surgeons. Assessment was subjective and relied on the opinions of the faculty as well as excessively on pure numbers of cases performed without a formalized system of technical training with constructive feedback. Attempts to substitute formalized objective written tests have not translated into better or more valid technical skills acquisition; measurement of cognitive capability has been shown to not correlate with technical competency.[10] Rather, the challenge has been to develop methods for not only teaching but also evaluating technical performance.[11] This forms the basis of modern technical training and evaluation.

As learning theory has progressed, methods of acquiring and refining motor skills have been applied to surgical training.[12] Early teaching of technical skills should take place away from the operating room, allowing practice until there is a basic fluidity in the mechanical performance of the task. Expertise is developed by repetitive deliberate practice, from which master technicians are formed.[13] Since the traditional apprenticeship model of training does not often offer this environment for learning, new methods of training and evaluating must be developed, validated, and applied in a formalized curriculum.

The Objective Structure Clinical Examination (OSCE) is a proven accepted method of assessing clinical competence of medical students. Utilizing the same basic philosophy, the University of Toronto developed the Objective Structured Assessment of Technical Skill (OSATS) for surgical residents, in which residents were observed performing various structured operative tasks.[14] Bench model simulation, which is less expensive and more widely applicable, provided equivalent results compared to the use of live animals. Since the initial descriptions of OSATS, it has been demonstrated to be consistently effective in imparting proficiency to surgical residents.[15,16]

With the Residency Review Committee in Surgery requirement for access to simulation and skills facilities in all general surgery residencies,[17] development and utilization of validated curricula for skills acquisition will assume central importance for surgical educators. Creation of a skills laboratory to accomplish training objectives for most surgery residencies need not be prohibitively expensive. Costs can be distributed over all of the intended users.[18,19]

Increasing frequency of the performance of laparoscopic surgical procedures has provided an impetus for the development of curricula and devices that provide basic skills prior to a trainee actually performing surgery on a patient. In fact, teaching laparoscopic skills in the simulation environment is very attractive and much easier than that with an open surgery. Various partial task training exercises have been used by the Society of American Gastrointestinal and Laparoscopic Surgeons (SAGES) to devise the Fundamentals of Laparoscopic Surgery (FLS) program.[5] This program, using box trainers and trained observers, teaches and evaluates five psychomotor skills of basic laparoscopy; it has been endorsed by the American College of Surgeons and the Association of Program Directors in Surgery; the American Board of Surgery requires FLS certification for all graduating general surgery residents. Other specialties involved in the performance of laparoscopic techniques will either use this program or develop their own.

Higher fidelity computer-based systems, although more costly, may provide more advanced procedural skills for residents and practicing surgeons. Students with experience in computer games are more adept at these types of exercises. As in the case of FLS training, which provides transferrable skills to the clinical setting, virtual reality simulators improve performance in the operating room.[20] The major shortcoming of these devices, which are image based, is the lack of haptic feedback; this also limits their application in open surgery.[21] More sophisticated computer applications, particularly with Internet2, are apt to eliminate these limitations in the future. At present, there are considerable challenges regarding validation of various protocols and devices for possible incorporation into a skills curriculum.

Highest fidelity simulation refers predominantly to immersion into an operating room or other interactive scenarios. Secrets to the success of these educational activities are the ability of the participants to suspend reality and a detailed debriefing among those involved after completion of the exercise.[5] In order to optimize the benefit of these activities, which are time intensive for the participants and expensive to provide, validation of the benefits must be built into each learning scenario. Whether a team-based activity, with nursing, operating room staff, anesthesia providers, and surgeons and their trainees, or an individual communication exercise using professional patients or retrospective evaluation of real patient/family interactions, it is clear that this type of learning will find greater application in the near future.

Endoscopy, including both upper endoscopy and colonoscopy, is now a requirement for general surgery graduates. Acquisition of endoscopic skills is facilitated by the use of endoscopy simulators, which can teach basic manipulation of the shaft and dials as well as steering maneuvers. Preparation of the novice endoscopist in the simulation lab accelerates the pace of the development of procedural adequacy.[22] At present, expert colonoscopists can be evaluated but are unlikely to benefit in terms of increased procedural proficiency.[23]

SAGES has parlayed their success in development of the FLS activity to develop a Fundamentals of Endoscopic Surgery (FES) program, which is nearly ready for beta testing. Presuming demonstration of validity of the FES curriculum, it is likely that it will also be adopted by major teaching organizations and the ABS.

Computer-based endoscopy simulators are expensive; their application in the training environment is more limited than that of basic laparoscopy trainers, making recuperation of the cost of the investment in these devices more difficult. Like all simulation exercises, however, they may find much broader applicability in ongoing credentialing and re-entry programs for practicing physicians. The American College of Surgeons has developed a program of accreditation for Basic Skills Labs and Comprehensive Education Institutes in order to extend research and education in teaching of surgeons and other physicians. The basic vision is to create regional education centers that concentrate expertise and share resources.

Challenges

The quality and safety movement, fueled by the highly publicized and excessively politicized report from the Institute of Medicine "To Err is Human: Building a Safer Health System,"[24] has leveraged the belief that exhausted and overworked residents and fellows are significant contributors to substandard patient safety into pressure to change the working environment for trainees. Publicity associated with the infamous "Libby Zion" incident in New York City ultimately resulted in the creation of the Bell Commission in the state of New York and ultimately the national adoption of the 80-h work-hour restrictions by the ACGME in 2003.[25] The currently required duty hours regulations include the following:[26]

1. Duty hours must be limited to 80 h per week.
2. One day in seven free from all educational and clinical responsibilities.

3. 10-h time period provided between all daily duty periods and after in-house call.
4. In-house call must occur no more frequently than every third night.
5. Continuous on-site duty, including in-house call, must not exceed 24 consecutive hours. Residents may remain on duty for up to six additional hours to participate in didactic activities, transfer care of patients, conduct outpatient clinics, and maintain continuity of medical and surgical care.
6. At-home call (or pager call).
   (a) The frequency of at-home call is not subject to the every-third-night, or 24+6 limitation. However, at-home call must not be so frequent as to preclude rest and reasonable personal time for each resident.
   (b) Residents taking at-home call must be provided with 1 day in seven completely free from all educational and clinical responsibilities, averaged over a 4-week period.
   (c) When residents are called into the hospital from home, the hours that residents spend in-house are counted toward the 80-h limit.

These regulations initially resulted in numerous violations, particularly by procedural specialties, resulting in the development of alternative patient care schemes. Night float rotations, nonphysician providers, and staggered shifts were creative ways devised to control hours of resident work; however, these efforts were met with objections that continuity of care would suffer as a result of adoption of a "shift" mentality.

Initial concerns that numbers of cases would be adversely affected by the 80-h rules have generally not been substantiated.[27] There has been a shift in operative experience, however. As the inpatients in the hospital have become more acutely ill, junior residents spend less time in the operating room. Expectations for acquisition of technical capabilities have been lowered for interns, who spend most of their time in the hospital outside of the operating room environment. Performance of complex cases is delayed until later in the residency, often resulting in residents who complete 5 years of training not having the skills or confidence to practice independently. As a result, a greater percentage of graduates seek additional fellowship training.[28–30]

Residents do appreciate the improved quality of life that they enjoy as a result of hours regulation; not all are equally enthusiastic about the effects on their training, with a potentially more adversarial relationship with their attendings, who must do extra work and hire physician extenders to perform tasks previously done by residents. Certainly, residents and attendings must be more resourceful in allocating index operative cases within defined time periods. While the benefits and detriments of the 80-h rules have been debated, a recent report from the surgical services at the University of Vermont has demonstrated a significant reduction in morbidity and mortality after adoption of the hour regulations.[31]

In fact, since the hour restrictions have been in effect for only 5 years (the duration of training of a general surgeon), the real end result of current regulations cannot yet be measured and is certainly more complex than some would suggest. Despite this uncertainty, in December 2008, the Institute of Medicine released a report and recommendations on resident duty hours.[32] This report recommends doing away with averaging of hours worked and in so doing, essentially reduces the number of hours that can be worked to much fewer than 80 h per week. It also does away with moonlighting during residency, which is a threat to residents in training who are often significantly in debt from student loans and who are expected to begin to repay these loans after completion of school and during residency. This most recent IOM report has resulted in a maelstrom of activity directed against adoption of the IOM recommendations predicated on the belief that we have not yet accurately assessed the effect of the 2003 regulations on training of physicians.[33–35] The ACGME has responded to the IOM by creating a task force with multiple stakeholder representation. Their work has recently been summarized as follows:[36]

1. The safety of patients is of utmost importance; the responsibility for safety resides with the resident, the attending and the systems of care.
2. Graded authority and responsibility on the part of residents are substantially diminished, with concerns for inadequate training.
3. There is a need for some flexibility in standards between specialties.
4. There are effects (in some instances unintended consequences) of alterations in training schemes on other specialties.
5. Residents are more rested and do have more satisfaction with their life.
6. Absolute rules and "substantial compliance" are very different in practice; rigid adherence to absolute rules often challenges professionalism and patient care.

Suffice it to say that multiple competing agendas must be acknowledged and resolved by reasonable compromise. Clearly, the training of surgeons is affected by the hours regulations.

Financing of graduate medical education from the Medicare budget is also an enormous long term challenge to the training of physicians. A summary of the method of federal payment for residents and fellows[37] indicates that the direct payment for residents has become inadequate to pay for resident training; an adjustment for teaching hospitals designed to reimburse the anticipated greater cost of care due to inefficiency and waste has been progressively reduced as the pressures on the Medicare trust fund have increased. With the exception of one redistribution of unused positions (which was not an absolute increase), the numbers of residency positions have been capped at 1997 levels by the Balanced

Budget Act; this is at a time when there is a public mandate to increase the number of graduates from medical school by 20–30% over 10 years and also during significant growth in the numbers of eligible Medicare recipients.[38]

Highly publicized Medicare fraud allegations resulting in substantial monetary fines and even the threat of prison have resulted in stricter requirements for documentation and supervision guidelines. Increasingly litigious and adversarial relationships among physician, attorneys, and patients have undermined confidence in the system of training physicians. The opportunity to provide an environment of progressive independent practice within a residency program has become difficult at best. Extension of the duration of training in ACGME recognized training programs is financially unattractive, since the initial period of full reimbursement for each resident/fellow is fixed by law and not likely to be lengthened; increasing the length of training is at the expense of institutional operating budgets.

Colon and Rectal Surgery

Needless to say, since general surgery residency is the foundation for colon and rectal surgery training, these factors that are challenging the quality of the 5-year trainee in general surgery have a substantial effect on colon and rectal surgical training. At present, the duration of training in colon and rectal surgery is 1 year beyond general surgery; in the past, this had been sufficient to essentially double the volume of cases done by a 5-year surgery trainee in the one additional year.[39] Competition for an increasing number of available residency positions in colon and rectal surgery is brisk, with 1.4 applicants per available position.[40] The changes in general surgery training just outlined have pressured colon and rectal surgeons to consider increasing the duration of training to 2 years, which may make the specialty less attractive to general surgery trainees who are considering advanced training.

In 2006, the primary constituents of the specialty, led by the American Board of Colon and Rectal Surgery (ABCRS) but also with representation from the RRC, the Program Directors Association (PDA) and the American Society of Colon and Rectal Surgeons (ASCRS), created a Blue Ribbon Committee. This was in response to the much heralded American Surgical Association Blue Ribbon Committee, which reported in 2004.[41] This latter committee also included major stakeholders in general surgery including the American Board of Surgery, the RRC and the American College of Surgeons as well as the American Surgical Association. Prompted by an apparent loss of interest by medical students in seeking a career in general surgery, this effort was an introspective examination of the factors that might make the specialty more attractive to medical students. The executive summary is a comprehensive document in which the foundation of traditional general surgery education is challenged at all levels. Proposed restructured training would provide for a basic core curriculum followed by advanced specialty and subspecialty training, divorced from practical considerations of funding of residency positions.

The American Board of Surgery has been the primary motivator of the development of the SCORE (Surgical Council on Resident Education) project.[42] Other members of this transformational project are the American College of Surgeons, the American Surgical Association, the Association of Program Directors in Surgery, the Association for Surgical Education and the RRC for Surgery. SCORE is in the process of developing specific learning objectives for each of the topics within 28 organ system-based categories. Operations and procedures are classified as Essential-common, Essential-uncommon and Complex. Procedural competency is not expected for complex procedures.

For colorectal procedures, total proctocolectomy including ileoanal reservoir, is considered complex.[42] For anorectal procedures, complex procedures include:

(a) Stapled hemorrhoidectomy
(b) Repair of complex anorectal fistulae
(c) Operation for incontinence/constipation
(d) Abdominal operations for rectal prolapse, both open and laparoscopic
(e) Perineal operations for rectal prolapse
(f) Operations for rectal cancer, including transanal resection and abdominoperineal resection

The implications of these changes in the anticipated experience for a general surgery trainee are obvious for colorectal surgeons. The colon and rectal surgeons must evaluate all aspects of colon and rectal training in light of possible significant future changes in general surgery residency.

One consideration has been to increase the duration of training from 1 to 2 years for colon and rectal surgery. A survey of graduates of colorectal training programs taking the ABCRS examination from 2005 to 2007 was administered and determined that general surgery residents decide relatively late in their training to pursue additional colorectal surgery residency positions.[43] This reflected the effect of mentoring and exposure to the field relatively late during general surgery residency. Shortening the overall duration of general surgery training was not favored by a 2:1 margin; if the general surgery training in preparation for colon and rectal surgery was diminished to 4 years, all acknowledge that colorectal training would extend to at least 2 years. Financial considerations for funding of 2 year residencies, as outlined above, would be a substantial impediment to this schema. Furthermore, a change to a 4/2 scheme would be disruptive to general surgery training programs, with the loss of approximately 80 chief residents.

An important factor to consider when evaluating a change in residency design/construct is that a significant percentage of practicing colon and rectal surgeons continue to perform some general surgery as part of their practice.[44] While the amount of non-colorectal tends to diminish as their practice matures, 48% of board certified colorectal surgeons still perform general surgery to some extent. Maintaining certification in both general and colorectal surgery may be unattractive unless there can be recognition of a shared body of knowledge and some reciprocity in the accreditation process; since the numbers of general surgeons are critically low, losing that percentage of general surgery performed by colorectal surgeons because of failure to maintain certification would have negative consequences.[45]

The Program Directors in Colon and Rectal Surgery have developed an essential curriculum, which has been ratified by the ABCRS. The ASCRS, which is the educational arm of the specialty, has arranged for the publication of this curriculum as a textbook, which is based on the agreed-upon curriculum. As a living document that reflects changes in core concepts of the specialty, the curriculum has formed the basis for didactic teaching and testing in colon and rectal surgery.

Technical requirements for satisfactory completion of a colon and rectal residency are in flux. For some time the ABCRS used 17 categories developed from the case lists of applicants for board certification.[45] Deficiencies in more than five operative categories were sufficient to prevent a candidate from qualifying for examination, with the presumption that the individual had not received adequate training to become a certified specialist. While the use of a rolling average acknowledged the changing practice patterns in tertiary centers, it has become increasingly clear that numbers of cases are a poor surrogate for technical competence. Furthermore, the rather liberal allowance of five category deficiencies allowed candidates with significant inadequacies in their overall education to sit for the examination. The Colon and Rectal Surgery Blue Ribbon Committee recommended to the ABCRS that absolute minimum standards be adopted and this is currently in transition as data are collected and analyzed; it is anticipated that these new more stringent requirements will be fully operational by 2011–2012.[46,47]

Since it is increasingly clear that numbers of operative cases performed do not necessarily equate to technical competence, considerable energy must be directed at the development of formative and summative evaluation instruments for assessment of procedural training. These efforts are cosponsored by all of the parties involved in training of colon and rectal surgeons. In addition, non-technical components of training must be scrutinized and, where necessary, altered to increase their overall contribution to training. If the primary aim of residency training is to prepare safe practitioners and protect the public, then all efforts must be directed at improving our ability to do so and to continue that capability for a professional lifetime.

Acknowledgment. This chapter was written by Clifford L. Simmang and Richard K. Reznick in the previous version of this textbook.

References

1. Halsted WS. The training of the surgeon. Bull Johns Hopkins Hosp. 1904;15:267–75.
2. Cameron JL. William Stewart Halsted: our surgical heritage. Ann Surg. 1997;225:445–58.
3. Grillo HC, Edward D. Churchill and the "rectangular" surgical residency. Surgery. 2004;136:947–52.
4. DaRosa DA, Bell RH. Graduate surgical education redesign: reflections on curriculum theory and practice. Surgery. 2004;136:966–74.
5. Tsuda S, Scott D, Doyle J, Jones DB. Surgical skills training and simulation. Curr Probl Surg. 2009;46:266–370.
6. Veldenz HC, Dovgan PS, Schinco MS, Tepas JJ. Morbidity and mortality conference: enhancing delivery of surgery residency curricula. Curr Surg. 2001;58:580–2.
7. http://www.acgme.org/Outcome/. Accessed 1/31/11.
8. Rosenfeld JC. Using the morbidity and mortality conference to teach and assess the ACGME general competencies. Curr Surg. 2005;62:664–9.
9. Sidhu RS, Grober ED, Musselman LJ, Reznick RK. Assessing competency in surgery: where to begin? Surgery. 2004;135: 6–20.
10. Scott DJ, Valentine J, Bergen PC, et al. Evaluating surgical competency with the American Board of Surgery In-training examination, skill testing, and intraoperative assessment. Surgery. 2000;128:612–22.
11. Reznick R, Regehr G, MacRae H, et al. Testing technical skill via an innovative "bench station" examination. Am J Surg. 1996;172:226–30.
12. Reznick RK, MacRae H. Teaching surgical skills-changes in the wind. N Engl J Med. 2006;355:2664–9.
13. Ericsson KA. Deliberate practice and the acquisition and maintenance of expert performance in medicine and related domains. Acad Med. 2004;79:S70–81.
14. Martin JA, Regehr G, Reznick R, Macrae H, et al. Objective structured assessment of technical skills (OSATS) for surgical residents. Br J Surg. 1997;84:273–8.
15. Grober ED, Hamstra SJ, Wanzel KR, Reznick RK, et al. The educational impact of bench model fidelity on the acquisition of technical skill. The use of clinically relevant outcome measures. Ann Surg. 2004;240:374–81.
16. Chipman JG, Schmitz CC. Using objective structured assessment of technical skills to evaluate a basic skills simulation curriculum for first-year surgical residents. J Am Coll Surg. 2009;209:364–70.
17. http://www.acgme.org/acWebsite/downloads/RRC_progReq/440_general_surgery_01012008_u08102008.pdf
18. Berg DA, Milner RE, Fisher CA, et al. A cost effective approach to establishing a surgical skills laboratory. Surgery. 2007;142:712–21.
19. Haluck RS, Satava RM, Fried G, et al. Establishing a simulation center for surgical skills: what to do and how to do it. Surg Endosc. 2007;21:1223–32.
20. Seymour NE, Gallagher AG, Roman SA, et al. Virtual reality training improves operating room performance. Results of a randomized, double-blinded study. Ann Surg. 2002;236:458–64.
21. Jakimowicz J, Fingerhut A. Simulation in surgery. Br J Surg. 2009;96:563–4.

22. Gerson LB. Evidence-based assessment of endoscopic simulators for training. Gastrointest Endosc Clin N Am. 2006;16: 489–509.
23. Koch AD, Buzink SN, Heemskerk J, et al. Expert and construct validity of the Simbionix GI Mentor II endoscopy simulator for colonoscopy. Surg Endosc. 2008;22:158–62.
24. To err is human: building a safer health system. Institute of Medicine Consensus Report, November 1999.
25. Killelea BK, Chao L, Scarpanito V, Wallack MK. The 80-hour workweek. Surg Clin North Am. 2004;84:1557–72.
26. http://www.acgme.org/acWebsite/dutyHours/dh_Lang703.pdf. Accessed 1/31/11.
27. Mendoza KA, Britt LD. Resident operative experience during transition to work-hour reform. Arch Surg. 2005;140: 137–45.
28. Gawande AA. Creating the educated surgeon in the 21st century. Am J Surg. 2001;181:551–6.
29. Doherty GM. Surgery resident education 1986–2008: effort, respect and advocacy. World J Surg. 2009;33:378–85.
30. Bell RH. Why Johnny cannot operate. Surgery. 2009;146: 533–42.
31. Shackford PAR, SR OT, et al. Implementation of resident work hour restrictions is associated with a reduction in mortality and provider-related complications on the surgical service. A concurrent analysis of 14,610 patients. Ann Surg. 2009;250:316–21.
32. Resident duty hours: enhancing sleep, supervision, and safety, December 2008.
33. Britt LD, Sachdeva AK, Healy GB, et al. Resident duty hours in surgery for ensuring patient safety, providing optimum resident education and training, and promoting resident well-being: a response from the American College of Surgeons to the report of the Institute of Medicine, "Resident Duty Hours: Enhancing Sleep, Supervision, and Safety". Surgery. 2009;146:398–409.
34. Lewis FR. Comment of the American Board of Surgery on the recommendation of the Institute of Medicine report, "Resident Duty Hours: Enhancing Sleep, Supervision, and Safety". Surgery. 2009;146:410–9.
35. Borman KR, Fuhrman GM. "Resident Duty Hours: Enhancing Sleep, Supervision, and Safety": Response of the Association of Program Directors in Surgery to the December 2008 Report of the Institute of Medicine. Surgery. 2009;146:420–42.
36. http://www.acgme.org/acWebsite/home/NascaLetterCommunity10_27_09.pdf. Accessed 1/31/11.
37. http://www.aamc.org/advocacy/library/gme/dgmebroc.pdf. Accessed 12/30/09.
38. http://www.aamc.org/advocacy/library/workforce/workforce-position.pdf. Accessed 12/30/09.
39. Schoetz DJ. Colon and rectal surgery: a true subspecialty. Dis Colon Rectum. 1998;41:1–10.
40. http://www.nrmp.org/data/resultsanddatasms2009.pdf. p. 26. Accessed 1/31/11.
41. Debas HT, Bass BL, Brennan MF, et al. American Surgical Association Blue Ribbon Committee Report on Surgical Education: 2004. Ann Surg. 2004;2005:50–7.
42. http://www.surgicalcore.org/patientcareoutline.html. Accessed 1/31/11.
43. Schmitz CC, Rothenberger DA, Trudel JL, Wolff BG. Career decisions and the structure of training. An American Board of Colon and Rectal Surgery survey of colorectal residents. Ann Surg. 2009;250:62–7.
44. Chu KM, Schoetz DJ. What impact might general surgery practice patters of colon and rectal surgeons have on future training? Dis Colon Rectum. 2007;50:1–5.
45. Williams TE, Satiani B, Thomas A, Ellison EC. The impending shortage and the estimated cost of training the surgical workforce. Ann Surg. 2009;250:590–7.
46. Schoetz DJ. Evolving practice patterns in colon and rectal surgery. J Am Coll Surg. 2006;203:322–7.
47. http://www.abcrs.org/html/emp/pdfs/min_op_standards.pdf. Accessed 1/31/11.

55 Continuing Medical Education

Martin Luchtefeld

Background

In today's world, the pace of increasing medical knowledge is unprecedented. The challenge for the practicing physician is to stay abreast of relevant new information in their field of practice. For the surgeon, there is the additional challenge of learning new techniques that have evolved since their surgical training period. The American Board of Medical Specialists and ACGME have attempted to define the competent physician by outlining six core competencies (Table 55-1).[1] This definition of the competent physician has gained widespread use in graduate medical education and several of these competencies speak directly to this issue of maintaining one's ability to practice medicine competently after residency: practice-based learning and improvement, medical knowledge, and patient care. Unfortunately, there is not a well-defined infrastructure to continue a practicing physician's education, such as that exists for medical students and residency/fellowship education.

In the surgical world, this problem is particularly acute. The consequences of performing procedures before being fully trained can be disastrous to the patient.

The relatively recent experience of the introduction of laparoscopic cholecystectomy illustrates the consequences of insufficient training and less-than-rigorous credentialing. When first introduced, there was a strong public demand for the laparoscopic approach to cholecystectomy. At the time, cholecystectomy was the most common procedure done by general surgeons at approximately 500,000 cases per year. A surgeon who could not do the procedure laparoscopically soon found that referrals diminished and practice suffered. As a consequence, there was a rush to provide training in the procedure. Unfortunately, there was no system in place to provide this training to the surgeon and surgical team. Courses were provided but were quite variable in the quality of education. The best courses included didactic sessions, videos, training in black boxes and procedures done in animal models that closely simulated the experience of laparoscopic cholecystectomy in humans. The courses certified attendance, but there were no specific guidelines to certify competence in the procedure. Hospitals faced the same economic pressures as the surgeons and credentialing standards and the awarding of privileges was lax. It was not uncommon for a surgeon to take a weekend course and schedule procedures the following week.[2] The result of this combination of unfortunate events was a great increase in the number of bile duct injuries.[3]

One of the concepts to emerge from this was that of the "learning curve." For cholecystectomy, the learning curve has been estimated to be 50 cases. This estimate is based on reports that 90% of bile duct injuries occur in the first 30 cases and that the calculated risk for injury is 1.7% on the first case and 0.17% on the fiftieth case.[4]

In an effort to avoid the problems encountered with the initiation of laparoscopic cholecystectomy, the American Society of Colon and Rectal Surgeons (ASCRS) approved a registry that was housed by the American College of Surgeons (ACS) Commission on Cancer and endorsed by the Society of Gastrointestinal and Endoscopic Surgeons (SAGES).[5] In addition, the ASCRS issued a position paper that colorectal cancer should best be treated laparoscopically only if the surgeon was participating in a trial or a prospective registry that would allow the evaluation of results at a later date.[6] Lastly, it was recommended that only surgeons who had performed at least 20 laparoscopic colon surgeries should attempt a laparoscopic colectomy for cancer with curative intent.[7]

Surgeons, with industry support, combined to provide a better mechanism for training and for the initiation and application of new technology. Over the past two decades, the laparoscopic approach was adopted for many procedures in addition to colectomy, such as Nissen fundoplication and bariatric surgery without the problems seen with laparoscopic cholecystectomy.

However, despite the successes of the introduction of various laparoscopic procedures, there is still a lack of a cohesive system to provide ongoing education for the practicing physician as well as lack of a defined curriculum and/or standards

D.E. Beck et al. (eds.), *The ASCRS Textbook of Colon and Rectal Surgery: Second Edition*,
DOI 10.1007/978-1-4419-1584-9_55, © Springer Science+Business Media, LLC 2011

TABLE 55-1. Six core competencies of the competent physician

1. Patient care
2. Medical knowledge
3. Practice-based learning and improvement
4. Interpersonal and communication skills
5. Professionalism
6. Systems-based practice

of accreditation. Most of the present system revolves around Continuing Medical Education (CME) credits.

CME, as defined by the Accreditation Council for Continuing Medical Education (ACCME), "constitutes educational activities that serve to maintain, develop, or increase the knowledge, skills, performance, and the relationships a physician uses to provide services for patients, the public, or the profession."[8]

History of Ongoing Education

The first requirements for CME began in 1934 when the American Board of Urology mandated this as a way to enhance specialist education of recent scientific advances.[9] CME remains the primary way that practicing physicians' document and continue their education outside of the university setting.[10] As of 2006, 56 of 68 state and territorial licensing boards require certain levels of completion of CME for recertification of their medical licenses, including all allopathic and osteopathic licensure boards in the USA and the US territories.[11]

Even though CME is a major venue for education for the practicing physician and one of the primary means of demonstrating competence, there is little evidence to support the effectiveness of CME as it is currently structured to improve patient care or outcomes.[12,13] Partially in response to this shortcoming, the AMA commissioned a task force called the "initiative to Transform Medical Education" to consider reform of all medical education, including CME. The stated goal of the initiative was to "…promote excellence in patient care by implementing reform in the medical education and training system across the continuum, from premedical preparation and medical school admission through continuing physician professional development."[14] Despite the efforts of this task force, to date, there has been very little change in the CME field.

The American College of Chest Physicians obtained support form the Agency for Healthcare Research and Quality (AHRQ) to review the data for the effectiveness of CME. The AHRQ awarded this funding to the Johns Hopkins Evidence-Based Practice Center (EPC) to do a systematic review and attempt to answer several key questions.

CME Effectiveness on Practice Performance

This review identified 105 studies that evaluated the impact of CME on physician practice performance, both short-term and long-term. A wide range of objectives was studied, including prescribing, screening, guideline adherence, and others. Even though the majority of studies reported positive outcomes, slightly less than 30% did not. Nine studies reported mixed results.[15]

This same review attempted to review the question of which media was most effective for CME. Nine of 20 studies that evaluated single live media had positive long-term outcomes. Of the remaining studies, three had mixed results, three did not change behavior, and four studies lacked a control group.

Single print media did not seem to be effective; eight of the nine studies evaluated did not meet their objectives, whereas 40 of the 57 studies using multiple media met their objective.[15]

The effects of specific educational techniques were also evaluated. Multiple techniques were included in this review: academic detailing, audience response systems, case-based learning, clinical experiences, demonstrations, discussion groups, feedback, lectures, mentoring or precepting programs, point-of-care techniques, problem-based learning, team-based learning, programed learning, readings, role play, simulations with standardized patients, and writing. Review of the eleven studies that evaluated the use of single technique suggested that there was not a positive impact on practice behavior. A number of reports evaluated either multiple techniques (76 studies) or compared multiple techniques to single technique (18 studies). While the evidence was not overwhelming, the data suggested that multiple techniques were more useful that single techniques in achieving a positive impact on practice behavior.[15]

The effect of a single exposure to CME was evaluated as was multiple exposures. Of the studies with a single exposure, just under half of the studies demonstrated a positive effect. In comparison, almost two-thirds of the studies that used multiple exposures to CME met their objectives.[15]

CME Effectiveness for Knowledge Application and Psychomotor Skills

The number of studies that are related to CME and physician knowledge application are few in number. In the EPC review, only 15 studies evaluated either knowledge application or psychomotor skills training. Even in these 15 studies, it was felt that the overall quality of evidence was low.[16] The studies on knowledge application were evaluated only in primary care physicians. Most studies (11 of 12) demonstrated effectiveness in improving knowledge application in the short term. As might be expected, multiple exposures and longer duration led to better results.

In the realm of psychomotor skills, there were only three studies to evaluate. In all three, the methods studied all improved psychomotor skills. However, the skills being taught were simple (knee injection, flexible sigmoidoscopy, and ankle/knee exam), and there was not enough information to make recommendations regarding the optimal methods.[16]

CME: Simulation Research

Included among possible forms of CME for a colon and rectal surgeon is simulation. Medical simulation is defined as "a person, device, or set of conditions which attempts to present [education and] evaluation problems authentically. The student or trainee is required to respond to the problems as he or she would under natural circumstances. Frequently the trainee receives performance feedback as if he or she were in the real situation."[17]

There is hope that simulation may give a practicing surgeon another alternative to develop the technical skills necessary to perform a new procedure before attempting this procedure on a patient. Simulation can be done in many ways: computer models, anatomical models, solitary or team performances. Although simulation can be valuable for certain aspects of medical education, the evidence for the effectiveness of simulation in the literature is relatively weak. AHRQ issued a report whose aim was to synthesize the results of nine literature reviews on simulation.[18] However, these reviews all evaluated simulation *outside* of CME.

While the authors of the AHRQ felt that simulation was an effective method of teaching, the overall strength of the evidence was weak due to there being only a small number of studies and not much quantitative data.[19] In addition, eight of the nine reviews had a narrow focus (single medical specialty, single simulation method) and the primary studies themselves were weak.[20]

One of the reviews cited by the AHRQ was the Best Evidence Medical Education (BEME) collaboration.[19] This review was broader in scope and evaluated all best educational practices in 670 journal articles. The studies were heterogeneous enough and weak methodologically so that rather than doing a quantitative meta-analysis instead a qualitative, narrative summary was done. The authors of the review stated that "the weight of the best available evidence suggests that high-fidelity medical simulations facilitate learning under the right conditions."[19] The conditions that facilitated learning are seen in Table 55-2.

There was a subset of 31 articles with enough data to allow a quantitative meta-analysis. These studies were designed to answer the question of whether or not there was an association between hours spent on simulation-based practice and learning outcomes. Perhaps not surprisingly, there was a highly significant "dose response" between practice time and achievement.[19]

Table 55-2. The 10 conditions to facilitate learning

1. Feedback is provided during learning experiences
2. Learners engage in repetitive practice
3. Simulation is integrated into an overall curriculum
4. Learners practice tasks with increasing levels of difficulty
5. Simulation is adaptable to multiple learning strategies
6. Clinical variation is built into simulation experiences
7. Simulation events occur in a controlled environment
8. Individualized learning is an option
9. Outcomes or benchmarks are clearly defined or measured
10. The simulation is a valid representation of clinical practice

Adapted from Issenberg SB, McGaghie WC, Petrusa ER et al. Features and uses of high-fidelity medical simulations that lead to effective learning: a BEME systematic review. Med Teach 2005;27:10–28.[19]

CME: Best Educational Practices

In a review of best educational practices, McGaghie et al.[20] suggested that CME best practices would have the following three elements: mastery learning, deliberate practice, and recognition that cultural barriers in the medical profession that inhibit best educational practices.

Mastery Learning

Mastery learning has a number of key elements (Table 55-3). The objective in mastery learning is to assure that the final educational objectives are met by all learners with little or no variation in outcome. It is recognized that not all learners reach these objectives at the same time. Mastery learning can be applied to technical/physical skills as well as knowledge gains, features of medical professionalism, and affective qualities.[20]

Deliberate Practice

Deliberate practice has at least nine requirements (Table 55-4) that can be considered an educational variable associated with strong education as part of the mastery learning model. Although deliberate practice is demanding of learners, it is well grounded in theories of skill acquisition and maintenance. Deliberate practice should enable constant improvement of a skill or knowledge rather than simply maintaining a certain level of competence.[20]

Cultural Barriers

There are a number of barriers to the implementation of best educational practices. Despite a paucity of research to suggest its efficacy, the current system of CME is well established,

TABLE 55-3. Elements of mastery learning

1. Baseline or diagnostic testing
2. Clear learning objectives, sequenced as units in increasing difficulty
3. Engagement in educational activities (e.g., skills practice, data interpretation, reading, focused on reaching the objectives)
4. A set minimum passing standard (e.g., test score) for each educational unit
5. Formative testing to gauge unit completion at a preset minimum passing standard for mastery
6. Advancement to the next educational unit given measured achievement at or above the mastery standard
7. Continued practice or study on an educational unit until the mastery standard is reached.

Adapted from McGaghie WC, Siddall VJ, Mazmanian PE, Myers J. Lessons for continuing medical education from simulation research in undergraduate and graduate medical education: effectiveness of continuing medical education: American College Of Chest Physicians evidence-based educational guidelines. Chest 2009;135:62S–8.[20]

TABLE 55-4. Deliberate practice requirements

1. Highly motivated learners with good concentration
2. Engagement with a well-defined learning objective or task
3. Appropriate level of difficulty
4. Focused, repetitive practice
5. Rigorous, precise measurements
6. Informative feedback from educational sources (e.g., simulators or teachers)
7. Monitoring, correction of errors, and more deliberate practice
8. Evaluation to reach a mastery standard
9. Advancement to another task or unit.

Adapted from McGaghie WC, Siddall VJ, Mazmanian PE, Myers J. Lessons for continuing medical education from simulation research in undergraduate and graduate medical education: effectiveness of continuing medical education: American College Of Chest Physicians evidence-based educational guidelines. Chest 2009;135:62S–8.[20]

and it would take considerable time, effort, and resources to overcome inertia and make significant change. Much of education in the past has been patient centered so the notion of simulation and deliberate practice is a relatively foreign idea. The practicing physician has had very little in the way of outside motivators to require the use of more demanding ongoing education.[20]

CME and Maintenance of Certification

The American Board of Opthalmic Examinations was founded in 1916 and administered its first board certification exam in 1917. Other specialty boards followed and then in 1933 the American Board of Medical Specialties was formed to "act in an advisory capacity to these boards" and to "stimulate improvement in postgraduate medical education." There are now 24 member boards of the ABMS. Certification was considered life-long but the issue of recertification was raised as early as 1936. Eventually, the rapid advance of medical knowledge lead to the recognition of the need for recertification although the first recertification examinations were not given until 1969.[11] The next evolution of this process is Maintenance of Certification (MOC), developed and introduced by the ABMS in 2000.[21] The implication is that the practitioner is *maintaining* competence and skills on a continuous basis rather than simply *recertifying* every 5–10 years. MOC has four elements (which are a distillation of the six elements of the competent physician):

Part I: Professional standing
Part II: Life-long learning and self-assessment
Part III: Cognitive expertise
Part IV: Practice performance assessment

In order to maintain certification, diplomats of the 24 member Boards (of which the American Board of Colon and Rectal Surgery is one) of the ABMS must satisfy all four parts of the MOC process. All member Boards require certain levels of CME to fulfill the requirements of lifelong learning (Part II). CME can also impact Part IV (practice performance assessment) helping physicians address their own practice performance by CME activities.

The Future of CME

It is clear that there is a need to improve the education system for practicing physicians. ACS has attempted to address this need in one way by accrediting Education Institutes. The stated goal of these Institutes is to "focus on competencies and to specifically address the teaching, learning, and assessment of technical skills using state-of-the-art educational methods and cutting-edge technology." The Institutes, to obtain certification, must plan to use a variety of methods, including bench models, simulation, simulators, and virtual reality to ensure that participants reach predetermined levels of skill by the completion of the course. There are also plans to do education research as well to better understand the science of acquisition and maintenance of surgical competence.[22]

The concept of mini-fellowships has also arisen as a way to fill the void for the practicing surgeon who desires to learn new skills or techniques. An internet search reveals that there are mini-fellowships for a vast array of technical skills. The sponsors can be industry, academic healthcare institutions, or in many cases a combination of both. The length of time commitment ranges from 3 days to 3 months. The experience almost always involves a combination of learning techniques, including didactics, simulation, cadaver labs, and video sessions. In some of these mini-fellowships, there is also opportunity to actually participate in surgery. These educational opportunities have not been studied but by using multiple techniques of teaching they are likely to be reasonably effective.

Parker and Parikh have recommended that CME in the future include the three following elements: assessment of learner needs, program design to meet those needs, and outcome assessment.[23] In the world of colon and rectal surgery, there are several learner needs. The most obvious of these is the need to learn technical skills related to new technology and new procedures. Another powerful driver of needs assessment is performance measures. Performance measures are drawn from a number of sources, including the American Medical Association's Physician Consortium for Performance Improvement, the National Committee for Quality Assurance, the Agency for Healthcare Research and Quality, the National Quality Forum and Centers for Medicare and Medicaid Services. Performance measures are usually derived from evidence-based clinical guidelines. CME providers should be aware of the participants' baseline knowledge of the science behind these guidelines.

In an ideal CME program, the practitioner could have learning opportunities based on their own practice performance. This would allow the physicians to compare their own data to established benchmarks and guidelines. Ultimately, this could lead to the improvement in quality and safety in the physicians' practice.

Technology has an evolving role in CME. It has already changed the way CME is delivered by way of CD-ROMs to computers to Internet-based podcasts. This has clearly made CME more accessible to the practitioner who is not based at a university or teaching facility. The emerging use of electronic medical records and computerized order entry facilitates the physicians' ability to track their own practice performance. For surgeons, the increasing complexity and fidelity of simulation enhance the learning of new techniques.

References

1. Accreditation Council for Graduate Medical Education. History of GME. http://www.acgme.org/acWebsite/home/home.asp.
2. Ellison EC, Carey LC. Lessons learned from the evolution of the laparoscopic revolution. Surg Clin N Am. 2009;88:927–41.
3. Ferguson CM, Rattner DW, Warshaw AL. Bile duct injuries in laparoscopic cholecystectomy. Surg Laparosc Endosc. 1992;2:1–7.
4. Moore MJ, Bennett CL. The learning curve for laparoscopic cholecystectomy. The Southern Surgeon Club. Am J Surg. 1995;170:55–9.
5. Ortega AE, Beart RW, Steele GD, et al. Laparoscopic bowel surgery registry: preliminary results. Dis Colon Rectum. 1995;38:681–6.
6. The American Society of Colon and Rectal Surgeons. Approved statement on laparoscopic colectomy. Dis Colon Rectum. 1994;37:8–12.
7. Laparoscopic Colectomy for Curable Cancer. Position Statement of the American Society of Colon and Rectal Surgeons (ASCRS) Endorsed by the Society of American Gastrointestinal Endoscopic Surgeons (SAGES). http://www.fascrs.org/physicians/position_statements/laparoscopic_colectomy/.
8. American Council for Continuing Medical Education CME Content. http://www.accme.org/index.cfm/fa/Policy.policy/Policy.
9. Josseron L, Chaperon J. History of continuing medical education in the United States. Presse Med. 2001;30(10):493–7 (in French).
10. ACCME. ACCME annual report data. Chicago;2004:1–12.
11. Schrock JW, Cydulka RK. Lifelong learning. Emerg Med Clin N Am. 2006;24:785–95.
12. Davis DA, Taylor-Vaisey A. Translating guidelines into practice. A systematic review of theoretic concepts, practical experience and research evidence in the adoption of clinical practice guidelines. CMAJ. 1997;157:408–16.
13. Grimshaw JM, Russell IT. Effect of clinical guidelines on medical practice: a systematic review of rigorous evaluations. Lancet. 1993;342:1317–22.
14. American Medical Association in *Initiative to transform medical education: phase 3: program implementation; recommendations for optimizing the medical education learning environment – final report of the December 2007 working conference*. http://www.ama-assn.org/ama1/pub/upload/mm/377/finalitme.pdf.
15. Davis D, Galbraith R. Continuing medical education: effectiveness of continuing medical education: American College of Chest Physicians evidence-based educational guidelines. Chest. 2009;135:42S–8.
16. O'Neil KM, Addrizzo-Harris DJ. Continuing medical education effect on physician knowledge application and psychomotor skills: effectiveness of continuing medical education: American College of Chest Physicians evidence-based educational guidelines. Chest. 2009;135:37S–41.
17. McGaghie WC. Innovative simulations for assessing professional competence. In: Tekian A, McGuire CH, McGaghie WC, editors. Simulation in professional competence assessment: basic considerations. Chicago, IL: Department of Medical Education, University of Illinois at Chicago; 1999. p. 7–22.
18. Marinopoulos SS, Dorman T, Ratanawongsa N, et al. (2007) *Effectiveness of continuing medical education* (Agency for Healthcare Research and Quality, Rockville, MD) Evidence Report/Technology Assessment No 149.
19. Issenberg SB, McGaghie WC, Petrusa ER, et al. Features and uses of high-fidelity medical simulations that lead to effective learning: a BEME systematic review. Med Teach. 2005;27:10–28.
20. McGaghie WC, Siddall VJ, Mazmanian PE, Myers J. Lessons for continuing medical education from simulation research in undergraduate and graduate medical education: effectiveness of continuing medical education: American College of Chest Physicians evidence-based educational guidelines. Chest. 2009;135:62S–8.
21. American Board of Medical Specialties ABMS maintenance of certification.http://www.abms.org/Maintenance_of_Certification/ABMS_MOC.aspx.
22. American College of Surgeons Website. http://www.facs.org/.
23. Parker K, Parikh SV. Applying Prochaska's model of change to needs assessment, programme planning and outcome measurement. J Eval Clin Pract. 2001;7:365–71.

56 Quality

Formosa Chen, Hiroko Kunitake, Elise Lawson, Joan Ryoo, and Clifford Y. Ko

Introduction

This topic is an interesting one, in that much research has been performed in this area and much policy has been enacted to improve quality of care. While an entire set of textbooks could be written on quality of care, the aims of this chapter are more focused on perhaps what would be interesting and important to a colon and rectal surgeon.

Thus, the specific aims of this chapter are to (1) familiarize the reader with the important principles and terminology in quality of care, (2) illustrate the application of these principles using colorectal surgery specific examples, and (3) provide a working knowledge to help today's surgeons navigate an environment where quality is increasingly being emphasized.

Background

The spotlight has been on health-care quality since the publication of the Institute of Medicine reports "*To Err is Human: Building a Safer Health System*" in 1999 and "*Crossing the Quality Chasm: A New Health System for the 21st Century*" in 2001. These reports brought to the public consciousness the issues of preventable medical errors and the gap between medical knowledge and medical practice.[1,2] What was surprising was not that errors occurred or that quality was suboptimal, but the frequency and degree to which they were found. The notion that in-hospital deaths due to preventable medical errors represented the eighth leading cause of death in the USA was alarming to providers and patients alike.

In the decade since the publication of these reports, the quality movement has intensified, and health-care quality measurement and assurance have become major topics at the forefront of health-care regulation and reform. Fueled by sensational stories in the popular media and the ready availability of information on the Internet, consumers are also learning to demand more from their health-care providers. Multiple stakeholders are involved in the quality movement, including the federal and state governments, insurance companies, employer groups, hospitals, physicians, and patients. Today, it is no longer possible to practice medicine without being confronted by the daily demands for higher quality care.

Defining "Quality" in Health Care

Defining quality of care is difficult because of the different viewpoints on what quality is and how it is defined. Avedis Donabedian wrote: "The definition of quality may be almost anything anyone wishes it to be, although it is, ordinarily, a reflection of values and goals current in the medical care system and in the larger society of which it is a part."[3] Currently, the most commonly cited definition of quality of care comes from the Institute of Medicine (IOM):

> Quality of care is the degree to which health services for individuals and populations increase the likelihood of desired health outcomes and are consistent with current professional knowledge.[4]

Even with such a concisely worded definition, challenging issues arise. Whose desired outcomes? Do the patient's or provider's desires matter more? How do we measure these outcomes? What is and who determines the current professional knowledge? To focus the agenda on quality improvement, the IOM has proposed six key dimensions of quality as areas for emphasis and additional research. They propose that a health system should be safe, effective, patient-centered, timely, efficient, and equitable. Each of these dimensions is addressed to some extent in this chapter.

Regardless of how each stakeholder and organization defines and prioritizes "quality," it is perhaps more important to understand how quality is conceptualized, how it is measured, and how these concepts and measurements impact patients, providers/surgeons, and the practice of health care. These themes provide the structure for the following sections of this chapter.

D.E. Beck et al. (eds.), *The ASCRS Textbook of Colon and Rectal Surgery: Second Edition*,
DOI 10.1007/978-1-4419-1584-9_56, © Springer Science+Business Media, LLC 2011

The History of Quality in Surgery

Despite the recent acceleration of the quality movement, awareness of the significance of quality of care in surgery arose nearly a century ago with Dr. Ernest Codman, a surgeon who began his career in Boston at the Massachusetts General Hospital. Dr. Codman proposed the "end result system" in which doctors would follow up their patients to determine the results and complications of treatment and make these findings public. He lost his staff privileges in 1914 when he proposed that surgeon competence should be evaluated, and he eventually established his own hospital to pursue performance measurement and improvement objectives. Dr. Codman was one of the founders of the American College of Surgeons and later the Joint Commission on the Accreditation of Hospitals. Dr. Codman's pursuit of surgical outcomes and his endorsement of transparency in medical care are now part of the foundation upon which we strive to improve surgical quality in the USA.

Influenced by Dr. Codman's efforts to improve the quality of care through the self-examination of clinical practice, in 1935, the Philadelphia County Medical Society established the Anesthesia Mortality Committee, the antecedent to the now familiar Morbidity and Mortality Conference.[5] Later renamed the Anesthesia Study Commission, they published a report in 1947 stating that at least two thirds of fatalities reviewed were classified as preventable.[6] Morbidity and Mortality conferences are now a required educational activity mandated by the Accreditation Council for Graduate Medical Education (ACGME) for all residency programs, although conferences vary in their effectiveness in terms of quality evaluation and improvement.

One century ago, surgeons who championed the need for examining their own quality of care were shunned. Today health-care quality improvement and assurance are incentivized and increasingly regulated. The methodologies used to evaluate care have evolved from the examination of experiential case series to the ability to perform complex and sophisticated statistical models and comparisons. Thus, one of the goals of this chapter is to try to simplify the state of the knowledge in health-care quality so that surgeons can apply it to their clinical practices. Instead of being driven by the external forces of change, surgeons should probably be drivers of quality improvement in their practices to benefit their patients.

A Conceptual Model of Quality of Care: The Donabedian Model of Quality of Care

Many have strived to develop means of understanding the multiple components of our complex and fragmented health-care system. One approach has been through the use of conceptual models. One of the most commonly used models for thinking about health-care quality is the Donabedian Model of Quality of Care, originally described by Avedis Donabedian as three *distinct* aspects of "outcome, process, and structure."[3] The model was later refined into a causal chain of the three interrelated components of (1) structure, (2) process, and (3) outcome (Figure 56-1). In this model, structure facilitates the processes of care, and both in turn impact outcomes. Each of these components is defined and discussed in further detail in the following sections.

The Donabedian Model (Part 1): Structure

"Structure" in the Donabedian model refers to the characteristics of the setting and providers in and through which health care takes place. Structural measures can describe entities as broad as the overall health care system or as specific as an individual physician.

Structural Measure at the Health System Level

An example of a structural measure that assesses quality at the level of the overall health-care system is the adequacy of the health-care workforce to meet the needs and demands of the population that it serves. An inadequate physician

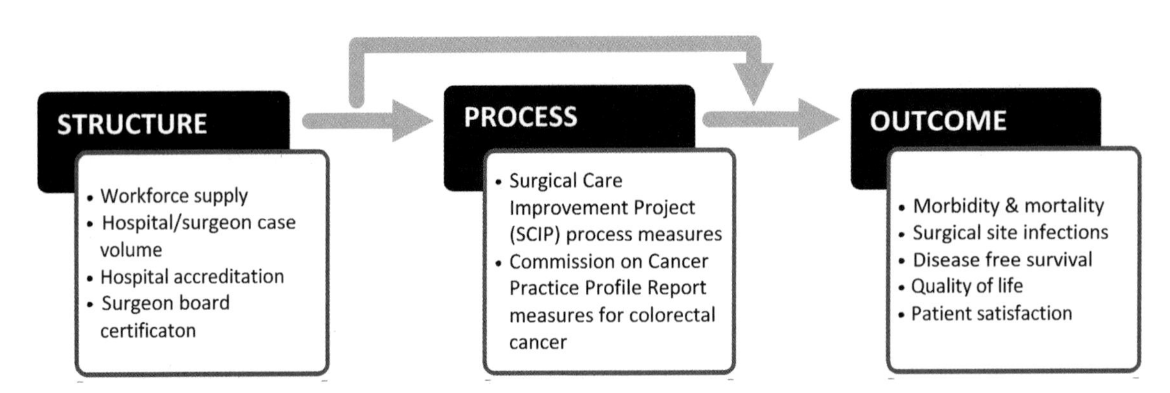

FIGURE 56-1. The Donabedian Model of Quality of Care: Interrelated components of structure, process, and outcome.

supply can lead to decreased access to appropriate specialists, delays in receipt of essential services, and worsened population health-related outcomes. The extremes of surgical workforce shortages are illustrated in developing countries such as Sierra Leone where there are four obstetricians in a country of 6 million (0.13 per 100,000 population)[7] or Uganda where there are 75 general surgeons serving a population of 30 million (0.25 per 100,000 population).[8] In contrast, on average there are 45 surgeons per 100,000 population in the USA. Despite this, surgical workforce shortages in the USA have been projected in multiple subspecialties by multiple studies.[9–14] A recent study by Williams et al.[11] has projected an imminent shortage of 1,300 general surgeons in the USA by 2010. The Association of American Medical Colleges (AAMC) also predicts a shortage of 124,000 physicians by 2025, with 33% of the shortage occurring in surgical specialties.[15] The AAMC has responded to the projected physician shortage by backing the Resident Physician Shortage Reduction Act of 2009, which proposes to increase the number of Medicare-supported residency positions by 15,000 slots, a 15% increase. However, this bill has stalled in Congress since its introduction in May 2009. While there are no studies specifically examining the projected workforce adequacy of colorectal surgeons, Etzioni et al.[10] projected a 47% increase in the number of oncologic colon and rectal resections between 2000 and 2020. Using different data sources, Etizioni et al.[16] also found that the demand for outpatient and inpatient colorectal procedures will increase by 21.3% and 40.6%, respectively, between 2005 and 2025.

Some researchers contend that overall there is no personnel shortage, but rather a misdistribution of surgeons between oversaturated and underserved areas.[17] Nevertheless, most studies agree that the growing elderly population will increase the demand for surgical services. Whether recent and upcoming policy changes to address the workforce shortage or whether market forces to affect the redistribution of surgeons can overcome the projected crisis is still to be seen. However, colorectal surgeons will certainly be faced with the challenge of providing more services to an expanding elderly population in an environment where surgeons will increasingly be held accountable for their outcomes. In the Donabedian model, the projected shortage of surgeons represents a potential structural flaw which will affect downstream processes and outcomes.

Structural Measure at the Institution Level

Examples of structural measures at the institution level include hospital accreditation status, nurse-to-patient ratios, availability of specialty services (e.g., interventional radiology, transplant services, etc.), teaching status or affiliation with academic institutions, and hospital volume.

Accreditation is a stamp of approval given to an institution, such as a hospital, or a cancer center by a respected authority, such as the Joint Commission on the Accreditation of Health Care Organizations or the Commission on Cancer of the American College of Surgeons, after a series of minimum qualifying criteria or benchmark standards have been met. Accredited institutions are believed to be of higher quality because they meet the stringent criteria of the accrediting body. From an institutional standpoint, accreditation activities are often integral to performance and quality improvement efforts. The pros of accreditation are as follows: (1) it provides a standardized evaluation of institutions that facilitates benchmarking and comparison; (2) preparing for and undergoing accreditation can promote organizational change and result in better cultures and systems for quality improvement; (3) being labeled "high quality" can lead to more patient referrals; and (4) some studies have found that accreditation is associated with higher quality care.[18] The cons of accreditation are as follows: (1) the process can be bureaucratic, administratively burdensome, and costly; and (2) some criticize accreditation as a superficial exercise with little bearing on actual quality. A systematic review of accreditation studies by Greenfield et al.[19] found no consistent relationship between accreditation status and quality indicators, with some studies showing a positive association and others showing no relationship between the two. In colorectal surgery, supporters of accreditation have proposed that accrediting programs for rectal cancer or inflammatory bowel disease may be beneficial in promoting higher quality and more standardized care for these patient populations. To date, potential programs such as these have remained solely in the "discussion" phase.

The topic of hospital volume, or the volume–outcome relationship, has also recently received increasing attention in the surgical literature. The volume–outcome relationship is the observed association between provider case volume and patient outcomes, usually with increasing provider volume (hospital or surgeon) associated with improved patient outcomes. This was first described in the surgical literature in 1979 by Luft et al.[20] who looked at mortality rates in 12 surgical procedures across 1,498 hospitals. The majority of studies examining the volume–outcome relationship have focused on short-term perioperative mortality, with fewer studies examining other outcomes such as long-term survival, cancer recurrence, length of stay, cost of care, and postoperative complications. A meta-analysis performed by Gruen et al.[21] examined the volume–outcome relationship between provider volume and mortality for six gastrointestinal cancers (esophagus, stomach, liver, pancreas, colon, and rectum). Using unadjusted mortality results from 101 publications, this group found a statistically significant inverse relationship between hospital volume and short-term perioperative mortality for all cancers except rectal cancer. However, they also noted that one-third of the reviewed studies found no association between hospital or surgeon volume and mortality. A systematic review performed by Killeen et al.[22] summarized the findings of 16 studies examining the volume–outcome relationship in colorectal cancer resection and concluded that the evidence supported a significant inverse relationship between volume and the outcomes of in-hospital mortality, 30-day mortality, and 5-year survival. However, the magnitude of the volume effect on mortality was small.

Other areas in colorectal surgery where a consistent volume–outcome relationship has been demonstrated include the increased use of laparoscopic and sphincter-sparing procedures by high-volume providers.[23–27] Most studies looking at the harvesting of lymph nodes in cancer procedures have found a significant volume–outcome relationship.[28–31] Studies examining postoperative complications have had mixed results.[29,31–37] With regard to benign colorectal diseases, two studies found that higher hospital volumes are associated with lower mortality following surgery for inflammatory bowel disease.[38,39] One study found that high-volume hospitals and surgeons were more likely to perform laparoscopic instead of open resections for diverticular disease. Studies examining cost of care have found that high-volume providers have shorter lengths of stay and in-hospital costs.[31,34,40,41]

Proponents of the volume–outcome relationship argue that regionalizing high-risk procedures to select high-volume providers can save patient lives. Critics argue that it is unclear whether increased volume leads to improved quality or whether high-quality care attracts more volume. They also argue that volume measures penalize low volume but high-quality providers. Regionalization policies may also adversely affect patient access to care and continuity of care if they are limited to select high-volume facilities that may be further away or outside of their list of usual providers. Given that the volume–outcome relationship is not consistently demonstrated across studies, some argue that volume is an imperfect proxy for quality.

Despite the ongoing controversy, health-care payers have incorporated structural measures into their criteria for "Centers of Excellence" to incentivize patients to utilize qualifying facilities or providers. A notable example is the Leapfrog Group's "Evidence-Based Hospital Referral" (EBHR) recommendations in which they establish a minimum annual hospital volume for seven higher-risk surgical procedures as a referral criteria and encourage purchasers, be they insurance companies or employer groups, to use their "leverage" to recognize and reward hospitals that meet EBHR standards.[1] Volume may solely be a proxy measure of quality, but it is increasingly being used by payers to determine referral patterns and may ultimately impact where surgeons choose to practice and the procedures they perform.

[1] The Leapfrog Group is a consortium of large employers that focuses on health-care quality. Their "Evidence-Based Hospital Referral" recommendations can be found at http://www.leapfrog-group.org/media/file/Leapfrog-Evidence-Based_Hospital_Referral_Fact_Sheet.pdf.

Structural Measure at the Practitioner Level

Examples of structural measures at the practitioner level include board certification and subspecialty training. Recently, there has been controversy surrounding the use of board certification as a colon and rectal surgeon as a marker for surgical quality in contrast to general surgeons. Board certification as a colon and rectal surgeon requires successful completion of an ACGME approved training program in general surgery and one additional year in an ACGME approved colon and rectal surgery residency. The candidate must then pass both the written (qualifying) and oral (certifying) examinations given by the American Board of Colon and Rectal Surgery. Overall, studies have generally shown improved outcomes for surgeons with specialty training.[42–45] A systematic review by Bilimoria et al.[43], which examined the effect of surgeon training and specialization on outcomes following colorectal cancer surgery, found lower recurrence rates in five out of the ten studies and improved long-term survival in seven of the ten studies for colorectal trained surgeons.[43] However, it was unclear if the additional training or having a specialized practice was responsible for the difference in outcomes. A study by Prystowsky et al.[46] found that American Board of Surgery (ABS) certification was associated with reduced mortality and morbidity but colorectal surgery training did not significantly affect outcomes. In this study, increasing years of experience was associated with reduced mortality. Board certification and specialty training are two examples of structural components which interact with structural components at the institutional and health-system level to influence process and outcome in the care of the colorectal surgery patient.

The Limitations of Structural Measures of Quality

There is a great deal of literature examining structural measures of quality and their association with patient outcomes. Evidence supporting the validity of these measures has prompted policy makers to adapt and apply these measures to influence health-care utilization patterns. However, the most significant downside to structural measures is their relative immutability, especially from the perspective of an individual surgeon. While structural measures may have an important role in policy discussions and population-based planning, there may be little that the surgeon can change in the structure of their practice to ultimately impact patient outcomes.

The Donabedian Model (Part 2): Process

Process refers to what providers do to the patient or do for the patient. Everything that occurs in the continuum of patient care constitutes a process of care. The literature contains numerous clinical practice guidelines that describe treatment processes and algorithms that comply with the standard of care or represent best practices. An example is the National Comprehensive Cancer Network

TABLE 56-1. An example of the distinction between a clinical guideline and a good measure

ASCRS practice parameter for the prevention of venous thrombosis[48]	Surgical care improvement project (SCIP) VTE prophylaxis process measure
Patients in the moderate-risk to high-risk categories for VTE undergoing abdominal surgery should receive prophylaxis with unfractionated (LDUH) or low-molecular-weight heparin (LMWH). Patients at risk for bleeding may receive mechanical prophylaxis instead.	*Numerator Statement*: Surgery patients who received appropriate venous thromboembolism (VTE) prophylaxis within 24 h prior to *Anesthesia Start Time* to 24 h after *Anesthesia End Time*. *Denominator Statement*: All selected surgery patients

TABLE 56-2. Examples of process measures in colorectal surgery

Name	Description and general application
Surgical Care Improvement Project (SCIP) process measures	Measures appropriate use of perioperative prophylactic antibiotics (selection, timing, and discontinuation), use of clippers for hair removal (instead of razors), immediate postoperative normothermia, use of venothromboembolism prophylaxis (selection and timing), continuation of perioperative beta-blockers, and removal of urinary catheters by postoperative day 2. Applicable to all surgical patients
National Quality Forum National Voluntary Consensus Standards for Quality of Cancer Care	Includes four colorectal cancer quality measures addressing the removal and examination of at least 12 lymph nodes in colon cancer resections, the completeness and quality of pathology reporting, and the timeliness of adjuvant chemotherapy in stage III colon cancer
National Initiative for Cancer Care Quality (NICCQ) quality indicators for colorectal cancer	Set of 25 indicators addressing multiple clinical domains. Measures cover diagnostic testing, pathology reporting, documentation, referrals to specialists, timing and receipt of treatment, technical quality of care, and respect for patient preferences. Applicable to stage II–III colorectal cancers

(NCCN) Practice Guidelines in Oncology.[2] Becoming more popular and commonplace are similar concepts – that being process measures or quality indicators. These are also processes that have been identified to be associated with high-quality care and have been developed into tools that can quantitatively measure how frequently these processes take place during patient care.

The difference between practice guidelines and process measures is that guidelines are often qualitative recommendations that often include gray areas of variable appropriateness, allowing for a physician's clinical judgment and patient preferences. In contrast, process measures are quantitative measurements, have simplistic measurement algorithms, and can be used to set standards of care.[47] Table 56-1 is an example of the distinction between a clinical guideline and a process measure.

The ASCRS practice parameter proposes the recommended care but uses words like "should" and "may," leaving the ultimate treatment decision up to the surgeon. The SCIP process measure on the other hand quantifies within a specific surgical population, the percentage of patients who actually received appropriate VTE prophylaxis within a defined 48 h window.

A good process measure has the following characteristics: (1) it is explicit in its inclusion and exclusion criteria (denominator); (2) it is rigid in its requirements for satisfying the process (numerator); and (3) it is linked to outcomes. Because good process measures are linked to quality of care, they are often called "quality indicators."

Examples of process measures or quality indicators include the Surgical Care Improvement Project (SCIP) process measures, the National Quality Forum National Consensus Standards for Quality of Cancer Care, and the National Initiative for Cancer Care Quality (NICCQ) quality indicators for colorectal cancers (Table 56-2).[48–50] These quality indicators establish the standard of care that patients should receive; they are explicit, quantitative, and evidence-based, and there is a growing trend by regulatory bodies and payers to use such quality indicators to set standards for appropriate care.

SCIP measures are reported to the Joint Commission and the Center for Medicare and Medicaid Services (CMS). These measures include the use of perioperative prophylactic antibiotics, the use of clippers for hair removal, immediate postoperative normothermia, the use of venothromboembolism prophylaxis, continuation of perioperative beta-blockers, and the removal of urinary catheters by postoperative day 2. Data collection on SCIP measures began in 2004 and has since become the focus of many institution-wide quality improvement (QI) efforts.

The utility of process measures or quality indicators lies in their ability to be measured and improved. As such, QI programs are often developed around indicators like the SCIP measures. Data collection and indicator measurement can be accomplished either prospectively or retrospectively and are often carried out by a nurse abstractor. Following baseline measurement of an organization's adherence to a set of quality indicators such as the SCIP measures, tailored

[2] The National Comprehensive Cancer Network (NCCN) Practice Guidelines in Oncology can be found at http://www.nccn.org/professionals/physician_gls/f_guidelines.asp.

interventions can then be designed and implemented to target areas of poor performance. The effectiveness of the QI program is demonstrated by improvement in adherence rates to the indicators. The ultimate goal of these QI programs is to improve patient outcomes by improving the delivery of specific processes of care.

The strength of the association between quality indicators and patient outcomes is based on the validity of the underlying scientific evidence. The development of process measures or quality indicators is often accomplished using Delphi methods that combine best evidence and expert opinion.[51] Follow-up studies examining the association between adherence to the quality indicators and patient outcomes are ultimately necessary to confirm the clinical validity of the measures. An example is a study by Pastor et al. examining the relationship between adherence to the SCIP measures and surgical site infections (SSI) in colorectal surgery patients. They found no significant reduction in the rate of SSI, despite significant improvements in compliance with the SCIP measures.[52] Studies like this raise the question of whether expending significant resources to improve performance in SCIP measures is actually improving patient outcomes. However, more studies are ultimately necessary to prove or disprove the validity of the SCIP measures.

One of the best ways to identify processes of care is through randomized controlled trials (RCTs). In point of fact, RCTs are considered the most reliable and impartial methods for determining which medical interventions work the best. Within colorectal surgery, the majority of clinical trials focus on new chemotherapy regimens or surgical techniques. Table 56-3 lists many of the colorectal-relevant randomized clinical trials published in the last 2 years. Although RCTs provide valuable information regarding specific treatment regimens, they are limited by the restricted selection of clinical trial participants, and therefore the results may not be absolutely generalizable to specific patients.

TABLE 56-3. Randomized controlled trials, Cochrane reviews, and protocols in colorectal surgery and colorectal diseases (2009–2010)

Study	Study description
Randomized clinical trials	
Laparoscopic vs. open	
Allardyce RA, et al. Br J Surg. 2010 Jan;97(1):86–91.	Australasian Laparoscopic Colon Cancer Study shows that elderly patients may benefit from lower postoperative complication rates following laparoscopic versus open resection
Cheung HY, et al. Arch Surg. 2009 Dec;144(12):1127–32.	Endolaparoscopic approach vs conventional open surgery in the treatment of obstructing left-sided colon cancer: a randomized controlled trial
Neudecker J, et al. Br J Surg. 2009 Dec;96(12):1458–67.	Short-term outcomes from a prospective randomized trial comparing laparoscopic and open surgery for colorectal cancer
Lujan J, et al. Br J Surg. 2009 Sep;96(9):982–9.	Randomized clinical trial comparing laparoscopic and open surgery in patients with rectal cancer
Buunen M, et al. Dan Med Bull. 2009 May;56(2):89–91.	COLOR II. A randomized clinical trial comparing laparoscopic and open surgery for rectal cancer
Ng SS, et al. Dis Colon Rectum. 2009 Apr;52(4):558–66.	Long-term morbidity and oncologic outcomes of laparoscopic-assisted anterior resection for upper rectal cancer: 10-year results of a prospective, randomized trial
Buunen M, et al. Lancet Oncol. 2009 Jan;10(1):44–52. Epub 2008 Dec 13.	Survival after laparoscopic surgery versus open surgery for colon cancer: long-term outcome of a randomised clinical trial
Allardyce RA, et al. ANZ J Surg. 2008 Oct;78(10):840–7.	Australian and New Zealand study comparing laparoscopic and open surgeries for colon cancer in adults: organization and conduct
Marcello PW, et al. Dis Colon Rectum. 2008 Jun;51(6):818–26; discussion 826–8. Epub 2008 Apr 17.	Hand-assisted laparoscopic vs. laparoscopic colorectal surgery: a multicenter, prospective, randomized trial
Rink AD, et al. Dis Colon Rectum. 2009 Oct;52(10): 1738–45.	Laparoscopic-assisted or laparoscopic-facilitated sigmoidectomy for diverticular disease? A prospective randomized trial on postoperative pain and analgesic consumption
Vignali A, et al. Dis Colon Rectum. 2009 Jun;52(6): 1080–8.	Effect of prednisolone on local and systemic response in laparoscopic vs. open colon surgery: a randomized, double-blind, placebo-controlled trial
Chemotherapy	
Braun MS, et al. J Clin Oncol. 2009 Nov 20;27(33): 5519–28. Epub 2009 Oct 26.	Association of molecular markers with toxicity outcomes in a randomized trial of chemotherapy for advanced colorectal cancer: the FOCUS trial
Okines A, et al. Br J Cancer. 2009 Oct 6;101(7):1033–8.	Surgery with curative-intent in patients treated with first-line chemotherapy plus bevacizumab for metastatic colorectal cancer First BEAT and the randomised phase-III NO16966 trial
Van Cutsem E, et al. N Engl J Med. 2009 Apr 2;360(14): 1408–17.	Cetuximab and chemotherapy as initial treatment for metastatic colorectal cancer
Jackson NA, et al. Cancer. 2009 Jun 15;115(12):2617–29.	Comparing safety and efficacy of first-line irinotecan/fluoropyrimidine combinations in elderly vs. nonelderly patients with metastatic colorectal cancer: findings from the bolus, infusional, or capecitabine with camptostar-celecoxib study

(Continued)

Table 56-3. (*Continued*)

Study	Study description
Kim GP, et al. J Clin Oncol. 2009 Jun 10;27(17):2848–54. Epub 2009 Apr 20.	Phase III noninferiority trial comparing irinotecan with oxaliplatin, fluorouracil, and leucovorin in patients with advanced colorectal carcinoma previously treated with fluorouracil: N9841
Roh MS, et al. J Clin Oncol. 2009 Nov 1;27(31):5124–30. Epub 2009 Sep 21.	Preoperative multimodality therapy improves disease-free survival in patients with carcinoma of the rectum: NSABP R-03
Debucquoy A, et al. Radiother Oncol. 2009 Nov;93(2): 273–8. Epub 2009 Sep 9.	Double blind randomized phase II study with radiation + 5-fluorouracil +/− celecoxib for resectable rectal cancer
Kono T, et al. Jpn J Clin Oncol. 2009 Dec;39(12):847–9. Epub 2009 Sep 4.	Preventive effect of goshajinkigan on peripheral neurotoxicity of FOLFOX therapy: a placebo-controlled double-blind randomized phase II study (the GONE Study)
Koda K, et al. Hepatogastroenterology. 2009 Jan–Feb; 56(89):116–9.	Randomized, controlled study of continuous 5-FU infusion starting immediately after curative surgery for advanced colorectal cancer
André T, et al. J Clin Oncol. 2009 Jul 1;27(19):3109–16. Epub 2009 May 18.	Improved overall survival with oxaliplatin, fluorouracil, and leucovorin as adjuvant treatment in stage II or III colon cancer in the MOSAIC trial
Van Cutsem E, et al. J Clin Oncol. 2009 Jul 1;27(19): 3117–25. Epub 2009 May 18.	Randomized phase III trial comparing biweekly infusional fluorouracil/leucovorin alone or with irinotecan in the adjuvant treatment of stage III colon cancer: PETACC-3
Kanemitsu Y, et al. Jpn J Clin Oncol. 2009 Jun;39(6): 406–9. Epub 2009 Apr 23.	A randomized phase II/III trial comparing hepatectomy followed by mFOLFOX6 with hepatectomy alone as treatment for liver metastasis from colorectal cancer: Japan Clinical Oncology Group Study JCOG0603
Skof E, et al. BMC Cancer. 2009 Apr 22;9:120.	Capecitabine plus Irinotecan (XELIRI regimen) compared to 5-FU/LV plus Irinotecan (FOLFIRI regimen) as neoadjuvant treatment for patients with unresectable liver-only metastases of metastatic colorectal cancer: a randomised prospective phase II trial
Bertagnolli MM, et al. J Clin Oncol. 2009 Apr 10;27(11): 1814–21. Epub 2009 Mar 9.	Microsatellite instability predicts improved response to adjuvant therapy with irinotecan, fluorouracil, and leucovorin in stage III colon cancer: Cancer and Leukemia Group B Protocol 89803
Fields AL, et al. J Clin Oncol. 2009 Apr 20;27(12):1941–7. Epub 2009 Mar 9.	Adjuvant therapy with the monoclonal antibody Edrecolomab plus fluorouracil-based therapy does not improve overall survival of patients with stage III colon cancer
Sebag-Montefiore D, et al. Lancet. 2009 Mar 7;373(9666): 811–20.	Preoperative radiotherapy versus selective postoperative chemoradiotherapy in patients with rectal cancer (MRC CR07 and NCIC-CTG C016): a multicentre, randomised trial
Dahl O, et al. Acta Oncol. 2009;48(3):368–76.	Final results of a randomised phase III study on adjuvant chemotherapy with 5 FU and levamisol in colon and rectum cancer stage II and III by the Norwegian Gastrointestinal Cancer Group
Robertson JD, et al. Clin Colorectal Cancer. 2009 Jan;8(1): 59–60.	Phase III trial of FOLFOX plus bevacizumab or cediranib (AZD2171) as first-line treatment of patients with metastatic colorectal cancer: HORIZON III
Siegel R, et al. BMC Cancer. 2009 Feb 6;9:50.	Preoperative short-course radiotherapy versus combined radiochemotherapy in locally advanced rectal cancer: a multi-centre prospectively randomised study of the Berlin Cancer Society
Ychou M, et al. Ann Oncol. 2009 Apr;20(4):674–80. Epub 2009 Jan 29.	A phase III randomised trial of LV5FU2 + irinotecan versus LV5FU2 alone in adjuvant high-risk colon cancer (FNCLCC Accord02/FFCD9802)
Adams RA, et al. Br J Cancer. 2009 Jan 27;100(2):251–8.	Toxicity associated with combination oxaliplatin plus fluoropyrimidine with or without cetuximab in the MRC COIN trial experience
Bidard FC, et al. Ann Oncol. 2009 Jun;20(6):1042–7. Epub 2009 Jan 19.	Efficacy of FOLFIRI-3 (irinotecan D1,D3 combined with LV5-FU) or other irinotecan-based regimens in oxaliplatin-pretreated metastatic colorectal cancer in the GERCOR OPTIMOX1 study
Hecht JR, et al. J Clin Oncol. 2009 Feb 10;27(5):672–80. Epub 2008 Dec 29.	A randomized phase IIIB trial of chemotherapy, bevacizumab, and panitumumab compared with chemotherapy and bevacizumab alone for metastatic colorectal cancer
Bokemeyer C, et al. J Clin Oncol. 2009 Feb 10;27(5): 663–71. Epub 2008 Dec 29.	Fluorouracil, leucovorin, and oxaliplatin with and without cetuximab in the first-line treatment of metastatic colorectal cancer
Sastre J, et al. Crit Rev Oncol Hematol. 2009 May;70(2):134–44. Epub 2008 Dec 25.PMID: 19111473.	Elderly patients with advanced colorectal cancer derive similar benefit without excessive toxicity after first-line chemotherapy with oxaliplatin-based combinations: comparative outcomes from the 03-TTD-01 phase III study
Kabbinavar FF, et al. J Clin Oncol. 2009 Jan 10;27(2): 199–205. Epub 2008 Dec 8.	Addition of bevacizumab to fluorouracil-based first-line treatment of metastatic colorectal cancer: pooled analysis of cohorts of older patients from two randomized clinical trials
Kaçar S, et al. Acta Chir Belg. 2008 Sep–Oct;108(5): 518–23.	Pre-operative radiochemotherapy for rectal cancer. A prospective randomized trial comparing pre-operative vs. postoperative radiochemotherapy in rectal cancer patients
Sanoff HK, et al. J Clin Oncol. 2008 Dec 10;26(35): 5721–7. Epub 2008 Nov 10.	Five-year data and prognostic factor analysis of oxaliplatin and irinotecan combinations for advanced colorectal cancer: N9741
Cunningham D, et al. Ann Oncol. 2009 Feb;20(2):244–50. Epub 2008 Oct 14.	Two different first-line 5-fluorouracil regimens with or without oxaliplatin in patients with metastatic colorectal cancer
Haller DG, et al. J Clin Oncol. 2008 Oct 1;26(28):4544–50.	Oxaliplatin plus irinotecan compared with irinotecan alone as second-line treatment after single-agent fluoropyrimidine therapy for metastatic colorectal carcinoma

(*Continued*)

TABLE 56-3. (*Continued*)

Study	Study description
Cancer screening	
Hol L, et al. Br J Cancer. 2009 Apr 7;100(7):1103–10.	Screening for colorectal cancer: random comparison of guaiac and immunochemical faecal occult blood testing at different cut-off levels
Paggi S, et al. Clin Gastroenterol Hepatol. 2009 Oct;7(10):1049–54. Epub 2009 Jul 1.	The impact of narrow band imaging in screening colonoscopy: a randomized controlled trial
Ling BS, et al. Arch Intern Med. 2009 Jan 12;169(1): 47–55.	Physicians encouraging colorectal screening: a randomized controlled trial of enhanced office and patient management on compliance with colorectal cancer screening
Adler A, et al. Gastroenterology. 2009 Feb;136(2): 410–6.e1; quiz 715. Epub 2008 Oct 15.	Narrow-band vs. white-light high definition television endoscopic imaging for screening colonoscopy: a prospective randomized trial
Other	
Morey MC, et al. JAMA. 2009 May 13;301(18):1883–91.	Effects of home-based diet and exercise on functional outcomes among older, overweight long-term cancer survivors: RENEW: a randomized controlled trial
Au HJ, et al. J Clin Oncol. 2009 Apr 10;27(11):1822–8. Epub 2009 Mar 9.	Health-related quality of life in patients with advanced colorectal cancer treated with cetuximab: overall and KRAS-specific results of the NCIC CTG and AGITG CO.17 Trial
Wright FC, et al. Arch Surg. 2008 Nov;143(11):1050–5; discussion 1055.	A randomized controlled trial to improve lymph node assessment in stage II colon cancer
Brisinda G, et al. J Surg Oncol. 2009 Jan 1;99(1):75–9.	End-to-end vs. end-to-side stapled anastomoses after anterior resection for rectal cancer
Contant CM, et al. Lancet. 2007 Dec 22;370(9605):2112–7.	Mechanical bowel preparation for elective colorectal surgery: a multicentre randomised trial
Finco C, et al. Surg Endosc. 2007 Jul;21(7):1175–9. Epub 2007 Mar 14.	Prospective randomized study on perioperative enteral immunonutrition in laparoscopic colorectal surgery
Pokala N, et al. Int J Colorectal Dis. 2007 Jun;22(6):683–7. Epub 2006 Oct 10.	A randomized controlled trial comparing simultaneous intra-operative vs. sequential prophylactic ureteric catheter insertion in re-operative and complicated colorectal surgery
Han-Geurts IJ, et al. Br J Surg. 2007 May;94(5):555–61. PMID: 17443854.	Randomized clinical trial of the impact of early enteral feeding on postoperative ileus and recovery
Parc Y, et al. Dis Colon Rectum. 2009 Dec;52(12): 2004–14.	Preoperative radiotherapy is associated with worse functional results after coloanal anastomosis for rectal cancer
Heymen S, et al. Dis Colon Rectum. 2009 Oct;52(10):1730–7.	Randomized controlled trial shows biofeedback to be superior to pelvic floor exercises for fecal incontinence
Tsunoda A, et al. Dis Colon Rectum. 2009 Sep;52(9): 1572–7.	Prospective randomized trial for determination of optimum size of side limb in low anterior resection with side-to-end anastomosis for rectal carcinoma
McLeod RS, et al. Dis Colon Rectum. 2009 May;52(5):919–27.	Recurrence of Crohn's disease after ileocolic resection is not affected by anastomotic type: results of a multicenter, randomized, controlled trial
Rimonda R, et al. Dis Colon Rectum. 2009 Apr;52(4): 657–61.	Electrothermal bipolar vessel sealing system vs. harmonic scalpel in colorectal laparoscopic surgery: a prospective, randomized study
Ng SS, et al. Dis Colon Rectum. 2009 Apr;52(4):558–66.	Long-term morbidity and oncologic outcomes of laparoscopic-assisted anterior resection for upper rectal cancer: 10-year results of a prospective, randomized trial
Garcia-Olmo D, et al. Dis Colon Rectum. 2009 Jan;52(1):79–86.	Expanded adipose-derived stem cells for the treatment of complex perianal fistula: a phase II clinical trial
Lehur PA, et al. ODS II Study Group. Dis Colon Rectum. 2008 Nov;51(11):1611–8. Epub 2008 Jul 19.	Outcomes of stapled transanal rectal resection vs. biofeedback for the treatment of outlet obstruction associated with rectal intussusception and rectocele: a multicenter, randomized, controlled trial
Bessa SS. Dis Colon Rectum. 2008 Jun;51(6):940–4. Epub 2008 Feb 14.	Ligasure vs. conventional diathermy in excisional hemorrhoidectomy: a prospective, randomized study
Michelsen HB, et al. Dis Colon Rectum. 2008 May;51(5):538–40. Epub 2008 Feb 26.	A prospective, randomized study: switch off the sacral nerve stimulator during the night
Tjandra JJ, et al. Dis Colon Rectum. 2008 May;51(5): 494–502. Epub 2008 Feb 16.	Sacral nerve stimulation is more effective than optimal medical therapy for severe fecal incontinence: a randomized, controlled study
Altomare DF, et al.; Ligasure for Hemorrhoids Study Group. Dis Colon Rectum. 2008 May;51(5):514–9. Epub 2008 Jan 30.	Ligasure Precise vs. conventional diathermy for Milligan-Morgan hemorrhoidectomy: a prospective, randomized, multicenter trial
Wong JC, et al. Dis Colon Rectum. 2008 Apr;51(4):397–403. Epub 2007 Dec 21.	Stapled technique for acute thrombosed hemorrhoids: a randomized, controlled trial with long-term results
Kang GS, et al. Dis Colon Rectum. 2008 Mar;51(3): 329–33. Epub 2008 Jan 4.	Evaluation of healing and complications after lateral internal sphincterotomy for chronic anal fissure: marginal suture of incision vs. open left incision: prospective, randomized, controlled study
Gupta PJ, et al. Dis Colon Rectum. 2008 Feb;51(2):231–4. Epub 2007 Dec 18.	Topical sucralfate decreases pain after hemorrhoidectomy and improves healing: a randomized, blinded, controlled study
Menteş BB, et al. Dis Colon Rectum. 2008 Jan;51(1): 128–33. Epub 2007 Dec 18.	Fine-tuning of the extent of lateral internal sphincterotomy: spasm-controlled vs. up to the fissure apex
Renzi A, et al. Dis Colon Rectum. 2008 Jan;51(1): 121–7. Epub 2007 Dec 15.	Clinical, manometric, and ultrasonographic results of pneumatic balloon dilatation vs. lateral internal sphincterotomy for chronic anal fissure: a prospective, randomized, controlled trial

(*Continued*)

Table 56-3. (*Continued*)

Study	Study description
Anesthesia	
Chen JY, et al. Clin J Pain. 2009 Jul-Aug;25(6):485–9.	Opioid-sparing effects of ketorolac and its correlation with the recovery of postoperative bowel function in colorectal surgery patients: a prospective randomized double-blinded study
Beaussier M, et al. Anesthesiology. 2007 Sep;107(3):461–8.PMID: 17721249.	Continuous preperitoneal infusion of ropivacaine provides effective analgesia and accelerates recovery after colorectal surgery: a randomized, double-blind, placebo-controlled study
Sim R, Cheong DM, et al. Colorectal Dis. 2007 Jan;9(1):52–60.	Prospective randomized, double-blind, placebo-controlled study of pre- and postoperative administration of a COX-2-specific inhibitor as opioid-sparing analgesia in major colorectal surgery
Cochrane reviews	
Ahmed N, et al. January 2010	Supportive care for patients with gastrointestinal cancer
Des Guetz G, et al. January 2010	Duration of adjuvant chemotherapy for patients with non-metastatic colorectal cancer
Devon KM, McLeod RS. January 2009	Pre and peri-operative erythropoeitin for reducing allogeneic blood transfusions in colorectal cancer surgery
Gurusamy KS, et al. January 2010	Surgical resection versus non-surgical treatment for hepatic node positive patients with colorectal liver metastases
McAlister V, et al. January 2010	Hypertonic saline for peri-operative fluid management
Nelson RL. January 2010	Operative procedures for fissure in ano
Nienhuijs SW, Hingh IH. October 2009	Conventional vs. LigaSure hemorrhoidectomy for patients with symptomatic Hemorrhoids
Traut U, et al. October 2009	Systemic prokinetic pharmacologic treatment for postoperative adynamic ileus following abdominal surgery in adults
De Haas-Kock, et al. July 2009	Concomitant hyperthermia and radiation therapy for treating locally advanced rectal cancer
Figuls MR, et al. April 2009	Second-line chemotherapy in advanced and metastatic CRC
Cochrane protocols	
Sagar J, Winslet M. July 2009	Colorectal stents for the management of malignant colonic obstructions
Des Guetz G, et al. April 2009	Neoadjuvant chemotherapy for patients having resection or ablation of liver metastases from colorectal cancer
Donghao LV, et al. January 2009	Chemotherapy with Camptothecin compounds for metastatic colorectal cancer
Herrle F, Schattenberg T. January 2009	Omentoplasty for the prevention of anastomotic leakage after colonic or rectal resection
Mishra SI, et al. January 2009	Exercise interventions on health related quality of life for cancer survivors
Montedori A, et al. January 2009	Covering ileo- or colostomy in anterior resection for rectal carcinoma

Limitations of Process Measures

One of the limitations of process measures is that it is often difficult to prove that performance of a process measure directly results in improved patient outcomes. Very few processes performed in clinical practice are substantiated by level I evidence (based on at least one well-designed randomized clinical trial). A second limitation is that there are no validated quality indicators for many areas in surgery where quality improvement may be warranted. The development of new and validated indicators can be an expensive, complex, and time-consuming process, making it prohibitive for some organizations wishing to develop their own tailored indicators. A third limitation is that data collection to measure adherence to process measures or quality indicators is often labor- and cost-intensive. Successful QI efforts require the buy-in of stakeholders at multiple levels within an organization, physician champions as well as adequate financial resources. Finally, outside of commonly used indicators such as the SCIP measures, there may be limited benchmarks against which an organization's performance can be compared. In the absence of benchmarks for comparison, QI programs often set an arbitrary goal of 85% or 90% compliance as their mark for success.

The Donabedian Model (Part 3): Outcomes

Outcomes are the end result of receiving health care. Traditionally, surgeons have examined their outcomes through morbidity and mortality conferences. In particular, these conferences focus on adverse outcomes of care. The objectives of outcome measurement are to evaluate and compare providers as a means to inform providers and patients, adjust financial compensation, and facilitate quality assurance and improvement.

In order to make valid comparisons between providers, appropriate patient risk adjustment must be performed. Risk-adjusted outcomes take into account the impact that patient characteristics and the context of care have on their outcomes. A simple way to think about risk adjustment is described by this equation by L.I. Iezzoni:

$$\text{Patient factors} + \text{Effectiveness of care}$$
$$+\text{Random variation} = \text{Outcome.}$$

"Patient factors" represent the patient's variables, such as their diagnosis, age, gender, socioeconomic status, comorbidities, and illness severity. "Effectiveness of care" relates to the nature of the intervention being studied. For example, surgical resection of a stage I cancer is more likely to result in a cure compared to surgical resection of stage IV cancer. The differential impact of the same treatment in different clinical contexts must also be considered when performing adequate risk adjustment. "Random variation" is perhaps best described by the saying: "You can do everything wrong and have a good outcome, and you can do everything right and have a bad outcome." The effect of random variation or "chance" is particularly significant when working with a small number of patients. An example where risk adjustment makes intuitive sense is when providers who care for older, sicker, and more complicated patients have higher mortality rates. Without appropriate risk adjustment to "level the playing field," it would be uninformative to compare outcomes across providers. The statistical methods for performing risk adjustment on outcomes data are sophisticated and complex and are beyond the scope of this chapter. For an in-depth examination of risk adjustment in measuring health-care outcomes, consider *Risk Adjustment for Measuring Healthcare Outcomes* edited by Lisa Iezzoni.[53]

Organizations often bypass the complexity of performing their own risk adjustment on outcomes data by relying on other organizations to do it for them. An example is the American College of Surgeons' National Surgical Quality Improvement Project (NSQIP). NSQIP first began as the National Veterans Administration Surgical Risk Study (NVASRS), which developed risk models for 30-day mortality and morbidity in nine surgical subspecialties to facilitate comparison of surgical outcomes at Veterans Administration (VA) hospitals to the national average. NVASRS allowed for the first time a comparison of surgical quality across surgical subspecialties and VA hospitals across the country. With its success, NVASRS then evolved into an ongoing quality improvement program known as the National Surgical Quality Improvement Project. In 1999, NSQIP was piloted in three non-VA hospitals, demonstrating that it was feasible to collect and analyze data using NSQIP risk-adjusted models in non-VA settings. Since 2001, with funding from the Agency for Healthcare Research and Quality (AHRQ), the American College of Surgeons has expanded NSQIP data collection to include over 250 private sector hospitals. NSQIP allows hospitals to submit their own data, compare their risk-adjusted outcomes to a national average, and identify areas in surgical care where their rates of mortality or complications are higher than expected based on their patient population.

In addition to objective or "hard" patient outcomes such as mortality or complications, there are also subjective patient-reported outcomes such as patient satisfaction, functional status, and quality of life. These areas of outcome measurement have received increasing attention in the era of patient-centered health care.

In the colorectal surgery literature, there are increasing numbers of studies focused on patient-reported sexual function, general health, quality of life, and satisfaction following colorectal surgery, given that many patients will favor quality of life over quantity of life.[54–62]

Using a multitude of survey instruments which address physical function, clinical symptoms, quality of life, and patient satisfaction, patient-reported outcomes aim to define the critical component of health care which is not captured in administrative or clinical data – the patient's perspective. Now, as we strive to improve quality, particularly in the context of pay-for-performance and patient-centered care, patient-reported outcomes have been recognized as a key component in the measurement of health-care quality. For the practicing surgeon, quality-of-life instruments and the results of quality of life studies highlight areas of importance to the patient which may need to be addressed during the provision of care.

There are many validated instruments available to evaluate physical function, clinical symptoms, and quality of life, and there are increasing numbers of instruments being developed for colorectal patients (Table 56-4).[63–79] Patient-reported outcomes survey instruments. For example, colorectal cancer-specific instruments include the European Organization for Research and Treatment of Cancer (EORTC) CR-38 and Functional Assessment of Cancer Therapy-Colorectal (FACT-C). To give a flavor of the content of these two instruments, they both are briefly discussed below.

The EORTC is one of the largest clinical trial groups in Europe which has focused on developing cancer-specific questionnaires and site-specific questionnaires to evaluate quality of life in cancer patients. The EORTC CR-38 was designed as a supplement to the core questionnaire, EORTC QLQ-C30, for use in colorectal cancer patients participating in international clinical trials. The EORTC CR-38 consists of 38 items covering symptoms and side effects related to different treatment modalities, body image, sexuality, and future perspective.[78,79] Nineteen questions are completed by all patients, and the remaining 19 questions are specific to certain subsamples of patients such as male or female gender or presence of a stoma. The CR-38 consists of two functional scales, body image and sexuality, and seven symptom scales: micturition, gastrointestinal, chemotherapy, defecation, stoma, male and female sexual problems. Together with the EORTC QLQ-C30, the CR-38 provides a comprehensive assessment of quality of life in colorectal cancer patients over a wide variety of stages and treatments.

The FACT-C combines the Functional Assessment of Cancer Therapy-General (FACT-G), a 27-item general questionnaire of health-related quality of life in patients with cancer or other chronic illness, with a nine-item Colorectal Cancer Subscale (CCS). The FACT-C contains five subscales, namely, EWB (Emotional Well-Being), SWB (Social Well-Being), FWB (Functional Well-Being), PWB (Physical Well-Being), and CCS (Colorectal Cancer Subscale), and assesses quality-of-life concerns pertinent to colorectal cancer patients.[72]

TABLE 56-4. Patient-reported outcomes survey instruments

Area	Survey instrument	Description	Specific for cancer patients?
Clinical symptoms	Fatigue Symptom Inventory [63,64]	Measurement of fatigue intensity, duration, and interference with daily functioning	Yes
Clinical symptoms	Brief Pain Inventory [65,66]	Assessment of pain severity, location, and impact on function	Yes
Clinical symptoms	Neurotoxicity Scale (NTX-12) [67]	Evaluate sensory and motor symptoms, auditory problems	Yes
Physical function	Instrumental Activities of Daily Living (IADL) [68]	Assessment of independent living skills (e.g., using the telephone, shopping, paying bills)	No
Quality of life	Impact of Cancer [69,70]	Measurement of positive and negative impacts of cancer	Yes
Quality of life	Life Orientation Test [71]	Measurement of optimism and pessimism	No
Quality of life	Functional Assessment of Cancer Therapy-Colorectal (FACT-C) [72]	Assessment of physical, mental, social well-being	Colorectal cancer specific
Quality of life Clinical symptoms Physical function	SF-36/SF-12 [73–77]	Summary physical health and summary mental health scores	No
Quality of life Physical function	European Organization for Research and Treatment of Cancer (EORTC) CR-38 [78,79]	Evaluate quality of life and function of colorectal cancer patients Y	Colorectal cancer specific

Overall, as quality of life becomes an increasingly evaluated outcome metric of quality of care, it is important that providers understand the instruments and their content.

Limitations to Outcome Measures

Ultimately, the goal of quality-of-care research, measurement, and improvement efforts is to improve patient outcomes. To this end, health-care researchers and providers often look directly to outcome measures which inform us only of the end result of care. The limitation of this is that when there are poor outcomes, outcome measures alone do not identify a specific structure or process that can be changed to alter the result of care. A thorough assessment of outcome measures must be performed in the context of structure and process to be completely understood. A second limitation of outcome measures, some argue, is that the overemphasis on adverse outcomes may encourage providers to "cherry pick" their patients. Proponents of risk-adjusted outcomes maintain that appropriately applied risk models can overcome the bias of patient selection. However, appropriate risk adjustment can be complex, costly, and prohibitively expensive for smaller organizations without the resources to obtain the necessary expertise or services.

Summarizing Structure, Process, and Outcome

Beauty lies in the eyes of the beholder. What is considered important or valid in quality depends on one's viewpoint. What health-policy planners or hospital administrators care about may be vastly different from what the surgeon or patient focuses on. Each component of the Donabedian model – structure, process, and outcome – describes and evaluates distinct aspects of quality within the overall health-care system. Quality measures have been developed, applied, and validated by different stakeholders in all three components for different purposes, each with its proponents and critics. Some would argue that the ultimate endpoint is patient outcomes. But others would counter that if doing the "wrong thing for the wrong patient at the wrong time in the wrong way" results in a good outcome, then that should not be considered good quality care. There is, unfortunately, no single perfect quality metric that serves as an adequate proxy for overall quality. Therefore, we will continue to utilize these imperfect measures of quality, with a full understanding of their strengths and limitations, even as we continue to develop and validate new ways of understanding and measuring quality of care.

Quality of the Data

Evaluating, measuring, and improving quality of care is important. Yet, one of the main difficulties with measuring and improving quality in all of health care, including colorectal surgery is the quality and availability of data. It remains important that all providers understand some of the intricacies of data – including the source of data, who collects the data, and what data are collected in the context of analysis. As all providers rely on data to define quality and to guide them in delivering better care, it is paramount that the data are of high quality. In point of fact, the well-known phrase, *Garbage In, Garbage Out*, reminds us that we absolutely need high-quality data to make valid conclusions and achieve high-quality care. Ideally, to evaluate the quality of colorectal surgery care, a database would capture comprehensive detailed information about the patient, their disease, the procedure and treatments they received, the provider, all outcomes from wound infection to disease recurrence and reoperation, patient's quality of life and function, mortality, and cost. However, creating such a database would be prohibitively expensive both in terms of manpower and cost. Instead, colorectal surgeons must depend on a large number of existing databases which capture different aspects of structure, process, and outcome, and assimilate the results from each to gauge what is quality care.

Currently available *sources* of data may be divided into two main types: administrative databases and clinical databases. Administrative databases such as the Medicare claims database, the National Hospital Discharge Database, and statewide hospital discharge databases (e.g., the California inpatient file, managed by the Office of Statewide Health Planning and Development, and the Statewide Planning and Research Cooperative System (SPARCS), managed by the New York Department of Health) record admissions, diagnoses, and procedures from administrative/billing claims. Clinical databases such as the Society of Thoracic Surgeons Registry, Surveillance Epidemiology End Result (SEER) of the National Cancer Institute, and National Surgical Quality Improvement Program (NSQIP) of the American College of Surgeons use chart abstractors and hospital registrars to record patient-level clinical data such as comorbidities and search for evidence of wound infections, urinary tract infections, cancer recurrence, and other clinical outcomes. There are also research-focused databases relevant to colorectal surgery such as the Cancer Care Outcomes Research and Surveillance Consortium (CanCORS) which combines medical record abstraction, patient surveys, and provider surveys in an attempt to provide a more complete assessment of the experience and outcomes of the colorectal surgery patient.

Advantages of administrative databases include access to large amounts of demographic and procedural data on large population-based samples which is easily compiled. However, administrative databases are limited by the lack of clinically meaningful data. Clinical databases provide clinical findings such as wound infections and patient outcomes. However, intensive resource expenditures are usually necessary to collect this data by chart abstraction and individual patient assessment.

An important issue to recognize in terms of data quality is identifying who is *collecting the data*. A number of databases or clinical registries have relied upon surgeons or other providers to collect the data. Other databases, such as cancer registries, rely upon a third party such as a trained and audited cancer registrar to collect the data. A number of studies have demonstrated that "third party" data collectors tend to have higher clinical accuracy. As increasingly more "clinical" data are being used to evaluate and improve quality, knowing the source of data, who collected the data, and what variables will be collected will be important.

Appropriateness and Appropriateness Criteria

Background

An appropriate procedure has been defined as one in which "the expected health benefit (e.g., increased life expectancy, relief of pain, reduction in anxiety, improved functional capacity) exceeds the expected negative consequences (e.g., mortality, morbidity, anxiety, pain, time lost from work) by a sufficiently wide margin that the procedure is worth doing, exclusive of cost."[80] Appropriateness criteria are a method of explicitly delineating and weighing these benefits and harms, based on evidence in the literature and the clinical judgment of a multidisciplinary panel of physicians. Once developed, the criteria can be retrospectively or prospectively applied to systematically assess the appropriateness or overuse and underuse of a procedure. They can also be used as clinical decision aides to guide shared decision making between the surgeon and patient. Numerous studies have shown that patients have better outcomes when they are treated according to appropriateness criteria.

Currently, a systematic review of the literature has identified a gap in the availability of appropriateness criteria in surgery, with criteria being formally developed for only 18 procedures including coronary artery bypass grafting, colonoscopy, cataract surgery, and carotid endarterectomy (unpublished data). Targets for appropriateness criteria development are typically procedures that are commonly performed, have elevated risk of morbidity and mortality, and/or utilize significant resources. Procedures with documented variation in use among different geographic areas have also been prioritized in the past. The amount and quality of scientific literature describing the procedure are also important considerations.

Development of Appropriateness Criteria

The gold standard for decision making in health care is the randomized controlled trial. Unfortunately, for most procedures, these trials have not been attempted, and if performed, they cannot be generalized to a wider patient population. Appropriateness criteria compensate for these gaps in the literature by combining available scientific evidence with expert clinical judgment. The RAND/UCLA Appropriateness Method (RAM) is a commonly used technique for the development of appropriateness criteria.[81]

Use of Appropriateness Criteria

Numerous studies have documented significant variations in health-care delivery across different patient populations. The Dartmouth Atlas, for example, reports geographic differences in rates of procedures performed that cannot be explained by differences in the patient population alone. It has been hypothesized that this variation may be due to the inappropriate overuse and underuse of procedures in different regions of the country. Appropriateness criteria have been applied retrospectively to systematically investigate this hypothesis. Although few studies have been performed in colorectal surgery, it is important to discuss and understand some of the seminal work that has been performed in other areas to inform this topic. Many future studies will likely be performed in colorectal surgery.

One of the earliest studies to use appropriateness criteria to study variations in procedure use was published in 1987 by Chassin et al.[82] who analyzed the use of coronary angiography, carotid endarterectomy, and upper gastrointestinal endoscopy in hospitals that were preidentified as being high, average, or low users of these procedures. By applying appropriateness criteria, the researchers found significant rates of inappropriate use for each procedure: 17% of cases for angiography, 32% for carotid endarterectomy, and 17% for endoscopy. Statistically significant differences in the rates of appropriate procedure performance were found for coronary angiography and endoscopy between high- and low-use hospitals, but the differences were small. Of note, the authors suggested that the variation between high- and low-use hospitals may be the result of both underuse and overuse.[82]

Studies have also been performed to determine if the use of appropriateness criteria affects clinical outcomes. Hemingway et al.[83] followed a cohort of consecutive patients undergoing coronary angiography at three London hospitals. Appropriateness criteria for percutaneous transluminal coronary angioplasty (PTCA) and coronary artery bypass grafting (CABG) were applied to these patients, and their treating physicians were blinded to the results. These patients were then followed for a median of 30 months, and their clinical outcomes were recorded. The researchers found that 34% of patients for whom PTCA was rated appropriate were treated medically instead. These patients were significantly more likely to experience angina compared to the patients treated with PTCA. Twenty-six percent of the patients for whom CABG was considered appropriate were treated medically. These patients were significantly more likely to die or have a nonfatal myocardial infarction compared to patients who underwent CABG. The researchers concluded that underuse was associated with adverse clinical outcomes.[83] Finally, a graded relationship between appropriateness rating and outcome was observed, meaning that patients who underwent a procedure and had received a high appropriateness score had better outcomes than those who underwent the procedure and had a lower score.

Apart from research and setting standards, appropriateness criteria are also developed for use as clinical decision aids. The American College of Cardiology Foundation, along with several partner societies, has published appropriateness criteria for coronary revascularization. These criteria are meant to provide guidance for patients and clinicians in discussions regarding revascularization and are also used for reviewing utilization patterns. They are explicitly not meant to replace clinical judgment and practice experience.

The American College of Radiology (ACR) has developed appropriateness criteria for a broad range of therapeutic and diagnostic topics to reduce inappropriate utilization of radiologic services. Radport is a decision support system that uses the ACR appropriateness criteria to guide the ordering of diagnostic imaging. A "utility score" is determined based on clinical information provided by the clinician and is meant to reduce the use of low-utility examinations.

Limitations of Appropriateness Criteria

A frequent criticism of appropriateness criteria is the reliance on expert opinion, which is inherently subjective. There will always be a role for clinical judgment in the consideration of appropriateness because it is not feasible to perform randomized controlled trials for every indication for every procedure. However, studies have shown that the results of appropriateness panels using the RAM are reproducible with new, independent panels. Furthermore, there is less variability in the development of appropriateness criteria than among the individual judgments of physicians.[84]

The utility and validity of appropriateness criteria are dependent upon the quality of the criteria, which in turn is dependent on both the available evidence base for the procedure as well as the judgment of the panel. The reliability of the RAM panel process will thus likely be lower when the scientific evidence base is minimal or weak. The panel itself is typically created by requesting nominations for panelists from various stakeholder societies. This ensures that panelists are well respected within their field for their clinical judgment and knowledge base and also provides face validity for the appropriateness criteria created through professional society endorsement.

Finally, concern is often raised regarding the clinical validity of appropriateness criteria. Despite efforts to create an exhaustive list of clinical indications for a procedure, there may still be patients for whom the criteria do not apply. Appropriateness criteria should thus be thought of as an aid in clinical decision making and should not replace a clinician's judgment. For utilization purposes, it may be helpful to continually review why patients rated inappropriate by the criteria are operated on (or vice versa) to ensure that the criteria are clinically valid.

Appropriateness Criteria and Guidelines in Colorectal Surgery

Appropriateness criteria have not been developed specifically for colorectal surgical procedures, although they do exist for colonoscopy. The American College of Radiology (ACR) has also developed appropriateness criteria to guide imaging decisions for screening and pretreatment staging of colorectal cancer as well as criteria to guide the treatment of rectal cancer (resectable, metastatic, or recurrent), anal cancer, and mesenteric ischemia. The ACR criteria are available online on their Web site.[3]

To date, what are generally available to colorectal surgeons are practice guidelines or practice parameters. The National Guideline Clearinghouse is an initiative of the Agency for Healthcare Research and Quality (AHRQ) and is a publicly available database of evidence-based clinical practice guidelines. The database includes practice parameters developed by the American Society of Colon and Rectal Surgeons (ASCRS) for topics including colon cancer, rectal cancer, anal squamous neoplasms, ulcerative colitis, Crohn's disease, sigmoid diverticulitis, constipation, fecal incontinence, anal fissures, hemorrhoids, perianal abscess, and fistula-in-ano. Though not formal appropriateness criteria, the ASCRS has developed guidelines for laparoscopic resection of colon and rectal cancer, a consensus document on bowel preparation before colonoscopy (in association with multiple other profession societies), and practice parameters for the prevention of venous thromboembolism. These guidelines contain elements of appropriateness but are not explicit enough to qualify as appropriateness criteria. This gap in the availability of appropriateness criteria, especially for surgical procedures, represents an opportunity for future research and development.

Comparative Effectiveness and Cost-Effectiveness

Background

If good quality care can be understood as "doing the right thing for the right patient at the right time the right way," part of evaluating and improving quality should include systematic and valid ways to define what is "right." Quality indicators and appropriateness criteria are two methods that have been presented in this chapter. Another method is comparative effectiveness. The focus of comparative effectiveness research (CER) is the *practical* comparison of different treatments or procedures to determine what works best for whom. Distinct from the traditional clinical trials that seek to determine efficacy (whether a treatment works or not), CER is geared toward delineating effectiveness – the relative benefits of treatment options in *routine* clinical practice.

The IOM has described six defining characteristics of CER: (1) it directly informs clinical decisions from the patient perspective or policy decisions from the population perspective; (2) it compares at least two treatment options, both of which could be considered "best practice"; (3) it describes results at the population and subgroup levels to inform more individualized decisions; (4) the outcomes measured are important to patients; (5) a variety of methods and data may be used, from observational studies and RCTs to meta-analyses or systematic literature reviews; and (6) the setting of CER should be similar to routine practice environments.[85]

CER has gained considerable interest at the national policy level as a means for maintaining quality while simultaneously addressing the "runaway" cost of health care, as spending is projected to reach 20% of the gross domestic product by 2016.[86] At the federal level, the American Recovery and Reinvestment Act of 2009 appropriated $1.1 billion dollars to CER.[87] In light of the emphasis placed on CER by the US government, CER is likely to affect clinical practice to a greater degree than in the past, regardless of misgivings raised by critics of this approach. Although cost-cutting is not the main focus of CER, a consequent benefit according to its proponents is cost reduction by the elimination of less effective, ineffective, or even harmful services. Extreme opponents have viewed CER as a means to limit treatment options and effect health-care rationing.[88] The reality is that the current expansion of health-care cost is not sustainable and we routinely lack sufficient information to make informed decisions about the risks and benefits of treatment options.[89] To this end, CER will help clinicians and patients make individualized and informed decisions based on sound clinical evidence.

Cost-Effectiveness

Cost-effectiveness is a specific subset of comparative effectiveness research that provides explicit comparisons of "the relative value of different interventions in creating better health and/or longer life."[89] What distinguishes cost-effectiveness from other types of comparative effectiveness studies is the explicit comparison of cost or values. For example, a study may compare laparoscopic to open colectomy for colon cancer. The comparison of postoperative complications, recurrence, and survival across the two modalities would constitute a comparative effectiveness study. The comparison of the associated cost or resource utilization, such as operating time, length of hospital stay, hospital charges, or time to return to work would constitute a cost-effectiveness study. There is often a considerable overlap between the two study types.

A reluctance to place a monetary value on health outcomes has lead to the widespread use of the cost-effectiveness ratio,

[3] The ACR appropriateness criteria can be found at http://www.acr.org/SecondaryMainMenuCategories/quality_safety/app_criteria.aspx.

which often takes the form of "incremental cost per quality-adjusted life year (QALY) gained." QALY is a measure of disease burden that takes into account both the quantity and quality of life lived. QALY values range from zero to one, with zero being death and one being 1 year of life lived in perfect health. But what "incremental cost" is one QALY worth and how much is considered cost-effective? While these values are somewhat arbitrary, researchers have often accepted a range of $50,000 to $100,000 per QALY gained as cost-effective. The value of $50,000 in US studies stems from the "dialysis standard," the approximate cost of taking care of a dialysis patient for one year. Using these definitions and standards, an intervention or treatment that costs less than $50,000 per QALY gained may be deemed cost-effective.

In theory, cost-effectiveness methodology provides the advantage of combining the best scientific evidence, available clinical outcomes, and cost data. Cost-effectiveness studies, however, are limited by their reliance on the use of appropriate assumptions in creating a model of care and accurate value and cost estimates. Predictably, the cost of providing surgical care is difficult to quantify, whether it be the direct or the indirect component. Direct cost involve near-term spending related to delivery of care, including that incurred secondary to complications of receiving that care. Indirect cost generally refer to economic and societal cost due to loss of productivity from health-care receipt, often estimated by measuring time to return to work following a surgical procedure. Studies assessing direct cost of care often use administrative billing or claims data as a proxy for cost. Such data is easy to obtain and can include large numbers of patients for population-based studies. However, hospital charges and claims data are "operator-dependent" and influenced by the person who bills or codes, thus not necessarily representing accurate or actual resources used in providing care. Studies that explicitly measure the cost of care by taking into account equipment, supplies, and labor, on the other hand, are usually limited to single institutions where medical charts and thorough accounting data are available for review. Despite these limitations, cost-effectiveness studies are a major component of ĈER and will play a role in determining appropriate cost-saving measures.

Comparative Effectiveness and Cost-Effectiveness in Colorectal Surgery

The impact of comparative effectiveness and cost-effectiveness studies on colorectal surgical practice has already been felt and will only increase over time, with the greatest effect anticipated on procedure choice and disease management. For example, debates on laparoscopic vs. open colectomy and "fast-track pathways" compared to traditional postoperative care in colorectal procedures have been informed by comparative effectiveness analyses and cost-effectiveness studies.

Laparoscopic surgery has been touted as equivalent in effectiveness and potentially superior to open colorectal surgery in both benign and malignant disease for its associated shorter postoperative recovery time, decreased pain associated with smaller incisions, and decreased length of hospitalization. Overall, the available literature suggests that short-term and long-term outcomes may be similar between the procedures but the heterogeneity of studies and the paucity of randomized controlled trials make comparing the two difficult, particularly when additionally attempting to assess cost.[90–92]

In a systematic review commissioned by the National Institute of Clinical Effectiveness (NICE) in the UK, laparoscopic surgery for nonmetastastic colorectal cancer was associated with a shorter recovery period and shorter length of hospital stay and no significant difference in 3-year disease-free survival or mortality compared with open resection. However, the authors noted longer operative times among laparoscopic cases as well as a fair number of laparoscopic to open conversions.[90] A Cochrane Database systematic review of 12 eligible randomized controlled trials involving nonmetastatic colorectal cancer patients found no differences in cancer-related mortality, port-site or wound recurrences, or recurrence rate at the site of the primary tumor, suggesting that laparoscopic and open resection of colon carcinoma are equivalent with regard to these long-term outcomes. The authors recommend further studies to adequately evaluate incisional hernia rates, postoperative adhesion rates, and upper rectal surgery long-term outcomes.[91]

Studies on the economic impact of laparoscopic vs. open colectomy have generally been few in number and plagued by the complexity of accurately determining cost. A systematic review by Dowson et al.[92] found that only two of 29 eligible randomized controlled trials between 1991 and 2005 had accounted for the indirect cost involved with both types of procedures. Thus, across all studies, operating room costs was higher, but there was no significant difference in total hospital cost. Length of hospital stay was uniformly shorter for laparoscopic surgery cases (median difference 2.8 days; $p<0.001$). The authors speculated that the "societal benefits" derived from the decreased indirect cost could potentially outweigh the greater up-front procedural cost, making laparoscopic surgery a viable alternative, particularly given the equivalence of short-term and long-term outcomes.[92]

On the basis of their systematic review, researchers from the NICE-commissioned study proceeded to a formal cost-effectiveness analysis of laparoscopic vs. open colon resection. Though the cost of laparoscopic surgery was £250–300 (approximately $390–470 USD) more than open colon resection, the analysis resulted in a 40% likelihood that laparoscopic surgery was more cost-effective than open surgery at the threshold of £30,000 ($46,800) per QALY gained in light of decreased length of hospitalization, faster recovery, and reduced pain. Given the "modest additional cost" of laparoscopy, the findings lead the authors to conclude that "a judgment [*sic*] is required as to whether the benefits associated with earlier recovery are worth this extra cost."[90]

A dearth of cost-effectiveness studies is noted in the evaluation of "fast-track" or "enhanced recovery" postoperative management following colorectal surgery. Several comparative effectiveness studies have been performed in which outcomes such as length of hospital stay, morbidity, mortality, and readmission rates were examined. Recent systematic reviews have suggested that enhanced recovery programs are safe and effective following colorectal surgery when compared with conventional postoperative care. Wind et al. found a significantly shorter index hospital stay, significantly less morbidity but no significant difference in readmission rates or mortality for fast-track patients compared with conventional postoperative care.[93] Similarly, a review by Walter et al.[94] showed decreased length of stay, decreased 30-day morbidity, and no increase in 30-day mortality between the two management modalities following colorectal resection. Thirty-day readmission rates were higher among fast-track patients compared with conventional management patients in the clinical controlled trials, although not in the randomized controlled trials. This last finding highlights an important caveat with regard to comparative effectiveness research and reviews of the evidence for fast-track care: some caution is warranted in adopting enhanced recovery measures outside of the study context given the limited number of studies available at this time (six studies with a total of 512 patients were eligible and analyzed in the former systematic review, and four studies with a total of 376 patients were eligible for analysis in the latter).

The opportunity for further research in the realm of comparative effectiveness and cost-effectiveness of colorectal surgical disease management is immense. All practitioners need awareness and some fluency with this type of evidence-based research. Inevitably, clinicians will encounter difficulty in decision making when confronted with the individual patient where population-based evidence provides a certain recommendation, but this intervention proves ineffective for the given person compared to the more costly alternative. From this perspective, the results of comparative effectiveness studies may prove a challenge to the practitioner, especially when such population-based data become matters of organizational or national policy. However, if we can take the best available evidence and make decisions rationally using an algorithm that at least begins with the most cost-effective option before moving to others, ultimately, we as a nation may see reduced cost and improvement in health outcomes.[88]

Attribution of Quality

There are a number of issues that have yet to be resolved, but remain important to recognize. One is attribution. It is a given that the evaluation of quality of surgical care may be measured at different levels. As an example, the rate of anastomotic leak or the rate of giving prophylactic antibiotics may be measured at the surgeon level, the facility level, the system level, or some other level altogether. There are a number of issues related to this topic that deserve discussion, but one of the more important aspects is the idea of accountability or attribution. In other words, who should be responsible for the performance/quality metric and who should be rewarded? Should it be an individual, a facility, or some sort of "team or service"? This is not such an easy determination because it is likely different for different metrics, and as the unit of measurement becomes smaller and smaller, the appropriateness of the measure becomes increasingly debatable. For example, there has been much discussion regarding the appropriateness of the number of nodes retrieved in a node negative colectomy. Whether one believes in the scientific merits of the measure or not, it provides an example of attribution, since attaining a sufficient number of lymph nodes in a colectomy specimen relies on both the surgeon and pathologist. Thus, if we were to have a metric that measures an individual, who should be rewarded for attaining a sufficient number of nodes – surgeon or pathologist? There are many metrics that are similar in nature, where it remains difficult to attribute a quality process or outcome to an individual provider.

Most of the common surgical metrics at the time of this writing are at the hospital level (e.g., surgical care improvement program); however, many "regulatory" groups are investigating how we might develop individual surgeon-based metrics.

Summary

It is difficult to say exactly what all of this quality-related information means for the practicing colorectal surgeon. It is fair to say, however, that quality evaluation is probably here to stay and that in an iterative fashion, quality measurement will likely continue to increase. Already, structural measures are being used for various surgical procedures, process measures are being measured at the hospital level with the Surgical Care Improvement Program (SCIP) and also at the individual surgeon level with the Patient Quality Reporting Initiative (PQRI). Outcomes are being measured in various programs (e.g., Hospital-Acquired Conditions). The American Board of Colon and Rectal Surgery has the Maintenance of Certification program, where the aim is to effect continuous professional development with ongoing education, assessment, and improvement. As the field of performance evaluation and quality improvement progresses, it will remain important for providers to be involved in the ongoing discussions and decisions. By being active stakeholders, providers can influence the development of quality improvement so that it continues to be fair, useful, applicable, and meaningful to surgeons and their patients.

References

1. Kohn LTC, Corrigan JM, Donaldson MS, editors. To err is human: building a safer health system. Washington, DC: National Academy Press; 1999.
2. America CoQoHCi. Crossing the quality chasm: a new health system for the 21st century. Washington, DC: National Academy Press; 2001.
3. Donabedian A. Evaluating the quality of medical care. Milbank Mem Fund Q. 1966;44(3):166–206.
4. Lohr KN. Medicare: a strategy for quality assurance. J Qual Assur. 1991;13(1):10–3.
5. Orlander JD, Barber TW, Fincke BG. The morbidity and mortality conference: the delicate nature of learning from error. Acad Med. 2002;77(10):1001–6.
6. Ruth HS, Haugen FP, Grove DD. Anesthesia Study Commission; findings of 11 years' activity. J Am Med Assoc. 1947;135(14): 881–4.
7. Kraft S. The crises begin at birth. Los Angeles Times. November 15, 2009:A1, A24–25.
8. Ozgediz D, Galukande M, Mabweijano J, et al. The neglect of the global surgical workforce: experience and evidence from Uganda. World J Surg. 2008;32(6):1208–15.
9. Nakayama DK, Burd RS, Newman KD. Pediatric surgery workforce: supply and demand. J Pediatr Surg. 2009;44(9): 1677–82.
10. Etzioni DA, Liu JH, Maggard MA, O'Connell JB, Ko CY. Workload projections for surgical oncology: will we need more surgeons? Ann Surg Oncol. 2003;10(9):1112–7.
11. Williams Jr TE, Ellison EC. Population analysis predicts a future critical shortage of general surgeons. Surgery. 2008;144(4):548–54. discussion 554–546.
12. Cohn SM, Price MA, Villarreal CL. Trauma and surgical critical care workforce in the United States: a severe surgeon shortage appears imminent. J Am Coll Surg. 2009;209(4): 446–52. e444.
13. Grover A, Gorman K, Dall TM, et al. Shortage of cardiothoracic surgeons is likely by 2020. Circulation. 2009;120(6):488–94.
14. Satiani B, Williams TE, Go MR. Predicted shortage of vascular surgeons in the United States: population and workload analysis. J Vasc Surg. 2009;50(4):946–52.
15. Dill MJS, Salsberg ES. The complexities of physician supply and demand: projections through 2025. Washington, DC: Association of American Medical Colleges; 2008.
16. Etzioni DA, Beart Jr RW, Madoff RD, Ault GT. Impact of the aging population on the demand for colorectal procedures. Dis Colon Rectum. 2009;52(4):583–90. discussion 590–591.
17. Voelker R. Experts say projected surgeon shortage a "looming crisis" for patient care. JAMA. 2009;302(14):1520–1.
18. Chen J, Rathore SS, Radford MJ, Krumholz HM. JCAHO accreditation and quality of care for acute myocardial infarction. Health Aff (Millwood). 2003;22(2):243–54.
19. Greenfield D, Braithwaite J. Health sector accreditation research: a systematic review. Int J Qual Health Care. 2008;20(3):172–83.
20. Luft HS, Bunker JP, Enthoven AC. Should operations be regionalized? The empirical relation between surgical volume and mortality. N Engl J Med. 1979;301(25):1364–9.
21. Gruen RL, Pitt V, Green S, Parkhill A, Campbell D, Jolley D. The effect of provider case volume on cancer mortality: systematic review and meta-analysis. CA Cancer J Clin. 2009;59(3):192–211.
22. Killeen SD, O'Sullivan MJ, Coffey JC, Kirwan WO, Redmond HP. Provider volume and outcomes for oncological procedures. Br J Surg. 2005;92(4):389–402.
23. Weber WP, Guller U, Jain NB, Pietrobon R, Oertli D. Impact of surgeon and hospital caseload on the likelihood of performing laparoscopic vs open sigmoid resection for diverticular disease: a study based on 55, 949 patients. Arch Surg. 2007;142(3): 253–9. discussion 259.
24. Borowski DW, Kelly SB, Bradburn DM, Wilson RG, Gunn A, Ratcliffe AA. Impact of surgeon volume and specialization on short-term outcomes in colorectal cancer surgery. Br J Surg. 2007;94(7):880–9.
25. Rogers Jr SO, Wolf RE, Zaslavsky AM, Wright WE, Ayanian JZ. Relation of surgeon and hospital volume to processes and outcomes of colorectal cancer surgery. Ann Surg. 2006;244(6):1003–11.
26. McGrath DR, Leong DC, Gibberd R, Armstrong B, Spigelman AD. Surgeon and hospital volume and the management of colorectal cancer patients in Australia. ANZ J Surg. 2005; 75(10):901–10.
27. Hodgson DC, Zhang W, Zaslavsky AM, Fuchs CS, Wright WE, Ayanian JZ. Relation of hospital volume to colostomy rates and survival for patients with rectal cancer. J Natl Cancer Inst. 2003;95(10):708–16.
28. Truong C, Wong JH, Lum SS, Morgan JW, Roy-Chowdhury S. The impact of hospital volume on the number of nodes retrieved and outcome in colorectal cancer. Am Surg. 2008;74(10): 944–7.
29. Larson DW, Marcello PW, Larach SW, et al. Surgeon volume does not predict outcomes in the setting of technical credentialing: results from a randomized trial in colon cancer. Ann Surg. 2008;248(5):746–50.
30. Bilimoria KY, Palis B, Stewart AK, et al. Impact of tumor location on nodal evaluation for colon cancer. Dis Colon Rectum. 2008;51(2):154–61.
31. Kuhry E, Bonjer HJ, Haglind E, et al. Impact of hospital case volume on short-term outcome after laparoscopic operation for colonic cancer. Surg Endosc. 2005;19(5):687–92.
32. Billingsley KG, Morris AM, Dominitz JA, et al. Surgeon and hospital characteristics as predictors of major adverse outcomes following colon cancer surgery: understanding the volume-outcome relationship. Arch Surg. 2007;142(1):23–31. discussion 32.
33. Kennedy ED, Rothwell DM, Cohen Z, McLeod RS. Increased experience and surgical technique lead to improved outcome after ileal pouch-anal anastomosis: a population-based study. Dis Colon Rectum. 2006;49(7):958–65.
34. Yasunaga H, Matsuyama Y, Ohe K. Volume-outcome relationship in rectal cancer surgery: a new perspective. Surg Today. 2009;39(8):663–8.
35. Salz T, Sandler RS. The effect of hospital and surgeon volume on outcomes for rectal cancer surgery. Clin Gastroenterol Hepatol. 2008;6(11):1185–93.
36. Billingsley KG, Morris AM, Green P, et al. Does surgeon case volume influence nonfatal adverse outcomes after rectal cancer resection? J Am Coll Surg. 2008;206(3):1167–77.
37. Harling H, Bulow S, Moller LN, Jorgensen T. Hospital volume and outcome of rectal cancer surgery in Denmark 1994–99. Colorectal Dis. 2005;7(1):90–5.

38. Ananthakrishnan AN, McGinley EL, Binion DG. Does it matter where you are hospitalized for inflammatory bowel disease? A nationwide analysis of hospital volume. Am J Gastroenterol. 2008;103(11):2789–98.
39. Kaplan GG, McCarthy EP, Ayanian JZ, Korzenik J, Hodin R, Sands BE. Impact of hospital volume on postoperative morbidity and mortality following a colectomy for ulcerative colitis. Gastroenterology. 2008;134(3):680–7.
40. Harmon JW, Tang DG, Gordon TA, et al. Hospital volume can serve as a surrogate for surgeon volume for achieving excellent outcomes in colorectal resection. Ann Surg. 1999;230(3): 404–11. discussion 411–413.
41. Kuwabara K, Matsuda S, Fushimi K, Ishikawa KB, Horiguchi H, Fujimori K. Impact of hospital case volume on the quality of laparoscopic colectomy in Japan. J Gastrointest Surg. 2009;13(9):1619–26.
42. Chowdhury M, Dagash H, Pierro A. a systematic review of the impact of volume of surgery and specialization on patient outcome. Br J Surg. 2007;94:145–61.
43. Bilimoria K, Phillips J, Rock C, Hayman A, Prystowsky J, Bentrem D. Effect of surgeon training, specialization, and experience on outcomes for cancer surgery: a systematic review of the literature. Ann Surg Oncol. 2009;16:1799–808.
44. Iversen L, Harling H, Laurberg S, Wille-Jorgensen P. Influence of caseload and surgical specialty on outcome following surgery for colorectal cancer: a review of evidence. Part 1: short-term outcome. Colorectal Dis. 2006;9:28–37.
45. Iversen L, Harling H, Laurberg S, Wille-Jorgensen P. Influence of caseload and surgical specialty on outcome following surgery for colorectal cancer: a review of evidence. Part 2: long-term outcome. Colorectal Dis. 2006;9:38–46.
46. Prystowsky J, Bordage G, Feinglass J. Patient outcomes for segmental colon resection according to surgeon's training, certification, and experience. Surgery. 2002;132:663–72.
47. Walter LC, Davidowitz NP, Heineken PA, Covinsky KE. Pitfalls of converting practice guidelines into quality measures: lessons learned from a VA performance measure. JAMA. 2004;291(20):2466–70.
48. Stahl TJ, Gregorcyk SG, Hyman NH, Buie WD. Practice parameters for the prevention of venous thrombosis. Dis Colon Rectum. 2006;49(10):1477–83.
49. National voluntary consensus standards for quality of cancer care: a consensus report. Washington, DC: National Quality Forum; 2009.
50. Malin JL, Schneider EC, Epstein AM, Adams J, Emanuel EJ, Kahn KL. Results of the National Initiative for Cancer Care Quality: how can we improve the quality of cancer care in the United States? J Clin Oncol. 2006;24(4):626–34.
51. McGory ML, Kao KK, Shekelle PG, et al. Developing quality indicators for elderly surgical patients. Ann Surg. 2009; 250(2):338–47.
52. Pastor C, Artinyan A, Varma MG, Kim E, Gibbs L, Garcia-Aguilar J. An increase in compliance with the Surgical Care Improvement Project measures does not prevent surgical site infection in colorectal surgery. Dis Colon Rectum. 2010;53(1):24–30.
53. Iezzoni LI, editor. Risk adjustment for measuring health care outcomes. 3rd ed. Chicago: Health Administration Press; 2003.
54. Koukouras D, Spiliotis J, Scopa CD, et al. Radical consequence in the sexuality of male patients operated for colorectal carcinoma. Eur J Surg Oncol. 1991;17(3):285–8.
55. Sailer M, Bussen D, Debus ES, Fuchs KH, Thiede A. Quality of life in patients with benign anorectal disorders. Br J Surg. 1998;85(12):1716–9.
56. Camilleri-Brennan J, Steele RJ. Prospective analysis of quality of life and survival following mesorectal excision for rectal cancer. Br J Surg. 2001;88(12):1617–22.
57. Ko CY, Rusin LC, Schoetz Jr DJ, et al. Long-term outcomes of the ileal pouch anal anastomosis: the association of bowel function and quality of life 5 years after surgery. J Surg Res. 2001;98(2):102–7.
58. Solomon MJ, Pager CK, Keshava A, et al. What do patients want? Patient preferences and surrogate decision making in the treatment of colorectal cancer. Dis Colon Rectum. 2003;46(10):1351–7.
59. Sokolovic E, Buchmann P, Schlomowitsch F, Szucs TD. Comparison of resource utilization and long-term quality-of-life outcomes between laparoscopic and conventional colorectal surgery. Surg Endosc. 2004;18(11):1663–7.
60. Efficace F, Bottomley A, Coens C, et al. Does a patient's self-reported health-related quality of life predict survival beyond key biomedical data in advanced colorectal cancer? Eur J Cancer. 2006;42(1):42–9.
61. Gall CA, Weller D, Esterman A, et al. Patient satisfaction and health-related quality of life after treatment for colon cancer. Dis Colon Rectum. 2007;50(6):801–9.
62. da Silva GM, Hull T, Roberts PL, et al. The effect of colorectal surgery in female sexual function, body image, self-esteem and general health: a prospective study. Ann Surg. 2008;248(2): 266–72.
63. Hann D, Denniston M, Baker F. Measurement of fatigue in cancer patients: further validation of the fatigue symptom inventory. Qual Life Res. 2000;9:847–54.
64. Hann D, Jacobsen P, Azzarello L, et al. Measurement of fatigue in cancer patients: development and validation of the fatigue symptom inventory. Qual Life Res. 1998;7:301–10.
65. Tan G, Jensen M, Thornby J, Shanti B. Validation of the brief pain inventory for chronic nonmalignant pain. J Pain. 2004;5(2):133–7.
66. Tittle M, McMillan S, Hagan S. Validating the brief pain inventory for use with surgical patients with cancer. Oncol Nurs Forum. 2003;30(2):325–30.
67. Kopec J, Land S, Cecchini R, et al. Validation of a self-reported neurotoxicity scale in patients with operable colon cancer receiving oxaliplatin. J Support Oncol. 2006;4(8):1–8.
68. Lawton M, Brody E. Assessment of older people: self-maintaining and instrumental activities of daily living. Gerontologist. 1969;9:179–86.
69. Zebrack B, Yi J, Petersen L, Ganz P. The impact of cancer and quality of life for long-term survivors. Psychooncology. 2008;17:891–900.
70. Crespi C, Ganz P, Petersen L, Castillo A, Caan B. Refinement and psychometric evaluation of the impact of cancer scale. J Natl Cancer Inst. 2008;100(21):1530–41.
71. Scheier M, Carver C, Bridges M. Distinguishing optimism from neuroticism (and trait anxiety, self-master, and self-esteem): a reevaluation of the life orientation test. J Pers Soc Psychol. 1994;67(6):1063–78.
72. Ward W, Hahn E, Mo F, Hernandez L, Tulsky D, Cella D. Reliability and validity of the functional assessment of cancer therapy-colorectal (FACT-C) quality of life instrument. Qual Life Res. 1999;8:181–95.

73. Gandek B, Ware J, Aaronson N, et al. Cross-validation of item selection and scoring for the SF-12 health survey in nine countries: results from the IQOLA Project. J Clin Epidemiol. 1998;51(11):1171–8.
74. Gandek B, Ware J. Methods for validating and norming translations of health status questionnaires: the IQOLA project approach. J Clin Epidemiol. 1998;51(11):953–9.
75. Ware J, Kosinski M, Keller S. A 12-item short-form health survey; construction of scales and preliminary tests of reliability and validity. Med Care. 1996;34(3):220–33.
76. Ware J, Kosinski M, Keller S. SF-36 physical and mental health summary scales: a user's manual. Boston, MA: Health Assessment Lab; 1994.
77. Ware J, Snow K, Kosinski M, Gandek B. SF-36 health survey manual and interpretation guide. Boston, MA: The Health Institute; 1993.
78. Sprangers M, te Velde A, Aaronson N. The construction and testing of the EORTC colorectal cancer-specific quality of Life questionnaire module (QLQ-CR38). European Organization for Research and Treatment of Cancer Study Group on Quality of Life. Eur J Cancer. 1999;35(2):238–47.
79. Gujral S, Conroy T, Fleissner C, et al. Assessing quality of life in patients with colorectal cancer: an update on the EORTC quality of life questionnaire. Eur J Cancer. 2007;43:1564–73.
80. Brook RH, Chassin MR, Fink A, Solomon DH, Kosecoff J, Park RE. A method for the detailed assessment of the appropriateness of medical technologies. Int J Technol Assess Health Care. 1986;2(1):53–63.
81. Fitch KB, Bernstein SJ, Aguilar MS, Burnand B, LaCalle JR, Lazaro P, et al. The Rand/UCLA appropriateness method user's manual. Santa Monica: Rand; 2000.
82. Chassin MR, Kosecoff J, Park RE, et al. Does inappropriate use explain geographic variations in the use of health care services? A study of three procedures. JAMA. 1987;258(18):2533–7.
83. Hemingway H, Crook AM, Feder G, et al. Underuse of coronary revascularization procedures in patients considered appropriate candidates for revascularization. N Engl J Med. 2001;344(9):645–54.
84. Shekelle PG, Kahan JP, Bernstein SJ, Leape LL, Kamberg CJ, Park RE. The reproducibility of a method to identify the overuse and underuse of medical procedures. N Engl J Med. 1998;338(26):1888–95.
85. Initial national priorities for comparative effectiveness research. Washington DC: Institute of Medicine; 2009.
86. Congressional Budget Office. Research on the comparative effectiveness of medical treatments; 2007.
87. Patwardhan M, Samsa G, McCrory D, et al. Cancer care quality measures: diagnosis and treatment of colorectal cancer. Evidence Report/Technology Assessment No. 138. AHRQ Publication No. 06-E002. 2006.
88. Weinstein MC, Skinner JA. Comparative effectiveness and health care spending – implications for reform. N Engl J Med. 2010;362(5):460–5.
89. Gold MR, Siegel JE, Russell LB, Weinstein MC. Cost-effectiveness in health and medicine. New York: Oxford University Press; 1996.
90. Murray A, Lourenco T, de Verteuil R, et al. Clinical effectiveness and cost-effectiveness of laparoscopic surgery for colorectal cancer: systematic reviews and economic evaluation. Health Technol Assess. 2006;10(45):1–141. iii–iv.
91. Kuhry E, Schwenk WF, Gaupset R, Romild U, Bonjer HJ. Long-term results of laparoscopic colorectal cancer resection. Cochrane Database Syst Rev. 2008(2):CD003432.
92. Dowson HM, Huang A, Soon Y, Gage H, Lovell DP, Rockall TA. Systematic review of the costs of laparoscopic colorectal surgery. Dis Colon Rectum. 2007;50(6):908–19.
93. Wind J, Polle SW, Fung Kon Jin PH, et al. Systematic review of enhanced recovery programmes in colonic surgery. Br J Surg. 2006;93(7):800–9.
94. Walter CJ, Collin J, Dumville JC, Drew PJ, Monson JR. Enhanced recovery in colorectal resections: a systematic review and meta-analysis. Colorectal Dis. 2009;11(4):344–53.

Index

D.E. Beck et al. (eds.), *The ASCRS Textbook of Colon and Rectal Surgery: Second Edition*, DOI 10.1007/978-1-4419-1584-9, © Springer Science+Business Media, LLC 2011

J

K

L

T

Printed in the United States of America